Oral and Maxillofacial Pathology

Oral and Maxillofacial Pathology

Fifth Edition

Brad W. Neville, DDS

Director of Oral and Maxillofacial Pathology
HCA South Atlantic Division
Trident Medical Center
Charleston, South Carolina

Distinguished University Professor Emeritus
James B. Edwards College of Dental Medicine
Medical University of South Carolina
Charleston, South Carolina

Douglas D. Damm, DDS

Emeritus Professor
Division of Oral & Maxillofacial Pathology
University of Kentucky College of Dentistry
Lexington, Kentucky

Oral & Maxillofacial Pathologist
Pathology & Cytology Laboratories
Lexington, Kentucky

Carl M. Allen, DDS, MSD

Emeritus Professor
Division of Oral and Maxillofacial Pathology and Radiology
College of Dentistry
The Ohio State University
Columbus, Ohio

Angela C. Chi, DMD

Professor
Woody L. Hunt School of Dental Medicine
Texas Tech University Health Sciences Center El Paso
El Paso, Texas

ELSEVIER

Elsevier
3251 Riverport Lane
St. Louis, Missouri 63043

ORAL AND MAXILLOFACIAL PATHOLOGY, FIFTH EDITION

ISBN: 978-0-323-78981-3

> **Notice**
>
> Practitioners and researchers must always rely on their own experience and knowledge in evaluating and using any information, methods, compounds or experiments described herein. Because of rapid advances in the medical sciences, in particular, independent verification of diagnoses and drug dosages should be made. To the fullest extent of the law, no responsibility is assumed by Elsevier, authors, editors or contributors for any injury and/or damage to persons or property as a matter of products liability, negligence or otherwise, or from any use or operation of any methods, products, instructions, or ideas contained in the material herein.

Previous editions copyrighted 2016, 2009, and 2002.

Senior Content Strategist: Lauren Boyle
Professional Content Development Manager: Jolynn Gower
Content Development Specialist: Meredith Madeira
Publishing Services Manager: Deepthi Unni
Project Manager: Nayagi Anandan
Design Direction: Bridget Hoette

Printed in India

Last digit is the print number: 9 8 7 6 5 4 3 2 1

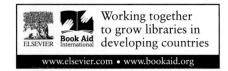

This book is dedicated to three of our mentors:

Charles A. Waldron
William G. Shafer
Robert J. Gorlin

in appreciation for all that they taught us and in recognition
of their contributions to the field of oral and maxillofacial pathology.

Contributors

Edward E. Herschaft, BA, DDS, MA
Professor
Woody L. Hunt School of Dental Medicine
Texas Tech University Health Sciences Center El Paso
El Paso, Texas

Professor Emeritus
James B. Edwards College of Dental Medicine
Medical University of South Carolina
Charleston, South Carolina

N. Lyn Wilson Westmark, DMD, MPH
Division of Oral Medicine and Hospital Dentistry
Division of Plastic, Maxillofacial, and Oral Surgery
Consulting Associate in the Department of Surgery
Duke University Hospital
Durham, North Carolina

Preface

The first edition of this textbook was published 29 years ago in 1995. At that time, we never could have dreamed that we would still be involved in writing updates of this text nearly three decades later. With this in mind, reaching our fifth edition represents somewhat of a milestone for us, and we are extremely grateful to have the opportunity to continue producing this work.

The basic format of the book remains the same. However, over the years, the content for many topics has changed dramatically due to the incredible explosion of new research and technology. One of the challenges with any new edition is deciding what new information should be included and what other information should be trimmed. This task becomes more difficult when one takes into account the diversity of our intended audience. For example, this new edition includes considerable new information about specific gene mutations and translocations that are associated with various hereditary diseases and neoplasms. Although the details of these specific molecular changes may seem of lesser importance to students taking their first course in oral pathology, they hold more significance for some of our other readers.

In addition to the updated information on existing topics, new entities in this fifth edition include molar root–incisor malformation, foreign body gingivitis, peri-implant diseases, coronavirus disease 2019 (COVID-19), lichenoid and granulomatous stomatitis, ectomesenchymal chondromyxoid tumor, central xanthoma of the jaws, and primordial odontogenic tumor. A total of 152 new images have been added, and we are greatly indebted to our many colleagues who generously shared their excellent clinical photographs and radiographs with us. We have attempted to be as thorough as possible in listing credit for these images. However, if someone's name has been inadvertently omitted, then please accept our apologies.

Our sincere thanks again go to Dr. Edward E. Herschaft, who updated his excellent chapter on forensic dentistry. We also welcome Dr. N. Lyn Wilson Westmark, who revised the chapter on facial pain and neuromuscular diseases. In addition, we must acknowledge the outstanding support and guidance provided by the staff at Elsevier in making this book a success. Special thanks go to Lauren Boyle, Joslyn Dumas, and Meredith Madeira for all of their assistance in the editorial process.

As always, our greatest appreciation goes to our families, who have once again provided us with their unconditional love and support during the countless hours spent working on this latest edition. (Although this new edition may have been somewhat of a milestone for us, we are worried that it may have seemed like a millstone to them!) We could never have accomplished it without you.

Contents

1 Developmental Defects of the Oral and Maxillofacial Region, 1

Orofacial Clefts, 1
Commissural Lip Pits, 4
Paramedian Lip Pits (Congenital Fistulas of the Lower Lip; Congenital Lip Pits), 4
Double Lip, 5
Fordyce Granules, 6
Leukoedema, 7
Microglossia (Hypoglossia), 8
Macroglossia, 8
Ankyloglossia (Tongue-Tie), 10
Lingual Thyroid, 10
Fissured Tongue (Scrotal Tongue; Lingua Plicata), 11
Hairy Tongue (Black Hairy Tongue; Coated Tongue), 12
Varicosities (Varices), 13
Caliber-Persistent Artery, 14
Lateral Soft Palate Fistulas, 15
Coronoid Hyperplasia, 15
Condylar Hyperplasia, 16
Condylar Hypoplasia, 17
Bifid Condyle, 19
Exostoses, 19
Torus Palatinus, 20
Torus Mandibularis, 21
Eagle Syndrome (Stylohyoid Syndrome; Stylocarotid Syndrome; Stylalgia), 23
Stafne Defect (Stafne Bone Cyst; Lingual Mandibular Salivary Gland Depression; Latent Bone Cyst; Static Bone Cyst; Static Bone Defect; Lingual Cortical Mandibular Defect), 23

DEVELOPMENTAL CYSTS, 25
Palatal Cysts of the Newborn (Epstein's Pearls; Bohn's Nodules), 25
Nasolabial Cyst (Nasoalveolar Cyst; Klestadt Cyst), 26
"Globulomaxillary Cyst", 27
Nasopalatine Duct Cyst (Incisive Canal Cyst), 27
Median Palatal (Palatine) Cyst, 30
"Median Mandibular Cyst", 31
Follicular Cysts of the Skin, 31
Dermoid Cyst (Dysontogenic Cyst), 32
Thyroglossal Duct Cyst (Thyroglossal Tract Cyst), 33
Branchial Cleft Cyst (Cervical Lymphoepithelial Cyst), 35
Oral Lymphoepithelial Cyst, 36

OTHER RARE DEVELOPMENTAL ANOMALIES, 37
Hemihyperplasia (Hemihypertrophy), 37
Progressive Hemifacial Atrophy (Progressive Facial Hemiatrophy; Romberg Syndrome; Parry-Romberg Syndrome), 38
Segmental Odontomaxillary Dysplasia (Hemimaxillofacial Dysplasia), 39
Crouzon Syndrome (Craniofacial Dysostosis), 40
Apert Syndrome (Acrocephalosyndactyly), 41
Mandibulofacial Dysostosis (Treacher Collins Syndrome; Franceschetti-Zwahlen-Klein Syndrome), 43

2 Abnormalities of Teeth, 51

General Considerations, 51

ENVIRONMENTAL ALTERATIONS OF TEETH, 51
Environmental Effects on Tooth Structure Development, 51
Postdevelopmental Loss of Tooth Structure, 58
Environmental Discoloration of Teeth, 67
Localized Disturbances in Eruption, 71

DEVELOPMENTAL ALTERATIONS OF TEETH, 74
Developmental Alterations in the Number of Teeth, 75
Developmental Alterations in the Size of Teeth, 81
Developmental Alterations in the Shape of Teeth, 82
Developmental Alterations in the Structure of Teeth, 98

3 Pulpal and Periapical Disease, 117

Pulpitis, 117
Secondary and Tertiary Dentin, 119
Pulpal Calcifications, 121
Periapical Granuloma (Chronic Apical Periodontitis), 123
Periapical Cyst (Radicular Cyst; Apical Periodontal Cyst), 126
Periapical Abscess, 129

Cellulitis, 132
Osteomyelitis, 134
Diffuse Sclerosing Osteomyelitis, 137
Chronic Nonbacterial Osteomyelitis, 138
Condensing Osteitis (Focal Sclerosing Osteomyelitis), 141
Osteomyelitis With Proliferative Periostitis (Periostitis Ossificans, Ossifying Periostitis), 141
Alveolar Osteitis (Dry Socket; Fibrinolytic Alveolitis), 143

4 Periodontal Diseases, 147
Gingivitis, 147
Spongiotic Gingival Hyperplasia (Spongiotic Gingivitis), 150
Necrotizing Gingivitis (Necrotizing Ulcerative Gingivitis, Vincent Infection; Trench Mouth), 151
Plasma Cell Gingivitis (Atypical Gingivostomatitis; Allergic Gingivostomatitis), 152
Foreign Body Gingivitis, 154
Desquamative Gingivitis, 155
Drug-Related Gingival Hyperplasia (Drug-Related Gingival Overgrowth), 156
Gingival Fibromatosis (Fibromatosis Gingivae; Elephantiasis Gingivae), 158
Periodontitis, 160
Peri-Implant Diseases, 167
Papillon-Lefèvre Syndrome, 167

5 Bacterial Infections, 172
Impetigo, 172
Erysipelas, 173
Streptococcal Tonsillitis and Pharyngitis, 174
Scarlet Fever (Scarlatina), 175
Tonsillar Plugs and Tonsillolithiasis, 176
Diphtheria, 177
Syphilis (Lues), 179
Gonorrhea, 184
Tuberculosis, 185
Leprosy (Hansen Disease), 188
Noma (Cancrum Oris; Orofacial Gangrene; Gangrenous Stomatitis; Necrotizing Stomatitis), 191
Actinomycosis, 192
Cat-Scratch Disease, 194
Rhinosinusitis (Sinusitis), 196

6 Fungal and Protozoal Diseases, 201
Candidiasis, 201
Histoplasmosis, 212
Blastomycosis, 214
Paracoccidioidomycosis (South American Blastomycosis), 216
Coccidioidomycosis (San Joaquin Valley Fever; Valley Fever; Cocci), 217
Cryptococcosis, 218
Mucormycosis (Zygomycosis; Phycomycosis), 219
Aspergillosis, 221
Toxoplasmosis, 222
Leishmaniasis, 224

7 Viral Infections, 229
Human Herpesviruses, 229
Herpes Simplex Virus, 229
Varicella (Chickenpox), 235
Herpes Zoster (Shingles), 238
Infectious Mononucleosis (Mono; Glandular Fever; "Kissing Disease"), 241
Cytomegalovirus, 242
Enteroviruses, 244
Measles (Rubeola), 246
Rubella (German Measles), 248
Mumps (Epidemic Parotitis), 249
Human Immunodeficiency Virus and Acquired Immunodeficiency Syndrome, 250
Coronavirus Disease 2019, 265

8 Physical and Chemical Injuries, 272
Linea Alba, 272
Morsicatio Mucosae Oris (Chronic Mucosal Chewing), 272
Traumatic Ulcerations, 273
Electrical and Thermal Burns, 276
Chemical Injuries of the Oral Mucosa, 278
Noninfectious Oral Complications of Antineoplastic Therapy, 280
Medication-Related Osteonecrosis of the Jaw (Bisphosphonate-Related Osteonecrosis; Antiresorptive-Related Osteonecrosis), 286
Orofacial Complications of Drug Abuse, 292
Anesthetic Necrosis, 294
Exfoliative Cheilitis, 294
Submucosal Hemorrhage, 296
Oral Trauma From Sexual Practices, 297
Amalgam Tattoo and Other Localized Exogenous Pigmentations, 298
Oral Piercings and Other Body Modifications, 300
Oral Lesions Associated With Cosmetic Fillers, 302
Systemic Metallic Intoxication, 304
Smoker's Melanosis, 306
Drug-Related Discolorations of the Oral Mucosa, 307
Reactive Osseous and Chondromatous Metaplasia (Cutright Lesion), 309
Oral Ulceration With Bone Sequestration (Spontaneous Sequestration; Traumatic Sequestration), 310
Antral Pseudocysts, 310

True Cysts of the Sinuses (Sinus Mucocele; Surgical Ciliated Cyst; Traumatic Ciliated Cyst; Postoperative Maxillary Cyst; Retention Cyst), 312
Cervicofacial Emphysema, 314
Myospherulosis, 315

9   Allergies and Immunologic Diseases, 321

Transient Lingual Papillitis, 321
Recurrent Aphthous Stomatitis (Recurrent Aphthous Ulcerations; Canker Sores), 321
Behçet Disease (Behçet Syndrome; Adamantiades Syndrome; Silk Road Disease), 326
Sarcoidosis, 328
Orofacial Granulomatosis, 330
Granulomatosis With Polyangiitis (Wegener Granulomatosis), 333
Lichenoid and Granulomatous Stomatitis, 336
Mucosal Reactions to Systemic Drug Administration, 337
Allergic Contact Stomatitis (Stomatitis Venenata), 342
Perioral Dermatitis (Periorificial Dermatitis), 343
Contact Stomatitis From Artificial Cinnamon Flavoring, 344
Lichenoid Contact Reaction From Dental Restorative Materials, 346
Angioedema (Angioneurotic Edema; Quincke Disease), 348

10   Epithelial Pathology, 354

Benign Epithelial Lesions Associated With Human Papillomavirus, 354
Molluscum Contagiosum, 364
Verruciform Xanthoma, 365
Seborrheic Keratosis, 366
Sebaceous Hyperplasia, 368
Ephelis (Freckle), 368
Actinic Lentigo (Lentigo Solaris; Solar Lentigo; Age Spot; Liver Spot; Senile Lentigo), 369
Lentigo Simplex, 370
Melasma (Mask of Pregnancy; Chloasma), 371
Oral Melanotic Macule (Focal Melanosis), 372
Oral Melanoacanthoma (Melanoacanthosis), 373
Melanocytic Nevus (Nevocellular Nevus; Mole), 374
Acquired Melanocytic Nevus, 375
Congenital Melanocytic Nevus, 379
Oral Potentially Malignant Disorders, 380
Leukoplakia (Leukokeratosis; Erythroleukoplakia), 381
Erythroplakia (Erythroplasia; Erythroplasia of Queyrat), 390
Smokeless Tobacco Use and Smokeless Tobacco Keratosis (Snuff Pouch; Snuff Dipper's Lesion; Tobacco Pouch Keratosis; Spit Tobacco Keratosis), 391

Oral Submucous Fibrosis, 393
Actinic Cheilosis (Actinic Cheilitis; Solar Cheilosis), 395
Actinic Keratosis (Solar Keratosis), 396
Nicotine Stomatitis (Nicotine Palatinus; Smoker's Palate), 397
Keratoacanthoma ("Self-Healing" Carcinoma; Pseudocarcinoma; Keratocarcinoma; Squamous Cell Carcinoma, Keratoacanthoma Type), 398
Squamous Cell Carcinoma, 401
Verrucous Carcinoma (Snuff Dipper's Cancer; Ackerman's Tumor), 421
Spindle Cell Carcinoma (Sarcomatoid Squamous Cell Carcinoma; Polypoid Squamous Cell Carcinoma; Carcinosarcoma; Pseudosarcoma), 423
Adenosquamous Carcinoma, 424
Basaloid Squamous Carcinoma (Basaloid Squamous Cell Carcinoma), 425
Carcinoma of the Maxillary Sinus, 426
Sinonasal Undifferentiated Carcinoma, 426
Nasopharyngeal Carcinoma, 428
Basal Cell Carcinoma (Basal Cell Epithelioma; Rodent Ulcer), 430
Merkel Cell Carcinoma (Merkel Cell Tumor; Primary Neuroendocrine Carcinoma of Skin; Small Cell Carcinoma of Skin; Trabecular Carcinoma of Skin; Toker Tumor), 432
Melanoma (Malignant Melanoma; Melanocarcinoma), 434

11   Salivary Gland Pathology, 460

Salivary Gland Aplasia/Hypoplasia, 460
Mucocele (Mucus Extravasation Phenomenon; Mucus Escape Reaction), 460
Ranula, 462
Salivary Duct Cyst (Mucus Retention Cyst; Mucus Duct Cyst; Sialocyst), 463
Sialolithiasis (Salivary Calculi; Salivary Stones), 465
Sialadenitis, 467
Cheilitis Glandularis, 468
Sialorrhea (Ptyalism), 469
Xerostomia, 470
IgG4-Related Disease, 471
Sjögren Syndrome, 472
Sialadenosis (Sialosis), 476
Adenomatoid Hyperplasia of the Minor Salivary Glands, 477
Necrotizing Sialometaplasia, 477

SALIVARY GLAND TUMORS, 479

General Considerations, 479
Pleomorphic Adenoma (Benign Mixed Tumor), 483
Oncocytoma (Oxyphilic Adenoma), 487

Oncocytosis (Multinodular Oncocytic Hyperplasia), 488

Warthin Tumor (Papillary Cystadenoma Lymphomatosum), 488

Monomorphic Adenoma, 490

Canalicular Adenoma, 490

Basal Cell Adenoma, 491

Ductal Papillomas (Sialadenoma Papilliferum; Intraductal Papilloma; Inverted Ductal Papilloma), 492

Mucoepidermoid Carcinoma, 493

Intraosseous Mucoepidermoid Carcinoma (Central Mucoepidermoid Carcinoma), 496

Acinic Cell Carcinoma, 497

Secretory Carcinoma (Mammary Analogue Secretory Carcinoma), 498

Malignant Mixed Tumors (Carcinoma Ex Pleomorphic Adenoma; Carcinoma Ex Mixed Tumor; Carcinosarcoma; Metastasizing Mixed Tumor), 499

Adenoid Cystic Carcinoma, 501

Polymorphous Adenocarcinoma (Polymorphous Low-Grade Adenocarcinoma), 503

Salivary Adenocarcinoma, Not Otherwise Specified, 505

12　Soft Tissue Tumors, 514

Fibroma (Irritation Fibroma; Traumatic Fibroma; Focal Fibrous Hyperplasia; Fibrous Nodule), 514

Giant Cell Fibroma, 514

Epulis Fissuratum (Inflammatory Fibrous Hyperplasia; Denture Injury Tumor; Denture Epulis), 517

Inflammatory Papillary Hyperplasia (Denture Papillomatosis), 519

Fibrous Histiocytoma, 520

Solitary Fibrous Tumor, 521

Fibromatosis (Desmoid-Type Fibromatosis), 523

Myofibroma (Myofibromatosis), 523

Oral Focal Mucinosis, 524

Pyogenic Granuloma (Lobular Capillary Hemangioma), 525

Peripheral Giant Cell Granuloma, 527

Peripheral Ossifying Fibroma (Ossifying Fibroid Epulis; Peripheral Fibroma with Calcification), 529

Lipoma, 530

Traumatic Neuroma (Amputation Neuroma), 532

Palisaded Encapsulated Neuroma (Solitary Circumscribed Neuroma), 533

Schwannoma (Neurilemoma), 534

Neurofibroma, 534

Neurofibromatosis Type I (von Recklinghausen Disease of the Skin), 537

Multiple Endocrine Neoplasia Type 2B, 540

Melanotic Neuroectodermal Tumor of Infancy, 541

Paraganglioma (Carotid Body Tumor; Chemodectoma; Glomus Jugulare Tumor; Glomus Tympanicum Tumor), 543

Granular Cell Tumor, 544

Congenital Epulis (Congenital Epulis of the Newborn; Congenital Granular Cell Lesion), 546

Hemangioma and Vascular Malformations, 547

Sturge-Weber Syndrome (Encephalotrigeminal Angiomatosis; Sturge-Weber Angiomatosis), 551

Nasopharyngeal Angiofibroma, 552

Lymphatic Malformations (Lymphangioma; Cystic Hygroma), 553

Leiomyoma, 555

Rhabdomyoma, 557

Ectomesenchymal Chondromyxoid Tumor, 558

Osseous and Cartilaginous Choristomas, 559

Fibrosarcoma, 559

Undifferentiated Pleomorphic Sarcoma (Malignant Fibrous Histiocytoma), 560

Liposarcoma, 561

Malignant Peripheral Nerve Sheath Tumor (Malignant Schwannoma; Neurofibrosarcoma; Neurogenic Sarcoma), 562

Olfactory Neuroblastoma (Esthesioneuroblastoma), 562

Angiosarcoma, 563

Kaposi Sarcoma, 564

Leiomyosarcoma, 565

Rhabdomyosarcoma, 566

Synovial Sarcoma, 567

Alveolar Soft-Part Sarcoma, 568

Metastases to the Oral Soft Tissues, 569

13　Hematologic Disorders, 578

Lymphoid Hyperplasia, 578

Hemophilia, 579

Plasminogen Deficiency (Ligneous Conjunctivitis; Hypoplasminogenemia), 581

Anemia, 582

Sickle Cell Anemia, 583

Thalassemia, 585

Aplastic Anemia, 586

Neutropenia, 587

Agranulocytosis, 589

Cyclic Neutropenia (Cyclic Hematopoiesis), 589

Thrombocytopenia, 590

Polycythemia Vera (Primary Polycythemia; Polycythemia Rubra Vera; Primary Acquired Erythrocytosis), 592

Leukemia, 593

Langerhans Cell Histiocytosis (Histiocytosis X; Langerhans Cell Disease; Idiopathic Histiocytosis; Eosinophilic Granuloma; Langerhans Cell Granuloma; Langerhans Cell Granulomatosis), 596

Hodgkin Lymphoma (Hodgkin Disease), 598
Non-Hodgkin Lymphoma, 600
Mycosis Fungoides (Cutaneous T-Cell Lymphoma), 604
Burkitt Lymphoma, 606
Extranodal NK/T-Cell Lymphoma, Nasal-Type (Angiocentric T-Cell Lymphoma; Midline Lethal Granuloma; Idiopathic Midline Destructive Disease; Polymorphic Reticulosis; Midline Malignant Reticulosis; Angiocentric Immunoproliferative Lesion), 607
Multiple Myeloma, 609
Plasmacytoma, 611

14   Bone Pathology, 618

Osteogenesis Imperfecta ("Brittle Bone Disease"), 618
Osteopetrosis (Albers-Schönberg Disease; Marble Bone Disease), 620
Cleidocranial Dysplasia (Cleidocranial Dysostosis; Scheuthauer-Marie-Sainton syndrome; Marie-Sainton Disease), 623
Focal Osteoporotic Marrow Defect, 625
Idiopathic Osteosclerosis, 626
Massive Osteolysis (Gorham Disease; Gorham-Stout Syndrome; Vanishing Bone Disease; Phantom Bone Disease; Idiopathic Osteolysis), 627
Paget Disease of Bone (Osteitis Deformans), 628
Central Giant Cell Granuloma (Giant Cell Lesion; Giant Cell Tumor), 631
Giant Cell Tumor ("True Giant Cell Tumor"), 633
Cherubism, 634
Simple Bone Cyst (Traumatic Bone Cyst; Hemorrhagic Bone Cyst; Solitary Bone Cyst; Idiopathic Bone Cavity; Unicameral Bone Cyst), 636
Aneurysmal Bone Cyst, 638
Central Xanthoma of the Jaws (Primary Xanthoma of Bone; Primary Intraosseous Xanthoma; Fibrous Xanthoma of Bone; Fibroxanthoma of Bone), 640

FIBRO-OSSEOUS LESIONS OF THE JAWS, 641
Fibrous Dysplasia, 641
Cemento-Osseous Dysplasias (Osseous Dysplasia), 645
Familial Gigantiform Cementoma (Familial Expansive Osseous Dysplasia), 650
Cemento-ossifying Fibroma (Conventional Ossifying Fibroma; Ossifying Fibroma; Cementifying Fibroma), 652
Juvenile Ossifying Fibroma (Juvenile Active Ossifying Fibroma; Juvenile Aggressive Ossifying Fibroma; Aggressive Ossifying Fibroma), 653

Osteoma, 655
Gardner Syndrome, 656
Osteoblastoma (Giant Osteoid Osteoma) and Osteoid Osteoma, 658
Cementoblastoma (True Cementoma), 659
Chondroma, 661
Chondromyxoid Fibroma, 661
Synovial Chondromatosis (Synovial Chondrometaplasia; Synovial Osteochondromatosis), 662
Desmoplastic Fibroma, 663
Osteosarcoma (Osteogenic Sarcoma), 665
Chondrosarcoma, 669
Ewing Sarcoma, 671
Metastatic Tumors to the Jaws, 673

15   Odontogenic Cysts and Tumors, 685
ODONTOGENIC CYSTS, 685
Dentigerous Cyst (Follicular Cyst), 685
Eruption Cyst (Eruption Hematoma), 688
Primordial Cyst, 689
Odontogenic Keratocyst (Keratocystic Odontogenic Tumor), 689
Orthokeratinized Odontogenic Cyst, 693
Nevoid Basal Cell Carcinoma Syndrome (Gorlin Syndrome), 694
Gingival (Alveolar) Cyst of the Newborn, 697
Gingival Cyst of the Adult, 698
Lateral Periodontal Cyst (Botryoid Odontogenic Cyst), 699
Calcifying Odontogenic Cyst (Calcifying Cystic Odontogenic Tumor; Gorlin Cyst; Dentinogenic Ghost Cell Tumor; Ghost Cell Odontogenic Carcinoma), 701
Glandular Odontogenic Cyst (Sialo-Odontogenic Cyst), 703
Buccal Bifurcation Cyst (Inflammatory Collateral Cyst), 704
Carcinoma Arising in Odontogenic Cysts, 705

ODONTOGENIC TUMORS, 707

TUMORS OF ODONTOGENIC EPITHELIUM, 707
Ameloblastoma, 707
Malignant Ameloblastoma and Ameloblastic Carcinoma, 716
Clear Cell Odontogenic Carcinoma (Clear Cell Odontogenic Tumor), 717
Adenomatoid Odontogenic Tumor, 718
Calcifying Epithelial Odontogenic Tumor (Pindborg Tumor), 720
Squamous Odontogenic Tumor, 723

MIXED ODONTOGENIC TUMORS, 724
Ameloblastic Fibroma, 724
Ameloblastic Fibro-Odontoma, 725
Ameloblastic Fibrosarcoma (Ameloblastic Sarcoma), 727

Odontoameloblastoma, 728
Odontoma, 729
Primordial Odontogenic Tumor, 731
**TUMORS OF ODONTOGENIC
    ECTOMESENCHYME, 731**
Central Odontogenic Fibroma, 731
Peripheral Odontogenic Fibroma, 733
Granular Cell Odontogenic Tumor (Granular Cell
    Odontogenic Fibroma), 734
Odontogenic Myxoma, 735
Cementoblastoma ("True Cementoma"), 737

16   Dermatologic Diseases, 747

Ectodermal Dysplasia, 747
White Sponge Nevus (Cannon Disease), 748
Hereditary Benign Intraepithelial Dyskeratosis
    (Witkop-Von Sallmann Syndrome), 749
Pachyonychia Congenita (Jadassohn-Lewandowsky
    Type; Jackson-Lawler Type), 750
Dyskeratosis Congenita (Cole-Engman Syndrome;
    Zinsser-Cole-Engman Syndrome), 752
Xeroderma Pigmentosum, 753
Hereditary Mucoepithelial Dysplasia, 754
Incontinentia Pigmenti (Bloch-Sulzberger
    Syndrome), 755
Darier Disease (Keratosis Follicularis; Dyskeratosis
    Follicularis; Darier-White Disease), 756
Warty Dyskeratoma (Isolated Darier Disease; Isolated
    Dyskeratosis Follicularis; Focal Acantholytic
    Dyskeratosis; Follicular Dyskeratoma), 757
Peutz-Jeghers Syndrome, 758
Hereditary Hemorrhagic Telangiectasia
    (Osler-Weber-Rendu Syndrome), 759
Ehlers-Danlos Syndromes, 760
Tuberous Sclerosis (Epiloia; Bourneville-Pringle
    Syndrome), 762
Multiple Hamartoma Syndrome (Cowden Syndrome;
    PTEN Hamartoma-Tumor Syndrome), 765
Epidermolysis Bullosa, 766
Pemphigus, 769
Paraneoplastic Pemphigus (Neoplasia-Induced
    Pemphigus; Paraneoplastic Autoimmune
    Multiorgan Syndrome), 774
Mucous Membrane Pemphigoid (Cicatricial
    Pemphigoid; Benign Mucous Membrane
    Pemphigoid), 775
Bullous Pemphigoid, 779
Erythema Multiforme, 781
Stevens-Johnson Syndrome and Toxic Epidermal
    Necrolysis, 783
Erythema Migrans (Geographic Tongue; Benign
    Migratory Glossitis; Wandering Rash of the
    Tongue; Erythema Areata Migrans; Stomatitis
    Areata Migrans), 784
Reactive Arthritis (Reiter
    Syndrome), 786

Lichen Planus, 787
Chronic Ulcerative
    Stomatitis, 792
Graft-Versus-Host Disease, 794
Psoriasis, 796
Lupus Erythematosus, 798
Systemic Sclerosis (Progressive Systemic Sclerosis;
    Scleroderma; Diffuse Cutaneous Systemic
    Sclerosis; Hide-Bound Disease), 801
CREST Syndrome (Acrosclerosis; Limited
    Scleroderma; Limited Cutaneous Systemic
    Sclerosis), 805
Acanthosis Nigricans, 806

**17   Oral Manifestations of Systemic
    Diseases, 819**

Mucopolysaccharidosis, 819
Lipid Reticuloendothelioses, 821
Lipoid Proteinosis (Hyalinosis Cutis Et Mucosae;
    Urbach-Wiethe Syndrome), 822
Jaundice (Icterus), 823
Amyloidosis, 824
Xanthelasma (Xanthelasma Palpebrarum), 827
Vitamin Deficiency, 827
Iron-Deficiency Anemia, 830
Plummer-Vinson Syndrome (Paterson-Kelly
    Syndrome; Sideropenic Dysphagia), 830
Pernicious Anemia, 831
Pituitary Dwarfism, 833
Gigantism, 834
Acromegaly, 834
Hypothyroidism (Cretinism; Myxedema), 835
Hyperthyroidism (Thyrotoxicosis; Graves
    Disease), 837
Hypoparathyroidism, 838
Pseudohypoparathyroidism (Albright Hereditary
    Osteodystrophy; Acrodysostosis), 839
Hyperparathyroidism, 840
Hypercortisolism (Cushing Syndrome), 842
Addison Disease (Hypoadrenocorticism), 843
Diabetes Mellitus, 844
Hypophosphatasia, 847
Vitamin D–Resistant Rickets (Hereditary
    Hypophosphatemia; Familial Hypophosphatemic
    Rickets), 848
Crohn Disease (Regional Ileitis; Regional
    Enteritis), 850
Pyostomatitis Vegetans, 851
Uremic Stomatitis, 852

**18   Facial Pain and Neuromuscular
    Diseases, 861**

N. Lyn Wilson Westmark
Bell Palsy (Idiopathic Seventh Nerve Paralysis;
    Idiopathic Facial Paralysis), 861

Frey Syndrome (Auriculotemporal Syndrome; Gustatory Sweating and Flushing), 862

HEAD AND NECK PAIN, 863

Trigeminal Neuralgia (Tic Douloureux; Tic), 864

Glossopharyngeal Neuralgia (Vagoglossopharyngeal Neuralgia), 866

Giant Cell Arteritis (Temporal Arteritis; Granulomatous Arteritis), 867

Burning Mouth Disorder (Burning Mouth Syndrome; Oral Dysesthesia; Oral Sensory Neuropathy; Stomatopyrosis; Stomatodynia; Glossopyrosis; Glossodynia; Burning Tongue Syndrome; Burning Mouth Syndrome), 868

Dysgeusia and Hypogeusia (Phantom Taste; Distorted Taste), 869

Osteoarthritis (Degenerative Arthritis; Degenerative Joint Disease), 871

Rheumatoid Arthritis, 872

Temporomandibular Disorders, 874

19   Forensic Dentistry, 881
Edward E. Herschaft
Record Management, 881
Identification, 883
Bite Pattern Evidence, 899
Human Abuse, 907
Dentists as Expert Witnesses, 910
Summary, 911

Appendix: Differential Diagnosis of Oral and Maxillofacial Diseases, 914

Index, 936

1

Developmental Defects of the Oral and Maxillofacial Region

◆ OROFACIAL CLEFTS

The formation of the face and oral cavity is complex in nature and involves the development of multiple tissue processes that must merge and fuse in a highly orchestrated fashion. Disturbances in the growth of these tissue processes or their fusion may result in the formation of **orofacial clefts**.

Development of the central face begins around the end of the fourth week of human development with the appearance of the nasal (olfactory) placodes on either side of the inferior aspect of the frontonasal process. Proliferation of ectomesenchyme on both sides of each placode results in the formation of the medial and lateral nasal processes. Between each pair of processes is a depression, or nasal pit, that represents the primitive nostril.

During the sixth and seventh weeks of development, the upper lip forms when the medial nasal processes merge with each other and with the maxillary processes of the first branchial arches. Thus the midportion of the upper lip is derived from the medial nasal processes, and the lateral portions are derived from the maxillary processes. The lateral nasal processes are not involved in the formation of the upper lip, but they give rise to the alae of the nose.

The **primary palate** also is formed by the merger of the medial nasal processes to form the intermaxillary segment. This segment gives rise to the premaxilla, a triangular-shaped piece of bone that will include the four incisor teeth and hard palate anterior to the incisive foramen. The **secondary palate,** which makes up 90% of the hard and soft palates, is formed from the maxillary processes of the first branchial arches.

During the sixth week, bilateral projections emerge from the medial aspects of the maxillary processes to form the palatal shelves. Initially, these shelves are oriented in a vertical position on each side of the developing tongue. As the mandible grows, the tongue drops down, allowing the palatal shelves to rotate to a horizontal position and grow toward one another. By the eighth to ninth week, sufficient growth has occurred to allow the anterior aspects of these shelves to begin fusion with one another. The palatal shelves also fuse with the primary palate and the nasal septum. The fusion of the palatal shelves begins in the anterior palate and progresses posteriorly; it is completed by the twelfth week.

Defective fusion of the medial nasal process with the maxillary process leads to **cleft lip (CL)**. Likewise, failure of the palatal shelves to fuse results in **cleft palate (CP)**. Frequently, CL and CP occur together. Approximately 45% of cases are CL + CP with 30% being CP only (CPO) and 25% being isolated CL. Both isolated CL and CL associated with CP are thought to be etiologically related conditions and can be considered as a group: CL, with or without CP (i.e., CL ± CP). Isolated CPO appears to represent a separate entity from CL ± CP.

The cause of CL ± CP and CPO is still being debated. First of all, distinguishing isolated clefts from cases associated with specific syndromes is important. Although many facial clefts are isolated anomalies, more than 400 developmental syndromes have been identified that may be associated with CL ± CP or CPO. Studies have suggested that up to 30% of patients with CL ± CP and 50% of those with CPO have associated anomalies. Some of these cases are single-gene syndromes that may follow autosomal dominant, autosomal recessive, or X-linked inheritance patterns. Other syndromes are the result of chromosome anomalies or are idiopathic. Anomalies frequently associated with CPO include congenital heart defects, hydrocephalus, and urinary tract defects.

The cause of nonsyndromic clefts does not follow any simple Mendelian pattern of inheritance but appears to be heterogeneous. Thus the propensity for cleft development may be related to a number of major genes, minor genes, and environmental factors that can combine to surpass a developmental threshold. Numerous candidate clefting genes and loci have been identified on different chromosome regions. Maternal alcohol consumption has been associated with an increased risk for both syndromic and nonsyndromic clefts. Maternal cigarette smoking at least doubles the frequency of cleft development compared with nonsmoking mothers. An increased frequency also has been related to anticonvulsant therapy, especially phenytoin, which causes a nearly tenfold greater risk of cleft formation. Although evidence has been mixed, a number of studies have suggested that folic acid supplementation may play a role in prevention of orofacial clefts.

CL ± CP and CPO represent the vast majority of orofacial clefts. However, other rare clefts also may occur.

The **lateral facial cleft** is caused by lack of fusion of the maxillary and mandibular processes and represents 0.3% of all facial clefts. This cleft may be unilateral or bilateral, extending from the commissure toward the ear, resulting in macrostomia. The lateral facial cleft may occur as an isolated defect, but more often it is associated with other disorders, such as the following:

- Mandibulofacial dysostosis (see page 43)
- Oculo-auriculo-vertebral spectrum (hemifacial microsomia)
- Nager acrofacial dysostosis
- Amniotic rupture sequence

The **oblique facial cleft** extends from the upper lip to the eye. It is nearly always associated with CP, and severe forms often are incompatible with life. The oblique facial cleft may involve the nostril, as in CL, or it may bypass the nose laterally as it extends to the eye. This cleft is rare, representing only 1 in 1300 facial clefts. Some of these clefts may represent failure of fusion of the lateral nasal process with the maxillary process; amniotic bands may cause others.

Median cleft of the upper lip is an extremely rare anomaly that results from failure of fusion of the medial nasal processes. It may be associated with a number of syndromes, including the oral-facial-digital syndromes and Ellis-van Creveld syndrome. Most apparent median clefts of the upper lip actually represent agenesis of the primary palate associated with holoprosencephaly.

Clinical and Radiographic Features

Clefting is one of the most common major congenital defects in humans. Considerable racial variation in prevalence is seen. In whites, CL ± CP occurs in 1 of every 700 to 1000 births. The frequency of CL ± CP in Asian populations is about 1.5 times higher than in whites. In contrast, the prevalence of CL ± CP in blacks is much lower, occurring in 0.4 of 1000 births. Native Americans appear to have the highest frequency, around 3.6 of 1000 births. CPO is less common than CL ± CP, with a frequency of 0.4 of 1000 births in whites and blacks.

CL ± CP is more common in males than in females. The more severe the defect, the greater the male predilection; the male-to-female ratio for isolated CL is 1.5:1; the ratio for CL +CP is 2:1. In contrast, CPO is more common in females. Likewise, the more severe the cleft, the greater the female predilection. Clefts of both the hard and soft palates are twice as common in females, but the ratio is nearly equal for clefts of the soft palate only.

Approximately 80% of cases of CL will be unilateral with 20% bilateral (Fig. 1.1). Approximately 70% of unilateral CLs occur on the left side. In addition, about 70% of unilateral CLs will be associated with CP, whereas the frequency of concomitant CP increases to 85% for patients with bilateral CL. CLs can be classified into three categories: microform, incomplete, and complete. A microform CL shows a notch or groove in the lip and vermilion junction, but all of the lip tissues are still present. An incomplete CL is more severe, exhibiting dehiscence of the orbicularis oris muscle with a

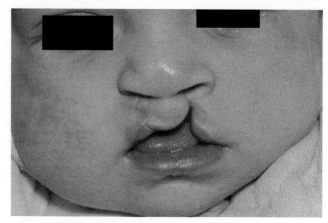

• **Fig. 1.1 Cleft Lip (CL).** Infant with bilateral cleft of the upper lip. (Courtesy of Dr. William Bruce.)

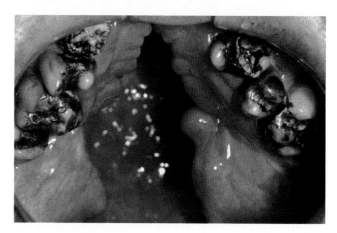

• **Fig. 1.2 Cleft Palate (CP).** Palatal defect resulting in communication with the nasal cavity.

variable degree of overlying skin involvement. A thin band of soft tissue (Simonart band) remains intact across the superior aspect of the cleft at the nasal sill. A complete CL extends through the length of the lip and across the nasal sill, resulting in abnormal insertion of the orbicularis oris into the nasal ala and columella. Complete clefts involving the alveolus usually occur between the lateral incisor and cuspid. It is not unusual for teeth, especially the lateral incisor, to be missing in the cleft area. Conversely, supernumerary teeth may be discovered. The bony defect can be observed on radiographs.

A CP shows considerable range in severity (Fig. 1.2). Clefts of the primary palate occur anterior to the incisive foramen and extend to the alveolar ridge. Clefts of the secondary palate occur posterior to the incisive foramen and may involve the hard and soft palates or the soft palate alone. Complete CPs involve both the primary and secondary palates. The minimal manifestation of CP is a **cleft** or **bifid uvula** (Fig. 1.3). The prevalence of cleft uvula is much higher than that of CP, with a frequency of 1 in every 80 white individuals. The frequency in Asian and Native American populations is as high as 1 in 10. Cleft uvula is less common in blacks, occurring in 1 out of every 250 persons.

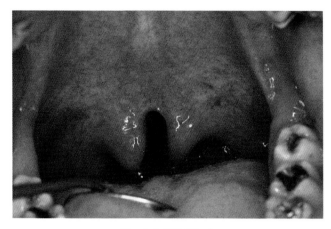

• **Fig. 1.3 Bifid Uvula.**

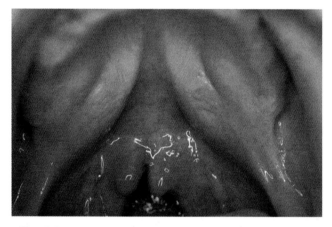

• **Fig. 1.4 Submucous Palatal Cleft.** A cleft of the midline palatal bone exists, but the overlying mucosa is intact. A bifid uvula also is present.

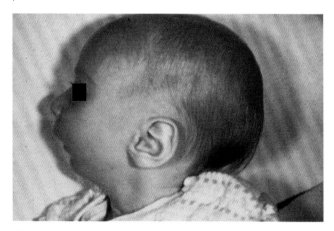

• **Fig. 1.5 Pierre Robin Sequence.** Micrognathic mandible in an infant with cleft palate (CP). (Courtesy of Dr. Robert Gorlin.)

In some instances a **submucous palatal cleft** develops. The surface mucosa is intact, but a defect exists in the underlying musculature of the soft palate (Fig. 1.4). Frequently a notch in the bone is present along the posterior margin of the hard palate. This incomplete cleft occasionally appears as a bluish midline discoloration but is best identified by palpation with a blunt instrument. An associated cleft uvula also usually is seen.

The **Pierre Robin sequence** (Fig. 1.5) is a well-recognized presentation characterized by CP, mandibular micrognathia, and glossoptosis (airway obstruction caused by lower, posterior displacement of the tongue). This condition may occur as an isolated phenomenon, or it may be associated with a wide variety of syndromes or other anomalies. Stickler syndrome and velocardiofacial syndrome (22q11.2 deletion syndrome) are the two most frequently associated genetic disorders. The prevalence of Pierre Robin sequence is estimated at 1 in 8000 to 14,000 births. Researchers have theorized that constraint of mandibular growth in utero results in failure of the tongue to descend, thus preventing fusion of the palatal shelves. The retruded mandible results in the following:
• Posterior displacement of the tongue
• Lack of support of the tongue musculature
• Airway obstruction

Respiratory difficulty, especially when the child is in a supine position, usually is noted from birth and can cause asphyxiation. The palatal cleft often is U-shaped and wider than isolated CP.

The patient with a cleft is burdened with a variety of problems, some obvious and some less so. The most obvious problem is the clinical appearance, which may lead to psychosocial difficulties. Feeding and speech difficulties are inherent, especially with CP. Malocclusion is caused by collapse of the maxillary arch, possibly along with missing teeth, supernumerary teeth, or both.

Treatment and Prognosis

The management of the patient with an orofacial cleft is challenging. Ideally, treatment should involve a multidisciplinary approach, including (but not limited to) a pediatrician, oral and maxillofacial surgeon, otolaryngologist, plastic surgeon, pediatric dentist, orthodontist, prosthodontist, speech pathologist, and geneticist.

During the neonatal period, lip taping and nasoalveolar molding may be utilized in an attempt to reduce the severity of the cleft deformity. Surgical repair often involves multiple primary and secondary procedures throughout childhood. The specific types of surgical procedures and their timing will vary, depending on the severity of the defect and the philosophy of the treatment team. A detailed discussion of these procedures is beyond the scope of this text. However, primary lip closure usually is accomplished during the first few months of life, followed by repair of the palate between 7 and 15 months of age. Secondary soft tissue, bone grafting, and orthognathic/orthodontic procedures often are used to improve function and cosmetic appearance. Distraction osteogenesis of the maxilla can prove useful in patients in whom palatal scarring limits the amount of advancement possible at the time of osteotomy.

Breathing difficulties in infants with Pierre Robin sequence are managed best with conservative measures, such as side and prone positioning. However, in children with significant airway obstruction, placement of a nasopharyngeal airway may be warranted. In more severe cases, mandibular distraction osteogenesis may be a preferable treatment alternative to tracheostomy. Death from isolated Pierre Robin sequence is uncommon (1.2%), but the mortality rate in infants who also have related syndromes can increase to as high as 26% due to central nervous system anomalies, cardiac anomalies, or respiratory difficulties.

Genetic counseling is important for the patient and family. In nonsyndromic cases of orofacial clefting, the risk for cleft development in a sibling or offspring of an affected person is 3%–5% if no other first-degree relatives also are affected. The risk increases to 10%–20% if other first-degree relatives are affected. The risk may be even higher for those with clefts that are associated with syndromes, depending on the possible inheritance pattern.

◆ COMMISSURAL LIP PITS

Commissural lip pits are small mucosal invaginations that occur at the corners of the mouth on the vermilion border. Their location suggests that they may represent a failure of normal fusion of the embryonal maxillary and mandibular processes.

Commissural lip pits appear to be common in adults, where they have been reported in 12%–20% of the population. Their prevalence in children is considerably lower, ranging from 0.2% to 0.7% of those examined.

Although commissural lip pits are generally considered to be congenital lesions, these figures suggest that these invaginations often develop later in life. Commissural pits are seen more often in males than in females. A family history suggestive of autosomal dominant transmission has been noted in some cases.

Clinical Features

Commissural lip pits usually are discovered on routine examination, and the patient often is unaware of their presence. These pits may be unilateral or bilateral. They manifest as blind fistulas that may extend to a depth of 1 to 4 mm (Fig. 1.6). In some cases, a small amount of fluid may be

expressed when the pit is squeezed, presumably representing saliva from minor salivary glands that drain into the depth of the invagination.

Unlike **paramedian lip pits** (described in the following section), commissural lip pits are not associated with facial or palatal clefts. However, there does appear to be a significantly higher prevalence of preauricular pits (aural sinuses) in these patients.

Histopathologic Features

Although biopsy rarely is performed for patients with commissural lip pits, microscopic examination reveals a narrow invagination lined by stratified squamous epithelium. Ducts from minor salivary glands may drain into this invagination.

Treatment and Prognosis

Because commissural lip pits are virtually always asymptomatic and innocuous, no treatment is usually necessary. In extremely rare instances, salivary secretions may be excessive or secondary infection may occur, necessitating surgical excision of the pit.

◆ PARAMEDIAN LIP PITS (CONGENITAL FISTULAS OF THE LOWER LIP; CONGENITAL LIP PITS)

Paramedian lip pits are rare congenital invaginations of the lower lip. They are believed to arise from persistent lateral sulci on the embryonic mandibular arch. These sulci normally disappear by 6 weeks of embryonic age.

Clinical Features

Paramedian lip pits typically appear as bilateral and symmetric fistulas on either side of the midline of the vermilion of the lower lip (Fig. 1.7). Their appearance can range from

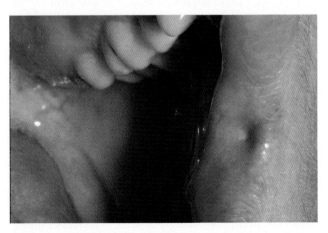

• **Fig. 1.6 Commissural Lip Pit.** Depression at the labial commissure.

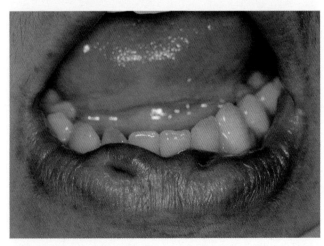

• **Fig. 1.7 Paramedian Lip Pits.** Bilateral pits on the lower lip in a patient with van der Woude syndrome. (Courtesy of Dr. Nadarajah Vigneswaran.)

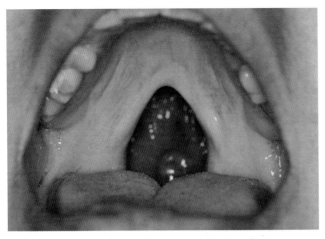

• **Fig. 1.8 Van der Woude Syndrome.** Same patient as depicted in Fig. 1.7 with a cleft of the soft palate. (Courtesy of Dr. Nadarajah Vigneswaran.)

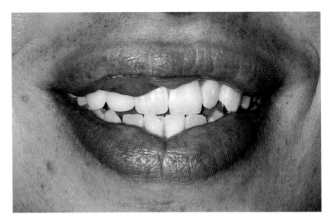

• **Fig. 1.9 Double Lip.** When the patient smiles, a redundant fold of tissue partially covers the right anterior maxillary teeth. (Courtesy of Dr. Logan Barnes.)

subtle depressions to prominent humps. These blind sinuses can extend down to a depth of 1.5 cm and may express salivary secretions. Occasionally, only a single pit is present that may be centrally located or lateral to the midline.

The greatest significance of paramedian lip pits is that they usually are inherited as an autosomal dominant trait in combination with cleft lip (CL) and/or cleft palate (CP) (**van der Woude syndrome**) (Fig. 1.8). Van der Woude syndrome is the most common form of syndromic clefting and accounts for 2% of all cases of CL and CP. Associated hypodontia also may be observed. Genetic studies have shown that this condition is caused by mutations in the gene that encodes interferon regulatory factor 6 (*IRF6*), which has been mapped to chromosome locus 1q32-q41. Some people who carry the trait may not demonstrate clefts or may have a submucous CP; however, they may pass the full syndrome to their offspring.

Paramedian lip pits also may be a feature of the **popliteal pterygium syndrome** and **Kabuki syndrome**. Popliteal webbing (**pterygia**), CL and/or CP, genital abnormalities, and congenital bands connecting the upper and lower jaws (**syngnathia**) characterize popliteal pterygium syndrome, which also is caused by mutation of the *IRF6* gene and is closely related to van der Woude syndrome. Kabuki syndrome is a separate condition that received its name because affected patients exhibit eversion of the lower lateral eyelids, which is reminiscent of the makeup used by actors in Kabuki, the traditional form of Japanese theater. Other common findings include intellectual disability, large ears, CL and/or CP, hypodontia, joint laxity, and various skeletal abnormalities.

Histopathologic Features

Microscopic examination of a paramedian lip pit shows a tract that is lined by stratified squamous epithelium. Minor salivary glands may communicate with the sinus. A chronic inflammatory cell infiltrate often is noted in the surrounding connective tissue.

Treatment and Prognosis

If necessary, the labial pits may be excised for cosmetic reasons. The most significant problems are related to associated congenital anomalies, such as CL and/or CP, and the potential for transmission of the trait to subsequent generations.

◆ DOUBLE LIP

Double lip is a rare oral anomaly characterized by a redundant fold of tissue on the mucosal side of the lip. Most often it is congenital in nature, but it may be acquired later in life. Congenital cases are believed to arise during the second to third month of gestation as a result of the persistence of the sulcus between the pars glabrosa and pars villosa of the lip. Acquired double lip may be a component of **Ascher syndrome,** or it may result from trauma or oral habits, such as sucking on the lip.

Clinical Features

In a patient with double lip, the upper lip is affected much more often than the lower lip; occasionally, both lips are involved. With the lips at rest, the condition is usually unnoticeable, but when the patient smiles or when the lips are tensed, the excess fold of tissue is visible (Fig. 1.9).

Ascher syndrome is characterized by a triad of features:
• Double lip
• Blepharochalasis
• Nontoxic thyroid enlargement

In a person with blepharochalasis, recurring edema of the upper eyelid leads to sagging of the lid at the outer canthus of the eye (Fig. 1.10). This drooping may be severe enough to interfere with vision. Both the double lip and blepharochalasis usually occur abruptly and simultaneously, but in some cases they develop more gradually.

The nontoxic thyroid enlargement occurs in as many as 50% of patients with Ascher syndrome and may be mild in degree. The cause of Ascher syndrome is not certain; autosomal dominant inheritance has been suggested in some cases.

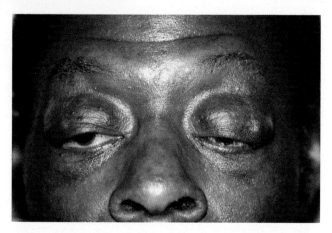

• **Fig. 1.10 Ascher Syndrome.** Edema of the upper eyelids (blepharochalasis).

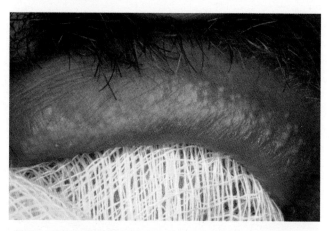

• **Fig. 1.11 Fordyce Granules.** Yellow papules on the vermilion of the upper lip.

Histopathologic Features

On microscopic examination, double lip shows essentially normal structures. Often there is an abundance of minor salivary glands. The blepharochalasis of Ascher syndrome usually shows hyperplasia of the lacrimal glands or prolapse of orbital fat.

Treatment and Prognosis

In mild cases of double lip, no treatment may be required. In more severe cases, simple surgical excision of the excess tissue can be performed for aesthetic purposes.

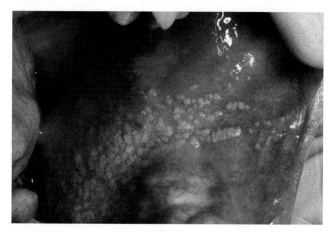

• **Fig. 1.12 Fordyce Granules.** Lesions on the buccal mucosa.

◆ FORDYCE GRANULES

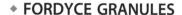

Fordyce granules are sebaceous glands that occur on the oral mucosa. Similar lesions also have been reported on the genital mucosa. Because sebaceous glands typically are considered to be dermal adnexal structures, those found in the oral cavity often have been considered to be "ectopic." However, because Fordyce granules have been reported in more than 80% of the population, their presence must be considered a normal anatomic variation.

Clinical Features

Fordyce granules appear as multiple yellow or yellow-white papules that are most common on the buccal mucosa and the lateral portion of the vermilion of the upper lip (Figs. 1.11 and 1.12). Occasionally, these glands also may appear in the retromolar area and anterior tonsillar pillar. They are more common in adults than in children, probably as a result of hormonal factors; puberty appears to stimulate their development. The lesions are typically asymptomatic, although patients may be able to feel a slight roughness to the mucosa. Considerable clinical variation may exist; some patients may have only a few lesions, whereas others may have literally hundreds of these "granules."

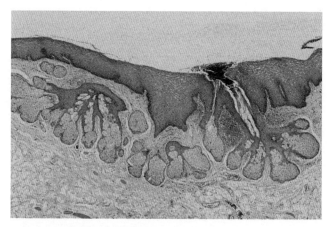

• **Fig. 1.13 Fordyce Granules.** Multiple sebaceous glands below the surface epithelium.

Histopathologic Features

Except for the absence of associated hair follicles, Fordyce granules closely resemble normal sebaceous glands found in the skin. Acinar lobules can be seen immediately beneath the epithelial surface, often communicating with the surface through a central duct (Fig. 1.13). The sebaceous cells in these lobules are polygonal in shape, containing centrally located nuclei and abundant foamy cytoplasm.

Treatment and Prognosis

Because Fordyce granules represent a normal anatomic variation and are asymptomatic, no treatment is indicated. Usually, the clinical appearance is characteristic and biopsy is not necessary for diagnosis.

On occasion, Fordyce granules may become hyperplastic or may form keratin-filled pseudocysts. Tumors arising from these glands are exceedingly rare.

◆ LEUKOEDEMA

Leukoedema is a common oral mucosal condition of unknown cause. It occurs more commonly in blacks than in whites, supporting the likelihood of an ethnic predisposition to its development. Leukoedema has been reported in 70%–90% of black adults and in 50% of black children. The prevalence in whites is considerably less, although published reports have ranged from less than 10% to more than 90%. This variation may reflect differing population groups, examination conditions, and stringency of criteria used to make the diagnosis. At any rate, leukoedema shows a much milder presentation in whites and often is hardly noticeable. The difference in racial predilection may be explained by the presence of background mucosal pigmentation in blacks that makes the edematous changes more noticeable.

Because leukoedema is so common, it can reasonably be argued that it represents a *variation of normal* rather than a disease. The finding of similar edematous mucosa in the vagina and larynx further supports this argument. Although leukoedema appears to be developmental in nature, some studies have indicated that it is more common and more severe in smokers and becomes less pronounced with cessation of smoking.

Clinical Features

Leukoedema is characterized by a diffuse, gray-white, milky, opalescent appearance of the mucosa (Fig. 1.14). The surface frequently appears folded, resulting in wrinkles or whitish streaks. The lesions do not rub off. Leukoedema typically occurs bilaterally on the buccal mucosa and may extend forward onto the labial mucosa. On rare occasions, it also can involve the floor of the mouth and palatopharyngeal tissues. Leukoedema can be easily diagnosed clinically because the white appearance greatly diminishes or disappears when the cheek is everted and stretched (Fig. 1.15).

Histopathologic Features

Biopsy specimens of leukoedema demonstrate an increase in thickness of the epithelium with striking intracellular edema of the spinous layer (Fig. 1.16). These vacuolated cells appear large and have pyknotic nuclei. The epithelial surface is frequently parakeratinized, and the rete ridges are broad and elongated.

Treatment and Prognosis

Leukoedema is a benign condition, and no treatment is required. The characteristic milky-white, opalescent lesions of the buccal mucosa that disappear when stretched help distinguish it from other common white lesions, such as leukoplakia, candidiasis, and lichen planus. The affected mucosa always should be stretched during clinical examination to

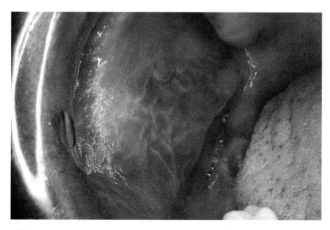

• **Fig. 1.14 Leukoedema.** White, wrinkled appearance of the buccal mucosa.

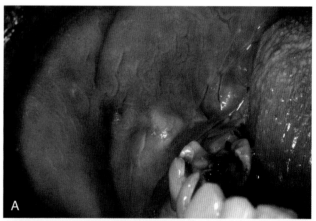

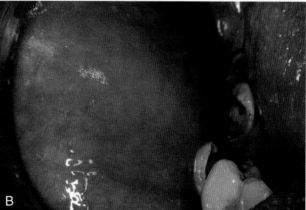

• **Fig. 1.15 Leukoedema. A,** Diffuse white appearance of the buccal mucosa. **B,** Whiteness disappears when the cheek is stretched.

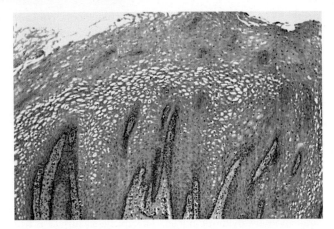

• **Fig. 1.16 Leukoedema.** Parakeratosis and intracellular edema of the spinous layer.

rule out any underlying lesions that may be hidden by the edematous change.

◆ MICROGLOSSIA (HYPOGLOSSIA)

Clinical Features

Microglossia is an uncommon developmental condition of unknown cause that is characterized by an abnormally small tongue. In rare instances, virtually the entire tongue may be missing **(aglossia)**. Isolated microglossia is known to occur, and mild degrees of microglossia may be difficult to detect and may go unnoticed. However, most reported cases have been associated with one of a group of overlapping conditions known as **oromandibular-limb hypogenesis syndromes**. These syndromes feature associated limb anomalies, such as **hypodactylia** (i.e., absence of digits) and **hypomelia** (i.e., hypoplasia of part or all of a limb). Other patients have had coexisting anomalies, such as cleft palate, intraoral bands, and *situs inversus*. Microglossia frequently is associated with hypoplasia of the mandible, and the lower incisors may be missing (Fig. 1.17).

Treatment and Prognosis

Treatment of the patient with microglossia depends on the nature and severity of the condition. Surgery and orthodontics may improve oral function. Surprisingly, speech development often is quite good but depends on tongue size.

◆ MACROGLOSSIA

Macroglossia is an uncommon condition characterized by enlargement of the tongue. The enlargement may be caused by a wide variety of conditions, including congenital malformations and acquired diseases. The most frequent causes are vascular malformations and muscular hypertrophy. Box 1.1 lists the most common and important causes of macroglossia. Many of these diseases are discussed in greater detail in subsequent chapters of this book.

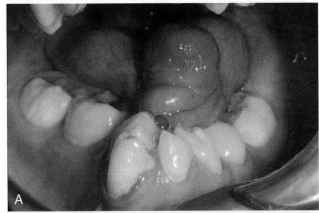
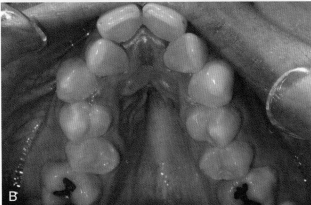

• **Fig. 1.17 Microglossia. A,** Abnormally small tongue associated with constricted mandibular arch. **B,** Same patient with associated constriction of the maxillary arch.

• BOX 1.1   Causes of Macroglossia

Congenital and Hereditary

- Vascular malformations
- Lymphangioma
- Hemangioma
- Hemihyperplasia
- Cretinism
- Beckwith-Wiedemann syndrome
- Down syndrome
- Duchenne muscular dystrophy
- Mucopolysaccharidoses
- Neurofibromatosis type I
- Multiple endocrine neoplasia, type 2B

Acquired

- Edentulous patients
- Amyloidosis
- Myxedema
- Acromegaly
- Angioedema
- Myasthenia gravis
- Amyotrophic lateral sclerosis
- Carcinoma and other tumors

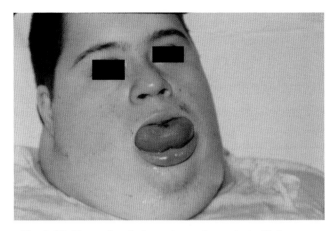

• **Fig. 1.18** **Macroglossia**. Large tongue in a patient with Down syndrome. (Courtesy of Dr. Sanford Fenton.)

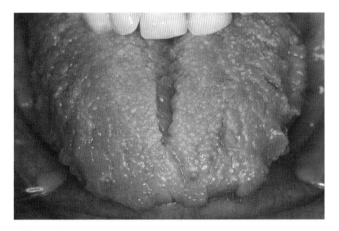

• **Fig. 1.19** **Macroglossia**. The tongue enlargement has resulted in a crenated border that corresponds to the embrasures between the teeth.

Clinical Features

Macroglossia most commonly occurs in children and can range from mild to severe (Fig. 1.18). In infants, macroglossia may be manifested first by noisy breathing, drooling, and difficulty in eating. The tongue enlargement may result in a lisping speech. The pressure of the tongue against the mandible and teeth can produce a crenated lateral border to the tongue (Fig. 1.19), open bite, and mandibular prognathism. If the tongue constantly protrudes from the mouth, it may ulcerate and become secondarily infected or may even undergo necrosis. Significant macroglossia can contribute to obstructive sleep apnea or, rarely, result in overt airway obstruction.

Macroglossia is a characteristic feature of **Beckwith-Wiedemann syndrome,** a rare hereditary condition that includes many other possible defects, such as the following:
• Omphalocele (i.e., protrusion of part of the intestine through a defect in the abdominal wall at the umbilicus)
• Visceromegaly
• Gigantism
• Neonatal hypoglycemia
Individuals with Beckwith-Wiedemann syndrome have an increased risk for several childhood visceral tumors,

including Wilms tumor, adrenal carcinoma, hepatoblastoma, rhabdomyosarcoma, and neuroblastoma. Facial features may include nevus flammeus of the forehead and eyelids, linear indentations of the earlobes, and maxillary hypoplasia (resulting in relative mandibular prognathism). Most examples of Beckwith-Wiedemann syndrome are sporadic, but 10%–15% of cases show autosomal dominant inheritance with preferential maternal transmission. The genetic basis is complex, involving a variety of alterations within two domains of imprinted growth-regulatory genes on chromosome 11p15.

In patients with **hypothyroidism** (see page 835), Beckwith-Wiedemann syndrome, or neuromuscular disorders, the tongue usually shows a diffuse, smooth, generalized enlargement. In those with other forms of macroglossia, the tongue usually has a multinodular appearance. Examples of this nodular type include **amyloidosis** (see page 824) and neoplastic conditions, such as **neurofibromatosis** (see page 537) and **multiple endocrine neoplasia, type 2B** (see page 540).

In patients with **lymphangiomas** (see page 553), the tongue surface is characteristically pebbly and exhibits multiple vesicle-like blebs that represent superficial dilated lymphatic channels. The enlarged tongue in those with **Down syndrome** typically demonstrates a papillary, fissured surface.

In patients with **hemifacial hyperplasia** (see page 37), the enlargement will be unilateral. Some patients with neurofibromatosis also can have unilateral lingual enlargement.

In edentulous patients, the tongue often appears elevated and tends to spread out laterally because of loss of the surrounding teeth; as a result, wearing a denture may become difficult.

Histopathologic Features

The microscopic appearance of macroglossia depends on the specific cause. In some cases, such as the tongue enlargement seen with Down syndrome or in edentulous patients, no histologic abnormality can be detected. When macroglossia is due to tumor, a neoplastic proliferation of a particular tissue can be found (e.g., lymphatic vessels, blood vessels, neural tissue). Muscular enlargement occurs in those with hemihyperplasia and Beckwith-Wiedemann syndrome. In neuromuscular disorders, such as myasthenia gravis or amyotrophic lateral sclerosis, tongue enlargement may result from muscular atrophy with prominent fatty replacement. In the patient with amyloidosis, an abnormal protein material is deposited in the tongue.

Treatment and Prognosis

The treatment and prognosis of macroglossia depend on the cause and severity of the condition. In mild cases, surgical treatment may not be necessary, although speech therapy may be helpful if speech is affected. In symptomatic patients, reduction glossectomy may be needed.

◆ ANKYLOGLOSSIA (TONGUE-TIE)

Ankyloglossia is a developmental anomaly of the tongue characterized by a short, thick lingual frenum resulting in limitation of tongue movement. It has been reported to occur in 0.1%–16% of neonates, being more common in boys than in girls. In adults, mild forms are not unusual, but severe ankyloglossia is a relatively uncommon condition that has been estimated to occur in about two to three of every 10,000 people. Most examples of ankyloglossia appear to be sporadic, although evidence suggests that there could be a genetic influence in some cases.

Clinical Features

Ankyloglossia can range in severity from mild cases with little clinical significance to rare examples of complete ankyloglossia in which the tongue is actually fused to the floor of the mouth (Fig. 1.20). The term *anterior ankyloglossia* is used when the frenum attachment extends toward the tip of the tongue. Sometimes slight clefting of the tongue tip may be seen. *Posterior ankyloglossia* is more subtle to detect, being related to short collagen bundles in the posterior midline floor of the mouth, which result in limitation of tongue movement.

With the increase in popularity of breast-feeding in recent decades, clinicians have related tongue-tie with feeding problems, such as nipple pain or difficulty in the baby attaching to the breast. Some investigators have speculated that ankyloglossia may lead to the development of an anterior open bite because the inability to raise the tongue to the roof of the mouth prevents development of the normal adult swallowing pattern. However, others have questioned this theory. It also is possible that a high mucogingival attachment of the lingual frenum may contribute to gingival recession, although a clear relationship has not been established.

It has been suggested that tongue-tie may result in speech defects. Usually, however, the shortened frenum results in only minor difficulties because most people can compensate for the limitation in tongue movement. Yet there are rare

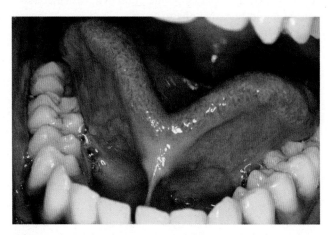

• **Fig. 1.20 Ankyloglossia.** Abnormal attachment of the lingual frenum, limiting tongue mobility.

examples of patients who have experienced an immediate noticeable improvement in speech after surgical correction of ankyloglossia.

Treatment and Prognosis

Because most cases of ankyloglossia result in few or no clinical problems, treatment is often unnecessary. For infants with specific breast-feeding problems, a frenotomy ("clipping" or simple release of the frenulum) can be performed, which has been shown to improve nipple pain and breast-feeding scores. In children or adults with associated functional or periodontal difficulties, a frenuloplasty (release with plastic repair) may allow greater freedom of tongue movement. In young children, it often is recommended that surgery be postponed until age 4 or 5. Because the tongue is always short at birth, assessing the degree of tongue limitation caused by ankyloglossia is difficult in the infant's early life. As the infant grows, the tongue becomes longer and thinner at the tip, often decreasing the severity of the tongue-tie. The condition probably is self-correcting in many cases because it is less common in adults.

◆ LINGUAL THYROID

During the third to fourth week of fetal life, the thyroid gland begins as an epithelial proliferation in the floor of the pharyngeal gut. By the seventh embryonic week, this thyroid bud normally descends into the neck to its final resting position anterior to the trachea and larynx. The site where this descending bud invaginates later becomes the foramen cecum, located at the junction of the anterior two-thirds and posterior third of the tongue in the midline. If the primitive gland does not descend normally, ectopic thyroid tissue may be found between the foramen cecum and the epiglottis. Of all ectopic thyroids, 90% are found in this region.

Clinical Features

Based on autopsy studies, small asymptomatic remnants of thyroid tissue can be discovered on the posterior dorsal tongue in about 10% of both men and women. However, clinically evident or symptomatic **lingual thyroids** are rare, with a prevalence of 1 per 100,000–300,000 persons. Such lesions are four to seven times more frequent in females, presumably because of hormonal influences. Symptoms most often develop during puberty, adolescence, pregnancy, or menopause. In 70% of cases, this ectopic gland is the patient's only thyroid tissue.

Lingual thyroids may range from small, asymptomatic, nodular lesions to large masses that can block the airway (Fig. 1.21). The most common clinical symptoms are dysphagia, dysphonia, and dyspnea. The mass often is vascular, but the physical appearance is variable, and there are no reliable features to distinguish it from other masses that might develop in this area. Hypothyroidism can develop in up to 72% of patients. Many authors say that lingual thyroid

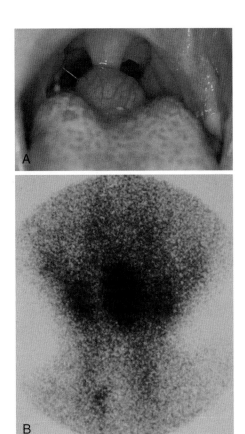

• **Fig. 1.21 Lingual Thyroid. A,** Nodular mass of the posterior dorsal midline of the tongue in a 4-year-old girl. **B,** Thyroid scan of the same patient. The scan shows localization (central dark zone) of iodine isotope in the tongue mass and minimal uptake in the neck.

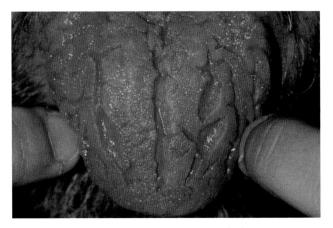

• **Fig. 1.22 Fissured Tongue**. Extensive fissuring involving the entire dorsal tongue surface. (Courtesy of Chris Neville.)

enlargement is a secondary phenomenon, compensating for thyroid hypofunction. Interestingly, from 25% to 75% of patients with infantile hypothyroidism have some ectopic thyroid tissue.

Diagnosis is best established by thyroid scan using iodine isotopes or technetium-99 m (^{99m}Tc). Computed tomography (CT), magnetic resonance imaging (MRI), and ultrasonography can be helpful in delineating the size and extent of the lesion. Biopsy is often avoided because of the risk of hemorrhage and because the mass may represent the patient's only functioning thyroid tissue. In some cases, incisional biopsy may be needed to confirm the diagnosis or to rule out malignant changes.

Treatment and Prognosis

No treatment except periodic follow-up is required for patients with asymptomatic lingual thyroids. In symptomatic patients, suppressive therapy with supplemental thyroid hormone often can reduce the size of the lesion. Some authors advise that this treatment also should be tried in asymptomatic patients to prevent possible subsequent enlargement. If hormone therapy does not eliminate symptoms, surgical removal or ablation with radioactive iodine-131 can be performed. If the mass is excised,

autotransplantation to another body site can be attempted to maintain functional thyroid tissue and to prevent hypothyroidism.

Rare examples of carcinomas arising in lingual thyroids have been reported; malignancy develops in about 1% of identified cases. Although lingual thyroids are decidedly more common in females, this predilection for females is less pronounced for lingual thyroid carcinomas. Because a disproportionate number of these malignancies have been documented in males, some authors have advocated prophylactic excision of lingual thyroids in men older than 30 years of age.

◆ FISSURED TONGUE (SCROTAL TONGUE; LINGUA PLICATA)

Fissured tongue is a relatively common condition that is characterized by the presence of numerous grooves, or fissures, on the dorsal tongue surface. The cause is uncertain, but heredity appears to play a significant role. Evidence indicates that the condition may be either a polygenic trait or an autosomal dominant trait with incomplete penetrance. A variety of other factors also may contribute to its development, including aging, smoking, and a history of psoriasis.

Clinical Features

Patients with fissured tongue exhibit multiple grooves, or furrows, on the surface of the tongue, ranging from 2 to 6 mm in depth (Fig. 1.22). Considerable variation can be seen. In the most severe cases, numerous fissures cover the entire dorsal surface and divide the tongue papillae into multiple separate "islands." Some patients have fissures that are located mostly on the dorsolateral areas of the tongue. Other patients exhibit a large central fissure with smaller fissures branching outward at right angles. The condition usually is asymptomatic, although some patients may complain of mild burning or soreness.

The prevalence of fissured tongue ranges from 2% to 5% of the overall population in some studies; however, other reports suggest prevalence rates as high as 20%–73%, probably related to the stringency of the diagnostic criteria. The condition may be seen in children or adults, but the prevalence and severity appear to increase with age, affecting as many as 30% of older adults. In some investigations, a male predilection has been noted.

A strong association has been found between fissured tongue and **geographic tongue** (see page 784) with many patients having both conditions. A hereditary basis also has been suggested for geographic tongue, and the same gene or genes may possibly be linked to both conditions. In fact, it even has been suggested that geographic tongue may *cause* fissured tongue. Fissured tongue also may be a component of **Melkersson-Rosenthal syndrome** (see page 330).

Histopathologic Features

Microscopic examination of fissured tongue reveals hyperplasia of the rete ridges and loss of the keratin "hairs" on the surface of the filiform papillae. The papillae vary in size and often are separated by deep grooves. Polymorphonuclear leukocytes can be seen migrating into the epithelium, often forming microabscesses in the upper epithelial layers. A mixed inflammatory cell infiltrate is present in the lamina propria. This overall pattern of inflammation is similar to that observed in erythema migrans and psoriasis.

Treatment and Prognosis

Fissured tongue is a benign condition, and no specific treatment is indicated. The patient should be encouraged to brush the tongue, because food or debris entrapped in the grooves may act as a source of irritation.

◆ HAIRY TONGUE (BLACK HAIRY TONGUE; COATED TONGUE)

Hairy tongue is characterized by marked accumulation of keratin on the filiform papillae of the dorsal tongue, resulting in a hairlike appearance. The condition apparently represents an increase in keratin production or a decrease in normal keratin desquamation. Depending on the population being studied, the prevalence of hairy tongue in adults ranges from 0.5% to 11.3%. Although the cause is uncertain, many affected people are heavy smokers. Other possible associated factors include general debilitation, poor oral hygiene, drugs that induce xerostomia, and a history of radiation therapy to the head and neck. Several reports have related transient development of hairy tongue with usage of the antibiotic linezolid.

Clinical Features

Hairy tongue most commonly affects the midline just anterior to the circumvallate papillae, sparing the lateral and anterior borders (Fig. 1.23). The elongated papillae are usually

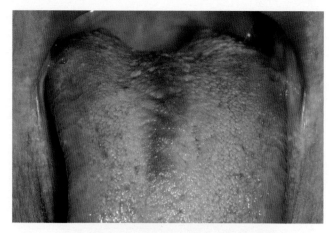

• **Fig. 1.23 Hairy Tongue.** Elongated, brown filiform papillae on the midline dorsal surface of the tongue.

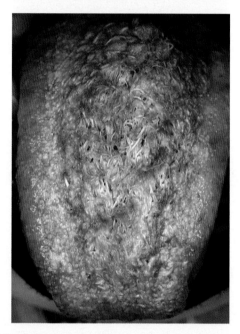

• **Fig. 1.24 Hairy Tongue.** Marked elongation and brown staining of the filiform papillae, resulting in a hairlike appearance.

brown, yellow, or black as a result of growth of pigment-producing bacteria or staining from tobacco and food. Sometimes most of the dorsal tongue may be involved, resulting in a thick, matted appearance (Fig. 1.24). Multiple individual elongated filiform papillae may be elevated by using gauze or a dental instrument. The condition is typically asymptomatic, although occasionally patients complain of a gagging sensation or a bad taste in the mouth. Because the diagnosis usually can be made from the clinical appearance, biopsy is unnecessary in most instances.

In some individuals, numerous bacteria and desquamated epithelial cells accumulate on the dorsal tongue surface, but without the hairlike filiform projections (Fig. 1.25). Such cases, which often are designated as a **coated tongue,** also may be a source of oral malodor. Coated tongue often is misdiagnosed as candidiasis and treated unnecessarily with antifungal medications.

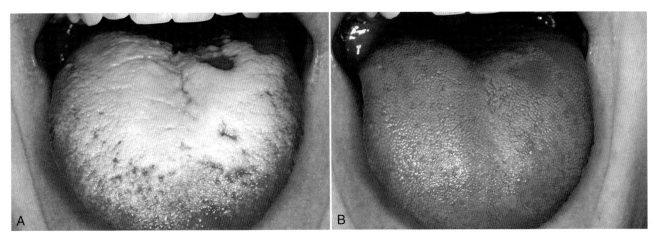

• **Fig. 1.25 Coated Tongue. A,** This patient had a severe outbreak of aphthous ulcers, which made routine oral hygiene difficult. The dorsal tongue has become white and markedly thickened from the accumulation of keratin and bacteria on the surface. **B,** After resolution of her oral ulcers plus improved hygiene, the tongue has returned to its normal appearance.

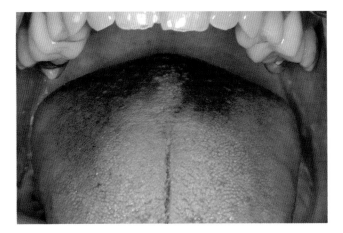

• **Fig. 1.26 Bismuth Staining.** Transitory staining of the posterior dorsal tongue after using bismuth subsalicylate for an upset stomach.

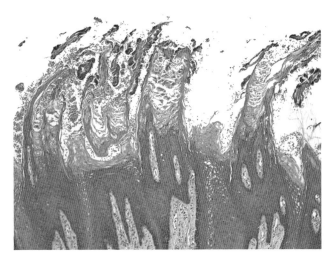

• **Fig. 1.27 Hairy Tongue.** Elongation and marked hyperkeratosis of the filiform papillae with bacterial accumulation on the surface.

Transitory black staining of the dorsal tongue without elongation of the filiform papillae sometimes can occur in patients who use bismuth subsalicylate to control upset stomach. The bismuth in such preparations can react with trace amounts of sulfur in the saliva to form bismuth sulfide, which accumulates on the tongue surface (Fig. 1.26). However, this discoloration rapidly resolves after discontinuation of the medication.

Histopathologic Features

On histopathologic examination, hairy tongue is characterized by marked elongation and hyperparakeratosis of the filiform papillae (Fig. 1.27). Usually, numerous bacteria can be seen growing on the epithelial surface.

Treatment and Prognosis

Hairy or coated tongue is a benign condition with no serious sequelae. The major concern is often the aesthetic appearance of the tongue along with possible associated bad breath. Any predisposing factors, such as tobacco, should be eliminated, and excellent oral hygiene should be encouraged. Periodic scraping or brushing with a toothbrush or tongue scraper can promote desquamation of the hyperkeratotic papillae and surface debris. Keratolytic agents, such as podophyllin, also have been tried with success, but for safety reasons their use probably should not be encouraged.

Because of the similarity in names, care should be taken to avoid confusing hairy tongue with **hairy leukoplakia** (see page 253), which typically occurs on the lateral border of the tongue. Hairy leukoplakia is caused by the Epstein-Barr virus and usually is associated with human immunodeficiency virus (HIV) infection or other immunosuppressive conditions.

◆ VARICOSITIES (VARICES)

Varicosities, or **varices,** are abnormally dilated and tortuous veins. Age appears to be an important etiologic factor because varices are rare in children but common in older adults. This suggests that their development may be an age-related degeneration manifested by weakening of blood vessel walls and loss of tone in the supporting connective tissues. One study found that people with varicose veins of the legs are more likely to have varicosities of the tongue. Other related factors include a history of smoking, cardiovascular disease, hypertension, and cirrhosis.

Clinical Features

The most common type of oral varicosity is the **sublingual varix,** which occurs in two-thirds of people older than 60 years of age. Sublingual varicosities classically present as multiple blue-purple, elevated or papular blebs on the ventral and lateral border of the tongue (Fig. 1.28). The lesions usually are asymptomatic, except in rare instances when secondary thrombosis occurs.

Less frequently, solitary varices occur in other areas of the mouth, especially the lips and buccal mucosa. These isolated varicosities often are first noticed after they have become thrombosed (Fig. 1.29). Clinically, a thrombosed varix presents as a firm, nontender, blue-purple nodule that may feel like a BB beneath the mucosal surface.

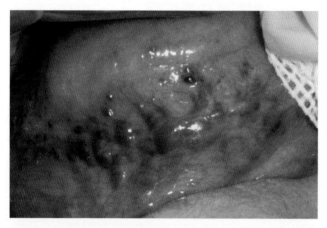

• **Fig. 1.28 Varicosities**. Multiple purple dilated veins on the ventral and lateral surface of the tongue.

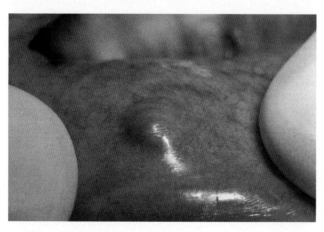

• **Fig. 1.29 Varicosity**. Firm, thrombosed varix on the lower lip.

Histopathologic Features

Microscopic examination of a varix reveals a dilated vein, the wall of which shows little smooth muscle and poorly developed elastic tissue. If secondary thrombosis has occurred, then the lumen may contain concentrically layered zones of platelets and erythrocytes (lines of Zahn). The clot can undergo organization via granulation tissue with subsequent recanalization. Older thrombi may exhibit dystrophic calcification, resulting in formation of a **phlebolith** (*phlebo* = vein; *lith* = stone).

Treatment and Prognosis

Sublingual varicosities typically are asymptomatic, and no treatment is indicated. Solitary varicosities of the lips and buccal mucosa may need to be surgically removed to confirm the diagnosis or for aesthetic purposes.

◆ CALIBER-PERSISTENT ARTERY

A **caliber-persistent artery** is a common vascular anomaly in which a main arterial branch extends up into the superficial submucosal tissues without a reduction in its diameter. Similar to oral varices, caliber-persistent arteries are seen more frequently in older adults. This suggests that their development may be an age-related degenerative phenomenon in which there is a loss of tone in the surrounding supporting connective tissue.

Clinical Features

The caliber-persistent artery occurs almost exclusively on the labial mucosa, especially on the upper lip. Some patients may have bilateral lesions or lesions on both lips. The average patient age is 58 years, and the gender ratio is nearly equal. The lesion presents as a linear, arcuate, or papular elevation that ranges from pale to normal to bluish in color (Fig. 1.30). Stretching the lip usually causes the artery to become inconspicuous. The unique feature is pulsation—not only vertically but also in a lateral direction. However, usually it is

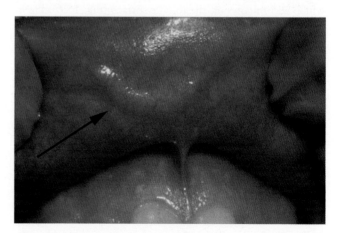

• **Fig. 1.30 Caliber-Persistent Artery**. Linear, arcuate lesion on the upper labial mucosa *(arrow)*. (Courtesy of Dr. John Lovas.)

not possible to feel a pulse in a caliber-persistent artery with gloved fingers.

The lesion is usually asymptomatic, being discovered as an incidental finding during an oral examination; rarely a patient may notice a pulsatile lip nodule. A few cases have been associated with ulceration of the overlying mucosa. In addition, a couple of examples have been found adjacent to labial squamous cell carcinomas, although this is probably coincidental.

Histopathologic Features

Microscopic examination shows a thick-walled artery situated close to the mucosal surface (Fig. 1.31).

Treatment and Prognosis

If the true nature of the caliber-persistent artery can be recognized clinically, no treatment is necessary. Oftentimes a biopsy is performed when the lesion is mistaken for a mucocele or another vascular lesion, such as a varix or hemangioma. Brisk bleeding typically is encountered if the lesion is removed.

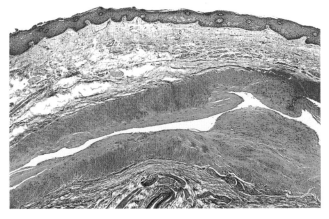

• **Fig. 1.31 Caliber-Persistent Artery.** Thick-walled artery located just beneath the mucosal surface.

◆ LATERAL SOFT PALATE FISTULAS

Lateral soft palate fistulas are rare anomalies of uncertain pathogenesis. Many cases appear to be congenital, possibly related to a defect in the development of the second pharyngeal pouch. Some fistulas may be the result of infection or surgery of the tonsillar region.

Clinical Features

Lateral soft palate fistulas usually are bilateral, but they may occur only on one side. They are more common on the anterior tonsillar pillar (Fig. 1.32), but they also may involve the posterior pillar. The perforations typically are asymptomatic, ranging from a few millimeters to more than 1 cm. A few cases have been associated with other anomalies, such as absence or hypoplasia of the palatine tonsils, hearing loss, and preauricular fistulas.

Treatment and Prognosis

The lesions are innocuous, and no treatment is necessary.

◆ CORONOID HYPERPLASIA

Hyperplasia of the coronoid process of the mandible is a rare developmental anomaly that may result in limitation of mandibular movement. The cause of **coronoid hyperplasia** is unknown, but the condition is three to five times more common in males than in females. Because most cases have been seen in pubertal males, an endocrine influence has been suggested. Heredity also may play a role, because cases have been noted in siblings.

Coronoid hyperplasia may be unilateral or bilateral, although bilateral cases are over four times more common than unilateral examples. Unilateral enlargement of the coronoid process also can result from a true tumor, such as an osteoma or osteochondroma, and such cases should be distinguished from pure coronoid hyperplasia. However, some

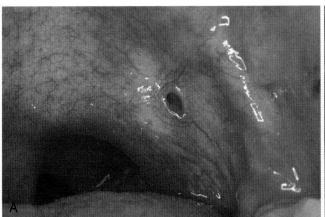
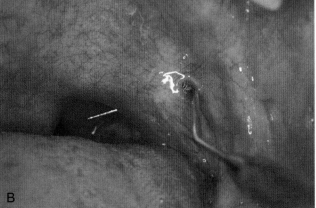

• **Fig. 1.32 Lateral Palatal Fistula. A,** Asymptomatic "hole" in the anterior tonsillar pillar. **B,** Periodontal probe has been used to demonstrate the communication of the lesion with the tonsillar fossa.

cases reported as tumors of the coronoid process actually may have been hyperplastic processes rather than true neoplasms.

Clinical and Radiographic Features

In a person with unilateral coronoid hyperplasia, the enlarged coronoid process impinges on the medial surface of the zygomatic arch, restricting mandibular opening. In addition, the mandible may deviate toward the affected side. Usually, there is no pain or associated abnormality in occlusion. Radiographs may reveal an irregular, nodular growth of the tip of the coronoid process.

In bilateral coronoid hyperplasia, the limitation of mandibular opening may progressively worsen over several

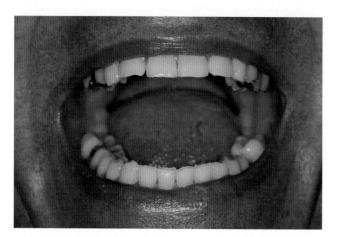

• **Fig. 1.33** **Coronoid Hyperplasia**. Limited ability to open the mouth in a young man with bilateral hyperplasia of the coronoid processes.

years during childhood, reaching maximum severity during the late teens (Fig. 1.33). The radiographic appearance is characterized by regular elongation of both processes (Fig. 1.34). Because the coronoid process often is superimposed on the zygoma on conventional radiographs, CT scans often demonstrate the hyperplasia more effectively.

Treatment and Prognosis

Treatment of coronoid hyperplasia consists of surgical removal of the elongated coronoid process or processes to allow freedom of mandibular motion. Coronoidectomy or coronoidotomy usually is accomplished via an intraoral approach. Although initial improvement in oral opening can be effected, the long-term results in some patients can be disappointing because of surgically induced fibrosis and the tendency for coronoid regrowth. Postoperative physiotherapy is important for reestablishing normal function.

◆ CONDYLAR HYPERPLASIA

Condylar hyperplasia is an uncommon malformation created by excessive growth of one or both of the mandibular condyles. The cause of this hyperplasia is unknown, but genetic factors, neoplasms, endocrine disturbances, and trauma have been suggested as possible etiologies. Table 1.1 summarizes two major classification systems.

Condylar hyperplasia can be difficult to distinguish from **hemifacial hyperplasia** (see page 37); however, in the latter condition the associated soft tissues and teeth also may be enlarged.

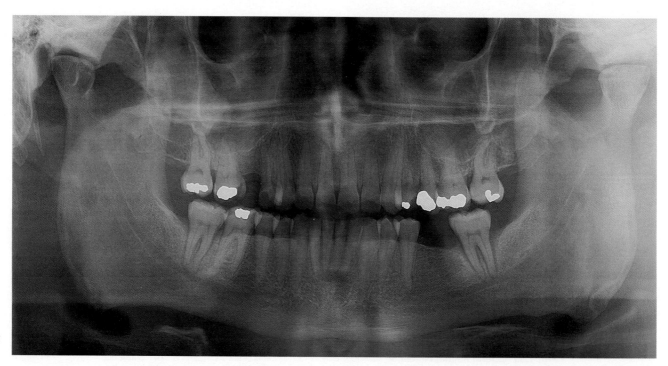

• **Fig. 1.34** **Coronoid Hyperplasia**. Panoramic radiograph of patient depicted in Fig. 1.33, which shows bilateral elongation of the coronoid processes.

TABLE 1.1	Classification of Condylar Hyperplasia		
Authors	**Category**	**Clinical Features**	
Obwegeser and Makek			
	Hemimandibular Hyperplasia	Primarily vertical overgrowth	
	Hemimandibular Elongation	Primarily horizontal overgrowth with lateral mandibular displacement	
	Hybrid	Combined features of both above types	
Wolford et al.			
	Type 1	Accelerated and prolonged aberration of "normal" condylar growth mechanism	
	Type 1A	Bilateral	
	Type 1B	Unilateral	
	Type 2	Unilateral condylar growth caused by an osteochondroma	
	Type 2A	Predominantly vertical elongation and enlargement of the condyle	
	Type 2B	Horizontal exophytic tumor growth from the condyle	
	Type 3	Other benign tumors causing condylar enlargement	
	Type 4	Malignant tumors causing enlargement of the condyle	

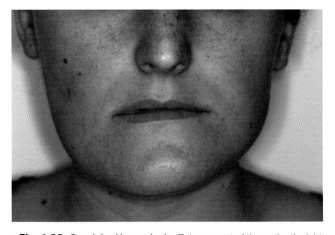

• **Fig. 1.35 Condylar Hyperplasia.** Enlargement of the patient's right condyle has resulted in facial asymmetry.

Clinical and Radiographic Features

Condylar hyperplasia may manifest itself in a variety of ways, including facial asymmetry, prognathism, crossbite, and open bite (Fig. 1.35). Sometimes compensatory maxillary growth and tilting of the occlusal plane occurs. The condition most commonly is discovered in adolescents and young adults. Several studies have shown a significant female predilection, with an overall female-to-male ratio of approximately 3:1.

The radiographic features are quite variable. Some patients have an enlargement of the condylar head, and others show elongation of the condylar neck (Fig. 1.36). Many cases also demonstrate hyperplasia of the entire ramus, suggesting that the condition sometimes affects more than just the condyle. Other examples show a tumorlike mass (e.g., osteochondroma) affecting the condylar head. Single-photon emission computed tomography (SPECT) and scintigraphy using ^{99m}Tc-methylenediphosphonate (MDP) have

been advocated as useful methods for assessing the degree of bone activity in condylar hyperplasia.

Histopathologic Features

Some cases will show an appearance that is similar to a normally growing condyle. Other examples will exhibit a nodular bony mass with a thickened cartilaginous cap consistent with an osteochondroma.

Treatment and Prognosis

Condylar hyperplasia is a self-limiting condition, and treatment is determined by the degree of functional difficulty and aesthetic change. Some patients can be treated with condylectomy, whereas others require unilateral or bilateral mandibular osteotomies. In patients with compensatory maxillary growth, a maxillary osteotomy also may be needed. Concomitant orthodontic therapy frequently is necessary.

◆ CONDYLAR HYPOPLASIA

Condylar hypoplasia, or underdevelopment of the mandibular condyle, can be either congenital or acquired. **Congenital condylar hypoplasia** often is associated with head and neck syndromes, including **mandibulofacial dysostosis** (see page 43), **oculoauriculovertebral syndrome (Goldenhar syndrome),** and **hemifacial microsomia.** In the most severe cases, complete agenesis of the condyle or ramus **(condylar aplasia)** is seen.

Acquired condylar hypoplasia results from disturbances of the growth center of the developing condyle. The most frequent cause is trauma to the condylar region during infancy or childhood. Other causes include infections, radiation therapy, and rheumatoid or degenerative arthritis.

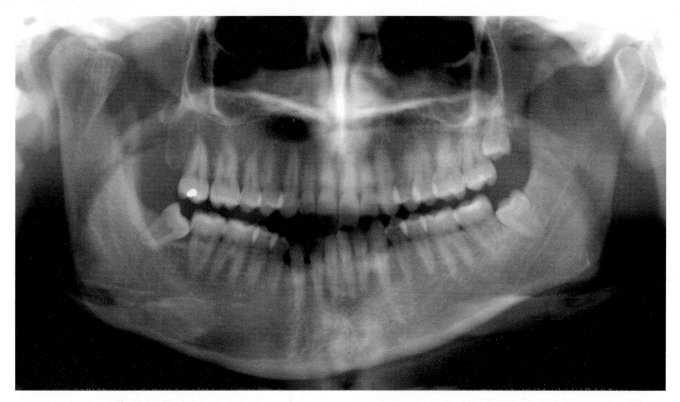

• **Fig. 1.36 Condylar Hyperplasia**. Panoramic radiograph of patient seen in Fig. 1.35, which shows prominent enlargement of the right mandibular condyle.

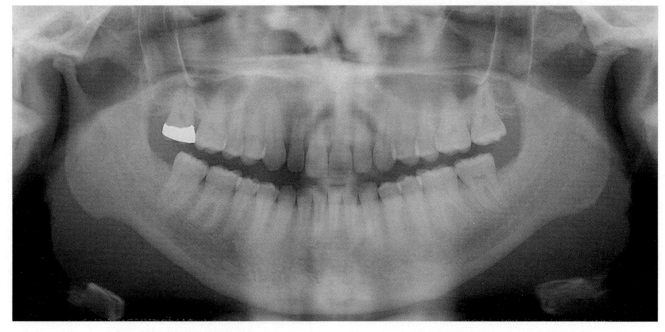

• **Fig. 1.37 Condylar Hypoplasia**. Panoramic radiograph showing bilateral hypoplasia of the mandibular condyles. (Courtesy of Dr. Rachel Sanyk.)

Clinical and Radiographic Features

Condylar hypoplasia can be unilateral or bilateral, producing a small mandible with a Class II malocclusion. Unilateral hypoplasia results in distortion and depression of the face on the affected side. The mandibular midline shifts to the involved side when the mouth is opened, accentuating the deformity. Ankylosis of the temporomandibular joint (TMJ) can develop in cases caused by trauma.

The deformity is observed easily on panoramic films and can range in severity (Fig. 1.37). In severe cases the condyle or ramus may be totally absent. Milder types demonstrate a short condylar process, shallow sigmoid notch, and poorly formed condylar head. A prominent antegonial notch may be present. CT scans may be helpful in evaluating the condyles.

Treatment and Prognosis

Treatment of the patient with condylar hypoplasia depends on the cause and severity of the defect, but surgery often is required. If the condyle is missing, then a costochondral rib graft can be placed to help establish an active growth center. In addition, osteotomies sometimes provide a cosmetically acceptable result. In certain instances, distraction osteogenesis can be used to stimulate new bone formation.

◆ BIFID CONDYLE

A **bifid condyle** is an uncommon developmental anomaly characterized by a double-headed mandibular condyle. The prevalence ranges from 0.31% to 1.82% in published reports. Most bifid condyles have a medial and lateral head divided by an anteroposterior groove. Some condyles may be divided into an anterior and posterior head.

The cause of bifid condyle is uncertain. Anteroposterior bifid condyles may be of traumatic origin, such as a childhood fracture. Mediolaterally divided condyles may result from trauma, abnormal muscle attachment, teratogenic agents, or persistence of a fibrous septum within the condylar cartilage.

Clinical and Radiographic Features

A bifid condyle usually is unilateral, but occasionally both sides may be affected. The malformation is often asymptomatic and may be discovered on routine radiographs, although some patients may have a "pop" or "click" of the TMJ when opening their mouths. Other patients may experience pain, hypomobility, or ankylosis. Panoramic radiographs and CT scans demonstrate a bilobed appearance of the condylar head (Fig. 1.38). Extremely rare examples of trifid and tetrafid condyles also have been reported.

Treatment and Prognosis

Because a bifid condyle is usually asymptomatic, no treatment is necessary in most instances. If the patient has joint complaints, the appropriate temporomandibular therapy may be required.

◆ EXOSTOSES

Exostoses are localized bony protuberances that arise from the cortical plate. These benign growths frequently affect the jaws and may be related to stresses placed on the bone from the function of teeth. The best-known oral exostoses, the **torus palatinus** and the **torus mandibularis,** are

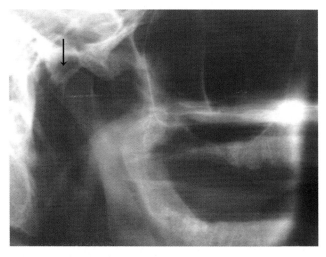

• **Fig. 1.38 Bifid Condyle**. Radiograph of the mandibular condyle showing a double head *(arrow)*.

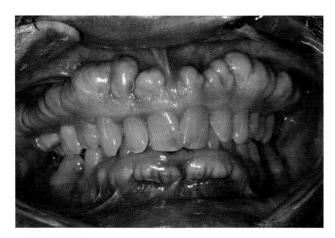

• **Fig. 1.39 Exostoses**. Multiple buccal exostoses of the maxillary and mandibular alveolar ridges.

described later in this chapter. Other types of exostoses also may affect the jaws and are considered here.

Clinical and Radiographic Features

Exostoses are discovered most often in adults. **Buccal exostoses** occur as a bilateral row of bony hard nodules along the facial aspect of the maxillary and/or mandibular alveolar ridge (Fig. 1.39). They usually are asymptomatic, unless the thin overlying mucosa becomes ulcerated from trauma. One study reported that buccal exostoses were found in nearly 1 of every 1000 adults (0.09%); however, a more recent survey found a much higher prevalence of nearly 19%. This variation may be due to the different populations being studied or to the clinical criteria used to make the diagnosis.

Palatal exostoses (palatal tubercles) are similar bony protuberances that develop from the lingual aspect of the maxillary tuberosities. These lesions usually are bilateral but may affect only one side (Fig. 1.40). They are more common in males and have been reported in 8%–69% of various

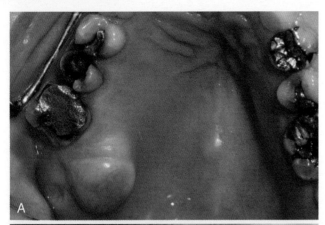

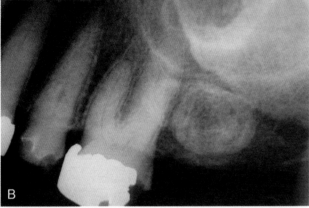

• **Fig. 1.40 Exostosis.** **A,** Secondarily ulcerated palatal exostosis. **B,** Radiograph shows an ovoid radiopacity distal to the molar.

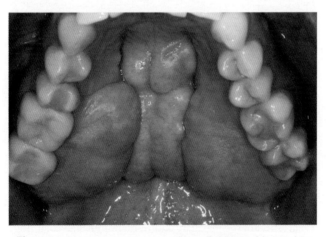

• **Fig. 1.41 Palatal Exostoses and Torus Palatinus.** Massive bilateral palatal exostoses in a patient with a large palatal torus.

populations. Many patients with buccal or palatal exostoses also will have palatal or mandibular tori (Fig. 1.41).

Less commonly, **solitary exostoses** may occur, possibly in response to local irritation. Such lesions may develop from the alveolar bone beneath free gingival grafts and skin grafts. Presumably placement of the graft acts as a stimulant to the periosteum to form new bone.

Another uncommon, interesting variant is the **reactive subpontine exostosis (subpontic osseous proliferation,**

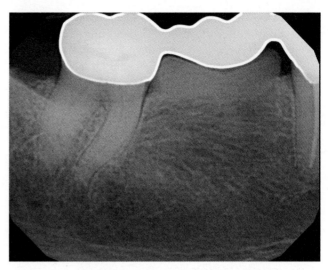

• **Fig. 1.42 Reactive Subpontine Exostosis.** Nodular growth of dense bone beneath the pontic of a posterior mandibular bridge. (Courtesy of Dr. Ed Murphy.)

subpontic osseous hyperplasia), which may develop from the alveolar crestal bone beneath the pontic of a posterior bridge (Fig. 1.42).

If enough excess bone is present, exostoses may exhibit a relative radiopacity on dental radiographs (see Fig. 1.40, *B*). In rare instances an exostosis may become so large that distinguishing it from a tumor, such as an osteoma, is difficult (see page 655).

Histopathologic Features

Microscopic examination reveals a mass of dense, lamellar, cortical bone with a small amount of fibrofatty marrow. In some cases an inner zone of trabecular bone also is present.

Treatment and Prognosis

Most exostoses are distinctive enough clinically to make biopsy unnecessary. If the diagnosis is uncertain, biopsy should be performed to rule out other bony pathosis. Sometimes the exostosis must be removed if it repeatedly has been exposed to trauma or has become ulcerated and painful. In addition, surgical removal may be required to accommodate a dental prosthesis or to allow for proper flap adaptation during periodontal surgery. Reactive subpontine exostoses may need to be removed if they interfere with oral hygiene or are associated with adjacent periodontal disease. Exostoses that develop secondary to adjacent tooth function may recur after removal if the teeth creating the stresses remain in place.

◆ TORUS PALATINUS

The **torus palatinus** is a common exostosis that occurs in the midline of the vault of the hard palate. The pathogenesis of these tori has long been debated with arguments centering on genetic versus environmental factors, such as masticatory stress. Some authorities have suggested that the torus palatinus is inherited as an autosomal dominant trait. However, others believe that the development of this lesion is multifactorial, including both genetic and environmental influences. In this model, patients are affected by a variety of hereditary and local environmental factors. If enough of these factors are present, then a "threshold" is surpassed and the trait (torus palatinus) is expressed.

Clinical and Radiographic Features

The torus palatinus presents as a bony hard mass that arises along the midline suture of the hard palate (Figs. 1.43 and 1.44). Tori sometimes are classified according to their morphologic appearance:

- The **flat torus** has a broad base and a slightly convex, smooth surface. It extends symmetrically onto both sides of the midline raphe.
- The **spindle torus** has a midline ridge along the palatal raphe. A median groove is sometimes present.
- The **nodular torus** arises as multiple protuberances, each with an individual base. These protuberances may coalesce, forming grooves between them.
- The **lobular torus** is also a multilobulated mass, but it rises from a single base. Lobular tori can be either sessile or pedunculated.

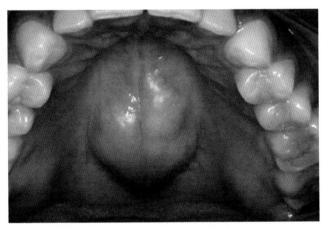

• **Fig. 1.43 Torus Palatinus**. Midline bony nodule of the palatal vault.

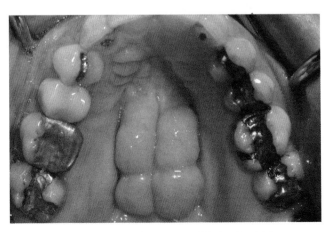

• **Fig. 1.44 Torus Palatinus**. Large, lobulated palatal mass.

Most palatal tori are small, measuring less than 2 cm in diameter; however, they can slowly increase in size throughout life—sometimes to the extent that they fill the entire palatal vault. Most tori cause no symptoms, but in some cases the thin overlying mucosa may become ulcerated secondary to trauma.

The torus palatinus usually does not appear on routine dental radiographs. Rarely, it may be seen as a radiopacity on periapical films if the film is placed behind the torus when the radiograph is taken.

The prevalence of palatal tori has varied widely in a number of population studies, ranging from 4% to 60%. Some of this variation may be due to the criteria used to make the diagnosis and also may be based on whether the study was conducted on live patients or skulls. There appear to be significant racial differences, however, with a higher prevalence in Asian and Inuit populations. In the United States, most studies have shown a prevalence of 20%–35%, although these figures likely include a significant number of relatively small lesions. Almost all studies from around the world have shown a pronounced female-to-male ratio of 2:1. The prevalence peaks during early adult life, tapering off in later years. This finding supports the theory that tori are dynamic lesions that are related, in part, to environmental factors; in later life, some may undergo resorption remodeling in response to decreased functional stresses.

Histopathologic Features

Microscopic examination of the torus shows a mass of dense, lamellar, cortical bone. An inner zone of trabecular bone sometimes is seen.

Treatment and Prognosis

Most palatal tori can be diagnosed clinically based on their characteristic appearance; therefore biopsy rarely is necessary. In edentulous patients, the torus may need to be removed surgically to accommodate a denture base. Surgical removal also may be indicated for palatal tori that repeatedly become ulcerated or that interfere with oral function. It also should be noted that palatal tori are prone to medication-related osteonecrosis (see page 286).

◆ TORUS MANDIBULARIS

The **torus mandibularis** is a common exostosis that develops along the lingual aspect of the mandible. As with torus palatinus, the cause of mandibular tori probably is multifactorial, including both genetic and environmental influences.

Clinical and Radiographic Features

The mandibular torus presents as a bony protuberance along the lingual aspect of the mandible above the mylohyoid line in the region of the premolars (Fig. 1.45). Bilateral involvement occurs in more than 90% of cases. Most mandibular

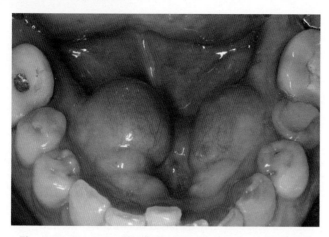

• **Fig. 1.45 Torus Mandibularis.** Bilateral lobulated bony protuberances of the mandibular lingual alveolar ridge.

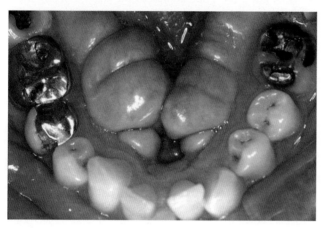

• **Fig. 1.46 Torus Mandibularis.** Massive "kissing" tori meet in the midline.

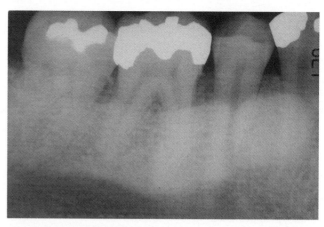

• **Fig. 1.47 Torus Mandibularis.** Torus is causing a radiopacity that is superimposed over the roots of the mandibular teeth.

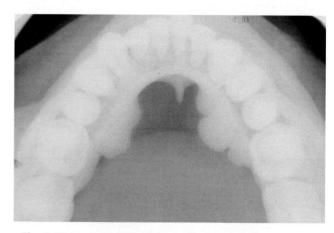

• **Fig. 1.48 Torus Mandibularis.** Occlusal radiograph showing bilateral mandibular tori.

tori occur as single nodules, although multiple lobules paralleling the teeth are not unusual. Patients often are unaware of their presence unless the overlying mucosa becomes ulcerated secondary to trauma. In rare instances, bilateral tori may become so large that they almost meet in the midline (Fig. 1.46). A large mandibular torus may appear on periapical radiographs as a radiopacity superimposed on the roots of the teeth (Fig. 1.47), especially on anterior films. Mandibular tori are easily visualized on occlusal radiographs (Fig. 1.48).

Most studies indicate that the torus mandibularis is not as common as the torus palatinus; the prevalence ranges from 3% to 58%. Like the torus palatinus, the mandibular torus appears to be more common in Asians and the Inuit. The prevalence in the United States ranges from 7% to 10% with little difference between blacks and whites. A slight male predilection has been noted.

The prevalence of mandibular torus peaks in early adult life, tapering slightly in later years. In addition, the prevalence has been correlated with both bruxism and the number of teeth remaining present. These findings support the theory that the torus mandibularis is multifactorial in development and responds to functional stresses.

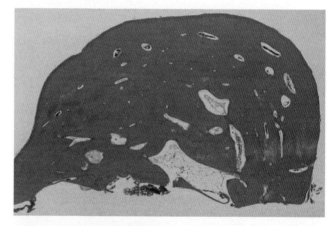

• **Fig. 1.49 Torus Mandibularis.** Nodular mass of dense, cortical bone. Some fatty marrow is visible at the base of the specimen.

Histopathologic Features

The histopathologic appearance of the torus mandibularis is similar to that of other exostoses, consisting primarily of a nodular mass of dense, cortical lamellar bone (Fig. 1.49). An inner zone of trabecular bone with associated fatty marrow sometimes is visible.

Treatment and Prognosis

Most mandibular tori are easily diagnosed clinically, and no treatment is necessary. However, surgical removal may be required to accommodate a lower full or partial denture. Occasionally, tori may recur if teeth are still present in the area.

◆ EAGLE SYNDROME (STYLOHYOID SYNDROME; STYLOCAROTID SYNDROME; STYLALGIA)

The styloid process is a slender bony projection that originates from the inferior aspect of the temporal bone, anterior and medial to the stylomastoid foramen. It is connected to the lesser cornu of the hyoid bone by the stylohyoid ligament. The external and internal carotid arteries lie on either side. Elongation of the styloid process or mineralization of the stylohyoid ligament complex is not unusual, having been reported in 18%–84% of the population with an increasing incidence with advancing age. Such mineralization is usually bilateral, but it may affect only one side. Most cases are asymptomatic; however, it is estimated that 4%–10% of patients with elongation of the styloid process experience symptoms of **Eagle syndrome,** caused by impingement or compression of adjacent nerves or blood vessels.

Clinical and Radiographic Features

Eagle syndrome most commonly affects adults, occurring more often in women than men. The patient experiences vague facial pain, especially while swallowing, turning the head, or opening the mouth. Other symptoms may include dysphagia, dysphonia, otalgia, headache, dizziness, syncope, and transient ischemic attacks.

Elongation of the styloid process or mineralization of the stylohyoid ligament complex can be seen on panoramic or lateral-jaw radiographs (Fig. 1.50). The mineralized stylohyoid complex may be palpated in the tonsillar fossa area, and pain often is elicited.

Classic Eagle syndrome occurs after a tonsillectomy. Development of scar tissue in the area of a mineralized stylohyoid complex then results in cervicopharyngeal pain in the region of cranial nerves V, VII, IX, and X, especially during swallowing. Some authors reserve the term *Eagle syndrome* only for those cases in which the ossification of the stylohyoid chain occurs as a result of the tonsillectomy or other neck trauma.

A second form of this condition unrelated to tonsillectomy is known as **stylocarotid syndrome**. The elongated, mineralized complex is thought to impinge on the internal or external carotid arteries and associated sympathetic nerve fibers. The patient may complain of pain in the neck when turning the head, and this pain may radiate to other sites in the head or neck. Less commonly, compression of the internal carotid artery can lead to transient ischemic attacks, stroke, and even internal carotid artery dissection.

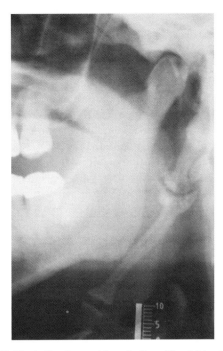

• **Fig. 1.50 Eagle Syndrome**. Mineralization of the stylohyoid ligament is visible posterior to the mandibular ramus.

Traumatic Eagle syndrome also has been reported, in which symptoms develop after fracture of a mineralized stylohyoid ligament.

Treatment and Prognosis

Treatment of Eagle syndrome depends on the severity of the symptoms. For mild cases, no treatment may be necessary (except reassurance of the patient). Local injection of corticosteroids sometimes provides relief. In more severe cases, partial surgical excision of the elongated styloid process or mineralized stylohyoid ligament is required. This can be accomplished via either an intraoral or transcervical approach. The prognosis is generally good. Rare examples of stylocarotid syndrome that result in internal carotid artery dissection may require balloon angioplasty and stent placement.

◆ STAFNE DEFECT (STAFNE BONE CYST; LINGUAL MANDIBULAR SALIVARY GLAND DEPRESSION; LATENT BONE CYST; STATIC BONE CYST; STATIC BONE DEFECT; LINGUAL CORTICAL MANDIBULAR DEFECT)

In 1942, Stafne described a series of asymptomatic radiolucent lesions located near the angle of the mandible. Subsequent reports of similar lesions have shown that this condition represents a focal concavity of the cortical bone on the lingual surface of the mandible. In most cases, biopsy has revealed histologically normal salivary gland tissue, suggesting that these lesions represent developmental defects containing a portion of the submandibular gland. However, a few of these defects have been reported to be devoid of contents or to contain muscle, fibrous connective tissue, blood vessels, fat, or lymphoid tissue.

Similar lingual cortical defects also have been noted more anteriorly in the mandible, in the area of the incisor, canine, or premolar teeth. These rare defects have been related to the sublingual gland or to aberrant salivary gland tissue. In addition, a few reports have implicated the parotid gland as the cause of an apparent cortical defect in the upper mandibular ramus. Therefore, all of the major salivary glands appear to be capable of causing such cortical concavities.

In rare examples, the radiolucent defect has been reported to be totally surrounded by intact bone. Such cases might be explained by entrapment of embryonic salivary gland tissue within the jawbone.

Clinical and Radiographic Features

The classic **Stafne defect** presents as an asymptomatic radiolucency below the mandibular canal in the posterior mandible, between the molar teeth and the angle of the mandible (Fig. 1.51). The lesion is typically well circumscribed and has a sclerotic border. Sometimes the defect may interrupt the continuity of the inferior border of the mandible, with a palpable notch observed clinically in this area. Most Stafne defects are unilateral, although bilateral cases may be seen. Anterior defects associated with the sublingual gland present as well-defined radiolucencies that may appear superimposed over the apices of the anterior or premolar teeth (Fig. 1.52). A parotid defect appears as a circumscribed radiolucency in the mandibular ramus (Fig. 1.53).

Stafne defects are not rare, having been reported in 0.08%–0.48% of panoramic radiographs. A striking male predilection is observed, with 80%–90% of all cases seen in men.

Although the defect is believed to be developmental in nature, it does not appear to be present from birth. Most cases have been reported in middle-aged and older adults, with children rarely affected; this implies that the lesion usually "develops" at a later age. Stafne defects typically remain stable in size; hence the name **static bone cyst**. In a few cases, however, the lesion has increased in size over time (Fig. 1.54). This also indicates that these lesions are not congenital.

The diagnosis usually can be made on a clinical basis by the typical radiographic location and lack of symptoms. If the clinical diagnosis is in doubt, then it can be confirmed by conventional CT scans, cone beam CT, MRI, or sialography. CT scans and MRIs show a well-defined concavity on the lingual surface of the mandible. Sialograms may be able to demonstrate the presence of salivary gland tissue in the area of the defect.

Histopathologic Features

Because of the typical radiographic appearance, biopsy usually is not necessary to establish the diagnosis of Stafne defects of the posterior mandible. If biopsy is performed,

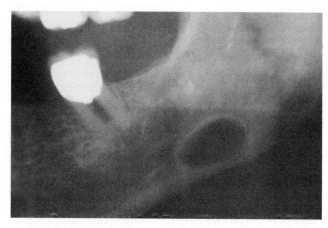

• **Fig. 1.51 Stafne Defect**. Radiolucency of the posterior mandible below the mandibular canal.

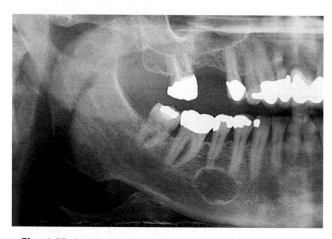

• **Fig. 1.52 Stafne Defect**. Well-circumscribed, corticated radiolucency of the right body of the mandible associated with the sublingual gland. (Courtesy of Dr. Sally Welch.)

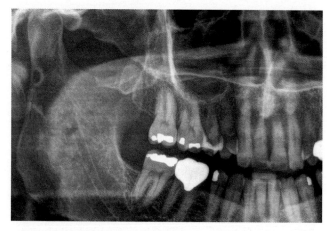

• **Fig. 1.53 Stafne Defect**. Small, circumscribed radiolucency along the posterior edge of the mandibular ramus in the region of the parotid gland. (Courtesy of Dr. Madison Bright.)

normal submandibular gland tissue often is found. However, some defects are devoid of tissue or contain muscle, blood vessels, fat, connective tissue, or lymphoid tissue. In cases reported to be devoid of contents, it is possible that the gland was simply displaced at the time of biopsy.

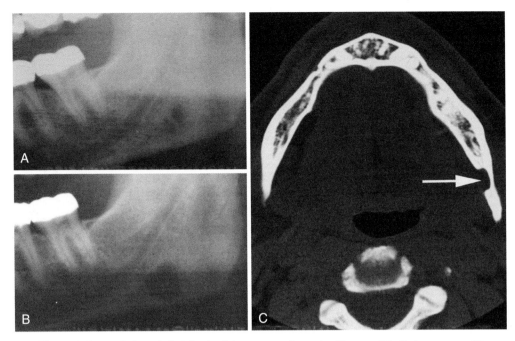

• **Fig. 1.54 Stafne Defect**. **A,** Ill-defined radiolucency near the angle of the mandible. **B,** Appearance of the same defect several years later showing enlargement of the lesion. **C,** Computed tomography (CT) image of the same lesion showing a left lingual cortical defect *(arrow)*. (Courtesy of Dr. Carroll Gallagher.)

Treatment and Prognosis

No treatment is necessary for patients with Stafne defects, and the prognosis is excellent. If the diagnosis is in question on plain films, appropriate CT imaging studies can confirm the presence of a well-defined, cupped-out lingual cortical defect, allowing a presumptive diagnosis to be made on a radiographic basis. Because anterior lingual salivary defects are more difficult to recognize, the diagnosis often is not suspected, and biopsy may be done to rule out other pathologic lesions.

DEVELOPMENTAL CYSTS

By definition, a **cyst** is a pathologic cavity (often fluid-filled) that is lined by epithelium. A number of different developmental cysts of the head and neck have been described. Some of these have been considered historically as "fissural" cysts because they were thought to arise from epithelium entrapped along embryonal lines of fusion. However, the concept of a fissural origin for many of these cysts has been questioned in more recent years. In many instances the exact pathogenesis of these lesions is still uncertain. Regardless of their origin, once cysts develop in the oral and maxillofacial region, they tend to slowly increase in size, possibly in response to a slightly elevated hydrostatic luminal pressure.

◆ PALATAL CYSTS OF THE NEWBORN (EPSTEIN'S PEARLS; BOHN'S NODULES)

Small developmental cysts are a common finding on the palate of newborn infants. Researchers have theorized that these "inclusion" cysts may arise in one of two ways. First, as the palatal shelves meet and fuse in the midline during embryonic life to form the secondary palate, small islands of epithelium may become entrapped below the surface along the median palatal raphe and form cysts. Second, these cysts may arise from epithelial remnants derived from the development of the minor salivary glands of the palate.

As originally described, **Epstein's pearls** occur along the median palatal raphe and presumably arise from epithelium entrapped along the line of fusion. **Bohn's nodules** reportedly arise along the lingual and buccal aspects of the alveolar ridge, often near the soft palate junction, and are believed to be derived from the minor salivary glands. However, these two terms have been used almost interchangeably in the literature and also have often been used to describe gingival cysts of the newborn (see page 697), similar-appearing lesions of dental lamina origin. Therefore, the term **palatal cysts of the newborn** may be preferable to help distinguish them from gingival cysts of the newborn. In addition, because these cysts are most common near the midline at the junction of the hard and soft palates, it is usually difficult to ascertain clinically whether they are arising from epithelium entrapped by fusion of the palate or from the developing minor salivary glands.

Clinical Features

Palatal cysts of the newborn are quite common and have been reported in as many as 55%–85% of neonates. The cysts are small, 1- to 3-mm, white or yellow-white papules that appear most often along the midline near the junction of the hard and soft palates (Fig. 1.55). Occasionally, they may occur in a more anterior location along the raphe or on the posterior palate lateral to the midline. Frequently a cluster of two to six cysts is observed, although the lesions also can occur singly.

Histopathologic Features

Microscopic examination reveals keratin-filled cysts that are lined by stratified squamous epithelium. Sometimes these cysts demonstrate a communication with the mucosal surface.

Treatment and Prognosis

Palatal cysts of the newborn are innocuous lesions, and no treatment is required. They are self-healing and rarely observable several weeks after birth. Presumably the epithelium degenerates, or the cysts rupture onto the mucosal surface and eliminate their keratin contents.

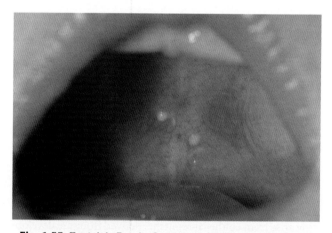

• **Fig. 1.55 Epstein's Pearls.** Small keratin-filled cysts at the junction of the hard and soft palates. (Courtesy of Tristan Neville.)

◆ NASOLABIAL CYST (NASOALVEOLAR CYST; KLESTADT CYST)

The **nasolabial cyst** is a rare developmental cyst that occurs in the upper lip lateral to the midline. The pathogenesis is uncertain, although there are two major theories. One theory considers the nasolabial cyst to be a "fissural" cyst arising from epithelial remnants entrapped along the line of fusion of the maxillary, medial nasal, and lateral nasal processes. A second theory suggests that these cysts develop from misplaced epithelium of the nasolacrimal duct because of their similar location and histologic appearance.

Clinical and Radiographic Features

The nasolabial cyst usually appears as a swelling of the upper lip lateral to the midline, resulting in elevation of the ala of the nose. The enlargement often elevates the mucosa of the nasal vestibule and obliterates the maxillary mucolabial fold (Fig. 1.56). On occasion, this expansion may result in nasal obstruction or may interfere with the wearing of a denture. Pain is uncommon unless the lesion is secondarily infected. The cyst may rupture spontaneously and may drain into the oral cavity or nose.

Nasolabial cysts are most commonly seen in adults, with peak prevalence in the fourth and fifth decades of life. A significant predilection exists for women, with a female-to-male ratio of 3.6 : 1. Approximately 10% of the reported cases have been bilateral.

Because the nasolabial cyst arises in soft tissues, in most cases no bony radiographic changes are seen. Occasionally, pressure resorption of the underlying bone may occur.

Histopathologic Features

The nasolabial cyst is characteristically lined by pseudostratified columnar epithelium, often demonstrating goblet cells and cilia (Fig. 1.57). Areas of cuboidal epithelium and squamous metaplasia are not unusual. Apocrine changes also have

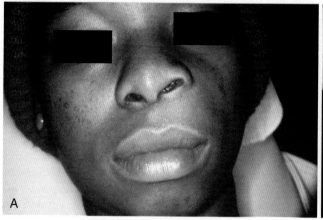
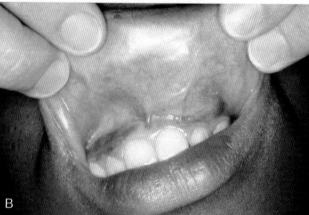

• **Fig. 1.56 Nasolabial Cyst. A,** Enlargement of the left upper lip with elevation of the ala of the nose. **B,** Intraoral swelling fills the maxillary labial fold. (Courtesy of Dr. Jim Weir.)

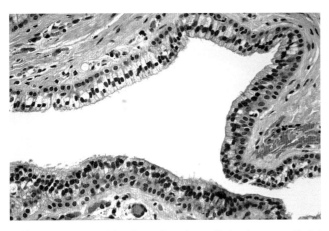

• **Fig. 1.57 Nasolabial Cyst**. Pseudostratified columnar epithelial lining.

been reported. The cyst wall is composed of fibrous connective tissue with adjacent skeletal muscle. Inflammation may be seen if the lesion is secondarily infected.

Treatment and Prognosis

Complete surgical excision of the cyst via an intraoral approach has been the traditional treatment of choice. Because the lesion is often close to the floor of the nose, it is sometimes necessary to sacrifice a portion of the nasal mucosa to ensure total removal. However, an alternative transnasal approach has been developed that allows endoscopic marsupialization of the lesion, converting the cyst into an air-containing sinus with its opening on the nasal floor. Recurrence is rare.

◆ "GLOBULOMAXILLARY CYST"

As originally described, the "**globulomaxillary cyst**" was purported to be a fissural cyst that arose from epithelium entrapped during fusion of the globular portion of the medial nasal process with the maxillary process. This concept has been questioned, however, because the globular portion of the medial nasal process is primarily united with the maxillary process and a fusion does not occur. Therefore, epithelial entrapment should not occur during embryologic development of this area.

Virtually all cysts in the globulomaxillary region (between the lateral incisor and canine teeth) can be explained on an odontogenic basis. Many are lined by inflamed stratified squamous epithelium and are consistent with **periapical cysts** (see page 126). Some exhibit specific histopathologic features of an **odontogenic keratocyst** (see page 689) or developmental **lateral periodontal cyst** (see page 699). On rare occasions, cysts in the globulomaxillary area may be lined by pseudostratified, ciliated, columnar epithelium. Such cases may lend credence to the fissural theory of origin. However, this epithelium may be explained by the close proximity of the sinus lining. In addition, respiratory epithelium also has been reported in periapical cysts, dentigerous cysts, and glandular odontogenic cysts found in other locations.

Because a fissural cyst in this region probably does not exist, the term *globulomaxillary cyst* should no longer be used. When a radiolucency between the maxillary lateral incisor and canine is encountered, the clinician should first consider an odontogenic origin for the lesion.

◆ NASOPALATINE DUCT CYST (INCISIVE CANAL CYST)

The **nasopalatine duct cyst** is the most common nonodontogenic cyst of the oral cavity, occurring in about 1% of the population. The cyst is believed to arise from remnants of the **nasopalatine duct,** an embryologic structure connecting the oral and nasal cavities in the area of the incisive canal.

In the 7-week-old fetus, the developing palate consists of the **primary palate,** which is formed by the fusion of the medial nasal processes. Behind the primary palate, downgrowth of the nasal septum produces two communications between the oral and nasal cavities, the primitive nasal choanae. Formation of the **secondary palate** begins around the eighth intrauterine week, with downward growth of the medial parts of the maxillary processes (palatine processes) to a location on either side of the tongue.

As the mandible develops and the tongue drops down, these palatine processes grow horizontally, fusing with the nasal septum in the midline and with the primary palate along their anterior aspect. Two passageways persist in the midline between the primary and secondary palates (the **incisive canals**). Also formed by this fusion and found within the incisive canals are epithelial structures—the **nasopalatine ducts**. These ducts normally degenerate in humans but may leave epithelial remnants behind in the incisive canals.

The incisive canals begin on the floor of the nasal cavity on either side of the nasal septum, coursing downward and forward to exit the palatal bone via a common foramen in the area of the incisive papilla. In addition to the nasopalatine ducts, these canals contain the nasopalatine nerve plus anastomosing branches of the descending palatine and sphenopalatine arteries. Occasionally, two smaller foramina carrying the nasopalatine nerves—the **canals of Scarpa**—are found within the incisive foramen.

In some mammals the nasopalatine ducts remain patent and provide communication between the oral and nasal cavities. On rare occasions, patent or partially patent nasopalatine ducts may be encountered in humans. In mammals the nasopalatine ducts may communicate with the vomer-nasal **organ of Jacobson,** acting as an accessory olfactory organ. However, in humans, Jacobson's organ usually recedes in uterine life to become a vestigial structure.

Researchers have suggested that the nasopalatine duct cyst may arise from the epithelium of Jacobson's organ, but this appears highly unlikely. Trauma or infection of the duct and mucous retention of adjacent minor salivary glands also have been mentioned as possible etiologic factors, but the role of each has been questioned. Although the pathogenesis of this lesion is still uncertain, the lesion most likely represents a spontaneous cystic degeneration of remnants of the nasopalatine duct.

Clinical and Radiographic Features

The nasopalatine duct cyst may develop at almost any age but is most common in the fourth to sixth decades of life. In spite of its being a "developmental" cyst, the nasopalatine duct cyst is rarely seen during the first decade. Most studies have shown a male predilection.

The most common presenting symptoms include swelling of the anterior palate, drainage, and pain (Fig. 1.58, *A*). Patients sometimes relate a long history of these symptoms, probably because of their intermittent nature. However, many lesions are asymptomatic and are discovered on routine radiographs. Rarely a large cyst may produce a "through-and-through" fluctuant expansion involving the anterior palate and labial alveolar mucosa.

Radiographs usually demonstrate a well-circumscribed radiolucency in or near the midline of the anterior maxilla, between and apical to the central incisor teeth (Figs. 1.58, *B* and 1.59). Root resorption rarely is noted. The lesion most often is round or oval with a sclerotic border. Some cysts may have an inverted pear shape, presumably because of resistance of adjacent tooth roots. Other examples may show a classic heart shape as a result of superimposition of the nasal spine or because they are notched by the nasal septum.

The radiographic diameter of nasopalatine duct cysts can range from small lesions, less than 6 mm, to destructive lesions as large as 6 cm. However, most cysts are in the range of 1.0 to 2.5 cm, with an average diameter of 1.5 to 1.7 cm. It may be difficult to distinguish a small nasopalatine duct cyst from a large incisive foramen. It is generally accepted that a diameter of 6 mm is the upper limit of normal size for the incisive foramen. Therefore, a radiolucency that is 6 mm or smaller in this area usually is considered a normal foramen unless other clinical signs or symptoms are present.

In rare instances, a nasopalatine duct cyst may develop in the soft tissues of the incisive papilla area without any bony involvement. Such lesions often are called **cysts of the incisive papilla**. These cysts frequently demonstrate bluish discoloration as a result of the fluid contents in the cyst lumen (Fig. 1.60).

Histopathologic Features

The epithelial lining of nasopalatine duct cysts is highly variable (Figs. 1.61 and 1.62). It may be composed of the following:

- Stratified squamous epithelium
- Pseudostratified columnar epithelium
- Simple columnar epithelium
- Simple cuboidal epithelium

Frequently, more than one epithelial type is found in the same cyst. Stratified squamous epithelium is most common, present in at least three-fourths of all cysts. Pseudostratified columnar epithelium has been reported in from one-third to three-fourths of all cases. Simple cuboidal or columnar epithelium is discovered less frequently.

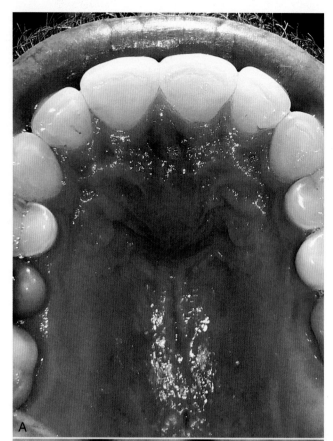

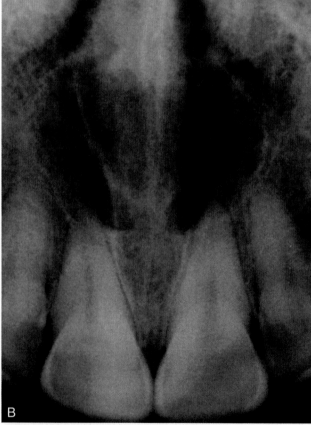

• **Fig. 1.58 Nasopalatine Duct Cyst. A,** Fluctuant swelling of the anterior hard palate. **B,** Periapical radiograph showing a well-circumscribed radiolucency apical to the roots of the maxillary central incisors. (Courtesy of Dr. Matt Koepke.)

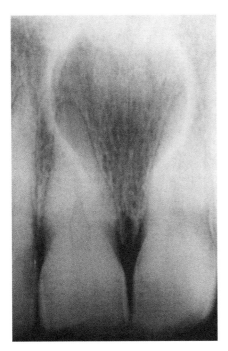

• **Fig. 1.59 Nasopalatine Duct Cyst**. Well-circumscribed radiolucency between and apical to the roots of the maxillary central incisors.

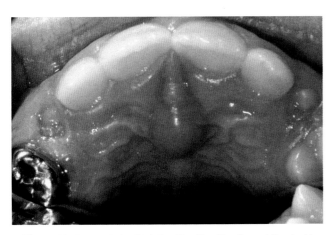

• **Fig. 1.60 Cyst of the Incisive Papilla**. Swelling of the incisive papilla.

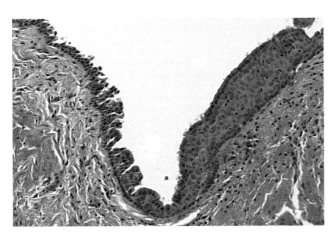

• **Fig. 1.61 Nasopalatine Duct Cyst**. Cystic lining showing transition from pseudostratified columnar to stratified squamous epithelium.

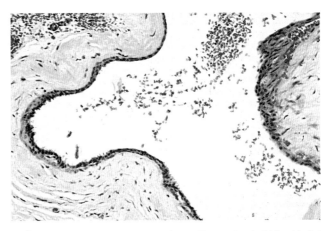

• **Fig. 1.62 Nasopalatine Duct Cyst**. Flattened cuboidal epithelial lining.

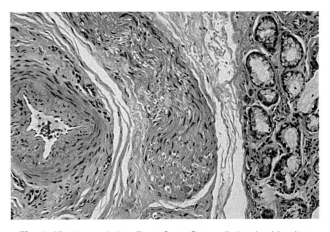

• **Fig. 1.63 Nasopalatine Duct Cyst**. Cyst wall showing blood vessels, nerve bundles, and minor salivary glands.

Cilia and goblet cells may be found in association with columnar linings. The type of epithelium may be related to the vertical position of the cyst within the incisive canal. Cysts developing within the superior aspect of the canal near the nasal cavity are more likely to demonstrate respiratory epithelium; those in an inferior position near the oral cavity are more likely to exhibit squamous epithelium.

The contents of the cyst wall can be a helpful diagnostic aid. Because the nasopalatine duct cyst arises within the incisive canal, moderate-sized nerves and small muscular arteries and veins usually are found in the wall of the cyst (Fig. 1.63). Small mucous glands have been reported in as many as one-third of cases. Occasionally, one may see small islands of hyaline cartilage. Frequently, an inflammatory response is noted in the cyst wall and may range from mild to heavy. This inflammation usually is chronic in nature and is composed of lymphocytes, plasma cells, and histiocytes. Associated acute inflammatory cells (neutrophils) sometimes may be seen.

Treatment and Prognosis

Nasopalatine duct cysts are treated by surgical enucleation. Biopsy is recommended because the lesion is not diagnostic radiographically; other benign and malignant lesions have been known to mimic the nasopalatine duct cyst. The lesion is best approached with a palatal flap that is reflected after an incision is made along the lingual gingival margin of the anterior maxillary teeth. Recurrence is rare. Malignant transformation has been reported in a couple of cases, but this is an extremely rare complication.

◆ MEDIAN PALATAL (PALATINE) CYST

The median palatal cyst is a rare fissural cyst that theoretically develops from epithelium entrapped along the embryonic line of fusion of the lateral palatal shelves of the maxilla. This cyst may be difficult to distinguish from a nasopalatine duct cyst. In fact, most "median palatal cysts" may represent posteriorly positioned nasopalatine duct cysts. Because the nasopalatine ducts course posteriorly and superiorly as they extend from the incisive canal to the nasal cavity, a nasopalatine duct cyst that arises from posterior remnants of this duct near the nasal cavity might be mistaken for a median palatal cyst. On the other hand, if a true median palatal cyst were to develop toward the anterior portion of the hard palate, then it could easily be mistaken for a nasopalatine duct cyst.

Clinical and Radiographic Features

The median palatal cyst presents as a firm or fluctuant swelling of the midline of the hard palate posterior to the palatine papilla (Fig. 1.64). The lesion appears most frequently in young adults. Often it is asymptomatic, but some patients complain of pain or expansion. The average size of this cyst is 2 × 2 cm, but sometimes it can become quite large. Occlusal radiographs demonstrate a well-circumscribed radiolucency in the midline of the hard palate (Fig. 1.65).

Occasional reported cases have been associated with divergence of the central incisors, although it may be difficult to rule out a nasopalatine duct cyst in these instances.

To differentiate the median palatal cyst from other cystic lesions of the maxilla, Gingell and associates suggested the following diagnostic criteria:
- Grossly appears symmetrical along the midline of the hard palate
- Located posterior to the palatine papilla
- Appears ovoid or circular radiographically
- Not intimately associated with a nonvital tooth
- Does not communicate with the incisive canal
- Shows no microscopic evidence of large neurovascular bundles, hyaline cartilage, or minor salivary glands in the cyst wall

It must be stressed that a true median palatal cyst should exhibit clinical enlargement of the palate. A midline radiolucency without clinical evidence of expansion is probably a nasopalatine duct cyst.

Histopathologic Features

Microscopic examination shows a cyst that usually is lined by stratified squamous epithelium. Areas of ciliated pseudostratified columnar epithelium have been reported in some cases. Chronic inflammation may be present in the cyst wall.

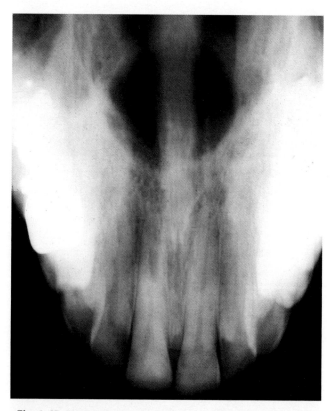

• **Fig. 1.65 Median Palatal Cyst**. Occlusal radiograph of same patient depicted in Fig. 1.64. A well-circumscribed midline radiolucent defect can be seen, which is separate from the incisive canal. (Courtesy of Dr. Craig Fowler.)

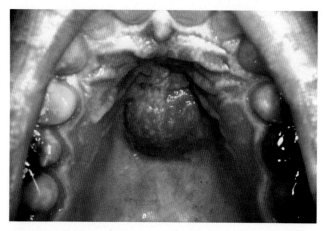

• **Fig. 1.64 Median Palatal Cyst**. Compressible mass in the midline of the hard palate posterior to the incisive papilla. (Courtesy of Dr. Craig Fowler.)

Treatment and Prognosis

The median palatal cyst is treated by surgical removal. Recurrence should not be expected.

◆ "MEDIAN MANDIBULAR CYST"

The **"median mandibular cyst"** is a controversial lesion of questionable existence. Theoretically, it represents a fissural cyst in the anterior midline of the mandible that develops from epithelium entrapped during fusion of the halves of the mandible during embryonic life. However, the mandible actually develops as a single bilobed proliferation of mesenchyme with a central isthmus in the midline. As the mandible grows, this isthmus is eliminated. Therefore, because no fusion of epithelium-lined processes occurs, entrapment of epithelium should not be possible.

Because respiratory prosoplasia is not uncommon in odontogenic cysts, it appears likely that most (if not all) of these midline cysts are of odontogenic origin. Many purported cases would be classified today as examples of the *glandular odontogenic cyst* (see page 703), which has a propensity for occurrence in the midline mandibular region. Others could be classified as *periapical cysts, odontogenic keratocysts,* or *lateral periodontal cysts.* Because a fissural cyst in this region probably does not exist, the term *median mandibular cyst* should no longer be used.

◆ FOLLICULAR CYSTS OF THE SKIN

Follicular cysts of the skin are common keratin-filled lesions that arise from one or more portions of the hair follicle. The most common type, which is derived from the follicular infundibulum, is known as an **epidermoid** or **infundibular cyst**. These cysts often arise after localized inflammation of the hair follicle and probably represent a nonneoplastic proliferation of the infundibular epithelium resulting from the healing process. The term **sebaceous cyst** sometimes is used mistakenly as a synonym for both the epidermoid cyst and another cyst of the scalp known as a **pilar, trichilemmal,** or **isthmus-catagen cyst**. However, because both the epidermoid cyst and pilar cyst are derived from the hair follicle rather than the sebaceous gland, the term *sebaceous cyst* should be avoided.

Keratin-filled cysts of the skin may occasionally arise after traumatic implantation of epithelium, although such lesions may be difficult to distinguish from an infundibular cyst. Rarely, such **epidermal inclusion (implantation) cysts** also can develop in the mouth. These small inclusion cysts should be distinguished from oral epidermoid cysts that occur in the midline floor of mouth region and represent the minimal manifestation of the teratoma-dermoid cyst-epidermoid cyst spectrum (see page 32).

Clinical Features

Epidermoid (infundibular) cysts account for approximately 80% of follicular cysts of the skin and are most common in the acne-prone areas of the head, neck, and back. They are unusual before puberty unless they are associated with **Gardner syndrome** (see page 656). Young adults are more likely to have cysts on the face, whereas older adults are more likely to have cysts on the back. Males are affected more frequently than females.

Epidermoid cysts present as nodular, fluctuant subcutaneous lesions that may or may not be associated with inflammation (Fig. 1.66). Sometimes the cyst may exhibit a small orifice or punctum that communicates with the skin surface. If a noninflamed lesion presents in an area of thin skin, such as the earlobe, then it may be white or yellow.

Pilar (trichilemmal) cysts comprise approximately 10%–15% of skin cysts, occurring most frequently on the scalp (Fig. 1.67). They are twice as common in women as in men. Some examples are inherited as an autosomal dominant trait, and affected patients can develop multiple cysts. The lesion is usually movable and shells out easily.

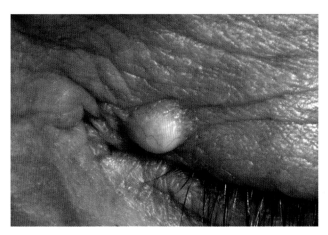

• **Fig. 1.66 Epidermoid Cyst.** Yellow nodule at the medial aspect of the eyelid.

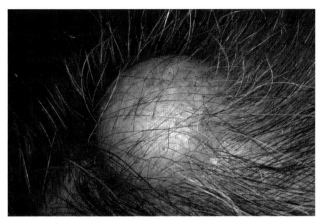

• **Fig. 1.67 Pilar Cyst.** Nodular mass on the scalp.

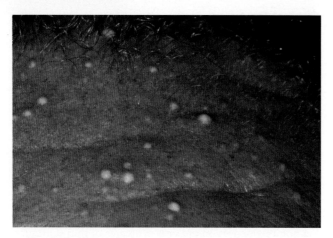

• **Fig. 1.68 Milia.** Multiple tiny keratin-filled cysts on the forehead.

Milia (singular: **milium**) are tiny keratin-filled cysts that resemble miniature epidermoid cysts (Fig. 1.68). A variety of such lesions have been described, including primary congenital milia, genodermatosis-associated milia, and milia that develop secondary to bullous disorders, trauma, or certain medications. Primary milia are thought to arise from the sebaceous collar of vellus hairs, whereas secondary milia may develop from eccrine ducts, hair follicles, or the overlying epidermis.

Histopathologic Features

Microscopic examination of an epidermoid cyst reveals a cavity that is lined by stratified squamous epithelium resembling epidermis (Fig. 1.69). A well-developed granular cell layer is seen, and the lumen is filled with degenerating orthokeratin. Not infrequently, the epithelial lining will be disrupted. When this occurs, a prominent granulomatous inflammatory reaction, including multinucleated giant cells, can be present in the cyst wall because the exposed keratin is recognized as a foreign material.

The pilar cyst also is lined by stratified squamous epithelium, although a granular cell layer usually is absent or greatly diminished (Fig. 1.70). The keratinocytes remain large in the

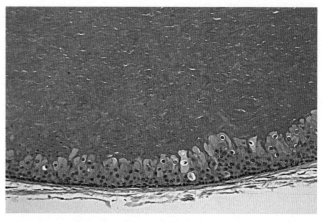

• **Fig. 1.70 Pilar Cyst.** Medium-power view showing an abrupt transition between the stratified squamous epithelial lining and compact keratin without the presence of a transitional granular cell layer.

upper epithelial layers with an abrupt transition to dense, compact keratin that fills the cyst lumen.

Treatment and Prognosis

Epidermoid and pilar cysts usually are treated by conservative surgical excision, and recurrence is uncommon. Malignant transformation has been reported but is exceedingly rare.

An individual milium can be removed by evacuation, in which the lesion is nicked by a scalpel blade, followed by application of pressure with a comedone extractor or curette. Multiple milia can be managed via electrocautery or application of topical retinoids.

◆ DERMOID CYST (DYSONTOGENIC CYST)

The **dermoid cyst** is an uncommon developmental cystic malformation. The cyst is lined by epidermis-like epithelium and contains dermal adnexal structures in the cyst wall. It is generally classified as a benign cystic form of **teratoma**.

By definition, a teratoma is a developmental tumor composed of tissue from more than one germ layer and

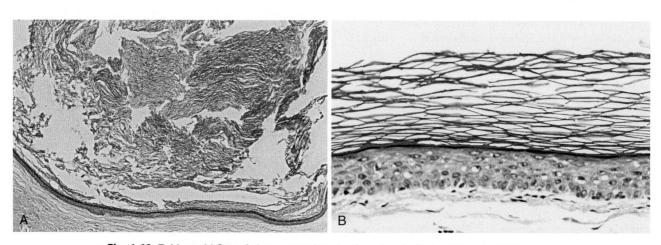

• **Fig. 1.69 Epidermoid Cyst. A,** Low-power view showing a keratin-filled cystic cavity. **B,** High-power view showing stratified squamous epithelial lining with orthokeratin production.

sometimes all three: (1) ectoderm, (2) mesoderm, and (3) endoderm. Such tumors are believed to arise from germ cells or entrapped totipotent blastomeres, which can produce derivatives of all three germ layers.

Teratomatous malformations have a spectrum of complexity. In their most complex form, these lesions produce multiple types of tissue that are arranged in a disorganized fashion. These "complex" teratomas are most common in the ovaries or testes and can be benign or malignant. Occasionally, ovarian teratomas (or "dermoids") produce well-formed teeth, or even partially complete jaws. Complex teratomas of the oral cavity are rare and usually are congenital in nature. When they occur, they usually extend through a cleft palate from the pituitary area via Rathke's pouch. Cervical teratomas also have been reported.

The term **teratoid cyst** has been used to describe a cystic form of teratoma that contains a variety of germ layer derivatives:

1. Skin appendages, including hair follicles, sebaceous glands, and sweat glands
2. Connective tissue elements, such as muscle, blood vessels, and bone
3. Endodermal structures, such as gastrointestinal lining

Rarely, oral cysts may be lined entirely by gastrointestinal epithelium. These **heterotopic oral gastrointestinal cysts (enterocystomas, enteric duplication cysts)** often are considered to be choristomas, or histologically normal tissue found in an abnormal location. However, these lesions probably can be included under the broad umbrella of teratomatous lesions, especially because they occasionally are found in combination with dermoid cysts.

Dermoid cysts are simpler in structure than complex teratomas or teratoid cysts. Although they do not contain tissue from all three germ layers, they probably represent a *forme fruste* of a teratoma. Similar cysts of the oral cavity can be seen that are lined by epidermis-like epithelium, but they contain no dermal appendages in the cyst wall. These lesions have been called **epidermoid cysts** and represent the simplest expression of the teratoma spectrum. These intraoral epidermoid cysts should not be confused with the more common **epidermoid cyst of the skin** (see page 31), a nonteratomatous lesion that arises from the hair follicle. Because the teratoid cyst/dermoid cyst/epidermoid cyst spectrum represents defective embryologic development, these cysts sometimes are known collectively as **dysontogenic cysts**.

Clinical and Radiographic Features

Dermoid cysts most commonly occur in the midline of the floor of the mouth (Fig. 1.71), although occasionally they are displaced laterally or develop in other locations. If the cyst develops above the geniohyoid muscle, then a sublingual swelling may displace the tongue toward the roof of the mouth and create difficulty in eating, speaking, or even breathing. Cysts that occur below the geniohyoid muscle often produce a submental swelling, with a "double-chin" appearance.

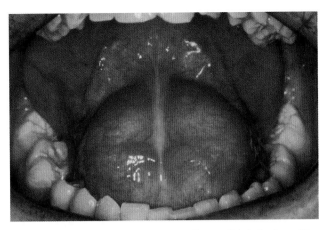

• **Fig. 1.71 Dermoid Cyst.** Fluctuant midline swelling in the floor of the mouth. (From Budnick SD: *Handbook of pediatric oral pathology*, Chicago, 1981, Year Book Medical.)

Oral dermoid cysts can vary in size from a few millimeters to 12 cm in diameter. They are most common in children and young adults; 15% of reported cases have been congenital. The lesion is usually slow growing and painless, presenting as a doughy or rubbery mass that frequently retains pitting after application of pressure. Secondary infection can occur, and the lesion may drain intraorally or onto the skin. MRIs, CT scans, or contrast medium radiographs may be helpful in delineating the extent of the lesion.

Histopathologic Features

Dermoid cysts are lined by orthokeratinized stratified squamous epithelium with a prominent granular cell layer. Abundant keratin often is found within the cyst lumen. On rare occasions, areas of respiratory epithelium can be seen. The cyst wall is composed of fibrous connective tissue that contains one or more skin appendages, such as sebaceous glands, hair follicles, or sweat glands (Fig. 1.72).

Treatment and Prognosis

Dermoid cysts are treated by surgical removal. Many examples can be removed by an intraoral incision, which avoids the creation of a scar on the skin. However, some lesions located below the geniohyoid muscle may require an extraoral approach. Recurrence is uncommon. Malignant transformation into squamous cell carcinoma has been reported only rarely.

◆ THYROGLOSSAL DUCT CYST (THYROGLOSSAL TRACT CYST)

The thyroid gland begins its development during the third to fourth week of embryonic life as a proliferation of endodermal cells from the ventral floor of the pharynx, between the tuberculum impar and copula of the developing tongue—a point that later becomes the foramen cecum. This thyroid anlage descends into the neck as a bilobed diverticulum

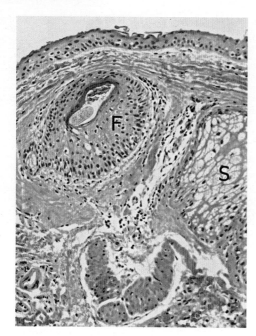

• **Fig. 1.72 Dermoid Cyst**. Squamous epithelial lining *(top)*, with hair follicle *(F)*, sebaceous glands *(S)* in the cyst wall.

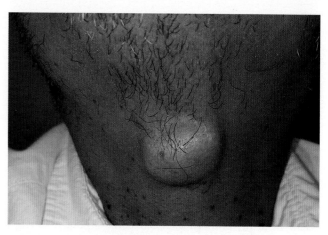

• **Fig. 1.73 Thyroglossal Duct Cyst**. Swelling of the anterior midline of the neck. (Courtesy of Dr. Steven B. Whitaker.)

anterior to the developing hyoid bone and reaches its definitive level below the thyroid cartilage by the seventh embryonic week. Along this path of descent, an epithelial tract or duct is formed, maintaining an attachment to the base of the tongue. This thyroglossal duct becomes intimately associated with the developing hyoid bone. As the hyoid matures and rotates to its adult position, the thyroglossal duct passes in front and beneath the hyoid, looping upward and behind it before curving downward again into the lower neck. The caudal segment of this duct often persists, forming the pyramidal lobe of the thyroid gland.

The thyroglossal duct epithelium normally undergoes atrophy and is obliterated, although autopsy studies have shown that as many as 7% of the population will have *thyroglossal tract remnants*. These epithelial remnants usually are asymptomatic, although some can give rise to cysts along this tract known as **thyroglossal duct cysts**. The impetus for cystic degeneration is uncertain. Inflammation is the most frequently suggested stimulus, especially from adjacent lymphoid tissue that may react to draining infections of the head and neck. Retention of secretions within the duct is another possible factor. In addition, there are several reports of familial occurrence of such cysts.

Clinical Features

Thyroglossal duct cysts classically develop in the midline and may occur anywhere from the foramen cecum area of the tongue to the suprasternal notch. Approximately 75% of cases develop inferior to the hyoid bone. Suprahyoid cysts may be submental in location. Cysts that develop in the area of the thyroid cartilage often are deflected lateral to the midline because of the sharp anterior margin of the thyroid cartilage. Intralingual cysts are rare.

Thyroglossal duct cysts may develop at any age, but they are most commonly diagnosed in children and young to middle-aged adults; about 40% of cases occur before the age of 20. There is no sex predilection. The cyst usually presents as a painless, fluctuant, movable swelling unless it is complicated by secondary infection (Fig. 1.73). Lesions that develop at the base of the tongue may cause laryngeal obstruction. Most thyroglossal duct cysts are smaller than 3 cm in diameter, but occasional cysts may reach 10 cm in size. If the cyst maintains an attachment to the hyoid bone or tongue, it will move vertically during swallowing or protrusion of the tongue. Sinus tracts to the skin or mucosa develop in as many as one-third of cases, usually from rupture of an infected cyst or as a sequela of surgery.

Histopathologic Features

Thyroglossal duct cysts usually are lined by respiratory or stratified squamous epithelium (Fig. 1.74). Sometimes a mixture of epithelial types is present, or an intact epithelial lining cannot be found due to secondary inflammation. Thyroid tissue may occur in the cyst wall, but this is not a constant finding.

Treatment and Prognosis

Thyroglossal duct cysts are best treated by a Sistrunk procedure. In this operation the cyst is removed in addition to the midline segment of the hyoid bone and a generous portion of muscular tissue along the entire thyroglossal tract. The recurrence rate associated with this procedure is less than 10%. A much higher recurrence rate can be expected with less aggressive surgery.

Carcinoma arising in a thyroglossal duct cyst is a rare complication that occurs in approximately 1%–3% of cases. Most of these have been papillary thyroid adenocarcinomas. Fortunately, metastases from thyroglossal carcinoma are rare, and the prognosis for people with these tumors is good.

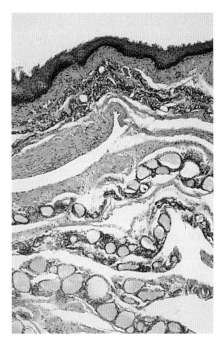

• **Fig. 1.74** **Thyroglossal Duct Cyst**. Cyst *(top)* lined by stratified squamous epithelium. Thyroid follicles can be seen in the cyst wall *(bottom)*.

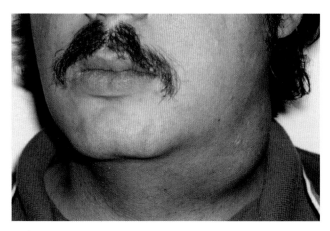

• **Fig. 1.75** **Branchial Cleft Cyst**. Fluctuant swelling of the lateral neck.

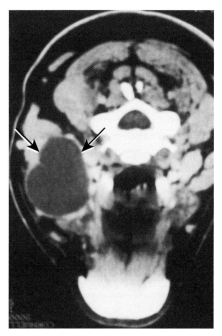

• **Fig. 1.76** **Branchial Cleft Cyst**. Imaging study of the same cyst depicted in Fig. 1.75, showing a well-circumscribed lesion of the lateral neck *(arrows)*.

◆ BRANCHIAL CLEFT CYST (CERVICAL LYMPHOEPITHELIAL CYST)

The **branchial cleft cyst** is a developmental cyst that is derived from remnants of the branchial arches. During the fourth to seventh week of gestation, the head and neck region of the embryo develops paired branchial arches, which are covered by ectoderm on the external surface and endoderm on the internal surface. The outer arch surfaces are separated by clefts and the inner surfaces are divided by pouches. In fish and amphibians, the branchial arches are destined to become the gill apparatus; in humans, the clefts and pouches gradually are eliminated during embryonic life by ingrowth of mesenchyme. However, incomplete obliteration of these pharyngeal clefts and pouches may give rise to branchial cleft anomalies, such as cysts, fistulae, or sinus tracts. About 95% of these anomalies are believed to arise from the second branchial arch, with the remaining 5% originating from the first, third, and fourth branchial arches.

Clinical Features

Branchial cleft cysts from the second arch occur in the upper lateral neck anterior or deep to the sternocleidomastoid muscle (Figs. 1.75 and 1.76). They most frequently develop in children and young adults between the ages of 10 and 40. Clinically, the cyst appears as a soft, fluctuant mass that can range from 1 to 10 cm in diameter. Associated tenderness or pain sometimes may occur with secondary infection. Occasionally, the lesion becomes evident after an upper respiratory tract infection or trauma. Some branchial cleft anomalies appear as sinuses or fistulae that may produce a mucoid discharge onto the skin. In rare instances, bilateral cysts may develop.

Anomalies from the first branchial arch comprise approximately 1% of branchial cleft malformations and usually are found in close proximity to the parotid gland. Third-cleft and fourth-cleft anomalies are rare and may develop in the lower neck or mediastinum.

Histopathologic Features

More than 90% of branchial cleft cysts are lined by stratified squamous epithelium that may or may not be keratinized (Fig. 1.77), although some cysts will exhibit respiratory epithelium. Those anomalies that present as sinus tracts or fistulae also will often have respiratory epithelium. The wall of the cyst typically contains lymphoid tissue, often

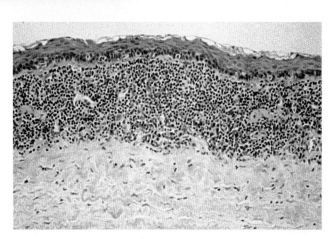

• **Fig. 1.77 Branchial Cleft Cyst**. Medium-power view showing a cyst lined by stratified squamous epithelium. Note the lymphoid tissue in the cyst wall.

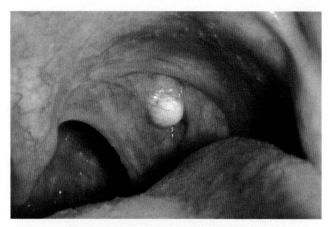

• **Fig. 1.78 Oral Lymphoepithelial Cyst**. Small yellow-white nodule of the tonsillar fossa.

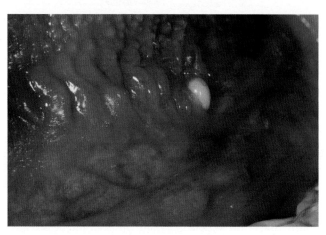

• **Fig. 1.79 Oral Lymphoepithelial Cyst**. Small yellow-white papule of the posterior lateral border of the tongue.

demonstrating germinal center formation. However, occasional cysts have been reported without lymphoid tissue.

Treatment and Prognosis

The branchial cleft cyst is treated by surgical removal. The lesion almost never recurs.

Rare examples of malignant transformation in these cysts have been reported. Although such an occurrence is theoretically possible, most suspected cases actually represent cystic metastases from previously undetected carcinomas of the head and neck region, especially human papillomavirus (HPV)-related tumors from the base of tongue, lingual tonsil, or palatine tonsil. When evaluating patients with cystic neck masses, fine-needle aspiration biopsy often is recommended to rule out the possibility of malignancy before surgery.

◆ ORAL LYMPHOEPITHELIAL CYST

The **oral lymphoepithelial cyst** is an uncommon lesion of the mouth that develops within oral lymphoid tissue. It is microscopically similar to the branchial cleft cyst (cervical lymphoepithelial cyst) but much smaller in size.

Lymphoid tissue is normally found in the oral cavity and pharynx, principally consisting of **Waldeyer ring,** which includes the palatine tonsils, lingual tonsils, and pharyngeal adenoids. In addition, accessory oral tonsils or lymphoid aggregates may occur in the floor of the mouth, ventral surface of the tongue, and soft palate.

Oral lymphoid tissue has a close relationship with the overlying mucosal epithelium. This epithelium demonstrates invaginations into the tonsillar tissue, resulting in blind pouches or tonsillar crypts that may fill up with keratin debris. The tonsillar crypt may become obstructed or pinched off from the surface, producing a keratin-filled cyst within the lymphoid tissue just below the mucosal surface. It also is possible that oral lymphoepithelial cysts may develop from salivary or surface mucosal epithelium that becomes

enclaved in lymphoid tissue during embryogenesis. It even has been suggested that these cysts may arise from the excretory ducts of the sublingual gland or minor salivary glands, and that the associated lymphoid tissue represents a secondary immune response.

Clinical Features

The oral lymphoepithelial cyst presents as a small submucosal mass that is usually less than 1 cm in diameter; rarely will the lesion be greater than 1.5 cm (Figs. 1.78 and 1.79). The cyst may feel firm or soft to palpation, and the overlying mucosa is smooth and nonulcerated. The lesion is typically white or yellow and often contains creamy or cheesy keratinous material in the lumen. The cyst is usually asymptomatic, although occasionally patients may complain of swelling or drainage. Pain is rare but may occur secondary to trauma.

Oral lymphoepithelial cysts may develop in people of almost any age, but they are most common in young adults. The most frequently reported locations are the floor of the mouth, ventral tongue, posterior lateral border of the tongue,

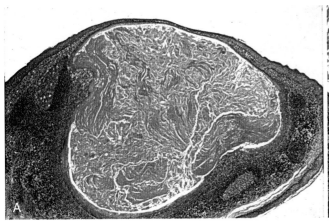
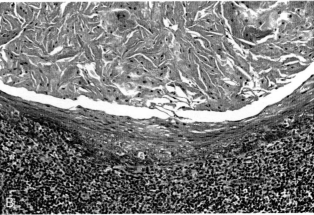

• **Fig. 1.80** **Oral Lymphoepithelial Cyst**. **A,** Low-power view showing a keratin-filled cyst below the mucosal surface. Lymphoid tissue is present in the cyst wall. **B,** High-power view showing lymphoid tissue adjacent to the cystic lining.

palatine tonsil, and soft palate. All of these locations represent sites of normal or accessory oral lymphoid tissue.

Histopathologic Features

Microscopic examination of the oral lymphoepithelial cyst demonstrates a cystic cavity that is lined by stratified squamous epithelium without rete ridges (Fig. 1.80). This epithelium is typically parakeratinized with desquamated epithelial cells seen filling the cyst lumen. In rare instances the epithelial lining also may contain mucous cells. Occasional cysts may communicate with the overlying mucosal surface.

The most striking feature is the presence of lymphoid tissue in the cyst wall. In most instances, this lymphoid tissue encircles the cyst, but sometimes it involves only a portion of the cyst wall. Germinal centers are usually, but not always, present.

Treatment and Prognosis

The oral lymphoepithelial cyst usually is treated with surgical excision and should not recur. Because the lesion is typically asymptomatic and innocuous, biopsy may not always be necessary if the lesion is distinctive enough to make the diagnosis on a clinical basis.

OTHER RARE DEVELOPMENTAL ANOMALIES

◆ HEMIHYPERPLASIA (HEMIHYPERTROPHY)

Hemihyperplasia is a rare developmental anomaly characterized by asymmetric overgrowth of one or more body parts. Although the condition sometimes is known as **hemihypertrophy,** it actually represents a hyperplasia of the tissues rather than a hypertrophy. Hemihyperplasia can be an isolated finding, but it also may be associated with a variety of malformation syndromes (Box 1.2).

• **BOX 1.2** **Malformation Syndromes Associated With Hemihyperplasia**

- Beckwith-Wiedemann syndrome
- Neurofibromatosis
- Klippel-Trénaunay-Weber syndrome
- Proteus syndrome
- Russell-Silver syndrome
- Sotos syndrome
- McCune-Albright syndrome
- Epidermal nevus syndrome
- Triploid/diploid mixoploidy
- Langer-Giedion syndrome
- Multiple exostoses syndrome
- Maffucci syndrome
- Ollier syndrome
- Segmental odontomaxillary dysplasia

Almost all cases of isolated hemihyperplasia are sporadic. A number of possible etiologic factors have been suggested, but the cause remains obscure. Various theories include vascular or lymphatic abnormalities, central nervous system disturbances, endocrine dysfunctions, and aberrant twinning mechanisms. Some cases are related to genetic defects in the 11p15 chromosomal region, the same locus that is associated with Beckwith-Wiedemann syndrome.

Clinical and Radiographic Features

In a person with hemihyperplasia, one entire side of the body **(complex hemihyperplasia)** may be affected or the enlargement may be limited to a single limb **(simple hemihyperplasia)**. If the enlargement is confined to one side of the face, the term **hemifacial hyperplasia** may apply. The condition occasionally can be crossed, involving different areas on both sides of the body. Hemihyperplasia shows a nearly 2:1 female-to-male predilection, and it occurs more often on the right side of the body.

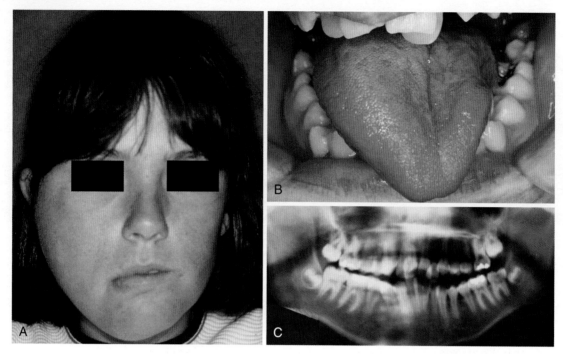

• **Fig. 1.81 Hemihyperplasia. A,** Enlargement of the right side of the face. **B,** Same patient with associated enlargement of the right half of the tongue. **C,** Panoramic radiograph of the same patient showing enlargement of the mandible and teeth on the right side. (Courtesy of Dr. George Blozis.)

Asymmetry often is noted at birth, although in some cases the condition may not become evident until later in childhood (Fig. 1.81). The enlargement becomes more accentuated with age, especially at puberty. This disproportionate growth continues until the patient's overall growth ceases, resulting in permanent asymmetry.

The changes may involve all the tissues on the affected side, including the underlying bone. Often the skin is thickened and may demonstrate increased pigmentation, hypertrichosis, telangiectasias, or nevus flammeus (see page 551). About 20% of those affected are intellectually disabled. One of the most significant features is an increased prevalence of abdominal tumors, especially Wilms tumor, adrenal cortical carcinoma, and hepatoblastoma. These tumors have been reported in 5.9% of patients with isolated hemihyperplasia, and they do not necessarily occur on the same side as the somatic enlargement.

Unilateral **macroglossia,** featuring prominent tongue papillae, is common. Enlargement of other oral soft tissues and bone can occur. The mandibular canal may be increased in size on radiographs. The crowns of the teeth on the affected side, especially the permanent cuspids, premolars, and first molars, can be larger. Premature development of these teeth, along with precocious eruption, may be obvious. The roots also may be larger, but some reports have described root resorption. Malocclusion with open bite is not unusual.

Histopathologic Features

Microscopic examination shows an increase in thickness of the epithelium with hyperplasia of the underlying connective tissues.

Treatment and Prognosis

A complete workup should be undertaken to rule out other possible causes of unilateral growth, such as Beckwith-Wiedemann syndrome, Proteus syndrome, and neurofibromatosis type I (see page 551), which can exhibit hemihyperplasia. During childhood, periodic ultrasound examination should be performed to rule out development of abdominal tumors. After the patient's growth has ceased, cosmetic surgery can be performed, including soft tissue debulking, face lifts, and orthognathic surgery. Orthodontic therapy also frequently is needed.

◆ PROGRESSIVE HEMIFACIAL ATROPHY (PROGRESSIVE FACIAL HEMIATROPHY; ROMBERG SYNDROME; PARRY-ROMBERG SYNDROME)

Progressive hemifacial atrophy is an uncommon and poorly understood degenerative condition characterized by atrophic changes affecting one side of the face. The cause of these changes remains obscure. Etiologic theories include an autoimmune disorder, neurovasculitis involving branches of the trigeminal nerve, or hyperactivity and dysregulation of the sympathetic nervous system. A history of trauma has been documented in some cases, and other reports have considered *Borrelia* spp. infection (Lyme disease) in the cause. Usually, the condition is sporadic, but a few familial cases have been reported, suggesting a possible hereditary influence. Progressive hemifacial atrophy exhibits many features similar to a localized form of **scleroderma** (see page 801), indicating a close relationship between these two disorders.

Clinical and Radiographic Features

The onset of the syndrome is usually during the first two decades of life. The condition begins as atrophy of the skin and subcutaneous structures in a localized area of the face (Fig. 1.82). This atrophy progresses at a variable rate and affects the dermatome of one or more branches of the trigeminal nerve. Hypoplasia of the underlying bone also may occur. Osseous hypoplasia is more common when the condition begins during the first decade. Occasionally, bilateral facial atrophy may occur, or the condition may affect one side of the entire body. Females are affected more often than males.

The overlying skin often exhibits dark pigmentation. Some patients have a sharp line of demarcation, resembling a large linear scar, between normal and abnormal skin near the midline of the forehead, known as *linear scleroderma "en coup de sabre"* (i.e., "strike of the sword"). Ocular involvement is common, and the most frequent manifestation is enophthalmos because of loss of periorbital fat. Local

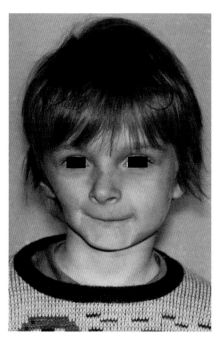

• **Fig. 1.82 Progressive Hemifacial Atrophy.** Young girl with right-sided facial atrophy.

alopecia may occur. Occasionally, trigeminal neuralgia, facial paresthesia, migraine, or epilepsy may develop. MRI studies may reveal a variety of central nervous system abnormalities.

The mouth and nose are deviated toward the affected side. Atrophy of the upper lip may expose the maxillary teeth. Unilateral atrophy of the tongue also can occur. Unilateral posterior open bite often develops as a result of mandibular hypoplasia and delayed eruption of the teeth. The teeth on the affected side may exhibit deficient root development or root resorption.

Histopathologic Features

Microscopic examination of the affected skin reveals atrophy of the epidermis and a variable perivascular infiltrate of lymphocytes and monocytes. In cases showing clinical features of linear scleroderma, dermal fibrosis can be seen. Degenerative changes in the vascular endothelium can be identified with electron microscopy.

Treatment and Prognosis

The atrophy typically progresses slowly for 2 to 20 years and then becomes stable. Active disease can be managed medically with methotrexate and systemic corticosteroids. Plastic surgery may be utilized to correct the cosmetic deformity, and orthodontic therapy may be helpful to treat any associated malocclusion.

◆ SEGMENTAL ODONTOMAXILLARY DYSPLASIA (HEMIMAXILLOFACIAL DYSPLASIA)

Segmental odontomaxillary dysplasia is a recently recognized developmental disorder that affects the jaw and (sometimes) the overlying facial tissues. The cause is unknown. Clinically, it is frequently mistaken for craniofacial fibrous dysplasia or hemifacial hyperplasia, but it represents a distinct and separate entity.

Clinical and Radiographic Features

Segmental odontomaxillary dysplasia usually is discovered during childhood and is characterized by painless, unilateral enlargement of the maxillary bone, along with fibrous hyperplasia of the overlying gingival soft tissues (Fig. 1.83). Mild facial asymmetry may be evident, often described as prominence of the upper lip. One or both maxillary premolars frequently are missing or impacted, and the primary teeth in the affected area may be hypoplastic or show enamel defects. Radiographic examination reveals thickened trabeculae that often are vertically oriented, which results in a relatively radiopaque, granular appearance. The maxillary sinus may be smaller on the affected side. Several cases have been associated with hypertrichosis, hyperpigmentation, or rough erythema of the overlying facial skin.

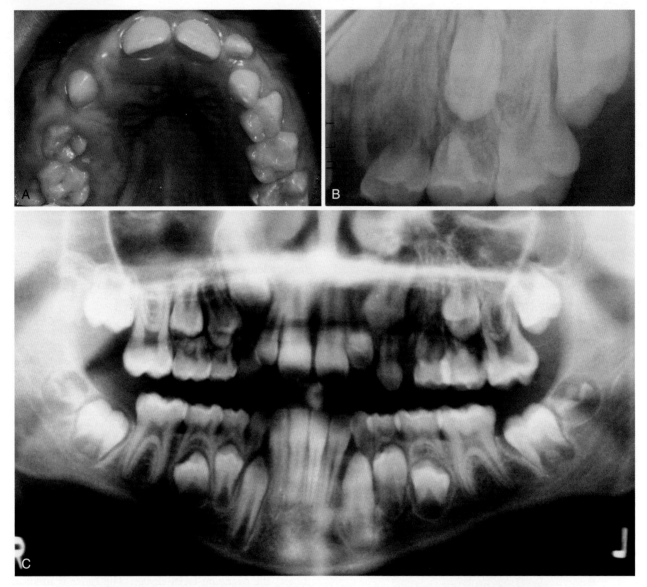

• **Fig. 1.83 Segmental Odontomaxillary Dysplasia. A,** Unilateral enlargement of the maxilla and overlying gingival soft tissues. **B,** Periapical radiograph showing coarse trabecular pattern with absence of the first premolar. **C,** Panoramic radiograph showing irregular bone pattern of the left maxilla expanding into the maxillary sinus.

Histopathologic Features

The gingival soft tissues may show nonspecific fibrosis. The affected maxillary bone consists of irregular trabeculae with a woven appearance. This bone shows numerous resting and reversal lines, but it lacks significant osteoblastic and osteoclastic activity. Deciduous teeth in the involved area may exhibit irregular dentinal tubules, a focally deficient odontoblastic layer, and external resorption.

Treatment and Prognosis

Once diagnosed, segmental odontomaxillary dysplasia remains relatively stable and may not require surgical intervention. Although the lesion can show gradual enlargement, the increase in size is proportional to the overall growth of the patient. When necessary, surgical recontouring can be performed for cosmetic purposes, to improve access for oral hygiene, or to facilitate tooth eruption. Both successful orthodontic therapy and placement of dental implants have been reported.

◆ CROUZON SYNDROME (CRANIOFACIAL DYSOSTOSIS)

Crouzon syndrome is one of a rare group of syndromes characterized by craniosynostosis, or premature closing of the cranial sutures. It is believed to be caused by one of a variety of mutations of the fibroblast growth factor receptor 2 (FGFR2) gene on chromosome 10q26. The condition occurs in about 1 of every 62,500 births and is inherited as an autosomal dominant trait. A significant number of cases, however, represent new mutations, often apparently related to increased paternal age.

Clinical and Radiographic Features

Crouzon syndrome exhibits a wide variability in expression. The premature sutural closing leads to cranial malformations, such as **brachycephaly** (short head), **scaphocephaly** (boat-shaped head), or **trigonocephaly** (triangle-shaped head). The most severely affected patients can demonstrate a "cloverleaf" skull (*kleeblattschädel* deformity). The orbits are shallow, resulting in characteristic ocular proptosis (Fig. 1.84). Visual impairment or total blindness and a hearing deficit may occur. Some patients report headaches, attributable to increased intracranial pressure. Marked mental deficiency is rarely seen. Skull radiographs typically show increased digital markings (i.e., "beaten-metal" pattern).

The maxilla is underdeveloped, resulting in midface hypoplasia and airway obstruction. Often the maxillary teeth are crowded, and occlusal disharmony usually occurs. Some patients will exhibit one or more congenitally missing teeth. Cleft lip and cleft palate are rare, but lateral palatal swellings may produce a midline maxillary pseudocleft.

Treatment and Prognosis

The clinical defects of Crouzon syndrome can be treated surgically, but multiple procedures may be necessary. Early craniectomy often is needed to alleviate the raised intracranial pressure. Fronto-orbital advancement can be performed to correct the ocular defects, with midfacial advancement used to correct the maxillary hypoplasia. Distraction osteogenesis can be a useful adjunct for these surgical procedures.

◆ APERT SYNDROME (ACROCEPHALOSYNDACTYLY)

Like Crouzon syndrome, **Apert syndrome** is a rare condition that is characterized by craniosynostosis. It occurs in about 1 of every 65,000 births and usually is caused by one of two point mutations in the *FGFR2* gene, which is located on chromosome 10q26. Although it is inherited as an autosomal dominant trait, most cases represent sporadic new mutations, which are thought to be exclusively of paternal origin and often associated with increased paternal age.

Clinical and Radiographic Features

Craniosynostosis typically produces **acrobrachycephaly** (tower skull); severe cases may demonstrate the *kleeblattschädel* deformity (cloverleaf skull). The occiput is flattened, and a tall appearance to the forehead is noted. Ocular proptosis is a characteristic finding, along with hypertelorism and downward-slanting lateral palpebral fissures (Fig. 1.85). Visual loss can result from the following:
- Chronic exposure of the unprotected eyes
- Increased intracranial pressure
- Compression of the optic nerves

Skull films may demonstrate digital impressions similar to those of Crouzon syndrome (Fig. 1.86). Fusion of two or more cervical vertebrae occurs in 68% of affected individuals.

The middle third of the face is significantly retruded and hypoplastic, resulting in a relative mandibular prognathism. The reduced size of the nasopharynx and narrowing of the posterior choanae can lead to respiratory distress in the young child. To compensate for this, most infants become mouth breathers, contributing to an "open-mouth" appearance. Sleep apnea may develop. Middle-ear infections are common, as is conductive hearing loss.

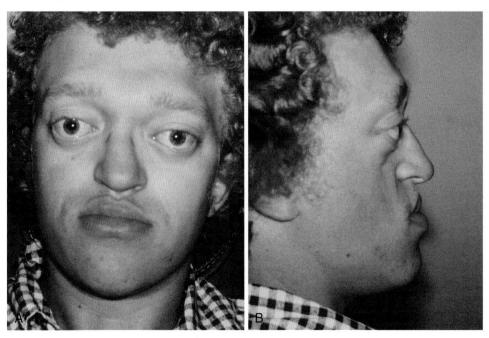

• **Fig. 1.84 Crouzon Syndrome**. Ocular proptosis and midface hypoplasia. (Courtesy of Dr. Robert Gorlin.)

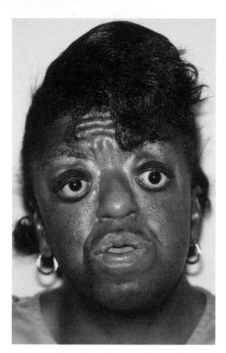

• **Fig. 1.85 Apert Syndrome**. Midface hypoplasia and ocular proptosis.

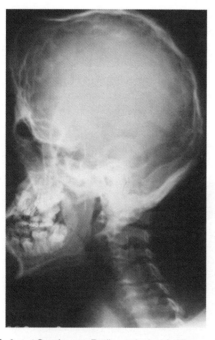

• **Fig. 1.86 Apert Syndrome**. Radiograph showing "tower skull," midface hypoplasia, and digital markings. Similar digital impressions are apparent in people with Crouzon syndrome. (Courtesy of Dr. Robert Gorlin.)

Characteristic limb defects help distinguish Apert syndrome from other craniosynostosis syndromes. Syndactyly of the second, third, and fourth digits of the hands and feet always is observed (Fig. 1.87). Associated synonychia also may occur. The first and fifth digits may be separate or joined to the middle digits. Synostosis of adjacent

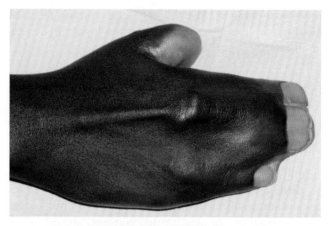

• **Fig. 1.87 Apert Syndrome**. Syndactyly of the hand.

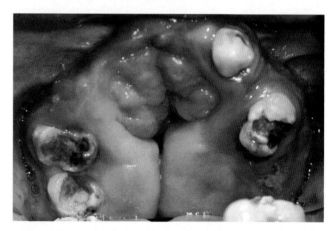

• **Fig. 1.88 Apert Syndrome**. Abnormal shape of the maxilla, with swellings of the posterior lateral hard palate, resulting in pseudocleft formation.

phalanges may be observed on radiographs. The average height of affected patients is below that of the general population.

Intellectual disability is reported in a large proportion of patients with Apert syndrome. An unusual acnelike eruption develops in most of the patients and involves the forearms.

Specific oral manifestations include a trapezoid-shaped appearance to the lips when they are relaxed, resulting from the midface hypoplasia and mouth breathing. Approximately 30% of patients exhibit either a cleft of the soft palate or a bifid uvula. The maxillary hypoplasia leads to a V-shaped arch and crowding of the teeth. Class III malocclusion typically occurs and may be associated with anterior open bite plus anterior and posterior crossbite. Swellings are observed along the lateral hard palate from the accumulation of glycosaminoglycans, especially hyaluronic acid (Fig. 1.88). These swellings often enlarge with age to produce a pseudocleft of the hard palate. Gingival thickening may be associated with delayed eruption of the teeth. One study showed that 35% of patients with Apert syndrome were missing one or two permanent teeth, especially maxillary lateral incisors or mandibular second premolars.

Treatment and Prognosis

The cosmetic and functional defects of Apert syndrome can be treated by an interdisciplinary approach using multiple surgical procedures. Although this condition historically has been associated with intellectual disability, early surgical intervention to allow for brain growth may contribute to greater intellectual and social development. Craniectomy often is performed during the first year of life to treat the craniosynostosis. Frontofacial advancement and midface advancement can be done later to correct the proptosis and midface hypoplasia. Coordinated orthodontic therapy often is necessary to bring unerupted teeth into place and to improve occlusion. Surgery also can be used to separate the fused fingers. Due to limitations in hand mobility, maintenance of proper oral hygiene may be difficult. Therefore, parental assistance with oral hygiene should be encouraged, as well as utilization of electric toothbrushes, floss holders, and fluoride rinses.

◆ MANDIBULOFACIAL DYSOSTOSIS (TREACHER COLLINS SYNDROME; FRANCESCHETTI-ZWAHLEN-KLEIN SYNDROME)

Mandibulofacial dysostosis is a rare syndrome that is characterized primarily by defects of structures derived from the first and second branchial arches. It usually is inherited as an autosomal dominant trait and occurs with a frequency of 1 in 50,000 live births. However, even rarer autosomal recessive forms have been identified. The condition has variable expressivity, and the severity of the clinical features often tends to be greater in subsequent generations of the same family. Approximately 60% of cases represent new mutations, and these often are associated with increased paternal age. Mutations of the *TCOF1* gene account for over 90% of autosomal dominant forms of mandibulofacial dysostosis, but occasional examples are associated with mutations of *POLR1D*. Rare autosomal recessive cases may be related to pathogenic variants of *POLR1C* or *POLR1D*.

Clinical and Radiographic Features

Individuals with mandibulofacial dysostosis exhibit a characteristic facies (Fig. 1.89), although the features occasionally can be so mild that they are easily overlooked. The zygomas are hypoplastic, resulting in a narrow face with depressed cheeks and downward-slanting palpebral fissures. In 75% of patients, a **coloboma,** or notch, occurs on the outer portion of the lower eyelid. Approximately half of the patients have no eyelashes medial to the coloboma. Often the sideburns show a tongue-shaped extension toward the cheek.

The ears may demonstrate a number of anomalies. The pinnae frequently are deformed or misplaced, and extra ear tags may be seen. Ossicle defects or absence of the external auditory canal often result in conductive hearing loss.

The mandible is underdeveloped, resulting in a markedly retruded chin. Radiographs often demonstrate hypoplasia of the condylar and coronoid processes with prominent antegonial notching. The mouth is downturned, and about 15% of patients have lateral facial clefting (see page 2) that produces macrostomia. Cleft palate is seen in about one-third of cases. The parotid glands may be hypoplastic or may be totally absent (see page 460).

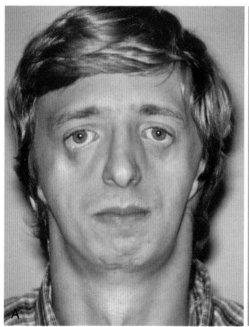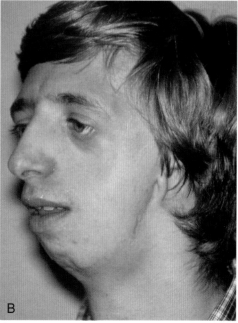

• **Fig. 1.89 Mandibulofacial Dysostosis**. Patient exhibits a hypoplastic mandible, downward-slanting palpebral fissures, and ear deformities. (Courtesy of Dr. Tom Brock.)

A number of infants may experience respiratory and feeding difficulties because of hypoplasia of the nasopharynx, oropharynx, and hypopharynx. Choanal atresia may be present, and the larynx and trachea are often narrow. Combined with the mandibular hypoplasia and resultant improper tongue position, these defects can lead to the infant's death from respiratory complications.

Treatment and Prognosis

Patients with mild forms of mandibulofacial dysostosis may not require treatment. In more severe cases the clinical appearance can be improved with cosmetic surgery. Because of the extent of facial reconstruction required, multiple surgical procedures usually are necessary. Individual operations may be needed for the eyes, zygomas, jaws, ears, and nose. Combined orthodontic therapy is needed along with the orthognathic surgery.

Bibliography

Orofacial Clefts

Côté A, Fanous A, Almajed A, et al.: Pierre Robin sequence: review of diagnostic and treatment challenges, *Int J Pediatr Otorhinolaryngol* 79:451–464, 2015.

Dixon MJ, Marazita ML, Beaty TH, et al.: Cleft lip and palate: synthesizing genetic and environmental influences, *Nat Rev Genet* 12:167–178, 2011.

Eppley BL, van Aalst JA, Robey A, et al.: The spectrum of orofacial clefting, *Plast Reconstr Surg* 115:101e–114e, 2005.

Evans CA: Orthodontic treatment for patients with clefts, *Clin Plast Surg* 31:271–290, 2004.

Gosain AK, Conley SF, Marks S, et al.: Submucous cleft palate: diagnostic methods and outcomes of surgical treatment, *Plast Reconstr Surg* 97:1497–1509, 1996.

Harada K, Sato M, Omura K: Long-term maxillomandibular skeletal and dental changes in children with cleft lip and palate after maxillary distraction, *Oral Surg Oral Med Oral Pathol Oral Radiol Endod* 102:292–299, 2006.

Hennekam RCM, Krantz ID, Allanson JE: Chapter 21. Orofacial clefting syndromes: General aspects, In *Gorlin's syndromes of the head and neck*, ed 5, New York, 2010, Oxford University Press, pp 943–972.

Hsieh ST, Woo AS: Pierre Robin sequence, *Clin Plast Surg* 46:249–259, 2019.

Krapels IP, Vermeij-Keers C, Müller M, et al.: Nutrition and genes in the development of orofacial clefting, *Nutr Rev* 64:280–288, 2006.

Logjes RJH, Haasnoot M, Lemmers PMA, et al.: Mortality in Robin sequence: identification of risk factors, *Eur J Pediatr* 177:781–789, 2018.

Murray JC: Gene/environment causes of cleft lip and/or palate, *Clin Genet* 61:248–256, 2002.

Rintala A, Leisti J, Liesmaa M, et al.: Oblique facial clefts, *Scand J Plast Reconstr Surg* 14:291–297, 1980.

Roy A-A, Rtshiladze MA, Stevens K, et al.: Orthognathic surgery for patients with cleft lip and palate, *Clin Plast Surg* 46:157–171, 2019.

Scott AR, Tibesar RJ, Sidman JD: Pierre Robin sequence: evaluation, management, indications for surgery, and pitfalls, *Otolaryngol Clin North Am* 45:695–710, 2012.

Shaye D, Liu CC, Tollefson TT: Cleft lip and palate. An evidence-based review, *Facial Plast Surg Clin N Am* 23:357–372, 2015.

Stoll C, Alembik Y, Dott B, et al.: Associated malformations in cases with oral clefts, *Cleft Palate Craniofac J* 37:41–47, 2000.

Wehby G, Murray JC: Folic acid and orofacial clefts: a review of the evidence, *Oral Dis* 16:11–19, 2010.

Weinberg SM, Neiswanger K, Martin RA, et al.: The Pittsburgh oral-facial cleft study: expanding the cleft phenotype. Background and justification, *Cleft Palate Craniofac J* 43:7–20, 2006.

Worley ML, Patel KG, Kilpatrick LA: Cleft lip and palate, *Clin Perinatol* 45:661–678, 2018.

Commissural Lip Pits

Baker BR: Pits of the lip commissures in Caucasoid males, *Oral Surg Oral Med Oral Pathol* 21:56–60, 1966.

Everett FG, Wescott WB: Commissural lip pits, *Oral Surg Oral Med Oral Pathol* 14:202–209, 1961.

Gorsky M, Buchner A, Cohen C: Commissural lip pits in Israeli jews of different ethnic origin, *Community Dent Oral Epidemiol* 13:195–196, 1985.

Paramedian Lip Pits

Hennekam RCM, Krantz ID, Allanson JE: Popliteal pterygium syndrome (facio-genito-popliteal syndrome), In *Gorlin's syndromes of the head and neck*, ed 5, New York, 2010, Oxford University Press, pp 862–865.

Kondo S, Schutte BC, Richardson RJ, et al.: Mutations in IRF6 cause Van der Woude and popliteal pterygium syndromes, *Nat Genet* 32:285–289, 2002.

Matsumoto N, Niikawa N: Kabuki make-up syndrome: a review, *Am J Med Genet C Semin Med Genet* 117:57–65, 2003.

Onofre MA, Brosco HB, Brosco JU, et al.: Congenital fistulae of the lower lip in van der Woude syndrome: a histomorphological study, *Cleft Palate Craniofac J* 36:79–85, 1999.

Richardson S, Khandeparker RV: Management of lip pits in van der Woude syndrome: a clinical classification with difficulty index, *J Oral Maxillofac Surg* 74:1849e1–1849e10, 2016.

Rizos M, Spyropoulos MN: Van der Woude syndrome: a review. Cardinal signs, epidemiology, associated features, differential diagnosis, expressivity, genetic counseling and treatment, *Eur J Orthod* 26:17–24, 2004.

Shotelersuk V, Punyashthiti R, Srivuthana S, et al.: Kabuki syndrome: report of six Thai children and further phenotypic and genetic delineation, *Am J Med Genet* 110:384–390, 2002.

Double Lip

Barnett ML, Bosshardt LL, Morgan AF: Double lip and double lip with blepharochalasis (Ascher's syndrome), *Oral Surg Oral Med Oral Pathol* 34:727–733, 1972.

Eski M, Nisanci M, Atkas A, et al.: Congenital double lip: review of 5 cases, *Br J Oral Maxillofac Surg* 45:68–70, 2007.

Gomez-Duaso AJ, Seoane J, Vazquez-Garcia J, et al.: Ascher syndrome: report of two cases, *J Oral Maxillofac Surg* 55:88–90, 1997.

Kalra N, Tyagi R, Khatri A, et al.: Double lip – an atypical facial anomaly: two case reports, *Int J Clin Pediatr Dent* 11:451–455, 2018.

Fordyce Granules

Azevedo RS, Almeida OP, Netto JNS, et al.: Comparative clinicopathological study of sebaceous hyperplasia and sebaceous adenoma, *Oral Surg Oral Med Oral Pathol Oral Radiol Endod* 107:100–104, 2009.

Daley TD: Pathology of intraoral sebaceous glands, *J Oral Pathol Med* 22:241–245, 1993.

Fordyce JA: A peculiar affection of the mucous membrane of the lips and oral cavity, *J Cutan Genito-Urin Dis* 14:413–419, 1896.

Halperin V, Kolas S, Jefferis KR, et al.: The occurrence of Fordyce spots, benign migratory glossitis, median rhomboid glossitis, and fissured tongue in 2,478 dental patients, *Oral Surg Oral Med Oral Pathol* 6:1072–1077, 1953.

Sewerin I: The sebaceous glands in the vermilion border of the lips and in the oral mucosa of man, *Acta Odontol Scand* 33(Suppl 68):13–226, 1975.

Leukoedema

Archard HO, Carlson KP, Stanley HR: Leukoedema of the human oral mucosa, *Oral Surg Oral Med Oral Pathol* 25:717–728, 1968.

Axéll T, Henricsson V: Leukoedema—an epidemiologic study with special reference to the influence of tobacco habits, *Community Dent Oral Epidemiol* 9:142–146, 1981.

Martin JL: Leukoedema: an epidemiological study in white and African Americans, *J Tenn Dent Assoc* 77:18–21, 1997.

Martin JL, Crump EP: Leukoedema of the buccal mucosa in negro children and youth, *Oral Surg Oral Med Oral Pathol* 34:49–58, 1972.

van Wyk CW, Ambrosio SC: Leukoedema: ultrastructural and histochemical observations, *J Oral Pathol* 12:319–329, 1983.

Microglossia

Dunham ME, Austin TL: Congenital aglossia and situs inversus, *Int J Pediatr Otorhinolaryngol* 19:163–168, 1990.

Hennekam RCM, Krantz ID, Allanson JE: Oromandibular-limb hypogenesis syndromes, In *Gorlin's syndromes of the head and neck*, ed 5, New York, 2010, Oxford University Press, pp 913–917.

Thorp MA, de Waal PJ, Prescott CAJ: Extreme microglossia, *Int J Pediatr Otorhinolaryngol* 67:473–477, 2003.

Voigt S, Park A, Scott A, et al.: Microglossia in a newborn. A case report and review of the literature, *Arch Otolaryngol Head Neck Surg* 138:759–761, 2012.

Yasuda Y, Kitai N, Fujii Y, et al.: Report of a patient with hypoglossia-hypodactylia syndrome and a review of the literature, *Cleft Palate Craniofac J* 40:196–202, 2003.

Macroglossia

Cielo CM, Duffy KA, Vyas A, et al.: Obstructive sleep apnoea and the role of tongue reduction surgery in children with Beckwith-Wiedemann syndrome, *Paediatr Respir Rev* 25:58–63, 2018.

Cohen MM Jr: Beckwith-Wiedemann syndrome: historical, clinico-pathological, and etiopathogenetic perspectives, *Pediatr Dev Pathol* 8:287–304, 2005.

McKee HR, Escott E, Damm D, et al.: Macroglossia in amyotrophic lateral sclerosis, *JAMA Neurol* 70:1432–1435, 2013.

Melville JC, Menegotto KD, Woernley TC, et al.: Unusual case of a massive macroglossia secondary to myxedema: a case report and literature review, *J Oral Maxillofac Surg* 76:119–127, 2018.

Morgan WE, Friedman EM, Duncan NO, et al.: Surgical management of macroglossia in children, *Arch Otolaryngol Head Neck Surg* 122:326–329, 1996.

Perkins JA: Overview of macroglossia and its treatment, *Curr Opin Otolaryngol Head Neck Surg* 17:460–465, 2009.

Vogel JE, Mulliken JB, Kaban LB: Macroglossia: a review of the condition and a new classification, *Plast Reconstr Surg* 78:715–723, 1986.

Wang J, Goodger NM, Pogrel MA: The role of tongue reduction, *Oral Surg Oral Med Oral Pathol Oral Radiol Endod* 95:269–273, 2003.

Weksberg R, Shuman C, Smith AC: Beckwith-Wiedemann syndrome, *Am J Med Genet C Semin Med Genet* 137:12–23, 2005.

Ankyloglossia

Buryk M, Bloom D, Shope T: Efficacy of neonatal release of ankyloglossia: a randomized trial, *Pediatrics* 128:280–288, 2011.

Dollberg S, Botzer E, Grunis E, et al.: Immediate nipple pain relief after frenotomy in breast-fed infants with ankyloglossia: a randomized, prospective study, *J Pediatr Surg* 41:1598–1600, 2006.

Suter VGA, Bornstein MM: Ankyloglossia: facts and myths in diagnosis and treatment, *J Periodontol* 80:1204–1219, 2009.

Walsh J, Benoit MM: Ankyloglossia and other oral ties, *Otolaryngol Clin North Am* 52:795–811, 2019.

Walsh J, Tunkel D: Diagnosis and treatment of ankyloglossia in newborns and infants: a review, *JAMA Otolaryngol Head Neck Surg* 143:1032–1039, 2017.

Lingual Thyroid

Baughman RA: Lingual thyroid and lingual thyroglossal tract remnants: a clinical and histopathologic study with review of the literature, *Oral Surg Oral Med Oral Pathol* 34:781–799, 1972.

Carranza Leon BG, Turcu A, Bahn R, et al.: Lingual thyroid: 35-year experience at a tertiary care referral center, *Endocr Pract* 22:343–349, 2016.

Gu T, Jiang B, Wang N, et al.: New insight into ectopic thyroid glands between the neck and maxillofacial region from a 42-case study, *BMC Endocr Disord* 15:70, 2015.

Majumdar I, Mastrandrea LD: Lingual thyroid as a cause of primary hypothyroidism: congenital hypothyroidism in the neonatal period and beyond, *Clin Pediatr* 49:885–888, 2010.

Montgomery ML: *Lingual thyroid: A comprehensive review, west J surg Obstet Gynecol* 43:661–669, 44:54–62, 122–128, 189–195, 237–247, 303–309, 373–379, 442–446, 1936.

Prasad KC, Bhat V: Surgical management of lingual thyroid: a report of four cases, *J Oral Maxillofac Surg* 58:223–227, 2000.

Stokes W, Interval E, Patel R: Lingual thyroid carcinoma: a case report and review of surgical approaches in the literature, *Ann Otol Rhinol Laryngol* 127:475–480, 2018.

Fissured Tongue

Al Qahtani NA, Deepthi A, Alhussain NM, et al.: Association of geographic tongue and fissured tongue with ABO blood type group among adult psoriasis patients: a novel study from a tertiary care hospital in Saudi Arabia, *Oral Surg Oral Med Oral Pathol Oral Radiol* 127:490–497, 2019.

Bouquot JE, Gundlach KKH: Odd tongues: the prevalence of common tongue lesions in 23,616 white Americans over 35 years of age, *Quintessence Int* 17:719–730, 1986.

Eidelman E, Chosack A, Cohen T: Scrotal tongue and geographic tongue: polygenic and associated traits, *Oral Surg Oral Med Oral Pathol* 42:591–596, 1976.

Halperin V, Kolas S, Jefferis KR: The occurrence of Fordyce spots, benign migratory glossitis, median rhomboid glossitis, and fissured tongue in 2,478 dental patients, *Oral Surg Oral Med Oral Pathol* 6:1072–1077, 1953.

Picciani BL, Souza TT, Santos Vde C, et al.: Geographic tongue and fissured tongue in 348 patients with psoriasis: correlation with disease severity, *ScientificWorldJournal* 2015:564326, 2015. https://doi.org/10.1155/2015/564326.

Hairy Tongue

Braggio C, Bocchialini G, Ventura L, et al.: Linezolid-induced black hairy tongue, *Acta Biomed* 89:408–410, 2018.

Danser MM, Gómez SM, Van der Weijden GA: Tongue coating and tongue brushing: a literature review, *Int J Dent Hygiene* 1:151–158, 2003.

Manabe M, Lim HW, Winzer M, et al.: Architectural organization of filiform papillae in normal and black hairy tongue epithelium, *Arch Dermatol* 135:177–181, 1999.

Sarti GM, Haddy RI, Schaffer D, et al.: Black hairy tongue, *Am Fam Physician* 41:1751–1755, 1990.

Schlager E, St. Claire C, Ashack K, et al.: Black hairy tongue: predisposing factors, diagnosis, and treatment, *Am J Clin Dermatol* 18:563–569, 2017.

Standish SM, Moorman WC: Treatment of hairy tongue with podophyllin resin, *J Am Dent Assoc* 68:535–540, 1964.

Thompson DF, Kessler TL: Drug-induced black hairy tongue, *Pharmacotherapy* 30:585–593, 2010.

Varicosities

Akkaya ÖD, Özkan G: Evaluation of the factors associated with sublingual varices: a descriptive clinical study, *Folia Morphol* 78:325–330, 2019.

Duarte NT, de Oliveira GA, da Rocha TJ, et al.: Prevalence of sublingual varices in patients with cirrhosis and the correlation with nitrogen compounds, *Oral Surg Oral Med Oral Pathol Oral Radiol* 129:39–44, 2020.

Hedström L, Albrektsson M, Bergh H: Is there a connection between sublingual varices and hypertension? *BMC Oral Health* 15:78, 2015.

Hedström L, Bergh H: Sublingual varices in relation to smoking and cardiovascular diseases, *Br J Oral Maxillofac Surg* 48:136–138, 2010.

Lazos JP, Piemonte ED, Panico RL: Oral varix: a review, *Gerodontology* 32:82–89, 2015.

Weathers DR, Fine RM: Thrombosed varix of oral cavity, *Arch Dermatol* 104:427–430, 1971.

Caliber-Persistent Artery

Awni S, Conn B: Caliber-persistent labial artery: a rarely recognized cause of lower lip swelling – report of 5 cases and review of the literature, *J Oral Maxillofac Surg* 74:1391–1395, 2016.

Lovas JG, Goodday RH: Clinical diagnosis of caliber-persistent labial artery of the lower lip, *Oral Surg Oral Med Oral Pathol* 76:480–483, 1993.

Lovas JGL, Rodu B, Hammond HL, et al.: Caliber-persistent labial artery: a common vascular anomaly, *Oral Surg Oral Med Oral Pathol Oral Radiol Endod* 86:308–312, 1998.

Miko T, Adler P, Endes P: Simulated cancer of the lower lip attributed to a "caliber persistent" artery, *J Oral Pathol* 9:137–144, 1980.

Rosdy NM, Firth NA, Rich AM: Calibre-persistent labial artery: often misdiagnosed as a mucocele, *Int J Oral Maxillofac Surg* 39:1230–1233, 2010.

Lateral Soft Palate Fistulas

Hennekam RCM, Krantz ID, Allanson JE: Fistulae of lateral soft palate and associated anomalies, In *Gorlin's syndromes of the head and neck*, ed 5, New York, 2010, Oxford University Press, p 1305.

Miller AS, Brookreson KR, Brody BA: Lateral soft-palate fistula: report of a case, *Arch Otolaryngol* 91:200, 1970.

Coronoid Hyperplasia

Farronato M, Lucchina AG, Mortellaro C, et al.: Bilateral hyperplasia of the coronoid process in pediatric patients: what is the gold standard for treatment? *J Craniofac Surg* 30:1058–1063, 2019.

Izumi M, Isobe M, Toyama M, et al.: Computed tomographic features of bilateral coronoid process hyperplasia with special emphasis on patients without interference between the process and the zygomatic bone, *Oral Surg Oral Med Oral Pathol Oral Radiol Endod* 99:93–100, 2005.

McLoughlin PM, Hopper C, Bowley NB: Hyperplasia of the mandibular coronoid process: an analysis of 31 cases and a review of the literature, *J Oral Maxillofac Surg* 53:250–255, 1995.

Mulder CH, Kalaykova SI, Gortzak RA: Coronoid process hyperplasia: a systematic review of the literature from 1995, *Int J Oral Maxillofac Surg* 41:1483–1489, 2012.

Condylar Hyperplasia

Eslami B, Behnia H, Javadi H, et al.: Histopathologic comparison of normal and hyperplastic condyles, *Oral Surg Oral Med Oral Pathol Oral Radiol Endod* 96:711–717, 2003.

Jones RHB, Tier GA: Correction of facial asymmetry as a result of unilateral condylar hyperplasia, *J Oral Maxillofac Surg* 70:1413–1425, 2012.

Nitzan DW, Katsnelson A, Bermanis I, et al.: The clinical characteristics of condylar hyperplasia: experience with 61 patients, *J Oral Maxillofac Surg* 66:312–318, 2008.

Nolte JW, Schreurs R, Karssemakers LHE, et al.: Demographic features in unilateral condylar hyperplasia: an overview of 309 asymmetric cases and presentation of an algorithm, *J Craniomaxillofac Surg* 46:1484–1492, 2018.

Obwegeser HL, Makek MS: Hemimandibular hyperplasia-hemimandibular elongation, *J Maxillofac Surg* 14:183–208, 1986.

Rodrigues DB, Castro V: Condylar hyperplasia of the temporomandibular joint: types, treatment, and surgical implications, *Oral Maxillofac Surg Clin N Am* 27:155–167, 2015.

Sun R, Sun L, Sun Z, et al.: A three-dimensional study of hemimandibular hyperplasia, hemimandibular elongation, solitary condylar hyperplasia, simple mandibular asymmetry and condylar osteoma or osteochondroma, *J Craniomaxillofac Surg* 47:1665–1674, 2019.

Wolford LM, Movahed R, Perez DE: A classification system for conditions causing condylar hyperplasia, *J Oral Maxillofac Surg* 72:567–595, 2014.

Condylar Hypoplasia

Arun T, Kayhan F, Kiziltan M: Treatment of condylar hypoplasia with distraction osteogenesis: a case report, *Angle Orthod* 72:371–376, 2002.

Berger SS, Stewart RE: Mandibular hypoplasia secondary to perinatal trauma: report of case, *J Oral Surg* 35:578–582, 1977.

Halle TR, Todd NW, Soares BP: Mandibular condylar hypoplasia in children with isolated unilateral congenital aural atresia, *Laryngoscope* 128:1191–1195, 2018.

Jerrell RG, Fuselier B, Mahan P: Acquired condylar hypoplasia: report of case, *ASDC J Dent Child* 58:147–153, 1991.

Svensson B, Larsson Å, Adell R: The mandibular condyle in juvenile chronic arthritis patients with mandibular hypoplasia: a clinical and histological study, *Int J Oral Maxillofac Surg* 30:306–312, 2001.

Bifid Condyle

Borrás-Ferreres J, Sánchez-Torres A, Gay-Escoda C: Bifid mandibular condyles: a systematic review, *Med Oral Patol Oral Cir Bucal* 23:e672–e680, 2018.

Güven O: A study on etiopathogenesis and clinical features of multi-headed (bifid and trifid) mandibular condyles and review of the literature, *J Craniomaxillofac Surg* 46:773–778, 2018.

Şahman H, Etöz OA, Şekerci AE, et al.: Tetrafid mandibular condyle: a unique case report and review of the literature, *Dentomaxillofac Radiol* 40:524–530, 2011.

Sala-Pérez S, Vázquez-Delgado E, Rodríguez-Baeza A, et al.: Bifid mandibular condyle: a disorder in its own right? *J Am Dent Assoc* 141:1076–1085, 2010.

Stefanou EP, Fanourakis IG, Vlastos K, et al.: Bilateral bifid mandibular condyles: report of four cases, *Dentomaxillofac Radiol* 27:186–188, 1998.

Exostoses

Bouquot JE, Gundlach KKH: Oral exophytic lesions in 23,616 white Americans over 35 years of age, *Oral Surg Oral Med Oral Pathol* 62:284–291, 1986.

Frazier KB, Baker PS, Abdelsayed R, et al.: A case report of subpontic osseous hyperplasia in the maxillary arch, *Oral Surg Oral Med Oral Pathol Oral Radiol Endod* 89:73–76, 2000.

Hegtvedt AK, Terry BC, Burkes EJ, et al.: Skin graft vestibuloplasty exostosis: a report of two cases, *Oral Surg Oral Med Oral Pathol* 69:149–152, 1990.

Jainkittivong A, Langlais RP: Buccal and palatal exostoses: prevalence and concurrence with tori, *Oral Surg Oral Med Oral Pathol Oral Radiol Endod* 90:48–53, 2000.

Morton TH Jr, Natkin E: Hyperostosis and fixed partial denture pontics: report of 16 patients and review of literature, *J Prosthet Dent* 64:539–547, 1990.

Pack ARC, Gaudie WM, Jennings AM: Bony exostosis as a sequela to free gingival grafting: two case reports, *J Periodontol* 62:269–271, 1991.

Sonnier KE, Horning GM, Cohen ME: Palatal tubercles, palatal tori, and mandibular tori: prevalence and anatomical features in a U.S. population, *J Periodontol* 70:329–336, 1999.

Torus Palatinus and Torus Mandibularis

Bertazzo-Silveira E, Stuginski-Barbosa J, Porporatti AL, et al.: Association between signs and symptoms of bruxism and presence of tori: a systematic review, *Clin Oral Investig* 21:2789–2799, 2017.

Eggen S: Torus mandibularis: an estimation of the degree of genetic determination, *Acta Odontol Scand* 47:409–415, 1989.

Eggen S, Natvig B: Relationship between torus mandibularis and number of present teeth, *Scand J Dent Res* 94:233–240, 1986.

Eggen S, Natvig B: Variation in torus mandibularis prevalence in Norway: a statistical analysis using logistic regression, *Community Dent Oral Epidemiol* 19:32–35, 1991.

Gorsky M, Bukai A, Shohat M: Genetic influence on the prevalence of torus palatinus, *Am J Med Genet* 75:138–140, 1998.

Jeong C-W, Kim K-H, Jang H-W, et al.: The relationship between oral tori and bite force, *Cranio* 37:246–253, 2019.

Kolas S, Halperin V, Jefferis K, et al.: The occurrence of torus palatinus and torus mandibularis in 2,478 dental patients, *Oral Surg Oral Med Oral Pathol* 6:1134–1141, 1953.

Morita K, Tsuka H, Shintani T, et al.: Prevalence of torus mandibularis in young healthy dentate adults, *J Oral Maxillofac Surg* 75:2593–2598, 2017.

Morrison MD, Tamimi F: Oral tori are associated with local mechanical and systemic factors: a case-control study, *J Oral Maxillofac Surg* 71:14–22, 2013.

Suzuki M, Sakai T: A familial study of torus palatinus and torus mandibularis, *Am J Phys Anthropol* 18:263–272, 1960.

Eagle Syndrome

Badhey A, Jategaonkar A, Kovacs AJA, et al.: Eagle syndrome: a comprehensive review, *Clin Neurol Neurosurg* 159:34–38, 2017.

Correll RW, Jensen JL, Taylor JB, et al.: Mineralization of the stylohyoid-stylomandibular ligament complex: a radiographic incidence study, *Oral Surg Oral Med Oral Pathol* 48:286–291, 1979.

Eagle WW: Elongated styloid processes: report of two cases, *Arch Otolaryngol* 25:584–587, 1937.

Hardin FM, Xiao R, Burkey BB: Surgical management of patients with Eagle syndrome, *Am J Otolaryngol* 39:481–484, 2018.

Öztaş B, Orhan K: Investigation of the incidence of stylohyoid ligament calcification with panoramic radiographs, *J Invest Clin Dent* 3:30–35, 2012.

Smoot TW, Taha A, Tarlov N, et al.: Eagle syndrome: a case report of stylocarotid syndrome with internal carotid artery dissection, *Interv Neuroradiol* 23:433–436, 2017.

Subedi R, Dean R, Baronos S, et al.: Carotid artery dissection: a rare complication of Eagle syndrome, *BMJ Case Rep*, 2017. https://doi.org/10.1136/bcr-2016-218184.

Todo T, Alexander M, Stokol C, et al.: Eagle syndrome revisited: cerebrovascular complications, *Ann Vasc Surg* 26:729e1–729e5, 2012.

Yavuz H, Caylakli F, Erkan AN, et al.: Modified intraoral approach for removal of an elongated styloid process, *J Otolaryngol Head Neck Surg* 40:86–90, 2011.

Stafne Defect

Barker GR: A radiolucency of the ascending ramus of the mandible associated with invested parotid salivary gland material and analogous with a Stafne bone cavity, *Br J Oral Maxillofac Surg* 26:81–84, 1988.

Buchner A, Carpenter WM, Merrell PW, et al.: Anterior lingual mandibular salivary gland defect. Evaluation of twenty-four cases, *Oral Surg Oral Med Oral Pathol* 71:131–136, 1991.

Correll RW, Jensen JL, Rhyne RR: Lingual cortical mandibular defects: a radiographic incidence study, *Oral Surg Oral Med Oral Pathol* 50:287–291, 1980.

Hisatomi M, Munhoz L, Asaumi J, et al.: Stafne bone defects radiographic features in panoramic radiographs: assessment of 91 cases, *Med Oral Patol Oral Cir Bucal* 24:e12–e19, 2019.

Lee KC, Yoon AJ, Philipone EM, et al.: Stafne bone defect involving the ascending ramus, *J Craniofac Surg* 30:e301–e303, 2019.

Nishimura S, Osawa K, Tanaka T, et al.: Multiple mandibular static bone depressions attached to the three major salivary glands, *Oral Radiol* 34:277–280, 2018.

Shimizu M, Osa N, Okamura K, et al.: CT analysis of the Stafne's bone defects of the mandible, *Dentomaxillofac Radiol* 35:95–102, 2006.

Sisman Y, Miloglu O, Sekerci AE, et al.: Radiographic evaluation on prevalence of Stafne bone defect: a study from two centres in Turkey, *Dentomaxillofac Radiol* 41:152–158, 2012.

Stafne EC: Bone cavities situated near the angle of the mandible, *J Am Dent Assoc* 29:1969–1972, 1942.

Turkoglu K, Orhan K: Stafne bone cavity in the anterior mandible, *J Craniofac Surg* 21:1769–1775, 2010.

Palatal Cysts of the Newborn

Cataldo E, Berkman MD: Cysts of the oral mucosa in newborns, *Am J Dis Child* 116:44–48, 1968.

Fromm A: Epstein's pearls, Bohn's nodules and inclusion-cysts of the oral cavity, *J Dent Child* 34:275–287, 1967.

George D, Bhat SS, Hegde SK: Oral findings in newborn children in and around Mangalore, Karnataka State, India, *Med Princ Pract* 17:385–389, 2008.

Jorgenson RJ, Shapiro SD, Salinas CF, et al.: Intraoral findings and anomalies in neonates, *Pediatrics* 69:577–582, 1982.

Paula JDR, Dezan CC, Frossard WTG, et al.: Oral and facial inclusion cysts in newborns, *J Clin Pediatr Dent* 31:127–129, 2006.

Perez-Aguirre B, Soto-Barreras U, Loyola-Rodriguez JP, et al.: Oral findings and its association with prenatal and perinatal factors in newborns, *Korean J Pediatr* 61:279–284, 2006.

Nasolabial Cyst

Allard RHB: Nasolabial cyst: review of the literature and report of 7 cases, *Int J Oral Surg* 11:351–359, 1982.

Chen C-N, Su C-Y, Lin H-C, et al.: Microdebrider-assisted endoscopic marsupialization for the nasolabial cyst: comparisons
between sublabial and transnasal approaches, *Am J Rhinol Allergy*
23:232–236, 2009.

Choi JH, Cho JH, Kang HJ, et al.: Nasolabial cyst: a retrospective analysis of 18 cases, *Ear Nose Throat J* 81:94–96, 2002.

Sheikh AB, Chin OY, Fang CH, et al.: Nasolabial cysts: a systematic
review of 311 cases, *Laryngoscope* 126:60–66, 2016.

Su C-Y, Chien C-Y, Hwang C-F: A new transnasal approach to endoscopic marsupialization of the nasolabial cyst, *Laryngoscope*
109:1116–1118, 1999.

Vasconcelos RF, Souza PE, Mesquita RA: Retrospective analysis of
15 cases of nasolabial cyst, *Quintessence Int* 30:629–632, 1999.

"Globulomaxillary Cyst"

Christ TF: The globulomaxillary cyst: an embryologic misconception,
Oral Surg Oral Med Oral Pathol 30:515–526, 1970.

Ferenczy K: The relationship of globulomaxillary cysts to the fusion of
embryonal processes and to cleft palates, *Oral Surg Oral Med Oral
Pathol* 11:1388–1393, 1958.

Vedtofte P, Holmstrup P: Inflammatory paradental cysts in the globulomaxillary region, *J Oral Pathol Med* 18:125–127, 1989.

Wysocki GP: The differential diagnosis of globulomaxillary radiolucencies, *Oral Surg Oral Med Oral Pathol* 51:281–286, 1981.

Wysocki GP, Goldblatt LI: The so-called "globulomaxillary cyst" is
extinct, *Oral Surg Oral Med Oral Pathol* 76:185–186, 1993.

Nasopalatine Duct Cyst

Anneroth G, Hall G, Stuge U: Nasopalatine duct cyst, *Int J Oral Maxillofac Surg* 15:572–580, 1986.

Barros CCDS, Santos HBP, Cavalcante IL, et al.: Clinical and histopathological features of nasopalatine duct cyst: a 47-year retrospective study and review of current concepts, *J Craniomaxillofac Surg*
46:264–268, 2018.

Brown FH, Houston GD, Lubow RM, et al.: Cyst of the incisive (palatine) papilla: report of a case, *J Periodontol* 58:274–275, 1987.

Chapple IL, Ord RA: Patent nasopalatine ducts: four case presentations and review of the literature, *Oral Surg Oral Med Oral Pathol*
69:554–558, 1990.

Suter VGA, Sendi P, Reichart PA, et al.: The nasopalatine duct cyst: an
analysis of the relation between clinical symptoms, cyst dimensions,
and involvement of neighboring anatomical structures using
cone beam computed tomography, *J Oral Maxillofac Surg* 69:
2595–2603, 2011.

Swanson KS, Kaugars GE, Gunsolley JC: Nasopalatine duct cyst: an
analysis of 334 cases, *J Oral Maxillofac Surg* 49:268–271, 1991.

Takagi R, Ohashi Y, Suzuki M: Squamous cell carcinoma in the maxilla probably originating from a nasopalatine duct cyst: report of
case, *J Oral Maxillofac Surg* 54:112–115, 1996.

Median Palatal Cyst

Donnelly JC, Koudelka BM, Hartwell GR: Median palatal cyst,
J Endod 12:546–549, 1986.

Gingell JC, Levy BA, DePaola LG: Median palatine cyst, *J Oral Maxillofac Surg* 43:47–51, 1985.

Manzon S, Graffeo M, Philbert R: Median palatal cyst: case report and
review of the literature, *J Oral Maxillofac Surg* 67:926–930, 2009.

Rangaswamy S, Singh M, Yumnum R: True median palatal cyst; a rare
case report, *J Oral Maxillofac Pathol* 22:286, 2018. https://doi.org/
10.4103/jomfp.JOMFP_199_17.

"Median Mandibular Cyst"

Gardner DG: An evaluation of reported cases of median mandibular
cysts, *Oral Surg Oral Med Oral Pathol* 65:208–213, 1988.

Soskolne WA, Shteyer A: Median mandibular cyst, *Oral Surg Oral Med
Oral Pathol* 44:84–88, 1977.

White DK, Lucas RM, Miller AS: Median mandibular cyst: review of
the literature and report of two cases, *J Oral Surg* 33:372–375,
1975.

Epidermoid Cyst

Berk DR, Bayliss SJ: Milia: a review and classification, *J Am Acad Dermatol* 59:1050–1063, 2008.

Golden BA, Zide MF: Cutaneous cysts of the head and neck, *J Oral
Maxillofac Surg* 63:1613–1619, 2005.

Hoang VT, Trinh CT, Nguyen CH, et al.: Overview of epidermoid
cyst, *Eur J Radiol Open* 6:291–301, 2019.

Hörer S, Marrakchi S, Radner FPW, et al.: A monoallelic two-hit
mechanism in PLCD1 explains the genetic pathogenesis of
hereditary trichilemmal cyst formation, *J Invest Dermatol* 139:
2154–2163, 2019.

McGavran MH, Binnington B: Keratinous cysts of the skin, *Arch Dermatol* 94:499–508, 1966.

Rajayogeswaran V, Eveson JW: Epidermoid cyst of the buccal mucosa,
Oral Surg Oral Med Oral Pathol 67:181–184, 1989.

Veenstra JJ, Choudhry S, Krajenta RJ, et al.: Squamous cell carcinoma
originating from cutaneous cysts: the Henry Ford experience and
review of the literature, *J Dermatolog Treat* 27:95–98, 2016.

Dermoid Cyst

Crivelini MM, Soubhia AM, Biazolla ÉR, et al.: Heterotopic gastrointestinal cyst partially lined with dermoid cyst epithelium, *Oral Surg
Oral Med Oral Pathol Oral Radiol Endod* 91:686–688, 2001.

Edwards PC, Lustrin L, Valderrama E: Dermoid cysts of the tongue:
report of five cases and review of the literature, *Pediatr Dev Pathol*
6:531–535, 2003.

Kim JP, Lee DK, Moon JH, et al.: Transoral dermoid cyst excision: a
multicenter prospective observational study, *Otolaryngol Head Neck
Surg* 159:981–986, 2018.

MacNeil SD, Moxham JP: Review of floor of mouth dysontogenic
cysts, *Ann Otol Rhinol Laryngol* 119:165–173, 2010.

Meyer I: Dermoid cysts (dermoids) of the floor of the mouth, *Oral Surg
Oral Med Oral Pathol* 8:1149–1164, 1955.

Said-Al-Naief N, Fantasia JE, Sciubba JJ, et al.: Heterotopic oral gastrointestinal cyst. report of 2 cases and review of the literature, *Oral
Surg Oral Med Oral Pathol Oral Radiol Endod* 88:80–86, 1999.

Şimşek-Kaya G, Özbudak IH, Kader D: Coexisting sublingual dermoid cyst and heterotopic gastrointestinal cyst: case report,
J Clin Exp Dent 10:e196–e199, 2018.

Teszler CB, El-Naaj IA, Emodi O, et al.: Dermoid cysts of the lateral
floor of the mouth: a comprehensive anatomo-surgical classification of cysts of the oral floor, *J Oral Maxillofac Surg* 65:327–332,
2007.

Thyroglossal Duct Cyst

Allard RHB: The thyroglossal cyst, *Head Neck Surg* 5:134–146, 1982.

Brousseau VJ, Solares CA, Xu M, et al.: Thyroglossal duct cysts: presentation and management in children versus adults, *Int J Pediatr
Otorhinolaryngol* 67:1285–1290, 2003.

Forest V-I, Murali R, Clark JR: Thyroglossal duct cyst carcinoma: case
series, *J Otolaryngol Head Neck Surg* 40:151–156, 2011.

Gioacchini FM, Alicandri-Ciufelli M, Kaleci S, et al.: Clinical presentation and treatment outcomes of thyroglossal duct cysts: a systematic review, *Int J Oral Maxillofac Surg* 44:119–126, 2015.

Mondin V, Ferlito A, Muzzi E, et al.: Thyroglossal duct cyst: personal
experience and literature review, *Auris Nasus Larynx* 35:11–25,
2008.

Rayess HM, Monk I, Svider PF, et al.: Thyroglossal duct cyst carcinoma: a systematic review of clinical features and outcomes, *Otolaryngol Head Neck Surg* 156:794–802, 2017.

Rohof D, Honings J, Theunisse HJ, et al.: Recurrences after thyroglossal duct cyst surgery: results in 207 consecutive cases and review of the literature, *Head Neck* 37:1699–1704, 2015.

Thompson LDR, Herrera HB, Lau SK: A clinicopathologic series of 685 thyroglossal duct remnant cysts, *Head Neck Pathol* 10:465–474, 2016.

Branchial Cleft Cyst

Adams A, Mankad K, Offiah C, et al.: Branchial cleft anomalies: a pictorial review of embryological development and spectrum of imaging findings, *Insights Imaging* 7:69–76, 2016.

Bajaj Y, Ifeacho S, Tweedie D, et al.: Branchial anomalies in children, *Int J Pediatr Otorhinolaryngol* 75:1020–1023, 2011.

Bhaskar SN, Bernier JL: Histogenesis of branchial cysts: a report of 468 cases, *Am J Pathol* 35:407–423, 1959.

Goldenberg D, Sciubba J, Koch WM: Cystic metastasis from head and neck squamous cell cancer: a distinct disease variant? *Head Neck* 28:633–638, 2006.

LaRiviere CA, Waldhausen JHT: Congenital cervical cysts, sinuses, and fistulae in pediatric surgery, *Surg Clin N Am* 92:583–597, 2012.

Muller S, Aiken A, Magliocca K, et al.: Second branchial cleft cyst, *Head Neck Pathol* 9:379–383, 2015.

Prosser JD, Myer CM 3rd: Branchial cleft anomalies and thymic cysts, *Otolaryngol Clin North Am* 48:1–14, 2015.

Thompson LD, Heffner DK: The clinical importance of cystic squamous cell carcinomas in the neck: a study of 136 cases, *Cancer* 82:944–956, 1998.

Oral Lymphoepithelial Cyst

Buchner A, Hansen LS: Lymphoepithelial cysts of the oral cavity, *Oral Surg Oral Med Oral Pathol* 50:441–449, 1980.

Chaudhry AP, Yamane GM, Scharlock SE, et al.: A clinicopathological study of intraoral lymphoepithelial cysts, *J Oral Med* 39:79–84, 1984.

Sykara M, Ntovas P, Kalogirou E-M, et al.: Oral lymphoepithelial cyst: a clinicopathological study of 26 cases and review of the literature, *J Clin Exp Dent* 9:e1035–e1043, 2017.

Yang X, Ow A, Zhang C-P, et al.: Clinical analysis of 120 cases of intraoral lymphoepithelial cyst, *Oral Surg Oral Med Oral Pathol Oral Radiol* 113:448–452, 2012.

Hemihyperplasia

Ballock RT, Wiesner GL, Myers MT, et al.: Hemihypertrophy. Concepts and controversies, *J Bone Joint Surg* 79:1731–1738, 1997.

Dalal AB, Phadke SR, Pradhan M, et al.: Hemihyperplasia syndromes, *Indian J Pediatr* 73:609–615, 2006.

Elliott M, Bayly R, Cole T, et al.: Clinical features and natural history of Beckwith-Wiedemann syndrome: presentation of 74 new cases, *Clin Genet* 46:168–174, 1994.

Hennekam RCM, Krantz ID, Allanson JE: Chapter 21. Hemihyperplasia, In *Gorlin's syndromes of the head and neck*, ed 5, New York, 2010, Oxford University Press, pp 477–480.

Hoyme HE, Seaver LH, Jones KL, et al.: Isolated hemihyperplasia (hemihypertrophy): report of a prospective multicenter study of the incidence of neoplasia and review, *Am J Med Genet* 79:274–278, 1998.

Vaiman M, Shilco P, Roitblat Y, et al.: Hemihyperplasia/hemihypertrophy in adolescents: prospective international study, *Int J Adolesc Med Health*, 2019. https://doi.org/10.1515/ijamh-2018-0066 (Epub ahead of print).

Yamada T, Sugiyama G, Higashimoto K, et al.: Beckwith-Wiedemann syndrome with asymmetric mosaic of paternal disomy causing hemihyperplasia, *Oral Surg Oral Med Oral Pathol Oral Radiol* 127:e84–e88, 2019.

Progressive Hemifacial Atrophy

El-Kehdy J, Abbas O, Rubeiz N: A review of Parry-Romberg syndrome, *J Am Acad Dermatol* 67:769–784, 2012.

Foster TD: The effects of hemifacial atrophy on dental growth, *Br Dent J* 146:148–150, 1979.

Orozco-Covarrubias L, Guzmán-Meza A, Ridaura-Sanz C, et al.: Scleroderma "en coup de sabre" and progressive facial hemiatrophy: is it possible to differentiate them? *J Eur Acad Dermatol Venereol* 16:361–366, 2002.

Schultz KP, Dong E, Truong TA, et al.: Parry Romberg syndrome, *Clin Plast Surg* 46:231–237, 2019.

Sommer A, Gambichler T, Bacharach-Buhles M, et al.: Clinical and serological characteristics of progressive facial hemiatrophy: a case series of 12 patients, *J Am Acad Dermatol* 54:227–233, 2006.

Tolkachjov SN, Patel NG, Tollefson MM: Progressive facial hemiatrophy: a review, *Orphanet J Rare Dis* 10:39, 2015. https://doi.org/10.1186/s13023-015-0250-9.

Wójcicki P, Zachara M: Surgical treatment of patients with Parry-Romberg syndrome, *Ann Plast Surg* 66:267–272, 2011.

Wong M, Phillips CD, Hagiwara M, et al.: Parry Romberg syndrome: 7 cases and literature review, *AJNR Am J Neuroradiol* 36:1355–1361, 2015.

Segmental Odontomaxillary Dysplasia

Armstrong C, Napier SS, Boyd RC, et al.: Histopathology of the teeth in segmental odontomaxillary dysplasia: new findings, *J Oral Pathol Med* 33:246–248, 2004.

Danforth RA, Melrose RJ, Abrams AM, et al.: Segmental odontomaxillary dysplasia. Report of eight cases and comparison with hemimaxillofacial dysplasia, *Oral Surg Oral Med Oral Pathol* 70:81–85, 1990.

Jones AC, Ford MJ: Simultaneous occurrence of segmental odontomaxillary dysplasia and Becker's nevus, *J Oral Maxillofac Surg* 57:1251–1254, 1999.

Miles DA, Lovas JL, Cohen MM Jr: Hemimaxillofacial dysplasia: a newly recognized disorder of facial asymmetry, hypertrichosis of the facial skin, unilateral enlargement of the maxilla, and hypoplastic teeth in two patients, *Oral Surg Oral Med Oral Pathol* 64:445–448, 1987.

Packota GV, Pharoah MJ, Petrikowski CG: Radiographic features of segmental odontomaxillary dysplasia. A study of 12 cases, *Oral Surg Oral Med Oral Pathol Oral Radiol Endod* 82:577–584, 1996.

Smith MH, Cohen DM, Katz J, et al.: Segmental odontomaxillary dysplasia. An underrecognized entity, *J Am Dent Assoc* 149:153–162, 2018.

Whitt JC, Rokos JW, Dunlap CL, et al.: Segmental odontomaxillary dysplasia: report of a series of 5 cases with long-term follow-up, *Oral Surg Oral Med Oral Pathol Oral Radiol Endod* 112:e29–e47, 2011.

Crouzon Syndrome

Helman SN, Badhey A, Kadakia S, et al.: Revisiting Crouzon syndrome: reviewing the background and management of a multifaceted disease, *Oral Maxillofac Surg* 18:373–379, 2014.

Hennekam RCM, Krantz ID, Allanson JE: Crouzon syndrome (craniofacial dysostosis), In *Gorlin's syndromes of the head and neck*, ed 5, New York, 2010, Oxford University Press, pp 736–738.

Kreiborg S: Crouzon syndrome, *Scand J Plast Reconstr Surg Suppl* 18:1–198, 1981.

Sawh-Martinez R, Steinbacher DM: Syndromic craniosynostosis, *Clin Plast Surg* 46:141–155, 2019.

Stavropoulos D, Bartzela T, Tarnow P, et al.: Dental agenesis patterns in Crouzon syndrome, *Swed Dent J* 35:195–201, 2011.

Wang JC, Nagy L, Demke JC: Syndromic craniosynostosis, *Facial Plast Surg Clin N Am* 24:531–543, 2016.

Apert Syndrome

Allam KA, Wan DC, Khwanngern K, et al.: Treatment of Apert syndrome: a long-term follow-up study, *Plast Reconstr Surg* 127:1601–1611, 2011.

Cohen MM Jr, Kreiborg S: A clinical study of the craniofacial features in Apert syndrome, *Int J Oral Maxillofac Surg* 25:45–53, 1996.

Hennekam RCM, Krantz ID, Allanson JE: Apert syndrome (acrocephalosyndactyly), In *Gorlin's syndromes of the head and neck*, ed 5, New York, 2010, Oxford University Press, pp 732–736.

Ibrahimi OA, Chiu ES, McCarthy JG, et al.: Understanding the molecular basis of Apert syndrome, *Plast Reconstr Surg* 115:264–270, 2005.

López-Estudillo AS, Rosales-Bérber MÁ, Ruiz-Rodriguez S, et al.: Dental approach for Apert syndrome in children: a systematic review, *Med Oral Patol Oral Cir Bucal* 22:e660–e668, 2017.

Stavropoulos D, Bartzela T, Bronkhorst E, et al.: Dental agenesis patterns of permanent teeth in Apert syndrome, *Eur J Oral Sci* 119:198–203, 2011.

Wenger TL, Hing AV, Evans KN: Apert syndrome, In Adam MP, Ardinger HH, Pagon RA, et al., editors: *GeneReviews® [Internet]*, Seattle (WA), 1993, University of Washington, Seattle, pp 2020–2019 May 30.

Mandibulofacial Dysostosis

Aljerian A, Gilardino MS: Treacher Collins syndrome, *Clin Plast Surg* 46:197–205, 2019.

Hennekam RCM, Krantz ID, Allanson JE: Mandibulofacial dysostosis (Treacher Collins syndrome, Franceschetti-Zwahlen-Klein syndrome), In *Gorlin's syndromes of the head and neck*, ed 5, New York, 2010, Oxford University Press, pp 889–892.

Katsanis SH, Jabs EW: Treacher Collins syndrome, In Adam MP, Ardinger HH, Pagon RA, et al., editors: *GeneReviews® [Internet]*, Seattle (WA), 2004, University of Washington, pp 1993–2020. Jul 20 [updated 2018 Sep 27].

Posnick JC, Ruiz RL: Treacher Collins syndrome: current evaluation, treatment, and future directions, *Cleft Palate Craniofac J* 37:434, 2000.

Thompson JT, Anderson PJ, David DJ: Treacher Collins syndrome: protocol management from birth to maturity, *J Craniofac Surg* 20:2028–2035, 2009.

Trainor PA, Dixon J, Dixon MJ: Treacher Collins syndrome: etiology, pathogenesis and prevention, *Eur J Hum Genet* 17:275–283, 2009.

2

Abnormalities of Teeth

Abnormalities of the teeth can be divided into those that are influenced by environmental forces and those that are idiopathic and appear hereditary in nature. Environmental alterations are discussed first, and later parts of this chapter delineate the idiopathic and hereditary alterations of teeth.

ENAMEL DEVELOPMENT

The enamel develops in three major stages: (1) **matrix formation,** (2) **mineralization,** and (3) **maturation.** During matrix formation that also is known as the *secretory phase*, the enamel proteins are laid down. In the next stage that is termed the *transition phase*, minerals are deposited and the majority of the original proteins are removed. During the final maturation period, the enamel undergoes final mineralization and the remnants of the original proteins are removed. In the early stage of mineralization, the enamel is dull, white, and relatively soft. During the late stage of maturation, the final hard translucent enamel replaces this diffuse opaque enamel.

Dental enamel is unique in that remodeling or repair does not occur after initial formation. Therefore, abnormalities in enamel formation are etched permanently on the tooth surface and the timing of the ameloblastic damage has a great effect on the location and appearance of the defect in the enamel. Deciduous enamel contains a neonatal ring, and the rate of enamel apposition is estimated to be 0.023 mm/day. Using this knowledge, the clinician can estimate accurately the timing of an insult to the deciduous teeth to within 1 week. In the permanent dentition, the position of the enamel defects provides a rough estimate of the time of damage; however, available data on the chronology of tooth development are derived from a relatively small sample size, and the ranges of normal values are wide. In addition, gender and racial variations are not established thoroughly.

Both systemic and local factors can result in enamel defects (Box 2.1), and many different local and systemic stimuli may result in defects that have similar clinical appearances. When multiple factors are active simultaneously, the severity of the enamel defects is worse. The ameloblasts in the developing tooth germ are extremely sensitive to external stimuli; environmental effects on enamel and other tooth structures are discussed in the following section. In addition, hereditary enamel defects may occur—either as an isolated finding (see **amelogenesis imperfecta** on page 98) or as part of a heritable syndrome.

ENVIRONMENTAL ALTERATIONS OF TEETH

Box 2.2 lists the major categories of tooth alteration that can be affected by environmental influences. In many cases, the cause and effect are obvious; in others, the primary nature of the problem is less distinct.

◆ **ENVIRONMENTAL EFFECTS ON TOOTH STRUCTURE DEVELOPMENT**

ENAMEL HYPOPLASIA, DIFFUSE OPACITIES, AND DEMARCATED OPACITIES

Clinical and Radiographic Features

Almost all visible environmental enamel defects can be classified into one of three patterns:
1. Hypoplasia
2. Diffuse opacities
3. Demarcated opacities

Subtle enamel defects can be masked by saliva, plaque, or poor illumination. When attempting to detect areas of altered enamel, the dentition should be cleaned thoroughly and dried with gauze. Dental operatory lights are an ideal light source (direct sunlight should be avoided). Plaque-disclosing solution can be used to highlight small defects. The altered enamel may be localized or present on numerous teeth, and all or part of the surfaces of each affected tooth may be involved. **Enamel hypoplasia** is a quantitative defect and occurs in the form of pits, grooves, or larger areas of missing enamel. **Enamel opacities** are a qualitative defect that may be diffuse or demarcated and appear as variations in the translucency of the enamel. The affected enamel is of normal thickness. **Diffuse opacities** often are associated with fluorosis (see page 57), and the affected teeth demonstrate an increased white opacity with no clear boundary with the adjacent normal enamel. In contrast, **demarcated opacities**

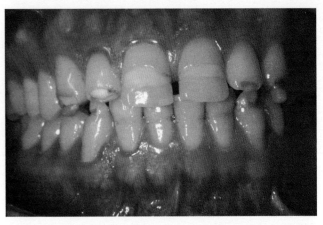

• **Fig. 2.1 Environmental Enamel Hypoplasia.** Bilaterally symmetrical pattern of horizontal enamel hypoplasia of the anterior dentition. Maxillary central incisors have been restored previously. (From Neville BW, Damm DD, White DK: *Color atlas of clinical oral pathology,* ed. 2, Hamilton, 1999, BC Decker.)

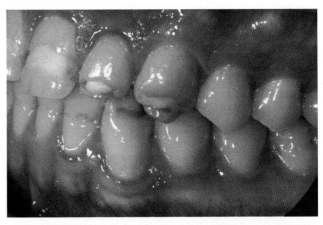

• **Fig. 2.2 Environmental Enamel Hypoplasia.** Same patient as depicted in Fig. 2.1. Note the lack of enamel damage on bicuspids. (From Neville BW, Damm DD, White DK: *Color atlas of clinical oral pathology,* ed. 2, Hamilton, 1999, BC Decker.)

exhibit a sharp boundary with the adjacent enamel. These opacities may be white, cream, yellow, or brown. Yellow or brown examples typically are more porous than white opacities and are associated more strongly with posteruptive loss of enamel.

The site of coronal damage correlates with the area of ameloblastic activity at the time of the injury; the affected enamel is restricted to the areas in which secretory activity or active maturation of the enamel matrix was occurring. The crowns of the deciduous dentition begin to develop at approximately the fourteenth week of gestation and continue until the child is 12 months of age. Development of the crowns of the permanent dentition occurs from approximately 6 months to 15 years of age.

Environmental enamel abnormalities are extremely common with a wide range of reported prevalence. In one review of more than 1500 children from 12 to 15 years of age in an industrialized nation, the prevalence of enamel defects in the permanent dentition was 68.4%. Within this group, 67.2% demonstrated opacities, 14.6% revealed hypoplasia, and both patterns were seen in 13.4% of the children. The average number of affected teeth per individual was 3.6, with greater than 10% of the children having 10 or more teeth involved.

A common pattern is seen as a result of systemic influences, such as exanthematous fevers, that occur during the first 2 years of life. Horizontal rows of pits or diminished enamel are present on the anterior teeth and first molars (Figs. 2.1 and 2.2). The enamel loss is bilaterally symmetric, and the location of the defects correlates well with the

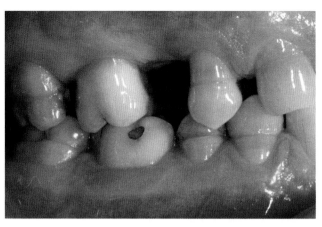

• **Fig. 2.3 Environmental Enamel Hypoplasia.** Horizontal enamel hypoplasia of the bicuspids and second molars. Note sparing of the first molars. (From Neville BW, Damm DD, White DK: *Color atlas of clinical oral pathology,* ed. 2, Hamilton, 1999, BC Decker.)

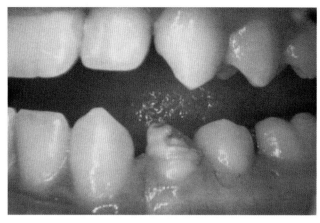

• **Fig. 2.4 Turner Hypoplasia.** Extensive enamel hypoplasia of mandibular first bicuspid secondary to previous inflammatory process associated with overlying first deciduous molar. (From Halstead CL, Blozis GG, Drinnan AJ, et al: *Physical evaluation of the dental patient,* St Louis, 1982, Mosby.)

developmental stage of the affected teeth. A similar pattern of enamel defects can be seen in the cuspids, bicuspids, and second molars when the inciting event occurs around the age of 4–5 years (Fig. 2.3).

In patients without fluorosis, demarcated opacities may demonstrate increased surface porosity and caries susceptibility. One study reported more than twice prevalence of decay in patients with localized enamel hypoplasia or hypomineralization compared to those without such defects. The areas prone to caries demonstrated full-thickness enamel defects.

Aesthetically or functionally defective teeth can be restored through a variety of cosmetically pleasing techniques, such as the following:
- Acid-etched composite resin restorations
- Labial veneers
- Full crowns

Turner Hypoplasia

Another pattern of enamel defects seen in permanent teeth is caused by traumatic injury or periapical inflammatory disease of the overlying deciduous tooth. The altered tooth is called a **Turner tooth** (after the clinician whose publications allowed this problem to be widely recognized). The appearance of the affected area varies according to the timing and severity of the insult. The enamel defects vary from focal areas of white, yellow, or brown discoloration to extensive hypoplasia, which can involve the entire crown.

When the process occurs secondary to periapical inflammatory disease, the permanent bicuspids are affected most frequently because of their relationship to the overlying deciduous molars (Figs. 2.4 and 2.5). Anterior teeth are involved less often because crown formation usually is complete before the development of any apical inflammatory disease in the relatively caries-resistant anterior deciduous dentition. Factors that determine the degree of damage to the permanent tooth by the overlying infection include the stage of tooth development, length of time the infection

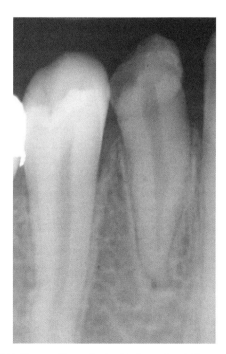

• **Fig. 2.5 Turner Hypoplasia.** Radiograph of the same tooth depicted in Fig. 2.4. Note the lack of significant enamel and irregularity of the dentin surface. (From Halstead CL, Blozis GG, Drinnan AJ, et al: *Physical evaluation of the dental patient,* St Louis, 1982, Mosby.)

remains untreated, the virulence of the infective organisms, and the host resistance to the infection.

In addition to classic Turner teeth, an increased prevalence of demarcated opacities has been reported in the permanent successors of carious primary teeth. In one report, if the primary tooth developed caries, the successor was twice as likely to demonstrate a circumscribed enamel defect. In addition, if the primary tooth was extracted for any reason other than trauma, then the prevalence of a demarcated enamel defect increased fivefold.

Formation of Turner teeth secondary to traumatic injury of deciduous teeth is not uncommon because up to 45% of all children sustain injuries to their primary teeth. In a prospective study of 114 children with 255 traumatized primary teeth, 23% of the corresponding permanent teeth demonstrated developmental disturbances. The maxillary central incisors are affected in the majority of the cases; the maxillary lateral incisors are altered less frequently (Fig. 2.6). In several large reviews, the prevalence of involvement of the posterior teeth or mandibular incisors was less than 10% of all cases.

The frequency of traumatic damage to the anterior maxillary dentition is not surprising, considering the common occurrence of trauma to the deciduous dentition of the prominent anterior maxilla and the close anatomic relationship between the developing tooth bud and the apices of the overlying primary incisors. As would be expected, the clinical appearance of the alteration varies according to the timing and severity of the damage. Avulsion and intrusive luxation are the types of trauma most strongly associated with formation of Turner teeth.

Because of the position of the primary apices relative to the tooth bud, the facial surface of the maxillary incisors is the location most frequently affected. Typically, the affected area appears as a zone of white or yellowish-brown discoloration with or without an area of horizontal enamel hypoplasia. The trauma also can cause displacement of the already formed hard-tooth substance in relation to the soft tissue of the remaining developing tooth. This results in a bend of the tooth known as **dilaceration** and can affect either the crown or the root of a tooth (see page 94). Dilaceration of the crown occurs most frequently between 1.5 and 3.5 years of age, whereas dilaceration of the root usually is seen in association with trauma that occurs between 4 and 5 years of age. Severe trauma early in the development of the tooth can result in such disorganization of the bud that the resultant product may resemble a complex odontoma (see page 729). Similar levels of damage late in the formative process can lead to partial or total arrest in root formation.

Molar-Incisor Hypomineralization

Molar-incisor hypomineralization (MIH) is a condition that presents with demarcated qualitative enamel defects involving one or more first permanent molars with or without involvement of incisors. The clinical pattern is asymmetrical and can involve one or more teeth with varying severity within the same patient. Although not described until the 1970s and not widely recognized in the United States beyond pediatric dentists, the disorder has proven to be very common; a study of 337 children in Indiana demonstrated a prevalence of 13%, a finding in agreement with a meta-analysis revealing an almost identical global prevalence of 13.1%.

The etiology of MIH remains unclear. Due to the timing of enamel maturation, involvement of the deciduous teeth most likely arises from prenatal or perinatal disorders such as maternal illness, medications used during pregnancy, prematurity, or birth complications; in contrast, involvement limited to the permanent teeth appears more strongly associated with early childhood illnesses, particularly those with fever, asthma, or pneumonia.

Patients affected with MIH have enamel defects of one or more first permanent molars, which demonstrate normal surface contour unless posteruptive enamel breakdown is present. The altered enamel may be white, yellow, or brown, with a sharp demarcation between the defective and surrounding normal enamel (Fig. 2.7). Yellow or brown opacities appear to be more porous and often are associated with posteruptive enamel loss. On a microscopic level, the enamel is the demarcated opacities has larger interprismatic spaces that provide bacterial access to the underlying dentin, frequently resulting in chronic inflammation of the adjacent pulp. Affected teeth with or without posteruptive enamel loss often are highly sensitive, leading to avoidance of proper oral hygiene with rapid caries development. During attempts at dental therapy, these teeth often are very difficult to anesthetize. There appears to be a spectrum of the disease in which only the molars may be affected or the incisors also may be

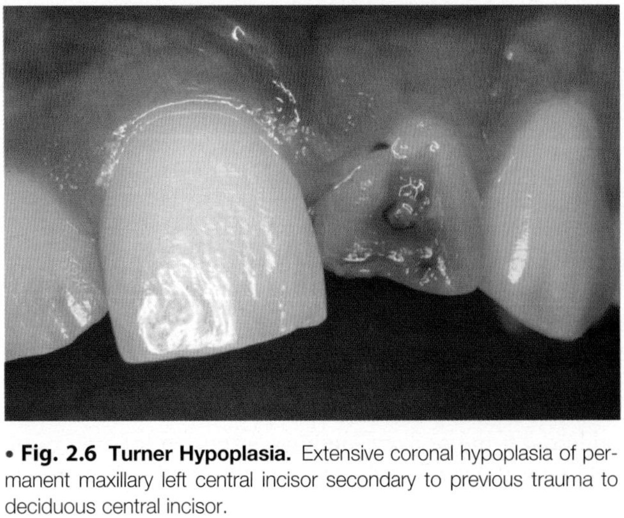

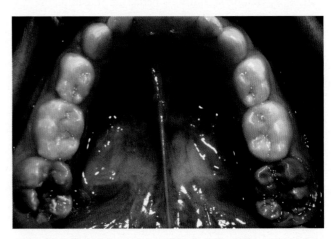

• **Fig. 2.6 Turner Hypoplasia.** Extensive coronal hypoplasia of permanent maxillary left central incisor secondary to previous trauma to deciduous central incisor.

• **Fig. 2.7 Molar-incisor hypomineralization (MIH).** First permanent mandibular molars demonstrating brown hypomaturation with areas of coronal breakdown.

involved. Affected incisors usually demonstrate only white opacities that primarily create aesthetic problems.

Similar alterations in primary cuspids and second molars have been termed *hypomineralized primary canines* (HPC) and *hypomineralized second primary molars* (HSPM). These alterations demonstrate a strong association with MIH in the permanent dentition. This association is not surprising because enamel maturation of the primary canines and second molars demonstrates significant overlap with enamel formation of the first permanent molar.

In a systematic review of **molar-incisor hypomineralizaion**, 27.4% of patients needed intervention due to pain, hypersensitivity, posteruptive breakdown, or caries. Casein phosphopeptide-amorphous calcium phosphate (CPP-ACP) can be used in mild cases to remineralize enamel and reduce sensitivity. Therapy for more advanced cases include adhesive restorations or sealants, preformed metal crowns followed by permanent indirect full crowns, or extraction often combined with orthodontic space closure. Amalgams are not ideal due to the atypically shaped cavities noted in MIH. Adhesive restorations also can be problematic due to cohesive failure related to poor quality enamel.

Molar Root-Incisor Malformation (Molar-Incisor Malformation)

Molar root-incisor malformation (MRIM) shares a number of features with **molar-incisor hypomineralization** (see previous section). Although the pathogenesis of both processes is uncertain, they are thought to be related to environmental stress early in life. In addition, the mandibular first molars and incisors are the predominant sites of involvement in both disorders.

All cases of MRIM appear sporadic with no family history of similar dental problems and almost all patients have a history of serious systemic health problems at birth or within the first 2 years of life. Although the health issues vary widely, a significant number represent central nervous system–related diseases such as meningitis, spina bifida, hydrocephalus, and seizures. Despite this, the timing of the health problems and the defining dental malformation often do not match. The primary alteration involves the roots of the first molars, which do not develop until approximately 3 years of age. Investigators speculate the environmental stressors damage or disorganize Hertwig's epithelial root sheath, leading to an abnormal function at a later date. The possibility of a genetic predisposition also has been suggested, but without any confirming evidence.

The defining feature of MRIM is the presence of short, narrow, spiked roots on all first molars with relatively normal overlying crowns (Figs. 2.8 and 2.9). The pulp chambers exhibit a reduced coronal-to-apical height with an ectopic mineralized plate between the chamber and the root canals. The malformed teeth often develop pain, mobility, and abscess formation without associated dental caries or trauma. This loss of vitality is thought to be secondary to the malformed pulp chamber or an abnormal periodontal attachment that allows formation of a combined periodontal-periapical inflammatory lesion. Similar involvement of the

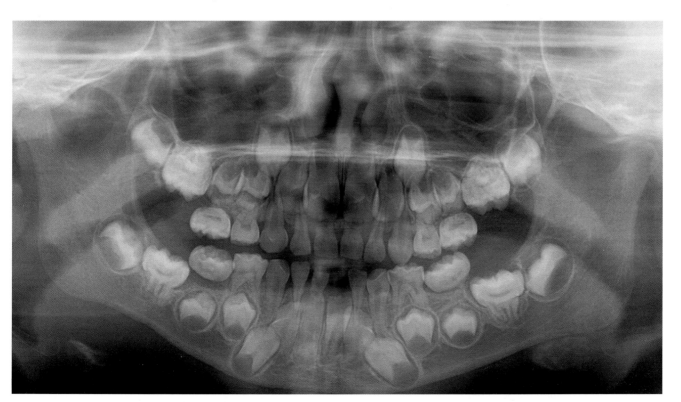

• **Fig. 2.8 Molar root-incisor malformation (MRIM).** Dentition exhibiting malformed roots on all permanent first molars with mineralized plates on the floor of the pulp chambers. Note involvement of the deciduous second molars and shallow dens invaginatus of the permanent maxillary central incisors. (Courtesy of Dr. Jeff Hall).

deciduous second molars may be seen, with rare involvement of the deciduous first molars. In about half of affected patients, one of more incisors will demonstrate marked constriction in the crown with a notch in the cervical third of the enamel. Shallow dens invaginatus (see page 88) also is seen frequently (Fig. 2.8).

In patients with **MRIM**, the anterior teeth should be inspected closely clinically and radiographically upon eruption to allow any teeth with dens invaginatus to be restored or sealed as soon as possible. Due to the high frequency of associated abscess, affected permanent first molars usually are extracted. Endodontic therapy is difficult due to the abnormal pulpal anatomy and the mineralized bridge present on the floor of the pulp. Following extraction, the healthy second and third molars may be guided into the edentulous first molar space as they develop. Alternatively, a space maintainer can be placed until the patient reaches an age that would allow successful implant placement.

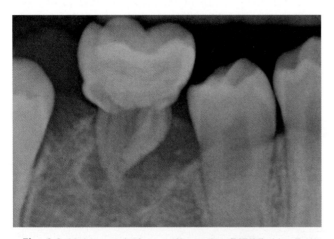

• **Fig. 2.9 Molar root-incisor malformation (MRIM).** Mandibular first molar exhibiting short spiky roots. (Courtesy of Dr. Michael Myers).

Hypoplasia Caused by Antineoplastic Therapy

As modern medicine improves the prognosis of childhood cancer, it has become evident that a number of developmental alterations arise secondary to use of therapeutic radiation or chemotherapy. It has been reported that greater than 90% of childhood cancer survivors will demonstrate at least one oral complication. As would be expected, developing teeth often are affected, with these antineoplastic therapies producing clinically obvious alterations most commonly in patients younger than 12 years and most extensively in those younger than 5 years. The degree and severity of the developmental alterations are related to the patient's age at treatment, the form of therapy, and the dose and field of radiation, if used.

Although both chemotherapeutic agents and radiation therapy can be responsible for developmental abnormalities, the most severe alterations are associated with radiation. A dose of 30 Gray (Gy) stops tooth development, and dental malformations are noted in patients with doses as low as 4 Gy. As the dose escalates, so does the effect on the developing dentition and jaws. Frequently observed alterations include hypodontia, microdontia, V-shaped hypoplastic roots, and enamel hypoplasia (Fig. 2.10). Tooth agenesis and microdontia are more common in patients exposed prior to 3 years of age, whereas radicular hypoplasia is more prevalent in older children. In addition, mandibular hypoplasia and a reduction of the vertical development of the lower third of the face are not rare. The mandibular hypoplasia may be caused by one or more of the following: direct effect of therapeutic radiation, reduced alveolar bone growth secondary to impaired root development, or growth failure due to pituitary hypofunction caused by therapeutic radiation involving the cranium. Chemotherapy can produce similar but less severe dental alterations including tooth agenesis, microdontia, root hypoplasia, and enamel hypoplasia.

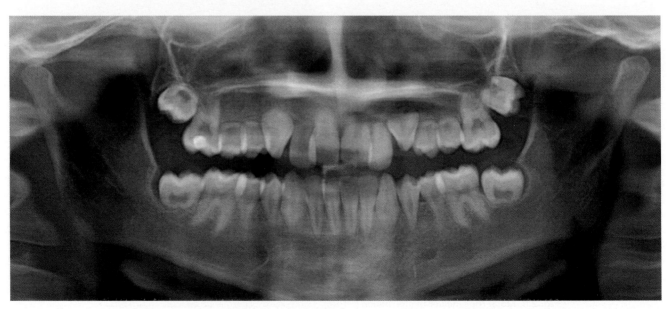

• **Fig. 2.10 Hypoplasia Caused by Antineoplastic Therapy.** Multiple teeth demonstrating radicular hypoplasia secondary to radiation and chemotherapy for cancer. (Courtesy of Dr. Bret Johnson.)

Dental Fluorosis

The ingestion of excess amounts of fluoride also can result in significant enamel defects known as **dental fluorosis.** Fluoride appears to create enamel defects through retention of the amelogenin proteins in the enamel structure. This leads to the formation of hypomineralized enamel that alters light reflection and creates the appearance of white, chalky areas. Most of the problems associated with dental fluorosis are aesthetic, particularly when the anterior teeth are affected.

The severity of dental fluorosis is dose dependent, with greater ingestion of fluoride during critical periods of tooth development causing more severe fluorosis. Interestingly, individuals who consume similar levels of fluoride may demonstrate varying degrees of dental fluorosis, suggesting a genetic influence. The affected teeth are caries resistant, and the altered tooth structure appears as areas of lusterless white and opaque enamel that may have zones of yellow to dark-brown discoloration (Figs. 2.11 and 2.12). In the past, areas of moderate-to-severe enamel fluorosis were termed **mottled enamel.** True enamel hypoplasia is

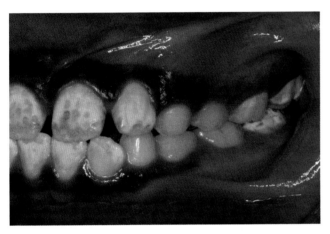

• **Fig. 2.11 Dental Fluorosis.** Dentition exhibiting lusterless, white, and opaque enamel with areas of chipping. Notice that the deciduous teeth are spared.

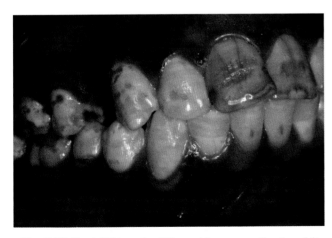

• **Fig. 2.12 Dental Fluorosis.** Diffuse white opaque alteration of the dentition with areas of brown enamel mottling. Patient spent his childhood in Kenya.

uncommon but can occur as deep, irregular, and brownish pits. Because other factors can result in a similar pattern of enamel damage, a definitive diagnosis requires that the defects be present in a bilaterally symmetric distribution, plus evidence of prior excessive fluoride intake or elevated levels of fluoride in the enamel or other tissues should be found.

Initially, fluoride's ability to reduce caries was thought to be secondary to its incorporation into developing enamel, resulting in a stronger and more acid-resistant fluorapatite crystal. Most investigators now agree that the posteruptive effects of fluoride are predominant and control caries by altering the demineralization and remineralization process that occurs at the tooth/bacterial biofilm interface. Nevertheless, fluoridated water remains an important topical source of application. Even though fluoride is present in numerous dental products, foods, and beverages, studies have shown that cessation of water fluoridation has been associated with an approximately 18% increase in dental caries. Consumption of optimally fluoridated water has been associated with a low frequency of altered enamel, which usually is mild in degree. However, an increased prevalence of dental fluorosis has been noted in recent years. The US Centers for Disease Control and Prevention reported that from 1986 to 1987, 22.6% of adolescents demonstrated some degree of fluorosis, whereas a similar group from 1999 to 2004 revealed a prevalence of 40.7%. Water fluoridation typically aims for a concentration between 0.7 and 1.2 ppm. In warm climates, the recommended concentration is 0.7 ppm due to higher consumption of water, whereas regions with more temperate climates use a concentration of 1 ppm. In 2011, the US Department of Health and Human Services recommended a nationwide standardized level of 0.7 ppm of fluoride.

The crowns of the maxillary central incisors are the most cosmetically important and their development is completed by age 3. Therefore, close monitoring of all sources of fluoride intake during the first 3 years of life is recommended strongly. Fluoride ingestion occurs primarily through four sources: drinking water, fluoride toothpaste, fluoride supplements, and infant formula. It has been reported that ingestion of fluoride dentifrices is responsible for approximately two-thirds of cases of fluorosis in the United States. A significant reduction in dental fluorosis can be seen if brushing with fluoride toothpaste does not start until after 12 months of age. Once initiated, close parental supervision with use of a rice-sized amount of toothpaste is recommended for children under 3 years of age, whereas a pea-sized amount is appropriate for children 3–6 years of age. In addition, reconstitution of infant formula with fluoridated water should be avoided. Because of the dissemination of fluoride through the food supply, the need for supplements in nonfluoridated areas is declining in many industrialized countries. Fluoride supplements are recommended only in nonfluoridated areas for children who are at high risk for rampant caries.

Although teeth affected by fluorosis have been treated with external bleaching, microabrasion, dental veneers or crowns, enamel infiltration with a low-viscosity light-cured resin has proven to be a successful approach to mask the altered enamel. Mild fluoride-associated opacities often fade over time, possibly due to surface tooth wear associated with daily activities.

Syphilitic Hypoplasia

Congenital syphilis (see page 181) results in a pattern of enamel hypoplasia that is well known but currently so rare that lengthy discussion is not warranted. Anterior teeth altered by syphilis are termed **Hutchinson incisors** and exhibit crowns that are shaped like straight-edge screwdrivers, with the greatest circumference present in the middle one-third of the crown and a constricted incisal edge. The middle portion of the incisal edge often demonstrates a central hypoplastic notch. Altered posterior teeth are termed **mulberry molars** and demonstrate constricted occlusal tables with a disorganized surface anatomy that resembles the bumpy surface of a mulberry.

◆ POSTDEVELOPMENTAL LOSS OF TOOTH STRUCTURE

Tooth structure can be lost after its formation by a variety of influences beyond the obvious cases related to caries or traumatic fractures. Destruction can begin on the enamel surface of the crown through abrasion, attrition, erosion, or abfraction. In addition, loss of tooth structure can begin on the dentin or cemental surfaces of the teeth by external or internal resorption.

TOOTH WEAR

Tooth wear, also termed *tooth surface loss,* is a normal physiologic process that occurs with aging but must be considered pathologic when the degree of destruction creates functional, aesthetic, or dental sensitivity problems. Although the four causes of tooth wear (i.e., **attrition, abrasion, erosion,** and **abfraction**), often are discussed as independent pathoses, most of these types of tooth loss are the result of a combination of influences. Many cases of attrition are accelerated by the presence of abrasive materials in the mouth. Erosion or abrasion often further damages areas of dentin exposed by attrition or abfraction. Areas softened by erosion are more susceptible to attrition, abrasion, and abfraction. The clinician should appreciate that acquired environmental loss of tooth structure often is multifactorial.

Most researchers agree that the reported prevalence of tooth wear is increasing. This is explained partly by a greater awareness among clinicians and by the adult population retaining more natural teeth as they age. In addition, younger individuals appear to exhibit an increased tooth surface loss that many believe may be caused by a more acidic diet (e.g., acidic soft drinks, diet foods, and fresh fruits). This belief is supported by the knowledge that consumption of acidic soft drinks in the United States has increased 300% over the past 20 years.

Attrition is the loss of tooth structure caused by tooth-to-tooth contact during occlusion and mastication. The term comes from the Latin verb *attritum,* which refers to the action of rubbing against another surface. Some degree of attrition is physiologic, and the process becomes more noticeable with age. When the amount of tooth loss is extensive and begins to affect aesthetic appearance and function, the process must be considered pathologic.

The following factors can accelerate tooth destruction:
- Poor-quality or absent enamel (e.g., fluorosis, environmental or hereditary enamel hypoplasia, or dentinogenesis imperfecta)
- Premature contacts (edge-to-edge occlusion)
- Intraoral abrasives, erosion, and grinding habits
- Medications or illicit drugs that induce bruxism

Abrasion is the pathologic wearing away of tooth structure or restorations secondary to the mechanical action of an external agent. The term arises from the Latin verb *abrasum,* which literally means *to scrape off* and implies wear or partial removal through a mechanical process. The most common cause of abrasion is toothbrushing that combines abrasive toothpaste with heavy pressure and a horizontal brushing stroke. Other items frequently associated with dental abrasion include pencils, toothpicks, pipe stems, and bobby pins. Chewing tobacco, cracking nuts and seeds, biting fingernails or thread, and using dental floss inappropriately also can cause clinically significant abrasion. When tooth wear is accelerated by chewing an abrasive substance between opposing teeth, the process has been termed **demastication** and exhibits features of both attrition and abrasion.

Erosion is the loss of tooth structure caused by a nonbacterial chemical process. The term is derived from the Latin verb *erosum,* which literally means *to corrode* and implies gradual destruction of a surface by a chemical or electrolytic process. Typically, exposure to an acid is to blame, but chelating agents are occasionally the primary cause. Although saliva aids remineralization and contains bicarbonate with a significant buffering ability, the bicarbonate level of saliva is directly correlated to salivary flow, with the buffering capability reduced in situations with low flow rates. Causes for salivary gland hypofunction include salivary gland aplasia, dehydration, therapeutic radiation, medications, and systemic conditions such as Sjögren syndrome, bulimia nervosa, and diabetes. The acidic source often is foods or drinks (especially acidic and carbonated soft drinks), but other causes include some medications and illicit drugs, swimming pools with poorly monitored pH, chronic involuntary regurgitation (e.g., hiatal hernia, esophagitis, chronic alcoholism, and pregnancy), voluntary regurgitation (e.g., psychologic problems, bulimia, and occupations that require low body weight), industrial environmental exposure, and occupations such as sommeliers. Erosion from dental exposure to gastric secretions is termed **perimolysis.** Because saliva has the ability to remineralize tooth surfaces exposed to acid, it appears that areas of erosive damage must have some abrasive component that removes the softened enamel before remineralization. The susceptibility to erosion varies among individuals and appears to be related to the quality of the enamel, the composition of the saliva, and the protective effect of the salivary pellicle.

Dental erosion appears associated strongly with both the frequency and duration of exposure to acidic foods and drinks. Due to the buffering abilities of saliva, acid clearance and pH stabilization typically occurs 2–13 minutes after exposure. Increased erosion is noted in individuals who ingest acidic foods in between meals or increase the exposure times by sipping drinks or slowly eating acidic fruits. Four or more daily dietary exposures to acid have been associated with a higher risk of erosive tooth wear. Use of straws positioned in the back of the mouth tend to bypass the teeth and reduce the erosive potential of acidic drinks, whereas straw placement in the labial vestibule increases the erosive effects. The erosive potential also is influenced by the calcium and phosphate concentration. Acidic foods with a significant calcium content, such as yogurt, demonstrate a low erosive potential.

Abfraction refers to the loss of tooth structure from occlusal stresses that create repeated tooth flexure with failure of enamel and dentin at a location away from the point of loading. The term is derived from the Latin words *ab* and *fractio,* which respectively translate into *away* and *breaking.* Dentin is able to withstand greater tensile stress than enamel. When occlusal forces are applied eccentrically to a tooth, the tensile stress is concentrated at the cervical fulcrum, leading to flexure that may produce disruption in the chemical bonds of the enamel crystals in the cervical areas. Once damaged, the cracked enamel can be lost or more easily removed by erosion or abrasion.

Agreement on the prevalence of abfraction does not exist. Some propose that abfraction causes most cervical tooth loss; others believe that little evidence exists to indicate that this sequence of events actually occurs in the mouth. A number of systematic reviews have found little support for occlusal forces being responsible for noncarious cervical tooth loss, bringing into question the validity of abfraction.

Clinical Features

Attrition

Attrition can occur in both the deciduous and the permanent dentitions. As would be expected, the surfaces predominantly affected are those that contact the opposing dentition. Most frequently, the incisal and occlusal surfaces are involved, in addition to the lingual of the anterior maxillary teeth and the labial of the anterior mandibular teeth. Large, flat, smooth, and shiny wear facets are found in a relationship that corresponds to the pattern of occlusion. The interproximal contact points also are affected from the vertical movement of the teeth during function. Over time, this interproximal loss can result in a shortening of the arch length. Pulp exposure and dentin sensitivity are rare because of the slow loss of tooth structure and the apposition of reparative secondary dentin within the pulp chamber (Fig. 2.13).

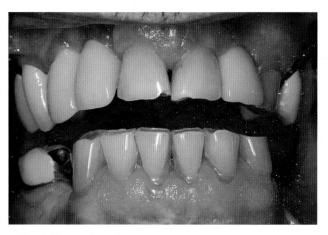

• **Fig. 2.13 Attrition.** Extensive loss of coronal tooth height without pulp exposure in patient with anterior edge-to-edge occlusion.

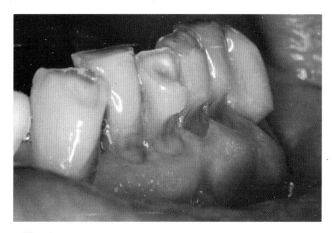

• **Fig. 2.14 Abrasion.** Horizontal cervical notches on the anterior mandibular dentition. Note visible pulp canals that have been filled with tertiary dentin.

Abrasion

Abrasion has a variety of patterns, depending on the cause. Toothbrush abrasion typically appears as horizontal cervical notches on the buccal surface of exposed radicular cementum and dentin (Fig. 2.14). The defects usually have sharply defined margins and a hard, smooth surface. If acid also is present, then the lesions are more rounded and shallower. The degree of loss is greatest on prominent teeth (i.e., cuspids, bicuspids, and teeth adjacent to edentulous areas) and occasionally is more advanced on the side of the arch opposite the dominant hand. Thread biting or the use of pipes or bobby pins usually produces rounded or V-shaped notches in the incisal edges of anterior teeth (Fig. 2.15). The inappropriate use of dental floss or toothpicks results in the loss of interproximal radicular cementum and dentin.

Erosion

In patients with **erosion,** the tooth loss does not correlate with functional wear patterns or with those typically associated with known abrasives. The predominant sites of tooth loss appear to correlate closely with those areas not protected

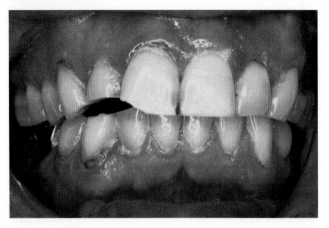

• **Fig. 2.15 Abrasion.** Notching of the anterior dentition on the right side caused by long-term use of tobacco pipe.

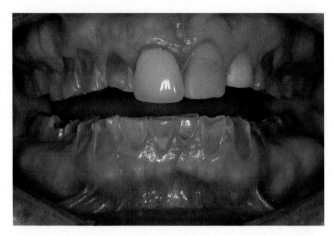

• **Fig. 2.17 Erosion.** Extensive tooth wear. Note spoon-shaped depressions in anterior teeth and depressed dentin adjacent to elevated ridges of enamel in more posterior teeth.

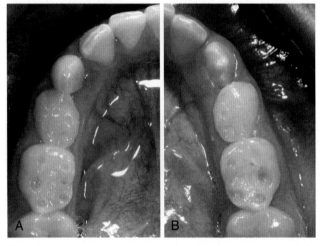

• **Fig. 2.16 Erosion.** Multiple cupped-out depressions corresponding to the cusp tips.

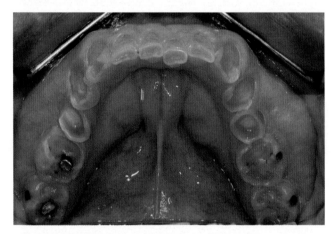

• **Fig. 2.18 Erosion.** Same patient as depicted in Fig. 2.17. Multiple mandibular teeth exhibiting depressions of dentin surrounded by elevated rims of enamel. Note the amalgam in the first molar that is raised above the surface of the surrounding depressed dentin.

by the serous secretions of the parotid and submandibular glands. The facial and palatal surfaces of the maxillary anterior teeth and the facial and occlusal surfaces of the mandibular posterior teeth are affected most frequently. Involvement of the lingual surfaces of the entire mandibular dentition is uncommon, possibly because of the protective buffering capacity of the submandibular serous saliva.

The classic pattern of dental erosion is the cupped lesion in which a central depression of dentin is surrounded by elevated enamel. Cupped areas are seen on the occlusal cusp tips, incisal edges, and marginal ridges (Fig. 2.16). In contrast to abrasion, erosion commonly affects the facial surfaces of the maxillary anteriors and appears as shallow spoon-shaped depressions in the cervical portion of the crown (Fig. 2.17). The posterior teeth frequently exhibit extensive loss of the occlusal surface, and the edges of metallic restorations subsequently may be above the level of the tooth structure (Fig. 2.18). After a portion of the cuspal enamel has been lost, the dentin is destroyed more rapidly than the remaining enamel, often resulting in a concave depression of the dentin surrounded by an elevated rim of enamel (see Fig. 2.18). The

more rapid dissolution of the dentin can lead to undermined enamel that often is lost easily by chipping. Occasionally, entire buccal cusps are lost and replaced by ski slope–like depressions that extend from the lingual cusp to the buccal cementoenamel junction (Fig. 2.19). When palatal surfaces are affected, the exposed dentin has a concave surface and shows a peripheral white line of enamel (Fig. 2.20). Active erosion typically reveals a clean, unstained surface, whereas inactive sites become stained and discolored.

Erosion limited to the facial surfaces of the maxillary anterior dentition often is associated with dietary sources of acid. When the tooth loss is confined to the incisal portions of the anterior dentition of both arches, an external environmental source is suggested. When erosion is located on the palatal surfaces of the maxillary anterior teeth and the occlusal surfaces of the posterior teeth of both dentitions, regurgitation of gastric secretions is a probable cause. The location of the tooth structure loss may suggest the cause of the damage but is not completely reliable.

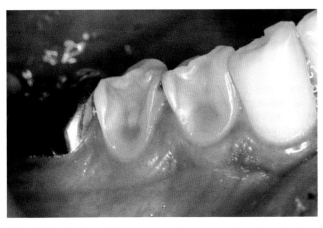

• **Fig. 2.19** **Erosion.** Extensive loss of enamel and dentin on the buccal surface of the maxillary bicuspids. The patient had sucked chronically on tamarinds (an acidic fruit).

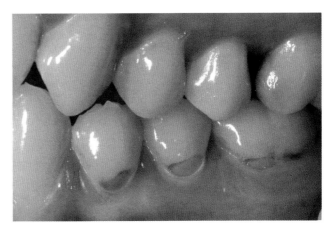

• **Fig. 2.21** **Abfraction.** Deep and narrow enamel cervical defects on the facial surface of the mandibular dentition. (From Neville BW, Damm DD, White DK: *Color atlas of clinical oral pathology,* ed 2, Hamilton, 1999, BC Decker.)

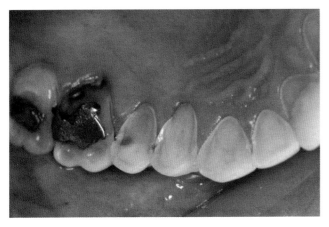

• **Fig. 2.20** **Erosion.** Palatal surfaces of the maxillary dentition in which the exposed dentin exhibits a concave surface and a peripheral white line of enamel. The patient had bulimia.

Abfraction

Abfraction appears as wedge-shaped defects limited to the cervical area of the teeth and may closely resemble cervical abrasion or erosion. Clues to the diagnosis include defects that are deep, narrow, and V-shaped (which do not allow the toothbrush to contact the base of the defect) and often affect a single tooth with adjacent unaffected teeth (Fig. 2.21). In addition, occasional lesions are subgingival, a site typically protected from abrasion and erosion. The lesions predominantly affect the facial surfaces of the bicuspids and molars.

In all forms of tooth wear, the process typically proceeds at a slow rate that allows deposition of tertiary dentin and prevents pulp exposure, even when extensive loss of tooth structure is present (see Fig. 2.14). In some cases, especially in the deciduous dentition, the tooth loss can proceed at a more accelerated rate, which results in a near or frank exposure of the pulp.

Treatment and Prognosis

Normal levels of attrition require no therapy, with intervention reserved for those cases that create a pathologic degree of tooth loss. Early diagnosis and intervention may assist in

preserving the permanent dentition. Before any definitive action, the clinician must remember that tooth wear almost invariably has a multifactorial cause. Failure to recognize the interrelationships of these pathoses can lead to inappropriate therapy and failure of any attempted repair. Intervention should emphasize detailed diagnosis, preventive measures, and long-term monitoring. Immediate therapy should be directed toward resolution of tooth sensitivity and pain, but identifying the causes of tooth structure loss and protecting the remaining dentition also are important goals.

In patients affected by dental erosion, preventive interventions should attempt not only to reduce the frequency and duration of acid exposure but also to improve the oral cavity's ability to resist the effects of acid. Upon exposure to an acid, the saliva has the ability to achieve remineralization with time, but teeth are vulnerable to abrasion before completion of this action. Although some investigators have recommended a minimum 1-hour interval between acid exposure and toothbrushing in an attempt to minimize abrasion of the weakened enamel, other studies have shown that a brushing delay is not warranted due to the inability of saliva to achieve complete remineralization. Low-abrasive toothpaste and professional guidance to prevent inappropriate, overzealous, or too frequent toothbrushing may assist in reducing associated abrasion. Consumption of buffering substances such as milk, cheese, and sugar-free antacids also is thought to be beneficial. Rinsing the mouth with water after acid exposure and proper hydration have been suggested to reduce the severity of demineralization and maintain sufficient salivary flow with appropriate buffering capability. A suspected common cause of tooth loss is decreased salivary flow secondary to dehydration, often associated with strenuous work or athletic activities and possibly complicated by use of acidic soft drinks or sports beverages in the place of water. Chewing xylitol gum has been suggested as a method for decreasing dental erosion by increasing salivary flow after acid exposure, but others have demonstrated that enamel softened by acid can be damaged by the adjacent soft tissues during the movements of chewing in this time of vulnerability. Patients should be informed of the potential for loss of tooth structure associated with the overuse of acidic foods and drinks (e.g., wine, carbonated beverages, foods pickled in acetic acid, and citrate-containing fruits, fruit juices, and candies), chronic regurgitation, and improper oral hygiene techniques. Mouth guards and occlusal adjustment can be used to slow nocturnal attrition and to protect the teeth from frequent exposure to acid from regurgitation or industrial sources. Dental sensitivity can be reduced through the use of varnishes, mouthwashes, or toothpastes containing strontium chloride, stannous fluoride, or monofluorophosphate. If initially unsuccessful, these agents can be combined with iontophoresis.

Active restorative therapy is premature in the presence of ongoing tooth wear and should be postponed until the patient expresses strong aesthetic concerns, exhibits dental sensitivity that is nonresponsive to conservative interventions, or demonstrates progressive and uncontrollable wear. Once indicated, the minimum treatment necessary to solve the problem should be implemented. In lesions thought to represent abfraction, glass ionomer materials are recommended because of their greater resilience that allows the material to flex with the tooth. In areas of abrasion, a material with optimum resistance to the abrasive process should be chosen. Replacement of lost posterior teeth and avoidance of edge-to-edge occlusion limit the effects of attrition. Lost tooth structure can be restored with composite resins, veneers, onlays, or full crowns. Restorative procedures that do not involve significant removal of remaining tooth structure are preferable in patients demonstrating extensive tooth wear.

INTERNAL AND EXTERNAL RESORPTION

In addition to loss of tooth structure that begins on the exposed coronal surfaces, destruction of teeth also can occur through resorption, which is accomplished by cells located in the dental pulp (i.e., **internal resorption**) or in the periodontal ligament (PDL) (i.e., **external resorption**). Internal resorption is a relatively rare occurrence, and most cases develop after injury to pulpal tissues, such as physical trauma or caries-related pulpitis. The resorption can continue as long as vital pulp tissue remains and may result in communication of the pulp with the PDL.

In contrast, external resorption is extremely common; with close examination, all patients are most likely to have root resorption on one or more teeth. In one radiographic review of 13,263 teeth, all patients showed evidence of root resorption, and 86.4% of the examined teeth demonstrated external resorption, with an average of 16 affected teeth per patient. Most areas of resorption are mild and of no clinical significance, but 10% of patients exhibit unusual amounts of external resorption.

The potential for resorption is inherent within the periodontal tissue of each patient, and this individual susceptibility to resorption is the most important factor in the degree of resorption that will occur after a stimulus. The factors

BOX 2.3 Factors Associated With External Resorption

- Cysts
- Dental trauma
- Excessive mechanical forces (e.g., orthodontic therapy)
- Excessive occlusal forces
- Grafting of alveolar clefts
- Hormonal imbalances
- Hyperparathyroidism
- Intracoronal bleaching of pulpless teeth
- Local involvement by herpes zoster
- Paget disease of bone
- Periodontal treatment
- Periradicular inflammation
- Pressure from impacted teeth
- Reimplantation of teeth
- Tumors

reported to increase the severity of external resorption are delineated in Box 2.3. Many cases have been termed *idiopathic* because no factor could be found to explain the accelerated resorption. Although local factors may exert a strong influence, many researchers believe genetic predisposition plays a strong role. One investigation demonstrated a 5.6-fold increase in root resorption during orthodontics in patients demonstrating homozygosity for the interleukin-1 beta (IL-1B) allele. In addition, examples of families with generalized idiopathic root resorption and monozygotic twins presenting with identical patterns of root resorption have been reported. Genetics appears to be a modifying factor that can increase the severity of external resorption when triggered by a secondary influence. When pretreatment radiographs of a given patient exhibit a degree of resorption beyond that which is normally seen, the clinician should realize the potential risks involved in initiating procedures (e.g., orthodontics) that are known to be associated with an increased risk of external resorption.

Clinical and Radiographic Features

Resorption of dentin or cementum can occur at any site that contacts vital soft tissue. **Internal resorption** usually is asymptomatic and discovered through routine radiographs. Pain may be reported if the process is associated with significant pulpal inflammation. Two main patterns are seen: (1) **inflammatory resorption** and (2) **replacement** or **metaplastic resorption** (Fig. 2.22). In inflammatory resorption, the resorbed dentin is replaced by inflamed granulation tissue. Although this pattern may involve any portion of the canal, the cervical zone is affected most frequently (and the pulpal inflammation usually is caused by bacterial invasion). The resorption continues as long as vital pulp remains; typically, the coronal pulp is necrotic with the apical portion remaining vital. The results of pulp testing are variable. In this pattern, the area of destruction usually appears as a uniform, well-circumscribed symmetric radiolucent enlargement of the

Internal resorption   External resorption

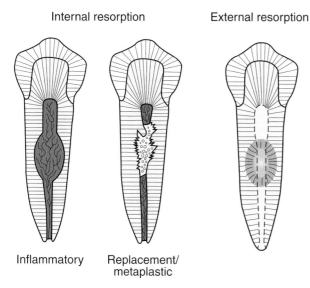

Inflammatory   Replacement/
                     metaplastic

• **Fig. 2.22 Tooth Resorption.** Illustration contrasting the common patterns of internal and external tooth resorption. Internal resorption will result in a radiolucent enlargement of the pulp chamber or canal. In external resorption, the radiolucency is superimposed on the pulp canal, which should not be enlarged.

pulp chamber or canal. When it affects the coronal pulp, the crown can display a pink discoloration (**pink tooth of Mummery**) as the vascular resorptive process approaches the surface (Fig. 2.23). When it occurs in the root, the original outline of the canal is lost and a balloon-like radiographic dilation of the canal is seen (Fig. 2.24). If the process continues, the destruction eventually can perforate the lateral root surface, which may be difficult to distinguish from external root resorption. Internal resorption secondary to infectious pulpitis may cease upon necrosis of the responsible cells within the pulp. Although many cases are progressive, some cases are self-limiting and usually arise in traumatized teeth or those that have recently undergone orthodontic or periodontal therapy.

In *replacement* or *metaplastic resorption*, portions of the pulpal dentinal walls are resorbed and replaced with bone or cementum-like bone (see Fig. 2.22). Radiographically, replacement resorption appears as an enlargement of the canal, which is filled with a material that is less radiodense than the surrounding dentin. Because a central zone of the pulp is replaced with bone, the radiographic appearance often demonstrates partial obliteration of the canal. The outline of destruction is less defined than that seen in inflammatory resorption.

External resorption demonstrates a wider variety of patterns and includes inflammatory, surface, replacement, and cervical resorption. **External inflammatory resorption** arises secondary to an inflammatory process, usually periapical inflammatory disease or periodontitis (Fig. 2.25). The affected teeth will demonstrate loss of root length, often with ragged apices. The results of vitality testing depend on the origin of the inflammatory process, and the resorption often ceases with elimination of the focus of infection.

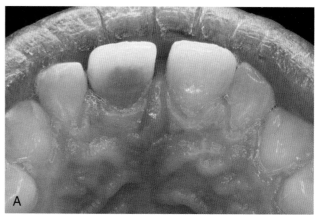

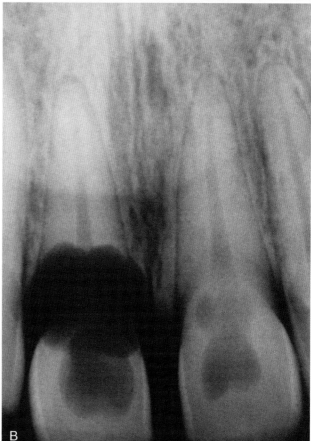

• **Fig. 2.23 Internal Resorption (Pink Tooth of Mummery).** **A,** Pink discoloration of the maxillary central incisor. **B,** Radiograph of same patient showing extensive resorption of both maxillary central incisors.

A variation of inflammatory resorption that occurs following luxation injuries is termed **transient apical breakdown** and presents with focal resorption of the root tip in association with widening of the apical periodontal ligament and loss or blurry appearance of the lamina dura encircling the apex. Vitality testing is variable and creates confusion with early periapical inflammatory disease. The resorption is followed quickly by repair, with the process resolving spontaneously within 12 months.

External surface resorption occurs secondary to pressure applied to the root surface. Orthodontic tooth movement,

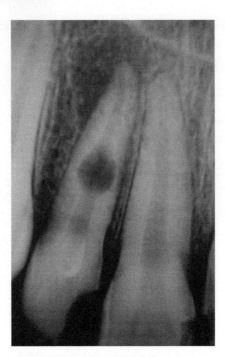

• **Fig. 2.24 Internal Resorption.** Balloonlike enlargement of the root canal.

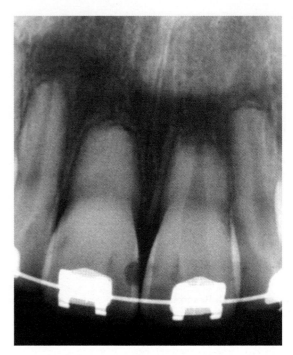

• **Fig. 2.26 External Surface Resorption.** Diffuse external resorption of radicular dentin of maxillary dentition. This process arose after initiation of orthodontics.

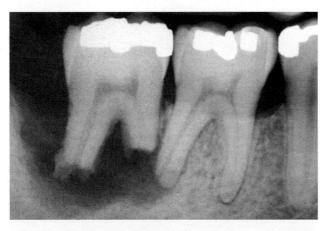

• **Fig. 2.25 External Inflammatory Resorption.** Extensive irregular destruction of both roots of the mandibular second molar associated with chronic periodontitis. (Courtesy of Dr. Tommy Shimer.)

adjacent impacted teeth, enlarging cysts, and tumors are common causes. Teeth affected by orthodontic treatment may demonstrate blunted or shortened roots (Fig. 2.26). Resorption secondary to impacted teeth, cysts, and tumors often will exhibit irregular or saucer-shaped area of tooth loss.

External resorption occurring during orthodontics appears to be influenced most strongly by the patient's individual susceptibility. However, heavy forces have been shown to induce a greater degree of resorption, and compressive forces appear more strongly related than tensile forces. The single most important local factor is the distance a tooth is moved during therapy. The maxillary anterior teeth typically are the most severely affected, particularly in patients who have been treated with premolar extractions. Movement

of teeth with an abnormal root shape (such as, dilaceration) also has been associated with an increased severity of external resorption. In patients who have demonstrated significant resorption during therapy, a 2- to 3-month treatment pause has been shown to reduce the final amount of treatment-associated external resorption.

External replacement resorption refers to osteoclastic removal of cementum and dentin with replacement by alveolar bone. This process usually occurs secondary to severe luxation or avulsion of the tooth. In reimplanted avulsed teeth, extensive external resorption of the root is extremely common without rapid and appropriate intervention (see Fig. 2.27). If the tooth remains outside of the socket without being placed in a proper storage medium, then the periodontal ligament cells undergo necrosis. Without vital periodontal ligament cells, the surrounding bone views the tooth as a foreign object and initiates resorption with replacement by bone. Affected teeth often will demonstrate ankylosis, with many surviving for years until almost the entire root is lost.

Invasive cervical resorption is an uncommon but rather troublesome pattern of external resorption that begins in the cervical cementum usually apical to the epithelial attachment (Fig. 2.28). Although the process may begin as a small perforation, the resorption often extends circumferentially into the dentin of the crown and a larger portion of the root. The destruction often will encircle the pulp chamber but typically will not invade the pulp until late in the course of tooth destruction. The pulp is surrounded by a protective resorption-resistant sheet containing a significant layer of predentin, a material that resists attachment of osteoclastic cells. As the process proceeds, portions of the granulation

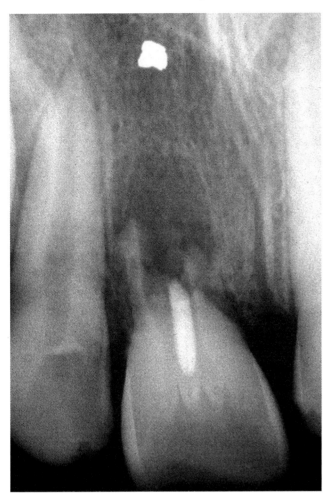

• **Fig. 2.27 External Replacement Resorption.** Complete loss of the root leaving only the metallic retrofill of the root tip. The tooth had been reimplanted after traumatic avulsion. (Courtesy of Dr. Lawrence Bean.)

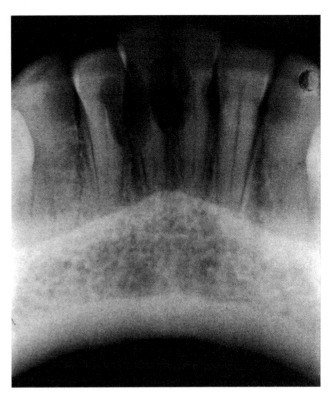

• **Fig. 2.28 Invasive Cervical Resorption.** Extensive cervical resorption of several anterior mandibular teeth. (Courtesy of Dr. Keith Lemmerman.)

tissue within the areas of resorption often are replaced by metaplastic bone. When the process involves more than three teeth, it is termed **multiple idiopathic cervical root resorption.** This condition typically exhibits an aggressive clinical course.

Although the cause of invasive cervical resorption is not known, it is believed that an initial injury leads to localized damage to the periodontal ligament with focal loss of cementum and exposure of the underlying dentin. With continued inflammation, granulation tissue forms and begins the resorptive process. As would be expected, the possible causes of the initial injury are diverse with orthodontic treatment, traumatic injury, removal of an adjacent tooth, periodontitis, malocclusion, and bruxism frequently mentioned as possible triggers. Cats develop a similar process termed *feline odonto-clastic resorptive lesions* that has been associated with a feline herpes virus. It has been suggested that some cases of invasive cervical resorption in humans may arise secondary to transmission of the feline virus from their cats, with reports of owners shown to demonstrate positive titers of neutralizing antibodies against the feline virus. Often, a combination of

factors appears to be involved in the initiation and propagation of the resorptive process. In addition to invasive cervical resorption, generalized and progressive external resorption also can affect the apical portion of the roots. Although this pattern can occur secondary to an endocrine disturbance or one of a small number of systemic conditions, many of these cases are idiopathic and difficult to arrest. On occasion, the idiopathic apical resorption demonstrates a bilaterally symmetrical pattern that suggests the possibility of occlusal interferences triggering resorption in a genetically predisposed patient (Fig. 2.29).

External resorption typically appears as a "moth-eaten" loss of tooth structure in which the radiolucency is less well defined and demonstrates variations in density. If the lesion overlies the pulp canal, then close examination demonstrates the retention of the unaltered canal through the area of the defect. Most cases involve the apical or midportions of the root. External resorption can create significant defects in the crowns of teeth before eruption (see Fig. 2.30). This pattern frequently is misdiagnosed as preeruptive caries and is thought by some investigators to be caused by defects in the enamel epithelium that allow connective tissue to come into direct contact with the enamel.

If difficulty arises in distinguishing external from internal resorption, then the mesial-buccal-distal rule can be used through two radiographic exposures. Although use of plain film techniques remains valid, the diagnostic accuracy of

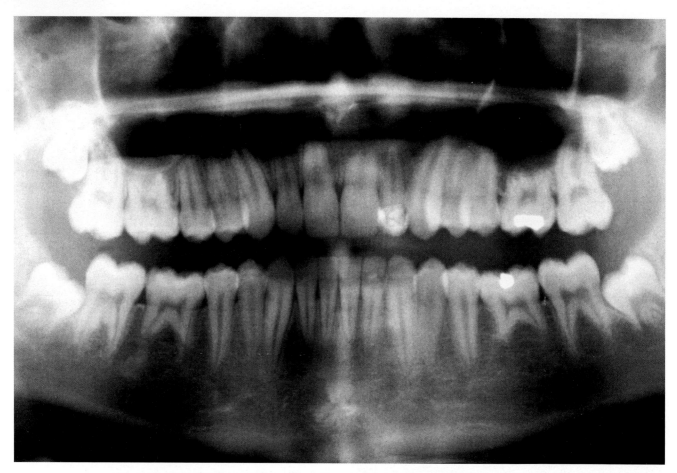

• **Fig. 2.29 Idiopathic External Resorption.** First molars in all four quadrants demonstrate extensive radicular external resorption.

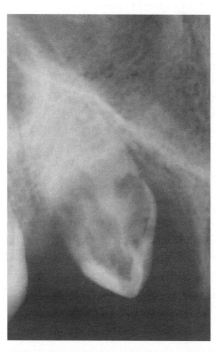

• **Fig. 2.30 External Resorption.** Extensive external resorption of the crown of the impacted right maxillary cuspid. Histopathologic examination revealed resorption without bacterial contamination or caries.

cone beam computed tomography (CBCT) has been shown to be superior and should be considered the standard of care for evaluation of the nature and extent of significant internal and external resorption.

Histopathologic Features

In patients with internal inflammatory resorption, the pulp tissue in the area of destruction is vascular and exhibits increased cellularity and collagenization. Immediately adjacent to the dentinal wall are numerous multinucleated dentinoclasts, which are histologically and functionally identical to osteoclasts (Fig. 2.31). An inflammatory infiltrate characterized by lymphocytes, histiocytes, and polymorphonuclear leukocytes is not uncommon. In replacement resorption, the normal pulp tissue is replaced by woven bone that fuses with the adjacent dentin. External resorption is similar in appearance, with numerous multinucleated dentinoclasts located in the areas of structure loss. Areas of resorption often are repaired through deposition of osteodentin. In large defects, external inflammatory resorption results in deposition of inflamed granulation tissue, and areas of replacement with woven bone may also be seen. Extensive bony replacement in areas of external resorption can lead to ankylosis.

Treatment and Prognosis

The treatment of internal and external resorption centers on the removal of all soft tissue from the sites of dental destruction. Internal resorption can be stopped consistently if endodontic therapy successfully removes all vital pulp tissue before the process perforates into the PDL. Once perforation occurs, therapy becomes more difficult, and the prognosis is poor. In such cases, initial placement of calcium hydroxide paste occasionally may result in remineralization of the site of perforation and stop the resorptive process. If remineralization of cervical sites of perforation is not successful, then surgical exposure and restoration of the defect may halt the process. Extraction often is necessary for radicular perforations that do not respond to therapy.

The first step in treating external resorption is the identification and elimination of any accelerating factor. Apically located sites cannot be approached without significant damage created by attempts at access. Because the cells responsible for the resorption are located within the PDL, endodontic therapy is not effective in stopping the process.

Treatment of invasive cervical resorption is difficult and varies according to the extent and location of the resorptive defects. Therapies include external repair with or without endodontics, internal repair with root canal therapy, repair with intentional reimplantation, periodic review without intervention, and extraction. In contrast to the isolated variant, therapy of multiple idiopathic cervical root resorption is unsatisfactory with the vast majority of reported cases demonstrating repeated recurrences of the resorptive process with ultimate loss of the affected teeth.

For avulsed teeth, the best way to prevent resorption is to maintain PDL vitality by immediate reimplantation or short-term use of a physiologic storage solution. Teeth reimplanted with an open apex should be monitored monthly; for teeth with a closed apex, endodontic therapy is necessary. Avulsed teeth with an open apex and nonvital PDL cells should not be implanted.

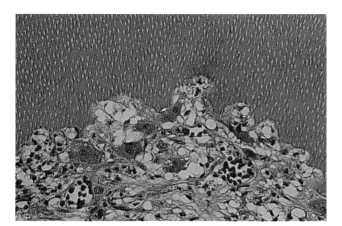

• Fig. 2.31 Internal Resorption. Resorption of the inner dentinal wall of the pulp. Note cellular and vascular fibrous connective tissue, which exhibits an adjacent inflammatory infiltrate and numerous dentinoclasts within resorptive lacunae.

◆ ENVIRONMENTAL DISCOLORATION OF TEETH

The color of normal teeth varies and depends on the shade, translucency, and thickness of the enamel. In primary teeth, the normal color is bluish white, whereas permanent teeth tend to be grayish white or yellowish white. With aging, the enamel thins and the dentin thickens, leading to teeth that are more yellow or grayish yellow. Abnormal colorations may be **extrinsic** or **intrinsic.** Extrinsic stains occur from surface accumulation of an exogenous pigment and typically can be removed with a surface treatment, whereas intrinsic discolorations arise from an endogenous material that is incorporated into the enamel or dentin and cannot be removed by prophylaxis with toothpaste or pumice. Box 2.4 lists the most frequently documented causes of tooth discolorations.

Dental fluorosis is discussed in the section on environmental effects on the structural development of the teeth (see page 57). The alterations associated with **amelogenesis imperfecta** (see page 98) and **dentinogenesis imperfecta (DGI)** (see page 104) are presented later in this chapter in the text devoted to primary developmental alterations of the teeth.

Clinical Features
Extrinsic Stains

Bacterial stains are a common cause of surface staining of exposed enamel, dentin, and cementum. Chromogenic bacteria can produce colorations that vary from green or black-brown to orange. The discoloration occurs most frequently in children and usually is seen initially on the labial surface of the maxillary anterior teeth in the gingival one-third. In contrast to most plaque-related discolorations, the black-brown stains most likely are not primarily of bacterial origin

---

• BOX 2.4   Tooth Discolorations

Extrinsic
- Bacterial stains
- Iron
- Tobacco
- Foods and beverages
- Gingival hemorrhage
- Restorative materials
- Medications

Intrinsic
- Amelogenesis imperfecta (AI)
- Dentinogenesis imperfecta (DGI)
- Dental fluorosis
- Erythropoietic porphyria
- Hyperbilirubinemia
- Ochronosis
- Trauma
- Localized red blood cell breakdown
- Medications

but are secondary to the formation of ferric sulfide from an interaction between bacterial hydrogen sulfide and iron in the saliva or gingival crevicular fluid.

Extensive use of **tobacco** products, betel quid, **tea,** or **coffee** often results in significant brown discoloration of the surface enamel (Fig. 2.32). The tar within the tobacco dissolves in the saliva and easily penetrates the pits and fissures of the enamel. Smokers (of tobacco or marijuana) most frequently exhibit involvement of the lingual surface of the mandibular incisors; users of smokeless tobacco often demonstrate involvement of the enamel in the area of tobacco placement. Stains from beverages also often involve the lingual surface of the anterior teeth, but the stains are usually more widespread and less intense. In addition, foods that contain abundant chlorophyll can produce a green discoloration of the enamel surface.

The green discoloration associated with chromogenic bacteria or the frequent consumption of chlorophyll-containing foods can resemble the pattern of green staining seen secondary to **gingival hemorrhage.** As would be expected, this pattern of discoloration occurs most frequently in patients with poor oral hygiene and erythematous, hemorrhagic, and enlarged gingiva. The color results from the breakdown of hemoglobin into green biliverdin.

A large number of **medications** may result in surface staining of the teeth. In the past, use of products containing high amounts of iron or iodine was associated with significant black pigmentation of the teeth. Exposure to sulfides, silver nitrate, or manganese can cause stains that vary from gray to yellow to brown to black. Copper, nickel, or ciprofloxacin may produce a green stain; cadmium, essential oils, doxycycline, linezolid, glibenclamide, and amoxicillin-clavulanic acid may be associated with a yellow to brown discoloration.

More recently, the most frequently reported culprits include **stannous fluoride** and **chlorhexidine.** Fluoride staining may be associated with the use of 8% stannous fluoride and is thought to be secondary to the combination of the stannous (tin) ion with bacterial sulfides. This black stain occurs predominantly in people with poor oral hygiene in areas of a tooth previously affected by early carious involvement. The labial surfaces of anterior teeth and the occlusal surfaces of posterior teeth are the most frequently affected. Chlorhexidine is associated with a yellow-brown stain that predominantly involves the interproximal surfaces near the gingival margins. The degree of staining varies with the concentration of the medication and the patient's susceptibility. Although an increased frequency has been associated with the use of tannin-containing beverages, such as tea and wine, effective brushing and flossing or frequent gum chewing can minimize staining. Chlorhexidine is not alone in its association with tooth staining; many oral antiseptics, such as Listerine and sanguinarine, also may produce similar changes.

Silver diamine fluoride has become a popular therapy for arresting and preventing caries in young children with childhood caries, especially for individuals with problems that interfere with routine dental care. Application of silver diamine fluoride is inexpensive and easy to apply, but it is associated with noticeable black discoloration. Although parents often will tolerate the discoloration on posterior teeth, the altered aesthetics limit its use on anterior teeth.

Intrinsic Stains

Congenital erythropoietic porphyria (Günther disease) is an autosomal recessive disorder of porphyrin metabolism that results in the increased synthesis and excretion of porphyrins and their related precursors. Significant diffuse discoloration of the dentition is noted as a result of the deposition of porphyrin in the teeth (Fig. 2.33). Affected teeth demonstrate a marked red-brown coloration that exhibits a red fluorescence when exposed to a Wood's ultraviolet (UV) light. The deciduous teeth demonstrate a more intense coloration because porphyrin is present in the enamel and the dentin; in the permanent teeth, only the dentin is affected. The discoloration is most intense along the cervical margin and decreases in intensity toward the occlusal surface. Excess porphyrins also are present in the urine, which typically is reddish-brown with a similar fluorescence when exposed to a Wood's light. Affected patients

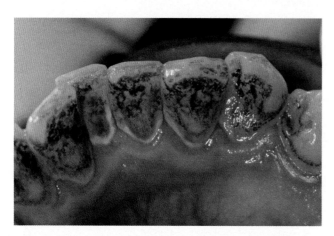

• **Fig. 2.32 Tobacco Discoloration.** Extrinsic brown stains of the enamel on the lingual surfaces of the anterior mandibular dentition secondary to long-term tobacco abuse.

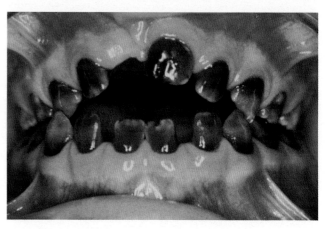

• **Fig. 2.33 Erythropoietic Porphyria–Related Discoloration.** Red-brown discoloration of the maxillary dentition.

also will demonstrate areas of cutaneous hyper- and hypo-pigmentation with bullae and vesicles on sun-exposed skin.

Another autosomal recessive metabolic disorder, **alkaptonuria,** is associated with a blue-black discoloration termed *ochronosis* that occurs in connective tissue, tendons, and cartilage. On rare occasions, a blue discoloration of the dentition may be seen in patients who also are affected with Parkinson disease.

Bilirubin is a breakdown product of red blood cells, and excess levels can be released into the blood in a number of conditions. The increased amount of bilirubin can accumulate in the interstitial fluid, mucosa, serosa, and skin, resulting in a yellow-green discoloration known as **jaundice** (see page 823). During periods of **hyperbilirubinemia,** developing teeth also may accumulate the pigment and become stained intrinsically. In most cases, the deciduous teeth are affected as a result of hyperbilirubinemia during the neonatal period. The two most common causes are **erythroblastosis fetalis** and **biliary atresia.** Other diseases that less frequently display intrinsic staining of this type include the following:

- Premature birth
- ABO incompatibility
- Neonatal respiratory distress
- Significant internal hemorrhage
- Congenital hypothyroidism
- Cholestasis
- Biliary hypoplasia
- Metabolic diseases (tyrosinemia, α1-antitrypsin deficiency)
- Neonatal hepatitis

The extent of the dental changes correlates with the period of hyperbilirubinemia, and most patients exhibit involvement limited to the primary dentition. Occasionally, the cusps of the permanent first molars may be affected. In addition to enamel hypoplasia, the affected teeth frequently demonstrate a green discoloration (**chlorodontia**). The color is the result of the deposition of biliverdin (the breakdown product of bilirubin that causes jaundice). Although the teeth often are dark green initially, the discoloration typically fades and becomes a less intense yellow-green or grayish (Fig. 2.34). The color of tooth structure formed after the resolution of the hyperbilirubinemia appears normal. The teeth often demonstrate a sharp dividing line, separating green portions (formed during hyperbilirubinemia) from normal-colored portions (formed after normal levels of bilirubin were restored).

Coronal discoloration is a frequent finding after **trauma,** especially in the deciduous dentition. Posttraumatic injuries may create pink, yellow, or dark-gray discoloration. Temporary pink discoloration that arises 1–3 weeks after trauma may represent localized vascular damage and often returns to normal in 1–3 weeks. In these instances, periapical radiographs are warranted to rule out internal resorption that may produce a similar clinical presentation. A yellow discoloration is indicative of pulpal obliteration, termed **calcific metamorphosis,** and is discussed more fully in Chapter 3 (see page 120). Occasionally, during a postmortem

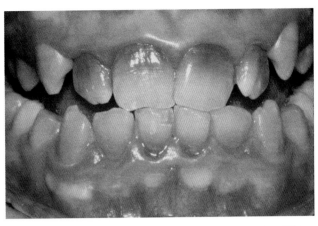

• **Fig. 2.34 Hyperbilirubinemia-Related Discoloration.** Diffuse grayish-blue discoloration of the dentition. Cervical portions are stained most intensely. (Courtesy of Dr. John Giunta.)

examination, a pink discoloration of teeth is found. The crowns and necks of the teeth are affected most frequently, and the process is thought to arise from hemoglobin breakdown within the necrotic pulp tissue in patients in whom blood has accumulated in the head.

A similar pink or red discoloration of the maxillary incisors has been reported in living patients with **lepromatous leprosy** (see page 188). Although controversial, some investigators believe these teeth are involved selectively because of the decreased temperature preferred by the causative organism. This process is thought to be secondary to infection-related necrosis and the rupture of numerous small blood vessels within the pulp, with a secondary release of hemoglobin into the adjacent dentinal tubules.

Dental **restorative materials,** especially amalgam, can result in black-gray discolorations of teeth. This most frequently arises in younger patients who presumably have more open dentinal tubules. Large Class II proximal restorations of posterior teeth can produce discoloration of the overlying facial surface. In addition, deep lingual metallic restorations on anterior incisors can significantly stain underlying dentin and produce visible grayish discoloration on the labial surface. To help reduce the possibility of discoloration, the clinician should not restore endodontically treated anterior teeth with amalgam (Fig. 2.35).

Regenerative endodontic therapy refers to treatment of permanent teeth with necrotic pulps and open apices, which are filled with a variety of materials to promote continued root maturation and apical closure. Discoloration of the treated tooth is a common complication that appears to be affected by the choice of filling materials. Significant discoloration has been noted with use of mineral trioxide aggregate or triple antibiotic paste containing minocycline, whereas calcium hydroxide or double antibiotic paste with metronidazole and ciprofloxacin has proven to be less problematic.

Several different **medications** can become incorporated into the developing tooth and result in clinically evident discoloration. The severity of the alterations is dependent on the time of administration, the dose, and the duration of the

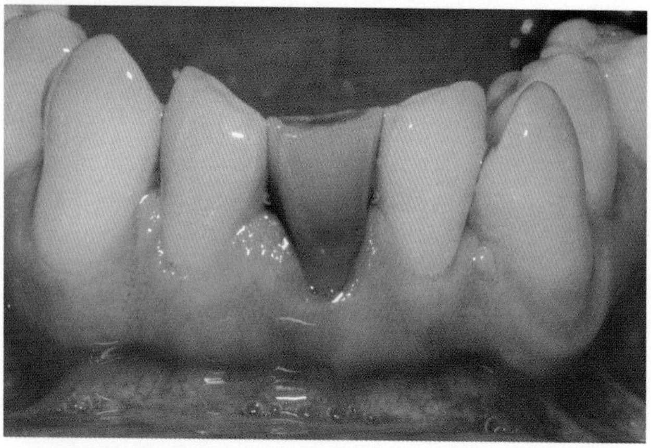

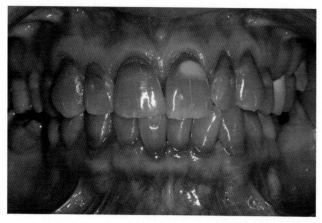

• **Fig. 2.35 Amalgam Discoloration.** Green-gray discoloration of mandibular central incisor, which had endodontic access preparation restored with amalgam.

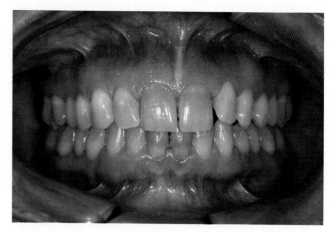

• **Fig. 2.37 Minocycline-Related Discoloration.** Dentition demonstrating grayish discoloration predominantly noted on the incisal half of the teeth. Note the horizontal bands of bluish alteration of the maxillary and mandibular alveolar ridges. (Courtesy of Dr. Roger Miller.)

• **Fig. 2.36 Tetracycline-Related Discoloration.** Diffuse brownish discoloration of the permanent dentition.

drug's use. The most infamous is **tetracycline,** with the affected teeth varying from bright yellow to dark brown and, in UV light, showing a bright yellow fluorescence (Fig. 2.36). After chronic exposure to ambient light, the fluorescent yellow discoloration fades over months to years into a nonfluorescent brown discoloration. Often the facial surfaces of the anterior teeth will darken while the posterior dentition and lingual surfaces remain a fluorescent yellow. The drug and its homologues can cross the placental barrier; therefore, administration should, if possible, be avoided during pregnancy and in children up to 8 years of age. All homologues of tetracycline are associated with discoloration and include chlortetracycline (gray-brown discoloration) and demethyl-chlortetracycline and oxytetracycline (yellow).

One semisynthetic derivative of tetracycline, **minocycline hydrochloride,** has been shown to produce significant discoloration of the dentition and also may affect teeth that are fully developed. Minocycline is a widely used medication for the treatment of acne and also is prescribed occasionally to treat rheumatoid arthritis. Its prevalence of use is increasing (and, presumably, so will the number of patients affected with discolored teeth and bone).

Although the mechanism is unknown, minocycline appears to bind preferentially to certain types of collagenous tissues (e.g., dental pulp, dentin, bone, and dermis). Once in these tissues, oxidation occurs and may produce the distinctive discoloration. Some investigators believe supplementation with ascorbic acid (an antioxidant) can block formation of the discoloration. No matter the cause, once the pulp tissues are stained, the coloration can be seen through the overlying translucent dentin and enamel. The staining is not universal; only 3%–6% of long-term users become affected. In those affected, the period of time before discoloration becomes evident can range from just 1 month to several years.

In susceptible individuals, minocycline creates discoloration in the skin, oral mucosa (see page 307), nails, sclera, conjunctiva, thyroid, bone, and teeth. Coloration of the bone occasionally results in a distinctive blue-gray appearance of the palate, mandibular tori, or anterior alveolar mucosa, which represents the black bone showing through the thin, translucent oral mucosa (Fig. 2.37). Several patterns of staining are noted in the dentition. Fully erupted teeth typically reveal a blue-gray discoloration of the incisal three-fourths, with the middle one-third being maximally involved (see Fig. 2.37). The exposed roots of erupted teeth demonstrate a dark-green discoloration, although the roots of developing teeth are stained dark black.

Another antibiotic, ciprofloxacin, is given intravenously to infants for *Klebsiella* spp. infections. Although less notable than tetracycline, this medication also has been associated with intrinsic tooth staining—usually a greenish discoloration.

Treatment and Prognosis

Careful polishing with fine pumice can remove most extrinsic stains on the teeth; typically, normal prophylaxis paste is insufficient. Stubborn stains often are resolved by mixing 3% hydrogen peroxide with the pumice or by using bicarbonate spray solutions. The use of jet prophylactic devices with a mild abrasive is the most effective. Recurrence of the stains is not uncommon unless the cause is reduced or eliminated. Improving the level of oral hygiene often minimizes the chance of recurrence.

Intrinsic discoloration is much more difficult to resolve because of the frequent extensive involvement of the dentin. Suggested aesthetic remedies include external bleaching of vital teeth, internal bleaching of nonvital teeth, bonded restorations, composite buildups, laminate veneer crowns, and full crowns. The treatment must be individualized to fulfill the unique needs of each patient and his or her specific pattern of discoloration.

◆ LOCALIZED DISTURBANCES IN ERUPTION

DELAYED ERUPTION

Eruption is the movement of a tooth from its position of development within the bone to its functional location in the mouth. After the tooth is in full occlusion, slight eruption continues in order to compensate for normal attrition and continued vertical growth of the face. Although delayed eruption is not a rare problem, few well-written reviews have been published on the subject.

Emergence is the moment of eruption when the first part of the cusp or crown is visible through the gingiva. This process normally occurs when the dental root is approximately two-thirds its final length. Emergence occurs over a broad chronologic age range and differs according to a number of influences, such as racial and gender variations. Eruption is considered delayed if emergence has not occurred within 12 months of the normal range or by the time 75% root formation is complete. Box 2.5 lists local conditions reported in the literature that can be associated with delayed eruption; Box 2.6 highlights systemic disorders associated with delayed eruption.

• BOX 2.5 Local Conditions Associated With Delayed Eruption

- Ankylosis of deciduous tooth
- Arch-length deficiency
- Ectopic eruption
- Enamel pearls
- Failure of resorption of deciduous tooth
- Gingival fibromatosis or hyperplasia
- Impaction of deciduous tooth
- Injury or infection of deciduous tooth
- Mucosal barriers, such as scar tissue
- Oral clefts
- Premature loss of deciduous tooth
- Radiation damage
- Regional odontodysplasia
- Segmental odontomaxillary dysplasia
- Supernumerary teeth
- Tumors, odontogenic and non-odontogenic

• BOX 2.6 Systemic Conditions Associated With Delayed Eruption

- Anemia
- Celiac disease
- Cerebral palsy
- Chemotherapy
- Dysosteosclerosis
- Drugs, such as phenytoin
- Endocrine disorders (e.g., hypothyroidism, hypopituitarism, hypoparathyroidism, pseudohypoparathyroidism)
- Genetic disorders
- Heavy metal intoxication
- Human immunodeficiency virus (HIV) infection
- Hypobaria
- Ichthyosis
- Inadequate nutrition
- Low birth weight
- Renal failure
- Tobacco smoke
- Vitamin D–resistant rickets

Clinical and Radiographic Features

The failure of eruption may be localized or diffuse. In many localized examples, the cause is readily apparent upon radiographic examination when objects are discovered in the path of eruption. In other cases, the cause is not obvious and may be discovered after surgical exploration (such as a small intramural odontogenic hamartoma within the follicular sac). Diffuse delayed eruption often is more problematic and frequently is associated with a systemic disorder (Fig. 2.38). An excellent example is presented during the discussion of hypothyroidism in Chapter 17 (see page 835).

Primary failure of eruption is a rare disease in which incomplete tooth eruption occurs despite a clear eruption pathway. The process most commonly affects the posterior teeth, and all teeth distal to the most mesially affected teeth will demonstrate lack of full eruption. Although the majority of cases are limited to the molars, the premolars also may be affected. The most common presentation is infraocclusion of the posterior teeth, with bilateral involvement noted frequently. Studies have demonstrated an association with a mutation in the *PTH1R* gene.

Treatment and Prognosis

For localized delayed emergence, removal of any pathosis in the path of eruption may be sufficient to allow eruption to occur. If eruption does not proceed, surgical exposure accompanied by orthodontic traction has been shown to be successful. In patients with primary failure of eruption localized to the posterior teeth, mild infraocclusion requires no treatment, whereas extraction with implant replacement is recommended for severely affected teeth. When the delayed eruption is generalized, the patient should be evaluated for systemic diseases known to be associated with the

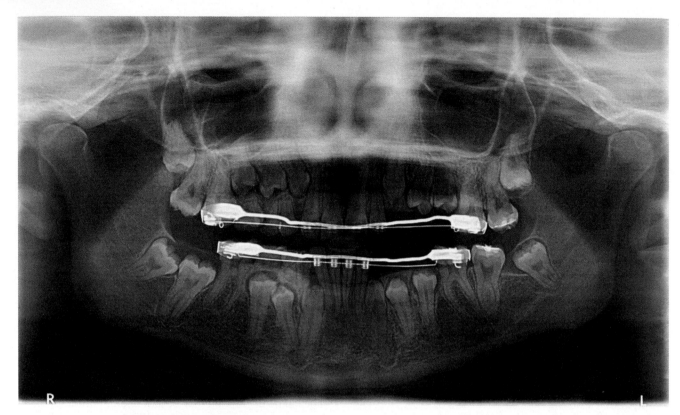

• **Fig. 2.38 Delayed Eruption.** Adult patient presenting with multiple unerupted permanent teeth without obvious causation. (Courtesy of Dr. Mark Lingen.)

process. Successful resolution of the underlying disorder often is followed by completion of eruption.

IMPACTION

Teeth that cease to erupt before emergence are **impacted.** Some authors subdivide these nonerupted teeth into those that are obstructed by a physical barrier (impacted) and those that appear to exhibit a lack of eruptive force (embedded). In many cases a tooth may appear to be embedded; however, on removal, a previously undetected overlying odontogenic hamartoma or neoplasm is discovered. Therefore, it appears appropriate to classify all these teeth as impacted.

Clinical and Radiographic Features

Impaction of deciduous teeth is extremely rare; when seen, it most commonly involves second molars. Analysis of cases suggests that ankylosis plays a major role in the pathogenesis. In the permanent dentition, the most frequently impacted teeth are the mandibular third molars, followed by maxillary third molars and maxillary cuspids. In decreasing order of frequency, impaction also may occur with mandibular premolars, mandibular canines, maxillary premolars, maxillary central incisors, maxillary lateral incisors, and mandibular second molars. First molars and maxillary second molars are rarely affected.

Lack of eruption most frequently is caused by crowding and insufficient maxillofacial development. Procedures that create more space, such as removal of bicuspids for orthodontic purposes, are associated with a decreased prevalence of third molar impaction. Impacted teeth are frequently diverted or angulated and eventually lose their potential to erupt (on completion of root development). Other factors known to be associated with impaction include the following:
- Overlying cysts or tumors
- Trauma
- Reconstructive surgery
- Thickened overlying bone or soft tissue
- A host of systemic disorders, diseases, and syndromes

Impacted teeth may be partially erupted or completely encased within the bone (i.e., full bony impaction). In addition, the impaction may be classified according to the angulation of the tooth in relationship to the remaining dentition: mesioangular, distoangular, vertical, horizontal, or inverted. On occasion, a small spicule of nonvital bone may be seen radiographically or clinically overlying the crown of partially erupted permanent posterior tooth (Fig. 2.39). The process is termed an **eruption sequestrum** and occurs when the osseous fragment becomes separated from the contiguous bone during eruption of the associated tooth. On occasion, mild sensitivity is noted in the area, especially during eating.

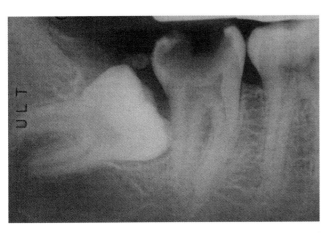

• **Fig. 2.39 Eruption Sequestrum.** A radiopaque fragment of sequestrating bone can be seen overlying an impacted third molar.

Treatment and Prognosis

The choices of treatment for impacted teeth include the following:
• Long-term observation
• Orthodontically assisted eruption
• Transplantation
• Surgical removal

Considerable evidence exists to support removal of impacted teeth associated with symptoms or the presence of clinically or radiographically obvious disease. The primary controversy surrounds appropriate therapy for asymptomatic and disease-free impactions. The British National Health Service instituted a restrictive policy toward removal of asymptomatic impacted third molars. This resulted in an initial decrease in third molar removal that was followed promptly by an increased need for extractions due to the development of caries, periodontal disease, and pericoronitis. If early prophylactic removal is discontinued, the number removed in elderly patients certainly will increase. Studies have demonstrated that removal in patients over the age of 65 is associated with significant increased morbidity and substantially worse surgical outcomes.

A 2016 Cochrane review found insufficient evidence to determine whether or not asymptomatic disease-free impacted teeth should be removed and stated that well-designed randomized controlled trials are unlikely to be feasible. The review stated that patient values and clinical expertise should be used to guide a shared decision. Patients deciding to retain their impacted teeth should obtain clinical assessment at regular intervals to prevent undesirable complications.

The risks associated with nonintervention include the following:
• Crowding of dentition
• Resorption, caries, and worsening of the periodontal status of adjacent teeth (Fig. 2.40)
• Development of pathologic conditions, such as infections, cysts, and tumors

The risks of intervention include the following:
• Transient or permanent sensory loss
• Alveolitis
• Trismus

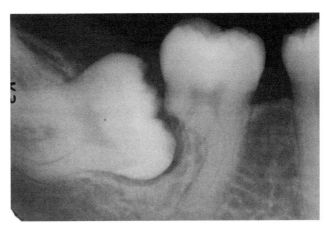

• **Fig. 2.40 Impaction-Related Tooth Resorption.** Mesioangular impaction of the right mandibular third molar associated with significant resorption of the distal root of the second molar. (Courtesy of Dr. Richard Brock.)

• Infection
• Fracture
• Temporomandibular joint (TMJ) injury
• Periodontal injury
• Injury to adjacent teeth

The eruption sequestrum requires no therapy and usually undergoes spontaneous resorption or exfoliation.

ANKYLOSIS

Eruption continues after the emergence of the teeth to compensate for masticatory wear and the growth of the jaws. The cessation of eruption after emergence is termed **ankylosis** and occurs from an anatomic fusion of tooth cementum or dentin with the alveolar bone. The process can be difficult to separate from primary failure of eruption (see page 71). Although the areas of union may be too subtle to be detected clinically and radiographically, histopathologic examination demonstrates fusion between the affected tooth and the adjacent bone in almost all cases. Other terms for this process within the literature include **infraocclusion, secondary retention, submergence, reimpaction,** and **reinclusion.** *Secondary retention* is an acceptable term but may be confused with *retained primary teeth,* which maintain their emergence. *Submergence, reimpaction,* and *reinclusion* connote an active depression, and this is not the case.

The pathogenesis of ankylosis is unknown and may be secondary to one of many factors. Disturbances from changes in local metabolism, trauma, injury, chemical or thermal irritation, local failure of bone growth, and abnormal pressure from the tongue have been suggested. The periodontal ligament (PDL) might act as a barrier that prevents osteoblasts from applying bone directly onto cementum. Ankylosis could arise from a variety of factors that result in a deficiency of this natural barrier. Such loss could arise from trauma or a genetically decreased PDL gap. Other theories point to a disturbance between normal root resorption and hard tissue repair. Several investigators believe genetic predisposition has a significant influence and point to monozygotic twins who demonstrate strikingly similar patterns of ankylosis to support this hypothesis.

Clinical and Radiographic Features

Ankylosis may occur at any age; however, clinically the condition is most obvious if the fusion develops during the first two decades of life. Most patients reported in the literature with obvious alterations in occlusion are between the ages of 7 and 18 years, with a peak prevalence occurring in 8- to 9-year-old children. The reported prevalence of clinically detectable ankylosis in children varies from 1.3% to 8.9% and has been reported to be as high as 44% in siblings of those affected.

Although any tooth may be affected, the most commonly involved teeth in order of frequency are the mandibular primary first molar, the mandibular primary second molar, the maxillary primary first molar, and the maxillary primary second molar. Ankylosis of permanent teeth is uncommon. In the deciduous dentition, mandibular teeth are affected ten times as often as the maxillary dentition. The occlusal plane of the involved tooth is below that of the adjacent dentition (infraocclusion) in a patient with a history of previous full occlusion (Fig. 2.41). A sharp, solid sound may be noted on percussion of the involved tooth but can be detected only when more than 20% of the root is fused to the bone. Radiographically, absence of the PDL space may be noted; however, the area of fusion is often in the bifurcation and interradicular root surface, making radiographic detection most difficult in plain films (Fig. 2.42). Cone beam computed tomography (CBCT) has proven to be a useful diagnostic adjunct and typically will demonstrate a focal loss of the periodontal ligament adjacent to a small area of external replacement resorption (page 64) on the adjacent tooth.

Ankylosed teeth that are allowed to remain in position can lead to a number of dental problems. The adjacent teeth often incline toward the affected tooth, frequently with the development of subsequent occlusal and periodontal problems. In addition, the opposing teeth often exhibit over-eruption. Occasionally, the ankylosed tooth leads to a

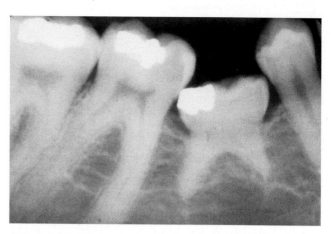

• **Fig. 2.42 Ankylosis.** Radiograph of an ankylosed deciduous molar. Note the lack of periodontal ligament (PDL) space.

localized deficiency of the alveolar ridge or impaction of the underlying permanent tooth. An increased frequency of lateral open bite and crossbite is seen.

Treatment and Prognosis

Because they are fused to the adjacent bone, ankylosed teeth fail to respond to normal orthodontic forces, with attempts to move the ankylosed tooth occasionally resulting in intrusion of the anchor teeth. Recommended therapy for ankylosis of primary molars is variable and often is determined by the severity and timing of the process. When an underlying permanent successor is present, extraction of the ankylosed primary molar should not be performed until it becomes obvious that exfoliation is not proceeding normally or adverse occlusal changes are developing. After extraction of an ankylosed molar, the permanent tooth will erupt spontaneously in the majority of cases. In permanent teeth or primary teeth without underlying successors, prosthetic buildup can be placed to augment the occlusal height. Severe cases in primary teeth are treated best with extraction and space maintenance. Luxation of affected permanent teeth may be attempted with extraction forceps in an effort to break the ankylosis. It is hoped that the subsequent inflammatory reaction results in the formation of a new fibrous ligament in the area of previous fusion. In these cases, reevaluation in 6 months is mandatory. Finally, several reports have documented successful repositioning of an ankylosed permanent tooth with a combination of orthodontics, segmental osteotomy, and distraction osteogenesis.

DEVELOPMENTAL ALTERATIONS OF TEETH

Numerous developmental alterations of teeth can occur. Box 2.7 delineates the major reported alterations, and the following text pertains to these entities. These alterations may be

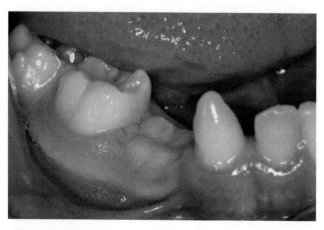

• **Fig. 2.41 Ankylosis.** Deciduous molar well below the occlusal plane of the adjacent teeth.

Number

- Tooth agenesis
- Hyperdontia

Size

- Microdontia
- Macrodontia

Shape

- Gemination
- Fusion
- Concrescence
- Accessory cusps
- Dens invaginatus
- Ectopic enamel
- Taurodontism
- Hypercementosis
- Accessory roots
- Dilaceration

Structure

- Amelogenesis imperfecta (AI)
- Dentinogenesis imperfecta (DGI)
- Radicular dentin dysplasia
- Regional odontodysplasia

primary or arise secondary to environmental influences (e.g., concrescence, hypercementosis, and dilaceration). For the sake of convenience, both the primary and the environmental forms will be discussed together.

◆ DEVELOPMENTAL ALTERATIONS IN THE NUMBER OF TEETH

Variations in the number of teeth that develop are common. Several terms are useful in the discussion of the numeric variations of teeth. **Tooth agenesis** refers to the failure of a tooth to develop. Varying degrees of severity are noted. **Hypodontia** denotes lack of development of one to five teeth, **oligodontia** indicates the developmental absence of six or more teeth (excluding third molars), and **anodontia** refers to a total lack of tooth development. **Hyperdontia** is the development of an increased number of teeth, and the additional teeth are termed **supernumerary.** Terms such as *partial anodontia* are oxymorons and should be avoided. In addition, these terms pertain to teeth that failed to develop and should not be applied to teeth that developed but are impacted or have been removed.

Genetic control appears to exert a strong influence on the development of teeth. Tooth agenesis and hyperdontia have been noted in patients with a variety of syndromes (Boxes 2.8 and 2.9). In all of these syndromes, an increased prevalence of tooth agenesis or hyperdontia exists, but the strength of the association varies. Furthermore, the actual genetic contribution to the increased or decreased number of teeth may be

unclear in some of these conditions. In addition to these syndromes, an increased prevalence of tooth agenesis is noted in patients with nonsyndromic cleft lip (CL) or cleft palate (CP).

Genetic influences still may affect nonsyndromic numeric alterations of teeth, because more than 200 genes are known to play a role in odontogenesis. Because of the complexity of the system, variations in tooth number arise in a wide variety of patterns. A large percentage of primary tooth agenesis cases appear to be inherited in an autosomal dominant fashion, with incomplete penetrance and variable expressivity, whereas a minority of examples presents an autosomal recessive or sex-linked pattern. The environment is not without its influence, with occasional examples suggesting multifactorial inheritance. Several investigators have reported variable expression of hypodontia in monozygotic twins (confirmed by DNA fingerprinting). This discordance confirms the occasional multifactorial nature of the process. Overall, dental agenesis most likely represents a variety of disorders caused by variable genetic and epigenetic factors.

Research has identified a gene mutation in only a small percentage of nonsyndromic tooth agenesis cases. Although this list will continue to lengthen over time, the most frequently implicated genes include the *WNT10A, PAX9, MSX1, EDA,* and the *AXIN2* genes, with one of these five genes involved in 50% of tooth agenesis in humans when the genetic mutation is known. Although variable expressivity is common, most of these examples represent oligodontia and exhibit numerous missing teeth. Interestingly, the affected gene tends to correlate to the pattern of missing teeth. It must be stressed that these genes are involved in only a very small number of affected patients with dental agenesis, and the genetic basis for the vast majority of missing teeth remains elusive.

Less information is available on the genetics of hyperdontia; however, like tooth agenesis, almost every possible pattern of inheritance has been suggested. In all likelihood, many cases are multifactorial and arise from a combination of genetics and environmental influences. Despite this, studies on certain kindreds have suggested an autosomal dominant pattern of inheritance with incomplete penetrance, autosomal recessive inheritance with lesser penetrance in females, and X-linked inheritance. Unlike dental agenesis, mutations of only a few genes have been linked to hyperdontia. Two of the best known examples are mutations in *RUNX2* (associated with cleidocranial dysplasia; see page 623) and *APC* (associated with Gardner syndrome; see page 656).

Some investigators have implied that tooth agenesis is a normal variant, suggesting that humans are in an intermediate stage of dentitional evolution. A proposed future dentition would contain one incisor, one canine, one premolar, and two molars per quadrant. Conversely, others have suggested that hyperdontia represents atavism—the reappearance of an ancestral condition. The latter hypothesis is difficult to accept because some patients have had as many as four premolars in one quadrant, a situation that has never

• BOX 2.8   Syndromes Associated With Tooth Agenesis

- Aarskog-Scott Syndrome
- ADULT syndrome
- Alagille syndrome
- Apert syndrome
- Axenfeld-Rieger syndrome, type 1
- Axenfeld-Rieger syndrome, type 2
- Blepharocheliodontic syndrome
- Böök syndrome
- Branchiootorenal syndrome, type 1
- Carvajal Naxos syndrome
- Char syndrome
- Charcot-Marie-Tooth syndrome
- Cleft lip/palate-ectodermal dysplasia
- Cockayne syndrome
- Coffin-Lowry syndrome
- Crouzon syndrome
- Crouzonodermoskeletal syndrome
- Diastrophic dysplasia
- Down syndrome
- Dubowitz syndrome
- Ectodermal dysplasia, hypohidrotic, autosomal dominant
- Ectodermal dysplasia, hypohidrotic, autosomal recessive
- Ectodermal dysplasia, hypohidrotic, X-linked
- Ectodermal dysplasia, trichoodontoonychial type
- Ectrodactyly, ectodermal dysplasia, and cleft lip/palate
- Ehlers-Danlos syndrome, type IV
- Ehlers-Danlos syndrome, type VIIC
- Ellis-van Creveld syndrome
- Fahr syndrome
- Fanconi renotubular syndrome 1
- Fraser syndrome
- Frontometaphyseal dysplasia
- GAPO syndrome
- Goldenhar syndrome
- Gorlin-Chaudhry-Moss syndrome
- Gorlin-Goltz syndrome
- Hallermann-Streiff syndrome
- Hanhart syndrome
- Hay-Wells syndrome
- Hypohidrotic ectodermal dysplasia with immune deficiency (HED-ID)
- Holoprosencephaly 3
- Hurler syndrome
- Incontinentia pigmenti
- Johanson-Blizzard syndrome
- Kabuki syndrome
- Kallmann syndrome
- Kartagener syndrome
- Kenny-Caffey syndrome, type 1
- Lacrimo-auriculo-dento-digital syndrome (LADD)
- Larsen syndrome
- Laurence-Moon syndrome
- Leukodystrophy, hypomyelinating, 7, with or without oligodontia and/or hypogonadotrophic hypogonadism
- Leukomelanoderma, infantilism, mental retardation, hypodontia, hypotrichosis
- Limb-mammary syndrome
- McCune-Albright syndrome
- Microphthalmia
- Moebius syndrome
- Mulvihill-Smith syndrome
- Nance-Horan syndrome
- Neu-Laxova syndrome
- Osteopetrosis and lymphedema-anhidrotic ectodermal dysplasia with immunodeficiency (OLEDAID)
- Odontoonychodermal dysplasia
- Oral-facial-digital syndrome type I
- Osteogenesis imperfecta, type 1
- Otodental dysplasia
- Pallister-Killian syndrome
- Phelan-McDermid syndrome
- Prune belly syndrome
- Pseudoxanthoma elasticum
- Rapp-Hodgkin syndrome
- Richieri-Costa-Pereira syndrome
- Rothmund-Thomson syndrome
- Rubinstein-Taybi syndrome
- Schimke immunoosseous dysplasia
- Schinzel syndrome
- Schopf-Schulz-Passarge syndrome
- Schwartz-Jampel syndrome, type 1
- Seckel syndrome
- Sickle cell anemia
- Simpson-Golabi-Behmel syndrome
- Sjogren-Larsson syndrome
- Smith-Magenis syndrome
- Solitary median maxillary central incisor syndrome
- Sotos syndrome
- Split-hand/foot malformation, type 1
- Sturge-Weber syndrome
- Treacher Collins-Franceschetti syndrome
- Tuomaala-Haapanen syndrome
- Van der Woude syndrome
- Velocardiofacial syndrome
- Waardenburg syndrome
- Weill-Marchesani syndrome
- Weyers acrofacial dysostosis
- Williams-Beuren syndrome
- Witkop syndrome
- Wolf-Hirschhorn syndrome
- Yunis-Varon syndrome

• BOX 2.9   Disorders Associated With Hyperdontia

- Apert syndrome
- Cleidocranial dysplasia
- Craniometaphyseal dysplasia
- Crouzon syndrome
- Curtius syndrome
- Down syndrome
- Ehlers-Danlos syndrome
- Ellis-van Creveld syndrome
- Fabry-Anderson syndrome
- Fucosidosis
- Gardner syndrome
- Hallermann-Streiff syndrome
- Incontinentia pigmenti
- Klippel-Trénaunay-Weber syndrome
- Laband syndrome
- Leopard syndrome
- Nance-Horan syndrome
- Oculofaciocardiodental syndrome
- Opitz BBB/G syndrome
- Oral-facial-digital syndrome, types I and III
- Robinow syndrome
- Rubinstein-Taybi syndrome
- Sturge-Weber syndrome
- Tricho-rhino-phalangeal syndrome

been reported in other mammals. The most widely accepted theory is that hyperdontia is the result of a localized and independent hyperactivity of dental lamina.

In contrast, tooth agenesis correlates with the absence of appropriate dental lamina. As discussed, the loss of the developing tooth buds in most instances appears to be genetically controlled. Despite this, the environment most likely influences the final result or, in some cases, may be responsible completely for the lack of tooth formation. The dental lamina is extremely sensitive to external stimuli, and damage before tooth formation can result in hypodontia. Trauma, infection, radiation, chemotherapeutic medications, endocrine disturbances, and severe intrauterine disturbances have been associated with missing teeth.

Clinical Features

Tooth Agenesis

Failure of teeth to form is one of the most common dental developmental abnormalities, with a reported prevalence of 3% to 10% in permanent teeth when absence of third molars is excluded. The prevalence increases to 23% if third molars are considered. A female predominance of approximately 1.5:1 is reported. Anodontia is rare, and most cases occur in the presence of hereditary hypohidrotic ectodermal dysplasia (see page 747). Indeed, when the number of missing teeth is high or involves the most stable teeth (i.e., maxillary central incisors or first molars), the patient should be evaluated for ectodermal dysplasia. Tooth agenesis is uncommon in the deciduous dentition with a prevalence of less than 1%. Absence of a deciduous tooth is associated strongly with an increased prevalence of a missing successor. Missing teeth in the permanent dentition are not rare, with third molars being the most commonly affected. After the third molars, the second premolars and lateral incisors are absent most frequently (Fig. 2.43). The teeth least likely to be missing are the maxillary central incisors and mandibular first molars and canines. In Caucasians with missing teeth, approximately 80% demonstrate loss of only one or two teeth. Ethnic differences have been documented, with Japanese and Chinese populations more frequently having absent mandibular central incisors when compared to Caucasians. In contrast, when compared to Caucasians, American blacks demonstrate a significantly decreased prevalence of tooth agenesis and a reduced average number of missing teeth per individual. In the deciduous dentition, 90% of missing teeth involve the maxillary lateral incisors and mandibular incisors. Tooth agenesis is associated positively with microdontia (see page 81), dental transposition (see page 79), reduced alveolar development, increased freeway space, anterior malocclusion, and retained primary teeth (Fig. 2.44).

Mutation of *PAX9* creates an autosomal dominant pattern of oligodontia that can involve various teeth but most commonly affects most of the permanent molars. In severe cases, loss of the primary molars, second premolars, and permanent mandibular central incisors also may be seen. Mutation of *MSX1* also is inherited as an autosomal dominant trait. Those affected tend to demonstrate loss of the distal tooth of each type, with more severely affected individuals also revealing anterior progression of the agenesis. In these patients, the most commonly missing teeth are the second premolars and third molars. In more severe cases, often the maxillary first premolars and maxillary lateral incisors also are missing. With the *MSX1* mutation, the degree of oligodontia is severe with an average of approximately 12 missing teeth per patient. *EDA* is associated with a nonsyndromic X-linked pattern of missing teeth, which primarily affects

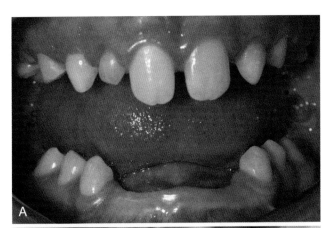
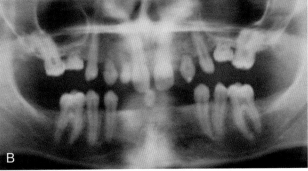

• **Fig. 2.44 Oligodontia. A,** Multiple developmentally missing permanent teeth and several retained deciduous teeth in a female adult. **B,** The panoramic radiograph shows no unerupted teeth in either jaw.

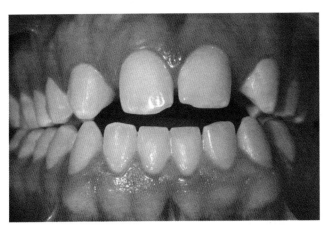

• **Fig. 2.43 Hypodontia.** Developmentally missing maxillary lateral incisors. Radiographs revealed no underlying teeth, and there was no history of trauma or extraction.

the maxillary and mandibular central incisors, lateral incisors, cuspids, and premolars. Tooth agenesis associated with nonsyndromic mutation of *WNT10A* appears limited to maxillary and mandibular lateral incisors and second premolars.

For dentists and their patients, the most critical discovery related to tooth agenesis revolves around the mutation of *AXIN2*. This pattern of oligodontia is inherited as an autosomal dominant disorder, with the most commonly missing teeth being the permanent second and third molars, second premolars, lower incisors, and maxillary lateral incisors. The maxillary central incisors always are present and usually accompanied by the canines, first premolars, and first molars. However, the number and type of missing teeth are highly variable, a typical finding of inheritable oligodontia. Although the missing teeth can produce a significant oral problem, the presence of the *AXIN2* mutation in these kindreds also has been associated with development of adenomatous polyps of the colon and colorectal carcinoma. This suggests that patients with similar examples of oligodontia should be questioned closely for a family history of colon cancer, with further medical evaluation recommended for those possibly at risk. An association between tooth agenesis and ovarian cancer also has been suggested, but no single mutation has been found that could explain the simultaneous occurrence of both conditions. In addition, close examination of affected patients often reveals two separate mutations that are independently responsible for the ovarian cancer and tooth agenesis.

Even in kindreds with an obviously inherited pattern of hypodontia or oligodontia, it must be stressed that, in the majority of the cases, the genes are yet to be discovered.

Hyperdontia

The prevalence of supernumerary permanent teeth in whites is between 0.1% and 3.8%, with a slightly higher rate seen in Asian populations. Although limited data is available, the prevalence in American blacks appears significantly higher with reports documenting an increased frequency up to nine times that seen in whites. The frequency in the deciduous dentition is much lower and varies from 0.3% to 0.8%. Approximately 76%–86% of cases represent single-tooth **hyperdontia,** with two supernumerary teeth noted in 12%–23%, and three or more extra teeth noted in less than 1% of cases. Single-tooth hyperdontia occurs more frequently in the permanent dentition, and approximately 95% present in the maxilla, with a strong predilection for the anterior region. However, these widely accepted data appear to be associated with a strong racial bias. Limited prevalence studies in American blacks reveal that fourth molars are the most common extra teeth, with a comparatively low frequency of supernumerary incisors. When all prevalence studies are combined, the most common site is the maxillary incisor region, followed by maxillary fourth molars and mandibular fourth molars, premolars, canines, and lateral incisors (Fig. 2.45). Supernumerary mandibular incisors are very rare. Although supernumerary teeth may

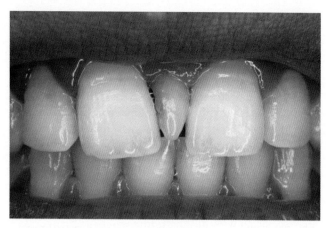

• **Fig. 2.45 Hyperdontia (Mesiodens).** Erupted supernumerary, rudimentary tooth of the anterior maxilla.

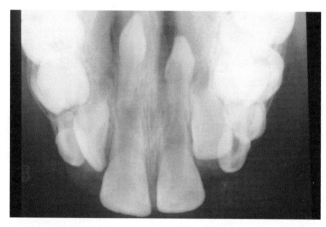

• **Fig. 2.46 Hyperdontia (Mesiodens).** Bilateral inverted supernumerary teeth of the anterior maxilla.

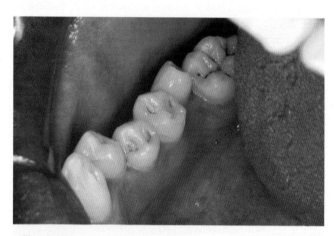

• **Fig. 2.47 Hyperdontia.** Right mandibular dentition exhibiting four erupted bicuspids.

be bilateral, most occur unilaterally (Fig. 2.46). In contrast to single-tooth hyperdontia, nonsyndromic multiple supernumerary teeth occur most frequently in the mandible. These multiple supernumerary teeth occur most often in the premolar region, followed by the molar and anterior regions, respectively (Fig. 2.47).

Although most supernumerary teeth occur in the jaws, examples have been reported in the gingiva, maxillary tuberosity, soft palate, maxillary sinus, sphenomaxillary fissure, nasal cavity, and between the orbit and the brain. The eruption of accessory teeth is variable and dependent on the degree of space available; 75% of supernumerary teeth in the anterior maxilla fail to erupt. Unlike hypodontia, hyperdontia is positively correlated with macrodontia (see page 81) and exhibits a 2:1 male predominance. Although examples may be identified in older adults, most supernumerary teeth develop during the first two decades of life.

Several terms have been used to describe supernumerary teeth, depending on their location. A supernumerary tooth in the maxillary anterior incisor region is termed a **mesiodens** (see Fig. 2.45); an accessory fourth molar is often called a **distomolar** or **distodens** (Fig. 2.48). A posterior supernumerary tooth situated lingually or buccally to a molar tooth is termed a **paramolar** (Fig. 2.49).

Supernumerary teeth are divided into **supplemental** (normal size and shape) or **rudimentary** (abnormal shape and smaller size) types. Rudimentary supernumerary teeth

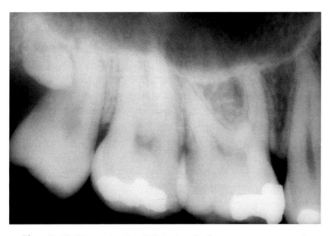

• **Fig. 2.48 Hyperdontia (Distodens).** Supernumerary maxillary fourth molar.

are classified further into **conical** (small, peg-shaped), **tuberculate** (barrel-shaped anterior with more than one cusp), and **molariform** (small premolar-like or molar-like). Although odontomas are considered hamartomas and could be placed within this classification, these lesions traditionally are included in the list of odontogenic neoplasms and are discussed in Chapter 15 (page 685). The conical mesiodens represents one of the more common supernumerary teeth and can erupt spontaneously, whereas tuberculate examples are less frequent and rarely erupt.

On rare occasions, an affected patient can present with both hypodontia and hyperdontia, which has been termed **hypohyperdontia.** The process most commonly involves missing mandibular incisors followed by second premolars; in contrast, supernumerary teeth are seen most frequently in the anterior maxilla followed by supplemental canines or maxillary premolars.

Occasionally, normal teeth may erupt into an inappropriate position (e.g., a canine present between two premolars). This pattern of abnormal eruption is called **dental transposition.** Such misplaced teeth have been confused with supernumerary teeth; but in reality, patients exhibiting dental transposition have been reported to exhibit an increased prevalence of hypodontia, not hyperdontia. The teeth involved most frequently in transposition are the maxillary canines and first premolars (Fig. 2.50). Crowding or malocclusion of these normal teeth may dictate reshaping, orthodontics, or extraction.

Accessory teeth may be present at or shortly after birth. Historically, teeth present in newborns have been called **natal teeth;** those arising within the first 30 days of life are designated **neonatal teeth.** The ratio of natal teeth to neonatal teeth is 3:1. The reported prevalence of such teeth ranges from 1:2000 to 1:3500 live births. (Fig. 2.51). Although some authors have suggested that these teeth may represent predeciduous supernumerary teeth, 90% are prematurely erupted deciduous teeth (not supernumerary teeth). Approximately 85% of natal teeth are mandibular

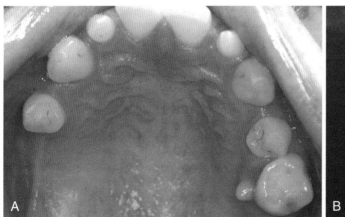
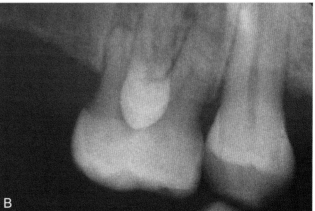

• **Fig. 2.49 Paramolar. A,** Rudimentary tooth situated palatal to a maxillary molar in a patient who also exhibits hypodontia. **B,** Radiograph of the same patient showing a fully formed tooth overlying the crown of the adjacent molar.

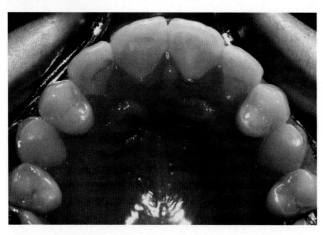

• **Fig. 2.50 Dental Transposition.** Maxillary dentition exhibiting cuspids and first bicuspids in inappropriate positions bilaterally. (Courtesy of Dr. Wendy Humphrey.)

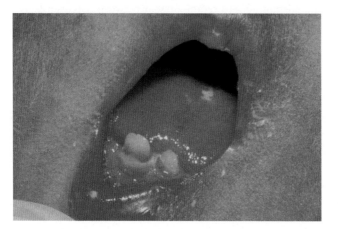

• **Fig. 2.51 Natal Teeth.** Mandibular central incisors that were erupted at birth.

incisors, 11% are maxillary incisors, and 4% are canines or posterior teeth. Often, the natal teeth erupt in pairs.

Treatment and Prognosis

Sequelae associated with tooth agenesis include abnormal spacing of teeth, delayed tooth formation, delayed deciduous tooth exfoliation, late permanent tooth eruption, and altered dimension of the associated gnathic regions. The management of the patient with missing teeth depends on the severity of the case. No treatment may be required for a single missing tooth; prosthetic replacement often is needed when multiple teeth are absent. Therapeutic options include removable partial dentures, traditional fixed prosthodontics, resin-bonded bridges, or osseointegrated implants with associated prosthetic crowns. Use of fixed prosthodontics typically is not recommended for children because of the risk of pulp exposure during abutment preparation and because further growth can lead to infraocclusion and ankylosis of teeth held together by the prosthesis. Likewise, because implants act more like ankylosed teeth than erupting teeth,

their use is not recommended before completion of skeletal growth except for patients with anodontia. For these reasons, a removable appliance or resin-bonded bridge often is appropriate in children and young adults while waiting for full dental and skeletal maturation.

In some cases of hypodontia and oligodontia, orthodontic therapy may improve the restorative treatment or even negate its need in selected patients. Patients with oligodontia exhibit an increased prevalence of orthodontics-associated external root resorption. This may be due to the altered root anatomy or to the extensive tooth movement that is required in some patients. Follow-up radiographs are recommended after 6–9 months of therapy to evaluate the root morphology for evidence of excessive resorption.

The presence of supernumerary teeth should be suspected if a significant delay is observed in the eruption of a localized portion of the dentition. Because of the decreased clarity in the anterior portion of a panoramic radiograph, this image should be combined with occlusal and periapical radiographs to fully visualize the area. Supernumerary teeth may develop long after eruption of the permanent dentition. Several publications have documented supernumerary bicuspids arising up to 11 years after completion of normal teeth development. In patients previously diagnosed with supernumerary teeth, or in those genetically predisposed, long-term monitoring for additional tooth development is warranted.

Early diagnosis and treatment often are crucial in minimizing the aesthetic and functional problems of the adjacent teeth. Because only 7% to 20% of supernumerary teeth exist without clinical complications, the standard of care is removal of the accessory tooth during the time of the early mixed dentition. Complications created by anterior supernumerary teeth tend to be more significant than those associated with extra teeth in the posterior regions. Reports have documented spontaneous eruption of the adjacent dentition in 75% of the cases if the supernumerary tooth is removed early. After removal of the supernumerary tooth, full eruption typically occurs within 18 months to 3 years. Impacted permanent teeth having closed apices or those associated with a tuberculate mesiodens may show a reduced tendency for spontaneous eruption. Permanent teeth that fail to erupt are treated best by surgical exposure with orthodontic eruption. Removal of unerupted deciduous teeth is not recommended, because most will erupt spontaneously.

A consequence of late therapy may include the delayed eruption, resorption of the adjacent teeth, displacement of the teeth with associated crowding, dilaceration, malocclusion, diastema formation, or eruption into the nasal cavity. Supernumerary teeth also predispose the area to subacute pericoronitis, gingivitis, periodontitis, abscess formation, and the development of any one of a large number of odontogenic cysts and tumors. In selected cases, clinical judgment may not dictate surgical removal, or patient resistance to therapy may be present. In these instances, regular monitoring is appropriate.

A study attempting to determine the optimum time for removal of mesiodens in a pediatric population suggested that removal after age 10 was associated with a higher prevalence of developmental defects of the adjacent permanent teeth such as dilaceration and root resorption. Although a cautious surgical approach is necessary to avoid damage to the adjacent developing incisor, removal of mesiodens prior to 6–7 years of age appears advantageous in decreasing local developmental complications.

Natal teeth must be approached individually with sound clinical judgment guiding appropriate therapy. Radiographs may be difficult to obtain but could be helpful in distinguishing premature eruption of a deciduous tooth from a supernumerary tooth. As stated, the erupted teeth in most cases represent the deciduous dentition, and removal should not be performed hastily. If the teeth are mobile and at risk for aspiration, removal is indicated. The surgical procedure must ensure complete removal of the associated dental papilla and epithelial root sheath to prevent formation of residual root fragments. If mobility is not a problem and the teeth are stable, then they should be retained. Traumatic ulcerations of the adjacent soft tissue (**Riga-Fede disease**) (see page 274) may occur during breast feeding but often can be resolved through use of a breastfeeding splint or grinding/smoothing of the incisal edges of the natal tooth. If the tooth is surgically removed during the first 10 days of life, vitamin K administration is advocated, because the infant's coagulation system may not be established sufficiently.

◆ DEVELOPMENTAL ALTERATIONS IN THE SIZE OF TEETH

Tooth size is variable among different races and between the sexes. The presence of unusually small teeth is termed **microdontia;** the presence of teeth larger than average is termed **macrodontia.** Although heredity is the major factor, both genetic and environmental influences affect the size of developing teeth. The deciduous dentition appears to be affected more by maternal intrauterine influences; the permanent teeth seem to be more affected by environment.

Clinical Features

Although the size of teeth from person to person is variable, the teeth on two sides of the jaws usually are symmetrical. Despite this, when significant size variation is present, the entire dentition rarely is affected. Typically, only a few teeth are altered significantly in size. Differences in tooth sizes may be related to other concurrent oral developmental anomalies. Microdontia is associated strongly with tooth agenesis (see page 75); macrodontia often is seen in association with hyperdontia (see page 75). Females demonstrate a higher frequency of microdontia and tooth agenesis; males have a greater prevalence of macrodontia and hyperdontia.

Microdontia

The term **microdontia** should be applied only when the teeth are physically smaller than usual. Normal-sized teeth may appear small when widely spaced within jaws that are

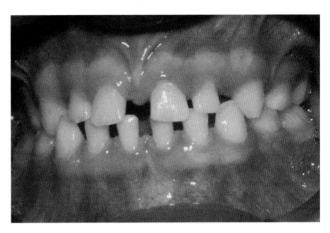

• **Fig. 2.52 Diffuse Microdontia.** Dentition in which the teeth are smaller than normal and widely spaced within the arch.

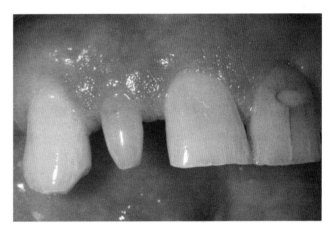

• **Fig. 2.53 Isolated Microdontia (Peg Lateral).** Small, cone-shaped right maxillary lateral incisor.

larger than normal. This appearance has been historically termed **relative microdontia,** but it represents **macrognathia** (not microdontia). Diffuse true microdontia is uncommon but may occur as an isolated finding in Down syndrome, in pituitary dwarfism, and in association with a small number of rare hereditary disorders that exhibit multiple abnormalities of the dentition (Fig. 2.52).

Isolated microdontia within an otherwise normal dentition is not uncommon. The maxillary lateral incisor is affected most frequently and typically appears as a peg-shaped crown overlying a root that often is of normal length (Fig. 2.53). The mesiodistal diameter is reduced, and the proximal surfaces converge toward the incisal edge. The reported prevalence varies from 0.8% to 8.4% of the population, and the alteration appears to be autosomal dominant with incomplete penetrance. In addition, isolated microdontia often affects third molars. Interestingly, the maxillary lateral incisors and the third molars are among the most frequent teeth to be congenitally missing. When a peg-shaped tooth is present, the remaining permanent teeth often exhibit a slightly smaller mesiodistal size.

Macrodontia

Analogous to microdontia, the term **macrodontia (megalo-dontia, megadontia)** should be applied only when teeth are physically larger than usual and should not include normal-sized teeth crowded within a small jaw (previously termed **relative macrodontia**). In addition, the term *macrodontia* should not be used to describe teeth that have been altered by fusion or gemination. Diffuse involvement is rare, and typically only a few teeth are abnormally large. Diffuse macrodontia has been noted in association with pituitary gigantism (see page 834), otodental syndrome, XYY males, and pineal hyperplasia with hyperinsulinism. Macrodontia with unilateral premature eruption is not rare in hemifacial hyperplasia (see page 37). Authors have postulated that the unilateral bone growth resulting from this condition may also affect developing teeth on the altered side. Isolated macrodontia is reported to occur most frequently in incisors or canines but also has been seen in second premolars and third molars (Fig. 2.54). In such situations, the alteration often occurs bilaterally.

In one distinctive pattern of macrodontia, the affected teeth demonstrate an extreme elongation of the roots known as **radiculomegaly**. The most commonly affected tooth is the cuspid with the roots often extending to the inferior border of the mandible and/or the floor of the orbit. Although radiculomegaly may be nonsyndromic, this finding is strongly suggestive of **oculo-facio-cardio-dental (OFCD) syndrome**. This X-linked dominant syndrome is characterized by ocular alterations (congenital cataracts, secondary glaucoma, microphthalmia) distinctive facies (narrow face, high nasal bridge, broad nasal tip, cleft palate), cardiac abnormalities (atrial or ventricular septal defects), and dental alterations (radiculomegaly, hypodontia, delayed eruption, retained deciduous teeth). The radiculomegaly is the most distinctive findings and does not become evident until the age of 15 due to the associated maturation time of the cuspid roots. The syndrome only occurs in females and is thought to demonstrate embryonic lethality in males. A novel mutation of the BCL-6 interacting corepressor gene (BCOR) is noted in affected patients.

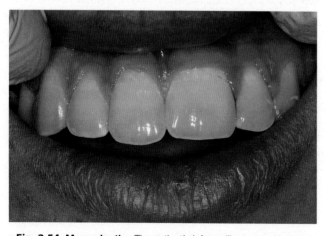

• **Fig. 2.54 Macrodontia.** The patient's left maxillary central incisor is abnormally large. (Courtesy of Dr. Peter Fam.)

Treatment and Prognosis

Treatment of the dentition is not necessary unless desired for aesthetic considerations. Maxillary peg laterals often are restored to full size by porcelain crowns.

◆ DEVELOPMENTAL ALTERATIONS IN THE SHAPE OF TEETH

GEMINATION, FUSION, AND CONCRESCENCE

Double teeth (connate teeth, conjoined teeth) are two separate teeth exhibiting union by dentin and (perhaps) their pulps. The union may be the result of fusion of two adjacent tooth buds or the partial splitting of one into two. The development of isolated large or joined (i.e., double) teeth is not rare, but the literature is confusing when the appropriate terminology is presented. Historically, *gemination* was defined as an attempt of a single tooth bud to divide, with the resultant formation of a tooth with a bifid crown and, usually, a common root and root canal. Conversely, *fusion* was considered the union of two normally separated tooth buds with the resultant formation of a joined tooth with confluence of dentin. Finally, *concrescence* was the union of two teeth by cementum without confluence of the dentin.

Many investigators have found these definitions confusing and open to debate. A double tooth found in the place of a maxillary permanent central incisor is a good example of the controversy. If the joined tooth is counted as one and the tooth number is correct, then the anomaly could result from the division of a single tooth bud or the fusion of the permanent tooth bud with the bud of an adjacent mesiodens. Some have suggested that the terms *gemination, fusion,* and *concrescence* should be discontinued, and all of these anomalies should be termed *twinning*. This also is confusing because other investigators use *twinning* to refer to the development of two separate teeth that arose from the complete separation of one tooth bud (this also is arguable).

Because of this confusion in terminology, the use of the term *twinning* cannot be recommended. Extra teeth are termed **supernumerary,** and another name is not necessary. Even though the exact pathogenesis may be questionable in some cases (whether caused by fusion of adjacent buds or partial split of one bud), the terms *gemination, fusion,* and *concrescence* serve a useful purpose because they are the most descriptive of the clinical presentation. **Gemination** is defined as a single enlarged tooth or joined (i.e., double) tooth in which the tooth count is normal when the anomalous tooth is counted as one. **Fusion** is defined as a single enlarged tooth or joined (i.e., double) tooth in which the tooth count reveals a missing tooth when the anomalous tooth is counted as one. **Concrescence** is union of two adjacent teeth by cementum alone, without confluence of the underlying dentin. Unlike fusion and gemination, concrescence may be developmental or post-inflammatory. When two teeth develop in close proximity, developmental union by cementum is possible. In addition, areas of inflammatory damage to the roots of teeth are repaired by cementum once the inciting process resolves. Concrescence of adjacent teeth may arise in initially separated teeth in which cementum deposition extends between two closely approximated roots in a previous area of damage.

Clinical Features

Gemination and Fusion

Double teeth (**gemination** and **fusion**) occur in both the primary and the permanent dentitions, with a higher frequency in the anterior and maxillary regions (Figs. 2.55–2.59). In the permanent dentition, the prevalence of double teeth in whites is approximately 0.3%–0.5%, whereas the frequency in deciduous teeth is greater, with a reported prevalence from 0.5% to 2.5%. Asian populations tend to

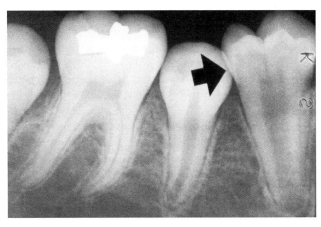

• **Fig. 2.57 Gemination.** Same patient as depicted in Fig. 2.56. Note the bifid crown and shared root canal.

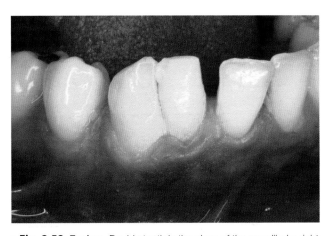

• **Fig. 2.58 Fusion.** Double tooth in the place of the mandibular right lateral incisor and cuspid.

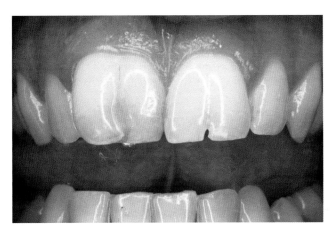

• **Fig. 2.55 Bilateral Gemination.** Two double teeth. The tooth count was normal when each anomalous tooth was counted as one.

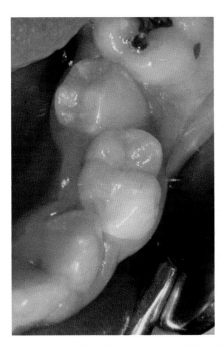

• **Fig. 2.56 Gemination.** Mandibular bicuspid exhibiting bifid crown.

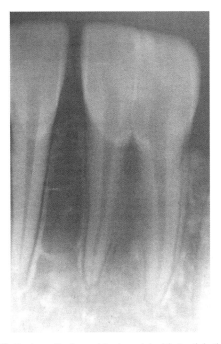

• **Fig. 2.59 Fusion.** Radiographic view of double tooth in the place of the mandibular central and lateral incisors. Note separate root canals.

demonstrate a higher occurrence that exceeds 5% in some studies. In both dentitions, incisors and canines are the most commonly affected teeth. Involvement of posterior primary teeth, premolars, and permanent molars also can occur. Gemination is more common in the maxilla, whereas fusion tends to occur more frequently in the mandible. Bilateral cases are uncommon (Fig. 2.60).

Gemination and fusion appear similar and may be differentiated by assessing the number of teeth in the dentition. Some authors have suggested that gemination demonstrates a single root canal whereas separate canals are present in fusion; but this does not hold true in all cases (Fig. 2.61). Fusion and gemination can be seen in one of four major patterns: a bifid crown with a single root, a large crown with a large root, two conjoined crowns with a double conical root, and two connected crowns with two linked roots.

Concrescence

Concrescence is two fully formed teeth, joined along the root surfaces by cementum. The process is noted more frequently in the posterior and maxillary regions. The developmental pattern often involves a second molar tooth in which its roots closely approximate the adjacent impacted third molar (Fig. 2.62). The post-inflammatory pattern frequently involves carious molars in which the apices overlie the roots of horizontally or distally angulated third molars. This latter pattern most frequently arises in a carious tooth that exhibits large coronal tooth loss. The resultant large pulpal exposure often permits pulpal drainage, leading to a resolution of a portion of the intrabony pathosis. Cemental repair then occurs (Figs. 2.63 and 2.64).

Treatment and Prognosis

The presence of double teeth (i.e., gemination or fusion) in the deciduous dentition can result in crowding, abnormal spacing, and delayed or ectopic eruption of the underlying permanent teeth. When detected, the progression of

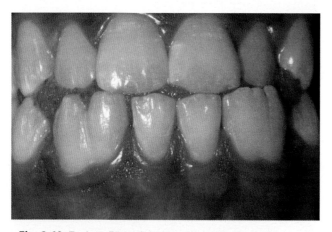

• **Fig. 2.60 Fusion.** Bilateral double teeth in the place of the mandibular lateral incisors and cuspids.

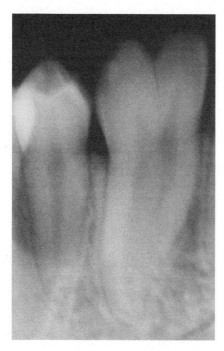

• **Fig. 2.61 Fusion.** Radiograph of the same patient depicted in Fig. 2.60. Note the bifid crown overlying the single root canal; the contralateral radiograph revealed a similar pattern.

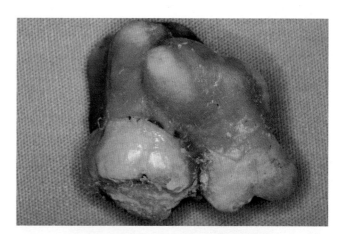

• **Fig. 2.62 Concrescence.** Union by cementum of adjacent maxillary molars.

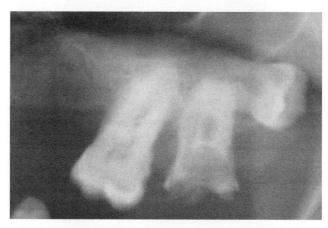

• **Fig. 2.63 Concrescence.** Union by cementum of maxillary second and third molars. Note the large carious defect of the second molar.

eruption of the permanent teeth should be monitored closely by careful clinical and radiographic observation. When appropriate, extraction may be necessary to prevent an abnormality in eruption. Occasionally, fusion in the primary dentition is associated with absence of the underlying permanent successor.

Several approaches are available for the treatment of joined teeth in the permanent dentition, and the treatment of choice is determined by the patient's particular needs. Cone beam computed tomography (CBCT) often proves beneficial during treatment planning due to its ability to define the level of the tooth union, the number of the roots, and the anatomy of the involved pulp chambers and canals more clearly. In gemination, if the double teeth have separate pulps, hemisection may be successful without root canal therapy. The separation may be done intraorally or require extraction with extraoral sectioning if the union extends close to the apex. If extraction is necessary, immediate (within 5 minutes) replantation of the desirable half may result in preservation of vitality and long-term survival of the tooth. In double teeth that share a common pulp, endodontic therapy is necessary if sectioning is considered. Selected shaping with or without placement of full crowns has been used in many cases. Other patients exhibit pulpal or coronal anatomic features that are resistant to reshaping and require surgical removal with prosthetic replacement. Double teeth often will demonstrate a pronounced labial or lingual groove that may be prone to develop caries. In such cases, placement of a fissure sealant or composite restoration is appropriate if the tooth is to be retained.

Patients with concrescence often require no therapy unless the union interferes with eruption; then surgical removal may be warranted. Post-inflammatory concrescence must be kept in mind whenever extraction is planned for nonvital teeth with apices that overlie the roots of an adjacent tooth. Significant extraction difficulties can be experienced on attempted removal of a tooth that is unexpectedly joined to its neighbor. Surgical separation often is required to complete the procedure without loss of a significant portion of the surrounding bone.

ACCESSORY CUSPS

The cuspal morphology of teeth exhibits minor variations among different populations; of these, three distinctive patterns deserve further discussion: (1) **cusp of Carabelli,** (2) **talon cusp,** and (3) **dens evaginatus.** When an accessory cusp is present, the other permanent teeth often exhibit a slightly increased tooth size.

Clinical and Radiographic Features

Cusp of Carabelli

The **cusp of Carabelli** is an accessory cusp located on the palatal surface of the mesiolingual cusp of a maxillary molar (Fig. 2.65). The cusp may be seen in the permanent or deciduous dentitions and varies from a definite cusp to a small indented pit or fissure. When present, the cusp is most pronounced on the first molar and is increasingly less obvious on the second and third molars. When a cusp of Carabelli is present, the remaining permanent teeth often are larger than normal mesiodistally, but a similar association in deciduous tooth size typically is not noted. A significant variation exists among different populations, with the prevalence reported to be as high as 90% in whites and rare in Asians. An analogous accessory cusp is seen occasionally on the mesiobuccal cusp of a mandibular permanent or deciduous molar and is termed a *protostylid.*

Talon Cusp

A **talon cusp** is a well-delineated additional cusp that is located on the surface of an anterior tooth and extends at least half the distance from the cementoenamel junction to

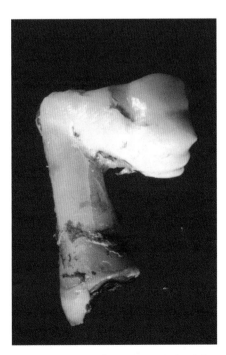

• **Fig. 2.64 Concrescence.** Gross photograph of the same teeth depicted in Fig. 2.63. Histopathologic examination revealed that union occurred in the area of cemental repair previously damaged by a periapical inflammatory lesion.

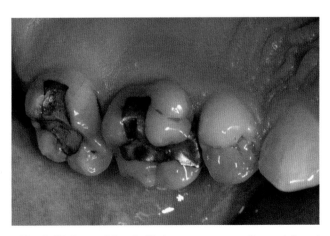

• **Fig. 2.65 Cusp of Carabelli.** Accessory cusp on the mesiolingual surface of the maxillary first molar.

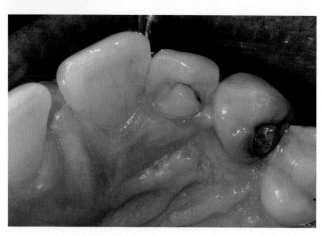

• **Fig. 2.66 Talon Cusp.** Accessory cusp present on the palatal surface of a maxillary lateral incisor. (Courtesy of Dr. S. Gabrielle Shuler).

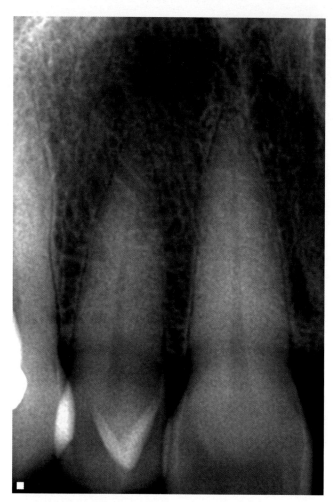

• **Fig. 2.67 Talon Cusp.** Radiograph of same patient shown in Fig. 2.66. Note the enamel and dentin layers within the accessory cusp. (Courtesy of Dr. Gabrielle Shuler).

the incisal edge. A talon cusp is thought to represent the end of a continuum that extends from a normal cingulum, to an enlarged cingulum, to a small accessory cusp, and, finally, to a full-formed talon cusp. Investigators have muddied the literature associated with this spectrum by categorizing all enlarged cingula as talon cusps and developing a classification system for the degree of enlargement. These classification systems make prevalence data difficult to evaluate and should be discouraged.

Three-fourths of all reported talon cusps are located in the permanent dentition. The cusps predominantly occur on permanent maxillary lateral (55%) or central (33%) incisors but have been seen less frequently on mandibular incisors (6%) and maxillary canines (4%) (Fig. 2.66). Their occurrence in the deciduous dentition is very rare, with the vast majority noted on maxillary central incisors. In almost all cases, the accessory cusp projects from the lingual surface of the affected tooth and forms a three-pronged pattern that resembles an eagle's talon. On rare occasions, the cusp may project from the facial surface or from both surfaces of a single tooth. A deep developmental groove may be present where the cusp fuses with the underlying surface of the affected tooth. Most, but not all, talon cusps contain a pulpal extension. Radiographically, the cusp is seen overlying the central portion of the crown and includes enamel and dentin (Fig. 2.67). Only a few cases demonstrate visible pulpal extensions on dental radiographs.

Talon cusps appear to occur more frequently in Asians, Native Americans, the Inuit, and those of Arab descent. Both sexes may be affected, and the occurrence may be unilateral or bilateral. In isolated cases, genetic influences appear to have an effect, because identical talon cusps occasionally have been documented in twins. Talon cusps also have been seen in patients with Rubinstein-Taybi syndrome, Mohr syndrome, Ellis-van Creveld syndrome, incontinentia pigmenti achromians, Berardinelli-Seip syndrome, and Sturge-Weber angiomatosis. Although the strength of association between the presence of talon cusps and these syndromes generally is not clear, Rubinstein-Taybi syndrome is correlated strongly

as demonstrated by a study of 45 affected patients in which 92% demonstrated talon cusps.

Dens Evaginatus

Dens evaginatus (central tubercle, tuberculated cusp, accessory tubercle, occlusal pearl, evaginated odontome, Leong premolar, tuberculated premolar) is a cusplike elevation of enamel located in the central groove or lingual ridge of the buccal cusp of premolar or molar teeth (Fig. 2.68). Although this pattern of accessory cusps has been reported on molars, dens evaginatus typically occurs on premolar teeth, usually is bilateral, and demonstrates a marked mandibular predominance. Deciduous molars are affected infrequently. The accessory cusp normally consists of enamel and dentin, with pulp present in about half of the cases. Although the prevalence is variable, most reviews suggest a frequency between 1% and 4%. The anomaly is encountered most frequently in Asians, the Inuit, and Native Americans but is rare in whites. Researchers expect an increased prevalence of this anomaly in the United States secondary to immigration by Asians and by Hispanics of mestizo heritage (i.e., those of mixed European and Native American ancestry). Radiographically, the occlusal surface exhibits a

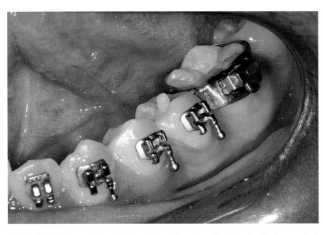

• **Fig. 2.68 Dens Evaginatus.** Cusplike elevation located in the central groove of mandibular second bicuspid. (Courtesy of Dr. Jason Latham).

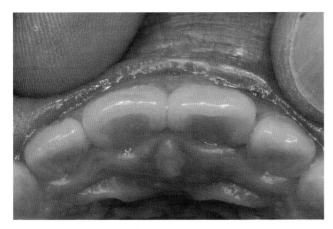

• **Fig. 2.69 Shovel-Shaped Incisors.** Chinese patient exhibiting maxillary incisors with prominent lateral margins, which create a hollowed lingual surface.

cusp-like structure often with a pulpal extension. The accessory cusp frequently creates occlusal interferences that are associated with significant clinical problems. In one large study, more than 80% of the tubercles were worn or fractured, with pulpal pathosis noted in more than 25% of patients. Pulpal necrosis is common and may occur through a direct exposure or invasion of patent, immature dentinal tubules. In addition to abnormal wear and pulpal pathosis, the accessory cusp also may result in dilaceration, displacement, tilting, or rotation of the tooth.

Frequently, dens evaginatus is seen in association with another variation of coronal anatomy, **shovel-shaped incisors.** This alteration also occurs predominantly in Asians, with a very high prevalence also noted in Native Americans and the Inuit. Affected incisors demonstrate prominent lateral margins, creating a hollowed lingual surface that resembles the scoop of a shovel (Fig. 2.69). Typically, the thickened marginal ridges converge at the cingulum; not uncommonly, a deep pit, fissure, or dens invaginatus is found at this junction. Maxillary lateral and central incisors most frequently are affected, with mandibular incisors and canines less commonly reported.

Treatment and Prognosis

Patients with cusps of Carabelli require no therapy unless a deep groove is present between the accessory cusp and the surface of the mesiolingual cusp of the molar. These deep grooves should be sealed to prevent carious involvement.

Patients with talon cusps on mandibular teeth often require no therapy; talon cusps on maxillary teeth frequently interfere with occlusion and should be removed. Other complications include compromised aesthetics, displacement of teeth, caries, periodontal problems, and irritation of the adjacent soft tissue (e.g., tongue or labial mucosa). Because many of these cusps contain pulp, rapid removal often results in pulpal exposure. Cone beam computed tomography (CBCT) can be used to determine the extent of pulp tissue within the cusp and assist in treatment planning. Often, removal without the loss of vitality may be accomplished through periodic grinding of the cusp, with time allowed for tertiary dentin deposition and pulpal recession. Successful reduction may be achieved with three visits spaced 6–8 weeks apart. At the end of each grinding session, the exposed dentin should be coated with a desensitizing agent such as fluoride varnish, which also may speed the rate of pulpal recession. Even with slow reduction and no direct pulp exposure, loss of vitality is possible when large numbers of immature dentin tubules are exposed. After successful removal of the cusp, the exposed dentin can be covered with calcium hydroxide, the peripheral enamel etched, and a composite resin placed. Alternatively, for large talon cusps or those with significant pulp tissue, the cusp can be removed in a single session with an intentional partial pulpotomy being performed in an attempt to maintain long-term vitality of the tooth.

On eruption, the affected tooth should be inspected for the presence of a deep fissure at the junction between the talon cusp and the surface of the tooth. If a fissure is present, it should be restored to avoid early carious extension into the nearby dental pulp. Reports also have documented the continuation of this fissure down the surface of the root, with subsequent development of lateral radicular inflammatory lesions secondary to the access provided to oral flora by the deep groove. In these latter cases, further surgery is required to expose the groove for appropriate cleansing.

Dens evaginatus typically results in occlusal problems and often leads to pulpal death. In affected teeth, removal of the cusp often is indicated, but attempts to maintain vitality have met with only partial success. Slow, periodic grinding of the cusp exposes immature patent dentinal tubules and may lead to irreversible pulpitis without direct exposure. To reduce the chance of pulpal pathosis, elimination of opposing occlusal interferences combined with removal of minimal dentin and treatment of the area with stannous fluoride has been recommended. More rapid cuspal removal with indirect or direct pulp capping also has proven beneficial in some patients. Other investigators support removal of occlusal interferences, protection of the cusp from fracture by the placement of surrounding resin reinforcement, and delaying cuspal removal until evidence of significant dentinal maturation, pulpal recession, and apical root closure are present.

If pulpal necrosis occurs in a tooth with an immature open apex, regenerative endodontic procedures can be employed to induce apical growth and promote increased thickness of the radicular dentinal walls. Another option for necrotic teeth with an immature open apex is revascularization. In this technique, the purulent pulp tissue is removed with sodium hypochlorite irrigation, placement of antimicrobial agents, and no use of endodontic instruments. Over several appointments, the necrotic tissue is eliminated and replaced with healing vascular pulp tissue. When the tooth is asymptomatic without evidence of continued infection, a ceramic cement plug (such as mineral trioxide aggregate) is placed over the top of the healing radicular pulp tissue with the access cavity restored with a glass ionomer cement and composite resin.

Shovel-shaped incisors should be inspected for surface defects at the point where the marginal ridges converge. Any deep fissures or invaginations should be restored shortly after eruption to prevent carious exposure of the adjacent pulp.

DENS INVAGINATUS (DENS IN DENTE)

Dens invaginatus is a deep surface invagination of the crown or root that is lined by enamel. Oehlers described this condition thoroughly in three classic articles published from 1957 to 1958. Two forms, coronal dens invaginatus and radicular dens invaginatus, are recognized. By a great margin, coronal dens invaginatus is seen more frequently.

Clinical and Radiographic Features
Coronal Dens Invaginatus

The reported prevalence of coronal dens invaginatus varies from 0.04% to 10% of all patients. In order of decreasing frequency, the teeth affected most often include the permanent lateral incisors, central incisors, premolars, canines, and molars. Involvement of deciduous teeth has been reported but is uncommon. A strong maxillary predominance is seen.

The crown of the affected tooth often will demonstrate clinical changes that suggest the need for radiographs to confirm the presence of an enamel-lined invagination. Suggestive clinical findings include a palatal pit or groove, a barrel or cone-shaped tooth, a crown that is dilated in comparison to the contralateral tooth, localized microdontia, a talon cusp, dens evaginatus, or a coronal labial groove.

The depth of the invagination varies from a slight enlargement of the cingulum pit to a deep infolding that extends to the apex. As would be expected, before eruption, the lumen of the invagination is filled with soft tissue similar to the dental follicle (i.e., reduced enamel epithelium with a fibrous connective tissue wall). On eruption, this soft tissue loses its vascular supply and becomes necrotic.

Historically, coronal dens invaginatus has been classified into three major types (Fig. 2.70). Type I exhibits an

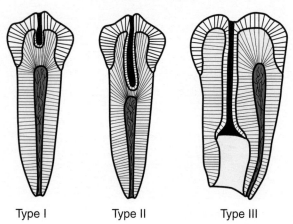

Coronal dens invaginatus

Type I   Type II   Type III

• **Fig. 2.70 Dens Invaginatus.** Illustration depicting the three types of coronal dens invaginatus.

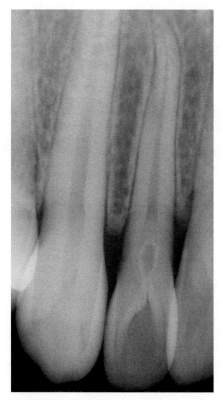

• **Fig. 2.71 Coronal Dens Invaginatus Type II.** Maxillary lateral incisor exhibiting invagination of the surface enamel that extends below the cementoenamel junction.

invagination that is confined to the crown. The invagination in type II extends below the cementoenamel junction and ends in a blind sac (Figs. 2.71 and 2.72). Large invaginations may become dilated and contain dystrophic enamel in the base of the dilatation (Fig. 2.73). In some cases, the enamel lining of the invagination is incomplete, and channels communicate between the invagination and the pulp. These connections can result in pulpal necrosis long before the apex has closed. Type III extends through the root and perforates in

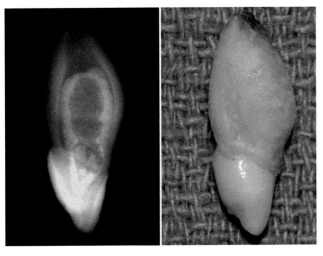

• **Fig. 2.72 Coronal Dens Invaginatus Type II. A,** Bulbous maxillary cuspid exhibiting a dilated invagination lined by enamel. **B,** Gross photograph demonstrating bulbous root and coronal notch.

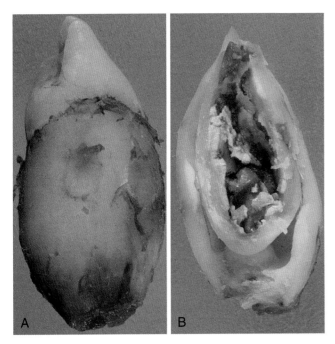

• **Fig. 2.73 Coronal Dens Invaginatus Type II.** Gross photograph of a sectioned tooth. Note the dilated invagination with apical accumulation of dystrophic enamel.

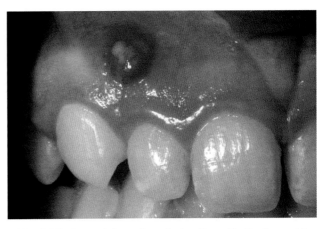

• **Fig. 2.74 Coronal Dens Invaginatus Type III.** Parulis overlying vital maxillary cuspid and lateral incisor. The cuspid contained a dens invaginatus that perforated the mesial surface of its root.

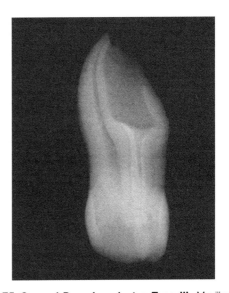

• **Fig. 2.75 Coronal Dens Invaginatus Type III.** Maxillary cuspid exhibiting an enamel invagination that parallels the pulp canal and perforates the lateral root surface. (Courtesy of Dr. Brian Blocher.)

the apical or lateral radicular area without any immediate communication with the pulp. In this latter type, the enamel that lines the invagination is often replaced by cementum close to the radicular perforation. This perforation provides direct communication from the oral cavity to the intraosseous periradicular tissues and often produces inflammatory lesions in the presence of a vital pulp (Figs. 2.74 and 2.75). Type I is by far the most common pattern (79%) followed by type II (15%) and type III (5%).

Occasionally, the invagination may be rather large and resemble a tooth within a tooth; hence the term **dens in dente.** In other cases, the invagination may be dilated and

disturb the formation of the tooth, resulting in anomalous tooth development termed **dilated odontome** (Fig. 2.76). Involvement may be singular, multiple, or bilateral.

Radicular Dens Invaginatus

Radicular dens invaginatus is rare and thought to arise secondary to a proliferation of Hertwig root sheath, with the formation of a strip of enamel that extends along the surface of the root. This pattern of enamel deposition is similar to that frequently seen in association with radicular **enamel pearls** (see Ectopic Enamel, page 90). Rather than protrude from the surface (as seen in an enamel pearl), the altered enamel forms a surface invagination into the dental papilla. Cementum-lined invaginations of the root have been reported, but these represent a simple variation of root morphology and should not be included under the term *radicular dens invaginatus.*

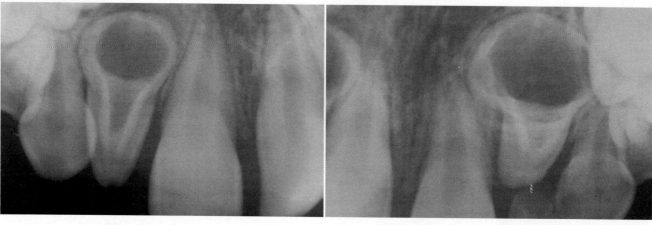

• **Fig. 2.76 Coronal Dens Invaginatus Type II.** Bilateral dilated dens invaginatus (dilated odontome) of the maxillary lateral incisors. (Courtesy of Dr. Mary Haigler).

Radiographically, the affected tooth demonstrates an enlargement of the root. Close examination often reveals a dilated invagination lined by enamel, with the opening of the invagination situated along the lateral aspect of the root.

Treatment and Prognosis

In small type I invaginations, the opening of the invagination should be restored after eruption in an attempt to prevent carious involvement and subsequent pulpal inflammation. If the invagination is not detected quickly, then pulpal necrosis frequently results. With larger type II invaginations, the contents of the lumen and any carious dentin must be removed; then a calcium hydroxide base may be placed to help treat any possible microcommunications with the adjacent pulp. In cases with obvious pulpal communication or signs of pulpal pathosis, both the invagination and the adjacent pulp canal require endodontic therapy. In teeth with open apices, regenerative endodontic procedures are recommended to obtain continued apexification.

Type III invaginations associated with periradicular inflammatory lesions require endodontic-like therapy of the perforating invagination. Once again, before final obturation with gutta-percha, temporary placement of calcium hydroxide helps to build dentinal bridges and maintain vitality of the adjacent pulp. If vitality is lost, endodontic therapy of the parallel root canal also becomes necessary. Some cases do not respond to conservative endodontic therapy and require periapical surgery and retrofill. Large and extremely dilated invaginations often have abnormal crowns and need to be extracted. Cone beam computed tomography (CBCT) has proven to be most beneficial in defining the complex anatomy of the invagination and the adjacent pulp, improving the accuracy of treatment planning decisions.

Among the few reported cases of true radicular dens invaginatus, the significantly altered anatomy has necessitated extraction in the vast majority.

ECTOPIC ENAMEL

Ectopic enamel refers to the presence of enamel in unusual locations, mainly the tooth root. The most widely known are **enamel pearls,** which are located on the external surface of the root apical to and separated from the cemento-enamel junction. Three patterns are seen: (1) *true enamel pearls* consisting entirely of enamel, (2) *composite pearls* demonstrating a core of dentin covered by enamel, and (3) *"E-D-P" pearls* containing enamel, dentin, and pulp. The vast majority of enamel pearls are the composite type. Instead of creating exophytic globes, ectopic enamel also may invaginate into the underlying radicular cementum and dentin, resulting in the extremely rare radicular form of dens invaginatus (see page 89).

In addition to enamel pearls, **cervical enamel extensions** also occur along the surface of dental roots. These extensions are thought to be more common than enamel pearls and represent a dipping of the enamel from the cementoenamel junction toward the bifurcation of molar teeth. This pattern of ectopic enamel forms a triangular extension of the coronal enamel that develops on the buccal surface of molar teeth directly overlying the bifurcation. The base of the triangle is continuous with the inferior portion of the coronal enamel; the leading point of the triangle extends directly toward the bifurcation of the tooth. These areas of ectopic enamel have been called *cervical enamel projections,* but this terminology is confusing because no significant exophytic projections are seen.

Clinical and Radiographic Features
Enamel Pearls

Enamel pearls usually develop on the roots of the maxillary permanent molars followed in prevalence by the mandibular permanent molars. Premolars and incisors rarely are affected. Involvement of deciduous molars has been reported but also is rare. The reported prevalence of enamel pearls varies (0.23%–4.82% of all patients) according to the population studied and is highest in Asians. In most cases, one pearl is found, but as many as four pearls have been documented on a single tooth. The majority occur on the roots at the furcation area or near the cementoenamel junction (Fig. 2.77). Radiographically, pearls appear as well-defined, radiopaque nodules along the root's surface (Fig. 2.78). Although they can be confused with dental calculus, cone beam computed tomography (CBCT) easily resolves this dilemma.

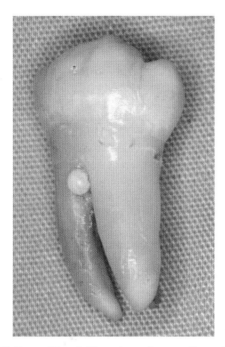

• **Fig. 2.77 Enamel Pearl.** Mass of ectopic enamel located in the furcation area of a molar tooth. (Courtesy of Dr. Joseph Beard.)

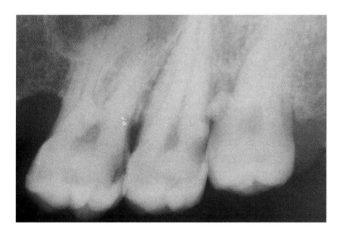

• **Fig. 2.78 Enamel Pearl.** Radiopaque nodule on the mesial surface of the root of the maxillary third molar. Another less distinct enamel pearl is present on the distal root of the second molar.

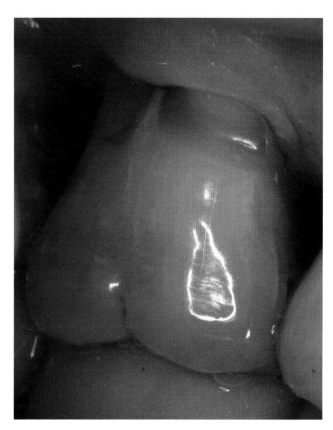

• **Fig. 2.79 Cervical Enamel Extension.** Flat V-shaped extension of enamel into the bifurcation of a maxillary molar. (Courtesy of Dr. Keith Lemmerman.)

The enamel surface of pearls precludes normal periodontal attachment with connective tissue, and a hemidesmosomal junction probably exists. This junction is less resistant to breakdown; once separation occurs, rapid loss of attachment is likely. In addition, the exophytic nature of the pearl is conducive to plaque retention and inadequate cleansing.

Cervical Enamel Extensions

As mentioned previously, **cervical enamel extensions** are located on the buccal surface of the root overlying the bifurcation (Fig. 2.79). Mandibular molars are affected slightly more frequently than maxillary molars. In reviews of extracted teeth in the lower 48 United States, the prevalence is surprisingly high, with approximately 20% of molars being affected. Similar studies demonstrate an even greater prevalence in other locations, such as Japan, China, and Alaska,

with cervical enamel extensions discovered in 50%–78% of extracted molars. Cervical enamel extensions may occur on any molar, but they are seen less frequently on third molars. Because connective tissue cannot attach to enamel, these extensions have been correlated positively with localized loss of periodontal attachment with furcation involvement. On review of a large number of dentitions with periodontal furcation involvement, a significantly higher frequency of cervical enamel extensions was found compared with dentitions without furcation involvement. In addition, the greater the degree of cervical extension, the higher the frequency of furcation involvement.

In addition to periodontal furcation involvement, cervical enamel extensions have been reported to be associated with the development of inflammatory cysts that are histopathologically identical to inflammatory periapical cysts. The cysts develop along the buccal surface over the bifurcation and most appropriately are called **buccal bifurcation cysts** (see page 704). The association between cervical enamel extensions and this unique inflammatory cyst is controversial.

Treatment and Prognosis

When enamel pearls are detected radiographically, most are incidental findings that require no therapy. Despite this, the area should be viewed as a weak point of periodontal attachment. Meticulous oral hygiene should be maintained in an effort to prevent localized loss of periodontal support and exposure of the enamel mass. If an enamel pearl becomes exposed and removal is contemplated, then the clinician must remember that the projection occasionally contains vital pulp tissue.

For teeth with cervical enamel extensions and associated periodontal furcation involvement, therapy is directed at achieving a more durable attachment and providing access to the area for appropriate cleaning. Reports have suggested that flattening or removing the enamel in combination with an excisional new attachment procedure and furcation plasty may accomplish this.

TAURODONTISM

Taurodontism is an enlargement of the body and pulp chamber of a multirooted tooth, with apical displacement of the pulpal floor and bifurcation of the roots. This pattern of molar formation was described initially by Keith in 1913 and has been found in earlier forms of prehistoric man such as the ancient Neanderthals. The morphologic pattern was termed taurodont due to its overall shape that resembles the molar teeth of cud-chewing animals (*tauro* = bull; *dont* = tooth).

Clinical and Radiographic Features

Affected teeth tend to be rectangular and exhibit pulp chambers with a dramatically increased apico-occlusal height and a bifurcation close to the apex (Fig. 2.80). The diagnosis usually is made subjectively from the radiographic appearance. The degree of taurodontism has been classified into *mild* (**hypotaurodontism**), *moderate* (**mesotaurodontism**), and *severe* (**hypertaurodontism**), according to the degree of apical displacement of the pulpal floor (Fig. 2.81). Witkop and colleagues and Shifman and Chanannel presented useful biometric criteria for the determination of taurodontism. These reports contain information that is useful in epidemiologic studies of the process.

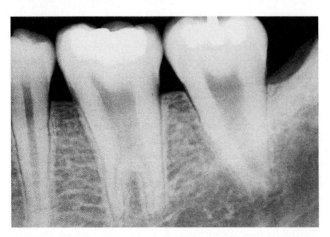

• **Fig. 2.80 Taurodontism.** Mandibular molar teeth exhibiting increased pulpal apico-occlusal height with apically positioned pulpal floor and bifurcation. (Courtesy of Dr. Michael Kahn.)

Patients with taurodonts often will demonstrate one or more additional molars with completely fused roots and a solitary enlarged canal. This developmental pattern is termed **pyramidal molars**. Some investigators believe taurodont molars represent an intermediate pattern on the continuum between normal and pyramidal molars.

Some authors include examples of taurodontism in premolar teeth; others argue that taurodontism is not shown by premolars. This argument is academic because the presence of taurodontism in premolars cannot be documented in situ. Investigations of taurodontism in premolar teeth require the examination of extracted teeth, because the necessary radiographs must depict the tooth in a mesiodistal orientation.

Taurodontism may be unilateral or bilateral and affects permanent teeth more frequently than deciduous teeth. There is no sex predilection. The reported prevalence is highly variable (0.5%–46%) and most likely is related to different diagnostic criteria and racial variations. In the United States, most reports indicate a prevalence of 2.5%–3.2% of the population. Some investigators believe the alteration is more of a variation of normal rather than a definitive pathologic anomaly. The process often demonstrates a field effect with the involvement of all molars. When this occurs, the first molar is usually affected least with increasing severity noted in the second and third molars, respectively.

Taurodontism may occur as an isolated trait or as a component of various syndromes (Box 2.10). An increased frequency of taurodontism has been reported in patients with hypodontia, cleft lip, and cleft palate. Investigations have shown that taurodontism may develop in the presence of any one of a large number of different genetic alterations. These findings suggest that chromosomal abnormalities may disrupt the development of the tooth's form and that taurodontism is not the result of a specific genetic abnormality.

Treatment and Prognosis

Patients with taurodontism require no specific therapy. Coronal extension of the pulp is not seen; therefore, the process does not interfere with routine restorative procedures. Some investigators have suggested the taurodontic shape may exhibit decreased stability and strength as an abutment tooth in prosthetic procedures due to decreased root surface area, but this hypothesis has not been verified. If endodontic therapy is required, the shape of the pulp chamber and the apically positioned pulpal floor frequently increase the difficulty of locating, instrumenting, and obturating the pulp canals. In addition, the presence of supernumerary roots and canals mandates careful exploration of all orifices and chamber grooves, with magnification being highly beneficial. Cone beam computed tomography (CBCT) has proven to be particularly useful in defining the highly variable canal morphologies encountered in taurodonts. One bit of good news is that patients have to demonstrate significant periodontal destruction before bifurcation involvement occurs.

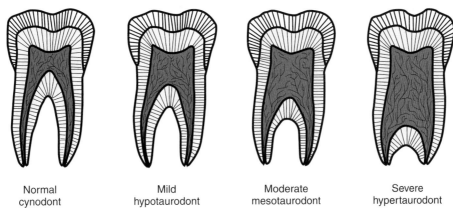

| Normal cynodont | Mild hypotaurodont | Moderate mesotaurodont | Severe hypertaurodont |

• **Fig. 2.81 Taurodontism.** Illustration exhibiting the classification of taurodontism according to the degree of apical displacement of the pulpal floor.

• **BOX 2.10   Syndromes Associated With Taurodontism**

- Amelogenesis imperfecta, hypoplastic type IE
- Amelogenesis imperfecta-taurodontism type IV
- Cranioectodermal dysplasia
- Down syndrome
- Ectodermal dysplasia
- Ellis-van Creveld syndrome
- Hyperphosphatasia-oligophrenia-taurodontism
- Hypophosphatasia
- Klinefelter syndrome
- Lowe syndrome
- Microcephalic dwarfism-taurodontism
- Microdontia-taurodontia-dens invaginatus
- Oculo-dento-digital dysplasia
- Oral-facial-digital syndrome type II
- Rapp-Hodgkin syndrome
- Scanty hair-oligodontia-taurodontia
- Sex chromosomal aberrations (e.g., XXX, XYY)
- Tricho-dento-osseous syndrome types I, II, and III
- Tricho-onycho-dental syndrome
- Wolf-Hirschhorn syndrome

• **BOX 2.11   Factors Associated With Hypercementosis**

Local Factors
- Abnormal occlusal trauma
- Adjacent inflammation (e.g., pulpal, periapical, periodontal)
- Unopposed teeth (e.g., impacted, embedded, without antagonist)
- Repair of vital root fracture

Systemic Factors
- Acromegaly and pituitary gigantism
- Arthritis
- Calcinosis
- Paget disease of bone
- Rheumatic fever
- Thyroid goiter
- Gardner syndrome
- Vitamin A deficiency (possibly)

HYPERCEMENTOSIS

Hypercementosis (cemental hyperplasia) is a nonneoplastic deposition of excessive cementum that is continuous with the normal radicular cementum.

Hypercementosis has been reported in association with a wide variety of disorders, Box 2.11 lists several of the most commonly mentioned local and systemic factors that have been associated with an increased frequency of the excessive cemental deposition. All of the listed systemic factors exhibit a weak association with hypercementosis except for **Paget disease of bone** (see page 628). Numerous authors have reported significant hypercementosis in patients with Paget disease, and this disorder should be considered whenever generalized hypercementosis is discovered in a patient of the appropriate age. Most localized cases of hypercementosis are not related to any systemic disturbance.

Clinical and Radiographic Features

Hypercementosis may be isolated, involve multiple teeth, or appear as a generalized process. The condition most frequently affects premolars and permanent molars with a mandibular predominance. Involvement of the deciduous dentition and permanent canines and incisors is uncommon.

Hypercementosis typically is identified in adults, and the frequency increases with age, which is most likely secondary to cumulative exposure to causative influences. Its occurrence has been reported in younger patients, and many of these cases demonstrate a familial clustering, suggesting hereditary influence.

Radiographically, affected teeth demonstrate a thickening or blunting of the root, but the exact amount of increased cementum often is difficult to ascertain because cementum and dentin demonstrate similar radiodensities (Figs. 2.82 and 2.83). The enlarged root is surrounded by the radiolucent PDL space and the adjacent intact lamina dura. On occasion, the enlargement may be significant enough to suggest the possibility of a cementoblastoma (see page 659). However, the

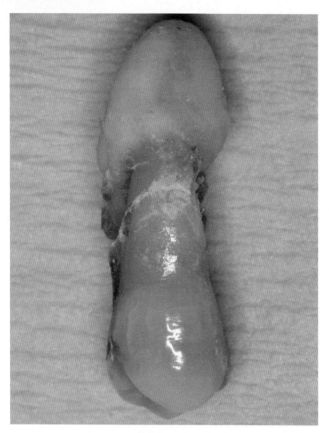

• **Fig. 2.82 Hypercementosis.** Gross photograph of a maxillary bicuspid that exhibits thickening and blunting of the apical portion of the root. (Courtesy of Dr. David Hicklin.)

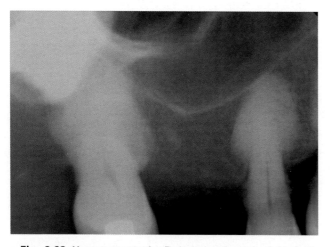

• **Fig. 2.83 Hypercementosis.** Periapical radiograph of the tooth depicted in Fig. 2.82. Note the radiopaque enlargement of the apical portion of the tooth. (Courtesy of Dr. David Hicklin.)

cementoblastoma usually can be distinguished on the basis of age (75% arise under the age of 30 years), associated pain, cortical expansion, and continued enlargement.

Histopathologic Features

The periphery of the root exhibits deposition of an excessive amount of cementum over the original layer of primary cementum. The excessive cementum may be hypocellular

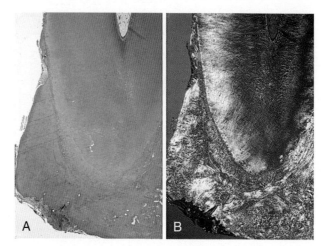

• **Fig. 2.84 Hypercementosis. A,** Dental root exhibiting excessive deposition of cellular and acellular cementum. The dividing line between dentin and cementum is indistinct. **B,** Polarized light demonstrating the sharp dividing line between the tubular dentin and osteocementum.

or exhibit areas of cellular cementum that resemble bone (osteocementum). Often the material is arranged in concentric layers and may be applied over the entire root or be limited to the apical portion. On routine light microscopy, distinguishing between dentin and cementum often is difficult, but viewing the section with polarized light helps to discriminate between the two different layers (Fig. 2.84).

Treatment and Prognosis

Patients with hypercementosis require no treatment. Because of a thickened root, occasional problems have been reported during the extraction of an affected tooth. Sectioning of the tooth may be necessary in certain cases to aid in removal. In addition, hypercementosis has been shown to alter the anatomy of the apical foramen and can complicate endodontic procedures.

DILACERATION

Dilaceration is an abnormal angulation or bend in the root or, less frequently, the crown of a tooth (Figs. 2.85 and 2.86). A large number of dilacerations present as idiopathic developmental alterations, predominantly in the posterior dentition. In addition, a number of teeth with dilaceration appear to arise after an injury that displaces the calcified portion of the tooth germ, and the remainder of the tooth is formed at an abnormal angle. Injury-related dilaceration more frequently affects the anterior dentition and often creates both a functional and a cosmetic dental problem. Less frequently the bend develops secondary to the presence of an adjacent anatomic structure, cyst, tumor, or odontogenic hamartoma (e.g., odontoma, supernumerary tooth) (Fig. 2.87).

Clinical and Radiographic Features

Dilacerations secondary to trauma usually arise following avulsion or intrusion of the overlying deciduous tooth and primarily affect the maxillary incisors. Dilaceration of the

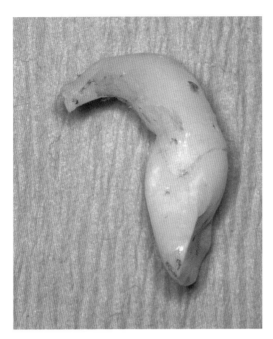

• **Fig. 2.85 Dilaceration.** Sharp curvature of the root of a maxillary central incisor.

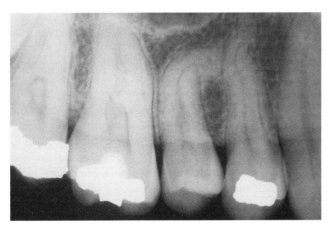

• **Fig. 2.86 Dilaceration.** Maxillary second bicuspid exhibiting mesial inclination of the root. The patient reported no history of injury to this area. (Courtesy of Dr. Lawrence Bean.)

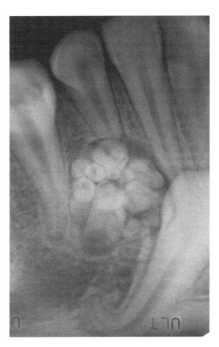

• **Fig. 2.87 Dilaceration.** Root angulation of a mandibular cuspid. Development has been altered by the presence of an adjacent compound odontoma. (Courtesy of Dr. Brent Bernard.)

crown is noted more frequently if the trauma occurs prior to the age of three, whereas radicular bends are associated with traumatic events occurring during the later years of tooth development. The maxillary central incisors are the most common teeth to demonstrate crown dilacerations, followed by the mandibular incisors. Impaction of the affected tooth occurs in approximately 50% of these cases.

Regarding dilacerated teeth not associated with trauma, the most commonly affected are mandibular third molars, followed by the maxillary second premolars and mandibular second molars. Although many reviews report a higher frequency of dilacerations in anterior teeth, the molars most likely demonstrate the highest prevalence but are not highlighted because of a lack of associated clinical problems in most instances. Occasionally, involvement of the deciduous teeth is reported, and some have been associated with prior trauma secondary to neonatal laryngoscopy and endotracheal intubation. Several publications have mentioned an increased prevalence associated with several syndromes, including Smith-Magenis syndrome, variants of Ehlers-Danlos syndrome, Axenfeld-Rieger syndrome, and congenital ichthyosis.

Dilaceration usually is radiographically obvious if the bend occurs in a mesial or distal direction. Roots that bend facially or lingually may be more difficult to detect. Often, the apical portion of these teeth will demonstrate a round increased radiodensity with a central radiolucent dark spot that correlates to the root canal of the bent tooth. The dilacerated portion of the root often may demonstrate a radiolucent halo that represents the associated periodontal ligament. Cone beam computed tomography (CBCT) has been shown to be vastly superior to plain films due to its ability to accurately depict the exact position of the tooth, the extent of root formation, and the degree of dilaceration.

Treatment and Prognosis

The treatment and prognosis vary according to the severity of the deformity. Altered deciduous teeth often demonstrate inappropriate resorption and result in delayed eruption of the permanent teeth. Extraction is indicated when necessary for the normal eruption of the succedaneous teeth. Patients with minor dilaceration of permanent teeth frequently require no therapy. Those teeth that exhibit delayed or abnormal eruption may be exposed and orthodontically moved into position. The possibility that orthodontic movement of severely dilacerated teeth may result in severe external root resorption must be considered during treatment planning. In some cases with extensive deformation of the affected tooth, perforation of the buccal alveolar ridge by the malpositioned root may occur on repositioning. In such cases, amputation of the root apex with subsequent endodontic therapy may be necessary. Grossly deformed teeth require surgical removal. The extraction of affected teeth may be difficult and result in root fracture on removal. When attempting to perform endodontic procedures, the clinician must use great care to avoid root perforation of teeth with significant dilaceration.

Root dilaceration concentrates stress if the affected tooth is used as an abutment for a dental prosthetic appliance. This increased stress may affect the stability and longevity of the abutment tooth. Splinting of the dilacerated tooth to an adjacent tooth results in a multirooted abutment and overcomes the stress-related problems.

SUPERNUMERARY ROOTS

The term **supernumerary roots** refers to the development of an increased number of roots on a tooth compared with that classically described in dental anatomy.

Clinical and Radiographic Features

Any tooth may develop accessory roots, and involvement has been reported in both the deciduous and the permanent dentitions. Data on the frequency of supernumerary roots are sparse, but the prevalence appears to vary significantly among different races. The most frequently affected teeth are the permanent molars (especially third molars) from either arch and mandibular cuspids and premolars (Fig. 2.88). In some instances, the supernumerary root is divergent and seen easily on radiographs; in other cases, the additional root is small, superimposed over other roots, and difficult to ascertain.

Treatment and Prognosis

No treatment is required for supernumerary roots, but the detection of the accessory root is of critical importance when endodontic therapy or exodontia is undertaken. Extracted teeth always should be examined closely to ensure that all roots have been removed successfully, because accessory roots may not be obvious on the presurgical radiographs. Just as important is the search for accessory canals during endodontic access procedures, because failure to discover these additional openings often results in a lack of resolution of the associated inflammatory process.

GLOBODONTIA

Otodental syndrome is a rare autosomal dominant disorder characterized by a distinctive pattern of dental malformation termed **globodontia** in association with high-frequency sensorineural hearing loss. This condition is thought to be due to haploinsufficiency of *FGF3*, which is localized at chromosome 11q13. Although both globodontia and hearing loss usually are present, variable expressivity is seen, with some family members exhibiting only hearing loss and others revealing globodontia without hearing loss.

Clinical and Radiographic Features

Both the deciduous and permanent dentitions are affected with the cuspids and molars demonstrating dramatically enlarged and bulbous crowns (Figs. 2.89 and 2.90). The normal cusp and groove anatomy of the molars is replaced by numerous developmental grooves that radiate from a central depression onto the facial, lingual, and proximal surfaces, resulting in an occlusal surface that has been described as resembling the *tied end of a sausage*. The canines are distorted similarly, often with three large bulbous projections separated by shallow grooves. The premolars often are missing or reduced in size; when present, they may demonstrate

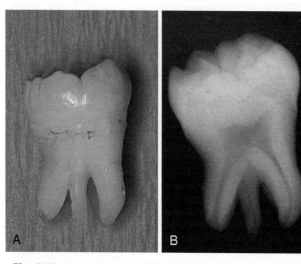

• **Fig. 2.88 Supernumerary Root. A,** Gross photograph showing a mandibular molar with a supernumerary root. **B,** Periapical radiograph of the extracted tooth.

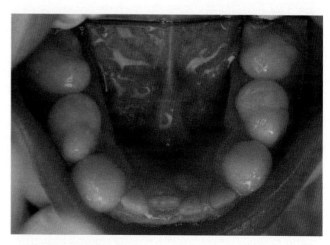

• **Fig. 2.89 Globodontia.** Dentition demonstrating clinically normal anterior teeth and posterior teeth with enlarged bulbous crowns. Patient had undiagnosed hearing loss that was discovered following identification of otodental syndrome by dentist. (Courtesy of Dr. John Eric Yezerski.)

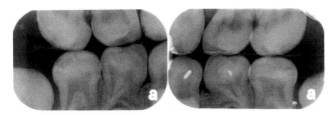

• **Fig. 2.90 Globodontia.** Bite-wing radiographs demonstrating posterior teeth with bulbous crowns and complex pulpal anatomy. (Courtesy of Dr. John Eric Yezerski.)

normal anatomy or appear conical. The incisors are unaffected and exhibit normal size and shape. The globodont roots are short, and the pulp chambers often appear bisected with vertical septa and occasional pulp stones. Focal areas of yellow coronal hypomaturation may occur, especially on the facial surfaces of the canines. In a number of patients, complex odontomas also have been noted. Delayed eruption of both dentitions frequently is seen.

The onset of the hearing loss varies from early childhood to middle age, but it often begins in infancy and progresses to a plateau in the fourth decade. A loss of approximately 65db is noted at all frequencies but is more pronounced at about 1000 Hz. In most patients, the hearing loss usually arises prior to the age of 20 years.

Treatment and Prognosis

Due to the grossly distorted anatomy, misalignment of the teeth and malocclusion are frequent problems. The bulbous molars have deep fissures that are prone to dental caries, stressing the need for regular professional dental care with preventive procedures such as topical fluorides and dental sealants. If an affected tooth develops dental caries, routine dental restorative treatment can be provided. Endodontic therapy can be very challenging in the molar teeth due to the complexity of the pulpal anatomy. Patients also have a propensity to develop endodontic-periodontic lesions, possibly due to the abnormal coronal and pulpal configuration.

LOBODONTIA

Lobodontia refers to a rare hereditary dental anomaly in which numerous teeth resemble those noted in carnivores. The term is derived from *lobo*, the Spanish word for wolf that arose from the Latin word *lupus*. The abnormality is extremely rare and is inherited as an autosomal dominant trait.

Clinical and Radiographic Features

The most distinctive features are the cuspids and premolars, which demonstrate pointed fang-like tritubercular cusps (Fig. 2.91). The middle of the three lobes of the cuspid crowns are conical with the lateral lobes being dramatically reduced. The premolars demonstrate prominent cone-shaped buccal cusps, often with diminutive lingual cusps.

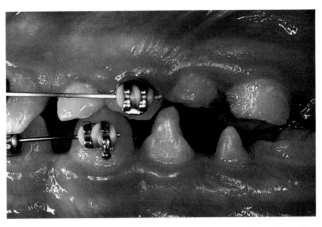

• **Fig. 2.91 Lobodontia.** Premolar demonstrating pointed fang-like cusps.

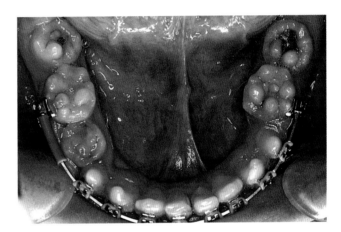

• **Fig. 2.92 Lobodontia.** Mandibular molars demonstrating a multitubercular appearance.

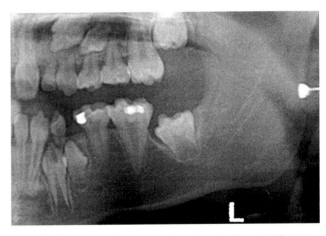

• **Fig. 2.93 Lobodontia.** Panoramic radiograph demonstrating pyramidal molars and tritubercular cusps on the premolars and cuspids.

The occlusal anatomy of the molars also is altered significantly and demonstrates a multitubercular appearance (Fig. 2.92). The molar roots are pyramidal with a single fused canal (Fig. 2.93). The incisors often are shovel-shaped with a prominent cingulum or shallow dens invaginatus. Hypodontia is common, most frequently involving the maxillary second premolars followed by the mandibular second premolars.

Treatment and Prognosis

Thorough radiographic examination is prudent to discover and restore teeth with dens invaginatus prior to devitalization. The abnormal occlusal cusps of the multitubercular molars often cause the same problems that are seen with dens evaginatus with traumatic occlusion, attrition, or fracture predisposing to loss of pulp vitality. Although definitive treatment has not been described, composite reinforcement of the prominent cusps may reduce cuspal damage and allow time for pulpal recession from the coronal protuberances.

♦ DEVELOPMENTAL ALTERATIONS IN THE STRUCTURE OF TEETH

AMELOGENESIS IMPERFECTA

Amelogenesis imperfecta (AI) encompasses a complicated group of conditions that demonstrate developmental alterations in the structure of the enamel in the absence of a systemic disorder or syndrome. Box 2.1 (see page 52) lists several systemic diseases associated with enamel disorders that are not considered isolated amelogenesis imperfecta. Although the definition of amelogenesis imperfecta excludes any association with a syndrome, a number of other dental anomalies are accepted within the spectrum of the disease: pulpal calcification, taurodontism, delayed eruption, gingival overgrowth, open-bite malocclusion, and rarely prognathism.

The formation of enamel is a multistep process, and problems may arise in any one of the steps. In general, the development of enamel can be divided into three major stages:
1. Secretory phase
2. Transition phase
3. Maturation phase

Enamel formation begins with secretion of a protein matrix in which immature hydroxyapatite crystals are deposited. The protein matrix subsequently is degraded and replaced almost completely with inorganic hydroxyapatite. During the secretory phase, the soft protein matrix is deposited. During the transition phase, the matrix deposition achieves the thickness of the final enamel, and the ameloblasts begin to undergo alterations that support the upcoming maturation of the enamel. In the final maturation stage, the protein matrix is degraded into a tissue fluid by proteases as the ameloblasts transport mineral ions into the fluid, leading to the growth of enamel crystals. During this time, the enamel becomes progressively more mineralized until the initial protein matrix is removed almost completely.

The nonsyndromic hereditary defects of the enamel formation are divided into two major patterns: hypoplastic, and hypomineralized. **Hypoplastic amelogenesis imperfecta** is characterized by inadequate deposition of the enamel matrix, which leads to deficient enamel development in the form of surface pits to thinned enamel to complete absence of enamel. **Hypomineralized amelogenesis imperfecta** presents with enamel of normal thickness that is weak and breaks down more rapidly. This pattern can be further subdivided into two presentations: **hypomaturation amelogenesis imperfecta** (characterized by incomplete protein removal resulting in brittle enamel) and **hypocalcified amelogenesis imperfecta** (characterized by insufficient calcium deposition leading to soft enamel that can be removed easily). Use of this classification often is problematic since clinical application of the terminology can be difficult due to mixed phenotypes.

An ideal classification system for amelogenesis imperfecta has not been established yet. Witkop's classification (Table 2.1) remains the most widely accepted and relies on the phenotype (clinical appearance) and the inheritance

TABLE 2.1	Classification of Amelogenesis Imperfecta		
Type	Pattern	Specific Features	Inheritance
IA	Hypoplastic	Generalized pitted	Autosomal dominant
IB	Hypoplastic	Localized pitted	Autosomal dominant
IC	Hypoplastic	Localized pitted	Autosomal recessive
ID	Hypoplastic	Diffuse smooth	Autosomal dominant
IE	Hypoplastic	Diffuse smooth	X-linked dominant
IF	Hypoplastic	Diffuse rough	Autosomal dominant
IG	Hypoplastic	Enamel agenesis	Autosomal recessive
IIA	Hypomaturation	Diffuse pigmented	Autosomal recessive
IIB	Hypomaturation	Diffuse	X-linked recessive
IIC	Hypomaturation	Snow-capped	X-linked
IID	Hypomaturation	Snow-capped	Autosomal dominant?
IIIA	Hypocalcified	Diffuse	Autosomal dominant
IIIB	Hypocalcified	Diffuse	Autosomal recessive
IVA	Hypomaturation-hypoplastic	Taurodontism present	Autosomal dominant
IVB	Hypoplastic-hypomaturation	Taurodontism present	Autosomal dominant

Modified from Witkop CJ Jr.: Amelogenesis imperfecta, dentinogenesis imperfecta and dentin dysplasia revisited: problems in classification, *J Oral Pathol* 17:547–553, 1988.

pattern. Classification by clinical appearance is problematic, because different phenotypes have been noted within a single affected family. In addition, similar phenotypes may be seen in individuals with very different molecular patterns of disease.

Although the molecular basis underlying many patterns of amelogenesis imperfecta remains poorly defined, the genetics associated with several variations of amelogenesis imperfecta has been clarified. This has led investigators to suggest a future classification system based primarily on the mode of inheritance with secondary discriminators that include the phenotype, molecular genetic basis (site and type of chromosomal mutation, when known), and the biochemical result (protein affected, when known). Although much remains to be discovered, the information necessary for this new

classification system is accumulating rapidly, with movement to this new pattern of classification being inevitable.

Whole-genome sequencing (WGS) and whole-exome sequencing (WES) are being replaced by next-generation sequencing (NGS), which has better molecular coverage, a cheaper cost, and greater ease in interpreting the results. NGS has benefitted researchers interested in amelogenesis imperfecta. During the time between the fourth and fifth editions of this text, the number of well-recognized altered genes associated with nonsyndromic AI increased from 7 to 16. Almost certainly, the number will continue to increase as NGS becomes a more standardized tool in research and clinical practice.

Table 2.2 attempts to associate these mutations with their associated phenotypic presentations.

TABLE 2.2 Modified Classification of Amelogenesis Imperfecta

Related Genes	Inheritance	Phenotype
AMELX	X-linked recessive	Heterozygous females: stripes of normal and affected enamel; Males: hypomaturation or diffuse smooth hypoplastic
ENAM	Autosomal dominant	Diffuse smooth hypoplastic
ENAM	Autosomal dominant	Localized hypoplastic
ENAM	Autosomal recessive	Homozygotes: Diffuse hypoplastic; Heterozygotes: Localized hypoplastic
AMBN	Autosomal recessive	Diffuse hypoplastic
MMP20	Autosomal recessive	Diffuse hypomaturation
KLK4	Autosomal recessive	Diffuse hypomaturation
ITGB6	Autosomal recessive	Hypomineralized/pitted hypoplastic
ITGB6	Autosomal recessive	Diffuse rough hypoplastic
LAMA3	Autosomal recessive Heterozygous carriers	Diffuse hypoplastic
LAMA3	Autosomal recessive Heterozygous carriers	Hypoplastic with grooving and pits
LAMB3	Autosomal recessive Heterozygous carriers	Diffuse hypoplastic
LAMB3	Autosomal recessive Heterozygous carriers	Hypoplastic with grooving and pits
COL17A1	Autosomal recessive Heterozygous carriers	Diffuse hypoplastic
AMTN	Autosomal dominant	Diffuse hypomineralized
FAM83H	Autosomal dominant	Diffuse hypocalcified
WDR72	Autosomal recessive	Diffuse hypomaturation
SLC24A4	Autosomal recessive	Hypomaturation/hypomineralized
GPR68	Autosomal recessive	Diffuse hypomineralized
C4orf26	Autosomal recessive	Diffuse hypomineralized
ACPT	Autosomal recessive	Diffuse hypoplastic
FAM20A	Autosomal recessive	Diffuse hypoplastic/enamel agenesis
DLX3	Autosomal dominant	Hypomaturation/hypoplastic with taurodontism

The altered genes may be grouped into those that affect enamel proteins (*AMELX, ENAM, AMBN*), enamel matrix proteases (*MMP20, KLK4*), cell-cell and cell-matrix adhesion (*ITGB6, LAMA3, LAMB3, COL17A1, AMTN, FAM83H*), matrix or ion transport (*WDR72, SLC24A4*), pH sensing (*GPR68*), crystal nucleation (*C4orf26*), control of gene expression (*FAM20A, DLX3*) and genes with unknown function (*ACPT*). In a study over 270 families with AI, just four genes were responsible for over 60% of all cases: *FAM83H, FAM20A, ENAM,* and *AMELX.*

Several genes deserve additional comment. *LAMA3, LAMB3,* and *COL17A1* are associated with autosomal recessive junctional epidermolysis bullosa. Heterozygous carriers sometimes have AI without evidence of any skin alterations, whereas the homozygous individuals would present with skin lesions and not be included in the nonsyndromic patterns of AI. Additionally, different mutations of *FAM20A* have been shown to cause not only AI but also gingival fibromatosis (see page 158) and enamel renal syndrome. Finally, various mutations of *DLX3* can cause nonsyndromic AI or tricho-dento-osseous syndrome (see page 103).

Clinical and Radiographic Features

Amelogenesis imperfecta may be inherited as an autosomal dominant, autosomal recessive, or X-linked disorder, with both the deciduous and the permanent dentitions diffusely involved in the vast majority. Due to differing gene pools, the rate of occurrence varies geographically with a prevalence of 1:700 in Sweden and a frequency in the United States of 1:14,000.

Hypoplastic Amelogenesis Imperfecta

In patients with hypoplastic amelogenesis imperfecta, the basic alteration centers on inadequate deposition of enamel matrix. Any matrix present is mineralized appropriately and radiographically contrasts well with the underlying dentin. In the **generalized pattern,** pinpoint-to-pinhead–sized pits are scattered across the surface of the teeth and do not correlate with a pattern of environmental damage (Fig. 2.94). The buccal surfaces of the teeth are affected more severely, and the pits may be arranged in rows or columns. Staining of the pits may occur. Variable expressivity is seen within groups of affected patients. The enamel between the pits is of normal thickness, hardness, and coloration.

In the **localized pattern,** the affected teeth demonstrate horizontal rows of pits, a linear depression, or one large area of hypoplastic enamel. Typically, the altered area is located in the middle third of the buccal surfaces of the teeth. The incisal edge or occlusal surface usually is not affected. Both dentitions or only the primary teeth may be affected. All of the teeth may be altered or only scattered teeth may be affected. When the involvement is not diffuse, the pattern of affected teeth does not correlate with a specific time in development. The autosomal recessive type is more severe and typically demonstrates involvement of all teeth in both dentitions.

In Witkop's phenotypic classification, amelogenesis imperfecta with diffusely reduced enamel thickness was subclassified as *smooth, rough,* and *enamel agenesis.* For many researchers, this separation is difficult in various kindreds; therefore, these phenotypic patterns have been merged by many into one category, **generalized thin hypoplastic amelogenesis imperfecta.**

In the **generalized thin variants,** the enamel is extremely thin with teeth that are shaped like crown preparations and demonstrate open contact points. The surface texture varies from smooth with or without shallow grooves to rough with or without scattered pits (Figs. 2.95 and 2.96). The color of the teeth varies from opaque white to yellow to brown. Anterior open bite is not rare. Radiographically, a thin peripheral outline of radiopaque enamel will be noted on many teeth. Often, unerupted teeth exhibiting resorption are seen.

The X-linked patterns of generalized thin amelogenesis imperfecta are a lesson in the lyonization effect. On approximately the sixteenth day of embryonic life in all individuals with two X chromosomes, one member of the pair is

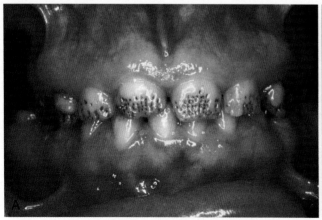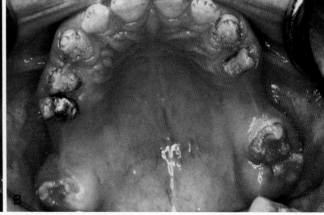

• **Fig. 2.94 Hypoplastic Amelogenesis Imperfecta, Generalized Pitted Pattern. A,** Note the numerous pinpoint pits scattered across the surface of the teeth. The enamel between the pits is of normal thickness, hardness, and coloration. **B,** Occlusal view of same patient showing diffuse involvement of all maxillary teeth, which would be inconsistent with environmental damage. (**A,** From Stewart RE, Prescott GH: *Oral facial genetics,* St Louis, 1976, Mosby. **B,** Courtesy of Dr. Joseph S. Giansanti.)

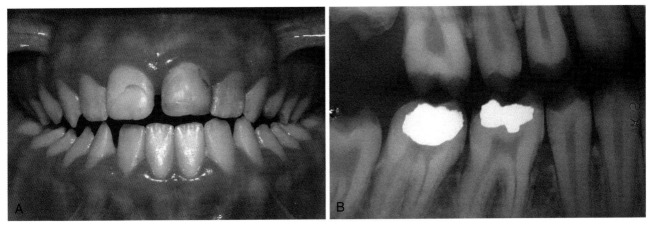

• **Fig. 2.95 Hypoplastic Amelogenesis Imperfecta, Autosomal Dominant Smooth Pattern (Generalized Thin Pattern). A,** Small, yellowish teeth exhibiting hard, glossy enamel with numerous open contact points and anterior open bite. **B,** Radiograph of the same patient demonstrating thin peripheral outline of radiopaque enamel. (**B,** Courtesy of Dr. John G. Stephenson.)

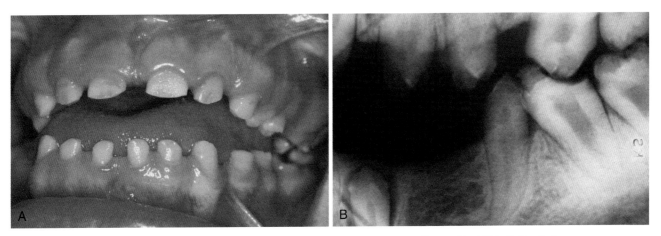

• **Fig. 2.96 Hypoplastic Amelogenesis Imperfecta, Rough Pattern (Generalized Thin Pattern). A,** Small, yellow teeth with rough enamel surface, open contact points, significant attrition, and anterior open bite. **B,** Radiograph of the same patient. Note the impacted tooth and the thin peripheral outline of radiodense enamel.

inactivated in each cell. As a result of this event, females are mosaics, with a mixture of cells, some with active maternal X chromosomes and others with active paternal X chromosomes. Usually, the mix is of approximately equal proportions. If one X were to direct the formation of defective enamel and the other X were to form normal enamel, then the teeth would exhibit alternating zones of normal and abnormal enamel. Hemizygous males exhibit diffuse thin enamel in both dentitions. On the other hand, heterozygous females exhibit vertical furrows of thin hypoplastic enamel alternating between bands of normal thickness. The banding often is detectable with dental radiographs.

Hypomaturation and Hypocalcification Variants of Amelogenesis Imperfecta (Hypomineralization Amelogenesis Imperfecta)

Classically, the hypomaturation pattern is associated with enamel that chips and fractures easily but does not demonstrate massive loss upon eruption. In contrast, the hypocalcification pattern has been associated with "cheesy" enamel that is lost rapidly and diffusely except for a residual band in the cervical portion of the teeth. In reality, the distinction is hazy with a spectrum of enamel quality encountered. At the ends of the spectrum, the separation between hypomaturation and hypocalcification can be made easily; however, the center of the spectrum contains numerous patterns that are difficult to classify on a phenotypic basis. For this reason, many investigators prefer the term **hypomineralization amelogenesis imperfecta** for both variants.

Prior to eruption, both forms of hypomineralization AI radiographically demonstrate enamel of normal thickness with a radiodensity that is similar to dentin. In a person with **hypomaturation amelogenesis imperfecta,** the affected teeth are normal in shape but exhibit white opaque enamel that may reveal areas of mottling. Upon eruption, variable degrees of brown discoloration and enamel chipping are seen. The presentation may closely resemble dental fluorosis, making definitive diagnosis difficult in many patients. On

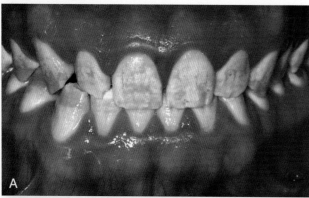

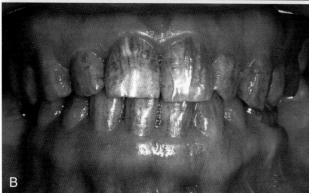

• **Fig. 2.97 Hypomaturation Amelogenesis Imperfecta, X-Linked. A,** Male patient exhibiting diffuse yellow-white dentition. **B,** The patient's mother exhibits vertical bands of white, opaque enamel and translucent enamel. (Courtesy of Dr. Carlos Salinas.)

occasion, fluorosis may demonstrate horizontal white banding that corresponds to periods of increased fluoride intake. If present, a chronological distribution also is helpful in interpreting the clinical appearance (such as sparing of the deciduous dentition or premolars and second molars [see Fig. 2.11, page 57]).

In the **pigmented hypomaturation pattern,** the surface enamel is mottled and agar-brown. The enamel often fractures from the underlying dentin and is soft enough to be punctured by a dental explorer. Anterior open bite and unerupted teeth exhibiting resorption are uncommon. Occasionally, the surface enamel may be affected severely and be similar in softness to that of hypocalcified patterns with rapid enamel loss upon eruption. These cases often demonstrate extensive calculus deposition. A combined hypomaturation and hypoplastic phenotype can be seen, but posteruption enamel loss can complicate classification.

The **X-linked hypomaturation pattern** is another lesson in lyonization; however, the lyonization is not as obvious as that seen in the X-linked hypoplastic pattern. Affected males exhibit different patterns in the deciduous and permanent dentitions. The deciduous teeth are opaque white with a translucent mottling, whereas the permanent teeth are opaque yellow and may darken with age (Fig. 2.97A). Heterozygous females exhibit a similar pattern in both dentitions. The teeth demonstrate vertical bands of white opaque enamel and translucent enamel; the bands are random and asymmetric (see

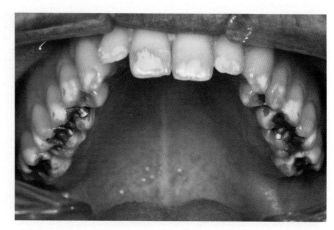

• **Fig. 2.98 Hypomaturation Amelogenesis Imperfecta, Snow-Capped Pattern.** Dentition exhibiting zone of white opaque enamel in the incisal and occlusal one-fourth of the enamel surface. (Courtesy of Dr. Heddie O. Sedano.)

Fig. 2.97B). The banding can be seen under regular lighting but is more obvious with transillumination.

The **snow-capped hypomaturation patterns** exhibit a zone of white opaque enamel on the incisal or occlusal one-quarter to one-third of the crown (Fig. 2.98). The altered areas do not exhibit a distribution that would support an environmental origin, and the surface lacks the iridescent sheen seen with mild fluorosis. The affected teeth often demonstrate an anterior-to-posterior distribution and have been compared with a denture dipped in white paint (only affected anteriors, the anteriors back to the bicuspids, or the anteriors back to the molars). Both the deciduous and the permanent dentitions are affected.

In **hypocalcified amelogenesis imperfecta,** the teeth are appropriately shaped on eruption, but the enamel is very soft and easily lost. On eruption, the enamel is yellow-brown or orange, but it often becomes stained brown to black and exhibits rapid calculus apposition (Fig. 2.99). With years of function much of the coronal enamel is removed, except for the cervical portion that is occasionally calcified better. Unerupted teeth and anterior open bite are not rare.

Amelogenesis Imperfecta with Taurodontism (Hypomaturation/Hypoplastic Amelogenesis Imperfecta)

This type of amelogenesis imperfecta exhibits enamel hypoplasia in combination with hypomaturation. The deciduous and the permanent dentitions are involved diffusely. Historically, two patterns have been recognized that are similar but differentiated by the thickness of the enamel and the overall tooth size. When studying a single kindred, phenotypic variation is seen that would place members of the same family in both divisions; therefore, many believe these divisions should be joined into one phenotype termed merely **amelogenesis imperfecta with taurodontism.**

In the presentation known as the **hypomaturation-hypoplastic pattern,** the predominant defect is one of enamel hypomaturation in which the enamel appears as

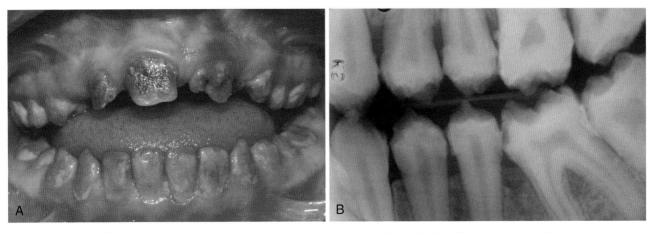

• **Fig. 2.99 Hypocalcified Amelogenesis Imperfecta. A,** Dentition exhibiting diffuse yellow-brown discoloration. Note numerous teeth with loss of coronal enamel except for the cervical portion. **B,** Radiograph of the same patient. Note the extensive loss of coronal enamel and the similar density of enamel and dentin.

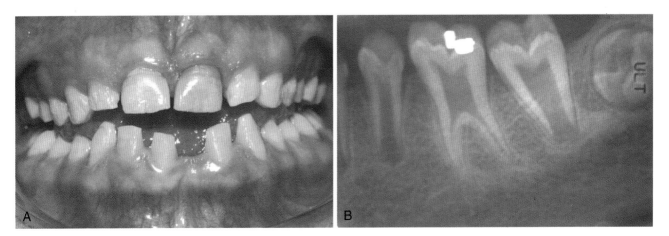

• **Fig. 2.100 Tricho-Dento-Osseous Syndrome. A,** Dentition exhibiting diffuse enamel hypoplasia and hypomaturation. At birth, the patient exhibited a kinky "steel wool" texture to her hair; with time, the hair straightened. A high index of suspicion was required to arrive at the diagnosis. **B,** Radiograph of the same patient showing significant taurodontism of the first molar and thin enamel, which is similar in density to the dentin.

mottled yellow-white to yellow-brown. Pits are seen frequently on the buccal surfaces of the teeth. Radiographically, the enamel appears similar to dentin in density, and large pulp chambers may be seen in single-rooted teeth in addition to varying degrees of taurodontism.

In the **hypoplastic-hypomaturation pattern,** the predominant defect is one of enamel hypoplasia in which the enamel is thin but also hypomature. Except for the decrease in the thickness of the enamel, this pattern is radiographically similar to the hypomaturation-hypoplastic variant.

A pattern of teeth alteration similar to amelogenesis imperfecta with taurodontism is seen in the systemic disorder, **tricho-dento-osseous syndrome.** This autosomal dominant disorder is mentioned here because the diagnosis may not be readily apparent without a high index of suspicion (Fig. 2.100). In addition to the dental findings, the predominant systemic changes are present variably and include kinky

hair, osteosclerosis, and brittle nails. The kinky hair is present at birth but may straighten with age. The osteosclerosis primarily affects the base of the skull and the mastoid process. The mandible often exhibits a shortened ramus and an obtuse angle.

Histopathologic Features

The histopathologic alterations present in amelogenesis imperfecta are not evident in routine preparations. Because decalcification of the teeth is necessary before processing to allow sectioning of paraffin-embedded specimens, all of the enamel is lost. To examine the enamel structure of altered teeth, ground sections of nondecalcified specimens are prepared. The alterations discovered are highly diverse and vary with each clinical type of amelogenesis imperfecta. Detailed descriptions of such alterations were provided by Witkop and Sauk.

Treatment and Prognosis

The clinical implications of amelogenesis imperfecta vary according to the subtype and its severity, but the main problems are aesthetics, dental sensitivity, and loss of vertical dimension. In addition, in some types of amelogenesis imperfecta there is an increased prevalence of caries, anterior open bite, delayed eruption, tooth impaction, or associated gingival inflammation.

Patients with generalized thin enamel hypoplasia demonstrate minimal normal enamel associated with rapid attrition. These variants require full coverage as soon as is practical; if the treatment is delayed, a loss of usable crown length occurs. In the deciduous dentition, stainless steel or composite crowns are appropriate, whereas all-ceramic materials are good choices for the permanent dentition. In young patients without sufficient crown lengths, full dentures (overdentures in some cases) often become the only satisfactory approach until the completion of skeletal growth allows placement of implant-supported prostheses.

The other types of amelogenesis imperfecta demonstrate less rapid tooth loss, and the aesthetic appearance often is the prime consideration. Many less severe cases can be improved by the placement of full crowns or facial veneers on cosmetically objectionable teeth. Problems with bonding restorations to the altered enamel may be overcome by the use of glass ionomer cements with dentinal adhesives.

Generalized delayed eruption and impaction of teeth affected by generalized thin hypoplastic amelogenesis imperfecta has been identified as a component of a very rare condition known as **enamel-renal syndrome** characterized by *FAM20A* mutations, nephrocalcinosis, and sometimes renal failure. The renal changes often are not clinically overt, and mortality associated with renal failure has been reported in affected patients. Such patients should be referred for renal evaluation.

HEREDITARY DISORDERS OF DENTIN

Hereditary disorders of dentin can occur in association with a number of syndromes or arise as an isolated disorder of teeth with no systemic manifestations. Osteogenesis imperfecta is the syndrome most frequently associated with dental manifestations that mimic dentinogenesis imperfecta, but Ehlers-Danlos syndrome, Goldblatt syndrome, and Schimke immuno-osseous dysplasia also have been associated with similar dental changes. In addition, sporadic reports of patients with dentinogenesis imperfecta–like alterations as part of an obviously systemic, but as yet undefined, syndrome have been noted. In addition to a dentinogenesis imperfecta–like phenotype, a variety of other dentin abnormalities have been noted in vitamin-D resistant rickets, vitamin-D dependent rickets, tumoral calcinosis, and calcinosis universalis. The following section concentrates on the nonsyndromic disorders of dentin.

Mature dentin is about 70% mineral, 20% organic matrix, and 10% water. About 85%–90% of the organic matrix is type I collagen, with two genes intimately involved in its production: *COL1A1* and *COL1A2*. The most abundant noncollagenous proteins in dentin are derived from dentin sialophosphoprotein (DSPP) that is cleaved to form three important dentin proteins: dentin sialoprotein (DSP), dentin glycoprotein (DGP), and dentin phosphoprotein (DPP). The primary gene guiding the formation of these proteins is the *DSPP* gene.

Dentinogenesis imperfecta (DGI) is a hereditary developmental disturbance of the dentin in the absence of any systemic disorder and has been shown to be associated with any one of 40 mutations of the *DSPP* gene. Similar dental changes can be seen in conjunction with the systemic hereditary disorder of bone, **osteogenesis imperfecta** (see page 618); but genetic studies have shown that the dental alterations are related to mutations in the *COL1A1* and *COL1A2* genes. Extensive pedigrees of individuals with DSPP-related dentinogenesis imperfecta have been studied, and none have exhibited other changes suggestive of osteogenesis imperfecta. This groundbreaking research has confirmed that osteogenesis imperfecta with opalescent teeth is clearly a separate disease from dentinogenesis imperfecta and should be removed from the classification of dentinogenesis imperfecta.

The classification of hereditary dentin disorders is much less complicated compared to the classification of amelogenesis imperfecta. However, the most widely used systems for classification of hereditary dentin disorders, one by Witkop and the other by Shields, remain widely is use, but in light of current knowledge, appear to be archaic (Table 2.3). Recent advances in genetics have made the Shields nomenclature problematic. The Online Mendelian Inheritance of Man (OMIM) database is the most current classification system for the molecular genetics of human pathoses. In the MIM system, dentinogenesis imperfecta type I as defined by the original Shield's classification (DGI-I) has been removed from the list of DGI and is classified appropriately as *osteogenesis imperfecta*. DGI-II has become DGI-I, whereas DGI-III and the dentin dysplasias (dentin dysplasia type I

TABLE 2.3	Dentinogenesis Imperfecta, Classical Nomenclature	
Shields	Clinical Presentation	Witkop
Dentinogenesis imperfecta I	Osteogenesis imperfecta with opalescent teeth	Dentinogenesis imperfecta
Dentinogenesis imperfecta II	Isolated opalescent teeth with pulpal obliteration	Hereditary opalescent teeth
Dentinogenesis imperfecta III	Isolated opalescent teeth with shell teeth	Brandywine isolate

Data from Shields ED: A new classification of heritable human enamel defects and a discussion of dentin defects. In Jorgenson RJ, Paul NW, editor: *Dentition: genetic effects (birth defects original article series)*, no 1, New York, 1983, Alan R Liss, pp. 107–127, vol 19; Witkop CJ Jr.: Amelogenesis imperfecta, dentinogenesis imperfecta and dentin dysplasia revisited: problems in classification, *J Oral Pathol* 17:547–553, 1988.

[DD-I] and dentin dysplasia type II [DD-II]) have retained their previous names. The Shields and OMIM systems currently are contradictory, resulting in confusion with respect to the definition of dentinogenesis imperfecta type I.

Dentinogenesis imperfecta formerly was divided into DGI-II (*hereditary opalescent dentin*) and DGI-III (*Brandywine isolate*). The defining phenotypic feature of the Brandywine isolate was the presence of unusual pulpal enlargement known as *shell teeth* with multiple pulp exposures seen primarily in the deciduous teeth. Current evidence has proven that DGI-III simply represents variable expression of dentinogenesis imperfecta. The original review of the isolate identified only 8% of the kindred with shell teeth. Investigators have documented enlarged pulps in affected individuals whose parents and children have classic dentinogenesis imperfecta. Identical patterns of expression also have been seen in other large kindreds with no connection to the Brandywine isolate. Finally, identical mutations of the *DSPP* gene have been shown to manifest as DGI-II and DGI-III in different families and in different members of the same family. It seems very clear that *dentinogenesis imperfecta type II* and *dentinogenesis imperfecta type III* represent a single disease with variable expressions.

The confusion does not end with DGI-II/III controversy. As mentioned, 40 different mutations of the *DSPP* gene have been discovered in patients of different ethnicities. Of these, 17 mutations affect the DSP region, whereas 23 variants involve the DPP region. No mutation of the DGP region has been discovered. In patients with DGI-II that are associated with mutation of DPP, the posterior region of the gene is altered. Numerous investigators have shown that DD-II arises from modification of the exact same gene but from alteration of the anterior region of the DPP. This clearly indicates that DD-II is allelic to DGI and not a separate disorder. With that understanding, DD-II, DGI-II, and DGI-III appear to represent a spectrum of the same disease, with DD-II being the mild end of the continuum and DGI-III representing the severe end. In a long overdue review of the outdated nomenclature systems, de La Dure-Molla proposed an updated classification system similar to the pattern utilized in the third edition of this text (Table 2.4). In this system, osteogenesis imperfecta with opalescent teeth is removed from the classification of dentinogenesis imperfecta, and the old DD-II, DGI-II, and DGI-III are designated as mild, moderate, and severe forms of DGI.

DENTIN SIALOPHOSPHOPROTEIN–ASSOCIATED DENTIN DEFECTS

Clinical and Radiographic Features

As the nomenclature of DSPP-associated dentin defects evolves, it is expected that the diseases will be listed in the order of phenotypic severity from the mildest to most severe (DD-II, DGI-II, and DGI-III). In spite of this, these disorders are described most efficiently when DGI-II is presented first.

TABLE 2.4	Modified Classification of Hereditary Disorders Affecting Dentin	
Shields	de La Dure-Molla	Involved Gene or Genes
Dentinogenesis imperfecta I	Osteogenesis imperfecta with opalescent teeth	COL1A1, COL1A2
• Dentin dysplasia type II • Dentinogenesis imperfecta II • Dentinogenesis imperfecta III	Dentinogenesis imperfecta • Mild form • Moderate form • Severe form	DSPP
Dentin dysplasia type I (DD-I)	Radicular dentin dysplasia	?? SMOC2, VPS4B, SSUH2

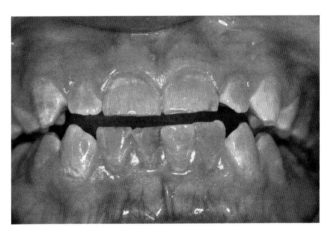

• **Fig. 2.101 Dentinogenesis Imperfecta (DGI), Moderate Form.** Dentition exhibiting diffuse brownish discoloration and slight translucence.

The prevalence of **dentinogenesis imperfecta** (hereditary opalescent dentin, Capdepont's teeth) is not distributed randomly throughout the United States and Europe. Most cases can be traced to whites (people of English or French ancestry) from communities close to the English Channel. The disorder is autosomal dominant and occurs in about 1:8000 whites in the United States. However, the condition is not limited to any race or geographic location.

Dentinogenesis imperfecta affects teeth in both dentitions with the severity of the dental alterations varying with the age at which the tooth develops. Deciduous teeth are affected most severely, followed by the permanent incisors and first molars, with the second and third molars being least altered.

The dentitions are discolored, often with a distinctive translucence (Fig. 2.101). The color varies from yellow-brown to light-brown to grayish-blue. Often, the color demonstrates minimal variation within a family but varies significantly among different families. The enamel fractures easily and frequently separates from the underlying defective

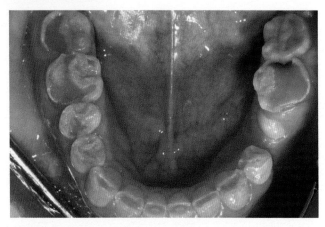

• **Fig. 2.102 Dentinogenesis Imperfecta (DGI), Moderate Form.** Dentition exhibiting grayish discoloration with significant enamel loss and attrition.

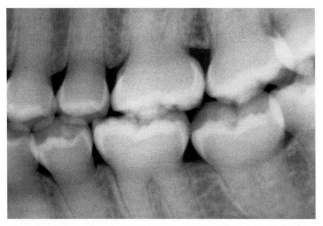

• **Fig. 2.103 Dentinogenesis Imperfecta (DGI), Moderate Form.** Radiograph of dentition exhibiting bulbous crowns, cervical constriction, and obliterated pulp canals and chambers.

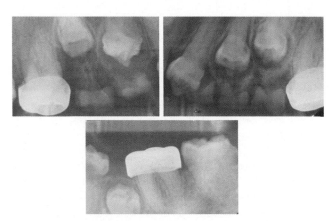

• **Fig. 2.104 Dentinogenesis Imperfecta (DGI), Severe Form.** Radiograph of dentition exhibiting bulbous crowns, early obliteration of the pulp, and enamel hypoplasia. (From Levin LS, Leaf SH, Jelmine RJ, et al: Dentinogenesis imperfecta in the Brandywine isolate (DI type III): clinical, radiologic, and scanning electron microscopic studies of the dentition, *Oral Surg Oral Med Oral Pathol* 56:267–274, 1983.)

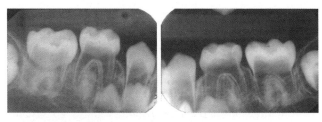

• **Fig. 2.105 Shell Teeth.** Dentition exhibiting normal thickness enamel, extremely thin dentin, and dramatically enlarged pulps.

dentin. Once exposed, the dentin often demonstrates significantly accelerated attrition (Fig. 2.102). Radiographically, the teeth have bulbous crowns, cervical constriction, and thin roots. In the **moderate form of DGI**, the pulp chambers and canals initially are very large but demonstrate rapid obliteration upon eruption (Fig. 2.103). Although the pulp appears totally obliterated, a network of interconnected vessels remains and can lead to periapical inflammatory disease when coronal vessels are invaded by bacteria in areas of exposed dentin. The deciduous teeth develop periapical inflammatory disease more often, possibly caused by advanced attrition secondary to thinner enamel.

The trait exhibits close to 100% penetrance but variable expressivity. Clinically obvious enamel hypoplasia is noted in some patients (Fig. 2.104). During the initial development of the dentinoenamel junction (DEJ), there is a temporary expression of enamel proteins by odontoblasts and a similar expression of dentin proteins by pre-ameloblasts. Some investigators have suggested that the enamel hypoplasia may be secondary to expression of mutant DSPP protein by preameloblasts during the early formative stage of the DEJ.

Although the pulps usually are obliterated by excess dentin production, the teeth in the **severe form of DGI** (shell teeth) demonstrate significant pulpal enlargement with normal-thickness enamel in association with extremely thin dentin and dramatically enlarged pulps (Fig. 2.105). The thin dentin may involve the entire tooth or be isolated to the root. Shell teeth have been seen most frequently in deciduous teeth in the setting of dentinogenesis imperfecta and the affected teeth often are associated with pulp exposures.

Shell teeth may be unassociated with dentinogenesis imperfecta as an isolated finding in both dentitions with normal tooth shape and coloration, a negative family history, and diffuse involvement. In this unrelated isolated variant, slow but progressive root resorption often occurs.

Several kindreds affected with dentinogenesis imperfecta also have been shown to demonstrate progressive, sensorineural, high-frequency hearing loss. Jaw position has been shown to affect the anatomy of the inner ear, and premature tooth loss has been associated with hearing deficits. At this time, it is unclear if the hearing loss is correlated with the *DSPP* mutation or represents an alteration secondary to the primary gnathic changes. All patients with dentinogenesis imperfecta should be evaluated for hearing loss.

The **mild form of Dentinogenesis imperfecta (dentin dysplasia type II; DD-II; coronal dentin dysplasia)** has dramatically different appearances in the primary and succedaneous dentitions. The primary teeth have a blue-

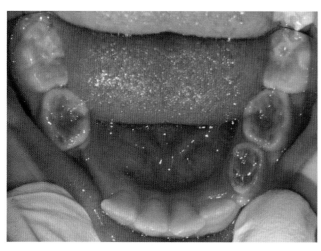

• **Fig. 2.106 Dentinogenesis Imperfecta, Mild Form.** Dentition demonstrating darkened and translucent deciduous molars in association with permanent incisors and first molars that appear clinically normal. (Courtesy of Dr. James Zettler.)

• **Fig. 2.108 Dentinogenesis Imperfecta (DGI).** Coronal dentin exhibiting short misshapen tubules within atypical granular dentin matrix.

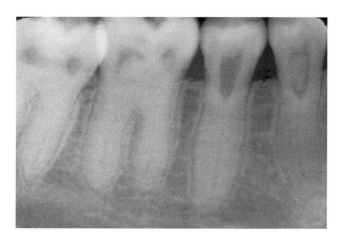

• **Fig. 2.107 Dentinogenesis Imperfecta, Mild Form.** Radiographic appearance of the permanent dentition exhibiting thistle tube–shaped enlargements of the pulp chambers and numerous pulp stones.

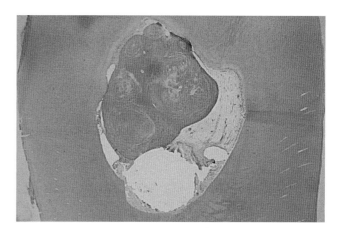

• **Fig. 2.109 Dentinogenesis Imperfecta, Mild Form.** Affected permanent tooth exhibiting large pulp stone within the pulp chamber.

to-amber-to-brown translucence, similar to classic dentinogenesis imperfecta (Fig. 2.106). Radiographically, the dental changes include bulbous crowns, cervical constriction, thin roots, and early obliteration of the pulp. The permanent teeth have a normal color clinically; however, radiographically, the pulp chambers exhibit significant enlargement and apical extension. These enlarged pulp chambers have been described as *thistle tube–shaped* or *flame-shaped* (Fig. 2.107). Pulp stones develop in the enlarged pulp chambers.

A similar but unrelated disorder is **pulpal dysplasia.** This process develops in teeth that are normal clinically. Radiographically, both dentitions exhibit thistle tube–shaped pulp chambers and multiple pulp stones.

Histopathologic Features

In dentinogenesis imperfecta, the dentin adjacent to the enamel junction appears similar to normal dentin, but the remainder is distinctly abnormal. Short misshapen tubules

course through an atypical granular dentin matrix, which often demonstrates interglobular calcification (Fig. 2.108). Scanty atypical odontoblasts line the pulp surface, and cells can be seen entrapped within the defective dentin. In ground sections the enamel is normal in most patients; however, about one-third of the patients have hypoplastic or hypocalcified defects.

In patients with the mild form of dentinogenesis imperfecta (formerly known as dentin dysplasia type II), the deciduous teeth demonstrate the same pattern noted in the moderate form. However, the permanent teeth exhibit normal enamel and coronal dentin. Adjacent to the pulp, numerous areas of interglobular dentin are seen. The radicular dentin is atubular, amorphous, and hypertrophic. Pulp stones develop in any portion of the chamber (Fig. 2.109).

Treatment and Prognosis

In dentinogenesis imperfecta, the entire dentition is at risk because of numerous problems. The root canals become threadlike and may develop microexposures, resulting in periapical inflammatory lesions. Despite the risk of enamel loss and significant attrition, the teeth often are not good candidates for full crowns because of cervical fracture. The success of full coverage is best in teeth with crowns and roots that exhibit close to a normal shape and size. Overlay dentures placed on teeth that are covered with fluoride-releasing glass ionomer cement have been used with success in some cases.

The success of therapy varies with the severity of the dental changes in individual patients. In those with extensive attrition, the vertical dimension can be rebuilt by placing nonprecious metal castings with adhesive luting agents on teeth that have received no preparation and are not subject to significant occlusal stress. The newer composites combined with a dentin-bonding agent have been used in areas subject to occlusal wear. When large kindreds have been followed over a long term, many of those affected are candidates for full dentures or implants by 30 years of age in spite of the numerous interventions. Newer materials and techniques may alter this outlook.

Deciduous teeth in the mild form of dentinogenesis imperfecta ("dentin dysplasia type II") can be approached in a manner similar to that described for the moderate form. Although not frequent, periapical inflammatory lesions have been seen in association with the permanent teeth of some affected patients. Because the pulp canals usually are not obliterated completely, endodontic therapy may be possible.

RADICULAR DENTIN DYSPLASIA (DENTIN DYSPLASIA TYPE I)

Dentin dysplasia was categorized initially in 1939. Historically, two major patterns have been described: type I (radicular dentin dysplasia; DD-I) and type II (coronal dentin dysplasia; DD-II). However, type II has been shown to be a variation of dentinogenesis imperfecta, and the discussion of this condition is included in the previous section. By definition, radicular dentin dysplasia should have no correlation with systemic disease. Systemic diseases reported to be associated with similar dentin changes are listed in Box 2.12.

The genetic changes associated with radicular dentin dysplasia currently are unsettled. Three separate investigations have reported different genes with diverse locations: *SMOC2* on 6q27 (autosomal recessive), *VPS4B* on 18q21.33 (autosomal dominant), and *SSUH2* on 3Q26.1 (autosomal dominant). Two possibilities exist: radicular dentin dysplasia exhibits genetic heterogeneity or several similar but different diseases exist. Subtle differences may be difficult to ascertain in diseases that are rare with so few cases to evaluate. In addition, the small image size in modern publications makes close inspection of these cases most difficult for researchers across the globe to interpret.

Clinical and Radiographic Features

Radicular dentin dysplasia (dentin dysplasia type I; DD-I); has been referred to as **rootless teeth,** because the loss of organization of the root dentin often leads to a shortened root length. Although an autosomal recessive example has been reported, the process typically exhibits an autosomal dominant pattern of inheritance and is one of the rarest forms of human dentin disorders with a prevalence of approximately 1:100,000. The enamel and coronal dentin are normal clinically and well formed (Fig. 2.110), but the radicular dentin loses all organization and subsequently is shortened dramatically (Fig. 2.111). Wide variation in root formation is produced because dentinal disorganization may occur during different stages of tooth development. If the dentin organization is lost early in tooth development,

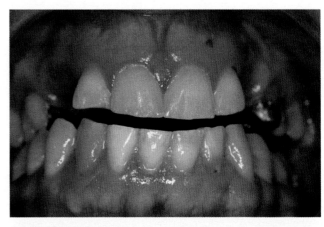

• **Fig. 2.110 Radicular Dentin Dysplasia.** Dentition exhibiting attrition but otherwise normal coronal coloration and morphology.

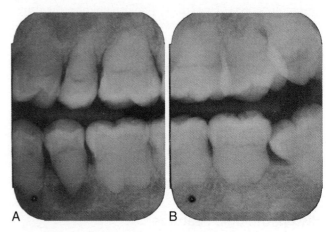

• **Fig. 2.111 Radicular Dentin Dysplasia.** Posterior dentition exhibiting dramatically shortened roots, absence of pulp canals, and small, crescent-shaped pulp chambers. Note radiolucency at apex of mandibular bicuspid. (Courtesy of Dr. Michael Quinn.)

• BOX 2.12 | **Systemic Diseases Correlated With Dentin Dysplasia-Like Alterations**

* Calcinosis universalis
* Rheumatoid arthritis and hypervitaminosis D
* Sclerotic bone and skeletal anomalies
* Tumoral calcinosis

markedly deficient roots are formed; later disorganization results in minimal root malformation. The variability is most pronounced in permanent teeth and may vary not only from patient to patient but also from tooth to tooth in a single patient. Because of the shortened roots, the initial clinical signs are extreme tooth mobility and premature exfoliation, spontaneously or secondary to minor trauma. Less frequently, delayed eruption is the presenting symptom. The strength of the radicular dentin is reduced, with the teeth being predisposed to fracture during extractions.

Radiographically, variations in radicular anatomy have been described, and a subclassification of radicular dentin dysplasia has been proposed (Box 2.13; Fig. 2.112). The deciduous teeth often are affected severely, with little or no detectable pulp, and roots that are markedly short or absent (similar to type DDIa). In most patients, the permanent teeth demonstrate short roots with no canals and a small crescent-shaped pulpal remnant parallel of the cementoenamel junction (types DDIb and DDIc). Type DDId is most unusual and should warn the clinician to rule out systemic diseases, such as tumoral calcinosis, that can produce identical changes.

• **BOX 2.13   Subclassification of Dentin Dysplasia Type I**

- DDIa: No pulp chambers, no root formation, and frequent periapical radiolucencies
- DDIb: A single small horizontally oriented and crescent-shaped pulp, roots only a few millimeters in length, and frequent periapical radiolucencies
- DDIc: Two horizontally oriented and crescent-shaped pulpal remnants surrounding a central island of dentin, significant but shortened root length, and variable periapical radiolucencies
- DDId: Visible pulp chambers and canals, near normal root length, enlarged pulp stones that are located in the coronal portion of the canal and create a localized bulging of the canal and root, constriction of the pulp canal apical to the stone, and few periapical radiolucencies

In general, the teeth without root canals are those that frequently develop periapical radiolucencies without obvious cause (see Fig. 2.111). The radiolucencies represent periapical inflammatory disease and appear secondary to caries or spontaneous coronal exposure of microscopic threads of pulpal remnants present within the defective dentin.

A similar but unrelated disorder is **fibrous dysplasia of dentin.** This autosomal dominant disorder exhibits teeth that are normal clinically. Radiographically the teeth are normal in shape but demonstrate a radiodense product filling the pulp chambers and canals. In contrast to dentinogenesis imperfecta, small foci of radiolucency can be seen in the pulp. Unlike radicular dentin dysplasia, no crescent pulp chambers or decrease in root length is seen. The radiodense intrapulpal material consists of fibrotic dentin.

Histopathologic Features

In patients with radicular dentin dysplasia, the coronal enamel and dentin are normal. Apical to the point of disorganization, the central portion of the root forms whorls of tubular dentin and atypical osteodentin. These whorls exhibit a peripheral layer of normal dentin, giving the root the appearance of a "stream flowing around boulders" (Fig. 2.113).

Treatment and Prognosis

In patients with radicular dentin dysplasia, preventive care is of foremost importance. Perhaps as a result of shortened roots, early loss from periodontitis is frequent. In addition, pulp vascular channels extend close to the dentinoenamel junction; therefore, even shallow occlusal restorations can result in pulpal necrosis. Meticulous oral hygiene must be established and maintained.

If periapical inflammatory lesions develop, the root length guides the therapeutic choice. Conventional endodontic therapy requires mechanical creation of canal paths and has been successful in teeth without extremely short roots. Teeth with short roots demonstrate pulpal ramifications that

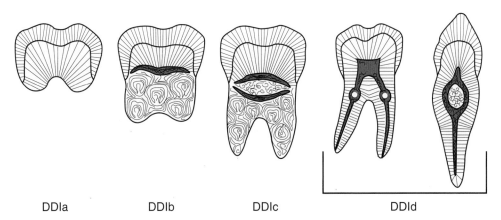

DDIa   DDIb   DDIc   DDId

• **Fig. 2.112 Radicular Dentin Dysplasia.** Illustration demonstrating the variability of the radiographic appearance according to the degree of dentin disorganization within the root.

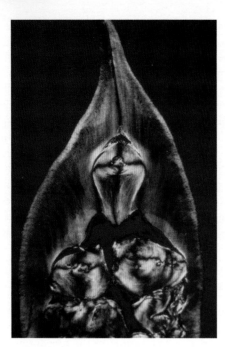

• **Fig. 2.113 Radicular Dentin Dysplasia.** Polarized light view of affected tooth demonstrating a classic "stream flowing around boulders" appearance.

• **BOX 2.14** **Pathoses Noted in Association With Regional Odontodysplasia**

- Ectodermal dysplasia
- Epidermal nevi
- Hydrocephalus
- Hypophosphatasia
- Ipsilateral facial hypoplasia
- Neurofibromatosis
- Orbital coloboma
- Rh factor incompatibility
- Vascular nevi

• **BOX 2.15** **Proposed Causations for Regional Odontodysplasia**

- Abnormal migration of neural crest cells
- Latent virus
- Local circulatory deficiency
- Local trauma or infection
- Hyperpyrexia
- Malnutrition
- Medication used during pregnancy
- Radiation therapy
- Somatic mutation

eliminate conventional endodontic treatment as an appropriate therapeutic option. Periapical curettage and retrograde amalgam seals have demonstrated short-term success. In patients with minimal root length, early tooth loss is typical and full dentures or implant-supported prostheses usually become necessary.

REGIONAL ODONTODYSPLASIA (GHOST TEETH)

Regional odontodysplasia is a localized, nonhereditary developmental abnormality of teeth with extensive adverse effects on the formation of enamel, dentin, and pulp. Most cases are idiopathic, but a number have been related to various syndromes, growth abnormalities, neural disorders, and vascular malformations (Box 2.14). A number of causes have been proposed (Box 2.15), but the most popular theory revolves around an alteration in the vascular supply. Several cases have occurred in patients with vascular nevi of the head and neck; in addition, similar changes have been induced in animals by restricting the vascular flow to an area of the jaws.

Clinical and Radiographic Features

Regional odontodysplasia is an uncommon finding that occurs in both dentitions and exhibits no racial predilection and a slight female predominance. A review of the age at the time of diagnosis reveals a bimodal peak that correlates with the normal time of eruption of the deciduous (2–4 years) and permanent (7–11 years) dentitions. Typically, the process affects a focal area of the dentition, with involvement of several contiguous teeth. A maxillary predominance exists with a predilection for the anterior teeth. Occasionally, an unaffected tooth may be intermixed within a row of altered teeth. Ipsilateral involvement of both arches and bilateral changes in the same jaw have been reported. Although rare generalized involvement has been documented, the presence of regional odontodysplasia in more than two quadrants is very uncommon. Involvement of the deciduous dentition typically is followed by similarly affected permanent teeth. In the area of altered teeth, the surrounding bone often exhibits a lower density; in addition, hyperplasia of the soft tissue may be noted overlying affected teeth that are impacted.

Many of the affected teeth fail to erupt. Erupted teeth demonstrate small irregular crowns that are yellow to brown, often with a very rough surface. Caries and associated periapical inflammatory lesions are fairly common. Because of dentinal clefts and very long pulp horns, pulpal necrosis is common (often in the absence of an obvious cause). Radiographically, the altered teeth demonstrate extremely thin enamel and dentin surrounding an enlarged radiolucent pulp, resulting in a pale wispy image of a tooth; hence the term **ghost teeth** (Fig. 2.114). A lack of contrast is seen between the dentin and the enamel, with an indistinct or "fuzzy" appearance of the coronal silhouette. Short roots and open apices may be seen. The enlarged pulps frequently demonstrate one or more prominent pulp stones. The most common presenting signs and symptoms include delayed or

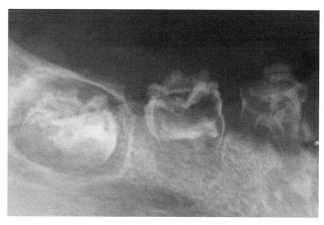

• **Fig. 2.114 Regional Odontodysplasia (Ghost Teeth).** Posterior mandibular dentition exhibiting enlarged pulps and extremely thin enamel and dentin. (Courtesy of Dr. John B. Perry.)

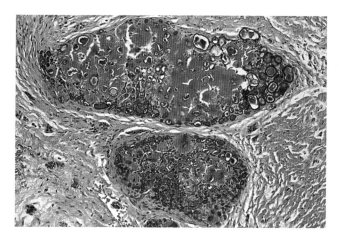

• **Fig. 2.115 Regional Odontodysplasia.** Follicular tissue contains scattered collections of enameloid conglomerates and islands of odontogenic epithelium.

failure of eruption, early exfoliation, abscess formation, malformed teeth, and non-inflammatory gingival enlargement.

Histopathologic Features

In ground sections the thickness of the enamel varies, resulting in an irregular surface. The prism structure of the enamel is irregular or lacking, with a laminated appearance. The dentin contains clefts scattered through a mixture of interglobular dentin and amorphous material. Globular areas of poorly organized tubular dentin and scattered cellular inclusions often are seen. The pulp tissue contains free or attached stones that may exhibit tubules or consist of laminated calcification. The follicular tissue surrounding the crown may be enlarged and typically exhibits focal collections of basophilic enamel-like calcifications called **enameloid conglomerates** (Fig. 2.115). This pattern of calcification is not specific for regional odontodysplasia and has been seen in

other processes with disturbed enamel formation, such as amelogenesis imperfecta. Scattered islands of odontogenic epithelium and other patterns of intramural calcification also are seen.

Treatment and Prognosis

Currently no therapeutic consensus exists with respect to management of patients affected by regional odontodysplasia. Careful evaluation of each patient's individual findings is important in order to develop the most appropriate treatment plan. Unerupted teeth should remain untouched, restoring function with a removable partial prosthesis until the skeletal growth period has passed in an effort to prevent atrophy of the alveolar ridge in the affected quadrant. Erupted teeth can be covered with etched-retained restorations or stainless steel crowns until final restorations can be placed after the completion of growth. Because of the fragile nature of the coronal hard tissue and the ease of pulp exposure, tooth preparation is contraindicated. Severely affected and infected teeth often are not salvageable and need to be removed.

Although vitality of the abnormal dentition often is difficult to maintain, such efforts may permit continued dentinal development of teeth affected by regional odontodysplasia. The resultant teeth tend to demonstrate hypoplastic crowns and short roots with more normal appearing canals and well-developed apices.

Following completion of skeletal growth, remaining defective teeth can be removed and replaced with implants. In patients with early loss of severely affected and erupted teeth, significant atrophy of the alveolar ridge can complicate implant placement. In such cases, surgical augmentation of the alveolar process can be used to improve the quality of the site prior to implant placement.

Bibliography

General References
Hennekam R, Allanson J, Krantz I: *Gorlin's syndromes of the head and neck,* ed 5, New York, 2010, Oxford University Press.
Stewart RE, Prescott GH: *Oral facial genetics,* St Louis, 1976, Mosby.
Witkop CJ: Clinical aspects of dental anomalies, *Int Dent J* 26:378–390, 1976.
Witkop CJ, Rao S: Inherited defects in tooth structure, In Bergsma D, editor: *Birth defects. Original article series,* vol. 7, Baltimore, 1971, Williams & Wilkins, pp 153–184. no 7.

Environmental Effects on Tooth Structure Development
Ahmed AT, Soto-Rojas AE, Dean JA, et al.: Prevalence of molar-incisor hypomineralization and other enamel defects and associated sociodemographic determinants in Indiana, *J Am Dent Assoc* 151:491–501, 2020.
Amirtham CV, Hirt T, Rutz G, et al.: Root malformation associated with a cervical mineralized diaphragm—a distinct form of tooth abnormality? *Oral Surg Oral Med Oral Pathol Oral Radiol* 117: e311–e319, 2014.

Andreasen JO, Sundström B, Ravn JJ: The effect of traumatic injuries to primary teeth on their permanent successors. 1. A clinical and histologic study of 117 injured permanent teeth, *Scand J Dent Res* 79:219–283, 1971.

Bardellini E, Amadori F, Pasini S, et al.: Dental anomalies in permanent teeth after trauma in primary dentition, *J Clin Pediatr Dent* 41:5–9, 2017.

Brook AH, Smith JM: Environmental causes of enamel defects, *CIBA Found Symp* 205:212–225, 1997.

Buzalaf MAR: Review of fluoride intake and appropriateness of current guidelines, *Adv Dent Res* 29:157–166, 2018.

Cortines AAO, Corrêa-Faria P, Paulsson L, et al.: Developmental defects of enamel in the deciduous incisors of infants born preterm: prospective cohort, *Oral Dis* 25:543–549, 2019.

da Silva Figueiredo Sé MJ, Ribeiro APD, Dos Santos-Pinto LAM, et al.: Are hypomineralized primary molars and canines associated with molar-incisor hypomineralization, *Pediatr Dent* 39:445–449, 2017.

Di Giovanni T, Eliades T, Papageorgiou SN: Interventions for dental fluorosis: a systematic review, *J Esthet Restor Dent* 30:502–508, 2018.

Elhennawy K, Schwendicke F: Managing molar-incisor hypomineralization: a systematic review, *J Dent* 55:16–24, 2016.

Garot E, Denis A, Delbos Y, et al.: Are hypomineralized lesions on second primary molars (HSPM) a predictive sign of molar incisor hypomineralization (MIH)? A systematic review and a meta-analysis, *J Dent* 72:8–13, 2018.

Gawade PL, Hudson MM, Kaste SC, et al.: A systematic review of dental late effects in survivors of childhood cancer, *Pediatr Blood Cancer* 61:407–416, 2014.

Kang C-M, Hahn SM, Kim HS, et al.: Clinical risk factors influencing dental developmental disturbances in childhood cancer survivors, *Cancer Res Treat* 50:926–935, 2018.

Kim JE, Hong JK, Yi WJ, et al.: Clinico-radiologic features of molar-incisor malformation in a case series of 38 patients. A retrospective observational study, *Medicine (Baltimore)*, 2019. https://doi.org/10.1097/MD.0000000000017356.

Lee HS, Ki SH, Kim SO, et al.: A new type of dental anomaly: molar-incisor malformation (MIM), *Oral Surg Oral Med Oral Pathol Oral Radiol* 118:101–109, 2014.

Pascon T, Barbosa AMP, Cordeiro RCL, et al.: Prenatal exposure to gestational diabetes mellitus increases developmental defects in the enamel of offspring, *PLoS One* 14:e0211771, 2019.

Pajari U, Lanning M: Developmental defects of teeth in survivors of childhood ALL are related to the therapy and age at diagnosis, *Med Pediatr Oncol* 24:310–314, 1995.

Schwendicke F, Elhennawy K, Reda S, et al.: Global burden of molar incisor hypomineralization, *J Dent* 68:10–18, 2018.

Silva MJ, Scurrah KJ, Craig JM, et al.: Etiology of molar incisor hypomineralization—a systemic review, *Community Dent Oral Epidemiol* 44:342–353, 2016.

Suckling GW: Developmental defects of enamel—historical and present day perspective of their pathogenesis, *Adv Dent Res* 3:87–94, 1989.

Turner JG: Injury to the teeth of succession by abscess of the temporary teeth, *Brit Dent J* 30:1233–1237, 1909.

Vargas-Ferreira F, Peres MA, Dumith SC, et al.: Association of pre- peri- and postnatal factors with developmental defects of enamel in schoolchildren, *J Clin Pediatr Dent* 42:125–134, 2018.

Von Arx T: Developmental disturbances of permanent teeth following trauma to the primary dentition, *Aust Dent J* 38:1–10, 1993.

Weerheijm KL: Molar incisor hypomineralisation (MIH), *Eur J Paediatr Dent* 4:114–120, 2003.

Wright JT, Curran A, Kim KJ, et al.: Molar root-incisor malformation: considerations of diverse developmental and etiologic factors, *Oral Surg Oral Med Oral Pathol Oral Radiol* 121:164–172, 2016.

Postdevelopmental Loss of Tooth Structure

Al-Qawasmi RA, Hartsfield JK Jr, Everett ET, et al.: Genetic predisposition to external apical root resorption, *Am J Orthod Dentofac Orthop* 123:242–252, 2003.

Bakland LK: Root resorption, *Dent Clin N Am* 36:491–507, 1992.

Bartlett DW, Shah P: A critical review of non-carious cervical (wear) lesions and the role of abfraction, erosion, and abrasion, *J Dent Res* 85:306–312, 2006.

Buzalaf MAR, Magalhães AC, Rios D: Prevention of erosive tooth wear: targeting nutritional and patient-related risks factors, *Br Dent J* 224:371–378, 2018.

Eccles JD: Tooth surface loss from abrasion, attrition and erosion, *Dent Update* 7:373–381, 1982.

Grippo JO: Abfractions: a new classification of hard tissue lesions of teeth, *J Esthet Dent* 3:14–19, 1991.

Grippo JO, Simring M, Coleman TA: Abfraction, abrasion, biocorrosion, and the enigma of noncarious cervical lesions: a 20-year perspective, *J Esthet Restor Dent* 24:10–25, 2012.

Heithersay GS: Clinical, radiologic, and histopathologic features of invasive cervical resorption, *Quintessence Int* 30:27–37, 1999.

Lee WC, Eakle WS: Possible role of tensile stress in the etiology of cervical erosive lesions of teeth, *J Prosthet Dent* 52:374–379, 1984.

Lee WC, Eakle WS: Stress-induced cervical lesions: review of advances in the past 10 years, *J Prosthet Dent* 75:487–494, 1996.

Litonjua LA, Andreana S, Patra AK, et al.: An assessment of stress analyses in the theory of abfraction, *Biomed Mater Eng* 14:311–321, 2004.

Mavridou AM, Bergmans L, Barendregt D, et al.: Descriptive analysis of factors associated with external cervical resorption, *J Endod* 43:1602–1610, 2017.

Mavridou AM, Hauben E, Wevers M, et al.: Understanding external cervical resorption in vital teeth, *J Endod* 42:1737–1751, 2016.

Michael JA, Townsend GC, Greenwood LF, et al.: Abfraction: separating fact from fiction, *Aust Dent J* 54:2–8, 2009.

Mummery JH: The pathology of "pink spots" on teeth, *Br Dent J* 41:301–311, 1920.

Newman WG: Possible etiologic factors in external root resorption, *Am J Orthod* 67:522–539, 1975.

O'Toole S, Bernabé E, Moazzez R, et al.: Timing of dietary acid intake and erosive tooth wear: a case-control study, *J Dent* 56:99–104, 2017.

Patel S, Dawood A, Wilson R, et al.: The detection and management of root resorption lesions using intraoral radiography and cone beam computed tomography—an *in vivo* investigation, *Int Endod J* 42:831–838, 2009.

Patel S, Foschi F, Condon R, et al.: External cervical resorption: part 2—management, *Int Endod J* 51:1224–1238, 2018.

Patel S, Mavridou AM, Lambrechts P, et al.: External cervical resorption—part 1: histopathology, distribution and presentation, *Int Endod J* 51:1205–1223, 2018.

Patel S, Saberi N: The ins and outs of root resorption, *Br Dent J* 224:691–699, 2018.

Rabinowitch BZ: Internal resorption, *Oral Surg Oral Med Oral Pathol* 33:263–282, 1972.

Ram D, Cohenca N: Therapeutic protocols for avulsed permanent teeth: review and clinical update, *Pediatr Dent* 26:251–255, 2004.

Ree JS, Somi S: A guide to the clinical management of attrition, *Br Dent J* 224:319–323, 2018.

Shah P, Razavi S, Bartlett DW: The prevalence of cervical tooth wear in patients with bruxism and other causes of wear, *J Prosthodont* 18:450–454, 2009.

Smith BGN, Bartlett DW, Robb ND: The prevalence, etiology and management of tooth wear in the United Kingdom, *J Prosthet Dent* 78:367–372, 1997.

Sneed WD: Noncarious cervical lesions: why on the facial? A theory, *J Esthet Restor Dent* 23:197–200, 2011.

Topkara A: External apical root resorption caused by orthodontic treatment: a review of the literature, *Eur J Paediatr Dent* 12:163–166, 2011.

Tronstad L: Root resorption—etiology, terminology and clinical manifestations, *Endod Dent Traumatol* 4:241–252, 1988.

Young WG: The oral medicine of tooth wear, *Aust Dent J* 46:236–250, 2001.

Young WG: Tooth wear: diet analysis and advice, *Int Dent J* 55:68–72, 2005.

Young WG, Khan F: Sites of dental erosion are saliva-dependent, *J Oral Rehabil* 29:35–43, 2002.

Discoloration of Teeth

Cabrerizo-Merino CC, Garcia-Ballesta C, Onate-Sanchez RE, et al.: Stomatological manifestations of Günther's disease, *J Pedod* 14:113–116, 1990.

Ciftci V, Kilavuz S, Bulut FD, et al.: Congenital erythropoietic porphyria with erythrodontia: a case report, *Int J Paediatr Dent* 29:542–548, 2019.

Crystal YO, Janal MN, Hamilton DS, et al.: Parental perceptions and acceptance of silver diamine fluoride staining, *JADA* 148:510–518, 2017.

Dayan D, Heifferman A, Gorski M, et al.: Tooth discoloration—extrinsic and intrinsic factors, *Quintessence Int* 14:195–199, 1983.

Eisenberg E, Bernick SM: Anomalies of the teeth with stains and discolorations, *J Prev Dent* 2:7–20, 1975.

Giunta JL, Tsamtsouris A: Stains and discolorations of teeth: review and case reports, *J Pedod* 2:175–182, 1978.

Kabler B, Rossi-Fedele G: A review of tooth discoloration after regenerative endodontic therapy, *J Endod* 42:563–569, 2016.

Kumar A, Kuma V, Singh J, et al.: Drug-induced discoloration of teeth: an updated review, *Clin Pediatr (Phila)* 51:181–185, 2012.

Rendall JR, McDougall AC: Reddening of the upper central incisors associated with periapical granuloma in lepromatous leprosy, *Br J Oral Surg* 13:271–277, 1976.

Seremidi K, Kavvadia K, Tosios K, et al.: Dental intrinsic green pigmentation from primary to mixed dentition: clinical and histological findings, *Eur J Paediatr Dent* 18:149–152, 2017.

Siekert RG, Gibilisco JA: Discoloration of the teeth in alkaptonuria (ochronosis) and parkinsonism, *Oral Surg Oral Med Oral Pathol* 29:197–199, 1970.

Tredwin CJ, Scully C, Bagan-Sebastian JV: Drug-induced disorders of teeth, *J Dent Res* 84:596–602, 2005.

Localized Disturbances in Eruption

Baensch F, Kriwalsky MS, Kleffmann W, et al.: Third molar complications in the elderly – a matched-pairs analysis, *J Oral Maxillofac Surg* 75:680–686, 2017.

Curran AE, Damm DD, Drummond JF: Pathologically significant pericoronal lesions in adults: histopathologic evaluation, *J Oral Maxillofac Surg* 60:613–617, 2002.

Douglass J, Tinanoff N: The etiology, prevalence, and sequelae of infraocclusion of primary molars, *J Dent Child* 58:481–483, 1991.

Ducommun F, Bornstein MM, Bosshardt D, et al.: Diagnosis of tooth ankylosis using panoramic views, cone beam computed tomography, and histological data: a retrospective observational case series study, *Eur J Orthod* 40:231–238, 2018.

Ekim SL, Hatibovic-Kofman S: A treatment decision-making model for infraoccluded primary molars, *Int J Paediatr Dent* 11:340–346, 2001.

Ghaeminia H, Perry J, Nienhuijs ME, et al.: Surgical removal versus retention for the management of asymptomatic disease-free impacted wisdom teeth, *Cochrane Database Syst Rev*, 2016. https://doi.org/10.1002/14651858.CD003879.pub4.

Hanisch M, Hanisch L, Kleinheinz J, et al.: Primary failure of eruption (PFE): a systemic review, *Head Face Med* 14:5, 2018. https://doi.org/10.1186/s13005-018-0163-7.

Karp JM: Delayed tooth emergence, *Pediatr Rev* 32:e4–e17, 2011.

Mercier P, Precious D: Risks and benefits of removal of impacted third molars, *J Oral Maxillofac Surg* 21:17–27, 1993.

Noffke CE, Chabikuli NJ, Nzima N: Impaired tooth eruption: a review, *SADJ* 60:422–425, 2005.

Suri L, Gagari E, Vastardis H: Delayed tooth eruption: pathogenesis, diagnosis, and treatment. A literature review, *Am J Orthod Dentofac Orthop* 126:432–445, 2004.

Developmental Alterations in Number of Teeth

Adekoya-Sofowora CA: Natal and neonatal teeth: a review, *Niger Postgrad Med J* 15:38–41, 2008.

Al-Ani AH, Antoun JS, Thomson WM, et al.: Hypodontia: an update on its etiology, classification, and clinical management, *Biomed Res Int*, 2017. https://doi.org/10.1155/2017/9378325.

Bodin I, Julin P, Thomsson M: Hyperdontia. I. Frequency and distribution of supernumerary teeth among 21,609 patients, *Dentomaxillofac Radiol* 7:15–17, 1978.

Bonds J, Pollan-White X, et al.: Is there a link between ovarian cancer and tooth agenesis? *Eur J Med Genet* 57:235–239, 2014.

De Santis D, Sinigaglia S, Faccioni P, et al.: Syndromes associated with dental agenesis, *Minerva Stomatol* 68:42–56, 2019.

Harris EF, Clark LL: Hypodontia: an epidemiologic study of American black and white people, *Am J Orthod Dentofac Orthop* 134:761–767, 2008.

Harris EF, Clark LL: An epidemiological study of hyperdontia in American blacks and whites, *Angle Orthod* 78:460–465, 2008.

Juuri E, Balic A: The biology underlying abnormalities of tooth number in humans, *J Dent Res* 96:1248–1256, 2017.

Kates GA, Needleman HL, Holmes LB: Natal and neonatal teeth: a clinical study, *J Am Dent Assoc* 109:441–443, 1984.

Lammi L, Arte S, Somer M, et al.: Mutations in AXIN2 cause familial tooth agenesis and predispose to colorectal cancer, *Am J Hum Genet* 74:1043–1050, 2004.

Lubinsky M, Kantaputra PN: Syndromes with supernumerary teeth, *Am J Med Genet, Part A* 170:2611–2616, 2016.

Nieminen P: Genetic basis of tooth agenesis, *J Exp Zool B Mol Dev Evol* 312B:320–342, 2009.

Omer RS, Anthonappa RP, King NM: Determination of the optimum time for surgical removal of unerupted anterior supernumerary teeth, *Pediatr Dent* 32:14–20, 2010.

Rajab LD, Hamdan MAM: Supernumerary teeth: review of the literature and a survey of 152 cases, *Int J Paediatr Dent* 12:244–254, 2002.

Rao PP, Chidzonga MM: Supernumerary teeth: literature review, *Cent Afr J Med* 47:22–26, 2001.

Shapira Y, Kuftinec MM: Tooth transposition—a review of the literature and treatment considerations, *Angle Orthod* 59:271–276, 1989.

Spouge JD, Feasby WH: Erupted teeth in the newborn, *Oral Surg Oral Med Oral Pathol* 22:198–208, 1966.

Yusof WZ: Non-syndrome multiple supernumerary teeth: literature review, *J Can Dent Assoc* 56:147–149, 1990.

Developmental Alterations in Size of Teeth
Bailit HL: Dental variation among populations. An anthropologic view, *Dent Clin N Am* 19:125–139, 1975.

Brook AH: A unifying aetiological explanation for anomalies of human tooth number and size, *Arch Oral Biol* 29:373–378, 1984.

Gorlin RJ, Marashi AH, Obwegeser HL: Oculo-facio-cardio-dental (OFCD) syndrome, *Am J Med Genet* 63:290–292, 1996.

Rushton MA: Partial gigantism of face and teeth, *Br Dent J* 62:572–578, 1937.

Schulze BRB, Horn D, Kobelt A, et al.: Rare dental abnormalities seen in oculo-facio-cardio-dental (OFCD) syndrome: three new cases and review of nine patients, *Am J Med Genet* 82:429–435, 1999.

Townsend GC: Hereditability of deciduous tooth size in Australian aboriginals, *Am J Phys Anthropol* 53:297–300, 1980.

Townsend GC, Brown T: Hereditability of permanent tooth size, *Am J Phys Anthropol* 49:497–504, 1978.

Gemination, Fusion, Concrescence
Brook AH, Winter GB: Double teeth: a retrospective study of "geminated" and "fused" teeth in children, *Br Dent J* 129:123–130, 1970.

Duncan WK, Helpin ML: Bilateral fusion and gemination: a literature analysis and case report, *Oral Surg Oral Med Oral Pathol* 64:82–87, 1987.

Levitas TC: Gemination, fusion, twinning and concrescence, *J Dent Child* 32:93–100, 1965.

Romito LM: Concrescence: report of a rare case, *Oral Surg Oral Med Oral Pathol Oral Radiol Endod* 97:325–327, 2004.

Ruprecht A, Batniji S, El-Neweihi E: Double teeth: the incidence of gemination and fusion, *J Pedod* 9:332–337, 1985.

Tuna EB, Yildirim M, Seymen F, et al.: Fused teeth: a review of the treatment options, *J Dent Child* 76:109–116, 2009.

Yuen SWH, Chan JCY, Wei SHY: Double primary teeth and their relationship with the permanent successors: a radiographic study of 376 cases, *Pediatr Dent* 9:42–48, 1987.

Accessory Cusps
Bailit HL: Dental variation among populations. An anthropologic view, *Dent Clin N Am* 19:125–139, 1975.

Bloch-Zupan A, Stachtou J, Emmanouil D, et al.: Oro-dental features as useful diagnostic tool in Rubinstein-Taybi syndrome, *Am J Med Genet A* 143A:570–573, 2007.

Chen J-W, Huang GT-J, Bakland LK: Dens evaginatus. Current treatment options, *JADA* 151:358–367, 2020.

Dankner E, Harari D, Rotstein I: Dens evaginatus of anterior teeth. Literature review and radiographic survey of 15,000 teeth, *Oral Surg Oral Med Oral Pathol Oral Radiol Endod* 81:472–476, 1996.

Falomo OO: The cusp of Carabelli: frequency, distribution, size and clinical significance in Nigeria, *West Afr J Med* 21:322–324, 2002.

Gaynor WN: Dens evaginatus—how does it present and how should it be managed? *N Z Dent J* 98:104–107, 2002.

Geist JR: Dens evaginatus: case report and review of the literature, *Oral Surg Oral Med Oral Pathol* 67:628–631, 1989.

Hattab FN, Yassin OM, Al-Nimri KS: Talon cusp in permanent dentition associated with other dental anomalies: review of literature and reports of seven cases, *J Dent Child* 63:368–376, 1996.

Leith R, O'Connell AC: Selective reduction of talon cusps—a case series, *J Clin Pediatr Dent* 42:1–5, 2018.

Levitan ME, Himel VT: Dens evaginatus: literature review, pathophysiology, and comprehensive treatment regimen, *J Endod* 32:1–9, 2006.

McCulloch KJ, Mills CM, Greenfeld RS, et al.: Dens evaginatus: review of the literature and report of several clinical cases, *J Can Dent Assoc* 64(104–106):110–113, 1998.

Ooshima T, Ishida R, Mishima K, et al.: The prevalence of developmental anomalies of teeth and their association with tooth size in the primary and permanent dentitions of 1650 children, *Int J Paediatr Dent* 6:87–94, 1996.

Saini TS, Kharat DU, Mokeem S: Prevalence of shovel-shaped incisors in Saudi Arabian dental patients, *Oral Surg Oral Med Oral Pathol* 70:540–544, 1990.

Tsujino K, Shintani S: Intentional partical pulpotomy for treatment of immature permanent maxillary incisor with talon cusp, *Bull Tokyo Dent Coll* 58:247–253, 2017.

Dens Invaginatus
Alani A, Bishop K: Dens invaginatus. Part 1: classification, prevalence and aetiology, *Int Endod J* 41:1123–1136, 2008.

Bishop K, Alani A: Dens invaginatus. Part 2: clinical, radiographic features and management options, *Int Endod J* 41:1137–1154, 2008.

Gallacher A, Ali R, Bhakta S: Dens invaginatus: diagnosis and management strategies, *Br Dent J* 221:383–387, 2016.

Hülsmann M: Dens invaginatus: aetiology, classification, prevalence, diagnosis, and treatment considerations, *Int Endod J* 30:79–90, 1997.

Oehlers FAC: Dens invaginatus (dilated composite odontome). I. Variations of the invagination process and associated anterior crown forms, *Oral Surg Oral Med Oral Pathol* 10:1204–1218, 1957.

Oehlers FAC: Dens invaginatus (dilated composite odontome). II. Associated posterior crown forms and pathogenesis, *Oral Surg Oral Med Oral Pathol* 10:1302–1316, 1957.

Oehlers FAC: The radicular variety of dens invaginatus, *Oral Surg Oral Med Oral Pathol* 11:1251–1260, 1958.

Zhu J, Wang X, Fang Y, et al.: An update on the diagnosis and treatment of dens invaginatus, *Aust Dent J* 62:261–275, 2017.

Ectopic Enamel
Cavanha AO: Enamel pearls, *Oral Surg Oral Med Oral Pathol* 19:373–382, 1965.

Fowler CB, Brannon RB: The paradental cyst: a clinicopathologic study of six new cases and review of the literature, *J Oral Maxillofac Surg* 47:243–348, 1989.

Grine FE, Holt S, Brink JS, et al.: Enamel pearls: their occurrence in recent human populations and earliest manifestations in the modern human lineage, *Arch Oral Biol* 101:147–155, 2019.

Hou G-L, Tsai C-C: Relationship between periodontal furcation involvement and molar cervical enamel projections, *J Periodontol* 58:715–721, 1987.

Moskow BS, Canut PM: Studies on root enamel: (2) enamel pearls—a review of their morphology, localization, nomenclature, occurrence, classification, histogenesis and incidence, *J Clin Periodontol* 17:275–281, 1990.

Pompura JR, Sándor GKB, Stoneman DW: The buccal bifurcation cyst: a prospective study of treatment outcomes in 44 sites, *Oral Surg Oral Med Oral Pathol Oral Radiol Endod* 83:215–221, 1997.

Risnes S: The prevalence, location, and size of enamel pearls on human molars, *Scand J Dent Res* 82:403–412, 1974.

Taurodontism
Jafarzadeh H, Azarpazhooh A, Mayhall JT: Taurodontism: a review of the condition and endodontic treatment challenges, *Int Endod J* 41:375–388, 2008.

Keith A: Problems relating to the teeth of the earlier forms of prehistoric man, *Proc R Soc Med* 6(Odontol sect):103–124, 1913.

Klein U, Palmagham B, Blumhagen R, et al.: Pyramidal and taurodont molars and their association with other tooth anomalies, *Pediatr Dent* 39:46–52, 2017.

Lim A, LeClerc J: Endodontic treatment of a hypertaurodontic mandibular left second molar in a patient with many taurodonts combined with multiple pulp stones, *Aust Endod J* 45:414–419, 2019.

Ruprecht A, Batniji S, El-Neweihi E: The incidence of taurodontism in dental patients, *Oral Surg Oral Med Oral Pathol* 63:743–747, 1987.

Shaw JCM: Taurodont teeth in south African races, *J Anat* 62:476–498, 1928.

Shifman A, Chanannel I: Prevalence of taurodontism found in radiographic dental examination of 1,200 young adult Israeli patients, *Community Dent Oral Epidemiol* 6:200–203, 1978.

Witkop CJ, Keenan KM, Cervenka J, et al.: Taurodontism: an anomaly of teeth reflecting disruptive developmental homeostasis, *Am J Med Genet* 4(Suppl):85–97, 1988.

Hypercementosis

Brooks JK, Ghita I, Vallee EM, et al.: Florid hypercementosis synchronous with periodontitis: a case report, *Quintessence Int* 50:478–485, 2019.

Eren Y, Erdal O, Serdar B, et al.: Evaluation of the frequency and characteristics of hypercementosis in the Turkish population with cone-beam computed tomography, *Niger J Clin Pract* 20:724–728, 2017.

Fox L: Paget's disease (osteitis deformans) and its effect on maxillary bones and teeth, *J Am Dent Assoc* 20:1823–1829, 1933.

Gardner BS, Goldstein H: The significance of hypercementosis, *Dent Cosmos* 73:1065–1069, 1931.

Leider AS, Garbarino VE: Generalized hypercementosis, *Oral Surg Oral Med Oral Pathol* 63:375–380, 1987.

Rao VM, Karasick D: Hypercementosis—an important clue to Paget disease of the maxilla, *Skelet Radiol* 9:126–128, 1982.

Dilaceration

de Amorim CS, Americano GCA, Martins LF, et al.: Frequency of crown and root dilacerations of permanent incisors after dental trauma to their predecessor teeth, *Dent Traumatol* 34:401–405, 2018.

Hamasha AA, Al-Khateeb T, Darwazeh A: Prevalence of dilacerations in Jordanian adults, *Int Endod J* 35:910–912, 2002.

Ligh RQ: Coronal dilacerations, *Oral Surg Oral Med Oral Pathol* 51:567, 1981.

Singh H, Kapoor P, Dudeja P, et al.: Interdisciplinary management of an impacted dilacerated maxillary central incisor, *Dent Press J Orthod* 23:37–46, 2018.

Topouzelis N, Tsaousoglou P, Pisoka V, et al.: Dilaceration of maxillary central incisor: a literature review, *Dent Traumatol* 26:427–433, 2010.

Van Gool AV: Injury to the permanent tooth germ after trauma to the deciduous predecessor, *Oral Surg Oral Med Oral Pathol* 35:2–12, 1973.

Supernumerary Roots

Kannan SK, Suganya SH: Supernumerary roots, *Indian J Dent Res* 13:116–119, 2002.

Younes SA, Al-Shammery AR, El-Angbawi MF: Three-rooted permanent mandibular first molars of Asian and black groups in the Middle East, *Oral Surg Oral Med Oral Pathol* 69:102–105, 1990.

Globodontia

Bloch-Zupan A, Goodman JR: Otodental syndrome, *Orphanet J Rare Dis* 1:5, 2006.

Gregory-Evans CY, Moosajee M, Hodges MD, et al.: SNP genome scanning localizes Oto-dental syndrome to chromosome 11q13 and microdeletions at this locus implicate FGF3 in dental and inner-ear disease and FADD in ocular coloboma, *Hum Mol Genet* 16:2482–2493, 2007.

Levin LS, Jorgenson RJ, Cook R: Otodental dysplasia: a new ectodermal dysplasia, *Clin Genet* 8:136–144, 1975.

Su JM, Zeng SJ, Ye XW, et al.: Three years follow-up of otodental syndrome in 3-year-old Chinese boy: rare case report, *BMC Oral Health*, 2019. https://doi.org/10.1186/s12903-019-0860-z.

Witkop CJ, Gundlach KKH, Streed WJ, et al.: Globdontia in the otodental syndrome, *Oral Surg Oral Med Oral Pathol* 41:472–483, 1976.

Lobodontia

Ather A, Ather H, Acharya SR, et al.: Lobodontia: the unraveling of the wolf teeth, *Romanian J Morphol Embryol* 54:215–217, 2013.

Brook AH, Winder M: Lobodontia—a rare inherited dental anomaly. Report of an affected family, *Br Dent J* 147:213–215, 1979.

Kiyan A, Allen C, Damm D, et al.: Lobodontia: report of a family with a rare inherited dental anomaly, *Oral Surg Oral Med Oral Pathol Oral Radiol* 116:e508–e509, 2013.

Robbins IM, Keene HJ: Multiple morphologic dental anomalies. Report of a case, *Oral Surg Oral Med Oral Pathol* 17:683–690, 1964.

Skrinjaric T, Gorseta K, Skrinjaric I: Lobodontia: genetic entity with specific pattern of dental dysmorphology, *Ann Anat* 203:100–107, 2016.

Amelogenesis Imperfecta

Aldred MJ, Crawford PJM: Amelogenesis imperfecta—toward a new classification, *Oral Dis* 1:2–5, 1995.

Aldred MJ, Crawford PJM: Molecular biology of hereditary enamel defects, *CIBA Found Symp* 205:200–209, 1997.

Aldred MJ, Savarirayan R, Crawford PJM: Amelogenesis imperfecta: a classification and catalogue for the 21st century, *Oral Dis* 9:19–23, 2003.

Crawford PJM, Aldred M, Bloch-Zupan A: Amelogenesis imperfecta, *Orphanet J Rare Dis* 2:17, 2007.

Hunter L, Addy LD, Knox J, et al.: Is amelogenesis imperfecta an indication for renal examination? *Int J Paediatr Dent* 17:62–65, 2007.

Nusier M, Yassin O, Hart TC, et al.: Phenotypic diversity and revision of the nomenclature for autosomal recessive amelogenesis imperfecta, *Oral Surg Oral Med Oral Pathol Oral Radiol Endod* 97:220–230, 2004.

Prasad MK, Geoffroy V, Vicaire S, et al.: A targeted next-generation sequencing assay for the molecular diagnosis of genetic disorders with orodental involvement, *J Med Genet* 53:98–110, 2016.

Sabandal MMI, Schäfer E: Amelogenesis imperfecta: review of diagnostic findings and treatment concepts, *Odontology* 104:245–256, 2016.

Smith CEL, Poulter JA, Antanaviciute A, et al.: Amelogenesis imperfecta; genes, proteins, and pathways, *Front Physiol*, 2017. https://doi.org/10.3389/fphys.2017.00435.

Seow WK: Clinical diagnosis and management strategies of amelogenesis imperfecta variants, *Pediatr Dent* 15:384–393, 1993.

Shields ED: A new classification of heritable human enamel defects and a discussion of dentin defects, In Jorgenson RJ, Paul NW, editors: *Dentition: genetic effects, birth defects*, vol. 19, New York, 1983, Alan R. Liss, pp 107–127. Original article series, no 1.

Witkop CJ Jr: Amelogenesis imperfecta, dentinogenesis imperfecta and dentin dysplasia revisited: problems in classification, *J Oral Pathol* 17:547–553, 1988.

Witkop CJ Jr, Sauk JJ Jr: Heritable defects of enamel, In Stewart RE, Prescott GH, editors: *Oral facial genetics*, St Louis, 1976, Mosby, pp 151–226.

Wright JT, Hart PS, Aldred MJ, et al.: Relationship of phenotype and genotype in X-linked amelogenesis imperfecta, *Connect Tissue Res* 44(Suppl 1):72–78, 2003.

Wright JT, Torain M, Long K, et al.: Amelogenesis imperfecta: genotype-phenotype studies in 71 patients, *Cells Tissues Organs* 194:279–283, 2011.

Dentinogenesis Imperfecta

Barron MJ, McDonnell ST, MacKie I, et al.: Hereditary dentine disorders: dentinogenesis imperfecta and dentine dysplasia, *Orphanet J Rare Dis* 3:31, 2008.

de La Dure-Molla M, Fournier BP, Berdal A: Isolated dentinogenesis imperfecta and dentin dysplasia: revision of the classification, *Eur J Hum Genet* 23:445–451, 2015.

Hart PS, Hart TC: Disorders of human dentin, *Cells Tissues Organs* 186:70–77, 2007.

Hursey RJ, Witkop CJ Jr, Miklashek D, et al.: Dentinogenesis imperfecta in a racial isolate with multiple hereditary defects, *Oral Surg Oral Med Oral Pathol* 9:641–658, 1956.

Levin LS, Leaf SH, Jelmini RJ, et al.: Dentinogenesis imperfecta in the Brandywine isolate (DI type III): clinical, radiologic, and scanning electron microscopic studies of the dentition, *Oral Surg Oral Med Oral Pathol* 56:267–274, 1983.

Li F, Liu Y, Yang J, et al.: Phenotype and genotype analyses in seven families with dentinogenesis imperfecta or dentin dysplasia, *Oral Dis* 23:360–366, 2017.

McKnight DA, Simmer JP, Hart PS, et al.: Overlapping DSPP mutations cause DD and DGI, *J Dent Res* 87:1108–1111, 2008.

Ranta H, Lukinmaa P-L, Waltimo J: Heritable dentin defects: nosology, pathology, and treatment, *Am J Med Genet* 45:193–200, 1993.

Rosenberg LR, Phelan JA: Dentin dysplasia type II: review of the literature and report of a family, *J Dent Child* 50:372–375, 1983.

Rushton MA: A new form of dentinal dysplasia: shell teeth, *Oral Surg Oral Med Oral Pathol* 7:543–549, 1954.

Shields ED, Bixler D, El-Kafrawy AM: A proposed classification for heritable human dentine defects with a description of a new entity, *Arch Oral Biol* 18:543–553, 1973.

Taleb K, Lauridsen E, Daugaard-Jensen J, et al.: Dentinogenesis imperfecta type II—genotype and phenotype analyses in three Danish families, *Mol Genet Genomic Med* 6:339–349, 2018.

Witkop CJ Jr: Amelogenesis imperfecta, dentinogenesis imperfecta and dentin dysplasia revisited: problems in classification, *J Oral Pathol* 17:547–553, 1988.

Witkop CJ Jr: Hereditary defects of dentin, *Dent Clin N Am* 19:25–45, 1975.

Radicular Dentin Dysplasia

Bixler D: Heritable disorders affecting dentin, In Stewart RE, Prescott GH, editors: *Oral facial genetics*, 1976, St Louis, pp 227–262.

Bloch-Zupan A, Jamet X, Etard C, et al.: Homozygosity mapping and candidate prioritization identify mutations, missed by whole-exome sequencing, in SMOC2, causing major dental developmental defects, *Am J Hum Genet* 89:773–781, 2011.

Chen D, Li X, Lu F, et al.: Dentin dysplasia type I—a dental disease with genetic heterogeneity, *Oral Dis* 25:439–446, 2018.

O'Carroll MK, Duncan WK, Perkins TM: Dentin dysplasia: review of the literature and a proposed subclassification based on radiographic findings, *Oral Surg Oral Med Oral Pathol* 72:119–125, 1991.

Rushton MA: A case of dentinal dysplasia, *Guys Hosp Rep* 89:369–373, 1939.

Tidwell E, Cunningham CJ: Dentinal dysplasia: endodontic treatment, with case report, *J Endod* 5:372–376, 1979.

Wesley RK, Wysocki GP, Mintz SM, et al.: Dentin dysplasia type I. Clinical, morphologic, and genetic studies of a case, *Oral Surg Oral Med Oral Pathol* 41:516–524, 1976.

Witkop CJ Jr: Manifestations of genetic diseases in the human pulp, *Oral Surg Oral Med Oral Pathol* 32:278–316, 1971.

Witkop CJ Jr: Hereditary defects of dentin, *Dent Clin N Am* 19:25–45, 1975.

Xiong F, Ji Z, Liu Y, et al.: Mutation in *SSUH2* causes autosomal dominant dentin dysplasia type I, *Hum Mutat* 38:95–104, 2017.

Yang Q, Chen D, Xiong F, et al.: A splicing mutation in *VPS4B* causes dentin dysplasia I, *J Med Genet* 53:624–633, 2016.

Regional Odontodysplasia

Abdel-Kader MA, Abdelazeem AF, Ahmed NEB, et al.: Oral rehabilitation of a case with regional odontodysplasia using a regenerative approach—a case report and a review of the literature, *Spec Care Dentist* 39:330–339, 2019.

Carlos R, Contreras-Vidaurre E, de Almeida OP, et al.: Regional odontodysplasia: morphological, ultrastructural, and immunohistochemical features of the affected teeth, connective tissue, and odontogenic remnants, *J Dent Child* 75:144–150, 2008.

Crawford PJM, Aldred MJ: Regional odontodysplasia: a bibliography, *J Oral Pathol Med* 18:251–263, 1989.

Kahn MA, Hinson RL: Regional odontodysplasia. Case report with etiologic and treatment considerations, *Oral Surg Oral Med Oral Pathol* 72:462–467, 1991.

Spini TH, Sargenti-Neto S, Cardoso SV, et al.: Progressive dental development in regional odontodysplasia, *Oral Surg Oral Med Oral Pathol Oral Radiol Endod* 104:e40–e45, 2007.

Tervonon SA, Stratmann U, Mokrys K, et al.: Regional odontodysplasia: a review of the literature and report of four cases, *Clin Oral Investig* 8:45–51, 2004.

Walton JL, Witkop CJ Jr, Walker PO: Odontodysplasia. Report of three cases with vascular nevi overlying the adjacent skin of the face, *Oral Surg Oral Med Oral Pathol* 46:676–684, 1978.

Zegarelli EV, Kutscher AH, Applebaum E, et al.: Odontodysplasia, *Oral Surg Oral Med Oral Pathol* 16:187–193, 1963.

3
Pulpal and Periapical Disease

◆ PULPITIS

Like the brain, the dental pulp is encased in hard tissue that can alter the response to local insults. The surrounding dentin provides rigid mechanical support and protection from the bacteria-rich oral cavity. A focal breach in this barrier can adversely affect the health of the dental pulp. Inflammatory vascular changes increase the pulpal volume, but swelling is restricted due to the surrounding dentinal walls, often triggering pain. Normal pulpal stroma is a resilient gelatin-like material that attempts to localize the increased pressures to the site of damage.

If the inflammatory process is not contained, the dental pulp is uniquely hampered in its response because the only source of vascularity enters through the apical foramen without a collateral blood supply. Upon exposure, the contaminated pulp space acts as a conduit between the oral cavity and the usually sterile alveolar bone. Spread of pulpal infection into bone can lead to serious complications, such as cavernous sinus thrombosis (see page 132), Ludwig angina (see page 132), or systemic sepsis with life-threatening complications. Pulpitis-related pain is an important defense mechanism that can lead to therapeutic intervention prior to serious complications.

Four main types of noxious stimuli are common causes of pulpal inflammation (**pulpitis**):
1. *Mechanical damage:* Mechanical sources of injury include traumatic accidents, iatrogenic damage from dental procedures, attrition, abrasion, and barometric changes.
2. *Thermal injury:* Severe thermal stimuli can be transmitted through large uninsulated metallic restorations or may occur from such dental procedures as cavity preparation, polishing, and exothermic chemical reactions of dental materials.
3. *Chemical irritation:* Chemical-related damage can arise from erosion or from the inappropriate use of acidic dental materials.
4. *Bacterial effects:* Bacteria can damage the pulp through toxins or directly after extension from caries or transportation via the vasculature.

The best classification system for pulpitis is one that guides the appropriate treatment. *Reversible pulpitis* denotes a level of pulpal inflammation in which the tissue is capable of returning to a normal state of health if the noxious stimuli are removed. *Irreversible pulpitis* implies that a higher level of inflammation has developed in which the dental pulp has been damaged beyond the point of recovery. Often, frank invasion by bacteria is the crossover point from reversible to irreversible pulpitis.

Clinical Features

Evaluation of pulpal pain (pulpalgia) includes a combination of the clinical presentation and the response of the tooth to a variety of vitality testing procedures. The predictive value of these tests is sometimes less than optimal. When the procedures demonstrate that the pulp is disease free, the results are highly reliable. However, when a pulp appears to test positively for irreversible pulpitis, histopathologic examination may demonstrate no obvious evidence of pulpal disease. The practitioner should use all available tests, clinical information, and personal judgment in an attempt to arrive at an appropriate diagnosis.

Clinically Normal Pulp

Clinically, a normal pulp exhibits no signs or symptoms that suggest pulpitis. These teeth respond to cold with mild pain that resolves in 1–2 seconds, whereas heat is not associated with pulpal discomfort. Pain to percussion will not be evident, and the radiographic examination of the periradicular bone will be within normal limits.

Reversible Pulpitis

A tooth with **reversible pulpitis** is acutely painful when a stimulus (usually cold or sweet foods, but sometimes heat) is applied, but the discomfort resolves within a few seconds after elimination of the stimulus. Typically, the tooth responds to electric pulp testing at lower levels of current than an appropriate control tooth. Mobility and sensitivity to percussion are absent. A cracked tooth or defective restoration often is present if this pattern of pulpal pain is noted in association with discomfort upon biting. If the pulpitis is allowed to progress, then the duration of the pain on stimulation can become longer and the pulp may become affected irreversibly.

A similar pattern of pulpal pain can occur when exposed dentin receives a thermal, chemical, or physical stimulus. **Dentin sensitivity** should be considered if exposed dentin is present and triggers for reversible pulpitis such as caries, tooth fractures, and defective or newly placed restorations are not present.

Irreversible Pulpitis

Patients with early **irreversible pulpitis** generally have sharp, severe pain on thermal stimulation, and the pain continues for a longer period of time after the stimulus is removed. Cold is especially uncomfortable, although heat or sweet and acidic foods also can elicit pain. In addition, the pain may be spontaneous or continuous and may be exacerbated when the patient lies down. The tooth responds to electric pulp testing at lower levels of current.

In the early stages of irreversible pulpitis, the pain often can be localized easily to the individual offending tooth; with increasing discomfort, however, the patient may be unable to identify the offending tooth within a quadrant. Although pulpal pain never crosses the midline, it can be referred from arch to arch, making pulp testing of both arches a necessity in difficult cases.

In the later stages of irreversible pulpitis, the pain increases in intensity and is experienced as a throbbing pressure that can keep patients awake at night. At this point, heat increases the pain; however, cold may produce relief. The tooth responds to electric pulp testing at higher levels of current or demonstrates no response. Mobility and sensitivity to percussion usually are absent because significant inflammation has not spread yet to the apical area. If pulpal drainage occurs (e.g., crown fracture, fistula formation), then the symptoms may resolve—only to return if the drainage ceases.

Pulpal Necrosis

Pulpal necrosis should be suspected when the tooth fails to respond to electric or thermal sensitivity testing. Partial pulpal necrosis (pulpal necrobiosis) often occurs and may be isolated to the coronal portion or one canal of a multi-rooted tooth. Teeth with necrotic pulps present with symptoms that vary from none to acute pain with or without bite sensitivity and hyperocclusion. Diagnosis of pulpal necrosis following tooth trauma often can be problematic due to frequent inaccurate results to electric and thermal pulp tests. These difficulties may arise from the subjective responses required by anxious patients or secondary to nerve damage in pulps with intact blood circulation. Pulse oximetry applied to the injured tooth using a custom stainless steel adapter has shown promise to be a more reliable method for testing pulp vitality over traditional methods.

Chronic Hyperplastic Pulpitis

One unique pattern of pulpal inflammation is **chronic hyperplastic pulpitis (pulp polyp).** This condition occurs in children and young adults who have large exposures of the pulp in which the entire dentinal roof often is missing. The most frequently involved teeth are the deciduous or succedaneous molars, which have large pulp chambers in these age groups. Mechanical irritation and bacterial invasion result in a level of chronic inflammation that produces hyperplastic granulation tissue that extrudes from the chamber and often fills the associated dentinal defect (Figs. 3.1–3.3). The apex may be open and reduces the chance of pulpal necrosis secondary to venous compression. The tooth is asymptomatic except for a possible feeling of pressure when it is placed into masticatory function.

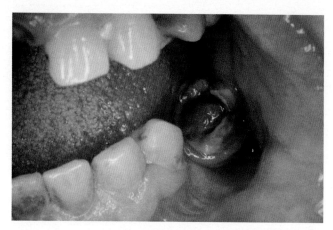

• **Fig. 3.1 Chronic Hyperplastic Pulpitis.** Erythematous granulation tissue extruding from the pulp chamber of the mandibular first molar.

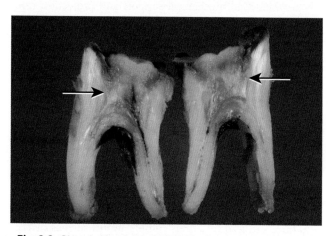

• **Fig. 3.2 Chronic Hyperplastic Pulpitis.** Gross photograph demonstrating hyperplastic pulp tissue filling a large coronal carious defect. *Arrows* delineate the previous roof of the pulp chamber.

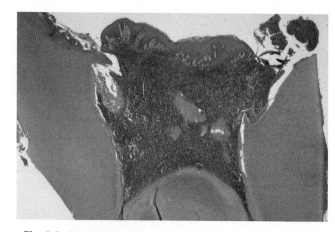

• **Fig. 3.3 Chronic Hyperplastic Pulpitis.** Same tooth as depicted in Fig. 3.2. Chronically inflamed granulation tissue fills the coronal defect. Note surface stratified squamous epithelium.

Histopathologic Features

Basically, the histopathology is primarily of academic interest and usually does not affect treatment significantly. Numerous investigations have shown a surprising lack of correlation between histopathologic findings and the clinical symptoms in the majority of pulps examined.

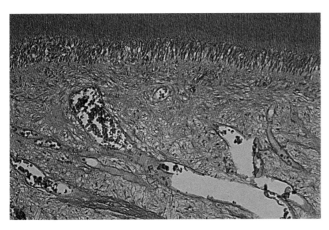

• **Fig. 3.4 Reversible Pulpitis.** Dental pulp exhibiting hyperemia and edema. The adjacent dentin was cut recently during placement of a dental restoration.

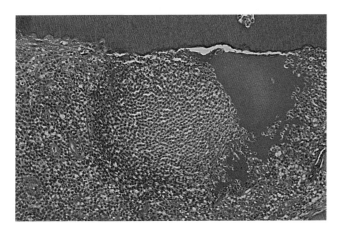

• **Fig. 3.5 Irreversible Pulpitis.** Dental pulp exhibiting acute inflammatory infiltrate consisting predominantly of polymorphonuclear leukocytes.

In patients with reversible pulpitis, the pulp usually shows hyperemia, edema, and a few inflammatory cells underlying the area of affected dentinal tubules (Fig. 3.4). Tertiary dentin may be noted in the adjacent dentinal wall, and scattered acute inflammatory cells are found occasionally.

Irreversible pulpitis often demonstrates congestion of the venules that results in focal necrosis. This necrotic zone contains polymorphonuclear leukocytes and histiocytes (Fig. 3.5). The surrounding pulp tissue usually exhibits fibrosis and a mixture of plasma cells, lymphocytes, and histiocytes (Fig. 3.6).

Chronic hyperplastic pulpitis demonstrates a cap of subacutely inflamed granulation tissue that fills the entire space of the original pulp chamber and histopathologically resembles a pyogenic granuloma (see page 525). The surface of the polyp may or may not be covered with stratified squamous epithelium, which migrates from the adjacent gingiva or arises from sloughed epithelium within the oral fluids (see Fig. 3.3). The deeper pulp tissue within the canals typically demonstrates fibrosis and a chronic inflammatory infiltrate. Pulpal calcifications are common in both the radicular and coronal portions. Often the apical portion of the pulp tissue is normal with minimal inflammation or fibrosis.

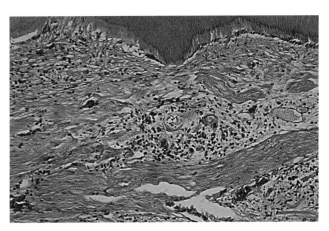

• **Fig. 3.6 Irreversible Pulpitis.** Same tooth as depicted in Fig. 3.5. The dental pulp exhibits an area of fibrosis and chronic inflammation peripheral to the zone of abscess formation.

Treatment and Prognosis

Reversible pulpitis is treated by removal of the local irritant. On occasion, analgesic medications sometimes are desirable. The prognosis of reversible pulpitis is good if action is taken early enough. The pulp status should be evaluated periodically over the next 3 months to ensure that healing has occurred and the process has not progressed to irreversible pulpitis or necrosis.

Irreversible and chronic hyperplastic pulpitis are treated by extraction of the tooth or by root canal therapy. During pulpectomy of mandibular teeth, profound dental anesthesia may be difficult to attain with an inferior alveolar nerve block. During access opening and instrumentation, patients may report pain despite having numbness of the lower lip and tip of the tongue. Premedication with greater than 400 mg of ibuprofen 30–60 minutes prior to the procedure has been shown to increase the likelihood of successful anesthesia. Similar results also have been obtained with 10 mg of ketorolac or 50 mg of diclofenac.

◆ SECONDARY AND TERTIARY DENTIN

Formation of dentin proceeds throughout life. The dentin formed before completion of the crown is called **primary dentin.** This process is followed by the formation of **secondary dentin.** The same odontoblasts that formed the primary dentin remain functional and produce secondary dentin. With advancing age in functioning teeth, dentin is deposited diffusely along the inner walls and leads to smaller pulp chambers and canals. This type of dentin is termed **physiologic secondary dentin** and exhibits slow and gradual deposition that increases after the age of 35–40 years. Significantly less secondary dentin has been described in impacted teeth, suggesting that functional forces of occlusion promote the deposition. Forensic scientists have suggested that the formation of secondary dentin occurs so consistently that its formation can be used for an estimate of age. Pulp/tooth area ratio, pulp/tooth width-length ratio, and pulpal volume have been performed with cone beam computed tomography increasing the accuracy and ease of the estimation of the secondary dentin deposition.

Physiologic secondary dentin is more advanced in males and has been associated positively with calcification-related diseases (e.g., arthritis, gout, kidney stones, gall stones, atherosclerosis, and hypertension). Early widespread formation of secondary dentin has been seen in association with **progeria,** a condition characterized by accelerated aging. On occasion, significant traumatic injury can lead to early obliteration of the pulp chamber and canal (**calcific metamorphosis**) in the affected tooth.

Localized new dentin also is laid down in areas of focal injury. This dentin is more haphazardly organized and is termed **tertiary (reactionary, reparative, irregular,** or **irritation) dentin.** This localized dentin formation may occur in response to the following:

- Attrition
- Fracture
- Erosion
- Abrasion
- Caries
- Periodontal disease
- Mechanical injury from dental procedures
- Irritation from dental materials

Injury of the peripheral odontoblastic processes is all that is required to initiate tertiary dentin formation. If the stimulus is mild to moderate, then the tertiary dentin typically is produced by surviving odontoblasts and is termed *reactionary dentin.* This type of tertiary dentin is more regular in appearance and continuous with the tubules of the primary and secondary dentin. If the stimulus is more severe and leads to the death of the primary odontoblasts, then a new generation of odontoblasts may arise from undifferentiated cells within the pulp and continue to form tertiary dentin that is termed *reparative dentin.* Demineralization of dentin during caries also releases significant amounts of calcium and phosphates. These minerals often diffuse toward the pulp and assist in sclerosis of the tubules as calcium phosphate.

The initial layer of reparative dentin is atubular and known as *interface dentin (fibrodentin).* This thin band may be acellular or exhibit scattered nuclear inclusions. After deposition of the interface dentin, the remainder of the reparative dentin is tubular but not continuous with the primary, secondary, or reactionary dentin. This lack of communication further assists in protecting the pulp from the external stimulus. When the primary odontoblasts die, their dentinal tubules are filled with degenerated odontoblastic processes and are termed *dead tracts.* These tubules usually are sealed off from the pulp by the reparative dentin.

Clinical and Radiographic Features

As noted on periapical radiographs, the deposition of secondary dentin results in diminishing size of pulp chambers and canals. Secondary dentin appears to reduce sensitivity of the affected teeth, susceptibility to dentinal caries, and the trauma of dental procedures. Although production of

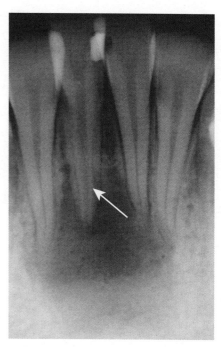

• **Fig. 3.7 Physiologic Secondary Dentin.** Periapical abscess with all four teeth nonresponsive to electric pulp testing. Decreased deposition of physiologic secondary dentin on the right central incisor *(arrow)* delineated the origin of the infection; endodontic treatment of this tooth resolved the lesion.

secondary dentin makes pulp exposure during operative procedures less likely, it also increases the difficulty of locating the pulp chamber and canals during endodontic therapy. On occasion, large inflammatory lesions may involve more than one apex; the size of the canals can be used to help determine the original focus of infection because the canal may be larger in the tooth that became nonvital earlier (Fig. 3.7). Teeth affected by calcific metamorphosis often are discovered clinically by a yellow discoloration of the crown; radiographically, the affected teeth exhibit an accelerated closure of the pulp chamber and canal when compared with adjacent or contralateral teeth (Fig. 3.8). In such cases, the pulpal space may appear to be obliterated completely or reduced dramatically. This alteration usually follows trauma to the tooth and may be seen as early as 3 months after the traumatic episode; however, usually the condition is not detected for about 1 year.

Histopathologic Features

Physiologic secondary dentin consists of regular tubular dentin that is applied onto the primary dentin. These two layers of dentin can be separated by a line of demarcation, often indicated by a bending of the tubules (Fig. 3.9). With advancing age, as the odontoblasts undergo degenerative changes, the physiologic secondary dentin becomes more irregular with fewer tubules.

The quality and appearance of tertiary dentin depend on the severity of the noxious stimulus that promoted its formation. Tertiary dentin is localized to the pulpal end of the

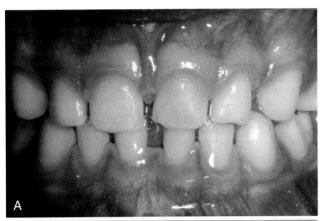

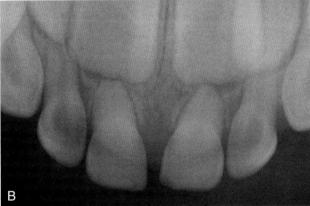

• **Fig. 3.8 Calcific Metamorphosis. A,** Left deciduous maxillary central incisor exhibiting yellow discoloration. **B,** Radiograph of the same patient showing total calcification of the pulp chambers and canals of the deciduous maxillary incisors. (Courtesy of Dr. Jackie L. Banahan.)

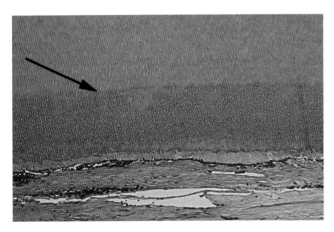

• **Fig. 3.9 Physiologic Secondary Dentin.** A distinct line of demarcation *(arrow)* separates the primary dentin and physiologic secondary dentin.

odontoblastic processes that were affected (Fig. 3.10). With a mild stimulus, such as abrasion or attrition, reactionary dentin exhibits slow deposition characterized by tubules that are continuous with the secondary dentin and only slightly irregular. With more severe damage (e.g., a rapidly progressing carious lesion), reparative dentin is formed, a process that occurs more rapidly and consists of a thin layer of interface

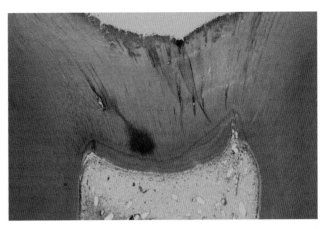

• **Fig. 3.10 Reparative Secondary Dentin.** Localized deposition of secondary dentin *(bottom)* at the pulpal end of the dentinal tubules affected by the carious process.

dentin on which is deposited irregular dentin with widely scattered, disorganized tubules.

Treatment and Prognosis

In studies of teeth exhibiting calcific metamorphosis, the vast majority of affected teeth never develop clinical or radiographic features suggestive of periapical inflammatory disease; therefore, endodontic therapy should be performed only if periapical pathosis or negative vitality testing is present. Even if a canal space cannot be identified radiographically, conventional root canal therapy usually can locate and negotiate the pulp canal. Because of the dramatically reduced canal space, location of the pulp canal can be difficult, and care must be exercised during access preparation to prevent perforation. If endodontic therapy is unsuccessful, then periapical surgery can be performed in those cases with evidence of periapical inflammatory disease. If vitality testing is positive, then periodic reevaluation appears prudent. To improve dental aesthetics, full coverage is recommended for discolored anterior teeth with large restorations. Otherwise, bleaching often effectively resolves the discoloration.

◆ PULPAL CALCIFICATIONS

Calcifications within the dental pulp are not rare. The prevalence of pulp stones reported in reviews of single cohorts varies widely, but a global meta-analysis of the frequency reported in the international dental literature revealed that 36.5% of all patients develop pulp stones, with approximately 10% of all teeth being affected. Because radiographically detectable pulp stones typically exceed 200 μm in diameter, the prevalence in a histopathologic review would be expected to be much higher. An increased prevalence of pulp stones has been reported in association with a variety of chronic pulpal irritants, such as attrition, abrasion, erosion, caries, periodontitis, dental restorative procedures, orthodontic tooth movement, and tooth injury. Pulp stones are noted more frequently in carious teeth or restored teeth, suggesting an inflammatory cause. Although many examples remain idiopathic, pulpal calcification also has been associated with aging, fluoride supplementation, hypervitaminosis D, and a few genetic disorders, such as the mild form of dentinogenesis imperfecta (see page 104).

The three types of pulpal calcifications are:
1. Denticles
2. Pulp stones
3. Diffuse linear calcifications

All pulpal calcifications start out as free bodies within the pulp tissue, but many may become attached or embedded in the dentinal walls of the pulp.

Denticles are believed to form as a result of an epithelio-mesenchymal interaction within the developing pulp. Epithelial strands originating from the root sheath, or cervical extensions into the pulp chamber adjacent to furcations, induce odontoblastic differentiation of the surrounding mesenchyme of the dental papilla, forming the core of the denticle. Odontoblasts deposit tubular dentin as they move away from the central epithelium and produce thimble-shaped structures surrounding the epithelium.

Pulp stones are believed to develop around a central nidus of pulp tissue (e.g., collagen fibril, ground substance, necrotic cell remnants). Initial calcification begins around the central nidus and extends outward in a concentric or radial pattern of regular calcified material. Pulp stones are formed within the coronal portions of the pulp and may arise as a part of age-related or local pathologic changes.

Diffuse linear calcifications do not demonstrate the lamellar organization of pulp stones; they exhibit areas of fine, fibrillar, irregular calcification that often parallel the vasculature. These calcifications may be present in the pulp chamber or canals, and the frequency increases with age.

Clinical and Radiographic Features

Denticles and pulp stones can reach sufficient size to be detected on intraoral radiographs as radiopaque enlargements within the pulp chamber or canal (Fig. 3.11). Diffuse calcifications are not detectable radiographically. Radiographically obvious pulp stones are noted most frequently in the molars followed by the premolars; a lower frequency is noted in the incisors. A maxillary and female predominance is noted. Although pulp stones can be seen at any age, there is an increased frequency over the age of 50 years.

Other than rare difficulties during endodontic procedures, pulpal calcifications are typically of little clinical significance. Some investigators associate the calcifications with dental neuralgias, but the high frequency of these lesions in the absence of clinical symptoms argues against this relationship. Others have suggested a relationship between pulpal calcification and carotid artery calcification, which potentially could be a marker for cardiovascular disease. Despite this, studies of the association by multiple groups have not proven a strong correlation. A similar association with kidney stones has been suggested. A systematic review and meta-analysis revealed patients with pulp stones are twice as likely to present with kidney stones. Prominent pulpal calcifications also have been noted in association with certain disease processes, such as the following:
- Radicular dentin dysplasia (Dentin dysplasia type Id) (see page 108)
- Dentinogenesis imperfecta, mild form (see page 104)
- Pulpal dysplasia (see page 107)
- Tumoral calcinosis
- Calcinosis universalis
- Ehlers-Danlos syndrome (see page 760)
- End-stage renal disease

Histopathologic Features

Denticles consist of tubular dentin surrounding a central nest of epithelium. With time, the central epithelium degenerates and the tubules undergo sclerosis, making their detection difficult. Most denticles are attached or embedded. Those that remain free in the pulp occasionally develop outer layers of irregular fibrillar calcification or lamellated layers of calcification similar to those seen in pulp stones.

Pulp stones demonstrate a central amorphous mass of irregular calcification surrounded by concentric lamellar rings of regular calcified material (Fig. 3.12). Occasionally,

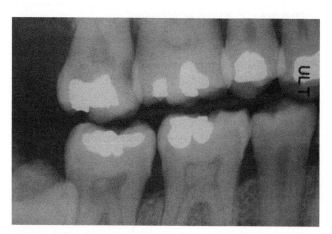

• **Fig. 3.11 Pulp Stones.** Multiple teeth demonstrating radiographically obvious calcifications within the pulp chambers.

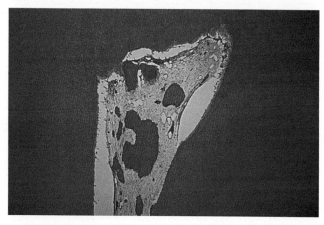

• **Fig. 3.12 Pulp Stones.** Multiple stones within the pulp chamber.

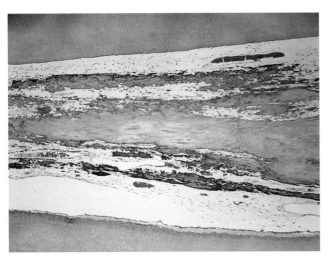

• **Fig. 3.13 Diffuse Linear Pulpal Calcifications.** Fine, fibrillar calcifications parallel the course of the neurovascular channels within the pulp canal.

a peripheral layer of tubular dentin may be applied by odontoblasts, which arise from the surrounding pulp tissue in response to the presence of the pulp stone. In addition, fibrillar irregular calcified material also may be evident on the periphery of pulp stones.

Diffuse linear calcifications consist entirely of fine, fibrillar, and irregular calcifications that develop in the pulp chambers and canals (Fig. 3.13). This material often is deposited in a linear fashion along the course of a blood vessel or nerve.

Treatment and Prognosis

No treatment is required. Most pulpal calcifications are not associated with any significant clinical alterations. In those teeth requiring root canal therapy, cone beam computed tomography has been helpful in discovering those cases in which the stone may obscure or totally block the root canal path.

◆ PERIAPICAL GRANULOMA (CHRONIC APICAL PERIODONTITIS)

The term **periapical granuloma** refers to a mass of chronically or subacutely inflamed granulation tissue at the apex of a nonvital tooth. This commonly used name is not totally accurate because the lesion does not show true granulomatous inflammation microscopically. Although the term **apical periodontitis** may be more appropriate, it may prove confusing to the clinician. Formation of apical inflammatory lesions represents a defensive reaction secondary to the presence of microbial infection in the root canal with spread of related toxic products into the apical zone. Initially, the defense reaction eliminates noxious substances that exit the canals. With time, however, the host reaction becomes less effective with microbial invasion or spread of toxins into the apical area.

In the early stages of infection, neutrophils predominate and radiographic alterations are not present; this phase of periapical inflammatory disease is termed *acute apical periodontitis.* The involved inflammatory cells are primarily neutrophils and release prostaglandins, which activate osteoclasts to resorb the surrounding bone, leading to a detectable periapical radiolucency. With time, chronic inflammatory cells begin to dominate the host response. Chronic lesions often are asymptomatic and demonstrate little additional change radiographically.

Periapical granulomas may arise after quiescence of a **periapical abscess** or may develop as the initial periapical pathosis. These lesions are not necessarily static. In addition to possible **periapical cyst** formation, a worsening of the pulpal infection can lead to a reappearance of inflammation, redevelopment of symptoms, and possible enlargement of the associated radiolucency. Secondary acute inflammatory changes within a periapical granuloma have been termed a *phoenix abscess,* after the mythical bird that would die, only to arise again from its own ashes. In progressive periapical granulomas, the enlargement often is not continuous but occurs in spurts associated with periodic acute exacerbations.

Clinical and Radiographic Features

The initial phase of periapical inflammatory disease—acute periapical periodontitis—creates a constant dull, throbbing pain. The associated tooth responds negatively to vitality testing or reveals a delayed positive result. Typically, pain on biting or percussion is present, and no obvious radiographic alterations are noted. If the acute inflammatory process evolves into a chronic pattern, then the associated symptoms diminish. In many instances, chronic periapical inflammatory disease is detected without any previous recollection of a prior acute phase.

Most periapical granulomas are asymptomatic, but pain and sensitivity can develop if acute exacerbation occurs. Typically, the involved tooth does not demonstrate mobility or significant sensitivity to percussion. The soft tissue overlying the apex may or may not be tender. The tooth does not respond to thermal or electric pulp tests unless the pulpal necrosis is limited to a single canal in a multirooted tooth.

Most lesions are discovered on routine radiographic examination. The associated radiolucencies are variable, ranging from small, barely perceptible lesions to lucencies exceeding 2 cm in diameter (Figs. 3.14–3.16). Affected teeth typically reveal loss of the apical lamina dura. The lesion may be circumscribed or ill-defined and may or may not demonstrate a surrounding radiopaque rim. Root resorption is not uncommon (Fig. 3.17). Although lesions greater than 200 mm² often represent periapical cysts, numerous investigators have been unable to distinguish periapical granulomas from periapical cysts simply on the basis of size and radiographic appearance. Cone-beam computed tomography (CBCT), magnetic resonance imaging (MRI), and high-resolution ultrasound have been reported to distinguish

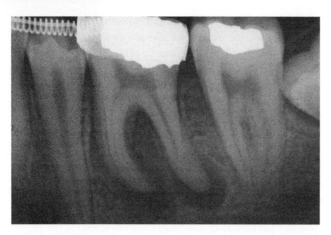

• **Fig. 3.14 Periapical Granulomas.** Discrete periapical radiolucencies associated with the apices of the mandibular first molar. (Courtesy of Dr. Garth Bobrowski.)

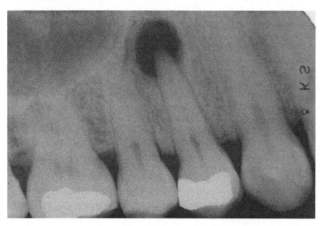

• **Fig. 3.15 Periapical Granuloma.** Well-defined radiolucency associated with the apex of the maxillary first bicuspid. (Courtesy of Dr. Frank Beylotte.)

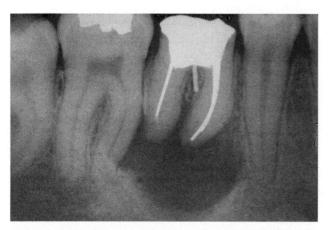

• **Fig. 3.16 Periapical Granuloma.** Large, well-defined radiolucency associated with the apices of the mandibular first molar. (Courtesy of Dr. Robert E. Loy.)

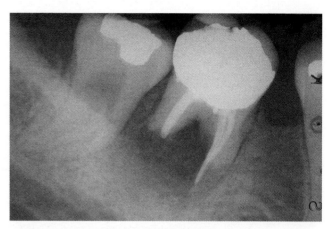

• **Fig. 3.17 Periapical Granuloma.** Ill-defined radiolucency associated with the mandibular first molar, which exhibits significant root resorption.

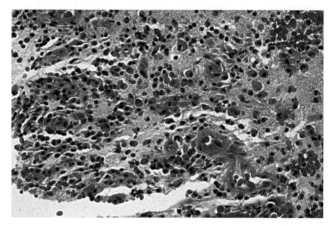

• **Fig. 3.18 Periapical Granuloma.** Granulation tissue exhibits mixed inflammatory infiltrate consisting of lymphocytes, plasma cells, and histiocytes.

periapical cysts from granulomas through features such as marginal circumscription, wall thickness, and presence or absence of a central fluid-filled cavity. Although these features may be helpful in many instances, the variations of periapical inflammatory disease continue to prevent definitive diagnosis solely by imaging. Cyst-like granulomas with luminal fluid but no epithelial lining are identified with some frequency by most oral pathologists. Conversely, relatively solid periapical cysts with an epithelial lining surrounding a small lumen can create a similar pattern to a periapical granuloma. Because periapical inflammatory disease is not static and granulomas can transform into cysts or abscesses (and vice versa) without significant radiographic change, it is not surprising that the radiographic and imaging features are not definitively diagnostic.

Histopathologic Features

Periapical granulomas consist of inflamed granulation tissue surrounded by a fibrous connective tissue wall. The granulation tissue demonstrates a variably dense lymphocytic infiltrate that is intermixed frequently with neutrophils, plasma cells, histiocytes, and, less frequently, mast cells and eosinophils (Fig. 3.18). When numerous plasma cells are present, scattered eosinophilic globules of gamma globulin (**Russell bodies**) may be seen. In addition, clusters of lightly basophilic particles (**pyronine bodies**) also may be present in association with the plasmacytic infiltrate. Both of these plasma cell products are not specific for the periapical granuloma and may be found within any accumulation of plasma cells. Epithelial rests of Malassez may be identified within the granulation tissue. Collections of cholesterol clefts, with associated multinucleated giant cells and areas of red blood cell extravasation with hemosiderin pigmentation, may be present. Small foci of acute inflammation with focal abscess formation may be seen but do not warrant the diagnosis of periapical abscess.

Treatment and Prognosis

Apical inflammatory lesions result from the presence of microorganisms or their toxic products in the root canal, the apical tissues, or both. Successful treatment depends on the reduction and control of the offending organisms. Because of the anatomic complexity of the root canal systems, some investigators believe absolute eradication of all microorganisms is unlikely; the goal of endodontics is to reduce the microbial load to a level that is insufficient to maintain periapical inflammation. If the tooth can be maintained, then root canal therapy can be performed. Nonrestorable teeth must be extracted, followed by curettage of all apical soft tissue. In symptomatic cases, nonsteroidal anti-inflammatory drugs (NSAIDs) are beneficial; use of systemic antibiotic medications is not recommended unless associated swelling or systemic changes are present.

Teeth treated endodontically should be evaluated at 1- and 2-year intervals (at a minimum) to rule out possible lesional enlargement and to ensure appropriate healing. In addition, many clinicians believe that evaluations at 1, 3, and 6 months are appropriate. Strong emphasis should be placed on the importance of the recall appointments.

Research has shown the most important factor for the successful treatment of periapical inflammatory disease is the quality of the endodontic treatment. In addition, the coronal restoration is critical, and failure can occur in cases with excellent endodontic therapy but poor coronal restoration.

If initial conventional therapy is unsuccessful, endodontic retreatment represents the best approach for minimizing the bacterial contamination and should be considered before periapical surgery. Periapical surgery remains an important tool for resolution of periapical inflammatory disease, but often it is reserved for lesions larger than 2 cm, those associated with teeth that are not appropriate for conventional endodontic therapy, and lesions that fail to respond to endodontic retreatment. Periapical surgery should include thorough curettage of all periradicular soft tissue, amputation of the apical portion of the root, and sealing the foramen of the canal. All soft tissue removed during periapical surgical procedures should be submitted for histopathologic examination. These surgical sites represent areas that have failed to respond to appropriate therapy; as such, histopathologic examination and diagnostic confirmation are mandatory. Although the vast majority of periradicular specimens represent periapical inflammatory disease, large reviews reveal a

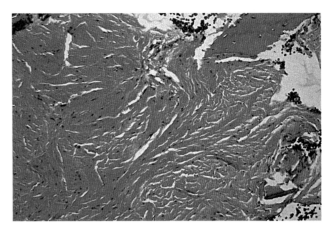

• **Fig. 3.19 Periapical Fibrous Scar.** Dense, fibrous connective tissue with vital bone and no significant inflammatory infiltrate.

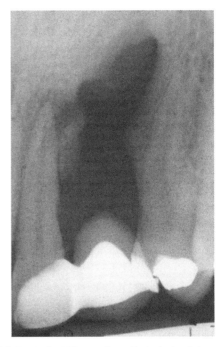

• **Fig. 3.20 Periapical Fibrous Scar.** Periapical radiolucency of maxilla at the previous site of extraction in which both cortical plates were lost. The site was filled with dense collagenous tissue. (Courtesy of Dr. James Tankersley.)

small but important percentage of other pathoses such as odontogenic keratocysts, fibro-osseous lesions, ameloblastomas, and giant cell granulomas.

On occasion, the defect created by periapical inflammatory lesions may fill with dense collagenous tissue rather than normal bone (Fig. 3.19). These **fibrous (periapical) scars** occur most frequently when both the facial and lingual cortical plates have been lost (Fig. 3.20); however, they occasionally arise in areas with intact cortical plates. If during surgery both plates are discovered to be missing, then the patient should be informed of the possibility of scar formation. The development of a periapical scar is not an indication for future surgery.

◆ PERIAPICAL CYST (RADICULAR CYST; APICAL PERIODONTAL CYST)

Epithelium at the apex of a nonvital tooth presumably can be stimulated by inflammation to form a true epithelium-lined cyst, or **periapical cyst.** The source of the epithelium is usually a rest of Malassez but also may be traced to crevicular epithelium, sinus lining, or epithelial lining of sinus tracts. Cyst development is common with a wide range of prevalence noted that most likely is related to the stringency of the diagnostic criteria used in a particular study.

When the cyst and root are removed totally, two variations of periapical cyst have been described. **Periapical pocket cysts** are characterized by an incomplete epithelial lining because of extension of the apical portion of the tooth into the cyst lumen. **Periapical true cysts** form a complete epithelium-lined baglike structure that is adjacent to, but separated from, the tooth apex. It is believed that pocket cysts often respond well to conventional endodontic therapy, whereas true cysts require periapical surgery for resolution. Studies have shown an inability to separate a "pocket" cyst from a "true" cyst unless the entire tooth and associated soft tissue are removed *in toto,* which makes the separation most impractical. Because distinguishing between an epithelialized periapical granuloma, a "pocket" cyst, or a "true" cyst has little postsurgical implications, laborious histopathologic examination and subclassification are impractical.

Periapical cysts represent a fibrous connective tissue wall lined by epithelium with a lumen containing fluid and cellular debris. Theoretically, as the epithelium desquamates into the lumen, the protein content is increased. Fluid enters the lumen in an attempt to equalize the osmotic pressure, and slow enlargement occurs. Most periapical cysts grow slowly and do not attain a large size.

On occasion, a similar cyst, best termed a **lateral radicular cyst,** may appear along the lateral aspect of the root. Like the periapical cyst, this lesion also usually arises from rests of Malassez, and the source of inflammation may be periodontal disease or pulpal necrosis with spread through a lateral foramen. Radiographically, these cysts mimic developmental **lateral periodontal cysts** (see page 699). Histopathologically, however, they are consistent with cysts of inflammatory origin.

Periapical inflammatory tissue that is not curetted at the time of tooth removal may give rise to an inflammatory cyst called a **residual periapical cyst.** With time, many of these cysts exhibit an overall reduction in size, and spontaneous resolution can occur from a lack of continued inflammatory stimulus.

Clinical and Radiographic Features
Periapical Cyst

Typically, patients with periapical cysts have no symptoms unless there is an acute inflammatory exacerbation. In addition, if the cyst reaches a large size, then swelling and mild sensitivity may be noted. Movement and mobility of adjacent teeth are possible as the cyst enlarges. The tooth from which the cyst originated does not respond to thermal and electric pulp testing.

The radiographic pattern is identical to that of a periapical granuloma. Cysts may develop even in small periapical radiolucencies, and the radiographic size cannot be used for the definitive diagnosis. A loss of the lamina dura is seen along the adjacent root, and a rounded radiolucency encircles the affected tooth apex (Fig. 3.21). Root resorption is common (Fig. 3.22). With enlargement, the radiolucency often flattens out as it approaches adjacent teeth. Significant growth is possible, and lesions occupying an entire quadrant

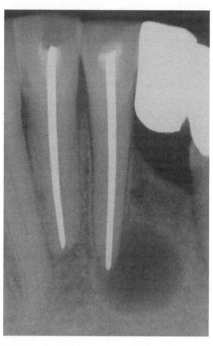

• **Fig. 3.21 Periapical Cyst.** Well-circumscribed radiolucency intimately associated with the apex of the mandibular central incisor. Note the loss of lamina dura in the area of the lesion.

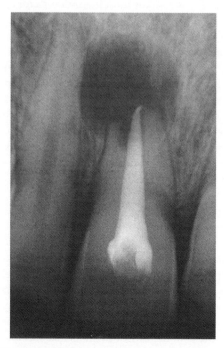

• **Fig. 3.22 Periapical Cyst.** Radiolucency associated with the maxillary central incisor, which exhibits significant root resorption.

have been noted (Fig. 3.23). Although periapical cysts more frequently achieve greater size than periapical granulomas, neither the size nor the shape of the lesion can be considered a definitive diagnostic criterion. The inability to separate these pathoses on a consistent basis holds true even with newer imaging techniques, such as cone-beam computed tomography (CBCT), magnetic resonance imaging (MRI), and high-resolution ultrasound (see similar discussion in Section "Periapical Granuloma"). Periapical cysts also are known to involve deciduous teeth. These are most frequently associated with molar teeth and appear as a radiolucent zone that surrounds the roots and fills the interradicular space at the bifurcation (Fig. 3.24).

Lateral Radicular Cyst

Lateral radicular cysts appear as discrete radiolucencies along the lateral aspect of the root (Fig. 3.25). Loss of lamina dura and an obvious source of inflammation may not be detected without a high index of suspicion. Before surgical exploration of laterally positioned radiolucencies, a thorough evaluation

of the periodontal status and vitality of adjacent teeth should be performed. Many examples of the so-called globulomaxillary cyst (see page 27) prove to be of inflammatory origin and represent lateral radicular cysts (Fig. 3.26).

Residual Periapical Cyst

The residual periapical cyst appears as a round-to-oval radiolucency of variable size within the alveolar ridge at the site of a previous tooth extraction (Fig. 3.27). As the cyst ages, degeneration of the cellular contents within the lumen occasionally leads to dystrophic calcification and central luminal radiopacity.

Histopathologic Features

The histopathologic features of all three types of inflammatory cysts are similar. The cyst is lined by stratified squamous epithelium, which may demonstrate exocytosis, spongiosis, or hyperplasia (Fig. 3.28). As seen in dentigerous cysts, scattered mucous cells or areas of ciliated pseudostratified columnar epithelium may be noted in periapical cysts (Fig. 3.29).

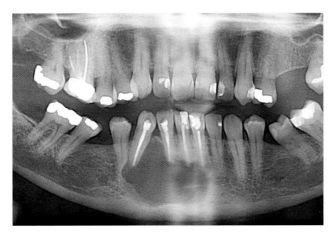

• **Fig. 3.23 Periapical Cyst.** Large unilocular radiolucency of the anterior mandible involving the apices of numerous endodontically treated teeth. (Courtesy of Dr. Enif Dominquez.)

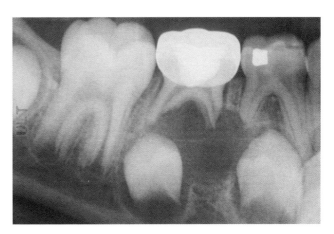

• **Fig. 3.24 Periapical Cyst.** Radiolucency involving the bifurcation and apices of the deciduous right mandibular second molar.

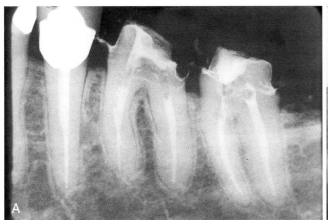

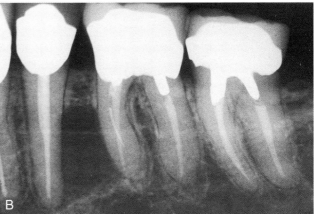

• **Fig. 3.25 Lateral Radicular Cyst. A,** Periapical radiograph of the left side of the posterior mandible taken at time of completion of endodontic therapy of the bicuspid and molars. **B,** Subsequent radiograph taken 27 months later. Note radiolucency between bicuspid and first molar extending laterally from the mesial root of the first molar. (Courtesy of Dr. Carroll Gallagher.)

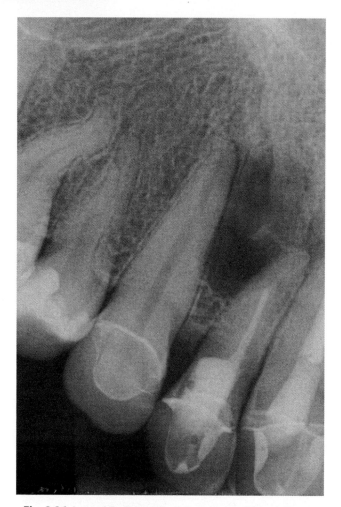

• **Fig. 3.26 Lateral Radicular Cyst.** Radiolucency between the maxillary lateral incisor and cuspid. (Courtesy of Dr. William Dunlap.)

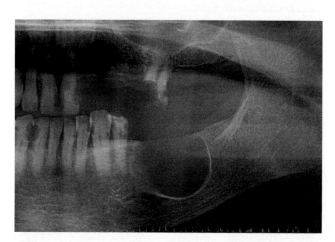

• **Fig. 3.27 Residual Periapical Cyst.** Well-circumscribed radiolucency of the left posterior mandible. (Courtesy of Dr. Jeff Wallen.)

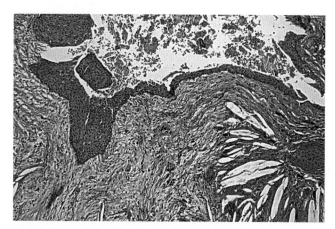

• **Fig. 3.28 Periapical Cyst.** Cyst lined by stratified squamous epithelium. Note connective tissue wall, which contains a chronic inflammatory infiltrate and numerous cholesterol clefts.

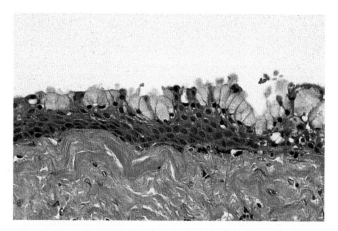

• **Fig. 3.29 Periapical Cyst.** Stratified squamous epithelial lining containing numerous mucous cells.

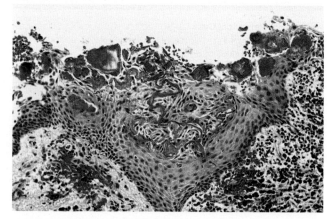

• **Fig. 3.30 Periapical Cyst.** Squamous epithelial cyst lining exhibiting numerous irregular and curvilinear Rushton bodies.

Although some maxillary periapical cysts lined by pseudostratified columnar epithelium may have originated from the adjacent sinus lining, the presence of mucous cells or respiratory-like epithelium also can be observed in mandibular cysts. The ability of odontogenic epithelium to demonstrate such specialized differentiation represents an example of *prosoplasia* (forward metaplasia) and highlights the diverse potential of odontogenic epithelium. The cyst lumen may be filled with fluid and cellular debris. On occasion, the lining epithelium may demonstrate linear or arch-shaped calcifications known as *Rushton bodies* (Fig. 3.30). The wall of the cyst consists of dense fibrous connective tissue—often with an

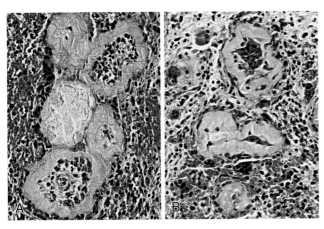

• **Fig. 3.31 Hyaline Bodies. A,** Multiple hyaline bodies appearing as corrugated collagenous rings surrounding lymphocytes and plasma cells; note early hyaline body filled with serum. **B,** Multiple hyaline bodies with numerous multinucleated giant cells within and around the corrugated collagenous rings.

inflammatory infiltrate containing lymphocytes variably intermixed with neutrophils, plasma cells, histiocytes, and (rarely) mast cells and eosinophils. Dystrophic calcification, cholesterol clefts with multinucleated giant cells, red blood cells, and areas of hemosiderin pigmentation may be present in the lumen, wall, or both. Due to the inability of macrophages and giant cells to remove cholesterol, its presence may be partially responsible for failure of healing of cysts in which the original focus of infection was treated appropriately.

Intramural islands of odontogenic epithelium that closely resemble squamous odontogenic tumor (see page 723) rarely have been noted, which could be misdiagnosed as a neoplastic process. Studies have shown these proliferations are not neoplastic and mandate no further treatment beyond the usual standard of care for periapical cysts.

Occasionally, the walls of inflammatory cysts will contain scattered **hyaline bodies (pulse granuloma, giant-cell hyaline angiopathy).** These bodies appear as small circumscribed pools of eosinophilic material that exhibits a corrugated periphery of condensed collagen often surrounded by lymphocytes and multinucleated giant cells (Fig. 3.31). Initially, these foci were thought to be a vascular degenerative process or a foreign body reaction to machinery oil or vegetable matter. Subsequently, these bodies have been shown to represent pools of inflammatory exudate (i.e., extravasated serum) that ultimately undergoes fibrosis and occasionally dystrophic calcification. The multinucleated giant cells are drawn to the site for removal of insoluble hemosiderin granules. Hyaline bodies may be found in any area of chronic intraosseous inflammation, especially periapical inflammatory disease.

Treatment and Prognosis

A periapical cyst is treated in the same manner as a periapical granuloma. When clinical and radiographic features indicate a periapical inflammatory lesion, extraction or conservative nonsurgical endodontic therapy is performed. Although

some authors believe that large cystic lesions cannot be resolved with conventional endodontics, experienced clinicians have successfully used nonsurgical root canal therapy for large areas of periapical inflammatory disease that approach 2 cm in diameter. Larger lesions associated with restorable teeth have been treated successfully with conservative endodontic therapy when combined with biopsy and marsupialization, decompression, or fenestration. As with any periapical inflammatory lesion, minimal follow-up at 1 and 2 years is advised strongly.

If the radiolucency fails to resolve, then the lesion often can be managed successfully by nonsurgical endodontic retreatment. As previously mentioned, periapical surgery typically is performed for lesions exceeding 2 cm, those associated with teeth that are not suitable for conventional endodontics, and lesions that fail to respond to endodontic retreatment. Biopsy is indicated to rule out other possible pathologic processes.

Because any number of odontogenic and non-odontogenic cysts and tumors can mimic the appearance of a residual periapical cyst, all of these cysts should be excised surgically. All inflammatory foci in the area of a lateral radicular cyst should be eliminated and the patient observed in a manner similar to that described for the periapical cyst. In some instances, lateral radicular cysts are removed before tooth vitality testing or periodontal evaluation for an adjacent focus of infection. If this diagnosis is made, then a thorough evaluation for an inflammatory source is mandatory.

◆ PERIAPICAL ABSCESS

The accumulation of acute inflammatory cells at the apex of a nonvital tooth is termed a **periapical abscess.** Acute inflammatory lesions with abscess formation may arise as the initial periapical pathosis or from an acute exacerbation of a chronic periapical inflammatory lesion (see discussion of *phoenix abscess,* page 123). Frequently, the source of the infection is obvious. On occasion, however, pulpal death may be trauma related, and the tooth may contain neither a cavity nor a restoration.

In the earliest stage of all forms of periapical inflammatory disease, the periapical periodontal ligament (PDL) fibers may exhibit acute inflammation but no frank abscess formation. This localized alteration, best termed **acute apical periodontitis,** may or may not proceed to abscess formation. Although this process often occurs in association with a nonvital tooth, acute apical periodontitis may be found in vital teeth secondary to trauma, high occlusal contacts, or wedging by a foreign object. The clinical presentation often closely resembles that of a periapical abscess and must be considered in the differential diagnosis.

Clinical and Radiographic Features

Many investigators subdivide periapical abscesses into **acute** and **chronic** types. However, these are misnomers because both types represent acute inflammatory reactions. Periapical abscesses should be designated as **symptomatic** or **asymptomatic** on the basis of their clinical presentations.

Periapical abscesses become symptomatic as the purulent material accumulates within the alveolus. The initial stages produce tenderness of the affected tooth that often is relieved by direct application of pressure. With progression, the pain becomes more intense, often with extreme sensitivity to percussion, extrusion of the tooth, and swelling of the tissues. The offending tooth does not respond to cold or electric pulp testing. Headache, malaise, fever, and chills may be present.

Radiographically, abscesses may demonstrate a thickening of the apical periodontal ligament, an ill-defined radiolucency, or both; however, often no appreciable alterations can be detected because insufficient time has occurred for significant bone destruction. Phoenix abscesses demonstrate the outline of the original chronic lesion, with or without an associated ill-defined bone loss.

With progression, the abscess spreads along the path of least resistance. The purulence may extend through the medullary spaces away from the apical area, resulting in **osteomyelitis,** or it may perforate the cortex and spread diffusely through the overlying soft tissue (as **cellulitis**). Each of these occurrences is described later in the chapter.

Once an abscess is in soft tissue, it can cause cellulitis or may channelize through the overlying soft tissue. The cortical plate may be perforated in a location that permits entrance into the oral cavity. The purulent material can accumulate in the connective tissue overlying the bone and can create a sessile swelling or perforate through the surface epithelium and drain through an intraoral sinus (Figs. 3.32 and 3.33). At the intraoral opening of a sinus tract, a mass of subacutely inflamed granulation tissue often is found, known as a **parulis** (**gum boil**) (Figs. 3.34 and 3.35). Occasionally, the nonvital tooth associated with the parulis may be difficult to determine, and insertion of a gutta-percha point into the tract can aid in detection of the offending tooth during radiographic examination (Fig. 3.36). Dental abscesses also may channelize through the overlying skin and drain via a **cutaneous sinus** (Fig. 3.37). As would be expected, asymptomatic abscesses associated with a sinus tract demonstrate an associated cortical fenestration. In contrast, symptomatic abscesses without a sinus tract typically will reveal cortical

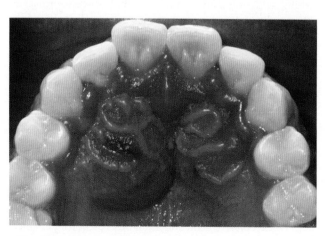

• **Fig. 3.32 Periapical Abscess.** Bilateral soft tissue swelling of the anterior palate.

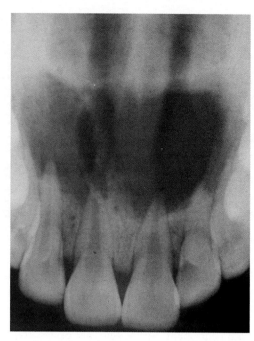

• **Fig. 3.33 Periapical Abscess.** Same patient as depicted in Fig. 3.32. Multiple, overlapping radiolucencies of the anterior maxilla are present. All four maxillary incisors exhibit pulpal necrosis.

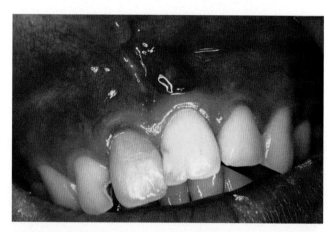

• **Fig. 3.34 Parulis.** Erythematous mass of granulation tissue overlying the left maxillary central incisor. Note discoloration of the maxillary right central incisor.

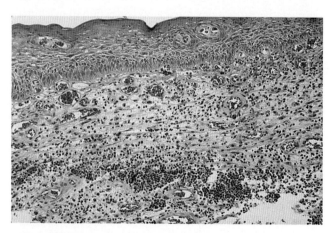

• **Fig. 3.35 Parulis.** Normal connective tissue has been replaced by acutely inflamed granulation tissue, which exhibits focal areas of neutrophilic abscess formation. Note the central sinus tract, which courses from the base of the specimen toward the surface epithelium.

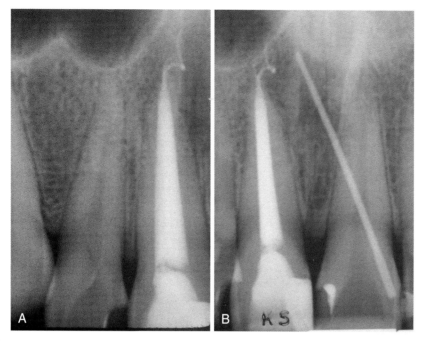

• **Fig. 3.36 Periapical Abscess. A,** Same patient as depicted in Fig. 3.34. None of the incisors demonstrates obvious periapical radiolucency. (The large radiolucency at the top is the anterior portion of the maxillary sinus.) **B,** Gutta-percha point revealed that the right maxillary incisor was the source of the infection.

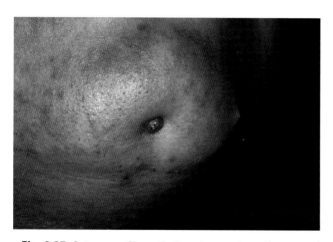

• **Fig. 3.37 Cutaneous Sinus.** Erythematous and sensitive mass of granulation tissue noted on the cutaneous surface of the chin.

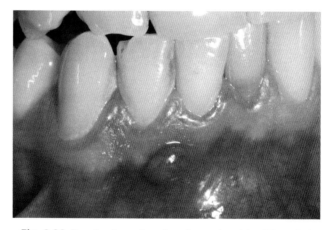

• **Fig. 3.38 Parulis.** Asymptomatic yellow-red nodule of the anterior mandibular alveolar mucosa. The adjacent teeth were asymptomatic and appeared clinically normal.

defects that are absent or smaller in size. When a sinus tract is noted, cone-beam computed tomography can identify the path of drainage through the cortical fenestration to the offending tooth.

Most dental-related abscesses perforate buccally because the bone is thinner on the buccal surface. However, infections associated with maxillary lateral incisors, the palatal roots of maxillary molars, and mandibular second and third molars typically drain through the lingual cortical plate.

If a chronic path of drainage is achieved, a periapical abscess typically becomes asymptomatic because of a lack of accumulation of purulent material within the alveolus. Occasionally, such infections are discovered during a routine oral examination after detection of a parulis or drainage

through a large carious defect (Figs. 3.38 and 3.39). If the drainage site becomes blocked, then signs and symptoms of the abscess frequently become evident in a short time. On occasion, periapical infections can spread through the bloodstream and result in systemic symptoms, such as fever, lymphadenopathy, and malaise. The risk of dissemination appears to be less for periapical abscesses that drain freely.

Histopathologic Features

Biopsy specimens from pure abscesses are uncommon because the material is in liquid form. Abscesses consist of a sea of polymorphonuclear leukocytes often intermixed with inflammatory exudate, cellular debris, necrotic material, bacterial colonies, or histiocytes (Fig. 3.40). Phoenix abscesses

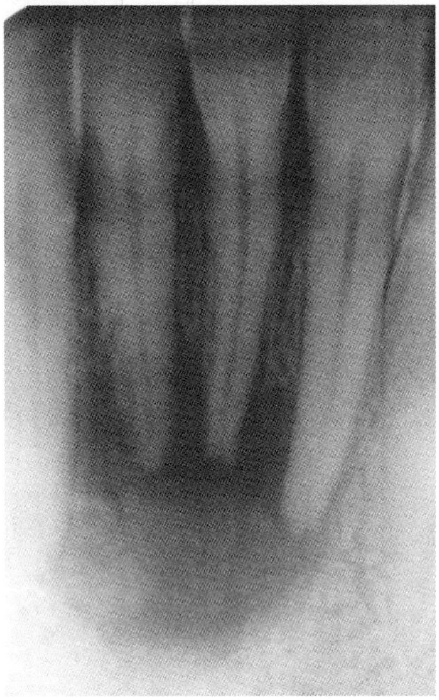

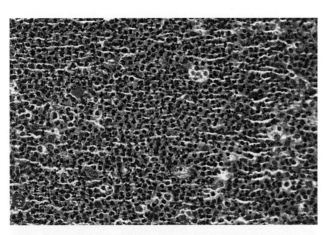

• **Fig. 3.39 Periapical Abscess.** Same patient as depicted in Fig. 3.38. Periapical radiolucency associated with the nonvital mandibular lateral incisor.

• **Fig. 3.40 Periapical Abscess.** Sheet of polymorphonuclear leukocytes intermixed with scattered histiocytes.

can maintain a soft tissue component; they present as subacutely inflamed periapical granulomas or cysts intermixed with areas of significant abscess formation. In these cases, the pathologist typically diagnoses the primary lesion but comments about the abscess formation.

Treatment and Prognosis

Treatment of the patient with a periapical abscess consists of drainage and elimination of the focus of infection. Those abscesses associated with a patent sinus tract may be asymptomatic but, nevertheless, should be treated. With localized periapical abscesses, the signs and symptoms typically diminish significantly within 48 hours of initiation of appropriate drainage. When the abscess causes clinical expansion of the bone or soft tissue adjacent to the apex of the affected tooth,

incisional drainage of the swelling should be considered because this technique appears to be associated with more rapid resolution of the inflammatory process when compared with drainage through the root canal. If the affected tooth is extruded, then reduction of the occlusion is recommended because chronic occlusal trauma has been shown to delay resolution of the inflammatory process. Unless contraindicated, treatment with NSAIDs usually is appropriate preoperatively, immediately postoperatively, and for subsequent pain control. Use of antibiotic medications for a well-localized and easily drained periapical abscess in a healthy patient is not recommended due to negligible benefits and potential harm associated with use of antibiotics. Antibiotic coverage should be reserved for patients without immediate access to dental care, the medically compromised, and patients with significant cellulitis (see next section) or clinical evidence of dissemination (i.e., fever, lymphadenopathy, malaise). Once the infection has been resolved by extraction or appropriate endodontic therapy, the affected bone typically heals.

Usually, a sinus tract resolves spontaneously after the offending tooth is extracted or endodontically treated. Sinus tracts that persist are thought to contain sufficient infectious material along the fistulous tract to maintain the surface granulation tissue, and surgical removal with curettage of the tract is required for resolution.

◆ CELLULITIS

If an abscess is not able to establish drainage through the surface of the skin or into the oral cavity, it may spread diffusely through fascial planes of the soft tissue. This acute and edematous spread of an acute inflammatory process is termed **cellulitis.** Although cellulitis may occur in otherwise healthy individuals, there is an increased prevalence in patients with variety of medical conditions, such as use of corticosteroid or cytotoxic medications, malignancy, diabetes mellitus, or immunosuppressive disorders including neutropenia, aplastic anemia, and acquired immunodeficiency syndrome (AIDS). Although numerous patterns of cellulitis can be seen from the spread of dental infections, two especially dangerous forms warrant further discussion: (1) **Ludwig angina** and (2) **cavernous sinus thrombosis.**

Ludwig angina, named after the German physician, Friedrich Wilhelm von Ludwig, who described the seriousness of the disorder in 1836, refers to cellulitis of the submandibular region. Angina comes from the Latin word *angere,* which means *to strangle* (an apt term, considering the clinical features described in the following section). In up to 90% of cases, Ludwig angina develops from spread of an acute infection from the lower molar teeth. Other situations associated with this clinical presentation are peritonsillar or parapharyngeal abscesses, tongue piercing, oral lacerations, fractures of the mandible, or submandibular sialadenitis.

The cavernous sinus is a group of thin-walled veins that are located lateral to the sella turcica and medial to the temporal bone. The trochlear and oculomotor nerves and the maxillary and ophthalmic branches of the trigeminal nerve course through the area. In addition, the internal carotid artery and abducens nerve travel within the sinus. The sinus receives venous drainage from the orbit via the superior and inferior ophthalmic veins. Infection of the sinus can produce a variety of clinical symptoms related to the numerous anatomic structures that course through this site.

The most common cause of cavernous sinus thrombosis is sinusitis, usually from the sphenoid sinus. Less common origins include infections of the middle ear, mastoid, mid-facial region, tonsils, and pharynx. Odontogenic infections are responsible in about 10% of the cases. Cavernous sinus thrombosis can occur via an anterior or posterior pathway. Infection from the maxillary anterior teeth can perforate the facial maxillary bone and spread to the canine space. A septic thrombus develops in the valveless facial veins located in this space, and retrograde propagation occurs from the angular vein to the inferior ophthalmic vein through the inferior orbital fissure into the cavernous sinus. The posterior pathway is followed by infections originating from maxillary premolar or molar teeth, which demonstrate buccal or infratemporal space involvement that may spread via the emissary veins from the pterygoid venous plexus to the inferior petrosal sinus and into the cavernous sinus. Thankfully, cavernous sinus thrombosis is relatively uncommon.

Clinical Features

Ludwig Angina

Ludwig angina is an aggressive and rapidly spreading cellulitis that involves the sublingual, submandibular, and submental spaces bilaterally. Once the infection enters the submandibular space, it may extend to the lateral pharyngeal space and then to the retropharyngeal space. This extension may result in spread to the mediastinum with several serious consequences.

Ludwig angina creates massive swelling of the neck that often extends close to the clavicles (Fig. 3.41). Involvement of the sublingual space results in elevation, posterior enlargement, and protrusion of the tongue (**woody tongue**), which can compromise the airway. In some cases, the elevation of the floor of the mouth creates a mass of tissue that elevates the tongue, creating a bifold appearance that has been termed **double tongue**. Submandibular space spread causes enlargement and tenderness of the neck above the level of the hyoid bone (**bull neck**). Although initially unilateral, spread to the contralateral neck typically occurs. Pain in the neck and floor of mouth may be seen in addition to restricted neck movement, dysphagia, dysphonia, dysarthria, drooling, and sore throat. Involvement of the lateral pharyngeal space can cause respiratory obstruction secondary to laryngeal edema. Tachypnea, dyspnea, tachycardia, stridor, restlessness, and the patient's need to maintain an erect position suggest airway obstruction. Fever, chills, leukocytosis, and an elevated sedimentation rate may be seen. Classically, obvious collections of pus are not present.

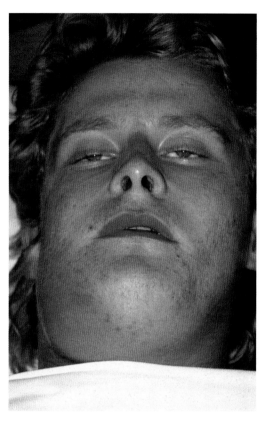

• **Fig. 3.41 Ludwig Angina.** Soft tissue swelling of the right submandibular region. (Courtesy of Dr. Brian Blocher.)

Cavernous Sinus Thrombosis

Cavernous sinus thrombosis appears as an edematous periorbital enlargement with involvement of the eyelids and conjunctiva. In cases involving the canine space, swelling also typically is present along the lateral border of the nose and may extend up to the medial aspect of the eye and periorbital area (Fig. 3.42). Protrusion and fixation of the eyeball often are evident, in addition to induration and swelling of the adjacent forehead and nose. Pupil dilation, lacrimation, photophobia, and loss of vision may occur. Pain over the eye and along the distribution of the ophthalmic and maxillary branches of the trigeminal nerve often is present. Proptosis, chemosis, and ptosis are noted in greater than 90% of affected patients. The cavernous sinuses freely communicate via the intercavernous sinus. Although many cases are initially unilateral, without appropriate therapy, the infection may spread to the contralateral side. Cranial magnetic resonance imaging (MRI), which will demonstrate cavernous sinus expansion in the majority of patients, is important to confirm the clinical diagnosis and allow prompt treatment.

Fever, chills, headache, sweating, tachycardia, nausea, and vomiting can occur. With progression, signs of central nervous system (CNS) involvement develop. Meningitis, tachycardia, tachypnea, irregular breathing, stiffening of the neck, and deepening stupor with or without delirium indicate advanced toxemia and meningeal involvement. Occasionally, brain abscesses may result.

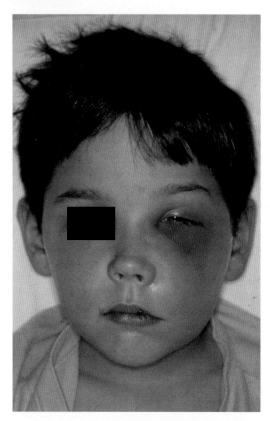

• **Fig. 3.42 Cellulitis Involving Canine Space.** Erythematous and edematous enlargement of the left side of the face with involvement of the eyelids and conjunctiva. Patients with odontogenic infections involving the canine space are at risk for cavernous sinus thrombosis. (Courtesy of Dr. Richard Ziegler.)

Treatment and Prognosis

Ludwig Angina

Treatment of Ludwig angina centers around two major priorities: maintenance of the airway and resolution of the infection. The choice of airway maintenance varies according to the severity of the obstruction. Choices include observation, orotracheal intubation, fiber-optic nasotracheal intubation, and tracheotomy. Orotracheal intubation often is very difficult because of the presence of trismus and swollen soft tissues. On occasion, cricothyroidotomy is performed instead of a tracheostomy because of a perceived lower risk of spreading the infection to the mediastinum.

Resolution of the infection involves elimination of the original focus of infection and intravenous (IV) antibiotic therapy. Penicillin with or without clindamycin or metronidazole frequently is the initial choice with culture and sensitivity testing used to guide final therapy. Although controversial, corticosteroids are prescribed by some clinicians to reduce swelling in order to protect the airway and augment antibiotic penetration.

Limited surgical incision and drainage is appropriate if collections of purulence can be identified. This decision is made best through a combination of physical examination and high-quality imaging. Contrast-enhanced computed tomography appears to be the best modality, but high resolution ultrasound also has been shown to be beneficial. Magnetic resonance imaging is utilized less frequently due to prolonged acquisition time, cost, and interaction with ferromagnetic materials such as implants. Cellulitis without identifiable pockets of purulence is managed medically after resolution of the original focus of infection. Before the use of modern antibiotic medications, the mortality from Ludwig angina often exceeded 50%. Although this rate has been reduced to less than 10%, deaths still occur as the result of complications such as pericarditis, pneumonia, mediastinitis, sepsis, empyema, and respiratory obstruction. The majority of deaths occur in patients over the age of 40 with complicating medical conditions such as diabetes, hypertension, and immunosuppression.

Cavernous Sinus Thrombosis

The therapeutic cornerstones for cavernous sinus thrombosis caused by dental infections are surgical drainage combined with high-dose broad-spectrum antibiotic medications exhibiting a good blood-brain-barrier penetration. The offending tooth should be extracted, and drainage is required if fluctuance is present. Administration of systemic corticosteroid drugs is indicated only in patients who have developed pituitary insufficiency in advanced cases of cavernous sinus thrombosis. Some investigators also prescribe anticoagulant medications to prevent thrombosis and septic emboli; conversely, others believe that thrombosis limits the infection and that the use of anticoagulant drugs may promote hemorrhagic lesions in the orbit and brain.

In older series the mortality rate approached 75%. Even with current medical advances and modern antibiotic medications, the mortality rate remains at approximately 20%–30% with many survivors demonstrating long-term disability such as permanent blindness, double vision, hemiparesis, and sixth cranial nerve palsy.

◆ OSTEOMYELITIS

Osteomyelitis is an acute or chronic inflammatory process in the medullary spaces or cortical surfaces of bone that extends away from the initial site of involvement. The term *osteomyelitis* arose from the ancient Greek words *osteon* (bone) and *muelinos* (marrow) and literally implies infection of the medullary segments of bone. This section describes the classic pattern of osteomyelitis.

The vast majority of osteomyelitis cases are caused by bacterial infections and result in an expanding lytic destruction of the involved bone, with suppuration and sequestra formation. Many believe that this condition is more appropriately termed *suppurative osteomyelitis, bacterial osteomyelitis,* or *secondary osteomyelitis*. This pattern of osseous pathosis is in contrast to an ill-defined group of idiopathic inflammatory disorders of bone that do not respond consistently to antibacterial medications and typically demonstrate ultimate sclerosis of bone without suppuration or sequestra formation. This second pattern of inflammatory bone disease is most appropriately termed *primary chronic osteomyelitis* but often is included under the term *diffuse sclerosing osteomyelitis*. This disorder and several other patterns of inflammatory bone disease (e.g., focal sclerosing osteomyelitis, proliferative periostitis, and alveolar osteitis) are unique and are covered separately later in the chapter. Osteoradionecrosis is excluded from this discussion because this is primarily a problem of hypoxia, hypocellularity, and hypovascularity in which the presence of bacteria represents a secondary colonization of nonhealing bone rather than a primary bacterial infection (see page 283). In addition, medication-related osteonecrosis represents another unique pattern that is discussed in a later chapter and appears more strongly related to altered bone metabolism (see page 286).

Suppurative osteomyelitis of the jaws is uncommon in developed countries, but it continues to be a source of significant difficulty in developing nations. In Europe and North America, most cases arise after odontogenic infections or traumatic fracture of the jaws. In addition, many cases reported in Africa occur in the presence of necrotizing gingivitis (NG, see page 151) or noma.

Chronic systemic diseases, immunocompromised status, and disorders associated with decreased vascularity of bone appear to predispose people to osteomyelitis. Tobacco use, alcohol abuse, IV drug abuse, diabetes mellitus, exanthematous fevers, malaria, sickle cell anemia, malnutrition, malignancy, collagen vascular diseases, and AIDS have been associated with an increased frequency of osteomyelitis. In addition to radiation, several osseous diseases (e.g., osteopetrosis, dysosteosclerosis, late Paget disease, end-stage cemento-osseous dysplasia) may result in hypovascularized bone that is predisposed to necrosis and inflammation.

Acute suppurative osteomyelitis exists when an acute inflammatory process spreads through the medullary spaces of the bone and insufficient time has passed for the body to react to the presence of the inflammatory infiltrate. **Chronic suppurative osteomyelitis** exists when the defensive response leads to the production of granulation tissue, which subsequently forms dense scar tissue in an attempt to wall off the infected area. The encircled dead space acts as a reservoir for bacteria, and antibiotic medications have great difficulty reaching the site. This pattern begins to evolve about 1 month after the spread of the initial acute infection and results in a smoldering process that is difficult to manage unless the problem is approached aggressively.

Clinical and Radiographic Features

Patients of all ages can be affected by osteomyelitis. There is a strong male predominance, approaching 75% in some reviews. Most cases involve the mandible due to its relatively poor vascular supply and dense cortical bone that is more susceptible to infection when compared to the maxilla. Maxillary disease becomes important primarily in pediatric patients and in cases that arise from NG or noma (in African populations).

Acute Suppurative Osteomyelitis

Patients with acute osteomyelitis have signs and symptoms of an acute inflammatory process that has typically been less than 1 month in duration. Fever, leukocytosis, lymphadenopathy, significant sensitivity, and soft tissue swelling of the affected area may be present. Plain dental or panoramic radiographs may demonstrate an ill-defined radiolucency (Fig. 3.43), occasionally combined with widening of the periodontal ligament, loss of lamina dura, or loss of circumscription of the inferior alveolar canal or mental foramen. Periosteal new bone formation also may be seen in response to subperiosteal spread of the infection. This proliferation is more common in young patients and presents as a single-layered linear radiopaque line separated from the normal cortex by an intervening radiolucent band. Because plain radiographs require loss of up to 50% of bone mineral density to demonstrate an obvious pathosis, such films often may be unremarkable early in the course of infection. Scintigraphy and magnetic resonance imaging (MRI) demonstrate high sensitivity but low specificity. Conventional CT is a better choice due to its good combination of sensitivity and specificity. Being specially designed for imaging the gnathic hard tissues, cone-beam CT represents another excellent alterative with shorter scanning times and lower doses of radiation when compared to conventional CT. On occasion, paresthesia of the lower lip, drainage, or exfoliation of fragments of necrotic bone may be discovered. A fragment of necrotic bone that has separated from the adjacent vital bone is termed a **sequestrum.** Sequestra often exhibit spontaneous exfoliation (Fig. 3.44). On occasion, fragments of necrotic bone may become surrounded by new vital bone, and the dead bone in this situation is known as an **involucrum.**

Chronic Suppurative Osteomyelitis

If acute osteomyelitis is not resolved expeditiously, the entrenchment of **chronic osteomyelitis** occurs, or the process may arise primarily without a previous acute episode. Swelling, pain, sinus formation, purulent discharge, sequestrum formation, tooth loss, or pathologic fracture may occur.

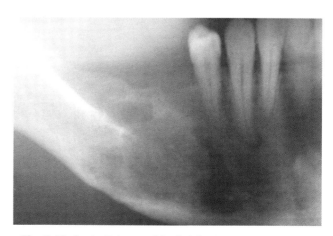

• **Fig. 3.43 Acute Osteomyelitis.** Ill-defined area of radiolucency of the right body of the mandible.

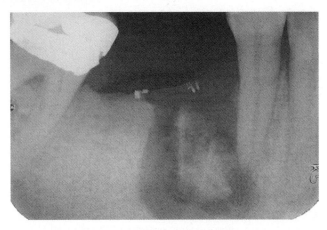

• **Fig. 3.44 Acute Osteomyelitis with Sequestrum.** Radiolucency of the right body of the mandible with central radiopaque mass of necrotic bone. (Courtesy of Dr. Michael Meyrowitz.)

Paresthesia of the lower lip is not uncommon in advanced cases. Patients may experience acute exacerbations or periods of decreased pain associated with chronic smoldering progression (Fig. 3.45).

Radiographs reveal a patchy, ragged, and ill-defined radiolucency that may contain central radiopaque sequestra and be intermixed with zones of radiodensity. Less frequently, the infection may be predominantly osteosclerotic or occasionally almost totally osteolytic. The osseous change is continuous and may exhibit spread to the periosteum, often triggering periosteal new bone formation.

Because of an anatomic peculiarity, large portions of each jawbone receive their blood supply through multiple arterial loops originating from a single vessel. Involvement of this single feeder vessel can lead to necrosis of a large portion of the affected bone. Sequestration that has involved an entire quadrant of the jaw has been reported in long-standing cases of chronic osteomyelitis.

Histopathologic Features
Acute Suppurative Osteomyelitis

Generation of biopsy material from patients with acute osteomyelitis is not common because of the predominantly liquid content and lack of a soft tissue component. When submitted, the material consists predominantly of necrotic bone. The bone shows a loss of the osteocytes from their lacunae, peripheral resorption, and bacterial colonization (Fig. 3.46). The periphery of the bone and the haversian canals contain necrotic debris and an acute inflammatory infiltrate consisting of polymorphonuclear leukocytes. The submitted material will be diagnosed as a sequestrum unless a good clinicopathologic correlation points to the appropriate diagnosis of acute osteomyelitis.

Chronic Suppurative Osteomyelitis

Biopsy material from patients with chronic osteomyelitis demonstrates a significant soft tissue component that consists of chronically or subacutely inflamed fibrous connective tissue filling the intertrabecular areas of the bone (Fig. 3.47). Scattered sequestra and pockets of abscess formation are common.

Treatment and Prognosis
Acute Suppurative Osteomyelitis

Therapy centers around surgical intervention to (1) resolve the source of infection, (2) establish drainage, (3) removal of obviously infected bone, and (4) obtain bacteriologic samples for culture and antibiotic sensitivity testing. While waiting on the bacteriologic evaluation, antibiotics are administered empirically, usually penicillin with metronidazole or clindamycin. Multiple procedures over days to weeks may be required for complete elimination of the infection and reconstruction of the gnathic defect.

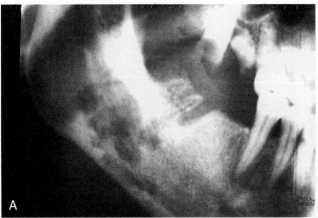
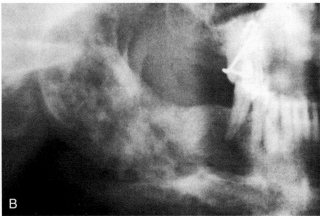

• **Fig. 3.45 Chronic Osteomyelitis. A,** Ill-defined area of radiolucency of the right body of the mandible adjacent to a recent extraction site. **B,** After the initial intervention, the patient failed to return for follow-up because of lack of significant pain. An enlarged, ill-defined radiolucency of the right body of the mandible was discovered 2 years after the initial surgery. (Courtesy of Dr. Charles Waldron.)

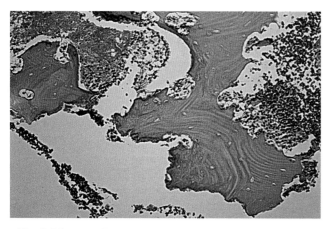

• **Fig. 3.46 Acute Osteomyelitis.** Nonvital bone exhibits loss of the osteocytes from the lacunae. Peripheral resorption, bacterial colonization, and surrounding inflammatory response also can be seen.

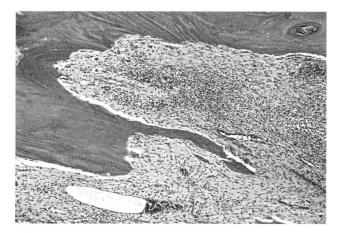

• **Fig. 3.47 Chronic Osteomyelitis.** Subacutely inflamed and reactive fibrous connective tissue filling the intertrabecular spaces with pockets of abscess formation and partially necrotic bone.

Chronic Suppurative Osteomyelitis

Chronic osteomyelitis is difficult to manage medically, presumably because pockets of dead bone and organisms are protected from antibiotic drugs by the surrounding wall of fibrous connective tissue. Surgical intervention is mandatory. The antibiotic medications are similar to those used in the acute form but must be given intravenously in high doses.

The extent of the surgical intervention depends on the spread of the process; removal of all infected material down to good bleeding bone is mandatory in all cases. For small lesions, curettage, removal of necrotic bone, and saucerization are sufficient. In patients with more extensive osteomyelitis, decortication or saucerization often is combined with transplantation of cancellous bone chips. In cases of persisting osteomyelitis, resection of the diseased bone followed by immediate reconstruction with an autologous graft is required. Weakened jawbones must be immobilized.

The goal of surgery is removal of all infected tissue. Persistence of chronic osteomyelitis is typically the result of incomplete removal of diseased tissue. On successful elimination of all infected material, resolution is expected.

Adjunctive procedures (e.g., hyperbaric oxygen) are rarely necessary if thorough surgical curettage and sequestrectomy have been accomplished.

Management of persistent cases of chronic osteomyelitis often requires use of more sophisticated techniques. Scintigraphic techniques with technetium-99m (^{99m}Tc)-labeled phosphorus compounds can be used to evaluate the therapeutic response and progress of treatment. Hyperbaric oxygen is recommended primarily for the rare patient who does not respond to standard therapy or for disease arising in hypovascularized bone (e.g., osteoradionecrosis, osteopetrosis, Paget disease, and cemento-osseous dysplasia).

◆ DIFFUSE SCLEROSING OSTEOMYELITIS

Diffuse sclerosing osteomyelitis (DSO) is characterized by more widespread infection associated with varying degrees of gnathic periosteal hyperplasia, sclerosis, and radiolucency. The term DSO should be used only when an obvious infectious process directly is responsible for sclerosis of bone. In these cases, a chronic intraosseous bacterial infection creates a smoldering mass of chronically inflamed granulation tissue that incites sclerosis of the surrounding bone.

Clinical and Radiographic Features

Diffuse sclerosing osteomyelitis is similar to the localized variant (condensing osteitis; see page 141); however, the disorder also is very different. It arises almost exclusively in adulthood, does not exhibit a sex predominance, and primarily occurs in the mandible. An increased radiodensity develops around sites of chronic infection (e.g., periodontitis, pericoronitis, and apical inflammatory disease) in a manner very similar to the increased radiodensity that may be seen surrounding areas of chronic suppurative osteomyelitis. Typically, the altered area is restricted to a single site but may be multifocal or extend to fill an entire quadrant.

The sclerosis centers on the crestal portions of the tooth-bearing alveolar ridge and does not appear to originate in the areas of attachment of the masseter or digastric muscle. The radiodensities do not develop from previously radiolucent fibro-osseous lesions and do not exhibit the predilection for black females, as is found in those patients with florid cemento-osseous dysplasia. Pain and swelling are not typical.

Histopathologic Features

Diffuse sclerosing osteomyelitis demonstrates sclerosis and remodeling of bone. The haversian canals are scattered widely and little marrow tissue can be found. Although the sclerosis occurs adjacent to areas of inflammation, the bone typically is not intermixed with a significant inflammatory soft tissue component. If the adjacent inflammatory process extends into the sclerotic bone, then necrosis often occurs. The necrotic bone separates from the adjacent vital tissue and becomes surrounded by subacutely inflamed granulation tissue. Secondary bacterial colonization often is visible.

Treatment and Prognosis

Diffuse sclerosing osteomyelitis is treated best through resolution of the adjacent foci of chronic infection. After resolution of the infection, the sclerosis remodels in some patients but remains in others. The persistent sclerotic bone is hypovascular, does not exhibit typical remodeling, and is very sensitive to inflammation. The patient and the clinician should work together to avoid future problems with periodontitis or apical inflammatory disease. With long-term alveolar resorption after denture placement, the altered bone does not exhibit typical resorption, and exposure of the bone through the overlying mucosa may occur with secondary osteomyelitis. These secondary lesions can be treated in the same way as a primary acute or chronic suppurative osteomyelitis (see page 136).

◆ CHRONIC NONBACTERIAL OSTEOMYELITIS

Chronic nonbacterial osteomyelitis (primary chronic osteomyelitis) often is confused with, but must be distinguished from, diffuse sclerosing osteomyelitis (DSO) and chronic suppurative osteomyelitis. In contrast to DSO and suppurative osteomyelitis, an association with a bacterial infection is not obvious, and suppuration with sequestration characteristically are absent. A number of causes have been proposed, such as a primary autoimmune disease or an altered immune response to an organism of low virulence, but no single theory has received widespread acceptance. In contrast to suppurative osteomyelitis, cultures are negative in almost all patients and the condition does not respond to long-term antibiotic therapy.

Chronic nonbacterial osteomyelitis (CNO) may be a primary disorder or represent **chronic tendoperiostitis**. Many clinicians believe chronic tendoperiostitis represents a reactive alteration of bone that is initiated and exacerbated by chronic overuse of the masticatory muscles, predominantly the masseter and digastric. In a large series of patients, parafunctional muscle habits (e.g., bruxism, clenching, nail biting, co-contraction, and inability to relax jaw musculature) were known or became evident during follow-up. In neurophysiologic studies, masseter inhibitory reflexes were abnormal in the vast majority of patients studied.

Although CNO may be isolated to the jaw, it could represent one focus of involvement in a patient with more widespread disease, such as **chronic recurrent multifocal osteomyelitis (CRMO)**, **SAPHO syndrome**, or **sternocostoclavicular hyperostosis (SCCH)**. Chronic recurrent multifocal osteomyelitis demonstrates involvement of multiple bones and is thought by many to represent a widespread variant of chronic nonbacterial osteomyelitis. SAPHO syndrome is closely related and an acronym for a complex clinical presentation that includes **S**ynovitis, **A**cne, **P**ustulosis, **H**yperostosis, and **O**steitis in which the osseous lesions mirror those of chronic nonbacterial osteomyelitis or CRMO. Sternocostoclavicular hyperostosis most likely represents a subset of CRMO and SAPHO in which the extragnathic bone involvement preferentially affects the sternum, medial end of the clavicle, and upper ribs. All three disorders are associated with an increased prevalence of autoimmune diseases (such as inflammatory bowel disease and seronegative spondyloarthropathies) and skin diseases such as psoriasis, palmoplantar pustulosis, acne fulminans, and acne conglobata. The cause of CRMO and SAPHO is unknown, but they possibly may arise in genetically predisposed individuals with apparent autoimmunity. In rare cases, dermatologic bacteria (most frequently *Propionibacterium acnes*) have been cultured from the osseous lesions, leading researchers to theorize that an abnormal immune response to the microorganism cross-reacts with normal bone or joint structures, leading to the variety of clinical manifestations. Despite this, no widely accepted explanation exists for these lesions.

Clinical and Radiographic Features

Chronic nonbacterial osteomyelitis (CNO) frequently is discovered as an isolated process that typically is localized to the mandible, although patients should be evaluated for extragnathic evidence of SAPHO syndrome or CRMO. The onset of symptoms tends to show two peaks, one in adolescence and the other in adults after the fifth decade of life. A female predominance is noted. Affected patients have recurrent episodes of pain, swelling, local induration, and limited mouth opening that is not associated with any obvious dental infection. Enlargement and tenderness of the overlying soft tissue and masseter muscle often are noted. During periods of disease activity, regional lymphadenopathy and reduced sensation in the distribution of the inferior alveolar nerve may be present. Laboratory testing often with show an elevation of the erythrocyte sedimentation rate and C-reactive protein levels, but the white blood cell count usually is within the normal reference range. Absence of fever, purulence, sequestration, and sinus formation are characteristic. The lack of an obvious association with an odontogenic infection and the nonsuppurative presentation clearly separate this condition from DSO and chronic suppurative osteomyelitis.

In the early stages of CNO, radiographs tend to demonstrate a mixed pattern, with areas of radiolucent osteolysis intermingled with zones of sclerosis (Fig. 3.48). In contrast to the pattern noted in CT images of suppurative osteomyelitis, the osteolytic areas are not continuous and alternate with zones of sclerosis. The affected area of the bone typically is thickened and demonstrates a periosteal proliferation that is more solid than the typical laminated proliferative periostitis of inflammatory origin. Facial asymmetry is not uncommon and often takes years to resolve secondary to slow remodeling. Over time, the affected area becomes predominantly sclerotic, but during subsequent periods of disease activity, new foci of osteolysis and cortical bone destruction appear. These newly affected areas subsequently undergo sclerosis, awaiting the next cycle of disease activity. With disease progression, the clinical symptoms typically diminish, and the affected bone demonstrates progressive sclerosis and a reduction in the volume. Radiolucent osteolytic areas may remain, but they tend to be relatively small and widely scattered. Overall, the predominant radiographic alteration of primary chronic osteomyelitis is medullary sclerosis, a pattern that is noted invariably in affected patients. Skeletal scintigraphy demonstrates significant uptake in the affected areas and should be performed in all patients in an effort to rule out extragnathic involvement. Alternatively, whole-body coronal magnetic resonance imaging (MRI) with a short tau inversion recovery sequence has proven to be valuable is discovering multifocal skeletal involvement.

Chronic Tendoperiostitis

Chronic tendoperiostitis may occur in people of all ages and there is no sex predilection. Recurrent pain, swelling of the cheek, trismus, and limited mouth opening are classic symptoms. Suppuration and an associated infectious cause are not found. Microbiologic cultures are typically negative, with the lesions failing to respond to appropriate antibiotic medications. Uncommon spontaneous resolution with development of radiographic normalcy has been noted.

In most instances, the sclerosis is limited to a single quadrant and centers on the anterior region of the mandibular angle and posterior portion of the mandibular body (i.e., attachment of the masseter muscle). Occasionally, the cuspid and premolar region and the anterior mandible (i.e., attachment of the digastric muscle) may be involved. Relatively radiolucent zones are apparent within the areas of radiodensity. The inferior border of the mandibular body may be affected with significant erosion of the inferior border appearing just anterior to the angle of the mandible (Fig. 3.49). Condylar process deformations are noted in occasional patients and have been suggested secondary to external forces of the masticatory muscles.

CRMO and SAPHO Syndrome

CRMO and SAPHO syndrome appear closely related, and many believe that CRMO represents the pediatric variant of SAPHO. CRMO presents in childhood with pain and swelling of multiple bones, particularly the metaphysis of

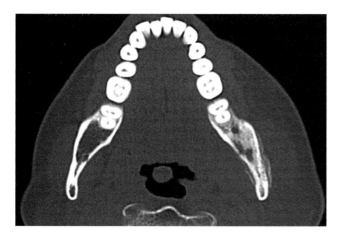

• **Fig. 3.48 Chronic Nonbacterial Osteomyelitis**. Sclerosis of the left posterior mandible intermixed with foci of radiolucency and overlying periosteal hyperplasia. No associated odontogenic infection was present. The patient also presented with trimus, tenderness, and soft tissue enlargement. (Courtesy of Dr. Benjamin Noblitt.)

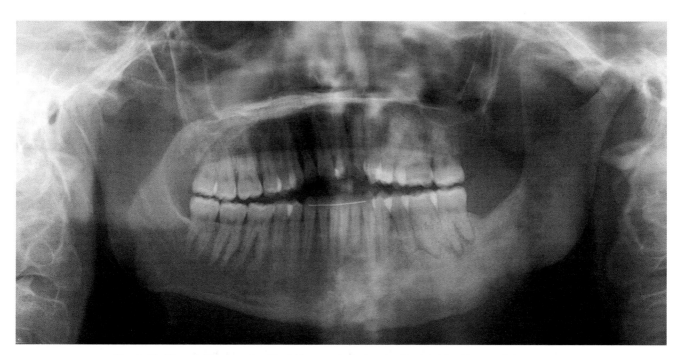

• **Fig. 3.49 Chronic Tendoperiostitis**. Diffuse mottled sclerosis of the left side of the mandible with erosion of the inferior border and focal radiolucent notching at the site of the masseter muscle insertion. Coronoid hyperplasia also is present, another sign of the temporomandibular disorder. (Courtesy of Dr. J. P. R. van Merkesteyn.)

long bones, the pelvis, spine, and clavicles. Affected bones typically demonstrate hyperostosis with osteitis that is associated with negative microbiologic cultures and lack of response to antibiotics. Many patients demonstrate concurrent or future neutrophilic skin diseases, such as palmoplantar pustulosis, severe acne, hidradenitis suppurativa, psoriasis, Sweet syndrome, or pyoderma gangrenosum. The dermatologic involvement may be absent, appear after some delay, or be so subtle as to escape detection. In contrast, SAPHO usually is noted in adults, classically affects the axial skeleton (anterior chest wall), and more frequently demonstrates concurrent neutrophilic skin lesions. Gnathic involvement has been reported in both CRMO and SAPHO, mandating full bone scan in any patient with an unexplained chronic nonbacterial osteomyelitis. In contrast to bacterial osteomyelitis, the osteolytic areas are scattered randomly within areas of sclerotic bone. Periosteal new bone formation is common but not related to cortical bone perforation. Investigation of the entire skeleton by bone scintigraphy or magnetic resonance imaging (MRI) classically reveals involvement of multiple sites.

In early gnathic lesions, diffuse osteolytic zones are more prominent than sclerosis, and the affected bone is enlarged because of significant production of periosteal new bone. With time, the bone becomes more sclerotic and decreases in size because of diminished periosteal apposition, while the osteolytic zones become smaller and fewer. External bone resorption and deformity of the mandible are characteristic in older lesions.

Histopathologic Features

Similar histopathologic features of the gnathic lesions are seen in isolated chronic nonbacterial osteomyelitis, SAPHO syndrome, CRMO, SCCH, and chronic tendoperiostitis. The periosteal proliferation reveals parallel and interconnecting thin trabeculae of bone with intervening strips of loose connective tissue. The medullary areas are filled with thin curvilinear trabeculae of cellular woven bone with a hypocellular fibroblastic stroma. These areas easily can be confused with immature fibrous dysplasia (see page 641). In other areas, the curvilinear bone may be lamellar with evidence of significant remodeling and an intermixed chronically inflamed and reactive stroma (Fig. 3.50). The radiolucent foci within the sclerotic bone represent areas of patchy and nodular fibrosis, often demonstrating a chronic inflammatory cellular infiltrate. Also noted with the areas of fibrosis and inflammation are irregular osseous trabeculae with atypical osteoid and significant cellularity that can be worrisome if observed out of context. In the areas of extensive sclerosis, numerous irregular trabeculae of pagetoid bone are present and demonstrate extensive evidence of remodeling with prominent reversal lines, osteoblastic rimming, and focal areas of osteoclastic activity. In obvious contrast to chronic suppurative osteomyelitis, bone necrosis, bacterial colonization, and frank purulence are absent.

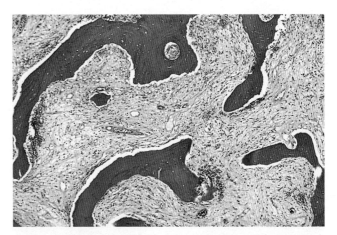

• **Fig. 3.50 Chronic Nonbacterial Osteomyelitis.** Curvilinear trabeculae of bone with numerous reversal lines and peripheral resorption intermixed with chronically inflamed and reactive connective tissue.

Treatment and Prognosis

This group of disorders is rare with a limited number of randomized and double-blind studies of the effectiveness of various therapeutic approaches. It can be difficult to ascertain if the clinical responses represent a true therapy-induced alteration or natural waxing and waning of disease activity in these patients.

The first step in patient management is whole body skeletal scintigraphy or MRI to rule out extragnathic bone involvement. If multifocal involvement is noted, the patient should be referred to a rheumatologist for thorough evaluation and systemic therapy. Therapies proven to be effective include nonsteroidal anti-inflammatory medications, corticosteroids, tumor necrosis factor α inhibitors, sulfasalazine, and methotrexate. If the lesions are restricted to bone without dermatologic or GI manifestation, bisphosphonates have proven successful in many patients. In spite of successful management of the majority of patients, recurrences have been noted, often leading to additional therapeutic interventions.

Most treatments directed toward elimination of infection have been proven ineffective. Long-term antibiotic treatment with or without hyperbaric oxygen therapy has not produced consistent long-term success. Surgical decortication has decreased the intensity and frequency of symptoms but has failed to resolve the process totally. Because of inconsistent results from surgical intervention, extensive surgery is contraindicated, especially in young, growing patients.

If the lesions are isolated to the mandible, the patient should be evaluated, and if appropriate, treated for **chronic tendoperiostitis**. The patients should be evaluated for persistent temporomandibular dysfunction symptoms and parafunctional habits. In patients with evidence of tendoperiostitis, nonsteroidal anti-inflammatory medications (etoricoxib or naproxen) combined with conservative therapy directed toward resolution of muscle overuse have resulted in significantly decreased symptoms in most patients and total resolution in a many. The ultimate goal of physical therapy is to make the patient aware of any parafunctional habits and to discontinue such movements through the following approaches:

- Muscular relaxation instructions (soft diet, avoidance of parafunctional habits)
- Rotation exercises
- Occlusal splint therapy
- Myofeedback
- Muscle relaxant drugs (e.g., diazepam)

If the patient fails after respond to 6–12 months of conservative therapy or demonstrates no evidence of chronic tendoperiostitis upon evaluation (such as TMJ dysfunction or parafunctional habits), bisphosphonate therapy (pamidronate) of short duration has proven beneficial in both pediatric and adult patients. Limited studies also have revealed a similar benefit to use of denosumab but with more frequent recurrences and the need for more extended therapy. If the antiresorptive medications prove ineffective, the systemic immune modulating medications described for use in patients with multifocal involvement should be considered.

◆ CONDENSING OSTEITIS (FOCAL SCLEROSING OSTEOMYELITIS)

Localized areas of bone sclerosis associated with the apices of teeth with pulpitis (from large carious lesions or deep coronal restorations) or pulpal necrosis are termed **condensing osteitis.** The association with an area of inflammation is critical because these lesions can resemble several other intrabony processes that produce a somewhat similar pattern.

Clinical and Radiographic Features

This secondary sclerosis of bone is seen most frequently in children and young adults but also can occur in older adults. The classic alteration consists of a localized, usually uniform zone of increased radiodensity adjacent to the apex of a tooth that exhibits a thickened periodontal ligament (PDL) space or an apical inflammatory lesion (Fig. 3.51). Clinical expansion should not be present. Most cases occur in the premolar and molar areas of the mandible, and the dental pulp of the involved tooth demonstrates pulpitis or necrosis. The lesion does not exhibit a radiolucent border, as is seen in cases of **focal cemento-osseous dysplasia** (see page 645), although an adjacent radiolucent inflammatory lesion may be present. In addition, the radiopacity is not separated from the apex as would be seen in **idiopathic osteosclerosis** (see page 626).

Treatment and Prognosis

Treatment of the patient with condensing osteitis consists of resolution of the odontogenic focus of infection. After extraction or appropriate endodontic therapy of the involved tooth, approximately 85% of cases of condensing osteitis will regress, either partially or totally. Typically, resolution of the lesion is associated with normalization of the associated periodontal membrane. If the lesion persists and the periodontal membrane remains wide, then reevaluation of the endodontic therapy should be considered. A residual area of condensing osteitis that remains after resolution of the inflammatory focus is termed a *bone scar* (Fig. 3.52). Root resorption has been noted during orthodontics if the sclerotic bone is the path of tooth movement.

◆ OSTEOMYELITIS WITH PROLIFERATIVE PERIOSTITIS (PERIOSTITIS OSSIFICANS, OSSIFYING PERIOSTITIS)

Bone formation within a periosteal reaction is a common finding that occurs in a wide variety of intraosseous pathoses and in all age groups. Causes of periosteal new bone formation include osteomyelitis, trauma, cysts, infantile cortical hyperostosis, fluorosis, avitaminosis C, hypertrophic osteoarthropathy, congenital syphilis, and neoplasms (such as, Ewing sarcoma, Langerhans cell histiocytosis, and osteogenic sarcoma). Of these, osteomyelitis and malignant neoplasms are associated most frequently with formation of bone within a periosteal reaction.

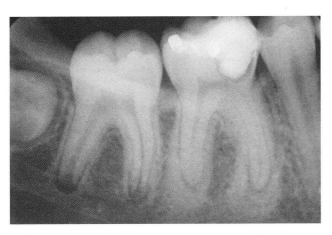

• **Fig. 3.51 Condensing Osteitis.** Increased areas of radiodensity surrounding the apices of the nonvital mandibular first molar.

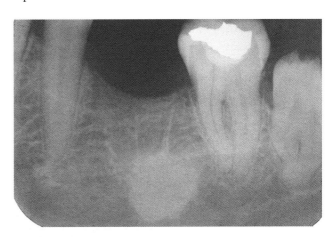

• **Fig. 3.52 Bone Scar.** Residual area of increased radiodensity in the area of extraction of the mandibular first molar. (Courtesy of Dr. Walter Blevins.)

In 1893 a Swiss physician, Carl Garrè, reported in the German literature on patterns of acute osteomyelitis. Since that time, numerous articles have been written that associate Garrè's report with a form of inflammatory periosteal hyperplasia demonstrating an onionskin-like reduplication of the cortical plate. (In these subsequent articles, Garrè's name was misspelled consistently as Garré, with an incorrect accent designation.) However, Garrè did not have any pathologic specimens for microscopic examination, and Roentgen did not discover X-rays until 2 years after Garrè's publication. Nowhere in the original publication is there any mention of periostitis, periosteal duplication, or "onionskinning." Although the term *Garrè osteomyelitis* often is used synonymously for this condition, it is an improper designation that should be disassociated with the entity described in the text that follows.

Clinical and Radiographic Features

Proliferative periostitis represents a periosteal reaction to the presence of inflammation. The affected periosteum forms several rows of reactive vital bone that parallel each other and expand the surface of the altered bone. Affected patients tend to be primarily children and young adults, with a mean age of 13 years. No sex predominance is noted.

As expected, the most frequent cause is dental caries with associated periapical inflammatory disease, although lesions have been reported secondary to periodontal infections, pericoronitis, tooth extractions, fractures, buccal bifurcation cysts, and non-odontogenic infections. Examples adjacent to an unerupted developing tooth also have been documented. Most cases arise in the premolar and molar area of the mandible. The hyperplasia is located most frequently along the lower border of the mandible, but buccal cortical involvement also is common. Isolated lingual cortical enlargement is infrequent. Most cases are unifocal, although multiple quadrants may be affected.

Appropriate radiographs demonstrate radiopaque laminations of bone that roughly parallel each other and the underlying cortical surface (Fig. 3.53). The laminations vary from 1 to 12 in number, and radiolucent separations often are present between the new bone and the original cortex. Less frequently, the new bone formation exhibits consolidation and contains numerous fine bony projections that radiate

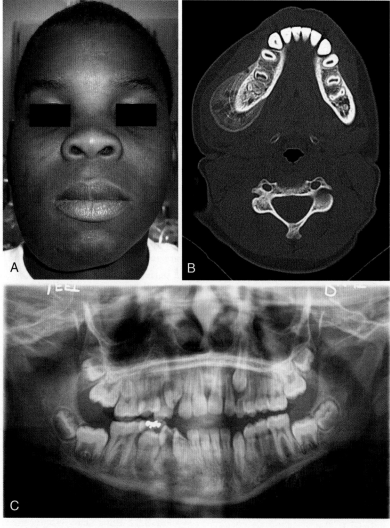

• **Fig. 3.53 Proliferative Periostitis. A,** Firm swelling of the lateral and inferior border of the right mandible that arose after traumatic injury. **B,** Computed tomography (CT) image demonstrating new periosteal bone growth with onionskin laminations. **C,** Panoramic radiograph exhibiting new periosteal bone formation along the right inferior border of the mandible. (Courtesy of Drs. Sherif Mekhail and Benjamin Lin.)

perpendicular from the underlying and intact periosteum. Within the new bone, areas of small sequestra or osteolytic radiolucencies may be found.

Because of difficulty in proper angulation and problems related to superimposition of the underlying bone, CT scanning has proved to be consistently superior to conventional radiography in demonstrating proliferative periostitis. On plain films, the alterations are typically seen best on a panoramic or lateral oblique radiograph. If lateral oblique radiographs fail to demonstrate the lesion, then occlusal views and, less frequently, posteroanterior radiographs may be successful.

Histopathologic Features

Usually, biopsy is not required unless the clinical diagnosis is in question. Specimens often reveal parallel rows of highly cellular and reactive woven bone in which the individual trabeculae are frequently oriented perpendicular to the surface. The trabeculae sometimes form an interconnecting meshwork of bone or are scattered more widely, resembling the pattern seen in immature fibrous dysplasia (Fig. 3.54). Between the cellular trabeculae, relatively uninflamed fibrous connective tissue is evident. Sequestra, if included, demonstrate the typical features of bone necrosis (see Osteomyelitis, page 134).

Treatment and Prognosis

Most cases of proliferative periostitis of the jaws are associated with periapical inflammatory lesions, and treatment in these cases (either extraction of the offending tooth or appropriate endodontic therapy) is directed toward eliminating the source of the infection. After the focus of infection has been eliminated and inflammation has resolved, the layers of bone will consolidate in 6–12 months as the overlying muscle action helps to remodel the bone to its original state.

If a unifocal periosteal reaction similar to proliferative periostitis appears in the absence of an obvious source of inflammation, biopsy is recommended because several neoplastic conditions can result in a similar pattern.

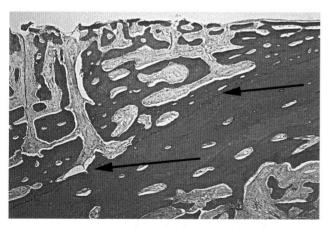

• **Fig. 3.54 Proliferative Periostitis.** Interconnecting trabeculae of new bone formation *(top left)* extending from the original cortical surface *(delineated by arrows)*.

◆ ALVEOLAR OSTEITIS (DRY SOCKET; FIBRINOLYTIC ALVEOLITIS)

After extraction of a tooth, a blood clot is formed at the site, with eventual organization of the clot by granulation tissue, gradual replacement by coarse fibrillar bone, and, finally, replacement by mature bone. Premature fibrinolysis of the initial clot is thought to be responsible for the clinical condition known as **alveolar osteitis.** Factors deemed to be associated with an increased prevalence include increasing age, oral contraceptive use, tobacco use, preoperative infection, difficult extraction, inexperienced surgeons, surgical flap design (envelope flap rather than modified triangular flap), use of a local anesthetic with vasoconstrictor, and inadequate postoperative irrigation. Of these factors, age, a preoperative infection, and difficulty of extraction have been shown in systematic reviews to be most strongly associated with the development of alveolar osteitis.

Clinical Features

The frequency of alveolar osteitis is higher in the mandible and the posterior areas. After oral contraceptive use is taken into account, there does not appear to be a significant sex predilection. The prevalence is between 1% and 3% of all extractions, but it increases to 25%–30% for impacted mandibular third molars. The frequency appears to be decreased when impacted teeth are removed prophylactically rather than for pericoronitis. The overall prevalence is highest between 20 and 40 years of age (when the majority of teeth are extracted), although the likelihood of developing alveolar osteitis appears greatest for extractions in the 40- to 45-year-old age group.

The affected extraction site is filled initially with a dirty gray clot that is lost and leaves a bare bony socket (**dry socket**). The detection of the bare socket may be hindered by partial retention of the clot or by overlying inflamed tissue that covers the site. The diagnosis is confirmed by probing of the socket, which reveals exposed and extremely sensitive bone. Typically, severe pain, foul odor, and (less frequently) swelling and lymphadenopathy develop 3–4 days after extraction of the tooth. On occasion, the pain radiates from the socket to the ipsilateral ear, temporal region, or eye. Rarely, trismus also may be noted. The signs and symptoms may last from 10 to 40 days.

Treatment and Prognosis

On evaluation of the patient complaining of postextraction pain, a radiograph should be taken of the affected area to rule out the possibility of a retained root tip or a foreign body. All sutures should be removed. The socket is irrigated with warm saline, followed by thorough clinical inspection of the socket for any unexpected pathosis. Curettage of the socket is not recommended, because this typically increases the associated pain. Potent oral analgesics should be prescribed, and the patient should be given a plastic syringe with instructions to keep the socket clean via home irrigation with a chlorhexidine or saline solution. This irrigation should continue until debris no longer collects within the healing socket (usually 3–4 weeks).

Use of an obtundent and antiseptic dressing, such as iodoform gauze containing eugenol, is controversial. Although the dressing may reduce the symptoms and help keep out food debris, many believe the dressing acts as foreign material and delays healing of the extraction socket. If a dressing is used, then it should be changed every 24 hours for the first 3 days, then every 2–3 days until granulation tissue covers the exposed bone. The dressing should be discontinued as soon as the patient is pain free. After that time, the patient should be given a plastic syringe with instructions for home irrigation.

Many investigators have studied preventive measures for alveolar osteitis including systemic and topical antibiotics, corticosteroids, cessation of smoking the day before and after surgery, copious surgical irrigation, antifibrinolytic agents, platelet-rich fibrin, chlorhexidine gel, and chlorhexidine rinses. Of these interventions, chlorhexidine in any formulation has been shown in multiple systematic reviews to be associated most consistently with a decreased frequency of alveolar osteitis. Chlorhexidine gel placed into the socket appears to be moderately more effective than rinses, with a possibly improved response if covered by a platelet-rich fibrin membrane. Any topical therapy should not be in an ointment form, because such use has resulted in chronic foreign body reactions (e.g., myospherulosis) (see page 315). Some investigators have suggested that debris in the healing socket could disturb wound healing and increase the prevalence of alveolar osteitis. To avoid this problem, gentle irrigation of socket with tap water beginning 48 hours after the surgery has been suggested by some. Finally, failure to follow the surgeon's postextraction instructions also may contribute and stresses the need for quality communication between the clinician and patient.

Bibliography

General References
Berman LH, Hargreaves KM: *Cohen's pathways of the pulp*, ed 12, St Louis, 2010, Elsevier.
Rotstein I, Ingle JI: *Ingle's endodontics*, ed 7, Beijing, China, 2019, PMPH USA.

Pulpitis
Abbott PV, Yu C: A clinical classification of the status of the pulp and the root canal system, *Aust Dent J* 52(1 Suppl):S17–S31, 2007.
Caldeira CL, Barletta FB, Ilha MC, et al.: Pulse oximetry: a useful test for evaluating pulp vitality in traumatized teeth, *Dent Traumatol* 32:385–389, 2016.
Hyman JL, Cohen ME: The predictive value of endodontic diagnostic tests, *Oral Surg Oral Med Oral Pathol* 58:343–346, 1984.
Levin LG, Law AS, Holland GR, et al.: Identify and define all diagnostic terms for pulpal health and disease states, *J Endod* 35:1645–1657, 2009.
Nagendrababu V, Pulillotil SJ, Veettil SK, et al.: Effect of nonsteroidal anti-inflammatory drug as an oral premedication on the anesthetic success of inferior alveolar nerve block in treatment of irreversible

pulpitis: a systematic review with meta-analysis and trial sequential analysis, *J Endod* 44:914–922, 2018.

Secondary and Tertiary Dentin
Amir FA, Gutmann JL, Witherspoon DE: Calcific metamorphosis: a challenge in endodontic diagnosis and treatment, *Quintessence Int* 32:447–455, 2001.
Kvall SI, Kolltveit KM, Thomsen IO, et al.: Age estimation of adults from dental radiographs, *Forensic Sci Int* 74:175–185, 1995.
Marroquin TY, Karkhanis S, Kvaal SI, et al.: Age estimation in adults by dental imaging assessment systematic review, *Forensic Sci Int* 275:203–211, 2017.
Morse DR: Age-related changes of the dental pulp complex and their relationship to systemic aging, *Oral Surg Oral Med Oral Pathol* 72:721–745, 1991.
Pashley DH, Pashley EL, Carvalho RM, et al.: The effects of dentin permeability on restorative dentistry, *Dent Clin N Am* 46:211–245, 2002.
Solheim T: Amount of secondary dentin as an indicator of age, *Scand J Dent Res* 100:193–199, 1992.
West JD: The aesthetics and endodontic dilemmas of calcific metamorphosis, *Pract Periodontics Aesthet Dent* 9:286–293, 1997.
Woods MA, Robinson QC, Harris EF: Age-progressive changes in pulp widths and root lengths during adulthood: a study of American blacks and whites, *Gerodontology* 9:41–50, 1990.

Pulpal Calcifications
Da Silva EJN, Prado MC, Queiroz PM, et al.: Assessing pulp stones by cone-beam computed tomography, *Clin Oral Investig* 21:2327–2333, 2017.
Gabardo MCL, Wambler LM, Rocha JS, et al.: Association between pulp stones and kidney stones: a systematic review and meta-analysis, *J Endod* 45:1099–1105, 2019.
Horsley SH, Beckstrom B, Clark SJ, et al.: Prevalence of carotid and pulp calcifications: a correlation using digital panoramic radiographs, *Int J Comput Assist Radiol Surg* 4:169–173, 2009.
Jannati R, Afshari M, Moosazadeh M, et al.: Prevalence of pulp stones: a systematic review and meta-analysis, *J Evid Based Med* 12:133–139, 2019.
Kansu O, Ozbek M, Avcu N, et al.: Can dental pulp calcification serve as a diagnostic marker for carotid artery calcification in patients with renal disease? *Dentomaxillofac Radiol* 38:542–545, 2009.
Morse DR: Age-related changes of the dental pulp complex and their relationship to systemic aging, *Oral Surg Oral Med Oral Pathol* 72:721–745, 1991.
Moss-Salentijn L, Hendricks-Klyvert M: Calcified structures in human dental pulps, *J Endod* 14:184–189, 1988.
Selden HS: Radiographic pulpal calcifications: normal or abnormal—a paradox, *J Endod* 17:34–37, 1991.

Periapical Inflammatory Disease (Granuloma; Cyst; Abscess)
Bhaskar SN: Periapical lesions—types, incidence, and clinical features, *Oral Surg Oral Med Oral Pathol* 21:657–671, 1966.
Cope AL, Francis N, Wood F, et al.: Systemic antibiotics for symptomatic apical periodontitis and acute apical abscess in adults, *Cochrane Database Syst Rev*, 2018. https://doi.org/10.1002/14651858.CD010136.pub3.
Estrela C, Bueno MR, Leles CR, et al.: Accuracy of cone beam computed tomography and panoramic and periapical radiography for detection of apical periodontitis, *J Endod* 34:273–279, 2008.
Jalali P, Tahmasbi M, Augsburger RA, et al.: Dynamics of bone loss in cases of acute and chronic apical abscess, *J Endod* 45:1114–1118, 2019.

Juerchott A, Pfefferle T, Flechtenmacher C, et al.: Differentiation of periapical granulomas and cysts using dental MRI: a pilot study, *Int J Oral Sci*, 2018. https://doi.org/10.1038/s41368-018-0017-y.

Lockhart PB, Tampi MP, Abt E, et al.: Evidence-based clinical practice guideline on antibiotic use for the urgent management of pulpal- and periapical-related dental pain and intraoral swelling. A report from the American Dental Association, *JADA* 150:906–921, 2019.

Lofthag-Hansen S, Huumonen S, Gröndahl K, et al.: Limited cone-beam CT and intraoral radiography of periapical pathology, *Oral Surg Oral Med Oral Pathol Oral Radiol Endod* 103:114–119, 2007.

Nair PNR: New perspectives on radicular cysts: do they heal? *Int Endod J* 31:155–160, 1998.

Nair PNR, Pajarola G, Schroeder HE: Types and incidence of human periapical lesions obtained with extracted teeth, *Oral Surg Oral Med Oral Pathol Oral Radiol Endod* 81:93–102, 1993.

Rosenberg PA, Frisbie J, Lee J: Evaluation of pathologists (histopathology) and radiologists (cone beam computed tomography) differentiating radicular cysts from granulomas, *J Endod* 36:423–428, 2010.

Schulz M, von Arx T, Altermatt HJ, et al.: Histology of periapical lesions obtained during apical surgery, *J Endod* 35:634–642, 2009.

Sönmez G, Kamburoğlu K, Yilmaz F, et al.: Versatility of high resolution ultrasonography in the assessment of granulomas and radicular cysts: a comparative in vivo study, *Dentomaxillofac Radiol* 48, 2019. https://doi.org/10.1259/dmfr.20190082.

Stockdale CR, Chandler NP: The nature of the periapical lesion—a review of 1108 cases, *J Dent* 16:123–129, 1988.

Sullivan M, Gallagher G, Noonan V: The root of the problem. Occurrence of typical and atypical periapical pathoses, *JADA* 147:646–649, 2016.

Tian F-C, Bergeron BE, Kalathingal S, et al.: Management of large radicular lesions using decompression: a case series and review of the literature, *J Endod* 45:651–659, 2019.

Tronstad L: Recent development in endodontic research, *Scand J Dent Res* 100:52–59, 1992.

Cellulitis

Busch RF, Shah D: Ludwig's angina: improved treatment, *Otolaryngol Head Neck Surg* 117:S172–S175, 1997.

Colbert S, Cameron M, Williams J: Septic thrombosis of the cavernous sinus and dental infection, *Br J Oral Maxillofac Surg* 49:e25–e26, 2011.

Hsu C-W, Tsai W-C, Lien C-Y, et al.: The clinical characteristics, implicated pathogens and therapeutic outcomes of culture-proven septic cavernous sinus thrombosis, *J Clin Neurosci* 68:111–116, 2019.

Iwu CO: Ludwig's angina: report of seven cases and review of the current concepts in management, *Br J Oral Maxillofac Surg* 28:189–193, 1990.

Ogundiya DA, Keith DA, Mirowski J: Cavernous sinus thrombosis and blindness as complication of an odontogenic infection, *J Oral Maxillofac Surg* 47:1317–1321, 1989.

Pynn BR, Sands T, Pharoah MJ: Odontogenic infections: part 1. Anatomy and radiology, *Oral Health* 85:7–21, 1995.

Sands T, Pynn BRT, Katsikeris N: Odontogenic infections: part 2. Microbiology, antibiotics and management, *Oral Health* 85:11–28, 1995.

Taub D, Yampolsky A, Diecidue R, et al.: Controversies in the management of oral and maxillofacial infections, *Oral Maxillofac Surg Clin N Am* 29:465–473, 2017.

Van der Poel NA, Mouritis MP, de Win MML, et al.: Prognosis of septic cavernous sinus thrombosis remarkably improved: a case series of 12 patients and literature review, *Eur Arch Otorhinolaryngol* 275:2387–2395, 2018.

Osteomyelitis

Adekeye EO, Cornah J: Osteomyelitis of the jaws: a review of 141 cases, *Br J Oral Maxillofac Surg* 23:24–35, 1985.

Daramola JO, Ajagbe HA: Chronic osteomyelitis of the mandible in adults: a clinical study of 34 cases, *Br J Oral Surg* 20:58–62, 1982.

Fullmer JM, Scarfe WC, Kushner GM, et al.: Cone beam computed tomographic findings in refractory chronic suppurative osteomyelitis of the mandible, *Br J Oral Maxillofac Surg* 45:364–371, 2007.

Hudson JW, Daly AP, Foster M: Treatment of osteomyelitis: a case for disruption of the affected adjacent periosteum, *J Oral Maxillofac Surg* 75:2127–2134, 2017.

Koorbusch GF, Deatherage JR, Curé JK: How can we diagnose and treat osteomyelitis of the jaws as early as possible? *Oral Maxillofac Surg Clin N Am* 23:557–567, 2011.

Koorbusch GF, Fotos P, Terhark K: Retrospective assessment of osteomyelitis: etiology, demographics, risk factors, and management in 35 cases, *Oral Surg Oral Med Oral Pathol* 74:149–154, 1992.

Marx RE: Chronic osteomyelitis of the jaws, *Oral Maxillofac Clin North Am* 3:367–381, 1991.

Diffuse Sclerosing Osteomyelitis

Groot RH, Ongerboer de Visser BW, van Merkesteyn JP, et al.: Changes in masseter inhibitory reflex responses in patients with diffuse sclerosing osteomyelitis of the mandible, *Oral Surg Oral Med Oral Pathol* 74:727–732, 1992.

Groot RH, van Merkesteyn JP, van Soest JJ, et al.: Diffuse sclerosing osteomyelitis (chronic tendoperiostitis) of the mandible: an 11-year follow-up report, *Oral Surg Oral Med Oral Pathol* 74:557–560, 1992.

Li X, Jia K, Zhang Y: Application of pamidronate disodium for the treatment of diffuse sclerosing osteomyelitis of the mandible: a clinical study, *Oral Surg Oral Med Oral Pathol Oral Radiol* 130:616–624, 2020.

Padwa BL, Dentino K, Robson CD, et al.: Pediatric chronic non-bacterial osteomyelitis of the jaw: clinical, radiographic, and histopathologic features, *J Oral Maxillofac Surg* 74:2393–2402, 2016.

Suei Y, Taguchi A, Tanimoto K: Diagnostic point and possible origin of osteomyelitis in synovitis, acne, pustulosis, hyperostosis and osteitis (SAPHO) syndrome: a radiographic study of 77 mandibular osteomyelitis cases, *J Rheumatol* 42:1398–1403, 2003.

Tlougan BE, Podjasek JO, O'Haver J, et al.: Chronic recurrent multifocal osteomyelitis (CRMO) and synovitis, acne, pustulosis, hyperostosis, and osteitis (SAPHO) syndrome with associated neutrophilic dermatoses: a report of seven cases and review of the literature, *Pediatr Dermatol* 26:497–505, 2009.

van de Meent MM, Meshkini H, Fiocco M, et al.: Conservative treatment of children with chronic diffuse sclerosing osteomyelitis/tendoperiostitis of the mandible, *J Craniomaxillofac Surg* 45:1938–1943, 2017.

van de Meent MM, Wetselaar-Glas MJM, Fiocco M, et al.: Non-surgical treatment of adults with chronic diffuse sclerosing osteomyelitis/tendoperiostitis of the mandible, *J Craniomaxillofac Surg* 47:1922–1928, 2019.

van Merkesteyn JPR, Groot RH, Bras J, et al.: Diffuse sclerosing osteomyelitis of the mandible: a new concept of its etiology, *Oral Surg Oral Med Oral Pathol* 70:414–419, 1990.

Condensing Osteitis

El-Beialy AR, Mostafa YA: Focal sclerosing osteomyelitis and orthodontic treatment planning, *J Clin Orthod* 43:269–271, 2009.

Eliasson S, Halvarsson C, Ljungheimer C: Periapical condensing osteitis and endodontic treatment, *Oral Surg Oral Med Oral Pathol* 57:195–199, 1984.

Eversole LR, Stone CE, Strub D: Focal sclerosing osteomyelitis/focal periapical osteopetrosis: radiographic patterns, *Oral Surg Oral Med Oral Pathol* 58:456–460, 1984.

Farman AG, de V Joubert JJ, Nortjé C: Focal osteosclerosis and apical periodontal pathoses in "European" and Cape Coloured dental outpatients, *Int J Oral Surg* 7:549–557, 1978.

Hedin M, Polhagen L: Follow-up study of periradicular bone condensation, *Scand J Dent Res* 79:436–440, 1979.

Osteomyelitis with Proliferative Periostitis

Fukuda M, Inoue K, Sakashita H: Periostitis ossificans arising in the mandibular bone of a young patient: report of an unusual case and review of the literature, *J Oral Maxillofac Surg* 75:1834.e1–1834.e8, 2017.

Kawai T, Hiranuma H, Kishino M, et al.: Gross periostitis ossificans in mandibular osteomyelitis. Review of the English language literature and radiographic variation, *Oral Surg Oral Med Oral Pathol Oral Radiol Endod* 86:376–381, 1998.

Kawai T, Murakami S, Sakuda M, et al.: Radiographic investigation of mandibular periostitis ossificans in 55 cases, *Oral Surg Oral Med Oral Pathol Oral Radiol Endod* 82:704–712, 1996.

Nortjé CJ, Wood RE, Grotepass F: Periostitis ossificans versus Garrè's osteomyelitis: part II. Radiologic analysis of 93 cases in the jaws, *Oral Surg Oral Med Oral Pathol* 66:249–260, 1988.

Wood RE, Nortjé CJ, Grotepass F, et al.: Periostitis ossificans versus Garrè's osteomyelitis: part I. What did Garrè really say? *Oral Surg Oral Med Oral Pathol* 65:773–777, 1988.

Alveolar Osteitis

Awang MN: The aetiology of dry socket: a review, *Int Dent J* 39:236–240, 1989.

Birn H: Etiology and pathogenesis of fibrinolytic alveolitis ("dry socket"), *Int J Oral Surg* 2:215–263, 1973.

Blum IR: Contemporary views on dry socket (alveolar osteitis): a clinical appraisal of standardization, aetiopathogenesis and management: a critical review, *Int J Oral Maxillofac Surg* 31:309–317, 2002.

Daley B., Sharif M.O., Newton T., et al: Local interventions for the management of alveolar osteitis (dry socket), *Cochrane Database Syst Rev* 2022, https://doi.org/10.1002/14651858.CD006968.pub2.

Eshghpour M, Danaeifar N, Kermani H, et al.: Does intra-alveolar application of chlorhexidine gel in combination with platelet-rich fibrin have an advantage over application of platelet-rich fibrin in decreasing alveolar osteitis after mandibular third molar surgery? A double-blinded randomized clinical trial, *J Oral Maxillofac Surg* 76:939.e1–939.e7, 2018.

Ghaeminia H, Hoppenreijs TJM, Xi T, et al.: Postoperative socket irrigation with drinking tap water reduces the risk of inflammatory complications following surgical removal of third molars: a multicenter randomized trial, *Clin Oral Investig* 21:71–83, 2017.

Houston JP, McCollum J, Pietz D, et al.: Alveolar osteitis: a review of its etiology, prevention, and treatment modalities, *Gen Dent* 50:457–463, 2002.

Noroozi A-R, Philbert RF: Modern concepts in understanding and management of the "dry socket" syndrome: comprehensive review of the literature, *Oral Surg Oral Med Oral Pathol Oral Radiol Endod* 107:30–35, 2009.

Taberner-Vallverdú M, Sánchez-Gareés MA, Gay-Escoda C: Efficacy of different methods used for dry socket prevention and risk factors analysis: a systematic review, *Med Oral Patol Cir Bucal* 6:e750–e758, 2017.

4

Periodontal Diseases

In this textbook of oral and maxillofacial pathology, the discussion of periodontal diseases is limited appropriately in scope. However, several fine textbooks are available on periodontology and can provide the reader with more information on the background, microbiology, clinical presentations, diagnostic procedures, and current therapies used to treat these diseases.

◆ GINGIVITIS

Gingivitis refers to inflammation limited to the soft tissues that surround the teeth. It does not include the inflammatory processes that may extend into the underlying alveolar ridge, periodontal ligament, or cementum. A similar pattern of inflammation has noted in the mucosa surrounding implants and has been termed **peri-implant mucositis** (see page 167). The primary types of gingivitis are listed in Box 4.1. This part of the text concentrates on the plaque-related types. **Necrotizing gingivitis, medication-influenced gingivitis,** and a specific type of allergic gingivitis **(plasma cell gingivitis)** are presented later in this chapter. Additional forms of allergic gingivitis are discussed in Chapter 9. The gingivitis associated with certain specific infections (e.g., herpes simplex, and human immunodeficiency virus [HIV]) is discussed in Chapters 5 and 7. The gingiva is a frequent site of involvement in several of the dermatologic vesiculoerosive diseases; these are well described in Chapter 16.

The rate, severity, and extent of gingivitis varies according to local and systemic risk factors. The primary local risk factor is the accumulation of plaque, which is related to the level of oral hygiene and anatomical factors such as subgingival restorations and tooth anomalies. Reduced salivary flow also increases the risk for gingivitis due to reduced cleansing of tooth surfaces. Systemic risk factors include metabolic conditions such as hyperglycemia, nutritional factors such as vitamin C deficiency, elevation of sex hormones as seen during puberty and pregnancy, hematologic disorders such as leukemia, and medications that may reduce salivary flow, induce gingival enlargement, or increase sex hormones. The first-generation high-dose oral contraceptives were associated with an increased prevalence of gingivitis, a finding not noted with the newer low-dose formulations. Surprisingly, due to associated vasoconstriction and fibrosis, smoking tends to mask clinical signs of gingivitis such as bleeding upon probing.

Clinical Features

Most cases of gingivitis occur from lack of proper oral hygiene, which leads to the accumulation of dental plaque and calculus; however, many other factors can affect the gingiva's susceptibility to the oral flora. The frequency of gingivitis is high in all age groups, with a prevalence that approaches 95%. Clinically detectable inflammatory changes of the gingiva begin in childhood and increase with age. With similar amounts of dental plaque, the severity of gingivitis is greater in adults than in prepubertal children. Around the time of puberty, there is a period of increased susceptibility to gingivitis **(puberty gingivitis),** with the peak prevalence of involvement occurring between the ages of 9 and 14 years. Between the ages of 11 and 17 years, the frequency declines; then a slow increase is seen until the prevalence approaches 100% in the sixth decade of life.

In most age groups, females demonstrate a lower frequency of gingivitis than do males (although females have periods of increased susceptibility). This may be due more to better oral hygiene in females than to a physiologic difference between the genders. In addition to the years of puberty, females exhibit a greater susceptibility to gingivitis when they are exposed to the high levels of progesterone associated with pregnancy or the older high-dose formulations of oral contraceptives. Several other systemic factors have been shown to increase the frequency of gingivitis and are listed in Box 4.2. In contrast, smoking and use of many antibiotic drugs, corticosteroid medications, and nonsteroidal anti-inflammatory drugs (NSAIDs) have been correlated with a reduced gingival response to plaque. Various local factors that can be related to gingivitis are shown in Box 4.3.

Injury to the gingiva from mastication, oral hygiene techniques, or other habits may result in a breach of the oral mucosa, with secondary infection from the local flora. Most such injuries result in transient areas of erythema. However, if the trauma follows a chronic pattern, then areas of persistently swollen, erythematous gingiva may result. Patients who are mouth breathers or demonstrate incomplete lip closure can display a unique pattern of gingivitis in which the anterior facial gingiva is smooth, swollen, and red (Fig. 4.1).

Susceptibility to plaque-related gingivitis appears to vary within the population, and the individual traits seem to determine the severity of gingivitis, independent of the degree of plaque accumulation. In addition, evidence

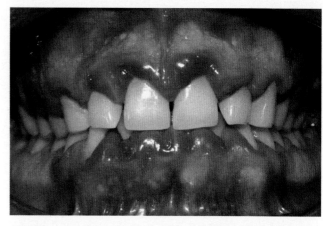

• Fig. 4.1 Mouth Breathing–Related Gingivitis. Slick, swollen, and red gingivitis of the anterior facial gingiva secondary to chronic mouth breathing.

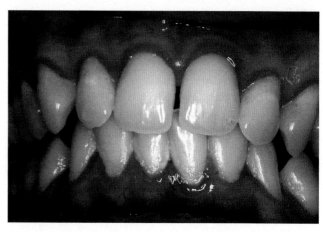

• Fig. 4.2 Marginal Gingivitis. Diffuse erythematous alteration of the free gingival margins.

suggests that susceptibility to gingivitis appears linked to susceptibility to future development of periodontitis.

Inflammation of the gingiva may be localized or generalized. If the altered gingiva is associated with less than 30% of the teeth, the process is considered localized, whereas generalized gingivitis demonstrates a wider degree of involvement. The inflammation may be diffuse or confined to the free gingival margins **(marginal gingivitis)** (Fig. 4.2) or the interdental papillae **(papillary gingivitis).** The earliest signs of gingivitis include a loss of stippling plus bleeding on gentle probing. Healthy gingiva is coral pink; with inflammation, the involved gingiva becomes light red. Moderate gingivitis demonstrates glazing, edema, an erythematous enlargement, and bleeding upon probing. Alterations noted in severe gingivitis include an overtly red and edematous appearance with a tendency to bleed easily upon light touching, often with margins that may be blunted, receded, or hyperplastic (Fig. 4.3). When chronic inflammation causes significant enlargement because of edema or fibrosis, the process is termed **chronic hyperplastic gingivitis** (Fig. 4.4). Bleeding

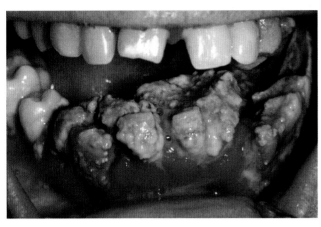

• **Fig. 4.3 Chronic Gingivitis.** Bright-red gingiva is blunted, receded, and hyperplastic secondary to a total lack of oral hygiene. Note the extensive calculus buildup.

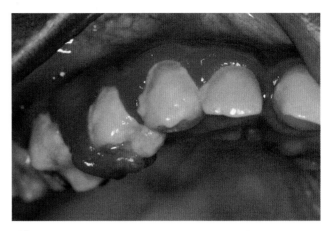

• **Fig. 4.5 Hyperplastic Gingivitis with Pyogenic Granuloma.** Diffuse erythematous enlargement of marginal and papillary gingiva with hemorrhagic, tumorlike proliferation (which arose during pregnancy) between the maxillary bicuspid and first molar.

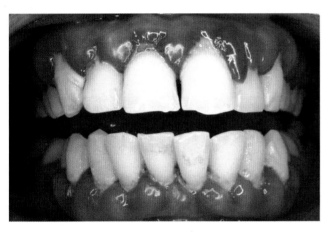

• **Fig. 4.4 Chronic Hyperplastic Gingivitis.** Diffuse erythema and enlargement of marginal and papillary gingiva.

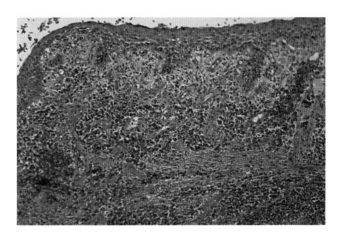

• **Fig. 4.6 Chronic Gingivitis.** Sulcular epithelium with exocytosis overlying connective tissue that contains inflammatory infiltrate consisting of lymphocytes, plasma cells, and polymorphonuclear leukocytes.

occurs easily, and exudate can be seen in the gingival sulcus. A localized tumorlike proliferation of subacutely inflamed granulation tissue, known as a **pyogenic granuloma** (see page 525), can develop on the gingiva of patients with severe gingivitis (Fig. 4.5).

Histopathologic Features

Incipient gingivitis demonstrates a light inflammatory infiltrate consisting of polymorphonuclear leukocytes that accumulate in the connective tissue adjacent to the sulcular epithelium. With progression, the infiltrate becomes more intense and demonstrates a mixture of lymphocytes, plasma cells, and acute inflammatory cells (Fig. 4.6). Areas of fibrosis, hyperemia, edema, and hemorrhage may be present.

Treatment and Prognosis

Although periodontitis always is preceded by gingivitis, most areas of gingivitis remain stable for years, and the number of affected sites that convert to periodontitis is small. Despite

this, optimal gingival health should be the goal of all clinicians and their patients. Even when attachment loss is not evident and the alterations appear restricted to the gingival soft tissues, improved oral hygiene practices are recommended to eliminate these areas of persistent inflammation during the early stages of disease.

Treatment of gingivitis consists of elimination (if possible) of any known cause of increased susceptibility and improvement in oral hygiene to decrease the dental plaque responsible for the inflammatory alterations. A further discussion of dental plaque and its relationship to gingival inflammation is presented in the discussion of periodontitis (see page 160). Most self-administered plaque control programs are ineffective unless periodic professional reinforcement of oral hygiene instructions also is provided. Research has shown that few individuals have the physical skills and motivation necessary to obtain and maintain ultimate oral hygiene. An analysis of multiple clinical trials revealed that use of a mechanical toothbrush was associated with plaque reduction of less than 50%. Although rechargeable rotation/oscillation-powered brushes have demonstrated the ability to remove an increased percentage of plaque, the best toothbrush remains the one that gets into the mouth. The average time individuals spend brushing their teeth is 45–70 seconds daily. To perform this task properly, the teeth should be brushed for 2 minutes twice each day.

Brushing fails to clean the interdental areas and should be supplemented by other cleaning aids, such as specialized wood sticks (not toothpicks), dental floss, or interdental brushes. Research has demonstrated that proper interdental cleansing is correlated directly with decreased caries, gingivitis, and periodontitis, along with an associated increased life span. Although critically important, the percentage of patients who perform daily interdental cleaning is estimated to be as low as 2%. A survey by the American Academy of Periodontology revealed that greater than 35% of respondents would rather complete an unpleasant task, such as file their tax returns or clean their toilets, than floss.

Mechanical removal of dental plaque can be aided by the use of numerous chemical agents, such as mouth rinses with chlorhexidine or essential oils, or dentifrices containing triclosan or stannous fluoride. On occasion, hyperplastic and fibrotic gingiva may have to be recontoured surgically to achieve total resolution of the altered anatomy after improvements in hygiene have been made. If the gingivitis does not resolve after improved plaque control and elimination of obvious contributing factors, then the patient should be evaluated for underlying systemic disorders that could be contributing to the process.

◆ SPONGIOTIC GINGIVAL HYPERPLASIA (SPONGIOTIC GINGIVITIS)

Spongiotic gingival hyperplasia is a clinically and histopathologically distinctive gingival pathosis that was described initially in 2007 as *juvenile spongiotic gingivitis*. Initial reports suggested the lesions were isolated and restricted to children, but it has become obvious that spongiotic gingival hyperplasia may be multifocal and can occur in adults. Although the disorder is idiopathic, many investigators believe the alteration represents an isolated patch of junctional or sulcular epithelium that may become irritated and exteriorized. Others have suggested the proliferation arises from epithelial rests left behind during odontogenesis. The changes do not appear to be plaque-related and fail to respond to improved oral hygiene.

Prior to the initial description, some of these cases were designed as puberty gingivitis, but several features dispute this contention. Numerous examples have been reported in prepubescent children or adults and, in contrast to puberty gingivitis, the lesions do not respond to improved oral hygiene. Additionally, an absence of estrogen and progesterone receptors has been documented in these lesions.

Clinical Features

The most common presentation of spongiotic gingival hyperplasia is a small bright red velvety or papillary alteration that often bleeds easily upon manipulation (Fig. 4.7). Due to the highly vascular appearance, the most common clinical impression is pyogenic granuloma. The facial gingiva overlying the root is affected most frequently, but involvement of the interproximal areas or lingual gingiva also may occur. The lesion typically is sessile, but some examples may be pedunculated with occasional extension into the gingival sulcus (Fig. 4.8). Although the lesion has been diagnosed in adulthood, approximately 90% have been documented during the first two decades of life with a mean age less than 15 years. The alteration demonstrates a strong predilection for the maxillary anterior facial gingiva with almost 80% documented in this region. Early reports suggested a female predominance, but a gender predilection has not been noted in later literature reviews. Although occasional multifocal involvement may be seen, most examples are isolated. The natural history of the lesion is difficult to ascertain due to therapeutic removal, but several examples have been noted for years prior to excision.

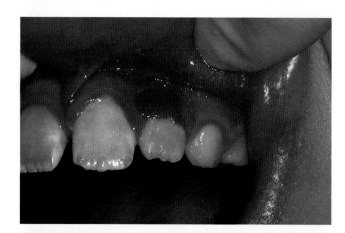

• **Fig. 4.7 Spongiotic Gingival Hyperplasia.** Bright red velvety alteration of maxillary facial gingiva in 9-year-old male. (Courtesy of Dr. Tom Ocheltree.)

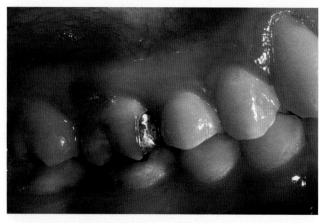

• **Fig. 4.8 Spongiotic Gingival Hyperplasia.** Red, papillary, and pedunculated lesion with a stalk that extends into the gingival sulcus in a 28-year-old female.

Histopathologic Features

Microscopically, the epithelium is variably hyperplastic and often demonstrates a pebbly to papillary surface. Occasional thinning of the interpapillary plates may be seen. Prominent intercellular edema (spongiosis) and exocytosis by neutrophils are noted consistently. Histopathologically, the epithelium is remarkably similar to junctional or sulcular areas. Upon immunoperoxidase evaluation, the epithelium typically demonstrates diffuse reactivity for CK 8/18 and CK19 with uncommon reactivity for CK1/10 and CK4. In contrast, gingival surface epithelium typically is reactive for CK1/10 and CK4 but without diffuse reactivity to CK8/18 and CK19 (basilar only). These results suggest that spongiotic gingival hyperplasia demonstrates an "*in-between phenotype*" with features that are much closer to junctional epithelium than gingival surface epithelium. In those rare cases that are noted in adults, CK19 can be utilized to confirm the diagnosis. Although many cases are papillary, spongiotic gingival hyperplasia has been shown to be negative for human papillomavirus (HPV) DNA by polymerase chain reaction. The associated stroma reveals vasodilation with congestion and a mixed inflammatory cellular infiltrate.

Treatment and Prognosis

Most of the reported examples have been removed conservatively with a scalpel or laser. Surgical removal from the anterior maxillary facial gingiva with an acceptable aesthetic result can be challenging. Successful elimination with cryotherapy also has been documented with excellent results. One report documented removal by mild cauterization combined with topical corticosteroids, but other cases have revealed an inconsistent response to topical corticosteroids. The reported recurrence rate varies from 6% to 28.6%. Successful elimination by low-energy laser ablation also has been documented in a small number of case reports. Although the lesion may persist for years, the possibility of spontaneous resolution is likely because the process is reported infrequently in adults. It has been suggested that the "*in-between phenotype*" noted in the cytokeratin expression may be junctional epithelium undergoing transition into gingival surface epithelium.

◆ NECROTIZING GINGIVITIS (NECROTIZING ULCERATIVE GINGIVITIS, VINCENT INFECTION; TRENCH MOUTH)

Necrotizing gingivitis (NG) has a distinctive pattern of gingival pathologic changes that have been recognized for hundreds of years. Until recently, the name of this process has been termed *acute necrotizing ulcerative gingivitis* (ANUG); however, several investigators have discontinued the use of acute, because there is no chronic form of the disease. In addition, others prefer the simplified term *necrotizing*

gingivitis with discontinuation of "ulcerative," since the ulceration occurs secondary to the necrosis.

In the 1890s, the French physician Jean Hyacinthe Vincent identified a fusiform bacterium, *Bacillus fusiformis* (currently *Fusobacterium nucleatum*), and a spirochete, *Borrelia vincentii*, after microscopic examination of plaque samples from affected sites. Vincent believed that the fusiform bacteria were principally responsible for the condition, and the spirochetes mainly were saprophytic opportunists. The spirochete and fusiform bacterium association remains true today, but more sophisticated techniques have implicated *Fusobacterium nucleatum*, *Prevotella intermedia*, *Porphyromonas gingivalis*, *Treponema* spp., and *Selenomonas* spp. Although the association with bacteria is strong, controversial research has suggested that viruses, such as cytomegalovirus, Epstein-Barr virus, and herpes simplex, may contribute to the onset and progression of the process.

The infection frequently occurs in the presence of psychologic stress. People in military service exhibit an increased frequency of NG; the disorder was so common in the battlefield trenches during World War I that the nickname *trench mouth* became well known.

In addition to stress, other factors have been related to an increased frequency of NG:
- Immunosuppression
- Smoking
- Local trauma
- Poor nutritional status
- Poor oral hygiene
- Inadequate sleep
- Recent illness

Several medications have been reported to cause agranulocytosis, a condition that may clinically present initially as NG. A thorough investigation of all currently utilized medications appears prudent and may lead to discovery of a significant associated immunosuppression. In addition, the immunocompromised status associated with acquired immunodeficiency syndrome (AIDS) (see page 257) or infectious mononucleosis (see page 241) has been related to the development of NG. The list of predisposing factors clearly supports the association between a depressed systemic immunity and the appearance of the disorder.

Clinical Features

NG may occur at any age; however, when encountered in the United States or Europe, it is seen most frequently in young and middle-aged adults. Several publications have reported a higher frequency in whites. The prevalence in the normal population is less than 0.1%; however, in stressed populations (e.g., military recruits), the frequency increases up to 7%. In developing countries, NG typically occurs in very young children suffering from malnutrition.

In a classic case of NG, the interdental papillae are highly inflamed, edematous, and hemorrhagic. Typically, the affected papillae are blunted and demonstrate areas of "punched-out," craterlike necrosis that are covered with a

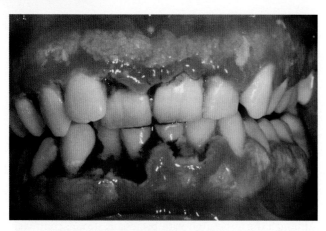

• **Fig. 4.9 Necrotizing Gingivitis (NG).** Gingiva is friable and hemorrhagic with necrosis of the interdental papillae.

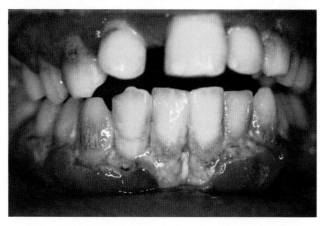

• **Fig. 4.10 Necrotizing Mucositis.** Gingiva exhibits epithelial necrosis that has extended between the adjacent interdental papillae and apically to the alveolar mucosa junction.

gray pseudomembrane (Fig. 4.9). Early cases may be missed easily because the ulceration initially involves only the tip of the interdental papilla. A fetid odor, exquisite pain, spontaneous hemorrhage, and accumulations of necrotic debris usually are noted. Although a bad odor is not always noted, its absence in a patient without predisposing factors should raise concern for other pathoses, such as gonorrhea (see page 184). Occasional ancillary clinical features include lymphadenopathy, fever, and malaise. The process sometimes can lead to a loss of attachment and the development of associated periodontitis (**necrotizing periodontitis**) or spread to adjacent soft tissue (**necrotizing mucositis, necrotizing stomatitis**) (Fig. 4.10). If the necrotizing infection extends through the mucosa to the skin of the face, then it is typically termed *noma* (**cancrum oris**) (see page 191).

Several investigators have suggested that NG, necrotizing periodontitis (NP), and necrotizing stomatitis are one disease process termed **necrotizing gingivostomatitis.** Evidence presented by numerous authors has shown the diseases to be similar clinically, histopathologically, and bacteriologically, with the only differences being underlying systemic factors and anatomic extension of the necrosis.

Histopathologic Features

The histopathologic features of NG are not specific. Typically, affected gingival papillae demonstrate surface ulceration that is covered by a thickened fibrinopurulent membrane. The underlying lamina propria demonstrates an intense acute or mixed inflammatory infiltrate and extensive hyperemia. In nonulcerated affected epithelium, often a loss of the typical surface keratinization occurs. Necrotic material and extensive bacterial colonization often are included in the material submitted for microscopic examination.

Treatment and Prognosis

In contrast to most forms of periodontal disease, NG typically demonstrates quick resolution after removal of the bacterial challenge. Even with conservative therapy, regeneration of the affected gingiva normally is seen. The affected area is treated best with débridement by scaling, curettage, or ultrasonic instrumentation (except when contraindicated, as in HIV-positive patients). Topical or local anesthetic often is required before the clinician can débride the tissues adequately. Frequent rinses with chlorhexidine, warm saltwater, or diluted hydrogen peroxide are beneficial in increasing the therapeutic response. Antibiotic medications (metronidazole and penicillin have been suggested as the drugs of choice) are a useful adjunct, especially in the presence of fever or lymphadenopathy.

Treatment should include instructions on oral hygiene and patient motivation; identification and resolution of any predisposing factors also are advantageous. Supportive therapy (e.g., rest, appropriate fluid intake, and soft nutritious diet) and smoking cessation often improve the clinical response. Follow-up appointments are necessary to reinforce the home care instructions and to rule out a recurrence of the process.

The clinician must be ever vigilant in the search for other clinical signs and symptoms of immunosuppression. Subtle palatal candidiasis or HIV-related oral hairy leukoplakia (see page 253) can be overlooked easily in a patient with NG. Appropriate attention must be directed toward the oral soft tissue examination, especially in patients with infections such as NG that are related to immunosuppression. In addition, a thorough investigation of underlying causes of immunosuppression should be performed on patients whose conditions are resistant to normal therapy.

◆ PLASMA CELL GINGIVITIS (ATYPICAL GINGIVOSTOMATITIS; ALLERGIC GINGIVOSTOMATITIS)

A distinctive pattern of gingival inflammation, **plasma cell gingivitis,** was brought to the attention of health care practitioners during the late 1960s and early 1970s. A rash of cases occurred during that time, and most appear to have been related to a hypersensitivity to a component of chewing gum. Since that time, the number of cases has dwindled, but similar gingival alterations are reported occasionally.

Although the association with chewing gum has decreased, allergy still is responsible for many reported cases. A brand of herbal toothpaste, a specific type of mint candy, and peppers used for cooking have all been implicated in more recent reports. The list of allergens appears to be variable, and a thorough evaluation often is required to rule out an allergic cause.

Clinical Features

Patients with plasma cell gingivitis experience a rapid onset of sore mouth, which often is intensified by dentifrices and hot or spicy foods. The entire free and attached gingiva demonstrates a diffuse enlargement with bright erythema and loss of normal stippling (Fig. 4.11). Extension onto the palate can occur, and edentulous areas typically exhibit less intense changes. On occasion, a similar localized gingival and vestibular alteration can occur from topical placement of a material that elicits a similar plasmacytic inflammatory reaction.

Additional sites of involvement may be seen, or the changes may be localized to the gingiva. In the chewing gum–related cases of the early 1970s, involvement of the lips and tongue was typical. The lips were dry, atrophic, occasionally fissured, and angular cheilitis was frequent. Tongue involvement resulted in erythematous enlargement with furrows, mild crenation, and loss of the typical dorsal coating.

More recent reports have described lesions often isolated to the gingiva without the classic lip and tongue involvement seen in the past. A larger percentage of these cases are idiopathic, and occasional extraoral involvement of sites such as the supraglottic region occurs.

Histopathologic Features

The cases of classic plasma cell gingivitis of the 1970s demonstrated psoriasiform hyperplasia and spongiosis of the surface epithelium with intense exocytosis and neutrophilic microabscesses. The underlying lamina propria contains numerous dilated vascular channels and an extremely dense chronic inflammatory infiltrate that is composed predominantly of plasma cells (Fig. 4.12). The more recent cases are similar but often demonstrate less involvement of the surface epithelium and a less dense underlying plasmacytic infiltrate.

Investigation of the clonality of the plasma cell infiltrate may be necessary to rule out the possibility of a monoclonal plasma cell neoplasm. All allergic and idiopathic cases of plasma cell gingivitis demonstrate a polyclonal mixture of plasma cells and a normal profile on plasma immunoelectrophoresis. In addition, the possibility of IgG4-related

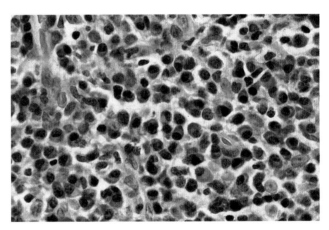

• **Fig. 4.12 Plasma Cell Gingivitis.** High-power photomicrograph exhibiting a dense inflammatory infiltrate consisting predominantly of plasma cells with scattered lymphocytes.

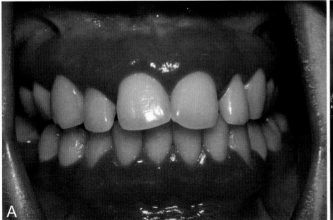
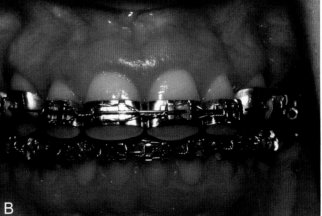

• **Fig. 4.11 Plasma Cell Gingivitis. A,** Diffuse, bright-red enlargement of the free and attached gingiva. **B,** Same patient as depicted in **A** 16 months later after elimination of the inciting allergen. (Courtesy of Dr. Phillip Sheridan).

disease (see page 471) should be considered. In IgG4-related disease, a storiform pattern of sclerosis and scattered eosinophils typically are present along with an IgG4/IgG plasma cell ratio greater than 40%, and elevation of the serum IgG4 level.

It must be remembered that an identical dense infiltrate of plasma cells can be seen in mouth breathing-related gingivitis, plaque-related gingival hyperplasia, and chronic periodontitis. The diagnosis depends on a strong clinical and histopathologic correlation in which the changes are associated with a rapid onset of sore mouth and do not resolve with improved oral hygiene. Reports of this entity that do not fulfill the diagnostic criteria still can be found in the dental and medical literature. Review of the original 1971 publication may be helpful for those contemplating the diagnosis.

Treatment and Prognosis

All patients with plasma cell gingivitis should be instructed to keep a complete dietary history with records of everything taken into the mouth (e.g., foods, dentifrice, mouthwash, tobacco, alcohol, chewing gum, candy, and medications). Possible allergens should be eliminated to discover the underlying cause. If an easy answer is not apparent, then extensive allergy testing and an elimination diet can be undertaken.

Many patients in whom no underlying cause could be discovered have been treated with topical or systemic immunosuppressive medications with variable results. Dexamethasone rinses, fluocinonide gel, topical triamcinolone, and topical fusidic acid are several of the reported choices. Despite all the evaluations and therapeutic interventions, some patients do not respond to treatment, and no cause for the disease can be identified.

◆ FOREIGN BODY GINGIVITIS

In 1990, Daley and Wysocki described an important pattern of recalcitrant gingivitis that remains surprisingly underrecognized. The alteration represents an inflammatory response to foreign material that has become embedded in the gingival tissues. Energy-dispersive X-ray microanalysis has shown that most of the foreign particles are of dental origin, with abrasives and restorative materials being identified most frequently. These materials appear to be introduced through disrupted gingival or sulcular epithelium during professional hygiene activities, restorative procedures, or during household use of oral hygiene or cosmetic products. The most discovered material is silicon, a major component of toothpaste, polishing paste, pumice, and carborundum disks. When introduced into the gingiva, silicon has been shown to activate fibroblasts, leading to increased levels of inflammatory cytokines. The gingival changes may become evident shortly after the introduction of the material or be delayed for months to years.

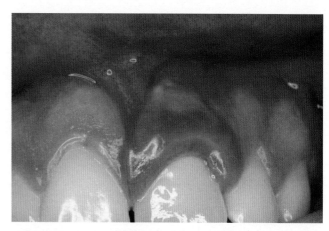

• **Fig. 4.13 Foreign Body Gingivitis.** Localized enlarged and erythematous gingiva associated with the maxillary left central incisor. The alterations developed shortly after placement of a porcelain-fused-to-metal (PFM) full crown and were not responsive to conservative local therapy. Biopsy revealed granulomatous inflammation intermixed with foreign material. (Courtesy of Dr. Timothy L. Gutierrez.)

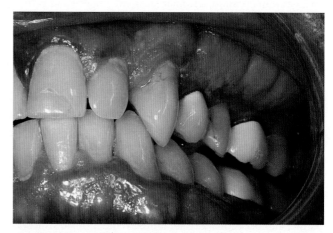

• **Fig. 4.14 Foreign Body Gingivitis.** Red, atrophic mucosa of the left maxillary facial gingiva. The alterations arose following placement of two porcelain-fused-to-metal (PFM) crowns. Biopsy revealed lichenoid mucositis with intermixed fragments of foreign material.

Clinical Features

Foreign body gingivitis presents as focal areas of gingival redness that may demonstrate peripheral radiating striae, intermixed white areas, zones of erosion, or enlargement (Figs. 4.13 and 4.14). Associated discomfort and multifocal involvement are common. The lesions frequently are confused with gingival lichen planus but fail to migrate or develop extra-gingival involvement. More recently, foreign body gingivitis has been associated with discrete gingival leukoplakias that may be verruciform in appearance, occasionally associated with varying degrees of dysplasia, and worrisome for an evolving proliferative verrucous leukoplakia (see page 384) (Fig. 4.15). Although the process may involve any gingival surface, the posterior areas of both arches and the anterior maxillary gingiva are affected most often. There is a female predominance, and most cases present in adulthood with a mean age of approximately 50 years.

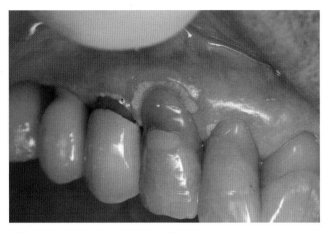

• **Fig. 4.15 Leukoplakic Foreign Body Gingivitis.** This clinical presentation exhibits features of both foreign body gingivitis and evolving proliferative verrucous leukoplakia. Biopsy should be extended to the sulcus to enhance the likelihood of including foreign material, if present. Even if foreign material is found, the definitive diagnosis requires a strong clinicopathologic correlation. (Courtesy of Dr. Fred Lucas.)

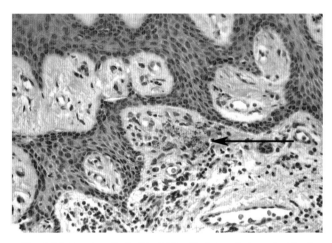

• **Fig. 4.16 Foreign Body Gingivitis.** Particles of pigmented foreign material *(arrow)* intermixed with lymphocytes and plasma cells.

Histopathologic Features

The histopathologic features are variable but consistently will demonstrate minute opaque grayish-black granules that may be intermixed with translucent crystalline structures (Fig. 4.16). The granules do not tend to polarize, whereas the crystals are highlighted by polarized light. The foreign material is subtle and may be missed without a high index of suspicion. The red variant of foreign body gingivitis tends to exhibit areas of epithelial atrophy often demonstrating degeneration of the basal cell layer, suggestive of gingival lichen planus. The superficial stroma typically reveals a dense lymphocytic band with a deeper patchy inflammatory cellular infiltrate composed predominantly of lymphocytes, plasma cells, and histiocytes. Scattered eosinophils occasionally may be present. The foreign material typically is intermixed within the deeper patchy infiltrate or noted within areas of intermixed granulomatous inflammation. The leukoplakic variant most frequently exhibits hyperorthokeratosis with

varying degrees of verruciform hyperplasia or dysplasia. The deeper stroma will demonstrate a similar patchy chronic inflammatory cellular infiltrate with lymphocytes, plasma cells, and histiocytes with or without granulomatous inflammation.

The diagnosis requires a strong clinicopathologic correlation. When foreign material is detected, it is impossible to ascertain if the material is coincidental or causative. In addition, superficial biopsies of foreign body gingivitis can miss the foreign material, because the granules often are deep and adjacent to the gingival sulcus. When presented with a focal lichenoid lesion with foreign material, **lichen planus** (see page 787) must be considered but typically will demonstrate migration and extragingival lesions. When presented with a verruciform leukoplakia with foreign material, the possibility of an evolving **proliferative verrucous leukoplakia** (see page 384) must be considered with appropriate therapy and close follow-up. When significant granulomatous inflammation is present but not intimately associated with the foreign material, the possibility of **orofacial granulomatosis** (see page 330) must be considered.

Treatment and Prognosis

Surgical excision of the affected tissue is the therapy of choice if the process is sufficiently symptomatic or presents as a thickened leukoplakia. In persistently atrophic or erosive areas of foreign body gingivitis, overlaying the damaged area with a graft from a healthy gingival donor site may be a better option than complete excision. Use of topical corticosteroids has produced temporary resolution of sensitivity in some patients, but symptoms typically return upon cessation of therapy. To prevent future introduction of iatrogenic foreign material, clinicians should use care during restorative and oral hygiene procedures that might introduce foreign material into a surgical wound. In addition, dental prophylaxis should be delayed for 2 days after scaling, root planing, and curettage procedures.

◆ DESQUAMATIVE GINGIVITIS

Desquamative gingivitis is a clinical term for gingiva that demonstrates superficial peeling of the epithelium characterized by formation and rupture of mucosal vesicles. The process almost always represents a manifestation of one of several different vesiculoerosive diseases, usually mucous membrane pemphigoid. Some clinicians broaden the definition to include patients with atrophic and erosive gingival lesions without true peeling of the epithelium. In such cases, lichen planus is diagnosed most frequently. Other diagnoses that are made less frequently include linear IgA disease, pemphigus vulgaris, epidermolysis bullosa acquisita, systemic lupus erythematosus (SLE), chronic ulcerative stomatitis, and paraneoplastic pemphigus. The gingival manifestations of these mucosal and dermatologic diseases are described in greater detail in Chapter 16, so further discussion here is not warranted.

◆ DRUG-RELATED GINGIVAL HYPERPLASIA (DRUG-RELATED GINGIVAL OVERGROWTH)

Drug-related gingival hyperplasia refers to an abnormal growth of the gingival tissues secondary to use of a systemic medication. A list of medications reported to be associated with gingival hyperplasia is provided in Box 4.4. Of these medications, a strong association has been noted only with cyclosporine (Fig. 4.17), phenytoin, and nifedipine

---

◆ BOX 4.4 Medications Reported to Be Associated With Gingival Hyperplasia

- Anticonvulsants
  - Carbamazepine
  - Ethosuximide
  - Ethotoin
  - Felbamate
  - Mephenytoin
  - Methsuximide
  - Phenobarbital
  - Phensuximide
  - Phenytoin
  - Primidone
  - Sodium valproate
  - Vigabatrin
- Calcium channel blockers
  - Amlodipine
  - Bepridil
  - Diltiazem
  - Felodipine
  - Isradipine
  - Lacidipine
  - Nicardipine
  - Nifedipine
  - Nitrendipine
  - Nisoldipine
  - Verapamil
- Cyclosporine
- Erythromycin
- Oral contraceptives

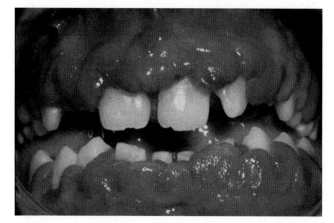

• **Fig. 4.17 Cyclosporine-Related Gingival Hyperplasia.** Diffuse, erythematous, and fibrotic gingival hyperplasia.

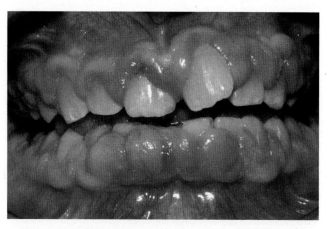

• **Fig. 4.18 Nifedipine-Related Gingival Hyperplasia.** Diffuse, fibrotic gingival hyperplasia after 1 month of intensive oral hygiene. Significant erythema, edema, and increased enlargement were present before intervention.

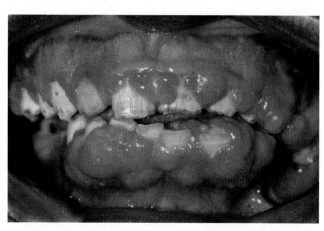

• **Fig. 4.19 Cyclosporine- and Nifedipine-Related Gingival Hyperplasia.** Dramatic gingival hyperplasia in a patient using two drugs associated with gingival enlargement.

(Fig. 4.18). In addition to nifedipine, a definitive but much weaker association has been documented with other calcium channel-blocking agents, such as diltiazem, amlodipine, and verapamil. In the remainder of these agents, the prevalence is much lower or the association is weak or anecdotal. Several calcium channel blockers exist that have not been associated with gingival hyperplasia and may represent safer alternatives. As new drugs are developed, the list of offending medications may grow. Cyclosporine is known to be associated with hypertension, often leading to utilization of a calcium channel blocker. When cyclosporine and nifedipine are used concurrently, the severity of the associated hyperplasia often is increased (Fig. 4.19).

Rare reports of gingival hyperplasia associated with use of vemurafenib have been noted. This medication is a targeted BRAF inhibitor utilized in the treatment of metastatic melanoma. It has demonstrated a number of proven cutaneous side effects including keratoacanthoma-like squamous cell carcinoma, keratosis pilaris, acanthopapillomas, and plantar hyperkeratosis. The exact nature of the gingival enlargement is unclear because none of the patients have had biopsy with histopathologic examination of these oral alterations.

The prevalence of these hyperplasias varies widely; however, as reported in one critical review of the literature, the prevalence related to use of phenytoin is approximately 50%. Cyclosporine and nifedipine each produce significant changes in about 25% of patients treated. Whether there is a relationship between the dose and the risk or severity of the hyperplasia is a controversial issue. Investigators have suggested that susceptibility to cyclosporine gingival hyperplasia is associated with certain histocompatibility antigen (HLA) types, whereas other HLA types appear to protect against hyperplasia. Whether similar correlations exist for the other forms of medication-associated gingival hyperplasia is unknown.

The degree of gingival enlargement appears to be related significantly to the patient's susceptibility and the level of oral hygiene. In observations of patients with excellent oral hygiene, gingival overgrowth (as ascertained by pseudopocket formation) is reduced dramatically or not present. Even with good oral hygiene, however, some degree of gingival enlargement can be discovered in susceptible individuals, although in many cases the changes are difficult to detect. Rigorous oral hygiene often can limit the severity to clinically insignificant levels. Of the medications discussed, cyclosporine appears to be the least responsive to the institution of a rigorous program of oral hygiene; even with this medication, however, the elimination of gingival inflammation results in noticeable clinical improvement. In addition, the degree of drug-associated gingival hyperplasia appears to be markedly higher in smokers.

Clinical Features

Because young patients use phenytoin most often, the gingival hyperplasia it induces is primarily a problem in people younger than age 25. Cases related to the calcium channel blockers occur mainly in middle-aged or older adults. Cyclosporine is used over a broad age range, and this correlates with the age of reported hyperplasia. A greater risk for gingival hyperplasia occurs when the drug is used in children, especially adolescents. No race predilection is present. A male predominance is noted with gingival hyperplasia associated with cyclosporine or calcium channel blockers but not with phenytoin.

After 1–3 months of drug use, the enlargements originate in the interdental papillae and spread across the tooth surfaces (Fig. 4.20). The anterior and facial segments are the most frequently involved areas. In extensive cases, the hyperplastic gingiva can cover a portion (or all) of the crowns of many of the involved teeth (Figs. 4.21 and 4.22). Extension lingually and occlusally can interfere with speech and mastication. Edentulous areas generally are not affected, but significant hyperplasia under poorly maintained dentures and around implants has been noted (Fig. 4.23).

Nongingival soft tissue growths that resemble pyogenic granulomas have been reported in allogeneic bone marrow

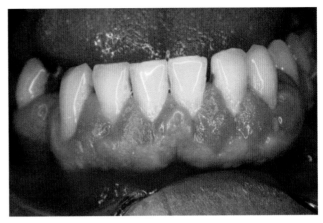

• **Fig. 4.20 Mild Phenytoin-Related Gingival Hyperplasia.** Gingival enlargement present predominantly in the interdental papillae.

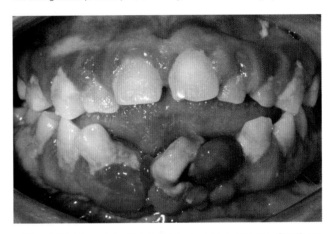

• **Fig. 4.21 Phenytoin-Related Gingival Hyperplasia.** Significant erythematous gingival hyperplasia is covering portions of the crowns of numerous teeth.

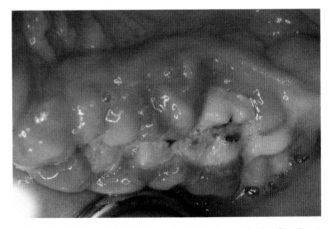

• **Fig. 4.22 Phenytoin-Related Gingival Hyperplasia.** Significant gingival hyperplasia almost totally covers the crowns of the posterior maxillary dentition. (Courtesy of Dr. Ann Drummond and Dr. Timothy Johnson.)

transplant recipients who are receiving cyclosporine for graft-versus-host disease (GVHD) (Fig. 4.24). It is thought that cyclosporine triggers the proliferations in areas chronically inflamed by GVHD.

In the absence of inflammation, the enlarged gingiva is normal in color and firm, with a surface that may be smooth,

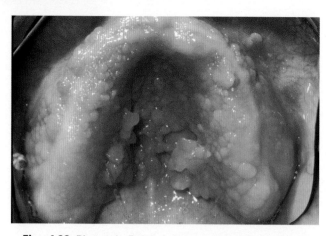

• **Fig. 4.23 Phenytoin-Related Palatal Hyperplasia.** Extensive hyperplasia of palatal mucosa in an edentulous patient with poor denture hygiene.

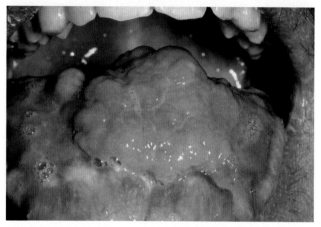

• **Fig. 4.24 Nongingival Cyclosporine Hyperplasia.** Exophytic and granulomatous-appearing mass of the dorsal surface of the tongue that arose in a bone marrow transplant patient who was receiving cyclosporine for graft-versus-host disease (GVHD).

stippled, or granular. With inflammation, the affected gingiva often becomes dark red and edematous, with a surface that is friable, bleeds easily, and occasionally is ulcerated. Pyogenic granuloma-like enlargements occasionally are seen in the presence of heavy inflammation.

Histopathologic Features

Upon histopathologic examination, the overlying surface epithelium may demonstrate elongation of the rete ridges, with long extensions into the underlying stroma. The lamina propria exhibits an increased amount of fibrous connective tissue that demonstrates a normal density of fibroblasts. In patients with secondary inflammation, there is increased vascularity and a chronic inflammatory cellular infiltrate that most frequently consists of lymphocytes and plasma cells. In patients with pyogenic granuloma-like overgrowths, the proliferations often demonstrate an increased vascularity and significant subacute inflammation.

Treatment and Prognosis

Discontinuation of the offending medication by the attending physician often results in cessation, and possibly some regression, of the gingival enlargement; even substitution of one medication for another in the same class may be beneficial. Often the response to medication substitution is not immediate. If the drug use is mandatory, then professional cleaning, frequent reevaluations, and home plaque control are important. Antiplaque agents, such as chlorhexidine, have been beneficial in the prevention of plaque buildup and the associated gingival hyperplasia.

Systemic or topical folic acid has been shown to ameliorate the gingival hyperplasia in some cases. In addition, several authors have documented significant resolution of cyclosporine-related gingival hyperplasia after a short course of metronidazole, azithromycin, or roxithromycin. Azithromycin also may be beneficial in resolving gingival hyperplasia related to nifedipine and phenytoin.

Although gingival hyperplasia is associated with increased probing depths, some investigators do not believe this necessarily leads to exaggerated attachment loss or an increased loss of teeth. Therefore, some clinicians exercise watchful waiting and do not perform invasive therapy without evidence of attachment loss, inappropriate aesthetics, or disruption of speech or mastication. When objectionable alterations are noted and all other interventions fail to achieve significant resolution, eradication of the excess gingival tissues by scalpel or laser remains the treatment of choice. Recurrence is not uncommon, however, especially in patients with inadequate oral hygiene. Due to increased rates of tooth loss in patients with recurrent and persistent drug-related gingival hyperplasia, substitution of the offending medication is the best approach if medically appropriate.

◆ GINGIVAL FIBROMATOSIS (FIBROMATOSIS GINGIVAE; ELEPHANTIASIS GINGIVAE)

Gingival fibromatosis is a slowly progressive gingival enlargement caused by a collagenous overgrowth of the gingival fibrous connective tissue. Despite the name, this disorder bears no relationship to the hypercellular and neoplastic fibromatoses that can occur in soft tissue and bone (see pages 523 and 663). Gingival fibromatosis is a rare condition with an estimated prevalence of 1:750,000.

Gingival fibromatosis may be familial or idiopathic. Other findings sometimes seen in conjunction with gingival fibromatosis include hypertrichosis (Fig. 4.25), generalized aggressive periodontitis, epilepsy, intellectual disability, sensorineural deafness, hypothyroidism, chondrodystrophia, and growth hormone deficiency. The familial variations may occur as an isolated finding or in association with one of several hereditary syndromes. Box 4.5 lists the syndromes that often have been associated with gingival fibromatosis.

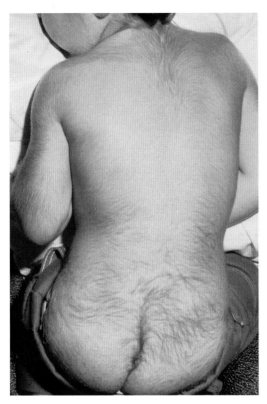

• **Fig. 4.25 Hypertrichosis in Association With Gingival Fibromatosis.** Dramatically increased body hair of the back and buttocks in a patient with gingival fibromatosis. (Courtesy of Dr. George Blozis.)

• BOX **4.5** **Syndromes Associated With Gingival Fibromatosis**

- Byars-Jurkiewicz syndrome
- Costello syndrome
- Cross syndrome
- Infantile systemic hyalinosis
- Jones-Hartsfield syndrome
- Murray-Puretic-Drescher syndrome
- Ramon syndrome
- Rutherford syndrome
- Zimmerman-Laband syndrome

In most cases of isolated gingival fibromatosis, an autosomal dominant pattern of inheritance is seen; however, autosomal recessive examples also have been noted. Incomplete penetrance and variable expressivity are seen. The phenotype of hereditary gingival fibromatosis demonstrates significant genetic heterogeneity with the existence of at least five genes that are responsible for similar patterns of clinical presentation.

Clinical Features

In most instances, the enlargement begins before age 20 and often is correlated with the eruption of the deciduous or permanent teeth (Fig. 4.26). Most investigators believe that the

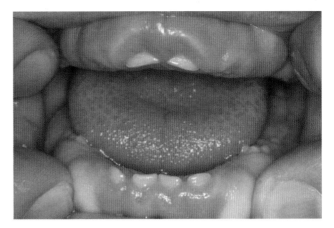

• **Fig. 4.26 Gingival Fibromatosis.** A young child with cheeks retracted by the parent. Note erythematous gingival hyperplasia arising in association with erupting deciduous dentition. (Courtesy of Dr. George Blozis.)

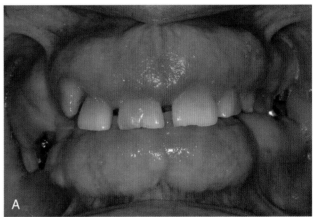

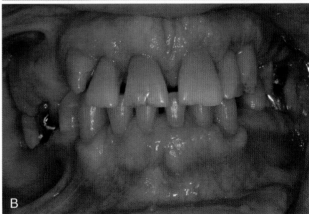

• **Fig. 4.27 Gingival Fibromatosis. A,** Dense fibrotic enlargement of the gingiva, which results in flaring of the dentition and open contact points. **B,** Same patient following surgical reduction of the excess fibrotic gingival tissue.

presence of teeth probably is necessary for the condition to occur. Despite this, rare patterns can present in infancy or even at birth. After the process has begun, it can overgrow the associated teeth and even interfere with lip closure. Failure or delay in eruption, or altered position of the erupted teeth, may be evident (Fig. 4.27). In some instances, a tooth

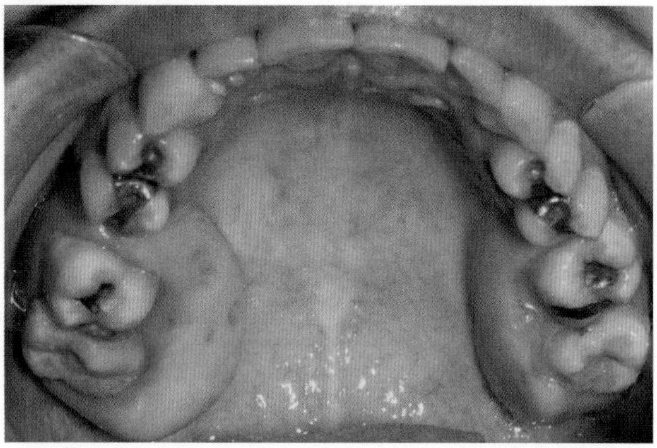

• **Fig. 4.28 Localized Gingival Fibromatosis.** Bilateral and symmetrical fibrotic enlargements of the palatal surfaces of the posterior maxillary alveolar ridges.

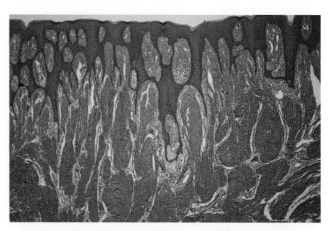

• **Fig. 4.29 Gingival Fibromatosis.** Surface stratified squamous epithelium exhibiting long, thin rete ridges and underlying dense, fibrous connective tissue.

may have erupted into a normal position, but the fibrous connective tissue continues to cover the crown and prevent visualization.

The gingival changes may be generalized or localized to one or more quadrants. Either jaw may be involved, but the maxilla is affected more frequently and demonstrates a greater degree of enlargement. Palatal surfaces typically are increased in thickness more than the buccal side. Typically, extension past the alveolar mucosal junction into the mucobuccal fold is not seen, but palatal extensions can cause significant distortion of the contour of the palate and, at times, almost can meet in the midline.

In localized cases, the hyperplasia may involve a group of teeth and remain stable or, later, may extend to other segments of one or both jaws. One distinctive and not uncommon pattern involves the posterior maxillary alveolar ridge. In this pattern, the hyperplastic tissue forms bilaterally symmetrical enlargements that extend posteriorly and palatally from the posterior alveolar ridges (Fig. 4.28). Less commonly, the overgrowth also may be isolated to the facial gingiva of the lower molars.

The gingiva is firm, normal in color, and covered by a surface that is smooth or finely stippled. In older patients, the surface may develop numerous papillary projections. The frenular attachments may appear to divide the gingival tissues of the alveolar ridge into lobules. Associated clinical problems include poor aesthetics, prolonged retention of deciduous teeth, abnormal occlusion, inadequate lip closure, and difficulty in eating and speaking.

Histopathologic Features

The enlargements of gingival fibromatosis consist of dense hypocellular, hypovascular collagenous tissue, which forms numerous interlacing bundles that generally are arranged mostly in a parallel pattern. The surface epithelium often is acanthotic and exhibits long, thin rete ridges that extend deeply into the underlying fibrous connective tissue (Fig. 4.29). Inflammation is absent to mild. On occasion,

scattered islands of odontogenic epithelium, foci of dystrophic calcification, or areas of osseous metaplasia may be seen.

Treatment and Prognosis

Mild cases often respond to scaling and root planing followed by close professional follow-up. For more advanced gingival thickening, conservative surgical removal is indicated. The rate of recurrence following excision is reduced if the removal is delayed until full eruption of the permanent dentition. Despite this, local and psychological benefits often exceed the downside of recurrence, warranting earlier removal. Although recurrence is common in dentulous patients, a rigorous program of oral hygiene often slows regrowth. In severe cases, selective extraction of teeth and gingivectomy often are required to achieve a normal gingival morphology.

◆ PERIODONTITIS

Periodontitis refers to an inflammation of the gingival tissues in association with some loss of both the attachment of the periodontal ligament and bony support. With progressive loss of attachment, significant destruction of the periodontal ligament and adjacent alveolar bone can occur. Apical migration of the crevicular epithelium along the root surface results in the formation of periodontal pockets. Loosening and eventual loss of teeth are possible. A patient is deemed to have periodontitis if one of two presentations is noted:
- Interdental clinical attachment loss in two or more nonadjacent teeth
- Buccal or oral clinical attachment loss of ≥3 mm with pocketing >3 mm at two or more teeth

A national health survey of adults aged 30–79 years conducted from 2009–2014 revealed the prevalence of periodontitis to be 42.2%, with 7.8% being severe. It is assumed that the prevalence is rising since the disease increases with age, the population is living longer, and a greater percentage of the population is retaining their teeth due to a reduction in dental caries.

For more than a century, the presence of the disease has been correlated with the accumulation of dental plaque on the tooth and under the gingiva. Despite this, some patients demonstrate extensive dental plaque but do not develop destructive lesions of the periodontium. Many investigators now believe that periodontitis represents a *microbial-shift disease*. Dramatic differences exist in the content of dental plaque in areas of healthy and diseased periodontium. Healthy sites are colonized primarily by facultative gram-positive organisms, whereas plaque within areas of active periodontitis contains anaerobic and microaerophilic gram-negative flora. Of the more than 500 types of bacteria that may reside in the oral cavity, only a few have been related to periodontitis, and the specific types often correlate with the clinical patterns of periodontitis. Chronic periodontitis is associated strongly with *Treponema denticola*, *Tannerella forsythensis*, and *Porphyromonas gingivalis*. Additional organisms frequently thought to be involved include *Aggregatibacter actinomycetemcomitans* (formerly *Actinobacillus actinomycetemcomitans*), *Prevotella intermedia*, *Campylobacter rectus*, and *Fusobacterium nucleatum*. Although controversial, some investigators also have suggested that human cytomegalovirus and other herpesviruses could play a contributing role.

The pathogenic organisms exist in an organized community termed a **biofilm**. Bacteria growing in biofilms are relatively protected from normal host defenses and exhibit an increased resistance to locally or systemically administered antibiotic medications. Lipopolysaccharides released from the biofilms are thought to trigger release of catabolic inflammatory mediators that lead to the loss of attachment. Mechanical disruption of this organized bacterial biofilm may be an important factor associated with successful treatment of periodontitis.

The 1999 classification of periodontitis was redefined in 2017 during the World Workshop on the Classification of Periodontal and Peri-implant Diseases and Conditions. The revised classification system identified three different forms of periodontitis:

- Necrotizing periodontitis
- Periodontitis as a direct manifestation of systemic diseases
- Periodontitis

This new classification system combines the old categories of "chronic periodontitis" and "aggressive periodontitis" into a single disease process. Since publication of the 1999 classification, clinicians and educators voiced concerns that the stipulated criteria to separate chronic from aggressive periodontitis were difficult to apply due to substantial overlap. In addition, there was no evidence of a specific pathophysiology that distinguishes the chronic from the aggressive forms of periodontitis. Despite the 2017 reclassification, significant controversy remains. Soon after publication of the findings from the 2017 world workshop, participating members submitted conflicting manuscripts supporting continued separation of chronic periodontitis of adulthood from aggressive periodontitis noted in children and young adults, especially the localized variant.

To stratify the variations within the current category of periodontitis, a staging and grading system was established during the World Workshop. The *staging* is a four-tier system (I–IV) that is meant to define the severity, extent, and complexity of the periodontitis in an individual and primarily utilizes the clinical attachment loss in association with the radiographic presentation and history of tooth loss. The grading is a three-tier system (A–C) that attempts to provide an estimate of the rate of progression, responsiveness to standard therapy, and the potential impact on systemic health. The grading system primarily utilizes the rate of clinical attachment loss over time combined with local factors (amount of biofilm) and grade modifiers such as diabetes and smoking.

Periodontitis associated with systemic disease is not rare, and Box 4.6 lists many of the disorders that may be associated with a premature loss of periodontal attachment. **Necrotizing periodontitis (NP)** represents the loss of attachment that often occurs in association with necrotizing gingivitis (NG) (see page 151). This form has been correlated with aggressive invasion by several spirochetes and *Prevotella intermedia*.

Clinical and Radiographic Features
Periodontitis

With the decline in caries, **periodontitis** has become the primary cause of tooth loss in patients older than 35 years of age. The disorder demonstrates an increased prevalence in males,

---

• BOX 4.6   Systemic Disorders With Premature Attachment Loss

1. Acatalasia
2. Acrodynia
3. Acquired immunodeficiency syndrome (AIDS)
4. Blood dyscrasias
   - Leukemia
   - Agranulocytosis
   - Cyclic neutropenia
5. Chédiak-Higashi syndrome
6. Chronic granulomatous disease
7. Cohen syndrome
8. Crohn disease
9. Down syndrome
10. Diabetes mellitus
11. Dyskeratosis congenita
12. Ehlers-Danlos syndrome, types IV and VIII
13. Glycogen storage disease
14. Haim-Munk syndrome
15. Hemochromatosis
16. Hypophosphatasia
17. Kindler syndrome
18. Langerhans cell disease
19. Leukocyte dysfunctions with associated extraoral infections
20. Oxalosis
21. Papillon-Lefèvre syndrome
22. Plasminogen deficiency
23. Sarcoidosis
24. Trisomy 21

although researchers believe that much of this effect is related to poorer oral hygiene and dental-visit behavior. In addition, an increased prevalence of periodontitis is associated with the following:

- Advancing age
- Smoking
- Diabetes mellitus
- Osteoporosis
- HIV infection
- Lower socioeconomic level

Local factors also may predispose patients to isolated periodontal defects; these include tooth shape and alignment, presence and quality of dental restorations, poor interdental contact, calculus formation, subgingival dental caries, traumatic occlusion, and abnormal alveolar bone or gingival anatomy.

Conversely, it has been suggested that the presence of significant periodontitis may place patients at risk for an increased prevalence or greater severity of certain medical disorders. Although controversial, periodontitis has been associated with an elevated risk for coronary artery disease, stroke, progressive diabetes mellitus, respiratory diseases, and delivery of low–birth weight babies. Although co-occurrence of periodontal disease with these serious medical conditions has been documented, these associations should not be interpreted to insinuate that periodontal disease is causing the medical condition to occur. Most of the supporting evidence arose from observational studies and would be strengthened by well-designed and randomized clinical trials. Since the current scientific evidence of an association between periodontal disease and these medical conditions is weak and without any strong proof of causality, the primary focus when treating periodontal disease should remain preserving the dentition to improve oral health and the quality of life.

In classic periodontitis of adulthood, no abnormalities of the immune system typically are found. Periodontitis begins in youth and early adulthood, takes years to decades to progress, and includes cyclic patterns of exacerbation and remission. The assumption that periodontitis is a disease of aging has been challenged, and most believe the increased periodontal destruction observed in older adults reflects a lifetime of disease accumulation rather than an age-specific disease.

In patients with periodontitis, gingivitis is present and precedes the development of significant periodontal lesions. Although many sites may demonstrate gingivitis and do not progress to attachment loss, lifelong local measures directed against sites of gingivitis represent an effective approach for prevention of chronic periodontitis. As loss of attachment occurs, blunting and apical positioning of the gingival margins typically are present (Fig. 4.30). Periodontal disease is present when a loss of attachment can be demonstrated using a periodontal probe. In the absence of significant gingival hyperplasia, a measurement of pocket depths greater than 3–4 mm indicates destruction of the periodontal ligament and resorption of adjacent alveolar bone; however, clinical

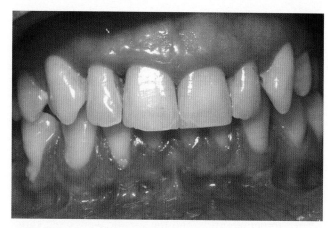

• **Fig. 4.30 Periodontitis.** Diffuse gingival erythema with blunting and apical positioning of the gingival margins. (Courtesy of Dr. Samuel Jasper.)

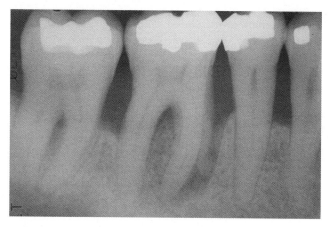

• **Fig. 4.31 Periodontitis.** Generalized horizontal bone loss with an isolated vertical defect involving the mesial root of the first molar.

attachment loss is the best measurement of accumulated periodontal destruction and represents the diagnostic gold standard. High-quality dental radiographs exhibit a decreased vertical height of the bone surrounding the affected teeth (Fig. 4.31). With advanced bone loss, tooth mobility is present. Although to date there are no confirmed biomarkers for periodontal disease, ongoing research is attempting to analyze saliva for genomic and microbial markers for the early diagnosis of periodontitis.

Although periodontitis is much more frequent in older adults, it also can be a significant problem in children and young adults. In such cases, an investigation for an association with a systemic disease process should be ruled out. Researchers believe that periodontitis arising in early age represents several different pathoses that have been grouped together because of similar clinical presentations. Most patients have a demonstrable neutrophil dysfunction but without systemic manifestations. Although this is a controversial topic, several investigators have suggested that this pattern of periodontitis requires specific bacterial flora and the presence of a selective immune dysfunction that allows these pathogens to flourish. This unique pattern of immune alteration may explain the failure to defend appropriately against certain periodontal pathogens without exhibiting systemic signs of immunodeficiency. Familial aggregation of patients with this pattern of periodontitis is noted and suggests an underlying genetic foundation. In all likelihood, high stage/grade periodontitis arising in younger patients is genetically heterogeneous, meaning the mutation of any one of several different gene loci can result in the disease.

When presenting in younger patients, the periodontitis may be localized or generalized. The localized variant often begins around 11–13 years of age with a strong familial history and a tendency to demonstrate attachment loss localized to the first molars and incisors. This pattern of periodontal disease demonstrates a 10-fold higher risk in adolescents of African or Middle Eastern descent. The periodontal destruction appears to localize around the first molars and the incisors, possibly because these teeth have been erupted for the longest duration (Fig. 4.32). In numerous clinical studies, minimal supragingival plaque or calculus has been documented; however, this finding is variable. The rate of bone destruction is three to five times faster than that seen in typical periodontitis of adulthood. In the 1999 classification, this pattern of disease was termed *localized aggressive periodontitis*; and many investigators continue to believe that this presentation deserves to be separated from classic chronic periodontitis of adulthood.

In the first molar regions, radiographs reveal vertical bone resorption that often is bilateral and symmetrical. In classic cases, an arc-shaped zone of bone loss extends from the distal aspect of the second bicuspid to the mesial aspect of the

second molar. Similar involvement is apparent around the anterior teeth. Tooth migration and mobility are common. If untreated, then the process often continues until the teeth are exfoliated. About one-third of patients affected with localized disease will progress to a more generalized pattern.

Of all the pathogens in dental plaque, *A. actinomycetemcomitans* appears to be predominant in the localized form of periodontitis seen in adolescents. This bacterium is present in disease sites in more than 90% of cases. Its ability to invade gingival tissue has created difficulties in mechanical eradication. Knowledge of its importance to the disease process has led to remarkable advances in therapy.

Generalized periodontitis also can be seen in younger patients but typically demonstrates a wider age range with most patients being between the ages of 12–32. In contrast to many examples of the localized variant, heavy plaque, calculus, and marked gingival inflammation may be present. Compared with the localized variant, more teeth are affected, and the bone loss is not restricted to specific areas of the jaws. In these cases, the pathogens active in the generalized variant are comprised of a wider variety of species, similar to chronic periodontitis seen in older adults.

Necrotizing Periodontitis (Necrotizing Ulcerative Periodontitis)

Necrotizing periodontitis (NP) has symptoms similar to NG (see page 151), but it also demonstrates loss of clinical attachment and alveolar bone. This destructive form of periodontitis may arise within a zone of preexisting periodontitis, or it may represent a sequela of a single or multiple episodes of NG. Many believe that NG and NP represent different

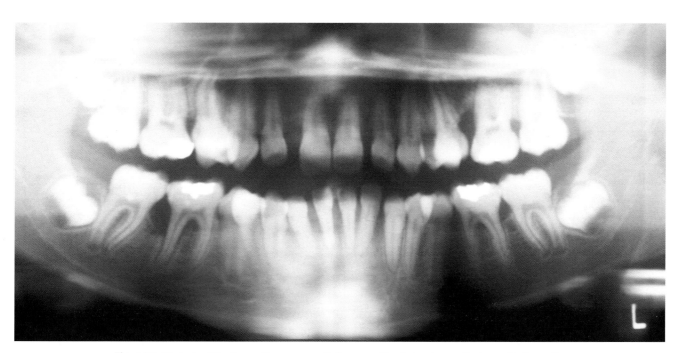

• **Fig. 4.32 Periodontitis.** Loss of bone support in the area of the first molars and incisors of both maxillary and mandibular arches in a 14-year-old patient. This pattern of periodontal destruction previously has been termed *localized aggressive periodontitis*.

stages of the same infection. Patients affected with this pattern frequently are younger than most patients affected with chronic periodontitis and often demonstrate immunosuppression or malnutrition.

Periodontal Abscess

A **periodontal abscess** (Figs. 4.33 and 4.34) is a localized purulent infection of the gingiva with involvement of the adjacent periodontal attachment and alveolar bone. On occasion, an abscess may be localized to the marginal or interdental gingiva without involvement of the adjacent periodontal ligament or alveolar bone. This lesion is termed a **gingival abscess** and often is secondary to plaque or foreign material that has become entrapped in the gingival sulcus.

A periodontal abscess often arises in a preexisting periodontal lesion and usually is precipitated by alterations in the subgingival flora, host resistance, or both. Factors frequently associated with abscess formation are closure of the entrance into a periodontal pocket, furcation involvement, or diabetes. Many cases arise in patients actively undergoing periodontal therapy, perhaps because of

incomplete removal of deep calculus with microbial penetration of the soft tissue surrounding the pocket or premature sealing of the coronal opening to the pocket. Other factors involved less frequently are trauma and anatomic dental anomalies, such as enamel pearls (see page 90) and dens invaginatus (see page 88). Most cases arise in adults; periodontal abscesses in children are rare and most frequently the result of a foreign body that has been introduced into previously healthy periodontal tissues.

On rare occasion, a periodontal abscess may be due a **cemental tear** in which there is a detachment of the cementum from the cementodentinal junction (Fig.4.35). These tears may be secondary to an inherent weakness in the cementum or due to excessive force causing a fracture to develop. Intermittent movement of the fragment during occlusal loading creates a localized inflammatory reaction with development of an associated radiolucency. If the tear is located on the proximal root surface, the inflammatory process may result in a purulent discharge from the periodontal sulcus; while abscesses associated with more apically-positioned lesions could drain through a sinus tract. In most instances, the pulp of the associated tooth remains

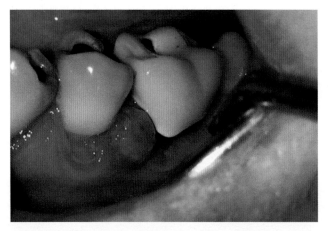

• **Fig. 4.33 Periodontal Abscess.** Localized erythematous enlargement of the interdental papilla between the mandibular first molar and second premolar. (Courtesy of Dr. Anthony Pecora.)

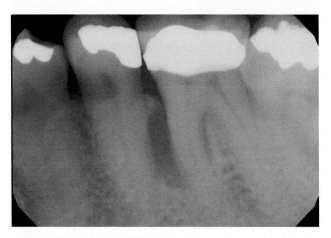

• **Fig. 4.34 Periodontal Abscess.** Same patient as depicted in Fig. 4.33. Note extensive loss of bone support associated with mesial root of the first molar. (Courtesy of Dr. Anthony Pecora.)

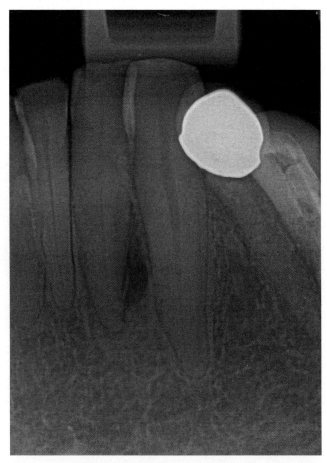

• **Fig. 4.35 Periodontal Abscess.** Cemental tear of the with associated radiolucency noted on the root of the mandibular left lateral incisor. The associated tooth was vital with no deep periodontal pockets noted upon probing. A sinus tract extended from the lesion to the surface of the facial gingiva. (Courtesy of Dr. Gregory Davis.)

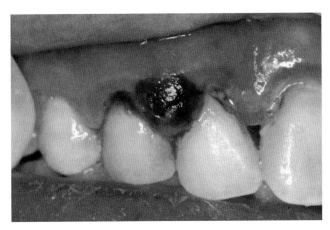

• **Fig. 4.36 Periodontal Abscess.** Dark-red and hemorrhagic enlargement of the interdental papilla between the maxillary right lateral incisor and cuspid.

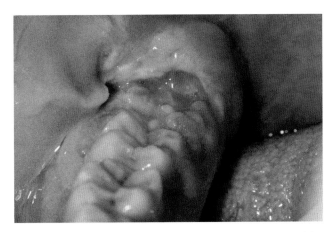

• **Fig. 4.37 Pericoronitis.** Painful erythematous enlargement of the soft tissues overlying the crown of the partially erupted right mandibular third molar.

vital unless the inflammatory lesion has been misdiagnosed, leading to inappropriate root canal therapy.

A periodontal abscess appears as a zone of gingival enlargement along the lateral aspect of a tooth. The involved gingiva may be erythematous and edematous with a slick, red surface, or it may be hemorrhagic with a dark-red coloration (Fig. 4.36). Common symptoms include the following:
• Throbbing pain
• Extreme sensitivity to palpation of the affected gingiva
• Sensitivity, mobility, or extrusion of the adjacent tooth
• Foul taste
• Lymphadenopathy
• Fever, leukocytosis, and malaise (occasionally)

Probing or gentle pressure on the affected gingiva often results in the expression of pus from the sulcus. The abscess may drain through an overlying sinus tract. With drainage, the abscess becomes asymptomatic but can demonstrate acute exacerbations if the mucosa heals over and the pressure builds again. Radiographs often demonstrate bone loss associated with the previous periodontal defect or additional radiolucency secondary to the current acute process. In some cases, the infection can spread into the periapical region and create a combined periodontal-endodontic lesion.

Pericoronitis

Pericoronitis is an inflammatory process that arises within the tissues surrounding the crown of a partially erupted tooth. The inflammatory reaction often arises when food debris and bacteria are present beneath the gingival flap overlying the crown. Other predisposing factors include stress and upper respiratory infections, especially tonsillitis or pharyngitis.

These gingival flaps can exhibit long periods of chronic inflammation without symptoms. If the debris and bacteria become entrapped deep within the gingival flap, then abscess formation develops. Abscess development is seen most frequently in association with the mandibular third molars, and the predominant symptoms are extreme pain in the area, a foul taste, and inability to close the jaws. The pain may radiate to the throat, ear, or floor of the mouth. The affected area is erythematous and edematous, and the patient often has lymphadenopathy, fever, leukocytosis, and malaise (Fig. 4.37). NG-like necrosis may develop in areas of persistent pericoronitis.

Histopathologic Features

When soft tissue from areas of periodontitis is examined microscopically, gingivitis is present and the crevicular epithelium lining the pocket is hyperplastic with extensive exocytosis of acute inflammatory cells. The adjacent connective tissue exhibits an increased vascularity and contains an inflammatory cellular infiltrate consisting predominantly of lymphocytes and plasma cells, but with a variable number of polymorphonuclear leukocytes. Frequently, large colonies of microorganisms, representing plaque and calculus, are noted.

Treatment and Prognosis
Periodontitis

Initial attention must be directed toward elimination of any existing risk factors. Once these influences have been managed, the treatment of periodontitis is directed toward stopping the loss of attachment. The foremost goal of this process is the elimination of the pathogenic bacterial plaque. Scaling, root planing, and curettage can be used to treat early periodontal lesions. In deeper pockets, a surgical flap may be required to gain access to the tooth for necessary débridement. At this time, the underlying bone may be recontoured (if necessary) to aid in the resolution of the periodontal pocket.

In some bony defects, regeneration of the attachment can be attempted through interdental denudation or the placement of autogenous bone grafts, allografts, or alloplastic materials. Often these grafts are used in conjunction with materials, such as polytetrafluoroethylene, to achieve guided tissue regeneration in moderate-to-advanced periodontal defects.

Systemic antibiotics are not warranted except in aggressive, severe, or refractory periodontitis. The organized biofilm is highly resistant to antimicrobials and does not respond to antibiotics administered with no other intervention. Antibiotics can be effective only if administered in association with nonsurgical periodontal therapy that disrupts the biofilm. Although a variety of antibiotics have proven to be effective, amoxicillin combined with metronidazole often is most beneficial.

Several forms of local antibiotic delivery have been developed. The antibiotic drugs are placed directly into sites of refractory periodontitis and consist of gels, ointments, nonresorbable fibers, and resorbable polymers. These antibiotic agents represent an adjunct to scaling and root planing and should be limited to sites that are resistant to conventional therapy alone.

In many cases, the prognosis for periodontitis correlates directly with the patient's desire to maintain oral health. Long-term studies show that periodontal health can be maintained after appropriate periodontal therapy if a program of rigorous oral hygiene and professional care is established. Patients should be encouraged to brush twice daily for at least 2 minutes with a fluoride-containing toothpaste. Rechargeable and oscillating/rotating electric toothbrushes have proven superior to manual or other types of powered toothbrushes. Daily interdental cleansing is important with interdental brushes proven superior to dental floss except in areas of tight contact that prevent utilization of brushes. Use of antiseptic rinses such as sodium hypochlorite, chlorhexidine, essential oils, cetylpyridinium chloride, or povidone-iodine has proven to be a useful adjunct to mechanical plaque removal. Sodium hypochlorite (bleach) has strong anti-plaque and anti-inflammatory properties without the staining and reduced effectiveness over time associated with use of chlorhexidine. Twice-weekly rinsing of a 0.25% solution of sodium hypochlorite has been associated with significantly reduced bleeding upon probing along with increased plaque-free tooth surfaces. The rinse also appears to reduce subgingival periodontopathic bacteria in periodontal pockets as deep as 7–9 mm.

Bacterial morphotypes return to pretreatment levels 42 days after professional prophylaxis, but pathogenic complexes capable of inducing attachment loss require approximately 3 months to be reestablished functionally. In patients with less-than-optimal oral hygiene or with isolated defects that cannot be self-cleaned, further loss of attachment can be prevented if professional scaling and root planing are performed at 3-month intervals.

In younger patients, scaling and root planning alone do not stop progression of the periodontitis. Defects in leukocyte function, in addition to the invasive capabilities of the involved pathogenic organisms, mandate the use of antibiotics in combination with mechanical removal of subgingival plaque and inflamed periodontal tissues. Although tetracycline, amoxicillin and clavulanate potassium, minocycline, and erythromycin can be used in selected patients, the combination of high-dose (500 mg three times per day)

amoxicillin and metronidazole has been shown to be most effective in controlling the involved periodontal pathogens, especially *A. actinomycetemcomitans*. The effectiveness of the antibiotics appears to be improved if initiated immediately after scaling and root planing. Continued therapy often is predicated on microbiologic testing to ensure selection of the most appropriate antimicrobial agent. Use of local antiseptic agents, such as sodium hypochlorite, chlorhexidine, or povidone-iodine has proven beneficial. Patients with active disease may be at increased risk for adverse peri-implant gingival infection.

A reevaluation with professional prophylaxis is performed once a month for 6 months and then every 3 months thereafter. Specimens for anaerobic cultures are obtained at each 3-month recall. Patients with refractory disease or significant colonization by pathogenic organisms receive additional courses of appropriate antibiotics. Long-term follow-up is mandatory because of the possibility of reinfection or incomplete elimination of the organisms. The presence of deep residual pockets is associated with disease progression. In such circumstances, periodontal surgery often is performed to eliminate these defects. This intervention is directed at any pocket consistently deeper than 5 mm and typically is performed after 2–6 months of nonsurgical therapy.

Necrotizing Periodontitis

Once any underlying influence (e.g., immunosuppression, malnutrition) has been resolved, NP often responds well to irrigation, débridement of the necrotic areas, effective oral hygiene measures, and administration of systemic antibiotic medications. Failure to respond to standard therapy mandates a thorough physical evaluation to rule out the possibility of an underlying disease.

Periodontal Abscess

A gingival or periodontal abscess is treated by drainage through the sulcus or by an incision through the overlying mucosa. Thorough cleansing of the area with removal of all foreign material, plaque, and calculus should be performed. Penicillin or other antibiotic drugs are prescribed when a fever is present. Analgesic agents are prescribed, and the patient receives a soft diet, is told to use warm salt-water rinses, and is instructed to return each day until the symptoms have resolved. After the acute phase has passed, the patient is treated for any underlying chronic pathologic periodontal condition.

Treatment of periodontal abscesses due to cemental tears involves complete removal of the fragment with the associated inflammatory tissue. If the tear is located along the coronal third of the root, the fragment often can be removed via nonsurgical scaling and root planing, while deeper lesions require a surgical periodontal approach.

Pericoronitis

Acute pericoronitis is treated with gentle antiseptic lavage under the gingival flap to remove gross food debris and bacteria. Systemic antibiotic agents are used if a fever or general symptoms are noted. The patient is instructed to use warm saltwater rinses and to return in 24 hours. Once the acute phase has subsided, the tooth can be extracted if long-term maintenance is contraindicated. If tooth retention is desirable, then the overlying gingival flap is removed surgically, which is followed by elimination of all food debris and bacterial colonies by thorough curettage.

◆ PERI-IMPLANT DISEASES

Brånemark's landmark work with osseointegration of titanium implants in the late 1950s has led to a revolution in dentistry with an estimated 12 million implants installed annually throughout the world. Despite a 10-year implant survival of 95%, biological complications related to local development of bacterial biofilms are noted and are very similar to gingivitis and periodontitis of the natural dentition. **Peri-implant mucositis** refers to inflammation of the soft tissues surrounding an implant without loss of associated bone, whereas **peri-implantitis** demonstrates inflammation of the soft tissues with loss of supporting bone. The reported prevalence of peri-implantitis is approximately 20% of all implant-treated patients and 10% of all implants. This frequency translates to development of peri-implantitis in over 1 million implants annually.

In contrast to natural dentition, the attachment of dental implants is much more fragile due to the lack of a periodontal ligament and normal junctional epithelium. Once established, peri-implantitis exhibits a more accelerated pattern of disease progression when compared to periodontitis. Strong risk factors include poor oral hygiene, no regular professional maintenance care, and a history or presence of periodontitis. Other possible negative influences include smoking, diabetes, implant design that prevents ease of cleansing, and cement remnants adjacent to the implant.

Clinical and Radiographic Features

Peri-implant mucositis is inflammation of the soft tissues surrounding a dental implant without additional bone loss after the initial remodeling that occurs during healing of the surgical placement. Healthy peri-implant soft tissues are fragile and often will demonstrate local dot-like bleeding upon gentle probing, but the mucosa will not demonstrate other evidence of inflammation. In contrast, peri-implant mucositis will demonstrate local swelling, redness, and shininess with or without sensitivity. Profuse (linear or drop-like) bleeding with or without purulence will be noted upon gentle probing. An increased probing depth without bone loss often is seen due to the soft tissue swelling.

Peri-implantitis will present with features of peri-implant mucositis combined with the presence of bone loss (Fig. 4.38). Although some degree of nonpathologic bone loss can be seen during the first year of function, any additional loss greater than 2 mm represents peri-implantitis. Increasing pockets depths also will be noted.

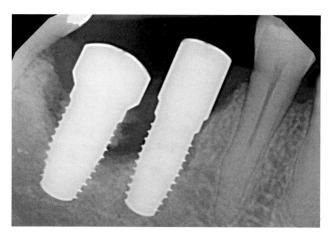

• **Fig. 4.38 Peri-implantitis.** Pathologic circumferential bone loss associated with mandibular implant. (Courtesy of Dr. Scott Price.)

Treatment and Prognosis

The treatment of the peri-implant diseases is very similar to that utilized for gingivitis and periodontitis. Peri-implant mucositis therapy should concentrate on improved patient oral hygiene and professionally administered plaque control with repeated oral hygiene instructions and close follow-up. Thorough removal of plaque with manual or electric toothbrushes and interdental cleansing with devices such as floss or interdental brushes must be stressed and may be supplemented with antiseptic agents such as chlorhexidine.

Treatment of peri-implantitis mirrors that of peri-implant mucositis but also includes thorough professional debridement often combined with antiseptics or locally delivered antibiotics. When the bone loss is severe, surgical intervention is necessary to debride and decontaminate the infected sites with hand instruments, ultrasonic tips, or lasers. Extensive intervention should be undertaken only if there is strong evidence the implant can remain functional and be maintainable. Patients at high risk for failure include those who are committed to smoking, have poor oral hygiene, a history of high stage/grade periodontitis, or evidence of rapidly progressing bone loss with mobility.

◆ PAPILLON-LEFÈVRE SYNDROME

In 1924, Papillon and Lefèvre initially described the syndrome that bears their names. This autosomal recessive disorder predominantly demonstrates oral and dermatologic manifestations; similar dermatologic changes can be seen in the absence of oral findings (**Unna-Thost syndrome, Howell-Evans syndrome, Vohwinkel syndrome, Gamborg Nielsen syndrome,** and **mal de Meleda**). Because of the autosomal recessive inheritance pattern, the parents typically are not affected; consanguinity is noted in approximately one-third of cases.

Genetic studies of patients with Papillon-Lefèvre syndrome have mapped the major gene locus to chromosome 11q14-q21 and revealed mutation and loss of function of the *cathepsin C* gene. This gene is important in the structural growth and development of the skin and is critical for appropriate immune response of myeloid and lymphoid cells. Researchers believe that the loss of appropriate function of the *cathepsin C* gene results in an altered immune response to infection. In addition, the altered gene may affect the integrity of the junctional epithelium surrounding the tooth.

A closely related disease, **Haim-Munk syndrome,** also exhibits palmoplantar keratosis, progressive periodontal disease, recurrent skin infections, and several skeletal malformations. In this syndrome, the skin manifestations are more severe, and the periodontal disease is milder. Studies have demonstrated that Haim-Munk syndrome and many examples of prepubertal periodontitis also exhibit mutation of the *cathepsin C* gene and represent allelic variants of the mutated gene responsible for Papillon-Lefèvre syndrome.

Clinical and Radiographic Features

Papillon-Lefèvre syndrome exhibits a prevalence of one to four per million people in the population, and carriers are thought to be present in two to four per thousand persons. In most cases, the dermatologic manifestations become clinically evident in the first 3 years of life. Diffuse transgredient (first occurs on the palms and soles and then spreads to the dorsa of the hands and feet) palmar-plantar keratosis develops, with occasional reports of diffuse follicular hyperkeratosis, nail dystrophy, hyperhidrosis, and keratosis on the elbows and knees (Fig. 4.39). Other less common sites of involvement include the legs, thighs, dorsal surface of the fingers and toes, and (rarely) the trunk. Although the appearance of the dermatologic manifestations is variable, the lesions typically present as white, light-yellow, brown, or red plaques and patches that develop crusts, cracks, or deep fissures.

The oral manifestations consist of dramatically advanced periodontitis that is seen in both the deciduous and the permanent dentitions. Upon eruption of the deciduous teeth, diffuse hemorrhagic and hyperplastic gingivitis develops in association with rapid loss of periodontal attachment (Fig. 4.40). The extensive loss of osseous support often results in teeth that radiographically appear to be floating in soft tissue (Fig. 4.41). At 4–5 years of age, all primary teeth typically have been lost or extracted. Once edentulous, the gingiva returns to a normal state of health until eruption of the permanent dentition restarts the cycle of rapidly progressive periodontal disease. By age 15, all the permanent teeth have been lost in most affected individuals. Although other pathogenic bacteria have been isolated from sites of active disease, *A. actinomycetemcomitans* has been related directly to the periodontal destruction.

In addition to the dermatologic and oral manifestations, numerous investigators have documented less frequent findings. Impaired somatic development and ectopic calcifications of the falx cerebri and choroid plexus have been reported, in addition to an increased susceptibility to

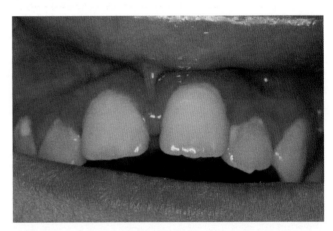

• **Fig. 4.40 Papillon-Lefèvre Syndrome.** Generalized erythematous gingivitis.

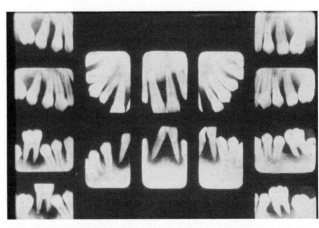

• **Fig. 4.41 Papillon-Lefèvre Syndrome.** Multifocal sites of bone loss in all four quadrants. (From Giansanti JS, Hrabak RP, Waldron CA: Palmoplantar hyperkeratosis and concomitant periodontal destruction [Papillon-Lefèvre syndrome], *Oral Surg Oral Med Oral Pathol* 36:40, 1973.)

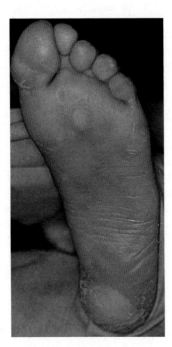

• **Fig. 4.39 Papillon-Lefèvre Syndrome.** Plantar keratosis of the foot.

infections beyond the oral cavity. Pyoderma, furunculosis, pneumonia, hepatic abscesses, cerebral abscesses, and other infections have been documented.

Sporadic cases of a Papillon-Lefèvre syndrome-like clinical phenotype has been reported. To confirm the diagnosis of Papillon-Lefèvre syndrome, gene sequencing usually is performed. It has been noted that active cathepsin C is excreted in the urine of normal individuals but is absent from those affected with Papillon-Lefèvre syndrome, making urinalysis a simple and inexpensive method for diagnostic confirmation.

Histopathologic Features

Once again, the histopathologic features of Papillon-Lefèvre syndrome are like those seen in chronic periodontitis and are not specific. Submitted tissue often contains hyperplastic crevicular epithelium with exocytosis. The underlying connective tissue exhibits increased vascularity and a mixed inflammatory cellular infiltrate consisting predominantly of plasma cells intermixed with polymorphonuclear leukocytes, lymphocytes, and histiocytes. Initially, histopathologic examination is recommended to rule out other pathologic causes of the periodontal destruction.

Treatment and Prognosis

Skin lesions in these patients have been treated most successfully using systemic retinoids, such as etretinate, acitretin, and isotretinoin. This approach has resulted in remarkable improvement with complete clearance in most patients. Surprisingly, a few authors have reported improvement of the associated periodontal disease during periods of retinoid use, but others have disputed this claim. Possible adverse reactions caused by retinoid administration include angular cheilitis, dry lips, hair loss, arthralgia, tendinous and ligamentous calcifications, and teratogenicity. To avoid these drug-related adverse reactions, patients with mild dermatologic manifestations often are treated with topical lubricants, keratolytic agents (salicylic or lactic acid), corticosteroids, or antibiotics.

Attempts at resolution of the periodontal disease often have been frustrating. Despite extensive periodontal therapy and antibiotic agents, in many patients, the disease progresses until all teeth are lost. However, several investigators have reported a cessation of attachment loss, and two different treatment approaches have been used.

Despite the use of numerous antibiotic medications, several reports document a difficulty in resolution of the infection associated with teeth that already exhibit attachment loss. Some clinicians recommend extraction of all deciduous teeth to eliminate the periodontal pathogens and reduce the risk of transmitting these organisms to the permanent dentition. Following eruption of the permanent teeth, antibiotics are utilized to prevent redevelopment of periodontitis.

The second approach revolves around a direct attack against *A. actinomycetemcomitans*. Therapy with high-dose amoxicillin and metronidazole has proven effective when combined with extraction of severely affected teeth, high patient compliance, and strong supportive periodontal therapy. In clinical studies, the progression of attachment loss of the erupted dentition and the periodontal destruction of the teeth that erupt after the initiation of therapy were slowed dramatically. Rigorous oral hygiene, chlorhexidine mouth rinses, frequent professional prophylaxis, and periodic appropriate antibiotic therapy are necessary for long-term maintenance.

Bibliography

Gingivitis

Chapple ILC, Mealey BL, Van Dyke TE, et al.: Periodontal health and gingival diseases and conditions on an intact and a reduced periodontium: consensus report of workgroup 1 of the 2017 world workshop on the classification of periodontal and peri-implant diseases and conditions, *J Periodontol* 89(Suppl 1):S74–S84, 2018.

Chapple ILC, Van der Weijden F, Doerfer C, et al.: Primary prevention of periodontitis: managing gingivitis, *J Clin Periodontol* 42(Suppl 16):S71–S76, 2015.

Darby I: Non-surgical management of periodontal disease, *Aust Dent J* 54(Suppl 1):S86–S95, 2009.

Geisinger ML, Ogdon D, Kaur M, et al.: Toss the floss? Evidenced-based oral hygiene recommendations for the periodontal patient in the age of "flossgate", *Clin Adv Periodontics* 9:83–90, 2019.

Gunsolley JC: A meta-analysis of six-month studies of antiplaque and antigingivitis agents, *J Am Dent Assoc* 137:1649–1657, 2006.

Murakami S, Mealey BL, Mariotti A, et al.: Dental plaque-induced gingival conditions, *J Periodontol* 89(Suppl 1):S17–S27, 2018.

Schätzle M, Löe H, Lang NP, et al.: The clinical course of chronic periodontitis. IV. Gingival inflammation as a risk factor in tooth mortality, *J Clin Periodontol* 31:1122–1127, 2004.

Tatakis DN, Trombelli L: Modulation of clinical expression of plaque-induced gingivitis. I. Background review and rationale, *J Clin Periodontol* 31:229–238, 2004.

Trombelli L: Susceptibility to gingivitis: a way to predict periodontal disease? *Oral Health Prev Dent* 2(Suppl 1):265–269, 2004.

Trombelli L, Scapoli C, Orlandini E, et al.: Modulation of clinical expression of plaque-induced gingivitis. III. Response of "high responders" and "low responders" to therapy, *J Clin Periodontol* 31:253–259, 2004.

van der Weijden F, Slot DE: Oral hygiene in the prevention of periodontal diseases: the evidence, *Periodontol* 2000(55):104–123, 2011.

Spongiotic Gingival Hyperplasia

Allon I, Lammert KM, Iwase R, et al.: Localized juvenile spongiotic gingival hyperplasia possibly originates from the junctional gingival epithelium – an immunohistochemical study, *Histopathology* 68:549–555, 2016.

Argyris PP, Nelson AC, Papanakou S, et al.: Localized juvenile spongiotic gingival hyperplasia featuring unusual p16INK4A labeling and negative human papillomavirus status by polymerase chain reaction, *J Oral Pathol Med* 44:37–44, 2015.

Chang JYF, Kessler HP, Wright JM: Localized juvenile spongiotic gingival hyperplasia, *Oral Surg Oral Med Oral Pathol Oral Radiol Endod* 106:411–418, 2008.

Darling MR, Daley TD, Wilson A, et al.: Juvenile spongiotic gingivitis, *J Periodontol* 78:1235–1240, 2007.

Nogueira VKC, Fernandes D, Navarro CM, et al.: Cryotherapy for localized juvenile spongiotic gingival hyperplasia: preliminary findings on two cases, *Int J Paediatr Dent* 27:231–235, 2017.

Roberts EP, Schuster GM, Haub S: Case report of spongiotic gingivitis in an adult male treated with novel 9,300-nanometer carbon dioxide laser low-energy ablation, *J Am Dent Assoc* 153:67–73, 2022.

Theofilou VI, Pettas E, Georgaki M, et al.: Localized juvenile spongiotic gingival hyperplasia: microscopic variations and proposed change to nomenclature, *Oral Surg Oral Med Oral Pathol Oral Radiol* 131:329–338, 2021.

Vargo RJ, Bilodeau A: Reappraising localized juvenile spongiotic gingival hyperplasia, *JADA* 150:147–153, 2019.

Necrotizing Gingivitis

Boliver I, Whiteson K, Stadelmann B, et al.: Bacterial diversity in oral samples of children in Niger with acute noma, acute necrotizing gingivitis, and healthy controls, *PLoS Negl Trop Dis* 6(3), 2012, e1556.

Dufty J, Gkranias N, Donos N: Necrotising ulcerative gingivitis: a literature review, *Oral Health Prev Dent* 15:321–327, 2017.

Herrera D, Alonso B, de Arriba L, et al.: Acute periodontal lesions, *Periodontol 2000*(65):149–177, 2014.

Herrera D, Retamal-Valdes B, Alonso B, et al.: Acute periodontal lesions (periodontal abscesses and necrotizing periodontal diseases) and endo-periodontal lesions, *J Periodontol* 89(Suppl 1):S85–S102, 2018.

Horning GM: Necrotizing gingivostomatitis-NUG to noma, *Compend Contin Educ Dent* 17:951–962, 1996.

Horning GM, Cohen ME: Necrotizing ulcerative gingivitis, periodontitis, and stomatitis: clinical staging and predisposing factors, *J Periodontol* 66:990–998, 1995.

Johnson BD, Engel D: Acute necrotizing ulcerative gingivitis: a review of diagnosis, etiology and treatment, *J Periodontol* 57:141–150, 1986.

Wade DN, Kerns DG: Acute necrotizing ulcerative gingivitis-periodontitis: a literature review, *Mil Med* 5:337–342, 1998.

Plasma Cell Gingivitis

Bhatavadekar N, Khandelwal N, Bouquot JE: Oral and maxillofacial pathology case of the month. Plasma cell gingivitis, *Tex Dent J* 125:372–373, 2008.

Jadwat Y, Meyerov R, Lemmer J, et al.: Plasma cell gingivitis: does it exist? Report of a case and review of the literature, *SADJ* 63:394–395, 2008.

Kerr DA, McClatchey KD, Regezi JA: Allergic gingivostomatitis (due to gum chewing), *J Periodontol* 42:709–712, 1971.

Kerr DA, McClatchey KD, Regezi JA: Idiopathic gingivostomatitis: cheilitis, glossitis, gingivitis syndrome: atypical gingivostomatitis plasma-cell gingivitis, plasmacytosis of gingiva, *Oral Surg Oral Med Oral Pathol* 32:402–423, 1971.

Owings JR: An atypical gingivostomatitis: report of four cases, *J Periodontol* 40:538–542, 1969.

Perry HO, Deffner NF, Sheridan PJ: Atypical gingivostomatitis: nineteen cases, *Arch Dermatol* 107:872–878, 1973.

Silverman S Jr, Lozada F: An epilogue to plasma-cell gingivostomatitis (allergic gingivostomatitis), *Oral Surg Oral Med Oral Pathol* 43:211–217, 1977.

Foreign Body Gingivitis

Daley TD, Wysocki GP: Foreign body gingivitis: an iatrogenic disease? *Oral Surg Oral Med Oral Pathol* 69:708–712, 1990.

Ferreira L, Peng H-H, Cox DP, et al.: Investigation of foreign materials in gingival lesions: a clinicopathologic, energy-dispersive microanalysis of the lesions and in vitro confirmation of pro-inflammatory effects of the foreign material, *Oral Surg Oral Med Oral Pathol Oral Radiol* 128:250–267, 2019.

Gordon SC, Daley TD: Foreign body gingivitis: clinical and microscopic features of 61 cases, *Oral Surg Oral Med Oral Pathol Oral Radiol Endod* 83:562–570, 1997.

Gordon SC, Daley TD: Foreign body gingivitis: identification of the foreign material by energy-dispersive x-ray microanalysis, *Oral Surg Oral Med Oral Pathol Oral Radiol Endod* 83:571–576, 1997.

Koppang HS, Roushan A, Srafilzadeh A, et al.: Foreign body gingival lesions: distribution, morphology, identification by x-ray energy dispersive analysis and possible origin of foreign material, *J Oral Pathol Med* 36:161–172, 2007.

Desquamative Gingivitis

Gagari E, Damoulis PD: Desquamative gingivitis as a manifestation of chronic mucocutaneous disease, *J Dtsch Dermatol Ges* 9:184–188, 2011.

Maderal AD, Salisbury PL, Jorizzo JL: Desquamative gingivitis. Clinical findings and diseases, *J Am Acad Dermatol* 78:839–848, 2018.

Russo LL, Fedele S, Guiglia R, et al.: Diagnostic pathways and clinical significance of desquamative gingivitis, *J Periodontol* 79:4–24, 2008.

Drug-Related Gingival Hyperplasia

Botha PJ: Drug-induced gingival hyperplasia and its management—a literature review, *J Dent Assoc S Afr* 52:659–664, 1997.

Condé SAP, Aarestrup FM, Vieira BJ, et al.: Roxithromycin reduces cyclosporine-induced gingival hyperplasia in renal transplant patients, *Transplant Proc* 40:1435–1438, 2007.

Desai P, Silver JG: Drug-induced gingival enlargements, *J Can Dent Assoc* 64:263–268, 1998.

Hall EE: Prevention and treatment considerations in patients with drug-induced gingival enlargement, *Curr Opin Periodontol* 4:59–63, 1997.

Livada R, Shiloah J: Calcium channel blocker-induced gingival hyperplasia, *J Hum Hypertens* 28:10–14, 2014.

Ramalho VLC, Ramalho HJ, Cipullo JP, et al.: Comparison of azithromycin and oral hygiene program in the treatment of cyclosporine-induced gingival hyperplasia, *Ren Fail* 29:265–270, 2007.

Salman A, Tekin B, Koca S, et al.: Another adverse effect of vemurafenib: gingival hyperplasia, *J Dermatol* 43:706–707, 2016.

Woo S-B, Allen CM, Orden A, et al.: Non-gingival soft tissue overgrowths after allogeneic marrow transplantation, *Bone Marrow Transplant* 17:1127–1132, 1996.

Zoheir N, Hughes FJ: The management of drug-influenced gingival enlargement, *Prim Dent J* 8:34–39, 2019.

Gingival Fibromatosis

Coletta RD, Graner E: Hereditary gingival fibromatosis: a systematic review, *J Periodontol* 77:753–764, 2006.

Häkkinen L, Csuszar A: Hereditary gingival fibromatosis: characteristics and novel putative pathogenic mechanisms, *J Dent Res* 86:25–34, 2007.

Ibrahim M, Abouzaid M, Mehrez M, et al.: Genetic disorders associated with gingival enlargement, In Panagakos F, editor: *Gingival diseases—Their aetiology, prevention and treatment*, New York, 2011, InTech, pp 189–194.

Ko YCK, Farr JB, Yoon A, et al.: Idiopathic gingival fibromatosis: case report and review of the literature, *Am J Dermatol* 38:e68–e71, 2016.

Rushton MA: Hereditary or idiopathic hyperplasia of the gums, *Dent Pract Dent Rec* 7:136–146, 1957.

Ye X, Shi L, Yin W, et al.: Further evidence of genetic heterogeneity segregating with hereditary gingival fibromatosis, *J Clin Periodontol* 36:627–633, 2009.

Periodontitis

Abt E, Kumar S, Weyant RJ: Periodontal disease and medical maladies. What do we really know? *JADA* 153:9–13, 2022.

Bataineh AB, Al Qudah MA: The predisposing factors of pericoronitis of mandibular third molars in a Jordanian population, *Quintessence Int* 34:227–231, 2003.

Cappuyns I, Gugerli P, Mombelli A: Viruses in periodontal disease—a review, *Oral Dis* 11:219–229, 2005.

Corbet EF: Diagnosis of acute periodontal lesions, *Periodontol* 2000(34):204–216, 2004.

Darveau RP: Periodontitis: a polymicrobial disruption of host homeostasis, *Nat Rev Microbiol* 8:481–490, 2010.

Deas DE, Mealey BL: Response of chronic and aggressive periodontitis to treatment, *Periodontol* 2000(53):154–166, 2010.

Eke PI, Borgnakke WS, Genco RJ: Recent epidemiologic trends in periodontitis in the USA, *Periodontol* 2000(82):257–267, 2020.

Feres M, Figueiredo LC: Current concepts in the microbial etiology and treatment of chronic periodontitis, *J Int Acad Periodontol* 11:234–249, 2009.

Fine DH, Armitage GC, Genco RJ, et al.: Unique etiologic, demographic, and pathologic characteristics of localized aggressive periodontitis support classification as a distinct subcategory of periodontitis, *JADA* 150:922–931, 2019.

Gaggl AJ, Rainer H, Grund E, et al.: Local oxygen therapy for treating acute necrotizing periodontal disease in smokers, *J Periodontol* 77:31–38, 2006.

Graziani F, Karapetsa D, Alonso B, et al.: Nonsurgical and surgical treatment of periodontitis: how many options for one disease, *Periodontol* 2000(75):152–188, 2017.

Herrera D, Alonso B, de Arriba L, et al.: Acute periodontal lesions, *Periodontol* 2000(65):149–177, 2014.

Jepsen S, Catron JG, Albandar JM, et al.: Periodontal manifestations of systemic diseases and developmental and acquired conditions: consensus report of workgroup 3 of the 2017 world workshop on the classification of periodontal and peri-implant diseases and conditions, *J Periodontol* 89(Suppl 1):S237–S248, 2018.

Kumar S: Evidence-based update on diagnosis and management of gingivitis and periodontitis, *Dent Clin N Am* 63:69–81, 2019.

Lee AHC, Neelakantan P, Dummer PMH, et al.: Cemental tear: literature review, proposed classification and recommendations for treatment, *Int Endod J* 54:2044–2073, 2021.

Lindhe J, Nyman S: Long-term maintenance of patients treated for advanced periodontal disease, *J Clin Periodontol* 11:504–514, 1984.

Meng HX: Periodontal abscess, *Ann Periodontol* 4:79–82, 1999.

Novak MJ: Necrotizing ulcerative periodontitis, *Ann Periodontol* 4:74–77, 1999.

Papapanou PN, Sanz M, Buduneli N, et al.: Periodontitis: consensus report of workgroup 2 of the 2017 world workshop on the classification of periodontal and peri-implant diseases and conditions, *J Periodontol* 89(Suppl 1):S173–S182, 2018.

Slots J: Herpesviruses in periodontal diseases, *Periodontol* 2000(38):33–62, 2005.

Slots J: Periodontitis: facts, fallacies, and the future, *Periodontol* 2000(75):7–23, 2017.

Tonetti MS, Greenwell H, Kornman KS: Staging and grading of periodontitis: framework and proposal of a new classification and case definition, *J Periodontol* 89(Suppl 1):S159–S172, 2018.

Peri-implant Diseases

Ephros H, Kim S, DeFalco R: Peri-implantitis. Evaluation and management, *Dent Clin N Am* 64:305–313, 2020.

Heitz-Mayfield LJA, Salvi GE: Peri-implant mucositis, *J Periodontol* 89(Suppl 1):S257–S266, 2018.

Klinge B, Klinge A, Bertl K, et al.: Peri-implant diseases, *Eur J Oral Sci* 126(Suppl 1):88–94, 2018.

Renvert S, Persson GR, Pirih FQ, et al.: Peri-implant health, peri-implant mucositis, and peri-implantitis: case definitions and diagnostic considerations, *J Periodontol* 89(Suppl 1):S304–S312, 2018.

Schwartz F, Derks J, Monje A, et al.: Peri-implantitis, *J Periodontol* 89(Suppl 1):S267–S290, 2018.

Papillon-Lefèvre Syndrome

Gelmetti C, Nazzaro V, Cerri D, et al.: Long-term preservation of permanent teeth in a patient with Papillon-Lefèvre syndrome treated with etretinate, *Pediatr Dermatol* 6:222–225, 1989.

Gorlin RJ, Sedano H, Anderson VE: The syndrome of palmar-plantar hyperkeratosis and premature destruction of the teeth: a clinical and genetic analysis of the Papillon-Lefèvre syndrome, *J Pediatr* 65:895–908, 1964.

Hart TC, Hart PS, Bowden DW, et al.: Mutations of the *cathepsin C* gene are responsible for Papillon-Lefèvre syndrome, *J Med Genet* 36:881–887, 1999.

Harmon Y, Legowska M, Fergelot P, et al.: Analysis of urinary cathepsin C for diagnosing Papillon-Lefèvre syndrome, *FEBS J* 283:498–509, 2016.

Hart TC, Hart PS, Michalec M, et al.: Haim-Munk syndrome and Papillon-Lefèvre syndrome are allelic mutations in *cathepsin C*, *J Med Genet* 37:88–94, 2000.

Hewitt C, McCormick D, Linden G: The role of *cathepsin C* in Papillon-Lefèvre syndrome, prepubertal periodontitis, and aggressive periodontitis, *Hum Mutat* 23:222–228, 2004.

Nickles K, Schacher B, Schuster G, et al.: Evaluation of two siblings with Papillon-Lefèvre syndrome 5 years after treatment of periodontitis in primary and mixed dentition, *J Periodontol* 82:1536–1547, 2011.

Upadhyaya JD, Pfundheller D, Islam MN, et al.: Papillon-Lefèvre syndrome: a series of three cases in the same family and a literature review, *Quintessence Int* 48:695–700, 2017.

Wiebe CB, Häkkinen L, Putnins EE, et al.: Successful periodontal maintenance of a case with Papillon-Lefèvre syndrome: 12-year follow-up and review of the literature, *J Periodontol* 72:824–830, 2001.

5

Bacterial Infections

◆ IMPETIGO

Impetigo is a superficial infection of the skin that is caused by *Staphylococcus aureus, Streptococcus pyogenes* (group A, β-hemolytic), or both. Two main patterns are seen. Seventy percent of the cases are **nonbullous impetigo** with *S. aureus* being most responsible in the industrialized world whereas *S. pyogenes* is predominant in developing nations. **Bullous impetigo** is less common and predominantly caused by *S. aureus.* The term *impetigo* is derived from a Latin word meaning "attack" because of its common presentation as a scabbing eruption. Intact epithelium normally is protective against infection; therefore, many cases arise in damaged skin, such as preexisting dermatitis, cuts, abrasions, or insect bites. Secondary involvement of an area of dermatitis has been termed **impetiginized dermatitis.** An increased prevalence is associated with debilitating systemic conditions, such as human immunodeficiency virus (HIV) infection, type 2 diabetes mellitus, or dialysis.

Clinical Features

Although impetigo may occur at any age, the infection is seen predominantly during childhood and represents the most common bacterial skin infection between the ages of 2 and 5. **Nonbullous impetigo (impetigo contagiosa)** is the more prevalent pattern and usually involves the face, the extremities, or trunk. The facial lesions usually develop around the nose and mouth. In many patients with facial involvement, the pathogenic bacteria are harbored in the nose and spread onto the skin into previously damaged sites, such as scratches or abrasions. Often, facial lesions will have a linear pattern that corresponds to previous fingernail scratches. The peak occurrence is during the summer or early fall in hot, moist climates. Impetigo is contagious and easily spread in crowded or unsanitary living conditions.

Nonbullous impetigo initially appears as red macules or papules, with the subsequent development of fragile vesicles. These vesicles quickly rupture and become covered with a thick, amber crust (Fig. 5.1). The crusts are adherent and have been described as honey-colored or like "cornflakes glued to the surface." Some cases may be confused with exfoliative cheilitis (see page 294) or recurrent herpes simplex (see page 231). Pruritus is common and scratching often causes the lesions to spread (Fig. 5.2). Lymphangitis, cellulitis, fever, anorexia, and malaise are uncommon, although leukocytosis occurs in about half of affected patients.

In an infrequent pattern of impetigo termed **ecthyma,** the central area of the crust becomes necrotic and forms a deep indurated ulceration. This lesion heals slowly and often is associated with a permanent scar.

Due to its strong association with *S. aureus,* **bullous impetigo** also has been termed **staphylococcal impetigo.** The lesions frequent the trunk and intertriginous areas (axilla, neck, groin); involvement of the buttocks and extremities is less common. *Blistering dactylitis* is a localized pattern of bullous impetigo that typically involves the distal portion of a finger or more rarely a toe. Infants and newborns are infected most commonly, but the disease also may occur in children and adults. The lesions are characterized by superficial vesicles that rapidly enlarge to form larger flaccid bullae. Initially, the bullae are filled with clear serous fluid, but the contents of the bullae quickly become more turbid and eventually purulent. Although the bullae may remain intact, they usually rupture and develop a thin brown crust that some describe as "lacquer." Weakness, fever, lymphadenopathy, and diarrhea may be seen. Although uncommon, spread of the infection can result in cellulitis, osteomyelitis, septic arthritis, and pneumonia. Associated scarlet fever, rheumatic heart disease, and poststreptococcal glomerulonephritis also have been noted.

Diagnosis

A strong presumptive diagnosis normally can be made from the clinical presentation. When the diagnosis is not obvious clinically or the infection fails to respond to standard therapy within 7 days, the definitive diagnosis requires isolation of *S. aureus* or *S. pyogenes* from cultures of the skin lesions and testing the isolate for antibiotic sensitivity.

Treatment and Prognosis

For patients with nonbullous impetigo involving only a small area with few lesions, topical mupirocin or fusidic acid (available in Canada and Europe, not in the United States) has been shown to be effective. Increasing reports of resistance to these medications are appearing, especially in infections associated with methicillin-resistant *S. aureus* (MRSA). In such cases, utilization of topical retapamulin or ozenoxacin has been proven effective in many patients. Removal of the crusts with a clean cloth soaked in warm soapy water is recommended before application of topical therapy, rather than placing the medication on inert,

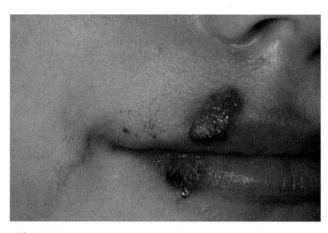

• **Fig. 5.1 Impetigo.** Amber crusts of the skin and vermilion border of the lips.

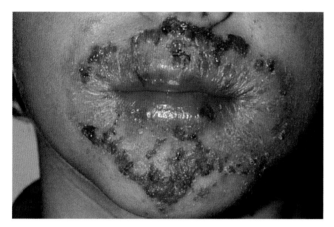

• **Fig. 5.2 Impetigo.** Scaly and amber-colored crusts of the perioral skin.

dried, exfoliating skin. For bullous or more extensive lesions, topical antibiotic drugs often are insufficient; the treatment of choice is a 1-week course of a systemic oral antibiotic. The best antibiotic is one that is effective against both *S. pyogenes* and penicillin-resistant *S. aureus*. Cephalexin, dicloxacillin, flucloxacillin, and amoxicillin-clavulanic acid represent good current choices. In communities frequented with MRSA, therapy with agents such as trimethoprim/sulfamethoxazole, clindamycin, tetracycline, or fluoroquinolones is recommended. For severe cases in which MRSA has been isolated, linezolid or vancomycin are most effective. Inappropriate diagnosis and treatment with topical corticosteroids may reduce the inflammatory host response to the bacterial infection and temporarily improve the appearance, but the causative organism will not be eliminated, allowing the infection to persist, or spread.

◆ ERYSIPELAS

Erysipelas is a superficial cellulitis of the skin that involves the dermis and the upper subcutaneous tissue. Although most cases are nonculturable, the infection most commonly is associated with β-hemolytic streptococci. Other organisms, such as *Staphylococcus aureus,* have been isolated from

the lesions, but it is unclear if these bacteria are causative or a contaminant. The infection rapidly spreads through the lymphatic channels, which become filled with fibrin, leukocytes, and streptococci. Although also associated with ergotism, the term *Saint Anthony's fire* has been used to describe erysipelas. Because the French House of St. Anthony, an 11th-century hospital, had fiery red walls like the color of erysipelas, the term *Saint Anthony's fire* was used to describe this disease. Today, with most cases noted in the lower legs, classical facial erysipelas often is a forgotten diagnosis. At times, the appropriate diagnosis has been delayed because of confusion with facial cellulitis from dental infections.

Clinical Features

Erysipelas tends to occur primarily in young and older adult patients or in those who are debilitated, diabetic, immunosuppressed, obese, or alcoholic. Patients who have areas of chronic lymphedema or large surgical scars (such as, postmastectomy or saphenous venectomy) also are susceptible to this disease. The infection may occur anywhere on the skin, especially in areas of previous trauma. Over 80% of the cases are noted in the lower legs, but involvement of the face, arm, and upper thigh is not rare. In facial erysipelas, an increased prevalence is noted in the winter and spring months, whereas summer is the peak period of involvement of the lower extremities.

When lesions occur on the face, they normally appear on the cheeks, eyelids, and bridge of the nose, at times producing a butterfly-shaped lesion that may resemble lupus erythematosus (see page 798). If the eyelids are involved, then they may become edematous and shut, thereby resembling angioedema (see page 348). The affected area is painful, bright red, well-circumscribed, swollen, indurated, and warm to the touch (Fig. 5.3). Often the affected skin will demonstrate a surface texture that resembles an orange peel *(peau d'orange).* Intermixed bullous or hemorrhagic lesions may be seen and often require more intensive antibiotic therapy. High fever and lymphadenopathy often are present. Lymphangitis, leukocytosis, nausea, and vomiting occur infrequently. Diagnostic confirmation is difficult because cultures usually are not beneficial.

Treatment and Prognosis

The treatment of choice is penicillin. Alternative antibiotic drugs include macrolides (such as, erythromycin), cephalosporins (such as, cephalexin), and fluoroquinolones (such as, ciprofloxacin). On initiation of therapy, the area of skin involvement often enlarges, probably secondary to the release of toxins from the dying streptococci. A rapid resolution is noted within 48 hours. Without appropriate therapy, possible complications include abscess formation, gangrene, necrotizing fasciitis, toxic shock syndrome with possible multiple organ failure, thrombophlebitis, acute glomerulonephritis, septicemia, endocarditis, and death. Recurrences may develop in the same area, most likely in a previous zone

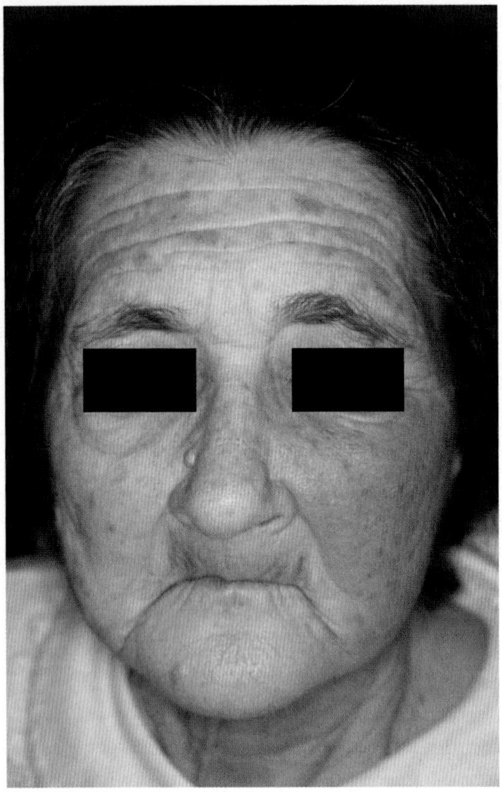

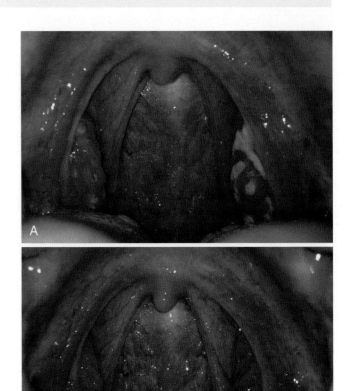

• **Fig. 5.3 Erysipelas.** Red, swollen area of the left cheek. (Courtesy of Dr. Arthur Gonty.)

• **Fig. 5.4 Tonsillitis. A,** Hyperplastic palatine tonsils with yellowish exudate of crypts. **B,** Same patient following successful therapy with amoxicillin/clavulanic acid. (Courtesy of Dr. Molly Smith.)

of damaged lymphatics or untreated athlete's foot. With repeated recurrences, permanent and disfiguring enlargements may result. In cases with multiple recurrences, prophylaxis with oral penicillin has been used.

◆ STREPTOCOCCAL TONSILLITIS AND PHARYNGITIS

Tonsillitis and **pharyngitis** are extremely common and may be caused by many different organisms. The most common causes are group A β-hemolytic streptococci, adenoviruses, enteroviruses, influenza, parainfluenza, and Epstein-Barr virus. Although a virus causes the majority of pharyngitis cases, infection with *S. pyogenes* (group A β-hemolytic streptococci) is responsible for 20%–30% of acute pharyngitis cases in children and 5%–15% of cases in adults. Spread is typically by person-to-person contact through respiratory droplets or oral secretions, with a short incubation period of 2–5 days.

Clinical Features

Although the infection can occur at any age, the greatest prevalence occurs in children 5–15 years old, with most cases in temperate climates arising in the winter or early spring. The signs and symptoms of **tonsillitis** and **pharyngitis** vary from mild to intense. Common findings include sudden onset of sore throat, temperature of 101–104°F, dysphagia, tonsillar hyperplasia, redness of the oropharynx and tonsils, palatal petechiae, cervical lymphadenopathy, and a yellowish tonsillar exudate that may be patchy or confluent (Fig. 5.4). Other occasional findings include a "beefy" red and swollen uvula, excoriated nares, and a scarlatiniform rash (see next topic). Conjunctivitis, coryza (rhinorrhea), cough, hoarseness, discrete ulcerative lesions, anterior stomatitis, absence of fever, a viral exanthem, and diarrhea typically are associated with the viral infections and normally are not present in streptococcal pharyngotonsillitis.

Diagnosis

Although the vast majority of pharyngitis cases are caused by a viral infection, reviews have shown that approximately 60% of patients with sore throats receive antibiotic therapy. To minimize overuse, antibiotics should not be prescribed without confirmation of bacterial infection. Except for very rare infections, such as *Corynebacterium diphtheriae* (see page 177) and *Neisseria gonorrhoeae* (see page 184), antibiotics are of no benefit for acute pharyngitis unless related to group A streptococci.

Current clinical guidelines in the United States recommend use of a rapid antigen detection kit (RADT). A positive result in patients with clinical evidence of pharyngitis supports antibiotic therapy. Due to the low sensitivity of RADT, bacterial culture is recommended upon a negative RADT in pediatric patients, resulting in a 1–5 day delay. In 2015, the FDA approved the first in-office nucleic acid amplification test (NAAT) that negates the need for a two-step algorithm and provides an answer within 15–25 minutes.

Although NAAT can significantly reduce the diagnostic delay in patients with pharyngitis, it does not resolve the diagnostic dilemma completely. Estimates suggest that approximately 20% of asymptomatic school-aged children are carriers of group A streptococci during the winter and spring seasons. When presenting with a viral pharyngitis, the carriers could demonstrate a false positive result to the NAAT tests. The gold standard for separating carriers from true streptococcal pharyngitis requires two serologic samples (titers of antistreptolysin and anti-DNase B) taken 2–4 weeks apart. Due to this extensive delay and associated cost, such extensive evaluation is not a part of standard clinical practice.

Treatment and Prognosis

Streptococcal pharyngitis usually is self-limited and resolves spontaneously within 3–4 days after onset of symptoms. The primary goals of therapy are to shorten the duration of symptoms, prevent the spread of infection, and prevent several rare complications. Possible suppurative complications include peritonsillar abscess, retropharyngeal abscess, cervical lymphadenitis, bacteremia (with resultant fever, nausea, and vomiting), necrotizing fasciitis, and toxic shock syndrome. Nonsuppurative complications also are seen and include acute rheumatic fever, rheumatic heart disease, and post-streptococcal glomerulonephritis. Initiation of appropriate therapy within the first 9 days after development of the pharyngitis prevents rheumatic fever. Patients are considered noncontagious 24 hours after initiation of appropriate antibiotic therapy.

The oral antibiotic of choice for group A streptococci is either penicillin V or amoxicillin. Common choices for patients allergic to penicillin are the first-generation cephalosporins such as cephalexin. Acetaminophen or ibuprofen can be utilized for moderate-to-severe pain, with ibuprofen being shown to be the superior of the two. Topical anesthetics such as lidocaine or benzocaine can be used for throat pain in older children and adolescents but should be avoided in younger children.

◆ SCARLET FEVER (SCARLATINA)

Scarlet fever is a systemic infection produced by specific strains of *S. pyogenes*, (group A, β-hemolytic streptococci). The disease begins as a streptococcal tonsillitis with pharyngitis in which the organisms elaborate an erythrogenic toxin that attacks the blood vessels and produces the characteristic skin rash. The condition occurs in susceptible patients who do not have antitoxin antibodies. The incubation period ranges from 1 to 7 days, and the significant clinical findings include fever, enanthem, and exanthem.

Scarlet fever was once a common cause of childhood death, but it nearly disappeared during the 20th century. Despite this, major outbreaks have occurred during the last decade, predominantly in the United Kingdom and eastern Asia. Between 2014 and 2016, the United Kingdom experienced its highest level of scarlet fever in 50 years. Although the subject of significant research, the cause for the resurgence remains unclear.

Clinical Features

Scarlet fever is most common in children from the ages of 3 to 12 years. The enanthem of the oral mucosa involves the tonsils, pharynx, soft palate, and tongue (see discussion of streptococcal pharyngotonsillitis in previous section). The tonsils, soft palate, and pharynx become erythematous and edematous, and the tonsillar crypts may be filled with a yellowish exudate. In severe cases, the exudates may become confluent and can resemble diphtheria (see page 177).

Scattered petechiae may be seen on the soft palate in up to 10% of affected patients. During the first 2 days, the dorsal surface of the tongue demonstrates a white coating through which only the fungiform papillae can be seen; this has been called **white strawberry tongue** (Fig. 5.5). By the fourth or fifth day, **red strawberry tongue** develops when the white coating desquamates to reveal an erythematous dorsal surface with hyperplastic fungiform papillae. These tongue findings are nonspecific and have been seen in multisystem inflammatory syndrome of COVID-19 (see page 265) and Kawasaki disease.

Classically, in untreated cases, fever develops abruptly around the second day. The patient's temperature peaks at approximately 103°F and returns to normal within 6 days. Abdominal pain, headache, malaise, nausea, and vomiting frequently are present. The exanthematous rash develops within the first 2 days and becomes widespread within 24 hours. The classic rash of scarlet fever is distinctive and often is described as a "sunburn with goose pimples." Pinhead punctate areas that are normal in color project through

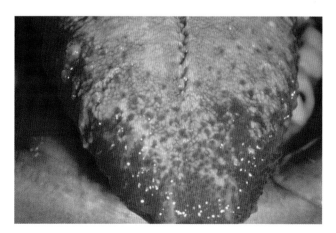

• **Fig. 5.5 Scarlet Fever.** Dorsal surface of the tongue exhibiting white coating in association with numerous enlarged and erythematous fungiform papillae (white strawberry tongue).

the erythema, giving the skin of the trunk and extremities a sandpaper texture. In heavily pigmented individuals, the rash may be more difficult to visualize, but the sandpaper texture remains palpable. The chest and stomach usually are involved initially with eventual spread to other parts of the body. The rash is more intense in areas of pressure and skin folds. Often, transverse red streaks, known as **Pastia lines,** occur in the skin folds secondary to the capillary fragility in these zones of stress. Frequently, the facial cheeks will appear flushed, and circumoral pallor will be noted.

The rash usually clears within 1 week, and then a period of desquamation of the skin occurs. This scaling begins on the face at the end of the first week and spreads to the rest of the skin by the third week, with the extremities being the last affected. The desquamation of the face produces small flakes; the skin of the trunk comes off in thicker, larger flakes. This period of desquamation may last from 3 to 8 weeks.

Diagnosis

As described in greater detail in the previous discussion of streptococcal pharyngotonsillitis, the diagnosis is made by use of a rapid antigen detection kit (RADT), which is followed by throat culture in patients whose RADT is negative. Alternatively, the single-step nucleic acid amplification test (NAAT) is replacing RADT in many clinics.

Treatment and Prognosis

Treatment of scarlet fever and the associated streptococcal pharyngitis is necessary to prevent the possibility of complications, such as peritonsillar or retropharyngeal abscess, sinusitis, or pneumonia. Late complications are rare and include otitis media, acute rheumatic fever, glomerulonephritis, arthralgia, meningitis, and hepatitis. The oral antibiotic of choice for group A streptococci is either penicillin V or amoxicillin. Other choices for penicillin-allergic patients are, the first-generation cephalosporins (such as, cefadroxil or cephalexin). Ibuprofen can be used to reduce the fever and relieve the associated discomfort. The fever and symptoms show dramatic improvement within 48 hours after the initiation of treatment. With appropriate therapy, the prognosis is excellent.

◆ TONSILLAR PLUGS AND TONSILLOLITHIASIS

Anatomically, Waldeyer's ring includes the palatine, lingual, pharyngeal and Eustachian tube tonsils. The tonsils demonstrate numerous deep, twisted, and epithelial-lined invaginations. The invaginations, which are termed *tonsillar crypts,* function to increase the surface area for interaction between the immune cells within the lymphoid tissue and the oral environment. These convoluted crypts commonly are filled with desquamated keratin showing secondary bacterial colonization. The contents of the invaginations often become compacted and form a mass of foul-smelling material known as a **tonsillar plug.** Occasionally, the condensed necrotic debris and bacteria undergo dystrophic calcification and form a **tonsillolith (tonsillar concretion).** These structures have been shown to contain a living biofilm of densely packed bacteria demonstrating a diversity of rods, cocci, and filamentous organisms embedded within an extracellular matrix.

Clinical and Radiographic Features

Tonsillar plugs and tonsilloliths are seen rather frequently. Reviews of panoramic radiographs reveal a prevalence of tonsilloliths within the palatine tonsils that ranges from 7.2% to 13.4%, with computed tomography demonstrating a much higher frequency of discovery (16% to 46.1%). Although more poorly recognized, concretions within the tonsillar tissue in the base of the tongue also are not rare with a reported frequency of 1.5% on panoramic radiographs and 4.8% on computed tomography. Affected palatine tonsils may demonstrate one or more enlarged crypts filled with yellow debris that varies in consistency from soft to friable to fully calcified. In contrast to acute tonsillitis, the surrounding tonsillar tissue is not acutely painful, dramatically inflamed, or significantly edematous. Tonsilloliths can develop over a wide age range, from childhood to old age, with a mean patient age in the early 40s. Although a male predominance has been reported, other studies have not noted a gender predilection. These calcifications vary from small clinically insignificant lesions to massive calcifications more than 14 cm in length. Tonsilloliths may be single or multiple, and bilateral cases are not rare.

Although many palatine tonsillar plugs and tonsilloliths are asymptomatic, they can promote recurrent tonsillar infections and may lead to pain, abscess formation, ulceration, dysphagia, chronic sore throat, irritable cough, or otalgia. Halitosis is a common complaint and not surprising because several of the bacteria within the associated biofilm are known to produce hydrogen sulfide and methyl mercaptan, both of which are associated strongly with oral malodor. Occasionally, patients report a dull ache or a sensation of a foreign object in the throat that is relieved on removal of the tonsillar plug. In patients with large stones, clinical examination often reveals a hard, yellow submucosal mass of the affected tonsil. In older adult patients, large tonsilloliths can be aspirated and produce significant pulmonary complications. Dyspnea, esophageal perforation, and mediastinitis have been reported in association with large tonsilloliths. When symptomatic, lingual tonsilloliths are reported to be associated with local discomfort, anterior neck pain, or sensation of a foreign body.

Most frequently, palatine tonsilloliths are discovered on panoramic radiographs as radiopaque objects superimposed on the midportion of the mandibular ramus (Fig. 5.6). In other cases, small radiopacities may be seen posterior or inferior to the angle of the mandible. Most lingual tonsilloliths

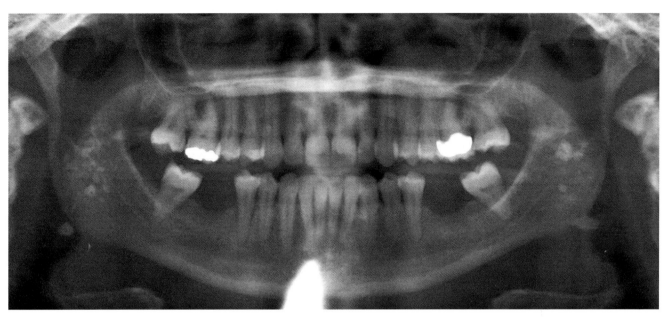

• **Fig. 5.6 Tonsilloliths.** Cluster of radiopacities noted bilaterally in the midportion of the ascending ramus. (Courtesy of Dr. Kim Nichols.)

are noted along the margin of the soft tissue shadow of the base of the tongue, primarily inferior and posteroinferior to the mandible on panoramic radiographs. When compared to palatine tonsilloliths, lingual concretions tend to be smaller in size and fewer in number.

Diagnosis

A strong presumptive diagnosis can be made through a combination of the clinical and radiographic features. After detection on a panoramic radiograph, if further diagnostic confirmation of tonsilloliths is deemed necessary, then their presence can be confirmed with computed tomography (CT), magnetic resonance imaging (MRI), or the demonstration of the calculi on removal of the affected tonsil.

Treatment and Prognosis

Tonsilloliths discovered incidentally during evaluation of a panoramic radiograph often are not treated unless associated with significant tonsillar hyperplasia or clinical symptoms. Affected individuals occasionally try to remove tonsillar plugs with instruments, such as straws, toothpicks, and dental instruments. Such therapy has the potential to damage the surrounding tonsillar tissue and should be discouraged. Patients should be educated to attempt removal by gargling warm salt water or using pulsating jets of water.

Superficial calculi can be enucleated or curetted; deeper symptomatic tonsilloliths require local excision. Redevelopment of removed concretions is common. Laser or coblation cryptolysis has been utilized successfully to reduce the extent of the tonsillar invaginations and stop the redevelopment of the concretions. If evidence of associated chronic tonsillitis is seen, then tonsillectomy provides definitive therapy.

◆ DIPHTHERIA

Diphtheria is a life-threatening infection most commonly produced by *Corynebacterium diphtheriae. C. ulcerans* and *C. pseudotuberculosis* are less common causes and usually discovered in individuals exhibiting contact with farm animals or dairy products. The name of the disease derives from the Greek word *diphthera* which translates to "leather hide" in reference to the tenacious pseudomembrane that is typical on the soft palate and pharynx of affected patients. The disease initially was described in 1826, and *C. diphtheriae* (also termed *Klebs-Löffler bacillus*) was discovered by Klebs in 1883 and isolated in pure culture by Löffler in 1884. Humans are the sole reservoir, and the infection is acquired through contact with an infected person or carrier usually through respiratory droplets.

The bacterium produces a lethal exotoxin that causes tissue necrosis, thereby providing nutrients for further growth and leading to peripheral spread. The exotoxin interferes with cellular protein synthesis. In addition to the death of affected cells, involvement of Schwann cells can lead to demyelination of peripheral nerves with significant associated neuropathies. The first effective antitoxin was discovered by the German physician, Emil von Behring, who was awarded the first Nobel Prize in medicine for this work. The antitoxin has been available since 1913, and immunization has been widespread in North America since 1922. The vaccination is an antitoxin that protects against toxin-related tissue damage but does not prevent infection by the bacteria.

Widespread vaccination led to a dramatically decreased prevalence of the infection until the 1990s when collapse of the Soviet Union produced inconsistent vaccination and localized outbreaks. The process finally was controlled by administration of vaccine to all children, adolescents, and adults (regardless of immunization histories). In addition, the disease remains endemic in areas of the globe such as south and southeast Asia and Africa where vaccination rates are less than 80%.

In addition to these pockets of disease, infections may occur in people who are immunosuppressed or who have failed to receive booster injections as required. Isolated outbreaks still are reported in the urban poor and Native American populations of North America. Overall, diphtheria currently is rare in the United States with only six reported cases between 2000 and 2015.

Clinical Features

The signs and symptoms of diphtheria arise 1–5 days after exposure to the organism. The initial systemic symptoms, which include low-grade fever, headache, malaise, anorexia, sore throat, and vomiting, arise gradually and may be mild. Although skin wounds may be involved, the infection predominantly affects mucosal surfaces and may produce exudates of the nasal, tonsillar, pharyngeal, laryngotracheal, or conjunctival areas. Urethritis from toxigenic *C. diphtheriae* has been noted secondary to orogenital contact. Involvement of the nasal cavity often is accompanied with prolonged mucoid or hemorrhagic discharge. The oropharyngeal exudate begins on one or both tonsils as a patchy, yellow-white, thin film that thickens to form an adherent gray covering. With time, the membrane may develop patches of green or black necrosis. The superficial epithelium is an integral portion of this exudate, and attempts at removal are difficult and may result in bleeding. The covering may continue to involve the entire soft palate, uvula, larynx, or trachea, resulting in stridor and respiratory difficulties. Palatal perforation can occur but is very uncommon. Rarely, the lesions have been isolated to the oral cavity.

The severity of the infection correlates with the spread of the membrane. Local obstruction of the airway can be lethal and historically was one of the most common causes of death, leading to the diphtheria nickname of "*strangling angel*." Involvement of the tonsils leads to significant cervical lymphadenopathy, which often is associated with an edematous neck enlargement known as *bull neck*. Toxin-related paralysis may affect oculomotor, facial, pharyngeal, diaphragmatic, and intercostal muscles. The soft palatal paralysis can lead to nasal regurgitation during swallowing. Oral or nasal involvement has been reported to spread to the adjacent skin of the face and lips.

Cutaneous diphtheria can occur anywhere on the body and is characterized by chronic skin ulcers that frequently are associated with infected insect bites and may harbor other pathogens, such as *S. aureus* or *S. pyogenes*. These skin lesions can arise even in vaccinated patients and typically are not associated with systemic toxic manifestations. When contracted by travelers from developed nations, the diagnosis often is delayed because of the nonspecific clinical presentation and a low index of suspicion. The cutaneous lesions represent an important reservoir of infection and can lead to more typical and lethal diphtheria in unprotected contacts.

Although bacteremia is rare, circulating toxin can result in systemic complications, such as myocarditis, neuropathy, thrombocytopenia, proteinuria, and renal failure. Myocarditis and neurologic difficulties are seen most frequently and usually are discovered in patients with severe nasopharyngeal diphtheria. Myocarditis may present as progressive weakness and dyspnea or lead to acute congestive heart failure. The neuropathy associated with diphtheria usually is biphasic. Initially, lower cranial neuropathies arise a few weeks after the pharyngeal infections and often present with dysphonia, dysphagia, palatal paralysis, and numbness of the face, tongue, and gingiva. Subsequently, polyneuropathy of the extremities becomes evident as the cranial neuropathies begin to fade. A significant number of patients become quadriplegic at the nadir. A peripheral polyneuritis resembling Guillain-Barré syndrome also may occur.

Diagnosis

Although the clinical presentation can be distinctive in severe cases, laboratory confirmation should be sought in all instances. Although culture remains the diagnostic gold standard, a polymerase chain reaction (PCR) analysis has become available and has reduced the time required to confirm the diagnosis. Except during an epidemic, the diagnosis can be difficult due to the rarity of the infection and the inexperience of many physicians with the disease.

Treatment and Prognosis

Treatment of the patient with diphtheria should be initiated at the time of the clinical diagnosis and should not be delayed until the results of the culture are received. Antitoxin should be administered in combination with antibiotics to prevent further toxin production, to stop the local infection, and to prevent transmission. Erythromycin, procaine penicillin, or intravenous (IV) penicillin may be used. Most patients are no longer infectious after 4 days of antibiotic therapy, but some may retain vital organisms. The patient is not considered to be cured until three consecutive negative culture specimens are obtained.

Because the antitoxin neutralizes only circulating toxin that is not bound to tissue, prompt administration is critical. This factor stresses the need for maintaining local stocks that have not reached their expiration date. Patients demonstrate improved outcomes if the antitoxin is administered within 48 hours of the first pharyngeal symptoms.

Before the development of the antitoxin, the mortality rate approached 50%, usually from cardiac or neurologic complications. Although the outcome is unpredictable, the current mortality rate is less than 5%, with most patients demonstrating a total or near-complete recovery with only mild residual deficits. Development of myocarditis is an important predictor of mortality.

Deaths still occur in the United States because of delays in therapy secondary to lack of suspicion. With worldwide travel and visitors from across the globe, prevention is paramount. Even in those vaccinated as children, it must be remembered that a booster inoculation is required every 10 years. Currently, the inoculation in adults has been combined into the *Tdap vaccine* that includes tetanus, diphtheria, and pertussis.

◆ SYPHILIS (LUES)

Syphilis is a worldwide chronic infection produced by *Treponema pallidum*. The organism is extremely vulnerable to drying; therefore, the primary modes of transmission are sexual contact or from mother to fetus. Humans are the only proven natural host for syphilis.

After the advent of penicillin therapy in the 1940s, the prevalence of syphilis slowly decreased for many years but often demonstrated peaks and troughs associated with sexual activity during that era. A peak occurred during the "sexual revolution" of the 1960s, but fear of acquired immunodeficiency syndrome (AIDS) in 2000 led to the fewest reported cases of primary and secondary syphilis since reporting began in 1941. As more effective therapy for AIDS has been developed, sexual activity has changed once again with an increasing prevalence of sexually transmitted diseases being reported, primarily because of increases among men who have sex with men (MSM). Congenital syphilis followed a similar trend and reached a low in 2012 only to increase by 38% over the next 2 years. This rapid increase in congenital syphilis was related directly to a 22% increase in syphilis noted in women during the same time period. Oral sex is thought to have played an increasingly important contribution to the recent surge in the number of sexually transmitted diseases, as many falsely believed that unprotected oral sex was a safe or no-risk sexual practice, representing a good replacement for other higher-risk behaviors. During the recent wave, it is estimated there are more than 12 million new syphilitic infections annually in the world.

In patients with syphilis, the infection undergoes a characteristic evolution that classically proceeds through three stages. A syphilitic patient is highly infectious only during the first two stages, but pregnant women also may transmit the infection to the fetus during the latent stage. Maternal transmission during the first two stages of infection almost always results in miscarriage, stillbirth, or an infant with congenital malformations. The longer the mother has had the infection, the less the chance of fetal infection. Infection of the fetus may occur at any time during pregnancy, but the stigmata do not begin to develop until after the fourth month of gestation. The clinical changes secondary to the fetal infection are known as **congenital syphilis.** Oral syphilitic lesions are uncommon but may occur in any stage. Due to the rarity of oral lesions and the nonspecific microscopic pattern, appropriate histopathologic diagnosis easily can be missed by pathologists inexperienced with the pathosis.

Clinical Features
Primary Syphilis

Primary syphilis is characterized by the **chancre** that develops at the site of inoculation, becoming clinically evident 3–90 days after the initial exposure. Most chancres are solitary and begin as papular lesions that develop a central ulceration. Approximately 85% arise in the genital areas, whereas 10% are anal, 4% are oral, and the remaining 1% affect other extragenital locations.

Intraoral lesions of primary syphilis are documented infrequently, because the symptoms associated with this stage tend to resolve within a few days with many patients not seeking therapy. The oral lesions are seen most commonly on the lip, but other sites include the buccal mucosa, tongue, palate, gingiva, and tonsils (Fig. 5.7). The upper lip is affected more frequently in males, whereas lower lip involvement is predominant in females. Some believe this selective labial distribution may reflect the surfaces most actively involved during fellatio and cunnilingus. The oral lesion appears as a painless, clean-based ulceration or, rarely, as a vascular proliferation resembling a pyogenic granuloma. Regional lymphadenopathy, which may be bilateral, is seen in most patients. At this time, the organism is spreading systemically through the lymphatic channels, setting the stage for future progression. If untreated, then the initial lesion heals within 3–8 weeks.

Secondary Syphilis

The next stage is known as *secondary* (disseminated) *syphilis* and is discovered clinically 4–10 weeks after the initial infection. The lesions of secondary syphilis may arise before the primary lesion has resolved completely. During secondary syphilis, systemic symptoms often arise. The most common are painless lymphadenopathy, sore throat, malaise, headache, weight loss, fever, and musculoskeletal pain. A consistent sign is a diffuse, painless, maculopapular cutaneous rash,

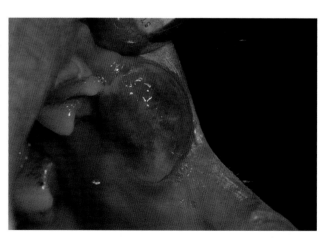

• **Fig. 5.7 Chancre of Primary Syphilis.** Erythematous and ulcerated mass of the right anterior buccal mucosa. (Courtesy of Dr. Benjamin Martinez.)

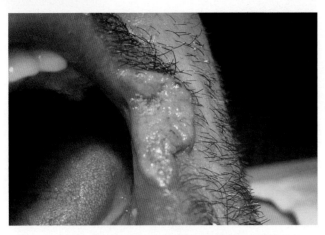

• **Fig. 5.8 Split Papule of Secondary Syphilis.** Ulcerated mass divided in half by the left oral commissure. (Courtesy of Dr. Chad Street.)

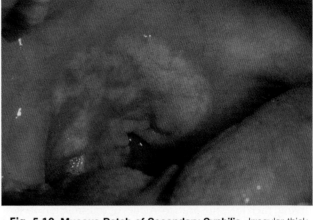

• **Fig. 5.10 Mucous Patch of Secondary Syphilis.** Irregular thickened white plaque of the right soft palate.

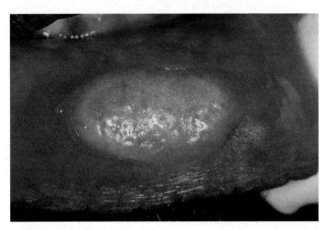

• **Fig. 5.9 Mucous Patch of Secondary Syphilis.** Circumscribed white plaque on the lower labial mucosa. (Courtesy of Dr. Pete Edmonds.)

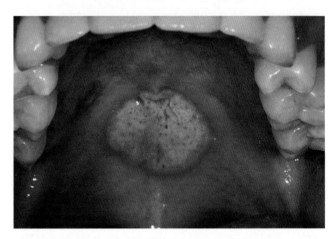

• **Fig. 5.11 Mucous Patch of Secondary Syphilis.** Circumscribed and thickened white plaque noted in the midline of the soft palate.

which is widespread and can even affect the palmar and plantar areas. On occasion, a cutaneous papule may develop in the crease of the nasal alar or the oral commissure and demonstrate a central fissure in association with the crease, forming the clinically distinctive lesion known as a **split papule** (Fig. 5.8). The rash also may involve the oral cavity and appear as red, maculopapular areas. Although the skin rash may result in areas of scarring and hyperpigmentation or hypopigmentation, it heals without scarring in most patients.

Most reported examples of intraoral syphilis are discovered during the secondary stage, and concurrent cutaneous lesions often are not described. Affected patients most often develop sensitive whitish and elevated plaques known as **mucous patches** that develop due to the intense inflammatory response to the spirochete infection (Figs. 5.9–5.11). Occasionally, several adjacent patches can fuse and form a serpentine or snail-track pattern. Subsequently, superficial epithelial necrosis may occur, leading to sloughing and exposure of the underlying raw connective tissue. Less often, thickened/corrugated leukoplakic plaques or erythematous patches like those seen in atrophic candidiasis may be present. Lesions of secondary syphilis may appear on any

mucosal surface but are found commonly on the tongue, lip, buccal mucosa, and palate. Occasionally, papillary lesions that may resemble viral papillomas arise during this time and are known as **condylomata lata.** Although these lesions typically occur in the genital or anal regions, rare oral examples occur (Fig. 5.12). In contrast to the isolated chancre noted in the primary stage, multiple lesions are typical of secondary syphilis. Spontaneous resolution usually occurs within 3–12 weeks; however, relapses may occur during the next year.

Tertiary Syphilis

After the second stage, patients enter a period in which they are free of lesions and symptoms, known as **latent syphilis.** This period of latency may last from 1 to 30 years; then the third stage known as *tertiary syphilis* develops in approximately 30% of affected individuals. This stage includes the most serious of all complications. The vascular system can be affected significantly through the effects of the earlier arteritis. Aneurysm of the ascending aorta, left ventricular hypertrophy, aortic regurgitation, and congestive heart failure may occur. Involvement of the central nervous system

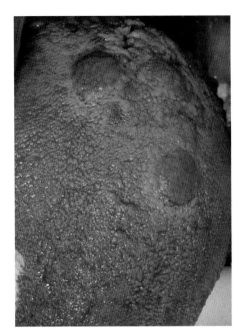

• **Fig. 5.12 Condyloma Lata.** Multiple indurated and slightly papillary nodules on the dorsal tongue. (Courtesy of Dr. Karen Novak.)

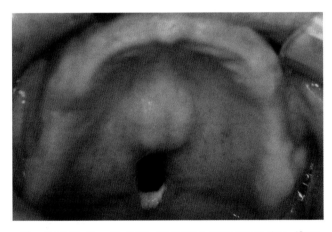

• **Fig. 5.13 Tertiary Syphilis.** Perforation of the hard palate. (Courtesy of Dr. George Blozis.)

(CNS) may result in tabes dorsalis, general paralysis, psychosis, dementia, paresis, and death. Ocular lesions such as iritis, choroidoretinitis, and Argyll Robertson pupil may occur. Argyll Robertson pupils constrict upon focusing, but they fail to respond to bright light. Less significant, but more characteristic, are scattered foci of granulomatous inflammation, which may affect the skin, mucosa, soft tissue, bones, and internal organs. This active site of granulomatous inflammation, known as a **gumma,** appears as an indurated, nodular, or ulcerated lesion that may produce extensive tissue destruction. Since the advent of successful antibiotic therapy, intraoral gummas are extremely uncommon; when seen, they usually affect the palate or tongue. When the palate is involved, the ulceration frequently perforates through to the nasal cavity (Fig. 5.13). The tongue may be involved diffusely with gummata and appear large, lobulated, and irregularly shaped. This lobulated pattern is termed **interstitial glossitis** and is thought to be the result of contracture of the lingual musculature after healing of gummas. Diffuse atrophy and loss of the dorsal tongue papillae produce a condition called **luetic glossitis.** In the past, this form of atrophic glossitis was thought to be precancerous, but several more recent publications dispute this concept.

Congenital Syphilis

In 1858, Sir Jonathan Hutchinson described the changes found in congenital syphilis and defined the following three pathognomonic diagnostic features, known as **Hutchinson triad:**

- Hutchinson teeth
- Ocular interstitial keratitis
- Eighth nerve deafness

Like many diagnostic triads, few patients exhibit all three features. In addition to Hutchinson triad, several other alterations may be seen, such as saddle-nose deformity, high-arched palate, frontal bossing, hydrocephalus, intellectual disability, gummas, and neurosyphilis. Table 5.1 delineates the prevalence rates of the stigmata of congenital syphilis in a cohort of affected patients.

TABLE 5.1	Stigmata of Congenital Syphilis		
Stigmata of Congenital Syphilis *		**Number of Patients**	**Percentage Affected**
Frontal bossing		235	86.7
Short maxilla		227	83.8
High-arched palate		207	76.4
Saddle nose		199	73.4
Mulberry molars		176	64.9
Hutchinson incisors		171	63.1
Higoumenaki sign[†]		107	39.4
Relative prognathism of mandible		70	25.8
Interstitial keratitis		24	8.8
Rhagades[‡]		19	7.0
Saber shin[§]		11	4.1
Eighth nerve deafness		9	3.3
Scaphoid scapulae[‖]		2	0.7
Clutton joint[¶]		1	0.3

*In a cohort of 271 patients.
[†]Enlargement of clavicle adjacent to the sternum.
[‡]Premature perioral fissuring.
[§]Anterior bowing of tibia as a result of periostitis.
[‖]Concavity of vertebral border of the scapulae.
[¶]Painless synovitis and enlargement of joints, usually the knee.
Modified from Fiumara NJ, Lessel S: Manifestations of late congenital syphilis: an analysis of 271 patients, *Arch Dermatol* 102:78–83, 1970.

Infants infected with syphilis can display signs within 2–3 weeks of birth. These early findings include growth impairment, fever, jaundice, anemia, hepatosplenomegaly, rhinitis, rhagades (circumoral radial skin fissures), and desquamative maculopapular, ulcerative, or vesiculobullous skin eruptions. Untreated infants who survive often develop tertiary syphilis with damage to the bones, teeth, eyes, ears, and brain. It is these findings that were described well by Hutchinson.

The infection alters the formation of both the anterior teeth **(Hutchinson incisors)** and the posterior dentition **(mulberry molars, Fournier molars, Moon molars).** Hutchinson incisors exhibit their greatest mesiodistal width in the middle third of the crown. The incisal third tapers to the incisal edge, and the resulting tooth resembles a straightedge screwdriver. The incisal edge often exhibits a central hypoplastic notch (Fig. 5.14). Mulberry molars taper toward the occlusal surface with a constricted grinding surface. The occlusal anatomy is abnormal, with numerous disorganized globular projections that resemble the surface of a mulberry (Fig. 5.15).

As mentioned previously, the prevalence of congenital syphilis is on the rise. To reverse this trend, all women should be screened for syphilis early in the pregnancy. In addition, women at high risk for syphilis should be tested again twice during the third trimester. Finally, any fetal death after 20 weeks of gestation should trigger testing of the mother.

Histopathologic Features

The histopathologic picture of the oral lesions in the syphilitic patient is not specific. During the first two stages, the pattern is similar. The surface epithelium is ulcerated in primary lesions and may be ulcerated or hyperplastic in the secondary stage. Extensive exocytosis typically is noted and represents a major clue to the diagnosis (Fig. 5.16). The

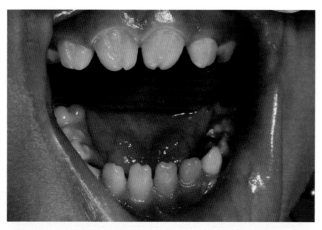

• **Fig. 5.14 Hutchinson Incisors of Congenital Syphilis.** Anterior dentition exhibiting crowns tapering toward the incisal edges that demonstrate with hypoplastic notching. (Courtesy of Dr. Roman Carlos.)

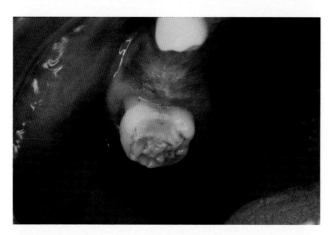

• **Fig. 5.15 Mulberry Molar of Congenital Syphilis.** Maxillary molar demonstrating occlusal surface with numerous globular projections.

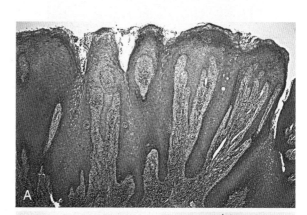

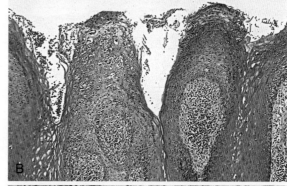

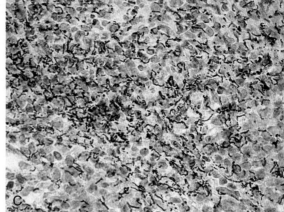

• **Fig. 5.16 Secondary Syphilis, Condyloma Lata. A,** Low-power photomicrograph of biopsy from patient in Fig. 5.12, which shows papillary epithelial hyperplasia and a heavy plasmacytic infiltrate in the connective tissue. **B,** High-power view showing intense exocytosis of neutrophils into the epithelium. **C,** Immunoperoxidase reaction for *Treponema pallidum* demonstrating numerous spirochetes in the epithelium.

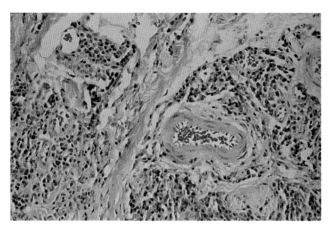

• **Fig. 5.17 Primary Syphilis.** A chronic perivascular inflammatory infiltrate of plasma cells and lymphocytes. (Courtesy of Dr. John Metcalf.)

underlying lamina propria exhibits an intense chronic inflammatory cellular infiltrate composed predominantly of lymphocytes and plasma cells, which is noted primarily in the superficial stroma and around deeper vascular channels (Fig. 5.17). Although the presence of plasma cells is commonplace within ulcerations and areas of oral mucositis, the combination of heavy exocytosis and an underlying dense lymphoplasmacytic infiltrate often raises the index of suspicion to a level that supports search for the organism. The use of special silver impregnation techniques, such as Warthin-Starry or Steiner stains, or immunoperoxidase reactions directed against the organism often show scattered corkscrew-like spirochetal organisms that frequently are found most easily within the surface epithelium and at the interface between the epithelium and the superficial stroma (see Fig. 5.16, *C*). The organism also can be detected in tissue through direct fluorescent antibody or nucleic acid amplification testing.

Oral tertiary lesions typically exhibit surface ulceration, with peripheral pseudoepitheliomatous hyperplasia. The underlying inflammatory infiltrate usually demonstrates foci of granulomatous inflammation with well-circumscribed collections of histiocytes and multinucleated giant cells. Even with special stains, the organisms are hard to demonstrate in the third stage; researchers believe the inflammatory response is an immune reaction, rather than a direct response to *T. pallidum.*

Diagnosis

The diagnosis of syphilis can be confirmed by demonstrating the spiral organism by biopsy or dark-field examination of a smear of an active lesion. False-positive results in smears are possible in the oral cavity because of morphologically similar oral inhabitants, such as *Treponema microdentium, T. macrodentium,* and *T. mucosum.* Demonstration of the organism on a smear or in biopsy material should be confirmed using specific immunofluorescent antibodies, nucleic acid amplification testing, or serologic evaluation.

Several nonspecific and not highly sensitive serologic screening tests for syphilis are available. These include the

Venereal Disease Research Laboratory (VDRL) and the rapid plasma reagin (RPR). The results of these screening tests are reported quantitatively with the serial antibody titers occasionally used to follow treatment response. Due to the delay associated with antibody development, the screening tests can be negative for up to 6 weeks after the initial infection. From this point, the tests remain strongly positive throughout the remainder of the primary stage and the entire secondary stage. This delay in serologic positivity must be remembered because biopsy results of an intraoral chancre could demonstrate definitive evidence of infection weeks before the screening tests reveal a positive result. After the development of latency, the positivity generally subsides with time. As part of appropriate prenatal care, all pregnant women should receive one of the nonspecific screening tests. Because these tests typically are negative in the early primary stage and may be falsely negative in immunosuppressed patients (such as, AIDS), tissue identification of the organism is critical in many patients.

Specific and highly sensitive serologic tests for syphilis also are available. These include the fluorescent treponemal antibody absorption (FTA-ABS), *T. pallidum* hemagglutination assay (TPHA), *T. pallidum* particle agglutination assay (TPPA), and microhemagglutination assay for antibody to *T. pallidum* (MHA-TP). These test results remain positive for life. This lifelong persistence of positivity limits their usefulness in the diagnosis of a second occurrence of infection. Therefore, in cases of possible reinfection, the organisms should be demonstrated within the tissue or exudates.

Treatment and Prognosis

The treatment for syphilis necessitates an individual evaluation and a customized therapeutic approach. The treatment of choice is parenteral penicillin G for all stages of syphilis. The type (benzathine, aqueous procaine, or aqueous crystalline), dosage, and length of treatment varies according to the stage and clinical manifestations. For the patient with a true penicillin allergy, doxycycline is second-line therapy, with tetracycline and ceftriaxone also demonstrating antitreponemal activity.

In some patients, the antibiotic therapy is associated with a release of endotoxin-like products from the dying spirochetes resulting in a symptom-complex termed *Jarisch-Herxheimer reaction.* Affected patients present with acute onset of fever, headache, myalgia, and other symptoms. The reaction is seen most frequently in the early stages of syphilis when the bacterial burden is high.

Even in patients who obtain a clinical and serologic "cure" with penicillin, it must be remembered that *T. pallidum* can escape the lethal effects of the antibiotic when the organism is located within the confines of lymph nodes or the CNS. Therefore, antibiotic therapy may not always result in a total cure in patients with neurologic involvement but may arrest only the clinical presentations of the infection. Patients with immunosuppression, such as those with AIDS, may not respond appropriately to standard antibiotic regimens, and numerous reports have documented a continuation to neurosyphilis despite seemingly appropriate single-dose therapy.

◆ GONORRHEA

Gonorrhea, a sexually transmitted disease that is produced by *Neisseria gonorrhoeae,* represents the second most common reportable bacterial infection in the United States (after chlamydia) with over 800,000 persons estimated to be infected each year. The disease is epidemic, especially in young adults residing in urban areas; worldwide, millions of people are infected each year. The rate in the United States remains the highest of any industrialized country, and certain segments of the population, such as those with a low socioeconomic or education level, injecting drug users, prostitutes, homosexual men, and military personnel, remain at high risk. In contrast to many other sexually transmitted diseases, women are affected slightly more frequently than men.

Clinical Features

The infection is spread through sexual contact, and most lesions occur in the genital areas. Indirect infection is rare because the organism is sensitive to drying and cannot penetrate intact stratified squamous epithelium. The incubation period is typically 2–5 days. Affected areas often demonstrate significant purulent discharge, but approximately 10% of men and up to 80% of women who contract gonorrhea are asymptomatic.

In men, the most frequent site of infection is the urethra, resulting in purulent discharge and dysuria. Less common primary sites include the anorectal and pharyngeal areas. The cervix is the primary site of involvement in women, and the chief complaints are increased vaginal discharge, intermenstrual bleeding, genital itching, and dysuria. The organism may ascend to involve the uterus and ovarian tubes leading to **pelvic inflammatory disease (PID)** with long-term complications that include ectopic pregnancies or infertility from tubal obstruction.

Between 0.5% and 3.0% of untreated patients with gonorrhea will have disseminated gonococcal infections from systemic bacteremia. The most common signs of dissemination are myalgia, arthralgia, polyarthritis, and dermatitis. In 75% of patients with disseminated disease, a characteristic skin rash develops. The dermatologic lesions consist of discrete papules and pustules that often exhibit a hemorrhagic component and occur primarily on the extremities. Less common alterations secondary to gonococcal septicemia include fever, endocarditis, pericarditis, meningitis, and oral mucosal lesions of the soft palate and oropharynx, which may be similar clinically to aphthous ulcerations.

Most cases of oral gonorrhea appear to be a result of fellatio, although oropharyngeal gonorrhea may be the result of gonococcal septicemia, kissing, or cunnilingus. Most cases are reported in women or homosexual men, with the most common sites being the pharynx, tonsils, and uvula. Although pharyngeal gonorrhea usually is asymptomatic, a mild-to-moderate sore throat may occur and be accompanied by nonspecific, diffuse oropharyngeal erythema. Involved tonsils typically demonstrate edema and erythema, often with scattered, small punctate pustules.

Although most cases of pharyngeal infection resolve spontaneously without adverse sequelae, new findings suggest the infection has important implications, which strongly support the need for treatment to reduce the potential for spreading the infection. Research also has suggested that pharyngeal involvement may play an important role in the development of antibiotic resistance. Several studies have shown that *N. gonorrhoeae* may undergo mutation by acquiring genetic material from other *Neisseria* species that frequent the throat, and drug penetration is low in the pharyngeal tissues. Oropharyngeal infection is associated with increased concern due to the typical lack of associated symptoms, difficulty in confirming infection (see Diagnosis), and resistance to therapy (see Treatment and Prognosis). Pharyngeal gonorrhea in the absence of a concomitant genital infection is relatively common among young people examined at STD clinics, with up to 28% of infections missed without pharyngeal testing. These findings have led to guidelines that recommend periodic extragenital testing among men who have sex with men (MSM). Several studies have suggested this screening should be extended to other high risk non-MSM populations such as commercial sex workers and young adults seeking care for a sexually transmitted disease (STD).

Rarely, lesions have been reported in the anterior portion of the oral cavity, with areas of infection appearing erythematous, pustular, erosive, or ulcerated. Occasionally, the infection may simulate **necrotizing gingivitis (NG),** but some clinicians have reported that the typical *fetor oris* is absent, providing an important clue to the actual cause (Fig. 5.18). Submandibular or cervical lymphadenopathy may be present.

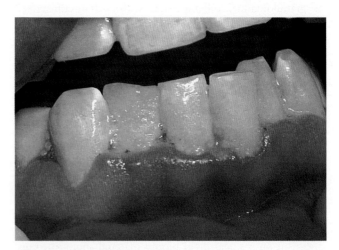

• **Fig. 5.18 Gonorrhea.** Necrosis, purulence, and hemorrhage of the anterior mandibular gingiva. (From Williams LN: The risks of oral-genital contact: a case report, *Gen Dent* 50:282–284, 2002. Published with permission by the Academy of General Dentistry. Copyright 2002 by the American Academy of General Dentistry. All rights reserved.)

During birth, infection of an infant may occur, even from an infected mother who is asymptomatic and possibly result in serious eye involvement, sepsis (associated with arthritis and meningitis), and less severe manifestations such as rhinitis, vaginitis, and urethritis. The eye involvement is called **gonococcal ophthalmia neonatorum** and rapidly can cause perforation of the globe of the eye and blindness. Common signs of infection include significant conjunctivitis and a mucopurulent discharge from the eye. As required by law in most states, erythromycin ophthalmic ointment is placed into both eyes of all newborn infants regardless if delivered vaginally or by caesarean section. Despite the ocular treatment, the best prevention of neonatal gonorrhea is prenatal screening and treatment of pregnant women.

Diagnosis

In males with a urethral discharge, a Gram stain of the purulent material can be used to demonstrate gram-negative diplococci within the neutrophils; additional testing usually is not indicated. Culture and nucleic acid amplification tests (NAATs) are available for diagnostic testing. Although culture has been the previous "gold standard" for diagnosis, the technique demonstrates a much lower sensitivity in the oropharynx with common false-negative results. NAAT is superior to culture in all urogenital and nongenital sites but has been shown to generate false positives in some anatomic sites and is not FDA-cleared for rectal, oropharyngeal, and conjunctival infection. Despite this, some laboratories have met expanded CLIA regulatory requirements to allow use of NAAT in these locations to assist in clinical management. Because up to 80% of women are asymptomatic, annual screening is recommended for all sexually-active women under the age of 25 and older women who are at high risk for infection. Since 90% of men are symptomatic and usually seek treatment, a similar recommendation has not been made for their gender.

Treatment and Prognosis

Treatment has been complicated due to the development of antibiotic resistance by *N. gonorrhoeae* and is becoming increasingly more worrisome. Only one class of antibiotics, the cephalosporins, is considered to be sufficiently effective by the Centers for Disease Control and Prevention (CDC). In addition, coinfection by *Chlamydia trachomatis* is common, leading to a suggested therapy that is effective against both organisms. Although the current cure rate for genital gonorrhea is high, oropharyngeal gonorrhea is harder to resolve and further complicated by the difficulty in diagnosis.

The currently recommended regimen is intramuscular ceftriaxone combined with oral azithromycin. Doxycycline can be used for those allergic to azithromycin, whereas gemifloxacin or gentamycin is recommended for patients allergic to ceftriaxone. Sadly, the effectiveness of cephalosporines appears to be waning, and this trend is expected to continue. Rescreening is recommended 3 months after therapy. The most common cause for treatment failure is reexposure to infected partners, who often are asymptomatic; therefore, the treatment of all recent sexual partners is recommended. Truly resistant infections should be cultured with antimicrobial testing and selection of an appropriate alternate antibiotic.

◆ TUBERCULOSIS

Tuberculosis (TB) is a chronic infectious disease caused by *Mycobacterium tuberculosis* and represents the leading cause of death worldwide related to a single bacterial infectious disease. It is estimated that over 10 million persons with incident tuberculosis and 1.5 million deaths occurred in 2018 with the highest number of affected persons in South-East Asia and Africa. In 1989, the United States embarked on a program to eliminate tuberculosis by rapidly identifying, treating, and contact tracing all cases of tuberculosis. In 2019 (the most recent complete data set available), the United States reported the lowest number of infections since recording began in 1953 with less than 9000 cases. The goal of nationwide elimination of the infection has been complicated by immigration as evidenced by the discovery that over 70% of the cases represented reactivation of latent tuberculosis acquired in the past among non-U.S.-born individuals. Current strategies are stressing increased diagnosis and treatment of latent tuberculosis infections. Worldwide, the prevalence of the infection declined with the introduction of effective antimicrobials, but in recent years it has demonstrated an increased frequency that appears to be associated with emergence of AIDS and drug-resistant strains. **Bacillus Calmette-Guérin (BCG) vaccine** for TB exists but is not available in the United States. The vaccine confers limited and highly variable protection along with several side effects, leading to its removal from the vaccination schedule of several countries.

Nontuberculous mycobacterial disease can occur from a variety of organisms. Before the tuberculin testing of dairy herds, many cases arose from the consumption of milk infected with *Mycobacterium bovis*. Except for HIV-infected individuals, most other cases of nontuberculous mycobacterial disease appear as localized chronic cervical lymphadenitis in otherwise healthy children, with calcification of the involved nodes leading to the diagnosis in some cases (Fig. 5.19). In patients with AIDS (see page 258), *Mycobacterium avium-intracellulare* is a common cause of opportunistic infections.

Infection must be distinguished from active disease. **Primary tuberculosis** occurs in previously unexposed people and almost always involves the lungs. Most infections are the result of direct person-to-person spread through airborne droplets from a patient with active disease. The organism initially elicits a nonspecific, chronic inflammatory reaction. In most individuals, the primary infection results only in a localized, fibrocalcific nodule at the initial site of involvement. However, viable organisms may be present in these nodules and remain dormant for years to life.

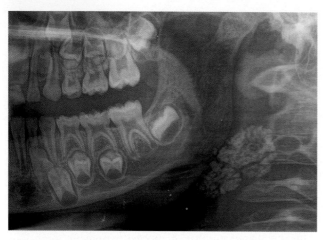

• **Fig. 5.19 Atypical Mycobacterial Infection.** Multiple matted and calcified left cervical lymph nodes noted posterior to the angle of the mandible. (Courtesy of Dr. Matt Dahar.)

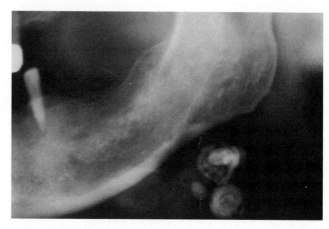

• **Fig. 5.20 Tuberculosis (TB).** Multiple calcified cervical lymph nodes.

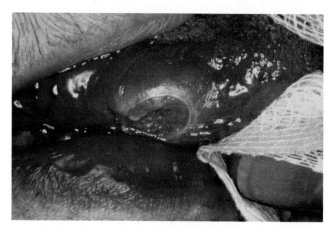

• **Fig. 5.21 Tuberculosis (TB).** Chronic mucosal ulceration of the ventral surface of the tongue on the right side. (Reprinted with permission from the American Dental Association.)

Only about 5%–10% of patients with TB progress from infection to active disease, and an existing state of immunosuppression often is responsible. In rare instances, active TB may ensue directly from the primary infection. However, active disease usually develops later in life from a reactivation of organisms in a previously infected person. This reactivation is typically associated with compromised host defenses and is called **secondary tuberculosis.** Diffuse dissemination through the vascular system may occur and often produces multiple small foci of infection that grossly and radiographically resemble millet seeds, resulting in the nickname, **miliary tuberculosis.** Secondary TB often is associated with immunosuppressive medications, diabetes, old age, poverty, and crowded living conditions. AIDS represents one of the strongest known risk factors for progression from infection to disease.

Clinical and Radiographic Features

Primary TB usually is asymptomatic. Occasionally, fever and pleural effusion may occur.

Classically, the lesions of secondary TB occur in the apex of the lungs but may spread to many different sites by expectorated infected material or through the lymphatic or vascular channels. Typically, patients have a low-grade fever, malaise, anorexia, weight loss, and night sweats. With pulmonary progression, a productive cough develops, often with hemoptysis or chest pain. Progressive TB may lead to a wasting syndrome that, in the past, was termed **consumption,** because it appeared that the patient's body was being consumed or destroyed.

Extrapulmonary TB is seen and represents an increasing proportion of the currently diagnosed cases. In patients with AIDS, more than 50% will have extrapulmonary lesions. Any organ system may be involved, including the lymphatic system, skin, skeletal system, CNS, kidneys, and gastrointestinal tract. Involvement of the skin may develop and has been called **lupus vulgaris.**

Head and neck involvement may occur. The most common extrapulmonary sites in the head and neck are the cervical lymph nodes followed by the larynx and middle ear. On occasion, calcification of involved cervical lymph nodes may lead to an unexpected diagnosis of tuberculosis (Fig. 5.20). Much less common sites include the nasal cavity, nasopharynx, oral cavity, parotid gland, esophagus, and spine.

Oral lesions of TB are uncommon. The most common presentations for oral involvement are chronic ulcerations or swellings (Fig. 5.21). Less frequent findings include nonhealing extraction sockets, areas of mucosal granularity, or diffuse zones of inflammation (Fig. 5.22). Chronic tongue ulcerations are seen most frequently and followed closely in prevalence by mandibular swellings associated with intrabony involvement. Other affected sites in order of decreasing frequency include the gingiva, lips, buccal mucosa, soft palate, and hard palate.

Often oral ulcerative lesions of TB coexist with palpable lymph nodes. Although this combination most strongly suggests squamous cell carcinoma, the possibility of TB also must be considered, especially in younger patients and those who reside in geographic areas with a high prevalence of the infection.

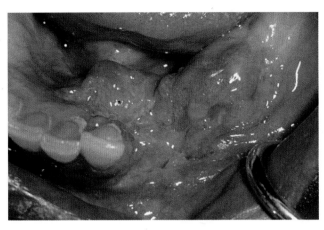

• **Fig. 5.22 Tuberculosis (TB).** Area of granularity and ulceration of the lower alveolar ridge and floor of mouth. (Courtesy of Dr. Brian Blocher.)

Most of the oral lesions represent secondary infection from the initial pulmonary foci, occurring most frequently in middle-aged adults. It is unclear whether these lesions develop from hematogenous spread or from exposure to infected sputum. The reported prevalence of clinically evident oral lesions varies from 0.5% to 5.0%. The discovery of pulmonary TB because of the investigation of oral lesions occurs but is unusual. Primary oral TB without pulmonary involvement is rare and is more common in children and adolescents.

Nontuberculous mycobacterial infections from contaminated milk currently are rare in the industrialized world because of pasteurization of milk, as well as rapid identification and elimination of infected cows. Drinking contaminated milk can result in a form of mycobacterial infection known as **scrofula.** Scrofula is characterized by enlargement of the oropharyngeal lymphoid tissues and cervical lymph nodes (Fig. 5.23). On occasion, the involved nodes may develop significant caseous necrosis and form numerous sinus tracts through the overlying skin (Fig. 5.24). In addition, areas of nodal involvement may radiographically appear as calcified lymph nodes that may be confused with sialoliths. Pulmonary involvement is unusual in patients with scrofula.

Histopathologic Features

The cell-mediated hypersensitivity reaction is responsible for the classic histopathologic presentation of TB. Areas of infection demonstrate the formation of granulomas, which are circumscribed collections of epithelioid histiocytes, lymphocytes, and multinucleated giant cells, often with central caseous necrosis (Fig. 5.25). The nuclei of the giant cells frequently are arranged along the periphery of the cell in a horseshoe or ring shape *(Langhans giant cells).* In a person with TB, one of these granulomas is called a **tubercle.** Special stains, such as the Ziehl-Neelsen or other acid-fast stains, are utilized to demonstrate the mycobacteria (Fig. 5.26). A newer technique, fluorescence microscopy of auramine-rhodamine stains, is employed by many institutions to increase the ease of finding the organisms. Because of the

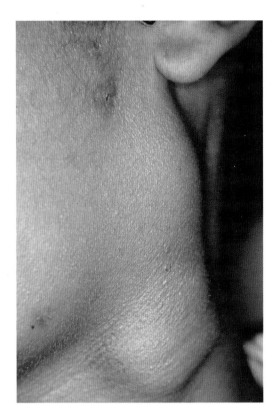

• **Fig. 5.23 Tuberculosis (TB).** Enlargement of numerous cervical lymph nodes. (Courtesy of Dr. George Blozis.)

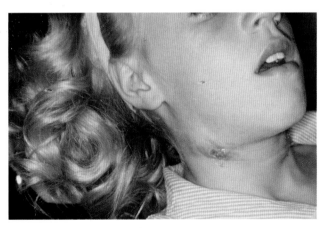

• **Fig. 5.24 Tuberculosis (TB).** Submandibular sinus tract secondary to involvement of underlying cervical lymph nodes.

relative scarcity of the organisms within tissue, the special stains successfully demonstrate the organism in only 27%–60% of cases. Therefore, a negative result does not completely rule out the possibility of TB.

Diagnosis

Approximately 2–4 weeks after initial exposure, a cell-mediated hypersensitivity reaction to tubercular antigens develops. This reaction is the basis for the purified protein derivative (PPD) skin test (i.e., tuberculin skin test), which uses a filtered precipitate of heat-sterilized broth cultures of

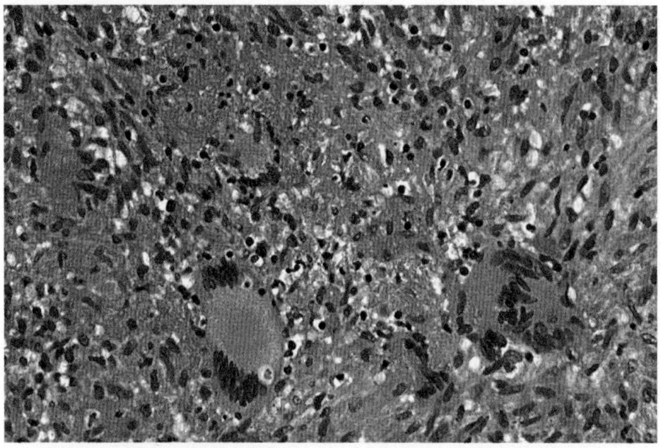

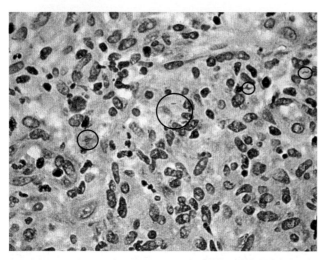

• **Fig. 5.25 Tuberculosis (TB).** Histopathologic presentation of the same lesion depicted in Fig. 5.22. Sheets of histiocytes are intermixed with multinucleated giant cells and areas of necrosis.

• **Fig. 5.26 Tuberculosis (TB).** Acid-fast stain of specimen depicted in Fig. 5.25 exhibiting scattered mycobacterial organisms presenting as small red rods.

M. tuberculosis. Positivity runs as high as 80% in developing nations; only 5%–10% of the population in the United States is positive. A positive tuberculin skin test result indicates exposure to the organism and does not distinguish infection from active disease. A negative tuberculin skin test result does not totally rule out the possibility of TB. False-negative reactions have been documented in older adults; the immunocompromised; patients with sarcoidosis, measles, or Hodgkin lymphoma; and when the antigen was placed intradermally. The false-negative rate may be as high as 66% in patients with AIDS.

In many areas, the skin test is being replaced with an interferon-gamma release assay (IGRA). This blood test provides results within 24 hours and does not require a second patient visit. In addition, the bacillus Calmette-Guérin vaccination does not cause a false-positive reaction as seen with the skin test.

Special mycobacterial stains and culture of infected sputum or tissue must be used to confirm the diagnosis of active disease. Even if detected with special stains, identification of the organism by culture is appropriate. This identification is important because some forms of nontuberculous mycobacteria have a high level of resistance to traditional antituberculous therapy and frequently require surgical excision. Because 2–6 weeks may be required to identify the organism in culture, antituberculous therapy often is initiated before definitive classification.

In order to reduce the time needed for confirmation of the diagnosis of tuberculosis, nucleic acid amplification tests (NAAT) have been developed to detect DNA of the mycobacterium much faster than the 2–6 weeks required for culture. In 2013, the FDA approved a revolutionary NAAT, the Xpert MTB/RIF assay that simultaneously detects the mycobacterium and determines its resistance to rifampin (a predictor of multidrug-resistant tuberculosis) in less than 2 hours.

Treatment and Prognosis

M. tuberculosis can mutate and develop resistance to single-agent medications. To combat this ability, multiagent therapy is the treatment of choice for an active infection, and treatment usually involves two or more active drugs for several months to years. A frequently used protocol consists of an 8-week course of pyrazinamide, isoniazid, rifampin, and ethambutol, followed by a 16-week course of isoniazid and rifampin. With an alteration of doses and the administration schedule, the response to therapy in patients with AIDS has been good, but relapses and progression of infection have been seen.

A different protocol termed *chemoprophylaxis* is used for patients who have a positive PPD skin test but no signs or symptoms of active disease. Although this situation does not mandate therapy, several investigators have demonstrated the value of therapy, especially in young individuals.

◆ LEPROSY (HANSEN DISEASE)

Leprosy is a chronic infectious disease produced by *Mycobacterium leprae*. Because of worldwide efforts coordinated by the World Health Organization (WHO), a dramatic decrease in the prevalence of leprosy has been seen over the past 20 years. In a 2014 review by the Centers for Disease Control and Prevention, a 17% decrease of new diagnoses was seen in the United States during 1994–2011. As seen with tuberculosis, over 70% of the cases arose in foreign-born persons, a rate 14 times higher than the rate of infection noted among U.S.-born individuals. Although immigrants are screened for clinical evidence of infection at the time of their admission into the United States, only 18% reported having symptoms prior to their arrival. In addition, individuals who did not apply for permanent residency and those who arrived without authorization do not undergo clinical screening. Despite the worldwide reduction in the prevalence of the infection, leprosy remains a public health problem in many areas of the world. Currently, most reported cases are noted in five countries: India, Brazil, Mozambique, Nepal, and Madagascar.

The organism has a low infectivity, and exposure rarely results in clinical disease. Small endemic areas of infection are present in Louisiana and Texas, but most patients in the United States have been infected abroad. Many believe that the organism requires a cool host body temperature for survival. Although the exact route of transmission is not known, the high number of organisms in nasal secretions suggests that in some cases the initial site of infection may be the nasal or oropharyngeal mucosa. Although humans are considered the major host, other animals (e.g., armadillo, chimpanzee, and mangabey monkey) may be additional possible reservoirs of infection.

For decades, leprologists have believed the bacillus is highly temperature dependent and produces lesions primarily in cooler parts of the body, such as the skin, nasal cavity, and palate. This concept has been questioned because the organism may be seen in significant numbers at sites of core body temperature, such as the liver and spleen. Recently, one investigator mapped common sites of oral involvement and compared this pattern to a map of the local temperature. This comparison demonstrated that the oral lesions tend to occur more frequently in the areas of the mouth with a lower surface temperature. The temperature-dependent theory of leprosy infection remains an area of interest and controversy.

The clinical manifestations appear to correlate with the immune response of the host to the mycobacterium, resulting in variability of disease severity and two main clinical presentations. The first, called **tuberculoid leprosy,** develops in patients with a high immune reaction. Typically, the organisms are not found in skin biopsy specimens, skin test results to heat-killed organisms (lepromin) are positive, and the disease usually is localized. The second form, **lepromatous leprosy,** is seen in patients who demonstrate a reduced cell-mediated immune response. These patients exhibit numerous organisms in the tissue, do not respond to lepromin skin tests, and exhibit diffuse disease. Many patients present with intermediate disease that can be divided into three subgroups: borderline-tuberculoid, borderline-borderline, and borderline-lepromatous. Active disease progresses through stages of invasion, proliferation, ulceration, and resolution with fibrosis. The incubation period is prolonged, with an average of 2–5 years for the tuberculoid type and 8–12 years for the lepromatous variant.

Clinical Features

Because laboratory services such as skin smears often are not available, patients increasingly are being classified on clinical grounds using the number of lesions (primarily skin) and the number of body areas affected.

Tuberculoid leprosy exhibits a small number of well-circumscribed, hypopigmented skin lesions. Nerve involvement usually results in anesthesia of the affected skin, often accompanied by a loss of sweating. Oral lesions are rare in this variant.

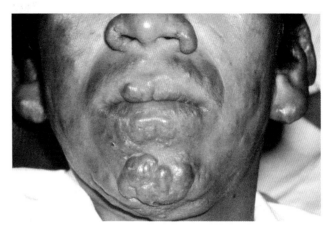

• **Fig. 5.27 Lepromatous Leprosy.** Numerous thickened facial nodules.

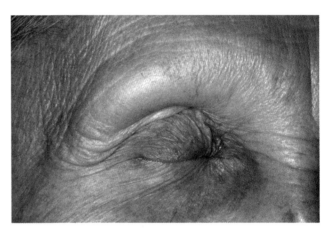

• **Fig. 5.28 Lepromatous Leprosy.** Loss of eyebrows and eyelashes.

Lepromatous leprosy begins slowly with numerous, ill-defined, hypopigmented macules or papules on the skin that, with time, become thickened (Fig. 5.27). The face is a common site of involvement, and the skin enlargements can lead to a distorted facial appearance **(leonine facies).** Hair, including the eyebrows and lashes, often is lost (Fig. 5.28). Nerve involvement leads to a loss of sweating and decreased light touch, pain, and temperature sensors. This sensory loss begins in the extremities and spreads to most of the body. Nasal involvement results in nosebleeds, stuffiness, and a loss of the sense of smell. The hard tissue of the floor, septum, and bridge of the nose may be affected. Collapse of the bridge of the nose is considered pathognomonic.

The reported prevalence of oral lesion varies from a complete absence of lesions to 60%. Several authors believe many reports document an artificially high frequency of oral lesions due to a failure to prove an association with the infection. Well-documented oral lesions occur predominantly in lepromatous leprosy and are rare in the tuberculoid and borderline variants.

The WHO mapped the frequency and distribution of oral lesions in leprosy patients. The sites that are cooled by the passage of air appear to be affected most frequently. The locations affected in order of frequency are the hard palate, soft palate, facial maxillary gingiva, tongue, lips, palatal gingiva, mandibular gingiva, and buccal mucosa. Affected soft tissue initially appears as yellowish to red, sessile, firm, enlarging papules that develop ulceration and necrosis, followed by attempted healing by secondary intention. Continuous infection of an area can lead to significant scarring and loss of tissue. Complete loss of the uvula and fixation of the soft palate may occur. The lingual lesions appear primarily in the anterior third and often begin as areas of erosion, which may develop into large nodules. Infection of the lip can result in significant macrocheilia, which can be confused clinically and microscopically with cheilitis granulomatosa (see page 330).

Direct infiltration of the inflammatory process associated with lepromatous leprosy can destroy the bone underlying the areas of soft tissue involvement. Often the infection creates a unique pattern of facial destruction that has been termed **facies leprosa** and demonstrates a triad of lesions consisting of atrophy of the anterior nasal spine, atrophy of the anterior maxillary alveolar ridge, and endonasal inflammatory changes. Involvement of the anterior maxilla can result in significant bone erosion with loss of the teeth in this area. Maxillary involvement in children can affect the developing teeth and produce enamel hypoplasia and short tapering roots. Dental pulp infection can lead to internal resorption or pulpal necrosis. Teeth with pulpal involvement may demonstrate a clinically obvious red discoloration of the crown. The cause of the discoloration is unknown but appears to be related to intrapulpal vascular damage secondary to the infection. Granulomatous involvement of the nasal cavity can erode through the palatal tissues and result in perforation.

Involvement of peripheral nerves is common, with leprosy considered one of the most common causes of treatable peripheral neuropathy in the world. The facial and trigeminal nerves can be involved with the infectious process. Facial paralysis may be unilateral or bilateral. Sensory deficits may affect any branch of the trigeminal nerve, but the maxillary division is the most commonly affected. In addition to sensory deficits, reports of disease-related orofacial pain may be confused with temporomandibular joint discomfort or tooth-related pain.

Histopathologic Features

Biopsy specimens of tuberculoid leprosy typically reveal granulomatous inflammation with well-formed clusters of epithelioid histiocytes, lymphocytes, and multinucleated giant cells (Fig. 5.29). A paucity of organisms exists; when present, they can be demonstrated only when stained with acid-fast stains, such as the Fite method. Lepromatous leprosy demonstrates no well-formed granulomas; the typical finding is sheets of lymphocytes intermixed with vacuolated histiocytes known as **lepra cells** (Fig. 5.30). Unlike tuberculoid leprosy, an abundance of organisms can be demonstrated with acid-fast stains in the lepromatous variant (Fig. 5.31). It has been reported that the organism can be found with special stains in 100% of lepromatous leprosy cases, 75% of borderline cases, and only 5% of tuberculoid cases.

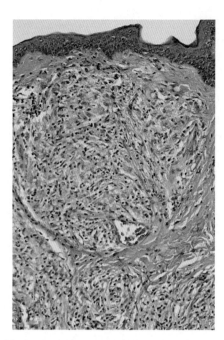

• **Fig. 5.29 Paucibacillary Leprosy.** Well-formed granulomatous inflammation demonstrating clusters of lymphocytes and histiocytes.

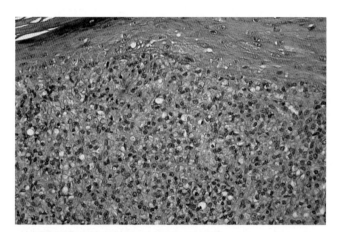

• **Fig. 5.30 Multibacillary Leprosy.** Sheets of lymphocytes and histiocytes exhibiting scattered vacuolated lepra cells.

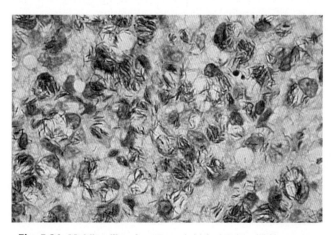

• **Fig. 5.31 Multibacillary Leprosy.** Acid-fast stain exhibiting numerous small mycobacterial organisms seen individually and in clusters.

Diagnosis

The definitive diagnosis is based on the clinical presentation and supported by the demonstration of acid-fast organisms on a smear or in the tissue. The diagnosis is complicated by the failure to demonstrate the organism in a slit-skin smear in almost 70% of all leprosy patients. In addition, the organism cannot be cultivated on artificial media. The search is ongoing to develop an accurate diagnostic test for leprosy, but none has been found that demonstrates the needed sensitivity and specificity to warrant widespread use.

Treatment and Prognosis

For therapeutic purposes, the WHO has developed a simple classification system based on the bacterial index noted upon biopsy. Those with an index less than 2+ are termed **paucibacillary,** whereas those greater than 2+ are designated **multibacillary.** Paucibacillary patients present clinically as tuberculoid or borderline-tuberculoid variants; multibacillary patients include borderline-borderline, borderline-lepromatous, and lepromatous variants. Patients with multibacillary leprosy receive a combination of rifampicin, clofazimine, and dapsone, whereas those presenting with paucibacillary leprosy receive rifampicin and dapsone. Use of dapsone or rifampicin alone has resulted in development of resistance to that respective drug. Since the introduction of multidrug therapy in 1981, an estimated 15 million patients have been cured, and disabilities have been prevented in another 2–3 million individuals. One of the major reasons for the decreasing prevalence of leprosy is the provision of an uninterrupted supply of free, high-quality medications in calendar blister packs to all patients regardless of the living conditions or remoteness of the location.

◆ NOMA (CANCRUM ORIS; OROFACIAL GANGRENE; GANGRENOUS STOMATITIS; NECROTIZING STOMATITIS)

The term **noma** is derived from the Greek word *nomein,* meaning *to devour.* Noma is a rapidly progressive, polymicrobial, opportunistic infection caused by components of the normal oral flora that become pathogenic during periods of compromised immune status. Historically, the process has been associated with organisms such as *Borrelia vincentii* and *Bacillus fusiformis,* but more recently, many believe the process may not be related to one or more aggressive bacteria but to a more diverse change in the oral microbiota. Some investigators have demonstrated a reduction of bacteria such as *Capnocytophaga* and *Fusobacteria* genera with an increased number of other organisms. *Prevotella intermedia* and *Peptostreptococcus* are thought by many to be key players, interacting with a variety of other bacterial organisms. Culture is thought to underestimate the variety of organisms involved due to the difficulties in growing many of these fastidious bacteria. Studies utilizing PCR for bacterial gene sequences

have failed to identify a specific causative organism because the plausible bacteria were noted in both affected and healthy subjects.

The reported predisposing factors include the following:
- Poverty
- Malnutrition or dehydration
- Poor oral hygiene
- Poor sanitation
- Unsafe drinking water
- Proximity to unkempt livestock
- Recent illness
- Malignancy
- An immunodeficiency disorder, including AIDS

In many cases a recent debilitating illness appears to set the stage for the development of noma. Measles most frequently precedes development of noma; other common but less frequent predisposing illnesses include herpes simplex, varicella, scarlet fever, malaria, typhus, tuberculosis, gastroenteritis, and bronchopneumonia. Cases associated with malignancies (e.g., leukemia) are not rare. In many instances, the infection begins as necrotizing gingivitis (NG) (see page 151), and several investigators believe that noma is merely an extension of the same process. Because the disease usually is well advanced at the time of initial presentation, descriptions of the initial stages of the disease are sketchy.

For centuries, noma was common in Europe and the United States but almost disappeared by the end of the 19th century except for victims in the Nazi concentration camps of World War II and an occasional case related to immunosuppressive conditions, such as HIV infection, severe combined immunodeficiency syndrome, or intense immunosuppressive therapy. Currently, most reported cases arise in the *"noma belt"* of sub-Saharan Africa that extends from Senegal to Ethiopia. The World Health Organization (WHO) estimates the global yearly incidence to be approximately 140,000. This number is thought by many to be a gross underestimation, because it is thought that fewer than 15% of acute cases present for therapy.

Clinical Features

Noma usually arises in children from 1 to 10 years of age, although it also can occur in adults with a major debilitating disease (e.g., diabetes mellitus, leukemia, lymphoma, or HIV infection). The infection often begins on the gingiva as necrotizing gingivitis, which may extend either facially or lingually to involve the adjacent soft tissue and form areas called **necrotizing mucositis.** Zones of necrosis also may develop in soft tissue not contiguous with the gingiva, particularly in areas of trauma (Fig. 5.32). The necrosis can extend into deeper tissues; over the next few days, zones of blue-black discoloration of the overlying skin surface may develop (Fig. 5.33). Often the necrotic zone is cone shaped, with a small point of cutaneous necrosis overlying a larger zone of oral mucosal destruction. Unlike other infections, the process does not follow tissue planes and

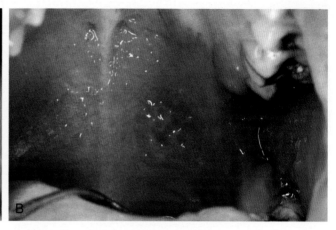

• **Fig. 5.32 Necrotizing Mucositis. A,** Large area of soft tissue necrosis of the posterior soft palate on the left side. **B,** Healing site of necrotizing mucositis 6 days after initiation of tetracycline therapy.

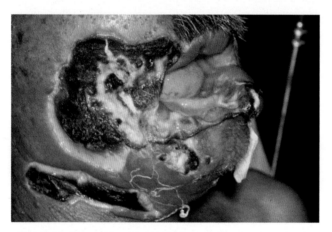

• **Fig. 5.33 Noma.** Extensive blackish orofacial necrosis of the right cheek in an immunocompromised patient.

tends to spread through anatomic barriers, such as muscle. These discolored zones break down into areas of yellowish necrosis that also frequently spreads into adjacent bone, with large areas of osteomyelitis possible. In most instances, the necrotic area is well defined and unilateral. Fetid odor, significant pain, fever, malaise, tachycardia, increased respiratory rate, anemia, leukocytosis, and regional lymphadenopathy are typical. Additional lesions also may occur in distant sites, such as the scalp, neck, ear, shoulders, chest, perineum, and vulva.

Treatment and Prognosis

In addition to using appropriate antibiotics to treat noma, the clinician must direct therapeutic attention not only to local wound care but also toward improving the patient's overall health status. Blood transfusion with intravenous fluids to correct dehydration and electrolyte imbalances is necessary along with a high protein diet and resolution of any associated disease such as malaria or measles. Ampicillin-cloxacillin and metronidazole are the first-line therapeutic antibiotics for necrotizing stomatitis. Conservative

débridement of gross necrotic areas is recommended, but aggressive removal is contraindicated because it does not stop the extension of the process and compounds the reconstruction problems.

Most affected children in developing countries have no access to quality health care and demonstrate a mortality rate of 85% due to lack of appropriate intervention. With quality health care, the survival is greater than 90%. Common causes of death include infectious complications, such as pneumonia, diarrhea, and septicemia. Most survivors will have extensive facial deformity with associated difficulties in growth and development, eating, speech, and social interactions. Reconstruction often is extremely challenging and should be delayed until healing is complete. Eradication of this disease is a major humanitarian concern that will require action from national and international organizations to eliminate the underlying extreme poverty, malnutrition, lack of immunizations, poor hygiene, inadequate sanitation, and insufficient oral health care.

◆ ACTINOMYCOSIS

Although the term **actinomycosis** seems to imply a fungal infection, it is an infection of filamentous, branching, gram-positive anaerobic bacteria. Actinomycetes are normal saprophytic components of the oral flora. Documented sites of colonization in healthy patients include the tonsillar crypts, dental plaque and calculus, carious dentin, bone sequestra, salivary calculi, gingival sulci, and periodontal pockets. The colonies within the tonsillar crypts may form plugs and become large enough for the patient to feel the firm masses of bacteria and desquamated keratin within the crypts (see page 176). In surveys of documented actinomycosis, *Actinomyces israelii* is the causative organism in the majority, with *A. viscosus* being a close second. Much less frequent causes of the infection are *A. naeslundii, A. odontolyticus, A. meyeri, A. pyogenes, A. viscosus,* and *A. bovis,* along with *Arachnia propionica* and *Bifidobacterium dentium.* In most such cases, the primary organism is combined synergistically with streptococci and staphylococci.

Clinical Features

Actinomycosis may be either an acute, rapidly progressing infection or a chronic, slowly spreading lesion that is associated with fibrosis. Approximately 55% of cases of actinomycosis are diagnosed in the cervicofacial region, with 25% occurring in the abdominal and pelvic region and 15% in the pulmonary system. The remaining 5% exhibits a variety of patterns, such as superficial skin infections, or infections of the genitourinary region (often linked to use of intrauterine contraceptive devices).

The suppurative reaction of the infection may discharge large yellowish flecks that represent colonies of the bacteria called **sulfur granules.** Although common, sulfur granules are not present invariably. In addition, another infection that also can produce sulfur granules and mimic actinomycosis is **botryomycosis,** an unrelated process that represents an unusual host reaction to *S. aureus* and other bacteria.

In the cervicofacial region, the organism typically enters tissue through an area of prior trauma, such as a soft tissue injury, periodontal pocket, nonvital tooth, extraction socket, or infected tonsil. The infection does not spread along the typical fascial planes and usually disregards the normal lymphatic and vascular routes. Direct extension through soft tissue is seen, and lymph nodes become involved only if they are in the path of the process. The classic description is of a "wooden" indurated area of fibrosis, which ultimately forms a central, softer area of abscess. The infection may extend to the surface, forming a sinus tract (Fig. 5.34). Pain often is minimal. The soft tissues of the submandibular, submental, and cheek areas are common areas of involvement, with the area overlying the angle of the mandible being the most frequently affected site.

Localized abscesses without the associated chronic fibrosing reaction have been reported in soft tissue that has received minor trauma. The tongue is the most frequently mentioned site, but any oral mucosal location is possible. Involvement of the tonsillar crypts may produce infectious symptoms; in most cases, however, the primary change is one of variable hyperplasia. Tonsillar hyperplasia thought

to be secondary to actinomycotic infestation of the crypts does not appear responsive to antibiotics, probably because of the superficial location of the bacterial colonies. Tonsillectomy is generally the most effective treatment for this situation.

Salivary gland involvement also is not unusual. Intraductal colonization by the organism may lead to infections in both the submandibular and parotid glands, resulting in abscess formation in the submandibular and masseter spaces, respectively. In addition, more localized infections occur in minor salivary gland ducts, which also may demonstrate mucous plugs or sialoliths.

Actinomycotic osteomyelitis of the mandible and maxilla has been reported. Trauma, periodontal infections, nonvital teeth, and extraction sites have all provided access. Ill-defined areas of radiolucency, often surrounded by radiopacity are noted on plain films. In cases examined by computed tomography or magnetic resonance imaging, an ill-defined and infiltrative lesion typically is present with a surrounding soft tissue inflammatory response that often extends to the skin. Sinus tract formation and intralesional gas are common, whereas lymphadenopathy usually is not noted (the organism spreads by direct invasion, not by the lymphatics).

Intrabony colonization of dentigerous cysts without other significant clinical or radiographic spread has been reported. Periapical inflammatory lesions involved by the bacteria can result in lesions that are difficult to resolve with standard endodontic treatment, but such lesions typically remain localized and do not evolve into invasive cervicofacial actinomycosis. In a retrospective review of a series of radicular cysts, the presence of actinomycotic colonies was not uncommon, but this finding usually was not associated with any clinical evidence of suppuration, abscess formation or draining sinus tracts. In such localized colonization with or without a focal inflammatory reaction, the investigators suggested the colonies may not have substantial clinical significance when there are no associated signs or symptoms.

Histopathologic Features

The tissue removed from areas of active infection demonstrates a peripheral band of fibrosis encasing a zone of chronically inflamed granulation tissue surrounding large collections of polymorphonuclear leukocytes and, with luck, colonies of organisms (Fig. 5.35). The colonies consist of club-shaped filaments that form a radiating rosette pattern (Fig. 5.36). With hematoxylin and eosin (H&E) stains, the central core stains basophilic and the peripheral portion is eosinophilic. Methenamine silver stains demonstrate the organisms well. If the colonies of actinomycetes become displaced from the exudate, then a rim of neutrophils typically clings to the periphery of the organisms. The histopathologic pattern in which masses of actinomycotic organisms are surrounded by a sea of neutrophils is known as the Splendore-Hoeppli phenomenon. When an actinomycotic infection is not spreading but remains localized within soft tissue, small

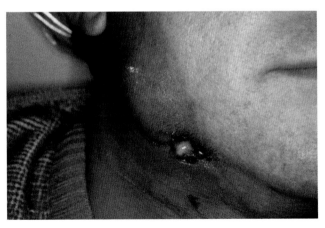

• **Fig. 5.34 Actinomycosis.** Draining sinus tract of the right submandibular area.

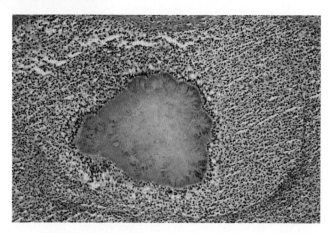

• **Fig. 5.35 Actinomycosis.** Colony of actinomycotic organisms surrounded by polymorphonuclear leukocytes.

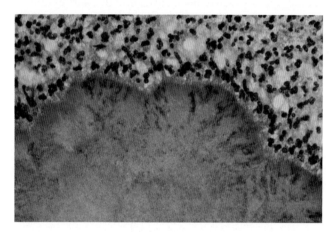

• **Fig. 5.36 Actinomycosis.** Actinomycotic colony exhibiting club-shaped filaments arranged in a radiating rosette pattern.

clusters of branching filamentous organisms often are surrounded by a thin rim of neutrophils that is encased in a thick band of granulomatous inflammation.

Diagnosis

The diagnosis of actinomycosis is achieved ideally by culture, but less than 50% of cases are positive because of the overgrowth of associated bacteria, prior antibiotic therapy, or improper anaerobic media conditions. Although a strong presumptive diagnosis can be obtained through a demonstration of the typical colonies in lesional biopsy material, molecular techniques such as PCR or DNA hybridization have been used to identify the bacterial species, with some of these techniques available for paraffin-embedded specimens. The material for culture and histopathologic examination typically is obtained during surgical exploration, with fine-needle aspiration being a satisfactory substitute in many cases. Sulfur granules in infections other than actinomycosis are so rare that their demonstration strongly supports the diagnosis. If desired, then fluorescein-conjugated antiserum can be used on the granules to specifically identify the *Actinomyces* species.

Treatment and Prognosis

The treatment of choice for actinomycosis in chronic fibrosing cases is prolonged high doses of antibiotics in association with abscess drainage and excision of the sinus tracts. A high antibiotic concentration is required to penetrate larger areas of suppuration and fibrosis. Although penicillin remains the standard of care with no documented *in vivo* resistance, some clinicians believe amoxicillin represents a better first-choice antibiotic. Other investigators have demonstrated *in vitro* resistance to penicillin and recommend tetracycline, which is as effective as penicillin and is the drug of choice for patients with a known allergy to penicillin. Early cervicofacial actinomycosis typically responds to a 5–6-week course of penicillin; patients with deep-seated infections may require up to 12 months.

In cases of osteomyelitis caused by actinomycetes, antibiotic therapy alone often is associated with persistent disease. Adequate débridement appears to be the cornerstone of therapy and ultimately determines the success of the subsequent antibiotic treatment. When combined with appropriate surgery, a 3-month course of penicillin usually is curative. In resistant cases, repeated débridement should be combined with cultures to direct future antibiotic therapy. Care should be taken to ensure that colonization of bony sequestra by actinomycotic colonies is not mistaken for invasive actinomycotic osteomyelitis.

Several authors have indicated that localized acute actinomycotic infections may be treated more conservatively than the deep, chronic cases of actinomycosis. Localized periapical and pericoronal actinomycosis, tongue abscesses, and focal subacute sialadenitis with intraductal involvement frequently respond well to surgical removal of infected tissue. It appears best to reserve antibiotics for patients in whom the microorganisms invade the surrounding structures and spread through the soft tissues.

CAT-SCRATCH DISEASE

Cat-scratch disease (CSD) is an infectious disorder that typically begins in the skin but classically spreads to the adjacent lymph nodes. This infection is the most common cause of chronic regional lymphadenopathy in children, with an estimated 24,000 cases occurring annually in the United States. This disease has been recognized since 1931, but the definitive cause was not determined until the 1980s. Isolation and culture of the organism were achieved finally in 1988. The causative organism was named initially *Rochalimaea henselae* but was reclassified as *Bartonella henselae* when the genera *Bartonella* and *Rochalimaea* were combined.

The infection is spread primarily through young kittens infested with the cat flea, *Ctenocephalides felis,* via a cat scratch, cat bite, cat saliva, or cat flea bite. A history of contact with cats has been noted in 90% of the cases, with 60% documenting an associated cat scratch or bite. The highest number of cases are seen between September through March in temperate climates. Kittens typically are born in spring with those under the age of 6 months most at risk of transmitting CSD. Cat fleas are most abundant during fall and winter with the highest risk of feline *B. henselae* bacteremia occurring during the winter. Uncommonly, CSD can arise from other species of *Bartonella* or from other mammal hosts, including dogs. Person-to-person transmission has not been documented.

Clinical Features

Eighty percent of the cases occur in patients younger than 21 years of age. Cat-scratch disease often begins as a papule that develops in 3–14 days along the initial scratch line (Fig. 5.37). The lesion typically progresses through erythematous, vesicular, and papular-crusted stages with resolution usually occurring within 1–3 weeks. About the time the skin lesion heals, lymph node changes arise and may be accompanied by fever or malaise (Fig. 5.38). In about half of the cases, a single node is involved. Multiple regional nodes are affected in about 20%, and nodal enlargement is discovered in multiple sites in about 33%. Suppuration is noted in approximately 10% of affected patients. The most frequently affected nodes are the axillary and epitrochlear (46%), head and neck (26%), and groin (17.5%).

Although most affected patients present with typical cat-scratch disease as described above, a variety of systemic manifestations are noted in 5%–20% of affected individuals, predominantly in older patients or those with immunosuppression. Of these, prolonged fever of unknown origin and hepatosplenic disease are the most common. Less common problems include cardiac, hematologic, neurologic, ocular, orthopedic, and pulmonary manifestations. Although necrotizing granulomas usually are noted in immunocompetent patients, vasoproliferative disorders, such as **bacillary angiomatosis** or **bacillary peliosis hepatis** (a specific form of hepatosplenic *Bartonella* disease) may be seen in immunocompromised patients. Bacillary angiomatosis is an unusual subcutaneous vascular proliferation that has been recognized in patients with AIDS. The affected areas often resemble Kaposi sarcoma (see page 254) and appear as variable

numbers of red-to-purple skin lesions. These may be macular, papular, or pedunculated and exhibit a widespread distribution on the skin. Pain and tenderness are common. The larger lesions are friable and bleed easily.

Histopathologic Features

The involved lymph nodes are enlarged because of significant cortical hyperplasia, which classically contains areas of stellate suppurative necrosis surrounded by a band of histiocytes and neutrophils (Fig. 5.39). Upon Warthin-Starry stains or

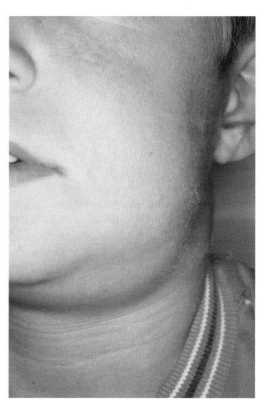

• **Fig. 5.38 Cat-Scratch Disease.** Submandibular lymphadenopathy has developed after initial trivial injury to skin. (Courtesy of Dr. George Blozis.)

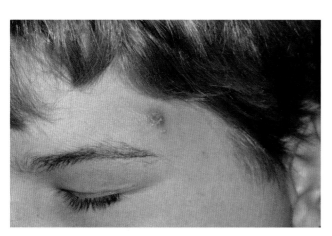

• **Fig. 5.37 Cat-Scratch Disease.** Papule that developed at initial site of injury.

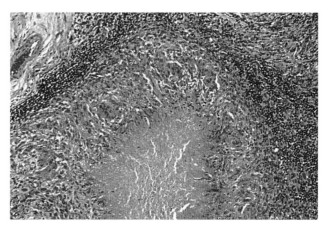

• **Fig. 5.39 Cat-Scratch Disease.** Intranodal area of necrosis surrounded by a band of epithelioid histiocytes and lymphocytes.

the Brown-Hopps method of Gram staining, cat-scratch bacilli may be found in areas without significant necrosis. As the disease progresses and necrosis increases, the organisms become more difficult to identify. A commercially available monoclonal antibody against *B. henselae* has been used to demonstrate the organisms via immunoperoxidase techniques on paraffin-embedded material. Upon immunostaining, the organisms are highlighted dramatically, an important advance over the previous special stains. Polymerase chain reaction (PCR) techniques also can be employed to detect the *Bartonella* DNA in tissue.

Bacillary angiomatosis reveals lobular proliferations of small blood vessels in an edematous to fibrotic stroma. The supporting connective tissue typically demonstrates a significant number of neutrophils and leukocytoclasis, important clues to the diagnosis. Also present are variably sized amphophilic and granular aggregates that upon Warthin-Starry staining prove to be masses of the causative bacteria.

Diagnosis

Today the diagnosis of cat-scratch disease usually is established by a combination of clinical and serologic criteria. Histopathology can confirm the clinical diagnosis but involves an invasive procedure. In patients with a suggestive clinical presentation, the diagnosis often can be confirmed by negative evaluations for other common causes of adenopathy, combined with positive serology. The most widely used tests are an indirect fluorescent assay (IFA) or enzyme-linked immunosorbent assay (ELISA) for detecting antibodies to *B. henselae*. These tests are somewhat problematic due to variable sensitivity and specificity. In addition, the type and titer of the associated antibody significantly impacts on the diagnosis. Even during the early stages of the infection, IgM antibodies against *B. henselae* seldom are present, and a negative result does not rule out CSD. IgG titers less than 1/64 do not support active disease. Titers between 1/64 and 1/256 are indeterminate and require repeated testing with evidence of rising titers to confirm a diagnosis of CSD. IgG titers over 1/256 strongly support a diagnosis of active CSD. If the serology is inconclusive, nodal biopsy can be performed to confirm or refute the diagnosis.

Treatment and Prognosis

Cat-scratch disease is a self-limiting condition and normally resolves within 4 months. The use of local heat, analgesics, and aspiration of the node on suppuration is the typical pattern of therapy. If persistent discomfort makes nodal aspiration necessary, then drainage should be achieved with a needle that is tunneled into the node laterally through normal skin 1–2 cm away from the lesion. Incision directly into the node could result in a chronic draining sinus.

Although the organism has demonstrated sensitivity to several antibiotics in culture, the results in immunocompetent patients have been inconsistent and difficult to evaluate because the disease is self-limited in most cases. In addition, lack of intracellular penetration and sequestration of the antibiotic within lymph nodes may be responsible for lack of effectiveness in patients despite positive results in culture. Antibiotics typically are reserved for those cases that demonstrate a prolonged course or severe involvement. Use of antibiotic drugs in patients with AIDS and bacillary angiomatosis has produced dramatic resolution within 2 days. Although a number of medications often in combination have been used successfully, the primary antibiotics used for cat-scratch disease or bacillary angiomatosis are azithromycin, trimethoprim-sulfamethoxazole, erythromycin, doxycycline, rifampin, ciprofloxacin, and gentamicin.

◆ RHINOSINUSITIS (SINUSITIS)

Rhinosinusitis is one of the most common health complaints in the United States with an associated annual incidence of 20 million doctor visits. To understand the problem, the clinician must first have some knowledge of sinus anatomy. Adults have bilateral maxillary, frontal, sphenoid, ethmoid, and mastoid sinuses. Except for the mastoid sinuses, these cavities drain into the nose through openings called **ostia**. The frontal, sphenoid, and maxillary sinuses must drain through the middle meatus. In addition, the ethmoids are located bilaterally in this area of the nose and present as a labyrinth of 3–15 small sinuses, which drain through smaller ostia. The ostiomeatal complex, with its numerous narrow openings (Fig. 5.40), is the key to sinus disease, because it is the primary nasal site for the deposition of foreign matter from inspired air.

Normal sinuses are lined by pseudostratified columnar epithelium with cilia. The cilia are necessary to move the

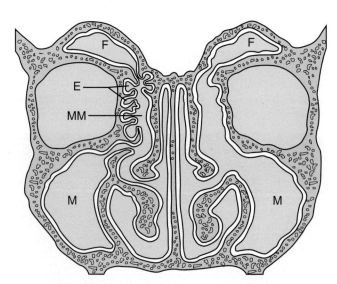

• **Fig. 5.40 The Paranasal Sinuses.** Illustration demonstrating the ostiomeatal complex and its importance to appropriate sinus drainage. The left side demonstrates the typical narrow middle meatus through which all sinus drainage must pass. The right side reveals enlargement of the middle meatus, such as that achieved through corrective endoscopic surgery. *M,* Maxillary sinus; *F,* frontal sinus; *E,* ethmoid sinuses; *MM,* middle meatus.

sinus secretions toward the ostia. Gravity also is beneficial in removing the secretions, except in the maxillary sinus where there is a superior location of the ostial opening and, therefore, the ciliary apparatus becomes even more important.

For a long time, researchers believed that primary inflammation of the lining of the maxillary antrum was the major cause of rhinosinusitis; however, advances have demonstrated that most sinus disease begins from a blockage of the ostiomeatal complex that disrupts normal drainage, decreases ventilation, and precipitates disease. Less common localized sinus infections can occur from focal areas of inflammation within a single sinus, such as a dental infection affecting the maxillary sinus.

Most acute rhinosinusitis cases are viral in origin and arise shortly after an upper respiratory tract infection. In contrast, most examples of chronic rhinosinusitis are bacterial. All the sinuses contain bacteria. With bacteria already present in the sinuses, changes as minor as a slight mucosal thickening in the ostiomeatal complex can lead to improper sinus drainage and infection. The most common predisposing factors for chronic rhinosinusitis are a recent upper respiratory viral infection, allergic rhinitis, or an adjacent odontogenic infection.

Historically, 10%–12% of maxillary rhinosinusitis cases were thought to arise from an odontogenic source, but many current investigators believe the prevalence is closer to 40%. In otherwise healthy patients, the most common bacterial organisms cultured from rhinosinusitis are aerobes such as *Streptococcus pneumoniae, Haemophilus influenzae,* and *Moraxella catarrhalis,* organisms typically unassociated with a dental origin. When rhinosinusitis arises secondary to an odontogenic infection, the causative organisms are usually those that predominate in periodontal or endodontic infections and include anaerobic bacteria, such as *Peptostreptococcus* spp., *Fusobacterium* spp., *Prevotella* spp., *Bacteroides* spp., and *Porphyromonas* spp.

Infrequently, in an environment of chronic rhinosinusitis, an area of dystrophic calcification (**antrolith**) may develop and be detected radiographically. The nidus for this calcification may be endogenous from materials, such as inflamed mucus, pus, or clots. In other cases, the source may be exogenous from tooth roots or foreign bodies, such as dental materials, vegetable matter, paper, glass, and stone. Focal antral calcification also has been seen in sinuses filled with a fungal ball of *Aspergillus fumigatus* (noninvasive mycetoma) (see page 221). A sinus that is unresponsive to therapy and exhibits focal antrolith formation within a diffuse soft tissue opacification is highly suggestive of noninvasive aspergillosis.

Clinical and Radiographic Features

Presenting symptoms of acute rhinosinusitis in adults include headache, fever, and facial pain over the affected sinus. Anorexia, photophobia, and malaise also may be seen. Anterior nasal or posterior pharyngeal discharge is present; it may be thick or thin in consistency and appear clear, mucoid, or purulent. Children, with their less complex sinuses, typically have only persistent cough, fever, and purulent

rhinorrhea. Localized involvement of the maxillary sinus can occur as pain over the cheekbone, toothache, periorbital pain, or temporal headache. Maxillary rhinosinusitis is associated with increased pain when the head is held upright and less discomfort when the patient is supine.

Chronic rhinosinusitis is less diagnostic, and radiographic imaging becomes more important. Frequent complaints include facial pressure, pain, or a sensation of obstruction. In some cases, nonspecific symptoms, such as headache, sore throat, lightheadedness, or generalized fatigue, also may be present or even dominate. Radiographically, the involved sinus has a cloudy, increased density

At times, rhinosinusitis can be confused with an odontogenic infection. In such cases, close examination of periapical radiographs, a thorough periodontal examination, and assessment of tooth vitality often may point to an odontogenic infection. A sinus infection should be strongly considered when patients complain of pain from several teeth, demonstrate tenderness over one or both of the maxillary sinuses, exhibit nasal congestion, or have a nasal discharge accompanied by a fever and headache.

As mentioned previously, up to 40% of maxillary rhinosinusitis cases are related to a dental origin such as tooth extraction, periapical inflammatory disease, advanced periodontitis, or iatrogenic causes such as oroantral fistulas, residual root tips, endodontic filling material, or complications secondary to implant placement or related sinus lift procedures. Odontogenic origin is more likely when unilateral sinus opacification is noted (>75%), and such infections are associated with the molars in more than 90% of the cases. Often, the unilateral opacification is combined with unilateral nasal obstruction, rhinorrhea and/or maxillary tenderness. Foul nasal drainage or extreme mouth odor also are strong clues.

In addition to the patient's symptoms, the diagnosis in the past often was made by procedures (such as, transillumination) and by plain radiographs (such as, periapical radiographs, panoramic images, and the Waters, Caldwell-Luc, lateral, and submental vertex views). Today, when the diagnosis is in question, many clinicians use nasal endoscopy, computed tomography (CT), or cone beam computed tomography (CBCT). Areas of infection and sites of improper drainage will be found. These techniques not only confirm the diagnosis but also pinpoint the primary pathologic alteration that led to the obstructive rhinosinusitis. In cases of odontogenic sinusitis, zones of antral mucosal thickening along the floor of the sinus often are associated with focal areas of bone loss, dehiscence, or foreign bodies adjacent to the offending tooth (Fig. 5.41).

An antrolith appears radiographically as a radiodense focus within the sinus. The calcification often is seen in association with a thickening of the antral lining or diffuse clouding of the affected sinus.

Treatment and Prognosis

Treatment options for acute rhinosinusitis include moisturizing sprays, decongestants, mucolytics, corticosteroids, antibiotics, or mechanical intervention, such as sinus puncture or

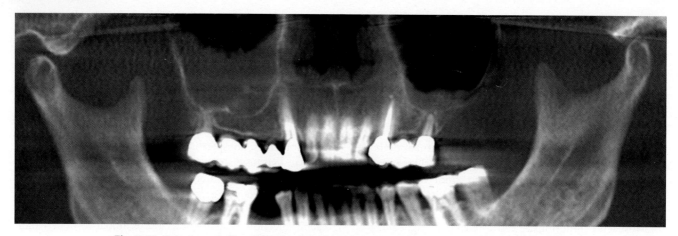

• **Fig. 5.41 Odontogenic Sinusitis.** Cloudy right maxillary antrum. The sinusitis is more noticeable on the patient's right side. However, less mucosal thickening is noted in the left antrum in association with the apices of the second premolar, which demonstrates thickening of the periodontal ligament with focal perforation of the sinus floor.

lavage. Although acute rhinosinusitis is usually a self-limiting disease, antibiotics frequently are prescribed. Most cases are viral in origin and resolve within 2 weeks, with or without antibiotic therapy. A Cochrane meta-analysis demonstrated a small benefit associated with antibiotic therapy, but this appeared to be overshadowed by adverse effects, such as diarrhea, abdominal pain, and vomiting.

If antibiotics are used, the first-line therapy for acute sinusitis in otherwise healthy patients is amoxicillin. Doxycycline or clarithromycin are alternatives for patients allergic to penicillin. If amoxicillin is associated with a poor clinical response, other choices include azithromycin, cefoxitin, ceftriaxone, cephalexin, clindamycin, and moxifloxacin. The choice of antibiotics should be guided by local resistance patterns and by appropriately collected cultures.

In otherwise healthy adult patients, chronic rhinosinusitis that is not responsive to typical medical management often is corrected surgically. When located in the maxillary sinus, such invasive therapy should be performed only after a thorough examination to rule out an association with an adjacent odontogenic infection.

Nasal endoscopy has shown that rhinosinusitis is a disease of obstruction, and that mucosal inflammation is usually a secondary development. Functional endoscopic sinus surgery (FESS) removes damaged antral mucosa, enlarges the ostial openings, and corrects blockages in the ostiomeatal complex, often with a rapid resolution of the signs and symptoms (see Fig. 5.38). The surgery is delicate because it extends close to the orbit and the CNS. Each patient's unique anatomy should be evaluated carefully by CT and nasal endoscopy before surgery.

Appropriate diagnosis of odontogenic sinusitis is critical due to several differences in the therapeutic approach. The maxillary sinus does not drain by gravity, because the ostia are located superior to the sinus floor. Healthy cilia must beat in a coordinated fashion to move the mucus up and through the ostia to clear the sinus cavity. It has been shown that impaired function of the ciliary epithelium is present in odontogenic sinusitis. This finding helps to explain why resolution of the dental inflammatory source often fails to resolve the process without medical therapy and FESS to eliminate the causative bacteria, remove the damaged mucosa, and restore proper cilia function. Due to differences in the bacteria involved in odontogenic sinusitis, the first-line antibiotic regimen is amoxicillin-clavulanate; levofloxacin, teicoplanin, or vancomycin is recommended for cases resistant to therapy. Doxycycline is the best choice for patients who are allergic to the penicillins. Although serious complications related to odontogenic sinusitis are rare, the infection can spread and result in pansinusitis, osteomyelitis, meningitis, blindness, and intracranial extension.

Bibliography

Streptococcal Infections (Impetigo, Erysipelas, Streptococcal Pharyngitis, Tonsillitis, and Scarlet Fever)

Bennett J, Moreland NJ, Oliver J, et al.: Understanding group A streptococcal pharyngitis and skin infections as causes of rheumatic fever: protocol for a prospective disease incidence study, *BMC Infect Dis* 19:633, 2019. https://doi.org/10.1186/s12879-019-4126-9.

Bialecki C, Feder HM, Grant-Kels JM: The six classic childhood exanthems: a review and update, *J Am Acad Dermatol* 21:891–903, 1989.

Bonnetblanc J-M, Bédane C: Erysipelas: recognition and management, *Am J Clin Dermatol* 4:157–163, 2003.

Drug and Therapeutics Bulletin: Managing scarlet fever, *BMJ* 362: k3005, 2018. https://doi.org/10.1136/bmj.k3005.

Galli L, Venturini E, Bassi A, et al.: Common community-acquired bacterial skin and soft-tissue infections in children: an intersociety consensus on impetigo, abscess, and cellulitis treatment, *Clin Ther* 41:532–551, 2019.

Giunta JL: Comparison of erysipelas and odontogenic cellulitis, *J Endod* 13:291–294, 1987.

Krasagakis K, Valachis A, Maniatakis P, et al.: Analysis of epidemiology, clinical features and management of erysipelas, *Int J Dermatol* 49:1012–1017, 2010.

Lamagni T, Guy R, Chand M, et al.: Resurgence of scarlet fever in England, 2014-16: a population-based surveillance study, *Lancet Infect Dis* 18:180–187, 2018.

Linke M, Booken N: Risk factors associated with a reduced response in the treatment of erysipelas, *J Dtsch Dermatol Ges* 13:217–225, 2015.

Luo R, Sickler J, Vahidnia F, et al.: Diagnosis and management of group A streptococcal pharyngitis in the United States, 2011-15, *BMC Infect Dis* 19:193, 2019. https://doi.org/10.1186/s12879-01903835-4.

Pavlotsky F, Amrani S, Trau H: Recurrent erysipelas: risk factors, *J Dtsch Dermatol Ges* 2:89–95, 2004.

Schachner L, Andriessen A, Bhatia N, et al.: Topical ozenoxacin cream 1% for impetigo: a review, *J Drugs Dermatol* 18:655–661, 2019.

Vazquez MN, Sanders JE: Diagnosis and management of group A streptococcal pharyngitis and associated complications, *Pediatr Emerg Med Pract* 14:1–20, 2017.

Tonsillar Plugs and Tonsillolithiasis

Chang CY, Thrasher R: Coblation cryptolysis to treat tonsil stones: a retrospective case series, *Ear Nose Throat J* 91:238–254, 2012.

Finkelstein Y, Talmi YP, Ophir D, et al.: Laser cryptolysis for the treatment of halitosis, *Otolaryngol Head Neck Surg* 131:372–377, 2004.

Kim M-J, Kim J-E, Huh K-H, et al.: Multidetector computed tomography imaging characteristics of asymptomatic palatine tonsilloliths: a retrospective study of 3886 examinations, *Oral Surg Oral Med Oral Pathol Oral Radiol* 125:693–698, 2018.

Stoodley P, deBeer D, Longwell M, et al.: Tonsillolith: not just a stone but a living biofilm, *Otolaryngol Head Neck Surg* 141:316–321, 2009.

Takahashi A, Sugawara C, Kudoh T, et al.: Prevalence and imaging characteristics of palatine tonsilloliths evaluated on 2244 pairs of panoramic radiographs and CT images, *Clin Oral Invest* 21:85–91, 2017.

Takahashi A, Sugawara C, Kudoh K, et al.: Lingual tonsillolith: prevalence and imaging characteristics evaluated on 2244 pairs of panoramic radiographs and CT images, *Dentomaxillofac Radiol* 47: 20170251, 2018.

Diphtheria

Berkowitz AL: Tetanus, botulism, and diphtheria, *Continuum (Minneap Minn)* 24:1459–1488, 2018.

Borba RCN, Vidal VM, Moreira LO: The re-emergency and persistence of vaccine preventable diseases, *An Acad Bras Cienc* 87(Suppl 2):1311–1322, 2015.

Galazka A: Implications of the diphtheria epidemic in the former Soviet Union for immunization programs, *J Infect Dis* 181 (Suppl 1): S244–S248, 2000.

Galazka A: The changing epidemiology of diphtheria in the vaccine era, *J Infect Dis* 181(Suppl 1):S2–S9, 2000.

Hadfield TL, McEvoy P, Polotsky Y, et al.: The pathology of diphtheria, *J Infect Dis* 181(Suppl 1):S116–S120, 2000.

Zibners L: Diphtheria, pertussis, and tetanus: evidence-based management of pediatric patients in the emergency department, *Pediatr Emer Med Pract* 14:1–24, 2017.

Syphilis

Bowen V, Su J, Torrone E, et al.: Increase in incidence of congenital syphilis—United States, 2012-2014, *MMWR Morb Mortal Wkly Rep* 64:1241–1245, 2015.

Ficarra G, Carlos R: The renaissance of an oral disease with oral implications, *Head Neck Pathol* 3:195–206, 2009.

Little JW: Syphilis: an update, *Oral Surg Oral Med Oral Pathol Oral Radiol Endod* 100:3–9, 2005.

Patton ME, Su JR, Nelson R, et al.: Primary and secondary syphilis—United States, 2005-2013, *MMWR Morb Mortal Wkly Rep* 63:402–406, 2014.

Schuch LF, da Silva KD, de Arruda AA, et al.: Forty cases of acquired oral syphilis and a review of the literature, *Int J Oral Maxillofac Surg* 48:635–643, 2019.

Workowski KA, Bolan GA: Sexually transmitted disease treatment guidelines, 2015, *MMWR Recomm Rep* 64:1–137, 2015.

Gonorrhea

Giunta JL, Fiumara NJ: Facts about gonorrhea and dentistry, *Oral Surg Oral Med Oral Pathol* 62:529–531, 1986.

Javanbakht M, Westmoreland D, Gorbach P: Factors associated with pharyngeal gonorrhea in young people: implications for prevention, *Sex Transm Dis* 45:588–593, 2018.

Lewis DA: Will targeting oropharyngeal gonorrhoea delay the further emergence of drug-resistant *Neisseria gonorrhoeae* strains? *Sex Transm Infect* 91:234–237, 2015.

Little JW: Gonorrhea: update, *Oral Surg Oral Med Oral Pathol Oral Radiol Endod* 101:137–143, 2006.

Regan DG, Hui BB, Wood JG, et al.: Treatment for pharyngeal gonorrhea under threat, *Lancet Infect Dis* 18:1175–1177, 2018.

Siegel MA: Syphilis and gonorrhea, *Dent Clin North Am* 40:369–383, 1996.

Williams LN: The risks of oral-genital contact: a case report, *Gen Dent* 50:282–284, 2002.

Workkowski KA, Bolan GA: Sexually transmitted diseases treatment guidelines, 2015, *MMWR Recomm Rep* 64:1–137, 2015.

Tuberculosis

Andrade NN, Mhatre TS: Orofacial tuberculosis—a 16-year experience with 46 cases, *J Oral Maxillofac Surg* 70:e12–e22, 2012.

Darlington CC, Salman I: Oral tuberculous lesions, *Am Rev Tuberc* 35:147–179, 1937.

Gupta S, Vats P, Jha A, et al.: Gingival manifestations of tuberculosis in pediatric patients: series of 4 cases, *Oral Surg Oral Med Oral Pathol Oral Radiol* 128:508–514, 2019.

Ju W-T, Fu Y, Liu Y, et al.: Clinical and pathologic analyses of tuberculosis in the oral cavity: report of 11 cases, *Oral Surg Oral Med Oral Pathol Oral Radiol* 125:44–51, 2018.

Kakisi OK, Kechagia AS, Kakisis IK, et al.: Tuberculosis of the oral cavity: a systematic review, *Eur J Oral Sci* 118:103–109, 2010.

MacNeil A, Glaziou P, Sismanidas C, et al.: Global epidemiology of tuberculosis and progress toward meeting global targets—worldwide, 2018, *MMWR Morb Mortal Wkly Rep* 69:281–285, 2020.

Phelan JA, Jimenez V, Tompkins DC: Tuberculosis, *Dent Clin North Am* 40:327–341, 1996.

Rinaggio J: Tuberculosis, *Dent Clin North Am* 47:449–465, 2003.

Schwartz NG, Price SF, Pratt RH, et al.: Tuberculosis—United States, 2019, *MMWR Morb Mortal Wkly Rep* 69:286–289, 2020.

Wang W-C, Chen J-Y, Chen Y-K, et al.: Tuberculosis of the head and neck: a review of 20 cases, *Oral Surg Oral Med Oral Pathol Oral Radiol Endod* 107:381–386, 2009.

Leprosy

Brand PW: Temperature variations and leprosy deformity, *Int J Lepr* 27:1–7, 1959.

Ghosh S, Gadda R-B, Vengal M, et al.: Oro-facial aspects of leprosy: report of two cases with literature review, *Med Oral Patol Oral Cir Bucal* 15:e459–e462, 2010.

Girdhar BK, Desikan KV: A clinical study of the mouth in untreated lepromatous patients, *Lepr Rev* 50:25–35, 1979.

Gupta B, Gupta S, Chaudhary M, et al.: Oro-facial manifestations in lepromatous leprosy patients in Central India: clinical findings from a cross-sectional study, *Clin Oral Investig*, 2019. https://doi.org/10.1007/S00784-019-03061-1 (Epub ahead of print).

Gurung P, Gomes CM, Vernal S, et al.: Diagnostic accuracy of tests for leprosy: a systematic review and meta-analysis, *Clin Microbiol Infect* 25:1315–1327, 2019.

Nolen L, Haberling D, Scollard D, et al.: Incidence of Hansen's disease—United States, 1994-2011, *MMWR Morb Mortal Wkly Rep* 63:969–972, 2014.

Prabhu SR, Daftary DK: Clinical evaluation of oro-facial lesions of leprosy, *Odontostomatol Trop* 4:83–95, 1981.

Reichart P: Facial and oral manifestations in leprosy: an evaluation of seventy cases, *Oral Surg Oral Med Oral Pathol* 41:385–399, 1976.

Rodrigues GA, Qualio NP, de Macedo LD, et al.: The oral cavity in leprosy: what clinicians need to know, *Oral Dis* 23:749–756, 2017.

Scheepers A: Correlation of oral surface temperature and the lesions of leprosy, *Int J Lepr* 66:214–217, 1998.

Scheepers A, Lemmer J, Lownie JF: Oral manifestations of leprosy, *Lepr Rev* 64:37–43, 1993.

World Health Organization: Chemotherapy of leprosy for control programmes, *World Health Organ Tech Rep Ser* 675:1–33, 1982.

World Health Organization: WHO expert committee on leprosy, *World Health Organ Tech Rep Ser* 968:1–61, 2012.

Noma

Adekeye EO, Ord RA: Cancrum oris: principles of management and reconstructive surgery, *J Maxillofac Surg* 11:160–170, 1983.

Ashok N, Tarakji B, Darwish S, et al.: A review of noma: a recent update, *Glob J Health Sci* 8:53–59, 2015.

Bourgeois DM, Leclercq MH: The World Health Organization initiative on noma, *Oral Dis* 5:172–174, 1999.

Enwonwu CO, Falkler WA Jr, Phillips RS: Noma (cancrum oris), *Lancet* 368:147–156, 2006.

Feller L, Khammissa RAG, Altini M, et al.: Noma (cancrum oris): an resolved global challenge, *Periodontol 2000* 80:189–199, 2019.

Srour ML, Marck K, Baratti-Mayer D: Noma: overview of a neglected disease and human rights violation, *Am J Trop Med Hyg* 96:268–274, 2017.

Actinomycosis

Bennhoff DF: Actinomycosis: diagnostic and therapeutic considerations and a review of 32 cases, *Laryngoscope* 94:1198–1217, 1984.

Gomes NR, Diniz MG, Pereira TD, et al.: *Actinomyces israelii* in radicular cysts: a molecular study, *Oral Surg Oral Med Oral Pathol Oral Radiol* 123:586–590, 2017.

Hirshberg A, Tsesis I, Metzger Z, et al.: Periapical actinomycosis: a clinicopathologic study, *Oral Surg Oral Med Oral Pathol Oral Radiol Endod* 95:614–620, 2003.

Miller M, Haddad AJ: Cervicofacial actinomycosis, *Oral Surg Oral Med Oral Pathol Oral Radiol Endod* 85:496–508, 1998.

Rush JR, Sulte HR, Cohen DM, et al.: Course of infection and case outcome in individuals diagnosed with microbial colonies morphologically consistent with *Actinomyces* species, *J Endod* 28:613–618, 2002.

Sadeghi S, Azaïs M, Ghannoum J: Actinomycosis presenting as macroglossia: case report and review of literature, *Head Neck Pathol* 13:327–330, 2019.

Sasaki Y, Kaneda T, Uyeda JW, et al.: Actinomycosis in the mandible: CT and MR findings, *AJNR Am J Neuroradiol* 35:390–394, 2014.

Sprague WG, Shafer WG: Presence of *Actinomyces* in dentigerous cyst: report of two cases, *J Oral Surg* 21:243–245, 1963.

Cat-Scratch Disease

Biswas S, Rolain J-M: *Bartonella* infection: treatment and drug resistance, *Future Microbiol* 5:1719–1731, 2010.

Carithers HA: Cat-scratch disease. An overview based on a study of 1,200 patients, *Am J Dis Child* 139:1124–1133, 1985.

Centers for Disease Control and Prevention: Cat-scratch disease in children—Texas, September 2000-August 2001, *MMWR Morb Mortal Wkly Rep* 51:212–214, 2002.

English CK, Wear DJ, Margileth AM, et al.: Cat-scratch disease: isolation and culture of the bacterial agent, *JAMA* 259:1347–1352, 1988.

Margileth AM, Wear DJ, English CK: Systemic cat scratch disease: report of 23 patients with prolonged or recurrent severe bacterial infection, *J Infect Dis* 155:390–402, 1987.

Nelson CA, Saha S, Mead PS: Cat-scratch disease in the United States, 2005-2013, *Emerg Infect Dis* 22:1741–1746, 2016.

Simonton K, Rupar D: Progressive cat scratch disease despite antimicrobial therapy, *J Pediatric Infect Dis Soc* 4:e45–e47, 2015.

Uluğ M: Evaluation of cat scratch disease cases reported from Turkey between 1996 and 2013 and review of the literature, *Cent Eur J Public Health* 23:170–175, 2015.

Wear DJ, Margileth AM, Hadfield TL, et al.: Cat scratch disease: a bacterial infection, *Science* 221:1403–1405, 1983.

Rhinosinusitis

Ahovuo-Saloranta A, Borisenko OV, Kovanen N, et al.: Antibiotics for acute maxillary sinusitis, *Cochrane Database Syst Rev* 2:CD000243, 2008.

Ogata Y, Okinaka Y, Takahashi M: Antrolith associated with aspergillosis of the maxillary sinus: report of a case, *J Oral Maxillofac Surg* 55:1339–1341, 1997.

Puglisi S, Privitera S, Maiolino L, et al.: Bacteriological findings and antimicrobial resistance in odontogenic and non-odontogenic chronic maxillary sinusitis, *J Med Microbiol* 60:1353–1359, 2011.

Raman A, Papagiannopoulos P, Kuhar HN, et al.: Histopathologic features of chronic sinusitis precipitated by odontogenic infection, *Am J Rhinol Allergy* 33:113–120, 2019.

Richtsmeier WJ: Medical and surgical management of sinusitis in adults, *Ann Otol Rhinol Laryngol* 101(Suppl 155):46–50, 1992.

Vidal F, Coutinho TM, Ferreira DC, et al.: Odontogenic sinusitis: a comprehensive review, *Acta Odontol Scand* 75:623–633, 2017.

Workman AD, Granquist EJ, Adappa ND: Odontogenic sinusitis: development in diagnosis, microbiology, and treatment, *Curr Opin Otolaryngol Head Neck Surg* 26:27–33, 2018.

6

Fungal and Protozoal Diseases

◆ CANDIDIASIS

Infection with the yeastlike fungal organism *Candida albicans* is termed **candidiasis** or, as the British prefer, **candidosis.** An older name for this disease is *moniliasis;* the use of this term should be discouraged because it is derived from the archaic designation *Monilia albicans.* Other members of the *Candida* genus, such as *C. tropicalis, C. krusei, C. parapsilosis,* and *C. guilliermondii,* may also be found intraorally, but they rarely cause disease.

Like many other pathogenic fungi, *C. albicans* may exist in two forms—a trait known as **dimorphism.** The yeast form of the organism is believed to be relatively innocuous, but the hyphal form is usually associated with invasion of host tissue.

Candidiasis is by far the most common oral fungal infection in humans and has a variety of clinical manifestations, making the diagnosis difficult at times. In fact, *C. albicans* may be a component of the normal oral microflora, with as many as 30%–50% of people simply carrying the organism in their mouths without clinical evidence of infection. This rate of carriage has been shown to increase with age, and *C. albicans* can be recovered from the mouths of nearly 60% of dentate patients older than 60 years who have no sign of oral mucosal lesions. At least three general factors may determine whether clinical evidence of infection exists:

1. The immune status of the host
2. The oral mucosal environment
3. The strain of *C. albicans*

In the past, candidiasis was considered to be only an opportunistic infection, affecting individuals who were debilitated by another disease. Certainly, such patients make up a large percentage of those with candidal infections today. However, now clinicians recognize that oral candidiasis may develop in people who are otherwise healthy. As a result of this complex host and organism interaction, candidal infection may range from mild, superficial mucosal involvement seen in most patients to fatal, disseminated disease in severely immunocompromised patients. This chapter focuses on those clinical presentations of candidiasis that affect the oral mucosa.

Clinical Features

Candidiasis of the oral mucosa may exhibit a variety of clinical patterns, which are summarized in Table 6.1. Many patients display a single pattern, although some individuals exhibit more than one clinical form of oral candidiasis.

Pseudomembranous Candidiasis

The best recognized form of candidal infection is **pseudomembranous candidiasis.** Also known as *thrush,* pseudomembranous candidiasis is characterized by the presence of adherent white plaques that resemble cottage cheese or curdled milk on the oral mucosa (Figs. 6.1 and 6.2). The white plaques are composed of tangled masses of hyphae, yeasts, desquamated epithelial cells, and debris. Scraping them with a tongue blade or rubbing them with a dry gauze sponge can remove these plaques. The underlying mucosa may appear normal or erythematous. If bleeding occurs, then the mucosa has probably also been affected by another process, such as erosive lichen planus or cancer chemotherapy.

Pseudomembranous candidiasis may be initiated by exposure of the patient to broad-spectrum antibiotics (thus eliminating competing bacteria) or by impairment of the patient's immune system. A common type of local immune impairment resulting in pseudomembranous candidiasis is use of topical corticosteroids for treatment of oral immune-mediated conditions, or inhaled corticosteroids for treatment of asthma. The immune dysfunctions seen in leukemic patients (see page 593) or those infected with human immunodeficiency virus (HIV) (see page 252) are often associated with pseudomembranous candidiasis. Infants may also be affected, ostensibly because of their underdeveloped immune systems. Antibiotic exposure is typically responsible for an acute (rapid) expression of the condition; immunologic problems usually produce a chronic (slow-onset, long-standing) form of pseudomembranous candidiasis.

Symptoms, if present at all, are usually relatively mild, consisting of a burning sensation of the oral mucosa or an unpleasant taste in the mouth, variably described as salty or bitter. Sometimes patients complain of "blisters," when in fact they feel the elevated plaques rather than true vesicles. The plaques are characteristically distributed on the buccal

TABLE 6.1	Clinical Forms of Oral Candidiasis		
Clinical Type	**Appearance and Symptoms**	**Common Sites**	**Associated Factors and Comments**
Pseudomembranous (thrush)	Creamy-white plaques, removable; burning sensation, foul taste	Buccal mucosa, tongue, palate	Antibiotic therapy, immunosuppression
Erythematous	Red macules, burning sensation	Posterior hard palate, buccal mucosa, dorsal tongue	Antibiotic therapy, xerostomia, immunosuppression, idiopathic
Central papillary atrophy (median rhomboid glossitis)	Red, atrophic mucosal areas; asymptomatic	Midline posterior dorsal tongue	Idiopathic, immunosuppression
Chronic multifocal	Red areas, often with removable white plaques; burning sensation, asymptomatic	Posterior palate, posterior dorsal tongue, angles of mouth	Immunosuppression, idiopathic
Angular cheilitis	Red, fissured lesions; irritated, raw feeling	Angles of mouth	Idiopathic, immunosuppression, loss of vertical dimension
Denture stomatitis (chronic atrophic candidiasis, denture sore mouth)	Red, asymptomatic	Confined to palatal denture-bearing mucosa	Probably not true infection; denture often is positive on culture but mucosa is not
Hyperplastic (candidal leukoplakia)	White plaques that are not removable; asymptomatic	Anterior buccal mucosa	Idiopathic, immunosuppression; care must be taken not to confuse this with other keratotic lesions with superimposed candidiasis
Mucocutaneous	White plaques, some of which may be removable; red areas	Tongue, buccal mucosa, palate	Rare; inherited or sporadic idiopathic immune dysfunction
Endocrine-candidiasis syndromes	White plaques, most of which are not removable	Tongue, buccal mucosa, palate	Rare; endocrine disorder develops after candidiasis

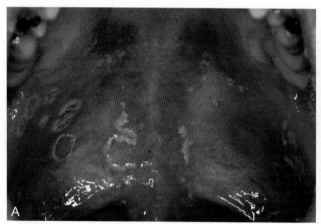 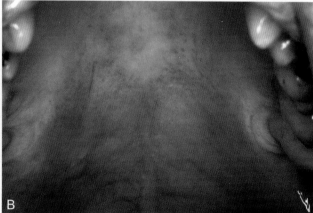

• **Fig. 6.1 Pseudomembranous Candidiasis. A,** Multiple white linear and circular plaques with associated erythema on the soft palate. **B,** Same patient, 2 weeks later, following a course of clotrimazole oral troches.

mucosa, palate, and dorsal tongue. Importantly, retention or over-production of keratin on the filiform papillae, producing a white appearance of the dorsal tongue (so-called coated or hairy tongue; see page 12) should not be confused with oral candidiasis.

Erythematous Candidiasis

In contrast to the pseudomembranous form, patients with erythematous candidiasis either do not show white flecks, or a white component is not a prominent feature. Erythematous candidiasis is undoubtedly more common than

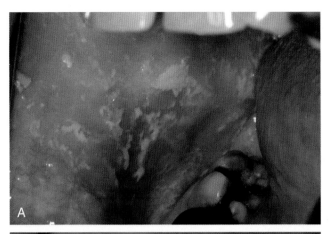

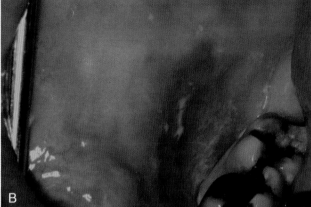

• **Fig. 6.2 Pseudomembranous Candidiasis. A,** White plaques on an erythematous base, characteristic of pseudomembranous candidiasis. **B,** Removal of several of the pseudomembranous plaques reveals a mildly erythematous mucosal surface but no evidence of bleeding.

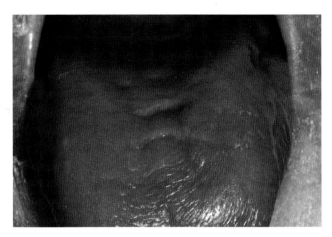

• **Fig. 6.3 Erythematous Candidiasis.** The diffuse erythema with a smooth atrophic appearance of the dorsal tongue represents erythematous candidiasis.

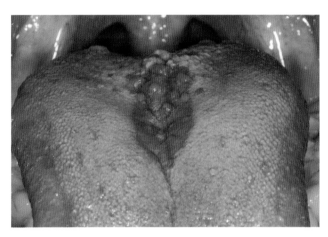

• **Fig. 6.4 Erythematous Candidiasis.** This asymptomatic, ovoid, erythematous patch on the posterior dorsal tongue is commonly caused by chronic infection by *Candida albicans.* The fungiform papillae appear prominent because the filiform papillae have been destroyed by the candidal infection. (Courtesy of Dr. Anthony Lotesto.)

pseudomembranous candidiasis, although it is often overlooked clinically. Several clinical presentations may be seen. **Acute atrophic candidiasis,** or "antibiotic sore mouth," typically follows a course of broad-spectrum antibiotic therapy. Patients often complain that the mouth feels as if a hot beverage had scalded it. This burning sensation is usually accompanied by a diffuse loss of the filiform papillae of the dorsal tongue, resulting in a reddened, "bald" appearance of the tongue (Fig. 6.3). Burning mouth syndrome (see page 868) frequently manifests with a scalded sensation of the tongue; however, the tongue appears normal in that condition. Patients who suffer from xerostomia for any reason (e.g., pharmacologic, postradiation therapy, or Sjögren syndrome) have an increased prevalence of erythematous candidiasis that is commonly symptomatic as well.

Other forms of erythematous candidiasis are usually asymptomatic and chronic. Included in this category is the condition known as **central papillary atrophy** of the tongue, or **median rhomboid glossitis** (Fig. 6.4). In the past, this was thought to be a developmental defect of the tongue, occurring in 0.01%–1.00% of adults. The lesion was supposed to have resulted from a failure of the embryologic tuberculum impar to be covered by the lateral processes of the tongue. Theoretically, the prevalence of central papillary

atrophy in children should be identical to that seen in adults; however, in one study in which 10,000 children were examined, not a single lesion was detected. Other investigators have noted a consistent relationship between the lesion and *C. albicans,* and similar lesions have been induced experimentally on the dorsal tongues of rats.

Clinically, central papillary atrophy appears as a well-demarcated erythematous zone that affects the midline, posterior dorsal tongue and often is asymptomatic (Fig. 6.5). The erythema is due in part to the loss of the filiform papillae in this area. The lesion is usually symmetrical, and its surface may range from smooth to lobulated. Often the mucosal alteration resolves with antifungal therapy, although occasionally only partial resolution can be achieved.

Some patients with central papillary atrophy may also exhibit signs of oral mucosal candidal infection at other sites. This presentation of erythematous candidiasis has been termed **chronic multifocal candidiasis.** In addition to the

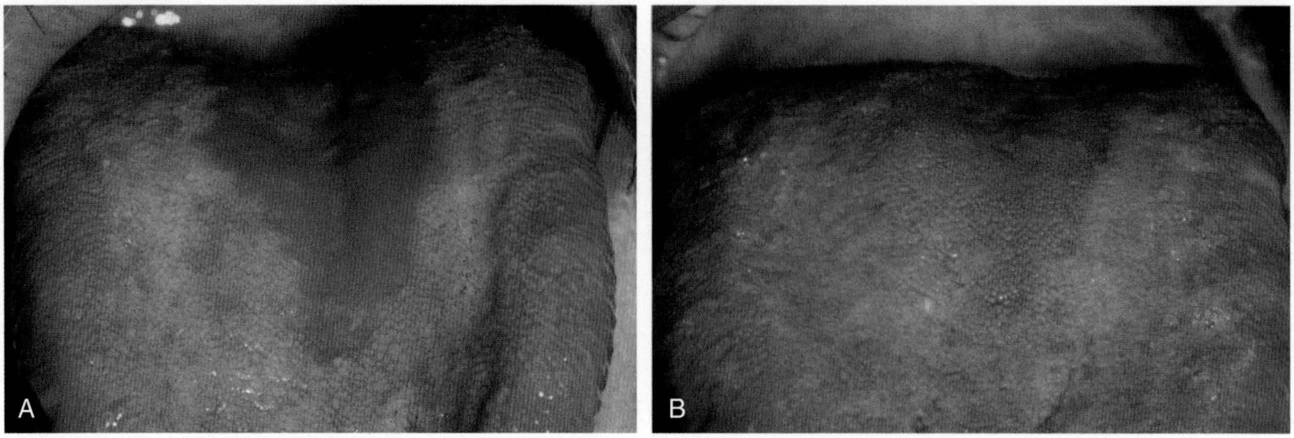

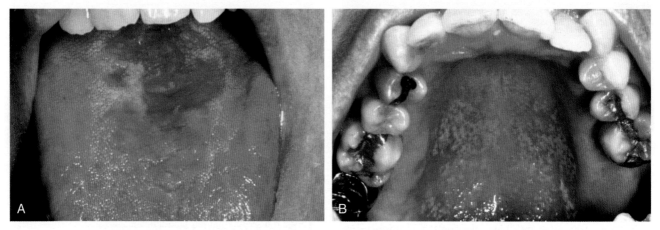

• **Fig. 6.5 Erythematous Candidiasis. A,** Severe presentation of central papillary atrophy. In this patient, the lesion was asymptomatic. **B,** Marked regeneration of the dorsal tongue papillae occurred 2 weeks after antifungal therapy with fluconazole.

• **Fig. 6.6 Candidiasis. A,** Multifocal oral candidiasis characterized by central papillary atrophy of the tongue and other areas of involvement. **B,** Same patient showing a "kissing" lesion of oral candidiasis on the hard palate.

dorsal tongue, the sites that show involvement include the junction of the hard and soft palate and the angles of the mouth. The palatal lesion appears as an erythematous area that, when the tongue is at rest, contacts the dorsal tongue lesion, resulting in what is called a "kissing lesion" because of the intimate proximity of the involved areas (Fig. 6.6).

The involvement of the angles of the mouth (**angular cheilitis, perlèche**) is characterized by erythema, fissuring, and scaling (Fig. 6.7). Sometimes this condition is seen as a component of chronic multifocal candidiasis, but it often occurs alone, typically in an older person with reduced vertical dimension of occlusion and accentuated folds at the corners of the mouth. Saliva tends to pool in these areas, keeping them moist and thus favoring a yeast infection. Patients often indicate that the severity of the lesions waxes and wanes. Microbiologic studies have suggested that 20% of these cases

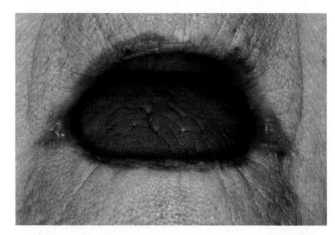

• **Fig. 6.7 Angular Cheilitis.** Characteristic lesions appear as mildly fissured, erythematous alterations of the skin at the corners of the mouth.

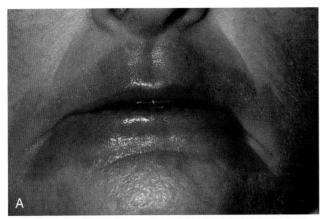

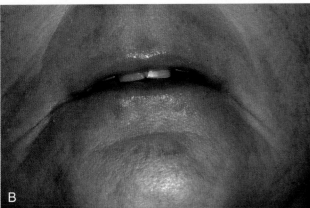

• **Fig. 6.8 Cheilocandidiasis. A,** Candidal infection of the perioral skin caused by use of a petrolatum-based product. The condition started as angular cheilitis, but the patient continuously applied petroleum jelly to the corners of the mouth and perioral skin, sealing moisture into the keratin layer of the epidermis, thereby allowing the candidal organisms to thrive. **B,** Two weeks after discontinuing the petroleum jelly and using topical iodoquinol with triamcinolone.

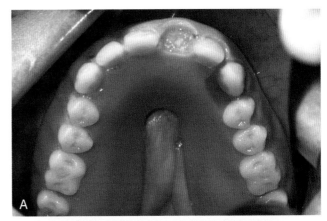

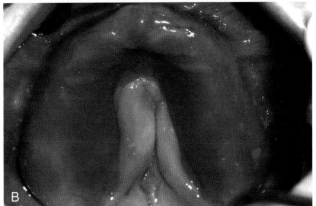

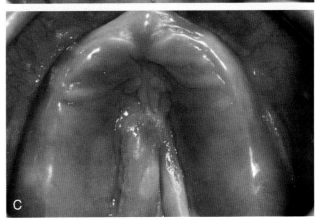

• **Fig. 6.9 Denture Stomatitis. A,** Maxillary denture with incomplete palatal vault associated with midline tissue hyperplasia. **B,** Mucositis corresponds to the outline of the prosthesis. **C,** Resolution of mucositis after antifungal therapy and appropriate denture cleansing.

are caused by *C. albicans* alone, 60% are due to a combined infection with *C. albicans* and *Staphylococcus aureus,* and 20% are associated with *S. aureus* alone. Infrequently, the candidal infection more extensively involves the perioral skin, usually secondary to actions that keep the skin moist (e.g., chronic lip licking, thumb sucking, chronic use of petrolatum-based salves), creating a clinical pattern known as **cheilocandidiasis** (Fig. 6.8). Other causes of exfoliative cheilitis often must be considered in the differential diagnosis (see page 294).

Denture stomatitis should be mentioned because it is often classified as a form of erythematous candidiasis, and some authors may use the term *chronic atrophic candidiasis* synonymously. This condition is characterized by varying degrees of erythema, sometimes accompanied by petechial hemorrhage, localized to the denture-bearing areas of a maxillary removable dental prosthesis (Figs. 6.9 and 6.10). Although the clinical appearance can be striking, the process is rarely symptomatic. Usually the patient admits to wearing the denture continuously, removing it only periodically to clean it. Whether this represents actual infection by *C. albicans* or is simply a tissue response by the host to the various microorganisms living

beneath the denture remains controversial. The clinician should also rule out the possibility that this reaction could be caused by improper design of the denture (which could cause unusual pressure on the mucosa), allergy to the denture base, or inadequate curing of the denture acrylic.

Although *C. albicans* is often associated with this condition, biopsy specimens of denture stomatitis seldom show candidal hyphae actually penetrating the keratin layer of the host epithelium. Therefore, this lesion does not meet one of the main defining criteria for the diagnosis of infection—host tissue invasion by the organism.

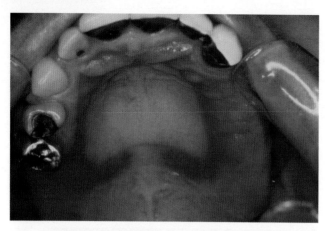

• **Fig. 6.10 Denture Stomatitis.** Denture stomatitis, not associated with *Candida albicans,* confined to the denture-bearing mucosa of a maxillary partial denture framework.

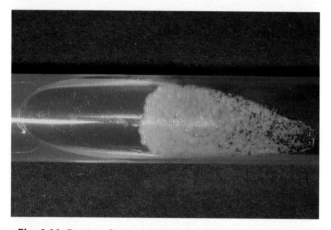

• **Fig. 6.11 Denture Stomatitis.** This Sabouraud agar slant has been streaked with swabs obtained from erythematous palatal mucosa *(left side of the slant)* and the tissue-bearing surface of the denture *(right side of the slant).* Extensive colonization of the denture is demonstrated, whereas little evidence of yeast associated with the mucosa is noted.

Furthermore, if the palatal mucosa and tissue-contacting surface of the denture are swabbed and separately streaked onto a Sabouraud agar slant, then the denture typically shows much heavier colonization by yeast (Fig. 6.11).

Chronic Hyperplastic Candidiasis (Candidal Leukoplakia)

In some patients with oral candidiasis, there may be a white patch that cannot be removed by scraping; in this case the term *chronic hyperplastic candidiasis* is appropriate. This form of candidiasis is the least common and is also somewhat controversial. Some investigators believe that this condition simply represents candidiasis that is superimposed on a preexisting leukoplakic lesion, a situation that may certainly exist at times. In some instances, however, the candidal organism alone may be capable of inducing a hyperkeratotic lesion. Such lesions are usually located on the anterior buccal mucosa and cannot clinically be distinguished from a routine leukoplakia (Fig. 6.12). Often the leukoplakic lesion associated with candidal infection has a fine intermingling of red fund white areas, resulting in a speckled leukoplakia (see page 384). Such lesions may have an increased frequency of epithelial dysplasia histopathologically.

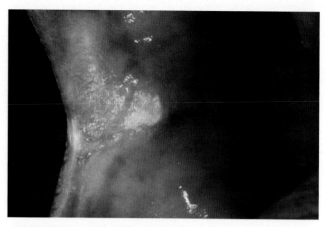

• **Fig. 6.12 Hyperplastic Candidiasis.** This lesion of the anterior buccal mucosa clinically resembles a leukoplakia because it is a white plaque that cannot be removed by rubbing. With antifungal therapy, such a lesion should resolve completely.

The diagnosis is confirmed by the presence of candidal hyphae associated with the lesion and, more importantly, by complete resolution of the lesion after antifungal therapy (Fig. 6.13). If the lesion remains following antifungal therapy, then biopsy of the persistent white patch is indicated.

Mucocutaneous Candidiasis

Severe oral candidiasis may also be seen as a component of a relatively rare group of immunologic disorders known as *mucocutaneous candidiasis.* Several distinct immunologic dysfunctions have been identified, and the severity of the candidal infection correlates with the severity of the immunologic defect. Most cases are sporadic, although an autosomal recessive pattern of inheritance has been identified in some families. Several studies have suggested that the cytokine IL-17 is critical in mucosal immunity related to *C. albicans,* and mutations of the gene responsible for producing this cytokine appear to cause some forms of mucocutaneous candidiasis. More recently, gain-of-function mutations in the STAT1 gene have been identified, resulting in abnormal Th1 and Th17 T-helper cell function. This increases the patient's susceptibility to candidiasis, as well as some bacterial infections. The STAT1 mutations now appear to be the genetic basis for the majority of mucocutaneous candidiasis cases. The immune problem usually becomes evident during the first few years of life, when the patient begins to have candidal infections of the mouth, nails, skin, and other mucosal surfaces. The oral lesions are usually described as thick, white plaques that typically do not rub off (essentially chronic hyperplastic candidiasis), although the other clinical forms of candidiasis may also be seen.

In some patients with mucocutaneous candidiasis, mutations in the autoimmune regulator (AIRE) gene have been documented, with the resultant formation of autoantibodies directed against the person's own tissues (Fig. 6.14). In most instances, the immunologic attack is directed against the endocrine glands; however, the reasons for this tissue specificity are currently unclear. Autoimmune destruction of the T-lymphocytes that produce interleukin-17 (IL-17) and

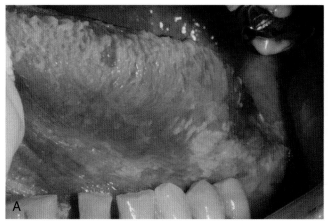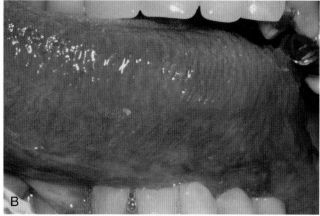

• **Fig. 6.13 Hyperplastic Candidiasis. A,** These diffuse white plaques clinically appear as leukoplakia, but they actually represent an unusual presentation of hyperplastic candidiasis. **B,** Treatment with clotrimazole oral troches shows complete resolution of the white lesions within 2 weeks, essentially confirming the diagnosis of hyperplastic candidiasis. If any white mucosal alteration had persisted, a biopsy of that area would have been mandatory.

IL-22 appears to be responsible for the candidal infections seen in these individuals. Young patients with mucocutaneous candidiasis should be evaluated periodically because any one of a variety of endocrine abnormalities (i.e., **endocrine-candidiasis syndrome**, **autoimmune polyendocrinopathy-candidiasis-ectodermal dystrophy [APECED] syndrome/autoimmune polyendocrine syndrome, type 1**), as well as iron-deficiency anemia, may develop in addition to the candidiasis. These endocrine disturbances include hypothyroidism, hypoparathyroidism, hypoadrenocorticism (Addison disease), and diabetes mellitus. Typically, the endocrine abnormality develops months or even years after the onset of the candidal infection. Two studies have documented increased prevalence of oral and esophageal carcinoma in this condition, with these malignancies affecting approximately 6%–10% of adults with APECED syndrome. The mean age of APECED patients with oral cancer was significantly younger than that of oral carcinoma patients in the general population. This finding of increased prevalence of oral and esophageal malignancies represents another justification for periodic reevaluation of these individuals, including esophageal endoscopy every 2–3 years.

Interestingly, the candidal infection remains relatively superficial rather than disseminating throughout the body. Both the oral lesions and any cutaneous involvement (usually presenting as roughened, foul-smelling cutaneous plaques and nodules) can be usually controlled with continuous use of relatively safe systemic antifungal drugs. As with any long-term antibiotic treatment, development of drug-resistant organisms can occur, however.

Histopathologic Features

The candidal organism can be seen microscopically in either an exfoliative cytologic preparation or in tissue sections obtained from a biopsy specimen. On staining with the periodic acid-Schiff (PAS) method or the Grocott-Gomori methenamine silver (GMS) method, the candidal hyphae

and yeasts can be readily identified (Fig. 6.15). Both techniques stain carbohydrates, contained in abundance by fungal cell walls; the organisms appear bright-magenta with the PAS stain or black with the GMS stain. To make a diagnosis of candidiasis, one must be able to see hyphae or pseudohyphae (which are essentially elongated yeast cells). These hyphae are approximately 2 μm in diameter, vary in their length, and may show branching. Often the hyphae are accompanied by variable numbers of yeasts, squamous epithelial cells, and inflammatory cells.

A 10%–20% potassium hydroxide (KOH) preparation may also be used to rapidly evaluate specimens for the presence of fungal organisms. With this technique, the KOH lyses the background of epithelial cells, allowing the more resistant yeasts and hyphae to be visualized.

The disadvantages of the KOH preparation include the following:
- Lack of a permanent record
- Greater difficulty in identifying the fungal organisms, compared with PAS staining
- Inability to assess the nature of the epithelial cell population with respect to other conditions, such as epithelial dysplasia or pemphigus vulgaris

The histopathologic pattern of oral candidiasis may vary slightly, depending on which clinical form of the infection has been submitted for biopsy. The features that are found in common include an increased thickness of parakeratin on the surface of the lesion in conjunction with elongation of the epithelial rete ridges (Fig. 6.16). Typically, a chronic inflammatory cell infiltrate can be seen in the connective tissue immediately subjacent to the infected epithelium, and small collections of neutrophils (microabscesses) are often identified in the parakeratin layer and the superficial spinous cell layer near the organisms (Fig. 6.17). The candidal hyphae are embedded in the parakeratin layer and, unless the patient is extremely immunocompromised, rarely penetrate into the viable cell layers of the epithelium. This is also

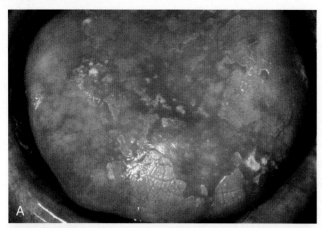

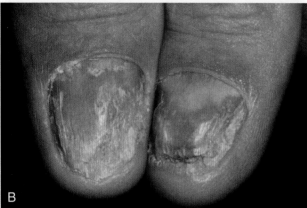

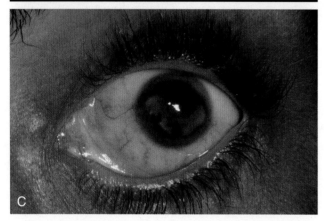

• **Fig. 6.14 Autoimmune Polyendocrinopathy-Candidiasis-Ectodermal Dystrophy (APECED) Syndrome. A,** Erythematous candidiasis diffusely involving the dorsal tongue of a 32-year-old man. **B,** Same patient showing nail dystrophy. **C,** Corneal keratopathy is also noted. Patient had a history of the onset of hypoparathyroidism and hypoadrenocorticism, which were both diagnosed in the second decade of life.

the finding in oral lesions of epithelial dysplasia or oral lichenoid lesions with superimposed candidiasis, suggesting that the organism is merely interested in "grazing" on the dead, keratinized surface cells. Sometimes this superficial infection will elicit the characteristic host response described above, but occasionally this response is lacking, which may be related to the candidal strain.

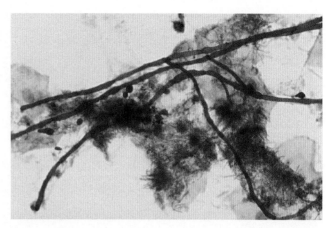

• **Fig. 6.15 Candidiasis.** This cytologic preparation demonstrates tubular-appearing fungal hyphae and ovoid yeasts of *Candida albicans*. (Periodic acid-Schiff [PAS] stain.)

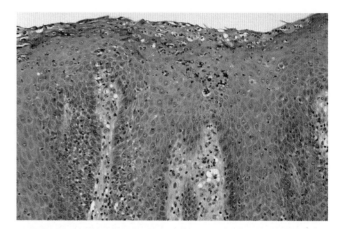

• **Fig. 6.16 Candidiasis.** This medium-power photomicrograph shows a characteristic pattern of parakeratosis, neutrophilic microabscesses, a thickened spinous layer, and chronic inflammation of the underlying connective tissue associated with long-standing candidal infection of the oral mucosa.

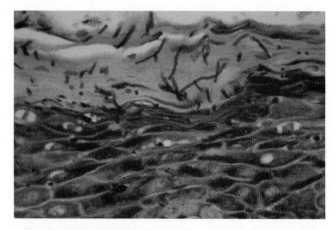

• **Fig. 6.17 Candidiasis.** This high-power photomicrograph shows the tubular hyphae of *Candida albicans* embedded in the parakeratin layer. (Periodic acid-Schiff [PAS] stain.)

Diagnosis

The diagnosis of candidiasis is usually established by the clinical signs in conjunction with exfoliative cytologic examination. Although a culture can definitively identify the organism as *C. albicans,* this process may not be practical in most office settings. The cytologic findings should demonstrate the hyphal phase of the organism, and antifungal therapy can then be instituted. If the lesion is clinically suggestive of chronic hyperplastic candidiasis but does not respond to antifungal therapy, then a biopsy should be performed to rule out the possibility of *C. albicans* superimposed on epithelial dysplasia, squamous cell carcinoma, or lichen planus.

The definitive identification of the organism can be made by means of culture. A specimen for culture is obtained by rubbing a sterile cotton swab over the lesion and then streaking the swab on the surface of a Sabouraud agar slant. *C. albicans* will grow as creamy, smooth-surfaced colonies after 2–3 days of incubation at room temperature.

Treatment and Prognosis

Several antifungal medications have been developed for managing oral candidiasis, each with its advantages and disadvantages (Table 6.2).

Polyene Agents

Nystatin

In the 1950s, the polyene antibiotic nystatin was the first effective treatment for oral candidiasis. Nystatin is formulated for oral use as a suspension or pastille (lozenge). Many patients report that nystatin has a very bitter taste, which may reduce patient compliance; therefore, the taste has to be disguised with sucrose and flavoring agents. If the candidiasis is due to xerostomia, the sucrose content of the nystatin preparation may contribute to xerostomia-related caries in these patients. The gastrointestinal tract poorly absorbs nystatin and the other polyene antibiotic, amphotericin; therefore, their effectiveness depends on direct contact with the candidal organisms. This necessitates multiple daily doses so that the yeasts are adequately exposed to the drug. Nystatin combined with triamcinolone acetonide cream or ointment can be applied topically and is effective for angular cheilitis that does not have a bacterial component.

Amphotericin B

For many years in the United States, the use of amphotericin B was restricted to intravenous (IV) treatment of life-threatening systemic fungal infections. This medication subsequently became available as an oral suspension for the management of oral candidiasis. Unfortunately, the interest in this formulation of the drug was scant, and it is no longer marketed in the United States.

Imidazole Agents

The imidazole-derived antifungal agents were developed during the 1970s and represented a major step forward in the management of candidiasis. The two drugs of this group that are used most frequently are clotrimazole and ketoconazole.

Clotrimazole

Like nystatin, clotrimazole is not well absorbed and must be administered several times each day. It is formulated as a pleasant-tasting troche (lozenge) and produces few side effects. The efficacy of this agent in treating oral candidiasis can be seen in Fig. 6.13. Clotrimazole cream is also effective treatment for angular cheilitis, because this drug has antibacterial and antifungal properties.

Ketoconazole

Ketoconazole was the first antifungal drug that could be absorbed across the gastrointestinal tract, thereby providing systemic therapy by an oral route of administration. Patients could not take antacids or H2-blocking agents, because an acidic environment is required for proper absorption. The single daily dose was much easier for patients to use; however, several significant disadvantages have been identified. The most serious is idiopathic liver toxicity caused by this drug, occurring in approximately 1 in 10,000 individuals. Furthermore, ketoconazole has been implicated in drug interactions with macrolide antibiotics (e.g., erythromycin), which may produce potentially life-threatening cardiac arrhythmias. For these reasons, the US Food and Drug Administration has stated that ketoconazole should not be used to treat routine oral candidiasis.

Triazoles

The triazoles are among the more recently developed antifungal drugs. Both fluconazole and itraconazole have been approved for treating candidiasis in the United States.

Fluconazole

Fluconazole appears to be more effective than ketoconazole; it is well absorbed systemically, and an acidic environment is not required for absorption. A relatively long half-life allows for once-daily dosing, and liver toxicity is rare at the doses used to treat oral candidiasis. Some reports have suggested that fluconazole may not be appropriate for long-term preventive therapy because resistance to the drug seems to develop in some instances. Known drug interactions include a potentiation of the effects of phenytoin (Dilantin), an antiseizure medication; warfarin compounds (anticoagulants); and sulfonylureas (oral hypoglycemic agents). Other drugs that may interact with fluconazole are summarized in Table 6.2.

Itraconazole

Itraconazole has proven efficacy against a variety of fungal diseases, including histoplasmosis, blastomycosis, and fungal conditions of the nails. Recently, itraconazole solution was approved for management of oropharyngeal candidiasis, and this appears to have an efficacy equivalent to clotrimazole and fluconazole. As with fluconazole, significant drug interactions are possible, and itraconazole is contraindicated for patients taking erythromycin, triazolam, and midazolam. (See Table 6.2 for other potential drug interactions.)

TABLE 6.2 Antifungal Medications

Generic Name	Trade Name	Indications	Dosage
Nystatin	Mycostatin oral suspension	Oral candidiasis	1–2 tsp as a mouthrinse, q.i.d., p.c. and h.s., for 10–14 days. Hold each dose in the mouth as long as possible
Clotrimazole	Mycelex oral troches	Oral candidiasis	Dissolve 1 troche (10 mg) slowly in the mouth, 5 times daily for 10–14 days
Ketoconazole	Nizoral tablets	Oral candidiasis Blastomycosis	Not to be used as initial therapy for oral candidiasis One tablet (200 mg) daily for 1–2 weeks for candidiasis
		Coccidioidomycosis Histoplasmosis Paracoccidioidomycosis	Minimum treatment period for systemic mycoses is 6 months
Fluconazole	Diflucan tablets	Oral candidiasis Cryptococcal meningitis	For oral candidiasis: two tablets (200 mg) on day 1 and then one tablet (100 mg) daily for 1–2 weeks
Itraconazole	Sporanox capsules	Blastomycosis Histoplasmosis Aspergillosis refractory to amphotericin B therapy	For blastomycosis and histoplasmosis: two capsules (200 mg) daily, increasing by 100-mg increments up to 400 mg daily in divided doses if no clinical response is noted For aspergillosis: 200–400 mg daily For life-threatening situations: loading dose of 200 mg t.i.d. for first 3 days, then dose can be reduced Treatment should continue for at least 3 months for all of the above
Itraconazole	Sporanox oral solution	Oral candidiasis	10 mL (100 mg) vigorously swished in the mouth and swallowed, twice daily for 1–2 weeks

h.s., Hora somni (at bedtime); *p.c.*, post cibum (after meals); *q.i.d.*, quarter in die (four times a day); *t.i.d.*, ter in die (three times a day).

Posaconazole

This triazole compound has been shown to be effective in the management of oropharyngeal candidiasis in patients with HIV infection. Given the cost of this drug and the proven effectiveness of other, less expensive, oral antifungal agents, the use of this medication for treatment of routine oral candidiasis would be difficult to justify.

Isavuconazole

This recently developed triazole is well absorbed as its pro-drug, isavuconazonium sulfate, and is converted by esterases in the serum to isavuconazole. Isavuconazole may have fewer drug interactions compared to other compounds in the triazole class.

Although this medication has a relatively wide spectrum of activity against a number of pathogenic fungi, it is currently approved in the United States only for treatment of invasive aspergillosis and invasive mucormycosis in adults.

Echinocandins

This relatively new class of antifungal drugs acts by interfering with candidal cell wall synthesis. The formation of β-1,3-glucan, which is a principal component of the candidal cell wall, is disrupted and results in permeability of the cell wall with subsequent demise of the candidal organism. These medications are not well absorbed; consequently they must be administered intravenously

Side Effects/Adverse Reactions	Drug Interactions
Usually well tolerated, although the taste may be unacceptable (bitter) for some patients	None known
Mild elevations of liver enzymes in 15% of patients Periodic assessment of liver function in patients with hepatic impairment Nausea, vomiting	No significant drug interactions
Serious hepatotoxicity in 1:10,000 patients Monitoring of liver function is indicated for patients with preexisting hepatic problems, patients who develop symptoms of hepatic failure, or patients treated for more than 28 days Serum testosterone is lowered Nausea, vomiting Anaphylaxis	Serious and/or life-threatening interactions with erythromycin Metabolism of cyclosporine, tacrolimus, methylprednisolone, midazolam, triazolam, coumarin-like drugs, phenytoin, and rifampin may be altered
Rare cases of hepatotoxicity, ranging from mild transient elevation of liver enzymes to hepatic failure Headache, nausea, vomiting, abdominal pain, diarrhea	Clinically or potentially significant side effects have been noted with the following medications: oral hypoglycemic agents, coumarin-like drugs, phenytoin, cyclosporine, rifampin, theophylline, rifabutin, and tacrolimus
Rare cases of hepatoxicity	Serious and/or life-threatening interactions with erythromycin, pimozide, quinidine, oral triazolam, and oral midazolam
Liver function should be monitored in patients with preexisting hepatic problems on therapy for more than 1 month Nausea, diarrhea, vomiting	Lovastatin and simvastatin should be discontinued Increased plasma concentrations may be seen with warfarin, ritonavir, indinavir, vinca alkaloid agents, diazepam, cyclosporine, dihydropyridine medications, tacrolimus, digoxin, and methylprednisolone
Rare cases of hepatotoxicity Liver function should be monitored in patients with preexisting hepatic problems on therapy for more than 1 month Nausea, diarrhea, vomiting	Serious and/or life-threatening interactions with erythromycin, oral triazolam, and oral midazolam Lovastatin and simvastatin should be discontinued

and are reserved for more life-threatening candidal infections. Examples include caspofungin, micafungin, and anidulafungin.

Other Antifungal Agents

Iodoquinol

Although not strictly an antifungal drug, iodoquinol has antifungal and antibacterial properties. When compounded in a cream base with a corticosteroid, this material is very effective as topical therapy for angular cheilitis.

In most cases, oral candidiasis is an annoying superficial infection that is easily resolved by antifungal therapy. If infection should recur after treatment, then a thorough

investigation of potential factors that could predispose to candidiasis may be necessary. Often the predisposing factor represents a contaminated acrylic mouth guard, bite plane, or maxillary denture, as candidal colonization of the tissue-bearing aspect of these appliances is common. Soaking the appliance in a dilute sodium hypochlorite (bleach) solution for an 8-hour period daily, during the period that the patient is treating their mucosal infection, is recommended. Immune suppression, in the form of topical, inhaled, or systemic corticosteroids, is also a common predisposing factor. Acquired immune suppression, such as that associated with HIV infection (see page 250) or uncontrolled diabetes mellitus, may need to be considered as well. In only the most

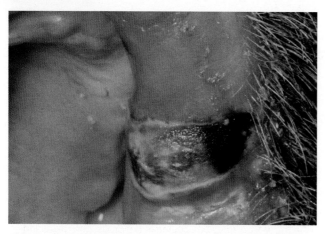

• **Fig. 6.18 Candidiasis.** This necrotic lesion of the upper lip developed in a man with uncontrolled type I diabetes mellitus. Biopsy and culture showed a rare example of invasive oral infection by *Candida albicans*.

severely compromised patient will candidiasis cause deeply invasive disease (Fig. 6.18).

◆ HISTOPLASMOSIS

Histoplasmosis, the most common systemic fungal infection in the United States, is caused by the organism *Histoplasma capsulatum*. Like several other pathogenic fungi, *H. capsulatum* is dimorphic, growing as a yeast at body temperature in the human host and as a mold in its natural environment. Humid areas with soil enriched by bird or bat excrement are especially suited to the growth of this organism. This habitat preference explains why histoplasmosis is seen endemically in fertile river valleys, such as the region drained by the Ohio and Mississippi Rivers in the United States. Airborne spores of the organism are inhaled, pass into the terminal passages of the lungs, and germinate.

Approximately 500,000 new cases of histoplasmosis are thought to develop annually in the United States. Other parts of the world, such as Central and South America, Europe, Asia, and Australia, also report numerous cases. Epidemiologic studies in endemic areas of the United States suggest that 80%–90% of the population in these regions has been infected.

Clinical and Radiographic Features

Most cases of histoplasmosis produce either no symptoms or such mild symptoms that the patient does not seek medical treatment. The expression of disease depends on the quantity of spores inhaled, the immune status of the host, and perhaps the strain of *H. capsulatum*. Most individuals who become exposed to the organism are relatively healthy and do not inhale a large number of spores; therefore, they have either no symptoms or they have a mild, flulike illness for 1–2 weeks. The inhaled spores are ingested by macrophages within 24–48 hours, and specific T-lymphocyte immunity develops in 2–3 weeks. Antibodies directed against the organism usually appear several weeks later. With these defense mechanisms, the host is usually able to destroy the

invading organism, although sometimes the macrophages simply surround and confine the fungus so that viable organisms can be recovered years later. Thus patients who formerly lived in an endemic area may have acquired the organism and later express the disease at some other geographic site if they become immunocompromised.

Acute histoplasmosis is a self-limited pulmonary infection that probably develops in only about 1% of people who are exposed to a low number of spores. With a high concentration of spores, as many as 50%–100% of individuals may experience acute symptoms. These symptoms (e.g., fever, headache, myalgia, nonproductive cough, and anorexia) result in a clinical picture similar to that of influenza. Patients are usually ill for 2 weeks, although calcification of the hilar lymph nodes may be detected as an incidental finding on chest radiographs years later.

Chronic histoplasmosis also primarily affects the lungs, although it is much less common than acute histoplasmosis. The chronic form usually affects older, emphysematous, white men or immunosuppressed patients. Clinically, it appears similar to tuberculosis. Patients typically exhibit cough, weight loss, fever, dyspnea, chest pain, hemoptysis, weakness, and fatigue. Chest roentgenograms show upper-lobe infiltrates and cavitation.

Disseminated histoplasmosis is even less common than the acute and chronic types. It occurs in 1 of 2000–5000 patients who have acute symptoms. This condition is characterized by the progressive spread of the infection to extrapulmonary sites. It usually occurs in either older, debilitated, or immunosuppressed patients. In some areas of the United States, 2%–10% of patients with **acquired immunodeficiency syndrome (AIDS)** (see page 262) develop disseminated histoplasmosis. Patients who are being treated with a tumor necrosis factor-alpha (TNF-α) inhibitor (such as, infliximab, etanercept, or adalimumab) and who live in endemic geographic regions also are at risk for disseminated disease, probably due to reactivation of the organism. Tissues that may be affected include the spleen, adrenal glands, liver, lymph nodes, gastrointestinal tract, central nervous system (CNS), kidneys, and oral mucosa. Adrenal involvement may produce hypoadrenocorticism **(Addison disease)** (see page 843).

Most oral lesions of histoplasmosis occur with the disseminated form of the disease. The most commonly affected sites are the tongue, palate, and buccal mucosa. The condition usually appears as a solitary, variably painful ulceration of several weeks' duration; however, some lesions may appear erythematous or white with an irregular surface (Fig. 6.19). The ulcerated lesions have firm, rolled margins, and they may be indistinguishable clinically from a malignancy (Fig. 6.20).

Histopathologic Features

Microscopic examination of lesional tissue shows either a diffuse infiltrate of macrophages or, more commonly, collections of macrophages organized into granulomas (Fig. 6.21). Multinucleated giant cells are usually seen in association with the

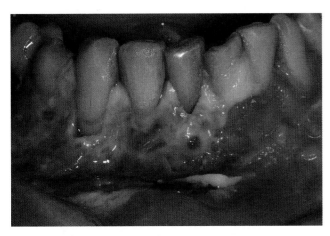

• **Fig. 6.19 Histoplasmosis.** This ulcerated granular lesion involves the right mandibular labial vestibule and gingivae, and is easily mistaken clinically for carcinoma. Biopsy established the diagnosis. (Courtesy of Douglas Damm, with appreciation to Dr. Robert Clark.)

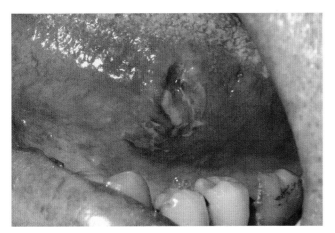

• **Fig. 6.20 Histoplasmosis.** This chronic ulceration of the ventral and lateral tongue represents an oral lesion of histoplasmosis that had disseminated from the lungs. The lesion clinically resembles carcinoma; because of this high-risk site, biopsy is mandatory.

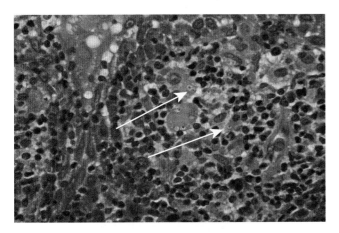

• **Fig. 6.21 Histoplasmosis.** This medium-power photomicrograph shows scattered epithelioid macrophages admixed with lymphocytes and plasma cells. Some macrophages contain organisms of *Histoplasma capsulatum (arrows)*.

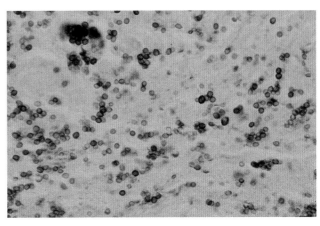

• **Fig. 6.22 Histoplasmosis.** This high-power photomicrograph of a tissue section readily demonstrates the small yeasts of *Histoplasma capsulatum*. (Grocott-Gomori methenamine silver stain.)

granulomatous inflammation. The causative organism can be identified with some difficulty in the routine hematoxylin and eosin (H&E)-stained section; however, special stains, such as the PAS and Grocott-Gomori methenamine silver methods, readily demonstrate the characteristic 1- to 3-μm yeasts of *H. capsulatum* (Fig. 6.22).

Diagnosis

The diagnosis of histoplasmosis can be made by histopathologic identification of the organism in tissue sections or by culture. Other helpful diagnostic studies include serologic testing in which antibodies directed against *H. capsulatum* are demonstrated and antigen produced by the yeast is identified.

Treatment and Prognosis

Acute histoplasmosis, because it is a self-limited process, generally warrants no specific treatment other than supportive care with analgesic and antipyretic agents. Often the disease is not treated because the symptoms are so nonspecific and the diagnosis is not readily evident.

Patients with chronic histoplasmosis require treatment, despite the fact that up to half of them may recover spontaneously. Often the pulmonary damage is progressive if it remains untreated, and death may result in up to 20% of these cases. For severe cases of chronic histoplasmosis, the treatment of choice is IV administration of one of the lipid preparations of amphotericin B, which are significantly less toxic than standard formulations of amphotericin B deoxycholate. Itraconazole may be used in nonimmunosuppressed patients because it is associated with even fewer side effects and is less expensive, but this medication requires daily dosing for 12–24 months.

Disseminated histoplasmosis occurring in an immunesuppressed individual is a very serious condition that results in death in 80%–90% of patients if they remain untreated. One of the lipid preparations of amphotericin B is indicated for such patients; once the life-threatening phase of the disease is under control, daily itraconazole is necessary for at least 12 months. Despite therapy, however, a mortality rate of 7%–23% is observed. Itraconazole alone may be used if the patient is nonimmunocompromised and has relatively mild to moderate disease; however, the response rate is slower than for patients receiving amphotericin B, and the relapse rate may be higher.

◆ BLASTOMYCOSIS

Blastomycosis is a relatively uncommon disease caused by two dimorphic fungi known as *Blastomyces dermatitidis*, and a more recently identified species, *Blastomyces gilchristii*. Although the organism is rarely isolated from its natural habitat, it seems to prefer rich, moist soil, where it grows as a mold. Much of the region in which it grows overlaps the territory associated with *H. capsulatum* (affecting the eastern half of the United States). The range of blastomycosis extends farther north, however, including Wisconsin, Minnesota, and the Canadian provinces surrounding the Great Lakes. Sporadic cases have also been reported in Africa, India, Europe, and South America. By way of comparison, histoplasmosis appears to be at least ten times more common than blastomycosis. In some series of cases, a prominent adult male predilection has been noted, often with a male-to-female ratio as high as 9:1. Although some researchers have attributed this to the greater degree of outdoor activity (e.g., hunting, fishing) by men in areas where the organism grows, others have noted that these series were typically reported from VA hospital data, which has an inherent male bias. The occurrence of blastomycosis in immunocompromised patients is relatively rare.

Clinical and Radiographic Features

Blastomycosis is almost always acquired by inhalation of spores, particularly after a rain. The spores reach the alveoli of the lungs, where they begin to grow as yeasts at body temperature. In most patients, the infection is probably halted and contained in the lungs, but it may become hematogenously disseminated in a few instances. In order of decreasing frequency, the sites of dissemination include skin, bone, prostate, meninges, oropharyngeal mucosa, and abdominal organs.

Although most cases of blastomycosis are either asymptomatic or produce only very mild symptoms, patients who do experience symptoms usually have pulmonary complaints. **Acute blastomycosis** resembles pneumonia, characterized by high fever, chest pain, malaise, night sweats, and productive cough with mucopurulent sputum. Rarely, the infection may precipitate life-threatening adult respiratory distress syndrome.

Chronic blastomycosis is more common than the acute form, and it may mimic tuberculosis; both conditions are often characterized by low-grade fever, night sweats, weight loss, and productive cough. Chest radiographs may appear normal, or

they may demonstrate diffuse infiltrates or one or more pulmonary or hilar masses. Unlike the situation with tuberculosis and histoplasmosis, calcification is not typically present. Cutaneous lesions usually represent the spread of infection from the lungs, although occasionally they are the only sign of disease. Such lesions begin as erythematous nodules that enlarge, becoming verrucous or ulcerated (Figs. 6.23 and 6.24).

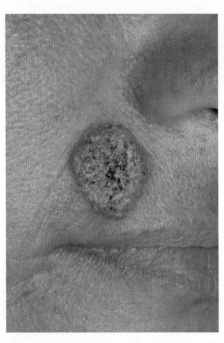

• **Fig. 6.23 Blastomycosis.** This granular erythematous plaque of cutaneous blastomycosis has affected the facial skin. (Courtesy of Dr. William Welton.)

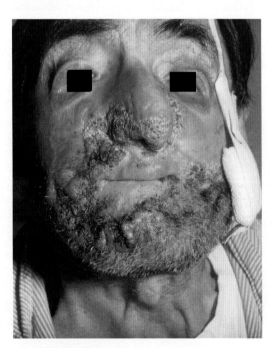

• **Fig. 6.24 Blastomycosis.** Severe cutaneous infection by *Blastomyces dermatitidis.* (Courtesy of Dr. Emmitt Costich.)

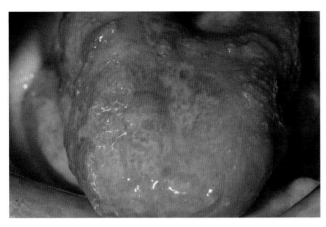

• **Fig. 6.25 Blastomycosis.** These irregular ulcerations of the tongue represent blastomycosis. Direct inoculation was thought to have occurred from the patient's habit of chewing dried horse manure ("Kentucky field candy"), in which the organism was probably growing.

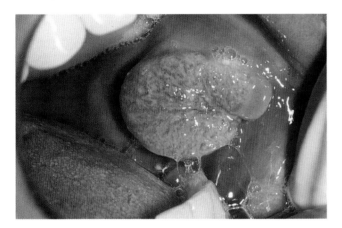

• **Fig. 6.26 Blastomycosis.** Granular exophytic and indurated mass on the buccal mucosa.

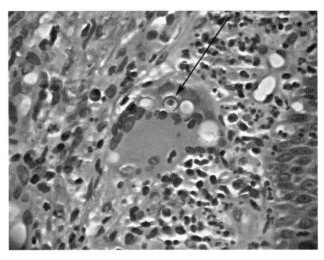

• **Fig. 6.27 Blastomycosis.** This high-power photomicrograph shows the large yeasts of *Blastomyces dermatitidis (arrow)* within a multinucleated giant cell.

Oral lesions of blastomycosis may result from either extrapulmonary dissemination or local inoculation with the organism. These lesions may have an irregular, erythematous, or white intact surface, or they may appear as ulcerations with irregular rolled borders and varying degrees of pain (Figs. 6.25 and 6.26). Clinically, because the lesions resemble squamous cell carcinoma, biopsy and histopathologic examination are required.

Histopathologic Features

Histopathologic examination of lesional tissue typically shows a mixture of acute inflammation and granulomatous inflammation surrounding variable numbers of yeasts. These organisms are 8–20 μm in diameter. They are characterized by a doubly refractile cell wall (Fig. 6.27) and a broad attachment between the budding daughter cell and the parent cell. Like many other fungal organisms, *B. dermatitidis* can be detected more easily using special stains, such as the Grocott-Gomori methenamine silver and PAS methods. Identification of these organisms is especially important,

because this infection often induces a benign reaction of the overlying epithelium in mucosal or skin lesions called **pseudoepitheliomatous (pseudocarcinomatous) hyperplasia.** Because this benign elongation of the epithelial rete ridges may look like squamous cell carcinoma at first glance under the microscope, careful inspection of the underlying inflamed lesional tissue is mandatory.

Diagnosis

Rapid diagnosis of blastomycosis can be performed by microscopic examination of either histopathologic sections or an alcohol-fixed cytologic preparation. The most rapid means of diagnosis, however, is the KOH preparation, which may be used for examining scrapings from a suspected lesion. The most accurate method of identifying *B. dermatitidis* is by obtaining a culture specimen from sputum or fresh biopsy material and growing the organism on Sabouraud agar. This can be a slow technique, however, sometimes taking as long as 3–4 weeks for the characteristic yeast-to-mycelium conversion to take place. A specific DNA probe has been developed, allowing immediate identification of the mycelial phase. Serologic studies and skin testing are usually not helpful because of lack of reactivity and specificity.

Treatment and Prognosis

As stated previously, most patients with blastomycosis are asymptomatic or have only mild symptoms, so treatment may not be given because the disease is often not suspected. In the case of documented symptomatic acute or chronic pulmonary blastomycosis, itraconazole should be prescribed for mild to moderate disease, whereas systemic administration of a lipid formulation of amphotericin B is indicated for severe cases.

Immunosuppressed patients or those with extrapulmonary lesions also need treatment with amphotericin B, followed by

6–12 months of itraconazole. Although ketoconazole and fluconazole are active against *B. dermatitidis,* these drugs have been shown to be less effective than itraconazole.

Disseminated blastomycosis occurs in only a small percentage of infected patients and, with proper treatment, the outlook for the patient is reasonably good. Still, mortality rates ranging from 4% to 22% have been described over the past 20 years, with men, blacks, and patients with HIV infection tending to have less favorable outcomes.

◆ PARACOCCIDIOIDOMYCOSIS (SOUTH AMERICAN BLASTOMYCOSIS)

Paracoccidioidomycosis is a deep fungal infection that is caused by either *Paracoccidioides brasiliensis* or *Paracoccidioides lutzii.* The condition is seen most frequently in patients who live in either South America (primarily Brazil, Colombia, Venezuela, Uruguay, and Argentina) or Central America. However, immigrants from those regions and visitors to those areas can acquire the infection. Within some endemic areas, the nine-banded armadillo has been shown to harbor *P. brasiliensis* (similar to the situation seen with leprosy) (see page 188). Although there is no evidence that the armadillo directly infects humans, it may be responsible for the spread of the organism in the environment.

Paracoccidioidomycosis has a distinct predilection for males, with a 13:1 male-to-female ratio typically reported. This striking difference is thought to be attributable to a protective effect of female hormones (because β-estradiol inhibits the transformation of the hyphal form of the organism to the pathogenic yeast form). This theory is supported by the finding of an equal number of men and women who have antibodies directed against the yeast.

Clinical Features

Patients with paracoccidioidomycosis are typically middle-aged at the time of diagnosis, and most are employed in agriculture. Most cases of paracoccidioidomycosis are thought to appear initially as pulmonary infections after exposure to the spores of the organism. Although infections are generally self-limiting, *P. brasiliensis* and *P. lutzii* may spread by a hematogenous or lymphatic route to a variety of tissues, including lymph nodes, skin, and adrenal glands. Adrenal involvement often results in hypoadrenocorticism (**Addison disease**) (see page 843).

Oral lesions are frequently observed and appear as mulberry-like ulcerations that most commonly affect the alveolar mucosa, gingiva, and palate (Fig. 6.28). The lips, tongue, oropharynx, and buccal mucosa are also involved in a significant percentage of cases. In most patients with oral lesions, more than one oral mucosal site is affected.

Histopathologic Features

Microscopic evaluation of tissue obtained from an oral lesion may reveal pseudoepitheliomatous hyperplasia in addition to ulceration of the overlying surface epithelium. These

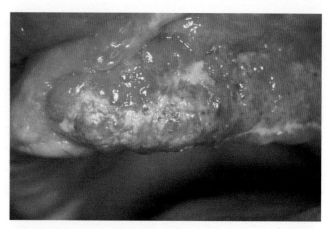

• **Fig. 6.28 Paracoccidioidomycosis.** This granular, erythematous, and ulcerated lesion of the maxillary alveolus represents infection by *Paracoccidioides brasiliensis.* (Courtesy of Dr. Ricardo Santiago Gomez.)

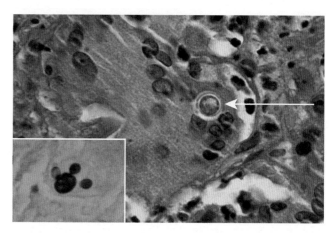

• **Fig. 6.29 Paracoccidioidomycosis.** This high-power photomicrograph shows a large yeast of *Paracoccidioides brasiliensis (arrow)* within the cytoplasm of a multinucleated giant cell. A section stained with the Grocott-Gomori methenamine silver method *(inset)* illustrates the characteristic "Mickey Mouse ears" appearance of the budding yeasts. (Courtesy of Dr. Ricardo Santiago Gomez.)

organisms elicit a granulomatous inflammatory host response that is characterized by collections of epithelioid macrophages and multinucleated giant cells (Fig. 6.29). Scattered, large (up to 30 μm in diameter) yeasts are readily identified after staining of the tissue sections with the Grocott-Gomori methenamine silver or PAS method. The organisms often show multiple daughter buds on the parent cell, resulting in an appearance that has been described as resembling "Mickey Mouse ears" or the spokes of a ship's steering wheel ("mariner's wheel").

Diagnosis

Demonstration of the characteristic multiple budding yeasts in the appropriate clinical setting is usually adequate to establish a diagnosis of paracoccidioidomycosis. Specimens for culture can be obtained, but *P. brasiliensis* and *P. lutzii* grow quite slowly.

Treatment and Prognosis

The method of management of patients with paracoccidioidomycosis depends on the severity of the disease presentation. Sulfonamide derivatives have been used since the 1940s to treat this infection. These drugs, such as trimethoprim/sulfamethoxazole, are still used today in many instances to treat mild-to-moderate cases, particularly in developing countries with limited access to the newer, more expensive antifungal agents. For severe involvement, IV amphotericin B is usually indicated, and this is followed by oral itraconazole. Non–life-threatening cases are best managed by oral itraconazole alone, although therapy may be needed for several months. Ketoconazole can also be used, although the side effects are typically greater than those associated with itraconazole.

◆ COCCIDIOIDOMYCOSIS (SAN JOAQUIN VALLEY FEVER; VALLEY FEVER; COCCI)

Molecular genetic studies have identified two species, *Coccidioides immitis* and *Coccidioides posadasii,* as the fungal organisms responsible for **coccidioidomycosis.** *C. immitis* grows saprophytically in the alkaline, semiarid, desert soil of the southwestern United States and Mexico primarily, whereas *C. posadasii* is generally found in similar isolated arid regions in Central and South America, with some overlap in their ranges. As with several other pathogenic fungi, *C. immitis* and *C. posadasii* are dimorphic organisms, appearing as a mold in the natural environment of the soil and as a yeast in tissues of the infected host. Arthrospores produced by the mold become airborne and can be inhaled into the lungs of the human host, producing infection. Both *Coccidioides* species produce clinically identical signs and symptoms.

Coccidioidomycosis is confined to the Western hemisphere and is endemic throughout the desert regions of southwestern United States and Mexico; however, with modern travel taking many visitors to and from the Sunbelt, this disease can be encountered virtually anywhere in the world. It is estimated that 100,000 people are infected annually in the United States, although 60% of this group are asymptomatic.

Clinical Features

Even though most infections with *C. immitis* are asymptomatic, approximately 40% of infected patients experience a flulike illness and pulmonary symptoms within 1–3 weeks after inhaling the arthrospores. Fatigue, cough, chest pain, myalgias, and headache are commonly reported, lasting several weeks with spontaneous resolution in most cases. Occasionally, the immune response may trigger a hypersensitivity reaction that causes the development of an erythema multiforme–like cutaneous eruption (see page 781) or erythema nodosum. Erythema nodosum is a condition that usually affects the skin of the legs and is characterized by the appearance of multiple painful erythematous inflammatory nodules in the subcutaneous connective tissue. This hypersensitivity reaction occurring in conjunction with coccidioidomycosis is termed **valley fever**, and it resolves as the host cell–mediated immune response controls the pulmonary infection.

Chronic progressive pulmonary coccidioidomycosis is relatively rare. It mimics tuberculosis, with its clinical presentation of persistent cough, hemoptysis, chest pain, low-grade fever, and weight loss.

Disseminated coccidioidomycosis occurs when the organism spreads hematogenously to extrapulmonary sites. This occurs in less than 1% of cases, but it is a more serious problem. The most commonly involved areas include skin, lymph nodes (including cervical lymph nodes), bone and joints, and the meninges. Immunosuppression greatly increases the risk of dissemination. The following groups are particularly susceptible:
- Patients taking large doses of systemic corticosteroids (e.g., organ transplant recipients)
- Patients who are being treated with cancer chemotherapy
- Patients who are being treated with TNF-α inhibitors
- Patients in the end stages of HIV infection
- Patients who are pregnant (especially in the third trimester or immediately postpartum)

Infants and older adult patients, both of whom may have suboptimally functioning immune systems, also may be at increased risk for disseminated disease. Persons of color (e.g., blacks, Filipinos, and Native Americans) also seem to have an increased risk, but it is unclear whether their susceptibility is due to genetic causes or socioeconomic factors, such as occupation or poor nutrition.

The cutaneous lesions may appear as papules, subcutaneous abscesses, verrucous plaques, and granulomatous nodules. Of prime significance to the clinician is the predilection for these lesions to develop in the area of the central face, especially the nasolabial fold. Oral lesions are distinctly uncommon, and these have been described as ulcerated granulomatous nodules (Fig. 6.30).

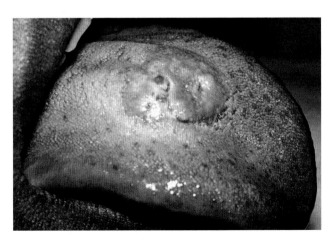

• **Fig. 6.30 Coccidioidomycosis.** This ulcerated nodule involving the mid-dorsal tongue represents disseminated coccidioidomycosis. (Courtesy of Dr. Craig Fowler.)

Histopathologic Features

Biopsy material shows large (20–60 μm), round spherules that may contain numerous endospores. The host response may be variable, ranging from a suppurative, neutrophilic infiltrate to a granulomatous inflammatory response. In some cases, the two patterns of inflammation are seen concurrently. Special stains, such as the PAS and Grocott-Gomori methenamine silver methods, enable the pathologist to identify the organism more readily.

Diagnosis

The diagnosis of coccidioidomycosis can be confirmed by culture or identification of characteristic organisms in biopsy material. If the organisms do not have a classic microscopic appearance, then *in situ* hybridization studies using specific complementary DNA probes for *C. immitis* can be performed to definitively identify the fungus. Cytologic preparations from bronchial swabbing or sputum samples may also reveal the organisms.

Serologic studies are helpful in supporting the diagnosis, and they may be performed at the same time as skin testing. Skin testing by itself may be of limited value in determining the diagnosis, because many patients in endemic areas have already been exposed to the organism and have positive test findings.

Treatment

The decision whether or not to treat a particular patient affected by coccidioidomycosis depends on the severity and extent of the infection and the patient's immune status. Relatively mild symptoms in an immunocompetent person do not warrant treatment. Amphotericin B is administered for the following groups:

- Immunosuppressed patients
- Patients with severe pulmonary infection
- Patients who have disseminated disease
- Patients who are pregnant
- Patients who appear to be in a life-threatening situation concerning the infection

For many cases of coccidioidomycosis, fluconazole or itraconazole is the drug of choice, usually given in high doses for an extended period of time. Although the response of the disease to these oral azole medications may be somewhat slower than that of amphotericin B, the side effects and complications of therapy are far fewer. Newer triazole medications, such as voriconazole, can be used if resolution is not seen with fluconazole or itraconazole.

◆ CRYPTOCOCCOSIS

Cryptococcosis is a relatively uncommon fungal disease caused primarily by the yeast *Cryptococcus neoformans* in North America. This organism normally causes no problem in immunocompetent people, but it can be devastating to the immunocompromised patient. The incidence of cryptococcosis increased dramatically during the 1990s, primarily because of the AIDS epidemic. At that time, this was the most common life-threatening fungal infection in these patients. However, with the advent of combination antiretroviral therapy (cART) (see page 264), this complication has become less of a problem in the United States. In countries where the population cannot afford cART, cryptococcosis remains a significant cause of death for AIDS patients. The disease has a worldwide distribution because of its association with the pigeon (with the organism living in the deposits of excreta left by the birds). Unlike many other pathogenic fungi, *C. neoformans* grows as a yeast both in the soil and in infected tissue. The organism usually produces a prominent mucopolysaccharide capsule that appears to protect it from host immune defenses.

The disease is acquired by inhalation of *C. neoformans* spores into the lungs, resulting in an immediate influx of neutrophils, which destroys most of the yeasts. Macrophages soon follow, although resolution of infection in the immunocompetent host ultimately depends on an intact cell-mediated immune system.

Over the past couple of decades, molecular genetic studies have identified another species of *Cryptococcus,* designated *Cryptococcus gattii,* which had initially been thought to be a serotype of *C. neoformans.* This organism seems to be more capable of producing infection in otherwise normal immunocompetent individuals. Although *C. gattii* is more commonly found in tropical and subtropical environments, outbreaks have been documented in the Pacific Northwest in North America. At the molecular level, microbiologists now recognize at least six different genotypes of these yeasts in what may be described as the *C. neoformans/gattii* species complex.

Clinical Features

Primary cryptococcal infection of the lungs is often asymptomatic; however, a mild flulike illness may develop. Patients complain of productive cough, chest pain, fever, and malaise. Most patients with a diagnosis of cryptococcosis have a significant underlying medical problem related to immune suppression (e.g., systemic corticosteroid therapy, cancer chemotherapy, malignancy, or AIDS). It is estimated that 5%–10% of AIDS patients acquire this infection (see page 250).

Dissemination of the infection is common in these immunocompromised patients, and the most frequent site of involvement is the meninges, followed by skin, bone, and the prostate gland.

Cryptococcal meningitis is characterized by headache, fever, vomiting, and neck stiffness. In many instances, this is the initial sign of the disease.

Cutaneous lesions develop in 10%–15% of patients with disseminated disease. These are of particular importance to the clinician, because the skin of the head and neck is often

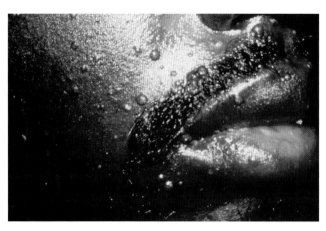

• **Fig. 6.31 Cryptococcosis.** These papules of the facial skin represent disseminated cryptococcal infection in a patient infected with human immunodeficiency virus (HIV). (Courtesy of Dr. Catherine Flaitz.)

involved. The lesions appear as erythematous papules or pustules that may ulcerate, discharging a puslike material rich in cryptococcal organisms (Fig. 6.31).

Although oral lesions are relatively rare, they have been described either as craterlike, nonhealing ulcers that are tender on palpation or as friable papillary erythematous plaques. Dissemination to salivary gland tissue also has been reported rarely.

Histopathologic Features

Microscopic sections of a cryptococcal lesion generally show a granulomatous inflammatory response to the organism. The extent of the response may vary, however, depending on the host's immune status and the strain of the organism. The yeast appears as a round-to-ovoid structure, 4–6 μm in diameter, surrounded by a clear halo that represents the capsule. Staining with the PAS or Grocott-Gomori methenamine silver method readily identifies the fungus; moreover, a mucicarmine stain uniquely demonstrates its mucopolysaccharide capsule.

Diagnosis

The diagnosis of cryptococcosis can be made by several methods, including biopsy and culture. Detection of cryptococcal polysaccharide antigen in the serum or cerebrospinal fluid is also useful as a diagnostic procedure.

Treatment and Prognosis

Management of cryptococcal infections can be very difficult because most of the affected patients have an underlying medical problem. Before amphotericin B was developed, cryptococcosis was almost uniformly fatal. For cryptococcal meningitis, a combination of systemic amphotericin B and another antifungal drug (flucytosine) is used initially for 2 weeks in most cases to treat this disease. Then, either

fluconazole or itraconazole is given for an additional minimal period of 10 weeks. For relatively mild cases of pulmonary cryptococcosis, only fluconazole or itraconazole may be used. These drugs produce far fewer side effects than do amphotericin B and flucytosine, and they have proven to be important therapeutic tools for managing this type of infection.

◆ MUCORMYCOSIS (ZYGOMYCOSIS; PHYCOMYCOSIS)

Mucormycosis is an opportunistic, frequently fulminant, fungal infection that is caused by normally saprobic organisms of the subphylum Mucoromycotina, including such genera as *Absidia, Mucor, Rhizomucor,* and *Rhizopus.* The term *zygomycosis* is still used extensively in the literature, although recent molecular genetic studies have indicated that the class Zygomycetes actually is comprised of several unrelated fungi. Mucoromycotina organisms are found throughout the world, growing in their natural state on a variety of decaying organic materials. Numerous spores may be liberated into the air and inhaled by the human host.

Mucormycosis may involve any one of several areas of the body, but the rhinocerebral form is most relevant to the oral health care provider. Mucormycosis is noted especially in insulin-dependent diabetics who have uncontrolled diabetes and are ketoacidotic; ketoacidosis inhibits the binding of iron to transferrin, allowing serum iron levels to rise. The growth of these fungi is enhanced by iron, and patients who are taking deferoxamine (an iron-chelating agent used in the treatment of diseases, such as thalassemia) are also at increased risk for developing mucormycosis. As with many other fungal diseases, this infection affects immunocompromised patients as well, including bone marrow transplant recipients, patients with AIDS, and those receiving systemic corticosteroid therapy. Only rarely has mucormycosis been reported in apparently healthy individuals in the oral region.

Clinical and Radiographic Features

The presenting symptoms of rhinocerebral mucormycosis may be exhibited in several ways. Patients may experience nasal obstruction, bloody nasal discharge, facial pain or headache, facial swelling or cellulitis, and visual disturbances with concurrent proptosis. Symptoms related to cranial nerve involvement (e.g., facial paralysis) are often present. With progression of disease into the cranial vault, blindness, lethargy, and seizures may develop, followed by death.

If the maxillary sinus is involved, the initial presentation may be seen as intraoral swelling of the maxillary alveolar process, the palate, or both. If the condition remains untreated, palatal ulceration may evolve, with the surface of the ulcer typically appearing black and necrotic. Massive tissue destruction may result if the condition is not treated (Figs. 6.32 and 6.33).

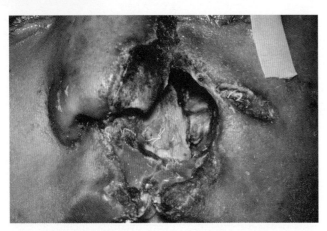

• **Fig. 6.32 Mucormycosis.** Diffuse tissue destruction involving the nasal and maxillary structures caused by a *Mucor* species. (Courtesy of Dr. Sadru Kabani.)

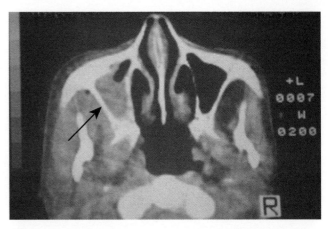

• **Fig. 6.34 Mucormycosis.** This computed tomography (CT) scan demonstrates the opacification of the left maxillary sinus *(arrow)*.

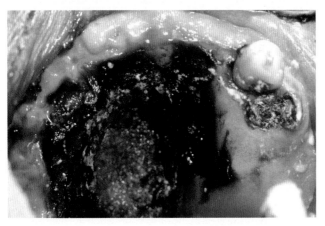

• **Fig. 6.33 Mucormycosis.** The extensive black, necrotic lesion of the palate represents mucormycotic infection that extended from the maxillary sinus in a patient with poorly controlled type I diabetes mellitus. (Courtesy of Dr. Michael Tabor.)

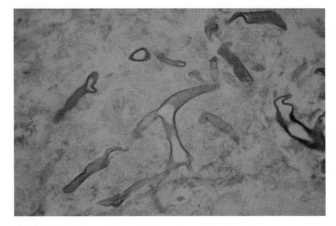

• **Fig. 6.35 Mucormycosis.** This high-power photomicrograph shows the large, nonseptate fungal hyphae characteristic of the mucormycotic organisms.

Radiographically, opacification of the sinuses may be observed in conjunction with patchy effacement of the bony walls of the sinuses (Fig. 6.34). Such a picture may be difficult to distinguish from that of a malignancy affecting the sinus area.

Histopathologic Features

Histopathologic examination of lesional tissue shows extensive necrosis with numerous large (6–30 μm in diameter), branching, nonseptate hyphae at the periphery (Fig. 6.35). The hyphae tend to branch at 90-degree angles. The extensive tissue destruction and necrosis associated with this disease are undoubtedly attributable to the preference of the fungi for invasion of small blood vessels. This disrupts normal blood flow to the tissue, resulting in infarction and necrosis. A neutrophilic infiltrate usually predominates in the viable tissue, but the host inflammatory cell response to the infection may be minimal, particularly if the patient is immunosuppressed.

Diagnosis

Diagnosis of mucormycosis is usually based on the histopathologic findings. Because of the grave nature of this infection, appropriate therapy must be instituted in a timely manner (often without the benefit of definitive culture results).

Treatment and Prognosis

Successful treatment of rhinocerebral mucormycosis consists of rapid accurate diagnosis of the condition, followed by radical surgical débridement of the infected, necrotic tissue and systemic administration of high doses of one of the lipid formulations of amphotericin B. Posaconazole or isavuconazole can be added for long-term treatment after initial control with amphotericin B. Recent studies have suggested that isavuconazole alone, given as initial therapy, may be as effective as amphotericin B for treatment of mucormycosis. Magnetic resonance imaging (MRI) of the head may be useful in determining the extent of disease involvement so that surgical margins can be planned. Evaluation of frozen sections of curetted tissue, which has been stained with Calcofluor white and examined with fluorescence microscopy, can also be used to guide the extent of débridement. In addition, control of the patient's underlying disease (e.g., diabetic ketoacidosis) must be attempted.

Despite such therapy, the prognosis is usually poor, with approximately 40%–50% of patients who develop rhinocerebral mucormycosis dying of their disease. Because their underlying systemic disease can usually be controlled, diabetic patients typically have a better prognosis than those who are immunosuppressed. If the patient survives, the massive tissue destruction that remains presents a challenge both functionally and aesthetically. Prosthetic obturation of palatal defects may be necessary.

◆ ASPERGILLOSIS

Aspergillosis is a fungal disease that is characterized by noninvasive and invasive forms. Noninvasive aspergillosis usually affects a normal host, appearing either as an allergic reaction or a cluster of fungal hyphae. Localized invasive infection of damaged tissue may be seen in a normal host, but a more extensive invasive infection is often evident in the immunocompromised patient. With the advent of intensive chemotherapeutic regimens, the AIDS epidemic, and both solid-organ and bone marrow transplantation, the prevalence of invasive aspergillosis has increased dramatically in the past 20 years. Patients with uncontrolled diabetes mellitus are also susceptible to *Aspergillus* spp. infections. Rarely, invasive aspergillosis has been reported to affect the paranasal sinuses of apparently normal immunocompetent individuals.

Normally, the various species of the *Aspergillus* genus reside worldwide as saprobic organisms in soil, water, or decaying organic debris. Resistant spores are released into the air and inhaled by the human host, resulting in opportunistic fungal infection second in frequency only to candidiasis. Interestingly, most species of *Aspergillus* cannot grow at 37°C; only the pathogenic species have the ability to replicate at body temperature.

The two most commonly encountered species of *Aspergillus* in the medical setting are *A. flavus* and *A. fumigatus,* with *A. fumigatus* being responsible for most cases of aspergillosis. The patient may acquire such infections in the hospital (**"nosocomial"** infection), especially if remodeling or building construction is being performed in the immediate area. Such activity often stirs up the spores, which are then inhaled by the patient.

Clinical Features

The clinical manifestations of aspergillosis vary, depending on the host immune status and the presence or absence of tissue damage. In the normal host, the disease may appear as an allergy affecting either the sinuses (**allergic fungal sinusitis**) or the bronchopulmonary tract. An asthma attack may be triggered by inhalation of spores by a susceptible person. Sometimes a low-grade infection becomes established in the maxillary sinus, resulting in a mass of fungal hyphae called a **fungus ball,** although **aspergilloma** and **mycetoma**

are terms that are also sometimes used (Fig. 6.36). Occasionally, the mass will undergo dystrophic calcification, producing a radiopaque body called an **antrolith** within the sinus.

Another presentation that may be encountered by the oral health care provider is aspergillosis after tooth extraction or endodontic treatment, especially in the maxillary posterior segments. Presumably, tissue damage predisposes the sinus to infection, resulting in symptoms of localized pain and tenderness accompanied by nasal discharge. Immunocompromised patients are particularly susceptible to oral aspergillosis, and some investigators have suggested that the portal of entry may be the marginal gingiva and gingival sulcus. Painful gingival ulcerations are initially noted, and peripherally the mucosa and soft tissue develops diffuse swelling with a gray or violaceous hue (Fig. 6.37). If the disease is not treated, extensive necrosis, which is seen clinically as a yellow or black ulcer, and facial swelling evolve.

Disseminated aspergillosis occurs principally in immunocompromised patients, particularly in those who have leukemia or who are taking high daily doses of corticosteroids. Such patients usually exhibit symptoms related to the primary site of inoculation: the lungs. The patient typically has chest pain, cough, and fever, but such symptoms are vague. Therefore, obtaining an early, accurate diagnosis may be difficult. Once the fungal organism obtains access

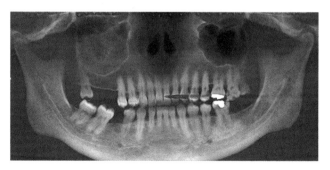

• **Fig. 6.36 Aspergillosis.** The opaque appearance of the right maxillary sinus is due to the presence of a fungus ball (aspergilloma). (Courtesy of Dr. Bart Farrell.)

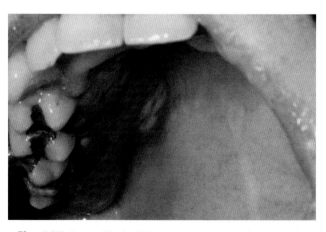

• **Fig. 6.37 Aspergillosis.** This young woman developed a painful purplish swelling of her hard palate after induction chemotherapy for leukemia.

to the bloodstream, infection can spread to such sites as the CNS, eye, skin, liver, gastrointestinal tract, bone, and thyroid gland.

Histopathologic Features

Tissue sections of invasive *Aspergillus* spp. lesions show varying numbers of branching, septate hyphae, 3–4 μm in diameter (Figs. 6.38 and 6.39). These hyphae show a tendency to branch at an acute angle and to invade adjacent small blood vessels. Occlusion of the vessels often results in the characteristic pattern of necrosis associated with this disease. In the immunocompetent host, a granulomatous inflammatory response—in addition to necrosis—can be expected. In the immunocompromised patient, however, the inflammatory response is often weak or absent, leading to extensive tissue destruction.

Noninvasive forms of aspergillosis have histopathologic features that differ from invasive aspergillosis, however. The fungus ball, for example, is characterized by a tangled mass of hyphae with no evidence of tissue invasion. Because the fungus ball develops in a paranasal sinus (where it is exposed to air), spore-bearing structures called *fruiting bodies* are formed (see Fig. 6.38). Allergic fungal

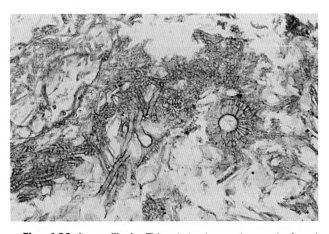

• **Fig. 6.38 Aspergillosis.** This photomicrograph reveals fungal hyphae and a fruiting body of an *Aspergillus* species.

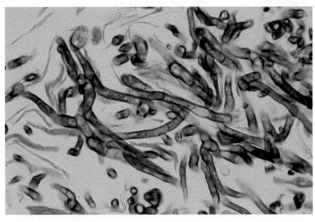

• **Fig. 6.39 Aspergillosis.** This high-power photomicrograph shows the characteristic septate hyphae of *Aspergillus* species. (Grocott-Gomori methenamine silver stain.)

sinusitis, on the other hand, histopathologically exhibits large pools of eosinophilic inspissated mucin with interspersed sheetlike collections of lymphocytes and eosinophils. Relatively few fungal hyphae are identified, and then only with careful examination after Grocott-Gomori methenamine silver staining.

Diagnosis

Although the diagnosis of fungal infection can be established by identification of hyphae within tissue sections, this finding is only suggestive of aspergillosis because other fungal organisms may appear similar microscopically. Ideally, the diagnosis should be supported by culture of the organism from the lesion; however, from a practical standpoint, treatment may need to be initiated immediately to prevent the patient's demise. Culture specimens of sputum and blood are of limited value, because they are often negative despite disseminated disease.

Treatment and Prognosis

Treatment depends on the clinical presentation of aspergillosis. For immunocompetent patients with a noninvasive aspergilloma, surgical débridement may be all that is necessary. Patients who have allergic fungal sinusitis are treated with débridement and corticosteroid drugs. For localized invasive aspergillosis in the immunocompetent host, débridement followed by antifungal medication is indicated. Although systemic amphotericin B deoxycholate therapy was considered appropriate in the past, studies have shown that voriconazole, a triazole antifungal agent, is more effective for treating these patients. In one large series of patients with invasive aspergillosis, 71% of those treated with voriconazole were alive after 12 weeks of therapy, compared with 58% survival in the group who received standard amphotericin B treatment. For patients who cannot tolerate voriconazole, alternative drugs include isavuconazole, liposomal amphotericin B, or one of the echinocandins, such as caspofungin or micafungin. Immunocompromised patients who have invasive aspergillosis should be treated by aggressive débridement of necrotic tissue, combined with systemic antifungal therapy as described previously.

The prognosis for immunocompromised patients is much worse compared with immunocompetent individuals, particularly if the infection is disseminated. Even with appropriate therapy, only about one third of these patients survive. Because aspergillosis in the immunocompromised patient usually develops while the individual is hospitalized, particular attention should be given to the ventilation system in the hospital to prevent patient exposure to the airborne spores of *Aspergillus* spp.

◆ TOXOPLASMOSIS

Toxoplasmosis is a relatively common disease caused by the obligate intracellular protozoal organism *Toxoplasma gondii*. For normal, healthy adults, the organism poses no problems, and an estimated 8%–22% of adults in the United States may have had asymptomatic infection, based on an epidemiologic study that examined serologic samples from more than 4000 randomized individuals. However, the prevalence of infection has considerable geographic variation around the world. Unfortunately, the disease can be devastating for the developing fetus or the immunocompromised patient. Other mammals, particularly members of the cat family, are vulnerable to infection, and cats are considered to be the definitive host. *T. gondii* multiplies in the intestinal tract of the cat by means of a sexual life cycle, discharging numerous oocysts in the cat feces. Another animal or human can ingest these oocysts, resulting in the production of disease.

Clinical Features

In the normal, immunocompetent individual, infection with *T. gondii* is often asymptomatic. If symptoms develop, they are usually mild and resemble infectious mononucleosis; patients may have a low-grade fever, cervical lymphadenopathy, fatigue, and muscle or joint pain. These symptoms may last from a few weeks to a few months, although the host typically recovers without therapy. Sometimes the lymphadenopathy involves one or more of the lymph nodes in the paraoral region, such as the buccal or submental lymph node. In such instances, the oral health care provider may discover the disease.

In immunosuppressed patients, toxoplasmosis may represent a new, primary infection or, more frequently, reactivation of previously encysted organisms. The principal groups at risk include the following:
- AIDS patients
- Transplant recipients
- Cancer patients

Manifestations of infection can include necrotizing encephalitis, pneumonia, and myositis or myocarditis. In the United States, it is estimated that from 3% to 10% of AIDS patients who are not being treated with combination antiretroviral therapy (cART) (see page 264) will experience CNS involvement. CNS infection is very serious. Clinically, the patient may complain of headache, lethargy, disorientation, and hemiparesis.

Congenital toxoplasmosis occurs when a non-immune mother contracts the disease during her pregnancy and the organism crosses the placental barrier, infecting the developing fetus. The potential effects of blindness, intellectual impairment, and delayed psychomotor development are most severe if the infection occurs during the first trimester of pregnancy.

Histopathologic Features

Histopathologic examination of a lymph node obtained from a patient with active toxoplasmosis shows characteristic reactive germinal centers exhibiting an accumulation of eosinophilic macrophages. The macrophages encroach on the germinal centers and accumulate within the subcapsular and sinusoidal regions of the node (Fig. 6.40).

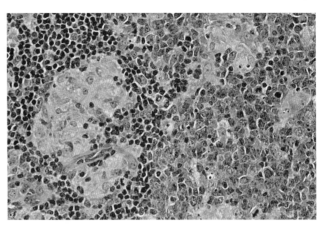

• **Fig. 6.40 Toxoplasmosis.** This high-power photomicrograph shows an accumulation of eosinophilic macrophages within a lymph node. (Courtesy of Dr. John Kalmar.)

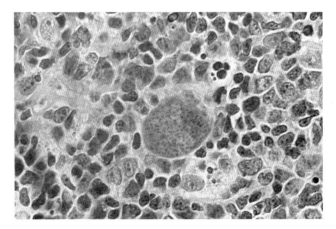

• **Fig. 6.41 Toxoplasmosis.** In this high-power photomicrograph, an encysted organism of toxoplasmosis is highlighted by an immunohistochemical study. (Courtesy of Dr. John Kalmar.)

Diagnosis

The diagnosis of toxoplasmosis is usually established by identification of rising serum antibody titers to *T. gondii* within 10–14 days after infection. Immunocompromised patients, however, may not be able to generate an antibody response; therefore, the diagnosis may rest on the clinical findings and the response of the patient to therapy.

Biopsy of an involved lymph node may suggest the diagnosis, and the causative organisms can sometimes be detected immunohistochemically using antibodies directed against *T. gondii*–specific antigens (Fig. 6.41). The diagnosis should also be confirmed by serologic studies, if possible.

Treatment and Prognosis

Most healthy adults with toxoplasmosis require no specific treatment because of the mild symptoms and self-limiting course. Perhaps more importantly, pregnant women should avoid situations that place them at risk for the disease. Handling or eating raw meat, eating raw, unpeeled fruits or vegetables, or cleaning a cat litter box should be avoided until after delivery. If exposure during pregnancy is suspected, treatment with a combination of sulfadiazine and pyrimethamine often prevents transmission of *T. gondii* to the fetus, although pyrimethamine is contraindicated in the first trimester due to its potential teratogenicity. Because these drugs act by inhibiting folate metabolism of the protozoan, folinic acid is given concurrently to help prevent hematologic complications in the patient. A similar drug regimen is used to treat immunosuppressed individuals with toxoplasmosis, although clindamycin may be substituted for sulfadiazine in managing patients who are allergic to sulfa drugs. Because most cases of toxoplasmosis in AIDS patients represent reactivation of encysted organisms, prophylactic administration of trimethoprim and sulfamethoxazole is generally recommended, particularly if the patient's CD4+ T-lymphocyte count is less than 100 cells/μL.

◆ LEISHMANIASIS

Leishmaniasis is a protozoal infection that is transmitted to humans by the bite of certain species of sandfly. Both Old World and New World forms of the disease are recognized, and they are caused by different species of sandfly as well as different species of *Leishmania*. Although the disease has been reported on every continent except Australia and Antarctica, most of the cases are found in relatively few countries, particularly India (Bihar State), Afghanistan, Saudi Arabia, Syria, Algeria, Peru, and Brazil. Of course, because of international travel to these areas, leishmaniasis can be seen in virtually every corner of the earth.

Dogs and other mammals are the primary reservoir for leishmaniasis, and in the mammalian host the organism is an obligate intracellular parasite. When an infected animal is bitten by the female sandfly, macrophages containing the amastigote (lacking flagella) phase of the organism are ingested by the fly as it drinks the animal's blood. In the gut of the sandfly, the amastigote organisms develop into free-living promastigotes (having flagella). When the fly later bites a human (or another mammal), the promastigote organisms are injected into the subcutaneous tissues, where they are phagocytosed by macrophages, neutrophils, or dendritic cells. Once ingested, the promastigote transforms into an amastigote, which multiplies within the host cells, completing the parasitic cycle. Sometimes the replication is so pronounced that the phagocytic host cells ruptures, releasing amastigotes into the bloodstream, and causing infection of more host cells.

Clinical Features

Depending on the *Leishmania* species and the immune status of the human host, at least three presentations of disease are generally recognized:
- Cutaneous—either Old World or New World; New World cases caused by *Leishmania mexicana* complex
- Mucocutaneous—primarily New World; caused by *Leishmania braziliensis* complex

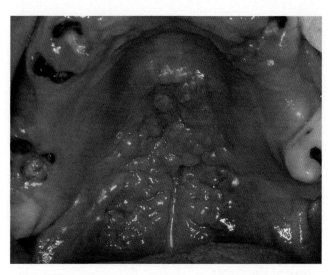

• **Fig. 6.42 Leishmaniasis.** Ulceration and granulomatous enlargement of the palatal mucosa in a patient with mucocutaneous leishmaniasis. (Courtesy of Dr. Ricardo Santiago Gomez.)

- Visceral ("kala-azar")—either Old World or New World; caused primarily by *Leishmania donovani* in the Old World; *L. braziliensis* in the New World

Cutaneous leishmaniasis is by far the most common form of the disease. Individual lesions develop 3–6 weeks after the person is bitten, presenting as an elevated erythematous papule or nodule with a depressed, ulcerated center, often said to resemble a volcano. Such lesions persist for months but often eventually heal. Significant scarring is usually noted, however.

Mucocutaneous leishmaniasis is not as common as cutaneous leishmaniasis, but it is much more destructive. Most of the *Leishmania* species responsible for this form of the disease are found in South America. The skin of affected patients shows more diffuse involvement, characterized by scaly and ulcerative plaques and nodules. From several months to as long as 5 years later, mucosal involvement develops. Typically this begins with the nasal mucosa, but oral, pharyngeal, tracheal, and laryngeal mucosa often are involved eventually (Fig. 6.42). Perforation of the nasal septum or the hard and soft palate, as well as destruction of the alveolar bone, may be present. The extent of the damage may be so severe that it can be a life-threatening process.

Visceral leishmaniasis (also known as *kala-azar,* which is Hindi for "black fever") is characterized by grayish discoloration of the skin in some patients, hepatosplenomegaly, fever (usually related to pancytopenia), and weight loss. The severity of disease expression is undoubtedly related to the health of the patient prior to infection.

Histopathologic Features

The amastigote *Leishmania* organisms can be detected within the cytoplasm of histiocytes in touch preparations of infected tissue or in histopathologic sections. The protozoans may be seen in routine H&E-stained sections, but other stains such as Giemsa, Brown-Hopps (a tissue Gram stain), or Leishman methods may aid identification. In older, chronic lesions, the organisms may be sparse, making the diagnosis more challenging.

Diagnosis

Although the diagnosis of leishmaniasis often can be made on the cytologic or histopathologic findings, it is sometimes necessary to obtain tissue for culture or polymerase chain reaction (PCR) studies. These latter techniques are usually available only at specialized laboratories. Serologic studies can be difficult to interpret at times because many individuals in endemic areas have had exposure to the organism, although they may not have active disease.

Treatment and Prognosis

Since the 1920s, antimony compounds have been used to treat leishmaniasis, but these drugs often have significant side effects because they are heavy metals. Liposomal amphotericin B is ideally the drug of choice, but this less toxic compound is often too expensive for widespread use in developing countries. Most leishmaniasis patients receive treatment with pentavalent antimonial compounds, with the antiprotozoal drug pentamidine used for patients who cannot tolerate antimonial compounds. Attempts to develop a vaccine have not met with success.

The prognosis of leishmaniasis can be affected by both host factors (e.g., malnutrition and immune suppression) and organism factors, which are related to the *Leishmania* species responsible for infection. Without treatment, visceral leishmaniasis has an ominous prognosis and often results in death, whereas cutaneous leishmaniasis is typically a chronic, bothersome superficial infection. Mucocutaneous leishmaniasis has an intermediate course, although significant morbidity results from tissue destruction by the infection. All forms of leishmaniasis generally require weeks to months of therapy, and relapses are relatively common.

Bibliography

Candidiasis
Allen CM: Diagnosing and managing oral candidiasis, *J Am Dent Assoc* 123:77–82, 1992.
Barbeau J, Séguin J, Goulet JP, et al.: Reassessing the presence of *Candida albicans* in denture-related stomatitis, *Oral Surg Oral Med Oral Pathol Oral Radiol Endod* 95:51–59, 2003.
Baughman RA: Median rhomboid glossitis: a developmental anomaly? *Oral Surg Oral Med Oral Pathol* 31:56–65, 1971.
Böckle BC, Wilhelm M, Müller H, et al.: Oral mucous squamous cell carcinoma—an anticipated consequence of autoimmune polyendocrinopathy-candidiasis-ectodermal dystrophy (APECED), *J Am Acad Dermatol* 62:864–868, 2010.
Carey B, Lambourne J, Porter S, et al.: Chronic mucocutaneous candidiasis due to gain-of-function mutation in STAT1, *Oral Dis* 25:684–692, 2019.

Carmona EM, Limper AH: Overview of treatment approaches for fungal infections, *Clin Chest Med* 38:393–402, 2017.
Fotos PG, Vincent SD, Hellstein JW: Oral candidosis: clinical, historical and therapeutic features of 100 cases, *Oral Surg Oral Med Oral Pathol* 74:41–49, 1992.
Gendreau L, Loewy ZG: Epidemiology and etiology of denture stomatitis, *J Prosthodont* 20:251–260, 2011.
Hellstein JW, Marek CL: Candidiasis: red and white manifestations in the oral cavity, *Head Neck Pathol* 13:25–32, 2019.
Humbert L, Cornu M, Proust-Lemoine E, et al.: Chronic mucocutaneous candidiasis in autoimmune polyendocrine syndrome type 1, *Front Immunol* 9:2570, 2018. https://doi.org/10.3389/fimmu.2018.02570.
Kisand K, Wolff ASB, Podkrajšek KT, et al.: Chronic mucocutaneous candidiasis in APECED or thymoma patients correlates with autoimmunity to Th17-associated cytokines, *J Exp Med* 207:299–308, 2010.
Lewis MAO, Williams DW: Diagnosis and management of oral candidosis, *Br Dent J* 223:675–681, 2017.
McManus BA, McGovern E, Moran GP, et al.: Microbiologic screening of Irish patients with autoimmune polyendocrinopathy-candidiasis-ectodermal dystrophy reveals persistence of *Candida albicans* strains, gradual reduction in susceptibility to azoles, and incidences of clinical signs of oral candidiasis without culture evidence, *J Clin Microbiol* 49:1879–1889, 2011.
Odds FC, Arai T, Disalvo AF, et al.: Nomenclature of fungal diseases: a report and recommendations from a sub-committee of the International Society for Human and Animal Mycology (ISHAM), *J Med Vet Mycol* 30:1–10, 1992.
Öhman S-C, Dahlen G, Moller A, et al.: Angular cheilitis: a clinical and microbial study, *J Oral Pathol* 15:213–217, 1986.
Quindós G, Gil-Alonso S, Marcos-Arias C, et al.: Therapeutic tools for oral candidiasis: current and new antifungal drugs, *Med Oral Patol Oral Cir Bucal* 24:e172–e180, 2019.
Samaranayake LP, Leung WK, Jin L: Oral mucosal fungal infections, *Periodontol 2000* 2000(49):39–59, 2009.
Sitheeque MAM, Samaranayake LP: Chronic hyperplastic candidosis/candidiasis (candidal leukoplakia), *Crit Rev Oral Biol Med* 14:253–267, 2003.
Williams DW, Kuriyama T, Silva S, et al.: *Candida* biofilms and oral candidosis: treatment and prevention, *Periodontol 2000* 2000(55):250–265, 2011.

Histoplasmosis
Antonello VS, Zaltron VF, Vial M, et al.: Oropharyngeal histoplasmosis: report of eleven cases and review of the literature, *Rev Soc Bras Med Trop* 44:26–29, 2011.
Ashraf N, Kubat RC, Poplin V, et al.: Re-drawing the maps for endemic mycoses, *Mycopathologia* 185:843–865, 2020. https://doi.org/10.1007/s11046-020-00431-2.
Azar MM, Hage CA: Laboratory diagnostics for histoplasmosis, *J Clin Microbiol* 55:1612–1620, 2017. https://doi.org/10.1128/JCM.02430-16.
Briody A, Santosh N, Allen CM, et al.: Chronic ulceration of the tongue, *J Am Dent Assoc* 147:744–748, 2016.
Deepe GS Jr: Outbreaks of histoplasmosis: the spores set sail, *PLoS Pathog* 14:e1007213, 2018. https://doi.org/10.1371/journal.ppat.1007213.
Folk GA, Nelson BL: Oral histoplasmosis, *Head Neck Pathol* 11:513–516, 2017.
Leal-Alcure M, Di Hipólito-Júnior O, Paes de Almeida O, et al.: Oral histoplasmosis in an HIV-negative patient, *Oral Surg Oral Med Oral Pathol Oral Radiol Endod* 101:e33–e36, 2006.

McKinsey DS, McKinsey JP: Pulmonary histoplasmosis, *Semin Respir Crit Care Med* 32:735–744, 2011.

Motta ACF, Galo R, Grupioni-Lourenço A, et al.: Unusual orofacial manifestations of histoplasmosis in renal transplanted patient, *Mycopathologia* 161:161–165, 2006.

Narayana N, Gifford R, Giannini P, et al.: Oral histoplasmosis: an unusual presentation, *Head Neck* 31:274–277, 2009.

Samaranayake LP: Oral mycoses in HIV infection, *Oral Surg Oral Med Oral Pathol* 73:171–180, 1992.

Singh A, Gauri M, Gautam P, et al.: Head and neck involvement with histoplasmosis; the great masquerader, *Am J Otolaryngol* 40:678–683, 2019.

Smith JA, Kauffman CA: Endemic fungal infections in patients receiving tumor necrosis factor-α inhibitor therapy, *Drugs* 69:1403–1415, 2009.

Wheat LJ, Azar MM, Bahr NC, et al.: Histoplasmosis, *Infect Dis Clin North Am* 30:207–227, 2016.

Blastomycosis

Albarillo FS, Varma GT, MacLeod SPR: Mandibular blastomycosis: a case report and review of the literature, *GERMS* 8(4):207–213, 2018. https://doi.org/10.18683/germs.2018.1148.

Ashraf N, Kubat RC, Poplin V, et al.: Re-drawing the maps for endemic mycoses, *Mycopathologia*, 2020 Feb 10. https://doi.org/10.1007/s11046-020-00431-2 (Epub ahead of print).

Bariola JR, Vyas KS: Pulmonary blastomycosis, *Semin Respir Crit Care Med* 32:745–753, 2011.

Bradsher RW: Pulmonary blastomycosis, *Semin Respir Crit Care Med* 29:174–181, 2008.

Castillo CG, Kauffman CA, Miceli MH: Blastomycosis, *Infect Dis Clin North Am* 30:247–264, 2016.

Brown EM, McTaggart LR, Zhang SX, et al.: Phylogenetic analysis reveals a cryptic species *Blastomyces gilchristii*, sp. nov. within the human pathogenic fungus *Blastomyces dermatitidis*, *PLoS One* 8:e59237, 2013.

Dworkin MS, Duckro AN, Proia L, et al.: The epidemiology of blastomycosis in Illinois and factors associated with death, *Clin Infect Dis* 41:e107–e111, 2005.

Gandhi V, Singh A, Woods GL, et al.: A 66-year-old woman with fever, cough, and a tongue lesion, *Chest* 147:e140–e147, 2015.

Klein BS, Vergeront JM, Weeks RJ, et al.: Isolation of *Blastomyces dermatitidis* in soil associated with a large outbreak of blastomycosis in Wisconsin, *N Engl J Med* 314:529–534, 1986.

Lemos LB, Baliga M, Guo M: Blastomycosis: the great pretender can also be an opportunist—initial clinical diagnosis and underlying diseases in 123 patients, *Ann Diagn Pathol* 6:194–203, 2002.

McBride JA, Gauthier GM, Klein BS: Clinical manifestations and treatment of blastomycosis, *Clin Chest Med* 38:435–449, 2017.

Paracoccidioidomycosis

Almeida de Arruda JA, Frenzel Schuch L, Guimarães Abreu L, et al.: A multicentre study of oral paracoccidioidomycosis: analysis of 320 cases and literature review, *Oral Dis* 24:1492–1502, 2018.

Aparecida Shikanai-Yasuda M, Pôncio Mendes R, Lopes Colombo A, et al.: Brazilian guidelines for the clinical management of paracoccidioidomycosis, *Rev Soc Bras Med Trop* 50:715–740, 2017.

Bagagli E, Franco M, Bosco S, et al.: High frequency of *Paracoccidioides brasiliensis* infection in armadillos (*Dasypus novemcinctus*): an ecological study, *Med Mycol* 41:217–223, 2003.

Costa MC, de Carvalho MM, Sperandio FF, et al.: Oral paracoccidioidomycosis affecting women: a systematic review, *Mycoses* 64:108–122, 2021.

de Oliveira GR, Mariano FV, dos Santos Silva AR, et al.: Single oral paracoccidioidomycosis mimicking other lesions: report of eight cases, *Mycopathologia* 173(1):47–52, 2012.

Gorete dos Santos-Nogueira M, Queiroz-Andrade GM, Tonelli E: Clinical evolution of paracoccidioidomycosis in 38 children and teenagers, *Mycopathologia* 161:73–81, 2006.

Paes de Almeida O, Jorge J, Scully C: Paracoccidioidomycosis of the mouth: an emerging deep mycosis, *Crit Rev Oral Biol Med* 14:268–274, 2003.

Queiroz-Telles F, Fahal AH, Falci DR, et al.: Fungal infections 4: neglected endemic mycoses, *Lancet Infect Dis* 17:e367–e377, 2017.

Shankar J, Restrepo A, Clemons KV, et al.: Hormones and the resistance of women to paracoccidioidomycosis, *Clin Microbiol Rev* 24:296–313, 2011.

Trindade AH, Meira HC, Pereira IF, et al.: Oral paracoccidioidomycosis: retrospective analysis of 55 Brazilian patients, *Mycoses* 60:521–525, 2017.

Vicente CR, Falqueto A: Differentiation of mucosal lesions in mucocutaneous leishmaniasis and paracoccidioidomycosis, *PLoS One* 13(11):e0208208, 2018. https://doi.org/10.1371/journal.pone.0208208.

Coccidioidomycosis

Arnold MG, Arnold JC, Bloom DC, et al.: Head and neck manifestations of disseminated coccidioidomycosis, *Laryngoscope* 114:747–752, 2004.

Ashraf N, Kubat RC, Poplin V, et al.: Re-drawing the maps for endemic mycoses, *Mycopathologia* 185:843–865, 2020. https://doi.org/10.1007/s11046-020-00431-2.

Gabe LM, Malo J, Knox KS: Diagnosis and management of coccidioidomycosis, *Clin Chest Med* 38:417–433, 2017.

Kollath DR, Miller KJ, Barker BM: The mysterious desert dwellers: *Coccidioides immitis* and *Coccidioides posadasii*, causative fungal agents of coccidioidomycosis, *Virulence* 10:222–233, 2019.

Laniado-Laborín R, Arathoon EG, Canteros C, et al.: Coccidioidomycosis in Latin America, *Med Mycol* 57:S46–S55, 2019.

McCotter OZ, Benedict K, Engelthaler DM, et al.: Update on the epidemiology of coccidioidomycosis in the United States, *Med Mycol* 57:S30–S40, 2019.

Rodriguez RA, Konia T: Coccidioidomycosis of the tongue, *Arch Pathol Lab Med* 129:e4–e6, 2005.

Ruddy BE, Mayer AP, Ko MG, et al.: Coccidioidomycosis in African Americans, *Mayo Clin Proc* 86:63–69, 2011.

Stockamp NW, Thompson GR III: Coccidioidomycosis, *Infect Dis Clin North Am* 30:229–246, 2016.

Thompson GR III, Lewis JS II, Nix DE, et al.: Current concepts and future directions in the pharmacology and treatment of coccidioidomycosis, *Med Mycol* 57:S76–S84, 2019.

Cryptococcosis

Christianson JC, Engber W, Andes D: Primary cutaneous cryptococcosis in immunocompetent and immunocompromised hosts, *Med Mycol* 41:177–188, 2003.

Maziarz EK, Perfect JR: Cryptococcosis, *Infect Dis Clin North Am* 30:179–206, 2016.

Mehrabi M, Bagheri S, Leonard MK, et al.: Mucocutaneous manifestation of cryptococcal infection: report of a case and review of the literature, *J Oral Maxillofac Surg* 63:1543–1549, 2005.

Namiq AL, Tollefson T, Fan F: Cryptococcal parotitis presenting as a cystic parotid mass: report of a case diagnosed by fine-needle aspiration cytology, *Diagn Cytopathol* 33:36–38, 2005.

Nosanchuk JD, Shoham S, Fries BC, et al.: Evidence of zoonotic transmission of *Cryptococcus neoformans* from a pet cockatoo to an immunocompromised patient, *Ann Intern Med* 132:205–208, 2000.

Ruhnke M: Mucosal and systemic fungal infections in patients with AIDS, *Drugs* 64:1163–1180, 2004.

Scully C, Paes De Almeida O: Orofacial manifestations of the systemic mycoses, *J Oral Pathol Med* 21:289–294, 1992.

Setianingrum F, Rautemaa-Richardson R, Denning DW: Pulmonary cryptococcosis: a review of pathobiology and clinical aspects, *Med Mycol* 57:133–150, 2019.

Skolnik K, Huston S, Mody CH: Cryptococcal lung infections, *Clin Chest Med* 38:451–464, 2017.

Mucormycosis

Akhrass FA, Debiane L, Abdallah L, et al.: Palatal mucormycosis in patients with hematologic malignancy and stem cell transplantation, *Med Mycol* 49:400–405, 2011.

Cheong HS, Kim SY, Ki HK, et al.: Oral mucormycosis in patients with haematologic malignancies in a bone marrow transplant unit, *Mycoses* 60:836–841, 2017.

Fanfair RN, Benedict K, Bos J, et al.: Necrotizing cutaneous mucormycosis after a tornado in Joplin, Missouri, in 2011, *N Engl J Med* 367:2214–2225, 2012.

Farmakiotis D, Kontoyiannis DP: Mucormycoses, *Infect Dis Clin North Am* 30:143–163, 2016.

Fattah SY, Hariri F, Ngui R, et al.: Tongue necrosis secondary to mucormycosis in a diabetic patient: a first case report in Malaysia, *J Mycol Méd* 28:519–522, 2018.

Jeong W, Keighley C, Wolfe R, et al.: Contemporary management and clinical outcomes of mucormycosis: a systematic review and meta-analysis of case reports, *Int J Antimicrob Agents* 53:589–597, 2019.

Jeong W, Keighley C, Wolfe R, et al.: The epidemiology and clinical manifestations of mucormycosis: a systematic review and meta-analysis of case reports, *Clin Microbiol Infect* 25:26–34, 2019.

Jones AC, Bentsen TY, Freedman PD: Mucormycosis of the oral cavity, *Oral Surg Oral Med Oral Pathol* 75:455–460, 1993.

Kwon-Chung KJ: Taxonomy of fungi causing mucormycosis and entomophthoramycosis (zygomycosis) and nomenclature of the disease: molecular mycologic perspectives, *Clin Infect Dis* 54(Suppl. 1):S8–S15, 2012.

Marty FM, Ostrosky-Zeichner L, Cornely OA, et al.: Isavuconazole treatment for mucormycosis: a single-arm open-label trial and case-control analysis, *Lancet Infect Dis* 16:828–837, 2016.

McDermott NE, Barrett J, Hipp J, et al.: Successful treatment of periodontal mucormycosis: report of a case and literature review, *Oral Surg Oral Med Oral Pathol Oral Radiol Endod* 109:e64–e69, 2010.

Nezafati S, Kazemi A, Asgari K, et al.: Rhinocerebral mucormycosis, risk factors and the type of oral manifestations in patients referred to a University Hospital in Tabriz, Iran 2007-2017, *Mycoses* 61:764–769, 2018.

Nucci M, Engelhardt M, Hamed K: Mucormycosis in South America: a review of 143 reported cases, *Mycoses* 62:730–738, 2019.

Prabhua S, Alqahtanib M, Al Shehabi M: A fatal case of rhinocerebral mucormycosis of the jaw after dental extractions and review of literature, *J Infect Public Health* 11:301–303, 2018.

Schütz P, Behbhani JH, Khan ZU, et al.: Fatal rhino-orbito-cerebral zygomycosis caused by *Apophysomyces elegans* in a healthy patient, *J Oral Maxillofac Surg* 64:1795–1802, 2006.

Song Y, Qiao J, Giovanni G, et al.: Mucormycosis in renal transplant recipients: review of 174 reported cases, *BMC Infect Dis* 17:283, 2017.

Vahabzadeh-Hagh AM, Chao KY, Blackwell KE: Invasive oral tongue mucormycosis rapidly presenting after orthotopic liver transplant, *Ear Nose Throat J* 98:268–270, 2019.

Aspergillosis

Cadena J, Thompson GR III, Patterson TF: Invasive aspergillosis: current strategies for diagnosis and management, *Infect Dis Clin North Am* 30:125–142, 2016.

Dykewicz MS, Rodrigues JM, Slavin RG: Allergic fungal rhinosinusitis, *J Allergy Clin Immunol* 142:341–351, 2018.

Ganesh P, Nagarjuna M, Shetty S, et al.: Invasive aspergillosis presenting as swelling of the buccal mucosa in an immunocompetent individual, *Oral Surg Oral Med Oral Pathol Oral Radiol* 119:e60–e64, 2015.

Gomesa CC, Costa Pinto LC, Loretti Victor F, et al.: Aspergillus in endodontic infection near the maxillary sinus, *Braz J Otorhinolaryngol* 81:527–532, 2015.

Haiduven D: Nosocomial aspergillosis and building construction, *Med Mycol* 47(Suppl. 1):S210–S216, 2009.

Kanj A, Abdallah N, Soubani AO: The spectrum of pulmonary aspergillosis, *Respir Med* 141:121–131, 2018.

Ledoux M-P, Denis J, Nivoix Y, et al.: Isavuconazole: a new broad-spectrum azole. Part 2: pharmacokinetics and clinical activity, *J Mycol Méd* 28:15–22, 2018.

Lee DH, Yoon TM, Lee JK, et al.: Computed tomography-based differential diagnosis of fungus balls in the maxillary sinus, *Oral Surg Oral Med Oral Pathol Oral Radiol* 129:277–281, 2020.

Myoken Y, Sugata T, Fujita Y, et al.: Early diagnosis and successful management of atypical invasive *Aspergillus* sinusitis in a hematopoietic cell transplant patient: a case report, *J Oral Maxillofac Surg* 64:860–863, 2006.

Scolozzi P, Perez A, Verdeja R, et al.: Association between maxillary sinus fungus ball and sinus bone grafting with deproteinized bovine bone substitutes: a case-control study, *Oral Surg Oral Med Oral Pathol Oral Radiol* 121:e143–e147, 2016.

Shah V, Rao J, Verma V, et al.: Invasive fungal rhinosinusitis with palatal erosion in an elderly edentulous patient with uncontrolled diabetes: report of a rare case, *Gerodontology* 34:144–146, 2017.

Shirley M, Scott LJ: Isavuconazole: a review in invasive aspergillosis and mucormycosis, *Drugs* 76:1647–1657, 2016.

Toxoplasmosis

Aguirre AA, Longcore T, Barbieri M, et al.: The one health approach to toxoplasmosis: epidemiology, control, and prevention strategies, *Ecohealth* 16:378–390, 2019.

Dunay IR, Gajurel K, Dhakal R, et al.: Treatment of toxoplasmosis: historical perspective, animal models, and current clinical practice, *Clin Microbiol Rev* 31:e00057-17, 2018.

García-Pola M-J, González-García M, García-Martín JM, et al.: Submaxillary adenopathy as sole manifestation of toxoplasmosis: case report and literature review, *J Otolaryngol* 31:122–125, 2002.

Innes EA: A brief history and overview of *Toxoplasma gondii*, *Zoonoses Public Health* 57(1):1–7, 2010.

Khan K, Khan W: Congenital toxoplasmosis: an overview of the neurological and ocular manifestations, *Parasitol Int* 67(2018):715–721, 2018.

Li B, Zou J, Wang W-Y, et al.: Toxoplasmosis presented as a submental mass: a common disease, uncommon presentation, *Int J Clin Exp Pathol* 8:3308–3311, 2015.

McAuley JB: Toxoplasmosis in children, *Pediatr Infect Dis J* 27:161–162, 2008.

Moran WJ, Tom DWK, King D, et al.: Toxoplasmosis lymphadenitis occurring in a parotid gland, *Otolaryngol Head Neck Surg* 94:237–240, 1986.

Rawal YB, Allen CM, Kalmar JR: A nodular submental mass, *Oral Surg Oral Med Oral Pathol Oral Radiol Endod* 104:734–737, 2007.

Robert-Gangneux F, Dardé M-L: Epidemiology of and diagnostic strategies for toxoplasmosis, *Clin Microbiol Rev* 25:264–296, 2012.

Sireci F, Bruno R, Martines F, et al.: A patient with toxoplasmosis as a cause of submental lymphadenopathy, *J Craniofac Surg* 30:e353–e355, 2019.

Leishmaniasis

Araujo Almeida TF, da Silveira EM, Rocha dos Santos CR, et al.: Exclusive primary lesion of oral leishmaniasis with immunohistochemical diagnosis, *Head Neck Pathol* 10:533–537, 2016.

Aronson NE, Joya CA: Cutaneous leishmaniasis: updates in diagnosis and management, *Infect Dis Clin North Am* 33:101–117, 2019.

Burza S, Croft SL, Boelaert M: Leishmaniasis, *Lancet* 392:951–970, 2018.

Chakravarty J, Sundar S: Current and emerging medications for the treatment of leishmaniasis, *Expert Opin Pharmacother* 20:1251–1265, 2019.

de Ruiter MHT, Stijnis C, Nolte JW, et al.: Fulminant presentation of oral mucosal leishmaniasis as severe stomatitis and periodontitis, *Neth J Med* 76:40–42, 2018.

Fernanda Cruz A, Gonçalves Resende R, Ricaldoni Albuquerque D, et al.: Mucosal leishmaniasis in Brazilian patients: two case reports with similar clinical presentation and different approaches, *Oral Surg Oral Med Oral Pathol Oral Radiol* 122:e199–e203, 2016.

Junqueira Pedras M, de Pina CJ, da Silva RE, et al.: Mucosal leishmaniasis: the experience of a Brazilian referral center, *Rev Soc Bras Med Trop* 51:318–323, 2018.

Kedzierski L: Leishmaniasis, *Hum Vaccin* 7:1204–1214, 2011.

Kevric I, Cappel MA, Keeling JH: New World and Old World Leishmania infections: a practical review, *Dermatol Clin* 33:579–593, 2015.

Mignogna MD, Celentano A, Leuci S, et al.: Mucosal leishmaniasis with primary oral involvement: a case series and a review of the literature, *Oral Dis* 21:e70–e78, 2015.

Mohammadpour I, Motazedian MH, Handjani F, et al.: Lip leishmaniasis: a case series with molecular identification and literature review, *BMC Infect Dis* 17:96, 2017.

Santos CR, Tuon FF, Cieslinski J, et al.: Comparative study on liposomal amphotericin B and other therapies in the treatment of mucosal leishmaniasis: a 15-year retrospective cohort study, *PLoS One* 14:e0218786, 2019. https://doi.org/10.1371/journal.pone.0218786.

Vicente CR, Falqueto A: Differentiation of mucosal lesions in mucocutaneous leishmaniasis and paracoccidioidomycosis, *PLoS One* 13:e0208208, 2018. https://doi.org/10.1371/journal.pone.0208208.

7

Viral Infections

❖ HUMAN HERPESVIRUSES

The human herpesvirus (HHV) family (**Herpetoviridae**) constitutes a large family of double-stranded DNA viruses. The best-known member of this family is **herpes simplex virus (HSV),** which includes HSV type 1 (HSV-1 or HHV-1) and HSV type 2 (HSV-2 or HHV-2). Other members of the HHV family include **varicella-zoster virus** (VZV or HHV-3), **Epstein–Barr virus** (EBV or HHV-4), **cyto-megalovirus** (CMV or HHV-5), and more recently discovered members, HHV-6, HHV-7, and HHV-8. Humans are the only natural reservoir for these viruses, which are endemic worldwide.

The term **herpes** derives from the ancient Greek word meaning to creep or crawl, which apparently alludes to a tendency for spreading, latent, or recurrent infection. All eight types cause a primary infection and remain latent within specific cell types for the life of the individual. On reactivation, these viruses cause recurrent infections that may be symptomatic or asymptomatic. The viruses are shed in saliva or other secretions, providing an avenue for infection of new hosts. Each type is known to transform cells in tissue culture, with several strongly associated with specific malignancies. The following sections concentrate on HSV, VZV, CMV, and EBV. Much less is known about herpesvirus types 6, 7, and 8.

Human herpesvirus 6 (HHV-6) and **7 (HHV-7)** are closely related, usually transmitted by saliva or respiratory droplets, and exhibit infection rates close to 90% by age 5 in the United States. Primary infection usually is asymptomatic but may cause an acute febrile illness followed by an erythematous maculopapular eruption. This pattern of symptomatic primary infection—termed **roseola (exanthema subitum, sixth disease)**—most often is caused by HHV-6 but also may be caused by HHV-7. Both viruses may replicate in salivary glands and establish latency in CD4+ T lymphocytes or other cell types. Reactivation occurs most frequently in immunocompromised patients and can result in widespread multiorgan infection, including encephalitis, pneumonitis, bone-marrow suppression, and hepatitis.

Human herpesvirus 8 (HHV-8) is involved in the pathogenesis of **Kaposi sarcoma (KS)** (see page 564) and has been termed **Kaposi sarcoma–associated herpesvirus (KSHV).** In immunocompetent persons, primary infection usually is asymptomatic, with male-to-male sexual contact being the most common mode of transmission in Western countries. The virus is found without difficulty in saliva, suggesting another possible pattern of transmission. Associated symptoms, such as transient fever, lymphadenopathy, and arthralgias, are rarely reported. Circulating B lymphocytes appear to be the major cell of latency. In addition to Kaposi sarcoma, HHV-8 is associated with certain types of lymphoma and a benign lymphoid proliferation known as *Castleman disease.*

❖ HERPES SIMPLEX VIRUS

The two herpes simplex viruses are similar in structure and disease mechanisms but differ in antigenicity, anatomic site predilection, and epidemiology. Differences in envelope glycoproteins account for their distinct antigenicity. Nevertheless, there is potential for antibody cross-reactivity, and antibodies directed against one type may decrease the likelihood or severity of infection with the other type.

HSV-1 is spread predominantly through infected saliva or active perioral lesions and adapted best to the oral, facial, and ocular areas. The pharynx, intraoral mucosa, lips, eyes, and skin above the waist are involved most frequently. In addition, transmission via sexual contact is possible. Over the past few decades, there has been an increase in the proportion of genital herpes caused by HSV-1 in developed nations; indeed, recent studies have attributed as many as 60% of new genital herpes cases to HSV-1 in some cohorts. This trend may reflect an increase in oral-genital sexual behavior and lower rates of nonsexual HSV-1 acquisition in childhood.

HSV-2 is adapted best to the genital zones, is transmitted predominantly through sexual contact, and typically involves the genitalia and skin below the waist. Oral and pharyngeal infection with HSV-2 is also possible but infrequent.

The natural history of HSV infection includes primary infection, latency, and recurrent infection. **Primary infection** refers to initial exposure of an individual without antibodies to the virus. The virus can infect a susceptible host through disturbances in the epithelial barrier, which may be induced by physical injury, other infections, or overgrowth of commensal organisms. Primary infection with HSV-1 typically occurs at a young age, may be asymptomatic, and usually does not cause significant morbidity. For symptomatic cases, the usual incubation period is 3–9 days.

After primary infection is established, the virus is taken up by sensory nerves and transported to the associated sensory or, less frequently, autonomic ganglia where the virus remains in a latent state. The most common site of latency for HSV-1 is the trigeminal ganglion, but other possible sites include the geniculate ganglion of the facial nerve, vestibular ganglion of the vestibulocochlear nerve, nodose ganglion of the vagus nerve, dorsal root ganglia, and brain. The virus uses the axons of the sensory neurons to travel back and forth to the skin or mucosa.

Recurrent (secondary) infection occurs with reactivation of the virus. Factors associated with reactivation include advanced age, ultraviolet light, physical or emotional stress, fatigue, heat, cold, pregnancy, allergy, trauma, dental treatment, respiratory illnesses, fever, menstruation, systemic diseases, and malignancy. Depending on the number of infected epithelial cells, secondary infection may manifest as asymptomatic viral shedding, prodromal symptoms without any detectable lesion (**false prodrome**), or clinically evident lesions (**recrudescence**) that may or may not be preceded by prodromal symptoms. Symptomatic recurrences are fairly common and affect the epithelium supplied by the sensory ganglion. However, reactivation with asymptomatic viral shedding greatly exceeds symptomatic cases. The reported frequency of asymptomatic viral shedding varies from 2 to 219 days per person per year, although this variation may reflect differences in study design and methods. Spread to an uninfected host can occur from symptomatic, active lesions or asymptomatic viral shedding. In addition, the virus may spread to other sites in the same host to establish residency at the sensory ganglion of the new location.

The estimated worldwide prevalence of HSV-1 infection is 67% among individuals younger than 50 years. Prevalence varies by region from approximately 45% in the Americas to 87% in Africa. Crowding and poor hygiene promote exposure to HSV-1. Furthermore, lower socioeconomic status correlates with earlier exposure. In Africa and Southeast Asia, most individuals are exposed via nonsexual oral transmission by 5 years of age, and virtually no new infections are seen in adulthood. In contrast, in the Americas, about half of new HSV-1 infections occur between the ages of 15 and 49 years, with approximately a fourth of these cases representing genital infection. The clinical presentation of symptomatic primary oral HSV-1 infection varies by age, with young individuals tending to exhibit gingivostomatitis and those exposed later in life often demonstrating pharyngotonsillitis.

HSV-2 infection represents one of the most common sexually transmitted infections worldwide. In the United States, HSV-2 seroprevalence among individuals between 14 and 49 years of age is approximately 12% and has been decreasing over the past few decades. Exposure increases linearly with age from 0.8% among adolescents 14–19 years to 21% among adults 40–49 years. Because many infected with HSV-2 refrain from sexual activity when active lesions are present, investigators believe that at least 70% of primary infections are contracted from individuals during asymptomatic viral shedding. Importantly, HSV-2 infection is associated with an increased risk for human immunodeficiency virus (HIV) infection (see page 250). It is uncertain whether this finding reflects sexual activity as a common risk factor for HIV and HSV-2 infection versus increased disease susceptibility due to biologic interactions between these viruses.

In addition to clinically evident infections, HSV has been implicated in several noninfectious processes. For example, more than 15% of cases of **erythema multiforme** are preceded by a symptomatic recurrence of HSV 3–10 days earlier (see page 781), and some investigators believe that up to 70% of mucosal erythema multiforme may be triggered by HSV. In some individuals, erythema multiforme outbreaks are frequent enough to warrant antiviral prophylaxis. In a small subset of patients, asymptomatic release of HSV coincides with attacks of aphthous stomatitis (see page 321). In these cases, the ulcerations are not infected with the virus. Instead the virus may be responsible for the initiation of immune dysregulation, or the immune dysregulation that produces aphthae may allow the release of virions. Nevertheless, the association between HSV and aphthae is weak, and prophylactic antiviral therapy generally does not decrease the recurrence of aphthous stomatitis. Furthermore, HSV and other herpesviruses have been associated with oral carcinomas, but much of the evidence is circumstantial. HSV DNA has been extracted from some tumors but not others, and elevated HSV-1 IgG antibodies have been detected in patients with oral cancer or precancer. HSV may aid carcinogenesis through the promotion of mutations, but its oncogenic role, if any, is uncertain.

Clinical Features

Acute herpetic gingivostomatitis (primary herpes) is the most common pattern of symptomatic primary HSV infection, and more than 90% of cases are caused by HSV-1. Most affected individuals are between the ages of 6 months and 5 years, with the peak prevalence occurring between 2 and 3 years of age. However, occasional cases have been reported in patients older than 60 years. Development before 6 months of age is rare because of protection by maternal anti-HSV antibodies. The onset is abrupt and often accompanied by anterior cervical lymphadenopathy, chills, fever (103 °F to 105 °F), nausea, anorexia, irritability, and sore mouth lesions. The manifestations vary from mild to severely debilitating.

Initially the affected mucosa develops numerous pinhead vesicles, which rapidly collapse to form numerous small, red lesions. These lesions enlarge slightly and develop central ulceration covered by yellow fibrin (Fig. 7.1). Adjacent ulcerations may coalesce to form larger, shallow, irregular ulcerations (Fig. 7.2). Both the movable and attached oral mucosa can be affected, and the number of lesions is highly variable. In all cases, the gingiva is enlarged, painful, and extremely erythematous (Fig. 7.3). In addition, the affected gingiva often exhibits distinctive punched-out erosions along the midfacial free gingival margins (Fig. 7.4). It is not

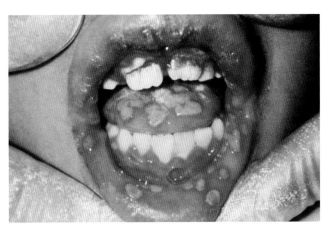

• **Fig. 7.1** **Acute Herpetic Gingivostomatitis.** Widespread yellowish mucosal ulcerations. (Courtesy of Dr. David Johnsen.)

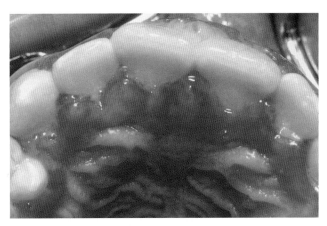

• **Fig. 7.3** **Acute Herpetic Gingivostomatitis.** Painful, enlarged, and erythematous palatal gingiva.

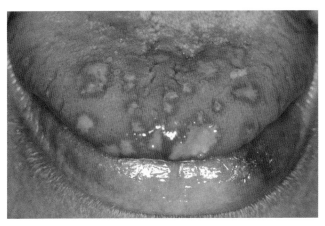

• **Fig. 7.2** **Acute Herpetic Gingivostomatitis.** Numerous coalescing, irregular, and yellowish ulcerations of the dorsal surface of the tongue.

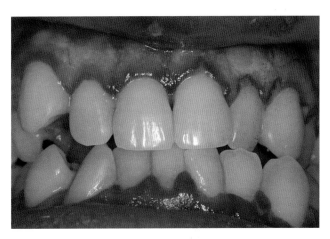

• **Fig. 7.4** **Acute Herpetic Gingivostomatitis.** Painful, enlarged, and erythematous facial gingiva. Note erosions of the free gingival margin. (Courtesy of Dr. Gina Liford.)

unusual for involvement of the labial mucosa to extend past the wet line to include the adjacent vermilion border. Satellite vesicles of the perioral skin are fairly common. Self-inoculation of the fingers, eyes, and genital areas can occur. Mild cases usually resolve within 5–7 days; severe cases may last 2 weeks. Rare complications include keratoconjunctivitis, esophagitis, pneumonitis, meningitis, and encephalitis.

As mentioned previously, primary infection in adults may cause **pharyngotonsillitis.** Sore throat, fever, malaise, and headache are the initial symptoms. Numerous small vesicles develop on the tonsils and posterior pharynx. The vesicles rapidly rupture to form shallow ulcers, which often coalesce and develop an overlying diffuse, gray-yellow exudate. Involvement of the oral mucosa anterior to Waldeyer ring occurs in less than 10% of cases. HSV appears to be a significant cause of pharyngotonsillitis in young adults who are from higher socioeconomic groups with previously negative test findings for HSV antibodies. Most cases are caused by HSV-1, but the proportion caused by HSV-2 is increasing. The clinical presentation closely resembles pharyngitis secondary to streptococci or infectious mononucleosis, making the true frequency difficult to determine.

Infrequently, primary HSV-1 infection may spread along nerve tracts beyond the trigeminal ganglion, especially if the host is immunocompromised. Spread via the lingual nerve to the geniculate ganglion of the facial nerve may result in Bell palsy (see page 861). In addition, the virus may reach the vestibular ganglion of the vestibulocochlear nerve, resulting in vestibular neuritis and sudden hearing loss.

Recurrent (secondary) herpes simplex infections may occur either at the site of primary inoculation or in adjacent areas of surface epithelium supplied by the involved ganglion. The most common clinical pattern of recurrent HSV-1 infection is **herpes labialis** ("cold sore" or "fever blister"), which involves the vermilion border and skin adjacent to the lips. Prevalence studies suggest that 15%–45% of the United States population has a history of herpes labialis. In some patients, ultraviolet light or trauma can trigger recurrences. Prodromal signs and symptoms (e.g., pain, burning, itching, tingling, localized warmth, erythema) arise 6–24 hours before the lesions appear. Multiple small, erythematous papules develop and form clusters of fluid-filled vesicles (Fig. 7.5). The vesicles rupture and crust within 2 days. Healing usually occurs within 7–10 days. Pain is

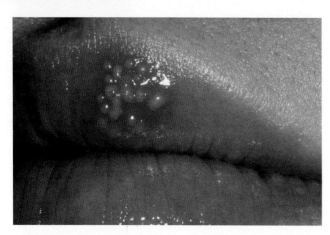

• **Fig. 7.5 Herpes Labialis.** Multiple fluid-filled vesicles on the lip vermilion.

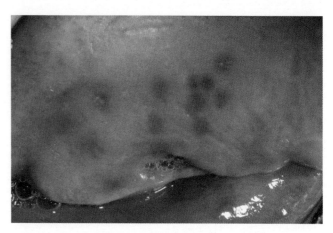

• **Fig. 7.7 Intraoral Recurrent Herpetic Infection.** Early lesions exhibiting as multiple erythematous macules on the hard palate. Lesions appeared a few days after extraction of a tooth.

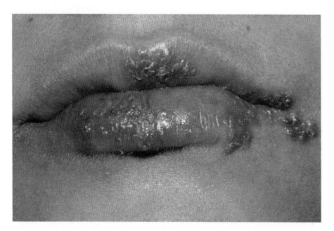

• **Fig. 7.6 Herpes Labialis.** Multiple sites of recurrent herpetic infection secondary to spread of viral fluid over cracked lips.

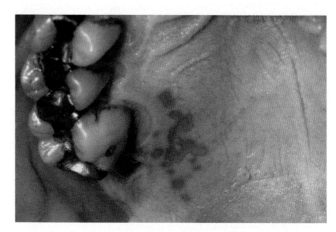

• **Fig. 7.8 Intraoral Recurrent Herpetic Infection.** Multiple coalescing ulcerations on the hard palate.

most severe in the first 8 hours and usually resolves within 4–5 days. Viral shedding is greatest upon vesicular rupture, and most active viral replication is complete within 48–72 hours. Rupture of vesicles and release of virus-filled fluid may result in spreading of the lesions on lips previously cracked from sun exposure (Fig. 7.6). Recurrences are observed less commonly on the skin of the nose, chin, or cheek. The majority of those affected experience approximately 2–4 recurrences annually, but a small percentage may experience outbreaks that occur monthly or even more frequently.

On occasion, some lesions arise almost immediately after a known trigger and appear without any preceding prodromal symptoms. These rapidly developing recurrences tend to respond less favorably to treatment.

Recurrences also can affect the intraoral mucosa. In the immunocompetent patient, **recurrent intraoral herpes (recurrent herpetic stomatitis)** almost always involves keratinized mucosa bound to bone (attached gingiva and hard palate). These sites often exhibit subtle changes, and the symptoms tend to be relatively mild. The lesions begin as 1- to 3-mm vesicles that rapidly collapse to form a cluster of erythematous macules that may coalesce or slightly enlarge

(Figs. 7.7 and 7.8). The damaged epithelium is lost, and a yellowish ulceration with irregular borders develops. Healing occurs within 7–10 days. In about a fourth of cases, recurrent intraoral herpes may be accompanied by recurrent herpes labialis.

Several less common presentations also exist. Primary or recurrent HSV infection of the fingers is known as **herpetic whitlow (herpetic paronychia)** (Fig. 7.9). This condition may result from self-inoculation in children with orofacial HSV-1 infection or adults with genital HSV-2 infection. Before the uniform use of gloves, medical and dental personnel could infect their digits from contact with infected patients and represented the most commonly affected group. Recurrent digital infection may result in paresthesia and permanent scarring.

Cutaneous herpetic infections also can arise in areas of previous epithelial damage. Parents kissing skin injuries in children represent one vector. Wrestlers and rugby players also may contaminate areas of abrasion and develop lesions known as **herpes gladiatorum** or **scrumpox.** On occasion, herpes simplex has been spread over the bearded region of the

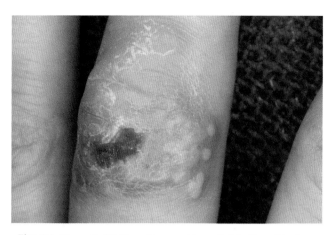

• **Fig. 7.9 Herpetic Whitlow.** Recurrent herpetic infection of the finger.

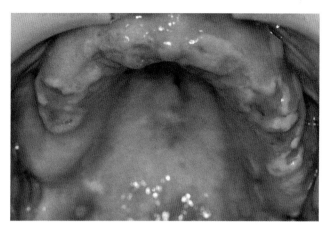

• **Fig. 7.11 Chronic Herpetic Infection.** Numerous shallow herpetic erosions with raised, yellow and circinate borders on the maxillary alveolar ridge in an immunocompromised patient.

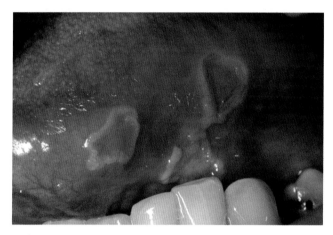

• **Fig. 7.10 Chronic Herpetic Infection.** Numerous mucosal erosions, each of which is surrounded by a slightly raised, yellow-white border, in a patient receiving systemic corticosteroid therapy for systemic sclerosis and rheumatoid arthritis.

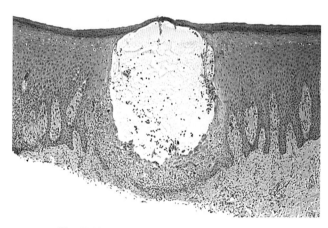

• **Fig. 7.12 Herpes Simplex.** Intraepithelial vesicle.

face into minor injuries created by daily shaving, leading to a condition known as **herpes barbae.** Ocular involvement may occur by self-inoculation in children and, with multiple recurrences, may result in blindness. Patients with diffuse, chronic skin diseases, such as eczema, pemphigus, and Darier disease, may develop diffuse life-threatening HSV infection, known as **eczema herpeticum (Kaposi varicelliform eruption).** Newborns may become infected after delivery through a birth canal contaminated with HSV, usually HSV-2. Without treatment, there is a greater than 50% mortality rate.

HSV recurrence in immunocompromised hosts can be significant. Without proper immune function, recurrent herpes can persist, spread, and potentially be fatal. Skin lesions may continue to enlarge with formation of broad zones of superficial erosion. Likewise, herpes labialis may be severe, with extensive areas of involvement. Intraoral lesions usually begin on bound mucosa but often spread to unbound mucosa as well. The lesions may appear as brownish, necrotic epithelium raised above the surface of the adjacent intact epithelium. Typically, these areas are much larger than the usual pinhead lesions in immunocompetent patients. With continued enlargement, a zone of superficial necrosis or erosion with a distinctive

circinate, raised, yellow border develops (Figs. 7.10 and 7.11). HSV infection in a chronic ulcer on the movable oral mucosa is ominous and should prompt thorough evaluation for possible immune dysfunction. In addition, immunocompromised patients may develop persistent oral ulcers that lack the distinctive curvilinear border, are nonspecific clinically, and may mimic aphthous stomatitis, necrotizing stomatitis, or ulcerative periodontal disease. Biopsy may reveal any of a number of infectious processes, such as HSV infection, at times combined with CMV or EBV infection.

Histopathologic Features

HSV-infected epithelial cells exhibit acantholysis, nuclear clearing, and nuclear enlargement (termed **ballooning degeneration**) (Fig. 7.12). The acantholytic epithelial cells may be referred to as **Tzanck cells.** (This term refers to free-floating epithelial cells in any intraepithelial vesicle and is not specific for herpes.) Nucleolar fragmentation occurs with a condensation of chromatin around the periphery of the nucleus. Multinucleated epithelial cells are formed by fusion between adjacent cells (see Fig. 7.12).

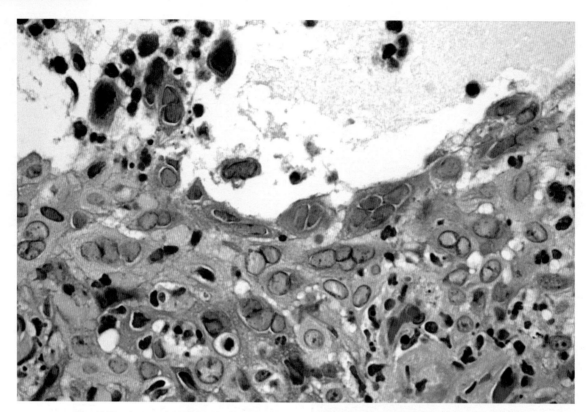

• **Fig. 7.13 Herpes Simplex.** Altered epithelial cells exhibiting ballooning degeneration, margination of chromatin, and multinucleation. (High-power magnification of the same case shown in Fig. 7.12.)

Intercellular edema develops and leads to the formation of an intraepithelial vesicle (Fig. 7.13). Mucosal vesicles rupture rapidly; those on the skin often persist and become infiltrated by inflammatory cells. Once they have ruptured, the mucosal lesions demonstrate a surface fibrinopurulent membrane. Often at the edge of the ulceration or mixed within the fibrinous exudate are the scattered Tzanck or multinucleated epithelial cells.

Diagnosis

The clinician often can make a strong presumptive clinical diagnosis of HSV infection. However, on occasion, HSV infection can be confused with other diseases, and laboratory confirmation is desirable.

The traditional method for diagnosis is viral isolation from tissue culture inoculated with the fluid of intact vesicles. However, intact vesicles are rare in the oral cavity, and culture of ruptured oral lesions is unreliable because of the potential for contamination with saliva that may contain coincidentally released HSV from asymptomatic viral shedding. Another problem with viral culture is that up to 2 weeks may be required for a definitive result.

The most commonly used sampling methods for diagnosis are the cytologic smear and tissue biopsy, with the former being the least invasive and most cost-effective. Microscopic examination shows characteristic changes in infected epithelial cells. Only VZV produces similar changes, but these two infections usually can be differentiated on a clinical basis. If

necessary, direct immunofluorescence, immunohistochemistry, in situ hybridization, or PCR may be performed for more definitive HSV detection and typing.

If diagnostic features of HSV are discovered in a biopsy of a persistent ulceration in an immunocompromised patient, additional studies should be performed to rule out coinfection with other viruses, such as CMV and EBV. The histopathologic features of CMV can be missed easily, resulting in patients not receiving the most appropriate therapy.

Serologic testing is useful in documenting recent or past exposure to HSV and is used primarily in epidemiologic studies. HSV antibodies typically begin to appear 4–8 days after initial exposure. Confirmation of primary infection by serology requires a negative sample obtained within 3 days of initial presentation and a positive sample obtained approximately 4 weeks later.

Treatment and Prognosis

In the past, primary herpetic gingivostomatitis was treated only symptomatically; however, if administered early, antiviral medications can be beneficial. Acyclovir suspension initiated during the first 3 symptomatic days and administered by a rinse-and-swallow technique five times daily for 5 days (children: 15 mg/kg up to the adult dose of 200 mg) results in significant acceleration of clinical resolution. Once therapy is initiated, development of new lesions ceases. In addition, associated eating and drinking difficulties, pain, healing time, duration of fever, and viral shedding are shortened dramatically. In conjunction with acyclovir, additional medications—such as dyclonine hydrochloride spray, tetracaine hydrochloride lollipops (prepared by a compounding pharmacist), or nonsteroidal anti-inflammatory drugs (NSAIDs)—may be used for more immediate pain relief. Viscous lidocaine and topical benzocaine should be avoided in pediatric patients because of reports of lidocaine-induced seizures in children and an association between topical benzocaine and methemoglobinemia. Intravenous fluids also may be administered to address fluid and electrolyte imbalances. In addition, patients should be instructed to restrict contact with active lesions to prevent autoinoculation or spread to others.

Recurrent herpes labialis has been treated with everything from ether to voodoo; nothing has solved the problem for all patients. Acyclovir ointment in polyethylene glycol was the first topical antiviral formulation available. Acyclovir ointment has been of limited benefit for herpes labialis in immunocompetent patients, because its base is thought to prevent significant absorption. Subsequently, penciclovir cream became available in a base that allows increased absorption through the vermilion border. This formulation has produced reduction in healing time and pain by approximately 1 day. Although the best results are obtained if penciclovir cream is initiated during the prodrome, late application also has produced a measurable clinical benefit. Additional choices are acyclovir cream and over-the-counter 10% docosanol cream. All three of these creams are associated with statistically significant, albeit clinically minimal, reduction in healing time and pain, with penciclovir exhibiting the greatest efficacy and docosanol the least efficacy.

Systemic acyclovir and two newer medications, valacyclovir and famciclovir, demonstrate similar effectiveness against HSV. However, valacyclovir and famciclovir exhibit improved bioavailability and more convenient oral dosing schedules. In particular, a valacyclovir regimen—consisting of 2 g during the prodrome followed by another 2 g 12 hours later—has been most successful in minimizing recurrences. The effects of this treatment are reduced significantly if it is not initiated during the prodrome. Although much less convenient, 400 mg of acyclovir taken five times daily for 5 days appears to produce similar results. For patients whose recurrences appear to be associated with dental procedures, a regimen of 2 g of valacyclovir taken twice on the day of the procedure and 1 g taken twice the next day may suppress or minimize an attack. In individuals with a known trigger that extends over a period of time (e.g., skiing or beach vacation), prophylactic short-term use of an antiviral (acyclovir, 400 mg twice daily; valacyclovir, 1 g daily; or famciclovir, 250 mg twice daily) has been shown to reduce the prevalence and severity of recurrences.

Long-term suppressive therapy with an antiviral medication typically is reserved for patients with more than six recurrences per year, HSV-triggered erythema multiforme, or an immunocompromised status. Over the past several decades, acyclovir-resistant strains of HSV have emerged, mainly among immunocompromised patients receiving long-term treatment

or prophylaxis. In immunocompromised patients, the viral load tends to be high and replication is not suppressed completely by antiviral therapy, creating a favorable environment for generating drug-resistant mutants. Although resistance is seen primarily in immunocompromised patients, cavalier use of antiviral medications for mild cases of recurrent herpes infection probably is inappropriate.

For the management of recurrent herpes labialis, some clinical trials suggest that low-level laser therapy may aid in decreasing pain and the recurrence rate. However, further studies are needed. Also, laser ablation of active lesions occasionally may cause worsening, and, thus, it may be advisable to limit the use of low-level laser therapy to areas in which lesions already have healed in an attempt to prevent additional recurrences.

The pain associated with intraoral secondary herpes usually is not intense, and many patients do not require treatment. Some studies have shown chlorhexidine to exert antiviral effects. In addition, acyclovir appears to function synergistically with chlorhexidine. Extensive clinical trials have not been performed, but chlorhexidine alone or in combination with acyclovir suspension may be beneficial for patients who desire or require therapy.

During dental treatment, precautions should be taken to prevent HSV transmission between patients and oral healthcare providers. Such precautions include wearing standard personal protective equipment, avoiding manipulation of tissues with clinically evident infection, minimizing aerosol production around HSV lesions, and refraining from application of petrolatum products to active, fluid-producing lesions (i.e., prior to the scab stage). In general, it is prudent to defer dental treatment until an HSV lesion is scabbed or completely healed.

Immunocompromised hosts with HSV infection often require intravenous (IV) antiviral medications. Furthermore, severely immunosuppressed individuals, such as bone marrow transplant patients and those with AIDS, often need prophylactic oral acyclovir, valacyclovir, or famciclovir. Herpes lesions that do not respond to appropriate therapy within 5–10 days most likely are the result of resistant strains. At this point, the initial antiviral therapy should be repeated at an elevated dose. If this intervention fails, additional alternatives include IV trisodium phosphonoformate hexahydrate (foscarnet) and IV cidofovir. Ulcerations that reveal coinfection with HSV and CMV respond well to ganciclovir, with foscarnet used in refractory cases. Research for a potential HSV vaccine is ongoing.

◆ VARICELLA (CHICKENPOX)

Varicella (chickenpox) represents primary infection with the varicella-zoster virus (VZV or HHV-3). Subsequently, latency ensues, and recurrence is possible as **herpes zoster** (see page 238), often after many decades. The virus may be spread through air droplets or direct contact with active lesions. In contrast to primary HSV infection, most cases of primary VZV infection are symptomatic. The incubation period is 10–21 days, with an average of 15 days.

In the prevaccine era, the annual incidence of chickenpox in the United States was approximately 4 million, with most cases arising in children younger than 10 years of age. However, since the introduction of universal varicella immunization in the United States in 1995, the incidence has declined across all age groups, and the age range of peak incidence has shifted to between 10 and 14 years. In surveillance areas with high vaccine coverage, the incidence of varicella decreased from 1995 to 2005 by approximately 90%; even further declines have occurred since 2006, when a two-dose vaccine regimen became routine. It is estimated that each year varicella vaccination prevents more than 3.5 million cases of chickenpox, 9000 hospitalizations, and 100 deaths in the United States.

Clinical Features

Because of high varicella vaccination rates in the United States, the majority of new varicella cases now represent **breakthrough infection** (i.e., infection with wild-type virus in a previously immunized patient). A maculopapular, cutaneous rash with only a small number of lesions, few or no vesicles, low or no fever, and a shortened disease course of approximately 4–6 days are characteristic findings. The atypical presentation of breakthrough disease may be difficult to recognize, with some cases mistaken for insect bites or poison ivy. Patients are contagious until no new lesions appear within a 24-hour period, although transmission is less frequent with mild breakthrough infection compared with symptomatic infection in unimmunized individuals.

Among unimmunized individuals, the symptomatic phase of primary VZV infection usually begins with malaise, pharyngitis, and rhinitis. In older children and adults, additional symptoms (e.g., headache, myalgia, nausea, anorexia, and vomiting) occasionally are seen. This is followed by a characteristic, intensely pruritic exanthem. The rash begins on the face and trunk and spreads to the extremities. Each lesion rapidly progresses through stages of erythema, vesicle, pustule, and hardened crust (Figs. 7.14 and 7.15). The vesicular stage is the classic presentation. Each vesicle is surrounded by a zone of erythema and has been described as "a dewdrop on a rose petal." In contrast to herpes simplex, the lesions typically continue to erupt for 4 or more days. Old crusted lesions intermixed with newly formed, intact vesicles are commonplace. Affected individuals are contagious from 2 days before the exanthem until all the lesions crust. Fever usually is present during the active phase of the exanthem.

Perioral and oral manifestations are fairly common and may precede the skin lesions. The vermilion border and palate are involved most often, followed by the buccal mucosa. Occasionally, gingival lesions resemble those noted in primary HSV infection, but distinguishing between the two is not difficult because the lesions of varicella tend to be relatively painless. The lesions begin as 3- to 4-mm, white,

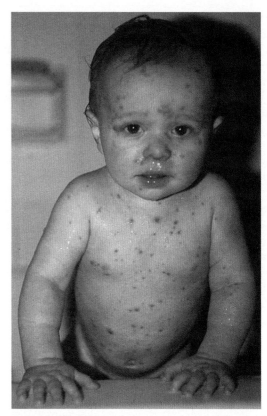

• **Fig. 7.14 Varicella.** Infant with diffuse erythematous and vesicular rash. (Courtesy of Dr. Sherry Parlanti.)

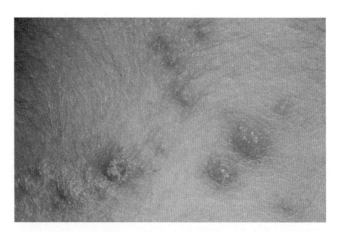

• **Fig. 7.15 Varicella.** Numerous vesicles with surrounding erythema and early crusting.

opaque vesicles that rupture to form 1- to 3-mm ulcerations (Fig. 7.16). The prevalence and number of oral lesions correlate with the severity of extraoral infection. In mild cases, oral lesions are present in about one-third of affected individuals; often there are only one or two oral ulcers that heal within 1–3 days. On the other hand, patients with severe infections almost always have oral ulcerations, often numbering up to 30 and persisting for 5–10 days.

Infants, adults, and immunocompromised individuals are at increased risk for severe disease and complications. In

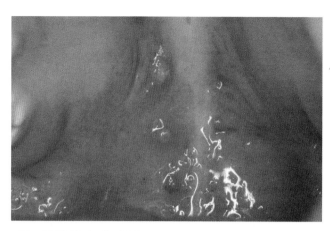

• **Fig. 7.16 Varicella.** White opaque vesicles on the hard palate. (Courtesy of Tristan Neville.)

addition, household members who become secondarily infected often suffer more severe disease than those initially infected.

In childhood, the most frequent complications of varicella are secondary skin infections, followed by encephalitis and pneumonia. In particular, secondary skin infection with group A, β-hemolytic streptococci may progress to necrotizing fasciitis, septicemia, toxic shock syndrome, or other life-threatening conditions. With enhanced public education and decreased use of aspirin in children, Reye syndrome (a potentially fatal condition characterized by acute encephalopathy, liver failure, and other major organ damage) is now rare.

The prevalence of complications in adults exceeds that in children. The most common and serious complication is pneumonitis, characterized by dry cough, tachypnea, dyspnea, hemoptysis, chest pain, and cyanosis. Other potential complications include pneumonia, encephalitis, gastrointestinal disturbance, and hematologic events (i.e., thrombocytopenia, pancytopenia, hemolytic anemia, sickle cell crisis). Central nervous system (CNS) involvement typically produces ataxia but also may result in headaches, drowsiness, convulsions, or coma. The risk of death is reported to be 15 times greater in adults compared with children, mostly because of an increased prevalence of encephalitis.

Infection during pregnancy can produce congenital or neonatal chickenpox. Involvement early in pregnancy can result in spontaneous abortion or congenital defects. When infection occurs before 20 weeks of gestation, the prevalence of congenital varicella syndrome is approximately 1%–2%. In addition, infection of the mother close to delivery can result in severe neonatal infection caused by a lack of maternal antibodies.

Infection in immunocompromised patients also can be severe. Cutaneous involvement typically is extensive and may be associated with secondary bacterial infection, high fever, hepatitis, pneumonitis, pancreatitis, gastrointestinal obstruction, and encephalitis. Before effective antiviral therapy, the mortality rate in immunocompromised individuals was approximately 7%.

Histopathologic Features

The cytologic alterations are virtually identical to those described for HSV. The virus causes acantholysis, with formation of numerous free-floating Tzanck cells, which exhibit nuclear margination of chromatin and occasional multinucleation.

Diagnosis

Since the institution of universal vaccination in the United States, the annual incidence of typical varicella disease has decreased, whereas the incidence of atypical breakthrough disease has increased; consequently, the need for laboratory confirmation has grown. Confirmation can be obtained through demonstration of viral cytopathologic effects present within epithelial cells harvested from vesicular fluid. These cytologic changes are identical to those found in HSV infection, although correlation with the clinical findings may aid in distinguishing between HSV and VZV infection. The most definitive method for diagnosis is PCR performed on vesicular fluid, cells from the base of a lesion, or a scab from a resolving skin lesion. During the acute phase, infection also may be detected by PCR assay of saliva or buccal swabs. PCR is preferred over viral isolation in cell culture and direct fluorescent antibody assay, because it is more sensitive and allows for distinction between wild-type and vaccine strains of VZV. In addition, a diagnosis can be made retrospectively in immunocompetent hosts by demonstrating a fourfold or greater increase in VZV antibody titers between acute and convalescent serum samples; however, in vaccinated persons an increase of this magnitude may not be evident.

Treatment and Prognosis

Before antiviral medications became available, the treatment of varicella primarily was symptomatic. Warm baths with soap, baking soda, or colloidal oatmeal; application of calamine lotion; and systemic diphenhydramine still are used to relieve pruritus. Diphenhydramine lotions are not recommended because of reports of toxicity secondary to percutaneous absorption. Acetaminophen is the preferred antipyretic for childhood cases. In this age group, aspirin should be avoided because of the risk of Reye syndrome, and NSAIDs are discouraged because they have been associated with an increased risk for severe skin and soft tissue complications.

Peroral antiviral medications (such as, acyclovir, valacyclovir, and famciclovir) have been shown to reduce the duration and severity of infection if administered within 24 hours of the rash. Routine use of antiviral medications is not recommended in immunocompetent children with uncomplicated chickenpox. Instead, such therapy is reserved for those at risk for more severe disease, such as unvaccinated individuals over 12 years of age, patients with chronic cutaneous or pulmonary disease, patients receiving long-term salicylate therapy, and those receiving short or intermittent courses of corticosteroids. In addition, some experts recommend antiviral therapy for individuals who contract the disease from a household member, because secondary household cases often are more severe than corresponding index cases. IV formulations are used in immunosuppressed patients or those exhibiting progressive, severe infection.

In patients who lack evidence of immunity and become exposed to VZV, postexposure immunization or purified varicella-zoster immune globulin (VariZIG) administration may be considered. Postexposure vaccination is appropriate for nonimmune individuals 12 months or older. Ideally it should be administered within 3 days, although it may be given up to 5 days after exposure in order to prevent or modify disease. A second dose of vaccine should be administered at the age-appropriate interval following the first dose. Alternatively, VariZIG can be given postexposure to nonimmune individuals at high risk for severe disease or complications and for whom vaccination is contraindicated. Individuals at elevated risk include immunocompromised patients, pregnant women without evidence of immunity, premature infants, and neonates of nonimmune mothers. VariZIG ideally should be administered as soon as possible, with the FDA approving administration up to 10 days postexposure.

In the United States, the FDA has approved a monovalent varicella virus vaccine (Varivax) as well as a quadrivalent measles, mumps, rubella, and varicella virus (MMRV) vaccine (ProQuad). The first dose of varicella-containing vaccine is recommended for children 12 through 15 months of age and a second dose for those 4 through 6 years. Either MMRV vaccine or separate injections of measles, mumps, and rubella (MMR) vaccine and monovalent varicella vaccine may be administered to toddlers receiving their first dose; the latter method minimizes the generally small risk of vaccine-related febrile seizures in this age group. For the second dose, MMRV is preferred over separate injections of MMR and varicella virus vaccines. In addition, the monovalent varicella vaccine is licensed for routine use in individuals 13 years or older without evidence of immunity; in this age group, two doses separated by at least 28 days are recommended. Children, adolescents, and adults who have received only one dose of varicella virus vaccine as per past recommendations should receive a second "catch-up" dose.

The varicella virus vaccine is a live, attenuated virus that can be spread to individuals in close contact. Therefore, vaccine recipients who develop a rash should avoid contact with those at risk, such as immunocompromised or pregnant individuals.

◆ HERPES ZOSTER (SHINGLES)

After primary infection with VZV (chickenpox), the virus is transported up the sensory nerves and establishes latency in corresponding dorsal root, cranial nerve, or autonomic ganglia. Clinically evident herpes zoster develops after reactivation of the virus, with involvement of the distribution of the affected sensory nerve. Unlike HSV, single rather than multiple recurrences are the rule. Herpes zoster occurs during the lifetime of approximately one in three individuals,

and it is estimated that 1 million new episodes of herpes zoster occur annually in the United States. The prevalence of attacks increases with age, apparently due to age-related decline in cell-mediated immunity. The incidence is low among young people but increases dramatically after 50 years of age, with studies suggesting that as many as 50% of individuals who live to 85 years of age will be affected at some time. Immunosuppression, HIV infection, treatment with cytotoxic or immunosuppressive drugs, radiation, malignancy, old age, alcohol abuse, stress (emotional or physical), and dental manipulation are additional predisposing factors for reactivation.

The long-term impact of varicella virus vaccination on herpes zoster prevalence is controversial and presently under evaluation. Interestingly, it is possible to develop herpes zoster by reactivation of either the wild-type or vaccine-strain virus, although the risk for vaccine-strain zoster seems to be much lower than that for wild-type zoster.

Clinical Features

The clinical features of herpes zoster can be grouped into three phases: prodrome, acute, and chronic. During initial viral replication, ganglionitis develops with resultant neuronal necrosis and severe neuralgia. This inflammatory reaction is responsible for the prodromal pain present in more than 90% of cases. As the virus travels down the nerve, the pain intensifies and has been described as burning, tingling, itching, boring, prickly, or knifelike. The pain develops in the area of epithelium innervated by the affected sensory nerve (dermatome) and may be accompanied by fever, malaise, and headache. Typically, one dermatome is affected, but involvement of two or more can occur. The thoracic dermatomes are affected in about two-thirds of cases. This prodromal pain normally precedes the acute phase rash by 1–4 days and, depending on which dermatome is affected, may masquerade as sensitive teeth, otitis media, migraine headache, myocardial infarction, or appendicitis.

The acute phase begins as the involved skin develops clusters of vesicles set on an erythematous base (Fig. 7.17). The

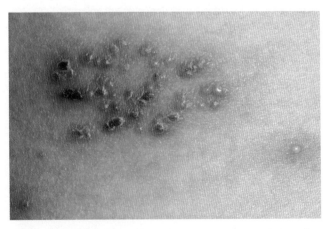

• **Fig. 7.17 Herpes Zoster.** Cluster of vesicles with surrounding erythema of the skin.

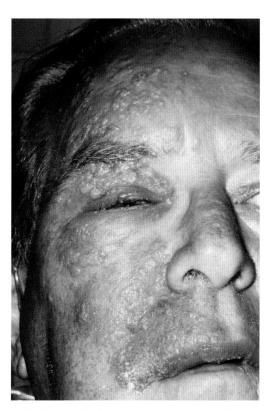

• **Fig. 7.18 Herpes Zoster.** Numerous crusting facial vesicles that extend to the midline.

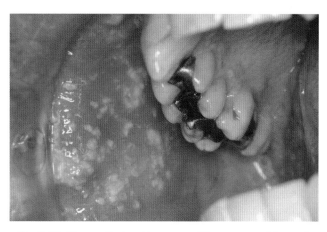

• **Fig. 7.19 Herpes Zoster.** Numerous white opaque vesicles on the right buccal mucosa of the same patient depicted in Fig. 7.18.

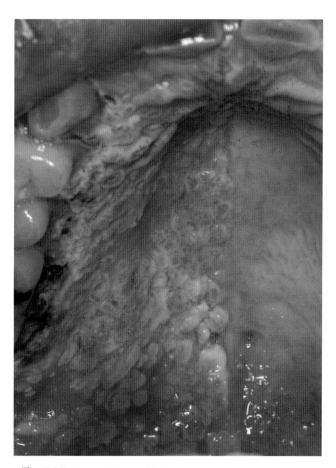

• **Fig. 7.20 Herpes Zoster.** White opaque to focally clear vesicles on the right palatal mucosa with extension to the midline. (Courtesy of Dr. Molly Rosebush.)

lesions tend to follow the path of the affected nerve and terminate at the midline (Fig. 7.18). Within 3–4 days, the vesicles become pustular and ulcerate, with crusts developing after 7–10 days. The lesions are contagious until they crust, although the rate of VZV transmission from herpes zoster lesions is lower than that from varicella lesions. The exanthem typically resolves within 2–3 weeks in otherwise healthy individuals. On healing, scarring with hypopigmentation or hyperpigmentation is not unusual. Infrequently, there is dermatomal pain without development of a rash; this pattern is called **zoster sine herpete** (zoster without rash).

Oral lesions occur with trigeminal nerve involvement and may be present on the movable or bound mucosa (Figs. 7.19 and 7.20). The lesions often extend to the midline and frequently are accompanied by involvement of the skin overlying the affected quadrant. Like varicella, the individual lesions manifest as 1- to 4-mm vesicles or pustules that rupture to form shallow ulcerations. The teeth in affected areas may develop pulpitis, pulpal necrosis, pulpal calcification, or root resorption. In addition, several reports have documented significant bone necrosis with tooth loss. It is postulated that gnathic osteonecrosis may be secondary to extension of inflammation from affected nerves to adjacent blood vessels, leading to ischemic necrosis. The osteonecrosis may develop either during or following the exanthem, with reported lag periods as long as 150 days.

Ocular involvement is present in approximately 10%–25% of cases and can cause significant morbidity, including permanent blindness. The ocular manifestations are highly variable and may arise from direct viral-mediated epithelial damage, neuropathy, immune-mediated damage, or secondary vasculopathy. Lesions on the tip of the nose (Hutchinson sign) indicate involvement of the nasociliary branch of the trigeminal nerve and an increased risk for severe ocular infection. In these cases, referral to an ophthalmologist is mandatory.

Reactivation of VZV in the geniculate ganglion may cause **Ramsay Hunt syndrome,** which is characterized by cutaneous lesions of the external auditory canal and involvement of the ipsilateral facial and auditory nerves. Affected individuals may exhibit facial paralysis as well as hearing deficits, vertigo, and other auditory and vestibular symptoms. In addition, some patients may develop loss of taste in the anterior two-thirds of the tongue. By using PCR or serology, investigators have detected active VZV infection in approximately 30% of patients thought to have Bell palsy (see page 861). Similar associations also have been demonstrated with HSV and EBV. These findings suggest an underlying viral cause for many cases of "idiopathic" facial paralysis.

Approximately 15% of patients progress to the chronic phase of herpes zoster (termed **postherpetic neuralgia**), which is characterized by persistent pain after resolution of the rash. In defining postherpetic neuralgia, there is a lack of consensus regarding the duration of pain persistence following the rash, although many investigators consider a minimum period of 1–3 months. Risk factors include female gender, older age, history of prodromal pain, moderate to severe rash and/or pain during the acute phase, and ophthalmic involvement. The pain is described as burning, throbbing, aching, itching, or stabbing, often with flares caused by light stroking or contact with clothing. Most of these neuralgias resolve within 1 year, with half of patients experiencing resolution after 2 months. Rare cases may last up to 20 years, and patients have been known to commit suicide because of the extreme pain. Although the cause is unknown, some investigators believe chronic VZV ganglionitis is responsible.

In rare cases, a potentially fatal ischemic stroke syndrome, termed **granulomatous angiitis,** may develop weeks to months after resolution of a zoster rash involving the trigeminal nerve distribution. This condition appears to result from direct extension of VZV and associated inflammation from the trigeminal ganglion to the internal carotid artery.

In immunocompromised individuals, herpes zoster is often severe, with an overall increased risk for complications. The cutaneous rash may become disseminated as a result of VZV viremia; in some cases, viremia may occur even without skin involvement. Potentially life-threatening complications include pneumonia, hepatitis, disseminated intravascular coagulopathy, meningitis, and encephalitis. However, immunocompromised status does not appear to increase the risk for developing postherpetic neuralgia significantly.

Histopathologic Features

The active vesicles of herpes zoster are microscopically identical to those seen in the primary infection, varicella. For more information, see the previous sections regarding the histopathologic features of varicella and herpes simplex.

Diagnosis

Herpes zoster often is diagnosed from the clinical presentation, but laboratory testing may be necessary for atypical cases or exclusion of zosteriform recurrent HSV infection. Viral culture can provide confirmation. However, the results take at least 24 hours, and false negatives often occur because it is difficult to recover viable virus from cutaneous lesions. Cytologic smears demonstrate viral cytopathologic effects, as seen in varicella and HSV infection. A rapid diagnosis can be obtained by direct staining of cytologic smears with fluorescent monoclonal VZV antibodies. Molecular techniques, such as dot-blot hybridization and PCR, also can be used to detect VZV.

Treatment and Prognosis

Supportive therapy for herpes zoster may include antipruritics, such as diphenhydramine, and nonaspirin antipyretics. Skin lesions should be kept dry, clean, and, if possible, covered to prevent secondary infection; antibiotics may be administered to treat such secondary infections.

Prompt therapy with antiviral medications, such as acyclovir, valacyclovir, and famciclovir, has been found to accelerate healing of mucocutaneous lesions and reduce pain during the acute phase. These medications are most effective if initiated within 72 hours after development of the first vesicle. Supplementation of antiviral agents with analgesics (such as, acetaminophen, NSAIDs, tramadol, and opioids), tricyclic antidepressants, antiepileptics (including gabapentin and pregabalin), or systemic corticosteroids may provide additional pain control.

Investigations regarding whether antiviral treatment administered alone or in combination with gabapentin during the acute phase may prevent or lessen the severity of postherpetic neuralgia have yielded variable results. Similarly, combination therapy with antivirals and corticosteroids may be helpful in the treatment of acute herpes zoster but does not appear to prevent postherpetic neuralgia.

In postherpetic neuralgia, tricyclic antidepressants, anticonvulsants (including gabapentin and pregabalin), and opioids may reduce pain. In addition, the FDA has approved the lidocaine patch, capsaicin patch, and capsaicin cream for the treatment of postherpetic neuralgia. However, the evidence in support of these topical therapies is of limited quality. Also, capsaicin—which is derived from peppers—may cause significant burning or stinging of the skin as a side effect. Non-pharmacologic treatments include nerve blocks and percutaneous electrical nerve stimulation, but there are few well-controlled studies to support these alternatives. Because postherpetic neuralgia often is difficult to treat, emphasis should be placed on herpes zoster prevention.

A recombinant, adjuvanted herpes zoster vaccine (Shingrix) has been approved by the FDA for use in adults 50 years and older. This vaccine consists of two doses administered 2–6 months apart. The recombinant vaccine is preferred by the Advisory Committee on Immunization

Practices over the live zoster vaccine (Zostavax) because it confers greater protection against herpes zoster and postherpetic neuralgia.

◆ INFECTIOUS MONONUCLEOSIS (MONO; GLANDULAR FEVER; "KISSING DISEASE")

Infectious mononucleosis is a symptomatic disease resulting from exposure to Epstein–Barr virus (EBV or HHV-4). The infection usually occurs by intimate contact. Intrafamilial spread is common, and once a person is exposed, EBV remains in the host for life. Children usually become infected through contaminated saliva on fingers, toys, or other objects. Adults usually contract the virus through direct salivary transfer, such as shared straws or kissing, hence, the nickname "kissing disease." In developing nations, exposure usually occurs by age 3 and is universal by adolescence. In contrast, in developed nations, EBV infection rates have been declining among children, and introduction to the virus often is delayed. According to some studies in the United States, approximately 50% of college students lack previous exposure. Infected children are typically asymptomatic, whereas adolescents and young adults who become infected are at greatest risk for symptomatic disease. Similar mononucleosis syndromes may be produced by other pathogens, including CMV (see page 242), HIV-1 (see page 250), and *Toxoplasma gondii* (see page 222).

Besides infectious mononucleosis, EBV is associated with **oral hairy leukoplakia (OHL)** (see page 253), various lymphomas (most notably Burkitt lymphoma [see page 606]) and lymphoproliferative disorders (such as the **EBV-positive mucocutaneous ulcer** [see page 601]), nasopharyngeal carcinoma (see page 428), salivary lymphoepithelial carcinoma, some gastric carcinomas, and occasional smooth muscle tumors.

Clinical Features

The clinical presentation varies by age. Most EBV infections in children are asymptomatic. In symptomatic children younger than 4 years, typical findings include fever, lymphadenopathy, pharyngitis, hepatosplenomegaly, and rhinitis or cough. Children 4 years and older are affected similarly but exhibit a much lower prevalence of hepatosplenomegaly, rhinitis, and cough. Most young adults experience fever, lymphadenopathy, pharyngitis, and tonsillitis. In adults older than 40 years, fever and pharyngitis are the predominant findings.

Complications are uncommon at any age but most frequently arise in children. Possible significant complications include splenic rupture, thrombocytopenia, autoimmune hemolytic anemia, aplastic anemia, neurologic problems, myocarditis, and hemophagocytic lymphohistiocytosis. The latter appears to be caused by massive activation of T lymphocytes and histiocytes and is often fatal without prompt treatment.

In classic infectious mononucleosis in a young adult, prodromal fatigue, malaise, and anorexia occur up to 2 weeks before the development of pyrexia. Fever may reach 104 °F and last from 2 to 14 days. Prominent lymphadenopathy is noted in more than 90% of cases and typically appears as symmetrically enlarged and tender nodes, with frequent involvement of the posterior and anterior cervical chains. Enlargement of parotid lymphoid tissue rarely has been reported and can be associated with facial nerve palsy. More than 80% of affected young adults have oropharyngeal tonsillar enlargement, sometimes with diffuse surface exudates and secondary abscesses (Fig. 7.21). The lingual tonsils, which are located on the base of the tongue and extend from the circumvallate papillae to the epiglottis, can become hyperplastic and compromise the airway. Rare fatalities have been reported from respiratory difficulties secondary to tonsillar hyperplasia, arytenoid hypertrophy, pharyngeal edema, and epiglottal swelling.

Oral lesions other than lymphoid enlargement also may be seen. Petechiae on the hard or soft palate are present in about 25% of patients (Fig. 7.22). The petechiae usually disappear within 24–48 hours. **Necrotizing gingivitis** (see page 151) also is fairly common. Necrotizing gingivitis-like pericoronitis (see page 165) and necrotizing mucositis (see page 152) occur less frequently. Cases of necrotizing gingivitis that

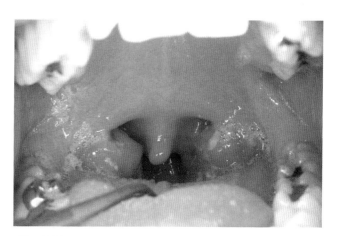

• **Fig. 7.21 Infectious Mononucleosis.** Hyperplastic pharyngeal tonsils with yellowish crypt exudates. (Courtesy of Dr. George Blozis.)

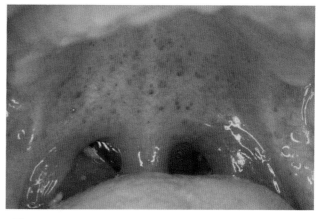

• **Fig. 7.22 Infectious Mononucleosis.** Numerous petechiae of the soft palate. (Courtesy of Dr. George Blozis.)

are refractory to conventional therapy should be evaluated to rule out the possibility of EBV infection.

In less than 10% of classic infectious mononucleosis cases, patients experience fatigue persisting for several weeks to months. However, active EBV infection beyond 4 months is rare. Several investigators have attempted to associate EBV with a controversial symptom complex called **chronic fatigue syndrome** (myalgic encephalomyelitis, systemic exertion intolerance disease), characterized by profound fatigue lasting more than 6 months, pharyngitis, myalgias, arthralgias, headaches, lymphadenopathy, postexertional malaise, unrestful sleep, and cognitive impairment. Nevertheless, current evidence does not support EBV as a specific cause of this condition, which likely may be triggered by a variety of illnesses or conditions.

Furthermore, some studies suggest that infectious mononucleosis increases the risk for developing multiple sclerosis later in life. However, it is uncertain whether EBV is a direct or indirect cause of multiple sclerosis versus an innocent bystander.

Diagnosis

The diagnosis of infectious mononucleosis commonly is based upon the clinical presentation combined with the presence of greater than 10% atypical lymphocytes on a peripheral blood smear and a positive heterophile antibody test. Heterophile antibodies are IgM antibodies that are directed against viral antigens and cross-react with sheep and horse erythrocytes. The Monospot test is a widely available assay for rapid detection of heterophile antibodies. However, false negative results are possible, especially during the first week of infection or among infected children younger than 4 years.

In suspected cases of EBV infection for which heterophile antibody testing is negative, EBV-specific antibody testing may be required. Immunoassays can be performed during various stages of infection and resolution in order to quantify antibodies directed against viral capsid antigens (VCA) and EBV nuclear antigens (EBNA).

Treatment and Prognosis

In most cases, infectious mononucleosis resolves within 4–6 weeks. NSAIDs can be used to minimize the most common symptoms. Adequate fluid intake and nutrition also are important. Patients with significant enlargement of the spleen should avoid contact sports to prevent the rare possibility of splenic rupture.

Tonsillar involvement may resemble streptococcal pharyngitis or tonsillitis (see page 174). However, ampicillin, amoxicillin, or other penicillins should be avoided because these antibiotics commonly cause nonallergic morbilliform skin rashes in patients with infectious mononucleosis.

Some clinicians advocate short-term corticosteroid administration in order to minimize acute symptoms. However, there is insufficient evidence from clinical studies to support the routine use of corticosteroid treatment for infectious mononucleosis. In addition, there is concern regarding an increased risk for complications, including encephalitis and myocarditis. In practice, most clinicians reserve corticosteroid treatment for management of severe complications, such as impending airway obstruction, hemolytic anemia, thrombocytopenia, or hemophagocytic lymphohistiocytosis. The latter also typically requires treatment with cyclosporine or etoposide.

Although antiviral medications, such as acyclovir, valacyclovir, and famciclovir, have been used successfully for temporary resolution of oral hairy leukoplakia (OHL), these medications do not demonstrate clinically obvious benefit for patients with infectious mononucleosis. These agents may block viral replication; however, the main clinical manifestations of infectious mononucleosis appear to be secondary to the immune response to EBV-infected B lymphocytes and are not altered by this intervention.

◆ CYTOMEGALOVIRUS

Similar to other human herpesviruses, **cytomegalovirus** (CMV or HHV-5) may establish latency after initial infection and reactivate under certain conditions. CMV can reside latently in salivary gland cells, endothelium, macrophages, and lymphocytes. The virus can be found in most bodily fluids, including saliva, blood, urine, tears, respiratory secretions, genital secretions, and breast milk. Most clinically evident disease is found in neonates or immunosuppressed adults. In infants, the virus is contracted through the placenta, during delivery, or during breast-feeding. The next peak of transmission occurs during adolescence, predominantly from sexual contact. Transmission also has been documented through blood transfusion and organ transplantation. Global CMV seroprevalence is estimated to be 83% in the general population. In the United States, seroprevalence is approximately 20% for children 1–5 years of age, 50% for individuals 6–49 years of age, and greater than 90% for those older than 80 years. In addition to increasing age, other risk factors for CMV seropositivity include female gender, low socioeconomic status, household crowding, and foreign birthplace.

Clinical Features

At any age, almost 90% of CMV infections are asymptomatic. In clinically evident congenital and neonatal infection, typical features include jaundice, hepatosplenomegaly, cutaneous erythropoiesis, and thrombocytopenia (often with associated petechiae and purpura). CNS involvement may cause microcephaly, seizures, and mental and motor impairment. In addition, CMV infection represents the most common cause of nonhereditary sensorineural hearing loss, with infected infants often developing hearing loss at birth or later in childhood.

Among immunocompetent individuals, symptomatic acute CMV infection is rare and exhibits nonspecific features, ranging from an infectious mononucleosis-like presentation to lethal multiorgan involvement. CMV mononucleosis typically is characterized by fever, chills, sore throat, headache, and fatigue. Compared with classic EBV mononucleosis, this condition is much less commonly associated with exudative pharyngitis, lymphadenopathy, and hepatosplenomegaly. Other possible findings in symptomatic CMV infection include joint and muscle pain, abdominal pain, nonproductive cough, maculopapular rash, and diarrhea. Persistent fever of unknown origin may be the primary finding in some cases. Rarely, immunocompetent patients may develop acute sialadenitis diffusely involving the major and minor salivary glands. In such cases, xerostomia often is noted, and the affected glands are painful and enlarged. Unusual complications include myocarditis, pericarditis, pneumonitis, anterior uveitis, and meningitis.

Clinically evident CMV involvement frequently arises in immunocompromised transplant patients. In some cases a temporary, mild fever is the only finding; in others, the infection becomes aggressive and is characterized by hepatitis, leukopenia, pneumonitis, gastroenteritis, and, more rarely, a progressive wasting syndrome.

Patients with AIDS (see page 250) also are at increased risk for symptomatic CMV disease, although a decrease in prevalence has been reported with the introduction of effective antiretroviral therapy (ART). The two most common manifestations of CMV infection in patients with AIDS are chorioretinitis and gastrointestinal involvement. The former may result in blindness, and the latter may cause bloody diarrhea or odynophagia.

Chronic oral ulcerations caused by CMV infection have been documented in association with HIV infection as well as other immunosuppressive conditions. Occasionally, such lesions may harbor coinfection with additional viruses, such as HSV and EBV. In addition, neonatal CMV infection can produce developmental tooth defects. In a study of 118 people with a history of neonatal CMV infection, examination revealed tooth defects in 40% of those with symptomatic infections and slightly more than 5% of those with asymptomatic infections. The teeth exhibited diffuse enamel hypoplasia, significant attrition, enamel hypomaturation, and yellow coloration from the underlying dentin.

Histopathologic Features

Biopsy specimens of intraoral CMV lesions may demonstrate changes within vascular endothelial cells or salivary duct epithelial cells (Fig. 7.23). Scattered infected cells are extremely swollen, showing both intracytoplasmic and intranuclear inclusions and prominent nucleoli. These enlarged cells have been called "owl eye" cells. Grocott-Gomori methenamine silver and periodic acid-Schiff (PAS) stains demonstrate the cytoplasmic inclusions but not the intranuclear changes.

Diagnosis

The diagnosis of CMV infection is based upon the clinical features combined with laboratory findings. Tissue biopsy may demonstrate cells with viral inclusions suggestive of

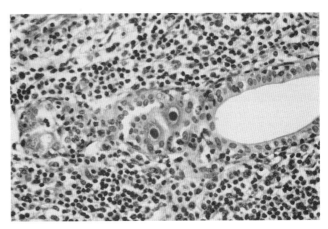

• **Fig. 7.23 Cytomegalovirus (CMV) Infection.** Salivary ductal epithelium exhibiting distinctive "owl eye" alterations.

CMV infection; however, these inclusions may be scant and difficult to demonstrate on routine light microscopy. More sensitive and specific methods for confirmation of CMV infection in biopsy specimens include immunohistochemistry and in situ hybridization. Because specific treatments exist for CMV infection in immunocompromised patients, biopsy is recommended for chronic ulcerations refractory to conservative therapy. In addition, in such cases HSV coinfection should be excluded.

Additional CMV detection methods include serology, viral culture, and PCR. Serologic testing by enzyme-linked immunosorbent assay (ELISA) is commonly available and relatively inexpensive. IgG seroconversion constitutes clear evidence of recent primary CMV infection but requires paired serum samples taken 1–3 months apart. Alternatively, recent primary infection may be diagnosed by positive IgM in combination with low IgG avidity (IgG antibodies with low binding strength to CMV). In transplant patients and other immunocompromised individuals, plasma viral load—determined by real-time quantitative PCR—may be monitored in order to assess the need for CMV treatment or response to CMV therapy.

In CMV mononucleosis, peripheral blood typically shows a 50% or greater relative lymphocytosis, with at least 10% atypical lymphocytes. Unlike EBV mononucleosis, this condition usually is heterophile antibody-negative.

Treatment and Prognosis

Although most CMV infections resolve spontaneously, therapy often is required in the immunosuppressed patient. Intravenous ganciclovir and oral valganciclovir are the most commonly used antiviral agents for CMV disease treatment and prevention in immunocompromised individuals. However, resistance to these agents has been reported; other effective treatments include foscarnet, cidofovir, combination antiviral therapy, and hyperimmune globulin. Nevertheless, the best preventive and interventional therapy in immunocompromised patients remains improvement of immune status, such as that achieved with antiretroviral therapy (ART) for HIV infection (see page 264).

Immunocompetent patients with clinically evident CMV infection usually are treated symptomatically with NSAIDs. Corticosteroids or IV gamma globulins have been used in patients with hemolytic anemia or severe thrombocytopenia. Use of antiviral agents in immunocompetent patients typically is reserved for severe disease because of the risk of drug-related toxicity.

No licensed vaccine is currently available for prevention of CMV infection; however, several vaccines are under investigation and may be used in the future to protect women of reproductive age and children.

◆ ENTEROVIRUSES

Human **enteroviruses** (family Picornaviridae, genus *Enterovirus*) traditionally have been classified into echoviruses, coxsackieviruses A and B, and polioviruses, with numerical designations for individual serotypes (e.g., Coxsackie virus A1). Beginning in the 1960s, newly discovered enterovirus serotypes have been designated numerically without being placed into one of the traditional groups (e.g., enterovirus 71). Current classification, based upon molecular and biologic features, divides the human enteroviruses into four species (A through D) but maintains the traditional names for individual serotypes. More than 100 serotypes have been identified. Also, a few enteroviruses (echoviruses 22 and 23) have been reclassified into the distinct *Parechovirus* genus. Polioviruses largely have been eradicated in developed countries by vaccination. However, the nonpolio enteroviruses continue to cause disease worldwide.

Most enterovirus infections are asymptomatic or subclinical. Among symptomatic cases, the clinical presentation is variable and may range from a minor febrile illness to a severe and potentially fatal infection. Death may be caused by neurologic or cardiopulmonary complications. In addition, more than 30 enteroviral subtypes are associated with skin rashes.

The estimated annual incidence of enterovirus infections in the United States is 10–15 million, with most cases affecting infants and young children. In many countries, epidemics occur every 2–3 years and primarily affect children 1–4 years old. The timing of the epidemics appears to correlate with the accumulation of a new population of susceptible young children.

The present discussion focuses upon the following clinical patterns of enteroviral infection: **herpangina, hand-foot-and-mouth disease,** and **acute lymphonodular pharyngitis.** These conditions are closely related and should not be considered entirely separate. In epidemics involving the same viral strain, the clinical presentations often vary and may include both herpangina and hand-foot-and-mouth disease. Also, many authorities regard acute lymphonodular pharyngitis as a variant of herpangina rather than a distinct entity.

Herpangina usually is produced by coxsackievirus A1 to A6, A8, A10, or A22. However, it also may represent infection by coxsackievirus A7, A9, or A16; coxsackievirus B2 to B6; echovirus 9, 16, or 17; or enterovirus 71. Hand-foot-and-mouth disease usually is caused by coxsackievirus A16 or enterovirus 71. In particular, in the Asia-Pacific region over the past few decades, enterovirus 71 has caused several large outbreaks of hand-foot-and-mouth disease, often associated with major neurologic complications. In addition, coxsackievirus A6 has emerged as a major cause of hand-foot-and-mouth disease in recent outbreaks in the United States and abroad. Other causative pathogens include coxsackievirus A5, A9, or A10 and echovirus 11. Acute lymphonodular pharyngitis is less recognized, and coxsackievirus A10 has been found in the few reported cases.

In nontropical areas, most cases arise in the summer or early fall, with crowding and poor hygiene aiding their spread. The fecal-oral route is the major mode of transmission, and frequent hand washing is important to diminish spread during epidemics. The incubation period is 4–7 days. During the acute phase, the virus also can be transmitted through saliva or respiratory droplets. Infection confers immunity against reinfection by a particular strain. Over time an individual may develop immunity against numerous enterovirus types but still remain susceptible to additional strains.

Clinical Features

In all three clinical patterns, the severity varies by strain. Most strains produce a self-limiting disease that requires no therapy, but some strains can produce epidemics with significant complications and occasional fatalities. Potential complications include pneumonia, pulmonary edema and hemorrhage, carditis, encephalitis, meningitis, and acute flaccid myelitis. In particular, the latter has been associated with several recent enterovirus outbreaks around the world and represents a severe neurologic illness characterized by profound muscle weakness, spinal cord gray matter abnormalities, and a predilection for children. In addition, infection with coxsackievirus B during pregnancy has been associated with fetal and neonatal death, whereas cardiac anomalies have been noted in infants who survive the initial infection.

Herpangina

Herpangina begins with an acute onset of sore throat, dysphagia, and fever, occasionally accompanied by cough, rhinorrhea, anorexia, vomiting, diarrhea, myalgia, and headache. Most cases, however, are mild or subclinical. Typically a small number of lesions (usually two to six) develop on the soft palate or tonsillar pillars (Fig. 7.24). The lesions begin as red macules, which form fragile vesicles that rapidly ulcerate. The ulcerations average 2–4 mm in diameter. The systemic symptoms resolve within a few days; the ulcerations usually take 7–10 days to heal.

Hand-Foot-and-Mouth Disease

Hand-foot-and-mouth disease is the best-known presentation of enterovirus infection. The name fairly well describes the location of the lesions. The oral lesions arise without

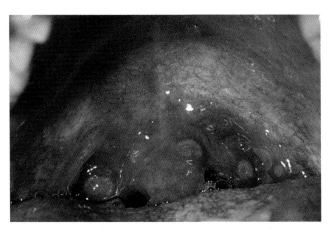

• **Fig. 7.24 Herpangina.** Numerous aphthous-like ulcerations of the soft palate.

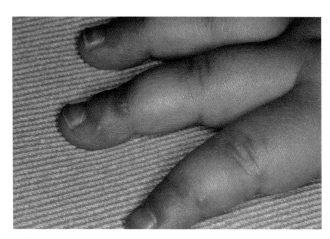

• **Fig. 7.26 Hand-foot-and-mouth Disease.** Numerous cutaneous vesicles on the sides of the fingers.

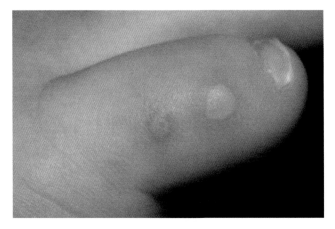

• **Fig. 7.25 Hand-foot-and-mouth Disease.** Multiple vesicles of the skin of the toe. (Courtesy of Dr. Samuel J. Jasper.)

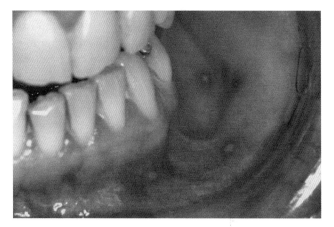

• **Fig. 7.27 Hand-foot-and-mouth Disease.** Multiple aphthous-like ulcerations of the mucobuccal fold.

prodromal symptoms and precede the development of the cutaneous lesions on the hands and feet. Sore throat, dysphagia, and mild fever usually are present also. Other possible findings include cough, rhinorrhea, anorexia, vomiting, diarrhea, myalgia, and headache.

The cutaneous lesions range from a few to dozens and primarily affect the borders of the palms and soles and the ventral surfaces and sides of the fingers and toes (Fig. 7.25). Rarely other sites, especially the buttocks, external genitals, and legs, may be involved. The cutaneous lesions begin as erythematous macules that develop central vesicles and heal without crusting (Fig. 7.26). In some cases, nail loss or ridges (Beau lines) may ensue after several weeks.

The oral lesions resemble those of herpangina but may be more numerous and more frequently involve anterior regions of the mouth. The number of lesions ranges from 1 to 30. The buccal mucosa, labial mucosa, and tongue are the most common sites, but any area of the oral mucosa may be involved (Fig. 7.27). The individual lesions typically measure 2–7 mm in diameter but may be larger than 1 cm. The lesions rapidly ulcerate and then typically heal within 1 week.

Coxsackie A6 infection may cause hand-foot-and-mouth disease with atypical features. Such cases occur over an

unusually broad age range, including children as well as adults. Compared to those with conventional disease, affected patients may exhibit a higher fever; more severe and widespread skin lesions (including vesicles, bullae, erosions, ulcers, and hemorrhagic lesions); and a longer disease course (approximately 2 weeks). Also, after recovery some patients exhibit delayed-onset palmar and plantar desquamation, nail loss, and Beau lines.

Acute Lymphonodular Pharyngitis

Acute lymphonodular pharyngitis is characterized by sore throat, fever, and mild headache, which may last from 4 to 14 days. Low numbers (one to five) of yellow to dark-pink nodules develop on the soft palate or tonsillar pillars (Fig. 7.28). The nodules represent hyperplastic lymphoid aggregates and resolve within 10 days without vesiculation or ulceration.

Histopathologic Features

In patients with herpangina and hand-foot-and-mouth disease, the affected epithelium exhibits intracellular and intercellular edema, which lead to the formation of an

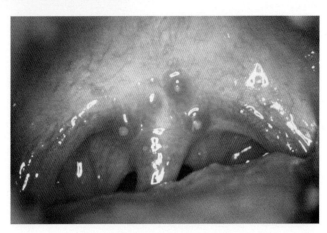

• **Fig. 7.28 Acute Lymphonodular Pharyngitis.** Numerous dark-pink and yellow lymphoid aggregates. (Courtesy of Dr. George Blozis.)

intraepithelial vesicle. The vesicle enlarges and ruptures through the epithelial basal cell layer, with formation of a subepithelial vesicle. Epithelial necrosis and ulceration soon follow. Inclusion bodies and multinucleated epithelial cells are absent.

Diagnosis

Herpangina, hand-foot-and-mouth disease, and acute lymphonodular pharyngitis usually are diagnosed based upon the clinical manifestations. In patients with atypical presentations, laboratory confirmation appears prudent. Reverse transcription polymerase chain reaction (RT-PCR) is preferred over viral culture because of its higher sensitivity. Testing can be performed on various specimen types, including throat swabs, rectal swabs, stool samples, and cutaneous vesicular fluid.

Treatment and Prognosis

In most instances, enterovirus infections are self-limiting and without significant complications. Therapy is directed toward symptomatic relief; nonaspirin antipyretics and topical anesthetics, such as dyclonine hydrochloride, often are beneficial.

Occasionally, certain strains produce infections with a more aggressive clinical course. Body temperature above 102 °F, fever for longer than 3 days, severe vomiting, and lethargy have been associated with increased risk for serious disease complications and warrant close patient monitoring.

◆ MEASLES (RUBEOLA)

Measles (rubeola) is a highly contagious infection produced by a virus in the family Paramyxoviridae and genus *Morbillivirus.* Prior to the development of an effective measles vaccine, the disease caused millions of deaths annually worldwide. In the pre-vaccine era in the United States, greater than 90% of individuals were infected by 15 years of age, with over 500,000 measles cases and about 500 measles-related deaths

reported annually. In susceptible populations, each infected person typically transmits the infection to 9–18 other individuals; there is a 90% chance that an exposed, nonimmune individual will contract the disease.

Eradication through widespread immunization is achievable yet remains a challenge. In the United States, following the introduction of universal measles vaccination in 1963, the annual incidence of measles decreased by more than 99%. A major resurgence occurred from 1989 to 1999, mainly among unvaccinated preschool-aged children. This resurgence led to the recommendation for a second vaccine dose and intensive, widespread immunization efforts. In 2000, the CDC declared that measles had been eliminated in the United States. Nevertheless, outbreaks of measles—often linked to importation of the virus from abroad with subsequent spread through undervaccinated subpopulations—continue to occur. Of particular concern, a major outbreak in 2019 represented the greatest number of reported annual cases in the United States in nearly three decades. Likewise, international efforts toward measles elimination have made progress but are ongoing. Despite an estimated 80% decrease in global measles deaths from 2000 to 2017, the disease continues to claim more than 100,000 lives per year worldwide. Political, financial, and logistical barriers as well as public complacency and concerns regarding vaccine safety have made measles control difficult.

Clinical Features

Most cases of measles arise in late winter or spring and are spread through respiratory droplets or aerosolized particles. The average incubation period is 10–14 days, and affected individuals are infectious from 4 days before until 4 days after appearance of the associated rash. The virus is associated with significant lymphoid hyperplasia that often involves the lymph nodes, tonsils, adenoids, and Peyer patches.

There are three stages of infection, with each stage lasting 3 days—hence the designation 9-day measles. The first 3 days are dominated by the "3 Cs": coryza (runny nose), cough (typically brassy and uncomfortable), and conjunctivitis (red, watery, and photophobic eyes). Fever typically accompanies these symptoms. During this initial stage, the most distinctive oral manifestation, **Koplik spots**, is seen. These lesions represent foci of epithelial necrosis and appear as numerous small, blue-white macules (or "grains of salt") surrounded by erythema (Fig. 7.29). Typical sites of involvement include the buccal and labial mucosa, and less often the soft palate.

As the second stage begins, the fever continues, the Koplik spots fade, and a maculopapular and erythematous (morbilliform) rash begins. The face is involved first, with eventual downward spread to the trunk and extremities. Ultimately, a diffuse erythematous eruption is formed, which tends to blanch on pressure (Fig. 7.30). Abdominal pain secondary to lymphatic involvement is not rare.

In the third stage, the fever ends. The rash begins to fade, with downward progression and replacement by brown

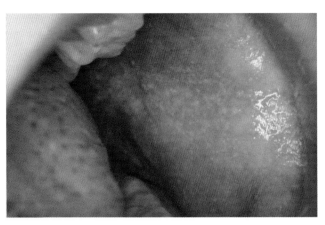

• **Fig. 7.29 Rubeola.** Numerous blue-white Koplik spots of buccal mucosa. (Courtesy of Dr. Robert J. Achterberg.)

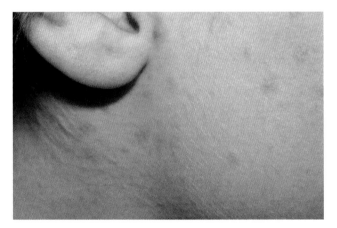

• **Fig. 7.30 Rubeola.** Erythematous maculopapular rash of the face. (Courtesy of Dr. Robert J. Achterberg.)

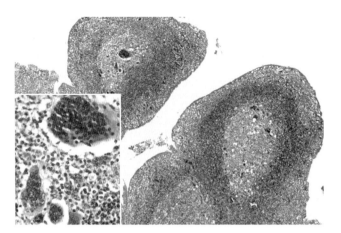

• **Fig. 7.31 Rubeola.** Histopathologic section of pharyngeal tonsil demonstrating lymphoid hyperplasia with scattered multinucleated giant cells. *Inset* reveals high-power magnification of Warthin-Finkeldey giant cells.

pigmentation. Ultimately, desquamation of the skin is noted in areas previously affected by the rash.

Complications affect approximately 30% of patients, especially those who are younger than 5 years, older than 20 years, malnourished, or immunocompromised. Common complications in young children are otitis media, pneumonia, laryngotracheobronchitis (croup), and diarrhea. Another fairly common sequela is keratoconjunctivitis, which tends to affect children with vitamin A deficiency and may cause blindness. Acute appendicitis occasionally is seen secondary to vascular obstruction created by the swelling of Peyer patches. Encephalitis develops in approximately 1 in 1000 cases, often resulting in death or permanent brain damage and intellectual disability. In about 1 in 10,000–100,000 cases, a delayed complication termed **subacute sclerosing panencephalitis (SSPE)** arises as late as 11 years after the initial infection. This degenerative CNS disorder leads to personality changes, seizures, coma, and death. During pregnancy, measles is associated with an increased risk for intrauterine fetal death, spontaneous abortion, low birthweight, and maternal death.

Measles in immunocompromised patients can be serious, with a high risk for complications and death. Most of these patients exhibit either an atypical rash or no exanthem. Pneumonitis is the primary complication.

Koplik spots are not the only oral manifestation that may be associated with measles. Candidiasis, necrotizing gingivitis, and necrotizing stomatitis may occur if significant malnutrition also is present. Severe measles in early childhood can cause pitted enamel hypoplasia of the developing permanent teeth. Enlargement of accessory lymphoid tissues, such as the lingual and pharyngeal tonsils, also may be noted.

Histopathologic Features

Because of the reduced prevalence of measles and the transient nature of Koplik spots, few oral and maxillofacial pathologists have had the opportunity to view these lesions microscopically. Initially, Koplik spots represent areas of hyperparakeratotic epithelium with spongiosis, dyskeratosis, and epithelial syncytial giant cells. The number of nuclei within these giant cells ranges from 3 to more than 25. Close examination of the epithelial cells often reveals pink-staining inclusions in the nuclei or, less commonly, cytoplasm. Electron microscopy has shown that the inclusions represent microtubular aggregates characteristic of paramyxovirus infection. As the spot ages, the epithelium exhibits heavy neutrophilic exocytosis leading to microabscess formation, epithelial necrosis, and, ultimately, ulceration. Frequently, examination of the epithelium adjacent to the ulceration reveals the suggestive syncytial giant cells.

Examination of hyperplastic lymphoid tissue during the prodromal stage of measles often reveals a similar alteration. In 1931, Warthin and Finkeldey, in two separate publications, reported an unusual finding in patients who had their tonsils removed within 1–5 days of the clinical appearance of measles. Within the hyperplastic lymphoid tissue, there were numerous multinucleated giant lymphocytes (Fig. 7.31). These multinucleated cells subsequently have been termed **Warthin-Finkeldey giant cells** and once were thought to be specific for measles. However, similar cells have been noted in a variety of conditions, such as lymphoma, Kimura disease, AIDS-related lymphoproliferative disease, and lupus erythematosus.

Diagnosis

The diagnosis of measles in an epidemic setting usually is based on the clinical features and history. Laboratory confirmation can be of value in isolated or atypical cases. The most commonly used method is IgM antibody assay performed on a single serum sample. The antibodies usually appear within 72 hours after onset of the exanthem and persist for 1–2 months. Confirmation by rising IgG titers, viral culture, and RT-PCR also are possible.

Treatment and Prognosis

Primary prevention is essential for reducing measles-associated morbidity and mortality. The measles vaccine is a live, attenuated virus, which is included in the widely used MMR (measles, mumps, and rubella) and MMRV (measles, mumps, rubella, and varicella) vaccines. Routine childhood measles vaccination is recommended, with the first dose administered between the ages of 12 and 15 months and a second dose between the ages of 4 and 6 years. The vaccine is highly effective, with over 99% of individuals developing long-term immunity after receiving two doses. In a given population, measles eradication typically is attained with 95% vaccine coverage. Despite controversy regarding vaccine safety, adverse reactions from measles vaccination are rare and typically mild or transient. Extensive research shows no increased risk of permanent neurologic sequelae, and no scientific evidence supports an increased risk for autism or inflammatory bowel disease.

In otherwise healthy patients with measles, fluids and nonaspirin antipyretics are recommended for symptomatic relief. Antibiotics may be prescribed for bacterial superinfections, such as bacterial otitis media or pneumonia. Children with measles also should receive vitamin A supplementation. For immunocompromised patients, ribavirin and interferon may be administered.

In developed nations, less than 1% of measles cases result in death, whereas in developing countries, the case-fatality rate is usually about 3% to 6%. However, mortality can be as high as 30% among displaced or isolated populations with poor vaccine coverage and approximately 50% among HIV-infected children. The most common causes of death are pneumonia and acute encephalitis.

◆ RUBELLA (GERMAN MEASLES)

Rubella is a mild illness caused by a virus in the family Togaviridae and genus *Rubivirus*. The greatest importance of this infection lies not in its effects on those who contract the acute illness but in its capacity to induce birth defects in the developing fetus. The infection occurs primarily in late winter and early spring. It is contracted through respiratory droplets, with nearly 100% transmission among individuals in close living conditions. The incubation time is from 12 to 23 days, and infected patients are contagious from 1 week before to 1 week after onset of the exanthem. Infants with congenital infection may release the virus for up to 1 year and, in some cases, may continue to harbor intraocular virus for decades.

In the past, this infection occurred in cycles, with localized epidemics every 6–9 years and pandemics every 10–30 years. The last pandemic occurred from 1962 to 1964. In 1964 and 1965, the United States alone had more than 12.5 million cases, which resulted in more than 11,000 spontaneous or therapeutic abortions, 2100 neonatal deaths, and 20,000 infants born with **congenital rubella syndrome (CRS)**.

An effective vaccine, first released in 1969, has dramatically affected the epidemiology of the infection and broken the cycle of occurrences. In the United States, during the two decades immediately following introduction of the vaccine, the number of rubella and CRS cases reported annually decreased 99% and 97%, respectively. Like rubeola, rubella exhibited a slight resurgence from 1989 to 1990, primarily due to a lack of vaccination diligence; this resurgence prompted intensification of vaccination efforts and a new two-dose schedule. These measures resulted in an overall decline in rubella cases but a shift in epidemiology. During the early 1990s, children younger than 15 years mainly were affected; however, since the mid-1990s, most reported rubella cases have occurred in patients 15 years and older, especially among Hispanic and foreign-born individuals. Notwithstanding, since 2001, the overall annual incidence has remained low (less than 1 per 10,000,000 population). In 2004, a panel of experts declared that rubella elimination (i.e., absence of endemic transmission) had been achieved in the United States. However, rubella remains endemic in several parts of the world, with more than 100,000 infants with CRS born annually worldwide.

Clinical Features

A large percentage of infections are asymptomatic; the frequency of symptoms is greater in adolescents and adults. Prodromal symptoms may be seen 1–5 days before the exanthem and include fever, headache, malaise, anorexia, myalgia, mild conjunctivitis, coryza, pharyngitis, cough, and lymphadenopathy. The lymphadenopathy may persist for weeks and is noted primarily in the suboccipital, postauricular, and cervical chains. The most common complication is arthritis, which increases in frequency with age and usually arises subsequent to the rash. Rare complications include encephalitis and thrombocytopenia.

The rash is often the first sign of the infection and begins on the face and neck, with spread to the entire body within 1–3 days. The exanthem forms discrete pink macules, then papules, and finally fades with flaky desquamation. Facial involvement often clears before the rash completes its spread into the lower body areas. Generally, the rash completely resolves by day 3—hence the designation 3-day measles.

Oral lesions, known as **Forchheimer sign,** have been reported in about 20% of cases. These lesions consist of small, discrete, dark-red papules that develop on the soft palate and may extend onto the hard palate. This enanthem arises simultaneously with the rash, becoming evident in about 6 hours after the first symptoms and not lasting longer than 12–14 hours. Palatal petechiae also may occur.

The risk of CRS correlates with the time of infection. The risk for fetal defects is as high as 90% when the infection occurs during the first 8–10 weeks of pregnancy, with the risk declining thereafter and becoming rare after 16 weeks of gestation. The classic triad of CRS consists of sensorineural deafness, heart disease, and cataracts. Hearing loss may not become evident until 2 years of age and usually is bilateral. Other frequently reported findings include microcephaly, microphthalmia, and hepatosplenomegaly. Among those who survive the neonatal period, there is an increased risk for developmental difficulties, such as autism. Less common, late-emerging complications include diabetes mellitus, thyroiditis, and progressive encephalopathy.

Diagnosis

The diagnosis of rubella is contingent on laboratory tests because the clinical presentation of the acquired infection is typically subclinical, mild, or nonspecific. Serologic analysis is the mainstay of diagnosis, although viral culture and RT-PCR also are possible.

Treatment and Prognosis

Rubella is mild, and therapy usually is not required. Nonaspirin antipyretics and antipruritics may be useful in patients with significant fever or symptomatic cutaneous involvement. Passive immunity may be provided by the administration of rubella immunoglobulin. If immunoglobulin is given within a few days of exposure, it decreases the severity of the infection. This therapy typically is reserved for pregnant patients who decline abortion.

High vaccination coverage—particularly among children, women of childbearing age, and foreign-born individuals—is essential for prevention of rubella. In the United States, both the MMR (measles, mumps, and rubella) and MMRV (measles, mumps, rubella, and varicella) vaccines are licensed for rubella prevention. Routine childhood administration of either MMR or MMRV is recommended, with the first dose at 12–15 months of age and the second dose at 4–6 years of age. In addition, in the absence of evidence of rubella immunity, the following groups should receive at least one dose of MMR: adults born during or after 1957, nonpregnant women of childbearing age, and health care personnel. Evidence of immunity may include serologic testing or documentation of at least one dose of rubella-containing vaccine at 12 months of age or older; immunity also generally can be presumed in those born before 1957, as long as the individual is not a health care worker. Contraindications for the MMR and MMRV vaccines include pregnancy, immunodeficiency, allergy to any of the vaccine components, and acute febrile illness. Pregnant women lacking immunity should be vaccinated immediately postpartum.

◆ MUMPS (EPIDEMIC PAROTITIS)

Mumps is an infection caused by a virus in the family Paramyxoviridae and genus *Rubulavirus*. This infection causes diffuse swelling of the exocrine glands; although the salivary glands are the best known sites of involvement, the pancreas, choroid plexus, and mature ovaries and testes also are affected frequently. The virus can be transmitted through respiratory droplets, saliva, and urine. The incubation period usually is 16–18 days, with a range of about 2–4 weeks. Patients are contagious from 1 day before the clinical appearance of infection to 14 days after its clinical resolution. In temperate climates, mumps most commonly occurs in winter and spring.

As with measles and rubella, the epidemiology has been affected dramatically by vaccination. Before the advent of widespread vaccination, mumps epidemics developed every 2–5 years; nearly everyone was exposed with 90% of infections occurring before age 15. In the United States, the mumps vaccine was licensed in 1967, although the Advisory Committee on Immunization Practices (ACIP) did not recommend universal childhood mumps vaccination until 1977. At that time, MMR (measles, mumps, and rubella) vaccine administration became the norm for children 12–15 months of age. Subsequently, the annual incidence of mumps decreased by 98% and reached an all-time low in 1985. In 1989, the ACIP issued a two-dose recommendation for MMR vaccination, primarily in response to a resurgence of measles. Compared with the prevaccine era, the two-dose vaccination schedule has reduced the prevalence of mumps by more than 99%.

Nevertheless, several mumps resurgences have occurred over the past several decades. These resurgences often have developed among adolescents and young adults, particularly in the college setting. This shift in peak age from childhood to adolescence and young adulthood is clinically significant, because certain disease complications, such as epididymoorchitis and oophoritis, primarily affect postpubertal patients. Although outbreaks in the mid-1980s to early 1990s were attributed to single-dose vaccine failure or a lack of vaccination, several outbreaks since the early 2000s have occurred despite high levels of two-dose vaccine coverage. The efficacy of the mumps component of the MMR vaccine is approximately 88% after two doses and is lower than that of the measles and rubella components. In 2017, the ACIP recommended a third dose of MMR vaccine for persons who have received 2 doses previously and are at increased risk for acquiring mumps during an outbreak.

Clinical Features

Approximately 30% of mumps infections are subclinical. In symptomatic cases, prodromal symptoms of low-grade fever, headache, malaise, anorexia, and myalgia develop first. These

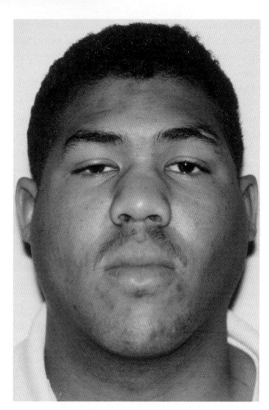

• **Fig. 7.32 Mumps.** Bilateral parotid enlargement. (From Neville BW, Damm DD, White DK: *Color atlas of clinical oral pathology,* ed 2, Hamilton, 1999, BC Decker.)

nonspecific findings typically are followed within a few days by significant salivary gland changes. The parotid glands are involved most often, but the sublingual and submandibular glands also can be affected. Discomfort and swelling develop in the tissues surrounding the lower half of the external ear and extending down along the posterior inferior border of the adjacent mandible (Fig. 7.32). The enlargement and pain typically peak within 2–3 days. Chewing movements of the jaw or eating saliva-stimulating foods tends to increase the pain. Enlargement of the glands usually begins on one side, followed by contralateral involvement within a few days. Unilateral involvement is seen in about 25% of patients.

The second most common finding is epididymo-orchitis, which occurs in about 25% of postpubertal males. The testicle exhibits rapid swelling, with significant pain and tenderness. The enlargement can range from a minimal swelling to a fourfold increase in size. Unilateral involvement is most common. Upon resolution of the swelling, testicular atrophy may occur; permanent sterility is rare, but subfertility develops in approximately 13% of patients with epididymyo-orchitis. Less commonly, oophoritis and mastitis can be seen in postpubertal females. In addition, spontaneous abortion occurs in approximately 25% of women who contract mumps during the first trimester of pregnancy.

Less commonly, meningoencephalitis, cerebellar ataxia, hearing loss, pancreatitis, arthritis, carditis, and decreased renal function may occur. The most common symptom associated with CNS involvement is headache, whereas involvement of the pancreas can lead to nausea and vomiting. Isolated changes, such as orchitis or meningitis, may occur in the absence of salivary gland involvement, thereby making diagnosis difficult in nonepidemic settings.

The most frequently reported oral manifestation is redness and enlargement of Wharton and Stensen salivary gland duct openings. In addition, involvement of the sublingual glands may produce bilateral enlargement of the floor of the mouth.

Diagnosis

Although the diagnosis of mumps in an epidemic setting usually can be made easily from the clinical presentation, isolated cases often require laboratory confirmation. Serologic tests include detection of either mumps-specific IgM or a fourfold rise of mumps-specific IgG titers between the acute and convalescent phases; however, false-negative results are common in previously vaccinated individuals. In addition, a swab of secretions obtained from parotid or other affected salivary gland ducts can be used for viral culture or RT-PCR.

Treatment and Prognosis

The treatment of mumps is palliative in nature. Frequently, nonaspirin analgesics and antipyretics are administered. In an attempt to minimize orchitis, bed rest is recommended for males until the fever breaks. Avoidance of sour foods and drinks helps to decrease the salivary gland discomfort. Mumps-related mortality is exceedingly rare and primarily associated with encephalitis.

As with measles and rubella, vaccination is important for controlling disease. The mumps vaccine is a live, attenuated virus, which is incorporated into the MMR and MMRV (measles, mumps, rubella, and varicella) vaccines. Monovalent mumps vaccine is no longer available in the United States. The current recommendation is for routine childhood administration of two doses of mumps-containing vaccine, with the first dose administered between the ages of 12 and 15 months and the second dose between the ages of 4 and 6 years. In addition, two doses of MMR vaccine should be administered to adults who lack immunity and fall into any of the following categories: health care workers born in or after 1957, college students, and international travelers. One dose of MMR vaccine is recommended for all other adults who lack evidence of immunity and were born in or after 1957.

◆ HUMAN IMMUNODEFICIENCY VIRUS AND ACQUIRED IMMUNODEFICIENCY SYNDROME

This section provides an overview of **human immunodeficiency virus (HIV)** and its related disease states, with an emphasis on manifestations in the oral region. For more detailed information regarding HIV infection and **acquired** immunodeficiency syndrome (AIDS), the reader may refer to a large body of scientific literature and entire texts dedicated to this topic.

HIV is a single-stranded RNA virus belonging to the family Retroviridae. There are two species: HIV-1 and HIV-2. The former exhibits a worldwide distribution and is responsible for the majority of cases, whereas the latter predominates in western Africa and is associated with a somewhat lower risk of transmission and slower disease progression.

In 1981, the CDC published the first scientific report of AIDS. This report detailed *Pneumocystis carinii* (since renamed *Pneumocystis jiroveci*) pneumonia in five previously healthy men from Los Angeles, California. A few years later, HIV was isolated and identified as the cause of AIDS. Since this initial description, more than 75 million individuals worldwide have become infected with HIV, and more than 32 million individuals have died of AIDS. Worldwide in 2020 alone, approximately 1.5 million new infections occurred, 38 million people were living with HIV, and 680,000 individuals died of AIDS-related illnesses. According to the most recent report by the Joint United Nations Programme on HIV/AIDS, HIV infection is most prevalent in Eastern and Southern Africa—which accounts for approximately 54% of people living with HIV worldwide and more than 40% of global AIDS deaths—followed by the Asia-Pacific region and Western and Central Africa. The toll has been devastating, although through global public health efforts and treatment advances, there has been an approximately 23% decline in the number of newly infected individuals worldwide over the past decade. Despite the considerable progress that has been made, HIV control efforts continue to be hampered by significant challenges, including socioeconomic disparities, social inequality, limited access to care, and disruption by the coronavirus disease 2019 (see page 265) pandemic.

The annual number of new HIV infections in the United States peaked in the mid-1980s at around 130,000 and subsequently sharply declined to about 50,000 in the early 1990s. In recent years, the number of new HIV infections diagnosed annually has remained relatively stable at around 36,000–38,000. Currently, it is estimated that 1.2 million individuals are living with HIV infection in the United States, and about 14% of them are unaware of their infection. At the beginning of the HIV/AIDS epidemic, the disease was nearly 100% fatal; however, since the introduction of effective antiretroviral therapy (ART) (see the Treatment and Prognosis section), there has been significant improvement in patient survival and, thus, an increased percentage of the population living with the virus.

Initially, in the United States, HIV primarily infected whites and male homosexuals. Today, male-to-male sexual contact remains the greatest risk factor; however, the epidemiology of the HIV/AIDS epidemic has shifted over time, with the highest incidence now recorded among blacks and Hispanics. In 2019, blacks represented only about 13% of the population but accounted for 44% of new HIV diagnoses. Similarly, Hispanics were disproportionately

affected, with this group accounting for about 18% of the population but 30% of new HIV infections. Factors contributing to these disparities may include poverty; limited access to health care and HIV education; cultural and language barriers; lack of awareness of HIV status; high rates of other sexually transmitted infections (such as HSV-2 infection) that may increase the risk of contracting HIV; and avoidance of testing and treatment for fear of discrimination. Among newly diagnosed cases of HIV in adults and adolescents in the United States in 2019, approximately 79% were male, 19% were female, and 2% were transgender. The latter group comprised a very small proportion of cases but recently exhibited a sharply increasing trend. With respect to age, the greatest incidence was noted among individuals 20 through 29 years old.

In infected individuals, the virus can be found in most bodily fluids, including serum, blood, saliva, semen, tears, urine, breast milk, ear secretions, and vaginal secretions. In the United States, the most frequent mode of transmission is male-to-male sexual contact (accounting for approximately two-thirds of HIV infections diagnosed annually), followed by heterosexual contact and injection drug use. Perinatal exposure and transfusion of blood or blood products account for a very small proportion (1% and less than 0.5%, respectively) of current cases; these modes of transmission have become rare due to improvements in perinatal testing, prophylactic use of antivirals, blood-screening methods, and availability of recombinant clotting factors. Infection by artificial insemination, breast-feeding from infected mothers, and organ transplantation also has been documented rarely.

Transmission by oral fluids is somewhat controversial and has been reported only anecdotally. In rare instances, transmission has occurred during breast-feeding from the oral fluids of postpartum infected infants to their previously noninfected mothers. Unusual cases of transmission from bites, oral cunnilingus, or repeated passionate kissing have been described as well. Saliva contains a number of HIV inhibitory factors, which appear to reduce the ability of the virus to infect its target cells. However, the presence of erosions, ulcerations, and hemorrhagic inflammatory pathoses (e.g., gingivitis, periodontitis) may predispose an individual to oral transmission. In summary, the best precaution is avoidance of all body fluids of infected patients.

The primary target cell of HIV is the CD4+ helper T lymphocyte, although other CD4+ cells (such as, macrophages and dendritic cells) may be infected as well. The virus binds to CD4 and additional cell surface molecules in order to gain entry, upon which the viral RNA genome is reverse transcribed into complementary DNA. This complementary DNA may become incorporated into the host cell DNA. Upon transmission, the virus initially takes hold in the mucosa, within days spreads to the lymphoid tissues, and by around day 10 becomes detectable within blood. Viremia usually peaks around a month after transmission; however, the incubation period is variable, and it may take anywhere from several weeks to months before antibodies are demonstrable. In people with HIV infection, antibodies against the virus are developed but are not protective. The virus then enters a latency period, during which replication may stabilize at a relatively low level but nevertheless continues. During this period, many patients are asymptomatic. The mean clinical latency among untreated individuals is 10 years; however, the duration is variable and typically can be maintained for much longer time periods by administration of ART. Among untreated individuals or those for whom therapy does not control the virus, there is a progressive loss of T-helper cells with resultant immunodeficiency. The normal response to viruses, fungi, and encapsulated bacteria is diminished. In addition, infection of macrophages and microglia in the CNS may lead to neurologic disease manifestations.

Clinical Features

The clinical stages of HIV infection include an acute phase, a chronic phase (or latency period), and AIDS. During the acute phase, the patient may be asymptomatic or exhibit a self-limited **acute retroviral syndrome.** This syndrome typically develops around 3–6 weeks after exposure in 50%–70% of infected patients. The symptoms resemble those of infectious mononucleosis (e.g., generalized lymphadenopathy, sore throat, fever, malaise, lethargy, maculopapular rash, headache, myalgia, arthralgia, diarrhea, photophobia, and peripheral neuropathies). Meningitis and encephalitis also are possible. Oral changes may include mucosal erythema and focal ulcerations. During this initial phase, HIV infection often is not considered or investigated, and HIV antibodies are not yet detectable. Nevertheless, during this period, patients exhibit high levels of viremia and are extremely infectious.

After infection is established, an immune response is developed, viremia declines, and the patient enters a clinical latency period. During this time, most patients are asymptomatic, but some exhibit persistent generalized lymphadenopathy (PGL). Without treatment, the immune system fails to control the virus, and the CD4+ cell count declines at an average rate of 50 per microliter per year. When the CD4+ cell count falls below a critical level (200 per microliter for individuals 6 years and older), there is severe immunodeficiency, resulting in the development of AIDS. During this stage, patients are at high risk for opportunistic infections or neoplasms. Such infections include *Pneumocystis jiroveci* pneumonia, disseminated cytomegalovirus infection, severe herpes simplex virus infection, atypical mycobacterial infection, cryptococcal meningitis, and CNS toxoplasmosis. In addition, persistent diarrhea is commonplace and may be bacterial or protozoal in origin. Neoplasms considered to be AIDS-defining conditions include Kaposi sarcoma, non-Hodgkin lymphoma, and invasive cancer of the uterine cervix. Furthermore, clinically significant neurologic dysfunction may result from a form of progressive encephalopathy known as HIV-associated dementia (AIDS-dementia complex).

Since the widespread use of effective ART and guidelines for the prevention of opportunistic infections, the spectrum of HIV disease has evolved. Opportunistic infections have become much less common compared to the early days of the HIV epidemic. Also, with increased longevity among the HIV-infected population, there have been shifts in cancer burden. The risk for AIDS-defining cancers has decreased—especially for Kaposi sarcoma and non-Hodgkin lymphoma—apparently because improvement of immune function with ART suppresses the viruses associated with these malignancies. In contrast, the risk for various non-AIDS-defining cancers as well as cardiovascular, renal, and hepatic disease has increased.

Oral manifestations of HIV disease also have been altered dramatically by the introduction of potent ART. In particular, there have been significant reductions in the frequency of oral candidiasis, OHL, and oral Kaposi sarcoma. In contrast, an increased prevalence of periodontitis has been reported, although this finding may be explained by aging of the patient population. Some researchers also have reported an increased prevalence of benign human papillomavirus (HPV)-induced pathoses and HIV-associated salivary gland disease, but other investigators have not confirmed these findings.

Importantly, the detection of oral manifestations may suggest possible HIV infection in an undiagnosed individual. In addition, the discovery of oral manifestations in a patient with known HIV infection may signal HIV disease progression and the need for initiation or adjustment of ART.

The following discussion of oral manifestations concentrates primarily on the clinical presentations and special treatment considerations for HIV-infected patients. (For more detailed information regarding these conditions in the general patient population, see the discussion of each disease elsewhere in this text.) Oral conditions most strongly associated with HIV infection are presented first, followed by a selection of less frequently encountered conditions.

Candidiasis

Candidiasis is the most common intraoral manifestation of HIV infection and often is the presenting sign that leads to the initial diagnosis (Fig. 7.33). Among studies performed

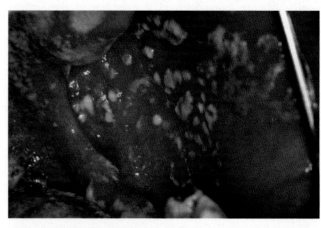

• **Fig. 7.33 HIV-associated Candidiasis.** Extensive removable white plaques of the left buccal mucosa.

in recent decades, the reported prevalence of oral candidiasis in HIV-infected individuals ranges from about 20% to 80%. The prevalence is lower in patients receiving ART compared to those not receiving such treatment. In particular, HIV protease inhibitors used in ART have been associated with reduced frequency and recurrence of oral candidiasis. For HIV-positive patients not receiving ART, the presence of oral candidiasis is predictive of progression to full-blown AIDS within 2 years. Compared to individuals with other types of immunocompromised status, those with HIV infection have a greater prevalence of oral candidiasis, suggesting that HIV may play a role in initiation of candidal infection. In addition, among HIV-infected groups in resource-limited settings, investigators have noted a strong association between oral candidiasis and tuberculosis—a leading cause of mortality in HIV-positive patients. The most common candidal species isolated from the oral mucosa of HIV-positive patients is *Candida albicans*, although various other *Candida* species may be encountered.

The following four clinical patterns are seen (see page 201):
1. Pseudomembranous candidiasis
2. Erythematous candidiasis
3. Hyperplastic candidiasis
4. Angular cheilitis

The first two variants constitute most cases. Although infrequently seen in immunocompetent patients, chronic multifocal oral involvement is common in HIV-infected patients. Erythematous candidiasis typically appears when the CD4+ lymphocyte count drops below 400 cells per microliter, whereas the pseudomembranous pattern usually develops when the count drops below 200 cells per microliter. Oral candidiasis can be painful and associated with a reduction in taste and smell, which may lead to decreased food intake and further wasting. In severe cases, patients may develop oral, oropharyngeal, and esophageal involvement; such individuals may experience retrosternal burning accompanied by odynophagia.

The diagnosis of candidiasis often is obvious from the clinical presentation but can be confirmed by cytologic smear or biopsy. Biopsy specimens of involved mucosa demonstrate the candidal organisms embedded in the superficial keratin, but the typical inflammatory reaction may be deficient (Fig. 7.34).

For the treatment of oral candidiasis in HIV-infected individuals, oral antifungal agents typically are preferred over topical therapy because they are more convenient, better tolerated, and associated with a lower risk for relapse. Fluconazole generally is the drug of choice and is prescribed for 1–2 weeks; for patients who also suffer from esophageal involvement, this medication is administered for 3 weeks. When there is concern regarding adverse side effects or drug interactions with systemic therapy, the patient may be treated with topical agents, such as miconazole mucoadhesive buccal tablets or clotrimazole troches. For patients with refractory disease, itraconazole oral solution, posoconazole oral suspension, amphotericin B oral solution (not available

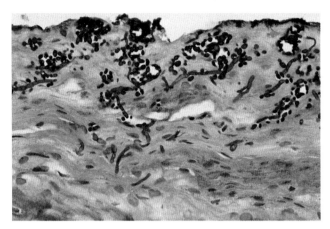

• **Fig. 7.34 HIV-associated Candidiasis.** Periodic acid-Schiff (PAS) stain of histopathologic section exhibiting numerous fungal organisms embedded in superficial keratin.

in the United States), or intravenous amphotericin B may be considered.

Routine prophylactic antifungal therapy is not recommended for patients with advanced HIV disease because acute oral candidiasis typically responds well to conventional treatment, prophylaxis is costly, and there is the potential for development of resistant candidal strains. Instead, immune reconstitution by ART is the best method for prevention of oral candidiasis in this patient population. However, for individuals with especially frequent and severe recurrences, prophylactic fluconazole may be considered.

Oral Hairy Leukoplakia

Although EBV is associated with several forms of lymphoma in HIV-infected patients, the most common EBV-related lesion in patients with AIDS is **oral hairy leukoplakia (OHL).** The prevalence of OHL among individuals with HIV has declined since the introduction of effective ART. The development of OHL may indicate HIV disease progression, a lack of compliance with ART, or antiretroviral drug resistance. Among HIV-infected individuals, OHL exhibits a predilection for males and tobacco users. OHL also has been reported in transplant recipients, steroid medication users, and aging individuals. Although the lesion occasionally occurs in relatively immunocompetent individuals, discovery of OHL in "normal" patients mandates a thorough physical evaluation to rule out immunocompromise.

OHL clinically presents as a white mucosal plaque that does not rub off. Most cases occur on the lateral border of the tongue and range in appearance from faint, white vertical streaks to thickened, furrowed areas of leukoplakia with a shaggy surface (Fig. 7.35). The lesions infrequently may extend to cover the entire dorsal and lateral surfaces of the tongue. Rarely, the buccal mucosa, soft palate, pharynx, or esophagus may be involved.

Histopathologically, OHL exhibits thickened parakeratin with surface corrugations or thin projections (Fig. 7.36). The epithelium is acanthotic and exhibits a bandlike zone of lightly stained cells with abundant cytoplasm ("balloon

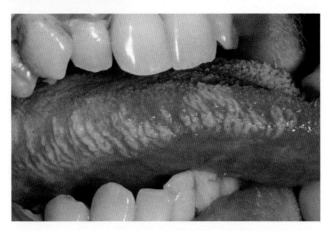

• **Fig. 7.35 HIV-associated Oral Hairy Leukoplakia (OHL).** Vertical streaks of keratin along the lateral border of the tongue.

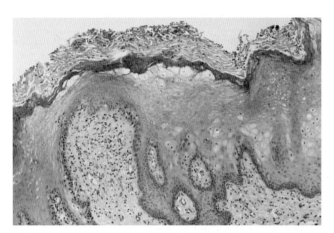

• **Fig. 7.36 HIV-associated Oral Hairy Leukoplakia (OHL).** Oral mucosa exhibiting hyperparakeratosis with surface corrugations.

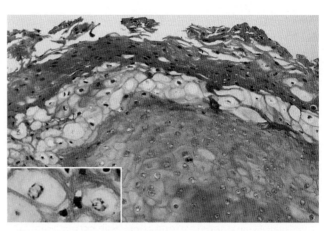

• **Fig. 7.37 HIV-associated Oral Hairy Leukoplakia (OHL).** Oral epithelium exhibiting hyperparakeratosis and layer of "balloon cells" in the upper spinous layer. *Inset* reveals high-power magnification of epithelial cells that demonstrate nuclear beading.

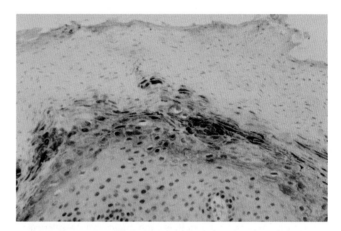

• **Fig. 7.38 HIV-associated Oral Hairy Leukoplakia (OHL).** Immunoperoxidase evaluation for Epstein–Barr virus (EBV) revealing positive reaction within numerous epithelial cells.

cells") in the upper spinous layer (Fig. 7.37). Close examination of the superficial epithelial cells reveals nuclear clearing and a characteristic pattern of peripheral margination of chromatin termed nuclear beading (see Fig. 7.38, *inset*), caused by extensive EBV replication that displaces the chromatin to the nuclear margin. Dysplasia is not noted. Heavy candidal infestation of the parakeratin layer may be seen, although the normal inflammatory reaction to the fungus usually is absent.

In a patient with known HIV infection, the clinical features of OHL typically are sufficient for a presumptive diagnosis. When definitive diagnosis is necessary, demonstration of EBV can be achieved by in situ hybridization, PCR, immunohistochemistry (Fig. 7.38), Southern blotting, or electron microscopy.

Treatment of OHL usually is not needed, although slight discomfort or aesthetic concerns may necessitate therapy. Systemic anti-herpesviral drugs produce rapid resolution, but recurrence is expected with discontinuation of therapy. Topical treatment with retinoids or podophyllum resin has resulted in temporary remissions. A few small-scale studies have demonstrated prolonged resolution after combined treatment with acyclovir cream and podophyllum resin. Surgical excision or cryotherapy also has been used by some.

Kaposi Sarcoma

Kaposi sarcoma (KS) is a vascular endothelial neoplasm caused by human herpesvirus 8 (HHV-8, Kaposi sarcoma–associated herpesvirus [KSHV]). Most cases in the United States have arisen in association with HIV infection. At the height of the AIDS epidemic in the early 1990s, the annual incidence of KS in the United States peaked at 4.7 cases per 100,000 population. However, since the introduction of combination ART in 1996, the annual incidence has declined substantially and currently is estimated at 0.5 cases per 100,000 population. Nevertheless, in the United States, HIV-infected individuals are 500 times more likely than the general population to be diagnosed with KS, and KS represents the second most common malignancy among people with AIDS.

In Western countries, KS has been reported primarily in HIV-infected, adult, male homosexuals and is thought to be related to sexual transmission of HHV-8. Some cases also have been reported in male homosexuals without HIV

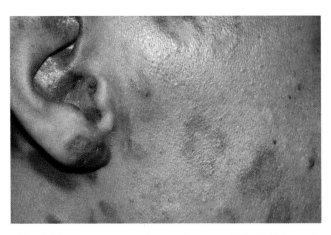

• **Fig. 7.39 HIV-associated Kaposi Sarcoma (KS).** Multiple purple macules on the right side of the face.

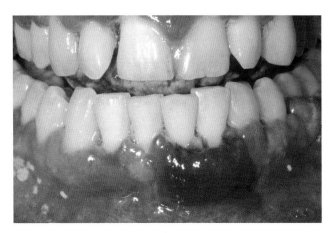

• **Fig. 7.41 HIV-associated Kaposi Sarcoma (KS).** Raised, dark-red enlargement of the left mandibular anterior facial gingiva.

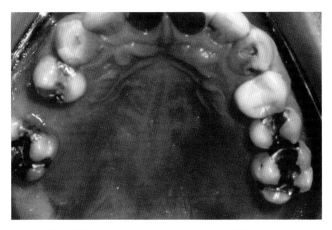

• **Fig. 7.40 HIV-associated Kaposi Sarcoma (KS).** Large zones of KS appearing as flat, brownish, and M-shaped discoloration of the hard palate.

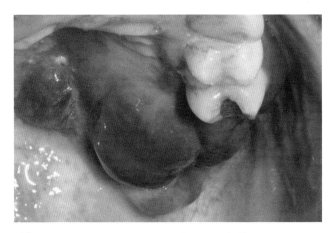

• **Fig. 7.42 HIV-associated Kaposi Sarcoma (KS).** Diffuse, red-blue nodular enlargement of the left hard palate.

infection. In Africa both AIDS-related and endemic types of KS frequently are seen, with no gender predilection and a significant number of children affected. Infection before sexual activity suggests alternate transmission pathways. Relatively high titers of HHV-8 have been found in saliva, and HHV-8 exhibits tropism for oral and oropharyngeal epithelial cells; these observations suggest that the oral cavity may represent an important reservoir of infectious virus and saliva may be a major transmission route.

KS mainly manifests as multiple lesions on the skin or oral mucosa, although visceral and lymph node involvement also may occur. Occasionally a solitary lesion is identified first. Among AIDS-related cases, the skin lesions exhibit a predilection for the face (Fig. 7.39) and lower extremities. The oral cavity is the initial site of involvement in 22% of patients with KS, and oral lesions are found more often in AIDS-related KS than other types of KS. Approximately 70% of individuals with AIDS-related KS demonstrate oral lesions at some point. The hard palate, gingiva, and tongue are the most frequently affected oral sites (Figs. 7.40 and 7.41). When present on the palate or gingiva, the neoplasm can invade bone and cause tooth mobility. The lesions

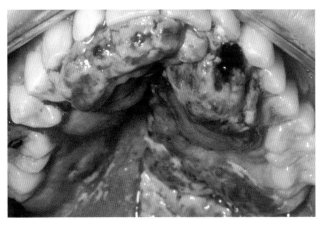

• **Fig. 7.43 HIV-associated Kaposi Sarcoma (KS).** Diffuse, red-blue gingival enlargement with widespread necrosis.

usually begin as erythematous blue or brown macules that do not blanch with pressure. Nonpigmented lesions have been reported very rarely. With time, the macules typically develop into plaques or nodules (Fig. 7.42), which may coalesce into a diffuse, exophytic mass (Fig. 7.43). Pain, bleeding, and necrosis may necessitate therapy. Uncommonly, advanced oral lesions may cause secondary lymphedema of the face and neck.

A biopsy is required for definitive diagnosis, although a presumptive clinical diagnosis sometimes is made. Other lesions can have a similar clinical appearance in HIV-infected patients, including bacillary angiomatosis (a multifocal vascular proliferation associated with the cat-scratch bacillus [see page 195]) and lymphoma.

Initiation of ART may induce regression of KS lesions, and patients who develop KS despite already receiving ART tend to have relatively mild disease without visceral involvement. Because KS typically regresses upon return of immunocompetence, many researchers question whether KS is a true sarcoma. However, in a small subset of patients, administration of ART causes immune reconstitution inflammatory syndrome (see Treatment and Prognosis section), which may induce paradoxical worsening of KS. Locoregional therapy may be used for limited, asymptomatic mucocutaneous lesions nonresponsive to ART or for palliation of advanced mucocutaneous lesions. Treatment options include topical therapy (e.g., alitretinoin gel or imiquimod cream for skin lesions), intralesional injection of chemotherapeutic or immunomodulatory agents (e.g., vinblastine, vincristine, bleomycin, and interferon-alpha), radiation, surgical excision, cryotherapy (for skin lesions), sclerotherapy, and laser therapy. Radiation therapy generally is not advised for oral lesions because of the potential for severe mucositis. For advanced AIDS-related KS, systemic chemotherapy (e.g., pegylated liposomal doxorubicin, paclitaxel) or immunomodulatory therapy in conjunction with ART is indicated. In addition, some authorities have suggested systemic therapy for oral lesions of AIDS-related KS even at the early macular stage, because progression to the exophytic stage in the oral cavity is associated with a poor prognosis.

Negative prognostic indicators for AIDS-related KS include tumor-associated edema, ulceration, extensive oral disease visceral involvement, CD4+ cell count below 150 per microliter, or other HIV-related illnesses. Interestingly, KS arising in lymph nodes does not necessarily represent metastasis or a poor prognosis. In the United States, the 5-year survival rate for individuals diagnosed with KS in recent years is approximately 70%. However, survival rates are much lower in regions where treatment is not widely available.

Persistent Generalized Lymphadenopathy

After seroconversion, HIV disease often remains silent except for **persistent generalized lymphadenopathy (PGL)**. The prevalence of this early clinical sign varies; however, in several studies it approaches 70%. PGL consists of lymphadenopathy that has been present for longer than 3 months and involves two or more extrainguinal sites. The most frequently involved sites are the posterior and anterior cervical, submandibular, occipital, and axillary nodes. Nodal enlargement fluctuates, usually is larger than 1 cm, and varies from 0.5 to 5.0 cm (Fig. 7.44).

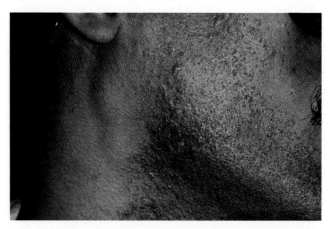

• **Fig. 7.44 HIV-associated Lymphadenopathy.** Enlarged cervical lymph nodes in a patient with persistent generalized lymphadenopathy (PGL).

Because lymphoma is known to occur in this population, a lymph node biopsy may be indicated for localized or bulky adenopathy, when cytopenia or an elevated erythrocyte sedimentation rate is present, or when requested for patient reassurance. Histopathologic examination reveals florid follicular hyperplasia. Although not as predictive as oral candidiasis or OHL, PGL does warn of progression to AIDS; almost one-third of affected and untreated patients will have diagnostic features of AIDS within 5 years.

Non-Hodgkin Lymphoma

Non-Hodgkin lymphoma (NHL) currently represents the most common malignancy among HIV-infected people in the United States, with an estimated lifetime risk of 4%. Similar to KS, NHL has become significantly less common among HIV-infected patients since the introduction of effective ART. Nevertheless, HIV-infected individuals in the United States are 12 times more likely to develop NHL compared to the general population. Factors implicated in the etiopathogenesis of these malignancies include suppressed immune surveillance, B-lymphocyte dysregulation, reactivation of oncogenic viruses (such as EBV and HHV-8), chronic antigen stimulation by viral coinfections (such as hepatitis B and hepatitis C), and possibly direct effects of HIV itself. Most cases represent high-grade, aggressive B-cell neoplasms. HIV-associated NHL can be categorized as follows:

1. Lymphomas also occurring in immunocompetent patients (most commonly Burkitt lymphoma and diffuse large B-cell lymphoma; rarely, extranodal marginal zone lymphoma of mucosa-associated lymphoid tissue [MALT lymphoma], peripheral T-cell, and natural killer cell lymphoma)
2. Lymphomas more specifically occurring in HIV-positive patients (e.g., primary effusion lymphoma; plasmablastic lymphoma; and HHV-8-positive diffuse large B-cell lymphoma, not otherwise specified)
3. Lymphoma also occurring in other immunodeficiency states (e.g., cases resembling post-transplant lymphoproliferative disorder [PTLD]).

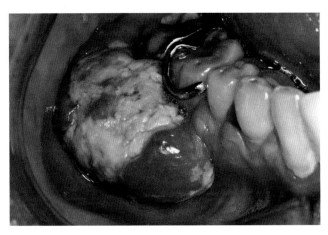

• **Fig. 7.45 HIV-associated Lymphoma.** Erythematous and ulcerated soft tissue mass involving the right posterior mandibular gingiva and mucobuccal fold.

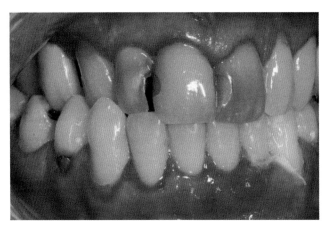

• **Fig. 7.46 HIV-associated Gingivitis.** Band of erythema involving the free gingival margin.

Lymphoma in patients with AIDS usually occurs in extranodal locations. Oral lesions are seen in approximately 4% of patients with AIDS-related NHL and most frequently involve the gingiva, palate, and tongue (Fig. 7.45). Intraosseous involvement also has been documented and may resemble diffuse progressive periodontitis with loss of periodontal attachment and loosening of teeth. In these cases, widening of the periodontal ligament and loss of lamina dura may represent radiographic clues to the diagnosis.

In order to prevent NHL in HIV-infected individuals, early and sustained ART is recommended. Treatment for HIV-associated NHL usually consists of combination chemotherapy in conjunction with ART. Early in the AIDS epidemic, people with AIDS typically suffered from severe opportunistic infections at the time of lymphoma diagnosis and, thus, could not tolerate intensive chemotherapy. However, with the introduction of ART, there has been a significant reduction in co-morbidity, thereby allowing for intensive lymphoma treatment. Current areas of investigation include immunotherapy and cellular therapies (e.g., chimeric antigen receptor T cells). Prognosis varies by specific lymphoma type. However, with the inclusion of ART, lymphoma survival for the HIV-infected population often approaches that for the general population.

HIV-Associated Periodontal Disease

Atypical patterns of periodontal disease strongly associated with poorly controlled HIV infection include linear gingival erythema, necrotizing gingivitis, and necrotizing periodontitis. These conditions also may arise in association with risk factors other than HIV infection.

Linear gingival erythema represents an unusual pattern of gingivitis, with a distinctive linear band of erythema involving the free gingival margin and extending 2–3 mm apically (Fig. 7.46). In addition, the alveolar mucosa and gingiva may demonstrate punctate or diffuse erythema in a significant percentage of cases. This diagnosis should be reserved for gingivitis that does not respond to improved plaque control and exhibits a greater degree of erythema than would be expected for the amount of plaque present. The literature related to linear gingival erythema is difficult to evaluate, because well-defined diagnostic criteria are lacking and the condition often is confused with conventional marginal gingivitis. Although some investigators believe linear gingival erythema results from an abnormal host immune response to subgingival bacteria, data suggest that this condition may represent an unusual pattern of candidiasis. Treatment may include débridement, povidone-iodine irrigation, chlorhexidine mouth rinse, and/or antifungal medication.

Necrotizing gingivitis (see page 151) and **necrotizing periodontitis** are conditions belonging to the broader category of necrotizing periodontal diseases. The microbial profile of necrotizing periodontal diseases in HIV-infected individuals includes organisms associated with disease in HIV-negative patients plus additional findings, such as *Candida albicans*, herpes viruses, and various types of bacterial superinfection. Among studies of sizeable patient cohorts with HIV/AIDS, reported prevalence is approximately 10%–11% for necrotizing gingivitis and 0.3%–9% for necrotizing periodontitis.

In necrotizing gingivitis, there is sudden onset of necrosis and ulceration involving one or more interdental papillae without periodontal attachment loss. Patients also exhibit gingival bleeding, pain, and halitosis (Fig. 7.47).

Necrotizing periodontitis is characterized by gingival necrosis and ulceration with rapidly progressing periodontal attachment loss. Although severe cases can affect all teeth, multiple isolated defects often are seen and contrast with the diffuse pattern associated with typical chronic periodontitis. Edema, severe pain, and spontaneous hemorrhage are common. Deep pocketing usually is not seen because extensive gingival necrosis typically coincides with loss of the adjacent alveolar bone (Fig. 7.48). Attachment loss may be especially rapid in patients with HIV infection, with some individuals exhibiting up to 10 mm of bone loss within a 6-month period.

HIV-infected patients also are at increased risk for developing **necrotizing stomatitis**, characterized by massive areas

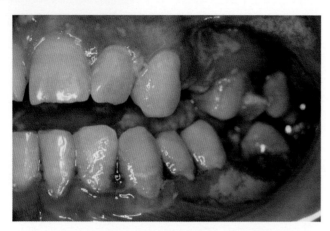

• **Fig. 7.47 HIV-associated Necrotizing Gingivitis.** Multiple punched-out interdental papillae of the mandibular gingiva. Note diffuse pseudomembranous candidiasis of the surrounding mucosa.

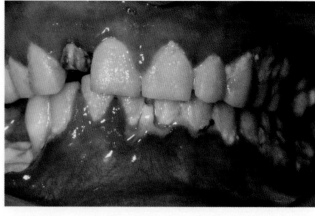

• **Fig. 7.49** HIV-associated Periodontitis with Necrotizing Stomatitis. Diffuse gingival necrosis with extension onto alveolar mucosa.

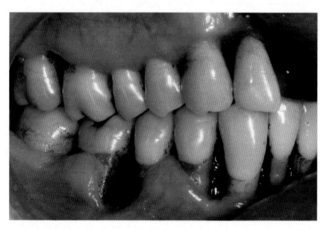

• **Fig. 7.48 HIV-associated Periodontitis.** Extensive loss of periodontal support without deep pocketing.

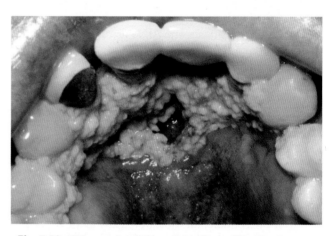

• **Fig. 7.50 HIV-associated Necrotizing Stomatitis.** Massive necrosis of soft tissue and bone of the anterior maxilla.

of tissue destruction beyond the alveolar ridges (Fig. 7.49). This process clinically resembles noma (see page 191) and may involve predominantly soft tissue or extend into the underlying bone, resulting in extensive sequestration (Fig. 7.50). Although necrotizing stomatitits often develops as an extension of necrotizing periodontitis, it also may arise in areas of the oral mucosa other than the gingiva. In the absence of gingival involvement, the clinical features of necrotizing stomatitis are nonspecific and mandate biopsy. In many instances, the areas of ulceration and necrosis demonstrate infection with one or more pathogens, such as HSV, CMV, and EBV.

Management of HIV-infected individuals with necrotizing periodontal diseases includes débridement, antimicrobial therapy, pain control, immediate follow-up care, and long-term maintenance in conjunction with ensuring that the patient is receiving appropriate ART. The initial removal of necrotic tissue typically is performed under local anesthesia and usually is combined with chlorhexidine or povidone-iodine irrigation. Additional débridement, scaling and root planning, and lavage are performed during follow-up visits. Systemic antibiotic therapy (such as metronidazole)

is reserved for patients with severe involvement, because of the risk for inducing secondary fungal or viral infection. Long-term maintenance considerations include oral hygiene reinforcement, chlorhexidine mouth rinse, nutritional counseling, and frequent recall visits.

In addition to linear gingival erythema and necrotizing periodontal diseases, HIV-infected patients may demonstrate conventional gingivitis, chronic periodontitis, and progressive nonnecrotizing periodontitis. Studies have shown that periodontal attachment loss can be combated successfully with regular professional scaling and root planing, plus optimization of oral hygiene. Recent evidence suggests that management of chronic periodontitis is important for reduction of systemic inflammatory mediators that may stimulate HIV activation.

Mycobacterial Infection

The best known mycobacterial infection is **tuberculosis (TB),** which is caused mainly by *Mycobacterium tuberculosis* (see page 185). Less common TB-causing mycobacteria include *M. bovis, M. africanum, M. canetti,* and *M. microti.* In addition, atypical mycobacterial infection with *Mycobacterium avium* and *Mycobacterium intracellulare* (*Mycobacterium* *avium-intracellulare* complex) can cause clinically evident disease, particularly in advanced stages of AIDS.

Approximately one-quarter of the world's population is infected with TB. Each year about 10 million people fall ill with TB worldwide, of which 9% represent HIV-positive individuals. Coinfection with HIV is associated with an increased risk for TB activation, and TB represents the leading cause of death in HIV-infected persons. Among 1.5 million TB deaths reported annually, approximately 250,000 occur in association with HIV. In the United States, HIV-related TB case rates are low, due in part to the widespread use of ART. Nevertheless, even with the beneficial effects of ART, HIV-infected individuals remain at increased risk for developing TB compared to the general population.

There is an unusual predilection for extrapulmonary involvement among HIV-infected individuals with TB. Nevertheless, oral lesions are uncommon and occur in less than 5% of all individuals with active TB. The tongue is the most frequently involved oral site, but lesions also can develop on the buccal mucosa, gingiva, floor of mouth, lips, and palate. The affected areas present as chronic ulcerations, granular leukoplakias, exophytic proliferative masses, or fissures. Jaw involvement also is possible and may present as tuberculous osteomyelitis, a periapical lesion, or an infected dental extraction socket.

Confirming TB often is difficult in AIDS patients, because tuberculin skin tests, microscopic examination of sputum smears for acid-fast bacilli, and chest radiographs lack sensitivity in this patient population. Liquid cultures, nucleic acid amplification tests, or urine lipoarabinomannan assay may facilitate diagnosis. In resource-limited settings, screening for a history of cough, fever, and/or night sweats is useful for identification of HIV-infected patients requiring diagnostic testing for TB.

In conjunction with ART, a regimen consisting of isoniazid, a rifamycin, pyrazinamide, and ethambutol for 2 months followed by isoniazid and a rifamycin for 4 months typically is effective for TB disease in HIV-infected adults. There is the potential for drug interactions between rifampin and some protease inhibitors or nonnucleoside reverse transcriptase inhibitors. Therefore, other rifamycins, such as rifabutin, may be selected.

Hyperpigmentation

Hyperpigmentation of the skin, nails, and mucosa has been reported in HIV-infected patients. The changes are similar microscopically to focal melanosis, with increased melanin pigmentation observed in the basal cell layer of the affected epithelium. Several medications taken by AIDS patients (e.g., ketoconazole, clofazimine, pyrimethamine, zidovudine, and emtricitabine) may cause increased melanin pigmentation. Adrenocortical destruction from several AIDS-associated opportunistic infections has been reported, resulting in an Addisonian pattern of pigmentation. Finally, some investigators have theorized that HIV-induced cytokine dysregulation may play a role in development of hyperpigmentation.

HIV-Associated Salivary Gland Disease

HIV-associated salivary gland disease can arise anytime during HIV infection. The condition is characterized by at least one of the following: (1) salivary hypofunction or subjective xerostomia, (2) diffuse enlargement of one or more major salivary glands. Irreversible salivary gland damage may result. The exact etiopathogenesis is unknown but has been linked to reactivation of BK polyomavirus (BKPyV) infection. Males are affected more often than females, and the disease occurs in both children and adults. Salivary gland enlargement most often affects the parotid. Bilateral involvement is seen in about 60% of cases and often is associated with cervical lymphadenopathy. Microscopic changes within the affected glands may include lymphocytic infiltration, hyperplasia of intraparotid lymph nodes, and lymphoepithelial cyst formation. Pathologic examination is important to rule out lymphoma.

Patients with mild HIV-associated salivary gland disease may require no specific treatment other than periodic monitoring. For more severe cases, management options include ART, aspiration, sclerotherapy, low-dose radiation therapy, and surgery. Some investigators have noted regression after initiation of ART, whereas others have reported increased prevalence with ART, possibly due to immune reconstitution inflammatory syndrome (see Treatment and Prognosis section).

Salivary gland enlargement within the setting of HIV infection also may be caused by **diffuse infiltrative lymphocytosis syndrome (DILS)** (also referred to as HIV-related sicca complex). This condition occurs in about 3%–8% of persons with HIV infection, although its frequency has declined since the introduction of effective ART. This syndrome mainly occurs in adults and is characterized by CD8+ lymphocytosis with diffuse lymphocytic infiltration of various sites, such as the major or minor salivary glands, lacrimal glands, lungs, kidneys, muscle, nerve, and liver. In particular, there may be massive parotid gland enlargement, which is more often bilateral than unilateral. Many patients also develop xerostomia, dry eyes, cervical lymphadenopathy, and interstitial pneumonia. There is an association between DILS and certain human leukocyte antigen (HLA) types. Labial salivary gland biopsy typically shows periductal CD8+ T-lymphocytic infiltration, acinar atrophy, ductal dilatation, and fibrosis. The most widely accepted treatments for DILS are ART and corticosteroids. DILS is associated with a relatively favorable HIV disease prognosis but also an increased risk for lymphoma; therefore, some authors recommend periodic monitoring for lymphoma development by fine-needle aspiration.

Interestingly, a few authors have reported ranulas (see page 462) and sialoliths (see page 465) in HIV-infected patients. However, the significance of these findings is uncertain, and a definitive association with HIV disease has not been established.

Thrombocytopenia

Thrombocytopenia (see page 590) is often an early manifestation of HIV infection but may occur at any time during the course of HIV disease. Among patients with untreated HIV infection, thrombocytopenia develops in approximately 3%

of those with CD4+ T cell counts at or above 400 per microliter and 10% of those with CD4+ T cell counts below 400 per microliter. The underlying mechanisms may include direct infection of platelet progenitor cells, platelet destruction by anti-HIV antibodies that cross-react with platelet glycoproteins, platelet destruction by nonspecific binding of immune complexes, and defective modulation of hematopoiesis by HIV-infected T lymphocytes. In addition, thrombocytopenia may develop secondary to medications, concurrent infections, or malignancy. Cutaneous lesions are present in most cases, but oral lesions also may occur; typical findings include petechiae, ecchymosis, and spontaneous gingival hemorrhage.

ART is considered first-line treatment for thrombocytopenia in HIV-infected patients. For severe or refractory cases, additional treatment options may include interferon-alpha, intravenous immunoglobulin (IVIG), IV anti-Rho immunoglobulin (anti-D), rituximab, platelet transfusion, and splenectomy.

Herpes Simplex Virus

The prevalence of oral recurrent HSV infection among HIV-infected individuals increases significantly once the CD4+ cell count drops below 50 per microliter. Within the setting of HIV infection, recurrent herpetic lesions may be widespread, occur in an atypical pattern, and persist for months (Fig. 7.51). Herpes labialis may extend to the facial skin and exhibit extensive lateral spread. Persistence of active HSV infection for more than 1 month in a patient infected with HIV is one accepted definition of AIDS. The clinical presentation and management of recurrent HSV infection in immunocompromised patients are discussed in the section on HSV (see page 235). Evaluation of persistent oral ulcerations in HIV-infected individuals should be performed in order to rule out HSV infection (at times combined with infection by CMV, EBV, or other viruses), deep fungal infection, neoplasia, or other processes.

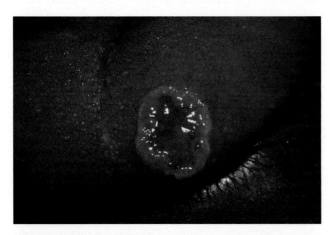

• **Fig. 7.51 HIV-associated Recurrent Herpetic Infection.** Mucosal erosion of the anterior dorsal surface of the tongue on the left side. Note the yellowish circinate border.

Varicella-Zoster Virus

During the ART era, the prevalence of recurrent varicella-zoster virus (VZV) infection (**herpes zoster**) in HIV-infected patients has decreased significantly but still remains greater than that in the general population. Some patients paradoxically develop herpes zoster shortly after initiating ART, as a result of immune reconstitution inflammatory syndrome (see Treatment and Prognosis section). Among patients with HIV infection, herpes zoster is often severe, with increased morbidity and mortality rates. Many of these patients are younger than 40 years, in contrast to immunocompetent patients who typically develop herpes zoster later in life. In patients with well-controlled HIV disease, herpes zoster usually is confined to a single dermatome but persists longer than usual. In full-blown AIDS, dissemination to multiple dermatomes is not unusual. Severe intraoral involvement may lead to bone sequestration and loss of teeth; these sequelae may be delayed a month or more after the initial onset of herpes zoster. Associated pain typically is intense.

For HIV-infected patients with acute, localized herpes zoster, treatment with oral valacyclovir, famciclovir, or acyclovir should be instituted as soon as possible. If there is more extensive disease, then IV acyclovir is indicated. Routine zoster vaccination for HIV-infected patients is not recommended currently; however, according to some experts, zoster vaccination may be considered for those with well-controlled HIV disease and CD4+ cell counts greater than 200 per microliter.

Human Papillomavirus

Among HIV-infected individuals, most human papillomavirus (HPV) lesions arise in the anogenital region, although oral involvement also is possible. Benign oral lesions caused by HPV (commonly referred to as "oral warts") include **oral squamous papilloma** (see page 355), **verruca vulgaris** (see page 357), **condyloma acuminatum** (see page 358), and **multifocal epithelial hyperplasia** (see page 360). The reported prevalence of these benign oral HPV lesions in various HIV-infected cohorts ranges from approximately 0.5% to 7%, and the prevalence is greater among HIV-positive individuals compared to the general population. Unusual HPV types (such as, HPV-7 [associated with butcher's warts], HPV-13, and HPV-32 [associated with multifocal epithelial hyperplasia]) frequently are identified in oral HPV lesions arising in HIV-infected patients.

A few retrospective studies have reported an increase in the frequency of benign oral lesions caused by HPV since the introduction of ART, and one prospective study noted an increase in oral HPV DNA among HIV-infected adults several months after initiation of ART. The reason for this apparent increase is unclear, although some authors have hypothesized that immune reconstitution by ART may lead to an inflammatory response that stimulates HPV activation (i.e., immune reconstitution inflammatory syndrome [see the Treatment and Prognosis section]). Also, some investigators have reported a positive correlation between oral HPV lesions, age, and duration of ART. Based on these findings, researchers have proposed that ART may extend patient survival without full restoration of HPV-specific immunity or that extended survival may allow increased cumulative risk for HPV infection acquisition over time despite restoration of immune function.

The oral lesions usually are multiple and may be located on any mucosal surface, with the labial mucosa, tongue, buccal mucosa, and gingiva most frequently involved. The lesions may exhibit a cluster of white, spikelike projections, pink cauliflower-like growths, or slightly elevated sessile papules (Fig. 7.52).

Histopathologically, the lesions may be sessile or papillary and covered by acanthotic or hyperplastic stratified squamous epithelium (Fig. 7.53). The affected epithelium often demonstrates vacuolization of numerous epithelial cells (i.e., koilocytosis) and occasionally may exhibit mild variation in nuclear size (Fig. 7.54). Immunohistochemistry or DNA in situ hybridization may be used to confirm the presence and type of HPV within histopathologic specimens (Fig. 7.55).

Surgical excision is the most commonly used treatment for benign oral HPV lesions; additional surgical options include cryosurgery, electrocautery, and laser ablation. However, all of these surgical methods are associated with frequent recurrence, and the latter two methods may expose the surgical team and patient to a plume containing

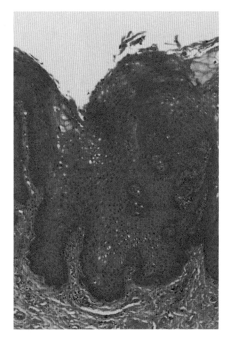

• **Fig. 7.53 HIV-associated Human Papillomavirus (HPV) Infection.** Oral mucosa exhibiting acanthosis and mild nuclear pleomorphism.

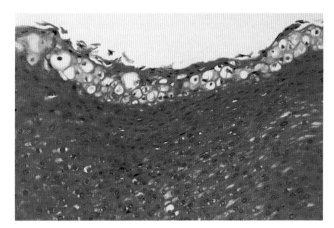

• **Fig. 7.54 HIV-associated Human Papillomavirus (HPV) Infection.** Oral mucosa exhibiting extensive koilocytosis in the superficial spinous cell layer.

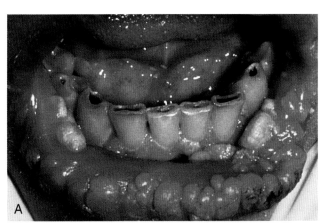

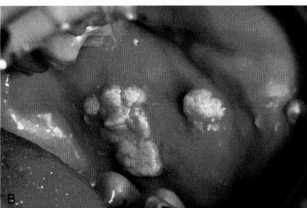

• **Fig. 7.52 HIV-associated Human Papillomavirus (HPV) Infection.** Multiple exophytic and somewhat papillary nodules of the lip, buccal mucosa, and gingiva.

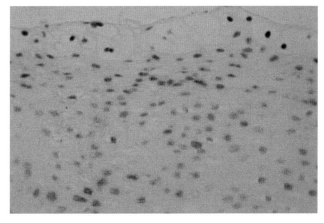

• **Fig. 7.55 HIV-associated Human Papillomavirus (HPV) Infection.** DNA in situ hybridization of oral mucosal biopsy that reveals diffuse cellular positivity for HPV.

infectious HPV. Alternative treatments with anecdotal evidence of efficacy include topical cidofovir, intralesional or systemic interferon-alpha, oral cimetidine, and topical podophyllin.

Dysplasia has been noted within HPV-related lesions in patients with AIDS and mandates close observation for development of squamous cell carcinoma. See the section below (page 263) for a discussion of oral and oropharyngeal squamous cell carcinoma within the setting of HIV infection.

Histoplasmosis

Histoplasmosis, the most common endemic respiratory fungal infection in the United States, is produced by *Histoplasma capsulatum* (see page 212). In healthy patients the infection typically is subclinical and self-limiting, but clinically evident infections often occur in immunocompromised individuals. Although a number of deep fungal infections are possible in patients with AIDS, histoplasmosis is the most common. In areas where the fungus is endemic, disseminated histoplasmosis affects approximately 2%–25% of HIV/AIDS patients and represents the initial AIDS-defining infection in as many as 50%–75% of these patients. Histoplasmosis also has been documented in nonendemic areas, possibly from reactivation of a previous subclinical infection.

The signs and symptoms associated with dissemination are nonspecific and include fever, weight loss, splenomegaly, and pulmonary infiltrates. Oral lesions are not uncommon and usually are caused by bloodborne organisms or spread from pulmonary involvement. On occasion, the initial diagnosis is made from the oral changes, with some patients demonstrating involvement isolated to the oral cavity. Although intrabony infection of the jaws has been reported, the most common oral presentation is a chronic, indurated mucosal ulceration with a raised border (Fig. 7.56). The oral lesions may be single or multiple and may involve any area of the mucosa.

First-line agents for progressive disseminated histoplasmosis in HIV-infected patients include IV liposomal amphotericin B and oral itraconazole. It is also important to ensure that these patients are receiving appropriate ART. Primary prophylaxis with itraconazole should be considered for HIV-infected patients who have CD4+ cell counts less than 150 per microliter and live in endemic areas with an especially high incidence of histoplasmosis.

Aphthous Stomatitis

Lesions that are clinically similar to **aphthous stomatitis** (see page 321) occur with increased frequency in patients infected with HIV. All three forms (minor, major, and herpetiform) are seen; surprisingly, however, almost two-thirds of affected patients have the usually uncommon herpetiform and major variants (Fig. 7.57). As immunosuppression becomes more profound, major aphthae demonstrate an increased prevalence.

Initiation of ART is important for inducing remission and limiting recurrences of aphthae. In addition, treatment with potent topical or intralesional corticosteroids has been successful in many patients. However, not all lesions respond, and recurrences are common. Systemic corticosteroid drugs also may prove beneficial but typically are avoided in order to prevent further immunosuppression. Secondary candidiasis may be a complication of topical or systemic corticosteroid therapy. For lesions nonresponsive to topical corticosteroids, thalidomide may be effective. However, thalidomide must be used cautiously because of its association with increased viral load and potentially serious adverse effects, including peripheral neuropathy, neutropenia, and thrombosis.

Biopsy of any chronic mucosal ulceration clinically diagnosed as an aphthous ulceration should be considered if the lesion is atypical clinically or does not respond to therapy (Fig. 7.58). In such cases, biopsy often reveals another cause, such as HSV, CMV, deep fungal infection, or neoplasia.

Molluscum Contagiosum

Molluscum contagiosum (see page 364) is an infection caused by the molluscum contagiosum virus (MCV), which is a member of the poxvirus family. The lesions classically appear on the skin and genitals as small, waxy, dome-shaped papules with central umbilication. In immunocompetent individuals, the lesions are usually localized and self-limiting. However, in patients with AIDS, the lesions may be

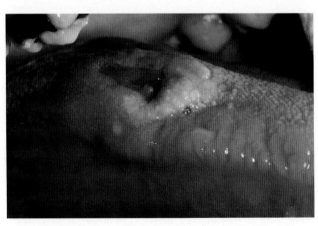

• **Fig. 7.56 HIV-associated Histoplasmosis.** Indurated ulceration with a rolled border on the dorsal surface of the tongue on the right side.

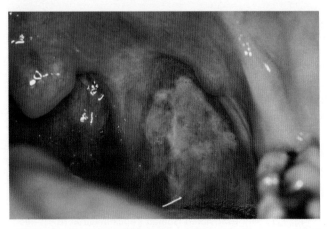

• **Fig. 7.57 HIV-associated Aphthous Ulceration.** Large superficial ulceration of the posterior soft palate.

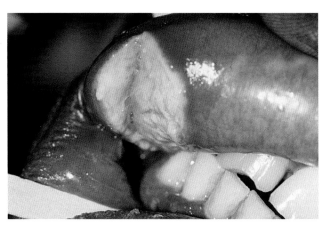

• **Fig. 7.58 HIV-associated Ulceration.** Atypical mucosal ulceration that mandates biopsy and may be attributable to a variety of causes.

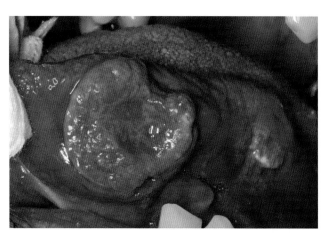

• **Fig. 7.60 HIV-associated Squamous Cell Carcinoma.** Ulcerated mass with raised, indurated borders on the ventrolateral tongue.

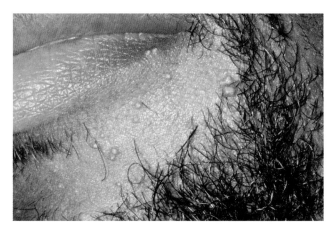

• **Fig. 7.59** HIV-associated Molluscum Contagiosum. Numerous perioral papules.

widespread, persistent, more numerous, and larger in size. Approximately 5% to 18% of HIV-infected patients are affected, and the facial skin commonly is involved (Fig. 7.59). Rare intraoral cases have been described as erythematous, white, or pink papules on either keratinized or nonkeratinized mucosa.

The most effective treatment for molluscum contagiosum in HIV-infected patients is ART. Paradoxical worsening of lesions shortly after initiation of ART due to immune reconstitution inflammatory syndrome (see Treatment and Prognosis section) is possible but typically is transient. For lesions that persist despite ART, there is limited evidence for treatment with topical imiquimod, topical or IV cidofovir, or intralesional interferon-alpha. Because MCV may be present in perilesional skin of HIV-infected patients, conventional local therapy (e.g., curettage, cryosurgery, cautery, or topical podophyllotoxin) often is associated with recurrence.

Oral and Oropharyngeal Squamous Cell Carcinoma

Relative to the general population, HIV-infected individuals are at modestly increased risk for developing squamous cell carcinoma of the oral cavity, pharynx, and other head and

neck sites. In developed countries, this increase in risk has been estimated to be 1.5- to 4-fold for head and neck cancers as a whole, with a similar increase in risk reported for oropharyngeal cancers in particular. A high prevalence of known risk factors (e.g., tobacco use and HPV infection) for oral and oropharyngeal cancers has been noted among various HIV/AIDS cohorts. In addition, an inverse relationship has been demonstrated between oral cavity/pharyngeal cancer risk and CD4+ cell count, and underlying immune dysfunction may account for an increased tendency for persistent oral HPV infection among HIV-infected individuals. Thus, investigators hypothesize that conventional risk factors as well as HIV-related immunosuppression may contribute to elevated cancer risk. However, one large-scale study based in California found no significant difference in the risk for oral cavity/pharyngeal cancer between HIV-positive and HIV-negative individuals after controlling for tobacco use, alcohol abuse, and other potential confounding factors.

Clinical presentation (Fig. 7.60) and treatment options for oral and oropharyngeal squamous cell carcinoma are similar among those with and without HIV infection. Although underlying immunosuppression is associated with aggressive behavior and poor patient outcomes for many cancer types, registry data in the United States for oral cavity/pharyngeal cancer show no significant difference in stage at diagnosis among HIV-infected individuals compared to the general population after adjusting for age, gender, and race. In addition, among individuals with HPV-positive head and neck cancers, one recent multi-center study did not find HIV infection to represent an adverse prognostic factor.

Screening and Diagnosis

The Centers for Disease Control and Prevention recommend that individuals between 13 and 64 years of age receive HIV testing as part of routine health care at least once and individuals with known HIV risk factors be tested at least annually. The standard screening tool is HIV antibody testing by enzyme immunoassay (EIA); in addition, there is a combination immunoassay for detection of both HIV anti-bodies and p24 antigen. False-positive antibody test results are possible, and a positive or indeterminate result should be confirmed by repeat EIA and a more specific assay, such as Western blot or plasma HIV RNA level. Seroconversion generally takes 3–12 weeks following infection; thus, repeat testing may be considered after a negative result, if there is a strong reason to suspect recent HIV infection. HIV home testing kits also are available. These kits allow the user to send a sample into a laboratory for antibody testing; however, pos-itive results still need to be confirmed by standard assays. For patients suspected of having acute retroviral syndrome, p24 antigen capture assay may be performed to detect the virus before the development of antibodies. Tests used to measure plasma HIV RNA levels include RT-PCR, branched DNA assay, transcription-mediated amplification, and nucleic acid sequence–based amplification. Although these tests may be performed for diagnosis, they more commonly are used to monitor response to therapy among patients already diagnosed.

AIDS is diagnosed based on the presence of any of the following criteria:
1. CD4+ T-lymphocyte count:
   - less than 200 per microliter for individuals 6 years or older
   - less than 500 per microliter for individuals 1–5 years of age
   - less than 750 per microliter for individuals less than 1 year old
2. Diagnosis of an AIDS-defining opportunistic illness (Box 7.1)

Treatment and Prognosis

Current guidelines recommend initiation of ART as soon as possible after HIV diagnosis regardless of CD4+ cell count—an approach known as "test and treat." There is strong evi-dence that early treatment reduces the risk for serious AIDS-related events (including AIDS-related cancer and opportu-nistic infection) as well as serious non-AIDS-related events (including non-AIDS-related cancer and major cardiovascu-lar, renal, and liver disease). With appropriate ART, a person newly diagnosed with HIV infection in North America is expected to have a nearly normal life expectancy. Further-more, early treatment is important to reduce the risk for viral transmission.

A wide variety of antiretroviral agents is available and con-tinues to expand. These agents are administered in combina-tion in order to reduce the emergence of viral resistance. Although numerous combinations are possible, ART often consists of two nucleoside reverse transcriptase inhibitors combined with a nonnucleoside reverse transcriptase inhib-itor, boosted protease inhibitor, or integrase inhibitor (2 NRTI + NNRTI/PI/II). With such treatment, viremia typ-ically declines to undetectable levels, and there is clinically significant immune reconstitution. Although ART works well for most patients, downsides of such therapy include

• BOX 7.1   AIDS-Defining Opportunistic Illnesses

1. Bacterial infections, multiple or recurrent*
2. Candidiasis of bronchi, trachea, or lungs
3. Candidiasis of esophagus
4. Cervical cancer, invasive[†]
5. Coccidioidomycosis, disseminated or extrapulmonary
6. Cryptococcosis, extrapulmonary
7. Cryptosporidiosis, chronic intestinal (more than 1 month duration)
8. CMV disease (other than liver, spleen, or nodes), onset at age of more than 1 month
9. CMV retinitis (with loss of vision)
10. Encephalopathy attributed to HIV
11. Herpes simplex: Chronic ulcer or ulcers (more than 1 month duration) or bronchitis, pneumonitis, or esophagitis (onset at age of more than 1 month)
12. Histoplasmosis, disseminated or extrapulmonary
13. Isosporiasis, chronic intestinal (more than 1 month duration)
14. Kaposi sarcoma (KS)
15. Lymphoma, Burkitt (or equivalent term)
16. Lymphoma, immunoblastic (or equivalent term)
17. Lymphoma, primary, of brain
18. *Mycobacterium avium* complex or *Mycobacterium kansasii*, disseminated or extrapulmonary
19. *Mycobacterium tuberculosis* of any site, pulmonary,[†] disseminated, or extrapulmonary
20. *Mycobacterium*, other species or unidentified species, disseminated, or extrapulmonary
21. *Pneumocystis jiroveci* pneumonia
22. Pneumonia, recurrent
23. Progressive multifocal leukoencephalopathy
24. *Salmonella* septicemia, recurrent
25. Toxoplasmosis of brain, onset at age of more than 1 month
26. Wasting syndrome attributed to HIV

*Only among children less than 6 years old.
[†]Only among adults, adolescents, and children aged 6 years or older.
AIDS, acquired immune deficiency syndrome; *CMV*, cytomegalovirus; *HIV*, human immunodeficiency virus.
Adapted from Centers for Disease Control and Prevention: Appendix stage-3-defining opportunistic illnesses in HIV infection, *MMWR Recomm Rep* 63(RR-03): 1–10, 2014.

cost, toxicity, adverse reactions, and difficulty with compli-ance. Some patients who receive ART during advanced stages of disease develop a paradoxical worsening of their condition—termed **immune reconstitution inflammatory syndrome**—despite decreasing viral load and increasing CD4+ cell counts. The underlying mechanism may be related to a hyper-inflammatory response to pathogens and pathogenic antigens present at the time of rapid immune reconstitution. ART is unable to cure HIV infection, appar-ently because of persistence of viral reservoirs in the periph-eral blood and lymphoid tissues. Therefore, lifelong treatment is necessary—discontinuation typically results in rebound of the virus within weeks.

Some health professionals have been concerned about the risk of occupational transmission of HIV. However, the risk appears to be very low, with only a paucity of confirmed cases of occupational transmission in the United States since the late 1990s. In the event of occupational exposure, postexposure prophylaxis with antiretroviral medications should be initiated as soon as possible (preferably within hours of the event) and continued for 4 weeks. Basic postexposure prophylaxis consists of a regimen containing three or more antiretroviral drugs. Because of the complexity of choosing and administering HIV postexposure prophylaxis, involvement of an infectious disease specialist or other physician experienced in ART is recommended.

◆ CORONAVIRUS DISEASE 2019

The emergence of the coronavirus disease 2019 (COVID-19) pandemic has created a massive global health challenge. As of this writing, hundreds of millions of individuals have been infected worldwide, with a rising death toll and widespread socioeconomic devastation. Our knowledge regarding this disease has evolved rapidly with intensive research efforts and the emergence of new variants of the virus; the discussion below represents a brief overview based on current knowledge, although the reader is encouraged to access additional resources for the most up-to-date information.

COVID-19 is caused by severe acute respiratory syndrome coronavirus 2 (SARS-CoV-2), which is a member of the family *Coronaviridae* and the genus *Betacoronavirus*. The virus is transmitted mainly by inhalation of contaminated respiratory droplets or aerosols; deposition of respiratory droplets or particles onto oral, nasal, or ocular mucous membranes; or touching mucous membranes with hands that have come into contact with respiratory fluids or contaminated surfaces. The incubation period ranges from about 2 to 14 days. The virus enters host cells by interaction between its spike protein and the host receptor, angiotensin-converting enzyme 2 (ACE2). Tissue types that highly express ACE2 include the lungs (particularly type II alveolar cells), myocardium, intestinal lining, renal proximal tubules, and tongue epithelium. Although the respiratory tract is the primary site of infection, various other tissue types may exhibit disease manifestations as well.

Clinical Features

The clinical presentation of individuals infected with SARS-CoV-2 is variable, ranging from no or minimal symptoms to severe, life-threatening illness. Clinical findings may include the following: fever, chills, cough, dyspnea, hypoxia, pneumonia, fatigue, myalgia, headache, sore throat, runny nose or nasal congestion, nausea, vomiting, and diarrhea. Critically ill patients may develop respiratory failure/acute respiratory distress syndrome, cardiac arrhythmia, acute cardiac injury, acute kidney injury, coagulopathy, septic shock, and multiple organ failure.

Interestingly, various skin eruptions also have been described in patients with COVID-19, although it is not entirely clear whether such lesions represent direct effects of the virus and/or adverse drug reactions. Reported skin findings include maculopapular rash, urticaria, vesicular eruption, petechiae, purpura, livedoid (reticular red-blue)/necrotic lesions, erythema multiforme-like lesions, and chilblain-like lesions (red to violaceous macules, plaques, and nodules at the distal aspects of toes and fingers with a pattern mimicking injury from cold temperatures). Such findings have been noted in patients with severe COVID-19 as well as those with no to mild symptoms.

A rare manifestation of COVID-19 is multisystem inflammatory disease in children (MIS-C). This condition bears some resemblance to Kawasaki disease (an acute-onset systemic vasculitis and febrile illness of unknown etiology). MIS-C typically develops 2–6 weeks after a SARS-CoV-2 infection that may be mild or asymptomatic. Characteristic features include age under 21 years; fever of 38°C or higher for at least 24 hours; laboratory evidence of inflammation (e.g., C-reactive protein, erythrocyte sedimentation rate, D-dimer); severe illness requiring hospitalization; and involvement of 2 or more organ systems. Reported oral manifestations of MIS-C include mucosal erythema, strawberry tongue (erythematous tongue with enlarged papillae), and cracked or swollen lips.

Among oral manifestations of COVID-19, taste disturbance is the most salient finding, with an overall prevalence of approximately 38% among reported patients according to a comprehensive systematic review of the literature. Hypogeusia and dysgeusia have been described more frequently than ageusia. In some cases, gustatory dysfunction is accompanied by olfactory dysfunction. Such taste and smell abnormalities exhibit a female predilection and may develop early in the course of mild to moderate disease—at times even in the absence of other signs or symptoms. Therefore, screening for new-onset smell and/or taste dysfunction may aid in the identification of patients with COVID-19. The underlying mechanism for COVID-19-related taste disturbance is uncertain, although it has been hypothesized that expression of ACE2 and transmembrane protease serine 2 (TMPRSS2) by taste bud cells facilitates viral entry and disruption of gustatory function. Furthermore, expression of these viral entry molecules by acinar and ductal epithelial cells within salivary glands has been proposed to explain reports of xerostomia, which has been noted in approximately 40% of patients and could contribute to taste disturbance as well.

Information regarding other potential oral manifestations of COVID-19 is limited. Anecdotal reports or series of patients with confirmed SARS-CoV-2 infection have noted various oral conditions, such as ulceration (including aphthous-like, herpes-like, necrotic, or nonspecific ulceration); tongue findings (including lingual papillitis or depapillated tongue); hemorrhagic lesions (such as petechiae, ecchymosis, spontaneous hemorrhage, and angina bullosa); vesiculobullous eruption; desquamative gingivitis; halitosis; orofacial pain; salivary gland abnormalities (including sialadenitis or ectasia); and erythematous plaques or macules (Fig. 7.61). However, it is uncertain whether such findings represent actual manifestations of COVID-19 versus secondary or incidental phenomena. Oral coinfections (e.g.,

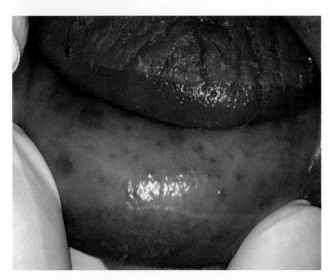

• **Fig. 7.61 Coronavirus Disease 2019.** Erythematous macules on the lower labial mucosa. (Courtesy of Dr. Bea Venturi.)

candidiasis/angular cheilitis, herpes simplex virus infection, mucormycosis) also have been reported in COVID-19 patients. Further studies are needed to determine the significance of such observations.

Histopathologic Features

Information regarding microscopic findings in oral mucosal lesions sampled from COVID-19 patients is limited. However, some investigators have noted paranuclear vacuolization in keratinocytes within the spinous cell layer of the surface epithelium, which may correlate with SARS-CoV-2 spike protein expression demonstrated by immunhistochemistry. Within the lamina propria, there may be inflammation (more often lymphohistiocytic than neutrophilic), thrombosis of small arteries or capillaries, and hemorrhage. Fibrinoid necrosis may be evident in patients with extensive ecchymosis.

Diagnosis

Current SARS-CoV-2 infection can be detected by antigen or nucleic acid amplification tests. Antigen tests are relatively easy to perform and typically can be used for at-home or point-of-care applications with rapid results. However, antigen tests have lower sensitivity than laboratory-based nuclei acid antigen tests (such as RT-PCR). Depending on test type, samples may be obtained from the nasopharynx, nasal cavity, oropharynx, saliva, or sputum.

Other laboratory test findings in patients with COVID-19 may include lymphopenia, prolonged prothrombin time, elevated lactate dehydrogenase, hypoalbuminemia, and elevated C-reactive protein. In patients with pneumonia, computed tomography (CT) typically exhibits bilateral ground-glass opacities of the lungs. In addition, this pattern has been documented in some asymptomatic patients with SARS-CoV-2 infection.

Treatment and Prognosis

Individuals with mild COVID-19 can be managed by home isolation and supportive care (i.e., acetaminophen, fluids, antibiotics for secondary infection, and supplemental oxygen). Drugs for nonhospitalized patients with mild to moderate disease and high risk of progression to serious disease represent an active area of investigation, and recommendations for various agents (e.g., oral antivirals, anti-SARS-CoV-2 monoclonal antibodies) have changed with the emergence of new variants of the virus. Patients with severe or critical disease require hospitalization for management of complications. Treatment may include antiviral agents (e.g., remdesivir), dexamethasone, IL-6 blockers, Janus kinase (JAK) inhibitors, respiratory support, and anticoagulants. MIS-C typically is treated by intravenous immunoglobulin with or without corticosteroids. Even with optimal care, fatality is >10% among hospitalized COVID-19 patients. Risk factors for severe disease and death include male gender, age over 60 years, hypertension, cardiovascular disease, diabetes, and obesity.

Several vaccines have been developed. Additional practices for disease prevention and mitigation include testing, isolation, contact tracing, and quarantine procedures; wearing face coverings; environmental disinfection and ventilation; frequent hand hygiene; and physical distancing from others.

Bibliography

Human Herpesviruses

Ballyram R, Wood NH, Khammissa RAG, et al.: Oral diseases associated with human herpes viruses: aetiology, clinical features, diagnosis and management, *SADJ* 6:253–259, 2016.

Binshabaib M, ALHarthi SS, Salehpoor D, et al.: Contribution of herpesviruses in the progression of periodontal and peri-implant diseases in systemically healthy individuals, *Rev Med Virol* 28: e1996, 2018.

Ferreira DC, Rôças IN, Paiva SS, et al.: Viral-bacterial associations in acute apical abscesses, *Oral Surg Oral Med Oral Pathol Oral Radiol Endod* 112:264–271, 2011.

Hernádi K, Csoma E, Adám B, et al.: Association of human herpesvirus 6 subtypes with symptomatic apical periodontitis, *Oral Surg Oral Med Oral Pathol Oral Radiol Endod* 112:401–406, 2011.

Popovic J, Gasic J, Zivkovic S, et al.: Prevalence of human cytomegalovirus and Epstein-Barr virus in chronic periapical lesions, *Intervirology* 58:271–277, 2015.

Slots J: Periodontal herpesviruses: prevalence, pathogenicity, systemic risk, *Periodontol* 2000(69):28–45, 2015.

Slots J, Slots H: Periodontal herpesvirus morbidity and treatment, *Periodontol* 2000(79):210–220, 2019.

Zhu C, Li F, Wong MCM, et al.: Association between herpesviruses and chronic periodontitis: a meta-analysis based on case-control studies, *PLoS One* 10:e0144319, 2015.

Herpes Simplex Virus

Ahluwalia J, Han A, Kusari A, et al.: Recurrent herpes labialis in the pediatric population: prevalence, therapeutic studies, and associated complications, *Pediatr Dermatol* 36:808–814, 2019.

Al-Maweri SA, Kalakonda B, AlAizari NA, et al.: Efficacy of low-level laser therapy in management of recurrent herpes labialis: a systematic review, *Lasers Med Sci* 33:1423–1430, 2018.

Arduino PG, Porter SR: Herpes simplex virus type 1 infection: overview on relevant clinico-pathological features, *J Oral Pathol Med* 37:107–121, 2008.

Ayoub HH, Chemaitelly H, Abu-Raddad LJ: Characterizing the transitioning epidemiology of herpes simplex virus type 1 in the USA: model-based predictions, *BMC Med* 17:57, 2019.

Belshe RB, Leone PA, Bernstein DI, et al.: Efficacy results of a trial of a herpes simplex vaccine, *N Engl J Med* 366:34–43, 2012.

Cernik C, Gallina K, Brodell RT: The treatment of herpes simplex infections: an evidence-based review, *Arch Intern Med* 168:1137–1144, 2008.

Chemaitelly H, Nagelkerke N, Omori R, et al.: Characterizing herpes simplex virus type 1 and type 2 seroprevalence declines and epidemiological association in the United States, *PLoS One* 14:e0214151, 2019.

Chen F, Xu H, Liu J, et al.: Efficacy and safety of nucleoside antiviral drugs for treatment of recurrent herpes labialis: a systematic review and meta-analysis, *J Oral Pathol Med* 46:561–568, 2017.

Chi CC, Wang SH, Delamere FM, et al.: Interventions for prevention of herpes simplex labialis (cold sores on the lips), *Cochrane Database Syst Rev* 2015:CD010095, 2015.

Crimi S, Fiorillo L, Bianchi A, et al.: Herpes virus, oral clinical signs and QoL: systematic review of recent data, *Viruses* 11:463, 2019.

Cunningham A, Griffiths P, Leone P, et al.: Current management and recommendations for access to antiviral therapy of herpes labialis, *J Clin Virol* 53:6–11, 2012.

El Hayderi L, Rübben A, Nikkels AF: The alpha-herpesviridae in dermatology: varicella zoster virus, *Hautarzt* 68(Suppl 1):6–10, 2017.

Jain M: Assessment of correlation of herpes simplex virus-1 with oral cancer and precancer—a comparative study, *J Clin Diagn Res* 10:ZC14–ZC17, 2016.

Kolokotronis A, Doumas S: Herpes simplex virus infection, with particular reference to the progression and complications of primary herpetic gingivostomatitis, *Clin Microbiol Infect* 12:202–211, 2006.

Looker KJ, Magaret AS, May MT, et al.: Global and regional estimates of prevalent and incident herpes simplex virus type 1 infections in 2012, *PLoS One* 10:e0140765, 2015.

Mainville GN, Marsh WL, Allen CM: Oral ulceration associated with concurrent herpes simplex virus, cytomegalovirus, and Epstein-Barr virus infection in an immunocompromised patient, *Oral Surg Oral Med Oral Pathol Oral Radiol* 119:e306–e314, 2015.

McQuillan G, Kruszon-Moran D, Flass EW, et al.: Prevalence of herpes simplex virus type 1 and type 2 in persons aged 14-49: United States, 2015–2016, *NCHS Data Brief* 304:1–8, 2018.

Miller CS: *AAOM clinical practice statement. Subject: dental care for the patient with an oral herpetic lesion*, https://www.aaom.com/index.php?option=com_content&view=article&id=161:clinical-practice-statement--dental-care-for-the-patient-with-an-oral-herpetic-lesion&catid=24:clinical-practice-statement. (Accessed 10 July 2020).

Petti S, Lodi G: The controversial natural history of oral herpes simplex virus type 1 infection, *Oral Dis* 25:1850–1865, 2019.

Rahini H, Mara T, Costella J, et al.: Effectiveness of antiviral agents for the prevention of recurrent herpes labialis: a systematic review and meta-analysis, *Oral Surg Oral Med Oral Pathol Oral Radiol* 113:618–627, 2012.

Starr JR, Daling JR, Fitzgibbons ED, et al.: Serologic evidence of herpes simplex virus 1 infection and oropharyngeal cancer risk, *Cancer Res* 61:8459–8464, 2001.

Woo SB, Challacombe SJ: Management of recurrent oral herpes simplex infections, *Oral Surg Oral Med Oral Pathol Oral Radiol Endod* 103(Suppl 1):S12.e1–S12.e18, 2007.

Infectious Mononucleosis

American Academy of Pediatrics: Epstein-Barr virus infections, In Kimberlin DW, Brady MT, Jackson MA, et al., editors: *Red book 2021–2024 report of the committee on infectious diseases*, ed 32, Itasca, 2021, American Academy of Pediatrics, pp 318–321.

Courant P, Sobkov T: Oral manifestations of infectious mononucleosis, *J Periodontol* 40:279–283, 1979.

De Paor M, O'Brien K, Fahey T, et al.: Antiviral agents for infectious mononucleosis (glandular fever), *Cochrane Database Syst Rev* 12:CD011487, 2016.

Dunmire SK, Verghese PS, Balfour HH Jr: Primary Epstein-Barr virus infection, *J Clin Virol* 102:84–92, 2018.

Fraser-Moodie W: Oral lesions in infectious mononucleosis, *Oral Surg Oral Med Oral Pathol* 12:685–691, 1959.

Guidry JT, Birdwell CE, Scott RS: Epstein-Barr virus in the pathogenesis of oral cancers, *Oral Dis* 24:497–508, 2018.

Okano M, Gross TG: Acute or chronic life-threatening diseases associated with Epstein-Barr virus infection, *Am J Med Sci* 343:483–489, 2012.

Rasa S, Nora-Krukle Z, Henning N, et al.: Chronic viral infections in myalgic encephalomyelitis/chronic fatigue syndrome (ME/CFS), *J Transl Med* 16:268, 2018.

Roberge RJ, Simon M, Russell M, et al.: Lingual tonsillitis: an unusual presentation of mononucleosis, *Am J Emerg Med* 19:173–175, 2001.

Slots J, Saygun I, Sabeti M, et al.: Epstein-Barr virus in oral diseases, *J Periodontol Res* 41:235–244, 2006.

Cytomegalovirus

American Academy of Pediatrics: Cytomegalovirus infection, In Kimberlin DW, Brady MT, Jackson MA, et al., editors: *Red book 2021–2024 report of the committee on infectious diseases*, ed 32, Itasca, 2021, American Academy of Pediatrics, pp 294–300.

Bate SL, Dollard SC, Cannon MJ: Cytomegalovirus seroprevalence in the United States: the National Health and Nutrition Examination Surveys, 1988–2004, *Clin Infect Dis* 50:1439–1447, 2010.

Epstein JB, Sherlock CH, Wolber RA: Oral manifestations of cytomegalovirus infection, *Oral Surg Oral Med Oral Pathol* 75:443–451, 1993.

Flaitz CM, Nichols CM, Hicks MJ: Herpesviridae-associated persistent mucocutaneous ulcers in acquired immunodeficiency syndrome: a clinicopathologic study, *Oral Surg Oral Med Oral Pathol Oral Radiol Endod* 81:433–441, 1996.

Jones AC, Freedman PD, Phelan JA, et al.: Cytomegalovirus infections of the oral cavity: a report of six cases and review of the literature, *Oral Surg Oral Med Oral Pathol* 75:76–85, 1993.

Lanzieri TM, Kruszon-Moran D, Amin MM, et al.: Seroprevalence of cytomegalovirus among children 1 to 5 years of age in the United States from the National Health and Nutrition Examination Survey of 2011 to 2012, *Clin Vaccine Immunol* 22:245–247, 2015.

Mainville GN, Marsh WL, Allen CM: Oral ulceration associated with concurrent herpes simplex virus, cytomegalovirus, and Epstein-Barr virus infection in an immunocompromised patient, *Oral Surg Oral Med Oral Pathol Oral Radiol* 119:e306–e314, 2015.

Regezi JA, Eversole LR, Barker BF, et al.: Herpes simplex and cytomegalovirus coinfected oral ulcers in HIV-infected patients, *Oral Surg Oral Med Oral Pathol Oral Radiol Endod* 81:55–62, 1996.

Schubert MM, Epstein JB, Lloid ME: Oral infections due to cytomegalovirus in immunocompromised patients, *J Oral Pathol Med* 22:268–273, 1993.

Stagno S, Pass RF, Thomas JP, et al.: Defects of tooth structure in congenital cytomegalovirus infection, *Pediatrics* 69:646–648, 1982.

Zuhair M, Smit GSA, Wallis G, et al.: Estimation of the worldwide seroprevalence of cytomegalovirus: a systematic review and meta-analysis, *Rev Med Virol* 29:e2034, 2019.

Enteroviruses

Abedi GR, Watson JT, Nix WA, et al.: Enterovirus and parechovirus surveillance—United States, 2014–2016, *MMWR Morb Mortal Wkly Rep* 67:515–518, 2018.

American Academy of Pediatrics: Enterovirus (nonpoliovirus), In Kimberlin DW, Brady MT, Jackson MA, et al., editors: *Red book 2021–2024 report of the committee on infectious diseases*, ed 32, Itasca, 2021, American Academy of Pediatrics, pp 315–317.

Centers for Disease Control and Prevention: Notes from the field: severe hand, foot, and mouth disease associated with coxsackievirus A6—Alabama, Connecticut, California, and Nevada, November 2011–February 2012, *MMWR Morb Mortal Wkly Rep* 61:213–214, 2012.

de Crom SC, Rossen JW, van Furth AM, et al.: Enterovirus and parechovirus infection in children: a brief overview, *Eur J Pediatr* 175:1023–1029, 2016.

Esposito S, Principi N: Hand, foot and mouth disease: current knowledge on clinical manifestations, epidemiology, aetiology and prevention, *Eur J Clin Microbiol Infect Dis* 37:391–398, 2018.

Khetsuriani N, Lamonte-Fowlkes A, Oberst S, et al.: Enterovirus surveillance—United States, 1970–2005, *MMWR Surveill Summ* 55:1–20, 2006.

Kimmis BD, Downing C, Tyring S: Hand-foot-and-mouth disease caused by coxsackievirus A6 on the rise, *Cutis* 102:353–356, 2018.

Murphy OC, Messacar K, Benson L, et al.: Acute flaccid myelitis: cause, diagnosis, and management, *Lancet* 397:334–346, 2021.

Ooi MH, Wong SC, Lewthwaite P, et al.: Clinical features, diagnosis, and management of enterovirus 71, *Lancet Neurol* 9:1097–1105, 2010.

Saguil A, Kane SF, Lauters R, et al.: Hand-foot-and-mouth disease: rapid evidence review, *Am Fam Physician* 100:408–414, 2019.

Steigman AJ, Lipton MM, Braspennickx H: Acute lymphonodular pharyngitis: a newly described condition due to Coxsackie A virus, *J Pediatr* 61:331–336, 1962.

Ventarola D, Bordone L, Silverberg N: Update on hand-foot-and-mouth disease, *Clin Dermatol* 33:340–346, 2015.

Varicella-Zoster Virus

American Academy of Pediatrics: Varicella zoster infections, In Kimberlin DW, Brady MT, Jackson MA, et al., editors: *Red Book 2021–2024 Report of the Committee on Infectious Diseases*, ed 32, Itasca, 2021, American Academy of Pediatrics, pp 831–842.

Barrett AP, Katelaris CH, Morris JGL, et al.: Zoster sine herpete of the trigeminal nerve, *Oral Surg Oral Med Oral Pathol* 75:173–175, 1993.

Bulilete O, Leiva A, Rullán M, et al.: Efficacy of gabapentin for the prevention of postherpetic neuralgia in patients with acute herpes zoster: a double blind, randomized controlled trial, *PLoS One* 14:e0217335, 2019.

Centers for Disease Control and Prevention: Updated recommendations for use of VariZIG—United States, 2013, *MMWR Morb Mortal Wkly Rep* 62:574–576, 2013.

Chen N, Li Q, Yang J, et al.: Antiviral treatment for preventing postherpetic neuralgia, *Cochrane Database Syst Rev* 2014:CD006866, 2014.

Dooling KL, Guo A, Patel M, et al.: Recommendations of the advisory committee on immunization practices for use of herpes zoster vaccines, *MMWR Morb Mortal Wkly Rep* 67:103–108, 2018.

Furuta Y, Ohtani F, Aizawa H, et al.: Varicella-zoster virus reactivation is an important cause of acute peripheral facial paralysis in children, *Pediatr Infect Dis* 24:97–101, 2005.

Gagliardi AM, Andriolo BN, Torloni MR, et al.: Vaccines for preventing herpes zoster in older adults, *Cochrane Database Syst Rev* 2019:CD008858, 2019.

Kolokotronis A, Louloudiadis K, Fotiou G, et al.: Oral manifestations of infections due to varicella zoster virus in otherwise healthy children, *J Clin Pediatr Dent* 25:107–112, 2001.

Jain MK, Manjunath KS, Jagadish SN: Unusual oral complications of zoster infection: report of a case and review of the literature, *Oral Surg Oral Med Oral Pathol Oral Radiol Endod* 110:e37–e41, 2010.

Lopez A, Leung J, Schmid S, et al.: Chapter 17: Varicella, In Roush SW, Baldy LM, Kirkconnell Hall MA, editors: *Manual for the surveillance of vaccine-preventable diseases, Atlanta, reviewed May 15*, 2018, Centers for Disease Control and Prevention. https://www.cdc.gov/vaccines/pubs/surv-manual/chpt17-varicella.pdf. (Accessed 11 July 2020).

Lopez AS, Zhang S, Marin M: Epidemiology of varicella during the 2-dose varicella vaccination program—United States, 2005–2014, *MMWR Morb Mortal Wkly Rep* 65:902–905, 2016.

Macartney K, Heywood A, McIntyre P: Vaccines for post-exposure prophylaxis against varicella (chickenpox) in children and adults, *Cochrane Database Syst Rev* 2014:CD001833, 2014.

Mauprivez C, Comte C, Labrousse M, et al.: Acute facial nerve palsy with ipsilateral soft palate ulcers, *J Oral Maxillofac Surg* 75:1906–1914, 2017.

Meer S, Coleman H, Altini M, et al.: Mandibular osteomyelitis and tooth exfoliation following zoster-CMV co-infection, *Oral Surg Oral Med Oral Pathol Oral Radiol Endod* 101:70–75, 2006.

Mustafa MB, Arduino PG, Porter SR: Varicella zoster virus: review of its management, *J Oral Pathol Med* 38:673–688, 2009.

Patel K, Schirru E, Niazi S, et al.: Multiple apical radiolucencies and external cervical resorption associated with varicella zoster virus: a case report, *J Endod* 42:978–983, 2016.

Talebzadeh B, Rahimi S, Abdollahi AA, et al.: Varicella zoster virus and internal root resorption: a case report, *J Endod* 41:1375–1381, 2015.

Measles

Dabbagh A, Laws RL, Steulet C, et al.: Progress toward regional measles elimination—worldwide, 2000–2017, *MMWR Morb Mortal Wkly Rep* 67:1323–1329, 2018.

Gastanaduy PA, Redd SB, Clemmons NS, et al.: Chapter 7: Measles, In Roush SW, Baldy LM, Kirkconnell Hall MA, editors: Manual for the surveillance of vaccine-preventable diseases, Atlanta, reviewed May 15. 2018, Centers for Disease Control and Prevention. https://www.cdc.gov/vaccines/pubs/surv-manual/chpt07-measles.html. (Accessed 13 July 2020).

Gupta K, Chen M, Rocker J: Measles: taking steps forward to prevent going backwards, *Curr Opin Pediatr* 32:436–445, 2020.

Koplik H: The diagnosis of the invasion of measles from a study of the exanthema as it appears on the buccal mucosa membrane, *Arch Pediatr* 13:918–922, 1896.

Moss WJ: Measles, *Lancet* 390:2490–2502, 2017.

Paules CI, Marston HD, Fauci AS: Measles in 2019—going backward, *N Engl J Med* 380:2185–2187, 2019.

Warthin AS: Occurrence of numerous large giant cells in the tonsils and pharyngeal mucosa in the prodromal stage of measles, *Arch Pathol* 11:864–874, 1931.

World Health Organization: Measles vaccines: WHO position paper—April 2017, *Wkly Epidemiol Rec* 92:205–227, 2017.

Rubella

Centers for Disease Control and Prevention: Elimination of rubella and congenital rubella syndrome—United States, 1969–2004, *MMWR Morb Mortal Wkly Rep* 54:279–282, 2005.

Forchheimer F: German measles (Rubella), In Stedman TL, editor: *Twentieth century practice, an international encyclopedia of modern medical science by leading authorities of Europe and America*, New York, 1898, W Wood, pp 175–188.

Grant GB, Desai S, Dumolard L, et al.: Progress toward rubella and congenital rubella syndrome control and elimination—worldwide, 2000–2018, *MMWR Morb Mortal Wkly Rep* 68:855–859, 2019.

Lambert N, Strebel P, Orenstein W, et al.: Rubella, *Lancet* 385:2297–2307, 2015.

Lanzieri T, Redd S, Abernathy E, et al.: Chapter 14: Rubella, In Roush SW, Baldy LM, Kirkconnell Hall MA, editors: Manual for the surveillance of vaccine-preventable diseases, Atlanta, reviewed May 15. 2018, Centers for Disease Control and Prevention. https://www.cdc.gov/vaccines/pubs/surv-manual/chpt14-rubella.html. (Accessed 13 July 2020).

Yazigi A, De Pecoulas AE, Vauloup-Fellous C, et al.: Fetal and neonatal abnormalities due to congenital rubella syndrome: a review of literature, *J Matern Fetal Neonatal Med* 30:274–278, 2017.

Young MK, Cripps AW, Nimmo GR, et al.: Post-exposure passive immunisation for preventing rubella and congenital rubella syndrome, *Cochrane Database Syst Rev*, 2015 (CD010586).

Mumps

Clemmons N, Hickman C, Lee A, et al.: Chapter 9: Mumps, In Roush SW, Baldy LM, Kirkconnell Hall MA, editors: Manual for the surveillance of vaccine-preventable diseases, Atlanta, reviewed May 15. 2018, Centers for Disease Control and Prevention. https://www.cdc.gov/vaccines/pubs/surv-manual/chpt09-mumps.html. (Accessed 11 July 2020).

Hviid A, Rubin S, Mühlemann K: Mumps, *Lancet* 371:932–944, 2008.

Lau RK, Turner MD: Viral mumps: increasing occurrences in the vaccinated population, *Oral Surg Oral Med Oral Pathol Oral Radiol* 128:386–392, 2019.

Linder TE, Brestel R, Schlegel C: Mumps virus infection: case report of an unusual head and neck manifestation, *Am J Otolaryngol* 17:420–423, 1996.

Marin M, Marlow M, Moore KL, et al.: Recommendation of the advisory committee on immunization practices for use of a third dose of mumps virus-containing vaccine in persons at increased risk for mumps during an outbreak, *MMWR Morb Mortal Wkly Rep* 67:33–38, 2018.

Marshall HS, Plotkin S: The changing epidemiology of mumps in a high vaccination era, *Lancet Infect Dis* 19:118–119, 2019.

Human Immunodeficiency Virus and Acquired Immunodeficiency Syndrome

Agaimy A, Mueller SK, Harrer T, et al.: Head and neck Kaposi sarcoma: clinicopathological analysis of 11 cases, *Head Neck Pathol* 12:511–516, 2018.

Almazyad A, Alabdulaaly L, Noonan V, et al.: Oral hairy leukoplakia: a series of 45 cases in immunocompetent patients, *Oral Surg Oral Med Oral Pathol Oral Radiol* 132:210–216, 2021.

Anaya-Saavedra G, Flores-Moreno B, García-Carrancá A, et al.: HPV oral lesions in HIV-infected patients: the impact of long-term HAART, *J Oral Pathol Med* 42:443–449, 2013.

Baccaglini L, Atkinson JC, Patton LL, et al.: Management of oral lesions in HIV-positive patients, *Oral Surg Oral Med Oral Pathol Oral Radiol* 103(Suppl 1):S50.e1–S50.e23, 2007.

Beachler DC, D'Souza G: Oral human papillomavirus infection and head and neck cancers in HIV-infected individuals, *Curr Opin Oncol* 25:503–510, 2013.

Blank LJ, Polydefkis MJ, Moore RD, et al.: Herpes zoster among persons living with HIV in the current antiretroviral therapy era, *J Acquir Immune Defic Syndr* 61:203–207, 2012.

Brooks JK, Jones JL, Price JB: Possible association of sialolithiasis with HIV infection and highly active antiretroviral therapy: a case report, *Spec Care Dentist* 40:298–302, 2020.

Butt FMA, Chindia ML, Rana F: Oral squamous cell carcinoma in human immunodeficiency virus positive patients: clinicopathological audit, *J Laryngol Otol* 126:276–278, 2012.

Cameron JE, Hagensee ME: Oral HPV complications in HIV-infected patients, *Current HIV/AIDS Reports* 5:126–131, 2008.

Centers for Disease Control and Prevention: Estimated HIV incidence and prevalence in the United States, 2014–2018, *HIV Surveillance Suppl Rep* 25(1), 2020. (PDF online): http://www.cdc.gov/hiv/library/reports/hiv-surveillance.html. (Accessed 14 July 2020.)

Centers for Disease Control and Prevention: *HIV surveillance report, 2019*, vol. 32, 2021. May 2021. (PDF online): https://www.cdc.gov/hiv/library/reports/vol-32/index.html. (Accessed 4 February 2022.)

Centers for Disease Control and Prevention: Revised surveillance case definition for HIV infection—United States, *MMWR Recomm Rep* 63:1–10, 2014.

Cesarman E, Damania B, Krown SE, et al.: Kaposi sarcoma, *Nat Rev Dis Prim* 5:9, 2019.

Chandran R, Feller L, Lemmer J, et al.: HIV-associated oral mucosal melanin hyperpigmentation: a clinical study in a South African population sample, *AIDS Res Treat* 2016:8389214, 2016.

Chen M, Yen YF, Lan YC, et al.: Risk of diffuse infiltrative lymphocytosis syndrome in HIV-infected patients: a nationwide population-based cohort study, *J Acquir Immune Defic Syndr* 79:158–163, 2018.

Coogan MM, Greenspan J, Challacombe SJ: Oral lesions in infection with human immunodeficiency virus, *Bull World Health Organ* 83:700–706, 2005.

Cresswell FV, Ellis J, Hartley J, et al.: A systematic review of risk of HIV transmission through biting or spitting: implications for policy, *HIV Med* 19:532–540, 2018.

Deeks SG, Overbaugh J, Phillips A, et al.: HIV infection, *Nat Rev Dis Prim* 1:15035, 2015.

Ebrahim S, Singh B, Ramklass SS: HIV-associated salivary gland enlargement: a clinical review, *SADJ* 69:400–403, 2014.

Anon: EC-Clearinghouse on Oral Problems Related to HIV Infection and WHO Collaborating Centre on Oral Manifestations of the Immunodeficiency Virus: classification and diagnostic criteria for oral lesions in HIV infection, *J Oral Pathol Med* 22:289–291, 1993.

El Howati A, Tappuni A: Systematic review of the changing pattern of the oral manifestations of HIV, *J Investig Clin Dent* 9:e12351, 2018.

Fauci AS, Folkers GK, Lane HC: Chapter 197: Human immunodeficiency virus disease: AIDS and related disorders, In Jameson JL, Fauci AS, Kasper DL, et al., editors: *Harrison's principles of internal medicine*, ed 20, 2018, McGraw-Hill. https://accessmedicine-mhmedical-com.ezproxy-v.musc.edu/content.aspx?bookid=2129&sectionid=159213747. (Accessed 18 July 2020).

Fornatora ML, Reich RF, Gray RG, et al.: Intraoral molluscum contagiosum: a report of a case and a review of the literature, *Oral Surg Oral Med Oral Pathol Oral Radiol Endod* 92:318–320, 2001.

Gabriela AS, Bertha FM, Alejandro GC, et al.: HPV oral lesions in HIV-infected patients: the impact of long-term HAART, *J Oral Pathol Med* 42:443–449, 2013.

Gaitán-Cepeda LA, Martínez-González M, Ceballos-Salobreña A: Oral candidosis as a clinical marker of immune failure in patients with HIV/AIDS on HAART, *AIDS Patient Care STDs* 19:70–77, 2005.

Ghosn J, Taiwo B, Seedat S, et al.: HIV, *Lancet* 392:685–697, 2018.

Ghrenassia E, Martis N, Boyer J, et al.: The diffuse infiltrative lymphocytosis syndrome (DILS). A comprehensive review, *J Autoimmun* 59:19–25, 2015.

Gillison ML: Oropharyngeal cancer: a potential consequence of concomitant HPV and HIV infection, *Curr Opin Oncol* 21:439–444, 2009.

Greenspan JS, Greenspan D, Webster-Cyriaque J: Hairy leukoplakia; lessons learned: 30-plus years, *Oral Dis* 22(Suppl 1):120–127, 2016.

Hernández-Ramírez RU, Qin L, Lin H, et al.: Association of immunosuppression and HIV viraemia with non-Hodgkin lymphoma risk overall and by subtype in people living with HIV in Canada and the USA: a multicentre cohort study, *Lancet HIV* 6: e240–e249, 2019.

Hernández-Ramírez RU, Shiels MS, et al.: Cancer risk in HIV-infected people in the USA from 1996 to 2012: a population-based, registry-linkage study, *Lancet HIV* 4:e495–e504, 2017.

Herrrera D, Retamal-Valdes B, Alonso B, et al.: Acute periodontal lesions (periodontal abscesses and necrotizing periodontal diseases) and endo-periodontal lesions, *J Periodontol* 89(Suppl 1):S85–S201, 2018.

INSIGHT START Study Group, Lundgren JD, Babiker AG, et al.: Initiation of antiretroviral therapy in early asymptomatic HIV Infection, *N Engl J Med* 373:795–807, 2015.

Islam NM, Bhattacharyya I, Cohen DM: Salivary gland pathology in HIV patients, *Diagn Histopathol* 18:366–372, 2012.

Joint United Nations Programme on HIV/AIDS (UNAIDS): *2020 global AIDS update—seizing the moment*, 2020. (PDF online): https://www.unaids.org/sites/default/files/media_asset/2020_global-aids-report_en.pdf. (Accessed 14 July 2020.)

Joyce MP, Kuhar D, Brooks JT: Notes from the field: occupationally acquired HIV infection among health care workers—United States, 1985–2013, *MMWR Morb Mortal Wkly Rep* 63:1245–1246, 2015.

Ju WT, Fu Y, Liu Y, et al.: Clinical and pathologic analyses of tuberculosis in the oral cavity: report of 11 cases, *Oral Surg Oral Med Oral Pathol Oral Radiol* 125:44–51, 2018.

Kaplan LD: HIV-associated lymphoma, *Best Pract Res Clin Haematol* 25:101–117, 2012.

Kimani SM, Painschab MS, Horner MJ, et al.: Epidemiology of hematological malignancies in people living with HIV, *Lancet HIV*, 2020. S2352-3018(20)30118-1 (online ahead of print August 10, 2020).

Kirti YK: Prevalence of oral candidiasis in Indian HIV sero-positive patients with CD4$^+$ cell count correlation, *Indian J Otolaryngol Head Neck Surg* 71:124–127, 2019.

Kuhar DT, Henderson DK, Struble KA, et al.: *Updated U.S. Public Health Service guidelines for the management of occupational exposures to HIV and recommendations for postexposure prophylaxis*, Atlanta, GA, 2013, U.S. Department of Health and Human Services, Centers for Disease Control and Prevention. PDF online https://stacks.cdc.gov/view/cdc/20711. (Accessed 14 July 2020.)

Kuteyi T, Okwundu CI: Topical treatments for HIV-related oral ulcers, *Cochrane Database Syst Rev* 1:CD007975, 2012.

Limper AH, Adenis A, Le T, et al.: Fungal infections in HIV/AIDS, *Lancet Infect Dis* 17:e334–e343, 2017.

Martin P: Interventions for molluscum contagiosum in people infected with human immunodeficiency virus: a systematic review, *Int J Dermatol* 55:956–966, 2016.

Meer S: Human immunodeficiency virus and salivary gland pathology: an update, *Oral Surg Oral Med Oral Pathol Oral Radiol* 128:52–59, 2019.

Narendran G, Swaminathan S: TB-HIV co-infection: a catastrophic comradeship, *Oral Dis* 22(Suppl 1):46–52, 2016.

National Cancer Institute: Kaposi sarcoma, In Howlader N, Noone AM, Krapcho M, et al., editors: *SEER cancer statistics review, 1975–2017*, Bethesda, MD, 2020, National Cancer Institute. Based on November 2019 SEER data submission (PDF online) https://seer.cancer.gov/csr/1975_2017/results_merged/sect_10_kaposi_sarcoma.pdf. (Accessed 3 August 2020).

Nittayananta W: Oral fungi in HIV: challenges in antifungal therapies, *Oral Dis* 22(Suppl 1):107–113, 2016.

Nobre ÁVV, Pólvora TLS, Silva LRM, et al.: Effects of non-surgical periodontal therapy on clinical and immunological profile and colonization of *Candida* spp in HIV-infected patients with chronic periodontitis, *J Periodontol* 90:167–176, 2019.

Noy A: HIV and lymphoma: from oncological futility to treatment, *Lancet HIV* 7:e598–e600, 2020.

Nwaiwu CA, Egro FM, Smith S, et al.: Seroconversion rate among health care workers exposed to HIV-contaminated body fluids: the University of Pittsburgh 13-year experience, *Am J Infect Control* 45:896–900, 2017.

Panel on Guidelines for the Prevention and Treatment of Opportunistic Infections in Adults and Adolescents with HIV: *Guidelines for the prevention and treatment of opportunistic infections in HIV-infected adults and adolescents: recommendations from the Centers for Disease Control and Prevention, the National Institutes of Health, and the HIV Medicine Association of the Infectious Diseases Society of America*, 2020. Available at: http://aidsinfo.nih.gov/contentfiles/lvguidelines/adult_oi.pdf. (Accessed 2 August 2020.)

Pantanowitz L, Khammissa RAG, Lemmer J, et al.: Oral HIV-associated Kaposi sarcoma, *J Oral Pathol Med* 42:201–207, 2013.

Pappas PG, Kauffman CA, Andes DR, et al.: Clinical practice guideline for the management of candidiasis: 2016 update by the Infectious Diseases Society of America, *Clin Infect Dis* 62:e1–e50, 2016.

Patil S, Majumdar B, Sarode SC, et al.: Oropharyngeal candidosis in HIV-Infected patients-an update, *Front Microbiol* 9:980, 2018.

Pienaar ED, Young T, Holmes H: Interventions for the prevention and management of oropharyngeal candidiasis associated with HIV infection in adults and children, *Cochrane Database Syst Rev* 11: CD003940, 2010.

Pólvora TLS, Nobre ÁVV, Tirapelli C, et al.: Relationship between human immunodeficiency virus (HIV-1) infection and chronic periodontitis, *Expert Rev Clin Immunol* 14:315–327, 2018.

Reid E, Suneja G, Ambinder RF, et al.: AIDS-related Kaposi sarcoma, version 2.2019, NCCN clinical practice guidelines in oncology, *J Natl Compr Cancer Netw* 17:171–189, 2019.

Said J, Cesarman E, Rosenwald A, et al.: Lymphomas associated with HIV infection, In Swerdlow SH, Campo E, Harris NL, editors: *WHO classification of tumours of the haematopoietic and lymphoid tissues*, ed 5, Lyon, 2017, IARC, pp 449–452.

Sharma S, Bajpai J, Pathak PK, et al.: Oral tuberculosis—current concepts, *J Family Med Prim Care* 8:1308–1312, 2019.

Shiboski CH, Lee A, Chen H, et al.: Human papillomavirus infection in the oral cavity of HIV patients is not reduced by initiating antiretroviral therapy, *AIDS* 30:1573–1582, 2016.

Shiels MS, Copeland G, Goodman MT, et al.: Cancer stage at diagnosis in patients infected with the human immunodeficiency virus and transplant recipients, *Cancer* 121:2063–2071, 2015.

Shiels MS, Islam JY, Rosenberg PS, et al.: Projected cancer incidence rates and burden of incident cancer cases in HIV-infected adults in the United States through 2030, *Ann Intern Med* 168:866–873, 2018.

Silverberg MJ, Chao C, Leyden WA, et al.: HIV infection, immunodeficiency, viral replication, and the risk of cancer, *Cancer Epidemiol Biomark Prev* 20:2551–2559, 2011.

Siwamogstham P, Kuanswan C, Reichart P: Herpes zoster in HIV infection with osteonecrosis of the jaw and tooth exfoliation, *Oral Dis* 12:500–505, 2006.

Speicher DJ, Ramirez-Amador V, Dittmer DP, et al.: Viral infections associated with oral cancers and diseases in the context of HIV: a workshop report, *Oral Dis* 22(Suppl 1):181–192, 2016.

Syrjänen S, Leimola-Virtanen R, Schmidt-Westhausen A, et al.: Oral ulcers in AIDS patients frequently associated with cytomegalovirus (CMV) and Epstein-Barr virus (EBV) infections, *J Oral Pathol Med* 28:204–209, 1999.

Tota JE, Engels EA, Madeleine MM, et al.: Risk of oral tongue cancer among immunocompromised transplant recipients and human immunodeficiency virus-infected individuals in the United States, *Cancer* 124:2515–2522, 2018.

Vale DA, Martins FM, Silva PH, et al.: Retrospective analysis of the clinical behavior of oral hairy leukoplakia in 215 HIV-seropositive patients, *Brazilian Oral Research* 30:e118, 2016.

Vidya KM, Rao UK, Nittayananta W, et al.: Oral mycoses and other opportunistic infections in HIV: therapy and emerging problems—a workshop report, *Oral Dis* 22(Suppl 1):158–165, 2016.

Vohra P, Jamatia K, Subhada B, et al.: Correlation of CD4 counts with oral and systemic manifestations in HIV patients, *J Family Med Prim Care* 8:3247–3252, 2019.

Walline HM, Carey TE, Goudsmit CM, et al.: High-risk HPV, biomarkers, and outcome in matched cohorts of head and neck cancer patients positive and negative for HIV, *Mol Cancer Res* 15:179–188, 2017.

World Health Organization: *Global tuberculosis report 2019*, Lyon, 2019, World Health Organization (PDF online) https://apps.who.int/iris/bitstream/handle/10665/329368/9789241565714-eng.pdf?ua=1. (Accessed 15 July 2020).

World Health Organization: *WHO case definitions of HIV for surveillance and revised clinical staging and immunologic classification of HIV-related disease in adults and children*, Geneva, 2007, World Health Organization. (PDF online): https://apps.who.int/iris/bitstream/handle/10665/43699/9789241595629_eng.pdf?sequence=1&isAllowed=y. (Accessed 15 July 2020.)

Coronavirus Disease 2019

Amorim Dos Santos J, Normando AGC, Carvalho da Silva RL, et al.: Oral manifestations in patients with COVID-19: a 6-month update, *J Dent Res* 100:1321–1329, 2021.

Amorim Dos Santos J, Normando AGC, Carvalho da Silva RL, et al.: Oral mucosal lesions in patients with COVID-19: a living systematic review, *J Dent Res* 100:141–154, 2021.

Aragoneses J, Suárez A, Algar J, et al.: Oral manifestations of COVID-19: updated systematic review with meta-analysis, *Front Med (Lausanne)* 8:726753, 2021.

Bhimraj A, Morgan RL, Shumaker AH, et al.: *Infectious Disease Society of America guidelines on the treatment and management of patients with COVID-19, version 6.0.1*, https://www.idsociety.org/practice-guideline/covid-19-guideline-treatment-and-management/. (Accessed 31 January 2022).

Bhujel N, Zaheer K, Singh RP: Oral mucosal lesions in patients with COVID-19: a systematic review, *Br J Oral Maxillofac Surg* 59:1024–1030, 2021.

Carrillo-Larco RM, Altez-Fernandez C: Anosmia and dysgeusia in COVID-19: a systematic review, *Wellcome Open Res* 5:94, 2020.

Centers for Disease Control and Prevention, National Center for Immunization and Respiratory Diseases, Division of Viral Diseases: *Interim clinical guidance for management of patients with confirmed coronavirus disease (COVID-19)*, 2022 https://www.cdc.gov/coronavirus/2019-ncov/hcp/clinical-guidance-management-patients.html. (Accessed 3 January 2022).

COVID-19 Treatment Guidelines Panel: Coronavirus Disease: *(COVID-19) treatment guidelines*, 2019, National Institutes of Health. https://www.covid19treatmentguidelines.nih.gov/. (Accessed 31 January 2022).

Cruz Tapia RO, Peraza Labrador AJ, Guimaraes DM, et al.: Oral mucosal lesions in patients with SARS-CoV-2 infection. Report of four cases. Are they a true sign of COVID-19 disease? *Spec Care Dentist* 40:555–560, 2020.

Fernandez-Nieto D, Jimenez-Cauhe J, Suarez-Valle A, et al.: Characterization of acute acral skin lesions in nonhospitalized patients: a case series of 132 patients during the COVID-19 outbreak, *J Am Acad Dermatol* 83:e61–e63, 2020.

Freeman EE, McMahon DE, Lipoff JB, et al.: The spectrum of COVID-19-associated dermatologic manifestations: an international registry of 716 patients from 31 countries, *J Am Acad Dermatol* 83:1118–1129, 2020.

Gherlone EF, Polizzi E, Tetè G, et al.: Frequent and persistent salivary gland ectasia and oral disease after COVID-19, *J Dent Res* 100:464–471, 2021.

Mutiawati E, Fahriani M, Mamada SS, et al.: Anosmia and dysgeusia in SARS-CoV-2 infection: incidence and effects on COVID-19 severity and mortality, and the possible pathobiology mechanisms—a systematic review and meta-analysis, *F1000Res* 10:40, 2021.

Nascimento RB, Araujo NS, Silva JC, et al.: Oral manifestations of multisystemic inflammatory syndrome in children (MIS-C) and Kawasaki disease associated to COVID-19: a systematic review, *Spec Care Dentist*, 2021. Nov 18:https://doi.org/10.1111/scd.12669, 2021.

Rodriguez-Morales AJ, Cardona-Ospina JA, Gutiérrez-Ocampo E, et al.: Clinical, laboratory and imaging features of COVID-19: a systematic review and meta-analysis, *Travel Med Infect Dis* 34:101623, 2020.

Soares CD, Souza LL, de Carvalho MGF, et al.: Oral manifestations of coronavirus disease 2019 (COVID-19). A comprehensive clinicopathologic and immunohistochemical study, *Am J Surg Pathol* 28, 2021. https://doi.org/10.1097/PAS.0000000000001825.

Thomas DC, Baddireddy SM, Kohli D: Anosmia: a review in the context of coronavirus disease 2019 and orofacial pain, *J Am Dent Assoc (1939)* 151:696–702, 2020.

Xu H, Zhong L, Deng J, et al.: High expression of ACE2 receptor of 2019-nCoV on the epithelial cells of oral mucosa, *Int J Oral Sci* 12:8, 2020.

8
Physical and Chemical Injuries

◆ LINEA ALBA

Linea alba ("white line") is a common alteration of the buccal mucosa that most likely is associated with pressure, frictional irritation, or sucking trauma from the facial surfaces of the teeth. No other associated problem, such as insufficient horizontal overlap or rough restorations of the teeth, is necessary for the development of linea alba.

Clinical Features

As the name implies, the alteration consists of a white line that usually is bilateral. It may be scalloped and is located on the buccal mucosa at the level of the occlusal plane of the adjacent teeth (Fig. 8.1). The line varies in prominence and usually extends from the corner of mouth posteriorly toward the pterygomandibular raphe with the alteration stopping adjacent to the most posterior teeth in occlusion. It often is more pronounced adjacent to the posterior teeth. In clinical surveys of oral alterations, linea alba appears to be one of the more common oral conditions. Several studies have reported a female predominance.

Histopathologic Features

Biopsy is rarely indicated. If a biopsy is performed, hyperkeratosis is seen overlying otherwise normal oral mucosa. On occasion, intracellular edema of the epithelium and mild chronic inflammation of the underlying connective tissue may be noted.

Treatment and Prognosis

No treatment is required for patients with linea alba, and no difficulties are documented because of its development. Spontaneous regression may occur.

◆ MORSICATIO MUCOSAE ORIS (CHRONIC MUCOSAL CHEWING)

Morsicatio mucosae oris is a classic example of medical terminology gone astray; it is the scientific term for chronic chewing of the oral mucosa. *Morsicatio* comes from the Latin word *morsus,* or *bite.* Chronic nibbling produces lesions that are located most frequently on the buccal mucosa (**morsicatio buccarum**); however, the labial mucosa (**morsicatio labiorum**) and the lateral border of the tongue (**morsicatio linguarum**) also may be involved. Similar changes have been seen because of suction and in glassblowers whose technique produces chronic irritation of the buccal mucosa.

Chronic cheek chewing is considered a body-focused repetitive behavior (BFRB) along with skin picking, hair pulling, and nail biting. When one of these behaviors is noted, the individual also has a greater chance to demonstrate anxiety, depression, obsessive-compulsive disorder, body dysmorphic disorder (BDD), or fear of negative evaluation. Chronic cheek biting also can be seen in patients with a mass in their cheek or in individuals whose anatomy has been altered during oncologic surgery. Most patients are aware of their habit, although many deny the self-inflicted injury or perform the act subconsciously. An increased prevalence has been noted in women and in patients older than 35 years.

Clinical Features

Most frequently, the lesions in patients with morsicatio are found bilaterally on the anterior buccal mucosa. They also may be unilateral, combined with lesions of the lips or the tongue, or isolated to the lips or tongue. Thickened, shredded, white areas may be combined with intervening zones of erythema, erosion, or focal traumatic ulceration (Figs. 8.2 and 8.3). The areas of white mucosa demonstrate an irregular ragged surface, and the patient may describe being able to remove shreds of white material from the involved area. Although dysplastic leukoplakias tend to have more sharply demarcated borders, the periphery of morsicatio-related lesions gradually blends with the adjacent mucosa.

The altered mucosa typically is in the midportion of the anterior buccal mucosa along the occlusal plane. Large lesions may extend some distance above or below the occlusal plane in patients whose habit involves pushing the cheek between the teeth with a finger.

Histopathologic Features

Biopsy reveals extensive hyperparakeratosis that often results in an extremely ragged surface with numerous projections of keratin. Surface bacterial colonization is typical (Fig. 8.4). On occasion, clusters of vacuolated cells are present in the

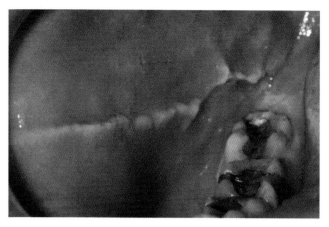

• **Fig. 8.1 Linea Alba.** White line of hyperkeratosis on the right buccal mucosa at the level of the occlusal plane.

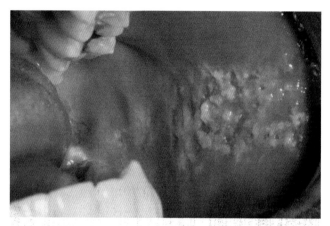

• **Fig. 8.2 Morsicatio Buccarum.** Thickened, shredded areas of white hyperkeratosis of the left buccal mucosa.

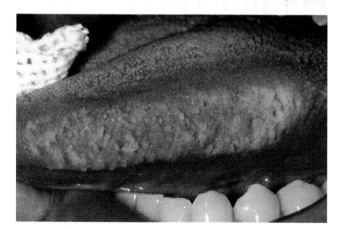

• **Fig. 8.3 Morsicatio Linguarum.** Thickened, rough areas of white hyperkeratosis of the lateral border of the tongue on the left side.

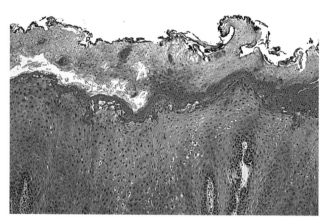

• **Fig. 8.4 Morsicatio Buccarum.** Oral mucosa exhibiting greatly thickened layer of parakeratin with ragged surface colonized by bacteria.

immunodeficiency virus (HIV) (see page 253), or to **uremic stomatitis** (see page 852). In contrast to OHL, the superficial epithelial cells will not demonstrate the characteristic nuclear beading associated with infection with Epstein-Barr virus. Lesions in patients who chronically chew betel quid (**betel chewer's mucosa;** see page 393) may resemble morsicatio microscopically. Similarities with linea alba and leukoedema also may be seen.

Diagnosis

In most cases, the clinical presentation of morsicatio is sufficient for a strong presumptive diagnosis, and clinicians familiar with these alterations rarely perform biopsy. Some cases of morsicatio may not be diagnostic from the clinical presentation, and biopsy may be necessary.

Treatment and Prognosis

No treatment of the oral lesions is required, and no long-term difficulties arise from the presence of the mucosal changes. For patients desiring either confirmation of the cause or preventive therapy, construction and use of acrylic shields to separate the teeth from the adjacent mucosa can provide quick resolution of the lesions. Alternatively, a maxillary splint with a facial cheek bumper can be constructed to increase the distance between the teeth and the adjacent buccal mucosa.

◆ TRAUMATIC ULCERATIONS

Acute and chronic injuries of the oral mucosa are common and may be associated with surface ulcerations. The ulcerations may remain for extended periods of time but most usually heal within days. A histopathologically unique type of chronic traumatic ulceration of the oral mucosa is the **eosinophilic ulceration (traumatic granuloma; traumatic ulcerative granuloma with stromal eosinophilia [TUGSE];**

superficial portion of the prickle cell layer. This histopathologic pattern is not pathognomonic of morsicatio and may bear a striking resemblance to **oral hairy leukoplakia (OHL),** a lesion that can be seen in a wide variety conditions associated with local and systemic immunosuppression (most notably patients infected with the **human**

eosinophilic granuloma of the tongue), which exhibits a deep pseudoinvasive inflammatory reaction and typically is slow to resolve. Interestingly, many of these traumatic granulomas undergo resolution after incisional biopsy. Lesions microscopically similar to eosinophilic ulceration have been reproduced in rat tongues after repeated crushing trauma and in traumatic lesions noted in patients with familial dysautonomia, a disorder characterized by indifference to pain. In addition, similar sublingual ulcerations may occur in infants because of chronic mucosal trauma from adjacent anterior primary teeth, often associated with nursing. An Italian physician, Antonio Riga, initially described the clinical presentation of the ulcerations in 1881, and Fede followed with a description of the associated histopathology in 1890. Accordingly, these distinctive ulcerations of infancy have been termed **Riga-Fede disease** and should be considered a variation of the traumatic eosinophilic ulceration.

In rare subsets of eosinophilic ulcerations, the lesion does not appear to be associated with trauma, and sheets of large, atypical cells intermixed with numerous eosinophils are seen histopathologically. The atypical cells have been shown to represent T lymphocytes with a strong immunoperoxidase reactivity for CD30. When T-cell clonality is demonstrated, many believe these cases represent the oral counterpart of the **primary cutaneous CD30+ lymphoproliferative disorder,** which also exhibits sequential ulceration, necrosis, and occasional self-regression. In these cases, a thorough physical evaluation appears prudent to rule out the possibility of a systemic lymphoproliferative process.

In most cases of traumatic ulceration, there is an adjacent source of irritation, although this is not present invariably. The clinical presentation often suggests the cause, but many cases resemble early ulcerative squamous cell carcinoma; biopsy is performed to rule out that possibility.

Clinical Features

As would be expected, simple chronic traumatic ulcerations occur most often on the tongue, lips, and buccal mucosa—sites that may be injured by the dentition (Fig. 8.5). Lesions of the gingiva, palate, and mucobuccal fold may occur from other sources of irritation. The individual lesions appear as areas of erythema surrounding a central removable, yellow fibrinopurulent membrane. In many instances, the lesion develops a rolled white border of hyperkeratosis immediately adjacent to the area of ulceration (Fig. 8.6).

Eosinophilic ulcerations are not uncommon but frequently are not reported. The lesions occur in people of all ages, with a significant male predominance. Most have been reported on the tongue, although cases have been seen on the gingiva, buccal mucosa, floor of mouth, palate, and lip. The lesion may last from 1 week to 8 months. The ulcerations appear very similar to the simple traumatic ulcerations; however, on occasion, underlying proliferative granulation tissue can result in a raised lesion similar to a pyogenic granuloma (see page 525) (Fig. 8.7).

Riga-Fede disease typically appears between 1 week and 1 year of age. The condition often develops in association with natal teeth (see page 79). The anterior ventral surface of the tongue is the most common site of involvement, although the dorsal surface also may be affected (Fig. 8.8). Ventral lesions contact the adjacent mandibular anterior

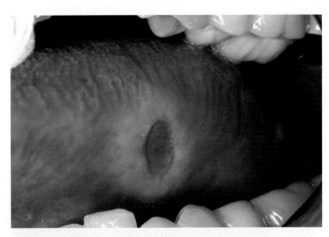

• **Fig. 8.6 Traumatic Ulceration.** Mucosal ulceration with a faintly hyperkeratotic collar located on the left ventral lateral surface of the tongue.

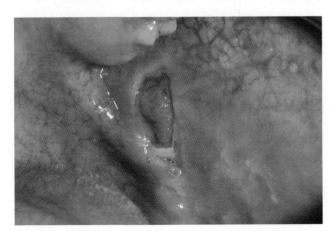

• **Fig. 8.5 Traumatic Ulceration.** Well-circumscribed ulceration of the posterior buccal mucosa on the left side.

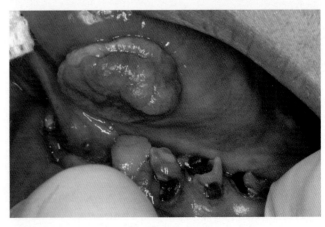

• **Fig. 8.7 Traumatic Granuloma.** Exophytic ulcerated mass on the ventrolateral tongue associated with multiple jagged teeth.

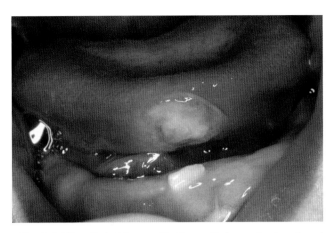

• **Fig. 8.8 Riga-Fede Disease.** Newborn with traumatic ulceration of anterior ventral surface of the tongue. Mucosal damage occurred from contact of tongue with adjacent tooth during breastfeeding.

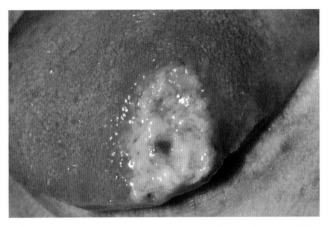

• **Fig. 8.9 Atypical Eosinophilic Ulceration.** Large ulceration of the anterior dorsal surface of the tongue.

incisors; lesions on the dorsal surface are associated with the maxillary incisors. A presentation similar to Riga-Fede disease can be the initial finding in a variety of neurologic conditions related to self-mutilation, such as familial dysautonomia (Riley-Day syndrome), congenital indifference to pain, Lesch-Nyhan syndrome, Gaucher disease, cerebral palsy, or Tourette syndrome.

The atypical eosinophilic ulceration occurs in older adults, with most cases developing in patients older than age 40. Surface ulceration is present, and an underlying tumefaction also is seen. The tongue is the most common site, although the gingiva, alveolar mucosa, mucobuccal fold, buccal mucosa, and lip may be affected (Fig. 8.9).

Histopathologic Features

Simple traumatic ulcerations are covered by a fibrinopurulent membrane that consists of fibrin intermixed with neutrophils. The membrane is of variable thickness, and the adjacent surface epithelium may be normal or may demonstrate slight hyperplasia with or without hyperkeratosis. The

ulcer bed consists of granulation tissue that supports a mixed inflammatory infiltrate of lymphocytes, histiocytes, neutrophils, and, occasionally, plasma cells. In patients with eosinophilic ulcerations, the pattern is very similar; however, the inflammatory infiltrate extends into the deeper tissues and exhibits sheets of lymphocytes and histiocytes intermixed with eosinophils. In addition, the vascular connective tissue deep to the ulceration may become hyperplastic and cause surface elevation.

Atypical eosinophilic ulcerations exhibit numerous features of the traumatic eosinophilic ulceration, but the deeper tissues are replaced by a highly cellular proliferation of large lymphoreticular cells. The infiltrate is pleomorphic, and mitotic features are somewhat common. Intermixed with the large atypical cells are mature lymphocytes and numerous eosinophils. Although an associated immunohistochemical profile rarely has been reported, several investigators have shown the large cells to be T lymphocytes, the majority of which react with CD30 (Ki-1). In many instances, molecular studies for T-cell clonality by polymerase chain reaction (PCR) have been performed on the CD30+ cells and demonstrated monoclonal rearrangement. Despite the clonality noted in many cases, the lymphoproliferative disorder typically demonstrates negative reactivity with anaplastic lymphoma kinase protein, a marker associated with large cell CD30+ lymphoma.

Treatment and Prognosis

For traumatic ulcerations that have an obvious source of injury, the irritating cause should be removed. A topical anesthetic or protective film can be applied for temporary pain relief. If the cause is not obvious, or if a patient does not respond to therapy, then biopsy is indicated. Rapid healing after a biopsy is typical even with large eosinophilic ulcerations (Fig. 8.10). Recurrence is not expected.

The use of corticosteroids in the management of traumatic ulcerations is controversial. Some clinicians have suggested that use of such medications may delay healing. Despite this, other investigators have reported success using corticosteroids to treat chronic traumatic ulcerations.

Although extraction of the anterior primary teeth is not recommended, this procedure has resolved the ulcerations in Riga-Fede disease. The teeth should be retained if they are stable. Grinding the incisal mamelons, coverage of the teeth with a light-cured composite or cellulose film, construction of a protective shield, or discontinuation of nursing have been tried with variable success.

In patients demonstrating histopathologic similarities to the cutaneous CD30+ lymphoproliferative disorder, a thorough evaluation for systemic lymphoma is mandatory, along with lifelong follow-up. Although recurrence frequently is seen, the ulcerations typically heal spontaneously, and most patients do not demonstrate dissemination of the process. Further documentation is critical to define more fully this poorly understood process.

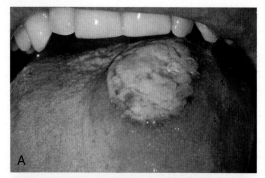

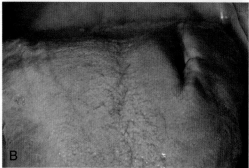

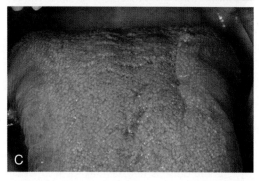

• **Fig. 8.10 Eosinophilic Ulceration. A,** Initial presentation of a large ulceration of the dorsal surface of the tongue. **B,** Significant resolution noted 2 weeks after incisional biopsy. **C,** Subsequent healing noted 4 weeks after biopsy.

◆ ELECTRICAL AND THERMAL BURNS

Electrical burns to the oral cavity are fairly common, constituting approximately 5% of all burn admissions to hospitals. Two types of electrical burns can be seen: (1) **contact** and (2) **arc.**

Contact burns require a good ground and involve electrical current passing through the body from the point of contact to the ground site. The electric current can cause cardiopulmonary arrest and may be fatal. Most electrical burns affecting the oral cavity are the arc type, in which the saliva acts as a conducting medium and an electrical arc flows between the electrical source and the mouth. Extreme heat, up to 3000°C, is possible with resultant significant tissue destruction. Most cases result from chewing on the female end of an extension cord or from biting through a live wire.

Most **thermal burns** of the oral cavity arise from ingestion of hot foods or beverages. Microwave ovens have been

associated with an increased frequency of thermal burns because of their ability to cook food that is cool on the exterior but extremely hot in the interior.

Since the early 2000s, a rash of thermal burns have been noted in association with use of electronic cigarettes (e-cigarettes). These devices were introduced in 2003 with availability in the United States and Europe beginning in 2007. E-cigarettes consist of a cartridge tank containing the vapor fluid, a heating element to vaporize the solution, and a lithium-ion battery to power the system. The heating systems can be triggered when the user inhales deeply or manually depresses a button on the side of the unit. The heating element can create temperatures up to 100–250°C (212–482°F). Over 450 brands exist and are largely unregulated because the devices are not required by law to undergo safety testing. During a two-year period in England, 105 house fires were linked to failures of e-cigarettes. Due to the risk of fire, electronic cigarettes are banned in checked baggage aboard aircraft.

Several different patterns of burns have been associated with use of e-cigarettes. Thermal burns with or without flames may be seen from thermal runaway of the lithium battery or overheating of the vaporizing system. In some cases of overheating, the battery seal at the ends of the device can fail and result in an explosive blast that launches the internal battery like a missile out of its case, combining physical injury with thermal burns. The e-cigarette also can release electrolyte solution, resulting in a chemical alkali burn.

Clinical Features

The hands are the most common site of electrical burns in adults. In contrast, the oral cavity is the most affected location in children, with 90% of these accidents occurring before age 4. The lips are affected most frequently, and the commissure commonly is involved. Initially, the burn appears as a painless, charred, yellow area that exhibits little to no bleeding (Fig. 8.11). Significant edema often develops within a few hours and may persist up to 12 days. Starting on the fourth day, the affected area becomes necrotic and begins to slough. Bleeding may develop during this period from exposure of the underlying vital vasculature, and the presence of this complication should be monitored closely. The adjacent mucobuccal fold, the tongue, or both also may be involved. On occasion, adjacent teeth may become nonvital, with or without necrosis of the surrounding alveolar bone. Malformation of developing teeth also has been documented. In patients receiving high-voltage electrical injury, resultant facial nerve paralysis is reported infrequently and typically resolves over several weeks to months. Focal enamel cavitation, which was thought to represent a high voltage exit point, also has been reported in association with an electrocution injury.

The injuries related to thermal food burns usually appear on the palate or posterior buccal mucosa (Fig. 8.12). The lesions appear as zones of erythema and ulceration that often exhibit remnants of necrotic epithelium at the periphery. If

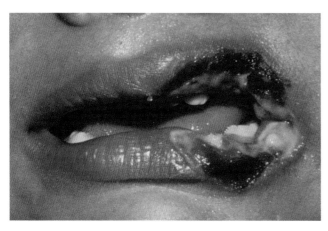

• **Fig. 8.11 Electrical Burn.** Yellow charred area of necrosis along the left oral commissure. (Courtesy of Dr. Patricia Hagen.)

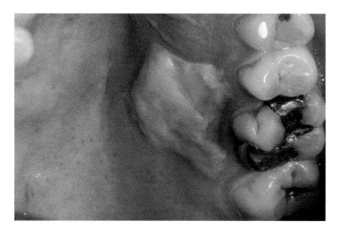

• **Fig. 8.12 Thermal Food Burn.** Area of yellow-white epithelial necrosis of the left posterior hard palate. Damage was the result of attempted ingestion of a hot pizza roll.

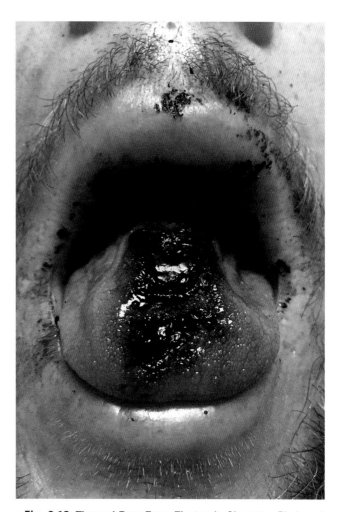

• **Fig. 8.13 Thermal Burn From Electronic Cigarette.** Blackened mucosal burn of the dorsal surface of the tongue. (Courtesy of Dr. Rebecca Pikos).

hot beverages are swallowed, swelling of the upper airway can occur and lead to dyspnea, which may develop several hours after the injury.

Burns related to electronic cigarettes most frequently affect the thigh, hands, face, and thorax. A significant percentage occur when the device fails while being carried in trouser pockets, resulting in significant burns of the thigh and the hands that are attempting to stop the fireball. Several oral injuries have been seen when the device explodes at the moment the user presses the heating button with the unit being held between their lips. In two surprisingly identical reports, the launching of the battery from its case into the mouth resulted in loss of the maxillary incisors with significant damage to the surrounding maxillary bone and the soft tissues of the hard palate, soft palate, lips, and tongue (Fig. 8.13).

Treatment and Prognosis

For patients with electrical burns of the oral cavity, tetanus immunization, if not current, is required. Most clinicians prescribe a prophylactic antibiotic, usually penicillin, to prevent secondary infection in severe cases. The primary problem with oral burns is contracture of the mouth opening during healing. Without intervention, significant microstomia can develop and may produce such restricted access to the mouth that hygiene and eating become impossible in severe cases. Extensive scarring and disfigurement are typical in untreated patients.

To prevent the disfigurement, a variety of microstomia prevention appliances can be used to eliminate or reduce the need for subsequent surgical reconstruction. Compliance is the most important consideration when choosing the most appropriate device. Tissue-supported appliances appear most effective for infants and young children; older, more cooperative patients usually benefit from tooth-supported devices. In most cases, splinting is maintained for 6–8 months to ensure proper scar maturation. Evaluation for possible surgical reconstruction usually is performed after a 1-year follow-up.

Most thermal burns are of little clinical consequence and resolve without treatment. When the upper airway is involved and associated with breathing difficulties, antibiotics and corticosteroids often are administered. In rare cases, swelling of the airway mandates intubation or tracheotomy to resolve the associated dyspnea. In these severe cases, oral intake of food often is discontinued temporarily with nutrition provided by a nasogastric tube.

In burns related to electronic cigarettes, the battery can deposit lithium cobalt oxides or lithium manganese into the damaged tissues. If irrigated with water, alkali lithium hydroxide and hydrogen gas can be generated in a vigorous exothermic reaction. For this reason, e-cigarette burns should be tested with pH paper and covered with mineral oil if an alkaline pH is confirmed; otherwise, the area can be irrigated with water, gently debrided of necrotic tissue, and treated with traditional burn therapy. Oral burns are treated with saline rinses, systemic analgesics, and a soft diet with avoidance of carbonated and alcoholic beverages. Lacerations of the oral soft tissues also may be present and must be repaired surgically. Computed tomographic imaging and radiographs are prudent to determine the degree of damage to the maxilla and inspect the oral cavity and gastrointestinal tract for foreign bodies. As expected, reconstruction of the maxillary dentition requires significant dental care, often with placement of implant prosthetics.

◆ CHEMICAL INJURIES OF THE ORAL MUCOSA

Many chemicals and drugs come into contact with the oral tissues. A percentage of these agents are caustic and can cause clinically significant damage.

Patients often can be their own worst enemies. The array of chemicals that have been placed within the mouth to resolve oral problems is amazing. Aspirin, sodium perborate, hydrogen peroxide, gasoline, turpentine, rubbing alcohol, and battery acid are just a few of the more interesting examples. In addition, mucosal damage has been documented from many of the topical medicaments sold as treatments for toothache or mouth sores. Over-the-counter products containing isopropyl alcohol, phenol, hydrogen peroxide, or eugenol have produced adverse reactions in patients. Tooth-whitening products also contain hydrogen peroxide or one of its precursors, carbamide peroxidase, which has been shown to create mucosal necrosis (Fig. 8.14). A surprising number of medications also are potentially caustic when held in the mouth long enough. Aspirin, bisphosphonates, and two psychoactive drugs, chlorpromazine and promazine, are well-documented examples.

Health care practitioners also are responsible for the use of many caustic materials. Silver nitrate, formocresol, sodium hypochlorite, paraformaldehyde, chromic acid, trichloroacetic acid, dental cavity varnishes, and acid-etch materials all can cause patient injury. Education and use of the rubber dam have reduced the frequency of such injuries.

Recreational drugs also can result in areas of mucosal necrosis. Cocaine has been applied directly to the gingiva or alveolar mucosa to judge the drug's purity and can result in areas of epithelial necrosis. Other drugs such as MDMA

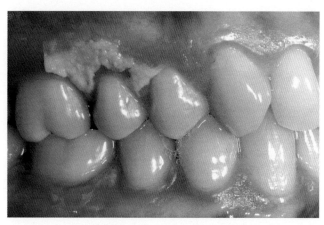

• **Fig. 8.14 Mucosal Burn From Tooth-whitening Strips.** Sharply demarcated zone of epithelial necrosis on the maxillary facial gingiva, which developed from the use of tooth-whitening strips. Less severe involvement also is present on the mandibular gingiva.

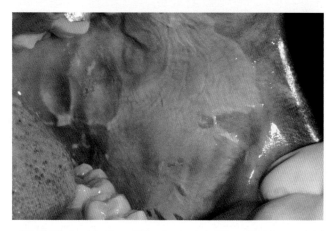

• **Fig. 8.15 Aspirin Burn.** Extensive area of white epithelial necrosis of the left buccal mucosa caused by aspirin placement in an attempt to alleviate dental pain.

(methylenedioxymethamphetamine) and amphetamine in association with cocaine also have been noted to damage oral mucosa. A later section of this chapter discusses further the orofacial complications of drug abuse.

The improper use of aspirin, hydrogen peroxide, silver nitrate, phenol, and certain endodontic materials deserves further discussion because of their frequency of misuse, the severity of related damage, and the lack of adequate documentation of these materials as harmful agents.

Aspirin

Mucosal necrosis from aspirin being held in the mouth is not rare (Fig. 8.15). Aspirin is available not only in the well-known tablets but also as powder.

Hydrogen Peroxide

Hydrogen peroxide became a popular intraoral medication for prevention of periodontitis in the late 1970s. Since that time, mucosal damage has been seen more frequently because of this application. Concentrations at 3% or greater are associated most often with adverse reactions. Epithelial necrosis has been noted with dilutions as low as 1%, and many over-the-counter oral medications exceed this concentration (Fig. 8.16).

Silver Nitrate

Silver nitrate remains a popular treatment for aphthous ulcerations because the chemical cautery brings about rapid pain relief by destroying nerve endings. Despite this, its use should be strongly discouraged. In all cases, the extent of mucosal damage is increased by its use. In some patients, an abnormal reaction is seen, with resultant significant damage and enhanced pain. In addition, rare reports have documented irreversible systemic argyria secondary to habitual intraoral use of topical silver nitrate after recommendation by a dentist (see page 304).

Phenol

Occasionally, phenol has been used in dentistry as a cavity-sterilizing agent and cauterizing material. It is extremely caustic, and judicious use is required. Over-the-counter agents advertised as "canker sore" treatments may contain low concentrations of phenol, often combined with high levels of alcohol. Extensive mucosal necrosis and rarely underlying bone loss have been seen in patients who placed this material (phenol concentration 0.5%) in attempts to resolve minor mucosal sore spots (Fig. 8.17).

A prescription therapy containing 50% sulfuric acid, 4% sulfonated phenol, and 24% sulfonated phenolic agents is being marketed heavily to dentists for treatment of aphthous ulcerations. Because extensive necrosis has been seen from use of medicaments containing 0.5% phenol, this product must be used with great care.

Endodontic Materials

Because of the past difficulty of obtaining profound anesthesia in some patients undergoing root canal therapy, some clinicians have used arsenical paste or paraformaldehyde formulations to devitalize the inflamed pulp. Gingival and bone necrosis have been documented because of leakage of this material from the pulp chamber into the surrounding tissues. Endodontic irrigants, such as formocresol (Fig. 8.18) or sodium hypochlorite, produce similar necrosis if the material leaks into the surrounding supporting tissues or is injected past the apex, leading some to suggest chlorhexidine as a safer irrigant. Because chlorhexidine lacks the tissue-dissolving properties of sodium hypochlorite, some clinicians have suggested alternating between chlorhexidine and sodium hypochlorite. Others have warned that contact of these two compounds results in formation of a precipitate, para-chloroaniline, which is thought to be potentially toxic and carcinogenic.

The following can reduce the chances of tissue damage during irrigation with sodium hypochlorite:
- Using a rubber dam
- Avoiding excessive pressure during application
- Keeping the syringe needle away from the apex

In some countries, clinicians have used recycled anesthetic cartridges to keep solutions of sodium hypochlorite for

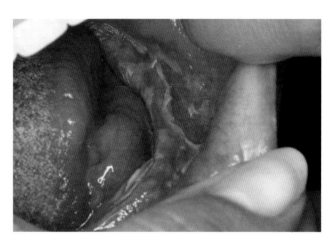

• **Fig. 8.17 Phenol Burn.** Extensive epithelial necrosis of the mandibular alveolar mucosa on the left side. Damage resulted from placement of an over-the-counter, phenol-containing, antiseptic and anesthetic gel under a denture. (Courtesy of Dr. Dean K. White.)

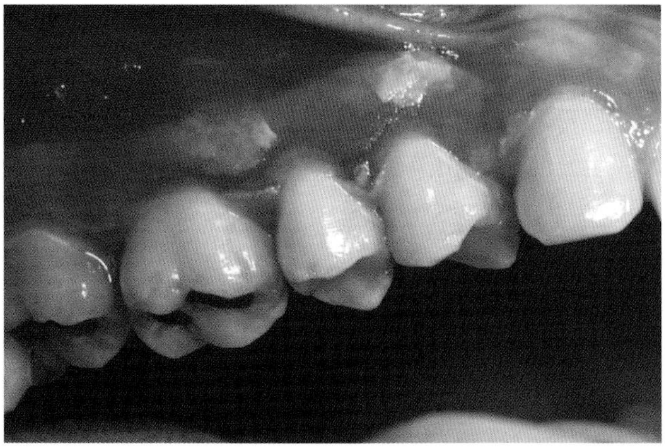

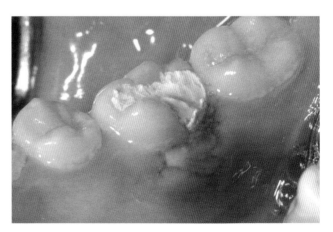

• **Fig. 8.18 Formocresol Burn.** Tissue necrosis secondary to leakage of endodontic material between a rubber dam clamp and the tooth.

• **Fig. 8.16 Hydrogen Peroxide Burn.** Extensive epithelial necrosis of the anterior maxillary gingiva secondary to interproximal placement of hydrogen peroxide with cotton swabs.

endodontic irrigation. Several reports have documented massive necrosis from inadvertent injection of sodium hypochlorite into soft tissue when these cartridges were mistaken for a local anesthetic.

For almost 100 years, calcium hydroxide has been utilized in the chemomechanical debridement of root canals due to its antimicrobial activity and its ability to dissolve uninstrumented fragments of pulpal tissue within the canal. The material is highly alkaline and overfill of the material can be toxic to periapical tissues. Numerous examples of chronic pain, numbness, or burning pain have been reported in patients in which calcium hydroxide escaped from the roots of lower molars and infiltrated the neurovascular canal.

Clinical Features

The previously discussed caustic agents produce similar damage. With short exposure, the affected mucosa exhibits a superficial white, wrinkled appearance. As the duration of exposure increases, the necrosis proceeds, and the affected epithelium becomes separated from the underlying tissue and can be desquamated easily. Removal of the necrotic epithelium reveals red, bleeding connective tissue that subsequently will be covered by a yellowish, fibrinopurulent membrane. Mucosa bound to bone is keratinized and more resistant to damage, whereas the nonkeratinized movable mucosa is destroyed more quickly. In addition to mucosal necrosis, significant tooth erosion has been seen in patients who chronically chew aspirin or hold the medication in their teeth as it dissolves.

The use of the rubber dam can dramatically reduce iatrogenic mucosal burns. When cotton rolls are used for moisture control during dental procedures, two problems may occur. On occasion, caustic materials can leak into the cotton roll and be held in place against the mucosa for an extended period, with mucosal injury resulting from the chemical absorbed by the cotton. In addition, oral mucosa can adhere to dry cotton rolls, and rapid removal of the rolls from the mouth often can cause stripping of the epithelium in the area. The latter pattern of mucosal injury has been termed **cotton roll burn (cotton roll stomatitis)** (Fig. 8.19).

Caustic materials injected into bone during endodontic procedures can result in significant bone necrosis, pain, and perforation into soft tissue. Necrotic surface ulceration and edema with underlying areas of soft tissue necrosis may occur adjacent to the site of perforation.

Histopathologic Features

Microscopic examination of the white slough removed from areas of mucosal chemical burns reveals coagulative necrosis of the epithelium, with only the outline of the individual epithelial cells and nuclei remaining. The necrosis begins on the surface and moves basally. The amount of epithelium affected depends on the duration of contact and the concentration of the offending agent. The underlying connective tissue contains a mixture of acute and chronic inflammatory cells.

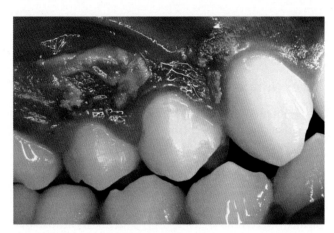

• **Fig. 8.19 Cotton Roll Burn.** Zone of white epithelial necrosis and erythema of the maxillary alveolar mucosa.

Treatment and Prognosis

The best treatment of chemical injuries is prevention of exposure of the oral mucosa to caustic materials. When prescribing potentially caustic drugs, the clinician must instruct the patient to swallow the medication and not allow it to remain in the oral cavity for any significant length of time. Children should not use chewable aspirin immediately before bedtime, and they should rinse after use.

Superficial areas of necrosis typically resolve completely without scarring within 10–14 days after discontinuation of the offending agent. For temporary protection, some clinicians have recommended coverage with a protective emollient paste or a hydroxypropyl cellulose film. Topical anesthetics also may be used to provide temporary pain relief. When large areas of necrosis are present, surgical débridement and antibiotic coverage often are required to promote healing and prevent spread of the necrosis.

In patients who report pain, numbness, or dysesthesia in association with a calcium hydroxide overfill into the inferior alveolar canal, referral to an oral surgeon or endodontist is recommended for possible surgical intervention with debridement to remove the material from the injured neurovascular tissue. The success of the surgical intervention is higher if performed within 72 hours of the injury.

◆ NONINFECTIOUS ORAL COMPLICATIONS OF ANTINEOPLASTIC THERAPY

No systemic anticancer therapy currently available can destroy tumor cells without causing the death of at least some normal cells, and tissues with rapid turnover (e.g., oral epithelium) are especially susceptible. The mouth is a common site (and one of the most visible areas) for complications related to cancer therapy. Both radiation therapy and systemic chemotherapy may cause significant oral problems—the more potent the treatment, the greater the risk of complications. Severe therapy-associated mucositis may require a decrease in dosage of the chemotherapy regimen or a break in the schedule of radiation treatment, both of which can negatively impact the long-term prognosis.

Clinical Features

A variety of noninfectious oral complications are seen regularly because of both radiation and chemotherapy. Two acute changes, **mucositis** and **hemorrhage,** are the predominant problems associated with chemotherapy, especially in cancers, such as leukemia, that involve high treatment doses.

Painful acute mucositis and dermatitis are the most frequently encountered side effects of radiation, but several chronic alterations continue to plague patients long after their courses of therapy are completed. Depending on the fields of radiation, the radiation dose, and the age of the patient, the following outcomes are possible:
- Xerostomia
- Loss of taste (hypogeusia)
- Osteoradionecrosis
- Trismus
- Chronic dermatitis
- Developmental abnormalities

Hemorrhage

Intraoral **hemorrhage** is typically secondary to thrombocytopenia, which develops from bone marrow suppression. Intestinal or hepatic damage, however, may cause lower vitamin K–dependent clotting factors, with resultant increased coagulation times. Conversely, tissue damage related to therapy may cause release of tissue thromboplastin at levels capable of producing potentially devastating disseminated intravascular coagulation (DIC). Oral petechiae and ecchymosis secondary to minor trauma are the most common presentations. Any mucosal site may be affected, but the labial mucosa, tongue, and gingiva are involved most frequently.

Mucositis

Oral mucositis has been shown to be the single most debilitating complication of high-dose chemotherapy and radiation therapy to the head and neck. In addition to significant local discomfort, the mucositis may be associated with an increased need for total parenteral nutrition, prolonged hospital stays, and most importantly, systemic bacteremia and sepsis.

Oral mucositis is seen in 20%–40% of patients receiving systemic chemotherapy, 80% of patients receiving high-dose chemotherapy, and almost all patients receiving radiation therapy to the head and neck for deeply seated neoplasms. The prevalence associated with chemotherapy is variable, depending on the regimen being used. Agents strongly associated with oral mucositis include methotrexate, 5-fluorouracil, etoposide, irinotecan, cytarabine, 6-mercaptopurine, 6-thioguanine, busulfan, melphalan, cyclophosphamide, idarubicin, doxorubicin (Adriamycin), daunorubicin, dactinomycin, bleomycin, and vinblastine. Beyond the direct effects of the antineoplastic agent, additional risk factors include young age, female gender, poor oral hygiene, oral foci of infection, poor nutrition, impaired salivary function, tobacco use, and alcohol consumption.

Cases of oral **mucositis** related to radiation or chemotherapy are similar in their clinical presentations. The manifestations of chemotherapy develop after a few days of treatment; radiation mucositis may begin to appear during the second week of therapy. Both chemotherapy and radiation-induced mucositis resolve slowly 2–3 weeks after cessation of treatment. Oral mucositis associated with chemotherapy typically involves the nonkeratinized surfaces (i.e., buccal mucosa, ventrolateral tongue, soft palate, and floor of the mouth), whereas radiation therapy primarily affects the mucosal surfaces within the direct portals of radiation.

The earliest manifestation is development of a whitish discoloration from a lack of sufficient desquamation of keratin. This is soon followed by loss of this layer with replacement by atrophic mucosa, which is edematous, erythematous, and friable. Subsequently, areas of ulceration develop with formation of a removable yellowish, fibrinopurulent surface membrane (Figs. 8.20–8.22). Pain, burning, and discomfort are significant and can be worsened by eating and oral hygiene procedures.

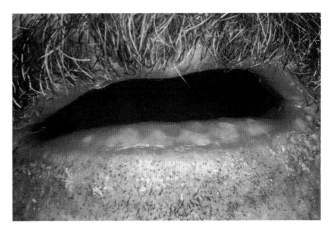

• **Fig. 8.20 Chemotherapy-Related Epithelial Necrosis.** Vermilion border of the lower lip exhibiting epithelial necrosis and ulceration in a patient receiving systemic chemotherapy.

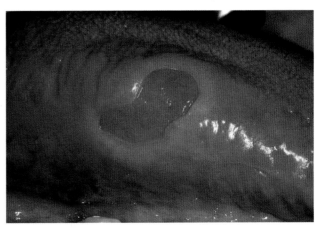

• **Fig. 8.21 Chemotherapy-Related Ulceration.** Ulceration of the right lateral border of the tongue in a patient receiving systemic chemotherapy.

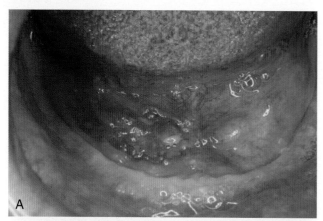

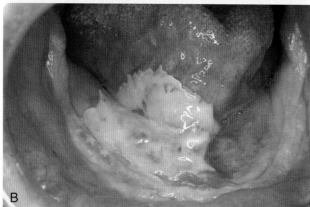

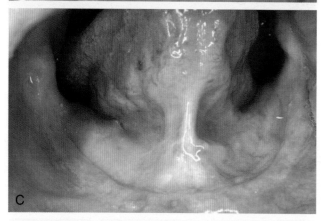

• **Fig. 8.22** **Radiation Mucositis. A,** Squamous cell carcinoma before radiation therapy. Granular erythroplakia of the floor of the mouth on the patient's right side. **B,** Same lesion after initiation of radiation therapy. Note the large, irregular area of epithelial necrosis and ulceration of the anterior floor of the mouth on the patient's right side. **C,** Normal oral mucosa after radiation therapy. Note resolution of the tumor and the radiation mucositis.

Dermatitis

Acute **dermatitis** of the skin in the fields of radiation is common and varies according to the intensity of the therapy. Patients with mild radiation dermatitis experience erythema, edema, burning, and pruritus. This condition resolves in 2–3 weeks after therapy and is replaced by hyperpigmentation and variable hair loss. Moderate radiation causes erythema and edema in combination with erosions and ulcerations. Within 3 months these alterations resolve, and permanent hair loss, hyperpigmentation, and scarring may ensue. Necrosis and

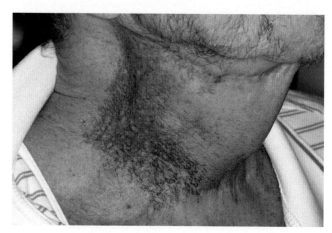

• **Fig. 8.23** **Radiation Dermatitis.** Cutaneous atrophy and telangiectasia secondary to radiation therapy. (Courtesy of Dr. Terry Day.)

deep ulcerations can occur in severe acute reactions. Radiation dermatitis also may become chronic and be characterized by dry, smooth, shiny, atrophic, necrotic, telangiectatic, depilated, or ulcerated areas (Fig. 8.23).

Xerostomia

Salivary glands are very sensitive to radiation, and **xerostomia** is a common complication. When a portion of the salivary glands is included in the fields of radiation, the remaining glands undergo compensatory hyperplasia to maintain function. The changes begin within 1 week of initiation of radiation therapy, with a dramatic decrease in salivary flow noted during the first 6 weeks of treatment. Even further decreases may be noted for up to 3 years.

Serous glands exhibit an increased radiosensitivity when compared with the mucous glands. On significant exposure, the parotid glands are affected dramatically and irreversibly. In contrast, the mucous glands partially recover and, over several months, may achieve flow that approaches 50% of preradiation levels. In addition to the discomfort of a mouth that lacks proper lubrication, diminished flow of saliva leads to a significant decrease of the bactericidal action and self-cleansing properties of saliva.

Without intervention, patients often develop symptomatic dry mouth that affects their ability to eat comfortably, wear dentures, speak, and sleep. In addition, there often is an increase in the caries index (**radiation-related caries),** regardless of the patient's past caries history (Fig. 8.24). The decay is predominantly cervical in location and often secondary to xerostomia. Radiation also causes biomechanical alterations in the teeth, resulting in reduced microhardness and decreased resistance to tensile and compressive stresses.

Several interventions to reduce radiation-related xerostomia have demonstrated promise. Intensity-modulated radiation therapy (IMRT) appears to be more gland-sparing than conventional radiation therapy and is emerging as the standard of care for head and neck cancer. Amifostine is a cytoprotective agent that has been shown to reduce the severity and duration of xerostomia in patients receiving radiotherapy (but not chemoradiotherapy) for head and neck cancer. On

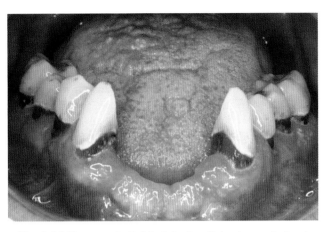

• **Fig. 8.24 Xerostomia-Related Caries.** Extensive cervical caries of mandibular dentition secondary to radiation-related xerostomia.

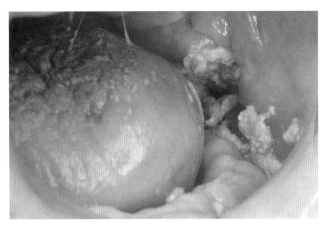

• **Fig. 8.25 Osteoradionecrosis (ORN).** Ulceration overlying left body of the mandible with exposure and sequestration of superficial alveolar bone.

the downside, this medication has significant side effects, and there are lingering concerns related to possible tumor protective effects. Surgical transfer of a single submandibular salivary gland outside of the radiation field to the submental space has proven successful in selected patients.

Taste Disorders

In a review of 1645 drugs, 282 were associated with **dysgeusia** (altered sense of taste) whereas 61 created **hypogeusia** (abnormally lowered sense of taste). Of these drugs, the most common group were antineoplastic medications. In addition, in patients who receive significant radiation to the oral cavity, a substantial loss of all four tastes often develops within several weeks. Although these tastes return within 4 months for most patients, some patients are left with permanent hypogeusia; others may have persistent dysgeusia (see page 869).

Osteoradionecrosis

Osteoradionecrosis (ORN) is defined as exposed nonvital irradiated bone that persists longer than 3 months in the absence of local neoplastic disease. It represents one of the most serious complications of radiation to the head and neck. In earlier studies, the prevalence approached 15%, but the risk has been reduced to less than 5% secondary to modern therapeutic advances such as intensity-modulated radiotherapy (IMRT) and three-dimensional conformal radiation therapy (3DCRT). These newer techniques can maintain therapeutic effectiveness but decrease the total maximum radiation to the jaw bones. Most cases of ORN occur in patients who have received greater than 60 Gy, with the majority of cases occurring between 4 months and 3 years after completion of radiation therapy. Although the rate of osteoradionecrosis appears to be decreasing due to advances in radiotherapy technique, the prevalence still appears to be increasing due to a greater percentage of head and neck cancer patients receiving radiation and the increasing numbers of surviving patients.

Two major etiologic theories for osteoradionecrosis remain popular. In 1983, Marx proposed that radiation

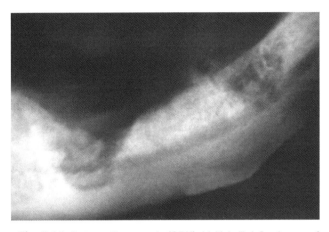

• **Fig. 8.26 Osteoradionecrosis (ORN).** Multiple ill-defined areas of radiolucency and radiopacity of the mandibular body.

produced hypovascularity, hypoxia, and hypocellularity with persistent hypoxia creating the primary disturbance leading to osteoradionecrosis. This theory laid the groundwork for use of hyperbaric oxygen in the management of affected patients. In 2002–2004, Delanian and Lefaix proposed the fibroatrophic theory that suggests radiation therapy causes activation and dysregulation of fibroblastic activity resulting in fibrotic tissue prone to breakdown. This theory has led to use of antioxidant and antifibrotic medications as a primary therapeutic approach.

Although most instances of ORN arise secondary to local trauma (such as, tooth extraction), a minority appear spontaneous. Seventy percent of osteoradionecrosis cases occur in the first three years following completion of radiation therapy, but patients remain at risk for trauma-induced ORN for the remainder of their lives. The mandible is involved 24 times more frequently than the maxilla (Fig. 8.25), and the process is three times more common in dentate patients. Affected areas of bone reveal ill-defined areas of radiolucency that may develop zones of relative radiopacity as the dead bone separates from the residual vital areas (Fig. 8.26). Intractable pain, cortical perforation, fistula formation, surface ulceration, and pathologic fracture may be present (Fig. 8.27).

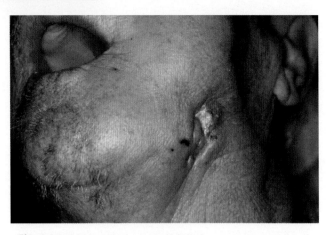

• **Fig. 8.27 Osteoradionecrosis (ORN).** Same patient as depicted in Fig. 8.26. Note fistula formation of the left submandibular area resulting from ORN of the mandibular body.

The radiation dose is the main factor associated with bone necrosis, although the proximity of the tumor to bone, the presence of remaining dentition, and the type of treatment also exert an effect. Additional factors associated with an increased prevalence include older age, male sex, poor health, or nutritional status, and continued use of tobacco or alcohol.

Prevention of bone necrosis is the best course of action. Before therapy, all unrestorable teeth and those with advanced periodontal disease should be extracted, all oral foci of infection should be eliminated, and excellent oral hygiene should be initiated and maintained. A healing time of at least 3 weeks between extensive dental procedures and the initiation of radiotherapy significantly decreases the chance of bone necrosis. Extraction of teeth or any bone trauma is strongly contraindicated during radiation therapy.

Trismus

Trismus may develop and can produce extensive difficulties concerning access for hygiene and dental treatment. Tonic muscle spasms with or without fibrosis of the muscles of mastication and the temporomandibular joint (TMJ) capsule can cause difficulties in jaw opening. When these structures are radiated heavily, jaw-opening exercises may help to decrease or prevent problems.

Developmental Abnormalities

Antineoplastic therapy during childhood can affect growth and development. The changes vary according to the age at treatment and the type and severity of therapy. Radiation can alter the facial bones and result in micrognathia, retrognathia, or malocclusion. Developing teeth are very sensitive and can exhibit several changes, such as root dwarfism, blunting of roots, dilaceration of roots, incomplete calcification, premature closure of pulp canals in deciduous teeth, enlarged canals in permanent teeth, microdontia, and hypodontia (see page 56).

Treatment and Prognosis

Optimal treatment planning involves the oral health practitioner before initiation of antineoplastic therapy. Elimination of all current or potential oral foci of infection is paramount, along with patient education about maintaining ultimate oral hygiene. Proper nutrition, cessation of tobacco use, and alcohol abstinence minimize oral complications. Once cancer therapy is initiated, efforts must be directed toward relieving pain, preventing dehydration, maintaining adequate nutrition, eliminating foci of infection, and ensuring continued appropriate oral hygiene.

Mucositis

Although therapy-related mucositis represents one of the most intensely studied toxicities related to cancer care, the current standard of care remains centered on palliative approaches combined with a small number of interventions that are available in specific situations. The best source of information originates from the Mucositis Study Group of the Multinational Association of Supportive Care in Cancer and International Society of Oral Oncology (MASCC/ISOO), with their guidelines being adopted by the European Society of Medical Oncology and the US National Comprehensive Cancer Network. As described in their most recent review, the number of interventions backed by strong science sadly is very low.

Palifermin is a keratinocyte growth factor and the only agent that has been approved by the FDA for prevention of oral mucositis. Although this agent has demonstrated significant effectiveness, its use is limited to patients receiving high-dose chemotherapy and total body irradiation prior to autologous stem cell transplantation for hematologic cancers. Concern remains that this epithelial growth factor may promote growth of tumor cells in patients with carcinoma.

Cryotherapy (placement of ice chips, ice-cold water, ice cream, or ice popsicles in the mouth 5 minutes before chemotherapy and continued for 30 minutes) has been shown to reduce significantly the prevalence and severity of oral mucositis caused by a bolus injection of 5 fluorouracil for solid cancers or high-dose melphalan before hematopoietic stem cell transplants (both are chemotherapeutic drugs with a short half-life). It has been suggested that the cold may produce local vasoconstriction leading to reduced exposure of the oral mucosa to the chemotherapeutic medications. Cryotherapy has no effect on the prevalence or severity of radiation mucositis.

Benzydamine is a nonsteroidal anti-inflammatory medication with topical analgesic and anesthetic effects. Although the medication is not marketed in the United States due to an association with hallucinations, it is available through compounding pharmacies. Benzydamine has been recommended by the MASCC/ISOO for prevention of oral mucositis in patients with head and neck cancer who are receiving radiotherapy up to 50 Gy without concomitant chemotherapy. Subsequently, a 2019 systematic review of anti-inflammatory agents in cancer patients suggested benzydamine also is effective in individuals receiving greater than 50 Gy and in those receiving chemoradiotherapy.

Zinc, in addition to being an antioxidant, favors the tissue repair process. In the MASCC/ISOO review, zinc supplementation demonstrated a reduction of oral mucositis in patients with oral cancer who were receiving radiation therapy or chemoradiation. Unfortunately, one study has suggested that cigarette smokers who use an antioxidant such as zinc may have a reduced therapeutic impact of their radiation therapy.

Low-level laser therapy also was associated with a decreased prevalence of oral mucositis in selected cancer patients. The strongest effect was seen in patients receiving high-dose chemotherapy prior to hematologic stem cell transplant with or without total body irradiation. In addition, a similar positive effect was seen in patients receiving head and neck radiation therapy without concomitant chemotherapy. In a systematic review and meta-analysis, prophylactic low-level laser therapy reduced the risk of severe oral mucositis; whereas its therapeutic use shortened the duration of severe oral mucositis in patients receiving chemotherapy or radiotherapy. In the most recent MASCC/ISOO guidelines, use of the mucosal coating agent sucralfate was not recommended. In addition, insufficient evidence was found to recommend use of the commonly utilized coating agent "magic mouthwash," a variable mixture of lidocaine, diphenhydramine, and milk of magnesia or kaopectate with or without an antifungal, antibiotic, or corticosteroid. Alternatively, the use of 0.5% doxepin mouthwash (tricyclic antidepressant with anesthetic and analgesic properties) or 2% morphine mouthwash has been recommended. Several additional coating agents exist but demonstrate insufficient scientific evidence of effectiveness to warrant a positive recommendation from MASCC/ISOO. If topical therapies are insufficient, patient-controlled analgesia with morphine or transdermal fentanyl is favored by the current guidelines.

One of the more effective mechanisms to reduce radiation-associated mucositis has been placement of midline radiation blocks or use of three-dimensional radiation treatment to limit the volume of irradiated mucosa. In addition, cotton rolls or custom splints have been used to cover metallic dental restorations to prevent localized enhanced scatter effect of the radiation.

Xerostomia

Xerostomic patients should be counseled to avoid all agents that may decrease salivation, especially the use of tobacco products and alcohol. To combat xerostomia-related caries, a regimen of daily topical fluoride (1.1% neutral sodium fluoride) application should be instituted.

The problem of chronic xerostomia has been approached using salivary substitutes and sialagogues. Use of liquids with a low pH or significant sugar content should be avoided as a mouth moistener. Because the mucous glands often demonstrate significant recovery after radiation, the sialagogues

show promise because they stimulate the residual functional glands. Moisturizing gels and sprays, sugar-free candies, chewing gum, and various artificial salivary substitutes are available. Gums and mints containing xylitol have an added benefit of inhibition of cariogenic bacteria. Many salivary substitutes are expensive and of short duration, with patients often alternatively choosing frequent use of water. In these cases, use of unfiltered fluoridated tap water is recommended over bottled water that may not contain sufficient fluoride. In controlled clinical studies, some of the most effective and longer-lasting products are one of the systemic sialagogues, such as pilocarpine, cevimeline, bethanechol, carbocholine, or anetholtrithione. Of these, the most widely used are pilocarpine and cevimeline. Although these drugs may be beneficial for many patients, they are contraindicated in patients with asthma, gastrointestinal ulcerations, labile hypertension, glaucoma, chronic obstructive pulmonary disease, and significant cardiovascular disease. Adverse reactions are uncommon but include excess sweating, rhinitis, headache, nausea, uropoiesis, flatulence, and circulatory disorders. Bethanechol also appears effective, is not contraindicated in patients with asthma and narrow angle glaucoma, and has been associated with fewer side effects than pilocarpine.

Radiation-related caries can be minimized through regular professional care, application of fluoride varnishes, and use of remineralizing toothpastes. Restoration of active areas of decay is achieved best through use of adhesive materials such as resin composites.

Taste Disorders

Although the taste buds often regenerate within 4 months after radiation therapy, the degree of long-term impairment is highly variable. In those with continuing symptoms, zinc sulfate supplements greater than the usual recommended daily doses may be beneficial.

Osteoradionecrosis

Although prevention must be stressed, cases of ORN do occur. The therapeutic approach is determined largely by the severity of the osteoradionecrosis. Early localized disease in asymptomatic or mildly symptomatic patients usually is approached conservatively with oral hygiene optimization and systemic antibiotics. In symptomatic patients with larger areas of involvement, the antioxidant and antifibrotic drugs pentoxifylline and tocopherol often are combined with sequestrectomy or saucerization to remove the necrotic bone and obtain primary mucosal closure. A meta-analysis of pentoxifylline and tocopherol has shown that the therapy is more effective than antibiotics or hyperbaric oxygen in patients with osteoradionecrosis. In resistant cases, addition of clodronate has been shown to lead to resolution in many patients. Clodronate is a unique first generation nonnitrogenous bisphosphonate that not only decreases osteoclastic activity but also stimulates osteoblastic function and reduces inflammatory cytokine expression; sadly, this

---

medication is not commercially available in the United States. Hyperbaric oxygen is expensive with numerous contraindications and possible adverse reactions. For these reasons, many reserve its use for high-risk patients with persistent osteoradionecrosis that is resistant to other forms of therapy. Some clinicians have begun use of ultrasound in place of hyperbaric oxygen due to its low adverse reaction profile and its ability to stimulate tissue regeneration and angiogenesis. For advanced cases that demonstrate extension to the lower border of the mandible, associated sinus formation, or pathologic fracture, the primary therapy is surgical resection with immediate reconstruction. The amount of bone removed is determined by clinical judgment, with the surgery extended until brightly bleeding edges are seen.

◆ MEDICATION-RELATED OSTEONECROSIS OF THE JAW (BISPHOSPHONATE-RELATED OSTEONECROSIS; ANTIRESORPTIVE-RELATED OSTEONECROSIS)

In 2003, a pattern of gnathic osteonecrosis began to be recognized, which was difficult to treat and appeared to be associated with certain medications. This process was correlated initially to bisphosphonates, leading to the name **bisphosphonate-related osteonecrosis of the jaw (BRONJ).** In the 2011 position paper of the American Dental Association (ADA), the name was modified to **antiresorptive-related osteonecrosis of the jaw (ARONJ)** due to the discovery of an association with a monoclonal antibody designed to prevent osteoclastic maturation (denosumab). Subsequently, the 2014 position paper of the American Association of Oral and Maxillofacial Surgeons (AAOMS) changed the name again to **medication-related osteonecrosis of the jaw (MRONJ)** due to the discovery that antiangiogenic therapies also may be implicated. In this update, the position paper provided a specific definition (Box 8.1) and updated the associated staging (Box 8.2). The name, medication-related osteonecrosis, is sufficiently generic and hopefully will stand the test of time. The name, definition, and associated staging remain unchanged in most recent 2022 update.

Antiangiogenic agents are prescribed for a variety of cancers and include tyrosine kinase inhibitors and monoclonal antibodies directed against vascular endothelial growth factor (Box 8.3). This risk is increased if these agents are combined

with bisphosphonates. Several additional medications also have been implicated in small series of cases including mTOR inhibitors (everolimus, temsirolimus), immunomodulators (adalimumab, infliximab, rituximab), and methotrexate; however, much more research is necessary to prove the association between these medications and MRONJ.

Currently, the medications most strongly associated with gnathic osteonecrosis include the aminobisphosphonates (nitrogen-containing bisphosphonates), denosumab, and a more recently developed medication, romosozumab. (Box 8.4). The bisphosphonates and denosumab are antiresorptives and used primarily to treat patients with osteoporosis or various cancers that involve bone (predominantly multiple myeloma, breast carcinoma, and prostate carcinoma). Less frequent uses include treatment for Paget disease, osteogenesis imperfecta, rheumatoid arthritis, and giant cell tumors of bone. Most osteonecrosis cases occur in patients receiving the medication as part of their therapy for cancer. Romosozumab is indicated primarily for patients with osteoporosis who are at high risk of fracture or have failed other osteoporosis therapy. The risk of osteonecrosis related to romosozumab use is comparable to that seen with alendronate.

Bisphosphonates, denosumab, and bevacizumab also are administered to children for a wide variety of diseases associated with childhood osteoporosis, osteogenesis imperfecta, hypercalcemia of malignancy, ectopic calcifications, chemotherapy-related osteonecrosis (such as corticosteroids), and several childhood malignancies. Despite the use of potent formulations, there have been no reports of osteonecrosis in children related to these medications. The reason for this is unclear, but investigators have speculated it may be due to the increased vascularity, high marrow cellularity, and greater bone turnover in this age group. Use of bisphosphonates in children with osteogenesis imperfecta identified a greater than 1.5-year delay in tooth eruption.

Once in the serum, 50% of bisphosphonates is cleared rapidly by the kidneys with the remainder going to bone. The medications are not distributed evenly throughout the skeleton. Osteocytes represent 85% of the cells associated with bone and do not retain the medication. In contrast, osteoclasts demonstrate an affinity eight times greater than osteocytes, but they release the drug for recycling at the end of their short 2-week life span. Osteoblasts exhibit four times the affinity of osteocytes and incorporate the medication into the bone matrix. Due to a half-life longer than 10 years, deposits of bisphosphonates can remain in place for over four decades. The effect of the medication on the bone varies with concentration. At low concentrations, the medication diminishes the ability of osteoclasts to resorb and degrade bone matrix, whereas high local concentration induces osteoclastic apoptosis. Therefore, bisphosphonates are selectively concentrated into areas of bone repair and remodeling, with potential effects over the patient's lifetime. In addition, the impact on the bone worsens as the local concentration is increased.

Denosumab is a monoclonal antibody that also reduces osteoclastic function, but it does this by inhibiting osteoclastic differentiation. Due to the short life span of osteoclasts, this medication quickly reduces osteoclastic activity by 85% with maximal reduction occurring within 1 month of an injection. The medication is not deposited in bone and has a half-life of 24.5 days, with complete clearance in 4–5 months.

Romosozumab is a monoclonal antibody that inhibits the action of the protein sclerostin. Bone cells release sclerostin which acts to decrease osteoblast-mediated bone formation and increase bone resorption. Administration of romosozumab blocks sclerostin activity, leading to increased bone formation with reduced bone resorption. The medication is administered monthly as an injection. Romosozumab use has shown rapid gains in bone mineral density with significant reductions in both vertebral and nonvertebral fractures. Serious adverse events related to its use are occasional hypersensitivity reactions and an increased frequency of serious cardiovascular events. Although rare, cases of gnathic osteonecrosis and atypical femoral fractures have been associated with its use. Less is known about this medication due to its late arrival and the reduction in its use due to the association with an increase in adverse cardiovascular events.

Any discussion of antiresorptive agents also must include information on bone healing. When a traumatic event such as an extraction occurs, the initial clot is replaced with granulation tissue and eventually woven bone. The remodeling period of this immature bone into structurally sound lamellar bone typically is 4 months but can range from 2–8 months. The final remodeling is performed by an organized synergism of osteoclasts, osteoblasts, and the local vascular supply, which work together in a cell packet known as the basic multicellular unit (BMU). This is a moving structure that requires continual replacement of participating cells at exactly the correct time and place in an ever-changing position. The osteoclasts are critical cells of the BMU and are

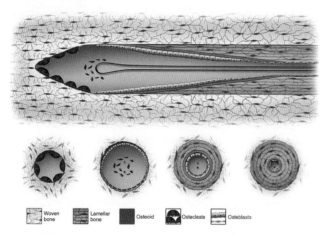

• **Fig. 8.28 Basic Multicellular Unit (BMU).** Organized synergy of osteoclasts, osteoblasts, and vasculature working together to transform immature woven bone into structural sound lamellar bone.

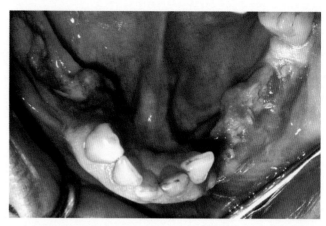

• **Fig. 8.29 Medication-Related Osteonecrosis.** Bilateral necrotic exposed bone of the mandible in a patient receiving zoledronic acid for metastatic breast cancer. (Courtesy of Dr. Brent Mortenson.)

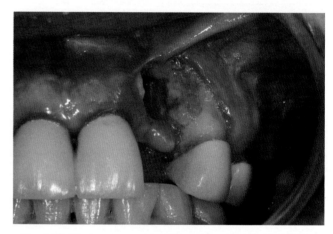

• **Fig. 8.30 Medication-Related Osteonecrosis.** Necrotic exposed bone of the left anterior maxilla in a cancer patient receiving denosumab. (Courtesy of Dr. Martin Steed).

largely responsible for the signaling necessary for the participation of the other cellular components (Fig. 8.28). Functional impairment or loss of the osteoclasts by antiresorptive drugs disrupts not only resorption but also new lamellar bone deposition and angiogenesis.

Although most osteonecrosis cases have occurred in the jaws, problems are beginning to surface elsewhere in the skeleton. Osteonecrosis of the ear has been documented following removal of an exostosis. More significantly, numerous orthopedic surgeons have reported an increased prevalence of subtrochanteric or femoral shaft fractures associated with aminobisphosphonates, leading the US Food and Drug Administration (FDA) to add this complication to the drug information.

Clinical and Radiographic Features

In an excellent comprehensive review of 2408 reported cases of BRONJ, 89% were discovered in patients who were treated with the IV formulations (primarily pamidronate and zoledronic acid) for cancer, with 43% being reported in patients with multiple myeloma. In another summary review, the prevalence of osteonecrosis associated with the IV formulations in cancer patients has been estimated to be 100 cases per 10,000 patients. Unfortunately, all the information now available is based on reported cases, and such reports frequently have inherent biases. Randomized prospective trials with appropriate controls will be necessary to obtain reliable data with respect to prevalence and management.

Osteonecrosis related to use of aminobisphosphonates for osteoporosis is most uncommon. A conservative estimate by the drug industry suggested an annual incidence of 0.7 per 100,000, but a more recent review suggested 10 cases occur per 100,000 patients (100 times less frequent than that seen in cancer patients treated with antiresorptive medications). In another systematic review with meta-analysis, the prevalence of osteonecrosis reported in patient receiving antiresorptives for osteoporosis was 0.01% whereas the frequency increased to 12% in patients receiving antiresorptive medications for cancer and 16% for those receiving both antiresorptives and antiangiogenics. However, well-designed prospective trials for the true frequency of this complication have yet to be performed. Additional risk factors for MRONJ include advanced patient age (older than 65 years), corticosteroid use, use of chemotherapy drugs, diabetes, smoking or alcohol use, poor oral hygiene, and duration of drug use exceeding 3 years. A predictive test for those at risk for bisphosphonate osteonecrosis has not been confirmed. Some investigators have suggested use of a serum marker for bone turnover, serum C-telopeptide (CTX), but the test has demonstrated insufficient reliability and accuracy in predicting the risk of developing of MRONJ.

In the previously mentioned comprehensive review, the mandible was involved in 65%, the maxilla in 27%, and both jaws in 8% (Fig. 8.29 and 8.30). In 67% of these patients, the necrosis followed a dental extraction, with another 26% arising spontaneously, and 7% associated with a variety of triggers such as denture pressure or minor trauma of a torus (Figs. 8.31 and 8.32). In patients with exposed bone, 16%

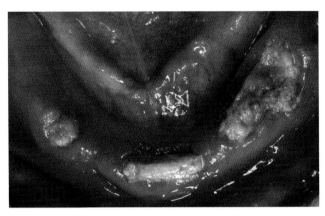

• **Fig. 8.31 Medication-Related Osteonecrosis.** Multifocal areas of exposed necrotic bone of the mandible in a patient receiving zoledronic acid for cancer.

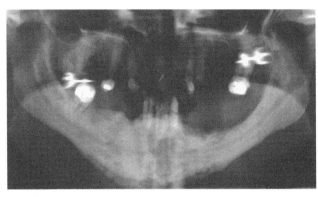

• **Fig. 8.33 Medication-Related Osteonecrosis.** Panoramic radiograph of patient depicted in Fig. 8.29. Note sclerosis of tooth-bearing areas along with multiple radiolucencies and periosteal hyperplasia of the lower border of the mandible. (Courtesy of Dr. Brent Mortenson.)

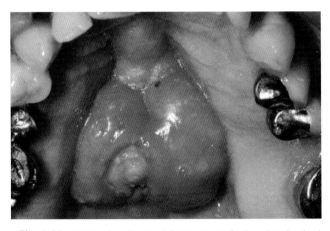

• **Fig. 8.32 Medication-Related Osteonecrosis.** Lobulated palatal torus with an area of exposed necrotic bone in a patient taking alendronate for osteoporosis.

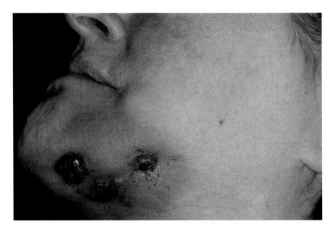

• **Fig. 8.34 Medication-Related Osteonecrosis.** Patient with multiple cutaneous sinuses associated with extensive necrosis of the left side of the mandible. The patient was taking zoledronic acid for multiple myeloma. (Courtesy of Dr. Molly Rosebush.)

were asymptomatic, 66% were painful, and another 18% demonstrated extensive involvement in which the associated pain was not responsive to antibiotics.

Research related to denosumab-associated osteonecrosis is in its infancy when compared to BRONJ, but reviews of cancer patients randomized to zoledronic acid or denosumab have demonstrated a similar frequency of osteonecrosis with these two medications. The frequency of MRONJ appears to range from 70 to 90 cases per 10,000 cancer patients receiving denosumab.

Investigators have suggested that bone at imminent risk for osteonecrosis often will demonstrate increased radiopacity before clinical evidence of frank necrosis. These changes typically occur predominantly in areas of increased bone remodeling, such as the alveolar ridges. Panoramic radiographs often will reveal a marked radiodensity of the crestal portions of each jaw, with a more normal appearance of the bone away from tooth-bearing portions. Periosteal hyperplasia also is not rare. In more severe cases, the osteonecrosis creates a moth-eaten and ill-defined radiolucency with or without central radiopaque sequestra (Fig. 8.33). In some cases, the necrosis can lead to development of a cutaneous sinus or pathologic fracture (Fig. 8.34).

Histopathologic Features

Biopsy of vital bone altered by aminobisphosphonates is not common. In such cases, the specimen often reveals irregular trabeculae of pagetoid bone, with adjacent enlarged and irregular osteoclasts that often demonstrate numerous intracytoplasmic vacuoles (Fig. 8.35). Specimens of active areas of MRONJ reveal trabeculae of sclerotic lamellar bone, which demonstrate loss of the osteocytes from their lacunae and frequent peripheral resorption with bacterial colonization (Fig. 8.36). Although the peripheral bacterial colonies often resemble actinomycetes, the infestation is not supportive of a diagnosis of invasive cervicofacial actinomycosis.

Treatment and Prognosis

Virtually all recommendations regarding management of patients who are taking or have been exposed to antiresorptive agents are empirical. No large, randomized, controlled studies have been done with respect to prevention or treatment of the complications of this therapy. The best therapeutic approach to MRONJ is prevention. In cancer patients evaluated before initiation of bisphosphonate

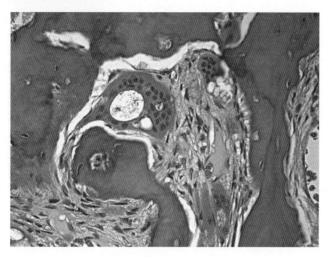

• **Fig. 8.35 Medication-Related Osseous Changes.** Pagetoid bone exhibiting enlarged, irregular osteoclasts that contain numerous intracytoplasmic vacuoles. (Courtesy of Dr. Don Cohen.)

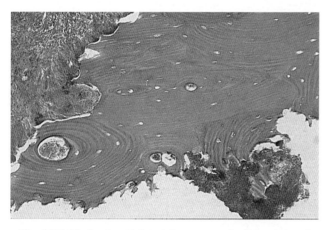

• **Fig. 8.36 Medication-Related Osteonecrosis.** Sclerotic lamellar bone exhibiting loss of the osteocytes from their lacunae and peripheral resorption with bacterial colonization.

therapy, the goal is to improve dental health to prevent future procedures that disrupt bone; this includes elimination of oral foci of infection and removal of large tori or partially impacted teeth. If only noninvasive oral care is indicated, then the initiation of the medication need not be delayed. If surgical procedures need to be performed, then a month-long delay in initiation of the medication is recommended, along with prophylactic antibiotic therapy. In an 18-year review of 273 patients presenting to the dental service of Memorial Sloan Kettering Cancer Center, a premedication dental evaluation was associated with a 0.9% prevalence of MRONJ; in contrast, patients who did not receive a premedication dental evaluation experienced a 10.5% frequency of MRONJ. This represents an almost 12-fold increase in the prevalence of MRONJ in those patients who did not have a dental evaluation prior to the start of their antiresorptive medication.

For cancer patients actively being treated with antiresorptive therapy, manipulation of bone should be avoided if possible. Conventional endodontics is a better option than extraction. If a nonvital tooth is not restorable, then endodontics should be performed and followed by crown amputation. Teeth with 1+ or 2+ mobility should be splinted; those with 3+ mobility can be extracted.

Despite the desire to avoid jaw surgery during IV therapy, occasional clinical situations may make surgical intervention unavoidable. Several investigators have suggested that the likelihood of osteonecrosis can be minimized by antibiotic prophylaxis starting 1 day prior and extending 3 days after any invasive dental procedure.

For patients with MRONJ, the primary goal of therapy is to minimize pain. Aggressive removal of dead bone typically results in further bone necrosis, and hyperbaric oxygen has not been significantly beneficial. Asymptomatic patients (Stage 1) should rinse daily with chlorhexidine and be monitored closely. Any rough edges of exposed bone should be smoothed and loose sequestra can be removed carefully. If the exposed bone irritates adjacent tissues, then coverage with a soft splint may provide some relief. In symptomatic patients (Stage 2), systemic antibiotic therapy and chlorhexidine usually reduce discomfort. If the antibiotics fail to stop the pain, then hospitalization with IV antibiotic therapy can be considered. In extensive cases with necrosis beyond the confines of the alveolus (Stage 3), the dead bone is removed surgically. Such removal may require segmental resection in the mandible and a partial or total maxillectomy of the upper jaw. Mandibular resection is reconstructed with a titanium osteosynthesis plate and may include a microsurgical free tissue transfer; whereas a prosthetic appliance is used for maxillary reconstruction. Because of the long half-life of bisphosphonates, discontinuation of the drug offers no short-term benefit. In isolated anecdotal reports of recalcitrant cases, discontinuation of the medication for 6–12 months occasionally has been associated with spontaneous sequestration and resolution.

The conservative predominantly nonsurgical therapeutic approach described in the preceding paragraph has been the subject of controversy with many surgeons supporting more aggressive intervention. Proponents of surgical intervention believe that conservative management translates to *palliation*; whereas surgical removal of necrotic and infected bone translates to *cure*. Both groups agree that Stage 3 is treated best with surgical resection, with the main controversy centering around therapy of patients presenting with Stage 1 and 2. Many believe that surgery represents the gold standard for MRONJ management in all stages with nonsurgical approaches reserved for patients who refuse surgery or are ineligible for surgery due to health reasons. These opinions are supported by numerous studies in which complete healing was achieved at a significantly higher rate in patients treated surgically. In addition, a 2019 longitudinal study of 92 patients with Stage 1 MRONJ treated with a standardized conservative nonsurgical protocol revealed 80% of the patients showed progression of the lesions with an upshift from Stage 1 to 2 or 3. This investigation suggests surgical intervention not only resolves symptoms but also prevents progression of the bone necrosis.

In a change from previous position papers, the 2022 update of the AAOMS position paper on medication-related osteonecrosis supports the value of earlier surgical intervention. Close clinical and radiographic follow-up is recommended for all stages of MRON with early operative intervention recommended for patients who fail nonoperative therapy or demonstrate worsening disease.

When surgery is performed, several adjunctive therapies in addition to antimicrobials occasionally are employed to improve the success of the procedure. These interventions include pentoxifylline and tocopherol, teriparatide, abaloparatide, hyperbaric oxygen, platelet rich plasma, and low-level laser therapy. Insufficient documentation of these interventions currently exists to warrant definitive inclusion into the current therapeutic protocols.

To eliminate all areas of necrotic bone, intraoperative fluorescence-guided debridement has been performed on bone labeled preoperatively with doxycycline. In this technique, necrotic bone appears pale bluish-white while vital bone appears brightly fluorescent. In a similar technique, the autofluorescence properties of vital bone are noted after exposure to 400–440-nm wavelengths of light. In this situation, vital bone demonstrates green fluorescence while necrotic bone reveals pale or no fluorescence.

Prevention also represents the best approach for patients taking antiresorptive medications for osteoporosis. In the original ADA position paper, a 3-month drug holiday before and after osseous surgery was suggested for any patient using bisphosphonates longer than 3 years. In the 2011 update, the ADA removed this suggestion due to the fear of increasing the skeletally related risks of low bone mass during the drug-free period. Despite this, the 2014 AAOMS update recommended use of a drug holiday for patients using bisphosphonates longer than 4 years or patients who also are utilizing systemic corticosteroids or antiangiogenic agents. In the 2022 AAOMS update, the working group was unable to reach a consensus on the use of drug holidays and was split evenly between those recommending temporary drug cessation and others who believed the risk of potential harm related to suspension of osteoporotic therapy outweighed the benefit of a drug holiday. Due to this controversy, AAOMS removed the 2014 recommendation for support of drug holidays because the benefit associated with operative intervention of MRON has not been substantiated.

A possible alternative in osteoporotic patients to minimize the risk of osteonecrosis **without a drug holiday** has been proposed. As previously mentioned, bisphosphonates concentrate in healing or remodeling bone. Once deposited, the medications remain for decades. As the concentration increases, the impact on the bone worsens. The best method to avoid osteonecrosis is to minimize the osseous deposition of bisphosphonates by ensuring the serum is free of the medication at the time of a surgical procedure and for the subsequent healing period. This can be accomplished in patients being treated for osteoporosis by suggesting use of annual IV administration of zoledronic acid and timing all surgical procedures to occur 2 months after the annual infusion. At this time, the serum will be essentially free of bisphosphonate with an additional 10 months of healing time prior to the next infusion. This is NOT a drug holiday; it selective scheduling of invasive procedures at a time when the serum is relatively free of bisphosphonate, reducing the chance of additional drug deposition into the healing bone. Alternatively, biannual injections with denosumab could be substituted for bisphosphonate therapy with any surgical procedure planned to occur 2 months after an injection (at which time 79.9% of the medication would be degraded) with 4 months of healing time prior to the next injection. Once again, this is NOT a drug holiday but would allow surgical healing during the period of lowest drug concentration. The worst approach would be to ignore totally the dates of drug administration. Surgery occurring close to the time of bisphosphonate infusion or denosumab injection would maximize the adverse effects on healing and future bone health. Due to the frequent administration pattern of the oral bisphosphonates, none of these medications can be utilized in a manner that would prevent concentration of the drug into surgical sites.

For patients with osteoporosis, all restorative, prosthodontic, conventional endodontic, and routine periodontic procedures can be implemented as needed. Although orthodontic treatment is not contraindicated, progress should be evaluated after 2–3 months of active therapy. At that point, therapy can proceed if the tooth movement is occurring predictably with normal forces. Invasive orthodontic techniques such as orthognathic surgery, four-tooth extraction cases, and miniscrew anchorage should be avoided, if possible.

When an osseous procedure is considered, the patient should be advised of the potential complications of antiresorptive use and the risk of MRONJ. Written informed consent and documentation of a discussion of the benefits, risks, and alternative therapies are highly advised.

Osteonecrosis associated with antiresorptive therapy for osteoporosis tends to be less extensive and more responsive to conservative therapy when compared to MRONJ in cancer patients. When the antiresorptive therapy can be discontinued, many cases of MRONJ resolve without surgical intervention. This spontaneous resolution occurs slowly over many months, but reports have documented greatly reduced healing times secondary to administration of teriparatide or abaloparatide (recombinant human parathyroid hormone).

The clinical approach to patients treated with antiresorptive medications varies according to the formulation of the drug, the disease being treated, and the duration of drug use. All patients who take these medications should be warned of the risks and instructed to obtain and maintain ultimate oral hygiene. The oral bisphosphonates are extremely caustic; patients should be warned to minimize oral mucosal contact and ensure the medication is swallowed completely.

Overall, the benefits of antiresorptive therapy for osteoporosis and metastatic cancer appear to greatly outweigh the risk of developing MRONJ. No patient should discontinue his or her medication against medical advice. An osteoporotic hip fracture is a life-altering event, with 75% of patients never fully recovering and a mortality rate of 20% in women and 30% in men. The antiresorptive medications reduce hip fractures by approximately 50%. A similar success has been seen in cancer patients where antiresorptive medications are associated with a significant reduction in skeletal-related adverse events.

Despite the obvious benefits of antiresorptive drugs, increased bone density does not correlate necessarily to good bone quality. The negative effects of oversuppression of bone metabolism must be considered. Reports are continuing to document spontaneous nontraumatic stress fractures with associated delayed healing in patients on long-term antiresorptive therapy for osteoporosis. Many physicians now believe that such therapy should be stopped after 5 years. Patients no longer osteoporotic could be removed from active therapy until bone density studies confirm redevelopment of significant osteoporosis. For those with continuing osteoporosis, alternatives such as teriparatide or raloxifene could be considered.

◆ OROFACIAL COMPLICATIONS OF DRUG ABUSE

Over the last decade, numerous reports have described significant oral manifestations of drug abuse, most commonly the illegal stimulants cocaine and methamphetamine.

After marijuana, cocaine represents one of the more commonly utilized illicit drugs with 1.4 million active (past month) users in the United States during 2011. Cocaine can be ingested by snorting, injecting, or smoking as free base or crack cocaine. Cocaine-laced *gummies* also are seen and can be associated with local oral changes. The drug is known by nicknames that include *blow, bump, C, candy, Charlie, coke, crack, flake, rock, snow,* and *toot.* Snorting is the main method of administration due to the associated euphoric high that lasts from 20 to 90 minutes. When snorted, cocaine is associated with a sympathetic-mediated vasoconstriction that can be associated with significant local ischemia combined with inflammation and ulceration secondary to the adulterants utilized to "cut" the cocaine.

Methamphetamine is a drug with stimulant effects on the central nervous system (CNS). In 1937, the drug was approved in the United States for the treatment of narcolepsy and attention deficit hyperactivity disorder. Within a few years, many began to use the drug to increase alertness, control weight, and combat depression. Because methamphetamine users perceive increased physical ability, greater energy, and euphoria, illegal use and manufacture of the drug began to develop. Because of greater control over the main ingredient, pseudoephedrine, production of homemade methamphetamine is decreasing but often being replaced by illegal importation of the finished product. Although illicit use of methamphetamine dropped in 2011 to 439,000 active users, the drug remains a serious problem in many areas of the nation. The drug is a powder that dissolves easily in liquid and can be snorted, injected, or taken orally. The powder form of the drug is known by nicknames that include *chalk, crank, crypto, fire, go fast, meth,* and *speed.* The powder can be purified into large crystals that can be smoked and are known as *crystal meth, crystal glass,* or *ice.*

Clinical Features

As mentioned, cocaine creates a feeling of euphoria and arousal. Other less desirable symptoms include aggressive behavior, blurred vision, dilated pupils, delirium, dizziness, light-headedness, restlessness, tinnitus, tremors, shivering, insomnia, and vomiting. Physical signs include tachycardia, tachypnea, hypertension, and hyperthermia. The sympathomimetic effects increase the oxygen demands of the myocardium, and the vasoconstrictive effects reduce oxygen delivery by the coronary arteries. This combination may trigger angina, myocardial infarction, or heart dysrhythmias.

One of the more common local complications to cocaine snorting is perforation of the nasal septum, a finding noted in approximately 5% of abusers. Loss of the nasal septum can lead to complete nasal collapse resulting in a saddle nose deformity. Less frequently, the necrosis can spread to the orbital wall, lateral nasal wall, or the hard palate and may cause palatal perforation that has been termed **cocaine-induced midline destructive lesion (CIMDL).** Associated findings include recurrent epistaxis, a nasal tone of voice (rhinolalia), regurgitation of food/drink, intranasal crusting, rhinitis, and sinusitis. Most of the reported palatal perforations are limited to the hard palate, followed by involvement of both the hard and soft palates. Perforation isolated to the soft palate is most uncommon. Although uncommon, similar nasal collapse and palatal perforations have been reported from intranasal abuse of narcotics, such as hydrocodone/acetaminophen or oxycodone/acetaminophen (Figs. 8.37 and 8.38). On occasion, mucosal burns of the lips may be seen in users of crack pipes (Fig. 8.39), and localized enamel erosion has been seen in habitual users of cocaine-laced gummies. Most cocaine in the United States is laced levamisole, an anthelminthic drug that is used to treat livestock. In humans, levamisole may cause scattered cutaneous hemorrhagic bullae and purpura.

The midline destructive process of CIMDL can mimic the clinical presentation of granulomatosis with polyangiitis (see page 333), and the confusion is complicated by the fact that approximately half of the CIMDL demonstrate antineutrophil cytoplasmic antibodies to PR3 (proteinase 3) and to a much lesser extent to MPO (myeloperoxidase). Although these similarities exist, granulomatosis with polyangiitis rarely perforates the hard palate and is negative for antineutrophil cytoplasmic antibodies against human neutrophil elastase, a finding often seen in CIMDL.

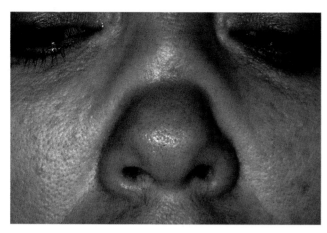

• **Fig. 8.37 Oxycodone-Related Saddle Nose Deformity.** Loss of nasal septum leading to nasal collapse in abuser of oxycodone.

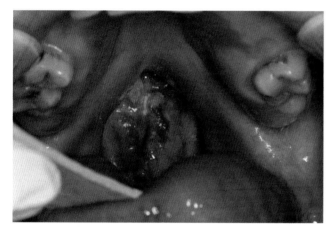

• **Fig. 8.38 Oxycodone-Related Palatal Perforation.** Midline perforation of the palate in abuser of oxycodone.

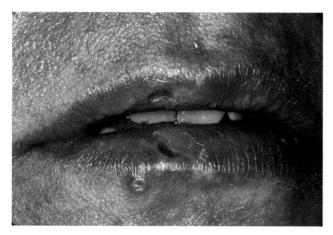

• **Fig. 8.39 Crack Pipe Burn.** Multiple erosions of the upper and lower vermilion borders secondary to burns inflicted by use of a crack pipe.

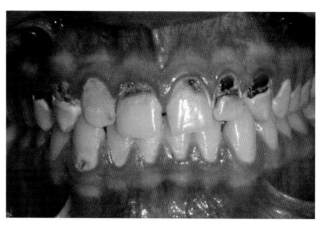

• **Fig. 8.40 Methamphetamine-Related Dental Caries.** Extensive smooth-surface decay of the anterior dentition.

Although methamphetamine abuse may occur throughout society, most users are men between the ages of 19 and 40 years. The effects of the medication last up to 12 hours, and the typical abuser reports use that exceeds 20 days per month, creating an almost continuous effect of the drug. The short-term effects of methamphetamine include insomnia, aggressiveness, agitation, hyperactivity, decreased appetite, tachycardia, tachypnea, hypertension, hyperthermia, vomiting, tremors, and xerostomia. Long-term effects additionally include strong psychologic addiction, violent behavior, anxiety, confusion, depression, paranoia, auditory hallucinations, delusions, mood changes, skin lesions, and several cardiovascular, CNS, hepatic, gastrointestinal, renal, and pulmonary disorders.

Many addicts develop delusions of **parasitosis** (**formication,** from the Latin word *formica,* which translates to *ant*), a neurosis that produces the sensation of snakes or insects crawling on or under the skin. This sensation causes the patient to attempt to remove the perceived parasites, usually by picking at the skin with fingernails, resulting in widespread traumatic injury. The factitial damage can alter dramatically the facial appearance in a short period of time, and these lesions have been nicknamed *speed bumps, meth mites, meth sores,* or *crank bugs.*

Rampant dental caries is another common manifestation and exhibits numerous similarities with milk-bottle caries. The carious destruction initially affects the facial smooth and interproximal surfaces, but without intervention, the coronal structure of the entire dentition can be destroyed (Fig. 8.40). Although it was theorized that the damage might have been secondary to corrosive agents in smoked crystal meth, a study of 571 meth users revealed that the tooth destruction is secondary to drug-related xerostomia combined with use of sugary soda, poor diet, infrequent toothbrushing, and lack of professional dental care. Of these, toothbrushing demonstrated the largest protective effect. Consumption of one or more sugary beverages daily was sufficient to contribute to decay; an increased number of sodas was not associated correspondingly to higher levels of caries. A similar degree of tooth destruction was noted in all forms of use: smoking, snorting, ingesting, and injecting.

Treatment and Prognosis

Cessation of illicit drug use is paramount in both cocaine and methamphetamine abuse. In patients with palatal perforation, complete cessation of cocaine use must be stopped 6 months prior to surgical reconstruction. If surgical reconstruction fails, a removable maxillary obturator can be constructed. Although cessation of the illicit drug use is critical, methamphetamine addicts should be encouraged during periods of xerostomia to discontinue use of highly acidic and sugar-filled soft drinks and to avoid diuretics, such as caffeine, tobacco, and alcohol. In addition, the importance of personal and oral hygiene should be stressed. Preventive measures such as topical fluorides may assist in protecting the remaining dentition.

The oral health practitioner should be alerted when an agitated, nervous adult presents with tachycardia, tachypnea, hypertension, and hyperthermia. Failure to recognize these signs can be serious. For up to 24 hours after ingestion, both cocaine and methamphetamine potentiate the effects of sympathomimetic amines. Use of local anesthetics with epinephrine or levonordefrin can lead to a hypertensive crisis, cerebrovascular accident, or myocardial infarction. Caution also should be exercised when administering sedatives, general anesthesia, nitrous oxide, or prescriptions for narcotics. A medical consultation with referral to a substance abuse center should be encouraged.

♦ ANESTHETIC NECROSIS

Administration of a local anesthetic agent can, on rare occasions, be followed by ulceration and necrosis at the site of injection. Researchers believe that this necrosis results from localized ischemia, although the exact cause is unknown and may vary from case to case. Faulty technique, such as subperiosteal injection or administration of excess solution in tissue firmly bound to bone, has been blamed. The epinephrine contained in many local anesthetics also has received attention as a possible cause of ischemia and secondary necrosis.

Clinical Features

Anesthetic necrosis usually develops several days after the procedure and most commonly appears on the hard palate (Fig. 8.41). A well-circumscribed area of ulceration develops at the site of injection.

Treatment and Prognosis

Treatment of anesthetic necrosis usually is not required unless the ulceration fails to heal. Minor trauma, such as that caused by performing a cytologic smear, has been reported to induce resolution in these chronic cases. Recurrence is unusual but has been reported in some patients in association with use of epinephrine-containing anesthetics. In these cases, the use of a local anesthetic without epinephrine is recommended.

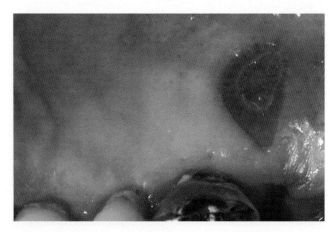

• **Fig. 8.41 Anesthetic Necrosis.** Mucosal necrosis of the hard palate secondary to palatal injection with a local anesthetic agent containing epinephrine.

♦ EXFOLIATIVE CHEILITIS

Exfoliative cheilitis is a persistent scaling and flaking of the vermilion border, usually involving both lips. The process arises from excessive production and subsequent desquamation of superficial keratin. A significant percentage of cases appear related to chronic injury secondary to habits, such as lip licking, biting, picking, or sucking. Those cases proven to arise from chronic injury are termed **factitious cheilitis**. A similar pattern also has been seen from accumulation of dried saliva intermixed with an overabundance of topically-applied medications, which results in a crusted surface. This process has been termed *ointment pseudo-cheilitis* and usually is noted in overconcerned patients, who also report a disproportionate amount of pain.

Many patients deny chronic self-irritation of the area. The patient may be experiencing associated personality disturbances, psychologic difficulties, or stress. In a review of 48 patients with exfoliative cheilitis, 87% exhibited psychiatric conditions and 47% also demonstrated abnormal thyroid function. Evidence suggests that there may be a link between thyroid dysfunction and some psychiatric disturbances.

In other cases, no evidence of chronic injury is evident. In these patients, other causes should be ruled out (e.g., atopy, chronic candidal infection, actinic cheilitis, cheilitis glandularis, hypervitaminosis A, and photosensitivity). In a review of 165 patients with acquired immunodeficiency syndrome (AIDS), more than one-quarter had alterations that resembled exfoliative cheilitis. In this group the lip alterations appeared secondary to chronic candidal infestation. The most common presentation of bacterial or fungal infections of the lips is **angular cheilitis** (see page 204). Diffuse primary infection of the entire lip is very unusual; most diffuse cases represent a secondary candidal infection in areas of low-grade trauma of the vermilion border of the lip **(cheilocandidiasis).**

In one review of 75 patients with chronic cheilitis, a thorough evaluation revealed that more than one-third represented irritant contact dermatitis (often secondary to chronic lip licking). In 25% of the patients, the cheilitis was discovered to be an allergic contact mucositis (see page 342). Atopic eczema was thought to be the cause in 19% of cases; the remaining portion was related to a wide variety of pathoses.

Despite a thorough investigation, there often remain a number of patients with classic exfoliative cheilitis for which no underlying cause can be found. These idiopathic cases are most troublesome and often resistant to a wide variety of interventions.

Clinical Features

A marked female predominance is seen in cases of factitious origin, with most cases affecting those younger than 30 years of age. Mild cases feature chronic dryness, scaling, or cracking of the vermilion border of the lip (Fig. 8.42). With progression, the vermilion can become covered with a thickened, yellowish hyperkeratotic crust that can be hemorrhagic or that may exhibit extensive fissuring. The perioral skin may become involved and exhibit areas of crusted erythema (Fig. 8.43). Although this pattern may be confused with perioral dermatitis (see page 343), the most appropriate

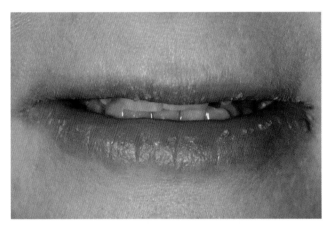

• **Fig. 8.42 Exfoliative Cheilitis.** Scaling and erythema of the vermilion border of the lower lip.

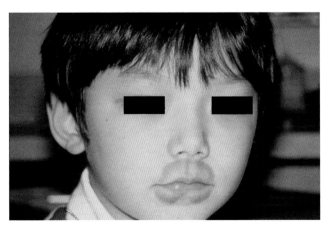

• **Fig. 8.43 Circumoral Dermatitis.** Crusting and erythema of the skin surface adjacent to the vermilion border in a child who chronically sucked on both lips.

name for this process is *circumoral dermatitis.* Both lips, or just the lower lip, may be involved. On occasion, the alterations can present in a cyclical pattern in which the changes resolve but subsequently redevelop over a relatively consistent period of time.

In patients with chronic cheilitis, development of fissures on the vermilion border is not rare. In a prevalence study of more than 20,000 patients, these fissures involved either lip and were slightly more common in the upper lip. In contrast to typical exfoliative cheilitis, these fissures demonstrate a significant male predilection and a prevalence rate of approximately 0.6%. The majority arise in young adults, with rare occurrence noted in children and older adults.

Although the cause is unknown, proposed contributing factors include overexposure to sun, wind, and cold weather; mouth breathing; bacterial or fungal infections; and smoking. An increased prevalence of lip fissures has been noted in patients with Down syndrome and may be the result of the high frequency of mouth breathing or the tendency to develop orofacial candidiasis. Application of lipstick or lip balm appears to be protective. Fissure occurrence also may be related to a physiologic weakness of the tissues. Those affecting the lower lip typically occur in the midline, whereas fissures on the upper vermilion most frequently involve a lateral position. These are the sites of prenatal merging of the mandibular and maxillary processes.

Treatment and Prognosis

In cases associated with an obvious cause, elimination of the trigger typically results in resolution of the changes. In cases with no underlying physical, infectious, or allergic cause, psychotherapy (often combined with mild tranquilization or stress reduction) may achieve resolution. In cases for which no cause can be found, therapeutic interventions often are not successful.

In patients with ointment pseudo-cheilitis, the crusted material can be removed easily when covered with a saline-soaked gauze, which then reveals an underlying normal mucosa. Although only simple reassurance and cessation of the topical medication is necessary for resolution, many patients refuse to accept this advice. Use of antidepressants such as fluoxetine in several patients has produced improvement in their symptoms with a decrease in their lip preoccupation and the associated labial crusting.

Cases that result from candidal infections often do not resolve until the chronic trauma also is eliminated. Initial topical antifungal agents, antibiotics, or both can be administered to patients in whom chronic trauma is not obvious or is denied. If the condition does not resolve, then further investigation is warranted to discover the true source of the lip alterations.

Hydrocortisone and iodoquinol (antibacterial and antimycotic) cream has been used to resolve chronic lip fissures in some patients (Fig. 8.44). Other reported therapies include various corticosteroid preparations, topical tacrolimus, sunscreens, and moisturizing preparations. In many

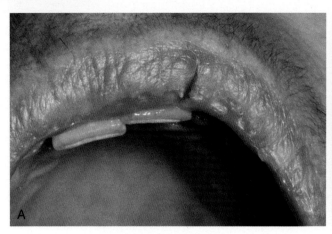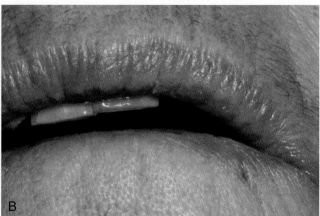

• **Fig. 8.44 Lip Fissure. A,** Chronic fissure of the vermilion border of the upper lip. **B,** Same site 2 weeks later, after use of hydrocortisone and iodoquinol cream.

cases, resistance to topical therapy or frequent recurrence is noted. In these cases, cryotherapy or excision with or without Z-plasty has been used successfully.

◆ SUBMUCOSAL HEMORRHAGE

Everyone has experienced a bruise from minor trauma. This occurs when a traumatic event results in hemorrhage and entrapment of blood within tissues. Different terms are used, depending on the size of the hemorrhage:

- Minute hemorrhages into skin, mucosa, or serosa are termed **petechiae.**
- If a slightly larger area is affected, the hemorrhage is termed a **purpura.**
- Any accumulation greater than 2 cm is termed an **ecchymosis.**
- If the accumulation of blood within tissue produces a mass, this is termed a **hematoma.**

Blunt trauma to the oral mucosa often results in hematoma formation. Less well known are petechiae and purpura, which can arise from repeated or prolonged increased intrathoracic pressure (Valsalva maneuver) associated with such activities as repeated coughing, vomiting, convulsions, or giving birth (Fig. 8.45). When considering a diagnosis of traumatic hemorrhage, the clinician should keep in mind that hemorrhages can result from nontraumatic causes, such as anticoagulant therapy, thrombocytopenia, disseminated intravascular coagulation (DIC), and several viral infections, especially infectious mononucleosis and measles.

Clinical Features

Submucosal hemorrhage appears as a nonblanching flat or elevated zone with a color that varies from red or purple to blue or blue-black (Fig. 8.46). As would be expected, traumatic lesions are located most frequently on the labial or buccal mucosa. Blunt facial trauma often is responsible, but injuries as minor as cheek biting may produce a hematoma or areas of purpura (Fig. 8.47). Mild pain may be present.

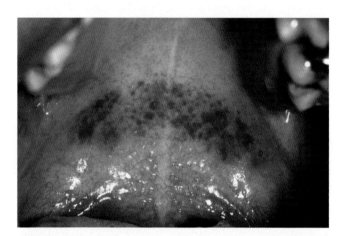

• **Fig. 8.45 Petechiae.** Submucosal hemorrhage of the soft palate caused by violent coughing.

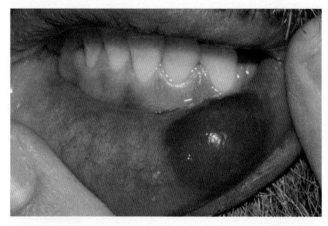

• **Fig. 8.46 Purpura.** Submucosal hemorrhage of the lower labial mucosa on the left side secondary to blunt trauma.

The hemorrhage associated with increased intrathoracic pressure usually is located on the skin of the face and neck and appears as widespread petechiae that clear within 24–72 hours. Although it has not been as well documented as the cutaneous lesions, mucosal hemorrhage can be seen in

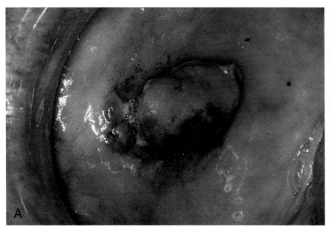
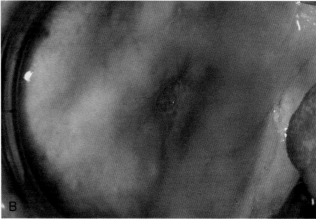

• **Fig. 8.47 Hematoma. A,** Dark-purple nodular mass of the buccal mucosa in a patient on Coumadin therapy. **B,** Near resolution of the lesion 8 days later after discontinuation of the medication. (Courtesy of Dr. Charles Ferguson.)

the same setting and most often appears as soft palatal petechiae or purpura.

Treatment and Prognosis

Often, no treatment is required if the hemorrhage is not associated with significant morbidity or related to systemic disease. The areas should resolve spontaneously. Large hematomas may require several weeks to resolve. If the hemorrhage occurs secondary to an underlying disorder, then treatment is directed toward control of the associated disease.

◆ ORAL TRAUMA FROM SEXUAL PRACTICES

Although orogenital sexual practices are illegal in many jurisdictions, they are extremely common. Among homosexual men and women, orogenital sexual activity almost is universal. For married heterosexual couples younger than age 25, the frequency has been reported to be as high as 90%. Considering the prevalence of these practices, the frequency of associated traumatic oral lesions is surprisingly low.

Clinical Features

The most reported lesion related to orogenital sex is submucosal palatal hemorrhage secondary to fellatio. The lesions appear as erythema, petechiae, purpura, or ecchymosis of the soft palate. The areas often are asymptomatic and resolve without treatment in 7–10 days (Fig. 8.48). Recurrences are possible with repetition of the inciting (exciting?) event. The erythrocytic extravasation is thought to result from the musculature of the soft palate elevating and tensing against an environment of negative pressure. Similar lesions have been induced from coughing, vomiting, or forceful sucking on drinking straws and glasses. Forceful thrusting against the vascular soft palate has been suggested as another possible cause.

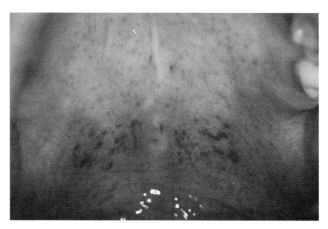

• **Fig. 8.48 Palatal Petechiae from Fellatio.** Submucosal hemorrhage of the soft palate resulting from the effects of negative pressure.

Oral lesions also can occur from performing cunnilingus, resulting in horizontal ulcerations of the lingual frenum. As the tongue is thrust forward, the taut frenum rubs or rakes across the incisal edges of the mandibular central incisors. The ulceration created coincides with sharp tooth edges when the tongue is in its most forward position. The lesions resolve in 7–10 days but may recur with repeated performances. Linear fibrous hyperplasia has been discovered in the same pattern in individuals who chronically perform the act (Fig. 8.49).

Histopathologic Features

With an appropriate index of suspicion, biopsy usually is not required; however, a biopsy has been performed in some cases of palatal lesions secondary to fellatio. These suction-related lesions reveal subepithelial accumulations of red blood cells that may be extensive enough to separate the surface epithelium from underlying connective tissue. Patchy degeneration of the epithelial basal cell layer can occur. The epithelium classically demonstrates migration of erythrocytes and leukocytes from the underlying lamina propria.

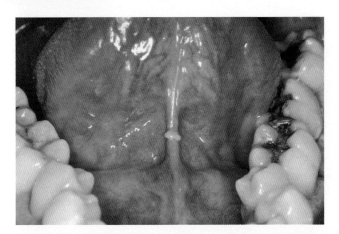

• **Fig. 8.49 Fibrous Hyperplasia From Repeated Cunnilingus.** Linear fibrous hyperplasia of the lingual frenum caused by repeated irritation from lower incisors.

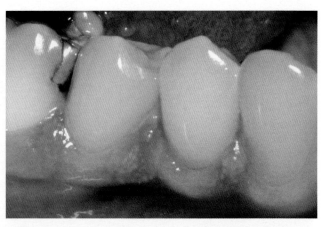

• **Fig. 8.50 Floss-Related Amalgam Implantation.** Linear strips of mucosal pigmentation that align with the interdental papillae. The patient used dental floss on the mandibular first molar immediately after the placement of the amalgam restoration. Because the area was still anesthetized, the patient impaled the floss on the gingiva and then continued forward using the amalgam-impregnated floss in the bicuspid area to create additional amalgam tattoos.

Treatment and Prognosis

No treatment is required, and the prognosis is good. In patients who request assistance, palatal petechiae can be prevented using less negative pressure and avoidance of forceful thrusting. Smoothing and polishing the rough incisal edges of the adjacent mandibular teeth can minimize the chance of lingual frenum ulceration.

◆ AMALGAM TATTOO AND OTHER LOCALIZED EXOGENOUS PIGMENTATIONS

Several pigmented materials can be implanted within the oral mucosa, resulting in clinically evident pigmentations. Implantation of dental amalgam (**amalgam tattoo**) occurs most often, with a frequency that far outdistances that for all other materials. *Localized argyrosis* has been used as another name for amalgam tattoo, but this nomenclature is inappropriate because amalgam contains not only silver but also mercury, tin, copper, zinc, and other metals.

Amalgam can be incorporated into the oral mucosa in several ways. Previous areas of mucosal abrasion can be contaminated by amalgam dust within the oral fluids. Broken amalgam pieces can fall into extraction sites. If dental floss becomes contaminated with amalgam particles of a recently placed restoration, then linear areas of pigmentation can be created in the gingival tissues as a result of hygiene procedures (Fig. 8.50). Amalgam from endodontic retrofill procedures can be left within the soft tissue at the surgical site (Fig. 8.51). Finally, fine metallic particles can be driven through the oral mucosa from the pressure of high-speed air turbines. Theoretically, the use of the rubber dam should decrease the risk; however, immediately after removal of the dam, the occlusion often is adjusted with the potential for amalgam contamination of any areas of mucosal damage.

In one interesting report, metal from silver solder on orthodontic brackets leached into adjacent gingival crevices and created discolorations that were thought to be secondary to formation of insoluble precipitates from metabolic

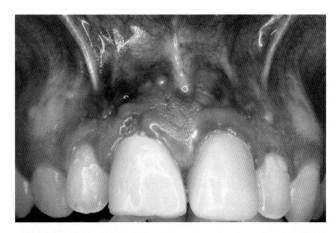

• **Fig. 8.51 Endodontic-Related Amalgam Implantation.** Multifocal areas of mucosal discoloration overlying the maxillary anterior incisors, which have been treated with apical retrofill procedures.

bacterial by-products. Submucosal implantation of pencil graphite, coal and metal dust, fragments of broken carborundum disks, dental burs, and, in the past, charcoal dentifrices, have resulted in similar-appearing areas of discoloration. Localized gingival discoloration also has been seen when fractured zirconia abutments abraded the associated titanium implant, releasing metallic fragments into the surrounding soft tissue.

Intentional tattooing, which can be found in approximately 25% of the world's population, also may be performed in the oral cavity. Although some cases are culturally related, health professionals also are responsible for several intentional oral and facial tattoos for the purpose of demonstrating landmarks, establishing progress of orthodontic treatment, marking sites of uncovered dental implants, judging tumor response to antineoplastic therapies, repigmenting areas of vitiligo, cosmetically disguising

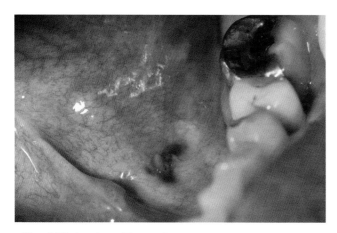

• **Fig. 8.52 Amalgam Tattoo.** Area of mucosal discoloration of the floor of the mouth on the patient's left side.

disfigured areas, and applying permanent cosmetic makeup. Injudicious intraoral use of these marking agents can cause diffusion of the pigment with discoloration of the adjacent skin surface.

Clinical and Radiographic Features

Amalgam tattoos appear as macules or, rarely, as slightly raised lesions. They may be black, blue, or gray. The borders can be well defined, irregular, or diffuse (Fig. 8.52). Lateral spread may occur for several months after the implantation. Any mucosal surface can be involved, but the most common sites are the gingiva, alveolar mucosa, and buccal mucosa (Fig. 8.53).

Periapical radiographs, when taken, are negative in many cases. When metallic fragments are visible radiographically, the clinical area of discoloration typically extends beyond the size of the fragment. The fragments are densely radiopaque, varying from several millimeters to pinpoint in size (see Fig. 8.53). On occasion, the pattern of the amalgam dispersal has been sufficiently unique to be used as a distinctive characteristic in the identification of unknown deceased individuals.

Cosmetic tattooing is gaining in popularity and may include injection of permanent cosmetic inks into the eyelids, eyebrows, and vermilion border of the upper and lower lips. On occasion, patients may react to the material and experience swelling, burning, and itching at the site, followed by enlargement and induration. These reactions are seen most frequently in association with red cosmetic tattoos and may arise days or several years after placement. In such cases, biopsy reveals a granulomatous, lichenoid, or rarely a pseudolymphomatous reaction to the foreign material. Reports also have documented development of squamous cell carcinoma or a keratoacanthoma-like proliferation of the vermilion border arising in patients with minimal sun exposure and prior placement of permanent red makeup tattoo.

Intentional intraoral tattoos occur most frequently on the anterior maxillary facial gingiva of individuals from several

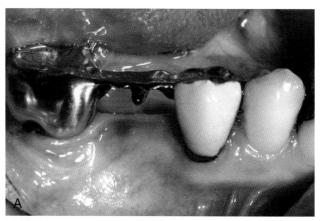

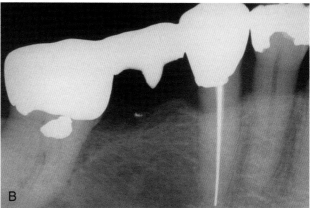

• **Fig. 8.53 Amalgam Tattoo. A,** Area of mucosal discoloration of the mandibular alveolar ridge immediately below the bridge pontic. **B,** Radiograph of the same patient showing radiopaque metallic fragment present at the site of mucosal discoloration.

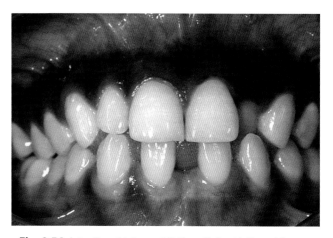

• **Fig. 8.54 Intentional Intraoral Tattoo.** Cultural tattoo of the maxillary facial gingiva in a patient from Senegal. (Courtesy of Dr. Kristin McNamara.)

African countries and have been documented at institutions in the United States (Fig. 8.54). In these cases, the anterior maxillary facial gingiva is given a blue-black discoloration that tends to fade to mostly gray over time. Occasionally, tattoos are placed on the labial mucosa of adults in the United States to convey a personal, often vulgar, message (Fig. 8.55).

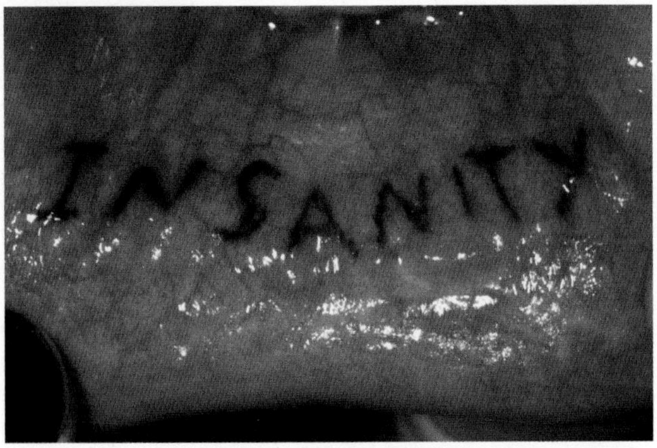

• **Fig. 8.55 Intentional Intraoral Tattoo.** Amateur tattoo of the lower labial mucosa. (Courtesy of Dr. Edward Herschaft.)

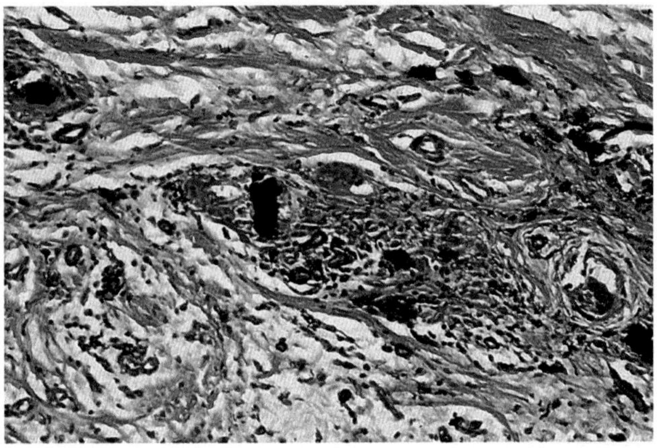

• **Fig. 8.56 Amalgam Tattoo.** Numerous dark, solid fragments of amalgam are surrounded by a lymphohistiocytic inflammatory infiltrate.

Histopathologic Features

Microscopic examination of amalgam tattoos reveals pigmented fragments of the metal within the connective tissue. Scattered, large, dark, solid fragments or numerous fine, black, or dark-brown granules may be seen (Fig. 8.56). The silver salts of the dental amalgam preferentially stain the reticulin fibers, especially those encircling nerves and vascular channels (Fig. 8.57).

The biologic response to amalgam appears related to particle size and the elemental composition of the amalgam. Large fragments often become surrounded by dense fibrous connective tissue with mild inflammation. Smaller particles typically are associated with a more significant inflammatory response that may be granulomatous or a mixture of lymphocytes and plasma cells. Graphite implantation appears similar microscopically to amalgam but usually presents as a coarser material that often can be differentiated by its pattern of birefringence after treatment with ammonium sulfide and by the lack of staining of the reticulin fibers. In addition, energy dispersive X-ray microanalysis can be used to identify the type of material present within areas of foreign body tattoos.

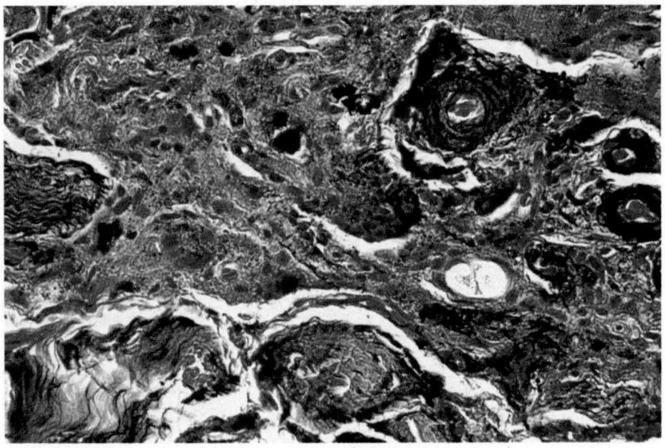

• **Fig. 8.57 Amalgam Tattoo.** Dark amalgam stain encircling numerous vascular channels.

Treatment and Prognosis

To confirm the diagnosis of amalgam tattoo, the clinician can obtain radiographs of the areas of mucosal discoloration to demonstrate the metallic fragments. The films should be capable of high detail, because many of the fragments are no larger than the point of a pin.

No treatment is required if the fragments can be detected radiographically. If no metallic fragments are found and the lesion cannot be diagnosed clinically, then biopsy may be needed to rule out the possibility of melanocytic neoplasia. On occasion, the amalgam implantation may create pigmentation in a cosmetically objectionable location such as the anterior maxillary facial gingiva. In such cases, conservative surgical excision can be performed; alternatively amalgam tattoos have been removed successfully with Q-switched ruby or alexandrite lasers. When located in a cosmetically sensitive location such as the anterior maxillary facial gingiva, a connective tissue graft often is combined with removal of the discolored soft tissue. With respect to the allergic reactions associated with cosmetic tattoos, a variety of treatments such as surgical removal, carbon dioxide laser, and corticosteroids have been used with variable results. In cosmetic tattoos associated with a granulomatous reaction, allopurinol or hydroxychloroquine also have been used successfully.

◆ ORAL PIERCINGS AND OTHER BODY MODIFICATIONS

Historical evidence from almost every continent shows that body piercing is an ancient practice with a strong association with religious, cultural, or superstitious beliefs. In the Western world, body piercing beyond the earlobes has become increasingly popular as a method of self-expression in recent years. In a survey of 481 college students in the United States, 51% admitted body piercing, and the prevalence still appears to be rising. Usually, the piercing is performed to place jewelry in sites such as the eyebrows, helix of the ears, nose, navel, nipples, genitals, and several intraoral sites.

Forked tongue (split tongue, bifid tongue) is a rather recent addition to the art of body modification, with few associated publications. In this practice, the anterior one-third of the tongue is split down the middle. This has been performed slowly by pulling fishing line through a pierced hole and tightening the loop over a period of 3 weeks or using a surgical instrument or laser to quickly separate the two halves. Some form of cautery is necessary to prevent the halves from reuniting. Forked tongue also has been reported as a complication of tongue piercing.

Another practice with unique orofacial manifestations is implantation of a form of **talisman** (magical charm) called **susuk (charm needles, charm pins).** This practice is common in Southeast Asia, especially Malaysia, Thailand, Singapore, Indonesia, and Brunei. The susuk is placed by a native magician or medicine man termed *bomoh* and is thought to enhance or preserve beauty, relieve pain, bring success in business, or provide protection against harm. Most of the individuals with susuk are Muslims, although Islam strictly prohibits black magic. Therefore, many affected individuals will deny placement of susuk, even when confronted directly with hard evidence.

Clinical and Radiographic Features

Intraoral piercings are noted most frequently in adolescents and young adults, with a female predominance. In a systematic review of the literature, oral and peri-oral piercings were seen in approximately 5.2% of young adults. The most affected sites are the tongue, lips, buccal mucosa, and, rarely, the uvula. If no complications occur, healing of the piercing site takes place within 4–6 weeks. Currently, the jewelry most often is niobium, surgical steel, or titanium; however, a wide variety of materials such as horn, ivory, plastic, stone, wood, aluminum, brass, copper wire, platinum, silver, and gold are used. In the tongue, the most frequent adornment is a **barbell** (Dumbbell might be a better name!) consisting of a metal rod with a ball that screws onto each end (Fig. 8.58). The lip jewelry is termed a **labret** and most often consists of a ring or a rod with a flat end attached to the mucosal side and a round ball for the cutaneous surface (Fig. 8.59).

In a review of US hospital emergency departments from 2002 to 2008, an estimated 24,459 patients presented with oral piercing-related injuries. Complications during the procedure include bleeding, nerve damage, localized infection,

and the risk of transmission of infectious diseases, such as hepatitis or HIV. Immediate postoperative complications include pain, swelling, hematoma formation, increased salivary flow, speech impediment, and a local allergic reaction. Serious complications such as Ludwig angina, infective endocarditis, and fatal brain abscesses have been documented. Chronic complications include mucosal or gingival trauma, chipped or fractured teeth, hypersalivation, aspiration or swallowing of jewelry, tissue hyperplasia around the posts, and embedded jewelry. Gingival recession (labrets, barbells) and tooth fracture (barbells) are extremely common, with the prevalence closely related to the duration of use. In a systematic review of previous publications, individuals with lip piercings were 4.14 times more likely to demonstrate gingival recession, whereas individuals with tongue piercing were 2.77 times more likely to exhibit recession and 2.44 times more likely to reveal tooth fracture. Habitual biting or chewing the jewelry often is associated with severe dental abrasion or movement of teeth. A fatal squamous cell carcinoma of the tongue arising at the site of a metal piercing has been reported in a 26-year-old patient.

In individuals with forked tongues, the anterior half of the tongue is split down the middle (Fig. 8.60). Risks of the

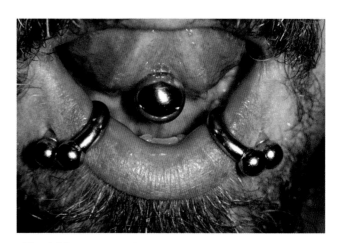

• **Fig. 8.59 Labial Piercing.** Lower lip pierced bilaterally with labrets consisting of a circular rod with terminating balls. The patient also has a lingual barbell.

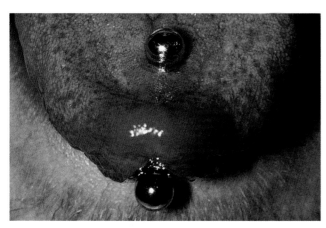

• **Fig. 8.58 Lingual Piercing.** Tongue pierced with a jewelry item known as a *barbell.*

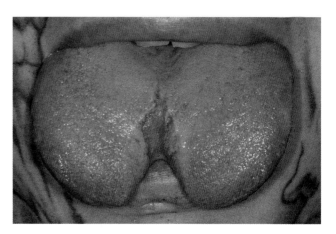

• **Fig. 8.60 Forked Tongue.** Anterior portion of the tongue divided into two separate lobes, each of which can be controlled independently. (Courtesy of Dr. Fleming Chisholm.)

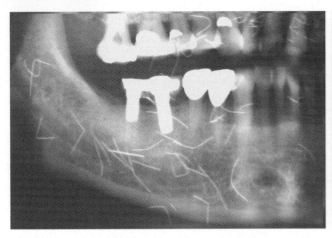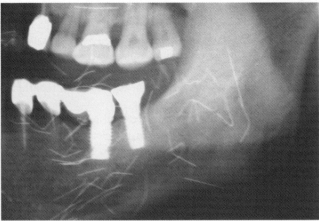

• **Fig. 8.61 Susuk (Charm Needles).** Panoramic radiograph showing multiple radiopaque needles superimposed on the jaws. (Courtesy of Dr. Jeff Bayme.)

procedure include inflammation, infection, profuse or prolonged hemorrhage, and permanent neurovascular damage. After healing, some individuals have developed the ability to control each half independently.

Susuk usually is shaped like a needle that is pointed on one end and blunt on the other. Most are made from silver or gold, measure 0.5 mm in diameter, and vary from 0.5 to 1.0 cm in length. Rarely, they are made from diamonds. The pins vary in number from one to many and are inserted subcutaneously, often in a symmetrical fashion. The orofacial region is the most common location (forehead, cheeks, and lips), but some choose the chest, arms, breasts, pubic region, and spinal area. In most instances, the individuals are middle-aged adults. Normally, no clinical evidence exists, either visually or by palpation, and the pins are discovered during routine radiography for unrelated medical or dental problems (Fig. 8.61).

Treatment and Prognosis

As mentioned, intraoral barbells and labrets are associated with an increasing prevalence of oral complications that relate closely with duration of use. The patient should be encouraged strongly to remove the jewelry. On removal, if the site demonstrates significant inflammation, local débridement, antibiotic therapy, and chlorhexidine mouthwash may be appropriate.

Except for slight sibilant distortions and shortening of the protrusive length of the tongue, few long-term adverse events have been noted in patients with forked tongues.

Susuk have not been associated with harmful effects, and no treatment is required. If the needles have a ferrous content, then magnetic resonance imaging (MRI) would be contraindicated. On occasion, affected individuals request removal of the susuk before they die because they believe their death will be excruciatingly painful. Despite this, the needles should not be removed without consent.

◆ ORAL LESIONS ASSOCIATED WITH COSMETIC FILLERS

In recent years, oral health care providers have encountered a variety of oral lesions secondary to injection of cosmetic fillers. These substances are used to augment the lips, cheeks, and chin or to minimize skin folds in the forehead, around the nose, and perioral surfaces. These fillers can be divided into temporary (collagen, hyaluronic acid), long-term (hyaluronic acid with dextranomer beads, poly-L-lactic acid, calcium hydroxyapatite) and permanent fillers (paraffin, silicon preparations, polymethylmethacrylate microspheres, hydroxyethyl-methacrylate, polyacrylamide gel, polyalkylimide gel, polyvinyl hydroxide microspheres in polyacrylamide gel, polytetrafluoroethylene). A number of these formulations are not approved for use in the United States, but patients may present with complications of fillers placed in other countries. The most encountered agents in an active oral pathology laboratory include hyaluronic acid (Restylane, Juvederm), poly-L-lactic acid (Sculptra), polymethylmethacrylate (Artecoll, ArteFill), and hydroxyapatite (Radiesse). Problems have occurred when these materials present as tumor-like masses in patients who do not make the connection to their previous cosmetic procedure or are reluctant to mention prior use of dermal filler. In order to help pathologists identify these various compounds, an online atlas of foreign materials has been established by the American Academy of Oral & Maxillofacial Pathology (AAOMP).

Clinical and Radiographic Features

The complications associated with dermal fillers can be divided into early and late. Early complications include ecchymosis, swelling/edema, infection, itching, pain, and rapid onset of dermal/mucosal nodules. Late or delayed complications include persistent ecchymosis, swelling/edema, neovascularization, hyperpigmentation, bluish discoloration from superficial placement of hyaluronic acid, chronic infection, and delayed formation of nodules. Patients also have been reported with recurring soft tissue swellings that mimic angioedema and orofacial granulomatosis several years after placement of cosmetic filler material.

Severe adverse reactions occur with some materials but are rare. These reactions include local allergic response, anaphylaxis, arthralgia, myalgia, retinal artery thrombosis, facial paralysis, and renal failure. The most common presentations in the dental office are latent tumor-like nodules usually presenting in the lips, anterior buccal mucosa, and mandibular vestibule (Fig. 8.62 and 8.63). These nodules often arise years after placement of the material. In patients with hydroxyapatite filler, clusters of radiopaque material have been discovered on panoramic and cone beam radiographs. In addition, head and neck cancer patients with dermal fillers sometimes have shown false positive uptake in oral tissues and adjacent lymph nodes during positron emission tomography/computed tomography (PET/CT) being used for pre-surgical staging of head and neck cancer.

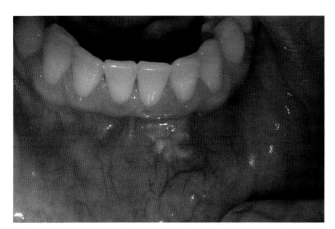

• **Fig. 8.62 Cosmetic Filler Material.** Yellow submucosal mass of the mandibular labial vestibule. Biopsy revealed hydroxyapatite (Radiesse) with fibrosis and granulomatous inflammation. (From Daley T, Damm DD, Haden JA, et al: Oral lesions associated with injected hydroxyapatite cosmetic filler, *Oral Surg Oral Med Oral Pathol Oral Radiol* 114:107–111, 2012.)

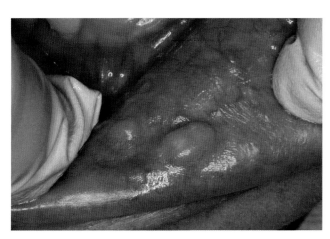

• **Fig. 8.63 Cosmetic Filler Material.** Firm submucosal mass of the right lower labial mucosa. Biopsy revealed stromal pools of hyaluronic acid (Restylane). (Courtesy of Dr. Walker Pendarvis).

Histopathologic Features

The histopathologic features are variable but often distinctive. In many cases, the identification of the specific material by the pathologist allows the clinician to present the patient with a brand name that often convinces the reluctant individual to admit a previous cosmetic procedure.

The nonpermanent filler, hyaluronic acid, often is nonimmunogenic and presents as pools of amorphous and lightly basophilic material surrounded by dense bands of collagen without a foreign body reaction although it may induce a remarkable granulomatous response in some patients. When removed due to formation of tumor-like nodules, most of the cosmetic filler materials are surrounded by dense collagen and granulomatous inflammation (Fig. 8.64). In many instances, the microscopic appearance of the material is sufficient for identification.

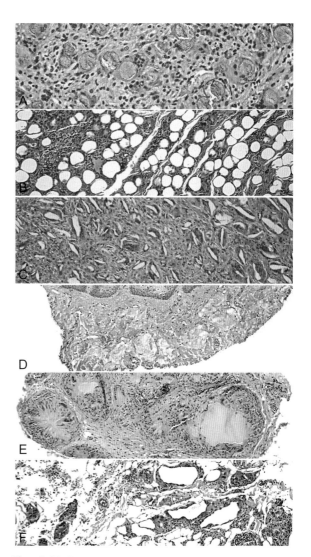

• **Fig. 8.64 Cosmetic Filler Material.** Cosmetic filler materials embedded in dense fibrous connective tissue with associated granulomatous inflammation. **A,** Hydroxyapatite (Radiesse) as seen in the biopsy of lesion depicted in Fig. 8.62. **B,** Different patient exhibiting polymethylmethacrylate (ArteFill). **C,** Different patient exhibiting poly-L-lactic acid (Sculptra). **D,** Different patient exhibiting hyaluronic acid (Restylane). **E,** Different patient exhibiting pools hyaluronic acid encased by granulomatous inflammation. **F,** Different patient exhibiting silicone.

Treatment and Prognosis

In many instances, the diagnostic biopsy is excisional and completely eradicates the problematic mass. In patients with larger lesions, surgical excision can be problematic due to numerous finger-like extensions of the material into the surrounding tissues. Additional therapeutic inventions have been employed and include a variety of antibiotics, hyaluronidase, injectable or systemic corticosteroids, antihistamines, antimalarial medications, 5-fluorouracil, imiquimod, allopurinol, colchicine, retinoic acid, calcineurin inhibitors, and laser removal.

◆ SYSTEMIC METALLIC INTOXICATION

Ingestion or exposure to any one of several heavy metals can cause significant systemic and oral abnormalities. Exposure to heavy metals may be massive, resulting in acute reactions, or it may be minimal over a longer period, producing chronic changes. Oral alterations from ingestion of lead, mercury, silver, bismuth, arsenic, and gold are rare but may occur and warrant discussion. Oral complications from excessive zinc, iron, tin, and manganese are extremely rare.

Lead

Little is known about the prevalence of lead poisoning **(plumbism),** but lead is one of the most widespread environmental toxins affecting children in the United States. Lead solder for plumbing was not banned until 1986. Homes built before then have the potential for significant water contamination, and one of the primary causes of lead intoxication in infants is formula preparation using tap water tainted by the metal.

Another significant source of lead poisoning in children is lead-based paint; children may ingest chips of the paint in older homes or be exposed to the fumes or dust during sanding and renovation. Paint with a high lead content was not restricted until 1977 and remains in many homes. Removal of lead from gasoline began in 1972 but was not completed in the United States until 1995.

Adult exposure also occurs and often is related to industry. The potential for exposure exists during handling of lead oxide batteries, in lead-processing industries, and from the welding of lead-covered surfaces. Some food and drink containers or vegetables grown in lead-contaminated soil also may contain inappropriate levels of the metal. Lead contamination in illicit alcohol has made the distinction between symptoms of lead intoxication and chronic alcohol abuse very difficult in certain sections of the American Deep South. Lead also can be found in pigments, books, brass fixtures, pottery, ceramics, crystal, electrical cable, radiation shielding, folk remedies, and cosmetics. Rarely, plumbism arises from retained lead bullet fragments in gunshot victims.

Mercury

The danger of mercury exposure is well known. Elemental mercury is poorly absorbed, and its ingestion is relatively harmless. In contrast, inhalation of mercury vapor is very hazardous, with a high rate of absorption and systemic retention. Ingestion of mercury salts (e.g., mercurous chloride) also is associated with significant adverse reactions. Exposure has occurred in association with the use of mercury in teething powders, baby powders, diapers, cathartic agents, and anthelmintic preparations. Investigators also have implicated thimerosal, an ethyl mercury antiseptic utilized in some vaccinations.

A great deal of attention has been directed toward the mercury released from dental amalgams, but no well-documented adverse health effects have been identified (except for relatively rare contact hypersensitivity to amalgams, see page 346). The level of mercury that is released from amalgams has been shown not to exceed the range expected from background exposure to environmental mercury. In 2009, the FDA issued a final regulation on dental amalgam, which stated the levels of mercury released by dental amalgam fillings are not high enough to cause harm in patients. To shed light on this controversy, the National Institutes of Health (NIH) funded two large randomized clinical trials that compared the neurologic and renal effects of dental amalgam in a 7-year study of a large cohort of children. In these pivotal investigations, no adverse effects from dental amalgam were seen. Interestingly, the control group that received only composite restorations demonstrated a 50% higher need for additional restorative treatment because of the failure of their restorations during the long-term study.

Silver

Silver has known antibacterial properties and has been associated with several additional health benefits. In the past, silver compounds were used topically in nose drops and systemically for a variety of disorders including mental illness, epilepsy, nicotine addition, common colds, sinusitis, gastrointestinal ulcerations, syphilis, and gonorrhea. Because of the numerous complications, including silver intoxication, in 1999 the FDA concluded that colloidal silver or silver salts generally are not recognized as safe and effective and are misbranded. Several silver nitrate and silver sulfadiazine formulations remain available by prescription. In addition, silver-impregnated dressings are used for their antimicrobial properties and the decreased frequency of dressing changes in patients with toxic epidermal necrolysis (see page 783). Although anecdotal descriptions of subsequent argyria have been reported secondary to use of these dressings, larger series have demonstrated a degree of systemic absorption of silver but no systemic adverse effects. These products should be used only under strict supervision. Well-documented examples of generalized argyria have been seen secondary to long-term treatment of aphthous ulcerations, denture sores, and minor gingival hemorrhage with topical silver nitrate.

Despite the efforts of the FDA, devices for production of homemade colloidal silver suspension and several colloidal silver formulations continue to be marketed over the Internet and in health food stores as essential mineral supplements for diseases such as arthritis, cancer, diabetes, AIDS, and herpes.

During the 2020 COVID-19 epidemic, the US Food and Drug Administration (FDA) and the Federal Trade Commission (FTC) had to issue several cease-and-desist orders to a number of internet vendors who were marketing colloidal silver as a miracle cure for coronavirus. These unregulated silver products have no known physiologic function, and their continued use cannot be supported.

Bismuth and Arsenic

In the United States, excess exposure to bismuth and arsenic currently is rare. The medical use of these metals has diminished dramatically. Most current cases arise from occupational exposure except for excessive arsenic in drinking water seen predominantly in isolated areas of India and Southeast Asia. Bismuth was used in the past for treatment of venereal diseases and various dermatoses, whereas arsenic compounds were prescribed for asthma and skin disorders, such as psoriasis. Bismuth iodoform paraffin paste continues to be used by otolaryngologists and oral surgeons as a surgical pack, with rare reports of associated toxicity. In addition, bismuth subsalicylate tablets (Pepto-Bismol) have been reported to produce localized mucosal discoloration. Chronic exposure to arsenic continues in some lesser developed areas of the world from drinking contaminated water.

Gold

Gold has been used in medical treatment in the past and continues to be used today in selected cases of active rheumatoid arthritis and other immunologically mediated diseases. In these cases, the side effects are well known, and physicians observe the patients closely. In reviews of large-scale skin testing, gold has been found to be among the top 10 most frequent allergens, with positive reactions seen in about 10% of the population, including increased prevalence in patients who have gold dental restorations.

Clinical Features

Lead

Lead poisoning results in nonspecific systemic signs and symptoms, thereby making the ultimate diagnosis very difficult. The presentation is extremely variable and determined by the type of lead and the age of the patient. Patients with acute cases most often have abdominal colic, which may occur along with anemia, fatigue, irritability, and weakness. Encephalopathy and renal dysfunction also may occur. Chronic exposure causes dysfunction of the nervous system, kidneys, marrow, bone, and joints. Symptoms generally include fatigue, musculoskeletal pain, and headache. Bones and teeth represent a major reservoir in patients with chronic plumbism, with 90% of the body's deposition being within bone. In radiographs of the long bones in infants, a radiopaque lead line often is noted along the epiphyseal plates.

Oral manifestations include ulcerative stomatitis and a gingival lead line **(Burton line).** The lead line appears as a bluish line along the marginal gingiva resulting from the action of bacterial hydrogen sulfide on lead in the gingival sulcus to produce a precipitate of lead sulfide. In a review of 187 lead-acid battery workers demonstrating chronic lead toxicity, 49.3% demonstrated a lead line along the gingival margins. As expected, this line was noted more frequently in individuals with poor oral hygiene and greater amounts of plaque. Gray areas also may be noted on the buccal mucosa and tongue.

Mercury

Mercury poisoning also may be acute or chronic. With acute cases, abdominal pain, vomiting, diarrhea, thirst, pharyngitis, and gingivitis typically are present. With chronic cases, gastrointestinal upset and numerous neurologic symptoms occur. The neurologic symptoms are termed **erethism** and include excitability, tremors, memory loss, insomnia, shyness, weakness, and delirium. Because mercury salts formerly were used in the processing of felt, hat makers in past centuries were exposed to the metal and experienced similar symptoms, giving rise to the phrase "mad as a hatter." Oral changes include a metallic taste and ulcerative stomatitis combined with inflammation and enlargement of the salivary glands, gingiva, and tongue. The gingiva may become blue-gray to black. Mercuric sulfide can be generated by the bacterial action on the metal and can cause significant destruction of the alveolar bone with resultant exfoliation of teeth.

Chronic mercury exposure in infants and children is termed **acrodynia (pink disease** or **Swift-Feer disease).** An erythematous and pruritic rash is present, often with desquamation of the palms and soles. Severe sweating, increased lacrimation, photophobia, neurologic symptoms, hypertension, tachycardia, and gastrointestinal upset also may be present. On occasion, these highly irritable children have torn out patches of their hair. Oral signs include excessive salivation, ulcerative gingivitis, bruxism, and premature loss of teeth. The triad of red, painful desquamating fingers and toes, neurologic symptoms, and hypertension should warn of the possibility of mercury intoxication. Overlap with Kawasaki disease has been noted, suggesting evaluation of 24-hour urine mercury levels when considering that diagnosis.

Silver

Acute silver intoxication can produce coma, pleural edema, hemolysis, and bone marrow failure. Chronic systemic silver intoxication is known as **argyria** and may have toxic effects on the liver, spleen, kidney, intestinal tract, and respiratory system. Silver is disseminated throughout the body with substantial amounts accumulating as subepithelial deposits in the skin. These deposits result in a diffuse grayish discoloration that develops primarily in the sun-exposed areas (Fig. 8.65). The conjunctivae, sclerae, and nails also may be pigmented. One of the first signs of argyria occurs in the oral cavity and appears as a slate-blue silver line along the gingival margins. This discoloration is secondary to deposition of metallic silver and silver sulfide pigments. In addition, the oral mucosa often exhibits a diffuse blue-black discoloration.

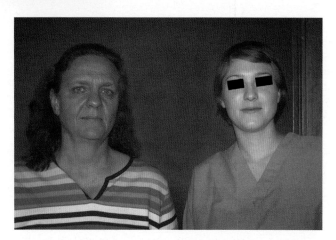

• **Fig. 8.65 Argyria.** Grayish discoloration of the face compared with a more normal facial complexion in an individual who used a silver-containing nutritional supplement. Before development of silver intoxication, this blue-eyed, red-haired individual had a very light complexion. (Courtesy of Bradford R. Williams.)

Bismuth

Systemic bismuth toxicity presents with confusion, encephalopathy, hepatorenal impairment, and methemoglobinemia. Chronic bismuth exposure also can result in a diffuse blue-gray discoloration of the skin, conjunctivae, or oral cavity. A blue-gray line along the gingival margin like that seen from lead intoxication is the most common intraoral presentation. Associated ptyalism, burning, stomatitis, and ulceration may be seen. Intoxication from bismuth-containing surgical packs has been associated with CNS symptoms, such as delirium. Chronic use of bismuth subsalicylate tablets can create a removable black discoloration of the otherwise normal filiform papillae (see Fig. 1.26, page 13).

Arsenic

Arsenic is a potent human carcinogen associated with cancers of the skin, lungs, kidney, urinary bladder, and possibly liver. Additional health effects from chronic excess arsenic include hypertension, diabetes mellitus, neurologic abnormalities, and disorders of the cardiovascular, pulmonary, hepatic, and renal systems. Progressive arterial occlusion can result in dry gangrene and spontaneous amputation of extremities, which has been termed "blackfoot disease." Significant cutaneous hyperkeratosis and a diffuse macular hyperpigmentation are seen frequently. The discoloration rarely may involve the oral mucosa and is due to both the presence of the metal and an increased melanin production. Additional oral manifestations are very uncommon and typically appear as excessive salivation and painful areas of necrotizing ulcerative stomatitis. In the past, extensive dorsal hyperkeratosis of the tongue was seen in patients with syphilis and may be related to arsenic therapy used before the advent of antibiotic therapy.

Gold

The most common complication of gold therapy is dermatitis, which often is preceded by a warning signal: pruritus. Although a generalized exfoliative dermatitis with resultant

alopecia and loss of nails can be seen, dermatitis about the face, eyelids, and at direct sites of skin contact is the most common presentation. Because of the high frequency of allergy to gold, skin testing often is performed before administration of gold drug therapy.

The second most common adverse reaction to gold is severe oral mucositis, which most frequently involves the buccal mucosa, lateral border of the tongue, palate, and pharynx. These mucosal changes represent a systemic allergic reaction and are different from intraoral contact gold hypersensitivity (see page 346). A metallic taste often precedes development of the oral lesions and should be considered another warning signal. Therapy with gold rarely can bring about a slate-blue discoloration of sun-exposed skin (**chrysiasis**).

Treatment and Prognosis

The management of heavy metal intoxication involves removal from further exposure to the agent, supportive care, decontamination, and use of chelating agents. In some cases, a medication may be responsible and can be discontinued; however, sometimes the source of the metal may be difficult to determine. In infants with radiographic evidence of gastrointestinal lead-containing paint chips, bowel irrigation with a polyethylene glycol electrolyte lavage solution may be warranted. In the past, two chelators, ethylenediaminetetraacetic acid (EDTA) (calcium disodium ethylenediaminetetraacetate) and BAL (2,3-dimercaptopropanol), were first-line therapy in the treatment of lead poisoning, whereas arsenic and mercury intoxication were treated with BAL. These medications may have significant side effects, and less toxic alternatives such as DMSA (2,3-dimercaptosuccinic acid) and DMPS (2,3-dimercaptopropane-1-sulfonate) now are available. No antidote exists for silver intoxication. Attempts to remove the bluish discoloration of facial argyria with dermabrasion have been unsuccessful. Sunscreen, avoiding sunlight, and cosmetics may be somewhat beneficial in minimizing the skin discoloration. Several publications have documented successful treatment of facial argyria with a low-fluence Q-switched 1064-nm Nd:YAG laser. Encephalopathy associated with use of bismuth-containing surgical packs clears on removal of the material, often combined with use of DMPS.

◆ SMOKER'S MELANOSIS

Oral pigmentations are increased significantly in heavy smokers. In one investigation of more than 31,000 whites, 21.5% of tobacco smokers exhibited areas of melanin pigmentation compared with 3% among those not using tobacco. In another study of an ethnically pigmented population, smokers had more oral surfaces exhibiting melanin pigmentation.

Melanin pigmentation in the skin exerts a well-known protective effect against ultraviolet (UV) damage. Investigations of melanocytes located away from sun-exposed areas have shown the ability of melanin to bind to noxious substances. Exposure to polycyclic amines (e.g., nicotine and benzpyrene) has been shown to stimulate melanin production by melanocytes that also are known to bind strongly to nicotine. Research has suggested that melanin production in the oral mucosa of smokers serves as a protective response against some of the harmful substances in tobacco smoke. This concept is supported by the findings in "reverse" smokers, who smoke with the lit end of the cigarette inside the mouth and demonstrate heavy melanin pigmentation of the palate. In some reverse smokers, areas of melanocytes are lost, and zones of depigmented red mucosa can develop. Cancer is found in 12% of patients with these red zones, further delineating the probable protective effects of melanocytes against toxic substances.

Clinical Features

Although any mucosal surface may be affected, smoker's melanosis most commonly affects the anterior facial gingiva (Fig. 8.66) followed by the buccal mucosa, tongue, and lip. Most people affected by this condition are cigarette users. In contrast, pipe smokers most frequently exhibit brown pigmentations located on the commissural and buccal mucosae, whereas reverse smokers show alterations of the hard palate. Increased oral pigmentation also has been noted in children because of passive smoking.

The areas of pigmentation significantly increase during the first year of smoking and appear correlated to the duration and number of cigarettes smoked each day. A higher frequency is seen in females, and researchers have suggested that female sex hormones exert a synergistic effect when combined with smoking. Reports from Sweden, Germany, and Japan have shown tobacco smoking to be the most common cause for mucosal pigmentation in light-skinned adult populations.

Histopathologic Features

Biopsy specimens of affected areas in people with smoker's melanosis reveal increased melanin pigmentation of the basal cell layer of the surface epithelium, similar to a melanotic macule (see page 372). In addition, collections of incontinent melanin pigmentation are seen free within the superficial connective tissue and in scattered melanophages.

Diagnosis

The clinician can make the diagnosis by correlating the smoking history with the clinical presentation and medical history. Other causes of melanin pigmentation, such as trauma, neurofibromatosis, Peutz-Jeghers syndrome, drug-related pigmentation, endocrine disturbances, hemochromatosis, chronic pulmonary disease, and racial pigmentation should be excluded.

Treatment and Prognosis

Cessation of smoking results in gradual disappearance of the areas of related pigmentation over a 3-year period. Biopsy should be considered when the pigmentation is in unexpected locations, such as the hard palate, or when there are unusual clinical changes, such as increased melanin density or surface elevation.

◆ DRUG-RELATED DISCOLORATIONS OF THE ORAL MUCOSA

An expanding number of medications have been implicated as a cause of oral mucosal discolorations. Although many medications stimulate melanin production by melanocytes, deposition of drug metabolites is responsible for the color change in others. These pigmentary alterations have been associated with use of retigabine, amiodarone, phenolphthalein, minocycline, tranquilizers, antimalarial medications, estrogen, chemotherapeutic agents, and some medications used in the treatment of patients with AIDS.

The antimalarial agents that are most frequently implicated are chloroquine, hydroxychloroquine, quinidine, and quinacrine; chlorpromazine represents the most frequently implicated tranquilizer. Besides treating malaria, antimalarial agents are used for many other disorders, including lupus erythematosus and rheumatoid arthritis.

Oral mucosal pigmentation also has been associated with the use of chemotherapeutic medications, such as doxorubicin, busulfan, cyclophosphamide, 5-fluorouracil, or imatinib. Although idiopathic hyperpigmentation also may occur, AIDS patients receiving zidovudine (AZT), clofazimine, or ketoconazole have demonstrated increased melanin pigmentation.

Clinical Features

The clinical presentations of pigmentations related to drug use vary. Most agents produce a diffuse melanosis of the skin and mucosal surfaces, but others may cause a unique pattern. As in many cases of increased melanin pigmentation, females are more sensitive, most likely because of an interaction with sex hormones.

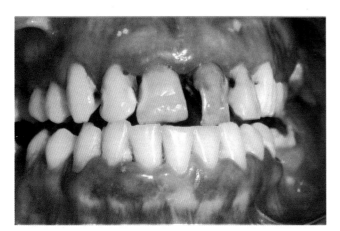

• **Fig. 8.66 Smoker's Melanosis.** Light, diffuse melanin pigmentation in a white female who is a heavy smoker. Pigmentary changes are limited to the anterior facial gingiva.

Use of phenolphthalein as a laxative has been associated with numerous small, well-circumscribed areas of hyperpigmentation on the skin. Similar areas of oral mucosal melanosis also can occur. Administration of peginterferon alfa in ethnically pigmented patients with hepatitis C has been associated with hyperpigmentation of the scattered filiform papillae on dorsal surface of the tongue.

Long-term use of minocycline, a semisynthetic derivative of tetracycline, results in discoloration of the bone and developing teeth. The affected bone is dark green but creates a blue-gray discoloration as seen through the translucent oral mucosa. The most common presentations include a linear band above the facial attached gingiva near the mucogingival junction and a broad zone of discoloration on the hard palate (Fig. 8.67). In addition, the dental pulp can become darkly stained, leading to clinically obvious darkened teeth (see page 70).

Minocycline-related pigmentation of the skin and oral mucosa unrelated to discoloration of the underlying bone also has been reported, with patients exhibiting either widespread increased melanosis or focal accumulations of iron-containing particles (Figs. 8.68 and 8.69). The cutaneous pigmentation

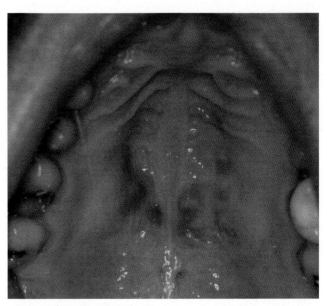

• **Fig. 8.69 Minocycline-Associated Pigmentation.** Multifocal areas of palatal pigmentation secondary to deposition of drug metabolites chelated to iron in association with long-term minocycline use. (From Treister NS, Magalnick D, Woo S-B: Oral mucosal pigmentation secondary to minocycline therapy: report of two cases and a review of the literature, *Oral Surg Oral Med Oral Pathol Oral Radiol Endod* 97:718–725, 2004.)

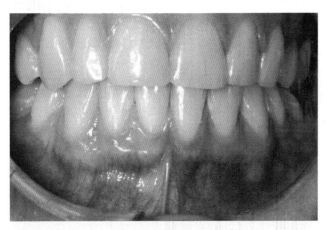

• **Fig. 8.67 Minocycline-Related Discoloration.** Blue-gray discoloration of the facial surface of the anterior mandibular alveolus because stained alveolar bone is visible through the thin mucosa.

appears to be dose-dependent and is seen in up to 15% of patients being treated for acne and as many as 70% of those treated for rheumatoid arthritis. Although the cutaneous and oral mucosal staining fades after discontinuation of the medication, the dental discoloration remains.

The classic presentation of intraoral pigmentation from use of antimalarial medications or tranquilizers is a blue-black discoloration limited to the hard palate (Fig. 8.70). In addition, the intake of antimalarial medications may occasionally lead to a more diffuse brown melanosis of the oral mucosa and skin. Imatinib (Gleevec™) is a tyrosine kinase inhibitor that is used to treat gastrointestinal stroma tumors and several leukemias. This medication is associated with a pattern of palatal

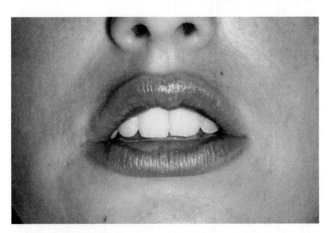

• **Fig. 8.68 Minocycline-Associated Pigmentation.** Sharply demarcated brown pigmentation on the vermilion border of the lips, which arose in association with long-term minocycline use and is the result of increased melanin deposition.

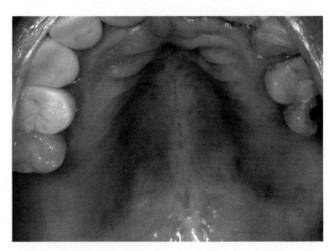

• **Fig. 8.70 Hydroxychloroquine Pigmentation.** Diffuse grayish pigmentation of the hard palate. (Courtesy of Dr. John Wright.)

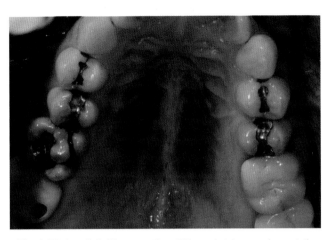

• **Fig. 8.71 Imatinib Pigmentation.** Diffuse, dark brown pigmentation of the palate caused by imatinib. (Courtesy of Dr. Walter Cólon).

discoloration that closely resembles the mucosal discoloration caused by antimalarial drugs (Fig. 8.71).

Estrogen, chemotherapeutic agents, and medications used in the treatment of AIDS patients may result in a diffuse brown melanosis of the skin and mucosal surfaces. Any mucosal surface may be involved, but the attached gingiva and buccal mucosa are affected most frequently. The pattern and appearance of the oral mucosal involvement are like those seen in racial pigmentation.

Treatment and Prognosis

Although the discolorations of the oral mucosa may be aesthetically displeasing, they cause no long-term problems. In most instances, discontinuing the medication results in gradual fading of the areas of hyperpigmentation.

◆ REACTIVE OSSEOUS AND CHONDROMATOUS METAPLASIA (CUTRIGHT LESION)

On occasion, cartilage or bone may be discovered within soft tissue specimens removed from the oral cavity. Cartilaginous rests are known to exist in the area of the nasopalatine duct. In the past, several investigators have reported the presence of cartilage within flabby soft tissue removed from maxillary edentulous alveolar ridges of long-term denture wearers. This finding was thought to represent cartilaginous metaplasia secondary to chronic denture trauma. In retrospect, the islands of cartilage within these cases most likely represent embryologic remnants, not traumatic metaplasia. These rests also are discovered occasionally during histopathologic examination of nasopalatine duct cysts and maxillary gingivectomy specimens.

Despite the suggestion that the anterior maxillary lesions are embryologic and not traumatic, development of **osseous** and **chondromatous metaplasia** from mechanical denture irritation does occur. Although such metaplasia is probably uncommon in the anterior maxilla, its development is not rare along the crest of the posterior mandibular alveolar ridge in long-term denture wearers with atrophic ridges.

Clinical and Radiographic Features

In patients with reactive osseous and chondromatous metaplasia, an extremely tender and localized area of the alveolar ridge typically is noted that may be associated with local enlargement (Fig. 8.72). These changes almost always arise in patients with extensive atrophy of the mandibular alveolar ridge leading to a knife edge–like crest. Although most examples involve the posterior mandible, similar areas rarely may be seen overlying the maxillary alveolar ridge or associated with anterior portions of the mandible. Because of significant associated symptoms and occasional enlargement, biopsy frequently is performed.

Histopathologic Features

Histopathologic examination of reactive osseous and chondromatous metaplasia typically demonstrates a mass of hypercellular periosteum that blends into areas of osseous and chondromatous tissue. The bone and cartilage frequently exhibit atypical features, such as hypercellularity, pleomorphism, nuclear hyperchromatism, and occasional binucleated or multinucleated cells (Fig. 8.73). These alterations are

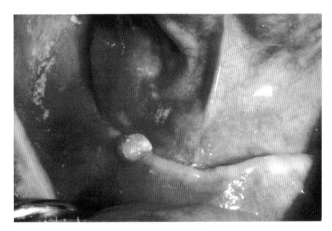

• **Fig. 8.72 Periosteal Hyperplasia With Osseous and Chondromatous Metaplasia.** Tender, elevated nodule along the thin crest of the mandibular alveolar ridge. (Courtesy of Dr. Steven Tucker.)

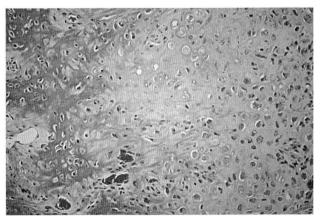

• **Fig. 8.73 Osseous and Chondromatous Metaplasia.** High-power photomicrograph demonstrating cellular woven bone and metaplastic cartilage.

worrisome for sarcoma, but the appropriate diagnosis can be made when an appropriate clinicopathologic correlation is made. In contrast, the cartilaginous rest discovered incidentally in maxillary specimens is usually very bland without any atypical features that would suggest malignancy.

Treatment and Prognosis

The thin mandibular ridges may be recontoured or supplemented with graft material to improve shape and to alleviate the symptoms associated with the localized periosteal hyperplasia. Implants also may reduce the traumatic injury to the ridge and lessen the chance of recurrence. If the ridge modification is not made, then the continued injury to the site occasionally results in recurrence of the lesion.

◆ ORAL ULCERATION WITH BONE SEQUESTRATION (SPONTANEOUS SEQUESTRATION; TRAUMATIC SEQUESTRATION)

Focal superficial sequestration of a fragment of cortical bone not related to systemic disease, infection, or a major traumatic event is uncommon. In such instances, the cause of the focal osteonecrosis is not known, although many believe the primary event is a traumatic or aphthous ulceration that leads to osteitis and necrosis of a small focus of adjacent cortical bone. Others have suggested the blood supply of the peripheral cortical plate may be delivered by the periosteal microvasculature, and loss of this supply leads to focal bone necrosis and sequestration. Such lesions tend to occur in anatomically unique sites in which a bony prominence is covered by a thin mucosal surface.

Clinical and Radiographic Features

In many instances, the focal bone necrosis follows a recent traumatic injury related to events such as toothbrushing trauma, excessive occlusal forces during mastication or bruxism, and iatrogenic injuries (trauma during periodontal scaling, dental impressions, intubation, or tooth extraction). On occasion, the lesion cannot be associated with a prior traumatic event or follows the development of an aphthous-like ulceration. The most frequent site of sequestrum development is the lingual surface of the posterior mandible along the mylohyoid ridge (Fig. 8.74). Focal involvement of exostoses also may occur. Although any exostosis may be involved, mandibular tori are affected most frequently. There is a male predominance and a predilection for middle age with rare cases seen under the age of 30.

The overlying mucosa typically demonstrates a focal area of ulceration that has been present for a period of time that varies from a few days to several months. The presence and intensity of associated pain are variable. Although most cases are unilateral, bilateral involvement may occur. On occasion,

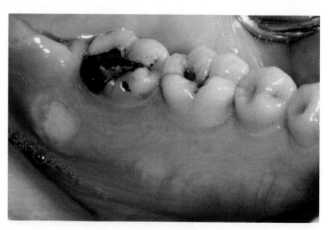

• **Fig. 8.74 Spontaneous Sequestration.** Mucosal ulceration with exposed bone of the posterior lingual surface of the mandible.

an occlusal radiograph will reveal a faint radiopaque mass superimposed and partially lingual to the intact cortical plate.

The mylohyoid ridge often is prominent but typically protected from trauma by the lingual inclination of the adjacent molars. Absence of the adjacent molars or restorations that do not replace the normal inclination could predispose the area to repeated trauma; such alterations have been noted in most affected patients.

Histopathologic Features

The sequestra consist of well-organized lamellar bone that exhibits loss of the osteocytes from their lacunae, along with peripheral resorption and bacterial colonization.

Treatment and Prognosis

Spontaneous loss of the dead bone or surgical removal of the sequestrum results in rapid healing. Recurrence is uncommon. In some instances, the dead bone is freely movable and easily removed. In other cases, the fragment is adherent to the underlying vital bone and must be surgically excised. To avoid surgery, some clinicians use a tetracycline rinse in addition to topical corticosteroids. Alternatively, these patients can be recalled weekly for 2–4 weeks, during which time the dead bone may exfoliate spontaneously without the need for invasive therapy.

◆ ANTRAL PSEUDOCYSTS

Antral pseudocysts are common findings on panoramic radiographs. The lesion appears as a dome-shaped, faintly radiopaque lesion often arising from the floor of the maxillary sinus. This condition continues to be misunderstood and is inappropriately termed **sinus mucocele** or **sinus retention cyst** by many clinicians (see next section). The antral pseudocyst develops due to an accumulation of an inflammatory exudate (serum, not mucus) beneath the maxillary sinus mucosa, causing a sessile elevation (Fig. 8.75). It must be stressed that the edematous fluid

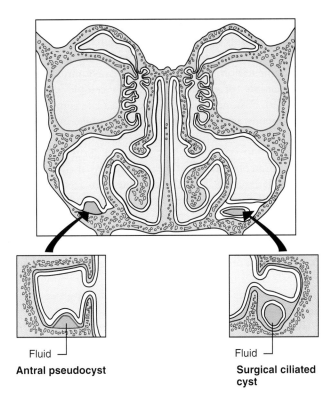

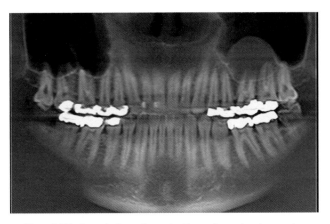

• **Fig. 8.76 Antral Pseudocyst.** Three-dimensional cone-beam radiograph showing dome-shaped radiopacity within the maxillary sinus. (Courtesy of Dr. Scott Jenkins and Dr. Nick Morrow.)

Fluid ⏌   Fluid ⏌

Antral pseudocyst   **Surgical ciliated cyst**

• **Fig. 8.75 Antral Pseudocyst and Surgical Ciliated Cyst.** An antral pseudocyst is an accumulation of serum beneath the sinus lining. A surgical ciliated cyst is an epithelium-lined cystic structure separate from the sinus.

is in the stroma underneath the epithelium, not surrounded by it.

Reviews of large numbers of radiographs have reported a prevalence that ranges from 1.5% to 14% of the population. The cause of the inflammatory infiltrate has not been determined definitively, but in a radiographic review, many cases showed a possible source from an adjacent odontogenic infection. Primary irritation of the sinus lining, such as that seen from a sinus infection or allergies, also can theoretically result in the inflammatory infiltrate.

An increased prevalence of pseudocysts has been noted during the cold winter months, leading some investigators to associate these lesions with an increased frequency of upper respiratory tract infections or irritation from dry, forced-air heating. This association is difficult to confirm because these lesions often are asymptomatic, making the timing of their development difficult to pinpoint. Although allergies have been proposed as a cause, no increased prevalence has been noted consistently during the time of peak pollen exposure.

Clinical and Radiographic Features

Most pseudocysts are asymptomatic. On occasion, affected patients report symptoms, such as headache, facial sinus pain, nasal obstruction, postnasal drip, and nasal discharge. Some studies have suggested these symptoms are secondary to other sinus disease and are not relieved by removal of the pseudocyst. Radiographically,

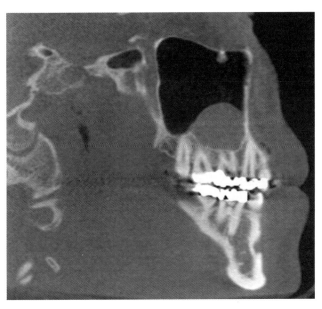

• **Fig. 8.77 Antral Pseudocyst.** Three-dimensional cone-beam sagittal section of same patient depicted in Fig. 8.76. Note that the floor of the sinus remains intact below the lesion. (Courtesy of Dr. Scott Jenkins and Dr. Nick Morrow.)

an antral pseudocyst typically presents as a uniform and spherical or dome-shaped radiodensity arising above the bony floor of the maxillary sinus (Figs. 8.76 and 8.77). Maxillary cysts and neoplasms can simulate the dome-shaped pattern of an antral pseudocyst, but close examination of a pseudocyst typically reveals the radiopaque floor of the sinus is not elevated and does not extend over the superior aspect of the lesion. Less frequently, pseudocysts also may arise from the lateral wall, medial wall, or roof of the antrum. A male predominance has been reported by some authors.

Histopathologic Features

Antral pseudocysts are covered by sinus epithelium and demonstrate a subepithelial inflammatory exudate that consists of serum, occasionally intermixed with inflammatory cells

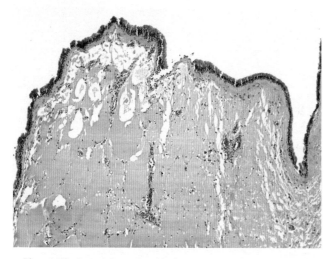

• **Fig. 8.78 Antral Pseudocyst.** Medium-power photomicrograph demonstrating sinus lining overlying edematous connective tissue.

(Fig. 8.78). Collections of cholesterol clefts and scattered small dystrophic calcifications may be seen.

Treatment and Prognosis

Typically, pseudocysts of the maxillary sinus are harmless, and no treatment is necessary. The adjacent teeth should be evaluated thoroughly, and any foci of infection should be eliminated. A few clinicians prefer to confirm their radiographic impression and rule out a tumor through drainage of the inflammatory exudate. Removal by means of a Caldwell-Luc operation endoscopic surgery should be performed on any radiographically diagnosed lesion that produces significant expansion or is associated definitively with symptoms.

◆ TRUE CYSTS OF THE SINUSES (SINUS MUCOCELE; SURGICAL CILIATED CYST; TRAUMATIC CILIATED CYST; POSTOPERATIVE MAXILLARY CYST; RETENTION CYST)

In contrast to the antral pseudocyst, which arises from subepithelial accumulation of edema fluid, true epithelium-lined cysts also may arise from the sinonasal mucosa and glands. They occur in three situations.

One type of cyst occurs after trauma or surgery to the sinus; this type is best known as a **surgical ciliated cyst, traumatic ciliated cyst**, or **postoperative maxillary cyst.** A portion of the sinus lining becomes separated from the main body of the sinus and forms an epithelium-lined cavity into which mucus is secreted. Alternatively, radical surgery may alter the anatomy of the sinus and block the drainage passage, resulting in an expanding cyst-like structure. The cyst most frequently originates after a Caldwell-Luc operation but may arise from difficult extraction of a maxillary

tooth in which the floor of the maxillary sinus is damaged. In addition, sinus or nasal epithelium rarely can be transplanted accidentally to the mandible during genioplasty, chin augmentation, or a sagittal split osteotomy and lead to formation of ciliated cysts in ectopic locations (Fig. 8.79). Postoperative cysts often are a late complication and frequently arise 10–30 years after the triggering surgical event.

The second type of cyst, known as a **sinus mucocele,** arises from an obstruction of the sinus ostium, thereby blocking normal drainage. This blocked sinus then acts like a separate cyst-like structure lined by epithelium and filled with mucus. Sinus mucoceles enlarge in size as the intraluminal pressure increases and can distend the walls of the sinus and erode through bone; they often clinically mimic malignancy of sinus origin. (It should be emphasized that a sinus mucocele is a distinct, separate pathologic entity that is unrelated to the common mucocele of minor salivary gland origin [see page 460]).

Retention cysts of the maxillary sinus are the third type of true cyst. These lesions arise from the partial blockage of a seromucous gland duct within the sinus wall, or from an invagination of the respiratory epithelium. Most retention cysts are located around the ostium or within antral polyps. The majority of retention cysts are small, not evident clinically, and discovered during histopathologic examination of antral polyps.

Postoperative surgical ciliated cysts appear to be uncommon in the United States and Europe but are reported more frequently in Japan due to the high prevalence of surgical therapy rather than antibiotic treatment for sinusitis prior to the 1970s. Sinus mucoceles arising from ostial obstruction are much more numerous and most frequently involve the frontal sinus, with the ethmoid and sphenoid sinuses being affected less often. Maxillary sinus mucoceles arising from blockage of the ostium are relatively rare and account for less than 10% of paranasal sinus mucoceles.

Clinical and Radiographic Features

Surgical ciliated cysts are spherical lesions that are separate from the sinus and lack the dome-shaped appearance of pseudocysts (Fig. 8.80). As these postoperative cysts enlarge, they can lead to perforation of the sinus walls. When the maxillary sinus is involved by a true sinus mucocele, the entire sinus will appear cloudy. As the lesion enlarges, the walls of the sinus may become thinned and eventually eroded. Retention cysts rarely reach a size that would produce detectable radiographic changes. Mandibular postoperative cysts secondary to genioplasty or chin augmentation present as a well-defined unilocular radiolucency in the midline, while those secondary to a sagittal split osteotomy arise in the ascending ramus.

Histopathologic Features

Surgical ciliated cysts and sinus mucoceles are true cystic structures lined by ciliated pseudostratified columnar epithelium, squamous epithelium with mucous cells, or metaplastic squamous epithelium (Fig. 8.81). A sinus retention cyst

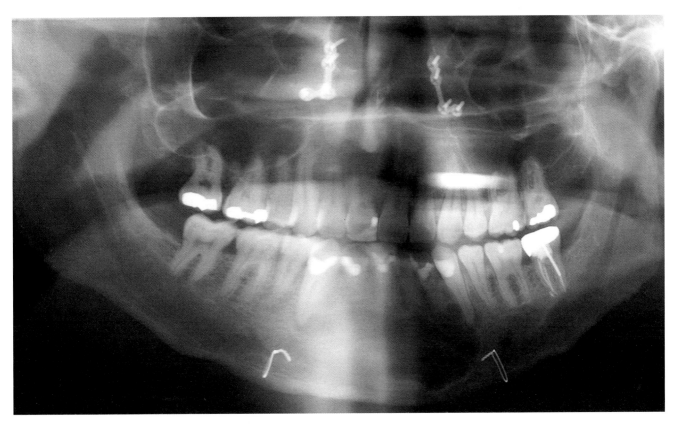

• **Fig. 8.79 Surgical Ciliated Cyst.** Ectopic ciliated cyst of the anterior mandible arising when respiratory epithelium was carried from LeFort 1 osteotomy site to mandible during gonioplasty procedure. (Courtesy of Dr. Adam Janette.)

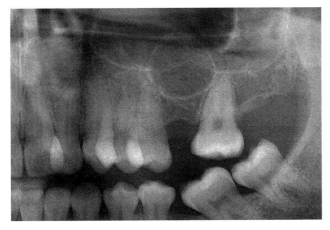

• **Fig. 8.80 Surgical Ciliated Cyst.** Well-defined radiolucency in area of previous extraction of the maxillary first molar. (Courtesy of Dr. Steven Anderson.)

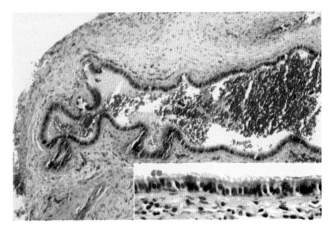

• **Fig. 8.81 Surgical Ciliated Cyst.** True cyst lined by respiratory epithelium. Inset provides high-power view of the ciliated pseudostratified columnar epithelium that lines the cyst.

shows focal dilation of a duct associated with the seromucous glands of the sinus lining. The lumen of the dilated duct is filled with thick mucus, often intermixed with chronic inflammatory cells.

Treatment and Prognosis

Because surgical ciliated cysts and sinus mucoceles are expansile and destructive lesions, surgical removal is necessary. Although many of the maxillary lesions are removed via a Caldwell-Luc operation, cysts close to the nasal cavity are treated best with transnasal endoscopic marsupialization. The mandibular lesions respond well to thorough curettage with marsupialization utilized in large cysts to reduce the size prior to definitive removal. Numerous investigators also have shown that sinus mucoceles arising from ostial obstruction often do not require surgical excision, but they respond well to endoscopic middle meatal antrostomy and marsupialization of the mucocele.

◆ CERVICOFACIAL EMPHYSEMA

Cervicofacial emphysema arises from the introduction of air into subcutaneous or fascial spaces of the face and neck. The forced air may spread through the spaces to the orbital, retropharyngeal, mediastinal, pleural, and peritoneal areas. A physician, Alexander Turnbull, reported the first case in 1900 that arose as a result of blowing into a bugle a short time after tooth extraction.

Cervicofacial emphysema of dental origin may arise in several ways:

- After the use of compressed air by the clinician
- After difficult or prolonged extractions
- As a result of increased intraoral pressure (e.g., vigorous nose blowing, sneezing, balloon blowing, playing wind instruments, habitual Valsalva maneuvers). The risks of these procedures are increased immediately after an oral surgical procedure
- Use of hydrogen peroxide for irrigation during an endodontic procedure
- From no obvious cause

Introduction of air within tissue has been seen after a large number of dental procedures, but most instances involve either surgical extraction of teeth, endodontic procedures, osteotomies, significant trauma, or the use of air or water syringes. In addition, the prevalence has increased because of the use of air-driven handpieces during oral surgery or use of lasers with compressed air systems designed to remove tissue debris from the operative field. On occasion, cervicofacial emphysema has resulted from compressed air being accidentally forced into small intraoral lacerations located away from the field of operation. An analogous problem termed **pneumoparotid** can arise when air enters the parotid duct, leading to enlargement of the parotid gland caused by air insufflation. This can be accidental, self-induced, or occupational (e.g., glassblowers and wind instrument players). Stensen duct has numerous redundant mucosal folds that seal as intraoral pressure is increased; in addition, contraction of the buccinator muscle further prevents entrance of air by compressing the duct. Despite this protection, dramatic increases in intraoral pressures can result in air filling the parotid ductal system.

Clinical and Radiographic Features

More than 90% of cases of cervicofacial emphysema develop during surgery or within the first postoperative hour. Cases with delayed onset are associated with increased postoperative pressure created by the patient. The initial change is one of soft tissue enlargement from the presence of the air in deeper tissues (Fig. 8.82). Pain usually is minimal, and crepitus is detected easily with gentle palpation. Subsequently, the enlargement increases and spreads because of secondary inflammation and edema. Variable pain, facial erythema, dysphagia, dysphonia, vision difficulties, and mild fever may occur. The facial enlargement often is confused with an angioedema, but the diagnosis can be made by identifying

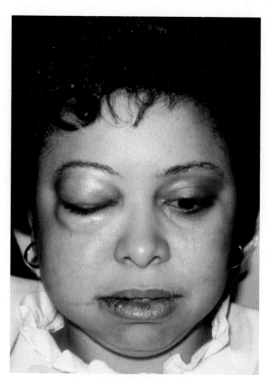

• **Fig. 8.82 Cervicofacial Emphysema.** Periorbital and facial enlargement caused by use of an air-driven handpiece during third molar removal.

crepitus within the swelling. In addition, computed tomography (CT) using the Hounsfield density measuring scale can confirm the presence of soft tissue air pockets.

Significant spread into the mediastinum can result in dysphonia, dysphagia, or dyspnea. Cardiac auscultation often reveals crepitus synchronous with the heartbeat (**Hamman's crunch**) in cases with mediastinal involvement. Pneumomediastinum can be confirmed on chest radiographs by observing displacement of the mediastinal pleura. Pericardial space involvement often can be detected through at 12-lead electrocardiogram that may demonstrate inverted T waves, ST segment elevation, and an electrical axis shift.

Pneumoparotid typically appears as a unilateral enlargement of the parotid that demonstrates crepitus on gentle palpation. Milking the parotid duct produces frothy, air-filled saliva, rather than the typical clear, water-like secretion.

Treatment and Prognosis

Broad-spectrum antibiotic coverage is recommended in all dental-related cases of cervicofacial emphysema. The body gradually removes the entrapped air during a 2- to 5-day period. Most cases spontaneously resolve without significant difficulty. Administration of 100% oxygen with a nonrebreather mask can shorten recovery, because the oxygen reduces the partial pressure of nitrogen in the lungs compared to the peripheral tissues with the resultant pressure gradient allowing nitrogen to diffuse more rapidly out of the peripheral tissues (the entrapped air is 78% nitrogen, 21%

oxygen). Rare cases of respiratory distress have been noted, and assisted ventilation was required. Associated deaths have been reported secondary to rare severe complications such as mediastinitis, tension pneumothorax, cardiac tamponade, cardiac failure, and air embolism.

The first goal of therapy for pneumoparotid is discovery of the inciting event. In occupation-related cases, such as those seen in trumpet players, the individual should be coached to compress the cheeks during playing. This procedure contracts the buccinator muscle and compresses the parotid duct. Acute symptoms are treated with antibiotics, massage, hydration, sialogogues, and warm compresses.

◆ MYOSPHERULOSIS

Placement of a topical antibiotic or hemostatic agent in a petrolatum or petroleum base into a surgical site occasionally may result in a unique foreign body reaction, known as **myospherulosis.** The resultant histopathologic pattern demonstrates spherical bodies initially thought to represent an endosporulating fungus but shown to be red blood cells altered by physical emulsion with the lipid-containing petrolatum.

Clinical and Radiographic Features

Myospherulosis may occur at any site within soft tissue or bone where the antibiotic has been placed. Most cases in the dental literature have occurred within bone at previous extraction sites where an antibiotic had been placed to prevent alveolar osteitis. Although maxillary and oral soft tissue examples have been documented, most cases have occurred within mandibular surgical sites. In addition, myospherulosis is reported occasionally in other anatomical sites, most often in the nose or a paranasal sinus following a surgical procedure in which a gauze packing coated with an antibiotic ointment was used. A similar microscopic pattern also has been seen in renal cell carcinoma, steatocystoma, cystic teratomas, breast tissue, and perirenal adipose tissue secondary to a reaction between endogenous lipid and blood.

Although rare cases may present as a multilocular lesion, myospherulosis classically presents as a circumscribed unilocular radiolucency in a site of previous surgery (Fig. 8.83). In some cases, swelling, pain, or purulent drainage may be present. On exploration of the lesion, a black, greasy, tarlike material is found.

Histopathologic Features

The histopathologic pattern demonstrates dense collagenous tissue intermixed with a granulomatous inflammatory response showing macrophages and multinucleated giant cells. Within the connective tissue are multiple cyst-like spaces that contain numerous brown-to-black-staining spherules (Fig. 8.84). The collections of spherules sometimes are surrounded by an outer membrane known as a *parent body,* forming structures that resemble a "bag of marbles."

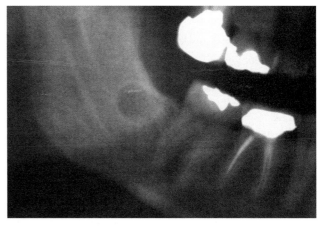

• **Fig. 8.83 Myospherulosis.** Radiolucency has persisted after extraction of the mandibular third molar. An antibiotic ointment was placed at the time of initial surgery.

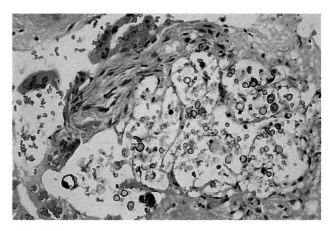

• **Fig. 8.84 Myospherulosis.** High-power photomicrograph exhibiting multiple cystlike spaces containing numerous brown-stained spherules.

The unusual dark coloration is due to the degradation of hemoglobin. To complicate matters, myospherulosis arising in a paranasal sinus occasionally is contaminated with respiratory fungal organisms, such as the Zygomycetes or *Aspergillus.*

Treatment and Prognosis

Myospherulosis is treated by surgical removal of the foreign material and associated tissue. Histopathologic examination of the altered tissue provides the definitive diagnosis. Recurrence is not expected. Those arising in a paranasal sinus and exhibiting fungal infestation respond well to local measures and do not require systemic antimicrobial therapy.

Bibliography

Linea Alba
Madani FM, Kuperstein AS: Normal variations of oral anatomy and common oral soft tissue lesions. Evaluation and management, *Med Clin N Am* 98:1281–1298, 2014.

Vieira-Andrade RG, Zuquim Guimarães Fde F, Vieira Cda S, et al.: Oral mucosa alterations in a socioeconomically deprived region: prevalence and associated factors, *Braz Oral Res* 25:393–400, 2011.

Morsicatio Buccarum
Hjørting-Hansen E, Holst E: Morsicatio mucosae oris and suctio mucosae oris: an analysis of oral mucosal changes due to biting and sucking habits, *Scand J Dent Res* 78:492–499, 1970.

Nanda A, Koli D, Sharma S, et al.: Checking the cheek bite injury: fabrication of an interim cheek guard appliance, *Spec Care Dentist* 34:208–211, 2014.

Romero M, Vicente A, Bravo LA: Prevention of habitual cheek biting: a case report, *Spec Care Dentist* 25:214–216, 2005.

Sewerin I: A clinical and epidemiologic study of morsicatio buccarum/labiorum, *Scand J Dent Res* 79:73–80, 1971.

Solley K, Turner C: Prevalence and correlates of clinical significant body-focused repetitive behaviors in a non-clinical sample, *Compr Psychiatry* 86:9–18, 2018.

Van Wyk CW, Staz J, Farman AG: The chewing lesion of the cheeks and lips: its features and the prevalence among a selected group of adolescents, *J Dent* 5:193–199, 1977.

Woo S-B, Lin D: Morsicatio mucosae oris—a chronic oral frictional keratosis, not a leukoplakia, *J Oral Maxillofac Surg* 67:140–146, 2009.

Eosinophilic Ulcerations
Aloebeid B, Pan L-X, Milligan L, et al.: Eosinophil-rich CD30+ lymphoproliferative disorder of the oral mucosa, *Am J Clin Pathol* 121:43–50, 2004.

Baldiwala M, Nayak R: Conservativee management of Riga-Fede disease, *J Dent Child* 81:103–106, 2014.

Benitez B, Mülli J, Tzankov A, et al.: Traumatic ulcerative granuloma with stromal eosinophilia – clinical case report, literature review, and differential diagnosis, *World J Surg Oncol* 17:184, 2019. https://doi.org/10.1186/s12957-019-1736-z.

Bhaskar SN, Lilly GE: Traumatic granuloma of the tongue (human and experimental), *Oral Surg Oral Med Oral Pathol* 18:206–218, 1964.

Elzay RP: Traumatic ulcerative granuloma with stromal eosinophilia (Riga-Fede's disease and traumatic eosinophilic granuloma), *Oral Surg Oral Med Oral Pathol* 55:497–506, 1983.

Ficarra G, Prignano F, Romagnoli P: Traumatic eosinophilic granuloma of the oral mucosa: a CD30+ (Ki-1) lymphoproliferative disorder, *Oral Oncol* 33:375–379, 1997.

Padmanabhan MY, Pandey RK, Aparna R, et al.: Neonatal sublingual traumatic ulceration—case report & review of the literature, *Dent Traumatol* 26:490–495, 2010.

Setti G, Martella E, Mancini C, et al.: Self-healing CD30 – T -clonal proliferation of the tongue: report of an extremely rare case, *BMC Oral Health* 19:186, 2019. https://doi.org/10.1186/s12903-019-0875-5.

Electrical and Thermal Burns
Czerepak CS: Oral splint therapy to manage electrical burns of the mouths in children, *Clin Plast Surg* 11:685–692, 1984.

Davidson CC, Orr DJ: An unusual exit point from an electrocution injury, *Burns* 36:e75–e77, 2010.

Harrison R, Hicklin D Jr: Electronic cigarette explosions involving the oral cavity, *JADA* 147:891–896, 2016.

Jones CD, Ho W, Gunn E, et al.: E-cigarette burn injuries: comprehensive review and management guideline proposal, *Burns* 45:763–771, 2019.

Rogér JM, Abayon M, Elad S, et al.: Oral trauma and tooth avulsion following explosion of e-cigarette, *J Oral Maxillofac Surg* 74:1181–1185, 2016.

Serror K, Chaouat M, Legrand MM, et al.: Burns caused by electronic vaping devices (e-cigarettes): a new classification proposal based on mechanisms, *Burns* 44:544–548, 2018.

Yeroshalmi F, Sidoti EJ Jr, Adamo AK, et al.: Oral electrical burns in children—a model of multidisciplinary care, *J Burn Car Res* 32:e25–e30, 2011.

Oral Adverse Reactions to Chemicals
Frost DE, Barkmeier WW, Abrams H: Aphthous ulcer—a treatment complication, *Oral Surg Oral Med Oral Pathol* 45:863–869, 1978.

Gilvette C, Porter SR, Fedele S: Traumatic chemical oral ulceration: a case report and review of the literature, *Br Dent J* 208:297–300, 2010.

Gluskin AH, Lai G, Peters CI, et al.: The double-edged sword of calcium hydroxide in endodontics. Precautions and preventative strategies for extrusion injuries into neurovascular anatomy, *JADA* 151:317–326, 2020.

Kleier DJ, Averbach RE, Mehdipour O: The sodium hypochlorite accident: experience of diplomates of the American Board of Endodontics, *J Endod* 34:1346–1350, 2008.

Pontes F, Pontes H, Adachi P, et al.: Gingival and bone necrosis caused by accidental sodium hypochlorite injection instead of anaesthetic solution, *Int Endod J* 41:267–270, 2008.

Rees TD, Orth CF: Oral ulcerations with use of hydrogen peroxide, *J Periodontol* 57:689–692, 1986.

Noninfectious Complications of Antineoplastic Therapy
Ariyawardana A, Cheng KKF, Kandwal A, et al.: Systematic review of anti-inflammatory agents for the management of oral mucositis in cancer patients and clinical practice guidelines, *Support Care Cancer* 27:3985–3995, 2019.

Bhide SA, Miah AB, Harrington KJ, et al.: Radiation-induced xerostomia: pathophysiology, prevention and treatment, *Clin Oncol* 21:737–744, 2009.

Costa DA, Costa TP, Netto EC, et al.: New perspectives on the conservative management of osteoradionecrosis of the mandible: a literature review, *Head Neck* 38:1708–1716, 2016.

Delanian S, Lefaix JL: The radiation-induced fibroatrophic process: therapeutic perspective via the antioxidant pathway, *Radiother Oncol* 73:119–131, 2004.

Haverman C, Huber M: Xerostomia management in the head and neck radiation patient, *Tex Dent J* 127:487–504, 2010.

Kolokythas A, Rasmussen JT, Reardon J, et al.: Management of osteoradionecrosis of the jaws with pentoxifylline-tocopheral: a systematic review of the literature and meta-analysis, *Int J Oral Maxillofac Surg* 48:173–180, 2019.

Lalla RV, Bowen J, Barasch A, et al.: MASCC/ISOO clinical practice guidelines for the management of mucositis secondary to cancer therapy, *Cancer* 120:1453–1461, 2014.

Lalla RV, Saunders DP, Peterson DE: Chemotherapy or radiation – induced oral mucositis, *Dent Clin N Am* 58:341–349, 2014.

Marx RE: A new concept in the treatment of osteoradionecrosis, *J Oral Maxillofac Surg* 41:351–357, 1983.

Palmier NR, Migliorati CA, Prado-Ribeiro AC, et al.: Radiation-related caries: current diagnostic, prognostic, and management paradigms, *Oral Surg Oral Med Oral Pathol Oral Radiol* 130:52–62, 2020.

Peng J, Shi Y, Wang J, et al.: Low-level laser therapy in the prevention and treatment of oral mucositis: a systematic review and meta-analysis, *Oral Surg Oral Med Oral Pathol Oral Radiol* 130:387–397, 2020.

Raggio BS, Winters R: Modern management of osteoradionecrosis, *Curr Opin Otolaryngol Head Neck Surg* 26:254–259, 2018.

Worthington HV, Clarkson JE, Bryan G, et al.: Interventions for preventing oral mucositis for patients with cancer receiving treatment, *Cochrane Database Syst Rev* (4):CD000978, 2011.

Zhang Z, Xiao W, Jia J, et al.: The effect of combined application of pentoxifylline and vitamin E for the treatment of osteoradionecrosis of the jaws: a meta-analysis, *Oral Surg Oral Med Oral Pathol Oral Radiol* 129:207–214, 2020.

Medication-Related Osteonecrosis of the Jaw

Carlson ER: Management of antiresorptive osteonecrosis of the jaws with primary surgical resection, *J Oral Maxillofac Surg* 72:655–657, 2014.

Carlson ER: Response to letter to the editor, *J Oral Maxillofac Surg* 72:1641–1642, 2014.

Damm DD, Jones DM: Bisphosphonate-related osteonecrosis of the jaws: a potential alternative to drug holidays, *Gen Dent* 61:33–38, 2013.

Eguia A, Bagan L, Cardona F: Review and update on drugs related to the development of osteonecrosis of the jaw, *Med Oral Patol Oral Cir Bucal* 25:E71–c83, 2020.

El-Rabbany M, Sgro A, Lam DK, et al.: Effectiveness of treatment for medication-related osteonecrosis of the jaw. A systematic review and meta-analysis, *JADA* 148:584–594, 2017.

Favia G, Tempesta A, Limongelli L, et al.: Medication-related osteonecrosis of the jaw: surgical or non-surgical treatment? *Oral Diseases* 24:238–242, 2018.

Filleul O, Crompot E, Saussez S: Bisphosphonate-induced osteonecrosis of the jaw: a review of 2,400 patient cases, *J Cancer Res Clin Oncol* 136:1117–1124, 2010.

Hellstein JW, Adler RA, Edwards B, et al.: Managing the care of patients receiving antiresorptive therapy for prevention and treatment of osteoporosis, *J Am Dent Assoc* 142:1243–1251, 2011.

Marx RE: Pamidronate (Aredia) and zoledronate (Zometa) induced avascular necrosis of the jaws: a growing epidemic (letter to the editor), *J Oral Maxillofac Surg* 61:1115–1117, 2003.

Marx RE, Cillo JE Jr, Ulloa JJ: Oral bisphosphonate-induced osteonecrosis: risk factors, prediction of risk using serum CTX testing, prevention, and treatment, *J Oral Maxillofac Surg* 65:2397–2410, 2007.

Nicolatou-Galitis O, Schiødt M, Mendes RA, et al.: Medication-related osteonecrosis of the jaw: definition and best practice for prevention, diagnosis, and treatment, *Oral Surg Oral Med Oral Pathol Oral Radiol* 127:117–135, 2019.

Otto S, Schnödt EM, Haidari S, et al.: Autofluorescence-guided surgery for the treatment of medication-related osteonecrosis of the jaw (MRONJ): a retrospective single-center study, *Oral Surg Oral Med Oral Pathol Oral Radiol* 131:519–526, 2021.

Owosho AA, Liang STY, Sax AZ, et al.: Medication-related osteonecrosis of the jaw: an update on the Memorial Sloan Kettering Cancer Center experience and the role of premedication dental evaluation in prevention, *Oral Surg Oral Med Oral Pathol Oral Radiol* 125:440–445, 2018.

Ristow O, Rückschloß T, Müller M, et al.: Is the conservative non-surgical management of medication-related osteonecrosis of the jaw an appropriate treatment option for early stages? A long-term single-center cohort study, *J Cranio Maxillo Fac Surg* 47:491–499, 2019.

Ruggiero SL, Dodson TB, Aghaloo T, et al.: American Association of Oral and Maxillofacial Surgeons' position paper on medication-related osteonecrosis of the jaw – 2022 update, *J Oral Maxillofac Surg* 80:920–943, 2022.

Ruggiero SL, Dodson TB, Fantasia J, et al.: American Association of Oral and Maxillofacial Surgeons position paper on medication-related osteonecrosis of the jaw—2014 update, *J Oral Maxillofac Surg* 72(10):1938–1956, 2014.

Ruggiero SL, Mehrotra B, Rosenberg TJ, et al.: Osteonecrosis of the jaws associated with the use of bisphosphonates: a review of 63 cases, *J Oral Maxillofac Surg* 62:527–534, 2004.

Saag KG, Petersen J, Brandi ML, et al.: Romosozumab or alendronate for fracture prevention in women with osteoporosis, *N Engl J Med* 377:1417–1427, 2017.

Schneider JP: Should bisphosphonates be continued indefinitely? An unusual fracture in a healthy woman on long-term alendronate, *Geriatrics* 61:31–33, 2006.

Williams WB, O'Ryan F: Management of medication-related osteonecrosis of the jaw, *Oral Maxillofacial Surg Clin N Am* 27:517–525, 2015.

Orofacial Complications of Drug Abuse

Clague J, Belin TR, Shetty V: Mechanisms underlying metamphetamine-related dental disease, *JADA* 148:377–386, 2017.

Goodchild JH, Donaldson M: Methamphetamine abuse and dentistry: a review of the literature and presentation of a clinical case, *Quintessence Int* 38:583–590, 2007.

Hamamoto DT, Rhodus NL: Methamphetamine abuse and dentistry, *Oral Dis* 15:27–37, 2009.

Silvestre FJ, Perez-Hervera A, Puente-Sandoval A, et al.: Hard palate perforation in cocaine abusers: a systematic review, *Clin Oral Invest* 14:621–628, 2010.

Trimarchi M, Bondi S, Torre ED, et al.: Palate perforation differentiates cocaine-induced midline destructive lesions from granulomatosis with polyangiitis, *Acta Otorhinolaryngol Ital* 37:281–285, 2017.

Anesthetic Necrosis

Carroll MJ: Tissue necrosis following a buccal infiltration, *Br Dent J* 149:209–210, 1980.

Giunta J, Tsamsouris A, Cataldo E, et al.: Postanesthetic necrotic defect, *Oral Surg Oral Med Oral Pathol* 40:590–593, 1975.

Schaffer J, Calman HI, Levy B: Changes in the palate color and form (case 9), *Dent Radiogr Photogr* 39(3–6):19–22, 1966.

Exfoliative Cheilitis

Axéll T, Skoglund A: Chronic lip fissures. Prevalence, pathology and treatment, *Int J Oral Surg* 10:354–358, 1981.

Connolly M, Kennedy C: Exfoliative cheilitis successfully treated with topical tacrolimus, *Br J Dermatol* 151:241–242, 2004.

Daley TD, Gupta AK: Exfoliative cheilitis, *J Oral Pathol Med* 24:177–179, 1995.

Freeman S, Stephens R: Cheilitis: analysis of 75 cases referred to a contact dermatitis clinic, *Am J Contact Dermat* 7:146–151, 1996.

Nico MMS, Dwan AJ, Lourenco SV, et al.: Ointment pseudo-cheilitis: a disease distinct from factitial cheilitis. A series of 13 patients from São Paulo, Brazil, *J Cutan Med Surg* 23:277–281, 2019.

Reade PC, Sim R: Exfoliative cheilitis—a factitious disorder? *Int J Oral Maxillofac Surg* 15:313–317, 1986.

Rosenquist B: Median lip fissure: etiology and suggested treatment, *Oral Surg Oral Med Oral Pathol* 72:10–14, 1991.

Taniguchi S, Kono T: Exfoliative cheilitis: a case report and review of the literature, *Dermatology* 196:253–255, 1998.

Submucosal Hemorrhage

Kravitz P: The clinical picture of "cough purpura," benign and non-thrombocytopenic eruption, *Va Med* 106:373–374, 1979.

Sundarajan D, Noonan V, Gallagher G: Oral submucosal hemorrhage, *J Mass Dent Soc* 65:31, 2016.

Oral Trauma from Sexual Practices

Damm DD, White DK, Brinker CM: Variations of palatal erythema secondary to fellatio, *Oral Surg Oral Med Oral Pathol* 52:417–421, 1981.

Elam AL: Sexually related trauma: a review, *Ann Emerg Med* 15:576–584, 1986.

Farman AG, Van Wyk CW: The features of non-infectious oral lesions caused by fellatio, *J Dent Assoc S Afr* 32:53–55, 1977.

Leider AS: Intraoral ulcers of questionable origin, *J Am Dent Assoc* 92:1177–1178, 1976.

Mader CL: Lingual frenum ulcer resulting from orogenital sex, *J Am Dent Assoc* 103:888–890, 1981.

Terezhalmy GT: Oral manifestations of sexually related diseases, *Ear Nose Throat J* 62:287–296, 1983.

Van Wyk CW: Oral lesions caused by habits, *Forensic Sci* 7:41–49, 1976.

Localized Exogenous Pigmentations

Aguirre-Zorzano LA, Garcia-De-La-Fuente AM, Estefanía-Fresco R: Treatment of amalgam tattoo with a new technique: mucoabrasion and free connective tissue graft, *Clin Adv Periodontics* 9:120–124, 2019.

Brooks JK, Reynolds MA: Ethnobotanical tattooing of the gingiva. Literature review and report of a case, *J Am Dent Assoc* 138:1097–2101, 2007.

Buchner A, Hansen LS: Amalgam pigmentation (amalgam tattoo) of the oral mucosa: a clinicopathologic study of 268 cases, *Oral Surg Oral Med Oral Pathol* 49:139–147, 1980.

Daley TD, Gibson D: Practical applications of energy dispersive x-ray microanalysis in diagnostic oral pathology, *Oral Surg Oral Med Oral Pathol* 69:339–344, 1990.

de Winter RW, van der Bent SAS, van Esch M, et al.: Allergic reaction to red cosmetic lip tattoo treated with hydroxychloroquine, *Dermatitis* 30:82–83, 2019.

Hussaini HM, Waddell JN, West LM, et al.: Silver solder "tattoo," a novel form of oral pigmentation identified with the use of field emission scanning electron microscopy and electron dispersive spectrography, *Oral Surg Oral Med Oral Pathol Oral Radiol Endod* 112:e6–e10, 2011.

Moraes RM, Gouvêa Lima GDM, Guilhermino M, et al.: Graphite oral tattoo: case report, *Dermatol Online J* 21, 2015. 13030/qt0z57p9xr.

Ortiz A, Yamauchi PS: Rapidly growing squamous cell carcinoma from permanent makeup tattoo, *J Am Acad Dermatol* 60:1073–1074, 2009.

Rawal SY, Burrell R, Hamidi CS, et al.: Diffuse pigmentation of maxillary attached gingiva: four cases of the culture practice of gingival tattoo, *J Periodontol* 78(1):170–176, 2007.

Taylor TD, Klotz MW, Lawton RA: Titanium tattooing associated with zirconia implant abutments: a clinical report of two cases, *Int J Oral Maxillofac Implants* 29:958–960, 2014.

Oral Piercings and Forked Tongue

Bressmann T: Self-inflicted cosmetic tongue split: a case report, *J Can Dent Assoc* 70:156–157, 2004.

Gill JB, Karp JM, Kopycha-Kedzierawski DT: Oral piercing injuries treated in United States Emergency departments, 2002–2008, *Pediatr Dent* 34:56–60, 2012.

Hennequin-Hoenderdos NL, Slot DE, Van der Weijen GA: The prevalence of oral and peri-oral piercings in young adults, a systematic review, *Int J Dent Hyg* 10:223–228, 2012.

Hennequin-Hoenderdos NL, Slot DE, Van der Weijen GA: The incidence of complications associated with lip and/or tongue piercings: a systematic review, *Int J Dent Hyg* 14:62–73, 2016.

Levin L, Zadik Y: Oral piercing: complications and side effects, *Am J Dent* 20:340–344, 2007.

Loh FC, Yeo JF: Talisman in the orofacial region, *Oral Surg Oral Med Oral Pathol* 68:252–255, 1989.

Nor MM, Yushar A, Razali M, et al.: Incidental radiologic findings of susuk in the orofacial region, *Dentomaxillofac Radiol* 35:473–474, 2006.

Stanko P, Poruban D, Mracna J, et al.: Squamous cell carcinoma and piercing of the tongue – a case report, *J Craniomaxillofac Surg* 40:329–331, 2012.

Ziebolz D, Stuehmer C, van Nüss K, et al.: Complications of tongue piercing: a review of the literature and three case reports, *J Contemp Dent Pract* 10:E65–E71, 2009.

Oral Lesions Associated with Cosmetic Fillers

Daley T, Damm DD, Haden JA, et al.: Oral lesions associated with injected hydroxyapatite cosmetic filler, *Oral Surg Oral Med Oral Pathol Oral Radiol* 114:107–111, 2012.

Dwivedi K, Prabhu IS, Bradley KM: Fluorodeoxyglucose activity associated with a cosmetic poly-L-lactide filler: a potential confounder on positron emission tomography and computed tomography, *Br J Oral Maxillofac Surg* 56:148–150, 2018.

Farahani SS, Sexton J, Stone JD, et al.: Lip nodules caused by hyaluronic acid filler injection: report of three cases, *Head Neck Pathol* 6:16–20, 2012.

Grippaudo FR, Di Girolamo M, Mattei M, et al.: Diagnosis and management of dermal filler complications in the perioral region, *J Cosmet Laser Ther* 16:246–252, 2014.

Gupta A, Miller PJ: Management of lip complications, *Facial Plast Surg Clin N Am* 27:565–570, 2019.

Karagozoglu KH, van der Waal I: Polyacrylamide soft tissue filler nodule mimicking a mucoepidermoid carcinoma, *Int J Oral Maxillofac Surg* 37:578–580, 2008.

Koka S, Shah K, Mallya S: Dermal filler presenting as lobular radiopacities in an edentulous patient: a clinical report, *J Prosthodont* 26:670–671, 2017.

Shahrabi-Farahani S, Lerman MA, Noonan V, et al.: Granulomatous foreign body reaction to dermal cosmetic fillers with intraoral migration, *Oral Surg Oral Med Oral Pathol Oral Radiol* 117:105–110, 2014.

Requena C, Requena L, Alegre V, et al.: Adverse reaction to silicone simulating orofacial granulomatosis, *Eur Acad Dermatol Venereol* 29:998–1001, 2015.

Valiyaparambil J, Rengasamy K, Mallya SM: An unusual soft tissue radiopacity—radiographic appearance of a dermal filler, *Br Dent J* 207:211–212, 2009.

Systemic Metal Intoxication

Ahnlide I, Ahlgren C, Björkner B, et al.: Gold concentration in blood in relation to the number of gold restorations and contact allergy to gold, *Acta Odontol Scand* 60:301–305, 2002.

Bellinger DC, Trachtenberg F, Barregard L, et al.: Neuropsychological and renal effects of dental amalgam in children: a randomized trial, *J Am Med Assoc* 295:1775–1783, 2006.

Burton H: On a remarkable effect on the human gums, produced by the absorption of lead, *Med Chir Trans* 23:63–79, 1840.

Choi H, Castillo B, Seminario-Vidal L: Silver absorption in patients with Steven-Johnson syndrome and toxic epidermal necrolysis treated with silver-impregnated dressings, a case series, *Int Wound J* 15:1049–1051, 2018.

DeRouen TA, Martin MD, Leroux BG, et al.: Neurobehavioral effects of dental amalgam in children, a randomized trial, *J Am Med Assoc* 295:1784–1792, 2006.

Drake PL, Hazelwood KJ: Exposure-repeated health effects of silver and silver compounds: a review, *Ann Occup Hyg* 49:575–585, 2005.

Dummet CO: Systemic significance of oral pigmentation and discoloration, *Postgrad Med J* 49(1):78–82, 1971.

Fowler J Jr, Taylor J, Storrs F, et al.: Gold allergy in North America, *Am J Contact Dermat* 12:3–5, 2001.

Garg A: Case presentation: the blue line, *Dent Implantol Update* 21:45–48, 2010.

Gaslin MT, Rubin C, Pribitkin EA: Silver nasal sprays: misleading internet marketing, *Ear Nose Throat J* 87:217–220, 2008.

Gordon NC, Brown S, Khosla VM, et al.: Lead poisoning: a comprehensive review and report of a case, *Oral Surg Oral Med Oral Pathol* 47:500–512, 1979.

Han TY, Chang HS, Lee HK, et al.: Successful treatment of argyria using a low-fluence Q-switched 1064-nm Nd:YAG laser, *Int J Dermatol* 50:751–753, 2011.

Harris RA, Poole A: Beware of bismuth: post maxillectomy delirium, *ANZ J Surg* 72:846–847, 2002.

Ioffreda MD, Gordon CA, Adams DR, et al.: Black tongue, *Arch Dermatol* 137:968–969, 2001.

Jacobs R: Argyria: my life story, *Clin Dermatol* 24:66–69, 2006.

Lee SM, Lee SH: Generalized argyria after habitual use of AgNO$_3$, *J Dermatol* 21:50–53, 1994.

Marshall JP, Schneider RP: Systemic argyria secondary to topical silver nitrate, *Arch Dermatol* 113:1077–1179, 1977.

Martin MD, Williams BJ, Charleston JD, et al.: Spontaneous exfoliation of teeth following severe elemental mercury poisoning: case report and histological investigation for mechanism, *Oral Surg Oral Med Oral Pathol Oral Radiol Endod* 84:495–501, 1997.

Mutter J, Yeter D: Kawasaki's disease, acrodynia, and mercury, *Curr Med Chem* 15:3000–3010, 2008.

Pimparkar BD, Bhave A: Arsenicosis: review of recent advances, *J Assoc Physicians India* 58:617–624, 2010.

Rerknimitr P, Kantikosum K, Chottawornsak N, et al.: Chronic occupational exposure to lead leads to significant mucocutaneous changes in lead factory workers, *J Eur Acad Dermatol Venereol* 33:1993–2000, 2019.

Su M, Barrueto F Jr, Hoffman RS: Childhood lead poisoning from paint chips: a continuing problem, *J Urban Health* 79:491–501, 2002.

Smoker's Melanosis

Axéll T, Hedin CA: Epidemiologic study of excessive oral melanin pigmentation with special reference to the influence of tobacco habits, *Scand J Dent Res* 90:434–442, 1982.

Hedin CA: Smokers' melanosis, *Arch Dermatol* 113:1533–1538, 1977.

Hedin CA, Axéll T: Oral melanin pigmentation in 467 Thai and Malaysian people with special emphasis on smoker's melanosis, *J Oral Pathol Med* 20:8–12, 1991.

Hedin CA, Larsson Å: The ultrastructure of the gingival epithelium in smokers' melanosis, *J Periodontal Res* 19:177–190, 1984.

Hedin CA, Pindborg JJ, Daftary DK, et al.: Melanin depigmentation of the palatal mucosa in reverse smokers: a preliminary study, *J Oral Pathol Med* 21:440–444, 1992.

Ramer M, Burakoff RP: Smoker's melanosis, *N Y State Dent J* 63:20–21, 1997.

Drug-Related Discolorations of the Oral Mucosa

Beacher N.G., Brodie M.J., Goodall C.: A case report: retigabine induced oral mucosal dyspigmentation of the hard palate, BMC Oral Health 15:122. https://doi.org/10.1186/s12903-015-0102-y.

Cale AE, Freedman PD, Lumerman H: Pigmentation of the jawbones and teeth secondary to minocycline hydrochloride therapy, *J Periodontol* 59:112–114, 1988.

Cockings JM, Savage NW: Minocycline and oral pigmentation, *Aust Dent J* 43:14–16, 1998.

Donnell CC, Walton RL, Carrozzo M: The blue palate – a case series of imatinib-related oral pigmentation and literature review, *Oral Surg Oral Med Oral Pathol Oral Radiol* 131:49–61, 2021.

Dummet CO: Oral mucosal discolorations related to pharmacotherapeutics, *J Oral Ther Pharmacol* 1:106–110, 1964.

Granstein RD, Sober AJ: Drug- and heavy metal-induced hyperpigmentation, *J Am Acad Dermatol* 5:1–18, 1981.

Hood AF: Cutaneous side effects of cancer chemotherapy, *Med Clin North Am* 70:187–209, 1986.

Langford A, Pohle H-D, Gelderblom H, et al.: Oral hyperpigmentation in HIV-infected patients, *Oral Surg Oral Med Oral Pathol* 67:301–307, 1989.

Lyne A, Creedon A, Bailey BMW: Mucosal pigmentation of the hard palate in a patient taking imatinib, *BMJ Case Rep*, 2015. https://doi.org/10.1136/bcr-2015-209335.

Rosebush MS, Briody AN, Cordell KG: Black and brown: non-neoplastic pigmentation of the oral mucosa, *Head Neck Pathol* 13:47–55, 2019.

Treister NS, Magalnick D, Woo S-B: Oral mucosal pigmentation secondary to minocycline therapy: report of two cases and a review of the literature, *Oral Surg Oral Med Oral Pathol Oral Radiol Endod* 97:718–725, 2004.

Reactive Osseous and Chondromatous Metaplasia

Cutright DE: Osseous and chondromatous metaplasia caused by dentures, *Oral Surg Oral Med Oral Pathol* 34:625–633, 1972.

Daley TD, Damm DD, Wysocki GP, et al.: Atypical cartilage in reactive osteocartilagenous metaplasia of the traumatized edentulous mandibular ridge, *Oral Surg Oral Med Oral Pathol Oral Radiol Endod* 83:26–29, 1997.

Lello GE, Makek M: Submucosal nodular chondrometaplasia in denture wearers, *J Prosthet Dent* 54:237–240, 1985.

Magnusson BC, Engström H, Kahnberg K-E: Metaplastic formation of bone and chondroid in flabby ridges, *Br J Oral Maxillofac Surg* 24:300–305, 1986.

Oral Ulceration with Bone Sequestration

Farah CS, Savage NW: Oral ulceration with bone sequestration, *Aust Dent J* 48:61–64, 2003.

Palla B, Burian E, Klecker JR, et al.: Systematic review of oral ulcerations with bone sequestration, *J Craniomaxillofac Surg* 44:257–264, 2016.

Peters E, Lovas GL, Wysocki GP: Lingual mandibular sequestration and ulceration, *Oral Surg Oral Med Oral Pathol Oral Radiol Endod* 75:739–743, 1993.

Scully C: Oral ulceration: a new and unusual complication, *Br Dent J* 192:139–140, 2002.

Sonnier KE, Horning GM: Spontaneous bony exposure: a report of 4 cases of idiopathic exposure and sequestration of alveolar bone, *J Periodontol* 68:758–762, 1997.

Thermos G, Kalogirou EM, Tosios K, et al.: Oral ulceration with bone sequestration: retrospective study of eight cases and literature review, *Oral Dis* 25:515–522, 2019.

Pseudocysts and True Cysts of the Maxillary Sinus

Allard RHB, van der Kwast WAM, van der Waal I: Mucosal antral cysts: review of the literature and report of a radiographic survey, *Oral Surg Oral Med Oral Pathol* 51:2–9, 1981.

Bourgeois SL, Nelson BL: Surgical ciliated cyst of the mandible secondary to simultaneous LeFort I osteotomy and genioplasty: report of case and review of the literature, *Oral Surg Oral Med Oral Pathol Oral Radiol Endod* 100:36–39, 2005.

Gardner DG: Pseudocysts and retention cysts of the maxillary sinus, *Oral Surg Oral Med Oral Pathol* 58:561–567, 1984.

Gardner DG, Gullane PJ: Mucoceles of the maxillary sinus, *Oral Surg Oral Med Oral Pathol* 62:538–543, 1986.

Kaneshiro S, Nakajima T, Yoshikawa Y, et al.: The postoperative maxillary cyst: report of 71 cases, *J Oral Surg* 39:191–198, 1981.

Li CC, Feinerman DM, MacCarthy KD, et al.: Rare mandibular surgical ciliated cysts: report of two new cases, *J Oral Maxillofac Surg* 72:1736–1743, 2014.

Sultan M, Haberland CM, Skrip L, et al.: Prevalence of antral pseudocysts in the pediatric population, *Pediatr Dent* 37:541–544, 2015.

Wang JH, Jang YJ, Lee B-J: Natural course of retention cysts of the maxillary sinus: long-term follow-up results, *Laryngoscope* 117:341–344, 2007.

Yang HC, Kang SH, Yoon SH, et al.: Transnasal endoscopic removal of bilateral postoperative maxillary cysts after aesthetic orthognathic surgery: differences from that of Caldwell-Luc operations, *Auris Nasus Larynx* 45:608–612, 2018.

Cervicofacial Emphysema

An GK, Zats B, Kunin M: Orbital, mediastinal, and cervicofacial subcutaneous emphysema after endodontic retreatment of a mandibular premolar: a case report, *J Endod* 40:880–883, 2014.

Heyman SN, Babayof I: Emphysematous complications in dentistry, 1960-1993: an illustrative case and review of the literature, *Quintessence Int* 26:535–543, 1995.

López-Peláez MF, Roldán J, Mateo S: Cervical emphysema, pneumomediastinum, and pneumothorax following self-induced oral injury: report of four cases and review of the literature, *Chest* 120:306–309, 2001.

Martìn-Granizo R, Herrera M, Garcìa-Gonzàlez D, et al.: Pneumoparotid in childhood: report of two cases, *J Oral Maxillofac Surg* 57:1468–1471, 1999.

McKenzie WS, Rosenberg M: Iatrogenic subcutaneous emphysema of dental and surgical origin: a literature review, *J Oral Maxillofac Surg* 67:1265–1268, 2009.

Patel N, Lazow SK, Berger J: Cervicofacial subcutaneous emphysema: case report and review of the literature, *J Oral Maxillofac Surg* 68:1976–1982, 2010.

Shovelton DS: Surgical emphysema as a complication of dental operation, *Br Med J* 102:125–129, 1957.

Turnbull A: A remarkable coincidence in dental surgery, *Br Med J* 1:1131, 1900.

Vargo RJ, Potluri A, Yeung AY, et al.: Cervicofacial subcutaneous emphysema: a clinical case and review of the literature, *Gen Dent* 64:68–71, 2016.

Myospherulosis

Dunlap CL, Barker BF: Myospherulosis of the jaws, *Oral Surg Oral Med Oral Pathol* 50:238–243, 1980.

LeBlanc P, Ghannoum JE: Myospherulosis of the mandible presenting as a multilocular lesion: a case report and review of the literature, *Head Neck Pathol* 10:221–224, 2016.

Lynch DP, Newland JR, McClendon JL: Myospherulosis of the oral hard and soft tissues, *J Oral Maxillofac Surg* 42:349–355, 1984.

Sarkar S, Gangane N, Sharma S: Myospherulosis of maxillary sinus—a case report with review of literature, *Indian J Pathol Microbiol* 41:491–493, 1998.

Wallace ML, Neville BW: Myospherulosis: report of a case, *J Periodontol* 61:55–57, 1990.

9

Allergies and Immunologic Diseases

◆ TRANSIENT LINGUAL PAPILLITIS

Transient lingual papillitis (lie bumps, tongue torches) represents a common oral pathosis that rarely has been documented. Affected patients experience clinical alterations that involve a variable number of fungiform papillae of the tongue. These papillae are covered with thin nonkeratinized epithelium containing scattered taste bud pores associated with a highly innervated stroma. This unique anatomy that appears relatively susceptible to injury has been proposed to be responsible for the selective involvement of fungiform papillae in transient papillitis. The pathogenesis currently is unknown, but the lesions most likely arise from a variety of influences. Suggested causes include local irritation, stress, gastrointestinal disease, hormonal fluctuation, upper respiratory tract infection, viral infection, and topical hypersensitivity to foods, drinks, or oral hygiene products.

Clinical Features

Three patterns of transient lingual papillitis have been documented. The first pattern is localized and involves one to several fungiform papillae that become enlarged and present as elevated papules that are red but may demonstrate a yellow, ulcerated cap (Fig. 9.1). The lesions appear most frequently on the anterior portion of the dorsal surface, are associated with mild to moderate pain, and resolve spontaneously within hours to several days. In a survey of 163 dental school staff members, 56% reported previous episodes of transient lingual papillitis. There was a female predominance, and the vast majority reported a single affected papilla. In one report, the occurrence of the lesions appeared to be associated with a food allergy.

In the second pattern, the involvement is more generalized and affects a large percentage of the fungiform papillae on the tip and lateral portions of the dorsal surface (Fig. 9.2). Individual papillae are very sensitive, enlarged, erythematous, and occasionally display focal surface erosion. Fever and cervical lymphadenopathy may be seen in some individuals. In such cases, spread of the process among family members has been reported, suggesting a possible correlation to an unknown virus. Spontaneous resolution occurs in about 7 days with occasional recurrences reported.

The third pattern of transient lingual papillitis also demonstrates more diffuse involvement. The altered papillae are asymptomatic, appear as elevated white to yellow papules, and have been termed the *papulokeratotic variant* because of a thickened parakeratotic cap (Fig. 9.3). Although these lesions could be the result of a topical allergy, the histopathology demonstrates features similar to chronic nibbling and suggests the possibility of an unusual pattern of frictional hyperkeratosis.

Histopathologic Features

On histopathologic examination of the first two variants, affected papillae demonstrate normal surface epithelium that may reveal focal areas of exocytosis or ulceration. The underlying lamina propria exhibits a proliferation of numerous small vascular channels and a mixed inflammatory cellular infiltrate. Investigation for evidence of human papillomavirus (HPV), herpes simplex, and fungal infestation has been negative. The papulokeratotic variant demonstrates marked hyperparakeratosis in which the surface is ragged and reveals bacterial colonization. A chronic lymphocytic infiltrate is noted in the superficial lamina propria with extension into the basilar portion of the adjacent epithelium.

Treatment and Prognosis

Although transient lingual papillitis resolves without therapy, topical corticosteroids, anesthetics, and coating agents have been used to reduce the pain or duration. In an attempt to eliminate the pain, occasional patients have reported removing the affected papillae with devices such as fingernail clippers. The papulokeratotic variant is asymptomatic and requires no therapy. Although frequently unsuccessful, search for a local or systemic triggering event seems prudent.

◆ RECURRENT APHTHOUS STOMATITIS (RECURRENT APHTHOUS ULCERATIONS; CANKER SORES)

Recurrent aphthous stomatitis (RAS) is one of the most common oral mucosal pathoses. The name arises from the Greek work *aphtha*, which refers to an ulcer of the mucosal surface. The reported prevalence in the general population varies from 5% to 66%, with a mean of 20%. Different subgroups of patients appear to have different causes for the

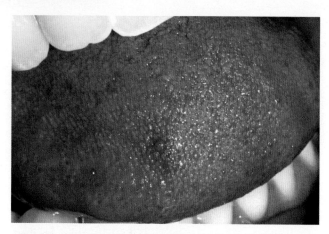

• **Fig. 9.1 Transient Lingual Papillitis.** Tender, yellow-pink papule on the dorsum of the tongue.

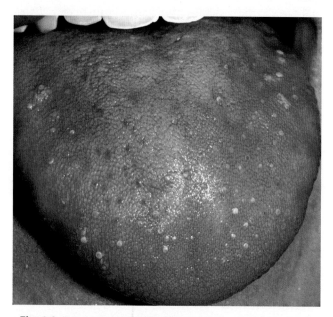

• **Fig. 9.2 Transient Lingual Papillitis.** Multiple painful white papules on the lateral dorsum and tip of tongue.

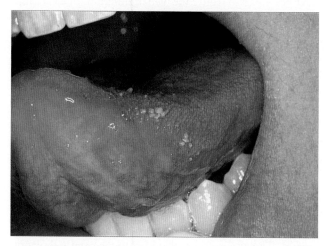

• **Fig. 9.3 Transient Lingual Papillitis.** Clusters of asymptomatic, elevated, yellow papules on the dorsolateral surface of the tongue. (Courtesy of Dr. Craig Fowler.)

occurrence of aphthae. These factors suggest a common disease process that may be initiated by a variety of causative agents, each of which can produce the disease in certain subgroups of patients. To state it simply, the cause appears to be "different things in different people."

Although no single triggering agent is responsible, the mucosal destruction appears to represent a T cell–mediated immunologic reaction with involvement of tumor necrosis factor-alpha (TNF-α). This factor is a major inflammatory cytokine and assists in the ultimate targeting of the surface epithelium for destruction by cytotoxic T cells (CD8+). Evidence of the destruction of the oral mucosa mediated by these lymphocytes is strong, but the initiating causes are elusive and most likely highly variable.

The following all have been reported to be responsible in certain subgroups of patients (and each discounted in other subgroups!):

• Allergies
• Genetic predisposition
• Hematologic abnormalities
• Hormonal influences
• Immunologic factors
• Infectious agents
• Nutritional deficiencies
• Smoking cessation
• Stress (mental and physical)
• Trauma

Investigators have theorized that aphthae develop from an immunologic reaction to an oral antigen. This reaction may arise due the presence of a highly antigenic reagent, a decrease in the mucosal barrier that previously masked the antigen, or immunodysregulation resulting in an abnormal response to a normally present antigen. All previously described triggers can be grouped into one of these three categories. One or more of these three factors may be involved in subgroups of patients.

Genetic predisposition appears to be important in many patients with approximately 40% of affected individuals reporting a positive family history. Children with a family history of RAS demonstrate a 90% chance of developing aphthae, whereas the prevalence drops to 20% in children without affected parents.

An antigenic stimulus appears to be the primary initiating factor in the immune-mediated cytotoxic destruction of the mucosa in many patients. The list seems endless, and every item on the list may be important in small subsets of patients. Commonly mentioned potential antigens include sodium lauryl sulfate in toothpaste, many systemic medications (e.g., nonsteroidal anti-inflammatory drugs [NSAIDs], bisphosphonates, various beta blockers, angiotensin receptor blockers, cyclooxygenase-2 inhibitors, rapamycin inhibitors, trimethoprim-sulfamethoxazole, and nicorandil), microbiologic agents (e.g., L forms of streptococci, *Helicobacter pylori*, herpes simplex virus [HSV], varicella-zoster virus [VZV], adenovirus, and cytomegalovirus [CMV]), and many foods (e.g., cheese, chocolate, coffee, cow's milk, gluten, nuts, strawberries, tomatoes, dyes, flavoring agents, and preservatives).

The mucosal barrier appears to be important in the prevention of aphthous stomatitis and might explain the almost exclusive presence of aphthous stomatitis on nonkeratinized mucosa. Numerous factors that decrease the mucosal barrier increase the frequency of occurrence (e.g., trauma, nutritional deficiencies, and smoking cessation); conversely, those associated with an increased mucosal barrier have been correlated with decreased ulcerations (e.g., smoking, hormonal changes, and marked absence of aphthae on mucosa bound to bone).

An increased prevalence of aphthous-like ulcerations has been noted in a variety of systemic disorders (Box 9.1). These ulcerations typically are identical clinically and histopathologically to those noted in otherwise healthy individuals. In many cases, resolution of the systemic disorder produces a decreased frequency and severity of the mucosal ulcerations.

Three clinical variations of aphthous stomatitis are recognized:
1. Minor
2. Major
3. Herpetiform

Minor aphthae (Mikulicz aphthae) are the most common and represent the pattern present in more than 80% of those affected. Major aphthae (Sutton disease or periadenitis mucosa necrotica recurrens [PMNR]) occur in approximately 10% of the patients referred for treatment. The remaining patients have herpetiform aphthae. The minor and major forms most likely represent variations of the same process, although herpetiform aphthae demonstrate a unique pattern. Some investigators differentiate the herpetiform variant because of supposed evidence of a viral cause, but the proof is weak and does not justify its distinction from the other aphthous ulcerations. Some authors include Behçet syndrome as an additional variation of aphthous stomatitis, but this multisystem disorder is more complex and is considered later in this chapter.

• BOX 9.1 Systemic Disorders Associated With Recurrent Aphthous Stomatitis

- Behçet syndrome
- Celiac disease
- Cyclic neutropenia
- Nutritional deficiencies (iron, folate, zinc, B_1, B_2, B_6, and B_{12})
- Immunoglobulin A (IgA) deficiency
- Immunocompromised conditions, including human immunodeficiency virus (HIV) disease
- Inflammatory bowel disease (ulcerative colitis, Crohn disease)
- MAGIC syndrome (mouth and genital ulcers with inflamed cartilage)
- PFAPA syndrome (periodic fever, aphthous stomatitis, pharyngitis, cervical adenitis)
- Systemic lupus erythematosus
- *H. pylori* disease
- Reactive arthritis
- Sweet syndrome
- Ulcus vulvae acutum

Clinical Features

Aphthous stomatitis is noted more frequently in children and young adults, with approximately 80% of affected individuals reporting their first ulceration before the age of 30. If persistent RAS arises after the third decade of life, there should be an increased suspicion of an association with a systemic condition such as a hematologic disorder, immune dysfunction, or Behçet syndrome.

Minor Aphthous Stomatitis

Patients with minor aphthae experience the fewest recurrences, and the individual lesions exhibit the shortest duration of the three variants. The ulcers arise almost exclusively on nonkeratinized mucosa and may be preceded by an erythematous macule in association with prodromal symptoms of burning, itching, or stinging. The ulceration demonstrates a yellow-white, removable fibrinopurulent membrane that is encircled by an erythematous halo (Fig. 9.4). Classically, the ulcerations measure between 3 and 10 mm in diameter, demonstrate a variable recurrence rate, and heal without scarring in 7–14 days (Fig. 9.5). Although scores of ulcerations

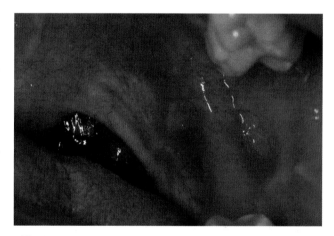

• **Fig. 9.4 Minor Aphthous Stomatitis.** Erythematous halo encircling a yellowish ulceration of the soft palate on the left side.

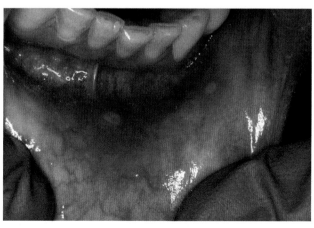

• **Fig. 9.5 Minor Aphthous Stomatitis.** Two ulcerations located on the mandibular labial mucosa.

may be present at once, from one to five lesions typically are present during a single episode, and the pain often is out of proportion for the size of the ulceration. The buccal and labial mucosae are affected most frequently, followed by the ventral surface of the tongue, mucobuccal fold, floor of the mouth, and soft palate (Fig. 9.6). Involvement of keratinized mucosa (e.g., hard palate, gingiva, dorsal surface of the tongue, and vermilion border) is rare and usually represents extension from adjacent nonkeratinized epithelium.

Major Aphthous Stomatitis

Major aphthae are larger than minor aphthae and demonstrate the longest duration per episode. The ulcerations are deeper than the minor variant, measure from 1 to 3 cm in diameter, take from 2 to 6 weeks to heal, and may cause scarring (Fig. 9.7). The number of lesions varies from 1 to 10. Any oral surface area may be affected, but the labial mucosa, soft palate, and tonsillar fauces are involved most commonly (Fig. 9.8). The onset of major aphthae is after puberty, and recurrent episodes may continue to develop for up to 20 years or more. With time, the associated scarring can become significant, and in rare instances may lead to a restricted mouth opening.

Herpetiform Aphthous Stomatitis

Herpetiform aphthae demonstrate the greatest number of lesions and the most frequent recurrences. The individual lesions are small, averaging 1–3 mm in diameter, with as many as 100 ulcers present in a single recurrence. Because of their small size and large number, the lesions bear a superficial resemblance to a primary HSV infection, leading to the confusing designation, **herpetiform.** It is common for individual lesions to coalesce into larger irregular ulcerations (Fig. 9.9). The ulcerations heal within 7–10 days, but the recurrences tend to be closely spaced. Although the nonkeratinized, movable mucosa is affected most frequently, any oral mucosal surface may be involved. There is a female predominance, and typically the onset is in adulthood.

Further classification of all three types is valuable when planning the most appropriate diagnostic evaluation and therapy. The lesions are diagnosed as **simple aphthosis** when they appear in patients with few lesions that heal within 1–2 weeks and recur infrequently. In contrast, patients with **complex aphthosis** have multiple (three or more) and almost constant oral ulcerations that often develop as older lesions resolve. Severe pain and large size

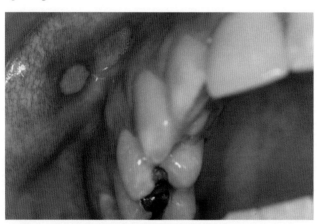

• **Fig. 9.6 Minor Aphthous Stomatitis.** Single ulceration of the anterior buccal mucosa.

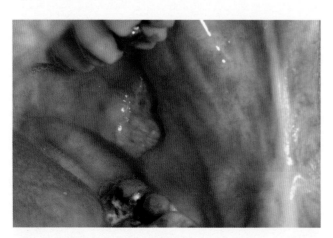

• **Fig. 9.7 Major Aphthous Stomatitis.** Large, deep, and irregular ulceration of the posterior buccal mucosa. Note extensive scarring of the anterior buccal mucosa from previous ulcerations.

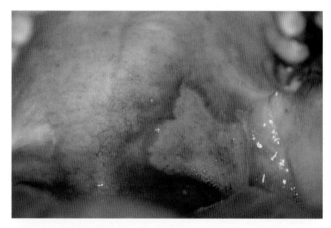

• **Fig. 9.8 Major Aphthous Stomatitis.** Large, irregular ulceration of the soft palate.

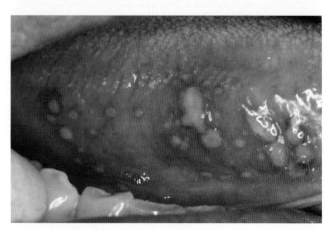

• **Fig. 9.9 Herpetiform Aphthous Stomatitis.** Numerous pinhead ulcerations of the ventral surface of the tongue, several of which have coalesced into larger, more irregular areas of ulceration.

are common. Although associated genital or perianal lesions also may be present, there is no other evidence of an associated systemic disease.

Histopathologic Features

The histopathologic picture of aphthous stomatitis is characteristic but not pathognomonic. The early ulcerative lesions demonstrate a central zone of ulceration, which is covered by a fibrinopurulent membrane. Deep to the area of ulceration, the connective tissue exhibits an increased vascularity and a mixed inflammatory cellular infiltrate that consists of lymphocytes, histiocytes, and polymorphonuclear leukocytes. The epithelium at the margin of the lesion demonstrates spongiosis and numerous mononuclear cells in the basilar one-third. A band of lymphocytes intermixed with histiocytes is present in the superficial connective tissue and surrounding deeper blood vessels.

Diagnosis

No laboratory procedure provides definitive diagnosis. The diagnosis is made from the clinical presentation and from exclusion of other diseases that produce ulcerations that closely resemble aphthae (see Box 9.1). In patients with complex aphthosis, a systematic evaluation for an underlying trigger or associated systemic condition is prudent. In a review of 244 patients with complex aphthosis, an associated triggering condition (e.g., hematologic deficiency, gastrointestinal disease, immunodeficiency, and drug reaction) was discovered in almost 60%. Because the histopathologic features are nonspecific, a biopsy is useful only in eliminating differential possibilities and is not beneficial in arriving at the definitive diagnosis.

Treatment and Prognosis

The patient's medical history should be reviewed for signs and symptoms of any systemic disorder that may be associated with aphthous-like ulcerations. Most patients with mild aphthosis receive either no treatment, therapy with several over-the-counter anesthetics or protective bioadhesive products, or periodic topical medicaments that minimize the frequency and severity of the attacks.

In patients with mild disease who fail or reject over-the-counter products, the mainstay of therapy is the use of topical corticosteroids, and the list of possible choices is long. Most patients with diffuse minor or herpetiform aphthae respond well to dexamethasone solution (0.5 mg/5 mL) used in a rinse-and-expectorate method. Patients with localized ulcerations can be treated successfully with 0.05% augmented betamethasone dipropionate gel or 0.05% fluocinonide gel. Adrenal suppression does not occur with appropriate use of these medications. Major aphthae are more resistant to therapy and often warrant more potent corticosteroids (Fig. 9.10). The individual lesions may be injected with triamcinolone acetonide or covered with 0.05% clobetasol propionate gel or 0.05% halobetasol propionate ointment. Triamcinolone tablets also can be dissolved directly over the lesions. In hard-to-reach areas, such as the tonsillar pillars, beclomethasone dipropionate aerosol spray can be used. In resistant cases, systemic corticosteroids may be required to supplement the topical medications and gain control. In such instances, prednisolone oral suspension in a swish-and-swallow method is preferable to prednisone tablets. In this way, the ulcerations receive both topical and systemic therapy.

An almost endless list of alternatives to corticosteroid agents has been used to treat patients suffering from aphthous stomatitis. Caution should be exercised, however, because many of these agents have not been examined in a double-blind, placebo-controlled fashion to assess the degree of effectiveness compared with placebo. Furthermore, some of these treatments may have significant side effects or may be quite expensive. Accepted topical alternatives include chlorhexidine, tetracycline oral suspension, and triclosan mouthrinse. In a Cochrane meta-analysis, no single systemic therapy was found to be effective in a wide variety of patients. Frequently mentioned systemic therapies include several

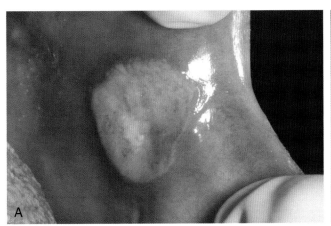
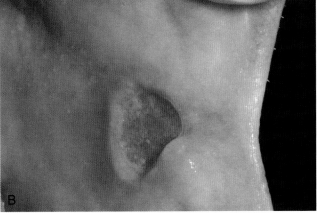

• **Fig. 9.10   Major Aphthous Stomatitis. A,** Large ulceration of the left anterior buccal mucosa. **B,** Same lesion after 5 days of therapy with betamethasone syrup used in a swish-and-swallow method. The patient was free of pain by the second day of therapy. The ulceration healed completely during the next week.

immunomodulatory agents, such as azathioprine, colchicine, dapsone, levamisole, pentoxifylline, and thalidomide. A growing list of medications that inhibit inflammatory cytokines such as TNF-α have been shown to be effective against RAS but often demonstrate significant adverse reactions and associated high cost. Included in this list are apremilast, adalimumab, etanercept, infliximab, and golimumab, with these therapies often reserved for complex aphthosis that has failed numerous more conservative therapies.

Although laser ablation shortens the duration and decreases associated symptoms, its use is of very limited practical benefit because patients cannot return on each recurrence. Chemical cautery with silver nitrate continues to be suggested as an effective therapy, but it can no longer be recommended because of the numerous safer alternatives and its rare association with massive necrosis (see page 279) and systemic argyria (see page 305). A cautery that uses sulfuric acid and phenolic agents is indicated in certain situations but must be used with caution due to the potential for significant local tissue necrosis related to its misuse.

The success of these different therapeutic approaches is variable from patient to patient. In addition, these interventions do not resolve the underlying problem and are merely an attempt to "beat back brush fires." Recurrences often continue, although breaking up the cycle may induce longer disease-free intervals between attacks. Surgical removal of aphthous ulcerations has been used but is an inappropriate therapy.

Patients with complex aphthosis require a more extensive evaluation for occult systemic disease and a search for possible triggers of the immune-mediated mucosal destruction. To go beyond the management of individual recurrences is difficult, expensive, and often frustrating. Despite this, patients with severe disease should be offered the opportunity to investigate the underlying causes.

◆ BEHÇET DISEASE (BEHÇET SYNDROME; ADAMANTIADES SYNDROME; SILK ROAD DISEASE)

The combination of chronic ocular inflammation and orogenital ulcerations was reported as early as the era of the ancient Greeks and later described in 1931 by a Greek ophthalmologist, Benedict Adamantiades. The classic triad was not delineated until 1937, when a Turkish dermatologist, Hulusi Behçet, defined the disease that bears his name. Although the disease traditionally has been thought primarily to affect the oral, genital, and ocular regions, it now is recognized to be a systemic vasculitis that also may demonstrate cutaneous, articular, vascular, gastrointestinal, and neurologic involvement.

Although no clear causation has been established, **Behçet disease** appears to represent an abnormal immune process triggered by an infectious or environmental antigen in a genetically predisposed individual. Investigators have correlated attacks to several environmental agents, including bacteria (especially streptococci), viruses (especially herpes simplex virus 1), pesticides, and heavy metals. Interestingly, reduction of oral bacterial load via periodontal therapy has been shown to reduce the prevalence of associated oral ulcerations in patients with Behçet disease. It is thought that antigens of some microorganisms exhibit a high homology with human proteins resulting in a cross-reaction that leads to the autoinflammatory response. Although the exact immune reactions have not been defined, T cells, neutrophils, and antigen-presenting cells appear to be involved significantly. Antigen-presenting cells are thought to trigger neutrophilic hyperactivity followed by stimulation of T helper cells with several cytokines released from neutrophils.

Histocompatibility antigen B-51 (HLA-B51) has been linked closely to Behçet disease, and the frequency of both the disease and this haplotype is high in Turkey, Japan, and the Eastern Mediterranean countries. This distribution appears correlated to the ancient trading route known as the "Silk Road" that extended from Japan to Rome and was traveled by the Turks. Sexual reproduction between immigrants and locals along the route appears to have spread the genetic vulnerability. Interestingly, when predisposed populations migrate to nonendemic locations, the prevalence decreases, suggesting environmental factors also are involved.

Clinical Features

Behçet disease is uncommon in blacks and usually arises in the third and fourth decades with the disease rarely presenting before puberty or beyond the age of 50. Men exhibit a slightly increased prevalence and tend to have a worse clinical course.

Virtually all affected patients demonstrate oral ulcerations that often herald the onset of the more generalized disease process. Other less frequently associated features in order of prevalence include genital ulcerations, cutaneous lesions, arthritis, uveitis, thrombophlebitis, gastrointestinal manifestations, and central nervous system (CNS) involvement.

The oral lesions are similar to aphthae occurring in otherwise healthy individuals and demonstrate the same duration and frequency. The individual lesions vary in size and are surrounded by a larger zone of diffuse erythema (Fig. 9.11). All three forms of oral aphthous stomatitis may be seen. Although most affected patients have lesions that resemble minor aphthae, some reports have documented a prevalence of major aphthae that approaches 40% in patients affected with Behçet disease. The herpetiform variant remains uncommon and is noted in approximately 3%. Although the lesions closely resemble conventional aphthae, the ulcerations in Behçet disease often are increased in number and frequently involve the soft palate and oropharynx.

The genital lesions occur in 75% of the patients. In males, approximately 90% of the lesions involve the scrotum, whereas those in females are most frequent on the vulva, vagina, or uterine cervix. Perineal, perianal, and groin involvement is seen in both genders (Fig. 9.12). These

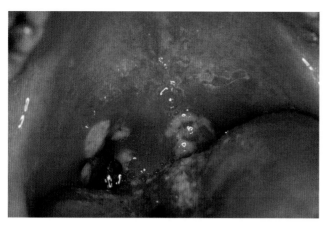

• **Fig. 9.11 Behçet Syndrome.** Diffuse erythema surrounding numerous irregular ulcerations of the soft palate.

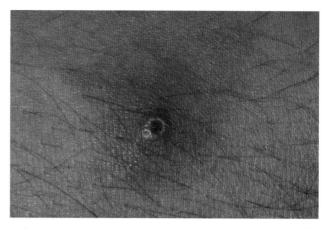

• **Fig. 9.13 Behçet Syndrome.** Sterile pustule of the skin that developed 1 day after injection of saline. This reaction is termed *cutaneous pathergy.*

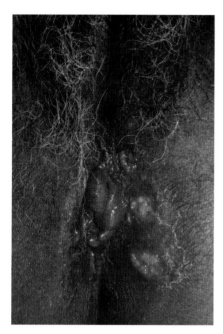

• **Fig. 9.12 Behçet Syndrome.** Numerous irregular ulcerations of the labia majora and perineum. (From Helm TN, Camisa C, Allen C, et al: Clinical features of Behçet's disease, *Oral Surg Oral Med Oral Pathol* 72:30, 1991.)

nondeforming. The knees, wrists, elbows, and ankles are affected most frequently.

Ocular involvement occurs in up to 70% of the cases and is more frequent and severe in males. The most common findings are posterior uveitis, conjunctivitis, corneal ulceration, papilledema, and arteritis. The most common secondary ocular complications are cataracts, glaucoma, and neovascularization of the iris and retina. Despite therapy, blindness occurs in 25% of patients with ocular involvement.

Although the vascular disease may involve arteries, veins are affected more frequently and present as superficial and deep thrombophlebitis. The thrombi tend to be adherent to the diseased veins without a tendency toward embolism. Behçet disease is a variable vessel vasculitis because it can affect vessels of any size with involvement of both the venous and arterial systems.

Gastrointestinal disease is variable and includes abdominal pain, anorexia, diarrhea, dyspepsia, and vomiting. CNS involvement is not common but, when present, is associated with a poor prognosis. From 10% to 25% of the patients demonstrate CNS involvement, and the alterations produced result in several changes that include paralysis and severe dementia.

Diagnosis

No laboratory finding is diagnostic of Behçet disease. To standardize diagnoses, definitive criteria have been developed. Table 9.1 delineates the requirements proposed by the Behçet International Study Group (ISG). Diagnostic criteria also were proposed by the International Criteria for Behçet Disease (ICBD Criteria). In this system, oral ulcerations, genital ulcerations, and ocular involvement are assigned 2 points for each site. Additional areas of involvement (cutaneous, articular, vascular, GI, CNS) are given 1 point. Patient involvement scoring 4 points or more is diagnosed as Behçet Disease. The ICBD criteria appear to be more sensitive but less specific than the ISG system and are thought possibly to be associated with overdiagnosis in some patients.

lesions recur less frequently than do the oral ulcerations, but they are deeper and tend to heal with scarring.

Common cutaneous lesions include erythema nodosum–like alterations, papulopustular lesions, pseudofolliculitis, and acneiform nodules. From a diagnostic standpoint, one of the most important skin manifestations is the presence of positive "pathergy." One or 2 days after the oblique insertion of a 20-gauge or smaller needle under sterile conditions, a tuberculin-like skin reaction or sterile pustule develops (Fig. 9.13). Positive pathergy is geographically variable with a prevalence of 60% in Middle Eastern patients but seen in only approximately 3% of affected Caucasian patients.

Arthritis is one of the more common minor manifestations of the disease and usually is self-limiting and

TABLE 9.1	International Study Group Criteria for the Diagnosis of Behçet Disease	
Criteria	**Description**	
Recurrent oral ulceration	Minor, major, or herpetiform aphthae	
Plus two of the following:		
Recurrent genital ulcerations	Aphthae-like ulcerations	
Eye lesions	Anterior or posterior uveitis, cells in vitreous on slit-lamp examination, or retinal vasculitis	
Skin lesions	Erythema nodosum, pseudofolliculitis or papulopustular lesions, or acneiform nodules noted in postadolescent patients not receiving corticosteroids	
Positive pathergy test	Read by physician at 24–48 hours	

Histopathologic Features

The histopathologic features are not specific for Behçet disease and can be seen in many disorders, including aphthous stomatitis. The pattern most frequently seen is called *leukocytoclastic vasculitis.* The ulceration is similar in appearance to that seen in aphthous stomatitis, but the small blood vessels classically demonstrate intramural invasion by neutrophils, karyorrhexis of neutrophils, extravasation of red blood cells, and fibrinoid necrosis of the vessel wall.

Treatment and Prognosis

Therapy is tailored to the disease severity and prognostic factors. Many patients are treated symptomatically, with the disease often going into remission as the patient ages. Females and older patients have a better prognosis than males or young patients. Ocular lesions and CNS involvement are associated with significant morbidity and mandate more aggressive therapy. Occasional disease-related mortality is noted and usually is associated with major vessel disease or central nervous system involvement.

The therapeutic regimens vary widely, depending on the involved sites and severity of disease. The oral lesions often respond to topical corticosteroids. Initial systemic treatment for mucocutaneous involvement is colchicine, with azathioprine, interferon (IFN) blockers and tumor necrosis factor (TNF) inhibitors suggested for refractory lesions. For patients who have ocular involvement, azathioprine and systemic steroids are first line therapies, and refractory cases are managed with cyclosporine, IFN blockers, and TNF inhibitors. Major vessel involvement is treated with immunosuppressive agents such as systemic steroids, azathioprine, cyclophosphamide, or cyclosporine. Methotrexate, IFN blockers, and TNF inhibitors are utilized in resistant cases. Gastrointestinal ulcerations are treated with 5-aminosalicylic acid with or without corticosteroids. Alternative therapy for refractory GI disease includes azathioprine, thalidomide, and TNF inhibitors. Neurologic involvement is treated with systemic corticosteroids and azathioprine with mycophenolate mofetil, methotrexate, and cyclophosphamide reserved for refractory cases.

In the future, wider use of a variety of biological treatments is expected in patients not responding to the current standard of care. These biologics include monoclonal antibodies against CD20, a growing list of tumor necrosis factor inhibitors, and many blocking agents directed against interleukins.

Behçet disease has a highly variable course. A relapsing and remitting pattern is typical, with attacks becoming more intermittent after 5–7 years. In the absence of CNS disease or significant vascular complications, the prognosis generally is good.

◆ SARCOIDOSIS

Sarcoidosis is a multisystem granulomatous disorder of unknown cause. Jonathan Hutchinson initially described the disease in 1875, but Boeck coined the term *sarcoidosis* (Greek meaning "flesh-like condition") 14 years later. The evidence implicates improper degradation of antigenic material with the formation of noncaseating granulomatous inflammation. The nature of the antigen is unknown, and probably several different antigens may be responsible. Possible involved antigens include infectious agents (e.g., mycobacterium, propionibacteria, Epstein-Barr virus, human herpesvirus 8 [HHV-8]), and several environmental factors (e.g., wood dust, pollen, clay, mold, and silica). Several investigators have confirmed a genetic predisposition and positive associations with certain HLA types.

Clinical Features

Sarcoidosis has a worldwide distribution with an increased prevalence in females and blacks. The process demonstrates a bimodal age distribution with one peak in young adults and another around 60 years of age. The disease may present acutely or demonstrate a chronic course with periods of remission and exacerbation. Acute cases often exhibit fever, fatigue, anorexia, or weight loss combined with other manifestations, such as respiratory symptoms, polyarthritis, visual problems, and skin lesions. In chronic cases, pulmonary symptoms are common and include dry cough, dyspnea, and chest discomfort. Approximately 20% of patients have no symptoms, and the disease is discovered on routine chest radiographs.

Although any organ may be affected, the lungs, lymph nodes, skin, eyes, and salivary glands are the predominant sites. Lymphoid tissue is involved in almost all cases. The mediastinal and paratracheal lymph nodes are involved commonly, and chest radiographs frequently reveal bilateral hilar

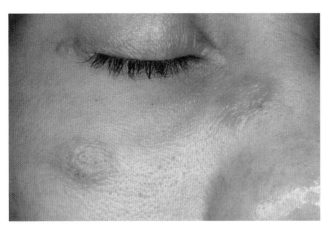

• **Fig. 9.14 Sarcoidosis.** Violaceous indurated plaques of the right malar area and bridge of nose. (Courtesy of Dr. George Blozis.)

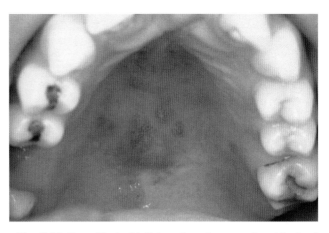

• **Fig. 9.15 Sarcoidosis.** Multiple erythematous macules of the hard palate. (Courtesy of Dr. George Blozis.)

lymphadenopathy. Approximately 90% of affected patients will reveal an abnormal chest radiograph sometime during the course of the disease. Cutaneous manifestations occur about 25% of the time. These often appear as chronic, violaceous, indurated lesions that are termed **lupus pernio** and frequent the nose, ears, lips, and face (Fig. 9.14). Scattered, nonspecific, tender erythematous nodules, known as **erythema nodosum,** frequently occur on the lower legs.

Ocular involvement is noted in 25% of the cases and most often appears as anterior uveitis. Lesions of the conjunctiva and retina may occur. Involvement of the lacrimal glands often produces keratoconjunctivitis sicca; the salivary glands can be altered similarly, with resultant clinical enlargement and xerostomia. The salivary gland enlargement, xerostomia, and keratoconjunctivitis sicca can combine to mimic Sjögren syndrome (see page 472).

Although lymphoid, pulmonary, cutaneous, and ocular lesions are most common, virtually any organ system may be affected. Other potential sites include the endocrine system, gastrointestinal tract, heart, kidneys, liver, nervous system, and spleen. Intraosseous lesions may occur and most commonly involve the phalanges, metacarpals, and metatarsals. Less frequently, the skull, nasal bones, ribs, and vertebrae are affected.

Two distinctive clinical syndromes are associated with acute sarcoidosis. **Löfgren syndrome** consists of erythema nodosum, bilateral hilar lymphadenopathy, and arthralgia. Patients with **Heerfordt syndrome (uveoparotid fever)** have parotid enlargement, anterior uveitis of the eye, facial paralysis, and fever.

If salivary gland and lymph node involvement are excluded, clinically evident oral manifestations in sarcoidosis are uncommon. Any oral mucosal site can be affected, most often appearing as a submucosal mass, an isolated papule, an area of granularity, or ulceration. The mucosal lesions may be normal in color, brown-red, violaceous, or hyperkeratotic (Figs. 9.15 and 9.16). The most frequently affected intraoral soft tissue site is the buccal mucosa, followed by the gingiva, lips, tongue, and palate. Lesions of the floor of the mouth occur but usually are secondary to

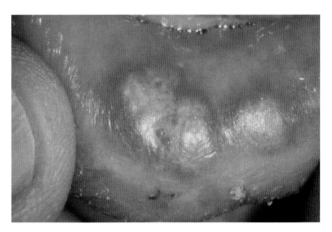

• **Fig. 9.16 Sarcoidosis.** Erythematous macules with central hyperkeratosis of the lower labial mucosa.

salivary gland involvement. Intraosseous lesions affect either jaw and represent approximately one-fourth of all reported intraoral cases. Of these cases, most appeared as ill-defined radiolucencies that occasionally eroded the cortex but never created expansion. In the previously reported intraoral cases, most patients demonstrated multisystem involvement, but the oral lesion was the initial manifestation in two-thirds of the patients.

Histopathologic Features

Microscopic examination of sarcoidosis exhibits a classic picture of granulomatous inflammation. Tightly clustered aggregates of epithelioid histiocytes are present, with a surrounding rim of lymphocytes. Intermixed with the histiocytes are scattered Langhans' or foreign body type giant cells (Fig. 9.17). The granulomas often contain laminated basophilic calcifications, known as **Schaumann bodies** (degenerated lysosomes), or stellate inclusions, known as **asteroid bodies** (entrapped fragments of collagen) (Fig. 9.18). None of these structures are specific for sarcoidosis. Special stains for fungal and bacterial organisms are negative. No polarizable, dissolvable, or pigmented foreign material can be detected.

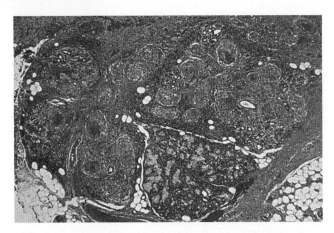

• **Fig. 9.17 Sarcoidosis.** Photomicrograph of a labial minor salivary gland demonstrating granulomatous inflammation characterized by circumscribed collections of histiocytes, lymphocytes, and multinucleated giant cells.

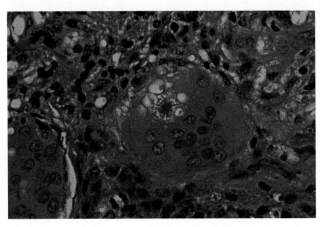

• **Fig. 9.18 Sarcoidosis.** Photomicrograph illustrating multinucleated giant cell with intracytoplasmic asteroid body.

Diagnosis

The diagnosis is established by the clinical and radiographic presentations, the histopathologic appearance, and the presence of negative findings with both special stains and cultures for organisms. Elevated serum angiotensin-converting enzyme (ACE) levels and appropriate documentation of pulmonary involvement strongly support the diagnosis. Despite this, elevated ACE is reported in only 60% of patients with sarcoidosis and in a minority of those with oral involvement. Other laboratory abnormalities that may be seen include eosinophilia; leukopenia; anemia; thrombocytopenia; and elevation of the serum alkaline phosphatase level, erythrocyte sedimentation rate, serum calcium concentration, and urinary calcium level.

In the past, a skin test for sarcoidosis, the **Kveim test,** was performed by intradermal injection of a sterilized suspension of human sarcoid tissue. However, this procedure is no longer used because of difficulty in obtaining material for the test, concern related to its accuracy, and the inability to guarantee the absence of contamination (e.g., prions) in this human tissue.

Minor salivary gland biopsy has been promoted as a diagnostic aid in suspected cases of sarcoidosis (see Fig. 9.17) but is less effective than a parotid biopsy. Previously, biopsy of the parotid was avoided because of the fear of salivary fistula formation and damage to the facial nerve. These concerns have been reduced through biopsy of the posterior superficial lobe of the parotid gland, and confirmation of sarcoidosis has been reported in 93% of patients from this procedure.

Treatment and Prognosis

In approximately 60% of patients with sarcoidosis, the symptoms resolve spontaneously within 2 years without treatment. Most initial diagnoses are followed by a 3- to 12-month period of observation to define the general course of the disease. Active intervention is recommended for progressive disease and patients with cardiac or neurologic involvement, hypercalcemia, disfiguring skin disease, or serious ocular lesions that do not respond to local therapy. In patients requiring treatment, corticosteroids remain first-line therapy, but resistance and relapses are common. Medications used in patients with refractory disease include methotrexate, azathioprine, chlorambucil, chloroquine, and cyclophosphamide. Several studies have shown promising results with TNF-α antagonists such as etanercept, infliximab, pentoxifylline, and thalidomide. In 10%–20% of those affected by sarcoidosis, resolution does not occur even with treatment. Approximately 4%–10% of patients die of pulmonary, cardiac, or CNS complications.

◆ OROFACIAL GRANULOMATOSIS

Since Wiesenfeld introduced it 1985, **orofacial granulomatosis** has become a well-accepted and unifying term encompassing a variety of clinical presentations that, on biopsy, reveal the presence of nonspecific granulomatous inflammation.

The disorder is idiopathic but appears to represent an abnormal immune reaction to a variety of inciting agents. In addition, similar lesions can be seen in association with several systemic diseases. Table 9.2 delineates systemic diseases that may mimic orofacial granulomatosis, and Table 9.3 lists several additional possible triggers.

Clinical Features

The clinical presentation of orofacial granulomatosis is highly variable. Most patients are adults; however, the process may occur at any age. By far, the most frequent site of involvement is the lips. The labial tissues demonstrate a nontender, persistent swelling that may involve one or both lips (Fig. 9.19). When these signs are combined with facial paralysis and a fissured tongue, the clinical presentation is called **Melkersson-Rosenthal syndrome** (Figs. 9.20 and 9.21). Involvement of the lips alone is called **cheilitis granulomatosa (of Miescher).** Neither of these two clinical

TABLE 9.2	Systemic Evaluation of Patients With Orofacial Granulomatosis
Systemic Cause	Preliminary Screening Procedure
Systemic drug reaction	Review medications, such as checkpoint inhibitors, highly active antiretroviral therapy, interferons, and tumor necrosis factor-α antagonists, which have been shown to trigger a sarcoid-like reaction
Chronic granulomatous disease	Neutrophil nitroblue tetrazolium reduction test (perform if medical history of chronic infections is noted)
Crohn disease	Hematologic evaluation for evidence of gastrointestinal malabsorption (e.g., low albumin, calcium, folate, iron, and red blood cell count; elevated erythrocyte sedimentation rate), serum IgA antibodies to *Saccharomyces cerevisiae*, leukocyte scintigraphy using ^{99m}Tc-HMPAO (hexamethyl propylene amine oxime), and fecal calprotectin; if initial screen is positive, then recommend esophagogastroduodenoscopy, ileocolonoscopy, and small-bowel radiographs
Sarcoidosis	Serum angiotensin–converting enzyme and chest radiograph (hilar lymphadenopathy)
Tuberculosis	Skin test and chest radiograph (negative acid-fast bacteria [AFB] stain on biopsy specimen does not rule out mycobacterial infection)

TABLE 9.3	Interventions to Rule Out Local Causes for Orofacial Granulomatosis
Local Cause	Intervention
Chronic oral infection	Eliminate all oral foci of infection.
Foreign material	The debris noted in foreign body gingivitis often is subtle and difficult to associate definitively with the diffuse inflammatory process. If lesions are nonmigrating and isolated to gingiva, then response to local excision of a single focus should be evaluated.
Allergy	Cosmetics, foods and food additives (aspartate, benzoate, carbone piperitone, carmoisine, carvone, chocolates, cinnamon, cocoa, dairy products, eggs, monosodium glutamate, peanuts, sun yellow dye, tartrazine, and wheat) flavorings, oral hygiene products (e.g., toothpaste and mouth rinses), and dental restorative metals have been implicated. Patch testing (i.e., contact dermatitis standard series with oral battery) or elimination diet may discover the offending antigen.

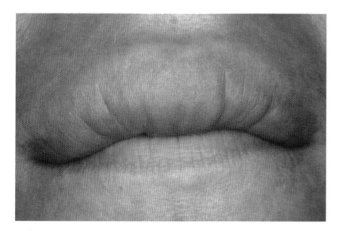

• **Fig. 9.19 Orofacial Granulomatosis (Cheilitis Granulomatosa).** Nontender, persistent enlargement of the upper lip. (From Allen CM, Camisa C: Diseases of the mouth and lips. In Sams WM, Lynch P, editors: *Principles of dermatology,* New York, 1990, Churchill Livingstone.)

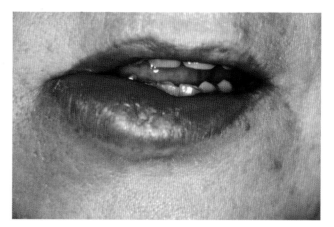

• **Fig. 9.20 Orofacial Granulomatosis (Melkersson-Rosenthal Syndrome).** Persistent enlargement of the lower lip. (Courtesy of Dr. Richard Ziegler.)

presentations represents a specific disease, and it appears best to include both under the term *orofacial granulomatosis.*

Intraoral sites also can be affected, and the predominant lesions are edema, ulcers, and papules. The tongue may develop fissures, edema, paresthesia, erosions, or taste alteration. The gingiva can develop swelling, erythema, pain, or erosions. The buccal mucosa often exhibits a cobblestone appearance of edematous mucosa or focal areas of submucosal enlargement. Linear hyperplastic folds may occur in the sulcus, often with elongated ulcerations in

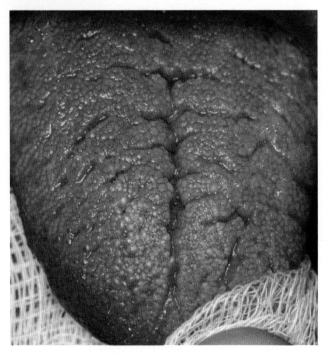

• **Fig. 9.21 Orofacial Granulomatosis (Melkersson-Rosenthal Syndrome).** Same patient as depicted in Fig. 9.20. Note numerous furrows on the dorsal surface of the tongue. (Courtesy of Dr. Richard Ziegler.)

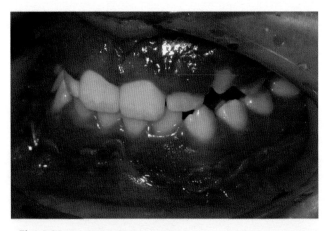

• **Fig. 9.22 Orofacial Granulomatosis.** Hyperplastic mucosa noted bilaterally in the mandibular mucobuccal fold. (Courtesy of Dr. Steven A. Anderson.)

the base of these folds (Fig. 9.22). The palate may have papules or large areas of hyperplastic tissue. Hyposalivation rarely is reported.

Histopathologic Features

In classic cases of cheilitis granulomatosa, edema is present in the superficial lamina propria with dilation of lymphatic vessels and scattered lymphocytes seen diffusely and in clusters. Fibrosis may be present in long-term lesions. Scattered aggregates of noncaseating granulomatous inflammation, consisting of lymphocytes and epithelioid histiocytes, are present,

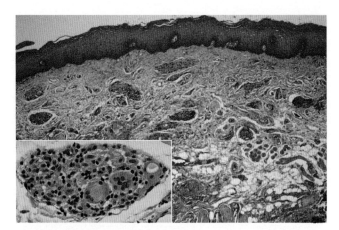

• **Fig. 9.23 Orofacial Granulomatosis.** Clusters of granulomatous inflammation around scattered vessels. The inset illustrates the histiocytes and multinucleated giant cells within the granulomas.

with or without multinucleated giant cells. Typically, the granulomas appear to cluster around scattered vessels and are not as well formed or discrete as those seen in sarcoidosis (Fig. 9.23).

Special stains for fungal organisms and acid-fast bacteria are negative. No dissolvable, pigmented, or polarizable foreign material should be present. When the lesions are confined to the gingiva, a thorough histopathologic evaluation search should be performed, because many cases of foreign body gingivitis are due to subtle collections of foreign material (see page 154).

Diagnosis

The initial diagnosis of orofacial granulomatosis is made on histopathologic demonstration of granulomatous inflammation that is associated with negative special stains for organisms and no foreign material. Because clinical and histopathologic features of orofacial granulomatosis can be produced by a variety of underlying causes, this diagnosis is the beginning, not the end, of the patient's evaluation. Prior to administering any medication or considering surgical intervention, the patient should be evaluated for the systemic diseases and local processes (see Tables 9.2 and 9.3) that may be responsible for similar oral lesions. If features diagnostic of one of these more specific disorders are discovered, then the oral lesions presumably would be related to that disease. If a specific diagnosis cannot be made, then potential foci of infection should be eliminated. If no resolution is noted after reducing local inflammatory factors, then referral of the patient for allergy testing should be considered.

Patients ultimately discovered to have Crohn disease often present at a younger age and have less lip swelling, although lesions of the buccal vestibule are more likely. Because gastrointestinal involvement has been discovered in up to 60% of patients with orofacial granulomatosis who have no intestinal symptoms, several investigators have suggested thorough gastrointestinal evaluation of all children and young adults presenting with orofacial granulomatosis. Conversely, others suggest evaluation for serum IgA antibodies to *Saccharomyces cerevisiae* and fecal calprotectin to assist in choosing those patients without intestinal symptoms who require further gastrointestinal evaluation.

The worldwide prevalence of allergy is estimated to be 15%–20%, whereas the frequency noted in patients with orofacial granulomatosis is up to 80% in several studies. Although allergy testing has been useful in many patients, diet restriction has been successful irrespective of patch test results in occasional individuals. Several investigators have suggested a cinnamon- and benzoate-free diet in all patients in whom an obvious trigger cannot be found.

Treatment and Prognosis

The first goal of management should be discovery of the initiating cause, although this may be difficult because the trigger often is elusive.

Oral lesions have been treated with a variety of interventions, with variable results. Topical or intralesional corticosteroids, topical tacrolimus, radiotherapy, sulfasalazine, hydroxychloroquine sulfate, azathioprine, cyclosporine A, methotrexate, danazol, dapsone, TNF-α antagonists (adalimumab, infliximab, and thalidomide), 5-aminosalicylic acid, clofazimine, metronidazole, and numerous other antibiotics have been tried. Currently, most investigators administer intralesional delayed-release high-concentrate triamcinolone to control the progression of this disease (Figs. 9.24 and 9.25). In those who have failed intralesional triamcinolone, a small number of reports have documented subsequent success with low-level laser therapy. In refractory cases, surgical recontouring has been used by some but carries a considerable risk of recurrence and rarely appears to be warranted.

The primary concern in affected patients is the cosmetically objectionable appearance, with the response to treatment being highly variable. No therapy has proved to be the "silver bullet" in resolving the individual lesions. In some cases, lesions resolve spontaneously, with or without therapy;

in others, they continue to progress despite a myriad of therapeutic attempts to stop the progression.

◆ GRANULOMATOSIS WITH POLYANGIITIS (WEGENER GRANULOMATOSIS)

Granulomatosis with polyangiitis is a well-recognized, although uncommon, disease process of unknown cause that was described initially in the German literature by Friedrich Wegener in 1936. The disorder has been termed **Wegener granulomatosis** until being renamed after discovery of Dr. Wegener's membership in a violent paramilitary branch of the Nazi party and his extensive activities in Jewish concentrations camps during the war. The disorder includes necrotizing granulomatous lesions of the respiratory tract, necrotizing glomerulonephritis, and systemic vasculitis of small arteries and veins. The pathogenesis of the disease is unknown but may be due to an abnormal immune reaction to an infectious, environmental, chemical, toxic, or pharmacological trigger in genetically predisposed individual.

Clinical Features

Granulomatosis with polyangiitis demonstrates a wide age range from childhood to old age, with a mean of age of 41 years and no sex predilection. Although most frequently presenting in adults, approximately 15% of the cases arise prior to age 20. A prevalence of 3 out of 100,000 has been reported, and 90% of the cases arise in Caucasians. The disease can involve almost every organ system in the body. With classic Wegener granulomatosis, patients initially show involvement of the upper and lower respiratory tract; if the condition remains untreated, then renal involvement often rapidly develops **(generalized Wegener granulomatosis).**

Limited Wegener granulomatosis is diagnosed when there is involvement of the respiratory system without rapid development of renal lesions. One subset of patients exhibits

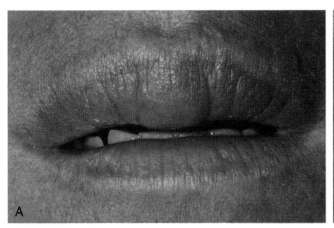 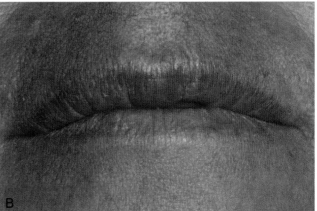

• **Fig. 9.24 Orofacial Granulomatosis. A,** Diffuse enlargement of the upper lip. **B,** Same patient after intralesional triamcinolone injections.

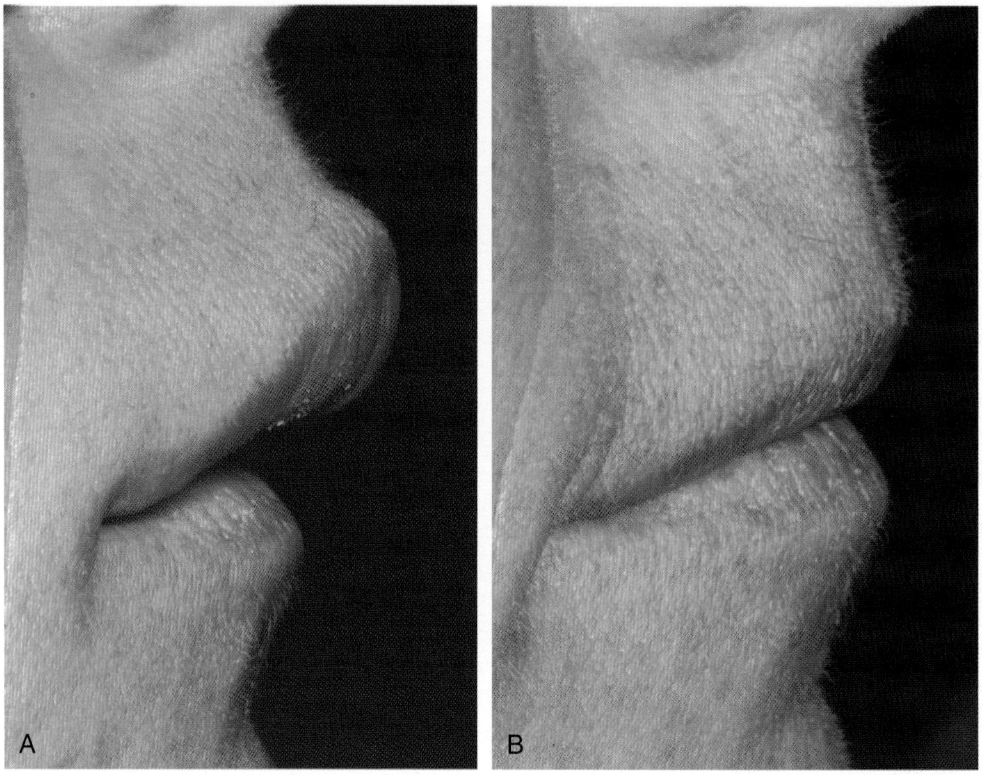

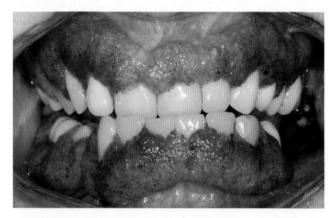

• **Fig. 9.25 Orofacial Granulomatosis.** Same patient depicted in Fig. 9.24. **A,** Clinical appearance before local therapy. **B,** Significant resolution after intralesional corticosteroid therapy.

lesions primarily of the skin and mucosa, a condition termed **superficial Wegener granulomatosis.** In this form of the disease, systemic involvement develops slowly. These three different clinical patterns highlight the variability of the clinical aggressiveness that can occur in patients with granulomatosis with polyangiitis.

Purulent nasal drainage, chronic sinus pain, nasal ulceration, congestion, and fever are frequent findings from upper respiratory tract involvement. Persistent otitis media, sore throat, and epistaxis also are reported. With progression, destruction of the nasal septum can result in a saddle-nose deformity. Patients with lower respiratory tract involvement may be asymptomatic, or they may have dry cough, hemoptysis, dyspnea, or chest pain. Renal involvement usually occurs late in the disease process and is the most frequent cause of death. The glomerulonephritis results in proteinuria and red blood cell casts. Occasionally, the eyes, ears, and skin also are involved.

The reported prevalence of oral lesions varies widely with oral involvement representing the initial presentation in 2% of affected patients. The most characteristic oral manifestation is **strawberry gingivitis.** This distinctive but uncommon pattern of gingival alteration appears to be an early manifestation of Wegener granulomatosis and has been documented before renal involvement in most cases. The affected gingiva demonstrates a florid and granular hyperplasia. The surface forms numerous short bulbous projections, which are hemorrhagic and friable; this red, bumpy surface is responsible for the strawberry-like

• **Fig. 9.26 Granulomatosis with Polyangiitis.** Hemorrhagic and friable gingiva (strawberry gingivitis). (Courtesy of Dr. Sam McKenna.)

appearance (Figs. 9.26 and 9.27). On occasion, scattered yellow papules correlating to subepithelial neutrophilic pustules may be noted intermixed with the hemorrhagic and hyperplastic gingiva. At the time of diagnosis, the involvement may be localized or generalized to multiple quadrants.

Oral ulceration also may be a manifestation of Wegener granulomatosis. These lesions are clinically nonspecific and may occur on any mucosal surface (Fig. 9.28). In contrast to the gingival changes, the oral ulcerations are diagnosed at a later stage of the disease, with more than 60% of the affected patients demonstrating renal involvement. Other less common orofacial manifestations include facial paralysis,

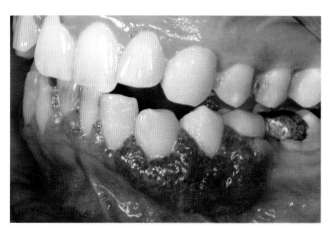

• **Fig. 9.27 Granulomatosis with Polyangiitis.** Hyperplastic and hemorrhagic mucosa of the facial mandibular gingiva on the left side. (Courtesy of Dr. James Wilson.)

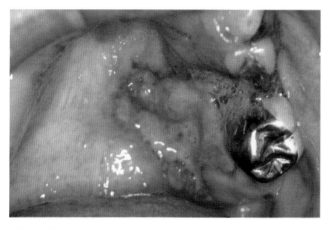

• **Fig. 9.28 Granulomatosis with Polyangiitis.** Deep, irregular ulceration of the hard palate on the left side. (From Allen CM, Camisa C, Salewski C, et al: Wegener's granulomatosis: report of three cases with oral lesions, *J Oral Maxillofac Surg* 49:294–298, 1991.)

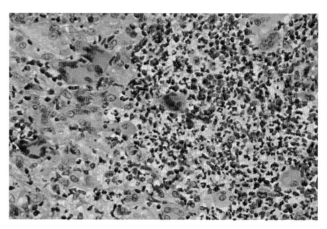

• **Fig. 9.29 Granulomatosis with Polyangiitis.** Connective tissue containing proliferation of numerous vascular channels and a heavy inflammatory infiltrate consisting of lymphocytes, neutrophils, eosinophils, and multinucleated giant cells.

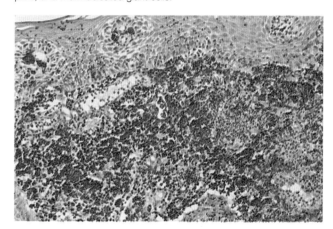

• **Fig. 9.30 Granulomatosis with Polyangiitis.** Gingival biopsy specimen showing a mixed inflammatory cellular infiltrate obscured by extensive extravasation of red blood cells.

labial mucosal nodules, sinusitis-related toothache, arthralgia of the temporomandibular joint (TMJ), jaw claudication, palatal ulceration from nasal extension, oral-antral fistulae, and poorly healing extraction sites.

Enlargement of one or more major salivary glands from primary involvement of the granulomatous process also has been reported. The glandular involvement also appears early in the course of the disease and may lead to early diagnosis and treatment.

Histopathologic Features

Granulomatosis with polyangiitis appears as a pattern of mixed inflammation centered around blood vessels. Involved vessels demonstrate transmural inflammation, often with areas of heavy neutrophilic infiltration, necrosis, and nuclear dust (leukocytoclastic vasculitis). The connective tissue adjacent to the vessel has an inflammatory cellular infiltrate, which contains a variable mixture of histiocytes, lymphocytes, eosinophils, and multinucleated giant cells (Fig. 9.29). Special stains for organisms are negative, and no foreign material can be found. In oral biopsy specimens, the mucosa may demonstrate pseudoepitheliomatous hyperplasia and subepithelial abscesses. Because of the paucity of large vessels in many oral mucosal biopsies, vasculitis may be difficult to demonstrate, and the histopathologic presentation may be one of ill-defined collections of epithelioid histiocytes intermixed with eosinophils, lymphocytes, and multinucleated giant cells. In addition, the lesions of strawberry gingivitis typically demonstrate prominent vascularity with extensive red blood cell extravasation (Fig. 9.30).

Diagnosis

The diagnosis of granulomatosis with polyangiitis is made from the combination of the clinical presentation and the microscopic finding of necrotizing and granulomatous vasculitis. The American College of Rheumatology proposed four diagnostic criteria with a minimum of two required for the diagnosis (Box 9.2). Radiographic evaluation of the chest and sinuses is recommended to document possible involvement of these areas. The serum creatinine and urinalysis results are used to rule out significant renal alterations.

Detection of antineutrophil cytoplasmic antibodies (ANCA) has proven to be an important laboratory marker for granulomatosis with polyangiitis and is performed by immunofluorescence and enzyme-linked immunosorbent assay (ELISA). Indirect immunofluorescence for ANCA reveals two patterns, cytoplasmic reactivity termed c-ANCA and perinuclear reactivity termed p-ANCA, which correlate respectively to antibodies directed against serine proteinase 3, (PR3-ANCA) and myeloperoxidase (MPO-ANCA). Serine proteinase 3 is a component of neutrophilic azurophilic cytoplasmic granules, whereas myeloperoxidase is present in neutrophilic lysosomal granules.

PR3-ANCA is most useful in the diagnosis of Wegener granulomatosis and is seen in approximately 85% of generalized Wegener granulomatosis and 60% of the early or localized cases. Immunofluorescence for ANCA should be ordered along with the specific enzyme-linked immunosorbent assay (ELISA) test for antibodies against proteinase 3 (PR3). These combined tests are associated with a sensitivity of 73% and a diagnostic specificity of 99% for Wegener granulomatosis. In contrast, MPO-ANCAs are detected in several vasculitides that typically do not present in the oral cavity and are positive in only 10% of patients with Wegener granulomatosis. False positives are uncommon and may be associated with a variety of other diseases. As mentioned in Chapter 8 (see page 292), a cocaine-induced midline destructive lesion (CIMDL) can be confused with Wegener granulomatosis due to similarities in the histopathologic findings and frequent positivity of PR3-ANCA. Although nasal involvement is common in Wegener granulomatosis, palatal perforation is rare. In addition, CIMDL often demonstrates antineutrophil cytoplasmic antibodies against human neutrophil elastase, a finding not seen in Wegener granulomatosis.

Treatment and Prognosis

The mean survival of untreated patients with disseminated classic granulomatosis with polyangiitis is 5 months; 80% of the patients are dead at 1 year and 90% within 2 years. The prognosis is better for the limited and superficial forms of the disease, although a proportion of patients with localized disease eventually will develop classic Wegener granulomatosis.

Treatment of granulomatosis with polyangiitis typically involves induction phase chemotherapy followed by a maintenance phase. The first line of therapy is oral prednisone and cyclophosphamide. On remission, the prednisone is gradually discontinued, with continuation of the cyclophosphamide for at least 1 year. Although high response rates are noted, serious side effects related to the therapy are not rare, especially those associated with cyclophosphamide. Rituximab is an effective and increasingly utilized alternative. Trimethoprim/sulfamethoxazole has been used successfully in localized cases. When added to the standard regimen, this antibiotic combination seems to reduce associated infections and to lower the relapse rate. Low-dose methotrexate and corticosteroids also have been used in patients whose disease is not immediately life threatening or has not responded appropriately to cyclophosphamide. Additional alternatives for the cyclophosphamide include cyclosporine, or infliximab. For maintenance therapy, cyclophosphamide often is replaced with rituximab, methotrexate, or azathioprine.

Treatment has a profound effect on the progression of the disease. With appropriate therapy, prolonged remission is noted in up to 75% of affected patients; a cure often is attainable when the disease is diagnosed and appropriately treated while the involvement is localized. Because of a relapse rate up to 30%, maintenance therapy is necessary in most patients. The PR3-ANCA levels can be used to monitor the disease activity. Patients appear less likely to have relapses if their antineutrophilic antibodies disappear during treatment; in contrast, patients whose levels of antibodies persist are at greater risk for relapse.

◆ LICHENOID AND GRANULOMATOUS STOMATITIS

For over two decades, a small number of publications have described a very distinctive clinical and histopathologic process known as **lichenoid and granulomatous stomatitis** which especially involves the upper labial mucosa. Although the cause currently is unknown, various proposed triggers include hypersensitivity to adjacent dental restorations, response to microbial agents such as local plaque/calculus, and a fixed allergic eruption to a medication or other systemic agent. Candidal infection often is superimposed and may be responsible for the associated symptoms. Treating the yeast often relieves any discomfort, but the erythematous lesion remains. A significant number of affected patients have reported use of drugs known to be associated with lichenoid reactions, most commonly nonsteroidal anti-inflammatory medications, angiotensin-converting enzyme inhibitors, and β-adrenoceptor blockers. Although the number of publications associated with this process is low, the unique clinical and microscopic presentation is not uncommon in an active practice of clinical and histopathologic oral pathology.

Clinical Features

Although the process may occur in both genders, most reported cases have been documented in women over 50 years of age. Affected individuals present with a chief complaint of mucosal burning that worsens with exposure

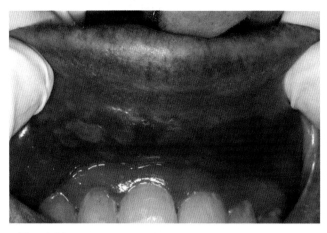

• **Fig. 9.31 Lichenoid and Granulomatous Stomatitis.** Diffuse erythema of the upper labial mucosa with intermixed erosions.

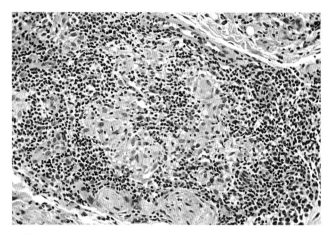

• **Fig. 9.33 Lichenoid and Granulomatous Stomatitis.** Deeper lymphoid nodule with clusters of epithelioid histiocytes.

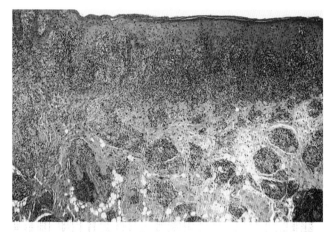

• **Fig. 9.32 Lichenoid and Granulomatous Stomatitis.** Biopsy of the labial mucosa demonstrating intense chronic interface mucositis with deeper perivascular/perineural lymphoid nodules.

Treatment and Prognosis

In the small number of cases reported to date, no consistently effective therapy has been documented. In individuals taking medications associated with lichenoid drug reactions, replacement with an alternative should be considered. In patients with composite resin restorations adjacent to the labial lesions, replacement with porcelain crowns has resolved the lesions in some patients. In other patients with extensive plaque/calculus, improved oral hygiene combined with chlorhexidine rinses may lead to resolution. In many patients, adjacent dental restorations and/or plaque are not noted. In these patients, use of topical corticosteroids has led to improvement in some individuals but has not been effective in others. Even in the absence of local plaque, antimicrobials such as antifungal medications, chlorhexidine rinses, or systemic clarithromycin with or without corticosteroids has been used successfully in small cohorts of patients.

◆ MUCOSAL REACTIONS TO SYSTEMIC DRUG ADMINISTRATION

The future of dentistry and medicine will involve a high volume of patients suffering from adverse drug reactions. By 2030, 20% of the population will be more than 65 years old. As the population ages and those affected with chronic diseases increase, patients taking multiple medications most likely will escalate. In the United States during the year 2000, more than 2.8 billion prescriptions were filled, enough to supply each inhabitant with 10 prescriptions annually. Although use of two medications is associated with a 6% risk of an adverse reaction, the frequency rises to 50% with five drugs and almost 100% when eight or more medications are used simultaneously.

Although difficult to confirm, oral mucosal reactions to systemic medications most likely are extremely common. In a review of 155 patients presenting with intraoral lesions consistent with lichen planus, 87.8% of the individuals were

to spicy foods. Oral examination reveals an erythematous alteration noted most frequently on the upper labial mucosa but with occasional involvement of the lower labial mucosa and buccal mucosa. The erythematous mucosa may be intermixed with small papules, white striae, or erosions (Fig. 9.31). In about half of the patients, the adjacent gingiva also is erythematous and tender.

Histopathologic Features

Biopsy of the labial mucosa typically demonstrates diffuse exocytosis of the epithelium with a thinned spinous cell layer and degeneration of many basal cells. Superficial candidiasis may be noted but not present in all patients. The superficial stroma reveals an intense band-like infiltrate of lymphocytes immediately adjacent to the surface epithelium. Deeper nodules of lymphocytes are noted in a perivascular/perineural distribution, often intermixed with clusters of epithelioid histiocytes (Figs. 9.32 and 9.33). Multinucleated giant cells are seen occasionally, but well-formed granulomas are not present.

taking medications known to be associated with lichen planus-like reactions. At one time, the clinical triad of oral lichen planus, diabetes mellitus, and hypertension was recognized under the historical term, *Grinspan syndrome*. However, this combination currently is believed to represent a lichen planus-like reaction secondary to the medications utilized to control the diabetes and hypertension. In all likelihood, a large percentage of patients presenting with lichen planus-like lesions in the oral cavity represent chronic drug reactions, not primary lichen planus.

Two types of adverse drug reactions are seen. Type A (augmented reactions) arise from an exaggerated but otherwise expected pharmacologic action of the prescribed medication (such as, bleeding associated with warfarin). Approximately 80% of the total adverse drug reactions are Type A. Type B (bizarre reactions) are idiosyncratic reactions that are not expected, the majority of which arise from immune-mediated effects, such as hypersensitivity reactions.

Lists of medications related to several patterns of drug-related mucosal alteration are provided. Because new drug reactions are being reported on a regular basis and large numbers of new medications continue to appear, these lists should be considered incomplete at the time of publication and additional investigation is prudent. When presented with a patient with a possible drug reaction, all medications, both prescribed and over-the-counter, that the patient is taking should be researched with a reputable pharmaceutical reference. This should include not only the information within the drug insert but also the constantly updated results of a complete search of the health care literature.

In addition to drug-related problems, such as aphthous stomatitis (see page 321), angioedema (see page 348), medication-related osteonecrosis (see page 286), cancer therapy-related mucositis (see page 281), cleft lip/palate (see page 1), erythema multiforme/Steven-Johnson Syndrome (see page 781), gingival hyperplasia (see page 156), methemoglobinemia, mucosal discolorations (see page 307), burning mouth disorder (see page 868), tardive dyskinesia, taste disturbances (see page 869), sialorrhea (see page 469), and xerostomia (see page 470), medications can induce a wide variety of mucosal ulcerations and erosions. A reaction of the oral mucosa to the systemic administration of a medication is called **stomatitis medicamentosa.** Several different patterns of oral mucosal disease can be seen:

- Anaphylactic stomatitis
- Intraoral fixed drug eruptions
- Lichenoid drug reactions
- Pemphigoid-like drug reactions
- Pemphigus-like drug reactions
- Lupus erythematosus–like eruptions
- Nonspecific erosive or ulcerative lesions

Anaphylactic stomatitis arises after the allergen enters the circulation and binds to immunoglobulin E (IgE)–mast cell complexes. Although systemic anaphylactic shock can result, localized alterations also occur. Fixed drug eruptions are inflammatory alterations of the mucosa or skin that recur at the same site after the administration of any allergen, often

a medication. Medications reported to be associated with fixed drug eruptions are listed in Box 9.3, lichenoid drug eruptions in Box 9.4, lupus erythematosus–like drug eruptions in Box 9.5, pemphigus-like drug reactions in Box 9.6, and mucosal pemphigoid–like eruptions in Box 9.7. In addition, a long list of medications is known to be associated with nonspecific erosive, ulcerative, or aphthae-like

---

• **BOX 9.3** **Medications Implicated in Fixed Drug Eruptions**

Acetaminophen	Levocetirizine
Analgin	Lidocaine
Barbiturates	Naproxen
Clarithromycin	Oxicams
Chlorhexidine	Oxyphenbutazone
Cotrimoxazole	Penicillamine
Dapsone	Phenazone derivatives
Fluconazole	Phenolphthalein
Gabapentin	Salicylates
Gold salts	Sulfonamides
Indomethacin	Tetracycline

• **BOX 9.4** **Medications Implicated in Lichenoid Eruptions**

Allopurinol	Imatinib
Amiphenazole	Imipramine
Amitriptyline	Immunoglobins
Amphotericin	Interferon-alpha
Angiotensin-converting	Isoniazid
enzyme (ACE) inhibitors	Ketoconazole
Antimalarials	Levamisole
Arsenicals	Levomepromazine
Barbiturates	Lincomycin
Beta-adrenoceptor	Lipid lowering drugs
blockers	Lithium
Bismuth	Lorazepam
Bleomycin	L-Thyroxin
Carbamazepine	Mepacrine
Carbimazole	Mercury
Chloral hydrate	Mesalamine
Chloroquine	Metformin
Chlorpromazine	Methopromazine
Chlorpropamide	Methyldopa
Cimetidine	Metronidazole
Cinnarizine	Nifedipine
Clofibrate	Niridazole
Colchicine	Nivolumab
Cyanamide	Nonsteroidal anti-
Dapsone	inflammatory drugs
Dipyridamole	(NSAIDs)
Ethambutol	Oral contraceptives
Ethionamide	Palladium
Fenclofenac	*para*-aminosalicylic acid
Flunarizine	Pembrolizumab
Furosemide	Penicillins
Gold salts	Penicillamine
Griseofulvin	Phenindione
Hepatitis B vaccine	Phenothiazines
Hydroxychloroquine	Phenylbutazone
Hydroxyurea	Phenytoin

Prazosin
Procainamide
Propylthiouracil
Protease inhibitors
Protionamide
Proton pump inhibitors
Pyrimethamine
Pyritinol
Quinidine
Quinine
Ranitidine
Rifampicin
Roxatidine
Sildenafil
Spironolactone

Streptomycin
Sulfasalazine
Sulfonamides
Sulfonylureas
Terbinafine
Tetracycline
Thiazide diuretics
Tocainide
Tolbutamide
Trihexyphenidyl
Triprolidine
Trovafloxacin
Tumor necrosis factor-α
   antagonists
Ursodeoxycholic acid

lesions, but is not included due to its length. Methotrexate is a well-known example that may trigger development of oral erosions that occasionally also are infested secondarily with Epstein-Barr virus due to the associated immunosuppression.

Clinical Features

The patterns of mucosal alterations associated with the systemic administration of medications are varied, almost as much as the number of drugs that result in these changes. Anaphylactic stomatitis may occur alone or in conjunction with urticarial skin lesions or other signs and symptoms of anaphylaxis (e.g., hoarseness, respiratory distress, and

• BOX 9.5 Medications Implicated in Lupus Erythematosus–like Eruptions

Systemic lupus-like reactions
Aminoglutethimide
Aminosalicylic acid
Angiotensin converting enzyme inhibitors
Beta-adrenoceptor blockers
Carbamazepine
Clonidine
Chlorpromazine
Chlorprothixene
Chlorthalidone
Disopyramide
D-Penicillamine
Ethosuximide
Hydralazine
Hydrochlorothiazide
Interferon-α
Interleukin 2
Isoniazid
Levodopa
Lipid lowering medications
Lithium carbonate
Methyldopa
Minocycline
Minoxidil
Nitrofurantoin
Perphenazine
Phenelzine
Phenylbutazone
Phenytoin
Prazosin
Primidone
Procainamide
Propafenone
Propylthiouracil
Quinidine
Sulfasalazine
Sulfonamide
Trimethadione
Tumor necrosis factor-α antagonists

Cutaneous lupus-like reactions
Allopurinol
Amoxicillin + Clavulanic acid
Anastrazole
Angiotensin converting enzyme inhibitors
Beta-adrenoceptor blockers
Brompheniramine
Buproprion
Calcium channel blockers
Capecitabine
Carbamazepine
Cinnarizine + Thiethylperazine
Ciprofloxacin
Docetaxel
Doxorubicin
Efalizumab
5-Fluorouracil
Gemcitabine
Griseofulvin
Interferon-α and β
Leflunomide
Leuprorelin
Lipid lowering medications
Masitinib
Naproxen
Nivolumab
Paclitaxil
Palbociclib
Pembrolizumab
Phenytoin
Piroxicam
Proton pump inhibitors
Ranitidine
Secukinumab
Tamoxifen
Terbinafine
Thiazide diuretics
Ticlopidine
Tiotropium
Tumor necrosis factor-α antagonists
Uracil-tegafur
Ustekinumab

Medications Implicated in Pemphigus-like Eruptions

Alpha-mercaptopropionyl
   glycine
Aspirin
Ampicillin
Benzylpenicillin
Captopril
Cefadroxil
Cephalexin
Diclofenac
Enalapril
Ethambutol
Fosinopril
Glibenclamide
Gold
Heroin
Ibuprofen
Interleukin-2
Interferon-α and β
Isotretinoin

Levodopa
Nifedipine
Norfloxacin
Oxyphenbutazone
Penicillamine
Penicillin
Phenobarbital
Phenylbutazone
Piroxicam
Practolol
Probenecid
Procaine penicillin
Progesterone
Propranolol
Pyritinol chlorhydrate
Ramipril
Rifampin
Thioproline

• BOX 9.7 **Medications Implicated in Mucosal Pemphigoid–like Eruptions**

Actinomycin
Angiotensin converting
   enzyme inhibitors
Angiotensin II antagonists
Amoxicillin
Ampicillin
Arsenic
Aspirin
Beta-adrenoceptor
   blockers
Calcium channel blockers
Cephalexin
Ciprofloxacin
Chloroquine
Clonidine
Dactinomycin
D-Penicillamine
Erlotinib
Fluoxetine
Flupenthixol
Furosemide
Gabapentin
Galantamine hydrobromide
Herpes zoster vaccine
Hexavalent combine
   vaccines
Interleukin-2
Influenza vaccine
Ipilimumab

Levetiracetam
Levofloxacin
Methyldopa
Nivolumab
Nonsteroidal
   anti-inflammatory
   medications (NSAIDs)
Omeprazole
Pembrolizumab
Penicillin
Placental extracts
Potassium iodide
Psoralens with UVA
Rifampicin
Risperidone
Salicylazosulfapyride
Sitagliptin
Spironolactone
Sulfasalazine
Sulfonamide
Swine flu vaccine
Terbinafine
Tetanus toxoid
Tiopronin
Tiobutarit
Tolbutamide
Tumor necrosis factor-α
   antagonists
Vildagliptin

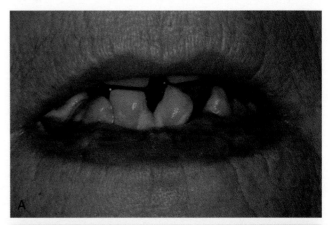

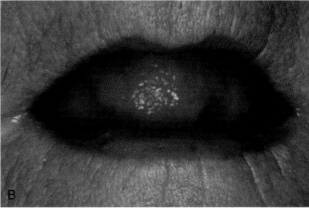

• **Fig. 9.34 Allergic Mucosal Reaction to Systemic Drug Administration. A,** Bilateral erosions of lower labial mucosa with intermixed striae. Biopsy revealed lichenoid pattern of mucositis but with numerous plasma cells intermixed with the lymphocytes. The erosions ultimately were proven to be associated with simvastatin. **B,** Same patient depicted in **A** after discontinuation of simvastatin.

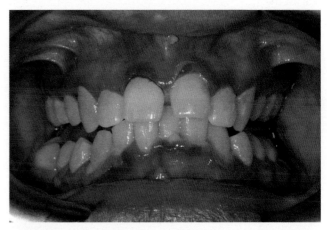

• **Fig. 9.35 Pemphigoid-like Drug Reaction to Ipilimumab—Nivolumab.** Multiple areas of gingival erythema with mucosal erosions and areas of epithelial sloughing. (Courtesy of Dr. James Woodyard.)

vomiting). The affected mucosa may exhibit multiple zones of erythema or numerous aphthae-like ulcerations. Mucosal fixed drug eruptions appear as localized areas of erythema and edema, which can develop into vesiculoerosive lesions and are located most frequently on the labial mucosa. Lichenoid, lupus-like, pemphigoid-like, and pemphigus-like drug reactions resemble their namesakes clinically, histopathologically, and immunologically (Figs. 9.34 and 9.35). These latter chronic drug reactions may involve any mucosal surface, but the most common sites are the posterior buccal mucosa and the lateral borders of the tongue (Figs. 9.36 and 9.37).

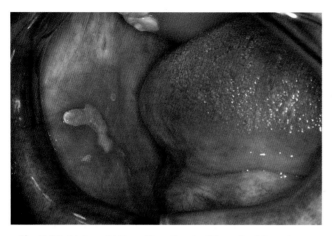

• **Fig. 9.36 Lichenoid Drug Reaction to Allopurinol.** Irregular area of superficial erosion of the right buccal mucosa.

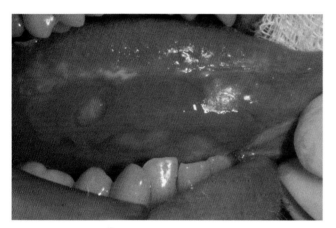

• **Fig. 9.37 Allergic Mucosal Reaction to Systemic Drug Administration.** Large irregular erosion of the right ventral surface of the tongue. The lesion arose secondary to use of oxaprozin, a nonsteroidal anti-inflammatory drug (NSAID).

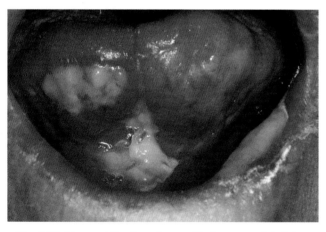

• **Fig. 9.38 Mucosal Erosions Due to Methotrexate Administration**. Multiple mucosal erosions of the ventral tongue, floor of mouth, and labial mucosa.

Bilateral and symmetrical lesions are common. In addition to drug reactions that mimic the patterns of classic vesiculoerosive diseases, nonspecific ulcerations and erosions arise secondary to a wide variety of medications such as methotrexate (Fig. 9.38).

Histopathologic Features

Anaphylactic stomatitis typically reveals a nonspecific pattern of subacute mucositis that contains lymphocytes intermixed with eosinophils and neutrophils. Fixed drug eruptions also reveal a mixed inflammatory cellular infiltrate that consists of lymphocytes, eosinophils, and neutrophils, often combined with spongiosis and exocytosis of the epithelium. Vacuolar change of the basal cell layer and individual necrotic epithelial cells occasionally are noted. The drug reactions that simulate lichen planus, lupus erythematosus, pemphigoid, and pemphigus resemble their namesakes. The histopathologic and immunologic features of these chronic drug reactions cannot be used reliably to separate them from their associated primary immunologic disease.

Immunofluorescence has been used to separate drug reactions from primary vesiculoerosive disease. In most instances, this technique has proven to be unsatisfactory. Despite these findings, a unique pattern of reaction has been seen when indirect immunofluorescence for IgG has been performed in patients with lichenoid drug reactions. In many of these patients, a distinctive annular fluorescent pattern, termed **string of pearls,** has been reported along the cell membrane of the basal cell layer of stratified squamous epithelium. The detected circulating antibody has been termed **basal cell cytoplasmic antibody.** Although further study is desirable, this technique may prove to be a useful adjunct during evaluation of oral lichenoid lesions.

Diagnosis

A definitive diagnosis of a chronic drug reaction of the oral mucosa is difficult because the initial clinical symptoms may arise months to years after initiation of offending medication. In addition, the clinical alterations may persist for months after cessation of the medication, occasionally requiring immunosuppressive therapy to achieve complete resolution. A detailed medical history must be obtained, and the patient should be questioned closely concerning the use of both prescription and over-the-counter medications. If the patient can provide an accurate history, all medications initiated after the oral lesions arose can be removed from the list of possible offenders. Once a potentially offending medication is discovered, a temporal relationship between the drug's use and the mucosal alteration should be investigated. The association may be acute and obvious, or the onset of the oral lesions may be delayed. If more than one medication is suspected, the most recently administered medication often is the culprit. If the last-to-be-introduced drug does not appear responsible, serial elimination of the medications can be performed in collaboration with the patient's physician until the offending agent is discovered.

In chronic drug reactions, definitive diagnosis can be made if the mucosal alterations resolve after discontinuation of the medication and recur on reintroduction of the agent. Presumptive diagnosis usually is sufficient and justified when the mucosal alterations clear after cessation of the offending medication. If immunosuppressive medications are necessary to achieve resolution, the mucosal alterations should not recur after removal of the medication and cessation of therapy. If the lesions recur following complete resolution, then the medication was not involved in the mucosal alteration.

In possible lupus-like drug reactions, serum evaluation for generic antinuclear antibodies (ANAs) and antibodies against double-stranded DNA and histones often can be beneficial. Lupus-like drug reactions typically are associated with circulating generic ANAs and antibodies against histones, whereas lupus erythematosus also reveals antibodies to double-stranded DNA (a finding not typically noted in drug reactions). This pattern does not hold true in reactions associated with the TNF-α antagonists, infliximab and etanercept, which simulate systemic lupus erythematosus (SLE) very closely and are associated with antibodies to double-stranded DNA.

Treatment and Prognosis

The responsible medication should be discontinued and, if necessary, replaced with another drug that provides a similar therapeutic result. Localized acute reactions can be resolved with topical corticosteroids. When systemic manifestations are present, anaphylactic stomatitis often warrants systemic administration of adrenaline (epinephrine), corticosteroids, or antihistamines. Chronic oral lesions often resolve on cessation of the offending drug, but topical corticosteroids may sometimes be required for complete resolution.

If discontinuation of the medication is contraindicated, palliative care can be provided; however, corticosteroids often are ineffective if the offending medication is continued.

◆ ALLERGIC CONTACT STOMATITIS (STOMATITIS VENENATA)

The list of agents reported to cause **allergic contact stomatitis** reactions in the oral cavity is extremely diverse. Numerous foods, food additives, chewing gums, candies, dentifrices, mouthwashes, glove and rubber dam materials, topical anesthetics, dental restorative materials, acrylic denture materials, dental impression materials, and denture adhesive preparations have been mentioned. Two types of allergens, cinnamon (see page 344) and dental restorative materials (see page 346), demonstrate clinical and histopathologic patterns that are sufficiently unique to justify separate descriptions.

Although the oral cavity is exposed to a wide variety of antigens, the frequency of a true allergic reaction to any one antigen from this contact appears to be rare. This was verified in a prospective study of 13,325 dental patients, in which only 7 acute and 15 chronic cases of adverse effects were attributed to dental materials. The oral mucosa is much less sensitive than the surface of the skin; this is most likely because of the following:

- The period of contact is often brief.
- The saliva dilutes, digests, and removes many antigens.
- The limited keratinization of oral mucosa makes hapten binding more difficult, and the high vascularity tends to remove any antigen quickly.
- The allergen may not be recognized (because of the lower density of Langerhans cells and T lymphocytes).

If the skin has been sensitized originally, the mucosa may or may not demonstrate future clinical sensitization. In contrast, if the mucosa is sensitized initially, then the skin usually demonstrates similar changes with future exposure. Long-term oral exposure may induce tolerance and reduce the prevalence of cutaneous sensitivity in some instances. For example, exposure to nickel-containing orthodontic hardware has been associated with a reduced prevalence of future cutaneous sensitivity to nickel jewelry.

In addition to oral lesions, allergic contact reactions may produce exfoliative cheilitis (see page 294) or perioral dermatitis (see next section). As mentioned in Chapter 8, most cases of chronic cheilitis represent local irritation, usually from chronic lip licking. Despite this, investigation has revealed that approximately 25% of affected cases are allergic contact cheilitis from a variety of antigens that include medications, lipsticks, sunscreens, toothpaste, dental floss, nail polishes, and cosmetics.

Clinical Features

Allergic contact stomatitis can be acute or chronic. Of those cases diagnosed, there is a distinct female predominance in both forms. After eliminating focal trauma, localized signs and symptoms suggest mucositis from an isolated allergen (e.g., dental metal); in contrast, widespread mouth pain suggests an association with a more diffuse trigger, such as food, drink, flavorings, or oral hygiene materials.

In patients with acute contact stomatitis, burning is the most frequent symptom. The appearance of the affected mucosa is variable, from a mild and barely visible redness to a brilliantly erythematous lesion with or without edema. Vesicles are seen rarely and, when present, rapidly rupture to form areas of erosion (Fig. 9.39). Superficial ulcerations that resemble aphthae occasionally arise. Itching, stinging, tingling, and edema may be noted.

In chronic cases the affected mucosa is typically in contact with the causative agent and may be erythematous or white and hyperkeratotic. Periodically, erosions may develop within the affected zones. Some allergens, especially toothpastes, can cause widespread erythema, with desquamation of the superficial layers of the epithelium (Fig. 9.40). Allergic contact cheilitis demonstrates clinical features identical to those cases created through chronic irritation, and it most frequently appears as chronic dryness, scaling, fissuring, or cracking of the vermilion border of the lip. Rarely, symptoms identical to orolingual paresthesia can be present without any clinically evident signs. One distinctive pattern, plasma cell gingivitis, is discussed elsewhere (see page 152).

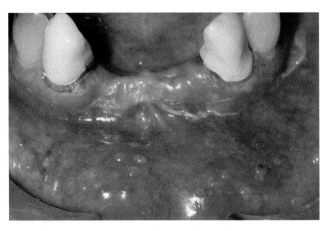

• **Fig. 9.39 Allergic Contact Stomatitis to Aluminum Chloride.** Mucosal erythema and vesicles of the lower labial mucosa caused by use of aluminum chloride on gingival retraction cord.

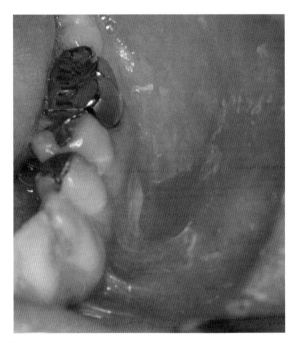

• **Fig. 9.40 Allergic Contact Stomatitis to Toothpaste.** Erythematous mucosa with superficial epithelial desquamation.

Diagnosis

Usually, the diagnosis of acute contact stomatitis is straightforward because of the temporal relationship between the use of the agent and the resultant eruption. If an acute oral or circumoral reaction is noted within 30 minutes of a dental visit, then allergy to all used dental materials, local anesthetics, and gloves should be investigated. In some cases, the clinical presentation of an allergic contact stomatitis can be difficult to distinguish from an irritant contact stomatitis in which the mucosal alteration is related to chemical or physical irritation rather than a hypersensitivity. Patch testing may prove beneficial in separating these contact reactions.

The diagnosis of chronic contact stomatitis is much more difficult. Most investigators require good oral health, elimination of all other possible causes, and visible oral signs,

together with a positive history of allergy and a positive skin test result to the suspected allergen. If allergic contact stomatitis is strongly suspected but skin test results are negative, then direct testing of the oral mucosa can be attempted. The antigen can be placed on the mucosa in a mixture with Orabase or in a rubber cup that is fixed to the mucosa.

Treatment and Prognosis

In mild cases of acute contact stomatitis, removal of the suspected allergen is all that is required. In more severe cases, antihistamine therapy, which is combined with topical anesthetics, usually is beneficial. Chronic reactions respond to removal of the antigenic source and application of a topical corticosteroid gel or oral suspension.

When attempting to discover the source of a diffuse allergic mucositis, use of plain baking soda or toothpaste that is free of flavoring or preservatives is recommended. The patient also should be instructed to avoid mouthwash, gum, mints, chocolate, cinnamon-containing products, carbonated drinks, and excessively salty, spicy, or acidic foods. If an association cannot be found, then cutaneous patch testing may provide helpful information.

◆ PERIORAL DERMATITIS (PERIORIFICIAL DERMATITIS)

Perioral dermatitis does not refer to every rash that occurs around the mouth but is specific for a unique inflammatory skin disease that involves the cutaneous surfaces surrounding the facial orifices. Because the disorder also often involves the paranasal and periorbital skin, **periorificial dermatitis** is the most appropriate designation. Although the process is idiopathic, the dermatitis is associated strongly with excessive use of potent topical corticosteroids on the facial skin. Many believe the corticosteroid use leads to local immunosuppression and infection in the hair follicles by organisms such as *Propionibacterium acnes* and *Fusobacterium* that release chemotactic factors for neutrophils leading to significant associated inflammation. Fluorinated toothpaste and overuse of heavy facial cosmetics, creams, and moisturizers also are implicated in some patients. Weaker correlations have been seen with systemic corticosteroids, corticosteroid inhalers, and nasal corticosteroids. Heavy exposure to ultraviolet light, heat, and wind appears to worsen the dermatitis. Some of these substances may initially induce an irritant or allergic contact dermatitis, whereas others are thought to produce inappropriate occlusion of the skin surface with subsequent proliferation of skin flora.

Clinical Features

Perioral dermatitis appears with persistent erythematous papules, vesicles, and pustules that involve the skin surrounding the vermilion border of the upper and lower lips. In addition, involvement of the perinasal skin is seen in approximately 40% of affected patients, and 25% have

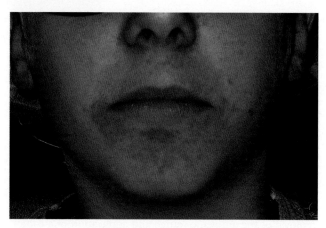

• **Fig. 9.41 Perioral Dermatitis.** Multiple erythematous papules of the skin surrounding the vermilion border of the lips. Note similar involvement around the nasal orifices (periorificial dermatitis). (Courtesy of Dr. Billy Millay.)

periorbital dermatitis (Fig. 9.41). Classically, there is a zone of spared skin immediately adjacent to the vermilion border. Cases related to fluoridated toothpaste often do not reveal sparing of the skin just outside the lip vermilion. Pruritus and burning are variable. Most of the cases are diagnosed in women between the ages of 20–45 years, lending further support to the association with cosmetic use. In some affected females, there appears to be a hormonal influence as evidenced by premenstrual flares or exacerbation associated with pregnancy or use of contraceptive pills. There is a less common pediatric variant that is seen between the age of 7 months to 13 years, which does not demonstrate the strong gender predilection observed in adults.

Histopathologic Features

Biopsy of perioral dermatitis demonstrates a variable pattern. In many cases there is a chronic lymphohistiocytic dermatitis that often exhibits spongiosis of the hair follicles. In other patients a rosacea-like pattern is noted in which there is perifollicular granulomatous inflammation. On occasion, this histopathologic pattern has been misdiagnosed as sarcoidosis.

Treatment and Prognosis

Most cases resolve with "zero therapy," which includes discontinuation of corticosteroids, cosmetics, facial creams, etc. Discontinuation of potent topical corticosteroid use often is followed by a period of exacerbation. Oral tetracycline is considered the therapeutic gold standard for perioral dermatitis but must be avoided during childhood and pregnancy. Alternative therapies include topical metronidazole, erythromycin, clindamycin, sulfacetamide, and pimecrolimus or systemic azithromycin, erythromycin, doxycycline, or clarithromycin. Isotretinoin has been used successfully in patients who are refractory to other therapies. The pathosis typically demonstrates significant improvement within several weeks and total resolution in a few months. Recurrence is uncommon.

◆ CONTACT STOMATITIS FROM ARTIFICIAL CINNAMON FLAVORING

Mucosal abnormalities secondary to the use of artificially flavored cinnamon products are fairly common, but the range of changes was not recognized widely until the late 1980s. Cinnamon oil is used as a flavoring agent in confectionery, ice cream, soft drinks, alcoholic beverages, processed meats, gum, candy, toothpaste, breath fresheners, mouthwashes, and even dental floss. Concentrations of the flavoring are up to 100 times that in the natural spice. The reactions are documented most in those products associated with prolonged or frequent contact, such as candy, chewing gum, mouthwash, and toothpaste. The anticalculus components of tartar-control toothpastes have a strong bitter flavor and require a significant concentration of flavoring agents including cinnamon to hide the taste, resulting in a greater chance these formulations will cause oral mucosal lesions. Although much less common, reactions to cinnamon in its natural spice form have been documented.

Clinical Features

The clinical presentations of contact stomatitis vary somewhat, according to the medium of delivery. Toothpaste and mouthwash often result in a more diffuse pattern; the signs associated with chewing gum and candy are more localized. Pain and burning are common symptoms in all cases. Anaphylaxis associated with cinnamon exposure has been reported but is rare.

The gingiva is the most frequent site affected by toothpaste, often resembling **plasma cell gingivitis** (see page 152); enlargement, edema, and erythema are common. Sloughing of the superficial oral epithelium without creation of an erosion is seen commonly. Erythematous mucositis, occasionally combined with erosion, has been reported on the buccal mucosa and tongue. Exfoliative cheilitis and circumoral dermatitis also may occur.

Reactions from chewing gum and candy are more localized and typically do not affect the lip vermilion or perioral skin. Most of the lesions appear on the buccal mucosa and lateral borders of the tongue. Buccal mucosal lesions often are oblong patches that are aligned along the occlusal plane (Fig. 9.42). Individual lesions have an erythematous base but often are predominantly white because of hyperkeratosis of the surface epithelium. Ulceration within the lesions may occur. Hyperkeratotic examples often exhibit a ragged surface and occasionally may resemble the pattern seen in morsicatio (see page 272). Lingual involvement may become extensive and spread to the dorsal surface (Fig. 9.43). Significant thickening of the surface epithelium can occur and may raise clinical concern for oral hairy leukoplakia (OHL) (see page 253) or carcinoma (Fig. 9.44).

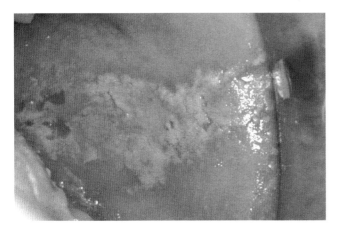

• **Fig. 9.42 Contact Stomatitis from Cinnamon Flavoring.** Oblong area of sensitive erythema with overlying shaggy hyperkeratosis.

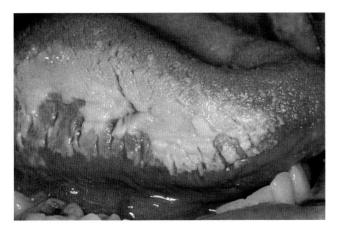

• **Fig. 9.43 Contact Stomatitis from Cinnamon Flavoring.** Sensitive and thickened hyperkeratosis of the lateral and dorsal surface of the tongue on the right side.

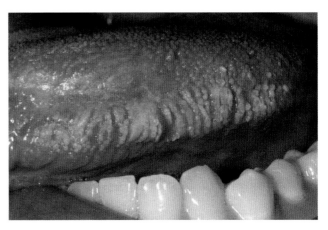

• **Fig. 9.44 Contact Stomatitis from Cinnamon Flavoring.** Left lateral border of the tongue demonstrating linear rows of hyperkeratosis that resemble oral hairy leukoplakia (OHL).

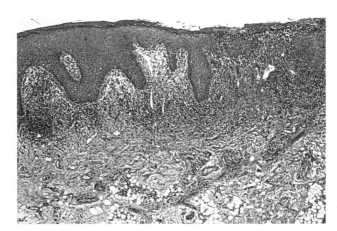

• **Fig. 9.45 Contact Stomatitis From Cinnamon Flavoring.** Oral mucosa demonstrating significant interface mucositis and deeper perivascular inflammation.

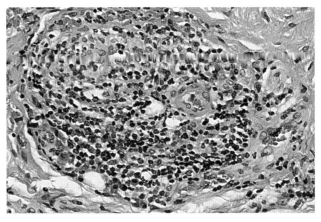

• **Fig. 9.46 Contact Stomatitis From Cinnamon Flavoring.** Perivascular inflammatory infiltrate consisting predominantly of lymphocytes and plasma cells.

Histopathologic Features

Usually, the epithelium in contact stomatitis from artificial cinnamon flavoring is acanthotic, often with elongated rete ridges and thinning of the suprapapillary plates. Hyperkeratosis and extensive neutrophilic exocytosis may be present. The superficial lamina propria demonstrates a heavy inflammatory cell infiltrate that consists predominantly of lymphocytes that may be intermixed with plasma cells, histiocytes, or eosinophils. This infiltrate often obscures the epithelium and connective tissue interface (Fig. 9.45). A characteristic feature in localized cases caused by gum, mints, or candies is the frequent presence of an obvious perivascular inflammatory infiltrate that extends well below the interface zone (Fig. 9.46).

Diagnosis

With a high index of suspicion and knowledge of the variations of the clinical pattern, the diagnosis of localized contact stomatitis often can be made from the clinical appearance and the history of cinnamon use. Occasionally, biopsies are performed for atypical or extensive cases because of the differential diagnosis, which includes several significant vesiculoerosive and neoplastic conditions. The histopathologic features are not specific, but they are sufficient to raise a high index of suspicion in an oral and maxillofacial pathologist who is familiar with the pattern. Use of cinnamon-containing toothpaste should be investigated in every patient with an atypical pattern of gingivitis. Diet-related examples often are the most difficult to diagnose and may necessitate cutaneous allergy patch testing or a diet diary to isolate the cause. Cutaneous patch testing often does not always correlate to the intraoral manifestations. Patients with positive patch testing may not demonstrate intraoral reactions, and patients with an obvious intraoral reaction to cinnamon may not exhibit positivity to cutaneous patch testing. The best method of diagnostic confirmation is elimination of the suspected allergen with rapid clearance of the mucosal alterations.

Treatment and Prognosis

Typically, the signs and symptoms disappear within 1 week after the discontinuation of the cinnamon product. If the patient resumes intake of the product, then the lesions reappear, usually within 24 hours. On occasion, resolution is more gradual; and the patient may benefit from short-term use of a topical corticosteroid.

◆ LICHENOID CONTACT REACTION FROM DENTAL RESTORATIVE MATERIALS

Dental amalgam has been in active use for over 180 years and has proven to be a durable and relatively inexpensive material that remains one of the most commonly placed dental restorations. Because of an associated low-level release of mercury from these fillings (an amount significantly less than the daily contribution from food and nondental sources), its use has been blamed for a wide variety of health concerns. Due to the controversy, several controlled studies were performed, showing no association between the presence of dental amalgams and systemic disease. Two oral pathoses, burning mouth syndrome and orofacial granulomatosis, also have been correlated with the presence of amalgams by some investigators, but no conclusive evidence exists to associate these disorders with the dental restorative material. The primary adverse effects that are well documented include acute and chronic hypersensitivity reactions.

Dental amalgams contain mercury, silver, tin, and copper, with some variations also including zinc, indium, palladium, or platinum. Most hypersensitivity reactions to dental restorative materials are to dental amalgam. Reactions have been seen much less frequently to other dental restorations containing materials such as gold, beryllium, chromium, cobalt, or composite resins.

Although rare acute reactions may be seen following placement of amalgam, the vast majority of adverse alterations represent chronic type IV hypersensitivity reactions that are seen most commonly associated with older and corroded amalgams. It is believed the metal ions released by corrosion haptenize with oral keratinocyte surface proteins and initiate a cell-mediated autoimmune response directed at the basal cell layer of the epithelium. Some

investigators have called these chronic alterations "galvanic lesions," but neither clinical nor experimental studies support the electrogalvanic hypothesis of origin.

These chronic contact reactions appear clinically and histopathologically similar to lichen planus (see page 787) but demonstrate a different mucosal distribution. When patients with true oral lichen planus are examined, the lesions migrate and exhibit no direct correlation to contact with dental materials. In addition, patients with lichen planus do not demonstrate a significantly increased positive patch testing to dental restorative materials and exhibit minimal-to-no clinical improvement on removal of their amalgams.

However, there is a subgroup of patients whose lichenoid lesions do not migrate and usually involve only the mucosa adjacent to a dental metal. On patch testing, most of these patients react to the offending metal, and the lesions resolve rapidly after removal of adjacent amalgams. Such lesions should be diagnosed as a **lichenoid contact reaction** to a dental restorative material, not as true lichen planus. Although many of these mucosal alterations appear to represent allergic contact reactions, occasional lesions may be secondary to a sharp cusp, a rough-surfaced restoration, or altered tooth anatomy that is difficult to clean and results in local accumulation of plaque.

Clinical Features

Acute reactions to dental amalgams are extremely rare and related to an immediate hypersensitivity reaction. The signs tend to arise within hours after placement of an amalgam and present with erythematous, pruritic, and urticarial lesions of the ipsilateral oral mucosa and facial skin. In severe reactions, soft tissue edema, tachycardia, and breathing difficulties also are seen.

Most chronic lichenoid contact reactions affect the posterior buccal mucosa and the ventral surface of the lateral borders of the tongue. In contrast to lichen planus, in which the mucosal alterations tend to be bilateral and symmetrical, lichenoid reactions to dental materials usually are confined to the area of contact and may be white or erythematous, with or without peripheral striae (Fig. 9.47). Most patients have no symptoms, but periodic erosion may be noted. In all likelihood, many of the lesions previously reported as the so-called plaque type of lichen planus were, in reality, lichenoid contact reactions or possibly evolving epithelial dysplasias or proliferative verrucous leukoplakia with an associated lichenoid immune response.

Diagnosis

The diagnosis of a lichenoid contact reaction is made from the clinical appearance of the lesion, the lack of lesional migration, and the correlation to adjacent dental metal (Fig. 9.48). Although the histopathologic features may be indistinguishable from lichen planus, biopsy occasionally is performed to confirm the clinical impression and to rule out other pathoses such as epithelial dysplasia. Although patch testing is positive

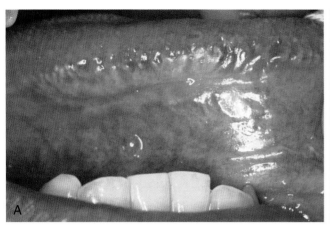
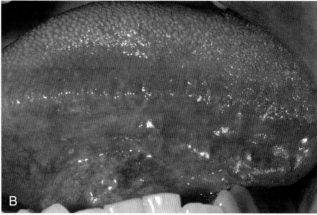

• **Fig. 9.47 Oral Mucosal Contact Reaction to Dental Amalgam. A,** Hyperkeratotic lesion with a peripheral radiating pattern on the lateral border of the tongue on the right side; the altered mucosa contacted the amalgams of the adjacent mandibular molar teeth. The lesion remained in the same location for 5 years and periodically became erosive and symptomatic. Smoothing and polishing of the adjacent restorations had no effect. **B,** Appearance of previously altered area of the tongue 14 days after removal of adjacent amalgams. Note total resolution of the mucosal alterations.

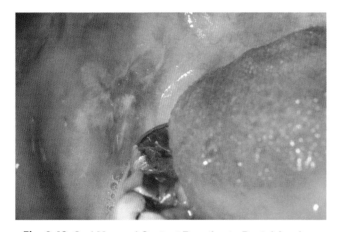

• **Fig. 9.48 Oral Mucosal Contact Reaction to Dental Amalgam.** Radiating pattern of hyperkeratotic striae on the posterior buccal mucosa that contacts a large distobuccal amalgam of the permanent mandibular second molar.

in up to 70% of patients with contact reactions and similarly reactive in less than 4% of patients with true lichen planus, the clinical presentation has proven to be a more reliable diagnostic indicator than patch testing. Many clinicians reserve patch testing for patients with large numbers of amalgams and extensive lichenoid lesions in which it is difficult clinically to distinguish lichen planus from lichenoid contact reactions. As an alternative to cutaneous patch testing in this situation, a single-test amalgam can be replaced to assess the response of the adjacent mucosa. If clearance is seen locally in the area of amalgam removal, then elimination of the remaining offending restorations is justified.

Histopathologic Features

Biopsy of allergic contact stomatitis from dental materials exhibits numerous features of lichen planus. The surface epithelium may be hyperkeratotic, atrophic, or ulcerated. Areas of hydropic degeneration of the basal cell layer often are present. The superficial lamina propria contains a dense band-like chronic inflammatory cellular infiltrate consisting predominantly of lymphocytes. In addition to the superficial lichenoid mucositis, some biopsies also reveal features typically not noted in classic lichen planus such as a deeper lymphocytic infiltrate often intermixed with plasma cells, occasional germinal centers, and variable numbers of eosinophils. Occasionally, the deeper infiltrate also will demonstrate a perivascular pattern.

Treatment and Prognosis

In patients with acute hypersensitivity reactions to an amalgam, the process usually is self-limiting and resolves spontaneously within 2–3 days. Despite this, systemic symptoms, such as significant breathing difficulties, may necessitate removal of the newly placed amalgam.

For chronic lichenoid reactions, local measures, such as improved oral hygiene, smoothing, polishing, and recontouring of the amalgam restoration, should be attempted before more aggressive measures, because clinically similar lesions have been noted because of surface plaque accumulation. If this is unsuccessful, then the amalgam in question should be replaced. Because patients rarely may exhibit hypersensitivity to composite resins, use of inert materials (such as glass ionomer, feldspathic ceramic, porcelain, or porcelain-fused-to-metal) is recommended. Like lichen planus, some investigators believe untreated lichenoid contact reactions rarely may evolve into carcinoma, although the possibility that some preneoplastic leukoplakias are mistaken for lichenoid contact reactions cannot be ruled out. Although this association is far from proven, removal of amalgams adjacent to possible lichenoid contact reactions appears prudent. Lichenoid lesions that fail to resolve following removal of the adjacent metal should be evaluated further.

◆ ANGIOEDEMA (ANGIONEUROTIC EDEMA; QUINCKE DISEASE)

Angioedema is a diffuse edematous swelling of the soft tissues that most commonly involves the subcutaneous and submucosal connective tissues but may affect the gastrointestinal or respiratory tract, occasionally with fatal results. The disorder has been referred to as **Quincke disease,** after the clinician who initially related the changes to an alteration in vascular permeability. The outdated term **angioneurotic edema** also has been used, because affected patients often complained of a choking sensation and were labeled neurotic.

The most common cause is mast cell degranulation, which leads to histamine release and the typical clinical alterations. IgE-mediated hypersensitivity reactions caused by drugs, foods, plants, dust, and inhalants produce mast cell degranulation and are common. Contact allergic reactions to foods, cosmetics, topical medications, and even dental rubber dams also have been responsible. Mast cell degranulation can even result from physical stimuli, such as heat, cold, exercise, emotional stress, sun exposure, and significant vibration. This latter pattern is termed **vibratory angioedema** with intraoral examples seen secondary to stimuli such as prolonged snoring or use of musical instruments with a mouthpiece.

An unusual pattern of drug reaction that can produce severe forms of angioedema that are not mediated by IgE is the type associated with use of drugs called *angiotensin-converting enzyme (ACE) inhibitors.* These medications represent one of the most frequently prescribed drugs, with 35–40 million patients currently taking these antihypertensives. Some of the most popular are captopril, enalapril, and lisinopril. The swelling associated with these drugs does not respond to antihistamines and is the result of excess bradykinin. As illustrated in Fig. 9.49, activation of coagulation factor XII causes conversion of plasma prekallikrein to kallikrein, with the kallikrein pathway leading to production of bradykinin. Angioedema results if the bradykinin is not degraded. Angiotensin converting enzyme plays a role in degrading bradykinin, and if significant inhibition of this enzyme by ACE inhibitors occurs, angioedema is seen.

To avoid this angioedema, a second generation of medications called *angiotensin II receptor blockers* (e.g., losartan and valsartan) was developed specifically to avoid any inhibition of bradykinin degradation. These newer medications lower the frequency of angioedema but do not eliminate the adverse reaction. The prevalence of this pattern of angioedema is estimated to be 0.1%–0.2% of those who use ACE inhibitors. In most affected patients, the angioedema arises within hours of initial use of the drug. In up to 30% of the cases, the angioedema is delayed, with the longest reported interval between drug use initiation and the initial attack being 10 years. Attacks precipitated by dental procedures have been reported in long-term users of ACE inhibitors. Many clinicians overlook the association between angioedema and ACE inhibitors, with studies demonstrating continued administration of the medication in more than 50% of affected patients.

As shown in Fig. 9.49, C1 esterase inhibitor (C1-INH) is antagonistic to bradykinin formation by actively blocking the formation of kallikrein and kininogen. Insufficient functional C1-INH predisposes to angioedema and may be hereditary or acquired. Two major autosomal dominant forms and an extremely rare third hereditary type are known. **Type I hereditary angioedema (HAE I)** accounts for approximately 85% of hereditary cases and is caused by a

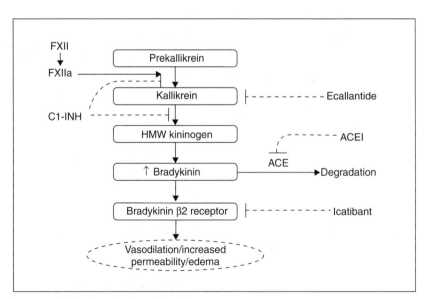

• **Fig. 9.49 Kallikrein Pathway in Angioedema.** Diagram demonstrating the kallikrein pathway with the over-production of bradykinin in angioedema. Note the blockage of bradykinin degradation by ACE inhibitors and the three medical interventions that can halt the process (C1-INH, ecallantide, icatibant). (From Craig TJ, Bernstein JA, Farkas H, et al.: Diagnosis and treatment of bradykinin-mediated angioedema expert consensus meeting, *Int Arch Allergy Immunol* 165:119–127, 2014).

quantitative reduction in C1-INH. **Type II hereditary angioedema (HAE II)** is responsible for 15% of hereditary cases and exhibits normal levels of C1-INH, but the inhibitor is dysfunctional. The third type is extremely rare and presents with normal levels of functional C1-INH. Previously this pattern was referred to as type III hereditary angioedema but currently is called **hereditary angioedema with normal C1-INH (HAE-nC1-INH).** In this rare pattern, the cause is unknown in the majority but 25% demonstrate a mutation in coagulation factor XII, the primary trigger of the kallikrein pathway. In HAE-nC1-INH, the major trigger is estrogen, with pregnancy or oral contraceptives associated with exacerbations and increased severity of attacks. High levels of estrogen are known to increase the levels of factor XII, and mutation of this clotting factor may be responsible for triggering the kallikrein pathway.

The acquired type of C1-INH deficiency is seen in association with certain types of lymphoproliferative diseases (Caldwell syndrome) or in patients who develop specific autoantibodies. In lymphoproliferative diseases, monoclonal antibodies directed against the tumor cells activate C1 and lead to consumption of C1-INH. In the autoimmune variant, the antibody attaches to the C1 receptor on the C1-INH molecule, leading to dysfunctional C1-INH and consumption of C1. In both the acquired and the hereditary forms of abnormal C1-INH activity, minor trauma, such as a dental procedure, can precipitate an attack.

A number of patients also have developed intraoral angioedema following administration of the clot buster tissue plasminogen (tPA, alteplase) for strokes, predominantly those arising in the frontal, insular, and peri-insular regions of the brain. Plasminogen leads to development of plasmin that triggers fibrinolysis and activates the complement cascade and kallikrein pathway with subsequent generation of bradykinin. The reason this reaction seems strongly correlated to use of tPA in specific patterns of stroke is unclear. The frequency of this complication is increased in patients utilizing ACE-inhibitors.

Finally, angioedema has been seen in the presence of high levels of antigen-antibody complexes (e.g., lupus erythematosus and viral or bacterial infections) and in patients with grossly elevated peripheral blood eosinophil counts.

Clinical Features

Angioedema is characterized by the relatively rapid onset of soft, nontender tissue swelling, which may be localized or diffuse (Fig. 9.50). In the hereditary forms, the initial onset typically is noted in childhood or adolescence except in the rare estrogen-related HAE-n-C1-INH pattern that usually arises in 20- to 30-year-old women. The episodes are unpredictable and intermixed with edema-free intervals. Recurrent skin swelling and abdominal pain are the most frequent presentations. The extremities are the most common cutaneous sites of involvement, although the face, genitals, trunk, and neck also can be affected. Although

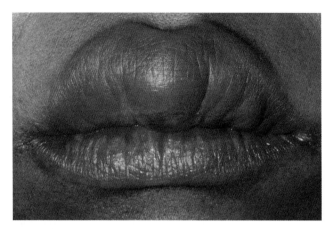

• **Fig. 9.50 Angioedema.** Diffuse upper lip swelling that arose rapidly.

not individually frequent, edema of the larynx, pharynx, uvula, or soft palate may be noted when patients are monitored for extended periods (and may be associated with respiratory distress). A deeper voice, hoarseness, aphonia, and dyspnea are important warning signs. Recurrent snoring-induced edema of the soft palate has been reported and associated with severe dyspnea. Isolated tongue involvement is uncommon. Involvement of the skin and mucous membranes can cause enlargements that may measure up to several centimeters in diameter (Fig. 9.51). Although pain is unusual, itching is common, and erythema may be present. The enlargement typically resolves over 24–72 hours. In contrast to the hereditary variants, the allergic, acquired, and ACE inhibitor–associated angioedemas demonstrate significant involvement of the head and neck, such as the face, lips, tongue, floor of mouth, pharynx, and larynx. The risk of angioedema associated with ACE inhibitors is significantly greater in blacks (three to four times that of other races), and this pattern is the type most frequently encountered by oral health practitioners.

Diagnosis

In cases of allergic causation, the diagnosis of angioedema often is made from the clinical presentation in conjunction with the known antigenic stimulus. When multiple antigenic exposures occur, the diagnosis of the offending agent can be difficult and involves dietary diaries and antigenic testing.

Those patients whose conditions cannot be related to antigenic exposure or medications should be evaluated for the presence of adequate functional C1-INH. Except for the estrogen-related pattern, the hereditary types exhibit normal levels of C1 and decreased levels of *functional* C1-INH. Type I demonstrates a decreased quantity of C1-INH; type II exhibits normal levels of the inhibitor, but it is dysfunctional. The acquired type associated with lymphoproliferative diseases demonstrates low C1 and low C1-INH, whereas the autoimmune variant exhibits low C1 and dysfunctional C1-INH.

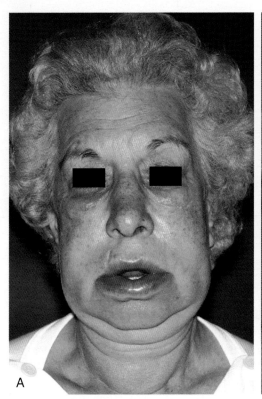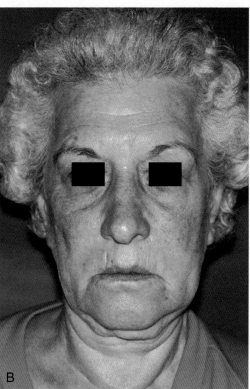

• **Fig. 9.51 Angioedema. A,** Soft, nontender tissue swelling of the face arose relatively rapidly after dental treatment. **B,** Facial appearance after resolution of edematous facial enlargement.

Treatment and Prognosis

The treatment of allergic angioedema usually consists of oral antihistamine therapy. If the attack is not controlled or if laryngeal involvement is present, then intramuscular epinephrine should be administered. If the epinephrine does not stop the attack, then intravenous corticosteroids and antihistamines should be given. Vibratory angioedema is treated via elimination of the triggering physical stimulus. In cases related to chronic snoring, use of a continuous positive airway pressure (C-PAP) unit has proven successful.

The hereditary types of angioedema, those related to ACE inhibitors, and cases related to tPA use in strokes do not respond to antihistamines and corticosteroids, because the primary cause is generation of bradykinin. As highlighted in Fig. 9.49, the kallikrein pathway can be blocked by administration of C1-INH concentrate or by either one of two medications: ecallantide or icatibant. If none of these interventions are available, fresh frozen plasma contains C1-INH and represents an acceptable substitute. Although significantly less expensive than the alternatives, some investigators do not recommend use of fresh frozen plasma, because there is a risk of transmitting infection. In addition, it replaces not only C1-INH but also potentially harmful C1 esterase, C1, C2, and C4. Laryngeal edema is the most common cause of death from angioedema and reinforces the need for intubation or tracheostomy in patients with serious airway blockage. Patients experiencing ACE inhibitor–associated angioedema

should avoid all medications in this class of drugs, and their physicians should consider alternative hypertension management strategies. Angiotensin II receptor blockers do not appear to be safe alternatives.

All patients with hereditary angioedema should carry medical warning cards that state the diagnosis and list elementary precautions. Prophylaxis for C1-INH deficiency is recommended in patients who have more than three attacks per year. Patients should avoid violent physical activity and trauma. Medical prophylaxis is recommended before any dental or surgical procedure, even interventions as minor as a dental impression. Current guidelines suggest administration of 1000 units of C1-INH concentrate as near as possible to the start of the procedure. Fresh frozen plasma also can be used but is less safe than C1-INH concentrate due to the problems delineated in the previous paragraph. Second-line prophylaxis is an attenuated androgen such as danazol or stanozolol which induces hepatic synthesis of C1-INH. Because epinephrine can trigger an attack, use of local anesthetic without a vasoconstrictor is recommended. Even with infusions of C1-INH concentrate prior to a dental procedure in a patient with the hereditary types, life-threatening angioedema remains possible with its occurrence possibly delayed up to 48 hours. For this reason, extended continuous monitoring of patients with hereditary angioedema is recommended following dental procedures. The autoimmune acquired type of angioedema is best prevented using corticosteroids.

Bibliography

Transient Lingual Papillitis

Brannon RB, Flaitz CM: Transient lingual papillitis: a papulokeratotic variant, *Oral Surgery, Oral Medicine, Oral Pathology, Oral Radiology, and Endodontics* 96:187–191, 2003.

Flaitz CM, Chavarria C: Painful tongue lesions associated with a food allergy, *Pediatric Dentistry* 23:506–507, 2001.

Kornerup IM, Senye M, Peters E: Transient lingual papillitis, *Quintessence International* 47:871–875, 2016.

Lacour J-P, Perrin C: Eruptive familial lingual papillitis: a new entity, *Pediatric Dermatology* 14:13–16, 1997.

Roux O, Lacour JP: Eruptive lingual papillitis with household transmission: a prospective clinical study, *The British Journal of Dermatology* 150:299–303, 2004.

Whitaker SB, Krupa JJ, Singh BB: Transient lingual papillitis, *Oral Surgery, Oral Medicine, Oral Pathology, Oral Radiology, and Endodontics* 82:441–445, 1996.

Recurrent Aphthous Stomatitis

Akintoye SO, Greenberg MS: Recurrent aphthous stomatitis, *Dental Clinics of North America* 58:281–297, 2014.

Brocklehurst P, Tickle M, Glenny AM, et al.: Systemic interventions for recurrent aphthous stomatitis (mouth ulcers), *Cochrane Database of Systematic Reviews* 9:CD005411, 2012.

Cui RZ, Bruce AJ, Rogers RS: Recurrent aphthous stomatitis, *Clinics in Dermatology* 34:475–481, 2016.

Liu C, Zhou Z, Liu G, et al.: Efficacy and safety of dexamethasone ointment on recurrent aphthous ulceration, *The American Journal of Medicine* 125:292–301, 2012.

Rogers RS: Complex aphthosis, *Advances in Experimental Medicine and Biology* 528:311–316, 2003.

Scully C, Porter S: Oral mucosal disease: recurrent aphthous stomatitis, *The British Journal of Oral & Maxillofacial Surgery* 46:198–206, 2008.

Ship JA: Recurrent aphthous stomatitis: an update, *Oral Surgery, Oral Medicine, Oral Pathology, Oral Radiology, and Endodontics* 81:141–147, 1996.

Subramanyam RV: Occurrence of recurrent aphthous ulcerations only on lining mucosa and its relationship to smoking—a possible hypothesis, *Medical Hypotheses* 77:185–187, 2011.

Vincent SD, Lilly GE: Clinical, historic, and therapeutic features of aphthous stomatitis: literature review and open clinical trial employing steroids, *Oral Surgery, Oral Medicine, and Oral Pathology* 74:79–86, 1992.

Behçet Disease

Alibaz-Oner F, Sawalha AH, Direskeneli H: Management of Behçet disease, *Current Opinion in Rheumatology* 30:238–242, 2018.

Alpsoy E: Behçet disease: a comprehensive review with a focus on epidemiology, etiology and clinical features, and management of mucocutaneous lesions, *The Journal of Dermatology* 43:620–632, 2016.

Bulur I, Onder M: Behçet disease: new aspects, *Clinics in Dermatology* 35:421–434, 2017.

Helm TN, Camisa C, Allen C, et al.: Clinical features of Behçet's disease: report of four cases, *Oral Surgery, Oral Medicine, and Oral Pathology* 72:30–34, 1991.

International Study Group for Behçet's Disease: Criteria for diagnosis for Behçet's disease, *Lancet* 335:1078–1080, 1990.

Karacayli U, Mumcu G, Simsek I, et al.: The close association between dental and periodontal treatments and oral ulcer course in Behçet's disease: a prospective clinical study, *Journal of Oral Pathology & Medicine* 38:410–415, 2009.

Sarcoidosis

Bagchi S, Shah N, Sheikh MA, et al.: Oral sarcoidosis aiding in diagnosis of underlying systemic disease, *BMJ Case Rep* 12:e232093, 2019. https://doi.org/10.1136/bcr-2019-232093.

Bouaziz A, LeScanff J, Chapelon-Abric C, et al.: Oral involvement in sarcoidosis: report of 12 cases, *The Quarterly Journal of Medicine* 105:755–767, 2012.

Motswaledi MH, Khammissa RAG, Jadwat Y, et al.: Oral sarcoidosis: a case report and review of the literature, *Australian Dental Journal* 59:389–394, 2014.

Poate TWJ, Sharma R, Moutasim KA, et al.: Orofacial presentations of sarcoidosis—a case series and review of the literature, *British Dental Journal* 205:437–442, 2008.

Suresh L, Radfar L: Oral sarcoidosis: a review of the literature, *Oral Diseases* 11:138–145, 2005.

Orofacial Granulomatosis

Al-Hamad A, Porter S, Fedele S: Orofacial granulomatosis, *Dermatologic Clinics* 33:433–446, 2015.

Campbell HE, Escudier MP, Patel P, et al.: Review article: cinnamon- and benzoate-free diet as a primary treatment for orofacial granulomatosis, *Alimentary Pharmacology & Therapeutics* 34:687–701, 2011.

Fedele S, Fung PPL, Bamashmous N, et al.: Long-term effectiveness of intralesional triamcinolone acetonide therapy in orofacial granulomatosis: an observational cohort study, *The British Journal of Dermatology* 170:794–801, 2014.

Grave B, McCullough M, Wiesenfeld D: Orofacial granulomatosis—a 20-year review, *Oral Diseases* 15:46–51, 2009.

Haaramo A, Alapulli H, Aine L, et al.: Detailed follow-up study of pediatric orofacial granulomatosis patients, *Journal of Pediatric Gastroenterology and Nutrition* 65:388–393, 2017.

Hullah EA, Escudier MP: The mouth in inflammatory bowel disease and aspects of orofacial granulomatosis, *Periodontology 2000* 2000 (80):61–76, 2019.

Jácome-Santos H, Resende RG, Silva AMB, et al.: Low-level laser as a complementary therapy in orofacial granulomatosis management: a case report, *Oral Surgery, Oral Medicine, Oral Pathology, Oral Radiology* 128:e1–e5, 2019.

Miest R, Bruce A, Rogers RS: Orofacial granulomatosis, *Clinics in Dermatology* 34:505–513, 2016.

Wiesenfeld D, Ferguson MM, Mitchell DN, et al.: Orofacial granulomatosis—a clinical and pathological analysis, *The Quarterly Journal of Medicine* 54:101–113, 1985.

Worsaae N, Christensen KC, Schiödt M, et al.: Melkersson-Rosenthal and cheilitis granulomatosa: a clinicopathologic study of thirty-three patients with special reference to their oral lesions, *Oral Surgery, Oral Medicine, and Oral Pathology* 54:404–413, 1982.

Granulomatosis with Polyangiitis

Allen CM, Camisa C, Salewski C, et al.: Wegener's granulomatosis: report of three cases with oral lesions, *Journal of Oral and Maxillofacial Surgery* 49:294–298, 1991.

Eufinger H, Machtens E, Akuamoa-Boateng E: Oral manifestations of Wegener's granulomatosis: review of the literature and report of a case, *International Journal of Oral and Maxillofacial Surgery* 21:50–53, 1992.

Fauci AS, Haynes BF, Katz P, et al.: Wegener's granulomatosis: prospective clinical and therapeutic experience with 85 patients for 21 years, *Annals of Internal Medicine* 98:76–85, 1983.

Ponniah I, Shaheen A, Shankar KA, et al.: Wegener's granulomatosis: the current understanding, *Oral Surgery, Oral Medicine, Oral Pathology, Oral Radiology, and Endodontics* 100:265–270, 2005.

Stewart C, Cohen D, Bhattacharyya I, et al.: Oral manifestations of Wegener's granulomatosis: a report of three cases and a literature review, *Journal of the American Dental Association (1939)* 138:338–348, 2007.

Thompson G, Benwell N, Hollingsworth P, et al.: Two cases of granulomatosis polyangiitis presenting with strawberry gingivitis and a review of the literature, *Seminars in Arthritis and Rheumatism* 47:520–523, 2018.

Weeda LW Jr, Coffey SA: Wegener's granulomatosis, *Oral and Maxillofacial Surgery Clinics of North America* 20:643–649, 2008.

Lichenoid and Granulomatous Stomatitis

Bäckman K, Jontell M: Microbial-associated oral lichenoid reactions, *Oral Diseases* 13:402–406, 2007.

Blomgren J, Axéll T, Sandahl O, et al.: Adverse reaction in oral mucosa associated with anterior composite restorations, *Journal of Oral Pathology & Medicine* 25:311–313, 1996.

Georgakopoulou EA, Achtari MD: Oral lichenoid lesions of the upper lip, *J Dermatol Case Rep* 11:16–19, 2017.

Georgakopoulos EA, Malamos D, Achtari MD: Oral lichenoid lesions of the upper lip and gingiva: what we know so far, *Oral Diseases* 24:135–137, 2018.

Katsoulas N, Tosios K, Sklavounou-Andrikopoulou A: Lichenoid lesions of the upper lip: a retrospective study of 24 cases, *Medicina Oral, Patología Oral y Cirugía Bucal* 23:e302–e307, 2018.

Mainville G, Sadeghi S, Rawal Y, et al.: Lichenoid and granulomatous stomatitis: 8 new cases and a decade of hindsight (abstract), *Oral Surgery, Oral Medicine, Oral Pathology, Oral Radiology* 124: e226–e227, 2017.

Robinson CM, Oxley JD, Weir J, et al.: Lichenoid and granulomatous stomatitis: an entity or a non-specific inflammatory process, *Journal of Oral Pathology & Medicine* 35:262–267, 2006.

Allergic Mucosal Reactions to Systemic Drug Administration

Alqahtani M, Woods TR, Smith MH, et al.: Medication use and medical history of 155 patients with oral lichenoid lesions: a retrospective study, *General Dentistry* 66:40–45, 2018.

Femiano F, Lanza A, Buonaiuto C, et al.: Oral manifestations of adverse drug reactions: guidelines, *Journal of the European Academy of Dermatology and Venereology* 22:681–691, 2008.

Lamey P-J, McCartan BE, MacDonald DG, et al.: Basal cell cytoplasmic autoantibodies in oral lichenoid reactions, *Oral Surgery, Oral Medicine, Oral Pathology, Oral Radiology, and Endodontics* 79:44–49, 1995.

Seymour RA, Rudralingham M: Oral and dental adverse drug reactions, *Periodontology 2000* 2000(46):9–26, 2008.

Teoh L, Moses G, McCullough MJ: A review and guide to drug-associated oral adverse effects—oral mucosal and lichenoid reactions. Part 2, *Journal of Oral Pathology & Medicine* 48:637–646, 2019.

Wright JM: Oral manifestations of drug reactions, *Dental Clinics of North America* 28:529–543, 1984.

Yuan A, Woo S-B: Adverse drug events in the oral cavity, *Oral Surg Oral Med Oral Pathol Oral Radiol* 119:35–47, 2015.

Allergic Contact Stomatitis

Cifuentes M, Davari P, Rogers RS: Contact stomatitis, *Clinics in Dermatology* 35:435–440, 2017.

De Rossi SS, Greenberg MS: Intraoral contact allergy: a literature review and case reports, *Journal of the American Dental Association (1939)* 129:1435–1441, 1998.

Fisher AA: Reactions of the mucous membrane to contactants, *Clinics in Dermatology* 5:123–136, 1987.

LeSueur BW, Yiannias JA: Contact stomatitis, *Dermatologic Clinics* 21:105–114, 2003.

Stoopler ET, DeRossi SS: AAOM clinical practice statement: Oral contact allergy, *Oral Surgery, Oral Medicine, Oral Pathology, Oral Radiology* 122:50–52, 2016.

Tosti A, Piraccini BM, Peluso AM: Contact and irritant stomatitis, *Seminars in Cutaneous Medicine and Surgery* 16:314–319, 1997.

van Loon LAJ, Bos JD, Davidson CL: Clinical evaluation of fifty-six patients referred with symptoms tentatively related to allergic contact stomatitis, *Oral Surgery, Oral Medicine, and Oral Pathology* 74:572–575, 1992.

Perioral Dermatitis

Goel NS, Burkhart CN, Morrell DS: Pediatric periorificial dermatitis: clinical course and treatment outcomes in 222 patients, *Pediatr Dermatol* 32:333–336, 2015.

Hall CD, Reichenberg J: Evidence based review of perioral dermatitis therapy, *Giornale Italiano di Dermatologia e Venereologia* 145:433–444, 2010.

Lipozenčić J, Hadžavdić SL: Perioral dermatitis, *Clinics in Dermatology* 32:125–130, 2014.

Tempark T, Shwayder TA: Perioral dermatitis: a review of the condition with special attention to treatment options, *American Journal of Clinical Dermatology* 15:101–113, 2014.

Vanderweil SG, Levin NA: Perioral dermatitis: it's not every rash that occurs around the mouth, *Dermatology Nursing* 21:317–320, 353, 2009.

Cinnamon-Induced Contact Stomatitis

Allen CM, Blozis GG: Oral mucosal reactions to cinnamon-flavored chewing gum, *Journal of the American Dental Association (1939)* 116:664–667, 1988.

Calapai G, Miroddi M, Minciullo PL, et al.: Oral adverse reactions due to cinnamon-flavored chewing gums consumption, *Oral Diseases* 20:637–643, 2014.

Drake TE, Maibach HI: Allergic contact dermatitis and stomatitis caused by a cinnamic aldehyde-flavored toothpaste, *Archives of Dermatology* 112:202–203, 1976.

Endo H, Rees TD: Clinical features of cinnamon-induced contact stomatitis, *The Compendium of Continuing Education in Dentistry* 27:403–409, 2006.

Isaac-Renton M, Li MK, Parsons LM: Cinnamon spice and everything not nice: many features of intraoral allergy to cinnamic aldehyde, *Dermatitis* 26:116–121, 2015.

Mihail RC: Oral leukoplakia caused by cinnamon food allergy, *The Journal of Otolaryngology* 21:366–367, 1992.

Miller RL, Gould AR, Bernstein ML: Cinnamon-induced stomatitis venenata: clinical and characteristic histopathologic features, *Oral Surgery, Oral Medicine, and Oral Pathology* 73:708–716, 1992.

Lichenoid Contact Reactions from Dental Restorative Materials

Holmstrup P: Reaction of the oral mucosa related to silver amalgam: a review, *Journal of Oral Pathology & Medicine* 20:1–7, 1991.

Jameson MW, Kardos TB, Kirk EE, et al.: Mucosal reactions to amalgam restorations, *Journal of Oral Rehabilitation* 17:293–301, 1990.

Kal BI, Evcin O, Dundar N, et al.: An unusual case of immediate hypersensitivity reaction associated with an amalgam restoration, *British Dental Journal* 205:547–550, 2008.

Luiz AC, Hirota SK, Dal Vechio A, et al.: Diagnosing oral lichenoid contact reaction: clinical judgment *versus* skin-patch test, *Minerva Stomatologica* 61:311–317, 2012.

Lynch M, Ryan A, Galvin S, et al.: Patch testing in oral lichenoid lesions of uncertain etiology, *Dermatitis* 26:89–93, 2015.

Mallo-Pérez L, Diaz-Donado C: Intraoral contact allergy to materials used in dental practice: a critical review, *Medicina Oral* 8:334–347, 2003.

Mårell L, Tillberg A, Widman L, et al.: Regression of oral lichenoid lesions after replacement of dental restorations, *Journal of Oral Rehabilitation* 41:381–391, 2014.

Suter VGA, Warnakulasuriya S: The role of patch testing in the management of oral lichenoid lesions, *Journal of Oral Pathology & Medicine* 45:48–57, 2016.

Thornhill MH, Pemberton MN, Simmons RK, et al.: Amalgam-contact hypersensitivity lesions and oral lichen planus, *Oral Surgery, Oral Medicine, Oral Pathology, Oral Radiology, and Endodontics* 95:291–299, 2003.

Angioedema

Al-Khudari S, Loochtan MJ, Peterson E, et al.: Management of angiotensin-converting enzyme inhibitor-induced angioedema, *Laryngoscope* 121:2327–2334, 2011.

Angostoni A, Cicardi M: Hereditary and acquired C1-inhibitor deficiency: biological and clinical characteristics in 235 patients, *Medicine* 71:206–215, 1992.

Craig TJ, Bernstein JA, Farkas H, et al.: Diagnosis and treatment of bradykinin-mediated angioedema: outcomes from an angioedema expert consensus meeting, *International Archives of Allergy and Immunology* 165:119–127, 2014.

Grant NN, Deeb ZE, Chia SH: Clinical experience with angiotensin-converting enzyme inhibitor-induced angioedema, *Otolaryngology and Head and Neck Surgery* 137:931–935, 2007.

Kalathoor I.: Snoring-induced vibratory angioedema, Am J Case Rep 16:700–2, https://doi.org/10.12659/AJCR.894636.

Pahs L, Droege C, Kneale H, et al.: A novel approach to the treatment of orolingual angioedema after tissue plasminogen activator administration, *Annals of Emergency Medicine* 68:345–348, 2016.

Nielsen EW, Gramstad S: Angioedema from angiotensin-converting enzyme (ACE) inhibitor treated with complement 1 (C1) inhibitor concentrate, *Acta Anaesthesiologica Scandinavica* 50:120–122, 2006.

Uzun T: Management of patients with hereditary angio-oedema in dental, oral, and maxillofacial surgery: a review, *The British Journal of Oral & Maxillofacial Surgery* 57:992–997, 2019.

10

Epithelial Pathology

◆ BENIGN EPITHELIAL LESIONS ASSOCIATED WITH HUMAN PAPILLOMAVIRUS

Human papillomavirus (HPV) comprises a large group of double-stranded DNA viruses, belonging to the family *Papillomaviridae*. HPV exhibits tropism for squamous epithelium and may infect skin or mucosa. Mucosal infection may arise in the anogenital region, upper aerodigestive tract, and other sites. More than 200 HPV types have been identified in humans, including more than 30 types known to infect the oral mucosa in particular.

HPV is associated with a variety of benign, potentially malignant, and malignant epithelial lesions, but most infected individuals are asymptomatic and lack clinically evident disease. Based upon oncogenic potential, mucosal HPV types are categorized as either *low-risk* (e.g., types 6, 11, 13, 32, 40, 42, 43, 44, 54, 55, 61, 62, 64, 67, 69, 70, 71, 72, 81, and others) or *high-risk* (e.g., types 16, 18, 31, 33, 35, 39, 45, 51, 52, 56, 58, 59, 66, 68, 73, and others).

The reported prevalence of asymptomatic oral HPV infection varies considerably, likely due to differences in sampling techniques, detection methods, and study cohorts. Many studies have analyzed shed epithelial cells in oral rinses, although such samples do not discriminate between oral cavity and oropharyngeal infection. Notwithstanding, meta-analyses and systematic reviews of the literature suggest that oral HPV infection is present in approximately 5%–8% of normal, healthy individuals worldwide. Most studies report a male predilection, although reported gender distribution is variable. In the United States, a population-based study conducted as part of the National Health and Nutrition Examination Survey (NHANES) for 2011–2014 estimated the prevalence of oral HPV infection among individuals 18–69 years old to be 11.5% among men and 3.2% among women. In this study, the age distribution for men with oral HPV infection exhibited a bimodal pattern, with peaks at 35–39 and 50–54 years. Notably, the prevalence of oral infection with high-risk HPV types was substantially greater among men compared to women (7.3% vs 1.4%, respectively). Also, there was an increased frequency of oral HPV infection among men with concurrent genital infection.

Factors associated with an increased prevalence of oral HPV infection include tobacco smoking, an increased number of lifetime sexual partners, an increased number of recent sexual partners, and human immunodeficiency virus (HIV) infection. In addition, some investigators have suggested possible associations with periodontitis, gingivitis, or poor oral hygiene, although the significance of these findings is uncertain.

Proposed modes of transmission for oral HPV infection include sexual and nonsexual person-to-person contact, salivary transfer, contaminated objects, autoinoculation, breast-feeding, perinatal transmission, and, possibly, prenatal transmission. In particular, orogenital transmission of the virus seems to be higher from women to men than from men to women. Among newborns, some studies have detected oral and nasopharyngeal HPV in as many as 23% and 37%, respectively, although most of these infections are cleared within the first few years of life. The exact route of transmission to newborns is uncertain, although exposure via the birth canal, umbilical cord blood, or amniotic fluid has been postulated.

The natural history of oral HPV infection is not well characterized. It appears that in most people the infection clears quickly, whereas in some individuals the infection persists. However, reported clearance rates are highly variable (range 0%–80%), probably due to differences in study design and methods. Factors associated with persistent oral infection include male gender, older age, human immunodeficiency virus (HIV) infection, and cigarette smoking.

HPV may enter the epithelium via microabrasion or trauma and initially infects the basal epithelial cells. Host cell entry occurs by endocytosis, and the episomal viral DNA (i.e., circular extrachromosomal molecule) is transported to the nucleus. In normal-appearing skin or mucosa, the virus may remain in a latent state within the nuclei of basal epithelial cells; in such cases, the episomal viral DNA is present in low copy numbers. In contrast, in benign and low-grade premalignant HPV-associated lesions, episomal HPV DNA typically is present within the various epithelial cell layers in increased copy numbers, with shedding of mature virions from the superficial cells. With division of each infected basal epithelial cell, one daughter cell remains in the basal layer to maintain a viral reservoir; the other daughter cell migrates into the suprabasal layers, interferes with cell cycle regulation, and uses the host cell machinery to synthesize proteins needed for viral replication. In the presence of high episomal numbers, viral DNA may become integrated into the host genome,

TABLE 10.1	Human Papillomavirus Types for Select Lesions		
Site Predilection	Lesion	Major HPV Types	Other Reported HPV Types
Oral/head and neck mucosa	Oral squamous papilloma	6, 11	5, 12, 16, 18, 22–24, 35, 51, 96, 110, 120, 121, 123, 130, 131, 156, 161
	Recurrent respiratory papillomatosis	6, 11	8, 16, 18, 31, 33, 35, 44, 45, 55, 70, 76, 84
	Exophytic sinonasal papilloma	6, 11	16, 57, 91
	Inverted sinonasal papilloma	6, 11, 16, 18	42, 57, 58, 83
	Multifocal epithelial hyperplasia	13, 32	1, 6, 11, 16, 18, 31, 39, 40, 51, 52, 55, 58, 66, 68, 69, 71, 74, 90
	Oropharyngeal squamous cell carcinoma	16	18, 26, 33, 35, 45, 52, 58, 67, 69
	Conjunctival papilloma	6, 11	5, 13, 16, 20, 23, 33, 45
Skin	Verruca vulgaris	2	1, 4, 6, 7, 10, 11, 26, 27, 29, 41, 57, 65, 75–77
	Verruca plana	3, 10	2, 5, 26–29, 38, 41, 49, 75, 76
	Palmoplantar wart	1, 4	2, 27, 41, 45, 57, 60, 63, 65, 66
	Butcher's wart	2, 7	1, 3, 4, 10, 28
Anogenital region	Condyloma acuminatum	6, 11	1, 2, 4, 6, 7, 9, 16, 18, 27, 31, 33, 35, 38–45, 51–59, 65, 66, 68, 70, 81
	Intraepithelial neoplasia	6, 11, 16, 18, 31, 33	26, 35, 39, 42, 43, 45, 51, 52, 53, 56, 58, 59, 66, 68, 70, 73, 81–83
	Cervical squamous cell carcinoma	16, 18	6, 11, 31, 33, 35, 39, 42, 45, 51, 52, 56, 58, 59, 66, 68, 73

HPV, Human papillomavirus.

leading to expression of oncoproteins and inactivation of tumor suppressor genes. Integrated HPV DNA often is found in HPV-associated malignancies and high-grade premalignant lesions, but it is not an absolute requirement for development of such lesions. Compared with HPV infection, HPV-induced malignant transformation is relatively rare. The incubation period for benign HPV disease is estimated to range from 3 weeks to 2 years, whereas the latency for development of HPV-associated malignancy may be 1 to several decades.

In the United States, routine HPV vaccination was introduced in 2006, with various modifications in vaccine policy, design, and licensing over the years. In current use is a 9-valent recombinant vaccine (Gardasil 9) targeting HPV types 6, 11, 16, 18, 31, 33, 45, 52, and 58. The Advisory Committee on Immunization Practices recommends routine HPV vaccination for adolescents 11–12 years of age and catch-up HPV vaccination for individuals through 26 years of age. In addition, HPV vaccination may be considered for inadequately vaccinated adults 27 through 45 years of age in consultation with a clinician. Two doses typically are administered 6–12 months apart for immunocompetent individuals under 15 years of age; three doses over 6 months are recommended for individuals 15 years of age or older and for immunocompromised patients at any age. The vaccine is indicated for prevention of genital warts; precancers and cancers of the uterine cervix, vulva, vagina, and anus; and oropharyngeal and other head and neck cancers. The latter indication was granted accelerated approval based

on surrogate efficacy data for HPV-related anogenital disease and is subject to post-approval confirmatory studies currently underway.

The following sections discuss benign HPV-associated lesions of the oral cavity and other head and neck sites. HPV-associated malignancies are addressed later in this chapter. Examples of HPV-related lesions and their corresponding virus types are listed in Table 10.1.

SQUAMOUS PAPILLOMA

The **squamous papilloma** is a benign proliferation of stratified squamous epithelium, resulting in a papillary or verruciform mass. In the upper aerodigestive tract, squamous papillomas most often involve the oral cavity, oropharynx, and larynx. The lesion generally is considered to be induced by HPV, with HPV types 6 and 11 identified most commonly. However, HPV detection rates vary considerably across studies, likely due to differences in detection methods and viral types assayed. HPV can be demonstrated in most laryngeal papillomas (approximately 90%–95% as per more recent studies) but in only a minority of oral cases. HPV testing typically is not needed for routine diagnosis and management of papillomas in the oral cavity, oropharynx, and larynx.

Oral squamous papillomas are relatively common and comprise approximately 3% of all oral lesions submitted for biopsy. In addition, researchers have estimated that squamous papillomas comprise 7%–8% of all oral masses or growths in children.

Clinical Features

Most studies have reported either no significant gender predilection or a slight male predominance. Some authors have asserted that the oral squamous papilloma develops predominantly in children; however, the lesion can arise at any age and, in fact, is diagnosed most often in persons 30–50 years old. Sites of predilection include the palate, tongue, and lips, but any oral surface may be affected. This lesion is the most common soft tissue mass arising from the soft palate.

The squamous papilloma is a soft, painless, usually pedunculated, exophytic nodule with numerous fingerlike surface projections that impart a "cauliflower" or wartlike appearance (Fig. 10.1). Projections may be pointed or blunted (Figs. 10.2 and 10.3), and the lesion may be white, slightly red, or normal in color, depending on the amount of surface keratinization. The papilloma is usually solitary and

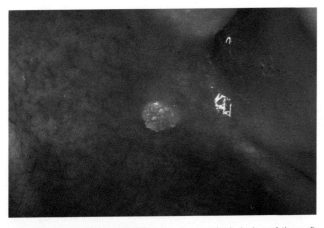

• **Fig. 10.1 Squamous Papilloma.** An exophytic lesion of the soft palate with multiple short, white surface projections.

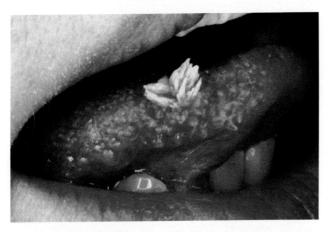

• **Fig. 10.2 Squamous Papilloma.** A pedunculated lingual mass with numerous long, pointed, and white surface projections. Note the smaller projections around the base of the lesion.

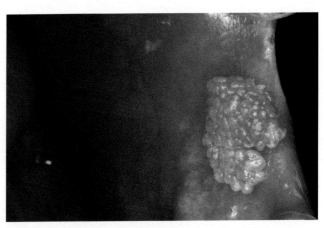

• **Fig. 10.3 Squamous Papilloma.** A pedunculated mass of the buccal commissure, exhibiting short or blunted surface projections and minimal white coloration.

enlarges rapidly to a maximum size of about 0.5 cm, with little or no change thereafter. However, lesions as large as 3.0 cm in greatest diameter have been reported.

It is sometimes difficult to distinguish this lesion clinically from verruca vulgaris (see page 357), condyloma acuminatum (see page 358), verruciform xanthoma (see page 365), multifocal epithelial hyperplasia (see page 360), or giant cell fibroma (see page 514). In addition, extensive coalescing papillary lesions (**papillomatosis**) of the orofacial region may be seen in several syndromes and skin disorders, including nevus unius lateris, acanthosis nigricans, focal dermal hypoplasia (Goltz-Gorlin) syndrome, Costello syndrome, and Down syndrome.

Also attributed mainly to HPV 6 and 11 infection, **recurrent respiratory papillomatosis (RRP)** is a rare and potentially devastating disease of the respiratory tract with a predilection for the larynx. RRP includes two distinct types: (1) **juvenile-onset** and (2) **adult-onset.** Hoarseness is the usual presenting feature, and rapidly proliferating papillomas in the juvenile-onset type may obstruct the airway. The strongest risk factor for juvenile-onset RRP is a maternal history of anogenital warts during pregnancy; HPV transmission via the birth canal, the placenta, or amniotic fluid has been hypothesized.

Histopathologic Features

The papilloma is characterized by a proliferation of keratinized stratified squamous epithelium arranged in fingerlike projections with fibrovascular connective tissue cores (Fig. 10.4). The connective tissue may show inflammation. The keratin layer is thickened in lesions with a white clinical appearance, and the epithelium typically exhibits a normal maturation pattern. However, some papillomas demonstrate basilar hyperplasia and mitotic activity, which can be mistaken for mild epithelial dysplasia. **Koilocytes** (virus-altered epithelial cells with crenated, pyknotic [small and dark] nuclei surrounded by clear halos) sometimes are evident high in the spinous cell layer. Similarities in microscopic features may make distinction of squamous papilloma from verruca vulgaris and condyloma acuminatum difficult.

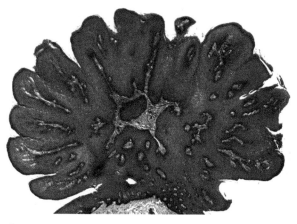

• **Fig. 10.4 Squamous Papilloma.** Low-power view showing a pedunculated squamous epithelial proliferation. There are multiple papillary projections with fibrovascular connective tissue cores.

Treatment and Prognosis

Conservative surgical excision, including the base of the lesion, is adequate treatment for the oral squamous papilloma, and recurrence is unlikely. Frequently, lesions have been left untreated for years with no reported malignant transformation, continuous enlargement, or dissemination to other parts of the oral cavity or orohparynx.

Although spontaneous remission is possible, juvenile-onset RRP tends to be continuously proliferative, sometimes leading to death by asphyxiation. Some investigators have noted especially aggressive behavior among cases associated with HPV 11 infection. The papillomatosis is treated by repeated surgical debulking procedures to relieve airway obstruction. Use of a microdebrider may decrease the risk for postsurgical scarring and loss of vocal cord function. Adjuvant therapy with interferon-alpha, cidofovir, bevacizumab, or other agents has yielded variable results. Adult-onset RRP typically is less aggressive and more localized. Conservative surgical removal may be necessary to eliminate hoarseness from vocal cord involvement. A few studies suggest that HPV vaccination may be beneficial for prevention and adjuvant treatment of RRP, although further investigation is needed. Transformation of RRP into squamous cell carcinoma is rare (occurring in <1% of juvenile-onset cases and about 3%–6% of adult-onset cases).

VERRUCA VULGARIS (COMMON WART)

Verruca vulgaris is a focal, benign, HPV-induced hyperplasia of stratified squamous epithelium. HPV 2 is present most often, although other HPV types may be found as well (see Table 10.1). Verruca vulgaris is contagious and can spread to other parts of a person's skin or mucosa by autoinoculation. It infrequently develops on oral mucosa but is extremely common on the skin.

Clinical Features

Verruca vulgaris most often arises in children but occasionally may develop even into middle age. The skin of the hands is the most commonly involved site (Fig. 10.5). Oral

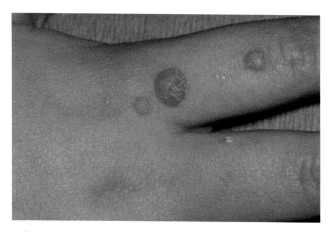

• **Fig. 10.5 Verruca Vulgaris.** Several warts on the finger, exhibiting a rough, papillary surface.

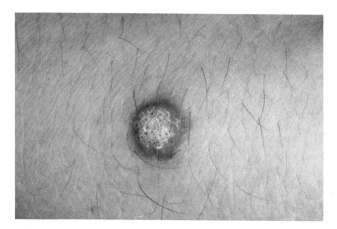

• **Fig. 10.6 Verruca Vulgaris.** Nodular lesion of the skin exhibiting numerous short papillary projections.

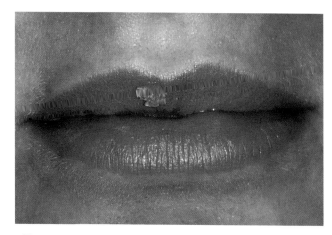

• **Fig. 10.7 Verruca Vulgaris.** White, papillary lesion on the upper lip vermilion. (Courtesy of Dr. Laura Summers.)

mucosal lesions usually are found on the vermilion border, labial mucosa, or anterior tongue.

Typically, the verruca appears as a painless papule or nodule with papillary projections or a rough, pebbly surface (Figs. 10.6 and 10.7). It may be pedunculated or sessile. Cutaneous lesions may be pink, yellow, or white; oral lesions are almost always white. Verruca vulgaris enlarges rapidly to its maximum size (usually <5 mm), and the size remains constant for months or years thereafter unless the lesion is irritated. Multiple or clustered lesions are common. On occasion, extreme accumulation of compact keratin may result in a hard surface projection, termed a **cutaneous horn** or **keratin horn.** Other cutaneous lesions, including seborrheic keratosis (see page 366), actinic keratosis (see page 396), and squamous cell carcinoma, also may create a cutaneous horn.

Histopathologic Features

Verruca vulgaris is characterized by a proliferation of hyperkeratotic stratified squamous epithelium arranged in fingerlike, pointed projections with connective tissue cores (Fig. 10.8). Chronic inflammatory cells often infiltrate the supporting connective tissue. Elongated rete ridges tend to converge toward the center of the lesion, producing a "cupping" effect. A prominent granular cell layer (hypergranulosis) exhibits coarse, clumped keratohyaline granules. Abundant koilocytes often are seen in the superficial spinous layer. Koilocytes are HPV-altered epithelial cells with perinuclear clearing and crenated, pyknotic nuclei. Eosinophilic intranuclear viral inclusions sometimes are noted within the cells of the granular layer.

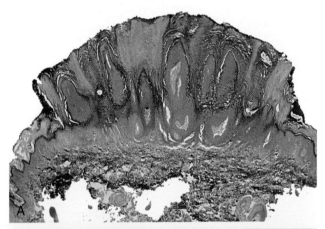

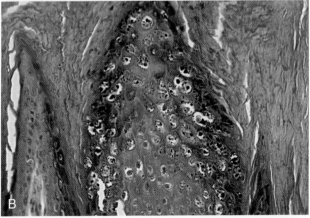

• **Fig. 10.8 Verruca Vulgaris. A,** Numerous papillary projections are covered by hyperkeratotic stratified squamous epithelium. Elongated rete ridges at the edge of the lesion converge toward the center. **B,** High-power view showing clear koilocytes in the upper epithelial layers.

Treatment and Prognosis

Verrucae often resolve spontaneously over time in immunocompetent individuals. Approximately two-thirds will disappear without treatment within 2 years, especially in children. However, removal may be considered for lesions that persist, spread, cause cosmetic concern, or produce discomfort. Commonly used treatments for cutaneous verrucae include topical salicylic acid, topical lactic acid, and cryotherapy. Surgical excision is indicated only for cases with an atypical clinical presentation in which the diagnosis is uncertain. Skin lesions that recur or are resistant to standard therapy may be treated by alternative methods, such as intralesional bleomycin, topical or intralesional 5-fluorouracil, cantharidin, immunotherapy with contact sensitizers (e.g., diphenylcyclopropenone, squaric acid dibutylester), intralesional immunotherapy (e.g., with *Candida* or mumps skin antigen, purified protein derivative), topical imiquimod, trichloroacetic acid, pulsed dye laser therapy, or photodynamic therapy.

Oral lesions usually are excised surgically, or they may be destroyed by laser, cryotherapy, or electrosurgery. Cryotherapy induces a subepithelial blister that lifts the infected epithelium from the underlying connective tissue, allowing it to slough away. All destructive or surgical treatments should extend to the base of the lesion.

Recurrence is seen in a small proportion of treated cases. There is no potential for malignant transformation.

CONDYLOMA ACUMINATUM (VENEREAL WART)

Condyloma acuminatum is a HPV-induced proliferation of stratified squamous epithelium of the anogenital region, mouth, and larynx. Approximately 90% of cases are attributed to HPV 6 and 11, although coinfection with various other types—including the high-risk types 16 and 18—is frequent (see Table 10.1).

Condyloma acuminatum represents a common sexually transmitted disease (STD), affecting about 1% of the sexually active population. However, since the introduction of HPV vaccination, significant reductions in incidence have been reported in many regions. Condyloma may be an indicator of sexual abuse when diagnosed in young children. In addition, studies of oral cavity and pharyngeal HPV infection in infants have suggested that vertical transmission from mothers with genital HPV infection may occur perinatally or perhaps *in utero*. Spread via contaminated environmental surfaces has been postulated as well. Oral and anogenital condylomata may be present concurrently. The incubation period is about 1–3 months, and autoinoculation of additional mucosal sites is possible.

Clinical Features

Condylomata usually are diagnosed in teenagers and young adults, but people of all ages are susceptible. Oral lesions most frequently occur on the labial mucosa and lingual frenum; the soft palate often is involved as well. The typical condyloma appears as a sessile, pink, well-demarcated, non-tender, exophytic mass with short, blunted surface projections (Fig. 10.9). The condyloma tends to be larger than the papilloma and characteristically is clustered with other condylomata. The average size is 1.0–1.5 cm, but oral lesions as large as 3 cm have been reported.

Histopathologic Features

Condyloma acuminatum appears as a benign proliferation of acanthotic stratified squamous epithelium with mildly keratotic, papillary surface projections (Fig. 10.10). Thin connective tissue cores support the papillary projections, which are more blunted and broader than those of squamous papilloma and verruca vulgaris. Keratin-filled crypts often are seen between the papillary projections. In some cases, lesions may extend from the surface mucosa to involve the underlying salivary ductal epithelium; such lesions should be distinguished from salivary ductal papillomas (see page 492).

The surface epithelium is mature and differentiated, but within the spinous cell layer, there are often **koilocytes** (HPV-altered cells with pyknotic, crinkled [or "raisin-like"] nuclei) (Fig. 10.11). Koilocytes may be less prominent in oral lesions compared with genital lesions, in which case distinction from squamous papilloma may be difficult. Ultrastructural examination reveals virions within the cytoplasm or nuclei of koilocytes, and the virus also can be demonstrated by immunohistochemical analysis, *in situ* hybridization (ISH), and polymerase chain reaction (PCR).

Treatment and Prognosis

Oral condylomata usually are treated by conservative surgical excision. Cryotherapy and laser ablation also may be used. However, there is some concern regarding the potential for laser therapy to produce an infectious plume that exposes the surgical team and patient to airborne HPV.

For anogenital condylomata, patient-applied topical agents (such as, imiquimod, podophyllotoxin, and sinecatechins) are becoming the mainstay of treatment. However, such treatments typically are not used for oral lesions. Anogenital warts that do not completely resolve with patient-applied treatment may be ablated by cryotherapy, laser, or electrosurgery. Additional treatment options include trichloroacetic acid, systemic, or intralesional interferon, and topical cidofovir. Interestingly, there are a few anecdotal reports of regression following HPV vaccination.

Regardless of the method used, condylomata should be treated because they are contagious and can spread by autoinoculation or to other persons. Notwithstanding, available treatments do not completely eradicate HPV infection or the potential for future viral transmission; recurrence has been reported in approximately 20%–50% of anogenital cases. Therefore, clinical follow-up is recommended.

Anogenital condylomata infected with HPV 16 or 18 are associated with an increased risk for malignant transformation to squamous cell carcinoma, but such transformation has not been well documented in oral lesions. Interestingly, a recent population-based study of Danish patients with

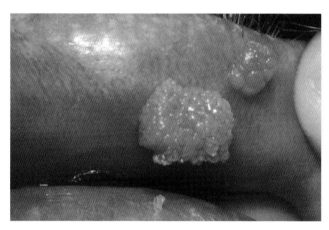

• **Fig. 10.9 Condyloma Acuminatum.** Two lesions of the upper lip mucosa exhibit short, blunted projections. (Courtesy of Dr. Brian Blocher.)

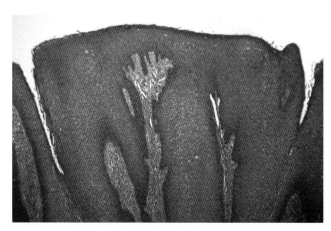

• **Fig. 10.10 Condyloma Acuminatum.** Medium-power photomicrograph showing acanthotic stratified squamous epithelium forming a blunted projection.

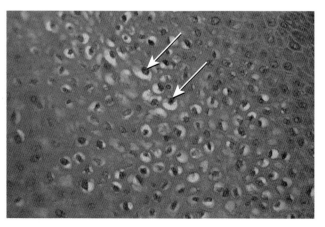

• **Fig. 10.11 Condyloma Acuminatum.** High-power photomicrograph demonstrating koilocytes *(arrows)* in the spinous layer.

genital condylomata reported a long-term, increased risk for not only anogenital but also head and neck cancer. Proposed explanations for this observation include an immunologic predisposition to persistent HPV infection (resulting in increased risk for HPV-related head and neck cancer) and behavioral cofactors (e.g., tobacco and alcohol consumption, male homosexual behavior).

HPV vaccination (see page 355) is useful for the prevention of anogenital condylomata; vaccination would be expected to aid in preventing oral lesions as well, although the impact of HPV vaccination on oral condylomata requires study.

MULTIFOCAL EPITHELIAL HYPERPLASIA (HECK DISEASE; MULTIFOCAL PAPILLOMA VIRUS EPITHELIAL HYPERPLASIA; FOCAL EPITHELIAL HYPERPLASIA)

Multifocal epithelial hyperplasia is a squamous epithelial proliferation primarily attributed to HPV 13 and 32. However, infection or co-infection with various other HPV types occasionally has been reported (Table 10.1). The condition initially was described in Native Americans and Inuits but subsequently has been noted in many populations and ethnic groups. A high proportion of reported cases have been from the Americas and Europe. In some populations, nearly 40% of children are affected. Multifocal epithelial hyperplasia often affects multiple members of a given family; this familial tendency may be related to either genetic susceptibility or HPV transmission between family members. An association with the HLA-DR4 (DRB1*0404) allele has been described, and transmission via saliva has been postulated (possibly through shared use of eating utensils or toothbrushes). Lower socioeconomic status, crowded living conditions, poor hygiene, malnutrition, and HIV infection or other immunodeficiency states appear to be additional risk factors. Although originally reported as "focal epithelial hyperplasia," the term *multifocal epithelial hyperplasia* is preferred because patients usually exhibit multiple lesions.

Clinical Features

Multifocal epithelial hyperplasia predominantly arises in young individuals, with a mean age of 23 years and a broad age range of 3–92 years. There is a slight female predilection. The most common sites of involvement include the labial, buccal, and lingual mucosa, but gingival, palatal, oral floor, and tonsillar lesions also are possible. In addition, involvement of the conjunctiva has been described very rarely.

There are two major clinical variants: papulonodular and papillomatous. The more common papulonodular variant is characterized by pink, smooth-surfaced papules and nodules, with a predilection for the buccal mucosa, labial mucosa, and commissure (Fig. 10.12). The papillomatous variant appears as white to pale pink, pebbly nodules on the tongue and attached gingiva (Fig. 10.13). In both variants, the individual

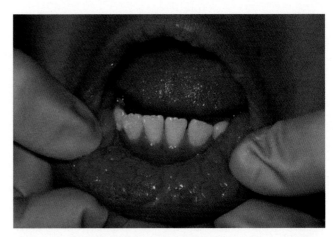

• **Fig. 10.12 Multifocal Epithelial Hyperplasia.** Multiple, flat-topped papules and nodules of normal coloration are seen on the lower lip of a child. (Courtesy of Dr. Mark Casafrancisco.)

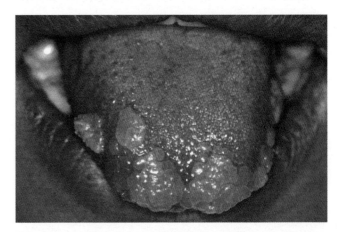

• **Fig. 10.13 Multifocal Epithelial Hyperplasia.** The lesions may demonstrate a papillary surface change and paleness, as demonstrated on this child's tongue. (Courtesy of Dr. Román Carlos.)

lesions are usually small (0.1–1.0 cm), discrete, and well-demarcated; however, they may coalesce to produce a cobblestone or fissured appearance, and individual lesions up to 3 cm in diameter are also possible. According to some authors, the lesions tend to be smaller, fewer in number, and less exophytic among older patients compared to younger patients; this observation may reflect spontaneous regression over time.

Histopathologic Features

The hallmark of multifocal epithelial hyperplasia is an abrupt and sometimes considerable acanthosis of the surface epithelium (Fig. 10.14). Because the thickened mucosa extends upward, the lesional rete ridges are at the same depth as the adjacent, normal rete ridges. The rete ridges are widened, often confluent, and sometimes club-shaped. Some superficial keratinocytes show koilocytic change similar to that seen in other HPV infections. Others occasionally demonstrate an altered nucleus that resembles a mitotic figure

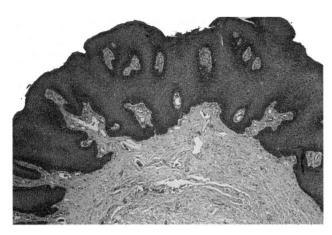

• **Fig. 10.14 Multifocal Epithelial Hyperplasia.** Prominent acanthosis of the epithelium with broad and elongated rete ridges. The slightly papillary surface alteration noted here may or may not be present.

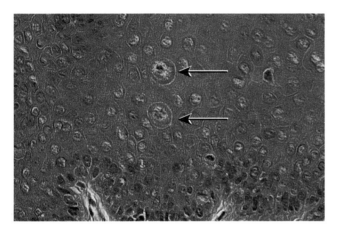

• **Fig. 10.15 Multifocal Epithelial Hyperplasia.** Mitosoid cells *(arrows)* contain altered nuclei in this otherwise mature and well-differentiated stratified squamous epithelium.

(mitosoid cell) (Fig. 10.15). Viruslike particles have been noted ultrastructurally within both the cytoplasm and the nuclei of cells within the prickle cell layer, and the presence of HPV has been demonstrated by DNA *in situ* hybridization, immunohistochemistry, and polymerase chain reaction (PCR).

Treatment and Prognosis

Spontaneous regression has been reported after months or years and is inferred from the rarity of the disease in adults. Conservative surgical excision may be performed for diagnostic or aesthetic purposes or for lesions subject to recurrent trauma. Lesions also can be removed by cryotherapy, carbon dioxide (CO_2) laser, or electrocoagulation. Alternative treatments include trichloroacetic acid, topical interferon-beta, systemic or intralesional interferon-alpha, and topical imiquimod. Recurrence (after either treatment or spontaneous regression) is possible. There seems to be no malignant transformation potential.

SINONASAL PAPILLOMAS (SCHNEIDERIAN PAPILLOMAS)

Sinonasal papillomas are benign, localized proliferations of the sinonasal mucosa and include three histomorphologically distinct types:
1. Exophytic
2. Inverted
3. Oncocytic

Lesions exhibiting features of both the inverted and the oncocytic types may be termed *mixed* or *hybrid* papillomas. In addition, a keratinizing **squamous papilloma,** similar to the oral squamous papilloma (see page 355), rarely may occur in the nasal vestibule.

Collectively, sinonasal papillomas represent 10%–25% of all sinonasal tumors. About half of sinonasal papillomas arise from the lateral nasal wall; the remainder predominantly involves the maxillary and ethmoid sinuses and the nasal septum. Multiple lesions may be present.

The etiopathogenesis of sinonasal papillomas remains unclear. Historically, numerous contributory factors—such as allergy, chronic sinusitis, nasal polyps, organic solvents, and tobacco smoke or other airborne pollutants—have been proposed but remain unsubstantiated. A variable association with HPV infection has been reported, with the strongest association noted for the exophytic type. According to a meta-analysis of studies using various HPV detection methods, approximately 39% of sinonasal papillomas are HPV-positive, with HPV prevalence rates for the exophytic, inverted, and oncocytic types of 65%, 38%, and 23%, respectively.

EXOPHYTIC (SEPTAL; SQUAMOUS; FUNGIFORM) SINONASAL PAPILLOMA

The **exophytic sinonasal papilloma** bears some similarity to the oral squamous papilloma, although it has a somewhat more aggressive biologic behavior and more varied epithelial types. It represents approximately 20%–25% of all sinonasal papillomas. The majority of cases are positive for HPV 6 or 11.

Clinical Features

The exophytic sinonasal papilloma arises almost exclusively on the nasal septum and is more common in men than women (2:1 to 10:1 male-to-female ratio). It occurs primarily in people 20–50 years of age. Typically, it causes unilateral nasal obstruction or epistaxis and appears as a pink or tan, broad-based nodule with papillary or warty surface projections (Fig. 10.16). Most lesions measure less than 2 cm in maximum diameter.

Histopathologic Features

The exophytic sinonasal papilloma has a microscopic appearance similar to that of the oral squamous papilloma, although the stratified squamous epithelium covering the fingerlike projections seldom is keratinized. Respiratory epithelium or "transitional" epithelium (intermediate between squamous and respiratory) may be seen in some lesions. Mucous (goblet) cells and intraepithelial microcysts containing mucus often are present. Intraepithelial neutrophils occasionally may be evident as well, and focal koilocytic changes may be noted in the superficial epithelial layers. Mitoses are infrequent, and dysplasia is rare. The lamina propria consists of delicate fibrous tissue with a minimal inflammatory component, unless it is irritated.

Treatment and Prognosis

Complete surgical excision is the treatment of choice for the exophytic sinonasal papilloma. Recurrence has been reported in approximately 20%–30% of cases; however, some of these cases may reflect incomplete excision rather than true recurrence. Most authorities consider this lesion to have minimal or no potential for malignant transformation.

INVERTED SINONASAL PAPILLOMA (INVERTED SCHNEIDERIAN PAPILLOMA; ENDOPHYTIC SINONASAL PAPILLOMA)

The **inverted sinonasal papilloma** is the most common sinonasal papilloma variant, comprising approximately 65%–75% of cases. It is also the variant with the greatest potential for local destruction and malignant transformation. The estimated incidence is 0.2–1.5 cases per 100,000 persons per year. As many as approximately 38% of cases are HPV-positive, with HPV 6, 11, 16, and 18 representing the most prevalent types.

Molecular genetic studies support that inverted papillomas represent true neoplasms of monoclonal origin (i.e., arising from a single progenitor cell). Investigators have identified activating *EGFR* mutations in a majority of cases examined, including lesions with or without malignant transformation; such mutations have not been found in exophytic or oncocytic sinonasal papillomas. Interestingly,

EGFR mutations and HPV tend to occur within inverted sinonasal papillomas in a mutually exclusive manner, which suggests the possibility of alternative mechanisms for lesion development and carcinogenesis. Furthermore, *TP53* and *CDKN2A* alterations may be early events in malignant transformation.

Clinical and Radiographic Features

The average age at presentation is 53 years, with a peak in the fifth and sixth decades. There is a male predilection (2:1 to 3:1 male-to-female ratio). Inverted sinonasal papillomas arise predominantly from the lateral nasal wall or a paranasal sinus, usually the antrum. Typical signs and symptoms include unilateral nasal obstruction, epistaxis, purulent discharge, hyposmia, headache, or local deformity. The lesion appears as a soft, pink-tan to reddish gray, polypoid, or nodular growth, often with a "mulberry-like" or cerebriform surface. Multiple lesions may be present. Bilateral involvement occurs in only about 5% of cases. The lesion has significant growth potential and, if neglected, may extend into the nasopharynx, middle ear, orbit, or cranial base.

Pressure erosion of the underlying bone often is evident radiographically. Primary sinus lesions may appear only as a soft tissue radiodensity or mucosal thickening on radiographs; sinus involvement generally represents extension from the nasal cavity. Focal hyperostosis demonstrated by computed tomography (CT) scan may indicate the site of lesion attachment, which is important for surgical planning. In addition, magnetic resonance imaging (MRI) can help to identify the extent of the lesion and often reveals a convoluted, cerebriform pattern (Fig. 10.17). Focal loss of this characteristic pattern may indicate malignant transformation.

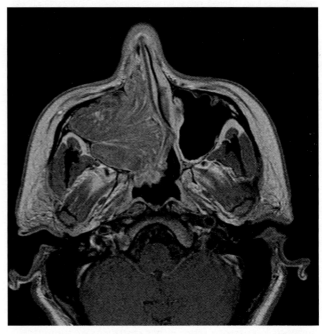

• **Fig. 10.17 Inverted Papilloma.** Magnetic resonance image (MRI) showing a tumor with a characteristic convoluted, cerebriform pattern. (Courtesy of Dr. Zoran Rumboldt.)

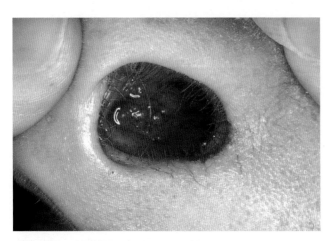

• **Fig. 10.16 Exophytic Sinonasal Papilloma.** Erythematous, papillary growth on the nasal septum.

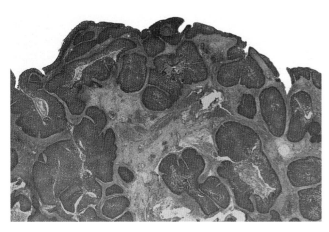

• **Fig. 10.18 Inverted Papilloma.** Low-power photomicrograph showing a squamous epithelial proliferation, with multiple "inverting" islands of epithelium extending into the underlying connective tissue.

Histopathologic Features

The inverted sinonasal papilloma microscopically exhibits downward proliferation of squamous or transitional epithelium into the stroma (Fig. 10.18). The basement membrane remains intact, and the epithelium appears to "push" into the underlying connective tissue. Goblet (mucous) cells, mucin-filled microcysts, transmigrating neutrophils, and neutrophilic microabscesses frequently are noted within the epithelium. Keratin production is uncommon, but thin surface keratinization may be seen. Mitoses often are noted within the basilar or parabasilar cells, and varying degrees of epithelial atypia may be evident. Papillary surface projections separated by deep clefts may be observed. The stroma consists of dense or myxomatous connective tissue with or without inflammatory cells. Destruction of underlying bone frequently is noted. Marked surface keratinization and moderate to severe dysplasia are worrisome histopathologic findings that warrant careful microscopic examination to rule out malignancy. Nonetheless, there are no histopathologic features that are reliably predictive of malignant transformation. Some studies suggest that the presence of HPV 16 or 18 may be associated with an increased risk for malignant transformation; however, RNA *in situ* hybridization for detection of transcriptionally active high-risk HPV has yielded mostly negative or minimal results in inverted sinonasal papillomas with or without associated carcinoma. Interestingly, a recent study suggests that there may be an increased risk for malignancy in a subset of nasal cavity inverted papillomas with transcriptionally active low-risk HPV infection, condyloma-like morphology, and no *EGFR* mutations. However, further studies are needed.

Treatment and Prognosis

Over the past few decades, the preferred treatment has shifted from traditional open surgery (i.e., medial maxillectomy with ethmoidectomy via a lateral rhinotomy or midfacial degloving approach) to transnasal endoscopic surgery.

Depending upon the extent and accessibility of disease, endoscopic and external surgical approaches may be combined. Average recurrence rates among studies conducted within the past few decades are approximately 11%–13% for patients treated by endoscopic or combined surgery and 18% for those treated by open surgery. Recurrences usually are noted within 2 years of treatment but can happen much later. Hence, long-term follow-up is essential. Frontal sinus involvement and continued tobacco smoking are associated with an increased risk for recurrence.

Approximately 5%–15% of inverted sinonasal papillomas transform into malignancy (usually squamous cell carcinoma). Malignancy may be synchronous or metachronous. When malignancy is present, treatment typically consists of radical surgery, with or without adjunctive radiotherapy. According to a recent systematic review and meta-analysis, the overall 5-year survival rate is higher for inverted papilloma-associated sinonasal squamous cell carcinoma compared to *de novo* sinonasal squamous cell carcinoma (65% vs 56%, respectively).

ONCOCYTIC SINONASAL PAPILLOMA (ONCOCYTIC SCHNEIDERIAN PAPILLOMA; CYLINDRICAL CELL PAPILLOMA)

The **oncocytic sinonasal papilloma** accounts for less than 7% of sinonasal papillomas. Some authorities consider this lesion to be a variant of the inverted type because of the similarity in clinicopathologic features and a similarly low frequency of HPV. Recent studies have detected activating *KRAS* mutations in the majority of cases examined, including a few associated with malignant transformation; such mutations have not been found in inverted or exophytic sinonasal papillomas.

Clinical Features

The oncocytic sinonasal papilloma most often occurs in adults older than 50 years. Most authors report either a male predominance or no significant gender bias. There is a predilection for the lateral nasal wall, maxillary antrum, and ethmoid sinus. The most common presenting symptom is unilateral nasal obstruction, and the lesion appears as a beefy-red or brown mass with a multinodular surface.

Histopathologic Features

Microscopically, the oncocytic sinonasal papilloma demonstrates both endophytic and exophytic growth. Surface papillary projections have a fibrovascular connective tissue core and are covered by a multilayered epithelium of tall columnar cells with small, dark nuclei and eosinophilic, occasionally granular cytoplasm. The lesional epithelial cell is similar to an oncocyte. Cilia may be seen on the surface, and there are numerous intraepithelial microcysts filled with mucin, neutrophils, or both.

Treatment and Prognosis

The treatment and recurrence potential for oncocytic sinonasal papilloma and inverted sinonasal papilloma (see previous topic) are similar. Reported malignant transformation rates for oncocytic sinonasal papilloma range from 4% to 17%.

◆ MOLLUSCUM CONTAGIOSUM

Molluscum contagiosum is an epithelial lesion induced by the molluscum contagiosum virus (MCV), a member of the DNA poxvirus group. At least 6% of the population (more in older age groups) has antibodies to this virus, although few ever develop lesions. In adults and adolescents, molluscum contagiosum is caused predominantly by MCV-2 via sexual contact, whereas in children it is caused mainly by MCV-1 via nonsexual contact (e.g., wrestling, sharing clothing, or towels). Autoinoculation of the virus is also possible. Warm, humid environments, such as communal baths or swimming pools, may encourage disease spread. Although infrequent, cases of molluscum contagiosum in infants have been reported, apparently resulting from vertical transmission of the virus from mother to infant.

After an incubation period of 14–50 days, multiple umbilicated papules may develop on the skin or, rarely, mucous membranes. The disease exhibits a predilection for warm portions of the skin and sites of recent injury. The lesions usually remain small for months or years and then spontaneously involute. However, florid cases have been reported in immunocompromised patients. Patients with atopic dermatitis and Darier disease also are at risk for developing severe, prolonged disease.

Clinical Features

Molluscum contagiosum mainly arises in children and young adults. There is no significant gender predilection. The lesions occur predominantly on the skin of the neck, face (particularly eyelids), trunk, and genitalia. Infrequently, oral involvement occurs, usually on the lips, buccal mucosa, palate, or gingiva. Congenital lesions may involve the scalp in a halo-like distribution.

The lesions typically appear as multiple clustered, pink or pearly white, smooth-surfaced, sessile papules measuring 2–4 mm in diameter (Fig. 10.19). Many show a small central indentation or plug from which a curd-like substance containing viral particles can be expressed. Most lesions are asymptomatic, although slight tenderness or pruritus is possible. Erythema and swelling may result from trauma or may be indicative of the host's immune response and ensuing spontaneous regression. In addition, eczematous eruptions occasionally may develop in the vicinity of molluscum contagiosum, particularly in patients with atopic dermatitis. Other possible secondary complications include bacterial superinfection and conjunctivitis.

In immunocompromised patients, the lesions may be unusually large, verrucous, or markedly hyperkeratotic.

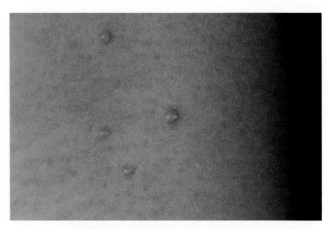

• **Fig. 10.19 Molluscum Contagiosum.** Multiple, smooth-surfaced papules, with several demonstrating small keratin-like plugs, are seen on the neck of a child.

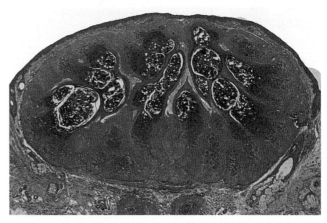

• **Fig. 10.20 Molluscum Contagiosum.** Well-defined epidermal proliferation demonstrating a central craterlike depression filled with virally altered keratinocytes.

Histopathologic Features

Molluscum contagiosum appears as a localized, lobular proliferation of surface stratified squamous epithelium (Fig. 10.20). The central portion of each lobule is filled with bloated keratinocytes that contain large, intranuclear, basophilic viral inclusions called **molluscum bodies** (or **Henderson-Paterson bodies**) (Fig. 10.21). These bodies begin as small, eosinophilic structures in cells just above the basal layer and enlarge as they approach the surface. A central crater is formed at the surface as stratum corneum cells disintegrate to release their molluscum bodies.

Treatment and Prognosis

Most cases of molluscum contagiosum undergo spontaneous remission, with a mean duration of 6.5–13 months. For immunocompetent patients, there is ongoing debate as to whether the disease should be treated or allowed to resolve on its own. Treatment may be performed to decrease the risk of disease transmission, prevent autoinoculation, provide symptomatic relief, or address cosmetic concerns.

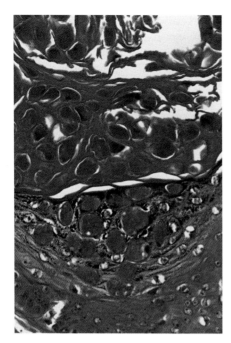

• **Fig. 10.21 Molluscum Contagiosum.** Higher-power photomicrograph showing keratinocytes with large, basophilic viral inclusions (molluscum bodies) being sloughed into the central crater *(top).*

Although there are few controlled studies of treatment efficacy, the lesions most commonly are removed by curettage or cryotherapy. Chemical destruction with cantharidin may be a preferable alternative for lesions in children. Additional treatment options include laser therapy, electrodesiccation, chemical destructive agents (e.g., salicylic acid, lactic acid, trichloroacetic acid, benzoyl peroxide, potassium hydroxide, and podophyllotoxin), topical tretinoin, topical imiquimod, intralesional injection of *Candida* antigen (which may stimulate a local immune response and MCV clearance), and oral cimetidine (most effective for lesions not involving the facial skin).

In immunosuppressed patients with recalcitrant lesions, interferon-alpha or cidofovir may be effective. Moreover, in HIV-infected patients, antiretroviral therapy indirectly counteracts MCV infection by increasing CD4+ T cell counts and improving the immune response.

Recurrence after initial clearing has been reported in up to one-third of patients. There is no apparent malignant transformation potential.

◆ VERRUCIFORM XANTHOMA

Verruciform xanthoma is a hyperplastic condition of the epithelium, with a characteristic subepithelial accumulation of lipid-laden histiocytes. It is primarily an oral disease, but skin and anogenital lesions also are possible. The cause is unknown. Although verruciform xanthoma is a papillary lesion, HPV has been identified in only a small number of cases, and no definitive pathogenetic role for this virus has been established. The lesion probably represents an unusual reaction or immune response to localized epithelial trauma or

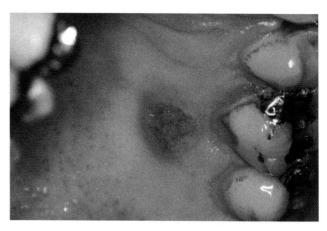

• **Fig. 10.22 Verruciform Xanthoma.** A well-demarcated, slightly elevated lesion of the hard palate that demonstrates a roughened or papillary surface.

damage. This hypothesis is supported by cases of verruciform xanthoma that have developed in association with disturbed epithelium (e.g., lichen planus, lupus erythematosus, epidermolysis bullosa, epithelial dysplasia, squamous cell carcinoma, pemphigus vulgaris, warty dyskeratoma, graft-vs-host disease [GVHD], candidiasis) and by a tendency for oral examples to involve the masticatory mucosa. The lesion is histopathologically similar to other dermal xanthomas, but it is not closely associated with diabetes or hyperlipidemia. Interestingly, in a few cutaneous and oral cases, investigators have identified somatic mutations in the *NSDHL* gene encoding 3-beta-hydroxysteroid dehydrogenase (an enzyme essential for cholesterol biosynthesis). Germline mutations in this gene are associated with CHILD (congenital hemidysplasia with ichthyosiform nevus and limb defects) syndrome.

Clinical Features

Verruciform xanthoma typically is seen in middle-aged to older adults but has been reported over a broad age range (2–94 years). There is a slight male predilection. Approximately half of intraoral lesions occur on the gingiva, but any oral site may be involved.

The lesion appears as a well-demarcated, soft, painless, sessile, slightly elevated mass with a white, yellow-white, pink, or red color and a papillary or roughened (verruciform) surface (Figs. 10.22 and 10.23). Rarely, flat-topped nodules are seen without surface projections. Most lesions are asymptomatic and smaller than 2 cm in greatest diameter, although large or "giant" examples have been reported infrequently. Multiple lesions occasionally have been described as well. Clinically, verruciform xanthoma may appear similar to squamous papilloma, verruca vulgaris, condyloma acuminatum, or early carcinoma.

Histopathologic Features

Verruciform xanthoma typically demonstrates papillary, acanthotic surface epithelium covered by a thickened layer of parakeratin. On routine hematoxylin and eosin (H&E)

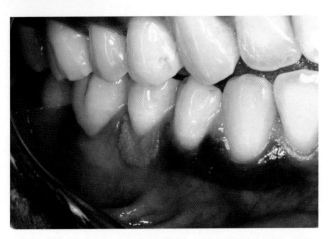

• **Fig. 10.23 Verruciform Xanthoma.** A gingival lesion with a papillary surface. (Courtesy of Dr. Ashleigh Briody.)

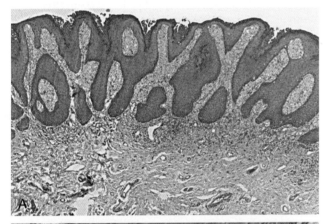

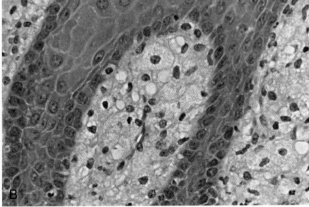

• **Fig. 10.24 Verruciform Xanthoma. A,** A slight papillary appearance is produced by hyperparakeratosis, and the rete ridges are elongated to a uniform depth. Note the parakeratin plugging between the papillary projections. **B,** The connective tissue papillae are composed almost exclusively of xanthoma cells—large macrophages with foamy cytoplasm.

staining, the keratin layer often exhibits a distinctive pinkish orange color (Fig. 10.24). Clefts or crypts between the epithelial projections are filled with parakeratin, and rete ridges are elongated to a uniform depth. However, some cases may exhibit a relatively flat surface with minimal keratinization. The most important diagnostic feature is the accumulation

of numerous large macrophages with foamy cytoplasm, which typically are confined to the connective tissue papillae. These foam cells, also known as **xanthoma cells,** contain lipid and periodic acid-Schiff (PAS)-positive, diastase-resistant granules. With immunohistochemical stains, the xanthoma cells are positive for markers consistent with monocyte-macrophage lineage, including CD68, CD63, CD163, and cathepsin B.

Treatment and Prognosis

The verruciform xanthoma is treated with conservative surgical excision. Recurrence after removal is rare, and no malignant transformation has been reported. However, there are a few reported cases of verruciform xanthoma arising in association with carcinoma *in situ* or squamous cell carcinoma. This observation does not necessarily imply that verruciform xanthoma is a potentially malignant lesion; however, it may indicate that hyperkeratotic or dysplastic oral lesions can undergo degenerative changes to form a verruciform xanthoma.

◆ SEBORRHEIC KERATOSIS

Seborrheic keratosis is an extremely common skin lesion of older people and represents an acquired, benign proliferation of epidermal basal cells. This lesion frequently affects the facial skin but does not occur in the mouth. The cause is unknown, although there is a positive correlation with chronic sun exposure, sometimes with a hereditary (autosomal dominant) tendency. In addition, somatic mutations in the *fibroblast growth factor receptor 3 (FGFR3)* and *phosphatidylinositol 3-kinase, catalytic subunit alpha (PIK3CA)* genes may contribute to the pathogenesis of these lesions. In some cases, HPV DNA or Merkel cell polyomavirus DNA has been detected, but these findings may be coincidental. Investigators recently have suggested that overexpression of amyloid precursor protein is a marker of aging, sun-damaged skin and may promote the development of seborrheic keratoses.

Clinical Features

Seborrheic keratoses begin to develop on the skin of the face, neck, trunk, and extremities during the fourth decade of life, and they become more prevalent with each passing decade. Lesions are usually multiple, beginning as small, tan to brown macules that are clinically indistinguishable from **actinic lentigines** (see page 369). Subsequently, the lesions gradually enlarge and elevate to form sharply demarcated plaques, with finely fissured, pitted, verrucous, waxy, or smooth surfaces (Figs. 10.25 and 10.26). The plaques appear "stuck onto" the skin and are usually less than 2 cm in diameter. Most examples are asymptomatic, although secondarily inflamed lesions may cause pain, discomfort, or pruritus.

Dermatosis papulosa nigra is a form of seborrheic keratosis that occurs in approximately 30%–77% of blacks and frequently has an autosomal dominant inheritance pattern.

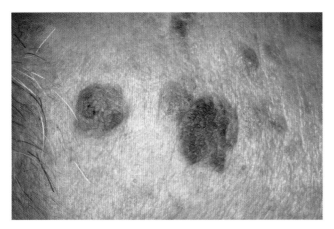

• **Fig. 10.25 Seborrheic Keratosis.** Multiple brown plaques on the face of an older man exhibit a fissured surface. They had been slowly enlarging for several years.

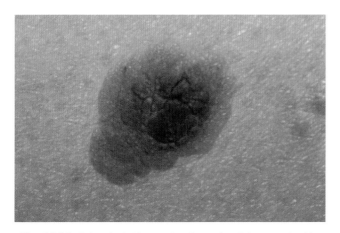

• **Fig. 10.26 Seborrheic Keratosis.** Crusted and pigmented epidermal plaque.

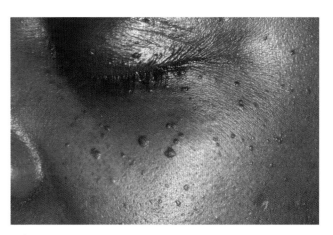

• **Fig. 10.27 Dermatosis Papulosa Nigra.** Multiple small pigmented papules of the malar area.

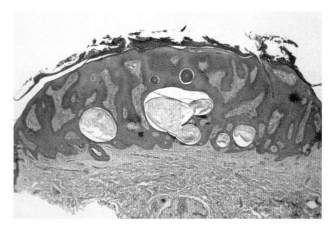

• **Fig. 10.28 Seborrheic Keratosis.** The acanthotic form demonstrates considerable acanthosis, surface hyperkeratosis, and numerous pseudocysts. The epidermal proliferation extends upward, above the normal epidermal surface.

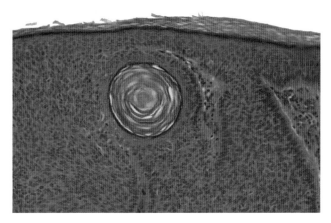

• **Fig. 10.29 Seborrheic Keratosis.** Pseudocysts are actually keratin-filled invaginations, as seen toward the left in this high-power photomicrograph. The surrounding epithelial cells are basaloid in appearance.

This condition typically appears as multiple small (1–4 mm), dark-brown to black papules scattered about the zygomatic and periorbital region (Fig. 10.27).

The sudden appearance of numerous seborrheic keratoses with pruritus may be associated with internal malignancy. This rare phenomenon is called the **Leser-Trélat sign.** In a similar phenomenon termed **pseudo-sign of Leser-Trélat**, there is drug-induced development of inflamed seborrheic keratoses; implicated medications include various biologic or antineoplastic agents (e.g., adalimumab, docetaxel, cytarabine, 5-fluorouracil, cisplatin).

Histopathologic Features

Seborrheic keratosis consists of an exophytic proliferation of basilar epithelial cells that exhibit varying degrees of surface keratinization, acanthosis, and papillomatosis (Fig. 10.28). Characteristically, the epithelial hyperplasia extends upward, above the normal epidermal surface. The lesion usually exhibits deep, keratin-filled invaginations that appear cystic on cross-section; hence, they are called **horn cysts** or **pseudo-horn cysts** (Fig. 10.29). Melanin pigmentation often is seen within the basal layer.

Several histopathologic patterns may be seen in seborrheic keratoses. The most common is the **acanthotic** form, which exhibits little papillomatosis and marked acanthosis with minimal surface keratinization. The **hyperkeratotic** form is characterized by prominent papillomatosis and hyperkeratosis with minimal acanthosis. The **adenoid** form consists of anastomosing trabeculae of lesional cells with little hyperkeratosis or papillomatosis. The lesions of dermatosis papulosa nigra are predominantly of the adenoid and acanthotic types.

Chronic trauma may alter these histopathologic features to produce an **irritated seborrheic keratosis (or inverted follicular keratosis of Helwig)**. This lesion shows a mild degree of proliferation into the connective tissue and an associated chronic inflammatory cell infiltrate. Squamous metaplasia of the lesional cells results in whorled epithelial patterns called **squamous eddies**. Inflamed seborrheic keratosis may exhibit enough nuclear atypia and mitotic activity to cause confusion with squamous cell carcinoma, but enough of the basic attributes of seborrheic keratosis typically remain to allow a proper diagnosis.

Treatment and Prognosis

Except to address aesthetic concerns or secondary irritation, seborrheic keratoses seldom are removed. Cryotherapy, electrodesiccation, curettage, and shave excision are the most common methods for removal. Laser therapy is more costly than traditional treatment methods but may be preferable for removal of a large number of lesions. Investigational treatments include various topical agents (e.g., nitric-zinc complex solution, 40% hydrogen peroxide, trichloroacetic acid).

The lesion exhibits no appreciable malignant potential. However, there are isolated reports of malignant skin lesions developing within or adjacent to seborrheic keratoses; it is unclear whether such cases are coincidental. Rarely, melanomas or other skin cancers may resemble seborrheic keratoses clinically; dermoscopy (a noninvasive *in vivo* imaging technique for visualization of subsurface skin structures) may aid in differentiating seborrheic keratoses from other lesions. It is important for a dermatologist or other qualified clinician to perform such evaluation and determine whether it is appropriate to treat a lesion by cryotherapy or to excise and submit it for histopathologic confirmation.

◆ SEBACEOUS HYPERPLASIA

Sebaceous hyperplasia is a localized proliferation of sebaceous glands, with a predilection for the facial skin. The exact cause is unknown, although investigators hypothesize that hormonal and genetic factors may be important. In addition, some reported cases have developed in association with cyclosporine administration in transplant recipients or with antiretroviral therapy for HIV-infected patients. It is uncertain whether such cases result from immunosuppression or direct medication effects. Furthermore, sebaceous hyperplasia may arise in association with *Muir-Torre syndrome* (a rare autosomal dominant disorder characterized by visceral malignancies, sebaceous adenomas and carcinomas, and keratoacanthomas) or X-linked hypohidrotic ectodermal dysplasia (see page 747). The major significance of sebaceous hyperplasia is its clinical similarity to more serious facial tumors, such as basal cell carcinoma.

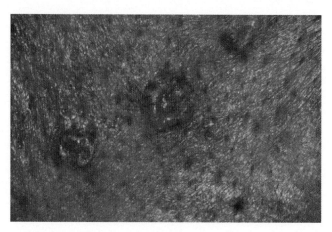

• **Fig. 10.30 Sebaceous Hyperplasia.** Multiple soft papules of the midface are umbilicated and small. Sebum can often be expressed from the central depressed area.

Clinical Features

Cutaneous sebaceous hyperplasia usually affects adults older than 40 years. It occurs most commonly on the skin of the face, especially the nose, cheeks, and forehead. Less commonly, lesions may involve the genital area, chest, and areola. The condition is characterized by one or more soft, nontender papules with white, yellow, or normal color (Fig. 10.30). Most lesions grow slowly and are smaller than 5 mm in greatest diameter. The lesions usually exhibit central umbilication, representing the area where the ducts of the involved sebaceous lobules terminate. The ability to express sebum (the thick, yellow-white product of the sebaceous gland) from this small, central depression aids in clinical distinction of sebaceous hyperplasia from basal cell carcinoma.

An oral counterpart, which probably has no relation to the skin lesion, appears as a white to yellow papule or nodular mass with a "cauliflower" appearance, usually involving the buccal mucosa or retromolar pad.

Histopathologic Features

Histopathologically, sebaceous hyperplasia is characterized by a collection of enlarged but otherwise normal sebaceous gland lobules grouped around one or more centrally located sebaceous ducts (Fig. 10.31).

Treatment and Prognosis

No treatment is necessary for sebaceous hyperplasia except for cosmetic reasons or unless basal cell carcinoma cannot be eliminated from the clinical differential diagnosis. Excisional biopsy is curative. Cryosurgery, electrodesiccation, laser therapy, photodynamic therapy, and isotretinoin are alternative treatment methods.

◆ EPHELIS (FRECKLE)

An **ephelis** is a common, small, hyperpigmented macule of the skin. The lesion results from increased melanin deposition in the epidermis, without an increase in the number

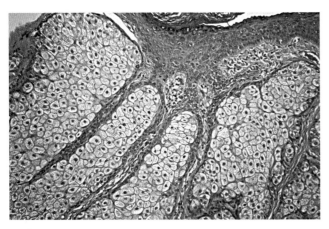

• **Fig. 10.31 Sebaceous Hyperplasia.** Sebaceous glands are enlarged and more numerous than normal, but they demonstrate no other pathologic changes.

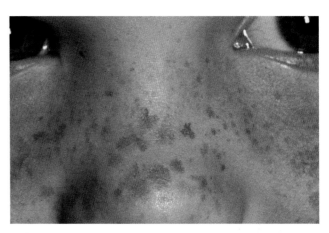

• **Fig. 10.32 Ephelides.** Multiple brown macules over the bridge of the nose.

of melanocytes. Ephelides may become more pronounced after sun exposure and are associated closely with a history of painful sunburns in childhood. There is a genetic predilection (autosomal dominant), and studies have demonstrated a strong relationship with certain variants of the *melanocortin 1 receptor (MC1R)* gene.

Clinical Features

Ephelides arise most often on the face, arms, and back of fair-skinned, blue-eyed, red- or blond-haired individuals. There is no gender predilection. The macules usually develop during the first decade of life, seldom arise after the teenage years, and become less prominent in adulthood.

Each lesion appears as a sharply demarcated, uniformly light brown, round or oval macule, measuring less than 3 mm in diameter (Fig. 10.32). There is great variability in the number of lesions present. Many individuals have less than 10, whereas some have hundreds. The brown color is not as dark as that seen in lentigo simplex (see page 370), and there is never elevation above the skin surface, as may occur in a melanocytic nevus (see page 374).

Histopathologic Features

The ephelis exhibits abundant melanin deposition in the basal cell layer of the epidermis. Despite increased melanin, the number of melanocytes is normal or slightly reduced. In contrast to lentigo simplex, there is no elongation of rete ridges.

Treatment and Prognosis

No treatment is necessary for ephelides. Cosmetically unpleasing lesions may be treated by cryotherapy, hydroquinone, chemical peels, or laser therapy. Sunscreens can prevent the appearance of new freckles and help prevent the darkening of existing lesions.

◆ ACTINIC LENTIGO (LENTIGO SOLARIS; SOLAR LENTIGO; AGE SPOT; LIVER SPOT; SENILE LENTIGO)

Actinic lentigo is a benign, brown macule that is considered a hallmark of photodamaged skin. The lesion is associated with both chronic and intermittent ultraviolet (UV) light exposure. A potential association with air pollutants also has been suggested. The lesion frequently arises on the facial skin but does not occur in the mouth. Actinic lentigo affects more than 90% of whites older than 70 years. The lesion rarely develops before age 40, although young adults with a history of severe sunburns may develop multiple large actinic lentigines on the upper back. Persons who have facial ephelides (freckles) in childhood are prone to developing actinic lentigines later in life.

Some authorities have proposed that actinic lentigo represents a precursor to adenoid seborrheic keratosis (see page 366). Interestingly, investigators have noted that at least some cases of both actinic lentigo and seborrheic keratosis exhibit mutations in the *FGFR3* and *PIK3CA* genes.

Clinical Features

Multiple lesions typically develop in older whites on sun-exposed skin, especially on the face, dorsa of the hands, forearms, shoulders, and upper back (Figs. 10.33 and 10.34). The lesions may appear more prominent and at a somewhat younger age among Asians compared to whites. The individual lesions appear as uniformly pigmented, brown to tan macules with well-demarcated but irregular borders. Most examples are smaller than 5 mm in diameter, although some lesions may measure more than 1 cm. Adjacent lesions may coalesce, and new ones continuously arise with age. Unlike ephelides, no change in color intensity is seen after UV light exposure.

Histopathologic Features

The rete ridges are elongated and club-shaped, with thinning of the epithelium above the connective tissue papillae

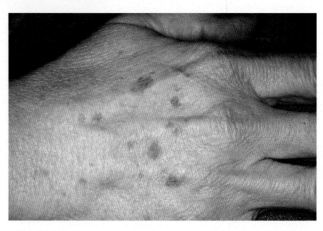

• **Fig. 10.33 Actinic Lentigines.** Multiple lesions on the sun-exposed skin of the hand of an older adult. Lesions are brown macules with irregular borders.

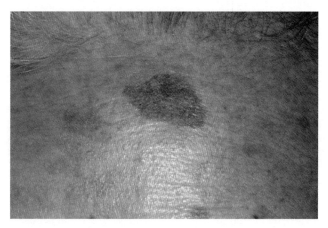

• **Fig. 10.34 Actinic Lentigo.** Large, flat, evenly pigmented lesion on the forehead of an older adult man.

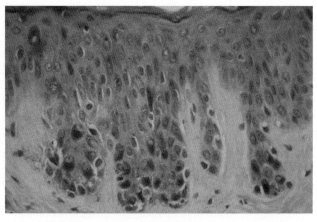

• **Fig. 10.35 Actinic Lentigo.** Rete ridges are elongated and occasionally intertwining. Pigmented melanocytes (with clear cytoplasm) are excessive and commingled with melanin-laden basilar cells.

(Fig. 10.35). The ridges sometimes coalesce with one another. Within each rete ridge, melanin-laden basilar cells are intermingled with excessive numbers of heavily pigmented melanocytes. Prominent solar elastosis typically is seen within the dermis.

Treatment and Prognosis

No treatment is required for actinic lentigo, except for aesthetic reasons. Ablative treatment methods include cryotherapy, laser therapy, intense pulsed light, and chemical peels. In addition, there is a wide range of topical therapies available, including hydroquinone, tretinoin, tazarotene, adapalene, and combined mequinol and tretinoin. Generally, sunscreens are recommended as preventive treatment and for maintenance of treatment success. Lesions rarely recur after removal, although new lesions may arise. Actinic lentigo does not undergo malignant transformation; however, the lesion represents a clinical marker of photodamage and may indicate an increased risk for developing skin cancer.

✦ LENTIGO SIMPLEX

Lentigo simplex is one of several forms of benign cutaneous melanocytic hyperplasia of unknown cause. In contrast to the ephelis (see page 368), lentigo simplex typically is found on skin that is not exposed to sunlight, appears somewhat darker in color, does not darken with sun exposure, and represents an increase in both local melanin production and the number of melanocytes. Oral lesions have been reported, but they are rare and may be examples of the oral melanotic macule (see page 372).

Some investigators believe that lentigo simplex represents the earliest stage of another common skin lesion, the melanocytic nevus (see page 374). However, lentigo simplex appears to lack *BRAF* mutations that are commonly found in conventional acquired melanocytic nevi. In addition, lentigo simplex does not appear to harbor *FGFR3* and *PIK3CA* mutations, which are frequently present in actinic lentigo.

Clinical Features

Lentigo simplex usually is seen in children, although it may occur at any age. The typical lesion is a sharply demarcated, uniformly tan to dark-brown macule smaller than 5 mm in diameter (Fig. 10.36). It is usually solitary, although some patients may have several lesions scattered on the skin of the trunk and extremities. Lentigo simplex reaches its maximum size in a matter of months and may remain unchanged indefinitely thereafter.

Clinically, individual lesions of lentigo simplex are indistinguishable from the nonelevated melanocytic nevus. With multiple lesions, conditions such as lentiginosis profusa, Peutz-Jeghers syndrome (see page 758), and LEOPARD[a] syndrome must be considered as diagnostic possibilities.

---

[a]**L**entigines (multiple), **e**lectrocardiographic abnormalities, **o**cular hypertelorism, **p**ulmonary stenosis, **a**bnormalities of genitalia, **r**etardation of growth, and **d**eafness (sensorineural).

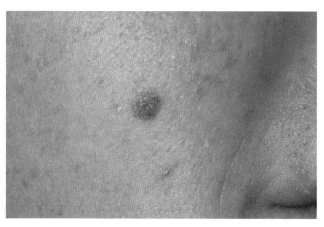

• **Fig. 10.36 Lentigo Simplex.** A sharply demarcated lesion of uniform brown coloration is seen on the midface.

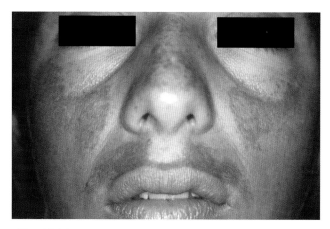

• **Fig. 10.37 Melasma.** Diffuse hyperpigmentation of the facial skin in a pregnant woman.

Histopathologic Features

Lentigo simplex shows an increased number of benign melanocytes within the basal layer of the epidermis. These melanocytes often are clustered at the tips of slightly to moderately elongated rete ridges. Abundant melanin is distributed among the melanocytes and basal keratinocytes, as well as within the papillary dermis in association with melanophages (**melanin incontinence**).

Treatment and Prognosis

Lentigo simplex may fade spontaneously after many years, but most lesions remain constant over time. Treatment is not required, except for cosmetic reasons. Treatment methods include conservative surgical excision, cryotherapy, and laser therapy. No malignant transformation potential has been documented.

◆ MELASMA (MASK OF PREGNANCY; CHLOASMA)

Melasma is an acquired, symmetrical hyperpigmentation of the sun-exposed skin of the face and neck. The exact etiopathogenesis is unknown, but UV light exposure, hormonal influences, and an underlying genetic predisposition appear to be important factors. The condition traditionally has been thought to arise primarily from the stimulatory effects of UV light on melanocytes; however, emerging evidence suggests that visible light, keratinocytes, dermal mast cells, extracellular matrix alterations, and angiogenesis may play important roles in disease development as well. Melasma classically is associated with pregnancy. In addition, an association with oral contraceptives, hormone replacement therapy, ovarian or thyroid disorders, liver dysfunction, malnutrition, phototoxic medications, antiepileptic agents, cosmetics, and air pollutants has been described. The condition most commonly affects medium- to dark-complexioned persons—particularly females of Asian, Hispanic, and Mediterranean descent. In some study populations it affects as many as 30%–40% of women. In the United States, melasma affects more than 5 million individuals.

Clinical Features

Melasma most often develops in females between the ages of 11–49 years, with an average age of approximately 30–38 years. Men are affected infrequently. The condition typically appears as bilateral brown or grayish cutaneous macules that range from a few millimeters to more than 2 cm in diameter (Fig. 10.37). The borders of the lesion tend to be ill-defined and irregular. Lesions develop slowly with sun exposure and primarily involve the skin of the midface, forehead, upper lip, chin, temporal, and mandibular ramus region. The condition only rarely affects extrafacial sites, such as the arms, sternal region, and back. The pigmentation may remain faint or darken over time.

Histopathologic Features

Melasma is characterized by increased melanin deposition and, possibly, an increased number of melanocytes in the epidermis. The melanocytes typically are plump, full of pigment, and highly dendritic. In addition, numerous melanophages (melanin-laden macrophages) may be seen in the dermis, especially around blood vessels. Some authors have noted that hallmarks of photoaging (including solar elastosis, increased numbers of dermal mast cells, increased vascularization, and basement membrane disruption) are more prominent in lesional skin compared to adjacent normal-appearing skin.

Treatment and Prognosis

Melasma is difficult to treat. In the United States, first-line therapy typically consists of topical triple-combination cream (Tri-Luma) containing 4% hydroquinone, 0.05% tretinoin, and 0.01% fluocinolone acetonide. Alternative treatments include dual-ingredient topical agents (e.g., hydroquinone combined with a retinoid, corticosteroid, or kojic acid) or single-ingredient topical agents (e.g., hydroquinone, retinoids, or azelaic acid). Recent studies suggest that microneedling may be a useful adjuvant to topical therapies. Oral tranexamic acid may be helpful for refractory cases.

Variable results have been reported with laser therapy, light therapy, chemical peels, or microdermabrasion. Because sun exposure is an important etiologic factor, sun avoidance, protective clothing, and the use of sunscreens containing zinc oxide or titanium dioxide are crucial for effective management. The lesions may resolve after parturition or after discontinuing oral contraceptives. There is no potential for malignant transformation.

◆ ORAL MELANOTIC MACULE (FOCAL MELANOSIS)

The **oral melanotic macule** is a flat, brown, mucosal discoloration produced by a focal increase in melanin deposition and, possibly, a concomitant increase in the number of melanocytes. The cause remains unclear. Unlike the cutaneous ephelis (freckle), the melanotic macule is not dependent on sun exposure. Some authorities have questioned the purported lack of an association with actinic irradiation for the melanotic macule located on the vermilion border and prefer to consider it a distinct entity **(labial melanotic macule).** Oral and labial melanotic macules are the most common oral melanocytic lesions submitted to oral pathology laboratories for histopathologic examination.

Clinical Features

The oral melanotic macule occurs over a broad age range, with a mean age at diagnosis of 42 years and a 2:1 female-to-male ratio. The lower lip vermilion is the most commonly involved site (33% of cases), followed by the buccal mucosa, gingiva, and palate. Rare examples have been reported on the tongue in newborns.

The typical lesion appears as a solitary (17% are multiple), well-demarcated, uniformly tan to dark-brown, asymptomatic, round or oval macule with a diameter less than 1 cm (Figs. 10.38–10.40). Occasional lesions may be blue or black. The maximum dimension is achieved rather rapidly and remains constant thereafter.

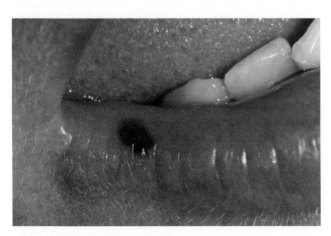

• **Fig. 10.38 Oral Melanotic Macule.** A single small, uniformly pigmented brown macule on the lower lip vermilion.

Histopathologic Features

The oral melanotic macule is characterized by an increase in melanin (and perhaps melanocytes) in the basal and parabasal layers of an otherwise normal stratified squamous epithelium (Fig. 10.41). Melanin also may be seen free **(melanin incontinence)** or within melanophages in the subepithelial connective tissue. Unlike actinic lentigo (see page 369), the melanotic macule typically does not show elongated rete ridges.

Treatment and Prognosis

The oral melanotic macule generally is considered a benign lesion with no malignant potential. However, a single case of apparent malignant transformation of an oral melanotic macule has been reported, and early melanoma can have a similar clinical appearance. Therefore, all oral pigmented macules of recent onset, large size, irregular pigmentation, unknown duration, or recent enlargement should be submitted for

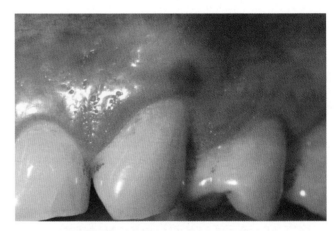

• **Fig. 10.39 Oral Melanotic Macule.** A well-demarcated brown macule of the gingival mucosa.

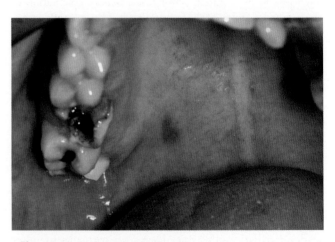

• **Fig. 10.40 Oral Melanotic Macule.** A brown macule on the soft palate. Smoker's melanosis may exhibit a similar clinical appearance and could be a consideration in the clinical differential diagnosis, although this patient denied any history of tobacco use.

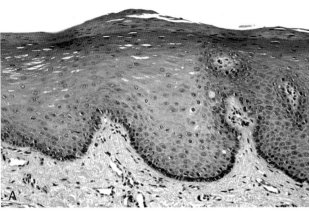

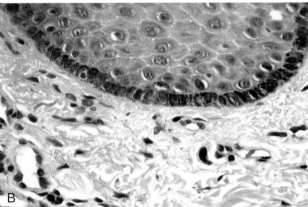

• Fig. 10.41 Oral Melanotic Macule. A, Low-power view showing increased melanin pigmentation distributed along basal epithelial layer. B, High-power view showing granular brown melanin pigment in the basilar cells.

Physiologic or Syndromic Associations

• Racial or physiologic pigmentation
• Peutz-Jeghers syndrome
• McCune-Albright syndrome
• LEOPARD syndrome (lentiginosis profusa, no intraoral melanosis)
• Laugier-Hunziker syndrome
• Cronkhite-Canada syndrome
• Bloom syndrome
• Dunnigan syndrome
• Dyskeratosis congenita
• Endocrine candidiasis syndrome
• Incontinentia pigmenti
• Oculo-cerebro-cutaneous syndrome
• Rothmund-Thomson syndrome
• Trisomy 14 mosaicism
• Unusual facies, vitiligo, spastic paraplegia syndrome
• Xeroderma pigmentosum
• Addison disease
• Neurofibromatosis type I
• Carney complex

Chronic Trauma or Irritation or Environmental Pollutant

• Chronic mucosal trauma or irritation (chronic cheek bite)
• Chronic autoimmune disease (erosive lichen planus, pemphigoid)
• Smoker's melanosis
• Yusho (chronic exposure to high levels of polychlorinated biphenyls [PCBs])

Systemic Medications

• Chloroquine and other quinine derivatives
• Phenolphthalein
• Estrogen
• AIDS-related medications

microscopic examination. In addition, because oral melanoma exhibits a predilection for the palatal and maxillary alveolar mucosa, it is advisable to submit pigmented macules in these locations for histopathologic examination. Furthermore, removal may be desirable for melanotic macules involving aesthetic areas. Excisional biopsy is the preferred treatment method. Electrocautery, laser ablation, or cryosurgery is effective, but no tissue remains for histopathologic examination after these procedures.

On occasion, flat pigmented lesions that are clinically and microscopically similar to the melanotic macule may occur in association with a systemic disease, a genetic disorder, chronic trauma/irritation, or certain medications. A list of these conditions is shown in Box 10.1.

◆ ORAL MELANOACANTHOMA (MELANOACANTHOSIS)

Oral melanoacanthoma is an uncommon, benign, acquired pigmentation of the oral mucosa characterized by dendritic melanocytes dispersed throughout the epithelium. The lesion appears to be a reactive process; in some cases an association with trauma or local irritation has been reported. Oral melanoacanthoma appears to be unrelated to the melanoacanthoma of skin, which most authorities believe represents a variant of seborrheic keratosis.

Clinical Features

Oral melanoacanthoma is seen primarily in blacks, although some cases also have been reported in Caucasians, Hispanics, and Asians. The lesion exhibits a female predilection and most commonly arises during the third and fourth decades of life. The buccal mucosa is the most common site of occurrence. The lips, palate, gingiva, and alveolar mucosa also may be involved. Most patients exhibit solitary lesions, although bilateral or multifocal involvement is possible. Oral melanoacanthomas typically are asymptomatic; however, pain, burning, and pruritus have been reported in a few cases. The lesion appears smooth, flat or slightly raised, and dark-brown to black (Fig. 10.42). Lesions often rapidly increase in size, and they occasionally reach a diameter of several centimeters within a few weeks.

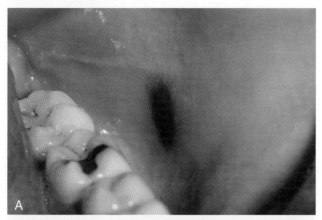

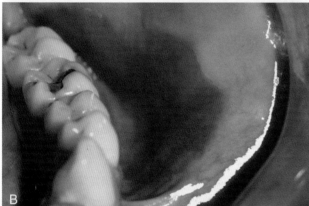

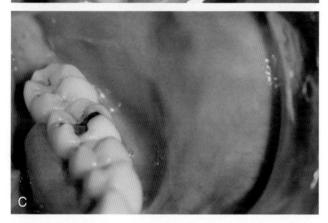

• **Fig. 10.42 Oral Melanoacanthoma. A,** Smooth, darkly pigmented macule of the buccal mucosa in a young adult. **B,** Appearance of the lesion 2 months later showing dramatic enlargement. **C,** Resolution of the lesion 3 months after incisional biopsy. (From Park SK, Neville BW: AAOMP case challenge: rapidly enlarging pigmented lesion of the buccal mucosa, *J Contemp Dent Pract* 3:69–73, 2002.)

Histopathologic Features

The oral melanoacanthoma is characterized by numerous benign dendritic melanocytes (cells that normally are confined to the basal layer) scattered throughout the lesional epithelium (Figs. 10.43 and 10.44). Basal layer melanocytes are also present in increased numbers. Spongiosis and mild acanthosis typically are evident. In addition, the underlying connective tissue often contains a mild to moderate chronic inflammatory cell infiltrate that may include eosinophils.

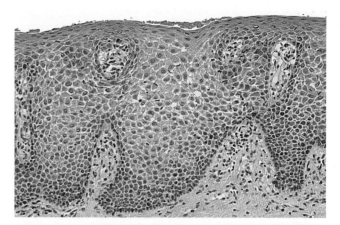

• **Fig. 10.43 Oral Melanoacanthoma.** Medium-power photomicrograph showing acanthosis of the epithelium. Spongiosis is demonstrated by intercellular spaces between the keratinocytes.

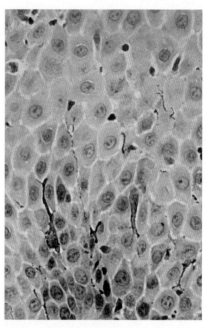

• **Fig. 10.44 Oral Melanoacanthoma.** High-power view showing numerous dendritic melanocytes extending between the spinous epithelial cells.

Treatment and Prognosis

Because of the alarming growth rate of oral melanoacanthoma, incisional biopsy usually is indicated to rule out melanoma. Once the diagnosis has been established, no further treatment is necessary. In several instances, lesions have undergone spontaneous resolution after incisional biopsy. Recurrence or development of additional lesions has been reported only rarely. There is no potential for malignant transformation.

◆ MELANOCYTIC NEVUS (NEVOCELLULAR NEVUS; MOLE)

The generic term *nevus* refers to congenital or developmental malformations of the skin (and mucosa). Nevi may arise from the surface epithelium or underlying connective tissue.

- Melanocytic nevus
- Acquired melanocytic nevus (e.g., conventional, blue, Spitz, and other subtypes)
- Congenital melanocytic nevus
- Epidermal nevus
- Nevus sebaceus
- Nevus flammeus (see page 551)
- Basal cell nevus (nevoid basal cell carcinoma) (see page 694)
- White sponge nevus (see page 748)

Melanocytic nevi represent benign proliferations of *nevus cells* (or *nevomelanocytes*). Such proliferations develop when an initiating genetic mutation arises within a melanocyte or melanocytic precursor cell. (Melanocytes are neural crest-derived cells that produce melanin pigment and colonize the skin, mucosa, and other sites.) The natural history of melanocytic nevi typically includes a period of clonal expansion followed by inhibition of further growth by cellular safeguard mechanisms. However, progression to malignant melanoma (see page 434) is possible if additional mutations arise in oncogenes or tumor suppressor genes.

Broadly speaking, melanocytic nevi can be classified as *congenital* (developing *in utero* and present at birth) or *acquired* (developing after birth). The most commonly recognized nevus is the **conventional acquired melanocytic nevus,** or **common mole**—so much so that the simple term *nevus* often is used synonymously for this pigmented lesion. However, many other types of nevi also are recognized (Box 10.2). The following sections will discuss acquired melanocytic nevi (including conventional and other subtypes) as well as congenital melanocytic nevi.

◆ ACQUIRED MELANOCYTIC NEVUS

CONVENTIONAL ACQUIRED MELANOCYTIC NEVUS (COMMON ACQUIRED NEVUS; BANAL NEVUS; COMMON MOLE)

The conventional acquired melanocytic nevus is probably the most common of all human "tumors," with an average of 10–40 cutaneous nevi per white adult. In contrast, oral examples are distinctly uncommon. One study based on a national pathology registry in the Netherlands reported an annual incidence of 4.35 excised oral melanocytic nevi per 10 million population. Some investigators have noted that oral melanocytic nevi represent only about 0.01%–0.2% of biopsies accessioned by oral pathology laboratories.

Activating mutations in *BRAF* (especially *BRAF* V600E) and *NRAS* have been identified in approximately 80% and 6% of conventional acquired melanocytic nevi, respectively; such mutations also have been detected frequently in cutaneous melanomas (see page 434). These *BRAF* and *NRAS* mutations result in stimulation of the mitogen-activated protein kinase (MAPK) signaling pathway, which mediates cell

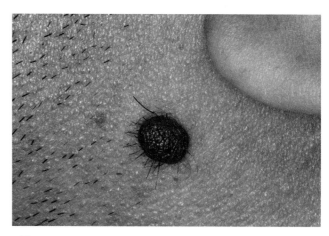

Fig. 10.45 Conventional Acquired Melanocytic Nevus, Intradermal. A brown nodule on the facial skin with a papillomatous surface and protruding hairs.

proliferation and differentiation. In addition, activated *NRAS* stimulates the phosphatidylinositol 3-kinase (PI3K)/Akt pathway, which regulates cell proliferation, growth, and survival. The life cycle of conventional acquired melanocytic nevi includes four stages: initiation (mutation development in a progenitor cell), promotion (activation and proliferation of the mutated progenitor cell), senescence (growth arrest), and involution.

Clinical Features

Conventional acquired melanocytic nevi begin to develop on the skin during childhood, and most cutaneous lesions are present before 35 years of age. Women usually have a few more nevi than men, and whites tend to have more than Asians or blacks. Most lesions are distributed above the waist, and the head and neck region commonly is involved.

Conventional acquired melanocytic nevi evolve through several developmental stages: junctional, compound, and intradermal. However, not all nevi pass through each stage. The **junctional nevus** clinically appears as a sharply demarcated, brown or black macule, typically less than 6 mm in diameter. Although this presentation may persist into adulthood, more often the nevus cells proliferate over a period of years to produce a slightly elevated, soft papule with a relatively smooth surface **(compound nevus).** The degree of pigmentation decreases; most lesions appear brown or tan. As time passes, the nevus gradually loses its pigmentation, the surface may become somewhat papillomatous, and hairs may be seen growing from the center **(intradermal nevus)** (Figs. 10.45 and 10.46). However, the nevus usually remains less than 6 mm in diameter. Ulceration is not a feature unless the lesion is traumatized. During the adult years, many conventional acquired melanocytic nevi involute and disappear; therefore, fewer lesions are detected in older persons.

Oral examples of conventional acquired melanocytic nevi are distinctly uncommon. Most arise on the palate, mucobuccal fold, lip vermilion, buccal mucosa, or gingiva, although any oral site may be affected (Fig. 10.47). Approximately two-thirds of cases are found in females, and the average

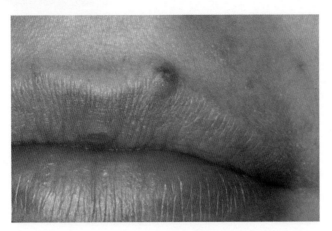

• **Fig. 10.46 Conventional Acquired Melanocytic Nevus, Intradermal.** A well-demarcated, lightly pigmented, dome-shaped papule is seen at the edge of the vermilion border of the upper lip.

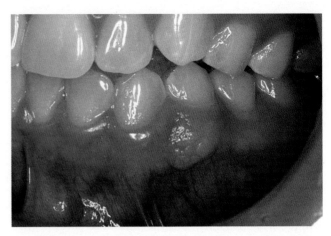

• **Fig. 10.48 Conventional Acquired Melanocytic Nevus, Intramucosal.** This intramucosal nevus of the mandibular gingiva is nonpigmented. (Courtesy of Dr. James Jacobs.)

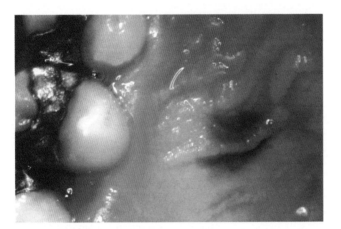

• **Fig. 10.47 Conventional Acquired Melanocytic Nevus, Intramucosal.** Pigmented lesion of the anterior hard palate. (Courtesy of Dr. Lewis Claman.)

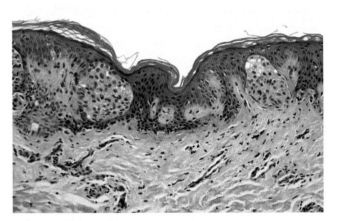

• **Fig. 10.49 Conventional Acquired Melanocytic Nevus, Junctional.** Nests of melanocytic nevus cells along the basal layer of the epithelium.

age at diagnosis is approximately 35 years. The mean lesion size is 0.9 cm in diameter. Intraoral lesions have an evolution and appearance similar to skin nevi but may not demonstrate a papillary surface as they mature. More than one in five intraoral nevi lack clinical pigmentation (Fig. 10.48).

Histopathologic Features

The conventional acquired melanocytic nevus is characterized by a benign, unencapsulated proliferation of nevus cells. Zones of differentiation often are seen among the lesional cells. Superficial nevus cells tend to be organized into small, round aggregates *(thèques)* and usually appear ovoid or epithelioid, with abundant cytoplasm and frequent intracellular melanin. Deeper nevus cells may have less cytoplasm, are seldom pigmented, and appear much like lymphocytes. The deepest nevus cells appear elongated and spindle-shaped, much like Schwann cells or fibroblasts. Some authorities classify these nevus cell variations as *types A* (epithelioid), *B* (lymphocyte-like), and *C* (spindle-shaped). Nevus cells typically lack the dendritic processes that melanocytes possess.

Melanocytic nevi are classified histopathologically according to their stage of development. The **junctional nevus** represents an early stage, in which thèques of nevus cells are confined to the junction of the epithelium and connective tissue (Fig. 10.49), especially at the tips of the rete ridges. As the nevus cells proliferate, they begin to drop off into the underlying dermis or lamina propria. When nevus cells are present along the junctional area and within the connective tissue, the lesion is called a **compound nevus** (Fig. 10.50). In later stages, the nevus cells are found only within the connective tissue. In the skin, this stage is called an **intradermal nevus;** the intraoral counterpart is called an **intramucosal nevus** (Fig. 10.51). At the time of diagnosis, most intraoral melanocytic nevi are classified as intramucosal nevi.

Treatment and Prognosis

No treatment is indicated for a conventional acquired melanocytic nevus on the skin unless it is cosmetically unacceptable, is chronically irritated by clothing, or changes in size or color. By midlife, cutaneous melanocytic nevi tend to regress; by age 90, very few remain. If removal is elected, then conservative surgical excision is the treatment of choice; recurrence is unlikely.

The lifetime risk of malignant transformation of an individual conventional acquired melanocytic nevus into cutaneous melanoma is low (approximately one in 3200 for men to one in 10,800 for women). Nevertheless, patients with a large number (>100) of cutaneous nevi are at increased risk for developing melanoma and should be monitored closely. According to a meta-analysis, about 30% of cutaneous melanomas arise in association with preexisting nevi, and the majority of nevus-associated melanomas occur on the skin of the trunk.

There is no definitive evidence that oral melanocytic nevi are a marker of increased risk for developing oral mucosal melanoma. However, early oral mucosal melanomas may appear clinically similar to oral melanocytic nevi or other benign pigmented lesions. Therefore, biopsy of all unexplained pigmented oral lesions generally is advised.

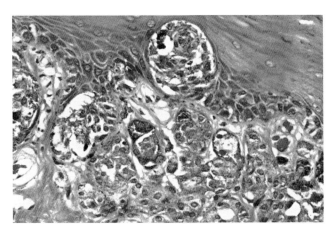

• **Fig. 10.50 Conventional Acquired Melanocytic Nevus, Compound.** High-power view showing nests of pigmented nevus cells within the epithelium and the superficial lamina propria.

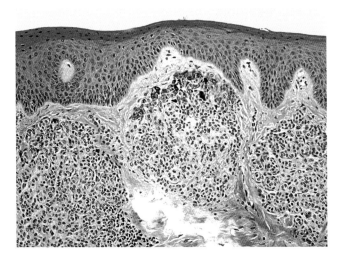

• **Fig. 10.51 Conventional Acquired Melanocytic Nevus, Intramucosal.** Collections of melanocytic nevus cells within the lamina propria.

BLUE NEVUS (DERMAL MELANOCYTOMA; JADASSOHN-TIÈCHE NEVUS)

The **blue nevus** is an uncommon, benign proliferation of dermal melanocytes, usually deep within the connective tissue. Two major types are recognized: (1) the **common** blue nevus and (2) the **cellular** blue nevus. The common blue nevus is the second most frequently encountered type of melanocytic nevus in the mouth. The blue color of this melanin-producing lesion can be explained by the **Tyndall effect**, which relates to the interaction of light with particles in a colloidal suspension. In the case of a blue nevus, the melanin particles are deep to the surface, so that light reflected back has to pass through the overlying tissue. Colors with long wavelengths (reds and yellows) tend to be absorbed more readily by the tissue; the shorter-wavelength blue light is more likely to be reflected back to the observer's eyes.

Most blue nevi are acquired, although congenital lesions are possible. Unlike conventional acquired melanocytic nevi, blue nevi only rarely harbor *BRAF* mutations. Instead, blue nevi tend to exhibit activating mutations in *GNAQ* or, to a lesser extent, *GNA11*; these genes encode G-protein alpha subunits important for signal transduction from cell-surface receptors. *GNAQ* or *GNA11* mutations in blue nevi and *BRAF* mutations in acquired melanocytic nevi both result in constitutive activation of the MAPK signaling pathway.

Clinical Features

The common blue nevus may affect any cutaneous or mucosal site, but it has a predilection for the hands and feet (mainly the dorsal aspect), the scalp, and the face. Mucosal lesions may involve the oral cavity, the conjunctiva, and, rarely, the sinonasal region. Oral examples almost always are found on the palate. The lesion exhibits a female predilection and usually occurs in children and young adults. It typically appears as a macular or dome-shaped, blue or blue-black lesion smaller than 1 cm in diameter (Fig. 10.52).

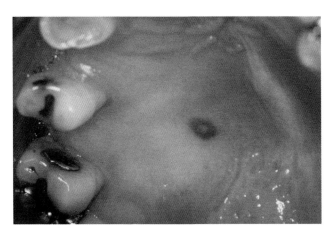

• **Fig. 10.52 Blue Nevus.** A well-circumscribed, deep-blue macular lesion on the palatal mucosa.

The cellular blue nevus is encountered much less frequently than the common type. It usually develops during the second to fourth decades of life but may be congenital. More than 50% of cellular blue nevi arise in the sacrococcygeal or buttock region, although other cutaneous or mucosal surfaces may be involved as well. Clinically, the lesion typically appears as a slow-growing, blue-black papule or nodule that sometimes attains a size of 2 cm or more. Occasional examples remain macular.

Histopathologic Features

Histopathologically, the common blue nevus consists of a collection of elongated, slender melanocytes with dendritic extensions and numerous melanin granules. These cells are located deep within the dermis or lamina propria (Fig. 10.53) and usually align themselves parallel to the surface epithelium. The cellular blue nevus appears as a well-circumscribed, highly cellular aggregate of plump, melanin-producing spindle cells within the dermis or submucosa. More typical pigmented dendritic spindle cells are seen at the periphery of the lesion. Occasionally, a blue nevus is found in conjunction with an overlying conventional acquired melanocytic nevus, in which case the term **combined nevus** is used.

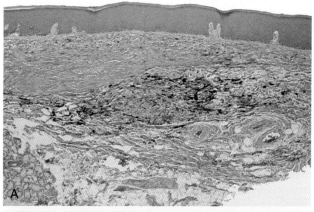
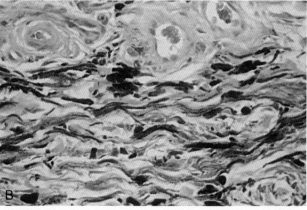

• **Fig. 10.53 Blue Nevus. A,** Abundant melanin is seen within spindle-shaped melanocytes located relatively deep within the lamina propria and parallel to the surface epithelium. **B,** High-power view showing heavily pigmented spindle-shaped cells.

Treatment and Prognosis

If clinically indicated, conservative surgical excision is the treatment of choice for blue nevi. Recurrence is minimal with such treatment. Malignant transformation of cutaneous or oral blue nevi to melanoma is rare but has been reported. Because an oral blue nevus clinically can mimic an early melanoma, biopsy of intraoral pigmented lesions is usually advisable.

SPITZ NEVUS (BENIGN JUVENILE MELANOMA; SPINDLE AND EPITHELIOID CELL NEVUS)

Spitz tumors represent a group of uncommon melanocytic lesions characterized by large, spindled and/or epithelioid melanocytes. Although initially described by Spitz in 1948 as "juvenile melanoma," these tumors currently are recognized as a spectrum of lesions ranging from benign to malignant. Herein we will focus on the **Spitz nevus**—a benign acquired melanocytic nevus variant, which accounts for about 1% of all cutaneous melanocytic nevi in children. Additional entities within this spectrum include the **atypical Spitz tumor** (an intermediate lesion with uncertain biologic behavior) and **Spitz melanoma** (a rare subset of malignant melanoma). Diagnosis of Spitz tumors can be challenging and represents an ongoing area of controversy.

Characteristic genetic findings in Spitz nevi include activating point mutations in *HRAS* (often accompanied by copy number gain in mutant *HRAS* due to chromosome 11p amplification), rearrangements involving the serine/threonine kinases *BRAF* and *MAP3K8*, and rearrangements of receptor tyrosine kinases (including *ROS1, NTRK1, ALK,* and others). These alterations result in activation of the MAPK signaling pathway. Whereas melanomas and conventional acquired melanocytic nevi tend to exhibit MAPK signaling activation via *BRAF* V600E and *NRAS* mutations, Spitz nevi demonstrate such mutations only infrequently.

Clinical Features

The Spitz nevus typically develops on the skin of the face, neck, or lower extremities during childhood. Oral examples have been reported rarely. White individuals are affected more often than blacks or Asians. The tumor usually appears as a solitary, dome-shaped, pink to reddish-brown papule smaller than 6 mm in greatest diameter. The young age at presentation and relatively small size help distinguish the Spitz nevus from melanoma. Spitz nevi may grow rapidly at first but usually stabilize after about 6 months.

Histopathologic Features

Most Spitz nevi are compound in architecture, with zonal differentiation from the superficial to deep aspects and good symmetry. Lesional cells are either spindle-shaped or plump (epithelioid), and the two cell types often are intermixed.

The epithelioid cells may be multinucleated and may appear somewhat bizarre, often lacking cohesiveness. Solitary or coalescent eosinophilic globules shown to be masses of basement membrane material (Kamino bodies) may be seen within the epidermis or at the junction of the epidermis and dermis. Ectatic blood vessels (imparting the reddish color of some lesions) and normal mitotic figures may be present in the superficial aspects of the lesion. Immunohistochemistry may show expression of various melanocytic antigens, such as S-100 protein, HMB-45 (usually positive in superficial areas of the tumor), and melan-A (MART-1).

Treatment and Prognosis

Conservative surgical excision is the most common treatment, and there is little chance of recurrence after removal. However, for lesions exhibiting typical clinical and dermoscopic features of Spitz nevus in children younger than 12 years, some authorities advocate close monitoring. Untreated lesions eventually may undergo involution or conversion to another nevus type.

HALO NEVUS (SUTTON NEVUS; LEUKODERMA ACQUISITUM CENTRIFUGUM)

The **halo nevus** is a melanocytic nevus with a hypopigmented border, apparently resulting from the destruction of nevus cells and melanocytes by the immune system. The cause of the immune attack is unknown, but regression of the nevus usually results. Most cases develop from preexisting acquired melanocytic nevi, although development from congenital nevi is possible as well. Some reports have suggested a possible association with vitiligo. Interestingly, multiple halo nevi may develop in patients who have had a recent excision of a melanoma. Infrequently, melanomas and basal cell carcinomas also may exhibit halo phenomena.

Clinical Features

Halo nevi most commonly occur on the skin of the trunk during the second decade of life. The lesion typically appears as a pigmented papule or macule, surrounded by a hypopigmented zone measuring 2–3 mm or wider (Fig. 10.54).

Histopathologic Features

Histopathologically, the halo nevus differs from the routine acquired melanocytic nevus only in the presence of an intense chronic inflammatory cell infiltrate.

Treatment and Prognosis

Most halo nevi regress and do not require treatment. If treatment is elected, then conservative surgical removal is curative and recurrence is unlikely.

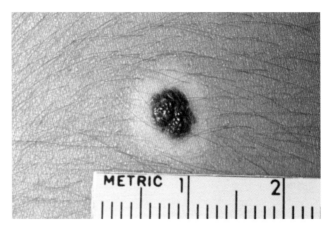

• **Fig. 10.54 Halo Nevus.** Elevated brown lesion of the skin showing surrounding depigmentation.

◆ CONGENITAL MELANOCYTIC NEVUS

The **congenital melanocytic nevus** affects approximately 1% of newborns in the United States. The trunk and extremities are involved most commonly, although about 15% of lesions arise in the head and neck area. Intraoral involvement is rare. Congenital melanocytic nevi usually are classified according to projected adult size as follows: small (<1.5 cm in diameter), medium (1.5–20 cm in diameter), or large (>20 cm in diameter). Especially large lesions may be termed "giant." Small to medium congenital melanocytic nevi are relatively common and often exhibit *BRAF* mutations, whereas large to giant lesions occur in only about 1 in 20,000–500,000 births and often harbor *NRAS* mutations. Growth of congenital nevi tends to mirror growth of the affected child; unlike conventional acquired melanocytic nevi, congenital lesions tend to persist into adulthood without regression.

Clinical Features

Small congenital melanocytic nevi may appear similar to acquired melanocytic nevi. However, most lesions are medium to large—appearing as light tan macules that over time develop into dark brown to black, rough-surfaced plaques or multinodular lesions (Figs. 10.55 and 10.56). A common feature is **hypertrichosis** (excess hair) within the lesion, which may become more prominent with age (**giant hairy nevus).** A very large congenital nevus sometimes may give the appearance that the patient is wearing an article of clothing and, thus, may be termed a **bathing trunk nevus** or **garment nevus**.

Patients with large, giant, or multiple congenital nevi are at risk for *neurocutaneous melanosis*. This rare and potentially fatal syndrome is characterized by congenital nevi in conjunction with melanotic neoplasms of the central nervous system (CNS), including leptomeningeal melanocytosis and melanoma. Associated findings may include seizures, paralysis, learning disorders, intellectual deficit, hydrocephalus, and brain malformations. MRI in early infancy may aid in screening at-risk patients for this condition.

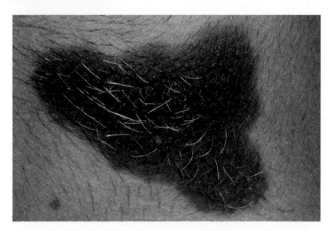

• **Fig. 10.55 Congenital Melanocytic Nevus.** Pigmented lesion of the skin showing hypertrichosis.

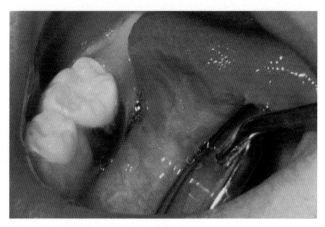

• **Fig. 10.56 Congenital Melanocytic Nevus.** Deeply pigmented lesion of the lingual mandibular gingiva in a 3-year-old child.

Histopathologic Features

The histopathologic appearance of the congenital melanocytic nevus is similar to that of the acquired melanocytic nevus, and some small congenital nevi cannot be distinguished microscopically from acquired nevi. Both congenital and acquired types are composed of nevus cells, which may have a junctional, compound, or intradermal pattern. The congenital nevus is usually of the compound or intradermal type. In contrast to the acquired melanocytic nevus, the congenital nevus often extends into deeper levels of the dermis, with "infiltration" of nevus cells between collagen bundles. In addition, congenital nevus cells often intermingle with neurovascular bundles in the reticular dermis and surround normal adnexal skin structures (e.g., hair follicles, sebaceous glands). Large congenital melanocytic nevi may extend into the subcutaneous fat.

Treatment and Prognosis

Many congenital melanocytic nevi are excised for aesthetic purposes. Systematic reviews of the literature suggest that approximately 2%–3% of large congenital nevi transform

- Leukoplakia
- Proliferative verrucous leukoplakia
- Erythroplakia
- Erythroleukoplakia
- Oral submucous fibrosis
- Actinic cheilosis
- Palatal lesions associated with reverse smoking
- Smokeless tobacco keratosis
- Oral lichenoid pathoses (including oral graft-vs-host disease, oral lupus erythematosus, oral lichen planus, and oral lichenoid lesions[†])
- Heritable conditions with cancer predisposition (including Fanconi anemia, dyskeratosis congenita, xeroderma pigmentosum, Li Fraumeni syndrome, Bloom syndrome, ataxia telangiectasia, and Cowden syndrome)

*Sources: (1) Warnakulasuriya S, Kujan O, Aguirre-Urizar JM, et al: Oral potentially malignant disorders: a consensus report from an international seminar on nomenclature and classification, convened by the WHO Collaborating Centre for Oral Cancer, Oral Dis 27:1862–1880, 2021. (2) Muller S, Tilakaratne WM: Oral potentially malignant disorders. In WHO Classification of Tumours Editorial Board, editors: World Health Organization Classification of Head and Neck Tumours, ed 5, Lyon, France, 2022, International Agency for Research on Cancer. Available at: https://tumourclassification.iarc.who.int/chaptercontent/52/103. Accessed March 30, 2022.
[†]Oral lesions with lichenoid features but lacking the typical clinical or histopathologic appearances of oral lichen planus.

into malignant melanoma. However, the efficacy of excision in reducing this slightly elevated risk for melanoma is unknown and remains controversial. Also, complete excision may not be feasible for large lesions. Alternative treatment options include partial surgical removal, dermabrasion, laser therapy, cryotherapy, and chemical peels. Close clinical follow-up is recommended regardless of whether or not treatment has been rendered.

◆ ORAL POTENTIALLY MALIGNANT DISORDERS

As defined by the World Health Organization, **oral potentially malignant disorders** represent "a heterogeneous group of clinically defined conditions associated with a variable risk of progression to oral squamous cell carcinoma." The true prevalence of these disorders is difficult to determine because of the limited availability of population-based data. However, a recent meta-analysis reported an estimated worldwide prevalence of 4.5%. Box 10.3 lists major types of oral potentially malignant disorders, and Box 10.4 provides definitions for various terms related to our discussion of these disorders. Most widely recognized among oral potentially malignant disorders is *leukoplakia*, with an estimated worldwide prevalence of 4.1%. In contrast, its counterpart, *erythroplakia*, is relatively rare (global prevalence <1%) but associated with a very high risk for harboring or transforming into malignancy. The following oral potentially malignant disorders are discussed in greater detail in the sections below:

- **Oral potentially malignant disorders.** A heterogeneous group of clinically defined conditions associated with a variable risk of progression to oral squamous cell carcinoma.
- **Malignant transformation potential.** The risk of cancer being present in a potentially malignant disorder, either at initial diagnosis or in the future (usually expressed in percentages).
- **Relative risk.** A specific epidemiologic measure of the association between exposure to a particular factor and the risk of acquiring a disease, expressed as a ratio of the incidence or prevalence of a disease among those exposed and those not exposed to the factor.
- **Hazard ratio.** A measure of how often an event (such as, cancer) occurs over time in one group compared to another group (e.g., patients in the treatment group vs the control group in a clinical trial, individuals exposed to a particular carcinogen compared to those not exposed).

leukoplakia, erythroplakia, smokeless tobacco keratosis, oral submucous fibrosis, and actinic cheilosis.

The phrase *potentially malignant* refers to the fact that the risk for cancer development is increased but not inevitable. In fact, the majority of patients with oral potentially malignant disorders do not progress to malignancy, although some will develop cancer or already may have cancer at initial presentation. According to a meta-analysis of the literature, the overall malignant transformation rate of oral potentially malignant disorders is approximately 8%. However, estimated malignant transformation rates vary considerably by disorder type (e.g., proliferative verrucous leukoplakia 44%–100%, leukoplakia 4%–22%, oral submucous fibrosis 4%–6%). With regard to erythroplakia, at least half of cases already represent carcinoma at initial presentation; after excluding the already malignant cases, the remainder mostly exhibit *high-grade dysplasia* (epithelial microscopic features associated with a high risk for progression to carcinoma), with estimated malignant transformation rates mostly in the range of 14%–50%.

There is some uncertainty regarding the malignant potential of lichen planus (see page 787) and other lichenoid pathoses, and their inclusion within the category of oral potentially malignant disorders has been debated. Considerable variation in reported malignant transformation rates for these conditions likely reflects difficulties with establishing definitive clinical and histopathologic criteria; however, the malignant transformation risk generally appears to be low (best estimates are less than 1%–3% for lichen planus and slightly higher for so-called oral lichenoid lesions). Some studies also suggest that the erosive form of lichen planus has greater potential for malignant progression compared to other subtypes.

◆ LEUKOPLAKIA (LEUKOKERATOSIS; ERYTHROLEUKOPLAKIA)

As defined by the World Health Organization, oral **leukoplakia** (*leuko* = white; *plakia* = patch) represents a white plaque that is of questionable risk for oral cancer and only can be diagnosed once having excluded other known diseases. The term is strictly a clinical one and does not imply a specific histopathologic tissue alteration. (As with most oral white lesions, the clinical color results from a thickened surface *keratin* layer, which appears white when wet, or a thickened *spinous* layer, which masks the normal vascularity [redness] of the underlying connective tissue.) Nonetheless, both clinical and microscopic examination may aid in ruling out other conditions that may appear as oral white plaques, such as lichen planus, morsicatio buccarum (chronic cheek nibbling), frictional keratosis, smokeless tobacco keratosis, nicotine stomatitis, leukoedema, and white sponge nevus. Thus, leukoplakia is somewhat unusual in that it represents a *diagnosis of exclusion*.

Prevalence

Based on pooled, weighted data from various studies, the worldwide prevalence of leukoplakia has been estimated to fall within a range of 1.5%–4.3%. Similarly, a recent meta-analysis of studies with clinical assessment and histopathologic confirmation reported an estimated worldwide prevalence of 4.1%.

Etiology

The cause of leukoplakia remains unknown, although hypotheses abound.

Tobacco

Among the various proposed contributory factors, tobacco smoking appears to be the most closely associated with leukoplakia. More than 80% of patients with leukoplakia are smokers, and smokers are much more likely to have leukoplakia than nonsmokers. Heavier smokers have greater numbers of lesions and larger lesions than do light smokers, especially after many years of tobacco use. In addition, leukoplakias often disappear or become smaller within the first year of smoking cessation.

Smokeless tobacco use frequently causes a clinically distinctive white oral plaque called **smokeless tobacco keratosis** (see page 391), which generally exhibits a very low malignant transformation risk. This lesion is considered an orally potentially malignant disorder but should not be classified as a true leukoplakia. In contrast, betel quid use (see page 393)—with or without smokeless tobacco—is associated with true leukoplakia; this habit is common in parts of Asia.

Alcohol

Alcohol exerts a strong synergistic effect with tobacco in oral cancer development. Nevertheless, there is conflicting evidence as to whether alcohol is associated independently with leukoplakia. People who excessively use mouth rinses with alcohol content greater than 25% may have grayish buccal mucosal plaques, but these lesions are not considered true leukoplakias.

Sanguinaria

Persons who use toothpaste or mouth rinses containing the herbal extract, sanguinaria, may develop a true leukoplakia

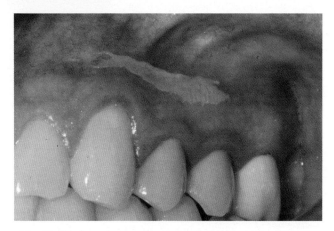

• **Fig. 10.57 Sanguinaria-associated Keratosis.** Thin white plaque on the maxillary alveolar mucosa.

called **sanguinaria-associated keratosis.** This lesion usually arises in the maxillary vestibule or on the maxillary alveolar mucosa (Fig. 10.57). More than 80% of individuals with maxillary vestibular or alveolar leukoplakia have a history of using products that contain sanguinaria, compared with 3% of the normal population.

The affected epithelium may demonstrate dysplasia identical to that seen in other leukoplakias, although the potential for cancer development is uncertain. The white plaque may persist for years even after the patient stops using the product.

Ultraviolet Radiation

UV radiation is a causative factor for leukoplakia of the lower lip vermilion. Such lesions typically represent actinic cheiloses (see page 395). Immunocompromised persons, such as transplant patients, are especially prone to developing leukoplakia and squamous cell carcinoma of the lower lip vermilion.

Microorganisms

Several microorganisms have been implicated in the etiology of leukoplakia. *Treponema pallidum,* for example, produces glossitis in the late stage of syphilis, with or without the arsenic therapy in popular use before the advent of modern antibiotics. The tongue is stiff and frequently has extensive dorsal leukoplakia.

Tertiary syphilis is rare today, but oral infection by *Candida albicans* is not. *C. albicans* can colonize the keratin layer of the oral mucosa, often producing a thick, granular, red and white plaque (Fig. 10.58). The terms **candidal leukoplakia** and **candidal hyperplasia** have been used to describe such a lesion, and biopsy may show epithelial dysplasia or hyperplasia. It is unknown whether this yeast produces dysplasia or secondarily infects previously altered epithelium; however, some of these lesions disappear, shrink, or become less severely dysplastic after antifungal therapy. In some cases, tobacco smoking may cause the leukoplakia and also may predispose the patient to develop candidiasis.

Some studies have detected HPV DNA about two to four times more often in oral leukoplakias than in

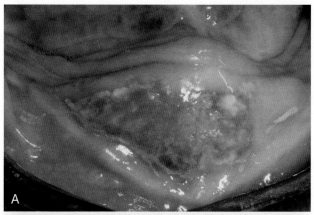

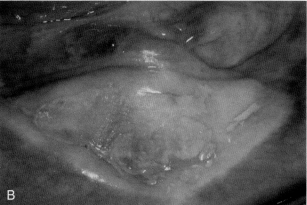

• **Fig. 10.58 Candidal Leukoplakia. A,** Well-circumscribed red and white plaque on the anterior floor of mouth, which showed candidal infestation on cytology smears. **B,** After antifungal therapy, the erythematous component resolved, resulting in a homogeneous white plaque.

clinically normal oral mucosa; in addition, recent meta-analyses have reported HPV DNA in about 20% of oral leukoplakias and 27% of oral epithelial dysplasias. However, the presence of HPV DNA alone cannot exclude the possibility of coincidental (or "bystander") infection. Additional investigations have identified a subset of dysplastic oral leukoplakias (and, more rarely, erythroplakias) positive for p16 by immunohistochemistry and positive for high-risk HPV DNA or mRNA by *in situ* hybridization (see page 405 for further discussion of these assays). These findings suggest that a small proportion of oral leukoplakias may be HPV-driven, although further studies are needed.

Recent advances in high-throughput sequencing technologies have enabled researchers to investigate the oral microbiome of patients with leukoplakia. Although results across studies have been variable, some researchers have noted decreased levels of commensal organisms (such as streptococci) and increased levels of anaerobic bacteria (such as *Fusobacterium nucleatum, Prevotella intermedia,* and *Porphyromonas gingivalis*) in patients with oral leukoplakia compared to healthy controls. Research in this field is still in its infancy, however, and more standardized studies are needed.

Chronic Trauma or Irritation

Several keratotic lesions, which until recently had been viewed as variants of leukoplakia, are now considered not to be precancers. Nicotine stomatitis is a generalized white palatal alteration that seems to be a hyperkeratotic response to the heat generated by tobacco smoking (usually a pipe), rather than a response to the carcinogens within the smoke (see page 397). Its malignant transformation potential is so low as to be about the same as that of normal palatal mucosa.

In addition, chronic mechanical irritation can produce a white lesion with a roughened keratotic surface, termed **frictional keratosis.** Although this lesion clinically appears similar to true leukoplakia, it is now thought to be no more than a normal hyperplastic response (similar to a callus on the skin). Keratoses of this type are readily reversible after elimination of the trauma, and obviously traumatic lesions—such as linea alba (see page 272), morsicatio (see page 272), and toothbrush gingival "abrasion"—have not been documented to transform into malignancy. **Alveolar ridge keratoses** (Fig. 10.59)—involving the retromolar pad or crest of an edentulous alveolar ridge—represent another form of frictional keratosis caused by masticatory function or denture trauma. Frictional keratosis should be differentiated from oral precancers.

Interestingly, a recent study noted an association between gingival white plaques and the presence of silicon-containing foreign particles. Potential sources of such particles include oral hygiene products and dental materials. Most of these leukoplakias exhibited a verrucous growth pattern; other frequent findings included chronic inflammation and hyperorthokeratosis. Epithelial dysplasia was evident in some cases as well. The clinicopathologic features resemble those seen in early stages of proliferative verrucous leukoplakia (see page 384).

Clinical Features

Oral leukoplakia exhibits a male predilection, with approximately 60%–80% of cases overall arising in men. However, there is a female predilection in some regions where women use tobacco products more than men. Oral leukoplakia usually affects persons older than 40 years, and prevalence increases rapidly with age. The average age (60 years) is similar to that for patients with oral cancer; however, in some studies, leukoplakia has been found to occur about 5 years earlier (on average) than oral squamous cell carcinoma.

Approximately 70% of oral leukoplakias are found on the lip vermilion, buccal mucosa, and gingiva. Lesions on the tongue, lip vermilion, and oral floor, however, account for more than 90% of those that show dysplasia or carcinoma. Among betel quid users, the buccal mucosa and commissure are the major sites for leukoplakia harboring carcinoma. Leukoplakia presents as a white plaque that cannot be wiped or scraped away. The inability to wipe the lesion away is a clinical finding that aids in distinguishing leukoplakia from other conditions, such as pseudomembranous candidiasis, chemical or thermal burns, and toothpaste-related allergic contact stomatitis.

Individual lesions may have a varied clinical appearance, and their features may change over time. **Homogeneous leukoplakia** refers to individual lesions with a relatively uniform appearance throughout. An early or mild lesion may present as **homogeneous thin leukoplakia**—a white to gray-white macule or plaque, which may be somewhat translucent, fissured, or wrinkled (Fig. 10.60). Such lesions usually are soft with sharply demarcated borders, but occasionally they may blend gradually into normal mucosa. Homogeneous thin leukoplakias may disappear or continue unchanged, and they seldom show dysplasia on biopsy. For tobacco smokers who do not reduce their habit, however, as many as two-thirds of

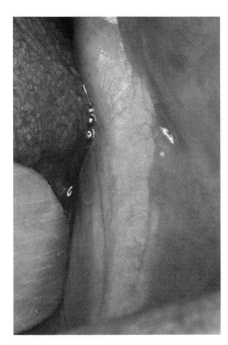

• **Fig. 10.59 Frictional Keratosis.** There is a rough, hyperkeratotic change to the posterior mandibular alveolar ridge ("alveolar ridge keratosis"), because this area is now edentulous and becomes traumatized from mastication. Such frictional keratoses should resolve when the source of irritation is eliminated and should not be mistaken for true leukoplakia.

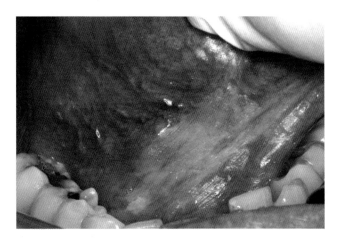

• **Fig. 10.60 Homogeneous Thin Leukoplakia.** A thin, white plaque on the right ventral tongue.

such lesions enlarge and progress to a stage called **homogeneous thick leukoplakia**, characterized by a thickened, leathery, distinctly white plaque with deepened fissures (Figs. 10.61 and 10.62). Most remain indefinitely at this stage, and as many as one-third regress or disappear. However, some lesions may progress to develop a nonhomogeneous appearance.

Nonhomogeneous leukoplakia refers to leukoplakia with a granular (Fig. 10.63), nodular, verrucous/verruciform, ulcerated, or red component. Notably, nonhomogeneous leukoplakia has a significantly greater risk for malignant transformation (or already harboring malignancy) compared to homogeneous leukoplakia. A nonhomogeneous leukoplakia with a mixture of red and white areas may be termed **erythroleukoplakia** or **speckled leukoplakia** (Fig. 10.64). The red areas tend to exhibit high-grade dysplasia or microinvasive carcinoma upon microscopic examination. The erythema may result from epithelium that is so immature that it no longer produces keratin and/or atrophic epithelium that allows underlying vascularity to be readily apparent. Lesions that become entirely red in appearance are known as **erythroplakias** (see page 390).

A special high-risk form of leukoplakia, **proliferative verrucous leukoplakia (PVL)** (or **proliferative leukoplakia**), is characterized by the development of multiple, slowly spreading, keratotic plaques with rough surface projections (Figs. 10.65–10.67). The gingiva frequently is involved, but other sites may be affected as well. Although the lesions typically begin as simple, flat hyperkeratoses that are indistinguishable from ordinary homogeneous leukoplakia, PVL exhibits persistent growth, with lesions eventually becoming exophytic and verrucous. As the lesions progress, they may go through a stage indistinguishable from **verrucous carcinoma** (see page 421), but they later usually develop dysplasia and transform into full-fledged **squamous cell carcinoma** (often within 8 years of initial PVL diagnosis). These lesions rarely regress despite therapy. PVL is unusual among the leukoplakia variants in having a strong female predilection (1:4 male-to-female ratio) and minimal association with tobacco use.

Many leukoplakic lesions are a mixture of the previously mentioned phases or subtypes. Figs. 10.68 and 10.69

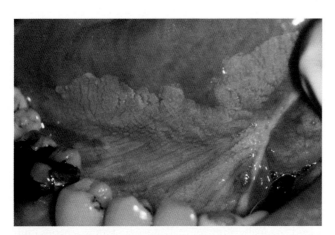

• **Fig. 10.61 Homogeneous Thick Leukoplakia.** A diffuse, corrugated white plaque on the right ventral surface of the tongue and floor of mouth.

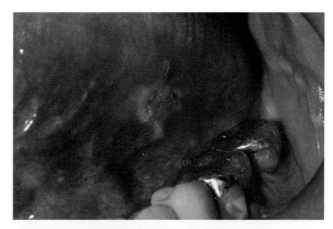

• **Fig. 10.63 Nonhomogeneous Leukoplakia.** Focal leukoplakic lesion with a rough, granular surface on the posterior lateral border of the tongue. Biopsy revealed early invasive squamous cell carcinoma.

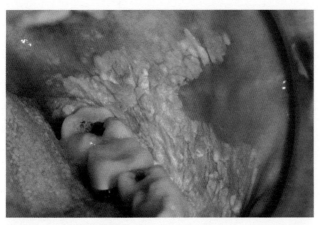

• **Fig. 10.62 Homogeneous Thick Leukoplakia.** Left buccal mucosa exhibiting an extensive thick, white plaque with associated fissures. Moderate epithelial dysplasia was noted on histopathologic evaluation, and squamous cell carcinoma later developed in this area.

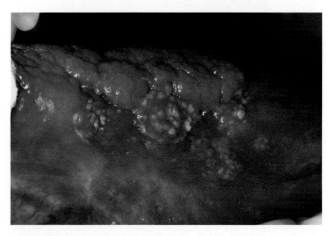

• **Fig. 10.64** Erythroleukoplakia (speckled leukoplakia). Red and white plaque on the ventrolateral tongue.

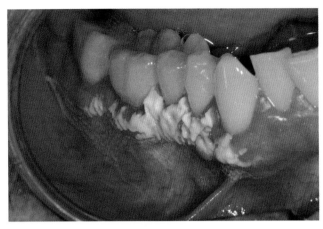

• **Fig. 10.65** **Proliferative Verrucous Leukoplakia (PVL).** Extensive white plaque with an irregular, rough surface on the mandibular facial gingiva and alveolar mucosa.

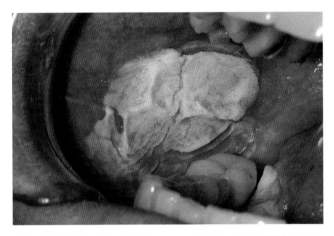

• **Fig. 10.66** **Proliferative Verrucous Leukoplakia (PVL).** Large, thickened white plaque on the buccal mucosa. Leukoplakia also is present on the ventrolateral tongue.

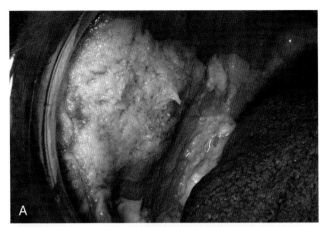

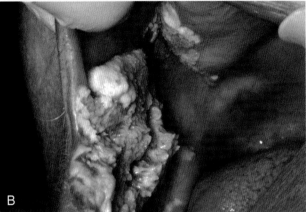

• **Fig. 10.67** **Proliferative Verrucous Leukoplakia (PVL). A,** An elderly white female developed extensive leukoplakia with rough surface projections on the buccal mucosa and mandibular alveolar ridge. **B,** After failing to comply with a recommendation for biopsy, the same patient returned 2 years later with a verrucous carcinoma.

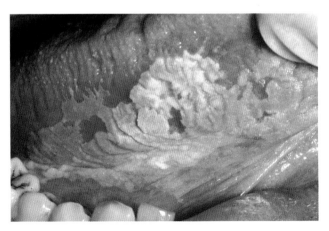

• **Fig. 10.68** **Leukoplakia.** Extensive ventral and lateral tongue lesion with areas representing various possible phases or clinical appearances (compare with Fig. 10.69).

provide a clinical and graphic representation of such a lesion. Biopsies should be taken from areas of a lesion most likely to harbor dysplasia or carcinoma (i.e., areas with a clinical appearance similar to those toward the right in Fig. 10.69).

Over the years, several techniques (e.g., vital dyes, brush cytology, chemiluminescence, autofluorescence, salivary bio-marker assays, *in vivo* microscopy) have been proposed to aid in the identification or diagnosis of premalignant and malignant oral lesions. However, there is currently insufficient evidence to support the use of such technologies in routine practice, and careful clinical evaluation with directed conventional biopsy remains the gold standard for assessment of oral leukoplakia (see Fig. 10.101).

Histopathologic Features

Microscopically, leukoplakia is characterized by a thickened keratin layer of the surface epithelium (**hyperkeratosis**), with or without a thickened spinous layer (**acanthosis**). Some leukoplakias demonstrate surface hyperkeratosis but show atrophy or thinning of the underlying epithelium.

Frequently, variable numbers of chronic inflammatory cells are noted within the subjacent connective tissue.

The keratin layer may consist of parakeratin (**hyperpar-akeratosis**), orthokeratin (**hyperorthokeratosis**), or a combination of both (Fig. 10.70). With parakeratin, there is no granular cell layer, and the epithelial nuclei are retained in the

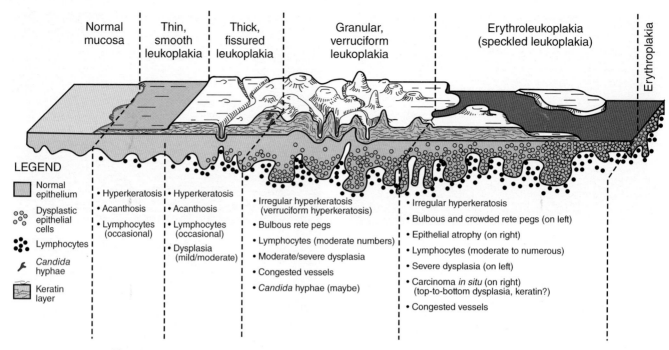

• **Fig. 10.69 Leukoplakia.** Composite representation of the various phases or clinical appearances of oral leukoplakia, with anticipated underlying histopathologic changes. Lesions have increasing malignant transformation potentials as their appearances approach those toward the right. (From Bouquot JE, Gnepp DR: Laryngeal precancer—a review of the literature, commentary and comparison with oral leukoplakia, *Head Neck* 13:488–497, 1991.)

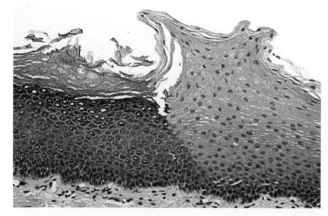

• **Fig. 10.70 Hyperorthokeratosis.** This medium-power photomicrograph demonstrates hyperorthokeratosis with a well-defined granular cell layer on the left side. The right side shows normal parakeratinized epithelium without a granular cell layer.

keratin layer. With orthokeratin, the epithelium demonstrates a granular cell layer, and the nuclei are lost in the keratin layer.

Oral epithelial dysplasia represents a spectrum of cytologic and architectural changes in oral epithelium that are associated with a risk for transformation into squamous cell carcinoma. These changes are evident at the light microscopic level and apparently result from accumulation of underlying genetic and epigenetic alterations. Epithelial dysplasia can be found in leukoplakia, erythroplakia (see next section), and other types of oral potentially malignant

disorders. The exact proportion of oral leukoplakias exhibiting dysplasia is difficult to determine due to variation in study design/bias, case definitions, and interobserver evaluation. In prior studies, epithelial dysplasia or carcinoma has been reported in only about 5%–25% of oral leukoplakias, although more recent analyses, with refined case definitions, have noted such changes in as many as 40%–46% of cases.

The histopathologic alterations of dysplastic epithelial cells are similar to those of squamous cell carcinoma and may include the following:

- Abnormal variation in size of nuclei and cells
- Abnormal variation in shape (pleomorphism) of nuclei and cells
- Increased nuclear-to-cytoplasmic ratio
- Increased nuclear size
- Hyperchromatic (excessively dark-staining) nuclei
- Increased number and size of nucleoli
- Dyskeratosis (premature keratinization of individual cells)
- Increased mitotic activity (excessive numbers of mitoses)
- Atypical mitotic figures (e.g., tripolar or star-shaped mitoses)
- Apoptotic mitoses

In addition, dysplastic epithelium may exhibit architectural alterations, including the following:

- Drop-shaped rete ridges
- Irregular epithelial stratification
- Basal cells exhibiting disorganization or loss of polarity
- Basal cell clustering or nesting
- Mitoses high in the epithelium; mitoses in maturing cells

- Keratin pearls (focal, round collections of concentrically layered keratinized cells) within rete ridges
- Generalized premature keratinization
- Altered keratin pattern for oral subsite
- Reduced keratinocyte cohesion
- Verrucous or papillary architecture
- Multifocal or "skip" lesions (areas of thick keratosis alternating with normal-appearing nonkeratinized epithelium)
- Sharply defined margins (between microscopically altered and "normal-appearing" epithelium)
- Extension of dysplastic changes into minor salivary gland ducts (Fig. 10.71) (This feature often is seen in the floor of mouth and is associated with an increased risk for recurrence.)
- Multiple different patterns of dysplasia

The grade of epithelial dysplasia refers to its "severity" or intensity. Traditionally, a 3-tier grading system has been applied as follows: (1) **mild epithelial dysplasia** (with alterations limited principally to the basal and parabasal layers) (Fig. 10.72), (2) **moderate epithelial dysplasia** (with alterations from the basal layer to the midportion of the spinous layer) (Fig. 10.73), and (3) **severe epithelial dysplasia** (with alterations from the basal layer to a level above the midpoint of the epithelium) (Fig. 10.74). However, this traditional definition does not reflect the full complexity of grading oral epithelial dysplasia. For example, cytologic atypia and architectural disturbances that are limited to the basal third of the epithelium but are especially marked or concerning may constitute severe epithelial dysplasia. Also note that architectural changes with minimal to no cytologic atypia may be sufficient for assigning the presence of dysplasia.

Alternatively, some authorities advocate a binary grading system (low-grade vs high-grade dysplasia). Such a 2-tier system may exhibit improved reproducibility compared to a 3-tier system. However, further validation and outcome studies are needed.

Carcinoma _in situ_ is defined as dysplasia involving the entire thickness of the epithelium (i.e., extending from the basal layer to the surface or "top-to-bottom" change) (Fig. 10.75). There may or may not be a thin layer of keratin on the surface. The epithelium may be hyperplastic or

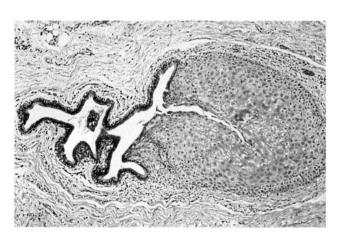

• **Fig. 10.71 Ductal Dysplasia.** Salivary gland duct exhibiting squamous metaplasia and dysplasia that originated from an overlying surface epithelial dysplasia.

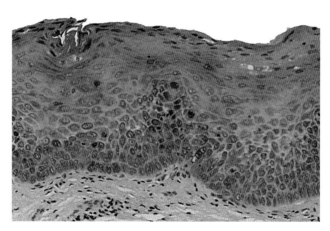

• **Fig. 10.73 Moderate Epithelial Dysplasia.** Dysplastic changes extend to the midpoint of the epithelium and are characterized by nuclear hyperchromatism, pleomorphism, and cellular crowding.

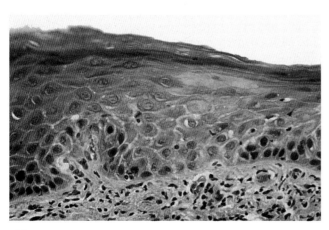

• **Fig. 10.72 Mild Epithelial Dysplasia.** Hyperchromatic and slightly pleomorphic nuclei are noted in the basal and parabasal cell layers of this stratified squamous epithelium.

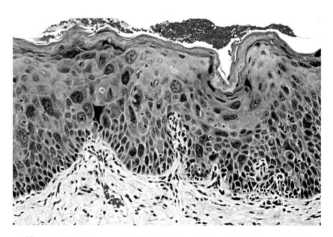

• **Fig. 10.74 Severe Epithelial Dysplasia.** Epithelium exhibiting marked pleomorphism, hyperchromatism, and scattered mitotic figures. Atypical cells involve most of the epithelial thickness.

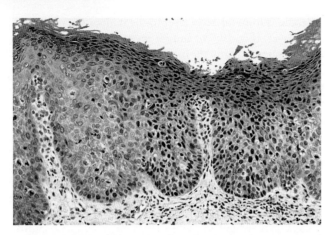

• **Fig. 10.75 Carcinoma *In Situ*.** Dysplastic changes extend throughout the entire thickness of the epithelium. Some authorities include carcinoma *in situ* within the category of severe epithelial dysplasia or high-grade dysplasia.

atrophic. Some authorities include carcinoma *in situ* within the category of severe epithelial dysplasia or high-grade dysplasia. Furthermore, some consider carcinoma *in situ* to be a precancerous lesion, whereas others believe that it represents a genuine malignancy discovered before invasion. Regardless, an important feature of carcinoma *in situ* is the absence of invasion, and without invasion, metastasis cannot occur. In this light, keratin pearl formation is rare in carcinoma *in situ* and may indicate focal invasive squamous cell carcinoma.

Proliferative verrucous leukoplakia exhibits microscopic features that vary by lesion stage. Early lesions may appear as relatively unremarkable hyperkeratoses that are indistinguishable from conventional leukoplakias. Such lesions typically lack cytologic atypia, but premature keratinization and sharply defined peripheral margins may be evident. With time, the condition progresses to form *corrugated hyperkeratotic lesions* with an architectural pattern marked by troughs/crests or undulation; alternatively, some lesions at this stage may be relatively flat with atrophic epithelium but disproportionate hyperkeratosis. Orthokeratosis usually predominates over parakeratosis. There is typically minimal to no cytologic atypia; abrupt transitions and "skip" lesions alternating between abnormal- and normal-appearing epithelium may be evident. Intermediate-stage disease is characterized by *bulky hyperkeratotic epithelial proliferation*. Such lesions exhibit a verrucous to papillary surface as well as exophytic and/or endophytic growth with broad, bulbous, and, at times, coalescing rete ridges. The total epithelial thickness may be many times greater than what is normally seen for a given oral subsite. All of the above stages may exhibit a secondary chronic inflammatory infiltrate within the superficial lamina propria; however, the presence of dysplasia (especially from an archictectural standpoint) should aid in avoiding misdiagnosis as lichen planus. Also, marked hyperorthokeratosis is a more frequent finding in proliferative verrucous leukoplakia compared to oral lichen planus. In the final stages, the epithelium becomes even more voluminous and proliferative; the lesions may develop into verrucous carcinoma, papillary squamous cell carcinoma, or frankly invasive conventional squamous cell carcinoma. Although characteristic disease stages have been described as above, individual lesions do not always progress in a stepwise manner through each stage. Overall, the diagnosis of PVL requires careful correlation of the variable clinical and microscopic findings.

Interestingly, investigators have identified a subset of oral epithelial dysplasias that harbor high-risk HPV (including HPV 16 and other types). Such lesions exhibit a predilection for the tongue and floor of mouth, and they tend to have distinctive microscopic features, including frequent apoptosis and karryorhexis. As per conventional grading criteria, the histopathologic findings often are compatible with high-grade dysplasia or carcinoma *in situ*; however, because there is a paucity of patient outcome data available at this time, some authorities advocate reporting these lesions as "HPV-associated dysplasia" without assigning a grade.

Treatment and Prognosis

The determination of management and prognosis for oral leukoplakia is guided by *histopathologic findings* (especially assessment and grading of oral epithelial dysplasia) as well as *clinical factors*. The identification of *biomarkers* predictive of malignant transformation risk represents an active area of research but remains investigational. The relevance of these factors with respect to treatment and prognosis are discussed in more detail below. Although several risk stratification models incorporating clinicopathologic parameters and/or molecular findings have been proposed, no single model has gained widespread acceptance, and further prospective clinical studies are needed.

Because leukoplakia represents a clinical term only, a biopsy is required to obtain a histopathologic diagnosis and to guide the appropriate management. Biopsies should be taken from the clinically most "severe" areas (with features toward the right of Fig. 10.69). Multiple biopsies may be needed for large or multifocal lesions.

Leukoplakia exhibiting moderate epithelial dysplasia or worse typically warrants complete destruction or removal, if feasible, and close clinical follow-up (e.g., at 1-, 3-, or 6-month intervals). Complete removal can be accomplished with equal effectiveness by surgical excision, electrocautery, cryosurgery, or laser ablation. An advantage of surgical excision is that it allows for optimal tissue preservation for histopathologic analysis, whereas the other methods may be preferable in some cases for limiting procedure-related morbidity.

The management of leukoplakia exhibiting less severe change may be guided by clinical surveillance, risk factor modification, and additional clinical factors. For example, leukoplakias with no or mild dysplasia and no adverse clinical factors (see below) often are managed conservatively by risk factor modification (e.g., tobacco counseling) and periodic clinical reevaluation (e.g., at 6- to 12-month intervals) rather than surgical excision. Some leukoplakias with no or minimal dysplasia may disappear or diminish in size within a few months after risk factor modification. However, if the clinical appearance of a lesion increases in severity over time, then additional biopsies may be performed. Also, for lesions with mild dysplasia plus adverse clinical predictors of outcome, surgical excision and/or short-interval clinical follow-up may be considered.

Clinical factors associated with an increased risk for malignant transformation of leukoplakia include female gender, older age, nonsmoking status, lesion persistence for several years, lesion size >200 mm², multifocal disease (e.g., proliferative verrucous leukoplakia), nonhomogeneous appearance, involvement of the ventrolateral tongue or floor of mouth, and a prior history of oral cancer. In particular, leukoplakias of the ventrolateral tongue and oral floor exhibit malignant transformation in 16%–39% of cases overall and in 47% of cases arising in females. Also, nonhomogeneous leukoplakia generally exhibits a greater risk for malignant transformation compared to homogeneous leukoplakia and warrants complete removal or destruction, if possible. According to one systematic review of observational studies, malignant transformation rates for nonhomogeneous and homogeneous lesions were 14.5% and 3%, respectively. Among nonhomogeneous leukoplakias, some studies have found cancer to develop in about 4%–15% of granular or verrucous lesions and 18%–47% of erythroleukoplakic lesions. In contrast, homogeneous thin leukoplakias seldom become malignant without demonstrating a clinical change, and malignant transformation occurs in only about 1%–7% of homogeneous thick leukoplakias. Notably, proliferative verrucous leukoplakia is associated with a very high risk for oral cancer development (>9% per year), and management is difficult. Patients with this condition typically are placed under close surveillance, with serial biopsies performed in an attempt to detect cancer development at an early stage.

Even after removal or apparent resolution of oral leukoplakia, reported overall recurrence rates range from 7% to 38%, and development of additional lesions is common. In particular, verruciform or granular leukoplakias exhibit an 83% recurrence rate and, thus, often undergo additional removal or destruction. There has been some disagreement in the literature regarding whether surgical excision of leukoplakia significantly reduces the risk for developing malignancy. Therefore, even after removal, long-term follow-up is extremely important.

Chemoprevention as an alternative treatment for oral leukoplakia remains experimental. Retinoid-based therapies (e.g., 13-*cis*-retinoic acid, vitamin A, beta-carotene alone or in combination with vitamin C) have reduced or eliminated some leukoplakic lesions in short-term studies. Toxic reactions to systemic retinoids are frequent, however, as is lesion recurrence after the conclusion of therapy. Additional potential chemopreventive agents of interest include nonsteroidal anti-inflammatory drugs (such as celecoxib and ketorolac), epidermal growth factor receptor (EGFR) inhibitors, immune checkpoint inhibitors, herbal extracts (such as green tea extract and freeze-dried black raspberry gel), and topical bleomycin. However, to date there is insufficient evidence to support the effectiveness of such medical therapies in preventing the progression of oral premalignant lesions to squamous cell carcinoma.

The transformation potential of oral leukoplakia is related closely to the degree of epithelial dysplasia present. According to one meta-analysis, the mean malignant progression rates for oral leukoplakia with mild/moderate dysplasia vs severe dysplasia/carcinoma *in situ* were approximately 10% and 24%, respectively. In addition, a population-based study of patients with oral leukoplakia reported overall hazard ratios of 4.9 for mild dysplasia vs 15.8 for severe dysplasia. Furthermore, a recent meta-analysis found a sixfold increased risk of malignant transformation for high-grade compared to low-grade oral epithelial dysplasia. Other large-scale studies of oral potentially malignant disorders have reported transformation rates of approximately 4%–12% for mild dysplasia, 9%–18% for moderate dysplasia, and 27%–39% for severe dysplasia. In the absence of oral epithelial dysplasia, the risk for malignant transformation is generally low but is not completely excluded.

Reported overall malignant transformation rates for oral leukoplakia vary, although most studies suggest rates in the range of about 1%–3% per year. Some of this variation may be due to patient selection bias, with lower rates typically reported among community-based than hospital-based studies. Additional confounding factors include variations in case definitions, statistical methodology, patient risk profiles, clinical management, and periods of observation. Typically, the latter extend for 5–10 years, but several studies have observed patients for more than 20 years. Carcinomatous transformation usually is noted 1–4 years after leukoplakia initially is identified, but it may occur within months or after decades.

An active area of investigation is the identification of chromosomal and molecular genetic alterations that may aid in predicting the risk of malignant transformation for oral leukoplakia. Cytogenetic studies have suggested that loss of heterozygosity (LOH) of chromosome arms 3p and 9p is associated with an increased risk of malignant transformation, and additional LOH at 4q, 8p, 11q, 13q, and 17p further increases this risk. A variable association with progression to malignancy has been reported for a host of other alterations—such as DNA aneuploidy, copy number variation, DNA methylation, microsatellite instability, increased or decreased levels of micro-RNAs, increased telomerase activity (important for cellular longevity), and changes in expression of various molecular markers (e.g., p53 and other regulators of apoptosis, p16 and other markers of cell cycle regulation, epidermal growth factor receptor [EGFR], Notch1, matrix metalloproteinases, vascular endothelial growth factor, podoplanin, regulators of DNA damage repair, stem cell markers). Interestingly, some investigators have noted an increased risk for cancer development among oral premalignant lesions with a "classical" profile (including LOH at 3p14 and 17p13 [the latter locus including *TP53*]) or an "immunological" profile (including downregulation of a certain micro-RNA type and decreased infiltration by T cells, monocytes, and myeloid dendritic cells). Moreover, differences in transcriptome profiles for dysplastic vs nondysplastic oral leukoplakias have been identified, and an intermediate group of hyperkeratoses without conventional dysplastic histomorphology but exhibiting some genomic or transcriptomic similarities to dysplastic lesions has been noted. Despite recent advances in biomarker research and molecular profiling for patients with oral leukoplakia, the standard method for predicting the risk of progression to malignancy remains histopathologic grading of oral epithelial dysplasia, along with consideration of clinical factors.

◆ ERYTHROPLAKIA (ERYTHROPLASIA; ERYTHROPLASIA OF QUEYRAT)

Similar to leukoplakia, **erythroplakia** is defined as a red patch that cannot be characterized clinically or pathologically as any other definable lesion. Queyrat originally used the term *erythroplasia* to describe a precancerous red lesion on the penis. Oral erythroplakia is clinically and histopathologically similar to the genital process. Almost all true erythroplakias demonstrate significant epithelial dysplasia, carcinoma *in situ,* or invasive squamous cell carcinoma. The causes of erythroplakia are presumed to be the same as those associated with oral squamous cell carcinoma (see page 402). The estimated point prevalence rate (number of persons with active lesions at a given point in time) of oral erythroplakia is 1 per 2500 adults, and the reported prevalence among several large-scale epidemiologic surveys— many of which were conducted in Asia and the United States—ranges from 0.01% to 0.83%.

Erythroplakia also may occur in conjunction with leukoplakia (see page 381) and has been found concurrently with a large proportion of early invasive oral carcinomas. Although erythroplakia is less common than leukoplakia, it is associated with a much greater risk for malignancy.

Clinical Features

Erythroplakia is predominantly a disease of middle-aged to older adults with no significant gender predilection. In the United States, a peak prevalence among individuals 65–74 years old has been reported. In India, the peak prevalence is in a somewhat younger age range of 45–54 years. The floor of mouth, tongue, soft palate, and buccal mucosa are among the most frequently described sites of involvement, and multiple lesions may be present.

The lesion typically appears as a well-demarcated, erythematous patch or plaque with a soft, velvety, or granular texture (Figs. 10.76 and 10.77). It is usually asymptomatic and may be associated with an adjacent leukoplakia (**erythroleukoplakia**). Some lesions may be somewhat depressed compared to the surrounding mucosa. Biopsy typically is required to distinguish erythroplakia from other conditions with a similar clinical appearance, such as nonspecific mucositis, candidiasis, psoriasis, or vascular lesions.

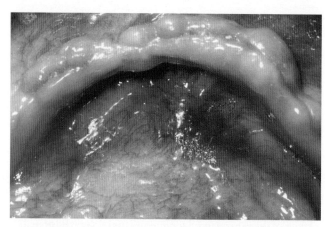

• **Fig. 10.76 Erythroplakia.** Erythematous macule on the right floor of the mouth. Biopsy showed early invasive squamous cell carcinoma.

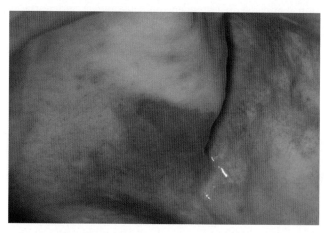

• **Fig. 10.77 Erythroplakia.** Well-circumscribed red patch on the posterior lateral hard and soft palate. (From Neville BW, Chi AC, Jeter M: Diagnostic challenge: a red lesion on the palate, *J Am Dent Assoc* 137:1537–1538, 2006.)

Histopathologic Features

In the majority of cases, histopathologic examination exhibits severe epithelial dysplasia (see page 385), carcinoma *in situ* (see page 387), or superficially invasive squamous cell carcinoma (see page 416). The epithelium lacks keratin production and often is atrophic, thereby allowing the underlying microvasculature to show through and produce a red appearance. The underlying connective tissue frequently demonstrates chronic inflammation.

Treatment and Prognosis

Red lesions of the oral mucosa, especially those of the oral floor and ventrolateral tongue, should be viewed with suspicion, and a biopsy should be performed. If a source of irritation can be identified and removed, then biopsy may be delayed for 2 weeks to allow a clinically similar inflammatory lesion time to regress.

As with leukoplakia, the treatment of erythroplakia is guided by the histopathologic diagnosis. Moderate dysplasia or worse typically warrants complete excision or destruction (see treatment methods for leukoplakia on page 388). Excision often is preferred, because it allows for microscopic examination to rule out invasive carcinoma. Recurrence and multifocal involvement are common; hence, long-term follow-up is suggested.

◆ SMOKELESS TOBACCO USE AND SMOKELESS TOBACCO KERATOSIS (SNUFF POUCH; SNUFF DIPPER'S LESION; TOBACCO POUCH KERATOSIS; SPIT TOBACCO KERATOSIS)

The three main types of smokeless tobacco used in the United States include chewing tobacco, dry snuff, and moist snuff. The latter is most popular, accounting for approximately 90% of smokeless tobacco sales nationwide. Chewing tobacco often is used by men in conjunction with outdoor activities, and dry snuff is used primarily by women in the southern United States. Smokeless tobacco users frequently develop the habit during adolescence.

According to the 2020 National Health Interview Survey, approximately 2.3% of adults (or 5.7 million individuals 18 years and older) in the United States use smokeless tobacco. The highest prevalence rates are seen in some Southeastern and Midwestern states. In recent years, smokeless tobacco consumption in the United States has been declining. This trend in part may reflect the impact of an increasingly diverse tobacco product marketplace (including the introduction of electronic cigarettes as another popular mode of nicotine delivery).

Although the present discussion focuses on major types of smokeless tobacco in the United States and other Western nations, various other forms are found around the world. For example, in India and other Asian countries, smokeless tobacco may be combined in a quid, composed of areca nut, slaked lime, and other ingredients wrapped in a betel leaf. Oral lesions associated with betel quid use are described separately (see page 393). In addition, in parts of Africa and the Middle East, many individuals use varieties of snuff known as toombak (tobacco with sodium bicarbonate) and shammah (tobacco with ash and lime).

Clinical Features

Several health and addiction hazards may be associated with smokeless tobacco use because of the ready absorption of nicotine and other molecules through the oral mucosa. A variety of local oral alterations also are found in chronic users. One of the most common local changes is painless gingival recession in the area of tobacco contact (Fig. 10.78), at times accompanied by destruction of the underlying facial alveolar bone. The severity of the defect correlates with the quantity and duration of smokeless tobacco use. Although the association between smokeless tobacco and gingival recession is well known, there is some variability across studies regarding

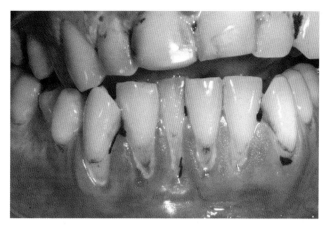

• **Fig. 10.78 Smokeless Tobacco–related Gingival Recession.** Extensive recession of the anterior mandibular facial gingiva.

the association between smokeless tobacco and periodontal bone loss. Researchers have suggested that this variability may be related to the specific type of smokeless tobacco used or confounding by concurrent cigarette smoking.

Dental caries also has been reported to be more prevalent in smokeless tobacco users, perhaps because of the high sugar content of some brands; other reports dispute caries susceptibility. Long-term use may lead to localized or generalized wear of occlusal and incisal surfaces, especially in those using the product in dusty environments. A brown-black extrinsic tobacco stain typically is found on the tooth surfaces adjacent to the tobacco. In addition, halitosis is a frequent finding.

Smokeless tobacco keratosis represents a characteristic white or gray plaque involving the mucosa in direct contact with snuff or chewing tobacco. In Western cultures, it affects 15% of chewing tobacco users and 60% of snuff users, if mild examples are included. Lesion development is influenced most strongly by habit duration and also by the brand of tobacco used, early onset of smokeless tobacco use, total hours of daily use, amount of tobacco consumed daily, and number of sites routinely used for tobacco placement. In Western populations, smokeless tobacco keratosis most often is noted in young adult men and men older than 65 years of age; however, in some subpopulations the prevalence is greatest among older women. Individual lesions begin to develop shortly after heavy tobacco use begins, and new lesions seldom arise in persons with a long history of use.

The altered mucosa typically is thin and almost translucent, with an indistinct border (Fig. 10.79). Sometimes mild peripheral erythema is present. Upon palpation, the lesion may feel soft and velvety. Stretching of the mucosa often reveals a distinct "pouch" (**snuff pouch, tobacco pouch**) caused by flaccidity in the area of chronic tobacco placement. The mucosa appears fissured or rippled, in a fashion resembling the sand on a beach after an ebbing tide. Similar alterations can occur when other bulky materials (e.g., hard candy, sunflower seeds, and beef jerky) are held chronically in the vestibule. Induration, ulceration, and pain are not associated with this lesion.

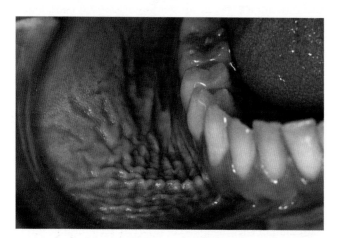

• **Fig. 10.79 Tobacco Pouch Keratosis, Mild.** A soft, fissured, gray-white lesion of the lower labial mucosa located in the area of chronic snuff placement. The gingival melanosis is racial pigmentation and not associated with the keratosis.

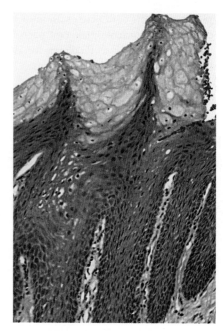

• **Fig. 10.81 Tobacco Pouch Keratosis.** Epithelium exhibiting acanthosis, hyperparakeratosis, and "chevron" formation.

• **Fig. 10.80 Tobacco Pouch Keratosis, Severe.** A somewhat leathery, white, fissured plaque of the right mandibular vestibule, which was located in the area of chronic chewing tobacco placement.

Smokeless tobacco keratosis usually takes 1–5 years to develop. Once it occurs, however, the keratosis typically remains unchanged indefinitely unless the daily tobacco contact time is altered. In some cases, the lesion gradually becomes thickened to the point of appearing leathery or nodular (Fig. 10.80).

Histopathologic Features

The histopathologic appearance of smokeless tobacco keratosis is not specific. The squamous epithelium is hyperkeratotic and acanthotic, with or without intracellular vacuolization or "edema" of glycogen-rich superficial cells. Parakeratin **chevrons** may be seen as pointed projections above or within superficial epithelial layers (Fig. 10.81. Increased subepithelial vascularity and vessel engorgement often are observed. In some cases, an unusual deposition of amorphous eosinophilic material is noted within the subjacent connective tissue and salivary glands (Fig. 10.82). Epithelial dysplasia is uncommon in smokeless tobacco keratosis and, when

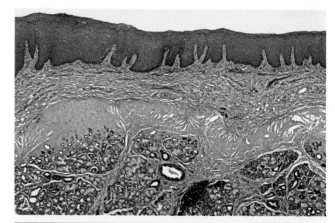

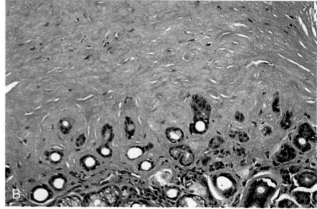

• **Fig. 10.82 Tobacco Pouch Keratosis. A,** Low-power view showing mild hyperkeratosis and acanthosis. Note linear deposition of amorphous, eosinophilic material in the lamina propria above the minor salivary glands. **B,** Higher-power view of the amorphous material.

present, is typically mild. Occasionally, however, significant dysplasia or squamous cell carcinoma may develop.

Treatment and Prognosis

Tobacco counseling should be provided. Biopsy is indicated for lesions with atypical findings (i.e., a granular or verruciform clinical appearance, ulceration, mass formation, induration, or hemorrhage) or intense whiteness. For lesions that are not atypical or intensely white, habit cessation leads to a normal mucosal appearance (usually within 2 weeks) in 98% of cases (Fig. 10.83). For patients unable to cease the habit, switching to a different tobacco-chewing site may be an alternative approach but may result in epithelial alteration or gingival and periodontal difficulties in two sites rather than one. A lesion that remains after 2 weeks without smokeless tobacco contact should be biopsied. Management depends on the histopathologic findings. Keratoses without dysplasia or malignancy may require only continued monitoring and tobacco cessation. Treatment considerations for patients with oral epithelial dysplasia or squamous cell carcinoma are discussed elsewhere (see pages 388 and 418).

Chronic use of smokeless tobacco in the United States is considered to be carcinogenic, although the risk is less than that associated with cigarette smoking and alcohol abuse. Squamous cell carcinoma (see page 391) related to smokeless tobacco use typically develops after a latency period of several decades. Most such cases represent conventional squamous cell carcinoma, although an uncommon low-grade variant known as **verrucous carcinoma ("snuff dipper's" cancer)** (see page 421) also is possible. In the United States, a pooled analysis of data from National Health Interview Surveys reported an association between current smokeless tobacco use and oral cavity cancer (approximate hazard ratio = 9) among individuals who had never used other forms of tobacco. In addition, case-control studies performed in the United States and Western Europe have noted lower risk associated with chewing tobacco and moist snuff and higher

risk associated with dry snuff. In particular, many of the early reports of malignant transformation described lesions among female dry snuff users in the southern United States. Studies from Sweden, however, have failed to show an increased oral cancer risk for users of Swedish moist snuff (also known as *snus*).

◆ ORAL SUBMUCOUS FIBROSIS

Oral submucous fibrosis is an oral potentially malignant disorder characterized by chronic, progressive scarring of the oral mucosa. The condition has an estimated global prevalence of approximately 5% and is seen primarily in the Indian subcontinent, Southeast Asia, Taiwan, southern China, Polynesia, and Micronesia. Cases among Asian communities in North America, Europe, and Africa also have been reported.

The etiology is linked to the use of betel quid (*paan*) and related products—a habit among up to 20% of the world's population. The quid consists of a betel leaf wrapped around a mixture of areca nut (from the *Areca catechu* palm tree), slaked lime, possibly tobacco, and sometimes sweeteners and spices. The slaked lime releases alkaloids from the areca nut to produce a feeling of euphoria in the user. Villagers habitually chew betel quid from an early age, frequently for 16–24 hours daily.

The annual incidence of oral submucous fibrosis has been increasing—especially among young persons—due to the growing popularity of commercially freeze-dried betel quid substitutes (such as, *pan masala, gutkha,* and *mawa*), conveniently packaged in portable sachets. These products contain a higher concentration of areca nut and may cause oral submucous fibrosis more rapidly than conventionally prepared betel quid.

The fibrosis appears to be induced by areca nut, whereas the epithelial alterations and carcinogenesis appear to result mainly from tobacco. However, several studies suggest that even betel quid without tobacco may be carcinogenic, albeit probably less so than when combined with tobacco. Nutritional deficiency increases the risk and severity of fibrosis.

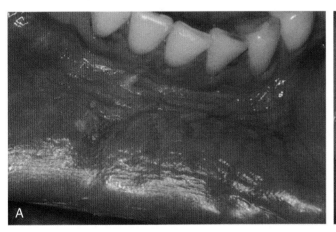 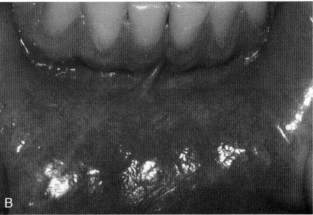

• **Fig. 10.83 Tobacco Pouch Keratosis. A,** Moderately severe lesion of the lower anterior vestibule and lip in a 15-year-old male. There is a gray-white, fissured surface. The patient had placed snuff in the area for several years. **B,** Two weeks after cessation of the tobacco habit, the mucosa returned to an almost normal appearance.

Furthermore, an underlying genetic predisposition has been proposed based on associations with certain human leukocyte antigen (HLA) types and various genetic polymorphisms, as well as the fact that only a small subset of betel quid or areca nut chewers develop this condition. Autoimmunity and other immunologic factors may contribute to disease development as well.

The pathogenesis of oral submucous fibrosis is hypothesized to involve the disruption of collagen metabolism by components of the areca nut. Alkaloids (especially arecoline) and polyphenols induce various downstream effects, including increased fibroblast proliferation, increased collagen production, and decreased collagen degradation. Arecoline also may suppress or damage endothelial cells, resulting in a loss of vascularity. In addition, there are considerable amounts of copper in areca nut products. Copper upregulates lysyl oxidase, which is an enzyme involved in collagen cross-linking; this process renders collagen fibrils resistant to degradation by collagenase. Various cytokines and growth factors may promote fibrosis as well.

Clinical Features

Oral submucous fibrosis often manifests in young adult users of betel quid or related areca nut products. Reported gender predilection varies by population. Typical chief complaints include an inability to open the mouth (**trismus**) and a generalized oral burning sensation (**stomatopyrosis**) with intolerance to spicy foods. An interincisal distance of less than 20 mm is considered severe; in advanced cases, the jaws may be inseparable.

Vesicles, petechiae, melanosis, xerostomia, and stomatopyrosis are usually the first signs and symptoms. The buccal mucosa, retromolar area, and soft palate are the most commonly affected sites. Subsequently, the mucosa develops a blotchy, marblelike pallor and progressive stiffness (Fig. 10.84). The tongue may become immobile, diminished in size, and devoid of papillae. Submucosal fibrous bands are palpable on the buccal mucosa, soft palate, and labial mucosa of fully developed cases. Involvement may extend to include the pharynx, larynx, and upper esophagus. **Leukoplakia** of the surface mucosa often is noted as well (see page 381).

Betel quid chewers also may exhibit a brown-red discoloration of the mucosa with an irregular surface that tends to desquamate. This particular change, known as **betel chewer's mucosa,** is not believed to be precancerous. In addition, some authors have reported **betel quid lichenoid lesions,** characterized by white, parallel, wavy striae resembling oral lichen planus (see page 787). Other possible sequelae include tooth staining, attrition, and periodontal disease.

Histopathologic Features

Oral submucous fibrosis is characterized by juxtaepithelial and submucosal deposition of densely collagenized connective tissue with variable numbers of chronic inflammatory cells (Fig. 10.85). In addition, early lesions may exhibit epithelial hyperplasia, hyperkeratosis, and dilated vessels, whereas more advanced lesions demonstrate epithelial atrophy and hypovascularity with constricted or occluded vessels. Epithelial dysplasia is found in about 10%–15% of cases submitted for biopsy, and carcinoma is found in at least 6% of sampled cases.

Betel chewer's mucosa appears histopathologically similar to morsicatio buccarum (see page 272), except the ragged keratinaceous surface is covered by encrusted betel quid ingredients.

Treatment and Prognosis

Unlike tobacco pouch keratosis, oral submucous fibrosis does not regress with habit cessation. Mild cases may be treated with intralesional corticosteroids to reduce symptoms and limit progression. Moderate to severe cases may require surgical excision or release of the fibrous bands, followed by lifelong physiotherapy; however, relapse is common. There is limited evidence for various alternative treatments, such as intralesional injection of interferon-gamma; topical or intralesional proteolytics (e.g., collagenase, hyaluronidase, chymotrypsin, papain); human placental extract; vitamins and

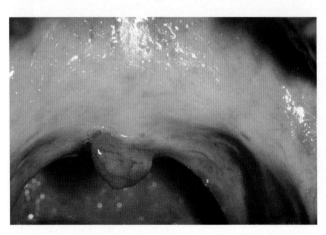

• **Fig. 10.84 Oral Submucous Fibrosis.** Pallor and fibrosis of the soft palate in a betel quid chewer. The uvula has retained its normal color.

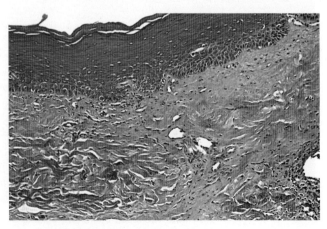

• **Fig. 10.85 Oral Submucous Fibrosis.** Mucosal biopsy exhibiting hyperparakeratosis, basilar hyperplasia, and fibrosis in the lamina propria.

minerals; antioxidants (e.g., lycopene); levamisole; vasodilators (e.g., pentoxifylline); and ayurvedic remedies (e.g., turmeric).

Frequent evaluation for development of oral squamous cell carcinoma is essential. Reported malignant transformation rates vary considerably (approximately 1%–23%), likely due to differences in study design and patient cohorts. However, according to recent meta-analyses and systematic reviews of the literature, approximately 4%–6% of patients with oral submucous fibrosis develop oral cancer, with an estimated annual malignant transformation rate of 0.73%–0.98%.

◆ ACTINIC CHEILOSIS (ACTINIC CHEILITIS; SOLAR CHEILOSIS)

Actinic cheilosis is a common premalignant alteration of the lower lip vermilion that results from chronic UV light exposure. Its etiopathogenesis is similar to that of **actinic keratosis** of the skin (see next topic). The incidence of actinic cheilosis increases with proximity to the equator, and there is a predilection among middle-aged to elderly, fair-complexioned men. Outdoor occupations are associated with this condition, leading to popular terms, such as *farmer's lip* and *sailor's lip*. In addition, there is increased susceptibility among patients with certain genetic disorders (e.g., xeroderma pigmentosum, albinism, and porphyria cutanea tarda). Furthermore, cofactors—such as immunosuppression and tobacco smoking—may increase the likelihood of progression to squamous cell carcinoma.

Clinical Features

Actinic cheilosis seldom occurs in persons younger than 45 years. There is a strong male predilection (reported male-to-female ratio as high as 10:1), which may reflect more outdoor occupational activity and less frequent use of lip protective agents among men compared to women.

The lesion develops so slowly that patients often are unaware of a change. Early clinical findings include atrophy (characterized by smooth, blotchy, pale areas), dryness, and fissures of the lower lip vermilion, with blurring of the margin between the vermilion and the adjacent skin. As the lesion progresses, rough, scaly areas develop on the drier portions of the vermilion. These areas may assume a leukoplakic appearance, especially when they extend near the wet line of the lip (Fig. 10.86). The patient may peel off the scale with some difficulty, only to see it reform within a few days.

Eventually, chronic ulceration may develop (Fig. 10.87). Such ulcerations may last for months and suggest progression to squamous cell carcinoma (Fig. 10.88).

Histopathologic Features

The surface epithelium exhibits varying degrees of dysplasia. There is usually hyperkeratosis, and the epithelium may be either atrophic or acanthotic. The underlying connective

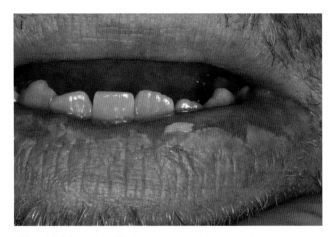

• **Fig. 10.86 Actinic Cheilosis.** Diffuse, irregular white plaque at the wet line of the lower lip vermilion.

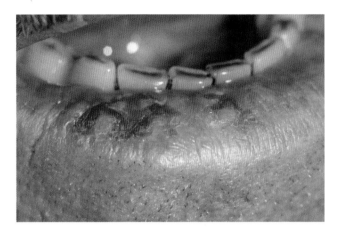

• **Fig. 10.87 Actinic Cheilosis.** Crusted and ulcerated lesions of the lower lip vermilion.

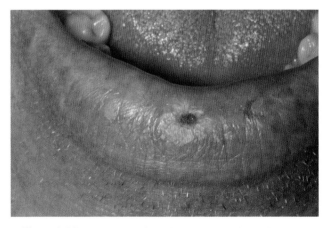

• **Fig. 10.88 Squamous Cell Carcinoma Arising in Actinic Cheilosis.** Patient with actinic cheilosis of the lower lip, who developed a small, chronic ulceration. Biopsy revealed early invasive squamous cell carcinoma.

tissue invariably demonstrates a band of amorphous, acellular, basophilic change known as **solar elastosis**, an UV light–induced alteration of collagen and elastic fibers (Fig. 10.89). A chronic inflammatory cell infiltrate and dilated blood vessels may be present as well.

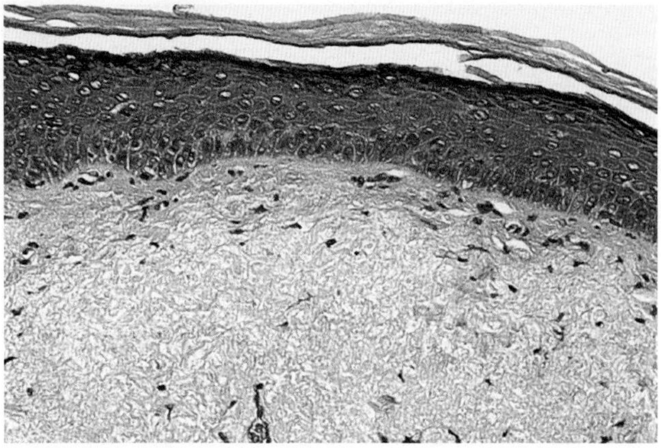

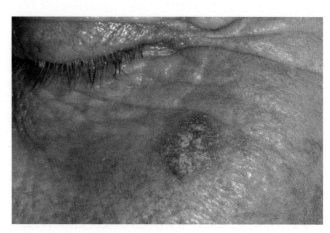

• **Fig. 10.89 Actinic Cheilosis.** Hyperorthokeratosis and epithelial atrophy. Note the striking underlying solar elastosis.

• **Fig. 10.90 Actinic Keratosis.** A plaque of the skin of the face with a rough, sandpaper-like surface.

Treatment and Prognosis

Many of the changes associated with actinic cheilosis are probably irreversible, but patients should be encouraged to reduce sun exposure, wear a wide-brimmed hat, and use sunscreen to prevent further damage. Areas of induration, thickening, ulceration, or leukoplakia should be submitted for biopsy to rule out carcinoma. In clinically severe cases without obvious malignant transformation, a lip shave procedure **(vermilionectomy)** may be performed. The vermilion mucosa is removed, and either a portion of the intraoral labial mucosa is pulled forward or the wound is allowed to heal by secondary intention. The advantage of this technique is that it provides tissue for histopathologic examination should areas of superficially invasive squamous cell carcinoma be present. Alternative treatments include CO_2 or erbium: YAG (Er:YAG) laser ablation, electrodesiccation, cryotherapy, 5-fluorouracil, topical imiquimod, topical diclofenac, and photodynamic therapy. Long-term follow-up is recommended. Of course, if a squamous cell carcinoma is identified, then the involved lip is treated accordingly.

The malignant transformation rate of actinic cheilosis is difficult to determine because of the lack of high-quality follow-up studies. However, it is estimated that actinic cheilosis more than doubles an individual's risk for developing squamous cell carcinoma of the lip. Also, the risk of malignant transformation is approximately 2.5 times greater for actinic cheilosis compared to actinic keratosis. However, it typically takes several decades for actinic cheilosis to transform into squamous cell carcinoma, and the resulting carcinoma usually is histopathologically well differentiated.

◆ ACTINIC KERATOSIS (SOLAR KERATOSIS)

Actinic keratosis is a common, cutaneous premalignant lesion that is caused by chronic, high-level exposure to UV radiation. A similar phenomenon, **actinic cheilosis,** is associated with sun damage to the lower lip vermilion (see previous section). UV light exposure can produce mutations in various genes, such as the tumor suppressor gene *TP53*.

Additional risk factors for actinic keratosis include fair skin, old age, severe male baldness, immunosuppression, arsenic exposure, and certain genetic abnormalities (e.g., albinism, Rothmund-Thompson syndrome, Cockayne syndrome, xeroderma pigmentosum [see page 753], and Bloom syndrome). Recent genomic analysis suggests associations with mutations in the *IRF4, MC1R,* and *TYR* genes, which have functions related to pigmentation and carcinogenesis. Furthermore, recent studies suggest that HPV infection may be a cofactor in some cases, especially those arising in immunosuppressed individuals.

Actinic keratosis affects more than 50% of white adults with significant lifetime sun exposure. In the United States, reported prevalence rates range from 14% to 27% for men and 6% to 10% for women. According to the National Ambulatory Medical Care Survey, more than 47 million physician office visits were conducted in the United States over a 10-year period for the diagnosis of actinic keratosis. Another study reported that actinic keratosis accounts for more than 5 million physician office visits per year in the United States.

Clinical Features

Actinic keratosis seldom occurs in persons younger than 40 years. Common sites of involvement include the face, neck, dorsum of the hands, forearms, and balding scalp. The lesions most often occur in clusters (apparently due to UV-induced *field cancerization* [see page 421]), although solitary lesions also are possible. Many patients are asymptomatic, but tenderness, pain, or pruritus is possible. The lesions appear as irregular, scaly plaques, which range in color from normal to white, gray, or brown, and may be superimposed on an erythematous background (Fig. 10.90). The keratotic scale peels off with varying degrees of difficulty. Palpation reveals a rough, "sandpaper-like" texture, and some lesions can be felt more easily than they can be seen. Each lesion typically is smaller than 7 mm in diameter, but some lesions may reach a size of 2 cm or more. Most lesions are minimally elevated above the skin surface, although occasional lesions

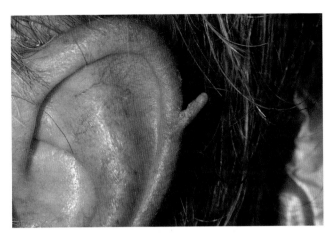

• **Fig. 10.91 Actinic Keratosis.** Skin lesion involving the helix of the ear. This example exhibits a prominent surface projection, termed a *cutaneous horn*, which results from an accumulation of keratin.

produce so much keratin that a central **cutaneous horn** (or **keratin horn**) may be evident (Fig. 10.91). Other skin lesions, such as verruca vulgaris or seborrheic keratosis, also may produce cutaneous horns.

Histopathologic Features

Histopathologically, actinic keratosis is characterized by hyperparakeratosis and acanthosis (Fig. 10.92). The epithelium often exhibits teardrop-shaped rete ridges, and by definition, some degree of epithelial dysplasia is present. When full-thickness dysplasia is noted, this is termed **bowenoid actinic keratosis.** Suprabasilar acantholysis may be seen, as well as melanosis and a lichenoid inflammatory infiltrate. The dermis exhibits a pale, basophilic band of sun-damaged collagen and elastic fibers **(solar elastosis).** In this band of sun-damaged connective tissue, there is a fourfold increase in the amount of elastic fibers, and band thickness increases with further exposure to actinic rays. Variable numbers of chronic inflammatory cells are typically present.

Treatment and Prognosis

Preventive measures include avoiding sun exposure, wearing protective clothing, and using sunscreen. Although studies suggest that more than half of actinic keratoses regress spontaneously, treatment is recommended because of the lesion's precancerous nature. For solitary lesions, the most common treatment is cryotherapy; additional treatment options include curettage, electrodesiccation, surgical excision, and laser therapy. Multifocal lesions or sun-damaged skin fields at risk for lesion development may be treated with topical agents (e.g., 5-fluorouracil, imiquimod, diclofenac, retinoids, and ingenol mebutate), chemical peels, laser therapy, or photodynamic therapy. Alternatively, cryotherapy may be combined with broader application of topical agents. Recurrence is rare, but fields of adjacent sun-damaged skin are at risk for development of cancer or additional actinic keratoses. Long-term follow-up, therefore, is recommended.

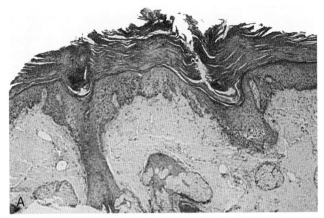

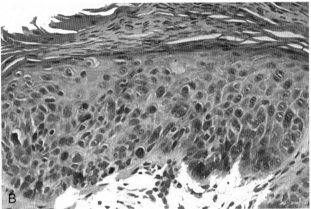

• **Fig. 10.92 Actinic Keratosis. A,** An extremely excessive amount of parakeratin is noted on the epidermal surface. **B,** High-power view showing hyperchromatism and pleomorphism of the epidermal cells.

The estimated malignant transformation rate for an individual lesion varies considerably (0.025%–16% per year) but generally is considered low. However, the risk increases significantly for a patient with a large number of lesions over an extended period. Longitudinal studies of larger patient groups suggest that malignancy develops on average within 2 years, and spontaneous regression may occur in about 20% of lesions within 12 months.

◆ NICOTINE STOMATITIS (NICOTINE PALATINUS; SMOKER'S PALATE)

Once a common mucosal change of the hard palate, **nicotine stomatitis** has become less common because cigar and pipe smoking have lost popularity. Although this hyperkeratotic lesion is associated with tobacco smoking, it does not appear to have a premalignant nature, perhaps because it develops in response to heat rather than the chemicals in tobacco smoke. In particular, pipe smoking appears to generate more heat on the palate than other forms of smoking. Similar changes also can be produced by the long-term use of extremely hot beverages. In addition, recent reports have suggested a potential association with electronic cigarette use.

In some South American and Asian cultures, hand-rolled cigarettes and cigars are smoked with the lit end held within

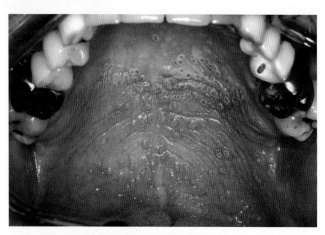

• **Fig. 10.93 Nicotine Stomatitis.** Palatal mucosa showing white change and numerous scattered papules with red punctate centers.

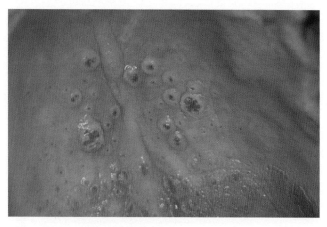

• **Fig. 10.94 Nicotine Stomatitis.** Close-up of the inflamed ductal openings of involved salivary glands of the hard palate. Note the white keratotic ring at the lip of many of the inflamed ducts.

the mouth. This "reverse smoking" habit produces a pronounced palatal keratosis, or **reverse smoker's palate,** which has a significant potential to develop dysplasia or carcinoma.

Clinical Features

Nicotine stomatitis most commonly affects men older than 45 years. With long-term exposure to heat, the palatal mucosa becomes diffusely gray or white; numerous slightly elevated papules are noted, usually with punctate red centers (Figs. 10.93 and 10.94). Such papules represent inflamed minor salivary glands and their ductal orifices.

The palatal keratin may become so thickened that a fissured or "dried mud" appearance is imparted. The whiteness also may involve the marginal gingiva and interdental papillae, and hyperkeratosis of the buccal mucosa occasionally is seen. A heavy brown or black tobacco stain may be present on the teeth.

Histopathologic Features

Nicotine stomatitis is characterized by hyperkeratosis and acanthosis of the palatal epithelium and mild, patchy, chronic inflammation of subepithelial connective tissue and mucous glands (Fig. 10.95). Squamous metaplasia of the excretory ducts is usually seen, and an inflammatory exudate may be noted within the duct lumina. In cases with papular elevation, hyperplastic ductal epithelium may be seen near the orifice. The degree of epithelial hyperplasia and hyperkeratosis appears to correlate positively with the duration and the level of heat exposure. Epithelial dysplasia rarely is seen.

Treatment and Prognosis

Nicotine stomatitis is completely reversible, even when it has been present for many decades. The palate usually returns to normal within 1–2 weeks of smoking cessation. Although this lesion is not precancerous and does not require treatment, the patient nevertheless should be encouraged to stop

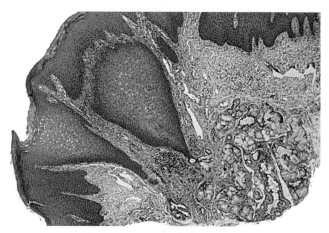

• **Fig. 10.95 Nicotine Stomatitis.** There is hyperkeratosis and acanthosis of the palatal epithelium. Note the squamous metaplasia of the minor salivary gland ducts.

smoking (and other high-risk areas should be examined closely). Any white lesion of the palatal mucosa that persists after 1 month of habit cessation should be considered a true leukoplakia and managed accordingly (see page 388).

◆ KERATOACANTHOMA ("SELF-HEALING" CARCINOMA; PSEUDOCARCINOMA; KERATOCARCINOMA; SQUAMOUS CELL CARCINOMA, KERATOACANTHOMA TYPE)

Keratoacanthoma is a self-limiting, epithelial proliferation with a strong clinical and histopathologic similarity to well-differentiated **squamous cell carcinoma.** Indeed, many dermatopathologists consider it to represent an extremely well-differentiated squamous cell carcinoma. Cutaneous lesions presumably arise from the epithelium of hair follicles. Intraoral lesions have been reported, but they are rare; in fact, some authorities do not accept keratoacanthoma as an intraoral disease.

Ultraviolet light exposure appears to be a major risk factor, with most solitary lesions arising on sun-exposed skin in older adults. Additional potential contributing factors include x-irradiation, tar exposure, immunosuppression, certain drugs (such as, *BRAF* inhibitors, hedgehog pathway inhibitors, and PD-1 inhibitors), foreign materials (such as, tattoos and cosmetic fillers), trauma (such as, burns and surgical procedures), other skin conditions (such as, lichen planus and psoriasis), and HPV or human polyomavirus 6 infection. Keratoacanthoma-like lesions have been produced in animals by the cutaneous application of carcinogens.

There appears to be a hereditary predisposition for multiple lesions, and the lesions occur with increased frequency in certain heritable conditions attributed to defects in DNA repair, including **Muir-Torre syndrome** (sebaceous neoplasms, keratoacanthomas, and gastrointestinal carcinomas) and **xeroderma pigmentosum** (see page 753).

Various underlying pathogenetic mechanisms have been proposed, including alterations in Wnt signaling, expression of cyclin-dependent kinase inhibitor p27, activation of the MAP kinase pathway, and *HRAS* mutations. Several studies have shown that keratoacanthomas and squamous cell carcinomas typically exhibit distinct genetic profiles.

Clinical Features

Keratoacanthoma shows a male predilection, with a peak between the ages of 65 and 71 years. Almost 95% of solitary lesions involve sun-exposed skin, and 8% of all cases involve the outer edge of the vermilion border of the lips, with equal frequency on the upper and lower lips.

Keratoacanthoma appears as a firm, well-demarcated, sessile, dome-shaped nodule with a central plug of keratin (Figs. 10.96 and 10.97), although lesions reported as intraoral keratoacanthoma usually have lacked a central plug. The outer portion of the nodule typically has a normal texture and color but may be erythematous. The central keratin plug is yellowish, brown, or black and has an irregular,

crusted, often verruciform surface. Most lesions are asymptomatic, although pruritus and mild tenderness are possible.

The evolution of keratoacanthoma can be divided into three phases: (1) growth phase, (2) stationary phase, and (3) involution phase. During the growth phase, rapid enlargement is typical, with the lesion usually attaining a diameter of 1–2 cm within 6 weeks (Fig. 10.98). This critical feature helps to distinguish it from the more slowly enlarging squamous cell carcinoma. The lesion stabilizes during the stationary phase, which usually is of similar duration as the growth phase. Most lesions regress spontaneously within 6–12 months of onset, frequently leaving behind a depressed scar. The regression of keratoacanthomas is a curious phenomenon, which some investigators have theorized is related to a cytotoxic immune response to the tumor or inactivation of the Wnt signaling pathway. Some authors also have described a subset of lesions (termed *abortive keratoacanthoma*) that involute after only 4–6 weeks.

Several other variants exist, including *giant keratoacanthoma* (greater than 2–3 cm in diameter), *keratoacanthoma centrifugum marginatum* (characterized by continuous peripheral growth and central scarring), *subungual keratoacanthoma* (involving the nail bed), and *mucosal keratoacanthoma* (involving the oral, nasal, genital, ocular, or other regions). These variants often do not regress.

In addition, early onset of multiple keratoacanthomas has been described in association with two rare, heritable conditions: **Ferguson-Smith syndrome (multiple self-healing squamous epitheliomas)** and **Witten-Zak syndrome**. The former is characterized by nodular lesions and primarily affects patients of Scottish descent; the latter typically exhibits a mixture of variably sized lesions. In contrast, the nonhereditary **Grzybowski syndrome (generalized eruptive keratoacanthomas)** manifests later in life as hundreds or thousands of small, pruritic papules of the skin and upper digestive tract and may be associated with internal malignancy.

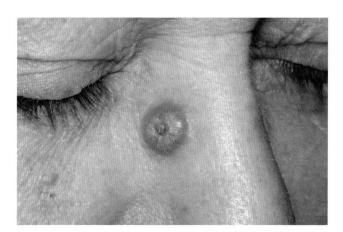

• **Fig. 10.96 Keratoacanthoma.** A nontender, well-demarcated nodule of the skin of the nose in an older woman. The nodule demonstrates a central keratin plug.

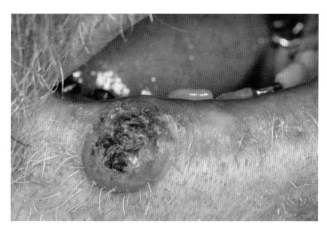

• **Fig. 10.97 Keratoacanthoma.** This lesion, which is located at the outer edge of the vermilion border of the lip, demonstrates a prominent core or plug of keratin.

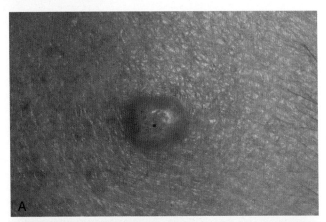

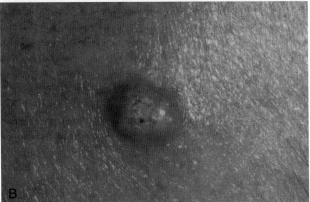

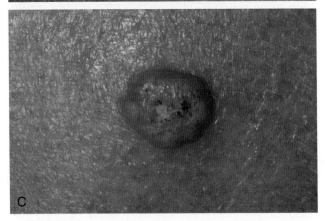

• **Fig. 10.98 Keratoacanthoma. A,** Appearance on initial presentation. Note small, central keratin-filled invagination. **B,** Same lesion 1 week later showing slight enlargement. **C,** Same lesion showing further growth 3 weeks after initial presentation. All three photographs were taken at the same magnification. (Courtesy of Dr. John Lovas.)

Histopathologic Features

Because the overall architectural pattern is crucial for the diagnosis of keratoacanthoma, excisional or large incisional biopsy with inclusion of adjacent, clinically normal skin is recommended for proper histopathologic interpretation. Microscopic examination with low-power magnification shows a generally symmetrical pattern. The surface epithelium at the edge of the tumor appears normal; at the lip of the central crater, however, a characteristic acute angle (or "buttress") is formed between the overlying epithelium

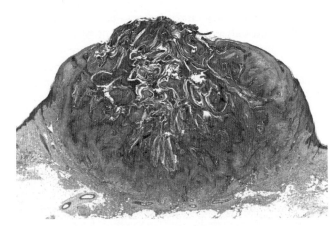

• **Fig. 10.99 Keratoacanthoma.** Low-power microscopic view showing extensive epidermal proliferation with a central keratin plug.

and the lesion. The crater is filled with keratin, and the epithelium at the base of the crater proliferates downward (Fig. 10.99), often with a pronounced chronic inflammatory cell response. Downward proliferation typically does not extend below the sweat glands in skin lesions or into underlying muscle in vermilion lesions. The tumor cells appear mature, although marked dyskeratosis (abnormal keratin production) typically is seen. Late-stage lesions show considerably more keratinization in the deeper aspects of the tumor than do early lesions; the deep tumor islands often contain enlarged cells with pale pink, "glassy" cytoplasm. Perineural and vascular invasion have been reported rarely; although worrisome, such features do not necessarily indicate a worse prognosis. Migration of eosinophils or neutrophils into the epithelium with resultant microabscess formation is a frequent finding. Regressing lesions tend to flatten, hollow out, and exhibit an underlying band of fibrosis.

Numerous immunohistochemical studies comparing keratoacanthoma and squamous cell carcinoma have been reported, but no reliable marker for discernment between these two lesions has been identified.

Treatment and Prognosis

Because of the difficulty in clinically and histopathologically distinguishing between keratoacanthoma and squamous cell carcinoma, many authorities advocate excision without waiting for spontaneous regression. Also, early treatment may prevent significant scarring. Approximately 4%–8% of lesions recur after excision. Although conventional surgical excision is preferred, alternative therapies include cryosurgery (reserved for small early lesions); electrodesiccation and curettage; Mohs micrographic surgery (especially for lesions that are large or involve cosmetic areas); laser therapy; photodynamic therapy; intralesional injection of various agents (e.g., 5-fluorouracil, bleomycin, methotrexate, interferon alpha); and topical agents (e.g., imiquimod, 5-fluorouracil). In addition, systemic retinoids may be used alone or in combination with local treatment for patients with multiple or especially large lesions.

Aggressive behavior and transformation into carcinoma have been reported in a small proportion of keratoacanthomas—particularly those occurring in the setting of immunosuppression. However, the close histopathologic similarities between this lesion and squamous cell carcinoma sometimes make it difficult to rule out the possibility of microscopic misinterpretation.

◆ SQUAMOUS CELL CARCINOMA

In the United States, approximately one of every two men and one of every three women will develop a malignancy (other than nonmelanoma skin cancer) at some point. It is estimated that for the year 2022, more than 1.9 million new cancer cases will be diagnosed in the United States, in addition to around 5.4 million nonmelanoma skin cancers. Although the relative 5-year cancer survival rate is approximately 68%, cancer still causes more than 609,000 deaths each year in the United States and represents the second leading cause of death after heart disease. From 1930 to 1991, the annual cancer death rate (excluding nonmelanoma skin cancer) increased and reached a peak of 215 per 100,000 population. This trend reflected an increase in the incidence of lung cancer as well as a decrease in mortality at an early age from other common disorders, such as cardiovascular disease and infection. Since 1991, however, the annual cancer death rate has declined to about 144 per 100,000 population. In part, this decline is related to a decrease in tobacco use and lung cancer deaths; in addition, improvements in detection and treatment have resulted in declines in breast, colorectal, and prostate cancer deaths.

Significant epidemiologic shifts also have occurred in head and neck cancer over the past several decades. In the United States and other developed nations, declining tobacco use has resulted in decreased annual incidence of laryngeal and floor of mouth cancers. In contrast, there has been a significant increase in the prevalence of oropharyngeal cancer associated with HPV infection.

Squamous cell carcinoma accounts for more than 90% of oral malignancies. Statistics for oral cancer can be difficult to review because of variations in terminology and reporting practices. In this section, we will use the term "oral" to refer to the oral cavity (including the intraoral mucosa and lip vermilion) as well as the oropharynx. However, some authors prefer to use the term "oral" when referring to the oral cavity only. Squamous cell carcinomas involving the intraoral mucosa, lip vermilion, and oropharynx exhibit different risk factors, clinical features, molecular profiles, and biologic behavior, although a clear distinction between these sites is not always made. Furthermore, cancer registries and investigators often report oral cavity and pharyngeal cancers in aggregate. (Among pharyngeal cancers, oropharyngeal lesions typically outnumber those arising from the nasopharynx and hypopharynx.) With that said, in the United States oral cavity and pharyngeal cancers combined account for less than 3% of all newly diagnosed cancers (excluding nonmelanoma skin cancers and *in situ* carcinomas for all sites but

urinary bladder) and represent the eighth most common cancer in males. Around 54,000 new oral cavity and pharyngeal cancer cases are diagnosed annually, and these cancers account for approximately 11,200 deaths per year.

In the United States, males overall have a much higher annual incidence of oral cavity and pharyngeal cancer than females, with a male-to-female ratio of approximately 2.7:1. According to Surveillance, Epidemiology, and End Results (SEER) Program data for 2000–2019, the age-adjusted annual incidence has been growing at a faster pace for males than females (0.7% vs 0.4% annual change, respectively). However, among young adults and pediatric patients, recent annual incidence rates are similar for both genders.

The risk for oral cavity and pharyngeal cancer increases with age, especially among males. According to SEER Program data, the 5-year age-adjusted incidence rate for oral cavity and pharyngeal cancer from 2014 to 2018 was 3 per 100,000 for males younger than 50 years, 43 per 100,000 for males 50–64 years, and 67 per 100,000 for males aged 65 years and older. Among individuals 50 years and older, the incidence was higher for white males than black males, whereas similar incidence rates were seen for black and white males younger than 50 years.

In the United States from 2000 to 2019, the age-adjusted incidence of oral cavity and pharyngeal cancer increased by 1% per year. Subsite analysis reveals that during this period there was a notable 3.1% annual increase in the number newly diagnosed oropharyngeal cancers. This growth in oropharyngeal cancer cases has been driven by HPV-related tumors (see discussion of etiology below), which exhibit a predilection for the palatine tonsils and base of tongue. In the early 2000s, HPV-related oropharyngeal cancer was characterized as an epidemic mainly affecting middle-aged white men. However, with aging of this original cohort, oropharyngeal cancer incidence has been increasing significantly among elderly as well as middle-aged men over the past two decades.

In the United States from 2009 to 2018, increased incidence also was observed for carcinomas arising from the oral tongue (anterior two-thirds of the tongue). Interestingly, in many developed nations, increased incidence of oral tongue cancer has been noted among individuals younger than 45 years; also, in some regions this patient subset has exhibited an unusual female predilection. The underlying cause for this trend is uncertain. Such cases often are not associated with the traditional risk factors of tobacco and alcohol use, and the oral tongue—unlike the base of tongue—is an infrequent site for HPV-positive carcinomas.

Carcinoma of the lip vermilion is somewhat different from intraoral carcinoma. It has a pathophysiology more akin to squamous cell carcinoma of sun-exposed skin. According to SEER data for 2015–2019, the overall 5-year age-adjusted incidence rate for lip cancer (including labial mucosa and lip vermilion lesions) in the United States is 0.5 per 100,000 population. The incidence increases with age, with rates among those 75 years and older of approximately 5.6 per 100,000 for males and 1.9 per 100,000 for females. White males are affected most commonly, although there has been a considerable decrease in the incidence of lip cancer in this group over the last several decades; this trend may be related to a decline in the number of white males engaged in outdoor occupations. Among women and non-white men, lip carcinoma is infrequent. The low incidence among women may be related to little outdoor occupational activity and prevalent use of lip protective agents. In non-whites, racial pigmentation may provide protection against sun exposure.

The worldwide incidence of oral cavity cancer is approximately 378,000 cases per year, with especially high rates reported in Melanesia, South-Central Asia, Australia/New Zealand, and Central/Eastern Europe. Much of the worldwide burden of oral cavity cancer is carried by low- and middle-income nations. Notably, Asia accounts for approximately two-thirds of newly diagnosed oral cavity cancer cases each year. For oropharyngeal cancer, the worldwide incidence is 98,000 cases per year, with the highest rates reported in Western Europe, Northern Europe, North America, Central/Eastern Europe, and Australia/New Zealand. Exceptionally wide variations in oral cancer incidence and mortality across regions likely results from differences in population habits, life expectancies, preventive education, and accuracy of disease reporting. Despite the difficulties involved in interpreting such data, these findings have been helpful in identifying potential causative factors.

Etiology of Oral Cancer

The cause of oral squamous cell carcinoma is multifactorial. Both extrinsic and intrinsic factors may be involved, and more than a single factor may be needed to produce such a malignancy. *Extrinsic* factors include tobacco smoke, alcohol, human papillomavirus (especially for oropharyngeal cancers), and sunlight (for vermilion cancers only). *Intrinsic* factors include systemic or generalized states, such as malnutrition or iron-deficiency anemia. Heredity does not appear to play a major causative role, although a few rare, heritable conditions (e.g., dyskeratosis congenita [see page 752], Fanconi anemia) have been associated with an increased risk for oral squamous cell carcinoma. Interestingly, a recent genome-wide association study reported that oral cavity and pharyngeal cancers were associated with certain HLA and other susceptibility loci.

Tobacco Smoking

More than 1 billion individuals currently smoke tobacco worldwide. Over the past 3 decades, smoking prevalence has decreased, although population growth has resulted in an increase in the total number of smokers. According to the 2019 Global Burden of Disease Study, tobacco smoking accounted for approximately 7.7 million deaths and was the leading risk factor for death among males. In the United States, tobacco smoking reached its greatest popularity during the 1940s, when at least 65% of white men smoked and other population subgroups were beginning to smoke in

large numbers. Today less than 20% of US adults use tobacco products and less than 13% smoke cigarettes. Although an overall decrease in smoking prevalence has been observed, intensive efforts will be required to meet the US Department of Health and Human Services' Healthy People objective to reduce cigarette smoking prevalence by the year 2030 to 5% or less.

Tobacco smoke contains more than 70 carcinogens, including polycyclic aromatic hydrocarbons (such as benzo[*a*]pyrene), *N*-nitrosamines, aromatic amines, formaldehyde, acetaldehyde, and benzene. In addition, smoking produces free radicals and oxidants that promote the destruction and counteract the protective effects of endogenous antioxidants (such as, glutathione-S-transferase, glutathione reductase, and superoxide dismutase).

Much indirect clinical evidence implicates tobacco smoking in the development of oral squamous cell carcinoma. The proportion of smokers (80%) among patients with oral carcinoma is about four times greater than that among the general population. For patients who quit smoking, the risk for developing oral cancer declines over time; approximately 10 years after cessation, the incidence of oral cancer approaches that of individuals who have never smoked. The risk for a second primary carcinoma of the upper aerodigestive tract is two to six times greater for treated patients with oral cancer who continue to smoke than for those who quit after diagnosis.

According to a meta-analysis of observational studies on tobacco smoking and cancer in various regions of the world, the pooled risk for oral cancer is approximately three times greater among smokers than nonsmokers. Moreover, the relative risk (smoker's risk for oral cancer compared with that of a nonsmoker) is dose-dependent. It is at least five for persons who smoke 40 cigarettes daily, but increases to as much as 17 for persons who smoke 80 or more cigarettes daily. The risk also increases the longer a person smokes. Furthermore, studies suggest that cigar or pipe smoking is associated with a similar or greater risk for oral cancer compared to cigarette smoking.

In India it is common to smoke bidi (small, hand-rolled cigarettes consisting of flaked tobacco rolled in a temburni or tendu leaf), and bidi smoking is associated with an approximately threefold greater risk of oral cancer compared to cigarette smoking. The highest risk of all probably is found in certain Indian and South American cultures in which the practice of reverse smoking is popular, especially among women. In reverse smoking, the burning end of a handmade cigar or cigarette is held inside the mouth. Where reverse smoking is practiced, as many as 50% of all oral malignancies are found on the hard palate, a site usually spared by this disease.

Smokeless Tobacco

Smokeless tobacco is used in a wide variety of forms by more than 350 million individuals worldwide. More than 80% of these individuals reside in Asia, including countries where smokeless tobacco often is incorporated into a betel quid (see next section). Based on evaluation of published scientific studies, the International Agency for Research on Cancer has concluded that smokeless tobacco—whether used alone or with betel quid—is carcinogenic to humans. Among systematic reviews and meta-analyses of smokeless tobacco use in the world literature, most reported oral cancer odds ratios vary from approximately 4 to 8 in Southeast Asia and less than 1 to 5 in the Americas and Europe. In addition, a recent pooled analysis of data from National Health Interview Surveys in the United States reported an association between current smokeless tobacco use and oral cavity cancer (with an approximate hazard ratio of 9) among individuals who had never used other forms of tobacco. Variation in reported risk may be influenced by study methodology as well as the types of smokeless tobacco used. A recent meta-analysis of studies from various world regions found that oral cancer risk among betel quid product users may be more than double that for users of oral snuff. In the United States, studies suggest a lower risk associated with moist snuff and chewing tobacco and a higher risk associated with dry snuff. This apparent increased risk associated with dry snuff is supported by clinicopathologic investigations that have found an abnormal male-to-female ratio for oral carcinoma (>1.0:1.5) in geographic areas, such as the southeastern United States, where the habit is more popular among women than among men. In addition, approximately 50% of all oral cancers in smokeless tobacco users occur at the site where the tobacco is habitually placed.

Betel Quid (Paan)

Betel quid (or *paan*) is a combination of natural substances (i.e., areca palm nuts, betel leaf, slaked lime, and perhaps tobacco leaf) chewed for their psychostimulating effects. The carcinogenicity of betel quid traditionally has been attributed to tobacco, although areca nut alone also appears to be carcinogenic. In addition, commercially freeze-dried betel quid substitutes (e.g., *pan masala* and *gutkha*) packaged in convenient sachets have become increasingly popular. Oral cancer risk estimates by various systematic reviews and meta-analyses range from about six- to ninefold for users of paan and gutkha. Among betel quid users in Asia, the lifetime risk of developing oral cancer is a remarkable 8%. Notably, as many as 80% of oral squamous cell carcinomas in the Indian subcontinent and Taiwan are associated with betel quid use. This habit also is associated with development of precancers, such as leukoplakia. As many as 600 million persons worldwide chew these quids on a regular basis.

Alcohol

Since 1998, the International Agency for Research on Cancer has classified alcohol as a carcinogen for the upper aerodigestive tract, including the oral cavity, oropharynx, hypopharynx, larynx, and esophagus. In particular, alcohol in combination with tobacco is a significant risk factor for oral cancer development, with a reported relative risk of 15 or more among heavy users of both substances. Furthermore, even after controlling for tobacco use, epidemiologic studies have reported a 2- to 14-fold increased risk for oral cancer among heavy drinkers (often defined as individuals who consume more than four alcoholic beverages or approximately 50 g of alcohol per day). The risk generally appears to be dose-dependent and time-dependent.

Indirect evidence for alcohol's role in oral cancer development includes the fact that approximately one-third of male patients with oral cancer are heavy alcohol users, whereas less than 10% of the general population can be classified as such. Likewise, cirrhosis of the liver is found in at least 20% of male patients with oral cancer.

The exact role of alcohol in oral carcinogenesis is not well understood, although several mechanisms have been proposed. Ethanol in alcoholic beverages is metabolized into acetaldehyde, which is a known carcinogen. In addition, carcinogenic impurities—such as, polycyclic aromatic hydrocarbons and nitrosamines—may be present in some alcoholic beverages. Moreover, alcohol may help solubilize other carcinogenic compounds and may increase the permeability of the oral epithelium to these compounds. Nutritional deficiencies and immunosuppression associated with heavy alcohol consumption may be contributory factors as well.

There is much debate in the literature regarding the potential for alcohol-containing mouthwashes to increase the risk for oral cancer. High-quality epidemiologic studies are limited, and inconsistent findings across studies have failed to establish a definite link.

Occupational Exposures and Environmental Pollutants

Some studies have reported an increased oral cancer risk for workers in the wood products industry chronically exposed to certain chemicals, such as phenoxyacetic acids. Such workers also are at increased risk for nasal and nasopharyngeal carcinoma. In addition, there is limited and inconsistent evidence for elevated oral cancer risk among metal workers, electrical workers, plumbers, machinists, painters, and other individuals with occupational exposure to solvents or metal dust.

In regions of Taiwan with a particularly high incidence of oral cancer, investigators have reported elevated levels of heavy metal pollutants (e.g., nickel, chromium, and arsenic) in farm soil and increased blood concentrations of some of these metals in affected patients.

Radiation

The effects of UV radiation on the lips are discussed elsewhere (actinic cheilosis, see page 395). Interestingly, several epidemiologic and other large-scale studies have reported an association between lip cancer and certain antihypertensive medications (e.g., hydrochlorothiazide, hydrochlorothiazide-triamterene, nifedipine). A similar association also has been noted for nonmelanoma skin cancers. Although further studies are needed to establish direct causality, it has been hypothesized that such medications may act as photosensitizers and may potentiate the development of UV-induced lip or skin cancer.

In addition, it is well known that **x-irradiation** decreases immune reactivity and produces chromosomal abnormalities. Indeed, radiotherapy to the head and neck area increases the risk for later development of a new primary oral malignancy, either a carcinoma or sarcoma. This effect is dose-dependent, but even low-dose radiotherapy for benign entities may increase the local risk somewhat. Although there has been controversy regarding whether dental radiography may pose an increased risk for developing various tumors, dental imaging has not been associated with oral carcinoma.

Vitamin/Mineral Deficiencies and Dietary Factors

Iron deficiency, especially the severe, chronic form known as the **Plummer-Vinson** or **Paterson-Kelly syndrome** (see page 830), is associated with an elevated risk for squamous cell carcinoma of the esophagus, oropharynx, and posterior mouth. Malignancies develop at an earlier age than in patients without iron deficiency anemia. Iron deficiency may cause impaired cell-mediated immunity. In addition, because the epithelium of the upper digestive tract has a relatively high turnover rate, rapid loss of iron-dependent enzymes may lead to degenerative changes, including mucosal atrophy and **esophageal webs** (intertwining fibrous bands of scar tissue), with heightened susceptibility to malignant transformation.

Vitamin-A deficiency produces excessive keratinization of the skin and mucous membranes, and researchers have suggested that this vitamin may help to prevent oral precancer and cancer. Some believe that blood levels of retinol and the amount of dietary betacarotene ingested are inversely proportional to the risk of oral squamous cell carcinoma and leukoplakia. Long-term therapy with retinoic acids and betacarotene also has been associated with regression of at least some leukoplakic lesions and a concomitant reduction in the severity of dysplasia within such lesions.

Several epidemiologic studies suggest that high intake of fruits and vegetables decreases the risk for numerous cancer types, including oral cancer. This finding may be related to the protective effects of not only vitamin A but also various other substances (e.g., vitamins C and E, folate, flavonoids, fiber, lycopene, and phytosterols) present within plant foods. However, tobacco and alcohol may represent confounding factors, because heavy tobacco and alcohol users often consume small amounts of fruits and vegetables. Also, some studies suggest that animal fats and processed or salted meat may increase the risk for oral cancer.

A few studies have reported an increased risk for oral cancer in association with drinking hot maté (an herbal tea mainly consumed in parts of South and Central America). Furthermore, there has been interest in the potential protective effects of green tea, coffee, and their associated polyphenols. However, further studies are needed to confirm and explain the carcinogenic or protective properties of such beverages.

Bacteria

The potential for microflora of the oral cavity to contribute to carcinogenesis represents a growing area of scientific investigation. Proposed mechanisms by which oral bacteria may contribute to oral cancer development include the following: (1) production of an inflammatory microenvironment that enhances cell proliferation and inhibits apoptosis, (2) disruption of immunosurveillance, and (3) metabolism of tobacco- and alcohol-related carcinogens (e.g., conversion of ethanol into the carcinogen acetaldehyde). Studies using traditional culture methods and molecular techniques have suggested potential associations between oral cancer and *Prevotella* species, *Fusobacterium* species, *P. gingivalis*, *Capnocytophaga gingivalis*, and certain streptococci. In addition, epidemiological studies have suggested associations with poor oral hygiene, poor dental status, and periodontal disease. More recently, there has been a surge in studies examining the microbiome of patients with oral cancer or oral potentially malignant disorders. Investigators hypothesize that shifts in the composition of complex microbial communities may be more important than individual bacterial pathogens in promoting cancer development. Although most such studies have found significant changes in bacterial flora among patients with disease as compared to controls, there is considerable heterogeneity in reported microbial profiles across studies. Further research with methodological standardization is needed.

Although rarely seen today, tertiary syphilis has been associated with a fourfold increased risk for development of dorsal tongue carcinoma. This risk may be due to the carcinogenic properties of the arsenical agents and other heavy metals that were used to treat syphilis before the advent of modern antibiotic therapy.

Candida

Hyperplastic candidiasis (see page 206) frequently is cited as an oral precancerous condition. Because this lesion appears as a white plaque that cannot be rubbed off, it also has been called *candidal leukoplakia*. Unfortunately, it is difficult both clinically and histopathologically to distinguish between a true hyperplastic candidiasis and a preexisting leukoplakia with superimposed candidiasis. Experimentally, some strains of *C. albicans* have produced hyperkeratotic lesions of the dorsal rat tongue without any other contributing factors. Other studies have demonstrated that certain strains may produce nitrosamines (carcinogens that can activate certain proto-oncogenes) or may convert ethanol into the carcinogen acetaldehyde. In addition, upregulation of pro-inflammatory cytokines may promote cell proliferation and inhibit apoptosis. Recent studies of the oral microbiome suggest that interactions between complex bacterial and fungal communities may promote cancer development as well. Decreased fungal diversity and increased abundance of certain fungi (such as *Candida*, *Hannaella*, and *Gibberrella*) may be seen in oral cancer patients compared to healthy individuals. However, the evidence for the promotion of oral carcinogenesis by fungi is largely circumstantial.

Oncogenic Viruses

Oncogenic (tumor producing) viruses may play a major role in a wide variety of cancers. Viral integration into the host's genetic material may result in abnormal cell growth and proliferation. The oncogenic viruses may immortalize the host cell, thereby facilitating malignant transformation. In the past, adenoviruses, Epstein-Barr virus (EBV), herpes simplex virus (HSV), human papillomavirus (HPV), and retroviruses (e.g., human immunodeficiency virus [HIV]) all have been suggested to play a role in the development of oral carcinoma. However, HPV and HIV are the only ones still implicated. HPV is discussed here; oral squamous cell carcinoma in the setting of HIV infection is discussed in the following section on immunosuppression and also on page 263.

HPV traditionally has been known for its role in the development of cancers of the anogenital region (especially the uterine cervix but also the anus, vulva, vagina, and penis). In addition, within the past few decades, a strong link between HPV and oropharyngeal carcinoma has been established, and the oropharynx has supplanted the uterine cervix as the most common site for HPV-attributable cancer in the United States. This epidemiologic shift has been hypothesized to result from an increase in oral sexual behavior and a decline in tobacco use. Significant increases in HPV-positive oropharyngeal cancer incidence also have been reported in other high-income nations. The proportion of oropharyngeal cancers attributable to HPV infection is estimated to be approximately 70% in the United States and 40% globally. In contrast, only a small subset of oral cavity carcinomas has been attributed to HPV infection.

The high-risk HPV types (see page 354) are most closely associated with dysplasia and squamous cell carcinoma. In particular, detection of HPV 16 in exfoliated oral epithelial cells or mouth rinse samples is associated with a nearly fourfold increased risk for oral cavity cancer and a 22-fold increased risk for oropharyngeal cancer. Investigators have proposed that persistent oral infection with HPV 16 and other high-risk HPV types increases the risk for eventual development of oropharyngeal cancer. HPV 16 has been identified in more than 90% of HPV-positive oropharyngeal squamous cell carcinomas. Similarly, in HPV-positive oral cavity squamous cell carcinomas, HPV 16 appears to be the most common type, although there may be a greater diversity of high-risk HPV types in oral cavity tumors compared to oropharyngeal ones. Most studies of HPV-positive oropharyngeal and oral cavity squamous cell carcinomas have focused on detection of HPV 16 and other high-risk types belonging to the genus *Alphapapillomavirus*; however, recent investigations using next-generation sequencing have suggested a possible role for certain *Betapapillomavirus* and *Gammapapillomavirus* types as well.

Meta-analyses of more recently published literature have estimated the prevalence of HPV DNA in oral squamous cell carcinomas to range from 13% to 58%; nonetheless, the presence of HPV DNA is not indicative of transcriptionally active HPV infection and cannot discriminate between biologically relevant vs bystander infection. Instead, detection of high-risk HPV E6/E7 mRNA is considered better evidence of HPV infection as a likely cause of tumor development. The primary mechanisms by which HPV is believed to contribute to carcinogenesis are linked to products of the *E6* and *E7* viral oncogenes: (1) E6 protein promotes degradation of the tumor suppressor protein p53 and (2) E7 increases

degradation of the tumor suppressor protein pRb, which leads to upregulation of p16 and downregulation of cyclin D1. Using assays for both high-risk HPV DNA and E6/E7 mRNA, a multicenter retrospective study in North America reported that only 6% of oral cavity squamous cell carcinomas analyzed could be attributed to HPV infection. Similarly, a large-scale study of archived samples from 29 countries using assays for high-risk HPV DNA and either E6 mRNA or p16 reported the HPV-attributable fraction for oral cavity cancers to be approximately 4%. In addition, according to a meta-analysis of studies from 44 countries using such assays, approximately 16% of oral cavity squamous cell carcinomas may be attributed to HPV infection. Overall, in contrast to oropharyngeal cancers, only a small subset of oral cavity cancers appears to be HPV-related.

The characteristic risk profiles for patients in the United States with HPV-positive vs HPV-negative oropharyngeal squamous cell carcinoma exhibit some similarities but also significant differences. In both patient groups, there is a male predilection. However, compared to HPV-negative cases, HPV-positive cases exhibit a greater predilection for white individuals and individuals of higher socioeconomic status. During the early 2000s, HPV-positive oropharyngeal squamous cell carcinoma was characterized as a disease mainly arising in middle-aged individuals, with a younger average age at diagnosis compared to the HPV-negative group. However, since that time, the average age at diagnosis for oropharyngeal cancer has been increasing; this aging trend has been thought to be driven preferentially by the HPV-positive group, although some investigators have proposed that both groups may be aging. Also, a continued shift toward an older HPV-positive oropharyngeal cancer patient population has been forecasted over the next couple of decades based on low HPV vaccine coverage in older cohorts. Compared to HPV-negative tumors, HPV-positive tumors are more strongly associated with certain parameters of sexual behavior (e.g., increased number of lifetime sexual or oral sexual partners, early age at sexual debut, increased intensity of oral sexual exposure [as measured by sex-years, or the number of oral sexual partners per 10 years since sexual debut]). In addition, among individuals who do not use tobacco or alcohol, HPV-positive disease is more prevalent than HPV-negative disease. Nevertheless, patients with HPV-positive oropharyngeal squamous cell carcinoma often have some history of tobacco and alcohol use, and recent population-based studies in the United States have demonstrated a significantly greater burden of HPV-positive oropharyngeal cancers among ever-smokers than never-smokers.

The reasons underlying the marked predilection of HPV-positive oropharyngeal squamous cell carcinomas for the palatine and lingual tonsils are uncertain. However, proposed explanations include the following: (1) the specialized reticular epithelium lining the tonsillar crypts represents a zone of weakness, with a discontinuous basement membrane permissive to viral infection and tumor invasion; (2) the deep invaginations of the tonsillar crypts act as a reservoir for pathogens (including HPV); and (3) decreased T-cell response (due to binding of PD-L1 on epithelial cells to the PD-1 receptor on T-cells) protects the tonsils from chronic antigen stimulation but also favors viral persistence and cancer development.

Immunosuppression

Immunosuppression may play a role in the development of at least some malignancies of the upper aerodigestive tract. Without effective immunologic surveillance and attack, it is thought that malignant cells cannot be recognized and destroyed at an early stage. Persons with HIV infection and those who are undergoing immunosuppressive therapy for malignancy or organ transplantation are at increased risk for oral squamous cell carcinoma and other head and neck malignancies, especially when tobacco smoking and alcohol abuse are present.

Oncogenes and Tumor Suppressor Genes

The molecular basis of carcinogenesis involves mutations or epigenetic changes in two broad classes of genes: proto-oncogenes and tumor suppressor genes. Proto-oncogenes may be transformed into activated oncogenes by environmental agents (e.g., viruses, irradiation, and chemical carcinogens) or inherited changes. Activated oncogenes promote uncontrolled cell division and are involved in the initiation and progression of a wide variety of malignancies. Tumor suppressor genes, on the other hand, inhibit cell division and indirectly allow tumor production when they become inactivated or mutated.

Traditionally, most authorities have proposed that sequential accumulation of several genetic aberrations is necessary before a cell expresses a malignant phenotype. On the other hand, based on recent analyses of transcriptomic functional pathways, copy number, and/or ultra-deep sequencing, some investigators have detected rather random molecular changes in oral precursor lesions. Further studies are needed to reconcile such findings.

Genetic aberrations commonly identified in head and neck squamous cell carcinomas include abnormalities of the *RAS*, *MYC*, *EGFR*, and *PIK3CA* oncogenes, and the *TP53*, *RB1*, *CDKN2A*, and E-cadherin–related tumor suppressor genes. Mutations also may be observed in genes that function as both oncogenes and tumor suppressor genes (e.g., *FAT1*, *NOTCH1*). Genetic alterations may result in dysregulation of various pathways (e.g., those involving Wnt/beta-catenin, PI3K/Akt/mTOR, JAK/STAT, RAS/RAF/MAPK, and TGF-beta) important for key cellular functions (e.g., cell cycle control, cell proliferation, and survival). Head and neck squamous cell carcinomas associated with tobacco and alcohol use often exhibit mutated *TP53*, overexpression of pRb (encoded by *RB1*), decreased expression of p16 (encoded by *CDKN2A*), and amplification of 3q26/28 and 11q13/22. In contrast, HPV-associated cases typically express exhibit wild-type *TP53*, low levels of pRb, and increased levels of p16. Additional alterations that tend to be found in HPV-positive tumors include those involving *PIK3CA*, *TRAF3*, *E2F1*, immune-related genes

(e.g., *HLA-A/B*), and genes encoding FGF and JAK/STAT signaling proteins.

Chronic Trauma or Irritation

The potential role of chronic trauma or irritation in promoting oral cancer is controversial. Frictional keratoses (see page 383), broken or sharp teeth, and overall denture use are not associated with a significantly increased risk for cancer. However, some studies have reported a markedly increased risk for oral cavity cancer among individuals with ill-fitting dentures (estimated odds ratio of 3.9)—even after controlling for confounding factors, such as tobacco, alcohol, and betel quid use. It is unclear whether this increased risk might reflect the direct effects of an inflammatory environment (with associated oxidative stress) or, possibly, altered microbiota in promoting carcinogenesis. Alternatively, this apparent risk may result from decreased opportunities for clinical detection of oral premalignancy due to infrequent professional dental care.

Clinical and Radiographic Features

Oral Cavity Carcinoma

Persons with oral cavity squamous cell carcinoma are most often older men who have been aware of an alteration for 4–8 months before seeking professional help (8–24 months among lower socioeconomic groups). There is minimal pain during the early growth phase, which may explain the delay in seeking professional care. If the health care professional does not have a high index of suspicion, then additional weeks or months may elapse before a biopsy is performed.

Oral cavity squamous cell carcinoma has a varied clinical presentation, including the following:
- Exophytic (mass-forming; fungating, papillary, and verruciform)
- Endophytic (invasive, burrowing, and ulcerated)
- Leukoplakic (white patch) (Fig. 10.100)
- Erythroplakic (red patch)
- Erythroleukoplakic (combined red-and-white patch) (Fig. 10.101)

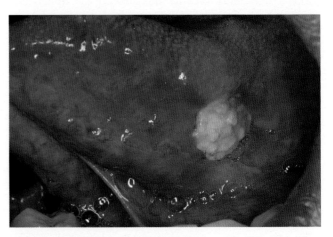

• **Fig. 10.100 Squamous Cell Carcinoma.** Leukoplakic lesion with a granular surface on the left ventrolateral tongue. (Courtesy of Dr. Larry Cunningham.)

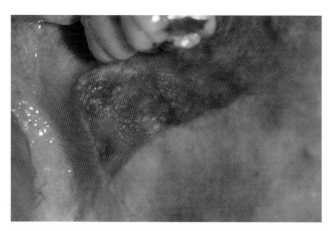

• **Fig. 10.101 Squamous Cell Carcinoma.** Speckled erythroplakia of the left posterior buccal mucosa. Brush sampling had been reported to be negative for epithelial abnormality, but incisional biopsy revealed invasive squamous cell carcinoma. (From Chi AC, Ravenel MC: AAOMP case challenge: a "speckled" lesion, *J Contemp Dent Pract* 6:168–172, 2005.)

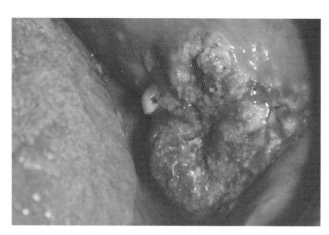

• **Fig. 10.103 Squamous Cell Carcinoma.** An exophytic buccal lesion shows a roughened and irregular surface with areas of erythema admixed with small areas of white keratosis. Surface ulceration is evident.

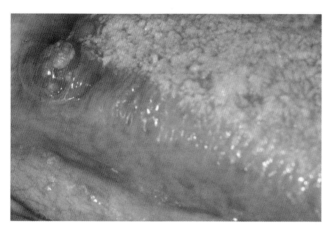

• **Fig. 10.102 Squamous Cell Carcinoma.** An exophytic lesion of the posterior lateral tongue demonstrates surface nodularity and minimal surface keratin production. It is painless and indurated.

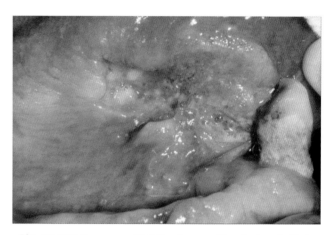

• **Fig. 10.104 Squamous Cell Carcinoma.** Chronic ulcerated lesion on the right ventral surface of the tongue. The rolled anterior margin felt indurated on palpation.

The *leukoplakic* and *erythroplakic* examples are probably early cases that have not yet produced a mass or ulceration, and the clinical features are identical to those described for leukoplakia and erythroplakia (see pages 381 and 390).

An *exophytic* lesion typically has a surface that is irregular, fungating, papillary, or verruciform, and its color may vary from normal to white or red, depending on the amount of keratin and vascularity (Figs. 10.102 and 10.103). The surface is often ulcerated, and the tumor feels hard (**indurated**) on palpation (Fig. 10.104).

The *endophytic* growth pattern has a central, depressed, irregularly shaped ulcer with a surrounding "rolled" border of pink, red, or white mucosa (Fig. 10.105). The rolled border results from invasion of the tumor downward and laterally under adjacent epithelium. Traumatic granulomas, deep fungal infections, tuberculosis, tertiary syphilis, and oral lesions of granulomatosis with polyangiitis (Wegener granulomatosis) or Crohn disease may exhibit a similar clinical appearance.

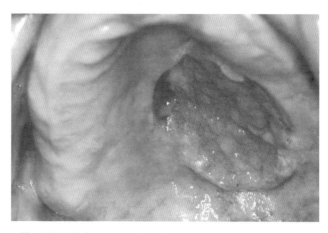

• **Fig. 10.105 Squamous Cell Carcinoma.** An ulcerated or endophytic lesion of the hard palate demonstrates rolled borders and a necrotic ulcer bed. This cancer was painless, although it had partially destroyed underlying palatal bone.

Destruction of underlying bone, when present, may be painful or completely painless; it appears on radiographs as a "moth-eaten" radiolucency with ill-defined or ragged margins (an appearance similar to osteomyelitis) (Fig. 10.106). Perineural invasion may cause paresthesia.

Lip Vermilion Carcinoma

Carcinoma of the lip vermilion typically is found in light-skinned persons with chronic exposure to UV radiation from sunlight. Seventy percent of affected individuals have outdoor occupations. It usually is associated with **actinic cheilosis** (see page 395) and may arise at the site where the patient holds a cigarette, cigar, or pipe. Almost 90% of lesions are located on the lower lip.

The typical vermilion carcinoma is a crusted, oozing, nontender, indurated ulceration that is usually less than 1 cm in greatest diameter when discovered (Figs. 10.107 and 10.108). The tumor usually grows slowly, and most patients are aware of a "problem" in the area for 12–16 months before diagnosis. Metastasis is a late event; at diagnosis, fewer than

10% of patients have lymph node metastasis, usually in the submental region. Perineural invasion may result in extension of the tumor into the mandible through the mental foramen. Although this tumor typically is diagnosed and treated at an early stage, patient neglect can result in considerable destruction of normal tissue (Fig. 10.109).

Intraoral Carcinoma

In the United States, the most common sites for intraoral carcinoma are the tongue (usually the posterior lateral and ventral surfaces) and floor of mouth. Other sites of involvement (in descending order of frequency) are the gingiva/alveolar mucosa, buccal mucosa, labial mucosa, and hard palate.

Carcinoma of the tongue accounts for more than 50% of intraoral cancers in the United States (Fig. 10.110). Two-thirds of lingual carcinomas appear as painless, indurated masses or ulcers of the posterior lateral border; 20% occur on anterior lateral or ventral surfaces, and only 4% occur on the dorsum. For unknown reasons, the oral tongue represents an increasingly common site of involvement in young patients.

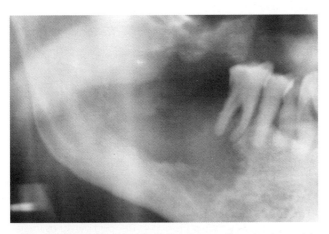

• **Fig. 10.106 Squamous Cell Carcinoma.** Bone involvement is characterized by an irregular, "moth-eaten" radiolucency with ragged margins—an appearance similar to that of osteomyelitis.

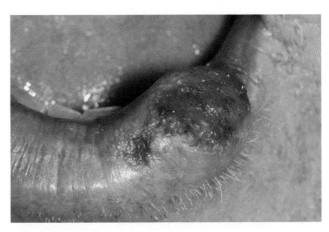

• **Fig. 10.108 Squamous Cell Carcinoma.** Ulcerated mass of the lower lip vermilion.

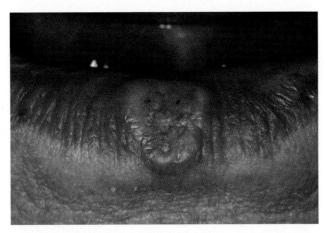

• **Fig. 10.107 Squamous Cell Carcinoma.** Crusted, ulcerated nodule of the lower lip vermilion. Risk factors in this patient included chronic sun exposure as well as immunosuppression due to bone marrow transplantation.

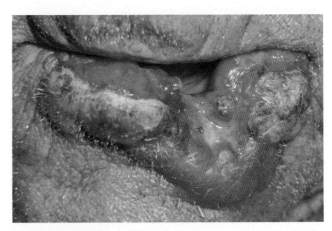

• **Fig. 10.109 Squamous Cell Carcinoma.** Patient neglect can result in extensive involvement, even in a readily visible site such as the lip vermilion. This ulcerating lesion of the lower lip had been present for more than 1 year before diagnosis.

Of all intraoral carcinomas, floor of mouth lesions are the most likely to arise from a preexisting leukoplakia or erythroplakia (Fig. 10.111). The floor of mouth also represents the oral cancer site most often associated with the development of a second primary malignancy, either elsewhere in the aerodigestive tract or in a distant organ. Floor of mouth carcinomas most often arise in the midline region near the frenum.

Gingival and alveolar carcinomas are usually painless and most frequently arise from keratinized, posterior mandibular mucosa (Fig. 10.112). Interestingly, among intraoral carcinomas, gingival lesions are least associated with tobacco smoking and have the greatest predilection for females. Gingival and alveolar carcinomas have a special propensity to mimic common, benign inflammatory and reactive lesions, such as the pyogenic granuloma, gingivitis (Fig. 10.113), periodontal disease, and peri-implantitis. Gingival tumors often destroy the underlying bone and cause tooth mobility. The lesion may go unrecognized until after tooth extraction, when it proliferates out of the socket to mimic the hyperplastic granulation tissue of an epulis granulomatosa (see page 526). Cancers that develop in an edentulous area may "wrap around" a denture flange and superficially resemble inflammatory fibrous hyperplasia (epulis fissuratum) (Fig. 10.114).

Tumors of the maxillary alveolar ridge may extend onto the hard palate. Some studies suggest that carcinomas involving the maxillary mucosa may be more aggressive than previously thought, with approximately 30% of cases harboring occult cervical lymph node metastasis.

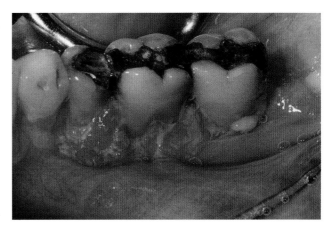

• **Fig. 10.112 Squamous Cell Carcinoma.** Red and white granular lesion of the posterior lingual mandibular gingiva.

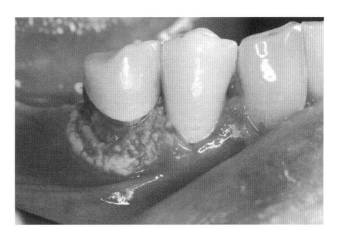

• **Fig. 10.113 Squamous Cell Carcinoma.** An innocuous, pebbled surface change of the gingiva was interpreted as inflammatory until multifocal white keratoses developed.

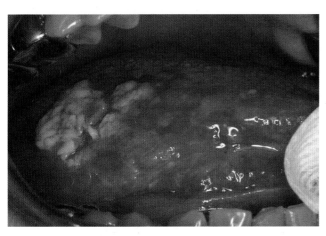

• **Fig. 10.110 Squamous Cell Carcinoma.** Diffuse, red and white lesion of the posterior lateral border of the tongue.

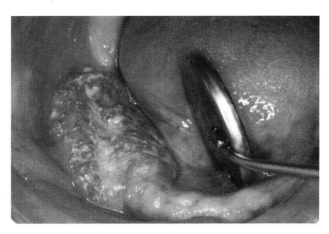

• **Fig. 10.114 Squamous Cell Carcinoma.** An exophytic lesion with an irregular and pebbled surface. There is a linear indentation along the facial aspect resulting from pressure from the patient's lower denture. The underlying alveolar bone was destroyed.

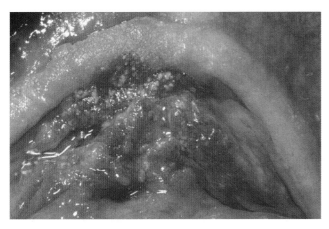

• **Fig. 10.111 Squamous Cell Carcinoma.** Granular red and white lesion in the anterior floor of mouth.

Similarly, some investigators suggest that carcinomas of the buccal mucosa may be more aggressive than previously suspected, with reported locoregional recurrence rates ranging from 30% to 80%. The buccal mucosa is an especially common site for intraoral carcinoma in regions of the world where betel quid use is prevalent.

Carcinomas of the retromolar trigone may spread to numerous adjacent structures, including the oropharynx, buccal mucosa, alveolar ridge, and pterygomandibular raphe (Fig. 10.115). Invasion of the pterygomandibular raphe may lead to involvement of the skull base, masticator space, and floor of mouth.

Oropharyngeal Carcinoma

Subsites for oropharyngeal carcinoma include the soft palate, posterior wall, palatine tonsil region (i.e., palatine tonsils, tonsillar fossa, and pillars), and base of tongue (including the lingual tonsils). In particular, the palatine tonsils and base of tongue are favored sites for HPV-positive tumors, and the majority of oropharyngeal carcinomas in the United States currently are attributed to HPV infection (Fig. 10.116A).

Oropharyngeal carcinomas may appear as an erythematous plaque, an ulcerated mass, or mucosal fullness. Small lesions arising from the tonsillar crypts may not be clinically apparent. Many patients have minimal symptoms at the time of diagnosis. HPV-positive oropharyngeal carcinomas tend to metastasize relatively early, and it is not unusual for patients to have a small, clinically evident or occult primary tumor yet prominent cervical metastasis (Fig. 10.117). Among patients with HPV-positive disease, the most common chief complaints at initial presentation are a neck mass followed by sore throat and **dysphagia** (difficulty in swallowing). In contrast, among patients with HPV-negative disease, the most common presenting complaints are sore throat followed by dysphagia and a neck mass. Other possible findings in patients with oropharyngeal cancer may include **globus sensation** (feeling of a lump) and **odynophagia** (pain on swallowing). The pain may be dull or sharp and frequently is referred to the ear.

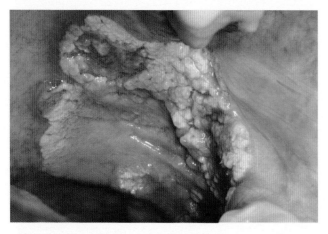

• **Fig. 10.115 Squamous Cell Carcinoma.** Carcinoma of the retromolar trigone with extension into the oropharynx (including the soft palate and anterior faucial pillar). Associated leukoplakia also extends anteriorly along the buccal mucosa.

Metastasis

Metastasis of oral squamous cell carcinoma occurs largely via the lymphatics to the cervical lymph nodes. Based on anatomic location, lymph nodes in the neck are divided into seven levels, as shown in Fig. 10.118. Regional metastasis is more often ipsilateral than contralateral or bilateral. Oral cavity carcinomas most frequently metastasize to the lymph nodes in levels I through III. Oropharyngeal carcinomas tend

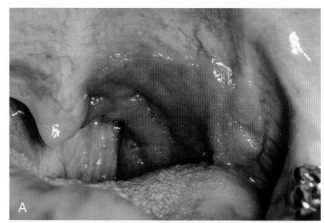

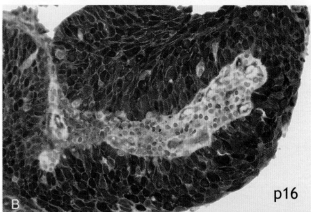

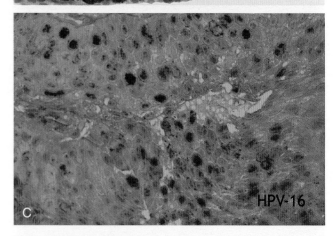

• **Fig. 10.116 Squamous Cell Carcinoma, Oropharyngeal. A,** Large, erythroplakic lesion involving the left soft palate and tonsillar region. **B,** Immunohistochemistry showed the tumor to be positive for p16, which is a surrogate marker for transcriptionally active, high-risk human papillomavirus (HPV) infection among oropharyngeal squamous cell carcinomas. **C,** In situ hybridization (ISH) demonstrated the presence of intranuclear HPV 16 DNA.

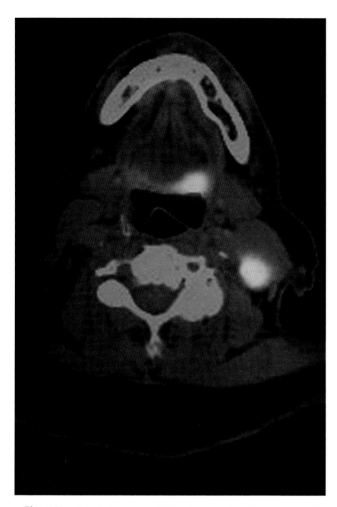

• **Fig. 10.117 Squamous Cell Carcinoma, Oropharyngeal with Regional Metastasis.** Computed tomography/positron emission tomography (CT/PET) fusion study of a patient with human papillomavirus-positive oropharyngeal squamous cell carcinoma. The scan highlights a relatively small (T1) primary tumor at the base of tongue/tonsillar region plus a prominent cervical lymph node metastasis in the lateral neck. (Courtesy of Dr. Terry Day).

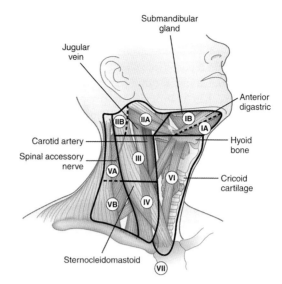

• **Fig. 10.118 Squamous Cell Carcinoma, Potential Sites for Cervical Lymph Node Metastasis.** Diagram demonstrating lymph node levels in the neck where metastatic deposits may be found:

  I. Submental/submandibular nodes
    IA. Submental nodes
    IB. Submandibular nodes
  II. Upper jugular nodes
    IIA. Anterior (medial) to the vertical plane defined by the spinal accessory nerve
    IIB. Posterior (lateral) to the vertical plane defined by the spinal accessory nerve
  III. Middle jugular nodes
  IV. Lower jugular nodes
  V. Posterior triangle nodes
    VA. Upper nodes extending from the skull base to bottom of the cricoid cartilage
    VB. Lower nodes extending from bottom of the cricoid cartilage to the clavicle
  VI. Anterior (central) compartment nodes
  VII. Superior mediastinal nodes

(From Thyroid. In Townsend CM, Daniel Beauchamp R, Mark Evers B, Mattox KL, Sabiston DC, editors: *Sabiston textbook of surgery: the biological basis of modern surgical practice*, 2022, Elsevier, pp 159–169.)

to metastasize to the lymph nodes in levels II and III. Involvement of other cervical lymph node groups is possible as well; in addition, oropharyngeal tumors may metastasize to the retropharyngeal nodes.

Upon clinical examination, a cervical lymph node that contains metastatic carcinoma is usually firm to stony hard, nontender, and enlarged (Fig. 10.119). If the malignant cells have perforated the capsule of the node and invaded into surrounding tissues, then the node will feel "fixed," or not easily movable. **Extranodal extension** (metastatic tumor present within the confines of the lymph node and extending through the capsule into the surrounding connective tissue, with or without an associated stromal reaction) is an adverse prognostic factor for intraoral and lip vermilion carcinomas. This feature is incorporated into the staging classification systems (see next section) for these tumors.

Distant metastasis also may occur—especially to the lungs, liver, and bones. Interestingly, recent studies have noted that post-treatment HPV-positive oropharyngeal carcinomas occasionally metastasize to atypical distant sites (e.g., kidneys, skin, skeletal muscle, axillary lymph nodes).

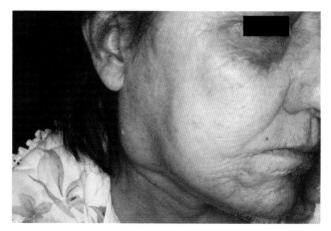

• **Fig. 10.119 Squamous Cell Carcinoma.** Metastatic deposits within cervical lymph nodes present as firm, painless enlargements as seen in this patient with metastasis to a superior jugular node from a posterior lateral tongue carcinoma.

Metastasis is not an early event for oral cavity carcinomas. However, because of delay in diagnosis, approximately 20%–30% of patients have cervical metastases evident at diagnosis (60% in reports from tertiary care medical centers). In contrast, oropharyngeal tumors are prone to early metastasis, with more than 50% of affected persons exhibiting cervical lymph node metastasis and 10% exhibiting distant metastasis at diagnosis. Furthermore, approximately 10%–40% of oral and oropharyngeal carcinoma patients who present without apparent cervical metastasis subsequently are found to have *occult* (subclinical) nodal disease.

Staging

The *tumor-node-metastasis (TNM) system* is used for **staging**, or describing the extent of cancer in the body. Staging is essential for guiding patient treatment and determining prognosis. The TNM system includes three basic parameters:
1. T—Size of the primary tumor, in centimeters
2. N—Regional lymph node involvement
3. M—Distant metastasis

Clinical staging is based on information obtained from procedures (e.g., physical examination, imaging, incisional biopsy) performed before initial definitive treatment of a cancer, whereas *pathologic staging* can be determined after additional information is obtained from pathologic examination of a surgically resected primary tumor and regional lymph nodes. Tables 10.2–10.7 summarize the tumor-node-metastasis (TNM) staging classification systems and corresponding prognostic stage groups for carcinomas of the oral cavity (including the intraoral lip mucosa), head and neck

TABLE 10.2	Tumor-Node-Metastasis (TNM) Staging Classification for Oral Cavity Carcinoma (Including Lip Mucosa)
Primary Tumor (T)	
TX	Primary tumor cannot be assessed
Tis	Carcinoma *in situ*
T1	Tumor 2 cm or less, with depth of invasion (DOI) no more than 5 mm
T2	Tumor 2 cm or less, with DOI more than 5 mm but no more than 10 mm *or* tumor more than 2 cm but no more than 4 cm, with DOI no more than 10 mm
T3	Tumor more than 2 cm but no more than 4 cm, with DOI more than 10 mm *or* Tumor more than 4 cm, with DOI no more than 10 mm
T4a	Moderately advanced local disease: Tumor more than 4 cm, with DOI more than 10 mm *or* tumor invades adjacent structures only (e.g., through cortical bone of the mandible or maxilla, or involves the maxillary sinus or skin of the face) *Note*: Superficial erosion of bone or tooth socket alone by a gingival primary is not sufficient to classify a tumor as T4.
T4b	Very advanced local disease: Tumor invades masticator space, pterygoid plates, or skull base and/or encases the internal carotid artery
Clinical Regional Lymph Node Involvement (cN)*	
NX	Regional lymph nodes cannot be assessed
N0	No regional lymph node metastasis
N1	Metastasis in a single ipsilateral node 3 cm or less in greatest dimension, and negative extranodal extension (ENE)
N2	Metastasis in a single ipsilateral lymph node, more than 3 cm but not more than 6 cm in greatest dimension, and negative ENE; *or* metastases in multiple ipsilateral lymph nodes, none more than 6 cm in greatest dimension, and negative ENE; *or* metastases in bilateral or contralateral lymph nodes, none more than 6 cm in greatest dimension, and negative ENE
N2a	Metastasis in a single ipsilateral node, more than 3 cm but not more than 6 cm in greatest dimension, and negative ENE
N2b	Metastases in multiple ipsilateral nodes, none more than 6 cm in greatest dimension, and negative ENE
N2c	Metastases in bilateral or contralateral nodes, none more than 6 cm in greatest dimension, and negative ENE
N3	Metastasis in a node more than 6 cm in greatest dimension and negative ENE; *or* metastasis in any node(s) and clinically overt ENE
N3a	Metastasis in a node more than 6 cm in greatest dimension and negative ENE
N3b	Metastasis in any node(s) and clinically overt ENE
Distant Metastasis (M)	
M0	No distant metastasis
M1	Distant metastasis

DOI, depth of invasion; ENE, extranodal extension.
*Note: A designation or "U" or "L" may be used for any N category to indicate metastasis above the lower border cricoid (U) or below the lower border of the cricoid (L).
(From Lip and Oral Cavity. In Edge SB, Byrd DR, Compton CC, et al, editors, *AJCC Cancer Staging Manual*, ed 7, New York, 2010, Springer, pp 29–40; Pharynx. In Edge SB, Byrd DR, Compton CC, et al, editors, *AJCC Cancer Staging Manual*, ed 7, New York, 2010, Springer, pp 41–56.)

TABLE 10.3 Tumor-Node-Metastasis (TNM) Staging Classification for Cutaneous Carcinoma of the Head and Neck (Including Lip Vermilion Carcinoma)

Primary Tumor (T)

TX	Primary tumor cannot be assessed
Tis	Carcinoma *in situ*
T1	Tumor 2 cm or less in greatest dimension
T2	Tumor more than 2 cm but no more than 4 cm in greatest dimension
T3	Tumor more than 4 cm in greatest dimension *or* Minor bone invasion *or* Perineural invasion* *or* Deep invasion[†]
T4	Tumor with gross cortical bone/marrow invasion, skull base invasion, and/or skull base foramen invasion
T4a	Tumor with gross cortical bone/marrow invasion
T4b	Tumor with skull base invasion and/or skull base foramen invasion

Clinical Regional Lymph Node Involvement (cN)[‡]

NX	Regional lymph nodes cannot be assessed
N0	No regional lymph node metastasis
N1	Metastasis in a single ipsilateral node, 3 cm or less in greatest dimension, and negative ENE
N2	Metastasis in a single ipsilateral lymph node, more than 3 cm but not more than 6 cm in greatest dimension, and negative ENE; *or* metastases in multiple ipsilateral lymph nodes, none more than 6 cm in greatest dimension, and negative ENE; *or* metastases in bilateral or contralateral lymph nodes, none more than 6 cm in greatest dimension, and negative ENE
N2a	Metastasis in a single ipsilateral node, more than 3 cm but not more than 6 cm in greatest dimension, and negative ENE
N2b	Metastases in multiple ipsilateral nodes, none more than 6 cm in greatest dimension, and negative ENE
N2c	Metastases in bilateral or contralateral nodes, none more than 6 cm in greatest dimension, and negative ENE
N3	Metastasis in a node more than 6 cm in greatest dimension and negative ENE; *or* metastasis in any node(s) and clinically overt ENE
N3a	Metastasis in a node more than 6 cm in greatest dimension and negative ENE
N3b	Metastasis in any node(s) and clinically overt ENE

Distant Metastasis (M)

M0	No distant metastasis
M1	Distant metastasis

ENE, extranodal extension.

*Perineural invasion for T3 classification is defined as tumor cells within the nerve sheath of a nerve lying deeper than the dermis or measuring 0.1 mm or larger in caliber, or presenting with clinical or radiographic involvement of named nerves without skull base invasion or transgression.

[†]Deep invasion is defined as invasion beyond the subcutaneous fat or more than 6 mm as measured from the granular layer of adjacent normal epidermis to the base of the tumor).

[‡]*Note:* A designation or "U" or "L" may be used for any N category to indicate metastasis above the lower border cricoid (U) or below the lower border of the cricoid (L). (From Califano JA, Lydiatt WM, Nehal KS, et al: Cutaneous carcinoma of the head and neck. In Amin MB, Edge SB, Greene FL, et al, editors, *AJCC cancer staging manual,* ed 8, Chicago, 2018, American College of Surgeons, pp. 171–181.)

skin (including the lip vermilion), and oropharynx. In general, the higher the stage, the worse the prognosis. In other words, a stage IV lesion is associated with a much worse prognosis than a stage I lesion. Note that different TNM staging classification systems are used for HPV-mediated oropharyngeal carcinoma and non-HPV-mediated oropharyngeal carcinoma (see the "Histopathologic Features" section for a discussion of p16 immunohistochemistry in the determination HPV status, and see the treatment and prognosis section for a discussion of HPV status as a key prognostic factor for oropharyngeal carcinoma). For oral cavity carcinomas, T category is based on primary tumor size as well as *depth of invasion* (as determined microscopically by measuring the distance from the level of the basement membrane of the adjacent normal surface epithelium to the deepest point of tumor invasion).

Summary (or *SEER*) *staging* represents a simplified system frequently used by tumor registries. This staging system uses basic categories (including localized, regional, and distant) to describe tumor spread. Table 10.8 provides survival rates by SEER stage for patients with oral cavity and pharyngeal cancer in the United States.

<table>
<tr><td>**TABLE 10.4**</td><td colspan="2">**Tumor-Node-Metastasis (TNM) Staging Classification for HPV-Mediated (p16-Positive) Oropharyngeal Carcinoma**</td></tr>
</table>

Primary Tumor (T)	
T0	No primary tumor identified
T1	Tumor 2 cm or less in greatest dimension
T2	Tumor more than 2 cm but not larger than 4 cm in greatest dimension
T3	Tumor more than 4 cm in greatest dimension *or* extension to lingual surface of the epiglottis
T4	Moderately advanced local disease: Tumor invades the larynx, extrinsic muscle of tongue, medial pterygoid, hard palate, mandible, or beyond
Clinical Regional Lymph Node Involvement (cN)	
NX	Regional lymph nodes cannot be assessed
N0	No regional lymph node metastasis
N1	Metastasis in one or more ipsilateral lymph nodes, none larger than 6 cm
N2	Metastasis in contralateral or bilateral lymph nodes, none larger than 6 cm
N3	Lymph node (s) larger than 6 cm
Distant Metastasis (M)	
M0	No distant metastasis
M1	Distant metastasis

From O'Sullivan B, Lydiatt WM, Haughey BH, et al: HPV-mediated oropharyngeal cancer. In Amin MB, Edge SB, Greene FL, et al, editors, *AJCC cancer staging manual,* ed 8, Chicago, 2018, American College of Surgeons, pp. 113–122.

<table>
<tr><td>**TABLE 10.5**</td><td>**Tumor-Node-Metastasis (TNM) Staging Classification for p16-Negative Oropharyngeal Carcinoma**</td></tr>
</table>

Primary Tumor (T)	
TX	Primary tumor cannot be assessed
Tis	Carcinoma *in situ*
T1	Tumor 2 cm or smaller in greatest dimension
T2	Tumor larger than 2 cm but not larger than 4 cm in greatest dimension
T3	Tumor larger than 4 cm in greatest dimension or extension to lingual surface of epiglottis
T4a	Moderately advanced local disease: Tumor invades the larynx, extrinsic muscle of tongue, medial pterygoid, hard palate, or mandible*
T4b	Very advanced local disease: Tumor invades lateral pterygoid muscle, pterygoid plates, lateral nasopharynx, or skull base and/or encases the carotid artery
Clinical Regional Lymph Node Involvement (cN)**	
NX	Regional lymph nodes cannot be assessed
N0	No regional lymph node metastasis
N1	Metastasis in a single ipsilateral lymph node, 3 cm or smaller in greatest dimension and negative ENE
N2	Metastasis in a single ipsilateral node larger than 3 cm but not larger than 6 cm in greatest dimension and negative ENE; or metastases in multiple ipsilateral lymph nodes, none larger than 6 cm in greatest dimension and negative ENE; or in bilateral or contralateral lymph nodes, none larger than 6 cm in greatest dimension and negative ENE
N2a	Metastasis in a single ipsilateral node larger than 3 cm but not larger than 6 cm in greatest dimension and negative ENE
N2b	Metastases in multiple ipsilateral nodes, none larger than 6 cm in greatest dimension and negative ENE

TABLE 10.5	Tumor-Node-Metastasis (TNM) Staging Classification for p16-Negative Oropharyngeal Carcinoma—cont'd
N2c	Metastases in bilateral or contralateral lymph nodes, none larger than 6 cm in greatest dimension and negative ENE
N3	Metastasis in a lymph node larger than 6 cm in greatest dimension and negative ENE; or metastasis in any node(s) and clinically overt positive ENE
N3a	Metastasis in a lymph node larger than 6 cm in greatest dimension and negative ENE
N3b	Metastasis in any node(s) and clinically overt positive ENE
Distant Metastasis (M)	
M0	No distant metastasis
M1	Distant metastasis

ENE, extranodal extension.

*Mucosal extension to the lingual surface of the epiglottis from primary tumors of the base of the tongue and vallecula does not constitute invasion of the larynx.

**A designation of "U" or "L" may be used for any N category to indicate metastasis above the lower border of the cricoid (U) or below the lower border of the cricoid (L). From Oropharynx (p16-) and Hypopharynx. In Amin MB, Edge SB, Greene FL, et al, editors, AJCC Cancer Staging Manual, ed 8, Chicago, 2018, American College of Surgeons, pp. 123–136.

TABLE 10.6	Prognostic Stage Groups for Oral Cavity Carcinoma and Cutaneous Carcinoma of the Head and Neck			
	Oral Cavity Carcinoma		**Cutaneous Carcinoma of the Head and Neck (Including Lip Vermilion Carcinoma)**	
Stage Group	**TNM Classification**		**Stage Group**	**TNM Classification**
Stage 0	Tis N0 M0		Stage 0	Tis N0 M0
Stage I	T1 N0 M0		Stage I	T1 N0 M0
Stage II	T2 N0 M0		Stage II	T2 N0 M0
Stage III	T3 N0 M0 T1 N1 M0 T2 N1 M0 T3 N1 M0		Stage III	T3 N0 M0 T1 N1 M0 T2 N1 M0 T3 N1 M0
Stage IVA	T4a N0 M0 T4a N1 M0 T1 N2 M0 T2 N2 M0 T3 N2 M0 T4a N2 M0		Stage IV	T1 N2 M0 T2 N2 M0 T3 N2 M0 Any T N3 M0 T4 Any N M0 Any T Any N M1
Stage IVB	Any T N3 M0 T4b Any N M0			
Stage IVC	Any T Any N M1			

From Ridge JA, Lydiatt WM, Patel SG, et al: Oral cavity. In Amin MB, Edge SB, Greene FL, et al, editors, *AJCC cancer staging manual*, ed 8, Chicago, 2018, American College of Surgeons, pp. 79–94. Califano JA, Lydiatt WM, Nehal KS, et al: Cutaneous Carcinoma of the Head and Neck. In Amin MB, Edge SB, Greene FL, et al, editors, *AJCC cancer staging manual*, ed 8, Chicago, 2018, American College of Surgeons, pp. 171–181.

Histopathologic Features

Squamous cell carcinoma typically arises from dysplastic surface epithelium and is characterized histopathologically by invasive islands and cords of malignant squamous epithelial cells. At the earliest moment of invasion, the adjectives *superficially invasive* or *microinvasive* often are used. The features of epithelial dysplasia are discussed in more detail in the section on leukoplakia (see page 381).

Invasion is represented by irregular extension of lesional epithelium through the basement membrane and into subepithelial connective tissue. Individual squamous cells and sheets or islands of cells proliferate within the connective tissue, without attachment to the surface epithelium. The invading tumor destroys normal tissue and may extend deeply into underlying adipose tissue, muscle, or bone. Lesional cells may breach the perineurium that encases nerve bundles (**perineural invasion**) or may invade the lumina of veins or

TABLE 10.7 Prognostic Stage Groups for Oropharyngeal Carcinoma

Non-HPV-Mediated (p16-Negative) Oropharyngeal Carcinoma		HPV-Mediated (p16-Positive) Oropharyngeal Carcinoma	
Stage Group	TNM Classification	Stage Group	TNM Classification
Stage 0	Tis N0 M0	Stage 0	Not applicable
Stage I	T1 N0 M0	Stage I	T0 N0 M0 T1 N0 M0 T2 N0 M0 T0 N1 M0 T1 N1 M0 T2 N1 M0
Stage II	T2 N0 M0	Stage II	T0 N2 M0 T1 N2 M0 T2 N2 M0 T3 N0 M0 T3 N1 M0 T3 N2 M0
Stage III	T3 N0 M0 T1 N1 M0 T2 N1 M0 T3 N1 M0 T4 N1 M0	Stage III	T0 N3 M0 T1 N3 M0 T2 N3 M0 T3 N3 M0 T4 N0 M0 T4 N1 M0 T4 N2 M0 T4 N3 M0
Stage IVA	T4a N0 M0 T4a N1 M0 T1 N2 M0 T2 N2 M0 T3 N2 M0 T4a N2 M0	Stage IV	Any T Any N M1
Stage IVB	Any T N3 M0 T4b Any N M0		
Stage IVC	Any T Any N M1		

From O'Sullivan B, Lydiatt WM, Haughey BH, et al: HPV-mediated oropharyngeal cancer. In Amin MB, Edge SB, Greene FL, et al, editors, *AJCC cancer staging manual*, ed 8, Chicago, 2018, American College of Surgeons, pp. 113–122. Lydiatt WM, Ridge JA, Patel SA, et al: Oropharynx (p16-) and hypopharynx. In Amin MB, Edge SB, Greene FL, et al, editors, *AJCC Cancer Staging Manual*, ed 8, Chicago, 2018, American College of Surgeons, pp. 123–136.

TABLE 10.8 Overall 5-Year Relative Survival Rates for Oral Cavity and Pharyngeal Cancers by SEER Stage*

SEER Stage at Diagnosis	Estimated 5-Year Relative Survival Rate				
	Oral Cavity and Pharynx	Lip	Tongue	Floor of Mouth	Oropharynx[†]
Localized	85%	93%	83%	73%	82%
Regional	68%	65%	69%	41%	76%
Distant	40%	33%	41%	23%	48%
All Stages	67%	91%	68%	52%	71%

*Based upon Surveillance Epidemiology and End Results (SEER) 18 data for patients diagnosed in 2011–2017. Source: Surveillance Research Program, National Cancer Institute. SEER*Explorer: an interactive website for SEER cancer statistics, http://seer.cancer.gov/explorer. Accessed November 23, 2021.
[†]Survival of oropharyngeal carcinoma is related to HPV status of the tumor. Some centers have reported overall 5-year survival rates of 54%–89% for HPV(+) oropharyngeal carcinomas and 33%–65% for HPV(−) tumors.

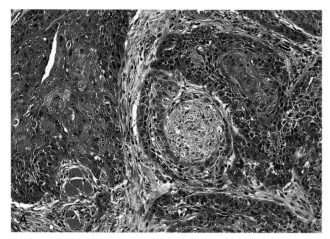

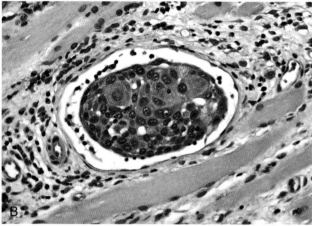

• **Fig. 10.120 Squamous Cell Carcinoma. A,** Perineural invasion. Tumor has breached the perineurium encasing this nerve fiber. **B,** Angioinvasion. Tumor is present within the lumen of this vessel.

lymphatics (**vascular invasion**) (Fig. 10.120). There is often a strong inflammatory or immune cell response to invading epithelium, and necrosis may be present. The tumor may induce dense fibrosis (**desmoplasia** or **scirrhous change**) and the formation of new blood vessels (**angiogenesis**).

The lesional cells generally show abundant eosinophilic cytoplasm with large, often darkly staining (**hyperchromatic**) nuclei and an increased nuclear-to-cytoplasmic ratio. Varying degrees of cellular and nuclear pleomorphism are seen. The normal product of squamous epithelium is keratin, and **keratin pearls** (a round focus of concentrically layered, keratinized cells) may be produced within lesional epithelium. Individual cells also may undergo keratinization.

HPV-positive squamous cell carcinomas of the oropharynx are rather distinctive in that they tend to arise from a specialized type of epithelium ("reticulated epithelium") lining the tonsillar crypts. Such tumors are not associated with dysplasia or keratosis of the surface epithelium, and there is often an abrupt transition between the adjacent surface epithelium and the endophytic tumor arising from the crypts. Features indicative of premalignancy in the reticulated epithelium are not well-defined. Reminiscent of the reticulated epithelium from which they usually arise, HPV-positive oropharyngeal squamous cell carcinomas tend to be nonkeratinizing with

basaloid cytologic features. Koilocytes generally are not evident. The invasive tumor islands and nests often are surrounded by lymphoid cells, and infiltration of tumor by lymphocytes is a variable finding. Prominent stromal desmoplasia tends to be lacking. Cystic degeneration may be evident in the primary tumor and is a common feature in cervical lymph node metastases. Similar features may be seen in HPV-positive tumors involving non-oropharyngeal head and neck sites (such as the oral cavity, larynx, and hypopharynx). Infrequent microscopic variants among this HPV-positive non-oropharyngeal subset include exophytic warty and conventional keratinizing types.

Histopathologic **grading** of squamous cell carcinoma is based upon the degree of resemblance to normal squamous epithelium and the amount of keratin production. Lesions typically are graded on a three-point (grades I–III) scale. The less differentiated tumors receive the higher numerals. The histopathologic grade of a tumor is related somewhat to its biologic behavior. In other words, a tumor that is mature enough to closely resemble its tissue of origin often grows at a slightly slower pace and metastasizes later in its course. Such a tumor is called *low-grade, grade I,* or *well-differentiated* (Fig. 10.121). In contrast, a tumor with marked pleomorphism and little or no keratin production may be so immature that it becomes difficult to identify

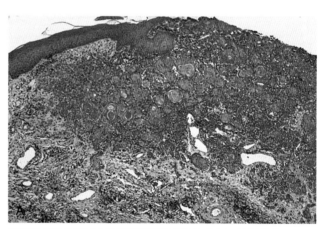

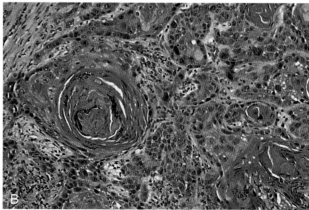

• **Fig. 10.121 Well-differentiated Squamous Cell Carcinoma. A,** Low-power photomicrograph showing islands of malignant squamous epithelium invading into the lamina propria. **B,** High-power view showing dysplastic epithelial cells with keratin pearl formation.

the tissue of origin. In such cases, immunohistochemical studies (e.g., for cytokeratins, p63, p40) may be needed to support an epithelial origin. Such tumors often enlarge rapidly, metastasize early, and are termed *high-grade, grade III/IV, poorly differentiated,* or *anaplastic* (Fig. 10.122). A tumor with a microscopic appearance somewhere between these two extremes is called *moderately differentiated* (Fig. 10.123). Histopathologic grading is performed for conventional oral cavity squamous cell carcinomas and for HPV-negative oropharyngeal squamous cell carcinomas but not for tumor variants that have an intrinsic biologic potential (e.g., HPV-positive oropharyngeal squamous cell carcinoma, verrucous carcinoma, spindle cell carcinoma, adenosquamous carcinoma, basaloid squamous carcinoma).

Grading is a somewhat subjective process, depending on the area of the tumor sampled and the individual pathologist's criteria for evaluation. Moreover, clinical staging correlates much better with the prognosis than microscopic grading. In the past, investigators have proposed various multi-parameter histopathologic assessment systems in an attempt to provide more objective criteria that correlate with prognosis. Variables such as pattern of invasion, tumor

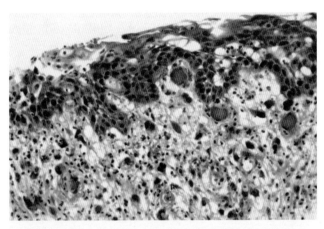

• **Fig. 10.122 Poorly Differentiated Squamous Cell Carcinoma.** The numerous pleomorphic cells within the lamina propria represent anaplastic carcinoma.

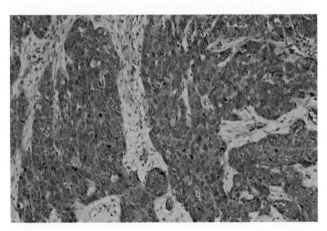

• **Fig. 10.123 Moderately Differentiated Squamous Cell Carcinoma.** Although no keratinization is seen in this medium-power view, these malignant cells are still easily recognizable as being of squamous epithelial origin.

thickness, degree of keratinization, nuclear pleomorphism, lymphocytic response, and mitotic rate have been included in such grading systems. However, widespread agreement regarding the use of such methods is lacking.

For oropharyngeal squamous cell carcinoma, HPV status is especially important in determining prognosis, and distinct staging systems have been developed for HPV-positive vs HPV-negative disease. HPV-positive oropharyngeal squamous cell carcinomas tend to metastasize to cervical lymph nodes relatively early during the course of disease. Nevertheless, HPV-positive cases tend to have better treatment outcomes compared to HPV-negative cases.

For newly diagnosed oropharyngeal squamous cell carcinomas, HPV status typically is assessed by using immunohistochemical expression of p16 as a surrogate marker for transcriptionally active, high-risk HPV infection (see Fig. 10.116B). (The molecular basis for this finding is that overexpression of p16 results from destabilization of the tumor suppressor pRB [retinoblastoma protein] by the HPV oncoprotein E7.) A positive result is defined as at least 70% nuclear and cytoplasmic expression of p16 with moderate to strong intensity. Also, in the case of a cervical lymph node with metastatic squamous cell carcinoma of unknown origin, p16 immunoreactivity may be useful in directing the search for the primary tumor to the oropharynx. The advantages of p16 immunohistochemistry include its cost effectiveness, wide availability, and ease of use on formalin-fixed paraffin-embedded tissue. Other types of HPV testing (e.g., DNA or RNA *in situ* hybridization [ISH] [see Fig. 10.116C], E6/E7 mRNA reverse transcriptase polymerase chain reaction [RT-PCR]) are generally more costly and not so widely available but may be performed in certain cases. For example, some authorities recommend second-line ISH for confirmation of HPV status in p16-positive cases. This recommendation is based on recent studies in which 8%–33% of oropharyngeal squamous cell carcinomas examined were found to be p16-positive yet HPV DNA-negative. Patients within this subset exhibit a worse prognosis than those with p16-positive/HPV DNA-positive disease.

In contrast to oropharyngeal squamous cell carcinomas, p16 immunohistochemistry performed on oral cavity squamous cell carcinomas exhibits low positive predictive value for transcriptionally active HPV infection and is not useful for prognostication. Furthermore, there is only limited data regarding high-risk HPV E6 and E7 expression in oral cavity squamous cell carcinoma, with no significant correlation with prognosis demonstrated thus far. Overall, routine p16 immunohistochemistry or HPV-specific testing is not recommended for non-oropharyngeal head and neck squamous cell carcinomas because of a lack of current evidence to support the prognostic significance of such findings.

Treatment and Prognosis

Clinical staging guides the treatment of squamous cell carcinoma. Most lip vermilion carcinomas are detected at an early stage and treated by surgical excision with excellent results. Surgery may be performed by conventional excision or Mohs micrographic surgery. More advanced cases may be treated by definitive radiation therapy or surgery combined with radiation or chemoradiation therapy. At diagnosis, less than 10% of all lip vermilion carcinomas have metastasized; therefore, neck dissection seldom is indicated. However, a notable exception is squamous cell carcinoma of the upper lip vermilion, which exhibits a high risk for regional lymph node metastasis (apparently related to the extensive lymphatic network in this location). Fortunately, squamous cell carcinoma only rarely occurs in the upper lip vermilion. Interestingly, recent studies also suggest that squamous cell carcinomas involving the lip vermilion exhibit a greater risk for metastasis compared to those limited to the skin adjacent to the lip vermilion.

For intraoral squamous cell carcinoma, early-stage lesions usually are treated with surgery; definitive radiation therapy may be an alternative for patients unable to tolerate surgery. Treatment options for patients with moderately advanced disease include surgery and clinical trials; after surgery, *adjuvant* treatment with radiation or combined radiation and systemic therapy may be considered. Adverse features that may indicate the need for adjuvant therapy include close or positive resection margins, extranodal extension, pathologic T3 or T4 primary, pathologic N2 or N3 nodal disease, nodal disease in levels IV or V of the neck, perineural invasion, and lymphovascular invasion. For individuals with very advanced disease, treatment options include clinical trials, radiation therapy, systemic therapy, *induction* (initial) systemic therapy followed by radiation or combined radiation and additional systemic therapy, supportive care, and palliative treatment.

In patients with intraoral carcinoma, cervical lymph node involvement is evident at presentation in approximately 30% of cases. In addition, approximately 10%–40% of patients initially presenting without apparent cervical metastasis subsequently are found to have occult nodal disease. However, the risk for regional metastasis varies considerably by subsite. In the past, **radical neck dissection** (*en bloc* removal of the lymphatics of the lateral triangle of the neck along with associated nonlymphatic structures, including the internal jugular vein, submandibular gland, sternocleidomastoid muscle, and spinal accessory nerve) was standard treatment for clinically evident or suspected cervical lymph node metastasis. However, over the past several decades, **modified radical neck dissection** (similar to radical neck dissection but with preservation of nonlymphatic structures) and **selective neck dissection** (removal of only select cervical lymph node groups) have gained favor; these techniques are associated with decreased morbidity and, depending upon the extent of disease, often allow for disease control comparable to that of classical radical neck dissection. Histopathologic findings (e.g., number and size of positive nodes, extranodal extension) in a selective neck dissection may aid in determining the need for postoperative radiation with or without systemic therapy. A current preference among some authorities is to classify cervical lymph node dissections as either *comprehensive* (including all lymph node groups of a classical radical neck dissection regardless of whether or not nonlymphatic structures are preserved) or *selective*. Another technique, **sentinel-node biopsy** (biopsy of the first lymph node in the lymphatic basin to receive drainage from the tumor), may be useful for identifying patients with occult neck metastasis. Also, microscopic measurement of primary tumor *depth of invasion* is predictive of occult cervical lymph node metastasis and may be considered when determining the need for *elective* selective neck dissection.

With regard to radiotherapy, *intensity-modulated radiation therapy (IMRT)* represents a technique used to target the treatment area while minimizing damage to neighboring tissue. Also, *brachytherapy* (placement of tiny, radioactive seeds) may be performed at experienced treatment centers for select applications (e.g., large superficial intraoral or lip tumors for which surgical removal would cause significant functional or cosmetic morbidity).

Systemic agents for the management of intraoral, oropharyngeal, and other head and neck squamous cell carcinomas include the following: (1) chemotherapy drugs, including platinum-containing compounds (e.g., cisplatin and carboplatin), 5-fluorouracil, and taxanes (e.g., paclitaxel and docetaxel); (2) targeted agents, including cetuximab (monoclonal antibody directed against epidermal growth factor receptor [EGFR]) and tipifarnib (farnesyltransferase inhibitor recently granted breakthrough therapy designation by the United States Food and Drug Administration for patients with recurrent or metastatic, *HRAS*-mutant tumors); and (3) immune checkpoint inhibitors (e.g., pembrolizumab, nivolumab) (at times considered for patients with recurrent, unresectable, or metastatic disease). In particular, cisplatin is the first-line agent for patients receiving adjuvant (postoperative) chemoradiation therapy for the management of head and neck mucosal squamous cell carcinomas (other than those involving the nasopharynx).

Induction or *neoadjuvant* chemotherapy may be administered initially to shrink a tumor prior to additional therapy. For locoregionally advanced head and neck cancers, some investigators have advocated this approach for enhanced organ preservation, reduced need for adjuvant radiation therapy, and decreased risk for distant metastasis. However, studies suggest that this approach may not result in a significant improvement in overall patient survival or disease control.

For oropharyngeal squamous cell carcinoma, treatment options generally include surgery or definitive radiation therapy for early-stage disease, combined-modality therapy for more advanced disease, and clinical trials. Notably, advances in minimally invasive surgical techniques—such as transoral robotic surgery (TORS) and transoral laser microsurgery (TLMS)—have allowed for reduced morbidity compared to conventional open surgery while still producing favorable outcomes in patients with early-stage disease. TORS or TLMS may be followed by adjuvant radiation therapy or combined radiation and systemic therapy. For patients with HPV-positive oropharyngeal squamous cell carcinoma, areas of interest among clinical trials include deintensified radiation or chemoradiation therapy protocols (aiming to reduce treatment-associated morbidity while maintaining acceptable survival rates) and therapeutic HPV vaccines (such as those targeting HPV 16 E6 and/or E7).

After head and neck cancer treatment, patients should be placed under surveillance to monitor for tumor recurrence or additional primary tumor development. As many as two-thirds of patients with head and neck squamous cell carcinoma develop recurrence, with most instances presenting within the first 2 years after completion of initial treatment. In addition to clinical examination and imaging, follow-up visits may include nutritional counseling, tobacco and alcohol counseling, speech/swallowing rehabilitation, and dental health assessment. Reevaluation typically is performed every few months (or sooner if needed) during the first 5 years, and at least yearly thereafter.

Based on SEER data in the United States for 2011–2017, the estimated 5-year relative survival rate for oral cavity and pharyngeal cancers combined is approximately 67%. Notably, there is a disparity in the 5-year survival rate for white compared to black patients (69% vs 51%, respectively); in part this finding may reflect a white male predilection for HPV-positive oropharyngeal carcinoma, which tends to exhibit more favorable outcomes compared to HPV-negative disease.

The prognosis varies considerably by tumor stage and subsite (Table 10.8). Because most lip vermilion carcinomas are diagnosed at an early stage, the overall 5-year relative survival rate is excellent (approximately 91%). In contrast, intraoral and oropharyngeal carcinomas often are diagnosed at later stages, with significantly lower 5-year relative survival rates (e.g., 52% for floor of mouth lesions and 71% for oropharyngeal lesions).

For oropharyngeal carcinoma, HPV-positive tumor status is a key favorable prognostic factor. Compared to patients with HPV-negative tumors, those with HPV-positive tumors typically exhibit a better response to chemotherapy and/or radiation therapy, with an approximately 60% reduction in risk of death and 30% greater 5-year absolute survival rate. (However, as the average age of HPV-positive group has been increasing, there has been a gradual uptick in mortality within the past decade.) The favorable survival rate for patients with HPV-positive oropharyngeal squamous cell carcinoma may reflect a unique underlying tumor biology, including an intact p53-mediated apoptotic response to radiation, upregulation of DNA repair proteins, a tendency for fewer genomic alterations, a distinctive immune microenvironment, and a lack of field cancerization (see next section). Unlike oropharyngeal squamous cell carcinoma, oral cavity squamous cell carcinoma does not exhibit a clear correlation between HPV tumor status and prognosis.

Current investigations aim to stratify head and neck cancer patients into subgroups based on HPV status, anatomic subsite, gene expression profiling, and cluster analysis for tailored treatment determination and improved prognostication. Studies evaluating the prognostic utility of individual molecular markers (e.g., p53, survivin) abound but lack sufficient evidence for routine clinical application.

Based on SEER data in the United States for 2015–2019, the 5-year age-adjusted mortality rate for oral cavity and pharyngeal cancers combined was 2.5 per 100,000 population. This finding represents a marked improvement over the age-adjusted mortality rate of 4.3 per 100,000 population in 1975. However, mortality increased by 0.4% per year from 2010 to 2019 apparently because of an uptick in deaths from HPV-related tumors. Notably, there was a 2.1% annual increase in incidence-based oropharyngeal cancer mortality among males compared to a 1.2% annual decrease among females from 2006 to 2017 according to data from the National Center for Health Statistics and the SEER Program. This growing trend in male mortality appears to reflect increased numbers of men diagnosed with oropharyngeal cancer in advanced stages of disease and in older age groups. Presumably, elderly individuals may have significant co-morbidities complicating treatment.

Current areas of investigational interest for addressing oral and pharyngeal cancer mortality include improvements in prevention, early diagnosis, and treatment. In particular, recent oropharyngeal cancer prevention efforts have focused on HPV vaccination. In the United States in 2020, the Food and Drug Administration granted accelerated approval for adding prevention of oropharyngeal and other head and neck cancers as an indication for the recombinant 9-valent HPV vaccine. Postapproval confirmatory studies are in process as of this writing. Unfortunately, immunization rates have been relatively low, with only 59% of US adolescents 13–17 years of age receiving the recommended doses of the vaccine in 2020. Notably, more than half of oropharyngeal cancer cases diagnosed in the US from 2001 to 2017 occurred in the Southeast and Midwest, where many states have some of the lowest HPV vaccination rates in the country. Nevertheless, some US studies have reported encouraging observations, including recent declines in absolute oropharyngeal cancer incidence among young white males and recent reductions in the number of vaccine-type oral HPV infections.

Secondary prevention of HPV-mediated oropharyngeal cancer through screening is complicated by the lack of a well-defined premalignant lesion in the tonsillar region. Investigational oropharyngeal cancer screening methods designed for certain patient groups include oral rinse/gargle testing for high-risk HPV DNA and blood-based assays for HPV-16 DNA or antibodies. Notwithstanding, further research is needed to demonstrate the clinical utility of such screening tests, and FDA approval has not been granted. In addition, some researchers have proposed risk prediction models for oropharyngeal or other head and neck cancers based on various parameters, such as age, sex, race, smoking, alcohol use, education, number of lifetime sexual partners, and high-risk HPV status. However, further studies are needed.

Multiple Carcinomas

Patients with one carcinoma of the oral cavity, oropharynx, or other head and neck mucosa are at increased risk for developing additional concurrent (synchronous) or, more commonly, later (metachronous) primary carcinomas of the head and neck mucosa, lungs, and esophagus. Indeed, about a third of head and neck squamous cell carcinoma patient deaths are attributed to second primary malignancies. According to a pooled analysis of data from 13 cancer registries, approximately 3%–7% of head and neck squamous cell carcinoma patients per year develop an additional primary malignancy, with a 20-year cumulative risk of 36%. Other studies have estimated the annual risk to be in the range of 2%–3%. In addition, analyses of SEER data for head and neck squamous cell carcinoma patients in the United States have shown that the risk for a second primary malignancy is greater for those with index tumors arising in non-oropharyngeal sites (which are mostly non-HPV-mediated) compared to those arising in the oropharynx (which are predominantly HPV-mediated).

This tendency for the development of multiple mucosal cancers is hypothesized to result from *field cancerization*—a process whereby exposure to carcinogens, such as tobacco and alcohol, creates a diffuse field of altered epithelial cells with increased potential for malignant transformation. Molecular analyses of various markers, including loss of heterozygosity (LOH), microsatellite alterations, *TP53* tumor suppressor gene mutations, and X-chromosome inactivation, have identified genetic alterations shared between tumor tissue and adjacent clinically normal-appearing tissue in one-third to one-half of cases examined. In addition, investigators have shown that a significant proportion of second primary tumors develop from the same preneoplastic precursor lesion or "field," with the remaining cases representing tumors that develop independently. Furthermore, researchers have proposed that patches of clonal cells can progress to develop additional mutations and give rise to subclones in a process known as *clonal divergence,* which would account for the genetic heterogeneity typically seen among these tumors. Interactions between mutant clones and the microenvironment appear to play an important role in field cancerization and carcinogenesis as well.

Interestingly, malignancies attributed to HPV infection do not appear to be associated with field cancerization. Nevertheless, there are emerging reports of patients with HPV-mediated head and neck squamous cell carcinoma who have developed additional primary tumors. A recent analysis combining a systematic review of the literature, SEER data, and institutional reports found that multiple tumors were present in approximately 0.5%–2.5% of individuals with HPV-mediated head and neck squamous cell carcinoma. In particular, this subset of individuals often exhibited small, synchronous, bilateral tonsillar tumors. The mechanism underlying this phenomenon is unknown, although proposed theories include the following: (1) intra-host spread of HPV infection via a lymphatic, hematogenous, or salivary route, (2) infection of different anatomic locations by different HPV strains, (3) infection of different anatomic locations by the same HPV strain upon initial or subsequent exposure, and (4) lymphatic intraoropharyngeal metastasis of tumor cells.

◆ VERRUCOUS CARCINOMA (SNUFF DIPPER'S CANCER; ACKERMAN'S TUMOR)

Verrucous carcinoma is a low-grade variant of oral squamous cell carcinoma. In 1948, Ackerman described this lesion in detail, although the term *verrucous carcinoma* had been used in 1944 in a series of cases reported by Burford,

Ackerman, and Robinson. Ackerman postulated that some of these lesions might be associated with smokeless tobacco use, because 11 of his 31 patients were "tobacco chewers." However, there was no mention of the type of smokeless tobacco used and no mention of whether any of these patients also had smoked tobacco. In addition to the oral mucosa, verrucous carcinoma has been identified at several extraoral sites, including laryngeal, vulvovaginal, penile, anorectal, sinonasal, and esophageal mucosa, as well as the skin of the breast, axilla, ear canal, and soles of the feet. Extraoral cases are unrelated to tobacco use. Several investigators have identified DNA from HPV types 6, 11, 16, and 18 in a minority of oral verrucous carcinomas, although the possibility that these cases represent coincidental HPV infection cannot be excluded.

Verrucous carcinoma represents less than 1%–16% of all oral squamous cell carcinomas, depending on the local popularity of smokeless tobacco use. The only epidemiologic assessment of this tumor in a Western culture reported an average annual incidence rate of one to three oral lesions per 1 million population each year. Among head and neck malignancies recorded in the SEER database from 1973 to 2015, only 0.5% of cases were diagnosed as verrucous carcinoma.

Some oral verrucous carcinomas arise in people who chronically use chewing tobacco, snuff, or betel quid. Cases also occur in those who combine habits (i.e., smokeless tobacco, smoking, and alcohol), exclusively smoke tobacco, or have no identifiable risk factors. However, exact figures are difficult to assess because patients often deny their habits. Nevertheless, among smokeless tobacco users, conventional squamous cell carcinoma is much more likely to develop than this low-grade variant.

Clinical Features

Verrucous carcinoma is found predominantly in older individuals (approximate average age: 65–70 years). Most studies report a male predilection or a nearly even gender distribution; however, in areas where women frequently use dry snuff, females may predominate. The most common sites of oral mucosal involvement include the mandibular vestibule, buccal mucosa, gingiva, tongue, and hard palate. The involved area often corresponds to the site of chronic tobacco placement. In cultural groups who keep the tobacco in the maxillary vestibule or under the tongue, these locations are involved most commonly.

Oral verrucous carcinoma is usually extensive by the time of diagnosis, and it is not unusual for a tumor to be present for 2–3 years before definitive diagnosis. The lesion appears as a diffuse, well-demarcated, painless, thick plaque with papillary or verruciform surface projections (Figs. 10.124 and 10.125). Lesions are typically white but also may appear erythematous or pink. The color depends on the amount of keratin produced and the degree of host inflammatory response to the tumor. When left untreated, the lesions may destroy underlying structures, such as bone, cartilage, muscle, and salivary glands. Enlarged cervical lymph nodes in patients with verrucous carcinoma usually represent inflammatory reactive changes rather than nodal metastasis.

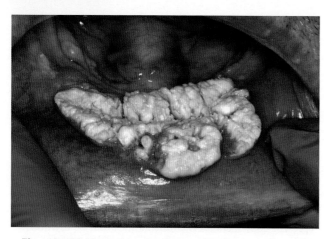

• **Fig. 10.124 Verrucous Carcinoma.** Extensive papillary, white mass of the lower labial mucosa and mandibular alveolar ridge. (Courtesy of Dr. Ashleigh Briody.)

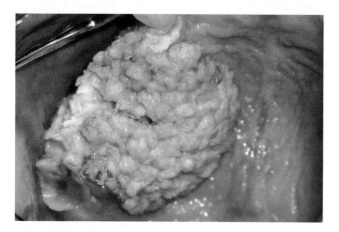

• **Fig. 10.125 Verrucous Carcinoma.** Large, exophytic, papillary mass of the maxillary alveolar ridge.

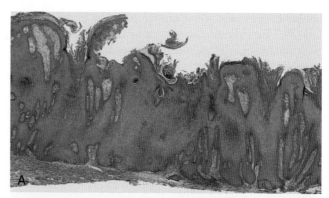

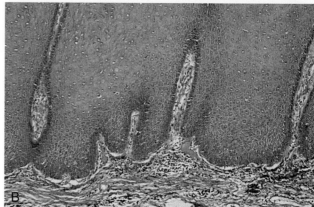

• **Fig. 10.126 Verrucous Carcinoma. A,** Low-power photomicrograph showing marked epithelial hyperplasia with a rough, papillary surface, and keratin plugging. **B,** High-power view showing bulbous rete ridges without significant dysplasia.

Leukoplakia or **tobacco pouch keratosis** may be seen on adjacent mucosal surfaces, and verrucous carcinoma is a lesion that may develop from the high-risk precancer, proliferative verrucous leukoplakia (PVL) (see page 384). PVL and verrucous carcinoma may have been reported in the past by the name **oral florid papillomatosis.**

Histopathologic Features

Verrucous carcinoma has a deceptively benign microscopic appearance; it is characterized by wide and elongated rete ridges that appear to "push" into the underlying connective tissue (Fig. 10.126). Lesions usually show abundant keratin (usually parakeratin) production and a papillary or verruciform surface. Parakeratin typically fills the depressions (**parakeratin clefts**) between the surface projections. These projections may be long and pointed or short and blunted. The lesional epithelial cells generally show no significant cytologic atypia. There is frequently an intense inflammatory cell infiltrate in the subjacent connective tissue. Sometimes this infiltrate exhibits "lichenoid" features (i.e., a superficial bandlike chronic inflammatory cell infiltrate).

The histopathologic diagnosis of verrucous carcinoma requires an adequate incisional biopsy. Because the individual cells are not very dysplastic, the pathologist must evaluate the overall histomorphologic configuration of the lesion to make the diagnosis. Adequate sampling also is important because conventional squamous cell carcinoma develops concurrently within up to 20% of verrucous carcinomas.

The microscopic differential diagnosis may include *carcinoma cuniculatum*—another well-differentiated variant of squamous cell carcinoma lacking significant cytologic atypia. This variant is characterized by deeply infiltrative tumor islands with branching, keratin-filled crypts resembling "rabbit burrows" and an often brisk inflammatory infiltrate (Fig. 10.127). This complex, infiltrative growth pattern differs from the broad, "pushing" rete seen in verrucous carcinoma. In carcinoma cuniculatum, the endophytic component predominates, and the surface is mildly exophytic with a subtle, papillary, or cobblestone-like architecture. In contrast, verrucous carcinoma exhibits a more prominent and warty exophytic component. Furthermore, some examples of carcinoma cuniculatum exhibit frank infiltration of bone to produce a "moth-eaten" lytic lesion on radiographs, whereas verrucous carcinoma typically causes no bony destruction or, at most, pressure resorption of the underlying bone. Both variants generally exhibit a favorable prognosis.

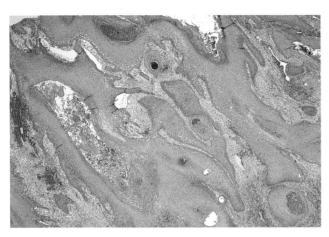

• **Fig. 10.127　Carcinoma Cuniculatum.** A well-differentiated carcinoma characterized by keratin-filled invaginations that burrow deep into the connective tissue.

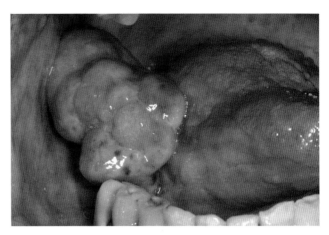

• **Fig. 10.128　Spindle Cell Carcinoma.** Large polypoid mass arising from the right lateral tongue.

Treatment and Prognosis

The treatment of choice is surgical excision. The surgery generally need not be as extensive as that required for conventional squamous cell carcinoma of a similar size. If cervical lymph node enlargement is clinically evident, then a selective neck dissection may be performed, although most such cases turn out to represent reactive lymphadenopathy rather than metastasis. Approximately 90% of patients are disease free 5 years after surgery, but some patients will require at least one additional surgical procedure during that time. The treatment failures usually occur in patients with the most extensive involvement or in those unable to tolerate extensive surgery because of unrelated systemic diseases. An additional cause of treatment failure is the initial inability to identify focal, concurrent conventional squamous cell carcinoma; such cases should be treated as conventional squamous cell carcinomas.

Radiotherapy is an alternative primary treatment modality but provides poorer local control and, thus, is considered less effective than surgery. In addition, radiotherapy has been unpopular because of published reports of poorly differentiated or anaplastic carcinoma developing within the lesion after treatment. However, more recent analysis suggests that this threat is overexaggerated. In a limited number of cases, tumor regression after chemotherapy, radiochemotherapy, or photodynamic therapy has been reported, although these treatment alternatives require further study.

◆ SPINDLE CELL CARCINOMA (SARCOMATOID SQUAMOUS CELL CARCINOMA; POLYPOID SQUAMOUS CELL CARCINOMA; CARCINOSARCOMA; PSEUDOSARCOMA)

Spindle cell carcinoma is a rare variant of squamous cell carcinoma characterized by dysplastic surface epithelium in conjunction with an invasive spindle cell element. With routine light microscopy, it may be indistinguishable from connective tissue sarcomas or other spindle cell malignancies. Spindle cell carcinoma of the upper aerodigestive tract is closely associated with tobacco and alcohol use. Some cases develop after radiotherapy for a more differentiated squamous cell carcinoma, a phenomenon known as **dedifferentiation.** Transcriptionally active HPV has been detected infrequently in this variant.

In the past, this biphasic lesion was thought to be a "collision" tumor between a carcinoma and sarcoma; however, current evidence supports a monoclonal origin for both tumor components. Electron microscopy, immunohistochemical analysis, and molecular genetic studies suggest that the lesional cells undergo a shift from a squamous epithelial to a mesenchymal-like phenotype (*epithelial-mesenchymal transition*), with decreased intercellular adhesion and increased infiltrative behavior.

Clinical Features

Spindle cell carcinoma tends to arise in older individuals and affects males more often than females. The lesion may develop anywhere within the upper aerodigestive tract, with a predilection for the larynx and oral cavity. In the mouth, the tongue, alveolar mucosa, oral floor, and lower lip are common sites, but other areas may be involved.

In contrast to other oral cancers, spindle cell carcinoma typically appears as a pedunculated, polypoid mass, but occasionally it may appear as a sessile, nodular, or fungating mass (Fig. 10.128). The surface often is ulcerated. Pain and paresthesia are prominent features. Lower lip lesions seem to have a special propensity to travel along nerves through the mental foramen and into the mandibular canal.

Histopathologic Features

Spindle cell carcinoma is composed predominantly of fascicles of anaplastic, spindle-shaped cells (Fig. 10.129). Some spindle cells may appear as obvious epithelial elements, but others strongly resemble atypical mesenchymal cells.

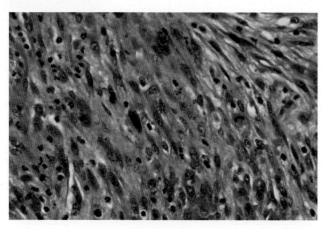

• **Fig. 10.129 Spindle Cell Carcinoma.** Streaming fascicles of pleomorphic spindle cells that represent anaplastic epithelial cells.

On rare occasions, bone, cartilage, or muscle differentiation may be seen. Numerous mitotic figures often are present. The overall picture is similar to that of an anaplastic fibrosarcoma (see page 559), except for the often-inconspicuous squamous element.

The squamous component usually consists of dysplasia or carcinoma *in situ* of the overlying surface epithelium but may appear as islands of atypical squamous epithelium among the spindle cells. Direct transition between the two cell types may be seen. Because of frequent surface ulceration, a neoplastic surface component may be difficult to discern. Tumors with a prominent inflammatory background may mimic granulation tissue. Metastatic lesions may show only spindle cells, only squamous cells, or a combination of spindle and squamous cells.

Serial sections may be needed to find areas of unequivocal squamous cell carcinoma, and immunohistochemical techniques can be particularly useful in distinguishing this tumor from mesenchymal spindle cell malignancies. Most mesenchymal tumors express vimentin but not epithelial markers. In contrast, most spindle cell carcinomas react with antibodies directed against at least one epithelial marker (such as cytokeratins, p63 with or without p40, and/or epithelial membrane antigen [EMA]). Nearly all cases express vimentin; immunoreactivity for other mesenchymal markers is possible but highly variable.

Treatment and Prognosis

The mainstay of treatment for oral spindle cell carcinoma is radical surgery, with neck dissection when clinically positive nodes are present. The benefit of radiotherapy and/or chemotherapy is unclear. However, adjuvant radiation therapy may be administered for patients with nodal metastasis or surgical margins positive for tumor. According to SEER data in the United States for 2004 through 2009, the 3-year disease-specific survival rate is approximately 50% for oral lesions; however, other studies have reported survival rates as low as 24%. Negative prognostic factors include endophytic (rather than polypoid) growth and an origin

from a previously irradiated carcinoma. Compared to conventional squamous cell carcinoma, spindle cell carcinoma appears to have a worse prognosis among oral cavity tumors but a more favorable prognosis among laryngeal tumors. The more favorable prognosis for laryngeal cases may reflect early detection due to symptoms from polypoid glottic lesions.

◆ ADENOSQUAMOUS CARCINOMA

Adenosquamous carcinoma is a rare squamous cell carcinoma variant that is characterized histopathologically by a combination of adenocarcinoma and squamous cell carcinoma. In the head and neck, this variant most often occurs in the larynx. The oral cavity, sinonasal tract, oropharynx, hypopharynx, and other subsites may be affected as well. This lesion generally is considered to represent a distinct clinicopathologic entity, although in the past some authorities considered it to be merely a high-grade **mucoepidermoid carcinoma** (see page 493). The histogenesis is not entirely certain. An origin from excretory ducts of minor glands, surface squamous epithelium, or both has been proposed. Tobacco and alcohol use have been implicated as causative factors. In addition, transcriptionally active HPV has been identified in a few cases involving the oropharynx and nasal cavity.

Clinical Features

Adenosquamous carcinoma exhibits a male predilection and usually occurs in older adults. In the oral cavity, the tumor may involve the tongue, floor of mouth, and other mucosal surfaces. The tumor typically presents as a nodular, broad-based, variably painful mass with or without ulceration. The majority of patients have cervical lymph node metastasis at diagnosis.

Histopathologic Features

Adenosquamous carcinoma appears as an admixture of a surface squamous cell carcinoma and an underlying adenocarcinoma. The glandular component tends to be most prominent in deeper portions of the tumor. Mucicarmine or Alcian blue staining demonstrates intracytoplasmic mucin in most cases, making differentiation from mucoepidermoid carcinoma difficult. However, features that may aid in distinction from mucoepidermoid carcinoma include the following: presence of dysplasia or carcinoma *in situ* in the surface epithelium, frank squamous differentiation (such as keratin pearl formation and intercellular bridges), and discrete adenocarcinomatous foci mainly found in deeper portions of the tumor. In addition, *MAML2* translocations may be detected in mucoepidermoid carcinoma but have not been noted in adenosquamous carcinoma. Squamous cell carcinoma with acantholysis or pseudoglandular degeneration also may be considered in the differential diagnosis but lacks intracytoplasmic mucin production and usually forms gland-like structures with irregular, rather than smooth and rounded, contours.

Both squamous and glandular components immunoreact with antibodies directed against high molecular–weight cytokeratins. In addition, the squamous component may express p63, whereas the glandular component may express CK7, CAM 5.2, and CEA. There is typically no immunoreactivity for CK20.

Treatment and Prognosis

Adenosquamous carcinoma typically is treated with radical surgical excision, at times supplemented with radiation or chemoradiation therapy. One review of previously reported head and neck cases noted local recurrence in 36%, regional metastasis in 47%, and distant metastasis in 25%; among cases for which outcomes were reported, 44% of patients died of disease. According to SEER data in the United States from 1973 through 2012, 5-year overall and disease-specific survival rates are 30% and 50%, respectively. Adenosquamous carcinoma generally has been considered to represent an aggressive variant of squamous cell carcinoma. However, after controlling for variables such as anatomic subsite, patient demographics, stage, treatment, and/or HPV status, a few studies suggest that outcomes for patients with adenosquamous carcinoma may not be substantially different from those for patients with conventional squamous cell carcinoma.

◆ BASALOID SQUAMOUS CARCINOMA (BASALOID SQUAMOUS CELL CARCINOMA)

Basaloid squamous carcinoma is a rare squamous cell carcinoma variant that arises primarily in the upper aerodigestive tract. Heavy tobacco and alcohol use appear to represent major risk factors. In addition, HPV may play an important role in the etiopathogenesis of a subset of basaloid squamous carcinomas—particularly those arising in the oropharynx.

Clinical Features

Basaloid squamous carcinoma tends to occur in older individuals (average age approximately 60 years) and arises more commonly in males than females. The most frequently involved sites within the head and neck include the oropharynx, larynx, oral cavity, and hypopharynx. Oral cavity tumors often arise in the floor of mouth, although other subsites may be affected as well. The lesion clinically appears as a fungating mass or ulcer and may be painful or interfere with swallowing **(dysphagia).** Most cases are diagnosed at an advanced clinical stage.

Histopathologic Features

As its name connotes, basaloid squamous carcinoma has two microscopic components. The first is a superficial, well-

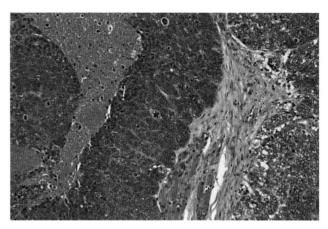

• **Fig. 10.130 Basaloid Squamous Carcinoma.** Sheets of basaloid squamous epithelium exhibiting a high mitotic index and tumor necrosis.

differentiated or moderately differentiated squamous cell carcinoma, often with surface ulceration, multifocal origin, and areas of carcinoma *in situ*. The second, deeper component is an invasive basaloid epithelium arranged in islands, cords, and glandlike lobules. This deeper tumor often shows palisading of peripheral cells, central necrosis, and occasional squamous differentiation (Fig. 10.130). This component appears similar to basal cell carcinoma, adenoid cystic carcinoma, basal cell adenocarcinoma, or neuroendocrine carcinoma. The interface between the two components is typically sharp and distinct, but gradual transition from squamous to basaloid cells may be seen occasionally. The tumor islands may be surrounded by hyalinized stroma and arranged in a "jigsaw puzzle" pattern. Microcystic spaces filled with PAS-positive basal lamina material may be interspersed among the tumor islands as well.

Treatment and Prognosis

Treatment typically consists of surgery, often followed by radiation or chemoradiation therapy. Studies based on cancer registry data in the United States for head and neck cases have reported 5- and 10-year survival rates of approximately 64% and 52%, respectively. This tumor generally has been considered an aggressive malignancy. However, several more recent investigations have noted that basaloid squamous carcinoma may have a similar outcome compared with conventional squamous cell carcinoma when controlling for variables such as clinical stage, anatomic location, and HPV status. Therefore, reports of poor outcomes for basaloid squamous carcinoma in part might reflect a tendency for these patients to be diagnosed with late-stage disease. In addition, studies suggest that oropharyngeal basaloid squamous carcinomas often harbor HPV, with significantly improved survival among HPV-positive cases compared to HPV-negative cases. Thus, conflicting reports in the literature regarding prognosis may reflect differences in subsite distribution and HPV tumor status among study cohorts.

◆ CARCINOMA OF THE MAXILLARY SINUS

Carcinoma of the maxillary sinus or antrum is an uncommon malignancy of largely unknown cause. It does not appear to be related to sinusitis or nasal polyps. Unlike squamous cell carcinomas in other head and neck sites, squamous cell carcinomas of the paranasal sinuses have been associated only weakly with tobacco use. A strong causal relationship to occupational wood and leather dust exposure has been established for the rarely occurring sinonasal intestinal type of adenocarcinoma. In addition, HPV may be an etiologic factor in some cases, with transcriptionally active high-risk HPV detected in approximately 25% of sinonasal squamous cell carcinomas examined.

Maxillary sinus carcinomas comprise only about 3% of all head and neck carcinomas; however, among paranasal sinus carcinomas, the maxillary sinus is the most common site (accounting for 80% of lesions). Most lesions remain asymptomatic or mimic sinusitis for long periods while the tumor grows to fill the sinus. Therefore, the diagnosis may not be made until the lesion has perforated through the surrounding bone.

The majority of maxillary sinus carcinomas represent squamous cell carcinomas. However, additional carcinomas that may arise in this location include sinonasal adenocarcinoma, **sinonasal undifferentiated carcinoma (SNUC)** (see next section), neuroendocrine (small cell undifferentiated) carcinoma, salivary gland-type adenocarcinoma, and sinonasal lymphoepithelial carcinoma. Rare examples of newly described carcinoma types (e.g., NUT carcinoma, SWI/SNF complex-deficient sinonasal carcinoma, HPV-related multiphenotypic carcinoma) may involve this location as well.

Clinical and Radiographic Features

Carcinoma of the maxillary sinus mainly affects older adults, with a slight male predilection. More than 80% of cases are advanced (stage III or IV) at the time of diagnosis. Patients generally complain of chronic unilateral nasal stuffiness or notice an ulceration or mass of the hard palate or alveolar bone (Fig. 10.131). When the second division of the trigeminal nerve is involved, intense pain or paresthesia of the midface or maxilla may occur, perhaps simulating a toothache. Adjacent teeth may become loose, and dental radiographs often reveal a "moth-eaten" destruction of the lamina dura and surrounding bone. A panoramic radiograph shows a cloudy sinus with destruction of its bony wall; however, the extent of the tumor is best visualized by CT or MRI.

If the tumor perforates the lateral wall of the sinus, unilateral facial swelling and pain are usually present. With medial extension, nasal obstruction and hemorrhage are common. Superior extension results in displacement or protrusion of the eyeball. Approximately 9%–14% of patients have regional lymph node metastasis at the time of diagnosis. Distant metastasis is uncommon until late in the progression of disease.

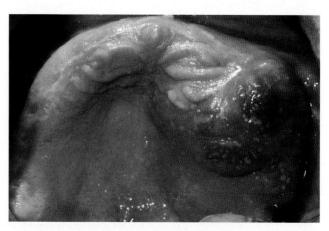

• **Fig. 10.131 Carcinoma of the Maxillary Sinus.** The tumor has produced a bulge of the posterior maxillary alveolar ridge and is beginning to ulcerate through the surface mucosa.

Histopathologic Features

Although the antrum is lined by respiratory epithelium, the great majority of maxillary sinus carcinomas are **squamous cell carcinomas,** usually moderately or poorly differentiated. Squamous cell carcinomas in the sinonasal tract may be subclassified as keratinizing, nonkeratinizing, or less frequent variants (such as, basaloid, papillary, adenosquamous, spindle cell, and verrucous).

Treatment and Prognosis

Treatment depends upon tumor type and stage. Most patients are treated by surgical resection, which may be combined with radiotherapy and/or chemotherapy. Neck dissection may be performed for patients with regional metastasis. Individuals with unresectable disease should consider clinical trial participation; treatment options for these patients typically include radiation therapy and/or chemotherapy. According to SEER data in the United States for 2010 through 2016, 5-year relative survival rates for cancer of the nasal cavity and paranasal sinuses are 82% for patients with localized disease, 52% for patients with regional metastasis, 43% for patients with distant metastasis, and 58% for all tumor stages combined. According to the National Cancer Database for 2004 through 2012, median survival for individuals with cancer of the maxillary sinus is 29 months. Death among patients with carcinoma of the maxillary sinus usually occurs from local destruction and the inability to control the primary disease. Some investigators have suggested that HPV-positive sinonasal carcinomas may exhibit improved clinical outcomes compared to HPV-negative cases; however, further studies are needed.

◆ SINONASAL UNDIFFERENTIATED CARCINOMA

Sinonasal undifferentiated carcinoma (SNUC) is a rare, highly aggressive neoplasm of the nasal cavity and paranasal sinuses. It comprises less than 3% of sinonasal malignancies.

The tumor initially was described in 1986, and fewer than 400 cases have been reported.

There has been some disagreement regarding whether SNUC constitutes a distinct clinicopathologic entity vs a diagnosis of exclusion. The recent identification of *IDH2* mutations in a significant proportion of cases combined with earlier descriptions of SNUC based on histomorphology and immunophenotyping would support classification as a distinct entity. Tumors within this category generally should lack the following features: (1) squamous, glandular, or other specific lines of cellular differentiation; (2) Epstein-Barr virus or human papillomavirus; (3) definite neuroendocrine differentiation; and (4) specific genotypes other than oncogenic *IDH* mutations.

In the earlier literature, these tumors probably were classified as anaplastic carcinomas or high-grade olfactory neuroblastomas. In more recent years, the definition of SNUC has been further refined as advanced molecular profiling techniques have led to the identification of novel tumor types excluded from this category. Such newly described entities, which have been distinguished from SNUC, include the following aggressive malignancies: *NUT carcinoma* (defined by balanced translocations involving the *NUTM1* gene on chromosome 15q14), *HPV-related multiphenotypic carcinoma* (associated with HPV33 and other high-risk HPV types), and *SWI/SNF complex-deficient sinonasal carcinoma* (i.e., *SMARCB1 [INI-1]-deficient sinonasal carcinoma* characterized *SMARCB1* inactivation and resultant loss of nuclear INI-1 protein expression, *SMARCA4-deficient sinonasal carcinoma* characterized by *SMARCA4* inactivation and resultant loss of SMARCA4 expression). SMARCB1 and SMARCA4 represent components of the SWI/SNF complex, which is involved in chromatin remodeling.

The histogenesis and etiopathogenesis of SNUC are poorly understood. Some investigators have theorized that the cell of origin may be related to the Schneiderian membrane or olfactory epithelium. In addition to characteristic *IDH2* mutations, many cases harbor concurrent alterations in *SOX9*, *SOX2*, PI3K pathway genes, *KIT*, *TP53*, *MYC*, and various other genes. There is only a weak association with tobacco smoking. In some instances, patients have developed SNUC secondary to radiation therapy for nasopharyngeal carcinoma or retinoblastoma.

Clinical and Radiographic Features

SNUC occurs over a broad age range (third through ninth decades), with a median age at presentation in the sixth decade. The male-to-female ratio is approximately 2:1 to 3:1.

The tumor is well known for rapid development of locally extensive disease. It typically appears as a large mass that can involve multiple regions of the sinonasal tract, including the nasal cavity, maxillary sinus, and ethmoid sinuses. In addition, extension into contiguous sites—such as, the nasopharynx, orbit, and cranial cavity—is common. Inferior penetration into the oral cavity is possible as well. There is often rapid development of multiple sinonasal symptoms, including nasal obstruction or discharge, epistaxis, swelling, and pain. Orbital involvement may lead to proptosis, periorbital swelling, diplopia, and vision loss. Cranial nerve palsies are common as well.

Tumor extent is best assessed by CT or MRI, which typically reveals a large, expansile sinonasal mass with bony destruction and invasion of adjacent structures (Fig. 10.132).

Histopathologic Features

SNUC is characterized by trabeculae, nests, islands, ribbons, and sheets of polygonal cells with minimal cytoplasm and pleomorphic, hyperchromatic to vesicular nuclei. No squamous or glandular differentiation should be observed. Mitotic figures are numerous. Tumor necrosis, apoptosis, and lymphovascular invasion usually are prominent. Lymphovascular invasion and perineural invasion often are noted. The surface epithelium overlying the tumor may exhibit dysplasia or carcinoma *in situ*. Immunohistochemistry for cytokeratins (such as AE1/AE3 and low molecular weight cytokeratins) or epithelial membrane antigen (EMA) typically is positive. Careful histopathologic examination, a broad immunohistochemical panel, and, at times, molecular studies are needed to rule out other entities, such as poorly differentiated squamous cell carcinoma, olfactory neuroblastoma, nasopharyngeal undifferentiated nonkeratinizing squamous cell carcinoma, neuroendocrine carcinoma, NUT carcinoma, SMARCB1-deficient sinonasal carcinoma, SMARCA4-deficient sinonasal carcinoma,

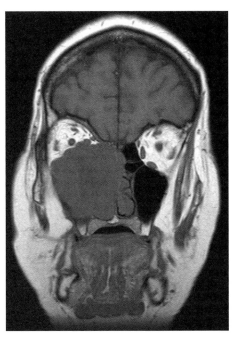

• **Fig. 10.132 Sinonasal Undifferentiated Carcinoma (SNUC).** T1-weighted magnetic resonance image (MRI) showing a large destructive mass filling the right maxillary sinus with extension into the orbital region and nasal cavity. (Courtesy of Dr. Zoran Rumboldt.)

melanoma, lymphoma, synovial sarcoma, Ewing sarcoma, and alveolar rhabdomyosarcoma.

Treatment and Prognosis

Most patients present with locally advanced disease. In such cases, the standard approach is aggressive multimodal therapy, including surgical resection, radiation therapy, and/or chemotherapy. Unresectable disease is treated by definitive chemoradiation therapy. When resectability is questionable, some authorities advocate induction chemotherapy in order to shrink the tumor prior to additional treatment. Clinical studies are needed to assess whether patients with *IDH*-mutant tumors may benefit from targeted IDH inhibitors.

The prognosis is generally poor, although several centers have reported improved outcomes with modern treatment approaches. An analysis of SEER data in the United States from 1973 to 2010 reported overall 5- and 10-year relative survival rates of about 35% and 31%, respectively; the overall median survival was 22 months. However, a recent multicenter collaborative study in France noted 62% overall survival among their patient cohort, with a majority exhibiting advanced disease at presentation. Local recurrence is common and is the major cause of morbidity and mortality. Metastasis is possible, usually to cervical lymph nodes, bone, liver, or brain. Some reports suggest that cases exhibiting *IDH2* mutations may have more favorable outcomes compared to those without such mutations.

◆ NASOPHARYNGEAL CARCINOMA

Nasopharyngeal carcinoma represents a group of malignancies that arise from the lining epithelium of the lymphoid tissue–rich nasopharynx; similar tumors are found in the palatine tonsil and base of tongue. These three anatomic sites are collectively called **Waldeyer tonsillar tissue** or **Waldeyer ring.**

Nasopharyngeal carcinoma is relatively uncommon. According to global data collected by the International Agency for Research on Cancer, there were approximately 133,000 new cases of nasopharyngeal cancer in the year 2020, which accounted for only about 0.7% of all cancers diagnosed during this period. Age-standardized annual incidence rates varied from less than 1 per 100,000 persons in the Americas and Europe to 5 per 100,000 persons in Southeast Asia. In southern Chinese men, however, the rate is a startling 25 per 100,000. Among southern Chinese men who migrate to the United States, the rate is intermediate, which suggests possible interactions between an environmental causative agent and host genetics. Intermediate rates also are observed among many indigenous people of Southeast Asia (including Thais, Vietnamese, Malays, and Filipinos), Inuits of Alaska and Canada, and Arabs of North Africa.

Both genetic and environmental factors have been implicated in the etiopathogenesis of nasopharyngeal carcinoma.

Linkage and genome-wide association studies have identified several susceptibility genes, particularly HLA genes residing at the MHC region on chromosome 6p21. Chief among environmental risk factors is Epstein-Barr virus (EBV) infection. Some studies also have implicated diets deficient in vitamin C, consumption of salted fish containing carcinogenic N-nitrosamines, and tobacco smoking. However, the risk for carcinoma development for a given level of tobacco exposure is lower in the nasopharynx than in other parts of the upper aerodigestive tract. Furthermore, investigators have detected high-risk HPV in a small subset of nasopharyngeal carcinomas with a predilection for white individuals.

Clinical Features

Nasopharyngeal carcinoma occurs in all age groups, with a peak between the ages of 40–59 years in high-incidence regions. In low-incidence regions, there is a modest peak during adolescence/young adulthood and a higher peak after 65 years of age. The disease occurs about two to three times more commonly in men than in women.

The primary tumor tends to arise in the fossa of Rosenmuller (a deep recess in the posterolateral nasopharyngeal wall). The lesion often is small and difficult to detect, even by endoscopy. In regions where nasopharyngeal carcinoma is endemic, plasma EBV DNA measurement may be combined with endocoscopic examination and MRI for detection of early-stage disease in asymptomatic patients. Serologic testing also may aid in diagnosis. The first sign of disease for 50%–60% of patients is an enlarged, firm to hard, cervical lymph node, which represents metastatic tumor (Fig. 10.133). Symptoms related to the ear are described by slightly less than half of patients. If the tumor obstructs the eustachian tube, then unilateral serous otitis media, otalgia, or hearing loss may be the presenting complaint. Epistaxis, nasal obstruction, and pharyngeal pain may be present as well. The tumor may invade through the foramen lacerum into the brain, producing CNS symptoms, or it may involve cranial nerves in the area, causing specific symptoms related to those nerves. Involvement of the pterygoid muscles can produce facial pain with limited jaw movement, thereby mimicking a temporomandibular joint disorder. Significantly, 5%–10% of patients also have distant metastasis at the time of diagnosis.

Histopathologic Features

The surgeon often has difficulty finding the primary lesion, and multiple systematic biopsy samples of the nasopharyngeal mucosa may be necessary for tumor identification and diagnosis. Nasopharyngeal carcinoma includes the following histopathologic types:
1. Keratinizing squamous cell carcinoma
2. Nonkeratinizing squamous cell carcinoma (including differentiated and undifferentiated variants)
3. Basaloid squamous cell carcinoma

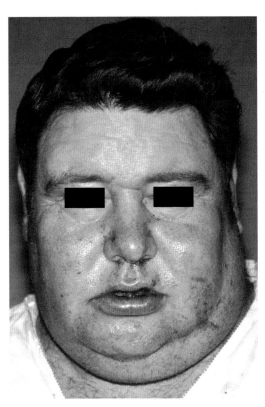

• **Fig. 10.133 Nasopharyngeal Carcinoma.** This patient initially appeared with metastatic carcinoma in the left lateral neck. Further evaluation revealed a primary tumor of the nasopharynx. (Courtesy of Dr. D. E. Kenady.)

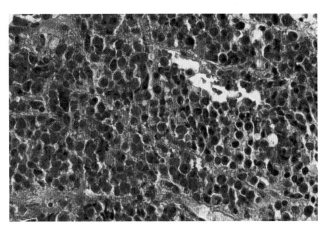

• **Fig. 10.134 Nasopharyngeal Carcinoma.** Poorly differentiated tumor exhibiting sheets of rounded tumor cells.

When more than one histopathologic type is present, the tumor is classified according to the predominant type.

The histopathologic features of **keratinizing squamous cell carcinoma** are identical to those of squamous cell carcinoma of other head and neck regions (see page 416). Keratinization must be evident at the light microscopic level.

Nonkeratinizing squamous cell carcinoma represents the most common type of nasopharyngeal carcinoma. This group can be further categorized as *differentiated* and *undifferentiated,* although these subtypes are of no clinical or prognostic significance. The lesional cells of **differentiated nonkeratinizing squamous cell carcinoma** are relatively mature and somewhat squamous in nature, but they produce no keratin. Broad interconnecting bands of oval or round cells are organized in plexiform and papillary patterns. **Undifferentiated nonkeratinizing squamous cell carcinoma** consists of sheets of undifferentiated cells with indistinct margins, very little cytoplasm, and large, vesicular nuclei (Fig. 10.134). These tumor cells are often intermixed with the lymphoid cells normally found at this anatomic site. The term **lymphoepithelioma** (or **lymphoepithelial carcinoma**) has been used to describe this variant because it was once thought to be a malignancy that originated from both epithelial and lymphoid tissues. This terminology should be discouraged, however, because the lymphoid tissue is not part of the neoplastic process. Such undifferentiated tumors may be difficult to distinguish from lymphoma by routine

light microscopic examination, and immunohistochemical studies often are used to demonstrate cytokeratins within the carcinoma cells. Occasional cases show neuroendocrine differentiation.

Basaloid squamous cell carcinoma is very rare in the nasopharynx. This tumor type is discussed in a separate section (see page 425).

The keratinizing type comprises less than 20% of nasopharyngeal carcinoma cases worldwide and is found more frequently in nonendemic than endemic areas. In contrast, the nonkeratinizing type comprises the vast majority (greater than 95%) of cases in endemic regions. In addition, the nonkeratinizing type is very closely associated with EBV infection (as best demonstrated by *in situ* hybridization for EBV-encoded early RNA [EBER]), whereas EBV status is variable in the keratinizing and basaloid squamous types. Among the small subset of HPV-positive cases, the keratinizing type is found more often than the nonkeratinizing type. Interestingly, according to an analysis of SEER data in the United States from 1973 through 2015, the annual incidence of nasopharyngeal cancer overall has been declining, but there has been a marked increase in the annual incidence of the nonkeratinizing type.

Treatment and Prognosis

Because of the inaccessibility of the nasopharynx and the keen radiosensitivity of nasopharyngeal carcinoma, radiotherapy is the mainstay of treatment. Early-stage disease typically is managed by radiotherapy alone. However, most patients present with locoregionally advanced disease, for which current evidence supports concurrent platinum-based systemic therapy and radiation therapy plus either induction or adjuvant chemotherapy. Clinical trial participation is encouraged for patients with locoregionally advanced or distant metastatic disease. Targeted therapies and immunotherapy (e.g., immune checkpoint inhibitors, EBV-directed vaccination, adoptive T-cell therapy) are currently under investigation.

In the United States, the relative 5-year survival rates for patients with localized, regional, and distant disease are 85%, 71%, and 49%, respectively. For all stages combined, the relative 5-year survival rate is 61%. A large-scale retrospective study performed in Asia for validation of the current TNM staging system reported 5-year overall survival rates of 98% for stage I disease, 92% for stage II disease, 83% for stage III disease, and 71% for stage IV disease. When treated with radiation therapy, the nonkeratinizing type exhibits a higher local control rate but a greater risk for distant metastasis compared with the keratinizing type. In the United States, higher survival rates have been observed among Asian-American patients compared with other ethnic groups. Additional favorable prognostic factors include age under 40 years, female gender, and low titers of circulating EBV DNA (determined pre-treatment and post-treatment by real-time PCR). The prognostic significance of HPV-positivity currently is unclear. Persons treated for nasopharyngeal carcinoma are also at increased risk for developing a second primary malignancy of the head and neck mucosa.

◆ BASAL CELL CARCINOMA (BASAL CELL EPITHELIOMA; RODENT ULCER)

Basal cell carcinoma represents the most common skin cancer, as well as the most common of all cancers. It is a locally invasive, slowly spreading, epithelial malignancy that arises from the basal cell layer of the skin and its appendages. About 80% are found on the skin of the head and neck.

The annual incidence is difficult to determine because basal cell carcinoma typically is not reported to cancer registries. However, researchers estimate that 5.4 million nonmelanoma skin cancers (basal and squamous cell carcinomas; "keratinocyte cancers") were treated in more than 3.3 million people in the United States in 2012. The worldwide incidence of basal cell carcinoma varies considerably by region, ranging from <1 per 100,000 person-years in Africa to >1000 per 100,000 person-years in Australia. The risk generally increases with age, proximity to the equator, and lighter skin pigmentation. Furthermore, the incidence has been increasing in many countries around the world; in part, this trend may be due to aging populations, although some investigators have reported a disproportionate increase among young adults (particularly women) as well.

This cancer mainly results from exposure to UV radiation—especially intense intermittent exposure but also cumulative exposure. Frequent sunburns and tendency for freckling in childhood are associated with an increased risk. Additional risk factors include outdoor occupational activity, psoralen and ultraviolet A (PUVA) treatment (often used for psoriasis), tanning device use, inability to tan, presence of nevi on the extremities, ionizing radiation exposure, immunosuppression, and arsenic ingestion. Allelic variations in genes related to DNA repair, pigmentation, tumor suppression, or other functions (e.g., the *melanocortin 1 receptor*

[MC1R] gene, *TP53*) also may confer increased susceptibility. Furthermore, several genodermatoses are associated with basal cell carcinoma, including the nevoid basal cell carcinoma syndrome (see page 694), xeroderma pigmentosum (see page 753), albinism, Rombo syndrome, Bazex Dupré-Christol syndrome, Bloom syndrome, Werner syndrome, Rothmund-Thomson syndrome, Muir-Torre syndrome, Cowden syndrome (see page 765), Brooke-Spiegler syndrome, and the Dowling-Meara subtype of epidermolysis bullosa simplex (see page 766).

Molecular genetic studies have shown that dysregulation of the hedgehog signaling pathway is a critical early event in the development of basal cell carcinoma. Inactivating mutations in the *patched 1 (PTCH1)* gene on chromosome 9q22 have been identified in both sporadic cases and patients with the nevoid basal cell carcinoma syndrome. Mutations in other genes participating in this pathway (e.g., *smoothened [SMO]*, *suppressor of fused [SUFU]*, *PTCH2*) may be found in sporadic cases as well. These mutations result in constitutive activation of hedgehog signaling and enhanced cellular proliferation. In addition, *TP53* mutations are found in about 60% of sporadic basal cell carcinomas and may represent a later event in tumor development.

Well-documented reports of oral basal cell carcinoma are rare. Many of the cases described in the literature actually represent misdiagnosed salivary or odontogenic neoplasms.

Clinical Features

Basal cell carcinoma most often affects white adults, especially those with fair complexions. Although most patients are older than 40 years at diagnosis, some lesions are detected as early as the second decade of life, particularly in patients with red or blonde hair and blue or green eyes. Males are affected about twice as often as females; however, among young patients, there is a female predilection (possibly due to tanning bed use). Approximately 80% of lesions occur on the head and neck, with the remainder involving the trunk and limbs. Lesions arising in the lip area most often involve the skin adjacent to the upper lip vermilion; upper lip vermilion tumors are more frequent than lower lip vermilion tumors.

The most common clinicopathologic variant, **nodular (noduloulcerative) basal cell carcinoma,** begins as a firm, painless papule that slowly enlarges and develops a central depression or umbilication. Telangiectatic blood vessels usually are evident within the rolled border surrounding the central depression (Figs. 10.135 and 10.136). When the lesion is pressed, a characteristic pearly opalescent quality is discerned. Expanding ulceration often develops in the central depression, and the patient may report intermittent bleeding followed by healing. Untreated lesions continue to enlarge slowly, with ulceration and destruction of underlying structures—hence the term **rodent ulcer** (Fig. 10.137). Destruction of underlying bone or cartilage may occur, but metastasis is extremely rare.

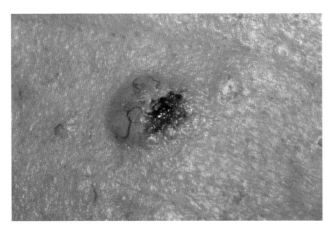

• **Fig. 10.135 Basal Cell Carcinoma.** Early noduloulcerative basal cell carcinoma of the forehead showing raised, rolled borders and focal ulceration. Fine, telangiectatic blood vessels can be seen on the surface.

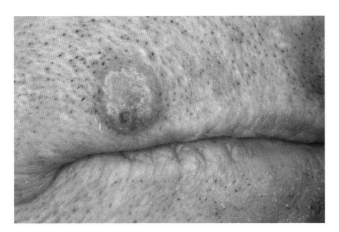

• **Fig. 10.136 Basal Cell Carcinoma.** Noduloulcerative lesion of the upper lip demonstrating telangiectasia and small ulceration.

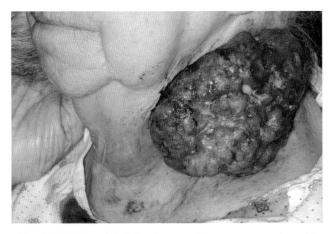

• **Fig. 10.137 Basal Cell Carcinoma.** This tumor was neglected for many years and became exceptionally large. (Courtesy of Dr. Terry Day.)

Several other variants have been described. **Pigmented basal cell carcinoma** represents a noduloulcerative tumor colonized by benign melanocytes (Fig. 10.138). The melanin production imparts a tan, brown, black, or even bluish color, and usually the pigment is not distributed uniformly, as it would be in a melanocytic nevus (see page 374).

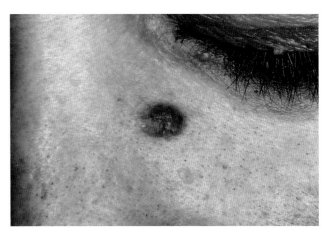

• **Fig. 10.138 Basal Cell Carcinoma.** Pigmented basal cell carcinoma of the cheek.

Sclerosing (morpheaform) basal cell carcinoma is an insidious lesion that often mimics scar tissue. The overlying skin appears pale and atrophic, and the lesion is firm to palpation with poorly demarcated borders. A slight elevation may be noted at the tumor edges. Often a great deal of invasion has occurred before the patient becomes aware of a problem.

Superficial basal cell carcinoma occurs primarily on the skin of the trunk and extremities. Often, lesions are multiple and appear as well-demarcated, erythematous, scaly patches that may be mistaken clinically for psoriasis or eczema. A fine, elevated, "threadlike" border is seen at the margins.

Some investigators believe that basal cell carcinomas associated with the **nevoid basal cell carcinoma syndrome** (see page 694) should be placed in a separate category. These lesions develop in both sun-exposed and protected areas of the skin and may number in the hundreds for a single patient. The tumors associated with this syndrome usually do not produce significant tissue destruction.

Histopathologic Features

Basal cell carcinoma displays considerable histopathologic diversity and includes the following microscopic patterns: noduloulcerative (nodulocystic), pigmented, keratotic, adenoid, superficial, infiltrative, sclerosing (morpheaform), and micronodular. The noduloulcerative, pigmented, and syndrome-related basal cell carcinomas are comprised of uniform, ovoid, dark-staining basaloid cells with medium-sized nuclei and little cytoplasm (Fig. 10.139). The cells are arranged in well-demarcated islands and strands, which appear to arise from the basal cell layer of the overlying epidermis and invade the underlying connective tissue. Epithelial islands typically demonstrate palisading of the peripheral cells; frequently, artifactual retraction is seen between the epithelial islands and the connective tissue. Although most of these neoplasms show no differentiation, some exhibit areas of keratin production, sebaceous differentiation, or interlacing strands of lesional cells that resemble duct

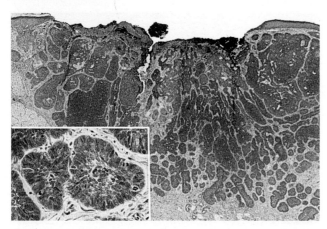

• **Fig. 10.139 Basal Cell Carcinoma.** Low-power photomicrograph showing ulceration of the epidermal surface associated with an invading tumor of hyperchromatic epithelial cells. *Inset* demonstrates islands of basophilic epithelium with peripheral palisading.

formation ("adenoid"). Necrosis of epithelial islands may produce a cystic appearance. Actinic damage in the form of **solar elastosis** almost always is seen in adjacent stroma.

Pigmented basal cell carcinoma demonstrates dendritic melanocytes within tumor islands, and melanophages may be seen in the surrounding stroma. Both the infiltrative and sclerosing types exhibit infiltrating thin strands of basaloid tumor cells; the latter type also shows a densely collagenous background. Superficial basal cell carcinoma includes lobules of tumor cells that drop from the epidermis in a multifocal pattern. Micronodular basal cell carcinoma exhibits small, round tumor nests less than 0.15 mm in diameter (or about the size of a hair follicle bulb). Occasionally, basal cell carcinoma is admixed with an independent primary squamous cell carcinoma of the skin. The resulting "collision" tumor is called **basosquamous carcinoma.** Some authorities consider basosquamous carcinoma to be a simple basal cell carcinoma with abundant squamous metaplasia.

Some studies suggest that immunohistochemical expression of Ber-EP4 (a cell surface glycoprotein preferentially expressed in cutaneous basal cell carcinoma) may help to distinguish extremely rare cases of intraoral basal cell carcinoma from peripheral ameloblastoma.

Treatment and Prognosis

The following features are associated with increased risk for recurrence among cutaneous basal cell carcinomas of the head and neck:

- Lesions of any size involving the cheeks, forehead, scalp, and neck
- For lesions involving subsites other than those above: (1) 6 mm or greater in size, or (2) less than 6 mm in size but unable to achieve clinically tumor-free margins of at least 4 mm
- Ill-defined clinical borders
- Micronodular, infiltrative, and sclerosing types
- Perineural invasion

- Recurrent lesions
- Lesions arising in immunosuppressed individuals or in a prior site of radiotherapy

Lesions with low risk for recurrence typically are treated by routine surgical excision or electrodesiccation and curettage, with 4-mm margins of clinically normal-appearing skin beyond the visible lesion. These methods result in a cure rate of 95%–98%. Head and neck lesions with a high risk for recurrence often are treated by **Mohs micrographic surgery.** This technique uses intraoperative, frozen-section evaluation of specially mapped and marked surgical specimens to ensure complete tumor removal. Radiotherapy may be an option for patients unable to tolerate surgery.

Alternative treatments—such as topical 5-fluorouracil, topical imiquimod, photodynamic therapy, or vigorous cryotherapy—may be effective for low-risk, superficial basal cell carcinomas. Such alternatives are associated with suboptimal but acceptable cure rates, and topical medical therapies may yield superior cosmetic outcomes. Patients with high-risk basal cell carcinomas for which curative surgery and radiation are not feasible may be treated with recently developed hedgehog pathway inhibitors (such as, vismodegib or sonidegib). Several other targeted agents are under development.

Recurrence of a properly managed basal cell carcinoma is uncommon, and metastasis is exceptionally rare. Unusual cases of metastatic disease may be treated with hedgehog pathway inhibitors or off-label use of PD-1 inhibitors. In patients with uncontrollable disease, death usually results from local invasion into vital structures. However, with early detection and the advent of Mohs surgery, such an outcome is unusual today.

Patients with a history of basal cell carcinoma must be evaluated periodically. There is an estimated 44% chance of a second basal cell carcinoma and 6% chance of a cutaneous squamous cell carcinoma developing within 3 years of treatment of the initial tumor. Some studies suggest that oral nicotinamide may be an effective chemopreventive agent for patients at high risk of developing additional nonmelanoma skin cancers.

◆ MERKEL CELL CARCINOMA (MERKEL CELL TUMOR; PRIMARY NEUROENDOCRINE CARCINOMA OF SKIN; SMALL CELL CARCINOMA OF SKIN; TRABECULAR CARCINOMA OF SKIN; TOKER TUMOR)

Merkel cell carcinoma is a rare, aggressive malignancy with neuroendocrine features. It most often occurs on the skin of the head and neck region in elderly individuals. The etiopathogenesis is driven by Merkel cell polyomavirus (MCPyV) infection and/or chronic UV light exposure. MCPyV is found in up to 80% of cases in North America and Europe, whereas most cases in regions of the southern hemisphere with high exposure to UV light (such as Australia) are negative for the virus. MCPyV-negative tumors tend to demonstrate a molecular UV signature (i.e., preponderance of C-to-T or CC-to-TT transitions in dipyrimidine sites), recurrent mutations in *TP53* and *RB1*, and an overall higher mutational burden than MCPyV-positive tumors. In addition, immunosuppression is a risk factor, with increased frequency of Merkel cell carcinoma noted among transplant recipients, patients receiving immunosuppressive therapy for autoimmune diseases, patients with other underlying malignancies (especially chronic lymphocytic leukemia), and patients with HIV infection.

In the United States, only about 2000 cases of Merkel cell carcinoma are diagnosed annually. However, the incidence has been increasing over the past few decades in this and other countries—a trend that may be caused by population aging, prolonged lifespan of individuals with conditions causing immunosuppression, and improved diagnosis and cancer registry tracking.

The exact cell of origin is uncertain. This neoplasm traditionally was thought to arise from Merkel cells (mechanoreceptor cells found primarily in skin, but also in other sites, including oral mucosa). However, this theory seems unlikely given that Merkel cells are terminally differentiated and mainly reside in the basal layer of the epidermis, whereas most Merkel cell carcinomas are dermal-based tumors without an intraepithelial component. A possible origin from dermal mesenchymal stem cells, epidermal stem cells, fibroblasts, or primitive B-cells also has been proposed.

Intraoral and lip vermilion cases have been reported rarely. However, some oral neuroendocrine malignancies previously reported as Merkel cell carcinomas actually may be more akin to high-grade small cell neuroendocrine carcinomas of the upper aerodigestive tract mucosa. The latter tumor type is closely associated with tobacco and alcohol abuse, is not associated with UV light exposure or MCPyV, exhibits microscopic features similar to small cell carcinoma of the lung, and may behave even more aggressively than Merkel cell carcinoma.

Clinical Features

Approximately 82% of cases are diagnosed in patients in their 7th through 9th decades of life. The tumor mainly affects whites (96% of cases) and exhibits a male predominance. It occurs primarily on sun-exposed areas of fair-skinned individuals, with a predilection for the skin of the face, upper limbs, and shoulders. The lip vermilion is also susceptible (Fig. 10.140). Extracutaneous lesions are rare and may involve the oral, nasal, pharyngeal, laryngeal, esophageal, and genital mucosa. The tumor usually appears as an asymptomatic, rapidly enlarging, smooth, dome-shaped nodule with prominent surface vessels (**telangiectasias**). Some authors have used the acronym **AEIOU** (**A**symptomatic, **E**xpanding rapidly, **I**mmunosuppression, **O**ld age, **U**ltraviolet-exposed fair skin) to summarize the salient clinical findings. The lesion typically is red, violaceous, or pink and ranges in size from 0.5 to 5.0 cm. An

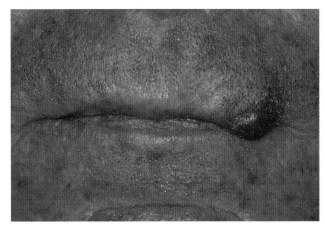

• **Fig. 10.140 Merkel Cell Carcinoma.** Red nodule on the vermilion border of the upper lip. (From Chang JYF, Stewart JM, Cheng YSL, et al: Upper lip nodule, *Oral Surg Oral Med Oral Pathol Oral Radiol Endod* 105:549–553, 2008.)

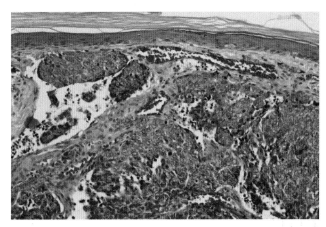

• **Fig. 10.141 Merkel Cell Carcinoma.** A sheet of undifferentiated basophilic cells is seen beneath the epidermal surface.

often innocuous clinical appearance may cause delay in diagnosis. Approximately 27% of cases demonstrate regional lymph node metastasis at diagnosis. In about 14% of cases, there is metastasis of unknown primary origin, presumably due to regression of the primary tumor. In addition, so-called high-grade neuroendocrine carcinoma of the salivary glands (especially the parotids) may represent metastasis from an occult or regressed cutaneous Merkel cell carcinoma.

Histopathologic Features

Merkel cell carcinoma consists of sheets, nodules, nests, and trabeculae of small to moderately sized, round, basophilic cells, which infiltrate the dermis and subcutis (Fig. 10.141). Epidermal involvement is infrequent. The tumor cells typically exhibit overlapping nuclei, finely granular ("salt and pepper") chromatin, scant cytoplasm, indistinct cell borders, brisk mitotic activity, and frequent apoptosis. MCPyV-positive lesions tend to have small to medium cells with uniformly round nuclei, whereas MCPyV-negative cases often exhibit irregular, elongated nuclei or large cells with clear cytoplasm. Intracytoplasmic argyrophilic granules may be demonstrated by the Grimelius stain, and immunohistochemical staining for cytokeratin 20 (CK20) usually shows a "perinuclear dot" pattern. Immunopositivity for neuroendocrine markers (e.g., chromogranin A, synaptophysin, neuron-specific enolase, and CD56), neurofilament, and SATB2 also may be helpful in establishing the diagnosis. In approximately 60%–80% of cases, MCPyV can be detected by polymerase chain reaction (PCR) for viral DNA or immunohistochemistry (using the CMB24 clone) for MCPyV large T-antigen. Lack of immunoreactivity for thyroid transcription factor 1 (TTF-1) may help to exclude metastatic small cell carcinoma of the lung, which may have similar histomorphologic features. The microscopic differential diagnosis also may include amelanotic melanoma, metastatic olfactory neuroblastoma, and other "round-cell" malignancies. Immunohistochemical studies and thorough physical examination may aid in excluding these other entities. Furthermore, Merkel cell carcinomas may occur in combination with other neoplasms, especially actinic keratosis and invasive or *in situ* squamous cell carcinoma.

Treatment and Prognosis

Treatment and prognosis are guided by staging. Surgery (i.e., wide local excision or Mohs micrographic surgery) is the mainstay of treatment and often is combined with adjuvant radiotherapy. Lymph node dissection is performed when clinically palpable nodes are found. Sentinel lymph node biopsy typically is used to determine whether regional lymph node dissection and/or radiation are indicated in patients with clinically negative nodes. Clinical trial participation is recommended for patients with regional or distant metastasis. Checkpoint immunotherapy using PD-1 or PD-L1 inhibitors recently has replaced chemotherapy as first-line treatment for advanced disease.

Recurrence develops in 55% of cases, most commonly within the draining lymph nodes. Monitoring titers of antibodies to MCPyV oncoproteins may aid in early detection of recurrent disease. Furthermore, approximately 25% of patients with Merkel cell carcinoma develop additional malignancies (e.g., squamous cell carcinomas of the skin, hematologic malignancies, or adenocarcinomas of the breast or ovary). Therefore, patients should be followed closely.

In the United States, a recent analysis of data from the National Cancer Database reported 5-year overall survival rates of 51% for patients with localized disease, 35% for patients with regional metastasis, and 14% for patients with distant metastasis. Female sex, upper limb involvement, and age under 70 years are positive predictors of survival. Primary mucosal lesions exhibit a worse prognosis than the more common, primary cutaneous lesions. Similarly, lip lesions may have a worse prognosis than those arising in more frequently involved head and neck sites. Additional adverse prognostic factors include immunosuppression and negative MCPyV tumor status.

◆ MELANOMA (MALIGNANT MELANOMA; MELANOCARCINOMA)

Melanoma is a malignant neoplasm of melanocytic origin; it may arise *de novo* or from a preexisting benign melanocytic lesion. Most cases occur on the skin, although mucosal lesions also are possible. UV radiation exposure from sunlight is a major etiologic factor, with increased incidence of melanoma among white populations as they approach the equator. Acute intermittent sun damage may be of greater causative importance than chronic exposure. Oral mucosal lesions, of course, are not related to sun exposure.

Risk factors for cutaneous melanoma include a fair complexion, light-colored hair and eyes, a tendency to sunburn or freckle easily, a history of severe sunburns in childhood, an indoor occupation with outdoor recreational habits, a personal or family history of melanoma, a personal history of dysplastic nevus or giant congenital nevus, a personal history of excessive (>100) conventional nevi, and presence of conventional nevi on the extremities. Associations with tanning device use, various childhood malignancies, and immunosuppressive therapy for organ transplantation also have been proposed.

Melanoma represents the third most common skin cancer. Invasive melanoma accounts for less than 5% of total skin cancer cases but the majority of skin cancer deaths. In the United States for the year 2022, the American Cancer Society estimates that over 99,000 new cases of cutaneous invasive melanoma will be diagnosed and more than 7000 people will die of the disease. However, within the past few years mortality rates have decreased in the United States by about 4% annually on average due to advances in treatment. According to the most recent estimate by the SEER Program, 1 in 50 persons in the United States will be diagnosed with cutaneous melanoma during his or her lifetime. Based on SEER data from 2015 through 2019, the age-adjusted annual incidence rates for skin melanoma are approximately 28 per 100,000 men and 17 per 100,000 women. The highest incidence rates are seen among elderly white men; however, women are affected more frequently than men among the younger patient subset. Over the past several decades, dramatic increases in the incidence of melanoma have been reported worldwide. Some investigators contend that this trend reflects increased numbers of skin biopsies and improved diagnosis of early-stage disease. However, others have demonstrated increased frequency of both early- and late-stage disease and, thus, propose that there is a true increase in disease rate.

According to the *National Cancer Database Report on Cutaneous and Noncutaneous Melanoma*, 91.2% of all melanomas arise on the skin, whereas ocular, mucosal, and unknown primaries account for 5.2%, 1.3%, and 2.2% of cases, respectively. Almost 25% of cutaneous melanomas arise in the head and neck area, 40% on the extremities, and the rest on the trunk. More than half of mucosal melanomas occur in the head and neck (including the oral and sinonasal regions).

Oral mucosal melanoma is very rare, accounting for only about 0.26%–0.5% of all oral cavity cancers. Several reports suggest that mucosal melanoma is more frequent in certain countries, such as Japan and Uganda; however, other investigators have suggested that the true annual incidence of mucosal melanoma is not greater in these countries but only appears so because of the comparatively low incidence of cutaneous melanoma in these racial groups. Potential associations with tobacco use, chronic trauma, and other environmental factors have been suggested by some authors but remain unsubstantiated.

There have been many discoveries regarding recurrent genetic alterations in melanomas, including those involving the MAPK and PI3K/Akt signaling pathways. In particular, researchers have identified the following four major types of somatic genetic abnormalities: (1) activating mutations in *BRAF* (identified in about half of cutaneous melanomas, especially *BRAF* V600E in tumors arising on the trunk and lower extremities of younger patients), (2) activating mutations in *NRAS* (identified in approximately 20% of cutaneous melanomas, especially those in the head and neck region of older patients), (3) *NF1* loss (identified in about 10% of cutaneous melanomas and strongly associated with severe sun exposure, older age, and desmoplastic tumors), and (4) "triple wild-type" (lacking the three aforementioned mutations but exhibiting alterations in *KIT, GNAQ, GNA11,* or other genes) (such as melanomas involving mucosa and acral skin). In addition to these major types of driver mutations, subsequent alterations typically develop in various other genes, such as *CDKN2A, PTEN, TERT, ARID2,* and *TP53.* Interestingly, mucosal melanomas tend to have a lower overall burden of somatic mutations compared to cutaneous lesions.

Molecular genetic studies focusing specifically on oral mucosal melanomas are limited. In several small-scale investigations, frequent *KIT* mutations have been noted. There are a few reports of infrequent mutations in other genes (e.g., *NRAS, FMNL2, BAP1*) as well. Unlike cutaneous melanoma, oral mucosal melanoma only rarely harbors *BRAF* mutations. Among some melanoma-prone kindreds, investigators have identified various germline mutations that confer a high risk for melanoma development. In particular, hereditary melanomas frequently are associated with *CDKN2A* mutations, and researchers have identified numerous other susceptibility loci.

Clinical Features

Cutaneous melanomas most commonly develop in white adults. Although the lesion occurs over a broad age range, most cases arise in individuals 45 through 84 years old, with a median age at diagnosis of 61 years. There is a female predilection among patients younger than 40 years (possibly related to tanning bed use); in contrast, a male predilection is seen among older patients. The most frequent primary site in men is the back, whereas in women the lower extremities are affected most commonly. Because many clinical similarities exist between cutaneous melanoma and its benign counterpart, the melanocytic nevus, an "ABCDE" clinical evaluation system has been developed to help distinguish between these two entities (Box 10.5). Referral for clinical assessment and dermoscopy by a dermatologist should be considered for patients with lesions exhibiting such atypical features.

Based on clinicopathologic, epidemiologic, and genetic findings, the World Health Organization's melanoma classification system (Box 10.6) delineates 9 "pathways" (or subtypes) and three major categories: (1) melanomas typically arising in skin with cumulative solar damage (pathways I-III) (including superficial spreading melanoma and lentigo maligna melanoma), (2) melanomas not consistently associated with cumulative solar damage (pathways IV-IX) (including acral and mucosal melanoma), and (3) melanomas that may arise in any pathway (including nodular melanoma). In particular, the following subtypes of melanoma are described below:
1. Superficial spreading melanoma
2. Nodular melanoma

• BOX 10.5 The "ABCDE" Clinical Features of Melanoma

- **A**symmetry (because of its **uncontrolled** growth pattern)
- **B**order irregularity (often with notching)
- **C**olor variegation (which varies from shades of brown to black, white, red, and blue, depending on the amount and depth of melanin pigmentation)
- **D**iameter greater than 6 mm (which is the diameter of a pencil eraser)
- **E**volving (lesions that have changed with respect to size, shape, color, surface, or symptoms over time)

• BOX 10.6 Melanoma Classification (Modified From the 2018 World Health Organization Classification)*

A. Melanomas typically associated with CSD
  - Pathway I: superficial spreading melanoma/low-CSD melanoma
  - Pathway II: lentigo maligna melanoma/high-CSD melanoma
  - Pathway III: desmoplastic melanoma
B. Melanomas not consistently associated with CSD
  - Pathway IV: Spitz melanoma
  - Pathway V: acral melanoma
  - Pathway VI: mucosal melanoma
  - Pathway VII: melanoma arising in a congenital nevus
  - Pathway VIII: melanoma arising in a blue nevus
  - Pathway IX: uveal melanoma
C. Melanomas arising in any pathway
  - Nodular melanoma
  - Nevoid melanoma

CSD, cumulative sun damage (as assessed by degree of solar elastosis on biopsy).
*Modified from Elder DE, Barnhill RL, Bastian BC, et al: Melanocytic tumor classification and the pathway concept of melanoma pathogenesis. In Elder DE, Massi D, Scolyer RA, et al, editors: *WHO classification of skin tumours*, ed 4, Lyon, 2018, IARC, pp. 66–71.

3. Lentigo maligna melanoma
4. Acral melanoma
5. Mucosal melanoma

Melanomas tend to exhibit two directional patterns of growth: (1) the **radial growth phase** and (2) the **vertical growth phase.** In the early stages, the radial growth phase tends to predominate in lentigo maligna melanoma, superficial spreading melanoma, and acral lentiginous melanoma. In these lesions, the malignant melanocytes have a propensity to spread horizontally through the basal layer of the epidermis. Eventually, however, the malignant cells begin to invade the underlying connective tissue, thus initiating the vertical growth phase. In nodular melanoma, the radial growth phase is very short or nonexistent, and the vertical growth phase predominates.

Superficial Spreading Melanoma

Superficial spreading melanoma is the most common subtype of melanoma, representing 70% of cutaneous lesions (Fig. 10.142). The most frequent sites of origin are the interscapular area of males and the back of the legs of females. The lesion appears as a macule or plaque with a variety of potential colors (i.e., tan, brown, gray, black, blue, white, and pink). Typically, the lesion is smaller than 3 cm in greatest diameter at diagnosis, but it may be several times that size. Clinically, invasion is indicated by the appearance of surface nodules or induration, and usually occurs within 1 year of discovery of the precursor macule. Satellites may develop around the primary lesion.

Nodular Melanoma

Nodular melanoma represents 15% of cutaneous melanomas, and one-third of such lesions develop in the head and neck. Nodular melanoma is thought to begin almost immediately in the vertical growth phase; therefore, it typically appears as a nodular elevation that rapidly invades the connective tissue. Nodular melanoma is usually deeply pigmented, although sometimes the melanoma cells are so poorly differentiated that they no longer can produce melanin, resulting in a nonpigmented **amelanotic melanoma.**

Lentigo Maligna Melanoma

Lentigo maligna melanoma, which accounts for 5%–10% of cutaneous melanomas, develops from a precursor lesion called **lentigo maligna (Hutchinson freckle).** Lentigo maligna occurs almost exclusively on heavily sun-exposed skin of fair-complexioned older adults, particularly in the midfacial region, and represents a **melanoma *in situ*** in a purely radial growth phase.

The lesion appears as a large, slowly expanding macule with irregular borders and a variety of colors, including tan, brown, black, and even white (Fig. 10.143). Patients usually indicate that the lesion has been present and has slowly expanded laterally for years. The average duration of the radial growth phase is 15 years. The appearance of nodularity within a lentigo maligna signals the onset of the invasive or vertical growth phase and the transition to lentigo maligna melanoma.

Acral Melanoma (Acral Lentiginous Melanoma)

Acral melanoma develops on glabrous (or non-hair-bearing) skin, such as the palms of the hands, soles of the feet, volar aspects of the fingers and toes, and subungual area. It represents the most frequent subtype of melanoma in individuals of African or Asian descent. The lesion typically begins as a dark, irregularly marginated macule or patch (*acral lentiginous melanoma*); a nodular invasive growth phase may develop after several months to years.

Mucosal Melanoma

Mucosal melanoma tends to arise in the mucosa of the sinonasal passages, oral cavity, urogenital tract, anorectal region, and conjunctiva, although various other primary sites are possible. Early lesions in the radial growth phase (*mucosal lentiginous melanomas*) typically appear flat. However, many examples are not recognized until they become nodular. Importantly, mucosal melanoma is much more aggressive than its cutaneous counterpart.

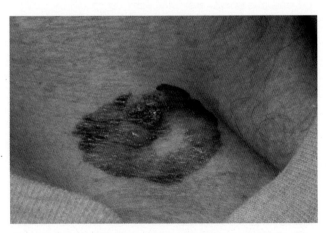

• **Fig. 10.142 Superficial Spreading Melanoma.** This lesion on the neck demonstrates the ABCDE warning signs of melanoma: **A**symmetry, **B**order irregularity, **C**olor variegation, **D**iameter larger than a pencil eraser, and **E**volving larger size. (Courtesy of Dr. Mark Bowden.)

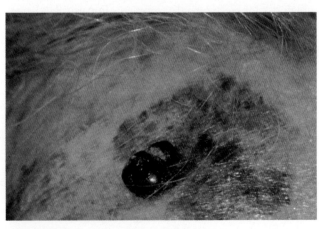

• **Fig. 10.143 Lentigo Maligna Melanoma.** A slowly evolving pigmented lesion of the facial skin in an older adult man.

Oral mucosal melanoma most often develops during the fifth through seventh decades of life. Most studies have reported either a slight male predilection or no significant gender predilection. Approximately 70%–80% of oral melanomas are found on the hard palate or maxillary alveolus. At least one in three patients with oral melanoma has a history of a pigmented macule in the tumor region for some time before melanoma diagnosis. The lesion typically begins as a brown to black macule with irregular borders (Figs. 10.144 and 10.145). However, some lesions contain little pigment and exhibit either a normal mucosal tint or a vascular appearance. The macule extends laterally, and a lobulated, exophytic mass develops once vertical growth is initiated (Fig. 10.146). Ulceration may develop early, but many lesions are not ulcerated at the time of diagnosis. Pain is uncommon except in ulcerated lesions, and most lesions remain relatively soft to palpation. Adjacent bone may show radiographic evidence of irregular or "moth-eaten" destruction. At the time of diagnosis, cervical lymph node metastasis is evident in about a third of cases, and distant metastasis is noted in about a quarter of cases.

In addition, melanoma occasionally affects the parotid gland, usually as a metastatic deposit from a scalp, conjunctival, or paranasal tumor.

Histopathologic Features

With cutaneous and oral melanomas, atypical melanocytes initially are seen at the epithelial and connective tissue junction. From here, they have the potential to proliferate throughout the epithelium, laterally along the basal cell layer, and downward into the connective tissue. In early stages, atypical melanocytes are seen either scattered singly among the basal epithelial cells or as nests within the basal cell layer. The atypical melanocytes are enlarged, with varying degrees of nuclear pleomorphism and hyperchromatism.

In superficial spreading melanoma, there is often *pagetoid spread* (i.e., single tumor cells infiltrating into the upper layers of the surface epithelium) (Fig. 10.147). This microscopic pattern resembles an intraepithelial adenocarcinoma known as *Paget's disease of skin*.

The spread of the lesional cells along the basal layer of the surface epithelium constitutes the radial growth phase. Appreciable lateral spread prior to invasion of the underlying connective tissue is characteristic of superficial spreading melanoma, lentigo maligna melanoma, acral lentiginous melanoma, and mucosal lentiginous melanoma. In acral and mucosal lentiginous melanomas, many of the melanocytes have prominent dendritic processes (Fig. 10.148).

The vertical growth phase is characterized by malignant melanocytes invading the connective tissue. In nodular melanoma, this vertical growth phase occurs early in the disease course. No radial growth can be observed in the overlying epithelium beyond the edge of the invasive tumor (Fig. 10.149). The tumor usually appears as pleomorphic, spindle-shaped or epithelioid cells arranged in loosely aggregated cords or sheets. Oral lesions show invasion of lymphatic and blood vessels more often than skin lesions. Several mucosal melanomas have been reported to contain unequivocal bone and cartilage, a feature that may cause

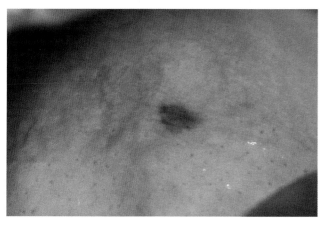

• **Fig. 10.144 Oral Melanoma.** This discrete area of pigmentation, measuring approximately 5 mm in diameter, was discovered on the posterior hard palate of a middle-aged woman during a routine oral examination. Biopsy revealed melanoma *in situ*.

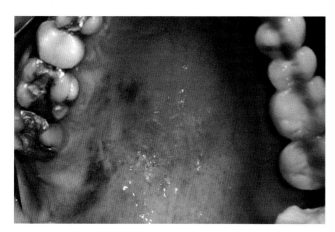

• **Fig. 10.145 Oral Melanoma.** Diffuse, splotchy area of pigmentation of the lateral hard palate. (Courtesy of Dr. Len Morrow.)

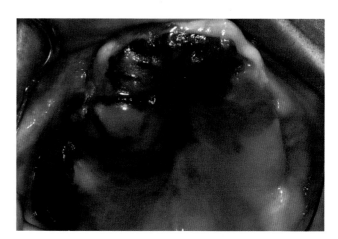

• **Fig. 10.146 Oral Melanoma.** Extensive, pigmented mass of the palate and maxillary alveolar ridge. An exophytic component is evident.

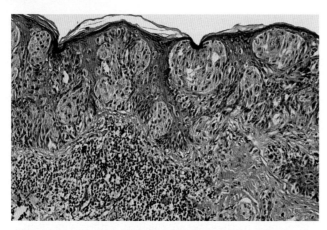

• **Fig. 10.147 Superficial Spreading Melanoma.** The radial growth phase is characterized by the spread of atypical melanocytes along the basilar portion of the epidermis. Also note the presence of individual melanocytes invading the higher levels of the epithelium.

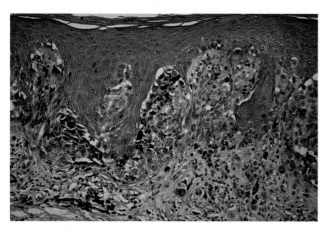

• **Fig. 10.148 Mucosal Lentiginous Melanoma.** This palatal melanoma demonstrates numerous atypical melanocytes in the basilar portion of the epithelium with invasion into the superficial lamina propria. This represents the biopsy specimen from Fig. 10.145.

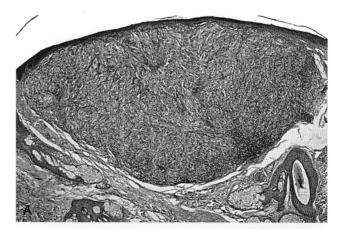

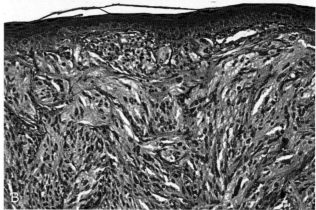

• **Fig. 10.149 Nodular Melanoma. A,** Low-power photomicrograph showing a nodular mass of malignant melanocytes invading into the dermis. Note the lack of radial growth in the adjacent overlying epidermis. **B,** Higher-power photomicrograph showing atypical spindle-shaped melanocytes.

diagnostic confusion with pleomorphic adenoma, sarcomatoid carcinoma, osteosarcoma, and mesenchymal chondrosarcoma.

Approximately 10% of oral melanomas are amelanotic. A lack of melanin production may cause diagnostic confusion with various other undifferentiated tumors at the light microscopic level. Immunohistochemical studies showing reactivity for S-100 protein, HMB-45, SOX10, and MART-1 (Melan-A) may aid in diagnosis.

Treatment and Prognosis

Depth of invasion is an important prognostic factor for cutaneous melanoma. The Clark system assigns a "level" corresponding to the deepest region that has been invaded by tumor cells (Table 10.9). The more recent Breslow classification, however, correlates more accurately with prognosis and is based on measurement of the distance from the top of the granular cell layer to the deepest identifiable point of tumor invasion.

TABLE 10.9	Clark Classification for Cutaneous Melanoma	
Clark Definition of Level of Tumor Invasion	**Clark Classification**
Cells confined to epithelium	Level I
Cells penetrating papillary dermis	Level II
Cells filling papillary dermis	Level III
Cells extending into reticular dermis	Level IV
Cells invading subcutaneous fat	Level V

Clinical staging for cutaneous melanoma is performed using a TNM classification system that takes into account Breslow tumor thickness, ulceration, regional lymph node metastasis, regional non-nodal lymphatic metastasis, and distant metastasis (Table 10.10). In addition, the serum level of lactate dehydrogenase (LDH) is considered in subclassifying cases with distant metastasis.

Wide surgical excision is the mainstay of treatment for patients with resectable disease. Current evidence indicates that a 1-cm margin is adequate for cutaneous tumors with

TABLE 10.10   Tumor-Node-Metastasis (TNM) Staging Classification and Prognostic Clinical Stage Groups for Cutaneous Melanoma

Primary Tumor (T)		
T Category	**Thickness (mm)**	**Ulceration Status**
TX	NA (Primary tumor thickness cannot be assessed [e.g., diagnosis by curettage])	NA
T0	NA (No evidence of primary tumor [e.g., unknown or completely regressed primary])	NA
Tis	NA (Melanoma *in situ*)	NA
T1	≤1.0 mm	Unknown or unspecified
T1a	<0.8 mm	Without ulceration
T1b	<0.8 mm 0.8–1.0 mm	With ulceration With or without ulceration
T2	>1.0–2.0 mm	Unknown or unspecified
T2a	>1.0–2.0 mm	Without ulceration
T2b	>1.0–2.0 mm	With ulceration
T3	>2.0–4.0 mm	Unknown or unspecified
T3a	>2.0–4.0 mm	Without ulceration
T3b	>2.0–4.0 mm	With ulceration
T4	>4.0 mm	Unknown or unspecified
T4a	>4.0 mm	Without ulceration
T4b	>4.0 mm	With ulceration

Regional Lymph Node Involvement and/or Lymphatic Metastasis (N)		
N Category	**No. of Metastatic Regional Lymph Nodes**	**Presence of In-transit, Satellite, and/or Microsatellite Metastasis**
NX	Regional lymph nodes cannot be assessed (e.g., sentinel lymph node biopsy not performed, regional lymph nodes previously removed for another reason)	No
N0	None detected	No
N1	1 node None	No Yes
N1a	1 clinically occult node (i.e., detected by sentinel lymph node biopsy)	No
N1b	1 clinically detected node	No
N1c	None	Yes
N2	2–3 nodes 1 node	No Yes
N2a	2–3 clinically occult nodes (i.e., detected by sentinel lymph node biopsy)	No
N2b	2–3 nodes, at least one of which was clinically detected	No
N2c	1 clinically occult or clinically detected node	Yes
N3	4 or more nodes 2 or more nodes Any number of matted nodes	No Yes Yes or no

Continued

TABLE 10.10	Tumor-Node-Metastasis (TNM) Staging Classification and Prognostic Clinical Stage Groups for Cutaneous Melanoma—cont'd

Regional Lymph Node Involvement and/or Lymphatic Metastasis (N)		
N Category	**No. of Metastatic Regional Lymph Nodes**	**Presence of In-transit, Satellite, and/or Microsatellite Metastasis**
N3a	4 or more clinically occult nodes (i.e., detected by sentinel lymph node biopsy)	No
N3b	4 or more nodes, at least 1 of which was clinically detected; *or* any number of matted nodes	No
N3c	2 or more clinically occult or clinically detected nodes; *and/or* any number of matted nodes	Yes

Distant Metastasis (M)		
M Category	**Anatomic Site**	**Serum Lactate Dehydrogenase Level**
M0	No evidence of distant metastases	NA
M1	Evidence of distant metastasis	
M1a	Distant metastasis to skin, soft tissue including muscle, and/or nonregional lymph node	Not recorded or unspecified
M1a(0)		Not elevated
M1a(1)		Elevated
M1b	Distant metastasis to lung with or without M1a sites of disease	Not recorded or unspecified
M1b(0)		Not elevated
M1b(1)		Elevated
M1c	Distant metastasis to non-CNS visceral sites with or without M1a or	Not recorded or unspecified
M1c(0)	M1b sites of disease	Not elevated
M1c(1)		Elevated
M1d	Distant metastasis to CNS with or without M1a, M1b, or M1c sites of disease	Not recorded or unspecified
M1d(0)		Not elevated
M1d(1)		Elevated

Clinical Stage Group	**TNM Classification**
Stage 0	Tis N0 M0
Stage IA	T1a N0 M0
Stage IB	T1b N0 M0 / T2a N0 M0
Stage IIA	T2b N0 M0 / T3a N0 M0
Stage IIB	T3b N0 M0 / T4a N0 M0
Stage IIC	T4b N0 M0
Stage III	Any T ≥ N1 M0
Stage IV	Any T Any N M1

CNS, central nervous system.
NA, not applicable.
In-transit metastasis is defined as clinically evident dermal and/or subcutaneous metastases occurring beyond 2 cm from the primary melanoma in the region between the primary and the regional lymph node basin.
Satellite metastasis is defined as grossly visible cutaneous and/or subcutaneous metastases occurring within 2 cm of and discontinuous from the primary melanoma.
Microsatellite metastasis is defined as microscopic cutaneous and/or subcutaneous metastasis adjacent or deep to a primary melanoma; the metastatic tumor cells must be discontinuous from the primary tumor and not separated only by fibrosis or inflammation, which could represent regression of the intervening tumor.
(From Gershenwald JE, Scolyer RA, Hess KR, et al: Melanoma of the skin. In Amin MB, Edge SB, Greene FL, et al, editors, *AJCC cancer staging manual*, ed 8, New York, 2018, American College of Surgeons, pp. 565–585.)

a thickness of 1 mm or less. For skin tumors with a thickness greater than 1 mm but not more than 2 mm, margins between 1 and 2 cm are recommended. Cutaneous tumors thicker than 2 mm typically require excision with 2-cm margins.

Lymph node dissection usually is performed on patients with clinically evident regional metastasis in the absence of distant metastasis. Because regional lymph node metastases are frequently occult, sentinel lymph node biopsy (biopsy of the first lymph node in the lymphatic basin to receive drainage from the tumor) often is performed to detect metastases that are not evident with clinical examination or imaging. If the sentinel lymph node biopsy is positive, completion lymphadenectomy may be performed. Additional treatment after surgery may include immunotherapy, targeted therapy, chemotherapy, or radiation therapy.

Recent discoveries regarding the role of the immune system in cancer and the molecular basis of melanoma and have led to novel approaches to therapy, particularly for patients with advanced disease. Newly developed immunotherapeutic agents include immune system checkpoint inhibitors against cytotoxic T-lymphocyte antigen-4 (CTLA-4), programmed death-1 (PD-1), or programmed death protein ligand-1 (PDL-1) (such as imiplimab, pembrolizumab, nivolumab, and atezolizumab). These agents represent significant improvements to the arsenal of immunotherapy, which also includes older agents such as interleukin-2 and interferon-alpha. For *BRAF*-mutant metastatic melanoma, recently approved targeted treatments include BRAF inhibitors (such as vemurafenib and dabrafenib), which may be used alone or in combination with MEK inhibitors. For patients with mucosal or acral melanomas exhibiting certain types of *KIT* mutations, targeted therapy with small molecule KIT inhibitors (such as imatinib, sunitinib, sorafenib, or nilotinib) may be of benefit. These recent developments in immunotherapy and genotype-directed therapy have led to significantly prolonged survival for patients with advanced cutaneous melanoma.

Primarily as a result of public education efforts, the clinical features of cutaneous melanoma are so widely known that the majority of lesions are discovered and treated at an early stage. Based on SEER data from 2011 through 2017, the 5-year relative survival rate for patients with localized cutaneous melanoma is approximately 99%, whereas patients with regional or distant metastasis exhibit survival rates of approximately 68% and 30%, respectively (see Table 10.11). However, in more recent years with major advances in treatment, many centers have reported 5-year survival rates greater than 50% for patients with distant metastasis.

Besides tumor stage, various other prognostic factors have been noted for cutaneous melanoma. Adverse microscopic findings include increased mitotic activity and minimal to absent tumor-infiltrating lymphocytes. For reasons that are unclear, cutaneous melanomas on the trunk, head,

TABLE 10.11	Overall 5-Year Relative Survival Rates for Cutaneous Melanoma by SEER Stage*	
SEER Stage at Diagnosis	Estimated 5-Year Relative Survival Rate
Localized	99%
Regional	68%
Distant	30%[†]
All Stages	93%

*Based upon Surveillance Epidemiology and End Results (SEER) 18 area data for patients diagnosed in 2011–2017. Source: Surveillance Research Program, National Cancer Institute. SEER*Explorer: an interactive website for SEER cancer statistics, http://seer.cancer.gov/explorer. Accessed November 23, 2021.
[†]In more recent years with the introduction of novel immunotherapeutic and targeted agents, many centers have reported 5-year survival rates of 50% or higher for patients with distant metastasis.

and neck carry a worse prognosis than those on the extremities. In particular, among head and neck lesions, those arising on the scalp and neck are associated with decreased survival rates. In contrast, favorable prognostic factors include age younger than 20 years and female gender. Follow-up after treatment is important not only to monitor for metastatic disease but also because, in 3%–5% of these patients, a second primary melanoma eventually will develop.

For mucosal melanomas of the head and neck, TNM classification takes into account the anatomic extent of the primary tumor (i.e., confined to mucosa or invading adjacent structures), regional lymph node metastasis, and distant metastasis (Table 10.12). Because head and neck mucosal lesions typically exhibit aggressive behavior, they are classified at a minimum as stage III. For patients with resectable disease, radical surgery is indicated and often is followed by adjunctive radiation with or without systemic agents (i.e., immunotherapy, targeted therapy, chemotherapy). Patients with very advanced disease should strongly consider clinical trial participation. Some clinical trials have shown promising results with recently developed immunotherapeutic or targeted agents; however, responses to such agents usually are more limited among mucosal than cutaneous melanomas, and further studies are needed.

The prognosis for oral mucosal melanoma is extremely poor. Most authors report 5-year survival rates in the range of only about 10%–25%, and median overall survival rarely exceeds 2 years after initial diagnosis. Death usually results from distant metastasis rather than lack of local control. The poor prognosis for oral mucosal melanoma appears to be related to difficulty in achieving wide resection and a tendency for early metastasis. Younger patients exhibit better survival than older ones, and patients with amelanotic lesions appear to have a particularly poor prognosis. Nodular lesions generally have a worse prognosis than macular lesions, and

TABLE 10.12	Tumor-Node-Metastasis (TNM) Staging Classification System and Prognostic Groups for Mucosal Melanoma of the Head and Neck	
Primary Tumor (T)		
T3	Tumors limited to the mucosa and immediately underlying soft tissue, regardless of thickness or greatest dimension (e.g., polypoid nasal disease; pigmented or nonpigmented lesions of the oral cavity, pharynx, or larynx)	
T4	Moderately advanced or very advanced disease	
T4a	Moderately advanced disease Tumor involving deep soft tissue, cartilage, bone, or overlying skin	
T4b	Very advanced disease Tumor involving brain, dura, skull base, lower cranial nerves (IX, X, XI, and XII), masticator space, carotid artery, prevertebral space, or mediastinal structures	
Regional Lymph Nodes (N)		
NX	Regional lymph nodes cannot be assessed	
N0	No regional lymph node metastases	
N1	Regional lymph node metastases present	
Distant Metastasis (M)		
M0	No distant metastasis	
M1	Distant metastasis present	
Prognostic Groups*		
Stage III	T3 N0 M0	
Stage IVA	T4a N0 M0 T3-4a N1 M0	
Stage IVB	T4b any N M0	
Stage IVC	Any T Any N M1	

*Prognostic groups shown here are from the 7th edition of the *AJCC Cancer Staging Manual*. No prognostic groups were proposed in the 8th edition.
(From: Mucosal melanoma of the head and neck. In Edge SB, Byrd DR, Compton CC, et al, editors: *AJCC cancer staging manual*, ed 7, New York, 2010, Springer, pp. 97–100. Mucosal melanoma of the head and neck. In Amin MB, Edge SB, Greene FL, et al, editors: *AJCC Cancer Staging Manual*, ed. 8, Chicago, 2018, American College Of Surgeons, pp. 163–170.)

ulceration appears to be an adverse prognostic factor. However, depth of invasion and presence of ulceration are not so closely correlated with prognosis of mucosal melanomas compared to cutaneous melanomas.

Bibliography

Benign Epithelial Lesions Associated with Human Papillomavirus

Ali A, Lassi ZS, Kapellas K, et al.: A systematic review and meta-analysis of the association between periodontitis and oral high-risk human papillomavirus infection, *J Public Health (Oxf)* 43: e610–e619, 2021.

Betz SJ: HPV-related papillary lesions of the oral mucosa: a review, *Head Neck Pathol* 13:80–90, 2019.

D'Souza G, Clemens G, Strickler HD, et al.: Long-term persistence of oral HPV over 7 years of follow-up, *JNCI Cancer Spectr* 4:pkaa047, 2020.

Graham SV: The human papillomavirus replication cycle, and its links to cancer progression: a comprehensive review, *Clin Sci (Lond)* 131:2201–2221, 2017.

Markowitz LE, Gee J, Chesson H, et al.: Ten years of human papillomavirus vaccination in the United States, *Acad Pediatr* 18(2S): S3–S10, 2018.

McBride AA: Human papillomaviruses: diversity, infection and host interactions, *Nat Rev Microbiol* 20:95–108, 2022.

Mena M, Taberna M, Monfil L, et al.: Might oral human papillomavirus (HPV) infection in healthy individuals explain differences in HPV-attributable fractions in oropharyngeal cancer? A systematic review and meta-analysis, *J Infect Dis* 219: 1574–1585, 2019.

Meites E, Gee J, Unger E, et al.: Human papillomavirus, In Hall E, Wodi AP, Hamborsky J, et al., editors: *Epidemiology and prevention of vaccine-preventable diseases*, ed 14, Washington, D.C., 2021, Public Health Foundation. (chapter 11).

Meites E, Szilagyi PG, Chesson HW, et al.: Human papillomavirus vaccination for adults: updated recommendations of the Advisory

Committee on Immunization Practices, *MMWR Morb Mortal Wkly Rep* 68:698–702, 2019.

Petrosky E, Bocchini JA Jr, Hariri S, et al.: Use of 9-valent human papillomavirus (HPV) vaccine: updated HPV vaccination recommendations of the Advisory Committee on Immunization Practices, *MMWR Morb Mortal Wkly Rep* 64:300–304, 2015.

Quinlan JD: Human papillomavirus: screening, testing, and prevention, *Am Fam Physician* 104:152–159, 2021.

Sanders AE, Slade GD, Patton LL: National prevalence of oral HPV infection and related risk factors in the U.S. adult population, *Oral Dis* 18:430–441, 2012.

Shigeishi H, Sugiyama M: Risk factors for oral human papillomavirus infection in healthy individuals: a systematic review and meta-analysis, *J Clin Med Res* 8:721–729, 2016.

Sonawane K, Suk R, Chiao EY, et al.: Oral human papillomavirus infection: differences in prevalence between sexes and concordance with genital human papillomavirus infection, NHANES 2011 to 2014, *Ann Intern Med* 167:714–724, 2017.

Syrjänen S: Oral manifestations of human papillomavirus infections, *Eur J Oral Sci* 126(Suppl. 1):49–66, 2018.

Syrjänen S, Rintala M, Sarkola M, et al.: Oral human papillomavirus infection in children during the first 6 years of life, Finland, *Emerg Infect Dis* 27:759–766, 2021.

Tam S, Fu S, Xu L, et al.: The epidemiology of oral human papillomavirus infection in healthy populations: a systematic review and meta-analysis, *Oral Oncol* 82:91–99, 2018.

Taylor S, Bunge E, Bakker M, et al.: The incidence, clearance and persistence of non-cervical human papillomavirus infections: a systematic review of the literature, *BMC Infect Dis* 16:293, 2016.

Villa A, Patton LL, Giuliano AR, et al.: Summary of the evidence on the safety, efficacy, and effectiveness of human papillomavirus vaccines: umbrella review of systematic reviews, *J Am Dent Assoc* 151:245–254.e24, 2020.

Wierzbicka M, Klussmann JP, San Giorgi MR, et al.: Oral and laryngeal HPV infection: incidence, prevalence and risk factors, with special regard to concurrent infection in head, neck and genitals, *Vaccine* 39:2344–2350, 2021.

Wood ZC, Bain CJ, Smith DD, et al.: Oral human papillomavirus infection incidence and clearance: a systematic review of the literature, *J Gen Virol* 98:519–526, 2017.

Squamous Papilloma

Abbey LM, Page DG, Sawyer DR: The clinical and histopathologic features of a series of 464 oral squamous cell papillomas, *Oral Surg Oral Med Oral Pathol* 49:419–428, 1980.

Ballestas SA, Shelly S, Soriano RM, et al.: Trends in recurrent respiratory papillomatosis treatment, *Acta Otorrinolaringol Esp (Engl Ed)* 72:109–120, 2021.

Bao Z, Yang X, Shi L, et al.: Clinicopathologic features of oral squamous papilloma and papillary squamous cell carcinoma: a study of 197 patients from eastern China, *Ann Diagn Pathol* 16:454–458, 2012.

Carneiro TE, Marinho SA, Verli FD, et al.: Oral squamous papilloma: clinical, histologic, and immunohistochemical analysis, *J Oral Sci* 51:367–372, 2009.

Derkay CS, Bluher AE: Update on recurrent respiratory papillomatosis, *Otolaryngol Clin North Am* 52:669–679, 2019.

Donà MG, Pichi B, Rollo F, et al.: Mucosal and cutaneous human papillomaviruses in head and neck squamous cell papillomas, *Head Neck* 39:254–259, 2017.

Gillison ML, Alemany L, Snijders PJF, et al.: Human papillomavirus and diseases of the upper airway: head and neck cancer and respiratory papillomatosis, *Vaccine* 30(Suppl. 5):F34–F54, 2012.

Kerge S, Vuorinen J, Hurme S, et al.: Benign proliferative epithelial lesions of oral mucosa are infrequently associated with α-, β-, or γ human papillomaviruses, *Laryngoscope Investig Otolaryngol* 4:43–48, 2018.

Rosenberg T, Philipsen BB, Mehlum CS, et al.: Therapeutic use of the human papillomavirus vaccine on recurrent respiratory papillomatosis: a systematic review and meta-analysis, *J Infect Dis* 219:1016–1025, 2019.

Syrjänen S, Syrjänen K: HPV-associated benign squamous cell papillomas in the upper aero-digestive tract and their malignant potential, *Viruses* 13:1624, 2021.

Trzcinska A, Zhang W, Gitman M, et al.: The prevalence, anatomic distribution and significance of HPV genotypes in head and neck squamous papillomas as detected by real-time PCR and Sanger sequencing, *Head Neck Pathol* 14:428–434, 2020.

Welschmeyer A, Berke GS: An updated review of the epidemiological factors associated with recurrent respiratory papillomatosis, *Laryngoscope Investig Otolaryngol* 6:226–233, 2021.

Verruca Vulgaris

Betz SJ: HPV-related papillary lesions of the oral mucosa: a review, *Head Neck Pathol* 13:80–90, 2019.

Green TL, Eversole LR, Leider AS: Oral and labial verruca vulgaris: clinical, histologic, and immunohistochemical evaluation, *Oral Surg Oral Med Oral Pathol* 62:410–416, 1986.

Kwok CS, Gibbs S, Bennett C, et al.: Topical treatment for cutaneous warts, *Cochrane Database Syst Rev* 9:CD001781, 2012.

Kwok CS, Holland R, Gibbs S: Efficacy of topical treatments for cutaneous warts: a meta-analysis and pooled analysis of randomized controlled trials, *Br J Dermatol* 165:233–246, 2011.

Mulhem E, Pinelis S: Treatment of nongenital cutaneous warts, *Am Fam Physician* 84:288–293, 2011.

Ringin SA: The effectiveness of cutaneous wart resolution with current treatment modalities, *J Cutan Aesthet Surg* 13:24–30, 2020.

Silverberg NB: Pediatric warts: update on interventions, *Cutis* 103(26–30):E2–E4, 2019.

Soenjoyo KR, Chua BWB, Wee LWY, et al.: Treatment of cutaneous viral warts in children: a review, *Dermatol Ther* 33, 2020, e14034.

Condyloma Acuminatum

Barton S, Wakefield V, O'Mahony C, et al.: Effectiveness of topical and ablative therapies in treatment of anogenital warts: a systematic review and network meta-analysis, *BMJ Open* 9:e027765, 2019.

Blomberg M, Friis S, Munk C, et al.: Genital warts and risk of cancer: a Danish study of nearly 50,000 patients with genital warts, *J Infect Dis* 205:1544–1553, 2012.

Bossart S, Gabutti MP, Seyed Jafari SM, et al.: Nonavalent human papillomavirus vaccination as alternative treatment for genital warts, *Dermatol Ther* 33:e13771, 2020.

Chaturvedi HT, Chaturevedi C: Oral condyloma acuminatum with changes in excretory duct of minor salivary gland: an unusual case report and review of literature, *J Oral Maxillofac Pathol* 24:588, 2020.

Giraldo P, Gonçalves AKS, Pereira SAS, et al.: Human papillomavirus in the oral mucosa of women with genital human papillomavirus lesions, *Eur J Obstet Gynecol Reprod Biol* 126:104–106, 2006.

Henley JD, Summerlin DJ, Tomich CE: Condyloma acuminatum and condyloma-like lesions of the oral cavity: a study of 11 cases with an intraductal component, *Histopathology* 44:216–221, 2004.

Thurgar E, Barton S, Karner C, et al.: Clinical effectiveness and cost-effectiveness of interventions for the treatment of anogenital warts:

systematic review and economic evaluation, *Health Technol Assess* 20(v–vi):1–486, 2016.

Tyros G, Mastraftsi S, Gregoriou S, et al.: Incidence of anogenital warts: epidemiological risk factors and real-life impact of human papillomavirus vaccination, *Int J STD AIDS* 32:4–13, 2021.

Workowski KA, Bachmann LH, Chan PA, et al.: Sexually transmitted infections treatment guidelines, 2021, *MMWR Recomm Rep* 70:1–187, 2021.

Multifocal Epithelial Hyperplasia

Bendtsen SK, Jakobsen KK, Carlander AF, et al.: Focal epithelial hyperplasia, *Viruses* 13:1529, 2021.

Cuberos V, Perez J, Lopez CJ, et al.: Molecular and serological evidence of the epidemiological association of HPV 13 with focal epithelial hyperplasia: a case–control study, *J Clin Virol* 37:21–26, 2006.

González-Losa MR, Suarez-Allén RE, Canul-Canche J, et al.: Multifocal epithelial hyperplasia in a community in the Mayan area of Mexico, *Int J Dermatol* 50:304–309, 2011.

González LV, Gaviria AM, Sanclemente G, et al.: Clinical, histopathological and virological findings in patients with focal epithelial hyperplasia from Colombia, *Int J Dermatol* 44:274–279, 2005.

Ledesma-Montes C, Garcés-Ortíz M, Hernández-Guerrero JC: Clinicopathological and immunocytochemical study of multifocal epithelial hyperplasia, *J Oral Maxillofac Surg* 65:2211–2217, 2007.

Ledesma-Montes C, Mendez-Mendoza A: Unusually high incidence of multifocal epithelial hyperplasia in children of the Nahuatl population of Mexico, *Indian J Dermatol Venereol Leprol* 83:663–666, 2017.

Ledesma-Montes C, Vega-Memije E, Garcés-Ortíz M, et al.: Multifocal epithelial hyperplasia. Report of nine cases, *Med Oral Patol Oral Cir Bucal* 10:394–401, 2005.

Lopez-Villanueva ME, Conde-Ferráez L, Ayora-Talavera G, et al.: Human papillomavirus 13 in a Mexican Mayan community with multifocal epithelial hyperplasia: could saliva be involved in household transmission? *Eur J Dermatol* 21:396–400, 2011.

Said AK, Leao JC, Fedele S, et al.: Focal epithelial hyperplasia—an update, *J Oral Pathol Med* 42:435–442, 2013.

Schwartz Z, Magro C, Nuovo G: The molecular-based differentiation of Heck's disease from its mimics including oral condyloma and white sponge nevus, *Ann Diagn Pathol* 43:151402, 2019.

Sethi S, Ali A, Ju X, et al.: An update on Heck's disease-a systematic review, *J Public Health (Oxf)* 27:fdaa256, 2021.

Witkop CJ Jr, Niswander JD: Focal epithelial hyperplasia in Central and South American Indians and Latinos, *Oral Surg Oral Med Oral Pathol* 20:213–217, 1965.

Sinonasal Papillomas

Bishop JA: OSPs and ESPs and ISPs, oh my! An update on sinonasal (Schneiderian) papillomas, *Head Neck Pathol* 11:269–277, 2017.

Brown NA, Plouffe KR, Yilmaz O, et al.: TP53 mutations and CDKN2A mutations/deletions are highly recurrent molecular alterations in the malignant progression of sinonasal papillomas, *Mod Pathol* 34:1133–1142, 2021.

Bugter O, Monserez DA, van Zijl FVWJ, et al.: Surgical management of inverted papilloma; a single-center analysis of 247 patients with long follow-up, *J Otolaryngol Head Neck Surg* 46:67, 2017.

Chawla A, Shenoy J, Chokkappan K, et al.: Imaging features of sinonasal inverted papilloma: a pictorial review, *Curr Probl Diagn Radiol* 45:347–353, 2016.

Coutinho G, Marques J, Leal M, et al.: Surgical outcomes of sinonasal inverted papilloma: a 17 year review, *Braz J Otorhinolaryngol* 86:315–320, 2020.

Ding R, Sun Q, Wang Y: Association between human papilloma virus infection and malignant sinonasal inverted papilloma, *Laryngoscope* 131:1200–1205, 2021.

Hongo T, Yamamoto H, Jiromaru R, et al.: Clinicopathologic significance of *EGFR* mutation and HPV infection in sinonasal squamous cell carcinoma, *Am J Surg Pathol* 45:108–118, 2021.

Hyams VJ: Papillomas of the nasal cavity and paranasal sinuses: a clinicopathological study of 315 cases, *Ann Otol Rhinol Laryngol* 80:192–206, 1971.

Goudakos JK, Blioskas S, Nikolaou A, et al.: Endoscopic resection of sinonasal inverted papilloma: systematic review and meta-analysis, *Am J Rhinol Allergy* 32:167–174, 2018.

Gupta R, Rady PL, Sikora AG, et al.: The role of human papillomavirus in the pathogenesis of sinonasal inverted papilloma: a narrative review, *Rev Med Virol* 31:e2178, 2021.

Kim JS, Kwon SH: Recurrence of sinonasal inverted papilloma following surgical approach: a meta-analysis, *Laryngoscope* 127:52–58, 2017.

Lawson W, Schlecht NF, Brandwein-Gensler M: The role of the human papillomavirus in the pathogenesis of Schneiderian inverted papillomas: an analytic overview of the evidence, *Head Neck Pathol* 2:49–59, 2008.

Lee JJ, Peterson AM, Embry TW, et al.: Survival outcomes of de novo vs inverted papilloma-associated sinonasal squamous cell carcinoma: a systematic review and meta-analysis, *JAMA Otolaryngol Head Neck Surg* 147:350–359, 2021.

Mehrad M, Stelow EB, Bishop JA, et al.: Transcriptionally active HPV and targetable *EGFR* mutations in sinonasal inverted papilloma: an association between low-risk HPV, condylomatous morphology, and cancer risk? *Am J Surg Pathol* 44:340–346, 2020.

Vor P, der Holte A, Fangk I, et al.: Prognostic factors and risk factors for development and recurrence of sinonasal papillomas: potential role of different HPV subtypes, *Eur Arch Otorhinolaryngol* 277:767–775, 2020.

Peng R, Thamboo A, Choby G, et al.: Outcomes of sinonasal inverted papilloma resection by surgical approach: an updated systematic review and meta-analysis, *Int Forum Allergy Rhinol* 9:573–581, 2019.

Re M, Gioacchini FM, Bajraktari A, et al.: Malignant transformation of sinonasal inverted papilloma and related genetic alterations: a systematic review, *Eur Arch Otorhinolaryngol* 274:2991–3000, 2017.

Stepp WH, Farzal Z, Kimple AJ, et al.: HPV in the malignant transformation of sinonasal inverted papillomas: a meta-analysis, *Int Forum Allergy Rhinol* 11:1461–1471, 2021.

Syrjänen K, Syrjänen S: Detection of human papillomavirus in sinonasal papillomas: systematic review and meta-analysis, *Laryngoscope* 123:181–192, 2013.

Udager AM, McHugh JB, Betz BL, et al.: Activating *KRAS* mutations are characteristic of oncocytic sinonasal papilloma and associated sinonasal squamous cell carcinoma, *J Pathol* 239:394–398, 2016.

Udager AM, McHugh JB, Goudsmit CM, et al.: Human papillomavirus (HPV) and somatic *EGFR* mutations are essential, mutually exclusive oncogenic mechanisms for inverted sinonasal papillomas and associated sinonasal squamous cell carcinomas, *Ann Oncol* 29:466–471, 2018.

Wang H, Li H, Hu L, et al.: *EGFR* and *KRAS* mutations in Chinese patients with sinonasal inverted papilloma and oncocytic papilloma, *Histopathology* 75:274–281, 2019.

Weindorf SC, Brown NA, McHugh JB, et al.: Sinonasal papillomas and carcinomas: a contemporary update with review of an emerging molecular classification, *Arch Pathol Lab Med* 143:1304–1316, 2019.

Molluscum Contagiosum

Fornatora ML, Reich RF, Gray RG, et al.: Intraoral molluscum contagiosum: report of a case and review of the literature, *Oral Surg Oral Med Oral Pathol Oral Radiol Endod* 92:318–320, 2001.

Lee R, Schwartz RA: Pediatric molluscum contagiosum: reflections on the last challenging poxvirus infection, part 1, *Cutis* 86:230–236, 2010.

Lee R, Schwartz RA: Pediatric molluscum contagiosum: reflections on the last challenging poxvirus infection, part 2, *Cutis* 86:287–292, 2010.

Leung AKC, Barankin B, Hon KLE: Molluscum contagiosum: an update, *Recent Pat Inflamm Allergy Drug Discov* 11:22–31, 2017.

Meza-Romero R, Navarrete-Dechent C, Downey C: Molluscum contagiosum: an update and review of new perspectives in etiology, diagnosis, and treatment, *Clin Cosmet Investig Dermatol* 12:373–381, 2019.

Oslo A, Deslandes E, Saada V, et al.: Clinical characteristics of molluscum contagiosum in children in a private dermatology practice in the greater Paris area, France: a prospective study in 661 patients, *Dermatol* 222:314–320, 2011.

van der Wouden JC, Koning S, Katz KA: Interventions for nongenital molluscum contagiosum in persons without immune deficiency, *JAMA Dermatol* 154:203–204, 2018.

van der Wouden JC, van der Sande R, Kruithof EJ, et al.: Interventions for cutaneous molluscum contagiosum, *Cochrane Database Syst Rev* 5:CD004767, 2017.

Verruciform Xanthoma

Bar O, Elad S, Avni B, et al.: Oral verruciform xanthoma in chronic graft-versus-host disease patients, *Support Care Cancer* 29:79–84, 2021.

Barrett AW, Boyapati RP, Bisase BS, et al.: Verruciform xanthoma of the oral mucosa: a series of eight typical and three anomalous cases, *Int J Surg Pathol* 27:492–498, 2019.

Belknap AN, Islam MN, Bhattacharyya I, et al.: Oral verruciform xanthoma: a series of 212 cases and review of the literature, *Head Neck Pathol* 14:742–748, 2020.

Farahani SS, Treister NS, Khan Z, et al.: Oral verruciform xanthoma associated with chronic graft-versus-host disease: a report of five cases and a review of the literature, *Head Neck Pathol* 5:193–198, 2011.

Getz GI, Parag-Sharma K, Reside J, et al.: Identification of *NSDHL* mutations associated with CHILD syndrome in oral verruciform xanthoma, *Oral Surg Oral Med Oral Pathol Oral Radiol* 128:60–69, 2019.

Ide F, Obara K, Yamada H, et al.: Cellular basis of verruciform xanthoma: immunohistochemical and ultrastructural characterization, *Oral Dis* 14:150–157, 2008.

Mehra S, Li L, Fan CY, et al.: A novel somatic mutation of the 3beta-hydroxysteroid dehydrogenase gene in sporadic cutaneous verruciform xanthoma, *Arch Dermatol* 141:1263–1267, 2005.

Nowparast B, Howell FV, Rick GM: Verruciform xanthoma: a clinicopathologic review and report of fifty-four cases, *Oral Surg Oral Med Oral Pathol* 51:619–625, 1981.

Philipsen HP, Reichart PA, Takata T, et al.: Verruciform xanthoma—biological profile of 282 oral lesions based on a literature survey with nine new cases from Japan, *Oral Oncol* 39:325–336, 2003.

Tamiolakis P, Theofilou VI, Tosios KI, et al.: Oral verruciform xanthoma: report of 13 new cases and review of the literature, *Med Oral Patol Oral Cir Bucal* 23:e429–e435, 2018.

Theofilou VI, Sklavounou A, Argyris PP, et al.: Oral verruciform xanthoma within lichen planus: a case report and literature review, *Case Rep Dent* 2018:1615086, 2018.

Seborrheic Keratosis

Izikson L, Sober AJ, Mihm MC, et al.: Prevalence of melanoma clinically resembling seborrheic keratosis: analysis of 9204 cases, *Arch Dermatol* 138:1562–1566, 2002.

Moscarella E, Brancaccio G, Briatico G, et al.: Differential diagnosis and management on seborrheic keratosis in elderly patients, *Clin Cosmet Investig Dermatol* 14:395–406, 2021.

Sun MD, Halpern AC: Advances in the etiology, detection, and clinical management of seborrheic keratosis, *Dermatology* 238:205–217, 2022.

Wade TR, Ackerman AB: The many faces of seborrheic keratoses, *J Dermatol Surg Oncol* 5:378–382, 1979.

Wollina U: Recent advances in managing and understanding seborrheic keratosis, *F1000Res* 8:F1000 Faculty Rev-1520, 2019.

Sebaceous Hyperplasia

Azevedo RS, Almeida OP, Netto JN, et al.: Comparative clinicopathological study of intraoral sebaceous hyperplasia and sebaceous adenoma, *Oral Surg Oral Med Oral Pathol Oral Radiol Endod* 107:100–104, 2009.

Daley TD: Intraoral sebaceous hyperplasia: diagnostic criteria, *Oral Surg Oral Med Oral Pathol* 75:343–347, 1993.

Dent CD, Hunter WE, Svirsky JA: Sebaceous gland hyperplasia: case report and literature review, *J Oral Maxillofac Surg* 53:936–938, 1995.

Eisen DB, Michael DJ: Sebaceous lesions and their associated syndromes: part I, *J Am Acad Dermatol* 61:549–560, 2009.

Hussein L, Perrett CM: Treatment of sebaceous gland hyperplasia: a review of the literature, *J Dermatolog Treat* 13:1–12, 2020.

Ephelis

Bastiaens M, ter Huurne J, Gruis N, et al.: The melanocortin-1-receptor gene is the major freckle gene, *Human Mol Genet* 10:1701–1708, 2001.

Bastiaens MT, Westendorp RG, Vermeer BJ, et al.: Ephelides are more related to pigmentary constitutional host factors than solar lentigines, *Pigment Cell Res* 12:316–322, 1999.

Bliss JM, Ford D, Swerdlow AJ, et al.: Risk of cutaneous melanoma associated with pigmentation characteristics and freckling: systematic overview of 10 case-control studies, *Int J Cancer* 62:367–372, 1995.

Plensdorf S, Martinez J: Common pigmentation disorders, *Am Fam Physician* 15(79):109–116, 2009.

Actinic Lentigo

Derancourt C, Bourdon-Lanoy E, Grob JJ, et al.: Multiple large solar lentigos on the upper back as clinical markers of past severe sunburn: a case-control study, *Dermatology* 214:25–31, 2007.

Hafner C, Stoehr R, van Oers JM, et al.: *FGFR3* and *PIK3CA* mutations are involved in the molecular pathogenesis of solar lentigo, *Br J Dermatol* 160:546–551, 2009.

Holm-Schou AS, Philipsen PA, Idorn LW, et al.: Lifetime UVR dose and skin cancer risk, determined by their common relation to solar lentigines, *Anticancer Res* 40:557–564, 2020.

Nakamura M, Morita A, Seité S, et al.: Environment-induced lentigines: formation of solar lentigines beyond ultraviolet radiation, *Exp Dermatol* 24:407–411, 2015.

Ortonne JP, Pandya AG, Lui H, et al.: Treatment of solar lentigines, *J Am Acad Dermatol* 54:S262–S271, 2006.

Peng F, Xue CH, Hwang SK, et al.: Exposure to fine particulate matter associated with senile lentigo in Chinese women: a cross-sectional study, *J Eur Acad Dermatol Venereol* 31:355–360, 2017.

Lentigo Simplex

Buchner A, Merrell PW, Hansen LS, et al.: Melanocytic hyperplasia of the oral mucosa, *Oral Surg Oral Med Oral Pathol* 71:58–62, 1991.

Cuda JD, Moore FJ, Busam KJ: Lentigo simplex, In Kang S, Amagai M, Bruckner AL, et al., editors: *Fitzpatrick's dermatology*, ed 9, New York, 2019, McGraw-Hill. Available at: https://accessmedicine-mhmedical-com.libraryaccess.elpaso.ttuhsc.edu/content.aspx?bookid=2570&sectionid=210,434,921. (Accessed 8 November 2021.)

Gorlin RJ, Andersen RC, Blaw M: Multiple lentigines syndrome, *Am J Dis Child* 117:652–662, 1969.

Hafner C, Stoehr R, van Oers JM, et al.: The absence of *BRAF*, *FGFR3*, and *PIK3CA* mutations differentiates lentigo simplex from melanocytic nevus and solar lentigo, *J Invest Dermatol* 129:2730–2735, 2009.

Melasma

Bailey AJM, Li HO, Tan MG, et al.: Microneedling as an adjuvant to topical therapies for melasma: a systematic review and meta-analysis, *J Am Acad Dermatol* 86:797–810, 2022.

Kwon SH, Hwang YJ, Lee SK, et al.: Heterogeneous pathology of melasma and its clinical implications, *Int J Mol Sci* 17:824, 2016.

Lee AY: Recent progress in melasma pathogenesis, *Pigment Cell Melanoma Res* 28:648–660, 2015.

Lee BW, Schwartz RA, Janniger CK: Melasma, *G Ital Dermatol Venereol* 152:36–45, 2017.

McKesey J, Tovar-Garza A, Pandya AG: Melasma treatment: an evidence-based review, *Am J Clin Dermatol* 21:173–225, 2020.

Passeron T, Picardo M: Melasma, a photoaging disorder, *Pigment Cell Melanoma Res* 31:461–465, 2018.

Rajanala S, Maymone MBC, Vashi NA: Melasma pathogenesis: a review of the latest research, pathological findings, and investigational therapies, *Dermatol Online J* 25:13030/qt47b7r28c, 2019.

Oral Melanotic Macule

Albuquerque DM, Cunha JL, Roza AL, et al.: Oral pigmented lesions: a retrospective analysis from Brazil, *Med Oral Patol Oral Cir Bucal* 26:e284–e291, 2021.

Axéll T: A prevalence study of oral mucosal lesions in an adult Swedish population, *Odontol Revy Supply* 36:1–103, 1976.

Bouquot JE: Common oral lesions found during a mass screening examination, *J Am Dent Assoc* 112:50–57, 1986.

Buchner A, Hansen LS: Melanotic macule of the oral mucosa: a clinicopathologic study of 105 cases, *Oral Surg Oral Med Oral Pathol* 48:244–249, 1979.

Buchner A, Merrell PW, Carpenter WM: Relative frequency of solitary melanocytic lesions of the oral mucosa, *J Oral Pathol Med* 33:550–557, 2004.

Kahn M, Weathers DR, Hoffman JG: Transformation of a benign oral pigmentation to primary oral mucosal melanoma, *Oral Surg Oral Med Oral Pathol Oral Radiol Endod* 100:454–459, 2005.

Kaugars GE, Heise AP, Riley WT, et al.: Oral melanotic macules: a review of 353 cases, *Oral Surg Oral Med Oral Pathol* 76:59–61, 1993.

Rosebush MS, Briody AN, Cordell KG: Black and brown: nonneoplastic pigmentation of the oral mucosa, *Head Neck Pathol* 13:47–55, 2019.

Shen ZY, Liu W, Bao ZX, et al.: Oral melanotic macule and primary oral malignant melanoma: epidemiology, location involved, and clinical implications, *Oral Surg Oral Med Oral Pathol Oral Radiol Endod* 112:e21–e25, 2011.

Tavares TS, Meirelles DP, de Aguiar MCF, et al.: Pigmented lesions of the oral mucosa: a cross-sectional study of 458 histopathological specimens, *Oral Dis* 24:1484–1491, 2018.

Oral Melanoacanthoma

Cantudo-Sanagustín E, Gutiérrez-Corrales A, Vigo-Martínez M, et al.: Pathogenesis and clinicohistopathological caracteristics [sic] of melanoacanthoma: a systematic review, *J Clin Exp Dent* 8: e327–e336, 2016.

Chandler K, Chaudhry Z, Kumar N, et al.: Melanoacanthoma: a rare cause of oral hyperpigmentation, *Oral Surg Oral Med Oral Pathol Oral Radiol Endod* 84:492–494, 1997.

Datta A, Lamba AK, Tandon S, et al.: A unique presentation of gingival melanoacanthoma: case report and review of literature, *Cureus* 12:e7315, 2020.

Fornatora ML, Reich RF, Haber S, et al.: Oral melanoacanthoma: a report of 10 cases, review of literature, and immunohistochemical analysis of HMB-45 reactivity, *Am J Dermatopathol* 25:12–15, 2003.

Galindo-Moreno P, Padial-Molina M, Gómez-Morales M, et al.: Multifocal oral melanoacanthoma and melanotic macula in a patient after dental implant surgery, *J Am Dent Assoc* 142: 817–824, 2011.

Gonçalves IM, Gomes DQ, Pereira JV, et al.: Clinical and histopathological study of the oral multifocal melanoacanthoma: a case report, *J Clin Exp Dent* 11:e391–e394, 2019.

Heine BT, Drummond JF, Damm DD, et al.: Bilateral oral melanoacanthoma, *Gen Dent* 44:451–452, 1996.

Yarom N, Hirshberg A, Buchner A: Solitary and multifocal oral melanoacanthoma, *Int J Dermatol* 46:1232–1236, 2007.

Melanocytic Nevus

Alikhan A, Ibrahimi OA, Eisen DB: Congenital melanocytic nevi: where are we now? Part I. Clinical presentation, epidemiology, pathogenesis, histology, malignant transformation, and neurocutaneous melanosis, *J Am Acad Dermatol* 67:495.e1–495.e17, 2012.

Amérigo-Góngora M, Machuca-Portillo G, Torres-Lagares D, et al.: Clinicopathological and immunohistochemical analysis of oral melanocytic nevi and review of the literature, *J Stomatol Oral Maxillofac Surg* 118:151–155, 2017.

Aouthmany M, Weinstein M, Zirwas MJ, et al.: The natural history of halo nevi: a retrospective case series, *J Am Acad Dermatol* 67:582–586, 2012.

Bauer J, Garbe C: Risk estimation for malignant transformation of melanocytic nevi, *Arch Dermatol* 140:127, 2004.

Bett BJ: Large or multiple congenital melanocytic nevi: occurrence of cutaneous melanoma in 1008 persons, *J Am Acad Dermatol* 52:793–797, 2005.

Brown A, Sawyer JD, Neumeister MW: Spitz nevus: review and update, *Clin Plast Surg* 48:677–686, 2021.

Buchner A, Hansen LS: Pigmented nevi of the oral mucosa: a clinicopathologic study of 36 new cases and review of 155 cases from the literature. Part I: a clinicopathologic study of 36 new cases, *Oral Surg Oral Med Oral Pathol* 63:566–572, 1987.

Buchner A, Hansen LS: Pigmented nevi of the oral mucosa: a clinicopathologic study of 36 new cases and review of 155 cases from the literature. Part II: analysis of 191 cases, *Oral Surg Oral Med Oral Pathol* 63:676–682, 1987.

Buchner A, Leider AS, Merrell PW, et al.: Melanocytic nevi of oral mucosa: a clinicopathologic study of 130 cases from northern California, *J Oral Pathol Med* 19:197–201, 1990.

Dhanuthai K, Theungtin N, Theungtin N, et al.: Pigmented oral lesions: a multicenter study, *Eur J Dent* 16:315–319, 2022.

Dorji T, Cavazza A, Nappi O, et al.: Spitz nevus of the tongue with pseudoepitheliomatous hyperplasia: report of three cases of a pseudomalignant condition, *Am J Surg Pathol* 26:774–777, 2002.

Eggen CAM, Lommerts JE, van Zuuren EJ, et al.: Laser treatment of congenital melanocytic naevi: a systematic review, *Br J Dermatol* 178:369–383, 2018.

Ferreira L, Jham B, Assi R, et al.: Oral melanocytic nevi: a clinicopathologic study of 100 cases, *Oral Surg Oral Med Oral Pathol Oral Radiol* 120:358–367, 2015.

Grichnik JM, Ross AL, Schneider SL, et al.: How, and from which cell sources, do nevi really develop? *Exp Dermatol* 23:310–313, 2014.

Hanna A, Rawal SY, Anderson KM, et al.: The epithelioid blue nevus: a rare intraoral nevomelanocytic tumor, *J Oral Maxillofac Pathol* 15:88–90, 2011.

Hauschild A, Egberts F, Garbe C, et al.: Melanocytic nevi, *J Dtsch Dermatol Ges* 9:723–734, 2011.

Ibrahimi OA, Alikhan A, Eisen DB: Congenital melanocytic nevi: where are we now? Part II. Treatment options and approach to treatment, *J Am Acad Dermatol* 67:515.e1–515.e13, 2012.

Lallas A, Apalla Z, Ioannides D, et al.: Update on dermoscopy of Spitz/Reed naevi and management guidelines by the International Dermoscopy Society, *Br J Dermatol* 177:645–655, 2017.

Lee HY, Na SY, Son YM, et al.: A malignant melanoma associated with a blue nevus of the lip, *Ann Dermatol* 22:119–124, 2010.

Li CC, Harrist TJ, Noonan VL, et al.: Intraoral Spitz nevus: case report and literature review, *Oral Surg Oral Med Oral Pathol Oral Radiol* 117:e320–e324, 2014.

Liu W, Wang Y, Du G, et al.: Potential association between oral mucosal nevus and melanoma: a preliminary clinicopathologic study, *Oral Dis*, 2023. Online ahead of print March 28, 2020.

Marangon Júnior H, Souza PE, Soares RV: Oral congenital melanocytic nevus: a rare case report and review of the literature, *Head Neck Pathol* 9:481–487, 2015.

Meleti M, Mooi WJ, Casparie MK, et al.: Melanocytic nevi of the oral mucosa—no evidence of an increased risk for oral malignant melanoma: an analysis of 119 cases, *Oral Oncol* 43:976–981, 2007.

Menezes FD, Mooi WJ: Spitz tumors of the skin, *Surg Pathol Clin* 10:281–298, 2017.

Moustafa D, Blundell AR, Hawryluk EB: Congenital melanocytic nevi, *Curr Opin Pediatr* 32:491–497, 2020.

Natarajan E: Black and brown oro-facial mucocutaneous neoplasms, *Head Neck Pathol* 13:56–70, 2019.

Nedelcu RI, Zurac SA, Brînzea A, et al.: Morphological features of melanocytic tumors with depigmented halo: review of the literature and personal results, *Rom J Morphol Embryol* 56(2 Suppl):659–663, 2015.

Ojha J, Akers JL, Akers JO, et al.: Intraoral cellular blue nevus: report of a unique histopathologic entity and review of the literature, *Cutis* 80:189–192, 2007.

Pampena R, Kyrgidis A, Lallas A, et al.: A meta-analysis of nevus-associated melanoma: prevalence and practical implications, *J Am Acad Dermatol* 77:938–945, 2017.

Price HN: Congenital melanocytic nevi: update in genetics and management, *Curr Opin Pediatr* 28:476–482, 2016.

Requena C, Requena L, Kutzner H, et al.: Spitz nevus: a clinicopathological study of 349 cases, *Am J Dermatopathol* 31:107–116, 2009.

Roh MR, Eliades P, Gupta S, et al.: Genetics of melanocytic nevi, *Pigment Cell Melanoma Res* 28:661–672, 2015.

Sainz-Gaspar L, Sánchez-Bernal J, Noguera-Morel L, et al.: Spitz nevus and other Spitzoid tumors in children—part 1: clinical, histopathologic, and immunohistochemical features, *Actas Dermosifiliogr (Engl Ed)* 111:7–19, 2020.

Sainz-Gaspar L, Sánchez-Bernal J, Noguera-Morel L, et al.: Spitz nevus and other Spitzoid tumors in children—part 2: cytogenetic and molecular features. Prognosis and treatment, *Actas Dermosifiliogr (Engl Ed)* 111:20–25, 2020.

Schaffer JV: Update on melanocytic nevi in children, *Clin Dermatol* 33:368–386, 2015.

Shain A, Bastian B: From melanocytes to melanomas, *Nat Rev Cancer* 16:345–358, 2016.

Sugianto JZ, Ralston JS, Metcalf JS, et al.: Blue nevus and "malignant blue nevus:" a concise review, *Semin Diagn Pathol* 33:219–224, 2016.

Shumway BS, Rawal YB, Allen CM, et al.: Oral atypical cellular blue nevus: an infiltrative melanocytic proliferation, *Head Neck Pathol* 7:171–177, 2013.

Tavares TS, Da Costa AAS, Aguiar MCF, et al.: Differential diagnoses of solitary and multiple pigmented lesions of the oral mucosa: evaluation of 905 specimens submitted to histopathological examination, *Head Neck* 43:3775–3787, 2021.

Weedon D, Little JH: Spindle and epithelioid cell nevi in children and adults: a review of 211 cases of the Spitz nevus, *Cancer* 40:217–225, 1977.

Wang DG, Huang FR, Chen W, et al.: Clinicopathological analysis of acquired melanocytic nevi and a preliminary study on the possible origin of nevus cells, *Am J Dermatopathol* 42:414–422, 2020.

Xavier RL, Vasconcelos MG, Galvão HC, et al.: Intra-oral Spitz naevus: a case report, *Clinics (Sao Paulo)* 63:140–142, 2008.

Yeh I: New and evolving concepts of melanocytic nevi and melanocytomas, *Mod Pathol* 33(Suppl. 1):1–14, 2020.

Zembowicz A: Blue nevi and related tumors, *Clin Lab Med* 37:401–415, 2017.

Oral Potentially Malignant Disorders

González-Moles MÁ, Ramos-García P, Warnakulasuriya S: An appraisal of highest quality studies reporting malignant transformation of oral lichen planus based on a systematic review, *Oral Dis* 27:1908–1918, 2021.

Idrees M, Kujan O, Shearston K, Farah CS: Oral lichen planus has a very low malignant transformation rate: a systematic review and meta-analysis using strict diagnostic and inclusion criteria, *J Oral Pathol Med* 50:287–298, 2021.

Iocca O, Sollecito TP, Alawi F, et al.: Potentially malignant disorders of the oral cavity and oral dysplasia: a systematic review and meta-analysis of malignant transformation rate by subtype, *Head Neck* 42:539–555, 2020.

Mello FW, Miguel AFP, Dutra KL, et al.: Prevalence of oral potentially malignant disorders: a systematic review and meta-analysis, *J Oral Pathol Med* 47:633–640, 2018.

Muller S, Tilakaratne WM: Oral potentially malignant disorders, In WHO classification of tumours editorial board, editor: *World Health Organization Classification of Head and Neck Tumours*, ed 5, Lyon, France, 2022, International Agency for Research on Cancer. Available at: https://tumourclassification.iarc.who.int/chaptercontent/52/103. (Accessed 30 March 2022.)

Ramos-García P, González-Moles MÁ, Mello FW, et al.: Malignant transformation of oral proliferative verrucous leukoplakia: a systematic review and meta-analysis, *Oral Dis* 27:1896–1907, 2021.

Ramos-García P, González-Moles MÁ, Warnakulasuriya S: Oral cancer development in lichen planus and related conditions-3.0 evidence level: a systematic review of systematic reviews, *Oral Dis* 27:1919–1935, 2021.

Speight PM, Khurram SA, Kujan O: Oral potentially malignant disorders: risk of progression to malignancy, *Oral Surg Oral Med Oral Pathol Oral Radiol* 125:612–627, 2018.

Warnakulasuriya S: Oral potentially malignant disorders: a comprehensive review on clinical aspects and management, *Oral Oncol* 102:104550, 2020.

Warnakulasuriya S, Kujan O, Aguirre-Urizar JM, et al.: Oral potentially malignant disorders: a consensus report from an international seminar on nomenclature and classification, convened by the WHO Collaborating Centre for Oral Cancer, *Oral Dis* 27:1862–1880, 2021.

Leukoplakia

Abadie WM, Partington EJ, Fowler CB, et al.: Optimal management of proliferative verrucous leukoplakia: a systematic review of the literature, *Otolaryngol Head Neck Surg* 153:504–511, 2015.

Aguirre-Urizar JM, Lafuente-Ibáñez de Mendoza I, Warnakulasuriya S: Malignant transformation of oral leukoplakia: systematic review and meta-analysis of the last 5 years, *Oral Dis* 27:1881–1895, 2021.

Arduino PG, Surace A, Carbone M, et al.: Outcome of oral dysplasia: a retrospective hospital-based study of 207 patients with a long follow-up, *J Oral Pathol Med* 38:540–544, 2009.

Awadallah M, Idle M, Patel K, et al.: Management update of potentially premalignant oral epithelial lesions, *Oral Surg Oral Med Oral Pathol Oral Radiol* 125:628–636, 2018.

Bagan JV, Jiménez-Soriano Y, Diaz-Fernandez JM, et al.: Malignant transformation of proliferative verrucous leukoplakia to oral squamous cell carcinoma: a series of 55 cases, *Oral Oncol* 47:732–735, 2011.

Bouquot JE, Gorlin RJ: Leukoplakia, lichen planus and other oral keratoses in 23,616 white Americans over the age of 35 years, *Oral Surg Oral Med Oral Pathol* 61:373–381, 1986.

Bouquot J, Kurland L, Weiland L: Leukoplakia of the head and neck: characteristics of 568 lesions with 6720 person-years of follow-up, *Oral Surg Oral Med Oral Pathol Oral Radiol Endod* 88:202, 1999.

Bouquot JE, Whitaker SB: Oral leukoplakia—rationale for diagnosis and prognosis of its clinical subtypes or phases, *Quintessence Int* 25:133–140, 1994.

Brouns E, Baart J, Karagozoglu KH, et al.: Malignant transformation of oral leukoplakia in a well-defined cohort of 144 patients, *Oral Dis* 20:e19–e24, 2014.

Cabay RJ, Morton TH, Epstein JB: Proliferative verrucous leukoplakia and its progression to oral carcinoma: a review of the literature, *J Oral Pathol Med* 36:255–261, 2007.

Celentano A, Glurich I, Borgnakke WS, et al.: World Workshop on Oral Medicine VII: prognostic biomarkers in oral leukoplakia and proliferative verrucous leukoplakia—a systematic review of retrospective studies, *Oral Dis* 27:848–880, 2021.

Chaturvedi AK, Udaltsova N, Engels EA, et al.: Oral leukoplakia and risk of progression to oral cancer: a population-based cohort study, *J Natl Cancer Inst* 112:1047–1054, 2020.

Chi AC, Lambert PR 3rd, Pan Y, et al.: Is alveolar ridge keratosis a true leukoplakia? A clinicopathologic comparison of 2153 lesions, *J Am Dent Assoc* 138:641–651, 2007.

de la Cour CD, Sperling CD, Belmonte F, et al.: Prevalence of human papillomavirus in oral epithelial dysplasia: systematic review and meta-analysis, *Head Neck* 42:2975–2984, 2020.

Eversole LR, Eversole GM, Kopcik J: Sanguinaria-associated oral leukoplakia: comparison with other benign and dysplastic leukoplakic lesions, *Oral Surg Oral Med Oral Pathol Oral Radiol Endod* 89:455–464, 2000.

Evren I, Brouns ER, Wils LJ, et al.: Annual malignant transformation rate of oral leukoplakia remains consistent: a long-term follow-up study, *Oral Oncol* 110:105014, 2020.

Farah CS: Molecular, genomic and mutational landscape of oral leukoplakia, *Oral Dis* 27:803–812, 2021.

Farah CS, Fox SA: Dysplastic oral leukoplakia is molecularly distinct from leukoplakia without dysplasia, *Oral Dis* 25:1715–1723, 2019.

Feller L, Lemmer J: Oral leukoplakia as it relates to HPV infection: a review, *Int J Dent* 2012:540561, 2012.

Ferreira L, Peng HH, Cox DP, et al.: Investigation of foreign materials in gingival lesions: a clinicopathologic, energy-dispersive micro-analysis of the lesions and in vitro confirmation of pro-inflammatory effects of the foreign materials, *Oral Surg Oral Med Oral Pathol Oral Radiol* 128:250–267, 2019.

Field EA, McCarthy CE, Ho MW, et al.: The management of oral epithelial dysplasia: the Liverpool algorithm, *Oral Oncol* 51:883–887, 2015.

Foy JP, Bertolus C, Ortiz-Cuaran S, et al.: Immunological and classical subtypes of oral premalignant lesions, *Oncoimmunology* 7:e1496880, 2018.

Gurizzan C, Lorini L, Bossi P: Oral potentially malignant disorders: new insights for future treatment, *Curr Opin Otolaryngol Head Neck Surg* 29:138–142, 2021.

Holmstrup P, Vedtofte P, Reibel J, et al.: Long-term treatment outcome of oral premalignant lesions, *Oral Oncol* 42:461–474, 2006.

Hsue SS, Wang WC, Chen CH, et al.: Malignant transformation in 1458 patients with potentially malignant oral mucosal disorders: a follow-up study based in a Taiwanese hospital, *J Oral Pathol Med* 36:25–29, 2007.

Jayaprakesh V, Reid M, Hatton E, et al.: Human papillomavirus type 16 and 18 in epithelial dysplasia of oral cavity and oropharynx: a meta-analysis, 1985–2010, *Oral Oncol* 47:1048–1054, 2011.

Kaugars GE, Burns JC, Gunsolley JC: Epithelial dysplasia of the oral cavity and lips, *Cancer* 62:2166–2170, 1988.

Kerr AR, Lodi G: Management of oral potentially malignant disorders, *Oral Dis* 27:2008–2025, 2021.

Khanal S, Trainor PJ, Zahin M, et al.: Histologic variation in high grade oral epithelial dysplasia when associated with high-risk human papillomavirus, *Oral Surg Oral Med Oral Pathol Oral Radiol* 123:566–585, 2017.

Kumar A, Cascarini L, McCaul JA, et al.: How should we manage oral leukoplakia? *Br J Oral Maxillofac Surg* 51:377–383, 2013.

Lee JJ, Hung CH, Cheng SJ, et al.: Carcinoma and dysplasia in oral leukoplakias in Taiwan: prevalence and risk factors, *Oral Surg Oral Med Oral Pathol Oral Radiol Endod* 110:472–480, 2006.

Lerman MA, Almazrooa S, Lindeman N, et al.: HPV-16 in a distinct subset of oral epithelial dysplasia, *Mod Pathol* 30:1646–1654, 2017.

Lingen MW, Abt E, Agrawal N, et al.: Evidence-based clinical practice guideline for the evaluation of potentially malignant disorders in the oral cavity: a report of the American Dental Association, *J Am Dent Assoc* 148:712–727, 2017.

Lingen MW, Tampi MP, Urquhart O, et al.: Adjuncts for the evaluation of potentially malignant disorders in the oral cavity: diagnostic test accuracy systematic review and meta-analysis—a report of the American Dental Association, *J Am Dent Assoc* 148:797–813, 2017.

Lingen M, Vigneswaran N, Kujan O, et al.: Oral epithelial dysplasia, In WHO classification of tumours editorial board, editor: *World Health Organization Classification of Head and Neck Tumours,* ed 5, Lyon, France, 2022, International Agency for Research on Cancer. Available at: https://tumourclassification.iarc.who.int/chaptercontent/52/106. (Accessed 30 March 2022.)

Liu W, Shi LJ, Wu L, et al.: Oral cancer development in patients with leukoplakia—clinicopathological factors affecting outcome, *PLoS ONE* 7:e34773, 2012.

Lodi G, Franchini R, Warnakulasuriya S, et al.: Interventions for treating oral leukoplakia to prevent oral cancer, *Cochrane Database Syst Rev* 7:CD001829, 2016.

Lodi G, Sardella A, Bez C, et al.: Interventions for treating oral leukoplakia, *Cochrane Database Syst Rev* 4:CD001829, 2006.

Macey R, Walsh T, Kerr AR, et al.: Diagnostic tests for oral cancer and potentially malignant disorders in patients presenting with clinically evident lesions, *Cochrane Database Syst Rev* 7:CD010276, 2021.

Mascarenhas AK, Allen CM, Moeschberger ML: The association between Viadent use and oral leukoplakia—results of a matched case–control study, *J Public Health Dent* 62:158–162, 2002.

Mehanna HM, Rattay T, Smith J, et al.: Treatment and follow-up of oral dysplasia—a systematic review, *Head Neck* 31:1600–1609, 2009.

Müller S: Oral epithelial dysplasia, atypical verrucous lesions and oral potentially malignant disorders: focus on histopathology, *Oral Surg Oral Med Oral Pathol Oral Radiol* 125:591–602, 2018.

Muller S, Tilakaratne WM: Oral potentially malignant disorders, In WHO classification of tumours editorial board, editor: *World Health Organization Classification of Head and Neck Tumours*, ed 5, Lyon, France, 2022, International Agency for Research on Cancer. Available at: https://tumourclassification.iarc.who.int/chaptercontent/52/103. (Accessed 30 March 2022.)

Nankivell P, Mehanna H: Oral dysplasia: biomarkers, treatment, and follow-up, *Curr Oncol Rep* 13:145–152, 2011.

Napier SS, Speight PM: Natural history of potentially malignant oral lesions and conditions: an overview of the literature, *J Oral Pathol Med* 37:1–10, 2008.

Odell EW: Aneuploidy and loss of heterozygosity as risk markers for malignant transformation in oral mucosa, *Oral Dis* 27:1993–2007, 2021.

Odell E, Kujan O, Warnakulasuriya S, et al.: Oral epithelial dysplasia: recognition, grading and clinical significance, *Oral Dis* 27:1947–1976, 2021.

Perdomo-Lara SJ, Buenahora MR, Álvarez E, et al.: Human papilloma virus genotypes in dysplasia and epithelial hyperplasia of oral cavity using the luminex xmap technology. A multicenter study, *Med Oral Patol Oral Cir Bucal* 25:e61–e70, 2020.

Petti S: Pooled estimate of world leukoplakia prevalence: a systematic review, *Oral Oncol* 39:770–780, 2003.

Pietrobon G, Tagliabue M, Stringa LM, et al.: Leukoplakia in the oral cavity and oral microbiota: a comprehensive review, *Cancers (Basel)* 13:4439, 2021.

Robledo-Sierra J, Ben-Amy DP, Varoni E, et al.: World Workshop on Oral Medicine VII: targeting the oral microbiome part 2: current knowledge on malignant and potentially malignant oral disorders, *Oral Dis* 25(Suppl. 1):28–48, 2019.

Rosin MP, Cheng X, Poh C, et al.: Use of allelic loss to predict malignant risk for low-grade oral epithelial dysplasia, *Clin Cancer Res* 6:357–362, 2000.

Roza ALOC, Kowalski LP, William WN Jr, et al.: Oral leukoplakia and erythroplakia in young patients: a systematic review, *Oral Surg Oral Med Oral Pathol Oral Radiol* 131:73–84, 2021.

Shepman KP, van der Meij EH, Smeele LE, et al.: Malignant transformation of oral leukoplakia: a follow-up study of a hospital-based population of 166 patients with oral leukoplakia from The Netherlands, *Oral Oncol* 34:270–275, 1998.

Shiu MN, Chen TH, Chang SH, et al.: Risk factors for leukoplakia and malignant transformation to oral carcinoma: a leukoplakia cohort in Taiwan, *Br J Cancer* 82:1871–1874, 2000.

Silverman S Jr, Gorsky M: Proliferative verrucous leukoplakia: a follow-up study of 54 cases, *Oral Surg Oral Med Oral Pathol Oral Radiol Endod* 84:154–157, 1997.

Silverman S Jr, Gorsky M, Lozada F: Oral leukoplakia and malignant transformation: a follow-up study of 257 patients, *Cancer* 53:563–568, 1984.

Syrjänen S, Lodi G, von Bültizingslöwen I, et al.: Human papillomaviruses in oral carcinoma and oral potentially malignant disorders: a systematic review, *Oral Dis* 17(Suppl. 1):58–72, 2011.

Thompson LDR, Fitzpatrick SG, Müller S, et al.: Proliferative verrucous leukoplakia: an expert consensus guideline for standardized assessment and reporting, *Head Neck Pathol* 15:572–587, 2021.

Tilakaratne WM, Jayasooriya PR, Jayasuriya NS, et al.: Oral epithelial dysplasia: causes, quantification, prognosis, and management challenges, *Periodontol* 2000(80):126–147, 2009.

Villa A, Celentano A, Glurich I, et al.: World Workshop on Oral Medicine VII: prognostic biomarkers in oral leukoplakia: a systematic review of longitudinal studies, *Oral Dis* 25(Suppl. 1):64–78, 2019.

Villa A, Menon RS, Kerr AR, et al.: Proliferative leukoplakia: proposed new clinical diagnostic criteria, *Oral Dis* 24:749–760, 2018.

Waldron CA, Shafer WG: Leukoplakia revisited: a clinicopathologic study of 3256 oral leukoplakias, *Cancer* 36:1386–1392, 1975.

Walsh T, Warnakulasuriya S, Lingen MW, et al.: Clinical assessment for the detection of oral cavity cancer and potentially malignant disorders in apparently healthy adults, *Cochrane Database Syst Rev* 12, 2021, CD010173.

Warnakulasuriya S, Ariyawardana A: Malignant transformation of oral leukoplakia: a systematic review of observational studies, *J Oral Pathol Med* 45:155–166, 2016.

Warnakulasuriya S, Kovacevic T, Madden P, et al.: Factors predicting malignant transformation in oral potentially malignant disorders among patients accrued over a 10-year period in South East England, *J Oral Pathol Med* 40:677–683, 2011.

Woo SB: Oral epithelial dysplasia and premalignancy, *Head Neck Pathol* 13:423–439, 2019.

Yan F, Reddy PD, Nguyen SA, et al.: Grading systems of oral cavity pre-malignancy: a systematic review and meta-analysis, *Eur Arch Otorhinolaryngol* 277:2967–2976, 2020.

Yang EC, Tan MT, Schwarz RA, et al.: Noninvasive diagnostic adjuncts for the evaluation of potentially premalignant oral epithelial lesions: current limitations and future directions, *Oral Surg Oral Med Oral Pathol Oral Radiol* 125:670–681, 2018.

Erythroplakia

Amagasa T, Yokoo E, Sata K, et al.: A study of the clinical characteristics and treatment of oral carcinoma in situ, *Oral Surg Oral Med Oral Pathol* 60:50–55, 1985.

Bouquot JE, Ephros H: Erythroplakia: the dangerous red mucosa, *Pract Periodontics Aesth Dent* 7:59–68, 1995.

de Azevedo AB, Dos Santos TCRB, Lopes MA, et al.: Oral leukoplakia, leukoerythroplakia, erythroplakia and actinic cheilitis: analysis of 953 patients focusing on oral epithelial dysplasia, *J Oral Pathol Med* 50:829–840, 2021.

Hashibe M, Mathew B, Kuruvilla B, et al.: Chewing tobacco, alcohol and the risk of erythroplakia, *Cancer Epidemiol Biomarkers Prev* 9:639–645, 2000.

Holmstrup P: Oral erythroplakia-what is it? *Oral Dis* 24:138–143, 2018.

Muller S, Tilakaratne WM: Oral potentially malignant disorders, In WHO classification of tumours editorial board, editor: *World Health Organization Classification of Head and Neck Tumours*, ed 5, Lyon, France, 2022, International Agency for Research on Cancer. Available at: https://tumourclassification.iarc.who.int/chaptercontent/52/103. (Accessed 30 March 2022.)

Reichart PA, Philipsen HP: Oral erythroplakia—a review, *Oral Oncol* 41:551–561, 2005.

Shafer WG, Waldron CA: Erythroplakia of the oral cavity, *Cancer* 36:1021–1028, 1975.

Villa A, Villa C, Abati S: Oral cancer and oral erythroplakia: an update and implication for clinicians, *Aust Dent J* 56:253–256, 2011.

Woo SB: Oral epithelial dysplasia and premalignancy, *Head Neck Pathol* 13:423–439, 2019.

Smokeless Tobacco Keratosis

Araghi M, Galanti MR, Lundberg M, et al.: No association between moist oral snuff (snus) use and oral cancer: pooled analysis of nine prospective observational studies, *Scand J Public Health* 49:833–840, 2021.

Bergström J, Keilani H, Lundholm C, et al.: Smokeless tobacco (snuff) use and periodontal bone loss, *J Clin Periodontol* 33:549–554, 2006.

Chu YH, Tatakis DN, Wee AG: Smokeless tobacco use and periodontal health in a rural male population, *J Periodontol* 81:848–854, 2010.

Cornelius ME, Loretan CG, Wang TW, et al.: Tobacco product use among adults—United States, 2020, *MMWR Morb Mortal Wkly Rep* 71:397–405, 2022.

Delnevo CD, Hrywna M, Miller Lo EJ, et al.: Examining market trends in smokeless tobacco sales in the United States: 2011–2019, *Nicotine Tob Res* 23:1420–1424, 2021.

Gentzke AS, Wang TW, Cornelius M, et al.: Tobacco product use and associated factors among middle and high school students—National Youth Tobacco Survey, United States, 2021, *MMWR Surveill Summ* 71:1–29, 2022.

Inoue-Choi M, Shiels MS, McNeel TS, et al.: Contemporary associations of exclusive cigarette, cigar, pipe, and smokeless tobacco use with overall and cause-specific mortality in the United States, *JNCI Cancer Spectr* 3:pkz036, 2019.

Müller S: Frictional keratosis, contact keratosis and smokeless tobacco keratosis: features of reactive white lesions of the oral mucosa, *Head Neck Pathol* 13:16–24, 2019.

Muthukrishnan A, Warnakulasuriya S: Oral health consequences of smokeless tobacco use, *Indian J Med Res* 148:35–40, 2018.

Rodu B: Smokeless tobacco and oral cancer: a review of the risks and determinants, *Crit Rev Oral Biol Med* 15:252–263, 2004.

Tomar SL, Hecht SS, Jaspers I, et al.: Oral health effects of combusted and smokeless tobacco products, *Adv Dent Res* 30:4–10, 2019.

Walsh PM, Epstein JB: The oral effects of smokeless tobacco, *J Can Dent Assoc* 66:22–25, 2000.

Warnakulasuriya KA, Ralhan R: Clinical, pathological, cellular and molecular lesions caused by oral smokeless tobacco—a review, *J Oral Pathol Med* 36:63–77, 2007.

Oral Submucous Fibrosis

Angadi PV, Rehka KP: Oral submucous fibrosis: a clinicopathologic review of 205 cases in Indians, *Oral Maxillofac Surg* 15:15–19, 2011.

Hazarey VK, Erlewad DM, Mundhe KA, et al.: Oral submucous fibrosis: study of 1000 cases from central India, *J Oral Pathol Med* 36:12–17, 2007.

Iocca O, Sollecito TP, Alawi F, et al.: Potentially malignant disorders of the oral cavity and oral dysplasia: a systematic review and meta-analysis of malignant transformation rate by subtype, *Head Neck* 42:539–555, 2020.

Isaac U, Issac JS, Ahmed Khoso N: Histopathologic features of oral submucous fibrosis: a study of 35 biopsy specimens, *Oral Surg Oral Med Oral Pathol Oral Radiol Endod* 106:556–560, 2008.

Kujan O, Mello FW, Warnakulasuriya S: Malignant transformation of oral submucous fibrosis: a systematic review and meta-analysis, *Oral Dis* 27:1936–1946, 2021.

More CB, Jatti Patil D, Rao NR: Medicinal management of oral submucous fibrosis in the past decade—a systematic review, *J Oral Biol Craniofac Res* 10:552–568, 2020.

Peng Q, Li H, Chen J, et al.: Oral submucous fibrosis in Asian countries, *J Oral Pathol Med* 49:294–304, 2020.

Ray JG, Chatterjee R, Chaudhuri K: Oral submucous fibrosis: a global challenge. Rising incidence, risk factors, management, and research priorities, *Periodontol* 2000(80):200–212, 2019.

Ray JG, Ranganathan K, Chattopadhyay A: Malignant transformation of oral submucous fibrosis: overview of histopathological aspects, *Oral Surg Oral Med Oral Pathol Oral Radiol* 122:200–209, 2016.

Reichart PA, Warnakulasuriya S: Oral lichenoid contact lesions induced by areca nut and betel quid chewing: a mini review, *J Investig Clin Dent* 3:163–166, 2012.

Shen YW, Shih YH, Fuh LJ, et al.: Oral submucous fibrosis: a review on biomarkers, pathogenic mechanisms, and treatments, *Int J Mol Sci* 21:7231, 2020.

Tilakaratne WM, Ekanayaka RP, Warnakulasuriya S: Oral submucous fibrosis: a historical perspective and a review on etiology and pathogenesis, *Oral Surg Oral Med Oral Pathol Oral Radiol* 122:178–191, 2016.

Warnakulasuriya S, Kerr AR: Oral submucous fibrosis: a review of the current management and possible directions for novel therapies, *Oral Surg Oral Med Oral Pathol Oral Radiol* 122:232–241, 2016.

World Health Organization International Agency for Research on Cancer: *IARC monographs on the evaluation of carcinogenic risks to humans, betel-quid and areca-nut chewing and some areca-nut-derived nitrosamines*, vol 85, Lyon, France, 2004, IARC Press.

Nicotine Stomatitis

Bardellini E, Amadori F, Conti G, et al.: Oral mucosal lesions in electronic cigarettes consumers versus former smokers, *Acta Odontol Scand* 76:226–228, 2018.

Ortiz GM, Pierce AM, Wilson DF: Palatal changes associated with reverse smoking in Filipino women, *Oral Dis* 2:232–237, 1996.

Rossie KM, Guggenheimer J: Thermally induced "nicotine" stomatitis: a case report, *Oral Surg Oral Med Oral Pathol* 70:597–599, 1990.

Saunders WH: Nicotine stomatitis of the palate, *Ann Otol Rhinol Laryngol* 67:618–627, 1958.

Schwartz DL: Stomatitis nicotina of the palate: report of two cases, *Oral Surg Oral Med Oral Pathol* 20:306–315, 1965.

Actinic Keratosis

Criscione VD, Weinstock MA, Naylor M, et al.: Actinic keratoses: natural history and risk of malignant transformation in the Veteran Affairs topical tretinoin chemoprevention trial, *Cancer* 115:2523–2530, 2009.

Eisen DB, Asgari MM, Bennett DD, et al.: Guidelines of care for the management of actinic keratosis, *J Am Acad Dermatol* 85:e209–e233, 2021.

Galati L, Brancaccio RN, Robitaille A, et al.: Detection of human papillomaviruses in paired healthy skin and actinic keratosis by next generation sequencing, *Papillomavirus Res* 9:100196, 2020.

Guorgis G, Anderson CD, Lyth J, et al.: Actinic keratosis diagnosis and increased risk of developing skin cancer: a 10-year cohort study of 17,651 patients in Sweden, *Acta Derm Venereol* 100:adv00128, 2020.

Gupta AK, Cooper EA, Feldman SR, et al.: A survey of office visits for actinic keratosis as reported by NAMCS, 1990–1999. National Ambulatory Medical Care Survey, *Cutis* 70(Suppl. 2):8–13, 2002.

Gupta AK, Paquet M, Villanueva E, et al.: Interventions for actinic keratoses, *Cochrane Database Syst Rev* 12:CD004415, 2012.

Moscarella E, Di Brizzi EV, Casari A, et al.: Italian expert consensus paper on the management of patients with actinic keratoses, *Dermatol Ther* 33:e13992, 2020.

Rosso JD, Armstrong AW, Berman B, et al.: Advances and considerations in the management of actinic keratosis: an expert consensus panel report, *J Drugs Dermatol* 20:888–893, 2021.

Siegel JA, Korgavkar K, Weinstock MA: Current perspective on actinic keratosis: a review, *Br J Dermatol* 177:350–358, 2017.

Actinic Cheilosis

Bakirtzi K, Papadimitriou I, Andreadis D, et al.: Treatment options and post-treatment malignant transformation rate of actinic cheilitis: a systematic review, *Cancers (Basel)* 13:3354, 2021.

Dancyger A, Heard V, Huang B, et al.: Malignant transformation of actinic cheilitis: a systematic review of observational studies, *J Investig Clin Dent* 9:e12343, 2018.

de Castro AT, Fonsêca TC, Cabral MG, et al.: Epithelial dysplasia in actinic cheilitis: microscopic study of 70 cases from Brazil, *Head Neck Pathol* 15:566–571, 2021.

Jadotte YT, Schwartz RA: Solar cheilosis: an ominous precursor: part I. Diagnostic insights, *J Am Acad Dermatol* 66:173–184, 2012.

Jadotte YT, Schwartz RA: Solar cheilosis: an ominous precursor: part II. Therapeutic perspectives, *J Am Acad Dermatol* 66:187–198, 2012.

Kaugars GE, Pillion T, Svirsky JA, et al.: Actinic cheilitis: a review of 152 cases, *Oral Surg Oral Med Oral Pathol Oral Radiol Endod* 88:181–186, 1999.

Lai M, Pampena R, Cornacchia L, et al.: Treatments of actinic cheilitis: a systematic review of the literature, *J Am Acad Dermatol* 83:876–887, 2020.

Markopoulos A, Albanidou-Farmaki E, Kayavis I: Actinic cheilitis: clinical and pathologic characteristics in 65 cases, *Oral Dis* 10:212–216, 2004.

Salgueiro AP, de Jesus LH, de Souza IF, et al.: Treatment of actinic cheilitis: a systematic review, *Clin Oral Investig* 23:2041–2053, 2019.

Silva LVO, de Arruda JAA, Abreu LG, et al.: Demographic and clinicopathologic features of actinic cheilitis and lip squamous cell carcinoma: a Brazilian multicentre study, *Head Neck Pathol* 14:899–908, 2020.

Trager MH, Farmer K, Ulrich C, et al.: Actinic cheilitis: a systematic review of treatment options, *J Eur Acad Dermatol Venereol* 35:815–823, 2021.

Keratoacanthoma

Chen YK, Lin LM, Lin CC, et al.: Keratoacanthoma of the tongue: a diagnostic problem, *Otolaryngol Head Neck Surg* 128:581–582, 2003.

de Visscher JG, van der Wal JE, Starink TM, et al.: Giant keratoacanthoma of the lower lip. Report of a case of spontaneous regression, *Oral Surg Oral Med Oral Pathol Oral Radiol Endod* 81:193–196, 1996.

Janette A, Pecaro B, Lonergan M, et al.: Solitary intraoral keratoacanthoma: report of a case, *J Oral Maxillofac Surg* 54:1026–1030, 1996.

Kwiek B, Schwartz RA: Keratoacanthoma (KA): an update and review, *J Am Acad Dermatol* 74:1220–1233, 2016.

Li J, Wang K, Gao F, et al.: Array comparative genomic hybridization of keratoacanthomas and squamous cell carcinomas: different patterns of genetic aberrations suggest two distinct entities, *J Invest Dermatol* 132:2060–2066, 2012.

Mandrell JC, Santa Cruz DJ: Keratoacanthoma: hyperplasia, benign neoplasm, or a type of squamous cell carcinoma? *Semin Diagn Pathol* 26:150–163, 2009.

Nirenberg A, Steinman H, Dixon A: Keratoacanthoma: update on the debate, *Am J Dermatopathol* 43:305–307, 2021.

Ra SH, Su A, Li X, et al.: Keratoacanthoma and squamous cell carcinoma are distinct from a molecular perspective, *Mod Pathol* 28:799–806, 2015.

Selmer J, Skov T, Spelman L, et al.: Squamous cell carcinoma and keratoacanthomas are biologically distinct and can be diagnosed by light microscopy: a review, *Histopathology* 69:535–541, 2016.

Tisack A, Fotouhi A, Fidai C, et al.: A clinical and biological review of keratoacanthoma, *Br J Dermatol* 185:487–498, 2021.

Weedon D, Brooks D, Malo J, et al.: Abortive keratoacanthoma: a hitherto unrecognised variant, *Pathology* 42:661–663, 2010.

Squamous Cell Carcinoma

Aceves Argemí R, González Navarro B, Ochoa García-Seisdedos P, et al.: Mouthwash with alcohol and oral carcinogenesis: systematic review and meta-analysis, *J Evid Based Dent Pract* 20:101407, 2020.

Adjei Boakye E, Buchanan P, Hinyard L, et al.: Incidence and risk of second primary malignant neoplasm after a first head and neck squamous cell carcinoma, *JAMA Otolaryngol Head Neck Surg* 144:727–737, 2018.

Agalliu I, Gapstur S, Chen Z, et al.: Associations of oral α-, β-, and γ-human papillomavirus types with risk of incident head and neck cancer, *JAMA Oncol* 2:599–606, 2016.

American Cancer Society: Cancer facts & figs. 2022, Atlanta, 2022, American Cancer Society, pp. 1–80.

Ang KK, Harris J, Wheeler R, et al.: Human papillomavirus and survival of patients with oropharyngeal cancer, *N Engl J Med* 363:24–35, 2010.

Asthana S, Labani S, Kailash U, et al.: Association of smokeless tobacco use and oral cancer: a systematic global review and meta-analysis, *Nicotine Tob Res* 21:1162–1171, 2019.

Asthana S, Vohra P, Labani S: Association of smokeless tobacco with oral cancer: a review of systematic reviews, *Tob Prev Cessat* 5:34, 2019.

Bagnardi V, Rota M, Botteri E, et al.: Alcohol consumption and site-specific cancer risk: a comprehensive dose–response meta-analysis, *Br J Cancer* 112:580–593, 2015.

Balachandra S, Kusin SB, Lee R, et al.: Blood-based biomarkers of human papillomavirus-associated cancers: a systematic review and meta-analysis, *Cancer* 127:850–864, 2021.

Bigelow EO, Seiwert TY, Fakhry C: Deintensification of treatment for human papillomavirus-related oropharyngeal cancer: current state and future directions, *Oral Oncol* 105:104652, 2020.

Bishop JA, Ma XJ, Wang H, et al.: Detection of transcriptionally active high risk HPV in patients with head and neck squamous cell carcinoma as visualized by a novel E6/E7 mRNA in situ hybridization method, *Am J Surg Pathol* 36:1874–1882, 2012.

Bishop JA, Montgomery EA, Westra WH: Use of p40 and p63 immunohistochemistry and human papillomavirus testing as ancillary tools for the recognition of head and neck sarcomatoid carcinoma and its distinction from benign and malignant mesenchymal processes, *Am J Surg Pathol* 38:257–264, 2014.

Boffetta P, Hayes RB, Sartori S, et al.: Mouthwash use and cancer of the head and neck: a pooled analysis from the International Head and Neck Cancer Epidemiology Consortium, *Eur J Cancer Prev* 25:344–348, 2016.

Bouquot JE: Common oral lesions found during a mass screening examination, *J Am Dent Assoc* 112:50–57, 1986.

Braakhuis BJM, Leemans CR, Brakenhoff RH: Expanding fields of genetically altered cells in head and neck squamous carcinogenesis, *Semin Cancer Biol* 15:113–120, 2005.

Brandwein-Gensler M, Teixeira MS, Lewis CM, et al.: Oral squamous cell carcinoma: histologic risk assessment, but not margin status, is strongly predictive of local disease-free and overall survival, *Am J Surg Pathol* 29:167–178, 2005.

Bravi F, Lee YA, Hashibe M, et al.: Lessons learned from the INHANCE consortium: an overview of recent results on head and neck cancer, *Oral Dis* 27:73–93, 2021.

Brugere J, Guenel P, Leclerc A, et al.: Differential effects of tobacco and alcohol in cancer of the larynx, pharynx, and mouth, *Cancer* 57:391–395, 1986.

Bulsara VM, Worthington HV, Glenny AM, et al.: Interventions for the treatment of oral and oropharyngeal cancers: surgical treatment, *Cochrane Database Syst Rev* 12:CD006205, 2018.

Califano JA, Lydiatt WM, Nehal KS, et al.: Cutaneous carcinoma of the head and neck, In Amin MB, Edge SB, Greene FL, et al., editors: *AJCC cancer staging manual*, ed 8, Chicago, 2018, American College of Surgeons, pp 171–181. (chapter 15).

Cancer Genome Atlas Network: Comprehensive genomic characterization of head and neck squamous cell carcinomas, *Nature* 17:576–582, 2015.

Castellsagué X, Alemany L, Quer M, et al.: HPV involvement in head and neck cancers: comprehensive assessment of biomarkers in 3680 patients, *J Natl Cancer Inst* 108:djv403, 2016.

Centers for Disease Control and Prevention: An update on cancer deaths in the United States. Atlanta: *United States Department of Health and Human Services*, 2022, Centers for Disease Control and Prevention, Division of Cancer Prevention and Control. Available at: https://www.cdc.gov/cancer/dcpc/research/update-on-cancer-deaths/index.htm. (Accessed 17 March 2022.)

Chakravarthy A, Henderson S, Thirdborough SM, et al.: Human papillomavirus drives tumor development throughout the head and neck: improved prognosis is associated with an immune response largely restricted to the oropharynx, *J Clin Oncol* 34:4132–4141, 2016.

Chaturvedi AK, D'Souza G, Gillison ML, et al.: Burden of HPV-positive oropharynx cancers among ever and never smokers in the U.S. population, *Oral Oncol* 60:61–67, 2016.

Chaturvedi AK, Engels EA, Pfeiffer RM, et al.: Human papillomavirus and rising oropharyngeal cancer incidence in the United States, *J Clin Oncol* 29:4294–4301, 2012.

Chaturvedi AK, Graubard BI, Broutian T, et al.: Effect of prophylactic human papillomavirus (HPV) vaccination on oral HPV infections among young adults in the United States, *J Clin Oncol* 36:262–267, 2018.

Chaturvedi AK, Graubard BI, Broutian T, et al.: Prevalence of oral HPV infection in unvaccinated men and women in the United States, 2009–2016, *JAMA* 322:977–979, 2019.

Chi AC, Day TA, Neville BW: Oral cavity and oropharyngeal squamous cell carcinoma—an update, *CA Cancer J Clin* 65:401–421, 2015.

Chuang SC, Scelo G, Tonita JM, et al.: Risk of second primary cancer among patients with head and neck cancers: a pooled analysis of 13 cancer registries, *Int J Cancer* 123:2390–2396, 2008.

Cianfriglia F, Di Gregorio DA, Manieri A: Multiple primary tumours in patients with oral squamous cell carcinoma, *Oral Oncol* 35:157–163, 1999.

Cline BJ, Simpson MC, Gropler M, et al.: Change in age at diagnosis of oropharyngeal cancer in the United States, 1975–2016, *Cancers (Basel)* 12:3191, 2020.

Coca-Pelaz A, Rodrigo JP, Suárez C, et al.: The risk of second primary tumors in head and neck cancer: a systematic review, *Head Neck* 42:456–466, 2020.

Cohen N, Fedewa S, Chen AY: Epidemiology and demographics of the head and neck cancer population, *Oral Maxillofac Surg Clin North Am* 30:381–395, 2018.

Cornelius ME, Loretan CG, Wang TW, et al.: Tobacco product use among adults—United States, 2020, *MMWR Morb Mortal Wkly Rep* 71:397–405, 2022.

Craig SG, Anderson LA, Schache AG, et al.: Recommendations for determining HPV status in patients with oropharyngeal cancers under TNM8 guidelines: a two-tier approach, *Br J Cancer* 120:827–833, 2019.

Curtius K, Wright NA, Graham TA: An evolutionary perspective on field cancerization, *Nat Rev Cancer* 18:19–32, 2018.

Damgacioglu H, Sonawane K, Zhu Y, et al.: Oropharyngeal cancer incidence and mortality trends in all 50 states in the US, 2001–2017, *JAMA Otolaryngol Head Neck Surg* 148:155–165, 2022.

Dasanayake AP, Silverman AJ, Warnakulasuriya S: Maté drinking and oral and oro-pharyngeal cancer: a systematic review and meta-analysis, *Oral Oncol* 46:82–86, 2010.

Day AT, Fakhry C, Tiro JA, et al.: Considerations in human papillomavirus-associated oropharyngeal cancer screening: a review, *JAMA Otolaryngol Head Neck Surg* 146:656–664, 2020.

D'Cruz AK, Vaish R, Dhar H: Oral cancers: current status, *Oral Oncol* 87:64–69, 2018.

Di Cosola M, Cazzolla AP, Charitos IA, et al.: *Candida albicans* and oral carcinogenesis. A brief review, *J Fungi (Basel)* 7:476, 2021.

Divaris K, Olshan AF, Smith J: Oral health and risk for head and neck squamous cell carcinoma: the Carolina Head and Neck Cancer Study, *Cancer Causes Control* 21:567–575, 2010.

Drake VE, Fakhry C, Windon MJ, et al.: Timing, number, and type of sexual partners associated with risk of oropharyngeal cancer, *Cancer* 127:1029–1038, 2021.

Ellington TD, Henley SJ, Senkomago V, et al.: Trends in incidence of cancers of the oral cavity and pharynx - United States 2007–2016, *MMWR Morb Mortal Wkly Rep* 69:433–438, 2020.

Fakhry C, Lacchetti C, Rooper LM, et al.: Human papillomavirus testing in head and neck carcinomas: ASCO clinical practice guideline endorsement summary of the CAP guideline, *J Oncol* 36:3152–3161, 2018.

Fakhry C, Westra WH, Li S, et al.: Improved survival of patients with human papillomavirus-positive head and neck squamous cell carcinoma in a prospective trial, *J Natl Cancer Inst* 100:261–269, 2010.

Farah CS: Molecular landscape of head and neck cancer and implications for therapy, *Ann Transl Med* 9:915, 2021.

Ferlay J, Ervik M, Lam F, et al.: *Global Cancer Observatory: cancer today*, Lyon, France, 2022, International Agency for Research on Cancer. Available at: https://gco.iarc.fr/today. (Accessed 17 March 2022.)

Fukuzawa K, Noguchi Y, Yoshikawa T, et al.: High incidence of synchronous cancer of the oral cavity and the upper gastrointestinal tract, *Cancer Lett* 144:145–151, 1999.

Gan SJ, Dahlstrom KR, Peck BW, et al.: Incidence and pattern of second primary malignancies in patients with index oropharyngeal cancers versus index nonoropharyngeal head and neck cancers, *Cancer* 119:2593–2601, 2013.

Gandini S, Botteri E, Iodice S: Tobacco smoking and cancer: a meta-analysis, *Int J Cancer* 122:155–164, 2008.

Gandini S, Negri E, Boffetta P, et al.: Mouthwash and oral cancer risk—quantitative meta-analysis of epidemiologic studies, *Ann Agric Environ Med* 19:173–180, 2012.

GBD: Tobacco Collaborators: Spatial, temporal, and demographic patterns in prevalence of smoking tobacco use and attributable disease burden in 204 countries and territories, 1990–2019: a systematic analysis from the Global Burden of Disease Study 2019, *Lancet* 397(2337–2360):2021, 2019.

Gillison ML, Alemany L, Snijders PJF, et al.: Human papillomavirus and diseases of the upper airway: head and neck cancer and respiratory papillomatosis, *Vaccine* 30(Suppl. 5):F34–F54, 2012.

Gillison ML, Chaturvedi AK, Anderson WF, et al.: Epidemiology of human papillomavirus-positive head and neck squamous cell carcinoma, *J Clin Oncol* 33:3235–3242, 2015.

Gillison ML, D'Souza G, Westra W, et al.: Distinct risk factor profiles for human papillomavirus type 16-positive and human papillomavirus type 16-negative head and neck cancers, *J Natl Cancer Inst* 100:407–420, 2008.

Goldstein BY, Chang SC, Hashibe M, et al.: Alcohol consumption and cancer of the oral cavity and pharynx from 1988 to 2009: an update, *Eur J Cancer Prev* 19:431–465, 2010.

Golusinski P, Corry J, Poorten VV, et al.: De-escalation studies in HPV-positive oropharyngeal cancer: how should we proceed? *Oral Oncol* 123:105620, 2021.

Ha PK, Califano JA: The molecular biology of mucosal field cancerization of the head and neck, *Crit Rev Oral Biol Med* 14:363–369, 2003.

Hayes RB, Ahn J, Fan X, et al.: Association of oral microbiome with risk for incident head and neck squamous cell cancer, *JAMA Oncol* 4:358–365, 2018.

Hecht SS, Hatsukami DK: Smokeless tobacco and cigarette smoking: chemical mechanisms and cancer prevention, *Nat Rev Cancer* 22:143–155, 2022.

Hjortdal O, Naess A, Berner A: Squamous cell carcinomas of the lower lip, *J Craniomaxillofac Surg* 23:34–37, 1995.

Ho AL, Brana I, Haddad R, et al.: Tipifarnib in head and neck squamous cell carcinoma with *HRAS* mutations, *J Clin Oncol* 39:1856–1864, 2021.

Hostiuc S, Ionescu IV, Drima E: Mouthwash use and the risk of oral, pharyngeal, and laryngeal cancer. A meta-analysis, *Int J Environ Res Public Health* 18:8215, 2021.

Hoxhaj I, Hysaj O, Vukovic V, et al.: Occurrence of metachronous second primary cancer in head and neck cancer survivors: a systematic review and meta-analysis of the literature, *Eur J Cancer Care (Engl)* 29:e13255, 2020.

Hussein AA, Helder MN, de Visscher JG, et al.: Global incidence of oral and oropharynx cancer in patients younger than 45 years versus older patients: a systematic review, *Eur J Cancer* 82:115–127, 2017.

IARC: *Working Group on the Evaluation of Carcinogenic Risks to Humans: IARC monographs on the evaluation of carcinogenic risks to humans, Alcohol drinking*, vol. 44, Lyon, France, 1988, IARC Press.

IARC: *Working Group on the Evaluation of Carcinogenic Risks to Humans: IARC monographs on the evaluation of carcinogenic risks to humans, Personal habits and indoor combustions*, vol. 100E, Lyon, France, 2012, IARC Press.

International Agency for Research on Cancer: *Lip, oral cavity (GLOBOCAN 2020 fact sheet)*, Lyon, France, 2020, IARC. Available at: https://gco.iarc.fr/today/data/factsheets/cancers/1-Lip-oral-cavity-fact-sheet.pdf. (Accessed 22 April 2022.)

International Agency for Research on Cancer: *Oropharynx (GLOBOCAN 2020 fact sheet)*, Lyon, France, 2020, IARC. Available at: https://gco.iarc.fr/today/data/factsheets/cancers/3-Oropharynx-fact-sheet.pdf. (Accessed 22 April 2022.)

Koyfman SA, Ismaila N, Crook D, et al.: Management of the neck in squamous cell carcinoma of the oral cavity and oropharynx: ASCO clinical practice guideline, *J Clin Oncol* 37:1753–1774, 2019.

La Vecchia C: Mouthwash and oral cancer risk: an update, *Oral Oncol* 45:198–200, 2009.

Lechner M, Liu J, Masterson L, et al.: HPV-associated oropharyngeal cancer: epidemiology, molecular biology and clinical management, *Nat Rev Clin Oncol* 19:306–327, 2022.

Lee YA, Al-Temimi M, Ying J, et al.: Risk prediction models for head and neck cancer in the US population from the INHANCE Consortium, *Am J Epidemiol* 189:330–342, 2020.

Leemans CR, Snijders PJF, Brakenhoff RH: The molecular landscape of head and neck cancer, *Nat Rev Cancer* 18:269–282, 2018.

Lesseur C, Diergaarde B, Olshan AF, et al.: Genome-wide association analyses identify new susceptibility loci for oral cavity and pharyngeal cancer, *Nat Genet* 48:1544–1550, 2016.

Liederbach E, Kyrillos A, Wang CH, et al.: The national landscape of human papillomavirus-associated oropharynx squamous cell carcinoma, *Int J Cancer* 140:504–512, 2017.

Lewis JS Jr: p16 immunohistochemistry as a standalone test for risk stratification in oropharyngeal squamous cell carcinoma, *Head Neck Pathol* 6(Suppl. 1):S75–S82, 2012.

Lingen MW, Xiao W, Schmitt A, et al.: Low etiologic fraction for high-risk human papillomavirus in oral cavity squamous cell carcinoma, *Oral Oncol* 49:1–8, 2013.

Lubek JE, Clayman L: An update on squamous carcinoma of the oral cavity, oropharynx, and maxillary sinus, *Oral Maxillofacial Surg Clin N Am* 24:307–316, 2012.

Lubin JH, Purdue M, Kelsey K, et al.: Total exposure and exposure rate effects for alcohol and smoking and risk of head and neck cancer: a pooled analysis of case–control studies, *Am J Epidemiol* 170:937–947, 2009.

Makarev E, Schubert AD, Kanherkar RR, et al.: *In silico* analysis of pathways activation landscape in oral squamous cell carcinoma and oral leukoplakia, *Cell Death Discov* 3:17022, 2017.

Maserejian NN, Joshipura KJ, Rosner BA, et al.: Prospective study of alcohol consumption as risk of oral premalignant lesions in men, *Cancer Epidemiol Biomarkers Prev* 15:774–781, 2006.

Miranda-Filho A, Bray F: Global patterns and trends in cancers of the lip, tongue and mouth, *Oral Oncol* 102:104551, 2020.

Mirghani H, Amen F, Moreau F, et al.: Do high-risk human papillomaviruses cause oral cavity squamous cell carcinoma? *Oral Oncol* 51:229–236, 2015.

Manoharan S, Nagaraja V, Eslick GD: Ill-fitting dentures and oral cancer: a meta-analysis, *Oral Oncol* 50:1058–1061, 2014.

Morales DR, Pacurariu A, Slattery J, et al.: Association between hydrochlorothiazide exposure and different incident skin, lip and oral cavity cancers: a series of population-based nested case–control studies, *Br J Clin Pharmacol* 86:1336–1345, 2020.

Morse DE, Psoter WJ, Cleveland D, et al.: Smoking and drinking in relation to oral cancer and oral epithelial dysplasia, *Cancer Causes Control* 18:919–929, 2007.

National Comprehensive Cancer Network: *NCCN Clinical Practice Guidelines in Oncology (NCCN Guidelines®): Head and Neck Cancers Version 2.2022*, Plymouth Meeting, PA, 2022, National Comprehensive Cancer Network. Available at: http://www.nccn.org/professionals/physician_gls/pdf/head-and-neck.pdf. (Accessed 24 April 2022.)

Nauta IH, Rietbergen MM, van Bokhoven AAJD, et al.: Evaluation of the eighth TNM classification on p16-positive oropharyngeal squamous cell carcinomas in the Netherlands and the importance of additional HPV DNA testing, *Ann Oncol* 29:1273–1279, 2018.

Ndiaye C, Mena M, Alemany L, et al.: HPV DNA, E6/E7 mRNA, and p16INK4a detection in head and neck cancers: a systematic review and meta-analysis, *Lancet Oncol* 15:1319–1331, 2014.

Ng JH, Iyer NG, Tan MH, et al.: Changing epidemiology of oral squamous cell carcinoma of the tongue: a global study, *Head Neck* 39:297–304, 2017.

Neville BW, Day TA: Oral cancer and precancerous lesions, *CA Cancer J Clin* 52:195–215, 2002.

O'Sullivan B, Lydiatt WM, Haughey BH, et al.: HPV-mediated oropharyngeal cancer, In Amin MB, Edge SB, Greene FL, et al., editors: *AJCC cancer staging manual*, ed 8, Chicago, 2018, American College of Surgeons, pp 113–122. (chapter 10).

Lydiatt WM, Ridge JA, Patel SA, et al.: Oropharynx (p16-) and hypopharynx, In Amin MB, Edge SB, Greene FL, et al., editors: *AJCC cancer staging manual*, ed 8, Chicago, 2018, American College of Surgeons, pp 123–136. (chapter 11).

Pan C, Issaeva N, Yarbrough WG: HPV-driven oropharyngeal cancer: current knowledge of molecular biology and mechanisms of carcinogenesis, *Cancers Head Neck* 3:12, 2018.

Parmar A, Macluskey M, Mc Goldrick N, et al.: Interventions for the treatment of oral cavity and oropharyngeal cancer: chemotherapy, *Cochrane Database Syst Rev* 12:CD006386, 2021.

Patel SC, Carpenter WR, Tyree S, et al.: Increasing incidence of oral tongue squamous cell carcinoma in young white women, age 18 to 44 years, *J Clin Oncol* 29:1488–1494, 2011.

Petti S: Lifestyle risk factors for oral cancer, *Oral Oncol* 43:340–350, 2009.

Pingali C, Yankey D, Elam-Evans LD, et al.: National, regional, state, and selected local area vaccination coverage among adolescents aged 13–17 years—United States, 2020, *MMWR Morb Mortal Wkly Rep* 70:1183–1190, 2021.

Rettig EM, Fakhry C, Khararjian A, et al.: Age profile of patients with oropharyngeal squamous cell carcinoma, *JAMA Otolaryngol Head Neck Surg* 144:538–539, 2018.

Ridge JA, Lydiatt WM, Patel SG, et al.: Oral cavity, In Amin MB, Edge SB, Greene FL, et al., editors: *AJCC cancer staging manual*, ed 8, Chicago, 2018, American College of Surgeons, pp 79–94. (chapter 7).

Robledo-Sierra J, Ben-Amy DP, Varoni E, et al.: World Workshop on Oral Medicine VII: targeting the oral microbiome part 2: current knowledge on malignant and potentially malignant oral disorders, *Oral Dis* 25(Suppl. 1):28–48, 2019.

Rodu B: Smokeless tobacco and oral cancer: a review of the risks and determinants, *Crit Rev Oral Biol Med* 15:252–263, 2004.

Rooper LM, Windon MJ, Hernandez T, et al.: HPV-positive squamous cell carcinoma of the larynx, oral cavity, and hypopharynx: clinicopathologic characterization with recognition of a novel warty variant, *Am J Surg Pathol* 44:691–702, 2020.

Satgunaseelan L, Allanson BM, Asher R, et al.: The incidence of squamous cell carcinoma of the oral tongue is rising in young non-smoking women: an international multi-institutional analysis, *Oral Oncol* 110:104875, 2020.

SEER*Explorer: an interactive website for SEER cancer statistics [Internet]. Surveillance Research Program, National Cancer Institute. Available at: https://seer.cancer.gov/explorer/. (Accessed 17 March 2022.)

Senkomago V, Henley SJ, Thomas CC, et al.: Human papillomavirus-attributable cancers—United States, 2012–2016, *MMWR Morb Mortal Wkly Rep* 68:724–728, 2019.

Siegel RL, Miller KD, Fuchs HE, et al.: Cancer statistics, 2022, *CA Cancer J Clin* 72:7–33, 2022.

Sinha DN, Gupta PC, Kumar A, et al.: The poorest of poor suffer the greatest burden from smokeless tobacco use: a study from 140 countries, *Nicotine Tob Res* 20:1529–1532, 2018.

Slaughter DP: The multiplicity of origin of malignant tumors: a collective review, *Internat Abstr Surg* 79:89–98, 1944.

Stransky N, Egloff AM, Tward AD, et al.: The mutational landscape of head and neck squamous cell carcinoma, *Science* 333:1157–1160, 2011.

Strober W, Shishido S, Wood B, et al.: Two for the price of one: prevalence, demographics and treatment implications of multiple HPV mediated head and neck cancers, *Oral Oncol* 100:104475, 2020.

Su CC, Tsai KY, Hsu YY, et al.: Chronic exposure to heavy metals and risk of oral cancer in Taiwanese males, *Oral Oncol* 46:586–590, 2010.

Su Mun L, Wye Lum S, Kong Yuiin Sze G, et al.: Association of microbiome with oral squamous cell carcinoma: a systematic review of the metagenomic studies, *Int J Environ Res Public Health* 18:7224, 2021.

Syrjänen S, Lodi G, von Bültizingslöwen I, et al.: Human papillomaviruses in oral carcinoma and oral potentially malignant disorders: a systematic review, *Oral Dis* 17(Suppl. 1):58–72, 2011.

Tota JE, Best AF, Zumsteg ZS, et al.: Evolution of the oropharynx cancer epidemic in the United States: moderation of increasing incidence in younger individuals and shift in the burden to older individuals, *J Clin Oncol* 37:1538–1546, 2019.

Tota JE, Gillison ML, Katki HA, et al.: Development and validation of an individualized risk prediction model for oropharynx cancer in the US population, *Cancer* 125:4407–4416, 2019.

Tramacere I, Negri E, Bagnardi V, et al.: A meta-analysis of alcohol drinking and oral and pharyngeal cancers. Part 2: results by sub-sites, *Oral Oncol* 46:720–726, 2010.

Trosman SJ, Koyfman SA, Ward MC, et al.: Effect of human papillomavirus on patterns of distant metastatic failure in oropharyngeal squamous cell carcinoma treated with chemoradiotherapy, *JAMA Otolaryngol Head Neck Surg* 141:457–462, 2015.

U.S. Department of Health and Human Services, Office of Disease Prevention and Health Promotion: *Healthy People 2030*, Washington, DC, 2010, U.S. Department of Health and Human Services. Available at: https://health.gov/healthypeople/objectives-and-data/browse-objectives/tobacco-use/reduce-current-cigarette-smoking-adults-tu-02. (Accessed 23 March 2022.)

Vallianou N, Kounatidis D, Christodoulatos GS, et al.: Mycobiome and cancer: what is the evidence? *Cancers (Basel)* 13:3149, 2021.

Van Dyne EA, Henley SJ, Saraiya M, et al.: Trends in human papillomavirus-associated cancers—United States, 1999–2015, *MMWR Morb Mortal Wkly Rep* 67:918–924, 2018.

van Oijen MG, Leppers VD, Straat FG, et al.: The origins of multiple squamous cell carcinomas in the aerodigestive tract, *Cancer* 88:884–893, 2000.

Wang DM, Kraft S, Rohani P, et al.: Association of nodal metastasis and mortality with vermilion vs cutaneous lip location in cutaneous squamous cell carcinoma of the lip, *JAMA Dermatol* 154:701–707, 2018.

Westra WH: The morphologic profile of HPV-related head and neck squamous carcinoma: implications for diagnosis, prognosis, and clinical management, *Head Neck Pathol* 6(Suppl. 1):S48–S54, 2012.

Windon MJ, D'Souza G, Rettig EM, et al.: Increasing prevalence of human papillomavirus-positive oropharyngeal cancers among older adults, *Cancer* 124:2993–2999, 2018.

Wood HM, Conway C, Daly C, et al.: The clonal relationships between pre-cancer and cancer revealed by ultra-deep sequencing, *J Pathol* 237:296–306, 2015.

World Health Organization International Agency for Research on Cancer: *IARC monographs on the evaluation and carcinogenic risks to humans, Betel-quid and areca-nut chewing and some areca-nut-derived nitrosamines*, vol. 85, Lyon, France, 2004, IARC Press.

Zhang Y, Fakhry C, D'Souza G: Projected association of human papillomavirus vaccination with oropharynx cancer incidence in the US, 2020–2045, *JAMA Oncol* 7:e212907, 2021.

Zhang WB, Peng X: Cervical metastases of oral maxillary squamous cell carcinoma: a systematic review and meta-analysis, *Head Neck* 38(Suppl. 1):E2335–E2342, 2016.

Zumsteg ZS, Cook-Wiens G, Yoshida E, et al.: Incidence of oropharyngeal cancer among elderly patients in the United States, *JAMA Oncol* 2:1617–1623, 2016.

Verrucous Carcinoma

Ackerman LV: Verrucous carcinoma of the oral cavity, *Surgery* 23:670–678, 1948.

Alonso JE, Kuan EC, Arshi A, et al.: A population-based analysis of verrucous carcinoma of the oral cavity, *Laryngoscope* 128:393–397, 2018.

Arduino PG, Carrozzo M, Pagano M, et al.: Verrucous oral carcinoma: clinical findings and treatment outcomes in 74 patients in Northwest Italy, *Minerva Stomatol* 57:335–341, 2008.

Burford WN, Ackerman LV, Robinson HBG: Symposium on twenty cases of benign and malignant lesions of the oral cavity, from the Ellis Fischel State Cancer Hospital, Columbia, Missouri, *Am J Orthod Oral Surg* 30:353–372, 1944.

Davidova LA, Fitzpatrick SG, Bhattacharyya I, et al.: Lichenoid characteristics in premalignant verrucous lesions and verrucous carcinoma of the oral cavity, *Head Neck Pathol* 13:573–579, 2019.

Farag AF, Abou-Alnour DA, Abu-Taleb NS: Oral carcinoma cuniculatum, an unacquainted variant of oral squamous cell carcinoma: a systematic review, *Imaging Sci Dent* 48:233–244, 2018.

Koch BB, Trask DK, Hoffman HT, et al.: National survey of head and neck verrucous carcinoma: patterns of presentation, care, and outcome, *Cancer* 92:110–120, 2001.

McCoy JM, Waldron CA: Verrucous carcinoma of the oral cavity: a review of forty-nine cases, *Oral Surg Oral Med Oral Pathol* 52:623–629, 1981.

Medina JE, Dichtel W, Luna MA: Verrucous-squamous carcinomas of the oral cavity: a clinicopathologic study of 104 cases, *Arch Otolaryngol* 110:437–440, 1984.

Mohan S, Pai SI, Bhattacharyya N: Adjuvant radiotherapy is not supported in patients with verrucous carcinoma of the oral cavity, *Laryngoscope* 127:1334–1338, 2017.

Naik AN, Silverman DA, Rygalski CJ, et al.: Postoperative radiation therapy in oral cavity verrucous carcinoma, *Laryngoscope* 132:1953–1961, 2022.

Padilla RJ, Murrah VA: Carcinoma cuniculatum of the oral mucosa: a potentially underdiagnosed entity in the absence of clinical correlation, *Oral Surg Oral Med Oral Pathol Oral Radiol* 118:684–693, 2014.

Peng Q, Wang Y, Quan H, et al.: Oral verrucous carcinoma: from multifactorial etiology to diverse treatment regimens (Review), *Int J Oncol* 49:59–73, 2016.

Walvekar RP, Chaukar DA, Deshpande MS, et al.: Verrucous carcinoma of the oral cavity: a clinical and pathological study of 101 cases, *Oral Oncol* 45:47–51, 2009.

Wang N, Huang M, Lv H: Head and neck verrucous carcinoma: a population-based analysis of incidence, treatment, and prognosis, *Medicine (Baltimore)* 99:e18660, 2020.

Yadav S, Bal M, Rane S, et al.: Carcinoma cuniculatum of the oral cavity: a series of 6 cases and review of literature, *Head Neck Pathol* 16:213–223, 2022.

Spindle Cell Carcinoma

Batsakis JG, Suarez P: Sarcomatoid carcinomas of the upper aerodigestive tracts, *Adv Anat Pathol* 7:282–293, 2000.

Bice TC, Tran V, Merkley MA, et al.: Disease-specific survival with spindle cell carcinoma of the head and neck, *Otolaryngol Head Neck Surg* 153:973–980, 2015.

Ding L, Bi ZF, Yuan H, et al.: Sarcomatoid carcinoma in the head and neck: a population-based analysis of outcome and survival, *Laryngoscope* 131:E489–E499, 2021.

Gerry D, Fritsch VA, Lentsch EJ: Spindle cell carcinoma of the upper aerodigestive tract: an analysis of 341 cases with comparison to conventional squamous cell carcinoma, *Ann Otol Rhinol Laryngol* 123:576–583, 2014.

Lewis JS Jr: Spindle cell lesions—neoplastic or non-neoplastic? Spindle cell carcinoma and other atypical spindle cell lesions of the head and neck, *Head Neck Pathol* 2:103–110, 2008.

Prieto-Granada CN, Xu B, Alzumaili B, et al.: Clinicopathologic features and outcome of head and neck mucosal spindle cell squamous cell carcinoma, *Virchows Arch* 479:729–739, 2021.

Romañach MJ, Azevedo RS, Carlos R, et al.: Clinicopathological and immunohistochemical features of oral spindle cell carcinoma, *J Oral Pathol Med* 39:335–341, 2010.

Spector ME, Wilson KF, Light E, et al.: Clinical and pathologic predictors of recurrence and survival in spindle cell squamous cell carcinoma, *Otolaryngol Head Neck Surg* 145:242–247, 2011.

Viswanathan S, Rahman K, Pallavi S, et al.: Sarcomatoid (spindle cell) carcinoma of the head and neck mucosal region: a clinicopathologic review of 103 cases from a tertiary referral cancer centre, *Head Neck Pathol* 4:265–275, 2010.

Watson RF, Chernock RD, Wang X, et al.: Spindle cell carcinomas of the head and neck rarely harbor transcriptionally-active human papillomavirus, *Head Neck Pathol* 7:250–257, 2013.

Adenosquamous Carcinoma

Fiacchini G, Benettini G, Tricò D, et al.: Human papillomavirus-related head and neck adenosquamous carcinoma: a systematic review and individual patient data meta-analysis, *Oral Oncol* 119:105252, 2021.

Kass JI, Lee SC, Abberbock S, et al.: Adenosquamous carcinoma of the head and neck: molecular analysis using CRTC-MAML FISH and survival comparison with paired conventional squamous cell carcinoma, *Laryngoscope* 125:E371–E376, 2015.

Keelawat S, Liu CZ, Roehm PC, et al.: Adenosquamous carcinoma of the upper aerodigestive tract: a clinicopathologic study of 12 cases and review of the literature, *Am J Otolaryngol* 23:160–168, 2002.

Lee RJ, Lin T, Lee SA, et al.: Importance of tumor extent in adenosquamous carcinoma of the head and neck: a retrospective cohort study, *Oral Surg Oral Med Oral Pathol Oral Radiol* 124:114–120, 2017.

Masand RP, El-Mofty SK, Ma XJ, et al.: Adenosquamous carcinoma of the head and neck: relationship to human papillomavirus and review of the literature, *Head Neck Pathol* 5:108–116, 2011.

Mehrad M, Trinkaus K, Lewis JS Jr: Adenosquamous carcinoma of the head and neck: a case–control study with conventional squamous cell carcinoma, *Head Neck Pathol* 10:486–493, 2016.

Schick U, Pusztaszeri M, Betz M, et al.: Adenosquamous carcinoma of the head and neck: report of 20 cases and review of the literature, *Oral Surg Oral Med Oral Pathol Oral Radiol* 116:313–320, 2013.

Sheahan P, Toner M, Timon CVI: Clinicopathologic features of head and neck adenosquamous carcinoma, *ORL J Otorhinolaryngol Relat Spec* 67:10–15, 2005.

Yoshimura Y, Mishimma K, Ohara S, et al.: Clinical characteristics of oral adenosquamous carcinoma: report of a case and an analysis of the reported Japanese cases, *Oral Oncol* 39:309–315, 2003.

Basaloid Squamous Carcinoma

Banks ER, Frierson HF Jr, Mills SE, et al.: Basaloid squamous cell carcinoma of the head and neck: a clinicopathologic and immunohistochemical study of 40 cases, *Am J Surg Pathol* 16:939–946, 1992.

Begum S, Westra WH: Basaloid squamous cell carcinoma of the head and neck is a mixed variant that can be further resolved by HPV status, *Am J Surg Pathol* 32:1044–1050, 2008.

Chernock RD, Lewis JS Jr, Zhang Q, et al.: Human papillomavirus positive basaloid squamous cell carcinomas of the upper aerodigestive tract: a distinct clinicopathologic and molecular subtype of basaloid squamous cell carcinoma, *Hum Pathol* 41:1016–1023, 2010.

Coletta RD, Cotrim P, Almeida OP, et al.: Basaloid squamous carcinoma of oral cavity: a histologic and immunohistochemical study, *Oral Oncol* 38:723–729, 2002.

Ereño C, Gaafar A, Garmendia M, et al.: Basaloid squamous cell carcinoma of the head and neck, *Head Neck Pathol* 2:83–91, 2008.

Fritsch VA, Lentsch EJ: Basaloid squamous cell carcinoma of the head and neck: location means everything, *J Surg Oncol* 109:616–622, 2014.

Gootee J, Patel M, Aurit S, et al.: The importance of adjuvant treatment and primary anatomical site in head and neck basaloid squamous cell carcinoma survival: an analysis of the National Cancer Database, *Clin Transl Oncol* 22:2264–2274, 2020.

Ide F, Shimoyama T, Horie N, et al.: Basaloid squamous cell carcinoma of the oral mucosa: a new case and review of 45 cases in the literature, *Oral Oncol* 38:120–124, 2002.

Jacobi C, Ayx I, Fritsche K, et al.: Potential impact of human papilloma virus on survival of basaloid squamous carcinoma of the head and neck, *Oncotarget* 6:3462–3470, 2015.

Linton OR, Moore MG, Brigance JS, et al.: Prognostic significance of basaloid squamous cell carcinoma in head and neck cancer, *JAMA Otolaryngol Head Neck Surg* 139:1306–1311, 2013.

Schuch LF, Nóbrega KHS, Gomes APN, et al.: Basaloid squamous cell carcinoma: a 31-year retrospective study and analysis of 214 cases reported in the literature, *Oral Maxillofac Surg* 24:103–108, 2020.

Shen W, Sakamoto N, Yang L: Cause-specific mortality prediction model for patients with basaloid squamous cell carcinomas of the head and neck: a competing risk analysis, *J Cancer* 9:4009–4017, 2018.

Carcinoma of the Maxillary Sinus

American Cancer Society: *Nasal cavity (nose) and paranasal sinus cancer*, 2022, https://www.cancer.org/cancer/nasal-cavity-and-paranasal-sinus-cancer.html. (Accessed 28 February 2022.)

Kılıç S, Kılıç SS, Kim ES, et al.: Significance of human papillomavirus positivity in sinonasal squamous cell carcinoma, *Int Forum Allergy Rhinol* 7:980–989, 2017.

Lewis JS Jr: Sinonasal squamous cell carcinoma: a review with emphasis on emerging histologic subtypes and the role of human papillomavirus, *Head Neck Pathol* 10:60–67, 2016.

National Comprehensive Cancer Network: *NCCN Clinical Practice Guidelines in Oncology (NCCN Guidelines®): Head and Neck Cancers Version 1.2022, Plymouth Meeting, PA*, 2022, National Comprehensive Cancer Network. Available at: https://www.nccn.org/professionals/physician_gls/pdf/head-and-neck.pdf. (Accessed 28 February 2022.)

Robin TP, Jones BL, Gordon OM, et al.: A comprehensive comparative analysis of treatment modalities for sinonasal malignancies, *Cancer* 123:3040–3049, 2017.

Svajdler M, Nemcova J, Dubinsky P, et al.: Significance of transcriptionally-active high-risk human papillomavirus in sinonasal squamous cell carcinoma: case series and a meta-analysis, *Neoplasma* 67:1456–1463, 2020.

Vazquez A, Khan MN, Blake DM, et al.: Sinonasal squamous cell carcinoma and the prognostic implications of its histologic variants: a population-based study, *Int Forum Allergy Rhinol* 5:85–91, 2015.

Wang Y, Yang R, Zhao M, et al.: Retrospective analysis of 98 cases of maxillary sinus squamous cell carcinoma and therapeutic exploration, *World J Surg Oncol* 18:90, 2020.

Sinonasal Undifferentiated Carcinoma

Abdelmeguid AS, Bell D, Hanna EY: Sinonasal undifferentiated carcinoma, *Curr Oncol Rep* 21:26, 2019.

Agaimy A, Bishop JA: SWI/SNF-deficient head and neck neoplasms: an overview, *Semin Diagn Pathol* 38:175–182, 2021.

Agaimy A, Franchi A, Lund VJ, et al.: Sinonasal undifferentiated carcinoma (SNUC): from an entity to morphologic pattern and back again—a historical perspective, *Adv Anat Pathol* 27:51–60, 2020.

Baraban E, Tong CCL, Adappa ND, et al.: A subset of sinonasal undifferentiated carcinoma is associated with transcriptionally active high-risk human papillomavirus by in situ hybridization: a clinical and pathologic analysis, *Hum Pathol* 101:64–69, 2020.

Chambers KJ, Lehmann AE, Remenschneider A, et al.: Incidence and survival patterns of sinonasal undifferentiated carcinoma in the United States, *J Neurol Surg B Skull Base* 76:94–100, 2015.

de Bonnecaze G, Verillaud B, Chaltiel L, et al: Clinical characteristics and prognostic factors of sinonasal undifferentiated carcinoma: a multicenter study, *Int Forum Allergy Rhinol* 8:1065–1072, 2018.

Dogan S, Chute DJ, Xu B, et al.: Frequent *IDH2* R172 mutations in undifferentiated and poorly-differentiated sinonasal carcinomas, *J Pathol* 242:400–408, 2017.

Jo VY, Chau NG, Hornick JL, et al.: Recurrent *IDH2* R172X mutations in sinonasal undifferentiated carcinoma, *Mod Pathol* 30:650–659, 2017.

Mito JK, Bishop JA, Sadow PM, et al.: Immunohistochemical detection and molecular characterization of *IDH*-mutant sinonasal undifferentiated carcinomas, *Am J Surg Pathol* 42:1067–1075, 2018.

Morand GB, Anderegg N, Vital D, et al.: Outcome by treatment modality in sinonasal undifferentiated carcinoma (SNUC): a case-series, systematic review and meta-analysis, *Oral Oncol* 75:28–34, 2017.

Riobello C, López-Hernández A, Cabal VN, et al.: IDH2 mutation analysis in undifferentiated and poorly differentiated sinonasal carcinomas for diagnosis and clinical management, *Am J Surg Pathol* 44:396–405, 2020.

Nasopharyngeal Carcinoma

American Cancer Society: Nasopharyngeal cancer: https://www.cancer.org/cancer/nasopharyngeal-cancer.html. (Accessed 17 February 2022.)

Argirion I, Zarins KR, Ruterbusch JJ, et al.: Increasing incidence of Epstein-Barr virus-related nasopharyngeal carcinoma in the United States, *Cancer* 26:121–130, 2020.

Bossi P, Chan AT, Licitra L, et al.: Nasopharyngeal carcinoma: ESMO-EURACAN clinical practice guidelines for diagnosis, treatment and follow-up, *Ann Oncol* 32:452–465, 2021.

KCA C, JKS W, King A, et al.: Analysis of plasma Epstein–Barr virus DNA to screen for nasopharyngeal cancer, *N Engl J Med* 377:513–522, 2017.

Chang ET, Ye W, Zeng YX, et al.: The evolving epidemiology of nasopharyngeal carcinoma, *Cancer Epidemiol Biomarkers Prev* 30:1035–1047, 2021.

Chen YP, Chan ATC, Le QT, et al.: Nasopharyngeal carcinoma, *Lancet* 394:64–80, 2019.

Du M, Nair R, Jamieson L, et al.: Incidence trends of lip, oral cavity, and pharyngeal cancers: global burden of disease 1990–2017, *J Dent Res* 99:143–151, 2020.

National Comprehensive Cancer Network: *NCCN Clinical Practice Guidelines in Oncology (NCCN Guidelines®): Head and Neck Cancers Version 3.2021, Plymouth Meeting, PA*, 2021, National Comprehensive Cancer Network. Available at: http://www.nccn.org/professionals/physician_gls/pdf/head-and-neck.pdf. (Accessed 24 November 2021.)

Pan JJ, Ng WT, Zong JF, et al.: Proposal for the 8th edition of the AJCC/UICC staging system for nasopharyngeal cancer in the era of intensity-modulated radiotherapy, *Cancer* 122:546–558, 2016.

Sung H, Ferlay J, Siegel RL, et al.: Global cancer statistics 2020: GLOBOCAN estimates of incidence and mortality worldwide for 36 cancers in 185 countries, *CA Cancer J Clin* 71:209–249, 2021.

Tham T, Machado R, Russo DP, et al.: Viral markers in nasopharyngeal carcinoma: a systematic review and meta-analysis on the detection of p16INK4a, human papillomavirus (HPV), and Ebstein-Barr virus (EBV), *Am J Otolaryngol* 42:102762, 2021.

Tham T, Teegala S, Bardash Y, et al.: Is human papillomavirus and p16 expression associated with survival outcomes in nasopharyngeal cancer?: a systematic review and meta-analysis, *Am J Otolaryngol* 39:764–770, 2018.

Wotman M, Oh EJ, Ahn S, et al.: HPV status in patients with nasopharyngeal carcinoma in the United States: a SEER database study, *Am J Otolaryngol* 40:705–710, 2019.

Zhou L, Shen N, Li G, et al.: The racial disparity of nasopharyngeal carcinoma based on the database analysis, *Am J Otolaryngol* 40:102288, 2019.

Basal Cell Carcinoma

Bath-Hextall FJ, Perkins W, Bong J, et al.: Interventions for basal cell carcinoma of the skin, *Cochrane Database Syst Rev* 1:CD003412, 2007.

Bauer A, Diepgen TL, Schmitt J: Is occupational solar ultraviolet irradiation a relevant risk factor for basal cell carcinoma? A systematic review and meta-analysis of the epidemiological literature, *Br J Dermatol* 165:612–625, 2011.

Chen AC, Martin AJ, Choy B, et al.: A phase 3 randomized trial of nicotinamide for skin-cancer chemoprevention, *N Engl J Med* 373:1618–1626, 2015.

Del Rosario RN, Barr RJ, Jensen JL, et al.: Basal cell carcinoma of the buccal mucosa, *Am J Dermatopathol* 23:203–205, 2001.

Firnhaber JM: Basal cell and cutaneous squamous cell carcinomas: diagnosis and treatment, *Am Fam Physician* 102:339–346, 2020.

Kilgour JM, Jia JL, Sarin KY: Review of the molecular genetics of basal cell carcinoma; inherited susceptibility, somatic mutations, and targeted therapeutics, *Cancers (Basel)* 13:3870, 2021.

Koutlas IG, Koch CA, Vickers RA, et al.: An unusual ostensible example of intraoral basal cell carcinoma, *J Cutan Pathol* 36:464–470, 2009.

Lomas A, Leonardi-Bee J, Bath-Hextall F: A systematic review of worldwide incidence of nonmelanoma skin cancer, *Br J Dermatol* 166:1069–1080, 2012.

National Cancer Institute: *Skin cancer treatment (PDQ®)—health professional version*, Bethesda, MD, 2022, National Cancer Institute. Available at: https://www.cancer.gov/types/skin/hp/skin-treatment-pdq.

National Comprehensive Cancer Network: *NCCN Clinical Practice Guidelines in Oncology (NCCN Guidelines®): Basal Cell Skin Cancer Version 2.2022, Plymouth Meeting, PA*, 2022, National Comprehensive Cancer Network. Available at: http://www.nccn.org/professionals/physician_gls/pdf/nmsc.pdf. (Accessed 29 April 2022.)

Nehal KS, Bichakjian CK: Update on keratinocyte carcinomas, *N Engl J Med* 379:363–374, 2018.

Peris K, Fargnoli MC, Garbe C, et al.: Diagnosis and treatment of basal cell carcinoma: European consensus-based interdisciplinary guidelines, *Eur J Cancer* 118:10–34, 2019.

Queen D, Knackstedt T, Polacco MA, et al.: Characteristics of nonmelanoma skin cancers of the cutaneous perioral and vermilion lip treated by Mohs micrographic surgery, *J Eur Acad Dermatol Venereol* 33:305–311, 2019.

Rogers HW, Weinstock MA, Feldman SR, et al.: Incidence estimate of nonmelanoma skin cancer (keratinocyte carcinomas) in the U.S. population, 2012, *JAMA Dermatol* 151:1081–1086, 2015.

Shumway BS, Kalmar JR, Allen CM, et al.: Basal cell carcinoma of the buccal mucosa in a patient with nevoid basal cell carcinoma syndrome, *Int J Surg Pathol* 19:348–354, 2011.

Thomson J, Hogan S, Leonardi-Bee J, et al.: Interventions for basal cell carcinoma of the skin, *Cochrane Database Syst Rev* 11:CD003412, 2020.

Verkouteren JAC, Ramdas KHR, Wakkee M, et al.: Epidemiology of basal cell carcinoma: scholarly review, *Br J Dermatol* 177:359–372, 2017.

Merkel Cell Carcinoma

Albores-Saavedra J, Batich K, Chable-Montero F, et al.: Merkel cell carcinoma demographics, morphology, and survival based on 3870 cases: a population based study, *J Cutan Pathol* 37:20–27, 2010.

American Cancer Society: *Merkel cell skin cancer*, 2022b. Available at: https://www.cancer.org/cancer/merkel-cell-skin-cancer.html. (Accessed 6 December 2021.)

Bichakjian CK, Nghiem P, Johnson T, et al.: Merkel cell carcinoma, In Amin MB, Edge SB, Greene FL, et al., editors: *AJCC cancer staging manual*, ed 8, Chicago, 2018, American College of Surgeons, pp 568–581. (chapter 46).

Feng H, Shuda M, Chang Y, et al.: Clonal integration of a polyomavirus in human Merkel cell carcinoma, *Science* 319:1096–1100, 2008.

Harms PW, Harms KL, Moore PS, et al.: The biology and treatment of Merkel cell carcinoma: current understanding and research priorities, *Nat Rev Clin Oncol* 15:763–776, 2018.

Harms KL, Healy MA, Nghiem P, et al.: Analysis of prognostic factors from 9387 Merkel cell carcinoma cases forms the basis for the new 8th edition AJCC staging system, *Ann Surg Oncol* 23:3564–3571, 2016.

Hendrikx SMGA, de Wilde PCM, Kaanders JHAM, et al.: Merkel cell carcinoma in the oral cavity: a case presentation and review of the literature, *Oral Oncol* 41:202–206, 2005.

Islam MN, Chehal H, Smith MH, et al.: Merkel cell carcinoma of the buccal mucosa and lower lip, *Head Neck Pathol* 12:279–285, 2018.

Kervarrec T, Tallet A, Miquelestorena-Standley E, et al.: Morphologic and immunophenotypical features distinguishing Merkel cell polyomavirus-positive and negative Merkel cell carcinoma, *Mod Pathol* 32:1601–1616, 2019.

National Comprehensive Cancer Network: *NCCN Clinical Practice Guidelines in Oncology (NCCN Guidelines®): Merkel Cell Carcinoma Version 1.2022*, Plymouth Meeting, PA, 2021, National Comprehensive Cancer Network. Available at: http://www.nccn.org/ professionals/physician_gls/pdf/mcc.pdf. (Accessed 3 December 2021.)

Sun L, Cliften PF, Duncavage EJ, et al.: UV signature mutations reclassify salivary high-grade neuroendocrine carcinomas as occult metastatic cutaneous Merkel cell carcinomas, *Am J Surg Pathol* 43:682–687, 2019.

Tetzlaff MT, Nagarajan P: Update on Merkel cell carcinoma, *Head Neck Pathol* 12:31–43, 2018.

Yom SS, Rosenthal DI, El-Naggar AK, et al.: Merkel cell carcinoma of the tongue and head and neck oral mucosal sites, *Oral Surg Oral Med Oral Pathol Oral Radiol Endod* 101:761–768, 2006.

Walsh NM, Cerroni L: Merkel cell carcinoma: a review, *J Cutan Pathol* 48:411–421, 2021.

Melanoma

Aguas SC, Quarracino MC, Lence AN, et al.: Primary melanoma of the oral cavity: ten cases and review of 177 cases from literature, *Med Oral Patol Oral Cir Bucal* 14:E265–E271, 2009.

American Cancer Society: Cancer facts & figs. 2022, Atlanta, 2022, American Cancer Society, pp. 1–78.

Bansal SP, Dhanawade SS, Arvandekar AS, et al.: Oral amelanotic melanoma: a systematic review of case reports and case series, *Head Neck Pathol* 16:513–524, 2022.

Barriera-Silvestrini P, Iacullo J, Knackstedt TJ: American Joint Committee on Cancer staging and other platforms to assess prognosis and risk, *Clin Plast Surg* 48:599–606, 2021.

Bobos M: Histopathologic classification and prognostic factors of melanoma: a 2021 update, *Ital J Dermatol Venerol* 156:300–321, 2021.

Chatzistefanou I, Kolokythas A, Vahtsevanos K, et al.: Primary mucosal melanoma of the oral cavity: current therapy and future directions, *Oral Surg Oral Med Oral Pathol Oral Radiol* 122:17–27, 2016.

Chen F, Zhang Q, Wang Y, et al.: *KIT, NRAS, BRAF* and *FMNL2* mutations in oral mucosal melanoma and a systematic review of the literature, *Oncol Lett* 15:9786–9792, 2018.

de Castro MS, Reis BSA, Nogueira DA, et al.: Primary oral melanoma: a clinicopathologic review and case presentation, *Quintessence Int* 48:815–827, 2017.

Dzwierzynski WW: Melanoma risk factors and prevention, *Clin Plast Surg* 48:543–550, 2021.

Elder DE, Barnhill RL, Bastian BC, et al.: Melanocytic tumour classification and the pathway concept of melanoma pathogenesis, In Elder DE, Massi D, Scolyer RA, et al., editors: *WHO classification of skin tumours*, ed 4, Lyon, 2018, IARC, pp 66–71.

Elder DE, Bastian BC, Cree IA, et al.: The 2018 World Health Organization classification of cutaneous, mucosal, and uveal melanoma: detailed analysis of 9 distinct subtypes defined by their evolutionary pathway, *Arch Pathol Lab Med* 144:500–522, 2020.

Gershenwald JE, Scolyer RA, Hess KR, et al.: Melanoma of the skin, In Amin MB, Edge SB, Greene FL, et al., editors: *AJCC cancer staging manual*, ed 8, Chicago, 2018, American College of Surgeons, pp 565–585. (chapter 47).

Hsieh R, Nico MM, Camillo CM, et al.: Mutational status of *NRAS* and *BRAF* genes and protein expression analysis in a series of primary oral mucosal melanoma, *Am J Dermatopathol* 39: 104–110, 2017.

Jing G, Wu Y, Song H, et al.: Primary malignant melanoma of the lip: a report of 48 cases, *J Oral Maxillofac Surg* 73:2232–2240, 2015.

Kahn M, Weathers DR, Hoffman JG: Transformation of a benign oral pigmentation to primary oral mucosal melanoma, *Oral Surg Oral Med Oral Pathol Oral Radiol Endod* 100:454–459, 2005.

Leonardi GC, Falzone L, Salemi R, et al.: Cutaneous melanoma: from pathogenesis to therapy (review), *Int J Oncol* 52:1071–1080, 2018.

Lourenzo SV, Sangüeza M, Sotto MN, et al.: Primary oral mucosal melanoma: a series of 35 new cases from South Africa, *Am J Dermatopathol* 31:323–330, 2009.

Lydiatt WM, Brandwein-Weber M, Kraus DH, et al.: Mucosal melanoma of the head and neck, In Amin MB, Edge SB, Greene FL, et al., editors: *AJCC cancer staging manual*, ed 8, Chicago, 2018, American College of Surgeons, pp 163–170. (chapter 14).

Lyu J, Wu Y, Li C, et al.: Mutation scanning of *BRAF, NRAS, KIT*, and *GNAQ/GNA11* in oral mucosal melanoma: a study of 57 cases, *J Oral Pathol Med* 45:295–301, 2016.

Maldonado-Mendoza J, Ramírez-Amador V, Anaya-Saavedra G, et al.: CD117 immunoexpression in oral and sinonasal mucosal melanoma does not correlate with somatic driver mutations in the MAPK pathway, *J Oral Pathol Med* 48:382–388, 2019.

Malinoski H, Reddy R, Cohen DM, et al.: Oral melanomas: a case series of a deadly neoplasm, *J Oral Maxillofac Surg* 77:1832–1836, 2019.

Massand S, Neves RI: Emerging therapies in the treatment of advanced melanoma, *Clin Plast Surg* 48:713–733, 2021.

Nassar KW, Tan AC: The mutational landscape of mucosal melanoma, *Semin Cancer Biol* 61:139–148, 2020.

National Cancer Institute: *Melanoma treatment (PDQ®)—health professional version*, Bethesda, MD, 2022, National Cancer Institute. Available at: https://www.cancer.gov/types/skin/hp/melanoma-treatment-pdq#_1.

National Cancer Institute SEER Program: *Cancer stat facts*, Bethesda, MD, 2022, National Cancer Institute. Available at: https://seer. cancer.gov/statfacts/html/melan.html. (Accessed 1 December 2021.)

National Comprehensive Cancer Network: *NCCN Clinical Practice Guidelines in Oncology (NCCN Guidelines®): Head and Neck Cancers Version 3.2021*, Plymouth Meeting, PA, 2021, National Comprehensive Cancer Network. Available at: http://www.nccn. org/professionals/physician_gls/pdf/head-and-neck.pdf. (Accessed 24 November 2021.)

National Comprehensive Cancer Network: *NCCN Clinical Practice Guidelines in Oncology (NCCN Guidelines®): Melanoma: Cutaneous Version 2.2021*, Plymouth Meeting, PA, 2021, National Comprehensive Cancer Network. Available at: http://www.nccn. org/professionals/physician_gls/pdf/cutaneous_melanoma.pdf. (Accessed 24 November 2021.)

Nisi M, Izzetti R, Gennai S, et al.: Oral mucosal melanoma, *J Craniofac Surg* 33:830–834, 2022.

Oranges CM, Sisti G, Nasioudis D, et al.: Hard palate melanoma: a population-based analysis of epidemiology and survival outcomes, *Anticancer Res* 38:5811–5817, 2018.

Öztürk Sari Ş, Yilmaz İ, Taşkin OÇ, et al.: *BRAF, NRAS, KIT, TERT, GNAQ/GNA11* mutation profile analysis of head and neck mucosal melanomas: a study of 42 cases, *Pathology* 49:55–61, 2017.

Patel PB, Wright JM, Kang DR, et al.: Longitudinal clinicopathologic data of the progression of oral mucosal melanoma-report of 2 cases and literature review, *Oral Surg Oral Med Oral Pathol Oral Radiol* 126:e21–e30, 2018.

Paulson KG, Gupta D, Kim TS, et al.: Age-specific incidence of melanoma in the United States, *JAMA Dermatol* 156:57–64, 2020.

Rambhia PH, Stojanov IJ, Arbesman J: Predominance of oral mucosal melanoma in areas of high mechanical stress, *J Am Acad Dermatol* 80:1133–1135, 2019.

Rapini RP, Golitz LE, Greer RO, et al.: Primary malignant melanoma of the oral cavity: a review of 177 cases, *Cancer* 55:1543–1551, 1985.

Rawal YB, Dodson TB, Bal HS: Oral melanoma: relevance to the dental team members, *J Am Dent Assoc* 148:113–119, 2017.

SEER*Explorer: an interactive website for SEER cancer statistics [Internet]. Surveillance Research Program, National Cancer Institute. Available at: https://seer.cancer.gov/explorer/. (Accessed 3 May 2022.)

Shain A, Bastian B: From melanocytes to melanomas, *Nat Rev Cancer* 16:345–358, 2016.

Siegel RL, Miller KD, Fuchs HE, et al.: Cancer statistics, 2022, *CA Cancer J Clin* 72:7–33, 2022.

Smith MH, Bhattacharyya I, Cohen DM, et al.: Melanoma of the oral cavity: an analysis of 46 new cases with emphasis on clinical and histopathologic characteristics, *Head Neck Pathol* 10:298–305, 2016.

Soares CD, Carlos R, Andrade BAB, et al.: Oral amelanotic melanomas: clinicopathologic features of 8 cases and review of the literature, *Int J Surg Pathol* 29:263–272, 2021.

Song H, Wang L, Lyu J, et al.: Loss of nuclear BAP1 expression is associated with poor prognosis in oral mucosal melanoma, *Oncotarget* 8:29080–29090, 2017.

Toussi A, Mans N, Welborn J, et al.: Germline mutations predisposing to melanoma, *J Cutan Pathol* 47:606–616, 2020.

Urso C: Melanocytic skin neoplasms: what lesson from genomic aberrations? *Am J Dermatopathol* 41:623–629, 2019.

Wu Y, Wang L, Ma X, et al.: The existence of early stage oral mucosal melanoma: a 10-year retrospective analysis of 170 patients in a single institute, *Oral Oncol* 87:70–76, 2018.

Yamada SI, Kurita H, Kamata T, et al.: Clinical investigation of 38 cases of oral mucosal melanoma: a multicentre retrospective analysis in Japan, *Australas J Dermatol* 58:e223–e227, 2017.

11

Salivary Gland Pathology

◆ SALIVARY GLAND APLASIA/HYPOPLASIA

Salivary gland aplasia or **hypoplasia** is a rare developmental anomaly that can affect one or more of the major salivary glands. The condition may occur alone, although agenesis or hypoplasia of the glands is often a component of one of several syndromes (Box 11.1).

Clinical and Radiographic Features

Salivary gland aplasia/hypoplasia has been reported more frequently in males than females by a 2:1 ratio. Some individuals are affected by agenesis of all four of the largest glands (both parotids and submandibular glands), but others may be missing only one to three of the four glands. In spite of the absence of the glands, the face often has a normal appearance because the sites are filled in by fat or connective tissue. Intraorally, the orifices of the missing glands are absent. Some patients also may exhibit absence of the lacrimal glands or lacrimal puncta.

As would be anticipated, the most significant symptom associated with salivary gland aplasia is severe xerostomia with its attendant problems (see page 470). The tongue may appear leathery, and the patient is at greater risk for developing dental caries and erosion (Fig. 11.1). However, some degree of moisture still may be present because of the continued activity of the minor salivary glands. Absence of the major glands can be confirmed by technetium-99m pertechnetate scintiscan, computed tomography (CT), magnetic resonance imaging (MRI), or ultrasonography.

Lacrimo-auriculo-dento-digital (LADD) syndrome is an autosomal dominant disorder that is caused by a mutation in one the following genes: fibroblast growth factor 10 (*FGF10*), fibroblast growth factor receptor 2 (*FGFR2*), or fibroblast growth factor receptor 3 (*FGFR3*). It is characterized by aplasia or hypoplasia of the lacrimal and salivary glands, cup-shaped ears, hearing loss, and dental and digital anomalies. Dental features may include hypodontia, microdontia, and mild enamel hypoplasia.

Treatment and Prognosis

Patient management is directed toward compensating for the saliva deficiency, and saliva substitutes are often necessary. If any residual functional salivary gland tissue is present, then sialagogue medications (such as, pilocarpine or cevimeline) may be used to increase saliva production. Salivary flow also may be stimulated via the use of sugarless gum or sour candy. Regular preventive dental care is important to avoid xerostomia-related caries and enamel breakdown.

◆ MUCOCELE (MUCUS EXTRAVASATION PHENOMENON; MUCUS ESCAPE REACTION)

The **mucocele** is a common lesion of the oral mucosa that results from rupture of a salivary gland duct and spillage of mucin into the surrounding soft tissues. This spillage is often the result of local trauma, although there is no known history of trauma in many cases. Unlike the salivary duct cyst (see page 463), the mucocele is not a true cyst because it lacks an epithelial lining. Some authors, however, have included true salivary duct cysts in their reported series of mucoceles, sometimes under the classification of *retention mucocele* or *mucus retention cyst*. Because these two entities exhibit distinctly different clinical and histopathologic features, they are discussed as separate topics in this chapter.

Clinical Features

Mucoceles typically appear as dome-shaped mucosal swellings that can range from 1 or 2 mm to several centimeters in size (Figs. 11.2–11.4). They are most common in children and young adults, perhaps because younger people are more likely to experience trauma that induces mucin spillage. However, mucoceles have been reported in patients of all ages, including infants and older adults. The spilled mucin below the mucosal surface often imparts a bluish translucent hue to the swelling, although deeper mucoceles may be normal in color. The lesion characteristically is fluctuant, but some mucoceles feel firmer to palpation. The reported duration of the lesion can vary from a few days to several years; most patients report that the lesion has been present for several weeks. Many patients relate a history of a recurrent swelling that periodically may rupture and release its fluid contents.

The lower lip is by far the most common site for the mucocele; a recent large study of 1715 cases found that 81.9% occurred at this one site (Table 11.1). Lower lip

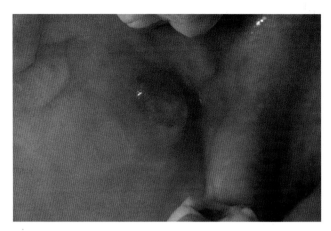

• **Fig. 11.3 Mucocele.** Nodule on the posterior buccal mucosa.

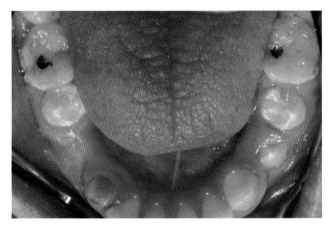

• **Fig. 11.1 Salivary Gland Aplasia.** Dry, leathery tongue and diffuse enamel erosion in a child with aplasia of the major salivary glands.

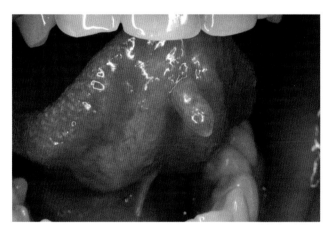

• **Fig. 11.4 Mucocele.** Exophytic lesion on the anterior ventral tongue.

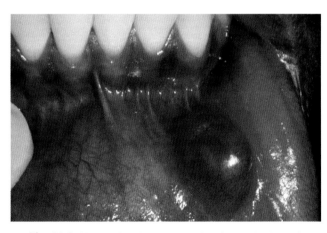

• **Fig. 11.2 Mucocele.** Blue-pigmented nodule on the lower lip.

	Location of Mucoceles	
TABLE 11.1		
Location	Number of Cases	Percentage of All Cases
Lower lip	1405	81.9
Floor of mouth	99	5.8
Ventral tongue	86	5.0
Buccal mucosa	82	4.8
Palate	23	1.3
Retromolar	9	0.5
Unknown	11	0.6
Upper lip	0	0.0
Total	**1715**	**100**

Data from Chi AC, Lambert PR 3rd, Richardson MS, et al: Oral mucoceles: a clinicopathologic review of 1,824 cases, including unusual variants, *J Oral Maxillofac Surg* 69:1086–1093, 2011.

mucoceles usually are found lateral to the midline. Less common sites include the floor of mouth (ranulas: 5.8%), anterior ventral tongue (from the glands of Blandin-Nuhn: 5.0%), buccal mucosa (4.8%), palate (1.3%), and retromolar pad (0.5%). Mucoceles rarely develop on the upper lip. In the large series summarized in Table 11.1, not a single example was identified from the upper lip. This is in contrast to salivary gland tumors, which are not unusual in the upper lip but are distinctly uncommon in the lower lip.

As noted, the soft palate and retromolar area are uncommon sites for mucoceles. However, one interesting variant, the **superficial mucocele,** does develop in these areas and

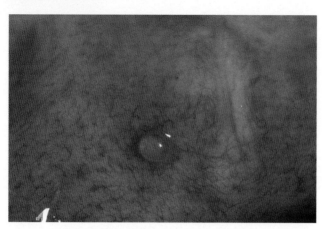

• **Fig. 11.5 Superficial Mucocele.** Vesicle-like lesion on the soft palate.

along the posterior buccal mucosa. Superficial mucoceles present as single or multiple tense vesicles that measure 1–4 mm in diameter (Fig. 11.5). The lesions often burst, leaving shallow, painful ulcers that heal within a few days. Repeated episodes at the same location are not unusual. Some patients relate the development of the lesions to mealtimes. Superficial mucoceles also have been reported to occur in association with lichenoid disorders, such as lichen planus, lichenoid drug eruptions, and chronic graft-versus-host disease (GVHD). The vesicular appearance is created by the superficial nature of the mucin spillage, which causes a separation of the epithelium from the connective tissue. The pathologist must be aware of this lesion and should not mistake it microscopically for a vesiculobullous disorder, especially mucous membrane pemphigoid.

Histopathologic Features

On microscopic examination, the mucocele shows an area of spilled mucin surrounded by a granulation tissue response (Figs. 11.6 and 11.7). The inflammation usually includes numerous foamy histiocytes (macrophages). In some cases, a ruptured salivary duct may be identified feeding into the area. The adjacent minor salivary glands often contain a chronic inflammatory cell infiltrate and dilated ducts.

Treatment and Prognosis

Some mucoceles are short-lived lesions that rupture and heal by themselves. Many lesions, however, are chronic in nature, and local surgical excision is necessary. To minimize the risk of recurrence, the surgeon should remove any adjacent minor salivary glands that may be feeding into the lesion when the area is excised. The excised tissue should be submitted for microscopic examination to confirm the diagnosis and rule out the possibility of a salivary gland tumor. The prognosis is excellent, although occasional mucoceles will recur, necessitating reexcision, especially if the feeding glands are not removed. Mucoceles on the anterior ventral tongue appear to have a higher recurrence rate, which likely is due to the deeper anatomic location of the glands of Blandin-Nuhn.

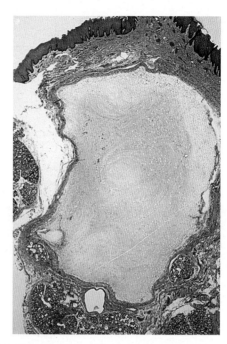

• **Fig. 11.6 Mucocele.** Mucin-filled cystlike cavity beneath the mucosal surface. Minor salivary glands are present below and lateral to the spilled mucin.

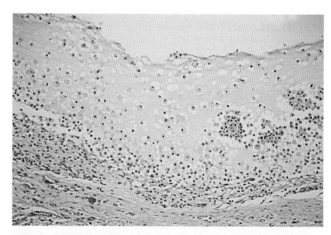

• **Fig. 11.7 Mucocele.** High-power view showing spilled mucin that is associated with granulation tissue containing foamy histiocytes.

◆ RANULA

Ranula is a term used for mucoceles that occur in the floor of the mouth, arising from the sublingual gland. The name is derived from the Latin word *rana,* which means "frog," because the swelling may resemble a frog's translucent underbelly. The term *ranula* also has been used to describe other similar swellings in the floor of the mouth, including true salivary duct cysts, dermoid cysts, and cystic hygromas. However, the term is best used for mucus escape reactions (mucoceles).

The sublingual gland has a complex anatomy. The lesser sublingual gland actually consists of 15–30 smaller glands, each secreting through a short duct of Rivinus to the sublingual plica. Some individuals also have a greater sublingual

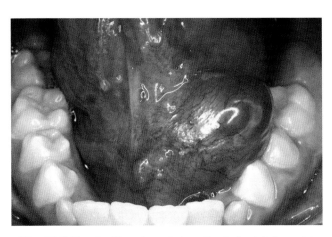

• **Fig. 11.8 Ranula.** Blue-pigmented swelling in the left floor of the mouth.

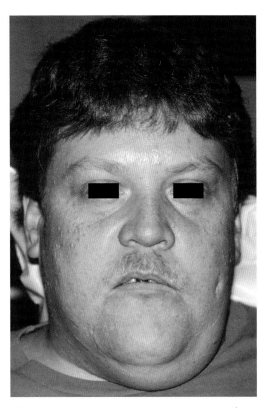

• **Fig. 11.9 Plunging Ranula.** Soft swelling in the neck.

gland with an excretory duct (Bartholin duct) that either joins with Wharton duct or opens next to it at the sublingual caruncle. Unlike the submandibular gland, the sublingual gland produces a continuous flow of mucus even in the absence of neural stimulation, which accounts for its ability to produce a ranula after rupture of one of its multiple ducts.

Clinical Features

The ranula usually appears as a blue, dome-shaped, fluctuant swelling in the floor of the mouth (Fig. 11.8), but deeper lesions may be normal in color. Ranulas are seen most frequently in children and young adults. They tend to be larger than mucoceles in other oral locations, often developing into large masses that fill the floor of the mouth and elevate the tongue. The ranula usually is located lateral to the midline, a feature that may help to distinguish it from a midline dermoid cyst (see page 32). Like other mucoceles, ranulas may rupture and release their mucin contents, only to re-form.

An unusual clinical variant, the **plunging** or **cervical ranula,** occurs when the spilled mucin dissects through the mylohyoid muscle and produces swelling within the neck (Fig. 11.9). A concomitant swelling in the floor of the mouth may or may not be present. If no lesion is produced in the mouth, then the clinical diagnosis of ranula may not be suspected. Imaging studies can be helpful in supporting a diagnosis of plunging ranula and in determining the origin of the lesion. CT, MRI, or ultrasound images of plunging ranulas from the sublingual gland may exhibit a slight extension of the lesion into the sublingual space, known as a "tail sign," although this feature is not always present.

Histopathologic Features

The microscopic appearance of a ranula is similar to that of a mucocele in other locations. The spilled mucin elicits a granulation tissue response that typically contains foamy histiocytes.

Treatment and Prognosis

Treatment of the ranula consists of removal of the feeding sublingual gland and/or marsupialization. Marsupialization (exteriorization) entails removal of the roof of the intraoral lesion, which often can be successful for small, superficial ranulas. However, marsupialization is often unsuccessful for larger ranulas, and most authors emphasize that removal of the offending gland is the most important consideration in preventing a recurrence of the lesion. If the gland is removed, then meticulous dissection of the lining of the lesion may not be necessary for the lesion to resolve, even for the plunging ranula. If the specific portion of the sublingual gland giving rise to the lesion can be identified, then partial excision of the gland may be successful.

◆ SALIVARY DUCT CYST (MUCUS RETENTION CYST; MUCUS DUCT CYST; SIALOCYST)

The **salivary duct cyst** is an epithelium-lined cavity that arises from salivary gland tissue. Unlike the more common mucocele (see page 460), it is a true developmental cyst that is lined by epithelium that is separate from the adjacent normal salivary ducts. The cause of such cysts is uncertain.

Cystlike dilatation of salivary ducts also may develop secondary to ductal obstruction (e.g., mucus plug), which creates increased intraluminal pressure. Some authors classify such lesions as salivary duct cysts (or *mucus retention cysts),* although others believe that these represent salivary ductal ectasia rather than true developmental cysts.

Clinical Features

Salivary duct cysts usually occur in adults and can arise within either the major or minor glands. Cysts of the major glands are most common within the parotid gland, presenting as slowly growing, asymptomatic swellings. Intraoral cysts can occur at any minor gland site, but most frequently they develop in the floor of the mouth, buccal mucosa, and lips (Fig. 11.10). They often look like mucoceles and are characterized by a soft, fluctuant swelling that may appear bluish, depending on the depth of the cyst below the surface. Some cysts may feel relatively firm to palpation. Cysts in the floor of the mouth often arise adjacent to the submandibular duct and sometimes have an amber color.

On rare occasions, patients have been observed to develop prominent ectasia of the excretory ducts of many of the minor salivary glands throughout the mouth. Such lesions have been termed *mucus retention cysts*, although they probably represent multifocal ductal dilatation. The individual lesions often present as painful nodules that demonstrate dilated ductal orifices on the mucosal surface. Mucus or pus may be expressed from these dilated ducts.

Histopathologic Features

The lining of the salivary duct cyst is variable and may consist of cuboidal, columnar, or atrophic squamous epithelium surrounding thin or mucoid secretions in the lumen (Fig. 11.11). Cystlike ductal ectasia secondary to salivary obstruction is characterized by oncocytic metaplasia of the epithelial lining. This epithelium often demonstrates papillary folds into the cystic lumen, somewhat reminiscent of a small Warthin tumor (see page 488) but without the prominent lymphoid stroma (Fig. 11.12). If this proliferation is extensive enough, then these lesions sometimes are diagnosed as **papillary cystadenoma,**

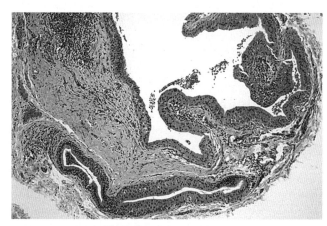

• **Fig. 11.12 Oncocytic Salivary Ductal Ectasia.** This dilated duct is lined by columnar eosinophilic oncocytes that exhibit papillary folds into the ductal lumen. Such lesions may develop secondary to ductal obstruction.

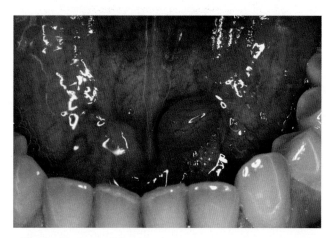

• **Fig. 11.10 Salivary Duct Cyst.** Nodular swelling overlying Wharton duct.

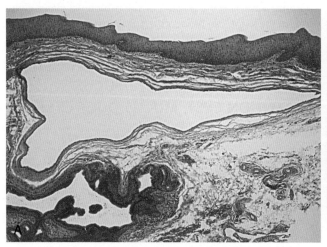

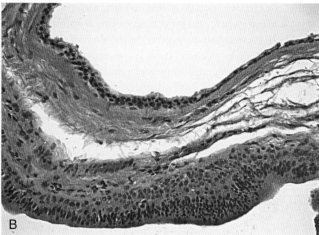

• **Fig. 11.11 Salivary Duct Cyst. A,** Low-power photomicrograph showing a cyst below the mucosal surface. **B,** High-power view of cystic cavity (*top*) lined by thin cuboidal epithelium. Adjacent to the cyst is an excretory salivary gland duct lined by columnar epithelium (*bottom*).

although it seems likely that most are not true neoplasms. The individual lesions of patients with multiple "mucus retention cysts" also show prominent oncocytic metaplasia of the epithelial lining.

Treatment and Prognosis

Isolated salivary duct cysts are treated by conservative surgical excision. For cysts in the major glands, partial or total removal of the gland may be necessary. The lesion should not recur. For patients with multifocal involvement, sialagogue medications may be helpful in stimulating salivary flow, thereby preventing the accumulation of inspissated mucus within the dilated excretory ducts.

◆ SIALOLITHIASIS (SALIVARY CALCULI; SALIVARY STONES)

Sialoliths are calcified structures that develop within the salivary ductal system. Researchers believe that they arise from deposition of calcium salts around a nidus of debris within the duct lumen. This debris may include inspissated mucus, bacteria, ductal epithelial cells, or foreign bodies. The cause of sialoliths is unclear, but their formation can be promoted by chronic sialadenitis and partial obstruction. Their development typically is not related to any systemic derangement in calcium and phosphorus metabolism.

Clinical and Radiographic Features

Sialoliths most often develop within the ductal system of the submandibular gland, which accounts for about 80% of cases; the formation of stones within the parotid gland system is distinctly less frequent. The long, tortuous, upward path of the submandibular (Wharton) duct and the thicker, mucoid secretions of this gland may be responsible for its greater tendency to form salivary calculi. Sialoliths also can form within the minor salivary glands, most often within the glands of the upper lip or buccal mucosa. Salivary stones can occur at almost any age, but they are most common in young and middle-aged adults.

Major gland sialoliths most frequently cause episodic pain or swelling of the affected gland, especially at mealtime. The severity of the symptoms varies, depending on the degree of obstruction and the amount of resultant backpressure produced within the gland. If the stone is located toward the terminal portion of the duct, then a hard mass may be palpated beneath the mucosa (Fig. 11.13).

Sialoliths typically appear as radiopaque masses on radiographic examination. However, not all stones are visible on standard radiographs (perhaps because of the degree of calcification of some lesions). They may be discovered anywhere along the length of the duct or within the gland itself (Fig. 11.14). Stones in the terminal portion of the submandibular duct are best demonstrated with an occlusal radiograph. On

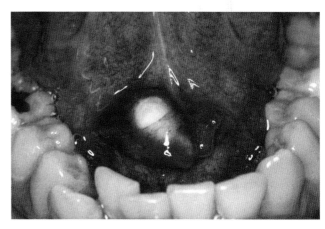

• **Fig. 11.13 Sialolithiasis.** Hard mass at the orifice of Wharton duct.

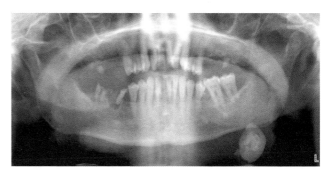

• **Fig. 11.14 Sialolithiasis.** Radiopaque mass located at the left angle of the mandible. (Courtesy of Dr. Roger Bryant.)

panoramic or periapical radiographs, the calcification may appear superimposed on the mandible and care must be exercised not to confuse it with an intrabony lesion (Fig. 11.15). Multiple parotid stones radiographically can mimic calcified parotid lymph nodes, such as might occur in tuberculosis. Ultrasound, CT scanning, and sialography may be helpful additional imaging studies for sialoliths. Diagnostic sialendoscopy also can be a valuable tool in the evaluation and diagnosis of ductal obstructions. In this technique, a miniaturized endoscope is inserted into the duct orifice, allowing visualization of the ductal system for any stones, strictures, or adhesions.

Minor gland sialoliths often are asymptomatic but may produce local swelling or tenderness of the affected gland (Fig. 11.16). A small radiopacity often can be demonstrated with a soft tissue radiograph.

Histopathologic Features

On gross examination, sialoliths appear as hard masses that are round, oval, or cylindrical. They are typically yellow, although they may be a white or yellow-brown color. Submandibular stones tend to be larger than those of the parotid or minor glands. Sialoliths are usually solitary, although occasionally two or more stones may be discovered at surgery.

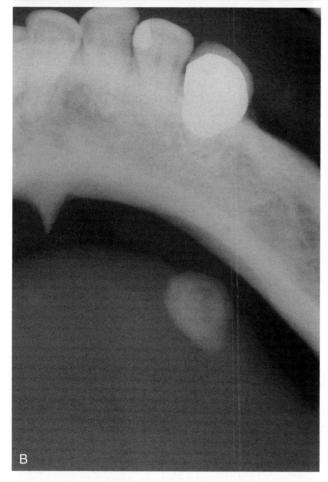

• **Fig. 11.15 Sialolithiasis. A,** Periapical film showing discrete radio-pacity (*arrow*) superimposed on the body of the mandible. Care must be taken not to confuse such lesions with intrabony pathosis. **B,** Occlusal radiograph of same patient demonstrating radiopaque stone in Wharton duct.

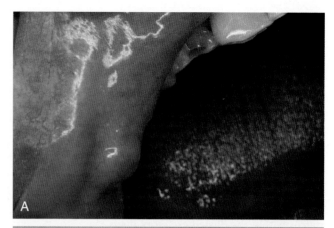

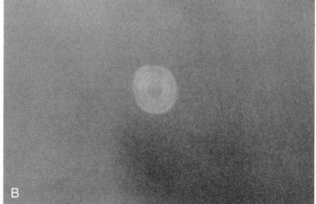

• **Fig. 11.16 Sialolithiasis. A,** Minor salivary gland sialolith presenting as a hard nodule in the upper lip. **B,** A soft tissue radiograph of the same lesion revealed a laminated calcified mass.

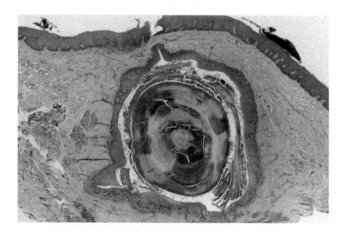

• **Fig. 11.17 Sialolithiasis.** Intraductal calcified mass showing concentric laminations. The duct exhibits squamous metaplasia.

Treatment and Prognosis

Microscopically, the calcified mass exhibits concentric laminations that may surround a nidus of amorphous debris (Fig. 11.17). If the associated duct also is removed, then it often demonstrates squamous, oncocytic, or mucous cell metaplasia. Periductal inflammation is also evident. The ductal obstruction frequently is associated with an acute or chronic sialadenitis of the feeding gland.

Small sialoliths of the major glands sometimes can be treated conservatively by gentle massage of the gland in an effort to milk the stone toward the duct orifice. Sialagogues (drugs that stimulate salivary flow), moist heat, and increased fluid intake also may promote passage of the stone. Interventional sialendoscopy (with basket retrieval) and lithotripsy are newer techniques that can be effective in the removal of sialoliths from the major glands. These minimally invasive techniques have low morbidity and may preclude the necessity of gland removal.

Larger sialoliths usually need to be removed surgically, sometimes with the assistance of sialendoscopy. If significant inflammatory damage has occurred within the feeding gland, then the gland may need to be removed. Minor gland sialoliths are best treated by surgical removal, including the associated gland.

◆ SIALADENITIS

Inflammation of the salivary glands **(sialadenitis)** can arise from various infectious and noninfectious causes. The most common viral infection is mumps (see page 249), although a number of other viruses also can involve the salivary glands, including Coxsackie A, ECHO, choriomeningitis, parainfluenza, human immunodeficiency virus (HIV), and cytomegalovirus (CMV) (in neonates). Most bacterial infections arise as a result of ductal obstruction or decreased salivary flow, allowing retrograde spread of bacteria throughout the ductal system. Blockage of the duct can be caused by sialolithiasis (see page 465), congenital strictures, or compression by an adjacent tumor. Decreased flow can result from dehydration, debilitation, or medications that inhibit secretions.

One of the more common causes of sialadenitis is recent surgery (especially abdominal surgery), after which an acute parotitis *(surgical mumps)* may arise because the patient has been kept without food or fluids (NPO) and has received atropine during the surgical procedure. Other medications that produce xerostomia as a side effect also can predispose patients to such an infection. Most community-acquired cases of acute bacterial sialadenitis are caused by *Staphylococcus aureus* or streptococcal species. Hospital-acquired infections are also most frequently associated with *S. aureus,* but they also may be caused by a variety of other species, including *Eikenella corrodens, Escherichia coli, Fusobacterium, Haemophilus influenzae, Klebsiella, Prevotella, Proteus, and Pseudomonas.* Noninfectious causes of salivary inflammation include Sjögren syndrome (see page 472), sarcoidosis (see page 328), external radiation therapy (see page 280), radioiodine therapy for thyroid disease, and various allergens.

Clinical and Radiographic Features

Acute bacterial sialadenitis is most common in the parotid gland and is bilateral in 10%–25% of cases. The affected gland is swollen and painful, and the overlying skin may be warm and erythematous (Fig. 11.18). An associated low-grade fever and trismus may be present. A purulent discharge often is observed from the duct orifice when the gland is massaged (Fig. 11.19).

Recurrent or persistent ductal obstruction (most commonly caused by sialoliths) can lead to a chronic sialadenitis. Periodic swelling and pain occur within the affected gland, usually developing at mealtime when salivary flow is

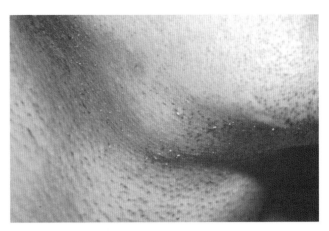

• **Fig. 11.18 Sialadenitis.** Tender swelling of the submandibular gland.

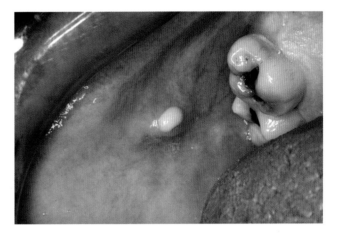

• **Fig. 11.19 Sialadenitis.** A purulent exudate can be seen arising from Stensen duct when the parotid gland is massaged.

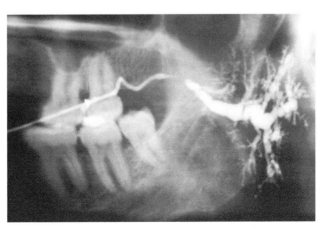

• **Fig. 11.20 Chronic Sialadenitis.** Parotid sialogram demonstrating ductal dilatation proximal to an area of obstruction. (Courtesy of Dr. George Blozis.)

stimulated. Sialography often demonstrates sialectasia (ductal dilatation) proximal to the area of obstruction (Fig. 11.20). In chronic parotitis, Stensen duct may show a characteristic sialographic pattern known as "sausaging," which reflects a combination of dilatation plus ductal strictures from scar formation. Chronic sialadenitis also can occur in the minor glands, possibly as a result of blockage of ductal flow or local trauma.

Juvenile recurrent parotitis is the most common inflammatory salivary disorder of children in the United States and the second most common such disorder worldwide (following mumps). It is characterized by recurring episodes of unilateral or bilateral, non-suppurative parotid swelling, usually beginning between the ages of 3 and 6 years. The exact cause is unknown, although congenital duct malformations, genetic factors, immunologic disorders, and dental malocclusion have been suggested as possible contributing factors. Although multiple recurrences often develop, the condition usually resolves around the time of puberty.

Subacute necrotizing sialadenitis is a form of salivary inflammation that occurs most commonly in teenagers and young adults. The lesion usually involves the minor salivary glands of the hard or soft palate, presenting as a painful nodule that is covered by intact, erythematous mucosa. Unlike necrotizing sialometaplasia (see page 477), the lesion does not ulcerate or slough necrotic tissue. An infectious or allergic cause has been hypothesized.

Histopathologic Features

In patients with acute sialadenitis, accumulation of neutrophils is observed within the ductal system and acini. Chronic sialadenitis is characterized by scattered or patchy infiltration of the salivary parenchyma by lymphocytes and plasma cells. Atrophy of the acini is common, as is ductal dilatation. If associated fibrosis is present, then the term **chronic sclerosing sialadenitis** is used (Fig. 11.21).

Subacute necrotizing sialadenitis is characterized by a heavy mixed inflammatory infiltrate consisting of neutrophils, lymphocytes, histiocytes, and eosinophils. There is loss of most of the acinar cells, and many of the remaining ones exhibit necrosis. The ducts tend to be atrophic and do not show hyperplasia or squamous metaplasia.

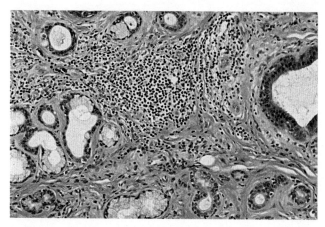

• **Fig. 11.21 Chronic Sclerosing Sialadenitis.** Chronic inflammatory infiltrate with associated acinar atrophy, ductal dilatation, and fibrosis.

Treatment and Prognosis

Patients with sialadenitis should have a screening panoramic radiograph to investigate for the presence of a sialolith. Additional imaging studies, such as ultrasound, CT, or MRI scans, also may be warranted. If purulence is noted at the duct orifice, then bacterial culture and sensitivity studies should be performed.

The treatment of acute sialadenitis includes appropriate antibiotic therapy and rehydration of the patient to stimulate salivary flow. Surgical drainage may be needed if there is abscess formation. Although this regimen is usually sufficient, a mortality rate as high as 20%–50% has been reported in debilitated patients because of the spread of the infection and sepsis.

The management of chronic sialadenitis depends on the severity of the condition and ranges from conservative therapy to surgical intervention. Initial management often includes antibiotics, analgesics, short-term corticosteroids, sialagogues, and glandular massage. Early cases that develop secondary to ductal blockage may respond to removal of the sialolith or other obstruction. However, if sialectasia is present, then the dilated ducts can lead to stasis of secretions and predispose the gland to further sialolith formation. Sialendoscopy and ductal irrigation often are employed to dilate ductal strictures and to eliminate sialoliths and mucus plugs. If necessary, a period of ductal stenting can also be performed. If conservative methods cannot control chronic sialadenitis, then surgical removal of the affected gland may be necessary.

Sialendoscopy with saline irrigation also has proven to be a useful technique for patients with juvenile recurrent parotitis, often greatly reducing the number of recurring episodes until the disorder resolves at puberty. Subacute necrotizing sialadenitis is a self-limiting condition that usually resolves within 2 weeks of diagnosis without treatment.

◆ CHEILITIS GLANDULARIS

Cheilitis glandularis is a rare inflammatory condition of the minor salivary glands. The cause is uncertain, although several etiologic factors have been suggested, including actinic damage, tobacco, poor hygiene, and heredity.

Clinical Features

Cheilitis glandularis characteristically occurs on the lower lip vermilion, although cases also have been reported to involve the upper lip and palate. Affected individuals experience swelling and eversion of the lower lip as a result of hypertrophy and inflammation of the glands (Fig. 11.22). The openings of the minor salivary ducts are inflamed and dilated, and pressure on the glands may produce mucopurulent secretions from the ductal openings. The condition most often has been reported in middle-aged and older men, although cases also have been described in women and children. However, some of the childhood cases may represent other entities,

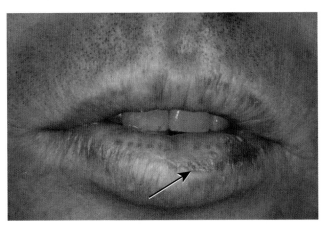

• **Fig. 11.22 Cheilitis Glandularis.** Prominent lower lip with inflamed openings of the minor salivary gland ducts. An early squamous cell carcinoma has developed on the patient's left side just lateral to the midline (*arrow*). (Courtesy of Dr. George Blozis.)

such as exfoliative cheilitis (see page 294). Examples also have been described in albino patients, presumably secondary to sun sensitivity.

Historically, cheilitis glandularis has been classified into three types, based on the severity of the disease:
1. Simple
2. Superficial suppurative (Baelz disease)
3. Deep suppurative (cheilitis glandularis apostematosa)

The latter two types represent progressive stages of the disease with bacterial involvement; they are characterized by increasing inflammation, suppuration, ulceration, and swelling of the lip.

Histopathologic Features

The microscopic findings of cheilitis glandularis may include chronic sialadenitis, ductal dilatation with mucin accumulation, and oncocytic ductal metaplasia. Concomitant dysplastic changes may be observed in the overlying surface epithelium in some cases.

Treatment and Prognosis

The treatment of choice for most cases of persistent cheilitis glandularis associated with actinic damage is vermilionectomy (lip shave), which usually produces a satisfactory cosmetic result. It has been noted that some cases have been associated with the development of squamous cell carcinoma of the overlying epithelium of the lip. Because actinic damage has been implicated in many cases of cheilitis glandularis, it is likely that this same solar radiation is responsible for the malignant degeneration.

◆ SIALORRHEA (PTYALISM)

Sialorrhea, or excessive salivation, is an uncommon condition that has various causes. Minor sialorrhea may result from local irritations, such as aphthous ulcers or ill-fitting dentures. Patients with new dentures often experience excess saliva production until they become accustomed to the prosthesis. Episodic hypersecretion of saliva, or "water brash," may occur as a protective buffering system to neutralize stomach acid in individuals with gastroesophageal reflux disease. Excessive salivation rarely develops in pregnant women (*ptyalism gravidarum*), sometimes in association with hyperemesis of pregnancy. Sialorrhea is a well-known clinical feature of rabies and heavy-metal poisoning (see page 304). It also may occur as a consequence of certain medications, such as antipsychotic agents, especially clozapine, and cholinergic agonists used to treat dementia of the Alzheimer type and myasthenia gravis.

Drooling can be a problem for patients who are intellectually disabled, who have undergone surgical resection of the mandible, or who have various neurologic disorders such as cerebral palsy, Parkinson disease, amyotrophic lateral sclerosis (ALS), or stroke. In these instances, the drooling is probably not caused by over-production of saliva but by poor neuromuscular control.

In addition, there is a second group of patients who report complaints of drooling; however, no obvious clinical evidence of excessive saliva production is observed, and they do not have any of the recognized causes for sialorrhea. Personality analysis has suggested that the complaint of drooling in such otherwise healthy patients does not have an organic basis but may be associated with high levels of neuroticism and a tendency to dissimulate.

Clinical Features

Excess saliva production typically produces drooling and choking, which may cause social embarrassment. In children with intellectual disability or cerebral palsy, uncontrolled salivary flow may lead to macerated sores around the mouth, chin, and neck that can become secondarily infected. The constant soiling of clothes and bed linens can be a significant problem for the parents and caretakers of these patients.

Treatment and Prognosis

Some causes of sialorrhea are transitory or mild, and no treatment is needed. For individuals with increased salivation associated with gastroesophageal reflux disease, medical management of their reflux problem may be beneficial.

For persistent severe drooling, therapeutic intervention may be indicated. Speech therapy can be used to improve neuromuscular control, but patient cooperation is necessary. Anticholinergic medications can decrease saliva production but may produce unacceptable side effects. Transdermal scopolamine has been tried with some success, but it should not be used in children younger than age 10. Intraglandular injection of botulinum toxin (type A or B) has been shown to be successful in reducing salivary secretions, with duration of action that varies from 6 weeks to 6 months. Salivary ablation also has been accomplished via image-guided injection of sodium tetradecyl sulfate and ethanol into the glands.

Several surgical techniques have been used successfully to control severe drooling in individuals with poor neuromuscular control:

- Relocation of the submandibular ducts to the base of the tongue or tonsillar fossa (sometimes along with excision of the sublingual glands)
- Relocation of the parotid ducts
- Submandibular gland excision plus parotid duct ligation
- Ligation of the parotid and submandibular ducts

◆ XEROSTOMIA

Xerostomia refers to a subjective sensation of a dry mouth; it is frequently, but not always, associated with salivary gland hypofunction. A number of factors may play a role in the cause of xerostomia, and these are listed in Box 11.2.

• BOX 11.2   Causes of Xerostomia

Developmental/Hereditary Origin

Salivary gland aplasia
Ectodermal dysplasia

Water/Metabolite Loss

Dehydration
Hemorrhage
Vomiting/diarrhea

Iatrogenic Origin

Medications
Radiation therapy to the head and neck
Chemotherapy

Infectious Diseases

Human immunodeficiency virus (HIV) infection
Hepatitis C infection
Cytomegalovirus infection

Autoimmune Disorders

Sjögren syndrome
Rheumatoid arthritis
Systemic lupus erythematosus
Systemic sclerosis
Primary biliary cirrhosis

Other Systemic Diseases

Diabetes mellitus
Diabetes insipidus
Sarcoidosis
Amyloidosis
    End-stage renal disease
Graft-versus-host disease (GVHD)
Psychogenic disorders

Local Factors

Decreased mastication
Smoking
Mouth breathing

Xerostomia is a common problem that has been reported in 25% of older adults. In the past, complaints of dry mouth in older patients often were ascribed to the predictable result of aging. However, it is now generally thought that any reductions in salivary function associated with age are modest and probably are not associated with any significant reduction in salivary function. Instead, xerostomia in older adults is more likely to be the result of other factors, especially medications. More than 500 drugs have been reported to produce xerostomia as a side effect, including 63% of the 200 most frequently prescribed medicines in the United States. A list of the most common and significant drugs associated with xerostomia is provided in Table 11.2. Not only are specific drugs known to produce dry mouth, but the prevalence of xerostomia also increases in relation to the total number of drugs that a person takes, regardless of whether the individual medications are xerogenic or not.

Clinical Features

Examination of the patient typically demonstrates a reduction in salivary secretions, and the residual saliva appears either foamy or thick and "ropey." The mucosa appears

---

TABLE 11.2   Medications That May Produce Xerostomia

Class of Drug	Example
Antihistamine agents	Diphenhydramine Chlorpheniramine
Decongestant agents	Pseudoephedrine Loratadine
Antidepressant agents	Amitriptyline Citalopram Duloxetine Fluoxetine Paroxetine Sertraline Bupropion
Antipsychotic agents	Phenothiazine derivatives Haloperidol Quetiapine
Sedatives and anxiolytic agents	Diazepam Lorazepam Alprazolam
Antihypertensive agents	Reserpine Methyldopa Chlorothiazide Furosemide Metoprolol Calcium channel blockers
Anticholinergic/antimuscarinic agents	Atropine Scopolamine Oxybutynin Solifenacin Tolterodine

dry, and the clinician may notice that the examining gloves stick to the mucosal surfaces. The dorsal tongue often is fissured with atrophy of the filiform papillae (see Fig. 11.1). The patient may complain of difficulty with mastication and swallowing, and they may even indicate that food adheres to the oral membranes during eating. The clinical findings, however, do not always correspond to the patient's symptoms. Some patients who complain of dry mouth may appear to have adequate salivary flow and oral moistness. For example, patients with burning mouth syndrome sometimes will describe dry mouth symptoms, despite having an apparently adequate flow of saliva upon examination. Such complaints may be related to the oral sensory neuropathy that underlies this condition (see page 868). Conversely, some patients who clinically appear to have a dry mouth have no complaints. The degree of saliva production can be assessed by measuring both resting and stimulated salivary flow.

There is an increased prevalence of oral candidiasis in patients with xerostomia because of the reduction in the cleansing and antimicrobial activity normally provided by saliva. In addition, these patients are more prone to dental decay, especially cervical and root caries. This problem has been associated more often with radiation therapy, and it is sometimes called *radiation-induced caries* but more appropriately should be called *xerostomia-related caries* (see page 282).

Treatment and Prognosis

The treatment of xerostomia is difficult and often unsatisfactory. Artificial salivas, moisturizing sprays, or gels may help make the patient more comfortable, as may continuous sips of water throughout the day. In addition, sugarless candy can be used in an effort to stimulate salivary flow. In recent years, use of miniaturized intraoral electrostimulating devices has been reported to be successful in improving dry mouth symptoms. If the dryness is secondary to the patient's medication, then discontinuation or dose modification in consultation with the patient's physician may be considered; a substitute drug also can be tried.

Systemic pilocarpine is a parasympathomimetic agonist that can be used as a sialagogue. At doses of 5–10 mg, three to four times daily, it can be an effective promoter of salivary secretion. Excess sweating is a common side effect, but more serious problems, such as increased heart rate and blood pressure, are uncommon. Cevimeline hydrochloride, a cholinergic agonist with affinity for muscarinic M_3 receptors, also has been proven to be an effective sialagogue. Both pilocarpine and cevimeline are contraindicated in patients with narrow-angle glaucoma.

Because of the increased potential for dental caries in patients with xerostomia, frequent dental visits are recommended. Office and daily home fluoride applications can be used to help prevent decay, and chlorhexidine mouth rinses minimize plaque buildup.

◆ IGG4-RELATED DISEASE

In the late 1800s, Johann von Mikulicz-Radecki described a patient with an unusual bilateral painless swelling of the lacrimal glands and all of the salivary glands, which was caused by an intense chronic inflammatory infiltrate. This clinical presentation became known as **Mikulicz disease.** Similar cases of parotid and lacrimal enlargement caused by other diseases (e.g., tuberculosis, sarcoidosis, and lymphoma) were considered to be different from Mikulicz disease and were termed **Mikulicz syndrome.** However, these two terms have become so confusing and ambiguous that they should no longer be used.

Although the true nature of his original patient's condition is uncertain, some examples of so-called Mikulicz disease likely have been benign lymphoepithelial lesions associated with Sjögren syndrome (see page 472). However, it is thought that other examples would be classified today as **IgG4-related disease,** a recently described fibroinflammatory disorder.

IgG4-related disease was first recognized as a sclerosing inflammatory process of the pancreas under the designation *autoimmune pancreatitis.* This condition later was linked to elevated serum levels of IgG4, as well as the presence of IgG4-positive plasma cells within pancreatic tissues. The systemic nature of IgG4-related disease was established when it was recognized that a variety of inflammatory lesions in other organs, including the salivary and lacrimal glands, represent the same disease process.

The pathogenesis of IgG4-related disease is uncertain, although both type 2 helper T-lymphocytes and B lymphocytes have been suggested to be involved. IgG4 actually is regarded as an anti-inflammatory and anti-allergic molecule, and its elevation likely represents a bystander phenomenon rather than a causative factor. Normally, IgG4 comprises less than 5% of the body's total IgG. In this condition, however, serum concentrations of polyclonal IgG4 can measure up to 25 times greater than normal levels, although 20%–40% of patients will show IgG4 levels within normal limits. Allergic disorders such as asthma, allergic rhinitis, and atopic dermatitis are common.

Clinical Features

IgG4-related disease typically occurs in middle-aged and older adults, with a mean age of approximately 60 years. Men are affected equally or slightly more often than women, although reports from Japan have shown a female predilection. Following the pancreas, the head and neck region is the second most common site affected by this condition. Orbital involvement may be characterized by swollen eyelids, lacrimal inflammation, proptosis, pain, and diplopia. Optic nerve involvement can lead to permanent visual loss. IgG4-related sialadenitis occurs most frequently in the submandibular gland and only rarely involves the parotid gland and minor salivary glands (Fig. 11.23). Patients present with

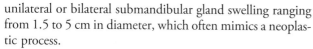

• **Fig. 11.23 IgG4-related Disease.** Bilateral enlargement of the sub-mandibular glands. (Courtesy of Dr. Benjamin Martinez.)

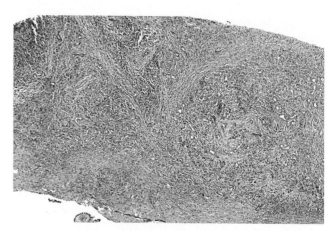

• **Fig. 11.24 IgG4-related Disease.** Diffuse lymphoplasmacytic inflammation in the submandibular gland with associated interlobular fibrosis. (Courtesy of Dr. Benjamin Martinez.)

unilateral or bilateral submandibular gland swelling ranging from 1.5 to 5 cm in diameter, which often mimics a neoplastic process.

Because IgG4-related disease can affect almost any tissue or organ within the body, the severity and course of the disorder depend on the specific site of involvement. Pancreatitis can lead to obstructive jaundice, weight loss, and abdominal discomfort. Sclerosing cholangitis can result in hepatic failure. Other complications include abdominal aortitis with aneurysm formation, inflammatory pseudotumors of the kidney, thyroid inflammation (Riedel thyroiditis), and lymphadenopathy.

Histopathologic Features

Microscopic examination of an affected submandibular gland reveals chronic sclerosing sialadenitis, which is characterized by a heavy lymphoplasmacytic infiltrate, hyperplastic lymphoid follicles, and acinar atrophy. Immunohistochemistry should reveal increased numbers of IgG4-positive plasma cells (greater than 30–50 per high-power field), plus the ratio of IgG4-positive plasma cells to total IgG-positive plasma cells should be greater than 40%. Prominent interlobular fibrosis results in a storiform pattern when the gland is viewed at low power (Fig. 11.24). Another common finding is obliterative phlebitis, which can be highlighted with an elastic stain. This overall pattern has sometimes been termed a **Küttner tumor.** Labial salivary gland biopsy has been suggested as a minimally invasive procedure for the diagnosis of IgG4-related sialadenitis; however, its sensitivity for the diagnosis is considered very low.

Treatment and Prognosis

IgG4-related disease often requires immediate, aggressive treatment with systemic corticosteroids to prevent significant organ damage and failure. Glucocorticoid-sparing agents,

such as azathioprine, mycophenolate mofetil, and methotrexate, also can be used. Most patients show a rapid response to immunosuppressive therapy and have a favorable prognosis. For patients with recurrent disease, B-cell depletion with rituximab can be effective. Submandibular gland lesions or highly fibrotic orbital pseudotumors sometimes are treated by surgical resection.

◆ SJÖGREN SYNDROME

Sjögren syndrome is a chronic, systemic autoimmune disorder that principally involves the salivary and lacrimal glands, resulting in xerostomia (dry mouth) and xerophthalmia (dry eyes). The effects on the eye often are called **keratoconjunctivitis sicca** (*sicca* means "dry"), and the clinical presentation of both xerostomia and xerophthalmia is also sometimes called the *sicca syndrome.* Traditionally, two forms of the disease are recognized:

1. *Primary* Sjögren syndrome (sicca syndrome alone; no other autoimmune disorder is present)
2. *Secondary* Sjögren syndrome (the patient manifests sicca syndrome in addition to another associated autoimmune disease)

The cause of Sjögren syndrome is unknown. Although it is not a hereditary disease *per se,* there is strong evidence of a genetic influence. Examples of Sjögren syndrome have been reported in twins or in two or more members of the same family. Relatives of affected patients have an increased frequency of other autoimmune diseases. A variety of candidate genes have been implicated in the pathogenesis, including those related to certain histocompatibility antigens (HLAs), interferon response, and B-lymphocyte function. Researchers have suggested that viruses, such as Epstein-Barr virus (EBV) or human T-cell lymphotropic virus, may play a pathogenetic role in Sjögren syndrome, but evidence for this is still speculative.

Clinical and Radiographic Features

Sjögren syndrome is considered to be the second most common autoimmune disorder, following rheumatoid arthritis. Although the exact prevalence depends on the clinical criteria used, current estimates place the population prevalence at 1% (0.1%–4.8%), with a 9:1 female-to-male ratio. It is seen predominantly in middle-aged adults, but rare examples have been described in children. The classification criteria adopted in 2016 by the American College of Rheumatology and European League Against Rheumatism are presented in Box 11.3.

When the condition is associated with another connective tissue disease, it is called *secondary Sjögren syndrome*. It can be associated with almost any other autoimmune disease, but the most common associated disorder is rheumatoid arthritis. About 15% of patients with rheumatoid arthritis have Sjögren syndrome. In addition, secondary Sjögren syndrome may develop in 30% of patients with systemic lupus erythematosus (SLE).

The principal oral symptom is xerostomia, which is caused by decreased salivary secretions; however, the severity of this dryness can vary widely from patient to patient. The saliva may appear frothy, with a lack of the usual pooling saliva in the floor of the mouth. Affected patients may complain of difficulty in swallowing, altered taste, or difficulty in wearing dentures. The tongue often becomes fissured and exhibits atrophy of the papillae (Fig. 11.25). The oral mucosa may be red and tender, usually as a result of secondary candidiasis. Related denture sore mouth and angular cheilitis are common. The lack of salivary cleansing action predisposes the patient to dental decay, especially cervical caries.

From one-third to one-half of patients have diffuse, firm enlargement of the major salivary glands during the course of their disease (Fig. 11.26). This swelling is usually bilateral, may be nonpainful or slightly tender, and may be intermittent or persistent in nature. The greater the severity of the disease, the greater the likelihood of this salivary enlargement. In addition, the reduced salivary flow places these individuals at increased risk for retrograde bacterial sialadenitis.

Although it is not diagnostic, sialographic examination often reveals punctate sialectasia and lack of normal arborization of the ductal system, typically demonstrating a "fruit-laden, branchless tree" pattern (Fig. 11.27). Scintigraphy with radioactive technetium-99m pertechnetate

---

• BOX 11.3   American College of Rheumatology/European League Against Rheumatism Classification Criteria for Primary Sjögren Syndrome

The classification of primary **Sjögren syndrome** applies to an individual who meets one or more *inclusion criteria*, does not have any of the conditions listed as *exclusion criteria*, and has total score of ≥4 when the weights from the following criteria items are added:

Item	Weight/Score
Labial salivary gland with focal lymphocytic sialadenitis and focus score of ≥1 foci/4 mm²	3
Anti-SSA/Ro-positive	3
Ocular staining score ≥5 (or van Bijsterveld score ≥4) in at least one eye^^^	1
Schirmer test ≤5 mm/5 minutes in at least one eye^^^	1
Unstimulated whole saliva flow rate ≤1 mL/minute (as described by Navazesh and Kumar)^^^	1

Inclusion criteria—patient has at least one symptom of ocular or oral dryness, defined as a positive response to at least one of the following questions:
(1) Have you had daily, persistent, troublesome dry eyes for more than 3 months?

(2) Do you have a recurrent sensation of sand or gravel in the eyes?
(3) Do you use tear substitutes more than three times a day?
(4) Have you had a daily feeling of dry mouth for more than 3 months?
(5) Do you frequently drink liquids to aid in swallowing dry food?
-or-
A patient in whom there is suspicion of Sjögren syndrome (SS) from the European League Against Rheumatism SS Disease Activity Index questionnaire (at least one domain with a positive item).

Exclusion criteria—patient with a prior diagnosis of any of the following conditions, which would exclude diagnosis of SS and participation in SS studies or therapeutic trials because of overlapping clinical features or interference with criteria tests:
(1) History of head and neck radiation treatment
(2) Active hepatitis C infection (with confirmation by PCR)
(3) Acquired immunodeficiency syndrome (AIDS)
(4) Sarcoidosis
(5) Amyloidosis
(6) Graft-versus-host disease
(7) IgG4-related disease

^^^Patients who are normally taking anticholinergic drugs should be evaluated for objective signs of salivary hypofunction and ocular dryness after a sufficient interval without these medications in order for these components to be a valid measure of oral and ocular dryness.

Source: Shiboski CH, Shiboski SC, Seror R, et al: 2016 American College of Rheumatology/European League Against Rheumatism classification criteria for primary Sjögren's syndrome. A consensus and data-driven methodology involving three international patient cohorts, Ann Rheum Dis 76:9–16, 2017.

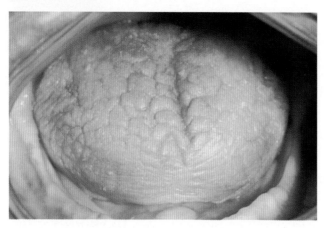

• **Fig. 11.25 Sjögren Syndrome.** Dry and fissured tongue. (Courtesy of Dr. David Schaffner.)

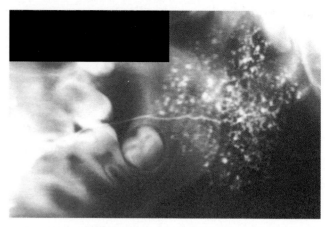

• **Fig. 11.27 Sjögren Syndrome.** Parotid sialogram demonstrating atrophy and punctate sialectasia ("fruit-laden, branchless tree"). (Courtesy of Dr. George Blozis.)

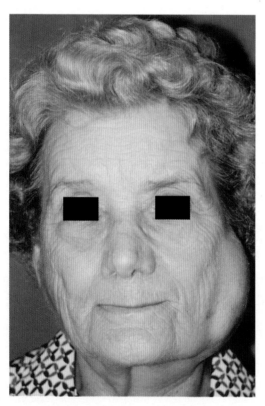

• **Fig. 11.26 Sjögren Syndrome.** Benign lymphoepithelial lesion of the parotid gland. (Courtesy of Dr. David Schaffner.)

characteristically shows decreased uptake and delayed emptying of the isotope. Ultrasonography may reveal multiple hypoechoic or anechoic areas in the parotid and submandibular glands.

The term **keratoconjunctivitis sicca** describes not only the reduced tear production by the lacrimal glands but also the pathologic effect on the epithelial cells of the ocular surface. As in xerostomia, the severity of xerophthalmia can vary widely from one patient to the next. The lacrimal inflammation causes a decrease of the aqueous layer of the tear film; however, mucin production is normal and may result in a

mucoid discharge. Patients often complain of a scratchy, gritty sensation or the perceived presence of a foreign body in the eye. Defects of the ocular surface epithelium develop, which may result in blurred vision and, sometimes, an aching pain. The ocular manifestations are least severe in the morning on wakening and become more pronounced as the day progresses.

A simple means to confirm the decreased tear secretion is the Schirmer test. A standardized strip of sterile filter paper is placed over the margin of the lower eyelid, so that the tabbed end rests just inside the lower lid. By measuring the length of wetting of the filter paper, tear production can be assessed. Values less than 5 mm (after a 5-minute period) are considered abnormal. In addition, the possibility of damage to the corneal and conjunctival surfaces can be assessed by slit lamp examination after rose bengal and lissamine green staining.

Sjögren syndrome is a systemic disease, and the inflammatory process also can affect various other body tissues. The skin is often dry, as are the nasal and vaginal mucosae. Fatigue is fairly common, and depression sometimes can occur. Other possible associated problems include lymphadenopathy, primary biliary cholangitis, Raynaud phenomenon, interstitial nephritis, interstitial lung fibrosis, vasculitis, and peripheral neuropathies (see Box 11.4).

Laboratory Values

In patients with Sjögren syndrome, the erythrocyte sedimentation rate often is high and serum immunoglobulin (Ig) levels, especially IgG, typically are elevated. A variety of autoantibodies can be produced, and although none of these is specifically diagnostic, their presence can be another helpful clue to the diagnosis. A positive rheumatoid factor (RF) is found in approximately 60% of cases, regardless of whether the patient has rheumatoid arthritis. Antinuclear antibodies (ANAs) are also present in 75%–85% of patients. Two particular nuclear autoantibodies—anti-SS-A (anti-Ro) and anti-SS-B (anti-La)—may be found, especially in patients

Site	Frequency
Constitutional	
Fatigue	70%–80%
Musculoskeletal	
Arthralgia	38%–75%
Arthritis	10%–30%
Inflammatory myositis	2%
Hematologic	
Anemia (usually mild)	30%–60%
Thrombocytopenia	5%–13%
Hypergammaglobulinemia	20%–50%
Elevated erythrocyte sedimentation rate	20%
Non-Hodgkin lymphoma (lifetime risk)	5%–10%
Gastrointestinal	
Dysphagia	65%
Gastroesophageal reflux	60%
Chronic diarrhea	9%
Constipation	23%
Liver enzyme abnormalities	10%–40%
Renal	
Interstitial nephritis	5%
Pulmonary	
Recurrent respiratory tract infections	10%–35%
Chronic cough	60%
Interstitial lung disease	3%–11%
Dermatologic	
Xerosis (dry skin)	50%
Raynaud phenomenon	15%–30%
Cutaneous vasculitis	10%
Annular erythema	10%
Neurologic (including peripheral neuropathies, cranial neuropathies, cognitive dysfunction, transverse myelitis)	20%

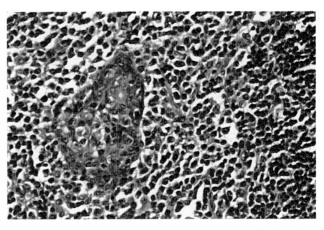

• **Fig. 11.28 Benign Lymphoepithelial Lesion in Sjögren Syndrome.** Lymphocytic infiltrate of the parotid gland with an associated epimyoepithelial island.

with primary Sjögren syndrome. Anti-SS-A antibodies have been detected in approximately 50%–76% of patients, whereas anti-SS-B antibodies have been discovered in 30%–60% of these individuals.

Histopathologic Features

The basic microscopic finding in Sjögren syndrome is a lymphocytic infiltration of the salivary glands, which leads to destruction of the acinar units. More advanced lesions result in a pattern known as a **benign lymphoepithelial lesion (myoepithelial sialadenitis).** Although the acini are destroyed, the ductal epithelium persists. The ductal cells and surrounding myoepithelial cells become hyperplastic, forming highly characteristic groups of cells, known as *epimyoepithelial islands,* throughout the lymphoid proliferation (Fig. 11.28). Germinal centers may or may not be seen. Lymphocytic infiltration of the minor glands also occurs, although epimyoepithelial islands are rarely seen in this location.

Biopsy of the minor salivary glands of the lower lip sometimes is used as a diagnostic test for Sjögren syndrome. A 1.5- to 2.0-cm incision is made on clinically normal lower labial mucosa, parallel to the vermilion border and lateral to the midline, allowing the harvest of five or more accessory glands. These glands then can be examined histopathologically for the presence of focal chronic inflammatory aggregates composed of 50 or more lymphocytes and plasma cells. The aggregates should be adjacent to normal-appearing acini and should be found consistently in most of the glands in the specimen. The following formula has been suggested:

$$\text{Focus score} = \frac{\text{Number of inflammatory aggregates} \times 4}{\text{Number of mm}^2 \text{ of salivary gland parenchyma}}$$

The focus score calculates the number of inflammatory aggregates per 4-mm^2 area of salivary gland tissue. A focus score ≥ 1 (i.e., one or more foci of 50 or more cells per 4-mm^2 area of glandular tissue) is considered supportive of the diagnosis of Sjögren syndrome (Fig. 11.29). The greater the number of foci (up to 12 or confluent foci) is, the greater is the correlation with this diagnosis. The focal nature of this chronic inflammation among otherwise normal acini is a highly suggestive pattern; in contrast, the finding of scattered inflammation with ductal dilatation and fibrosis (chronic sclerosing sialadenitis) does not support the diagnosis of Sjögren syndrome.

Although labial salivary gland biopsy has become a widely used test in the diagnosis of Sjögren syndrome, it is not 100% reliable. Some patients diagnosed with Sjögren syndrome will show no significant labial gland inflammation; conversely, examination of labial glands removed incidentally from non-Sjögren patients sometimes will show focal lymphocytic infiltrates. Sjögren syndrome patients who smoke have been shown to have a significantly lower frequency of abnormal lymphocytic foci scores in their labial gland specimens. It also is important that a pathologist experienced in the analysis of these specimens examines the labial gland biopsies. One study showed that slightly more than half of labial gland specimens required a revised diagnosis after being reviewed by a second pathologist.

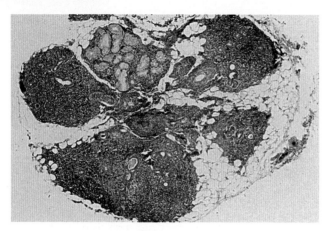

• **Fig. 11.29 Sjögren Syndrome.** Labial gland biopsy showing multiple lymphocytic foci.

Other authors have advocated incisional biopsy of the parotid gland through a posterior/inferior auricular approach instead of a labial salivary gland biopsy. One study has shown this technique to be more sensitive in demonstrating inflammatory changes that support the diagnosis of Sjögren syndrome; however, other authors think that this technique confers no increased benefit over labial gland biopsy. Parotid biopsy may enable the clinician to evaluate an enlarged gland for the development of lymphoma and rule out the possibility of sialadenosis or sarcoidosis.

Treatment and Prognosis

The treatment of the patient with Sjögren syndrome is mostly supportive. The dry eyes are best managed by periodic use of artificial tears. Thicker ocular gels or ointments may be utilized at bedtime for longer lasting relief. For more severe eye disease, short-term topical corticosteroids or 0.05% cyclosporine can be prescribed to decrease ocular inflammation. In addition, the FDA recently has approved topical lifitegrast for treatment of dry eye symptoms.

Artificial salivas are available for the treatment of xerostomia; sugarless candy or gum can help to keep the mouth moist. Sialagogue medications, such as pilocarpine and cevimeline, can be useful to stimulate salivary flow if enough functional salivary tissue still remains. Medications known to diminish secretions should be avoided, if at all possible. Because of the increased risk of dental caries, daily fluoride applications may be indicated in dentulous patients. Antifungal therapy often is needed to treat secondary candidiasis.

Patients with Sjögren syndrome have a lifetime risk for lymphoma of 5%–10%, which is estimated to be about 15–20 times greater than the general population. These tumors may arise initially within the salivary glands or within lymph nodes. With the advent of modern molecular pathology techniques to detect B-cell monoclonality (e.g., *in situ* hybridization, polymerase chain reaction [PCR]), many salivary gland infiltrates formerly thought to represent benign lymphoepithelial lesions are now being diagnosed as

lymphomas. These tumors are predominantly low-grade non-Hodgkin B-cell lymphomas of the mucosa-associated lymphoid tissue (i.e., **MALT lymphomas, extranodal marginal zone B-cell lymphomas**), although occasionally, high-grade lymphomas can develop that demonstrate more aggressive behavior. Prognostic risk factors for lymphoma development include persistent parotid gland enlargement, lymphadenopathy, splenomegaly, neutropenia, low C4 complement levels, cryoglobulinemia, and palpable purpura. The detection of immunoglobulin gene rearrangements in labial salivary gland biopsies may prove to be a useful marker for predicting the development of lymphoma.

◆ SIALADENOSIS (SIALOSIS)

Sialadenosis is an unusual non-inflammatory disorder characterized by salivary gland enlargement, particularly involving the parotid glands. The condition frequently is associated with an underlying systemic problem, which may be endocrine, nutritional, or neurogenic in origin (Box 11.5). The best known of these conditions include diabetes mellitus, general malnutrition, alcoholism, and bulimia.

These conditions are believed to result in dysregulation of the autonomic innervation of the salivary acini, causing an aberrant intracellular secretory cycle. This leads to excessive accumulation of secretory granules, with marked enlargement of the acinar cells. In addition, reduced innervation of myoepithelial cells may lead to atrophy of the supporting myofilaments around the acinar cells.

Clinical and Radiographic Features

Sialadenosis usually appears as a slowly evolving swelling of the parotid glands, which may or may not be painful (Fig. 11.30). The condition is usually bilateral, but it also

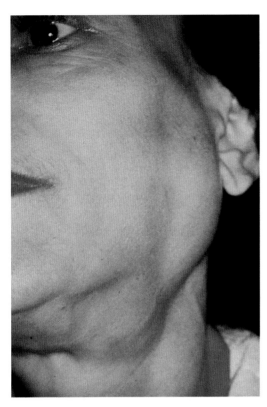

• **Fig. 11.30 Sialadenosis.** Enlargement of the parotid and submandibular glands secondary to alcoholism. (Courtesy of Dr. George Blozis.)

can be unilateral. In some patients, the submandibular glands may be affected, but involvement of minor salivary glands is distinctly rare. Decreased salivary secretion may occur. Sialography demonstrates a "leafless tree" pattern, which is thought to be caused by compression of the finer ducts by hypertrophic acinar cells.

Histopathologic Features

Microscopic examination reveals hypertrophy of the acinar cells, sometimes two to three times greater than normal size. The nuclei are displaced to the cell base, and the cytoplasm is engorged with zymogen granules. In cases associated with long-standing diabetes or alcoholism, there may be acinar atrophy and fatty infiltration. Significant inflammation is not observed.

Treatment and Prognosis

The clinical management of sialadenosis is often unsatisfactory because it is closely related to the control of the underlying cause. Mild examples may cause few problems. If the swelling becomes a cosmetic concern, then partial parotidectomy can be performed. Pilocarpine has been reported to be beneficial in reducing salivary gland enlargement in bulimic patients.

♦ ADENOMATOID HYPERPLASIA OF THE MINOR SALIVARY GLANDS

Clinical Features

Adenomatoid hyperplasia is a rare lesion of the minor salivary glands characterized by localized swelling that mimics a neoplasm. This pseudotumor most often occurs on the hard or soft palate, although it also has been reported in other oral minor salivary gland sites. The pathogenesis of adenomatoid hyperplasia is uncertain, but it has been speculated that local trauma may play a role. It is most common in the fourth to sixth decades of life. Most examples present as sessile, painless masses that may be soft or firm to palpation. They usually are normal in color, although a few lesions are red or bluish.

Histopathologic Features

Microscopic examination demonstrates lobular aggregates of relatively normal-appearing mucous acini that are greater in number than normally would be found in the area. These glands also sometimes appear to be increased in size. In some instances, the glands are situated close to the mucosal surface. Chronic inflammation occasionally is seen, but it usually is mild and localized.

Treatment and Prognosis

Because the clinical presentation of adenomatoid hyperplasia mimics a tumor, biopsy is necessary to establish the diagnosis. Once the diagnosis has been established, no further treatment is indicated and the lesion should not recur.

The pathologist should be wary of making a diagnosis of adenomatoid hyperplasia without good clinical correlation. On occasion, attempted biopsy of a true salivary gland tumor may harvest only adjacent normal salivary tissue, which might be misinterpreted as adenomatoid hyperplasia. Good communication between the clinician and pathologist is important.

♦ NECROTIZING SIALOMETAPLASIA

Necrotizing sialometaplasia is an uncommon, locally destructive inflammatory condition of the salivary glands. Although the cause is uncertain, most authors believe it is the result of ischemia of the salivary tissue that leads to local infarction. The importance of this lesion rests in the fact that it mimics a malignant process, both clinically and microscopically.

A number of potential predisposing factors have been suggested, including the following:
• Traumatic injuries
• Dental injections
• Ill-fitting dentures
• Upper respiratory infections

- Adjacent tumors
- Previous surgery
- Eating disorders with binge-purging

Researchers have suggested that these factors may play a role in compromising the blood supply to the involved glands, resulting in ischemic necrosis. However, many cases occur without any known predisposing factors.

Clinical Features

Necrotizing sialometaplasia most frequently develops in the palatal salivary glands; more than 75% of all cases occur on the posterior palate. The hard palate is affected more often than the soft palate. About two-thirds of palatal cases are unilateral, with the rest being bilateral or midline in location. Necrotizing sialometaplasia also has been reported in other minor salivary gland sites and, occasionally, in the parotid gland. The submandibular and sublingual glands are rarely affected. Although it can occur at almost any age, necrotizing sialometaplasia is most common in adults; the mean age of onset is 46 years. Males are affected nearly twice as often as females.

The condition appears initially as a nonulcerated swelling, often associated with pain or paresthesia (Fig. 11.31). Within 2–3 weeks, necrotic tissue sloughs out, leaving a craterlike ulcer that can range from less than 1 cm to more than 5 cm in diameter (Fig. 11.32). The patient may report that "a part of my palate fell out." At this point, the pain often subsides. In rare instances, there can be destruction of the underlying palatal bone.

Histopathologic Features

The microscopic appearance of necrotizing sialometaplasia is characterized by acinar necrosis in early lesions, followed by associated squamous metaplasia of the salivary ducts (Fig. 11.33). Although the mucous acinar cells are necrotic, the overall lobular architecture of the involved glands is still preserved—a helpful histopathologic clue. There may be liberation of mucin, with an associated inflammatory response. The squamous metaplasia of the salivary ducts can be striking and produce a pattern that is easily misdiagnosed as squamous cell carcinoma or mucoepidermoid carcinoma. The frequent association of pseudoepitheliomatous hyperplasia of the overlying epithelium may further compound this mistaken impression. In most cases, however, the squamous proliferation has a bland cytologic appearance. In examples that are difficult to distinguish from carcinoma, low immunoreactivity for p53 protein and Ki-67 may help to support a diagnosis of necrotizing sialometaplasia.

Treatment and Prognosis

Because of the worrisome clinical presentation of necrotizing sialometaplasia, biopsy usually is indicated to rule out the possibility of malignant disease. Once the diagnosis has been established, no specific treatment is indicated or necessary. The lesion typically resolves on its own accord, with an average healing time of 5–6 weeks.

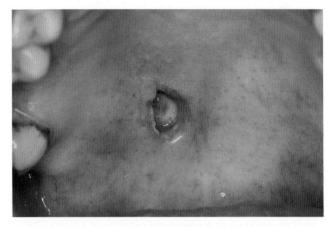

• **Fig. 11.32 Necrotizing Sialometaplasia.** Later-stage lesion showing craterlike defect of the posterior palate.

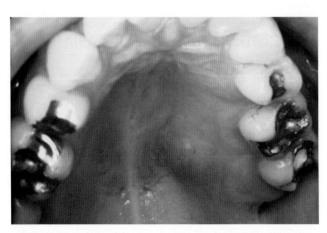

• **Fig. 11.31 Necrotizing Sialometaplasia.** Early lesion demonstrating swelling of the posterior lateral hard palate. (From Allen CM, Camisa C: Diseases of the mouth and lips. In Sams WM, Lynch P, editors: *Principles of dermatology,* New York, 1990, Churchill Livingstone.)

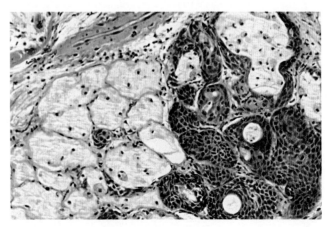

• **Fig. 11.33 Necrotizing Sialometaplasia.** Necrotic mucous acini (*left*) and adjacent ductal squamous metaplasia (*right*).

On rare occasions, necrotizing sialometaplasia has been described occurring adjacent to salivary gland tumors. Therefore, care should be taken to ensure that such glandular necrosis is not masking the presence of an adjacent true neoplasm.

SALIVARY GLAND TUMORS

◆ GENERAL CONSIDERATIONS

Tumors of the salivary glands constitute an important area in the field of oral and maxillofacial pathology. Although such tumors are uncommon, they are by no means rare. The annual incidence of salivary gland tumors around the world ranges from about 1.0 to 6.5 cases per 100,000 people. Although soft tissue neoplasms (e.g., hemangioma), lymphoma, and metastatic tumors can occur within the salivary glands, the discussion in this chapter is limited to primary epithelial neoplasms.

An often-bewildering array of salivary tumors has been identified and categorized. In addition, the classification scheme is a dynamic one that changes as clinicians learn more about these lesions. Box 11.6 includes most of the currently recognized tumors. Some of the tumors on this list are not specifically discussed because their rarity places them outside the scope of this text.

A number of investigators have published their findings on salivary gland neoplasia, but a comparison of these studies is often difficult. Some studies have been limited to only the major glands or have not included all the minor salivary gland sites. In addition, the ever-evolving classification system makes an evaluation of some older studies difficult, especially when researchers attempt to compare them with more recent analyses. Notwithstanding these difficulties, it is still helpful to compare these studies because they provide a good overview of salivary neoplasia in general. An evaluation of various studies shows fairly consistent trends (with minor variations) with regard to salivary gland tumors.

Tables 11.3 and 11.4 summarize five large series of primary epithelial salivary gland tumors, analyzed by sites of occurrence and frequency of malignancy, respectively. Some variations between studies may represent differences in diagnostic criteria, geographic differences, or referral bias in the cases seen. (Some centers may tend to see more malignant tumors on referral from other sources.)

The most common site for salivary gland tumors is the parotid gland, accounting for 61%–80% of all cases. Fortunately, a relatively low percentage of parotid tumors are malignant, ranging from 15% to 32%. Overall, it can be stated that two-thirds to three-quarters of all salivary tumors occur in the parotid gland, and two-thirds to three-quarters of these parotid tumors are benign.

Table 11.5 summarizes four large series of parotid neoplasms. The pleomorphic adenoma is overwhelmingly the most common tumor (45%–63% of all cases in the parotid gland). Warthin tumors are also fairly common; they

---

● BOX 11.6 Classification of Salivary Gland Tumors

Benign

- Pleomorphic adenoma (mixed tumor)
- Myoepithelioma
- Basal cell adenoma
- Canalicular adenoma
- Warthin tumor (papillary cystadenoma lymphomatosum)
- Oncocytoma
- Sebaceous adenoma
- Sebaceous lymphadenoma
- Ductal papillomas
  - Sialadenoma papilliferum
  - Intraductal papilloma
  - Inverted ductal papilloma
- Papillary cystadenoma

Malignant

- Malignant mixed tumors
  - Carcinoma ex pleomorphic adenoma
  - Carcinosarcoma
  - Metastasizing mixed tumor
- Mucoepidermoid carcinoma
- Acinic cell carcinoma
- Adenoid cystic carcinoma
- Polymorphous adenocarcinoma
- Basal cell adenocarcinoma
- Epithelial-myoepithelial carcinoma
- Secretory carcinoma
- Microsecretory adenocarcinoma
- Sclerosing microcystic adenocarcinoma
- Salivary duct carcinoma
- Myoepithelial carcinoma
- Cystadenocarcinoma
- Sebaceous adenocarcinoma
- Sebaceous lymphadenocarcinoma
- Clear cell adenocarcinoma
- Oncocytic carcinoma
- Squamous cell carcinoma
- Malignant lymphoepithelial lesion (lymphoepithelial carcinoma)
- Small cell neuroendocrine carcinoma
- Large cell neuroendocrine carcinoma
- Undifferentiated carcinoma
- Sialoblastoma
- Adenocarcinoma, not otherwise specified (NOS)

---

account for 8%–22% of cases. A variety of malignant tumors occur, with the mucoepidermoid carcinoma appearing to be the most frequent overall. Although previous studies suggested that the United Kingdom may have a lower frequency of this tumor, a more recent series showed prevalence numbers equivalent to other countries.

Approximately 10% of all salivary tumors occur in the submandibular gland, but the frequency of malignancy in this gland is much greater than that of the parotid gland, ranging from 26% to 45%. However, as shown in Table 11.6, the pleomorphic adenoma is still the most common tumor and makes up 53%–72% of all neoplasms. Unlike its occurrence in the parotid gland, the Warthin

TABLE 11.3　Sites of Occurrence of Primary Epithelial Salivary Gland Tumors

Author (Year)	Number of Cases	Parotid	Submandibular	Sublingual	Minor
Eveson and Cawson (1985a)	2410	73%	11%	0.3%	14%
Seifert et al. (1986)	2579	80%	10%	1.0%	9%
Ellis et al. (1991)	13,749	64%	10%	0.3%	23%
Tian et al. (2010)	6982	61%	10%	1.0%	28%
Gao et al. (2017)	7190	63%	10%	2.6%	25%

TABLE 11.4　Frequency of Malignancy for Salivary Tumors at Different Sites

Author (Year)	Number of Cases	Parotid	Submandibular	Sublingual	Minor
Eveson and Cawson (1985a)	2410	15%	37%	86%	46%
Seifert et al. (1986)	2579	20%	45%	90%	45%
Ellis et al. (1991)	13,749	32%	41%	70%	49%
Tian et al. (2010)	6982	18%	26%	95%	62%
Gao et al. (2017)	7190	22%	36%	93%	62%

TABLE 11.5　Parotid Tumors

	Gao et al. (China, 2017)	Tian et al. (China, 2010)	Ellis et al. (United States, 1991)	Eveson & Cawson (Great Britain, 1985a)
Total number of cases	4505	4264	8222	1756
Benign Tumors				
Pleomorphic adenoma	45.4%	49.9%	53.0%	63.3%
Warthin tumor	20.6%	22.4%	7.7%	14.0%
Oncocytoma	0.7%	0.5%	1.9%	0.9%
Basal cell adenoma	7.2%	5.8%	1.4%	—
Other benign tumors	3.8%	3.4%	3.7%	7.1%*
Total	77.7%	82.1%	67.7%	85.3%
Malignant Tumors				
Mucoepidermoid carcinoma	7.2%	4.3%	9.6%	1.5%
Acinic cell carcinoma	2.5%	3.2%	8.6%	2.5%
Adenoid cystic carcinoma	2.8%	1.8%	2.0%	2.0%
Malignant mixed tumor	2.4%	2.3%	2.5%	3.2%
Squamous cell carcinoma	0.7%	0.7%	2.1%	1.1%
Other malignant tumors	6.7%	5.6%	7.5%	4.4%
Total	22.3%	17.9%	32.3%	14.7%

*Includes all "other monomorphic adenomas."

TABLE 11.6   Submandibular Tumors

	Gao et al. (China, 2017)	Tian et al. (China, 2010)	Ellis et al. (United States, 1991)	Eveson & Cawson (Great Britain, 1985a)
Total number of cases	713	663	1235	257
Benign Tumors				
Pleomorphic adenoma	61.4%	72.2%	53.3%	59.5%
Warthin tumor	0.6%	0.6%	1.3%	0.8%
Oncocytoma	0.1%	0.2%	1.5%	0.4%
Basal cell adenoma	0.7%	0.3%	1.0%	—
Other benign tumors	1.4%	0.6%	1.7%	1.9%*
Total	64.2%	73.9%	58.8%	62.6%
Malignant Tumors				
Mucoepidermoid carcinoma	5.3%	4.2%	9.1%	1.6%
Acinic cell carcinoma	0.6%	1.1%	2.7%	0.4%
Adenoid cystic carcinoma	15.0%	11.2%	11.7%	16.8%
Malignant mixed tumor	3.2%	4.1%	3.5%	7.8%
Squamous cell carcinoma	0.1%	1.1%	3.4%	1.9%
Other malignant tumors	11.5%	4.5%	10.8%	8.9%
Total	35.8%	26.1%	41.2%	37.4%

*Includes all "other monomorphic adenomas."

tumor is unusual in the submandibular gland, making up about 1% of all tumors. Adenoid cystic carcinoma is the most common malignancy, ranging from 11% to 17% of all cases.

Tumors of the sublingual gland are rare, comprising about 1% of all salivary neoplasms. However, 70%–97% of sublingual tumors are malignant.

Tumors of the various smaller minor salivary glands make up 9%–28% of all tumors, which makes this group the second most common site for salivary neoplasia. Table 11.7 summarizes the findings of five large surveys of minor gland tumors. Unfortunately, relatively high proportions (38%–54%) of these have been malignant in most studies. Excluding rare sublingual tumors, it can be stated that the smaller the gland is, the greater is the likelihood of malignancy for a salivary gland tumor.

As observed in the major glands, the pleomorphic adenoma is the most common minor gland tumor and accounts for about 33%–41% of all cases. Mucoepidermoid carcinoma is the most frequent malignancy of minor gland origin, comprising 13%–23% of all tumors. Adenoid cystic carcinoma and polymorphous adenocarcinoma are also

recognized as relatively common malignant tumors arising from the minor salivary glands.

The palate is the most frequent site for minor salivary gland tumors, with 42%–57% of all cases found there (Table 11.8). Most of these occur on the posterior lateral hard or soft palate, which have the greatest concentration of glands. Table 11.9 shows the relative prevalence of various tumors on the palate. The lips are the second most common location for minor gland tumors (15%–24% of cases), followed by the buccal mucosa (12%–15% of cases). Labial tumors are significantly more common in the upper lip, which accounts for 74%–87% of all lip tumors (Table 11.10). Although mucoceles are commonly found on the lower lip, this is a surprisingly rare site for salivary gland tumors.

Significant differences in the percentage of malignancies and the relative frequency of various tumors can be noted for different minor salivary gland sites. As shown in Table 11.11, 41%–51% of palatal tumors and 30%–59% of buccal mucosa tumors are malignant, similar to the overall prevalence of malignancy in all minor salivary gland sites combined. In the upper lip, however, only 9%–25% of

TABLE 11.7 Minor Salivary Gland Tumors

	da Silva et al. (Brazil, 2018)	Jones et al. (United Kingdom, 2008)	Pires et al. (United States, 2007)	Ellis et al. (United States, 1991)	Waldron et al. (United States, 1988)
Total number of cases	1114	455	546	3355	426
Benign Tumors					
Pleomorphic adenoma	35.5%	40.4%	33.2%	38.1%	40.8%
"Monomorphic" adenoma (canalicular and basal cell adenoma)	3.0%	15.2%	9.2%	4.5%	10.8%
Other benign tumors	7.7%	6.6%	13.5%	8.8%	5.9%
Total	46.2%	62.2%	55.9%	51.3%	57.5%
Malignant Tumors					
Mucoepidermoid carcinoma	18.0%	13.0%	22.9%	21.5%	15.3%
Acinic cell carcinoma*	1.6%	1.3%	3.8%	3.5%	3.5%
Adenoid cystic carcinoma	12.6%	11.4%	6.4%	7.7%	9.4%
Malignant mixed tumor	1.4%	2.4%	0.4%	1.7%	1.4%
Polymorphous adenocarcinoma	13.9%	6.2%	5.1%	2.2%	11.0%
Other malignant tumors	6.2%	3.5%	5.5%	12.1%	1.9%
Total	53.8%	37.8%	44.1%	48.7%	42.5%

*Incidence numbers for acinic cell carcinoma are probably high because they often predate recognition of secretory carcinoma, which has similar features.

TABLE 11.8 Location of Minor Salivary Gland Tumors

Author (Year)	Number of Cases	Palate	Lips	Buccal	Retromolar	Floor of Mouth	Tongue	Other
Waldron et al. (1988)	426	42%	22%	15%	5%	5%	1%	9%
Ellis et al. (1991)	3355	44%	21%	12%	2%	3%	5%	12%
Buchner et al. (2007)	380	54%	22%	14%	5%	3%	1%	0%
Jones et al. (2008)	455	51%	24%	12%	2%	2%	2%	8%
da Silva et al. (2018)	1114	57%	15%	13%	4%	2%	3%	6%

tumors are malignant because of the high prevalence of the canalicular adenoma, which has a special affinity for this location. In contrast, although lower lip tumors are uncommon, 43%– 86% are malignant (mostly mucoepidermoid carcinomas). Up to 95% of retromolar tumors are malignant, also because of a predominance of mucoepidermoid carcinomas. Unfortunately, most tumors in the floor of the mouth and tongue are also malignant.

Salivary tumor pathology has been revolutionized over the past decade by the identification of a variety of genetic mutations in these neoplasms. Not only do such genetic abnormalities help us to understand the pathogenesis of these tumors, the specificity of such mutations often plays a critical role in helping to establish the final diagnosis and subsequent treatment. Table 11.12 lists a number of genetic abnormalities that have been associated with various salivary tumors.

TABLE 11.9 Palatal Salivary Gland Tumors

	da Silva et al. (Brazil, 2018)	Gao et al. (China, 2017)	Buchner et al. (United States, 2007)	Pires et al. (United States, 2007)	Ellis et al. (United States, 1991)
Total number of cases	631	1105	206	181	1478
Benign Tumors					
Pleomorphic adenoma	42.8%	39.0%	46.6%	39.8%	48.2%
Other benign tumors	5.9%	6.8%	10.2%	13.2%	5.0%
Total	48.7%	45.8%	56.8%	53.0%	53.2%
Malignant Tumors					
Mucoepidermoid carcinoma	17.1%	18.2%	18.9%	23.8%	20.7%
Acinic cell carcinoma*	1.1%	2.0%	0.0%	2.2%	1.4%
Adenoid cystic carcinoma	13.0%	17.2%	8.7%	7.7%	8.3%
Malignant mixed tumor	1.6%	4.9%	0.5%	0.0%	2.4%
Polymorphous adenocarcinoma	14.4%	2.5%	10.2%	6.1%	3.0%
Other malignant tumors	4.1%	9.4%	4.9%	7.2%	11.0%
Total	51.3%	54.2%	43.2%	47.0%	46.8%

*Incidence numbers for acinic cell carcinoma are probably high because they predate recognition of secretory carcinoma, which has similar features.

TABLE 11.10 Location of Labial Salivary Gland Tumors

Author (Year)	Number of Cases	Upper Lip	Lower Lip
Waldron et al. (1988)	93	85%	15%
Neville et al. (1988)	103	84%	16%
Ellis et al. (1991)	536	77%	23%
Pires et al. (2007)	144	74%	26%
Jones et al. (2008)	107	87%	13%
da Silva et al. (2018)	163	82%	18%

◆ PLEOMORPHIC ADENOMA (BENIGN MIXED TUMOR)

The **pleomorphic adenoma,** or **benign mixed tumor,** is easily the most common salivary neoplasm. It accounts for 45%– 63% of parotid tumors, 53%–72% of submandibular tumors, and 33%–41% of minor gland tumors.

Pleomorphic adenomas are epithelial tumors characterized by a mixture of ductal cells, myoepithelium-like cells, and mesenchymal metaplasia. A remarkable microscopic diversity can exist from one tumor to the next, as well as in different areas of the same tumor. The terms *pleomorphic adenoma* and *mixed tumor* both represent attempts to describe this tumor's unusual histopathologic features, but neither term is entirely accurate. Although the basic tumor pattern is highly variable, rarely are the individual cells actually pleomorphic. (However, focal minor atypia is acceptable.) Likewise, although the tumor often has a prominent mesenchyme-appearing "stromal" component, it is not truly a mixed neoplasm that is derived from more than one germ layer. Cytogenetic analysis has shown translocations in approximately 70% of pleomorphic adenomas, primarily involving *pleomorphic adenoma gene 1 (PLAG1)* or the *high-mobility group AT-hook 2 gene (HMGA2).*

Clinical and Radiographic Features

Regardless of the site of origin, the pleomorphic adenoma typically appears as a painless, slowly growing, firm mass (Figs. 11.34–11.36). The patient may be aware of the lesion for many months or years before seeking a diagnosis. The

TABLE 11.11 Intraoral Minor Salivary Gland Tumors: Percentage Malignant by Site

Author (Year)	Palate	Upper Lip	Lower Lip	Buccal	Retromolar	Floor of Mouth	Tongue
Waldron et al. (1988)	42%	14%	86%	46%	91%	80%	75%
Ellis et al. (1991)	47%	22%	60%	50%	90%	88%	86%
Buchner et al. (2007)	43%	9%	56%	37%	95%	69%	60%
Jones et al. (2008)	41%	15%	43%	30%	88%	75%	71%
da Silva et al. (2018)	51%	25%	48%	59%	93%	64%	89%

TABLE 11.12 Genetic Abnormalities of Various Salivary Gland Tumors

Tumor	Associated Gene Mutation/ Translocation/Rearrangement	Note
Pleomorphic adenoma	*PLAG1* or *HMGA2* gene rearrangement	
Basal cell adenoma	*CTNNB1* mutation	
Sialadenoma papilliferum	*BRAF* V600E mutation	Not seen in oncocytic variants
Mucoepidermoid carcinoma	*MAML2* fusion with *CRTC1* or *CRTC3*	
Secretory carcinoma	*ETV6::NTRK3* gene fusion	*ETV6::RET* or *ETV6::MET* fusions are less common
Carcinoma ex pleomorphic adenoma	*PLAG1* or *HMGA2* gene rearrangement	
Adenoid cystic carcinoma	*MYB::NFIB* gene fusion	
Polymorphous adenocarcinoma	*PRKD1* hotspot mutation	
Cribriform adenocarcinoma of salivary gland	*PRKD1, PRKD2,* or *PRKD3* gene rearrangement	
Clear cell carcinoma	*EWSR1* gene rearrangement	
Microsecretory adenocarcinoma	*MEF2C::SS18* gene fusion	

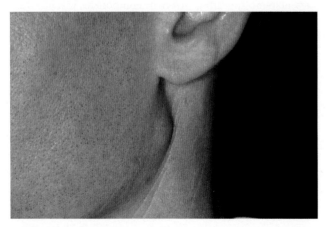

• **Fig. 11.34 Pleomorphic Adenoma.** Small, firm nodule located below the left ear in the parotid gland. (Courtesy of Dr. Mike Hansen.)

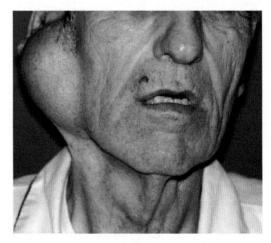

• **Fig. 11.35 Pleomorphic adenoma.** Slowly growing tumor of the parotid gland.

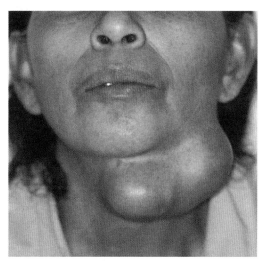

• **Fig. 11.36 Pleomorphic Adenoma.** Tumor of the submandibular gland. (Courtesy of Dr. Román Carlos.)

tumor can occur at any age but is most common in young and middle-aged adults between the ages of 30 and 60. Pleomorphic adenoma is also the most common primary salivary gland tumor to develop during childhood. There is a slight female predilection.

Most pleomorphic adenomas of the parotid gland occur in the superficial lobe and present as a swelling overlying the mandibular ramus in front of the ear. Facial nerve palsy and pain are rare. Initially, the tumor is movable but becomes less mobile as it grows larger. If neglected, then the lesion can grow to grotesque proportions. About 10% of parotid mixed tumors develop within the deep lobe of the gland beneath the facial nerve (Fig. 11.37). Sometimes these lesions grow in a medial direction between the ascending ramus and stylomandibular ligament, resulting in a dumbbell-shaped tumor that appears as a mass of the lateral pharyngeal wall or soft palate. On rare occasions, bilateral pleomorphic adenomas of the parotid glands have been reported, developing in either a synchronous or metachronous fashion.

The palate is the most common site for minor gland mixed tumors, accounting for approximately 50%–65% of intraoral examples. This is followed by the upper lip (19%–27%) and buccal mucosa (13%– 17%). Palatal tumors almost always are found on the posterior lateral aspect of the palate, presenting as smooth-surfaced, dome-shaped masses (Fig. 11.38). If the tumor is traumatized, then secondary ulceration may occur. Because of the tightly bound nature of the hard palate mucosa, tumors in this location are not movable, although those in the lip or buccal mucosa frequently are mobile (Fig. 11.39).

Histopathologic Features

The pleomorphic adenoma is typically a well-circumscribed, encapsulated tumor (Fig. 11.40). However, the capsule may be incomplete or show infiltration by tumor cells. This lack of complete encapsulation is more common for minor gland

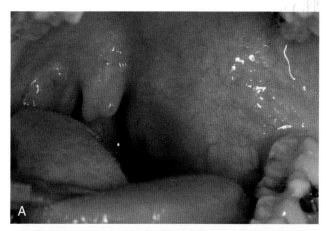
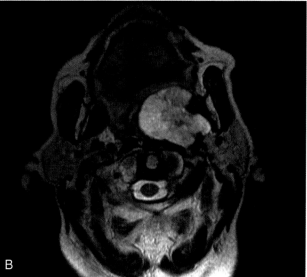

• **Fig. 11.37 Pleomorphic Adenoma. A,** Large tumor from the deep lobe of the parotid gland, which has resulted in a firm mass of the lateral soft palate. **B,** Contrast-enhanced axial magnetic resonance image (MRI) of a tumor of the deep lobe of the parotid gland. (Courtesy of Dr. Terry Day.)

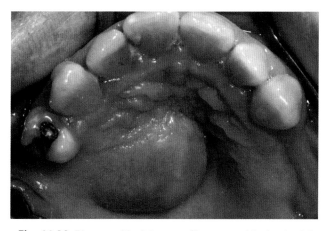

• **Fig. 11.38 Pleomorphic Adenoma.** Firm mass of the hard palate lateral to the midline.

tumors, especially along the superficial aspect of palatal tumors beneath the epithelial surface.

The tumor is composed of a mixture of glandular epithelium and myoepithelium-like cells within a mesenchyme-like background. The ratio of the epithelial elements and

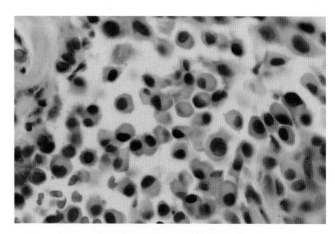

• **Fig. 11.39 Pleomorphic Adenoma.** Nodular mass of the right upper lip/buccal mucosa. (Courtesy of Dr. Manuel LaRosa.)

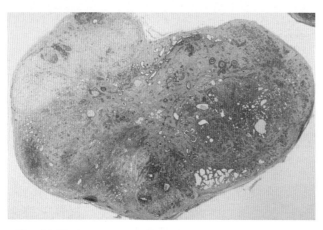

• **Fig. 11.40 Pleomorphic Adenoma.** Low-power view showing a well-circumscribed, encapsulated tumor mass. Even at this power, the variable microscopic pattern of the tumor is evident.

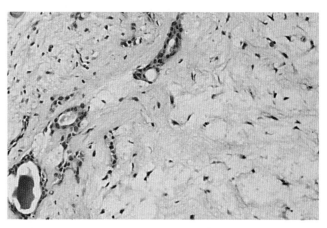

• **Fig. 11.41 Pleomorphic Adenoma.** Plasmacytoid myoepithelial cells.

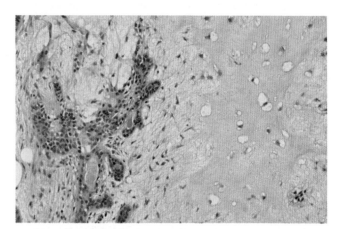

• **Fig. 11.42 Pleomorphic Adenoma.** Ductal structures *(left)* with associated myxomatous background *(right)*.

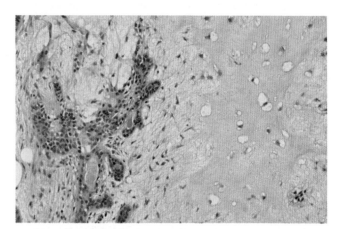

• **Fig. 11.43 Pleomorphic Adenoma.** Chondroid material *(right)* with adjacent ductal epithelium and myoepithelial cells.

the mesenchyme-like component is highly variable among different tumors. Some tumors may consist almost entirely of background "stroma." Others are highly cellular with little background alteration.

The epithelium often forms ducts and cystic structures or may occur as islands or sheets of cells. Keratinizing squamous cells and mucus-producing cells also can be seen. Myoepithelial cells often make up a large percentage of the tumor cells and have a variable morphology, sometimes appearing angular or spindled. Some myoepithelial cells are rounded and demonstrate an eccentric nucleus and eosinophilic hyalinized cytoplasm, thus resembling plasma cells (Fig. 11.41). These characteristic plasmacytoid myoepithelial cells are more prominent in tumors arising in the minor glands.

The highly characteristic "stromal" changes are believed to be produced by the myoepithelial cells. Extensive accumulation of mucoid material may occur between the tumor cells, resulting in a myxomatous background (Fig. 11.42). Vacuolar degeneration of cells in these areas can produce a chondroid appearance (Fig. 11.43). In many tumors, the stroma exhibits areas of an eosinophilic, hyalinized change (Fig. 11.44). At times, fat or osteoid also is seen.

Occasionally, salivary tumors are seen that are composed almost entirely of myoepithelial cells with no ductal elements. Such tumors often are called **myoepitheliomas,** although they probably represent one end of the spectrum of mixed tumors.

Treatment and Prognosis

Pleomorphic adenomas are best treated by surgical excision. For lesions in the superficial lobe of the parotid gland, superficial parotidectomy with identification and preservation of the facial nerve traditionally has been recommended, although some surgeons may opt for less aggressive partial superficial parotidectomy or extracapsular dissection. However, local enucleation should be avoided because the entire tumor may not be removed or the capsule may be violated, resulting in seeding of the tumor bed. For tumors of the deep lobe of the parotid, total parotidectomy is usually necessary, also with preservation of the facial nerve, if possible. Submandibular tumors are best treated by total removal of the gland with the tumor. Tumors of the hard palate usually are excised down to periosteum, including the overlying mucosa. In other oral sites the lesion often enucleates easily through the incision site.

With adequate surgery the prognosis is excellent, with a cure rate of more than 95%. The risk of recurrence appears to be lower for tumors of the minor glands. Conservative enucleation of parotid tumors often results in recurrence, with management of these cases made difficult as a result of multifocal seeding of the primary tumor bed. In such cases, multiple recurrences are not unusual and may necessitate adjuvant radiation therapy. Tumors with a predominantly myxoid appearance are more susceptible to recur than those with other microscopic patterns.

Malignant degeneration is a potential complication, resulting in a **carcinoma ex pleomorphic adenoma** (see page 499). The risk of malignant transformation is probably small, but it may occur in as many as 3%–4% of all cases. This risk increases with the duration of the tumor.

◆ ONCOCYTOMA (OXYPHILIC ADENOMA)

The **oncocytoma** is a benign salivary gland tumor composed of large epithelial cells known as **oncocytes.** The prefix *onco-* is derived from the Greek word *onkoustai,* which means *to swell.* The swollen granular cytoplasm of oncocytes is due to excessive accumulation of mitochondria. Focal oncocytic metaplasia of salivary ductal and acinar cells is a common finding that is related to patient age; oncocytes are uncommon in persons younger than 50, but they can be found in almost all individuals by age 70. In addition to salivary glands, oncocytes have been identified in a number of other organs, especially the thyroid, parathyroid, and kidney. The oncocytoma is a rare neoplasm, representing approximately 1% of all salivary tumors.

Clinical Features

The oncocytoma is predominantly a tumor of older adults, with peak prevalence in the sixth to eighth decades of life. No significant sex predilection has been observed. Oncocytomas occur primarily in the major salivary glands, especially the parotid gland, which accounts for about 85%–90% of all cases. Oncocytomas of the minor salivary glands are exceedingly rare.

The tumor appears as a firm, slowly growing, painless mass that rarely exceeds 4 cm in diameter. Parotid oncocytomas usually are found in the superficial lobe and are clinically indistinguishable from other benign tumors. On occasion, bilateral tumors can occur, although these may represent examples of **oncocytosis (multinodular oncocytic hyperplasia)** (see next topic).

Histopathologic Features

The oncocytoma is usually a well-circumscribed tumor that is composed of sheets of large polyhedral cells (oncocytes), with abundant granular, eosinophilic cytoplasm (Fig. 11.45). Sometimes these cells form an alveolar or glandular pattern.

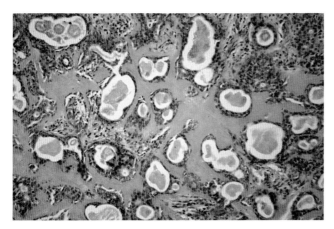

• **Fig. 11.44 Pleomorphic Adenoma.** Many of the ducts and myoepithelial cells are surrounded by a hyalinized, eosinophilic background alteration.

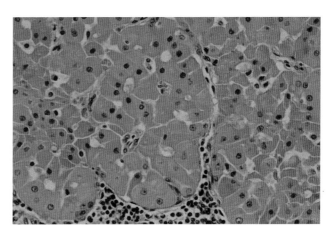

• **Fig. 11.45 Oncocytoma.** Sheet of large, eosinophilic oncocytes.

The cells have centrally located nuclei that can vary from small and hyperchromatic to large and vesicular. Little stroma is present, usually in the form of thin fibrovascular septa. An associated lymphocytic infiltrate may be noted.

The granularity of the cells corresponds to an overabundance of mitochondria, which can be demonstrated by electron microscopy. These granules also can be identified on light microscopic examination with a phosphotungstic acid hematoxylin (PTAH) stain. The cells also contain glycogen, as evidenced by their positive staining with the periodic acid-Schiff (PAS) technique but by negative PAS staining after digestion with diastase.

Oncocytomas may contain variable numbers of cells with a clear cytoplasm. In rare instances, these clear cells may compose most of the lesion and create difficulty in distinguishing the tumor from low-grade salivary clear cell adenocarcinoma or metastatic renal cell carcinoma.

Treatment and Prognosis

Oncocytomas are best treated by surgical excision. In the parotid gland, this usually entails partial parotidectomy (lobectomy) to avoid violation of the tumor capsule. The facial nerve should be preserved whenever possible. For tumors in the submandibular gland, treatment consists of total removal of the gland. Oncocytomas of the oral minor salivary glands should be removed with a small margin of normal surrounding tissue.

The prognosis after removal is good, with a low rate of recurrence. However, oncocytomas of the sinonasal glands can be locally aggressive and have been considered to be low-grade malignancies. Rare examples of histopathologically malignant oncocytomas (**oncocytic carcinoma**) also have been reported. Unfortunately, these carcinomas have a relatively poor prognosis.

◆ ONCOCYTOSIS (MULTINODULAR ONCOCYTIC HYPERPLASIA)

Oncocytic metaplasia is the transformation of ductal and acinar cells to oncocytes. Such cells are uncommon before the age of 50; however, as people get older, occasional oncocytes are common findings in the salivary glands. Focal oncocytic metaplasia also may be a feature of other salivary gland tumors. **Oncocytosis** refers to both the proliferation and the accumulation of oncocytes within salivary gland tissue. It may mimic a tumor, both clinically and microscopically, but it also is considered to be a metaplastic process rather than a neoplastic one.

Clinical Features

Oncocytosis is found primarily in the parotid gland; however, in rare instances, it may involve the submandibular or minor salivary glands. It can be an incidental finding in otherwise normal salivary gland tissue, but it may be

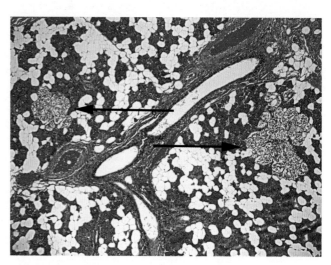

• **Fig. 11.46 Oncocytosis.** Multifocal collections of clear oncocytes *(arrows)* in the parotid gland.

extensive enough to produce clinical swelling. Usually the proliferation is multifocal and nodular, but sometimes the entire gland can be replaced by oncocytes (**diffuse hyperplastic oncocytosis).** As with other oncocytic proliferations, oncocytosis occurs most frequently in older adults.

Histopathologic Features

Microscopic examination usually reveals focal nodular collections of oncocytes within the salivary gland tissue. These enlarged cells are polyhedral and demonstrate abundant granular, eosinophilic cytoplasm as a result of the proliferation of mitochondria. On occasion, these cells may have a clear cytoplasm from the accumulation of glycogen (Fig. 11.46). The multifocal nature of the proliferation may be confused with that of a metastatic tumor, especially when the oncocytes are clear in appearance.

Treatment and Prognosis

Oncocytosis is a benign condition and often is discovered only as an incidental finding. No further treatment is necessary, and the prognosis is excellent.

◆ WARTHIN TUMOR (PAPILLARY CYSTADENOMA LYMPHOMATOSUM)

Warthin tumor is a benign neoplasm that occurs almost exclusively in the parotid gland. Although it is less common than the pleomorphic adenoma, it represents the second most common benign parotid tumor, accounting for 7.7%–22.4% of all parotid neoplasms in large surveys (Table 11.5). However, several papers from central Europe have reported an increased incidence of Warthin tumor in recent years, surpassing that of pleomorphic adenoma in this region. The name **adenolymphoma** also has been used for this tumor, but this term should be avoided because it overemphasizes the lymphoid component and may give the mistaken impression that the lesion is a type of lymphoma. Analyses of the epithelial and lymphoid components of the Warthin tumor usually have shown both to be polyclonal; this suggests that this lesion may not represent a neoplasm but would be better classified as a tumorlike process. Only 10% of tumors show genetic alterations.

The pathogenesis of Warthin tumor is uncertain. The traditional hypothesis suggests that it arises from heterotopic salivary gland tissue found within parotid lymph nodes. However, researchers have also suggested that these tumors may develop from a proliferation of salivary gland ductal epithelium that is associated with secondary formation of lymphoid tissue. A number of studies have demonstrated a strong association between the development of this tumor and smoking. Smokers have an eightfold greater risk for Warthin tumor than do nonsmokers. Obesity recently has been shown to be another potential risk factor.

Clinical Features

The Warthin tumor usually appears as a slowly growing, painless, nodular mass of the parotid gland (Fig. 11.47). It may be firm or fluctuant to palpation. The tumor most frequently occurs in the tail of the parotid near the angle of the mandible, and it may be noted for many months before the patient seeks a diagnosis. One unique feature is the tendency of Warthin tumor to occur bilaterally, which has been noted in 5%–17% of reported cases. Most of these bilateral tumors do not occur simultaneously but are metachronous (occurring at different times).

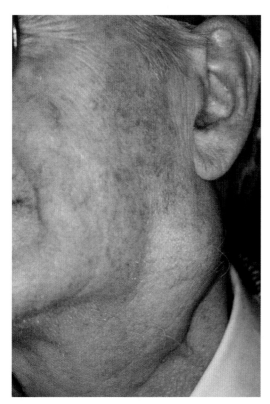

• **Fig. 11.47 Warthin Tumor.** Mass in the tail of the parotid gland. (Courtesy of Dr. George Blozis.)

In rare instances, the Warthin tumor has been reported within the submandibular gland or minor salivary glands. However, because the lymphoid component is often less pronounced in these extraparotid sites, the pathologist should exercise caution to avoid overdiagnosis of a lesion better classified as a papillary cystadenoma or a salivary duct cyst with oncocytic ductal metaplasia.

Warthin tumor most often occurs in older adults, with peak prevalence in the sixth and seventh decades of life. The observed frequency of this tumor is much lower in blacks than in whites. Most studies show a decided male predilection, with some early studies demonstrating a male-to-female ratio up to 10:1. However, more recent investigations show a more balanced sex ratio. Because Warthin tumors have been associated with cigarette smoking, this changing sex ratio may be a reflection of a more equal prevalence of smoking in women over the past few decades. This association with smoking also may help explain the frequent bilaterality of the tumor, because any tumorigenic effects of smoking would be manifested in both parotids.

Histopathologic Features

The Warthin tumor has one of the most distinctive histopathologic patterns of any tumor in the body. Although the term **papillary cystadenoma lymphomatosum** is cumbersome, it accurately describes the salient microscopic features.

The tumor is composed of a mixture of ductal epithelium and a lymphoid stroma (Figs. 11.48 and 11.49). The epithelium is oncocytic in nature, forming uniform rows of cells surrounding cystic spaces. The cells have abundant, finely granular eosinophilic cytoplasm and are arranged in two layers. The inner luminal layer consists of tall columnar cells with centrally placed, palisaded, and slightly hyperchromatic nuclei. Beneath this is a second layer of cuboidal or polygonal cells with more vesicular nuclei. The lining epithelium demonstrates multiple papillary infoldings that protrude into the cystic spaces. Focal areas of squamous metaplasia or mucous cell prosoplasia may be seen. The epithelium is supported by

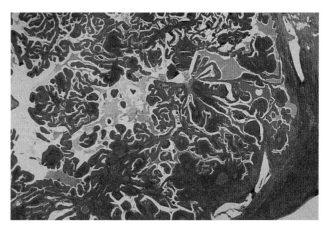

• **Fig. 11.48 Warthin Tumor.** Low-power view showing a papillary cystic tumor with a lymphoid stroma.

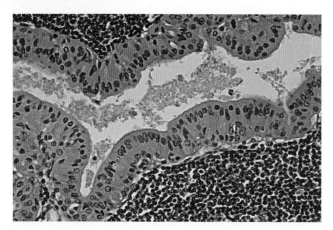

• **Fig. 11.49 Warthin Tumor.** High-power view of epithelial lining showing double row of oncocytes with adjacent lymphoid stroma.

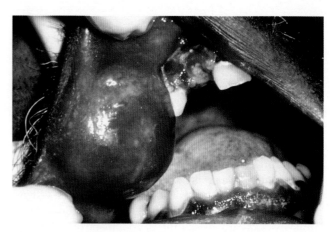

• **Fig. 11.50 Canalicular Adenoma.** Mass in the upper lip. (Courtesy of Dr. John Fantasia.)

a lymphoid stroma that frequently shows germinal center formation.

Treatment and Prognosis

Surgical removal is the treatment of choice for most patients with Warthin tumor. The procedure usually is easily accomplished because of the superficial location of the tumor. Some surgeons prefer local resection with minimal surrounding tissue; others opt for superficial parotidectomy to avoid violating the tumor capsule and because a tentative diagnosis may not be known preoperatively. If a confident diagnosis of Warthin tumor can be made by fine-needle aspiration cytology of a non-suspicious parotid growth, some clinicians will elect to manage the patient conservatively with regular follow-up visits rather than surgery.

A 2%–6% recurrence rate has been reported following surgery. Many authors, however, believe that the tumor is frequently multicentric in nature; therefore, it is difficult to determine whether these are true recurrences or secondary tumor sites. Malignant Warthin tumors (**carcinoma ex papillary cystadenoma lymphomatosum**) have been reported but are exceedingly rare.

◆ MONOMORPHIC ADENOMA

The term **monomorphic adenoma** originally was used to describe a group of benign salivary gland tumors demonstrating a more uniform histopathologic pattern than the common pleomorphic adenoma. In some classification schemes, a variety of tumors were included under the broad heading of monomorphic adenoma, including Warthin tumor, oncocytoma, basal cell adenoma, and canalicular adenoma. Other authors have used this term more specifically as a synonym just for the basal cell adenoma or canalicular adenoma. Because of its ambiguous nature, the term *monomorphic adenoma* probably should be avoided, and each of the tumors mentioned should be referred to by its more specific name.

◆ CANALICULAR ADENOMA

The **canalicular adenoma** is an uncommon tumor that occurs almost exclusively in the minor salivary glands. Because of its uniform microscopic pattern, the canalicular adenoma also has been called a *monomorphic adenoma.* However, because this term also has been applied to other tumors, its use probably should be discontinued. Likewise, the term **basal cell adenoma** sometimes has been used synonymously for this tumor but should be avoided because it refers to a separate tumor with different clinical features (see next topic). Based on its immunohistochemical profile, the canalicular adenoma may arise from intercalated duct luminal cells.

Clinical Features

The canalicular adenoma shows a striking predilection for the upper lip, with 66%–78% occurring in this location. It represents the first or second most common tumor (along with pleomorphic adenoma) of the upper lip. The buccal mucosa is the second most common site. Occurrence in other minor salivary glands is uncommon, and canalicular adenomas of the parotid gland are rare.

The tumor nearly always occurs in older adults, with peak prevalence in the seventh decade of life. There is a definite female predominance, ranging from 1.5 to 1.8 females for each male.

The canalicular adenoma appears as a slowly growing, painless mass that usually ranges from several millimeters to 2 cm (Fig. 11.50). It may be firm or somewhat fluctuant to palpation. The overlying mucosa may be normal in color or bluish and can be mistaken for a mucocele. However, mucoceles of the upper lip are rare. In some instances, the lesion has been noted to be multifocal, with multiple separate tumors discovered in the upper lip or buccal mucosa.

Histopathologic Features

The microscopic pattern of canalicular adenoma is monomorphic in nature. This pattern is characterized by single-layered cords of columnar or cuboidal epithelial cells with

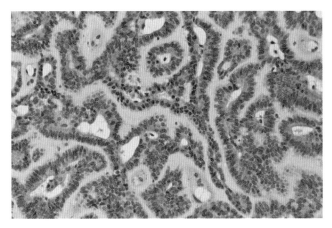

• **Fig. 11.51 Canalicular Adenoma.** Uniform columnar cells forming canal-like ductal structures.

deeply basophilic nuclei (Fig. 11.51). In some areas, adjacent parallel rows of cells may be seen, resulting in a bilayered appearance of the tumor cords. These cells enclose ductal structures, sometimes in the form of long canals. Larger cystic spaces often are created, and the epithelium may demonstrate papillary projections into the cystic lumina. Small groups of metaplastic cells, known as squamous balls or morules, sometimes are found in the cystic spaces. The tumor cells are supported by a loose connective tissue stroma with prominent vascularity. Unlike the appearance in pleomorphic adenomas, stromal alterations, such as chondroid metaplasia, do not occur. A thin, fibrous capsule often surrounds the tumor, although satellite islands are observed in the surrounding salivary gland tissue in approximately 13%–24% of cases, which explains the tendency for multifocal tumors.

Treatment and Prognosis

The canalicular adenoma is best treated by local surgical excision. Recurrence is uncommon and actually may represent cases that are multifocal in nature.

◆ BASAL CELL ADENOMA

The **basal cell adenoma** is a benign salivary tumor that derives its name from the basaloid appearance of the tumor cells. It is an uncommon neoplasm that represents only 1%–4% of all salivary tumors. Because of its uniform histopathologic appearance, it often has been classified as one of the monomorphic adenomas. However, as mentioned previously, this term probably should be avoided because of its imprecise and frequently confusing definition. In addition, ultrastructural and immunohistochemical studies have shown that basal cell adenomas are not necessarily composed of only one cell type but sometimes of a combination of salivary ductal epithelium and myoepithelial cells. The basal cell adenoma shows some histopathologic similarity to the canalicular adenoma; in the past, these two terms sometimes were used synonymously. However, histopathologic and clinical differences warrant that they be considered as distinct entities.

Clinical Features

Unlike the canalicular adenoma, the basal cell adenoma is primarily a tumor of the parotid gland, with around 75% of all cases occurring there. However, the minor glands represent the second most common site, specifically the glands of the upper lip and buccal mucosa. The tumor can occur at any age but is most common in middle-aged and older adults, with peak prevalence in the seventh decade of life. The tumor appears to be more common in women, with some studies showing as high as a 2:1 female-to-male ratio.

Clinically, the basal cell adenoma appears as a slowly growing, freely movable mass similar to a pleomorphic adenoma. Most tumors are less than 3 cm in diameter. Parotid tumors usually are located within the superficial lobe of the gland.

One subtype, the **membranous basal cell adenoma,** deserves separate mention. This form of the tumor appears to be hereditary, often occurring in combination with skin appendage tumors, such as **dermal cylindromas** and **trichoepitheliomas (Brooke-Spiegler syndrome).** Multiple bilateral tumors may develop within the parotids. Because these tumors often bear a histopathologic resemblance to the skin tumors, they also have been called **dermal analogue tumors.**

Histopathologic Features

The basal cell adenoma is usually encapsulated or well circumscribed. The most common subtype is the solid variant, which consists of multiple islands and cords of epithelial cells that are supported by a small amount of fibrous stroma. The peripheral cells of these islands are palisaded and cuboidal to columnar in shape, similar to the microscopic appearance of basal cell carcinoma. These peripheral cells are frequently hyperchromatic; the central cells of the islands tend to have paler staining nuclei. The central cells occasionally form eddies or keratin pearls.

The trabecular subtype demonstrates narrow cordlike epithelial strands (Fig. 11.52). The tubular subtype is characterized by the formation of small, round, ductlike structures. Some basal cell adenomas demonstrate zones with a cribriform pattern that can mimic adenoid cystic carcinoma. Frequently, a mixture of histopathologic subtypes is seen. Immunohistochemical expression of nuclear β-catenin in the basal cell adenoma can help to distinguish this tumor from adenoid cystic carcinoma. One recent study found that 60% of basal cell adenomas harbored mutations of the *CTNNB1* gene.

The membranous basal cell adenoma exhibits multiple large lobular islands of tumor that are molded together in a jigsaw puzzle fashion. These islands are surrounded by a thick layer of hyaline material, which represents reduplicated

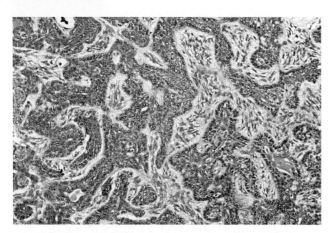

• **Fig. 11.52 Basal Cell Adenoma.** Parotid tumor showing cords of basaloid cells arranged in a trabecular pattern.

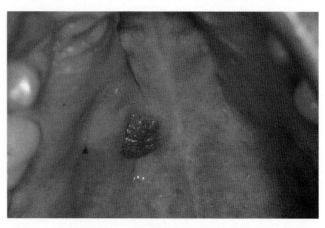

• **Fig. 11.53 Sialadenoma Papilliferum.** Exophytic papillary mass on the palate. (Courtesy of Dr. Peter Lyu.)

basement membrane. Similar hyaline droplets also are often found among the epithelial cells. The microscopic appearance is similar to that of a dermal cylindroma, one of the skin tumors with which it is often associated.

Treatment and Prognosis

The treatment of basal cell adenoma is similar to that of pleomorphic adenoma and consists of complete surgical removal. Recurrence is rare for most histopathologic subtypes. However, the membranous subtype has a 25%–37% recurrence rate, possibly related to its multifocal nature.

The malignant counterpart of the basal cell adenoma is the **basal cell adenocarcinoma.** Most basal cell adenocarcinomas arise *de novo,* but some examples develop from malignant degeneration of a preexisting basal cell adenoma. Fortunately, these tumors have a relatively good prognosis; although local recurrence is common, the tumor rarely metastasizes or results in death.

◆ DUCTAL PAPILLOMAS (SIALADENOMA PAPILLIFERUM; INTRADUCTAL PAPILLOMA; INVERTED DUCTAL PAPILLOMA)

A number of salivary gland tumors can be characterized microscopically by a papillomatous pattern, the most common being Warthin tumor (papillary cystadenoma lymphomatosum). The **sialadenoma papilliferum, intraductal papilloma,** and **inverted ductal papilloma** are three rare salivary tumors that also show unique papillomatous features.

It also should be mentioned that, on occasion, the common squamous papilloma (see page 355) of the oral mucosa will arise at the site where a minor salivary gland duct merges with the surface epithelium. Because of this location, such squamous papillomas may contain scattered mucous cells within the exophytic papillary growth, and these lesions have sometimes been called *ductal papillomas.* However, it should be emphasized that these lesions are surface papillomas and not primary salivary gland tumors.

Clinical Features

The sialadenoma papilliferum occurs almost exclusively in the minor salivary glands, especially on the palate (80% of all cases), although it also has been reported in the parotid gland. It usually is seen in middle-aged and older adults and has a 1.7:1 male-to-female ratio. The tumor appears as an exophytic, papillary surface growth that is clinically similar to the common squamous papilloma (Fig. 11.53).

The intraductal papilloma is an ill-defined lesion that often has been confused with other salivary gland lesions, such as the papillary cystadenoma. It usually occurs in adults and is most common in the minor salivary glands, where it appears as a submucosal swelling.

The inverted ductal papilloma is a rare tumor that has been described only in the minor salivary glands of adults. The lower lip and mandibular vestibule are the most common locations. The lesion usually appears as an asymptomatic nodule, which sometimes may show a pit or indentation in the overlying surface mucosa (Fig. 11.54).

Histopathologic Features

At low-power magnification, the sialadenoma papilliferum is somewhat similar to the squamous papilloma, exhibiting multiple exophytic papillary projections that are covered by stratified squamous epithelium. This epithelium is contiguous with a proliferation of papillomatous ductal epithelium found below the surface and extending downward into the deeper connective tissues (Fig. 11.55). Multiple ductal lumina are formed, which characteristically are lined by a double-rowed layer of cells consisting of a luminal layer of tall columnar cells and a basilar layer of smaller cuboidal cells. These ductal cells sometimes have an oncocytic appearance. An inflammatory infiltrate of plasma cells, lymphocytes, and neutrophils is characteristically present.

Because of their microscopic similarity, the sialadenoma papilliferum has been considered to be an analogue of the cutaneous syringocystadenoma papilliferum. This concept is supported by the consistent finding of *BRAF* V600E mutations in classic sialadenoma papilliferum, which also have

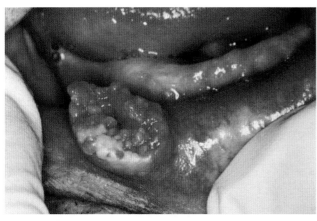

• **Fig. 11.54 Inverted Ductal Papilloma.** Exophytic mass with central papillary projections on the lower labial mucosa. (Courtesy of Dr. Amy Bogardus.)

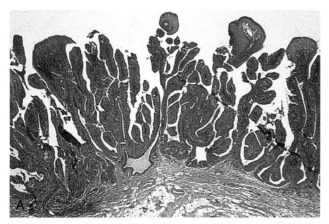

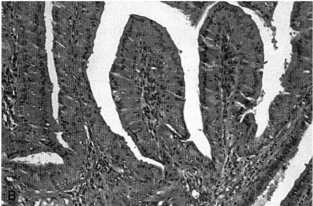

• **Fig. 11.55 Sialadenoma Papilliferum. A,** Low-power view showing a papillary surface tumor with associated ductal structures in the superficial lamina propria. **B,** High-power view of cystic areas lined by papillary, oncocytic epithelium.

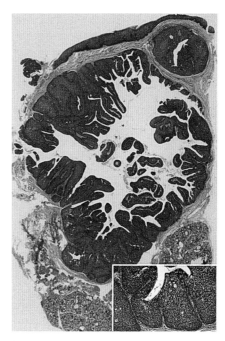

• **Fig. 11.56 Inverted Ductal Papilloma.** Papillary intraductal proliferation located beneath the mucosal surface. Higher-power view shows both squamous cells and mucous cells *(inset)*. (Courtesy of Dr. Dean K. White.)

into the cystic lumen. In contrast, the inverted ductal papilloma is composed primarily of a proliferation of squamoid epithelium with multiple thick, bulbous papillary projections that fill the ductal lumen (Fig. 11.56). This epithelium may be contiguous with the overlying mucosal epithelium, communicating with the surface through a small pore-like opening. Although the tumor is primarily squamous in nature, the luminal lining cells of the papillary projections are often cuboidal or columnar in shape, with scattered mucus-producing cells. *In situ* hybridization analysis has shown positivity for human papillomavirus (HPV) types 6 and 11 in both the surface and inverted epithelium of some inverted ductal papillomas.

Treatment and Prognosis

All three forms of ductal papilloma are best treated by conservative surgical excision. Recurrence is rare.

◆ MUCOEPIDERMOID CARCINOMA

Mucoepidermoid carcinoma is the most common salivary gland malignancy. Because of its highly variable biologic potential, it was originally called **mucoepidermoid tumor.** The term recognized one subset that acted in a malignant fashion and a second group that appeared to behave in a benign fashion with favorable prognosis. However, researchers later recognized that even low-grade tumors occasionally will exhibit malignant behavior; therefore, the term *mucoepidermoid carcinoma* is the preferred designation.

been identified in 52% of cases of syringocystadenoma papilliferum. However, oncocytic variants of sialadenoma papilliferum do not exhibit this mutation, suggesting that this pattern may represent a distinctly different lesion or subtype.

The intraductal papilloma exhibits a dilated, unicystic structure that is located below the mucosal surface. It is lined by a single or double row of cuboidal or columnar epithelium, which has multiple arborizing papillary projections

The pathogenesis of this tumor is uncertain, although radiation exposure may be one risk factor. Recent series have reported that 59%–86% of mucoepidermoid carcinomas will show *MAML2* rearrangements, resulting in the production of *CRTC1::MAML2* or *CRTC3::MAML2* gene fusions. Such gene rearrangements have been identified more frequently in low- and intermediate-grade tumors.

Clinical Features

Most large series show mucoepidermoid carcinoma to be the most common malignant salivary gland neoplasm, comprising 4%–10% of all major gland tumors and 13%–23% of minor gland tumors. The tumor occurs fairly evenly over a wide age range, extending from the second to seventh decades of life. Rarely is it seen in the first decade of life. However, mucoepidermoid carcinoma is the most common malignant salivary gland tumor in children.

The mucoepidermoid carcinoma is most common in the parotid gland and usually appears as an asymptomatic swelling. Most patients are aware of the lesion for 1 year or less, although some report a mass of many years' duration. Pain or facial nerve palsy may develop, usually in association with high-grade tumors. The minor glands constitute the second most common site, especially the palate (Fig. 11.57). Minor gland tumors also typically appear as asymptomatic swellings, which are sometimes fluctuant and have a blue or red color that can be mistaken clinically for a mucocele. Although the lower lip, floor of mouth, tongue, and retromolar pad areas are uncommon locations for salivary gland neoplasia, the mucoepidermoid carcinoma is the most common salivary tumor in each of these sites (Fig. 11.58). Intraosseous tumors also may develop in the jaws (see page 496).

Histopathologic Features

As its name implies, the *mucoepidermoid carcinoma* is composed of a mixture of mucus-producing cells and squamous (epidermoid) cells (Figs. 11.59–11.61). The mucous cells vary in shape but contain abundant foamy cytoplasm that stains positively with mucin stains. The epidermoid cells are characterized by squamoid features, often demonstrating a polygonal shape, abundant eosinophilic cytoplasm, and intercellular bridges, but rarely overt keratinization. In addition, a third type of cell—the intermediate cell—is typically present and

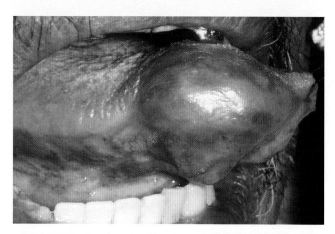

• **Fig. 11.58 Mucoepidermoid Carcinoma.** Mass of the tongue.

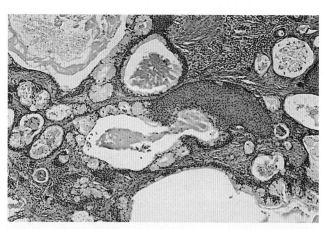

• **Fig. 11.59 Mucoepidermoid Carcinoma.** Low-power view of a moderately well-differentiated tumor showing ductal and cystic spaces surrounded by mucous and squamous cells.

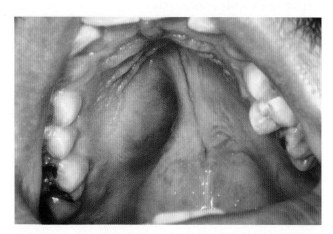

• **Fig. 11.57 Mucoepidermoid Carcinoma.** Blue-pigmented mass of the posterior lateral hard palate. (Courtesy of Dr. James F. Drummond.)

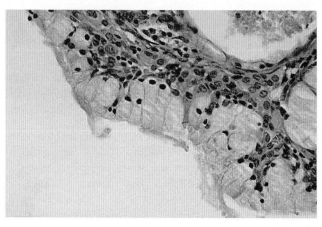

• **Fig. 11.60 Mucoepidermoid Carcinoma.** This low-grade tumor shows numerous large mucous cells surrounding a cystic space.

is believed to be a progenitor of both the mucous and the epidermoid cells. Intermediate cells vary in appearance from small, basaloid ("maternal") cells to slightly larger ovoid cells with scant, pale eosinophilic cytoplasm. Some tumors also show variable numbers of clear cells, which sometimes can predominate the microscopic picture (Fig. 11.62). An associated lymphoid infiltrate is not unusual and may be so prominent in some cases that the lesion can be mistaken for a metastatic tumor within a lymph node. Other variants of mucoepidermoid carcinoma can demonstrate numerous oncocytes or prominent sclerosis of the tumor stroma.

Traditionally, mucoepidermoid carcinomas have been categorized into one of three histopathologic grades based on the following:
1. Amount of cyst formation
2. Degree of cytologic atypia
3. Relative numbers of mucous, epidermoid, and intermediate cells

Low-grade tumors show prominent cyst formation, minimal cellular atypia, and a relatively high proportion of mucous cells. **High-grade** tumors consist of solid islands of squamous and intermediate cells, which can demonstrate considerable pleomorphism and mitotic activity (Fig. 11.63). Mucus-

producing cells may be infrequent, and the tumor sometimes can be difficult to distinguish from squamous cell carcinoma.

Intermediate-grade tumors show features that fall between those of the low-grade and high-grade neoplasms. Cyst formation occurs but is less prominent than that observed in low-grade tumors. All three major cell types are present, but the intermediate cells usually predominate. Cellular atypia may or may not be observed.

However, some authors have found that the relative proportion of the three different cell types does not necessarily correlate with prognosis. To overcome this, two expert groups have proposed evaluation schemes based on significant microscopic parameters, to which relative point values have been assigned to determine the grade of the tumor (Table 11.13).

Treatment and Prognosis

The treatment of mucoepidermoid carcinoma is predicated by the location, histopathologic grade, and clinical stage of the tumor. Early-stage tumors of the parotid often can be treated by subtotal parotidectomy with preservation of the facial nerve. Advanced tumors may necessitate total removal of the parotid gland, with sacrifice of the facial nerve. Submandibular gland tumors are treated by total removal of the gland. Mucoepidermoid carcinomas of the minor glands usually are treated by assured surgical excision. For low-grade neoplasms, only a modest margin of surrounding normal tissue may need to be removed, but high-grade or large tumors warrant wider resection, similar to that required for squamous cell carcinomas. If there is underlying bone destruction, then the involved bone must be excised.

Neck dissection is indicated for patients with clinical evidence of metastatic disease and also may be considered for patients with larger or high-grade tumors. Postoperative radiation therapy also may be used for more aggressive tumors.

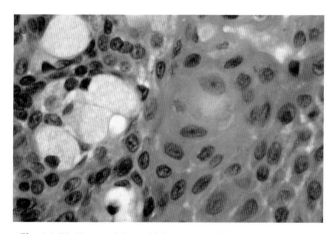

• **Fig. 11.61 Mucoepidermoid Carcinoma.** High-power view showing a sheet of squamous cells with focal mucus-producing cells *(left)*.

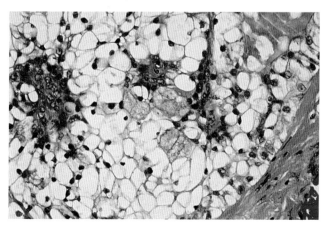

• **Fig. 11.62 Mucoepidermoid Carcinoma.** Clear cell mucoepidermoid carcinoma.

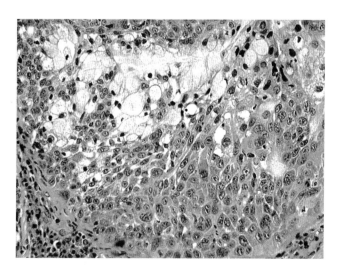

• **Fig. 11.63 Mucoepidermoid Carcinoma.** High-power view showing a sheet of pleomorphic squamous epithelial cells intermixed with mucous and intermediate cells.

TABLE 11.13	Mucoepidermoid Carcinoma: Comparison of Two Grading Systems	
Parameter		**Point Value**
Auclair et al. (1992)		
Intracystic component <20%		2
Neural invasion present		2
Necrosis present		3
Four or more mitoses per 10 high-power fields		3
Anaplasia present		4
Grade		**Total Point Score**
Low		0–4
Intermediate		5–6
High		7–14
Brandwein et al. (2001)		
Intracystic component <25%		2
Tumor front invades in small nests and islands		2
Pronounced nuclear atypia		2
Lymphatic or vascular invasion		3
Bony invasion		3
Greater than four mitoses per 10 high-power fields		3
Perineural spread		3
Necrosis		3
Grade		**Total Point Score**
I		0
II		2–3
III		4 or more

From Auclair PL, Goode RK, Ellis GL: Mucoepidermoid carcinoma of intraoral salivary glands: evaluation and application of grading criteria in 143 cases, *Cancer* 69:2021–2030, 1992; Brandwein MS, Ivanov K, Wallace DI, et al: Mucoepidermoid carcinoma: a clinicopathologic study of 80 patients with special reference to histological grading, *Am J Surg Pathol* 25:835–845, 2001.

The prognosis depends on the grade and stage of the tumor. Patients with low-grade tumors generally have a good prognosis. For most primary sites, local recurrences or regional metastases are uncommon, and around 90%–98% of patients are cured. The prognosis for those with intermediate-grade tumors is only slightly worse than that for low-grade tumors. The outlook for patients with high-grade tumors is more guarded, with only 30%64% of patients surviving. Historically, tumors that exhibit *CRTC1::MAML2* or *CRTC3::MAML2* fusion genes have shown a better prognosis than tumors without such translocations. However, some recent articles have questioned the prognostic significance of this finding.

For unknown reasons, submandibular gland tumors are associated with a poorer outlook than those in the parotid gland. Mucoepidermoid carcinomas of the oral minor salivary glands generally have a good prognosis, probably because they are mostly low- to intermediate-grade tumors. However, tumors of the tongue, floor of the mouth, and oropharynx are less predictable and may exhibit more aggressive behavior.

◆ INTRAOSSEOUS MUCOEPIDERMOID CARCINOMA (CENTRAL MUCOEPIDERMOID CARCINOMA)

On rare occasions, salivary gland tumors arise centrally within the jaws. The most common and best-recognized intrabony salivary tumor is the **intraosseous mucoepidermoid carcinoma**, which comprises about 2%–3% of all mucoepidermoid carcinomas. However, other salivary tumors have been reported to develop within the jaws, including adenoid cystic carcinoma, benign and malignant mixed tumors, adenocarcinoma, acinic cell adenocarcinoma, epithelial-myoepithelial carcinoma, and monomorphic adenoma.

Several hypotheses have been proposed to explain the pathogenesis of intraosseous salivary tumors. One theory suggests that they may arise from ectopic salivary gland tissue that was developmentally entrapped within the jaws. However, the discovery of ectopic salivary tissue is uncommon in biopsy specimens from the jaws; therefore, this seems an unlikely source for most intrabony salivary tumors. Some maxillary tumors may arise from glands of the sinus lining, but this is often difficult to prove or disprove. The most likely source for most intraosseous tumors is odontogenic epithelium. Mucus-producing cells are common in odontogenic cyst linings, especially dentigerous cysts (see page 685). In addition, many intraosseous mucoepidermoid carcinomas develop in association with impacted teeth or odontogenic cysts.

Clinical and Radiographic Features

Intraosseous mucoepidermoid carcinomas are most common in middle-aged adults and affect women twice as often as men. They are more common in the mandible than in the maxilla and are most often seen in the molar-ramus area. The most frequent presenting symptom is cortical swelling, although some lesions may be discovered as incidental findings on radiographs. Pain, trismus, and paresthesia are reported less frequently.

Radiographs usually reveal either a unilocular or multilocular radiolucency with well-defined borders (Fig. 11.64). However, some examples are characterized by a more irregular and ill-defined area of bone destruction. Some cases are associated with an unerupted tooth and, therefore, clinically may suggest an odontogenic cyst or tumor.

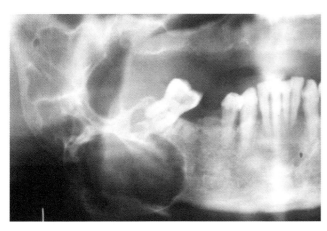

• **Fig. 11.64 Intraosseous Mucoepidermoid Carcinoma.** Multi-locular lesion of the posterior mandible. (Courtesy of Dr. Joseph F. Finelli.)

Histopathologic Features

The microscopic appearance of intraosseous mucoepidermoid carcinoma is similar to that of its soft tissue counterpart. Most tumors are low-grade lesions, although high-grade mucoepidermoid carcinomas also have been reported within the jaws.

Treatment and Prognosis

The primary treatment modality for patients with intraosseous mucoepidermoid carcinoma is surgery; adjunctive radiation therapy also sometimes is used. Radical surgical resection offers a better chance for cure than do more conservative procedures, such as enucleation or curettage. The local recurrence rate with conservative treatment is 40%, in contrast to 11%–13% for more radical treatment. Metastasis has been reported in about 9% of cases. The overall prognosis is fairly good; around 10% of patients die, usually as a result of local recurrence of the tumor.

◆ ACINIC CELL CARCINOMA

The **acinic cell carcinoma** is a salivary gland malignancy with cells that show serous acinar differentiation. Because many of these tumors act in a nonaggressive fashion and are associated with a good prognosis, this neoplasm formerly was called **acinic cell tumor,** a nonspecific designation that did not indicate whether the lesion was benign or malignant. However, because some of these tumors do metastasize or recur and cause death, it is generally agreed today that acinic cell carcinoma should be considered a malignancy.

Many cases previously reported as acinic cell carcinoma, but which are poor in zymogen granules, would be reclassified today as examples of a recently delineated salivary neoplasm—secretory carcinoma (see next topic). This is especially true for purported acinic cell carcinomas in nonparotid sites. Therefore, evaluation of the literature and data on acinic cell carcinoma prior to 2010 is made more difficult.

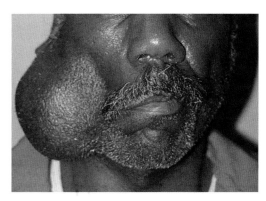

• **Fig. 11.65 Acinic Cell Carcinoma.** Large, firm mass of the right parotid gland.

Clinical Features

Around 85%–90% of all acinic cell carcinomas occur in the parotid gland, a logical finding because this is the largest gland and one that is composed entirely of serous elements (Fig. 11.65). Most surveys have shown that this neoplasm makes up 2%–3% of all parotid tumors, although one study showed it represented 8.6% of all parotid tumors (see Table 11.5). It is much less common in the submandibular gland, which is the site for only 2.7%–5% of these tumors. About 9% of all acinic cell carcinomas reportedly develop in the oral minor salivary glands, with the buccal mucosa, lips, and palate being the most common sites. Overall, around 1.3%–3.8% of all minor salivary gland tumors have been reported to be acinic cell carcinomas, although it is likely that many of these cases would be reclassified today as secretory carcinoma.

The tumor occurs over a broad age range, with a relatively even peak prevalence stretching from the second to the seventh decades of life; the mean age is in the middle 40s to early 50s. The tumor usually appears as a slowly growing mass, and the lesion often is present for many months or years before a diagnosis is made. The tumor may be otherwise asymptomatic, although associated pain or tenderness sometimes is reported. Facial nerve paralysis is an infrequent but ominous sign for parotid tumors.

Histopathologic Features

Acinic cell carcinomas are highly variable in their microscopic appearance. The tumor often is well circumscribed and sometimes may even appear encapsulated; however, some tumors exhibit an infiltrative growth pattern. The most characteristic cell is one with features of the serous acinar cell, with abundant granular basophilic cytoplasm and a round, darkly stained eccentric nucleus. These cells are fairly uniform in appearance, and mitotic activity is uncommon. Other cells may resemble intercalated duct cells, and some tumors also have cells with a clear, vacuolated cytoplasm. On rare occasions, the tumor may demonstrate features of high-grade transformation, including pleomorphism, increased mitotic activity, and necrosis.

Several growth patterns have been described. The **solid** variety consists of numerous well-differentiated acinar cells arranged in a pattern that resembles normal parotid gland tissue (Figs. 11.66 and 11.67). In the **microcystic** variety, multiple small cystic spaces are created that may contain some mucinous or eosinophilic material. In the **papillary-cystic** variety, larger cystic areas are formed that are lined by epithelium having papillary projections into the cystic spaces. The **follicular** variety has an appearance similar to that of thyroid tissue. A lymphoid infiltrate, sometimes with germinal center formation, is not unusual.

Acinic cell carcinoma shows a positive immunohistochemical reaction for DOG1, which can be helpful in distinguishing it from other salivary tumors, especially secretory carcinoma. In addition, nuclear NR4A3 immunostaining recently has been reported to be a sensitive and specific marker for acinic cell carcinoma.

Treatment and Prognosis

Acinic cell carcinomas confined to the superficial lobe of the parotid gland are best treated by lobectomy; for those in the deep lobe, total parotidectomy is usually necessary. The facial nerve may need to be sacrificed if it is involved by tumor. Submandibular tumors are managed by total removal of the gland, and minor gland tumors are treated with assured surgical excision. Lymph node dissection is not indicated unless there is clinical evidence of metastatic disease. Adjunctive radiation therapy may be considered for uncontrolled local disease.

The acinic cell carcinoma is associated with one of the better overall prognoses of any of the malignant salivary gland tumors. Approximately 10%–20% of patients have recurrences locally, and metastases develop in 8%–11% of patients. However, the tumor sometimes exhibits a protracted course, with recurrences noted years or decades after initial treatment. About 10% of patients with low- and intermediate-grade tumors will die of their disease; however, high-grade tumors show a much worse prognosis with a death rate of approximately 60%.

◆ SECRETORY CARCINOMA (MAMMARY ANALOGUE SECRETORY CARCINOMA)

Secretory carcinoma is a recently recognized salivary gland malignancy with histopathologic and molecular features that are similar to secretory carcinoma of the breast. Both of these tumors harbor a balanced chromosomal translocation, t(12;15)(p13;q25), which results in the formation of an *ETV6::NTRK3* fusion gene. Recently, some examples have been associated with other molecular abnormalities, such as *ETV6::RET*, *ETV6::MET*, or other unknown fusion partners. Prior to its recognition in 2010, many examples of secretory carcinoma probably were diagnosed as acinic cell carcinoma, which has overlapping light microscopic features (see legend for Fig. 11.68).

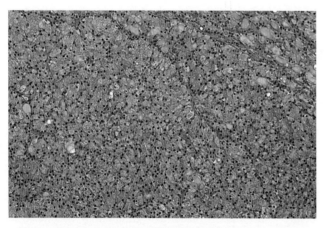

• **Fig. 11.66 Acinic Cell Carcinoma.** Parotid tumor demonstrating sheet of granular, basophilic serous acinar cells.

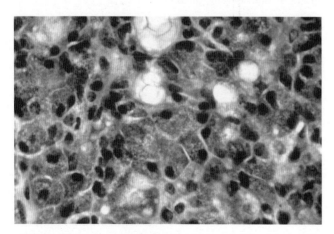

• **Fig. 11.67 Acinic Cell Carcinoma.** High-power view of serous cells with basophilic, granular cytoplasm.

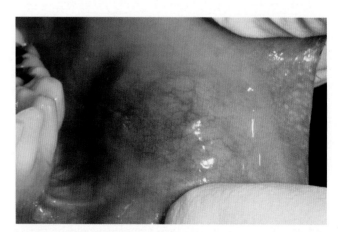

• **Fig. 11.68 Secretory Carcinoma.** Bluish swelling of the anterior buccal mucosa, which could be mistaken clinically for a mucocele. (This tumor originally was diagnosed as acinic cell carcinoma before secretory carcinoma was recognized as a distinct entity. This same image was used to illustrate an acinic cell carcinoma in the third edition of this text!)

Clinical Features

The most common site of origin for the secretory carcinoma is the parotid gland, which accounts for 68% of reported cases. The minor salivary glands (24%) and submandibular gland (8%) are less frequent sites. The lips, buccal mucosa, and palate are the most common intraoral subsites (Fig. 11.68). The mean age is 47 years, and the tumor has been reported to occur slightly more often in males than in females. The lesion usually presents as a slowly growing, painless mass, which the patient may have noticed for months or many years. Occasional examples have been associated with some degree of discomfort.

Histopathologic Features

Secretory carcinoma of salivary gland origin shows microscopic features that are similar to those of secretory carcinoma of the breast. The tumor cells typically exhibit bland, vesicular nuclei surrounded by slightly granular or vacuolated cytoplasm. These cells are variably arranged as solid, tubular, microcystic, or macrocystic structures. Larger cystic spaces may exhibit papillary infolding of tumor cells with a "hobnail" appearance (Fig. 11.69). Mitotic figures are usually rare. However, occasional examples can show high-grade transformation characterized by nuclear pleomorphism, atypical mitoses, perineural invasion, and necrosis.

The tumor cells show diffuse immunoreactivity for S-100 protein, vimentin, and mammaglobin. The *ETV6* translocation and fusion gene can be confirmed via fluorescent *in situ* hybridization (FISH), reverse transcription-polymerase chain reaction (RT-PCR), or next-generation sequencing (NGS). Recent studies have shown that pan-Trk immunohistochemistry can reliably identify tumors with the *ETV6::NTRK3* fusion.

Treatment and Prognosis

Although data on treatment and outcome are limited, secretory carcinoma usually appears to be a low-grade malignancy with a generally favorable prognosis. However, examples

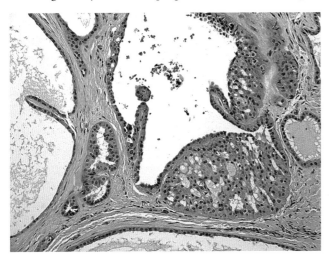

• **Fig. 11.69 Secretory Carcinoma.** Medium-power view showing papillary-cystic spaces and small solid islands.

with high-grade transformation may demonstrate a more aggressive course, with local tumor recurrence and/or metastases resulting in patient death. Treatment most often consists of surgical resection, sometimes supplemented by adjuvant radiation therapy, especially for more aggressive tumors. It has been suggested that tumors with less common, unusual molecular features may be associated with a worse prognosis.

◆ MALIGNANT MIXED TUMORS (CARCINOMA EX PLEOMORPHIC ADENOMA; CARCINOMA EX MIXED TUMOR; CARCINOSARCOMA; METASTASIZING MIXED TUMOR)

Malignant mixed tumors represent malignant counterparts to the benign mixed tumor or pleomorphic adenoma. These uncommon neoplasms constitute 2%–4% of all salivary tumors and can be divided into three categories:

1. Carcinoma ex pleomorphic adenoma (carcinoma ex mixed tumor)
2. Carcinosarcoma
3. Metastasizing mixed tumor

The most common of these is the **carcinoma ex pleomorphic adenoma,** which is characterized by malignant transformation of the epithelial component of a previously benign pleomorphic adenoma. The **carcinosarcoma** is a rare "mixed" tumor in which both carcinomatous and sarcomatous elements are present. The **metastasizing mixed tumor** has histopathologic features that are identical to the common pleomorphic adenoma (mixed tumor). In spite of its benign appearance, however, the lesion metastasizes. The metastatic tumor also has a benign microscopic appearance, usually similar to that of the primary lesion.

Clinical Features

Carcinoma Ex Pleomorphic Adenoma

There is fairly convincing evidence that the carcinoma ex pleomorphic adenoma represents a malignant transformation within what was previously a benign neoplasm. First of all, the mean age of patients with this tumor is about 10–15 years older than that for the benign pleomorphic adenoma. It is most common in middle-aged and older adults, with peak prevalence in the sixth to eighth decades of life. In addition, patients may report that a mass has been present for many years, sometimes undergoing a recent rapid growth with associated pain or ulceration. However, some tumors may have a short duration. The histopathologic features, which are discussed later, also support malignant transformation of a benign pleomorphic adenoma. It has been noted that the risk for malignant change in a pleomorphic adenoma increases with the duration of the tumor.

More than 80% of cases of carcinoma ex pleomorphic adenoma are seen within the major glands, primarily the parotid gland (Fig. 11.70). Nearly two-thirds of minor salivary gland

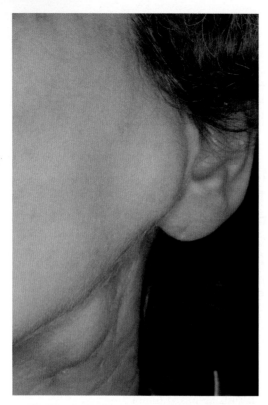

• **Fig. 11.70 Carcinoma Ex Pleomorphic Adenoma.** Mass of the parotid gland.

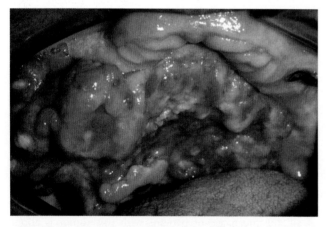

• **Fig. 11.71 Carcinoma Ex Pleomorphic Adenoma.** Granular exophytic and ulcerated mass filling the vault of the palate.

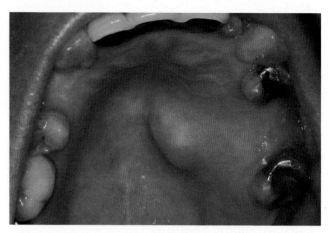

• **Fig. 11.72 Carcinoma Ex Pleomorphic Adenoma.** Smooth-surfaced nodular mass of the left posterior hard palate.

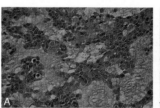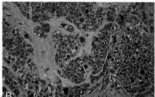

• **Fig. 11.73 Carcinoma Ex Pleomorphic Adenoma. A,** Medium-power view of the benign portion of the tumor showing sheets of plasmacytoid myoepithelial cells within a myxoid background. **B,** Malignant portion of the tumor showing epithelial cells with pleomorphic nuclei.

cases occur on the palate (Fig. 11.71). Although pain or recent rapid growth is not unusual, many cases present as a painless mass that is indistinguishable from a benign tumor (Fig. 11.72). Parotid tumors may produce facial nerve palsy.

Carcinosarcoma

The carcinosarcoma is an extremely rare tumor. Most cases have been reported in the parotid gland, but the lesion also has been seen in the submandibular gland and minor salivary glands. The clinical signs and symptoms are similar to those of the carcinoma ex pleomorphic adenoma. Some patients have a previous history of a benign pleomorphic adenoma, although other cases appear to arise *de novo*.

Metastasizing Mixed Tumor

The metastasizing mixed tumor is also quite rare. As with other malignant mixed tumors, most cases originate in the parotid gland, but the primary tumor also may occur in the submandibular gland or minor salivary glands. Metastases have been found most frequently in the bones or lung, but they also can occur in other sites, such as regional lymph nodes, skin, or the liver. Most patients have a history of a benign mixed tumor, which may have been excised many years earlier. Many times the primary tumor exhibits multiple recurrences before metastasis occurs.

Histopathologic Features
Carcinoma Ex Pleomorphic Adenoma

The carcinoma ex pleomorphic adenoma shows a variable microscopic appearance. Areas of typical benign pleomorphic adenoma usually can be found and may constitute most or only a small portion of the lesion. However, extensive sampling may be required to identify the benign component in some cases. Within the tumor are areas of malignant degeneration of the epithelial component, characterized by cellular pleomorphism and abnormal mitotic activity (Fig. 11.73). This change is most often in the form of a poorly differentiated adenocarcinoma (such as, salivary duct carcinoma), but other patterns also can develop, including myoepithelial carcinoma, polymorphous low-grade adenocarcinoma, mucoepidermoid carcinoma, and adenoid cystic carcinoma.

Based on the pattern of growth, carcinoma ex pleomorphic adenoma can be divided into three subcategories: *invasive, minimally invasive,* or *noninvasive.* Invasive carcinoma ex pleomorphic adenoma shows malignant cells penetrating greater than 1.5 mm from the tumor capsule into adjacent tissues. Minimally invasive tumors show extracapsular invasion that measures 1.5 mm or less. Noninvasive tumors may be discovered as a small malignant focus within the center of an encapsulated pleomorphic adenoma but without violation of the tumor capsule. Because such tumors have a markedly better prognosis than invasive tumors, they also have been designated as **carcinoma in situ ex mixed tumor** or **intracapsular carcinoma ex pleomorphic adenoma.**

Carcinosarcoma

The carcinosarcoma is a biphasic tumor, demonstrating both carcinomatous and sarcomatous areas. The epithelial component usually consists of a poorly differentiated adenocarcinoma or an undifferentiated carcinoma. The sarcomatous portion often predominates the tumor and is usually in the form of chondrosarcoma but also may show characteristics of osteosarcoma, fibrosarcoma, liposarcoma, rhabdomyosarcoma, or malignant fibrous histiocytoma. Some lesions have evidence of an origin from a benign mixed tumor.

Metastasizing Mixed Tumor

The metastasizing mixed tumor has microscopic features of a benign pleomorphic adenoma, within both the primary and the metastatic sites. Malignant histopathologic changes are not observed.

Treatment and Prognosis
Carcinoma Ex Pleomorphic Adenoma

Invasive carcinoma ex pleomorphic adenoma usually is best treated by wide excision, possibly in conjunction with local lymph node dissection and adjunctive radiation therapy. The prognosis is guarded; the overall 5-year survival rate ranges from 25% to 69%, but this rate drops to 10%–35% at 15 years. The prognosis is related to the histopathologic subtype of the malignant component. One study showed that well-differentiated carcinomas, such as polymorphous low-grade adenocarcinoma, have nearly a 90% 5-year survival rate. However, the outlook is much worse for patients with tumors that are poorly differentiated or that have invaded more than 6 mm beyond the residual capsule or benign residual tumor. In contrast, the prognosis for noninvasive or minimally invasive carcinoma ex pleomorphic adenoma approaches that for benign mixed tumor. However, rare examples of metastasis or tumor death have been documented in these latter groups.

Carcinosarcoma

Carcinosarcomas are treated by radical surgical excision, which may be combined with radiation therapy and chemotherapy. The prognosis is poor, with around 60% of patients dying from local recurrence or metastatic disease.

Metastasizing Mixed Tumor

The treatment for a metastasizing mixed tumor consists of surgical excision of both the primary tumor and the metastatic sites. A mortality rate of approximately 40% has been reported.

◆ ADENOID CYSTIC CARCINOMA

The **adenoid cystic carcinoma** is one of the more common and best-recognized salivary malignancies. Because of its distinctive histopathologic features, it originally was called a **cylindroma,** and this term still is heard sometimes as a synonym for this neoplasm. However, use of the term *cylindroma* should be avoided because it does not convey the malignant nature of the tumor, and also because this same term is used for a skin adnexal tumor that has a markedly different clinical presentation and prognosis. Over 80% of adenoid cystic carcinomas will exhibit overexpression of the *MYB* oncogene, frequently in association with a chromosomal translocation, t(6;9)(q22-23;p23-24), and resultant *MYB::NFIB* fusion gene.

Clinical and Radiographic Features

The adenoid cystic carcinoma can occur in any salivary gland site, but approximately 60% develop within the various minor salivary glands. The parotid gland is the second most common location, followed by the submandibular gland. The palate is the most common site for minor gland tumors (Figs. 11.74 and 11.75). Rare intraosseous examples also have been reported in the jaws. On an individual basis,

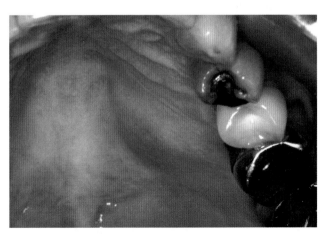

• **Fig. 11.74 Adenoid Cystic Carcinoma.** Subtle nodular swelling of the left hard palate.

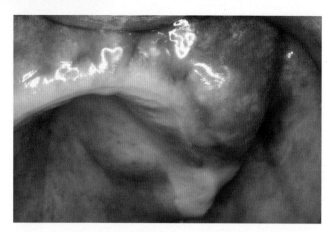

• **Fig. 11.75 Adenoid Cystic Carcinoma.** Painful mass of the hard palate and maxillary alveolar ridge. (Courtesy of Dr. George Blozis.)

however, a striking difference can be seen among the various glands. In the parotid gland, the adenoid cystic carcinoma is relatively rare, constituting only 2% of all tumors. In the submandibular gland, this tumor accounts for 11%–17% of all tumors and is the most common malignancy. It is also relatively common among palatal salivary neoplasms; it represents 8%–17% of all such tumors. The lesion is most common in middle-aged adults and is rare in people younger than age 20. There is a slight female predilection.

The adenoid cystic carcinoma usually appears as a slowly growing mass. Pain is a common and important finding, occasionally occurring early in the course of the disease before there is a noticeable swelling. Patients often complain of a constant, low-grade, dull ache, which gradually increases in intensity. Facial nerve paralysis may develop with parotid tumors. Palatal tumors can be smooth surfaced or ulcerated. Tumors arising in the palate or maxillary sinus often show radiographic evidence of bone destruction (Fig. 11.76).

Histopathologic Features

The adenoid cystic carcinoma is composed of a mixture of abluminal myoepithelial cells and luminal ductal cells that can have a varied arrangement (Fig. 11.77). Three major patterns are recognized: (1) cribriform, (2) tubular, and (3) solid. Usually a combination of these is seen, and the tumor is classified based on the predominant pattern.

The **cribriform pattern** is the most classic and best-recognized appearance, characterized by islands of basaloid epithelial cells that contain multiple cylindrical, cystlike spaces resembling Swiss cheese. These spaces often contain a mildly basophilic mucoid material, a hyalinized eosinophilic product, or a combined mucoid-hyalinized appearance. Sometimes the hyalinized material also surrounds these cribriform islands (Fig. 11.78), or small strands of tumor are found embedded within this hyalinized "stroma." The tumor cells are small and cuboidal, exhibiting deeply basophilic nuclei and little cytoplasm. These cells are fairly uniform in appearance, and mitotic activity is rarely seen. The pathologist should be mindful that other salivary tumors, especially polymorphous

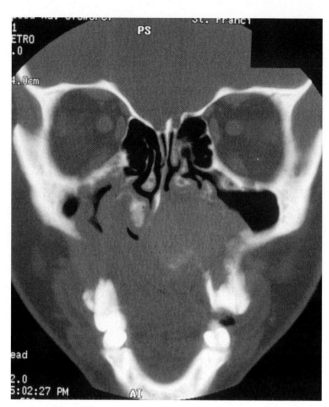

• **Fig. 11.76 Adenoid Cystic Carcinoma.** Computed tomography (CT) scan of this massive palatal tumor shows extensive destruction of the hard palate with extension of the tumor into the nasal cavity and both maxillary sinuses. (Courtesy of Dr. Kevin Riker.)

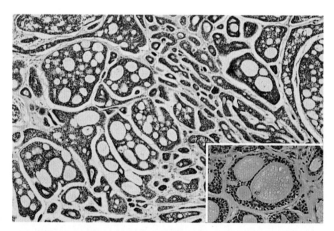

• **Fig. 11.77 Adenoid Cystic Carcinoma.** Islands of hyperchromatic cells forming cribriform and tubular structures. *Inset* shows a high-power view of a small cribriform island.

low-grade adenocarcinoma, also may exhibit areas with a cribriform pattern.

In the **tubular pattern,** the tumor cells are similar but occur as multiple small ducts or tubules within a hyalinized stroma. The tubular lumina can be lined by one to several layers of cells, and sometimes both a layer of ductal cells and myoepithelial cells can be discerned.

The **solid variant** consists of larger islands or sheets of tumor cells that demonstrate little tendency toward duct or cyst formation. Unlike the cribriform and tubular patterns,

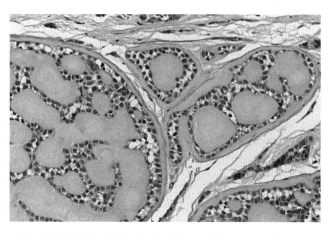

• **Fig. 11.78 Adenoid Cystic Carcinoma.** The tumor cells are surrounded by hyalinized material.

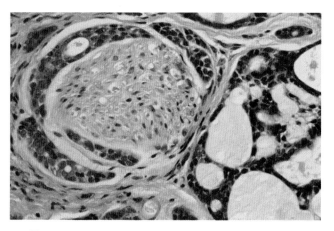

• **Fig. 11.79 Adenoid Cystic Carcinoma.** Perineural invasion.

cellular pleomorphism and mitotic activity, as well as focal necrosis in the center of the tumor islands, may be observed.

A highly characteristic feature of adenoid cystic carcinoma is its tendency to show perineural invasion (Fig. 11.79), which probably corresponds to the common clinical finding of pain in these patients. Sometimes the cells appear to have a swirling arrangement around nerve bundles. However, perineural invasion is not pathognomonic for adenoid cystic carcinoma; it also may be seen in other salivary malignancies, especially polymorphous low-grade adenocarcinomas.

Positive immunostaining reactions for CD43 and c-kit (CD117) in adenoid cystic carcinoma have been reported to be useful diagnostic features that can help to distinguish this tumor from polymorphous adenocarcinoma, basal cell adenoma, and canalicular adenoma. However, other authors have questioned the utility of c-kit immunostaining. The combination of p63 and p40 immunostaining has been shown to be helpful in differentiating adenoid cystic carcinoma from polymorphous adenocarcinoma (next topic). The myoepithelial cells of adenoid cystic carcinoma almost always are positive for both markers, whereas the lesional cells of polymorphous adenocarcinoma typically are positive for p63, but negative for p40. In addition, the Ki-67 cell

proliferation index of adenoid cystic carcinoma is significantly greater than that observed in polymorphous adenocarcinoma (21.4% vs 2.4%). In cases where the diagnosis is uncertain, molecular testing to confirm *MYB* rearrangement can be helpful.

Treatment and Prognosis

Adenoid cystic carcinoma is a relentless tumor that is prone to local recurrence and eventual distant metastasis. Surgical resection is usually the primary treatment of choice. Adjuvant radiation therapy may slightly improve patient survival in some cases, especially for advanced stage tumors.. Because metastasis to regional lymph nodes is uncommon (6%–19% of cases), neck dissection usually is not indicated. However, elective neck dissection may be warranted for patients with a higher risk of local metastasis, such as those with larger T3 or T4 tumors, or tumors of the tongue.

Because the tumor is prone to late recurrence and metastasis, the 5-year survival rate has limited significance and does not equate to a cure. The 5-year survival rate may be as high as 68%–89%, but this rate continues to decrease over time. The 10-year survival currently ranges from 60% to 68%, and by 20 years, only 25%–40% of patients are still alive. Tumors with a solid histopathologic pattern are associated with a worse outlook than those with a cribriform or tubular arrangement. The presence of perineural invasion also is associated with a poorer prognosis. With respect to site, the prognosis is poorest for tumors arising in the maxillary sinus and submandibular gland. Better survival is observed in females, younger patients, and patients with localized disease at the time of diagnosis. Tumor DNA ploidy analysis may help to predict the prognosis of adenoid cystic carcinoma; patients with diploid tumors have been shown to have a significantly better outcome than patients with aneuploid tumors. It also has been suggested that tumors showing *MYB::NFIB* fusion may have a slightly worse prognosis.

Death usually results from local recurrence or distant metastases. Tumors of the palate or maxillary sinus may invade upward to the base of the brain. Metastases eventually occur in approximately 40%–50% of patients, most frequently involving the lungs, bone, and brain.

◆ POLYMORPHOUS ADENOCARCINOMA (POLYMORPHOUS LOW-GRADE ADENOCARCINOMA)

The **polymorphous adenocarcinoma** was first described in 1983. Before its identification as a distinct entity, examples of this tumor were categorized as pleomorphic adenoma, an unspecified form of adenocarcinoma, or sometimes as adenoid cystic carcinoma. Once recognized as a specific entity, however, it was realized that this lesion possesses distinct clinicopathologic features and is one of the more common minor salivary gland malignancies. This tumor originally was termed *polymorphous low-grade adenocarcinoma* because it usually behaves as a low-grade malignancy. However, occasional examples have shown high-grade transformation; therefore, the "low-grade" designation has been dropped from the name in the most recent WHO classification scheme. Recent molecular studies have shown that over 70% of polymorphous adenocarcinomas exhibit *PRKD1* hotspot mutations.

Clinical Features

The polymorphous adenocarcinoma is almost exclusively a tumor of the minor salivary glands. However, rare examples also have been reported in the major glands, either arising *de novo* or as the malignant component of a carcinoma ex pleomorphic adenoma. Sixty-five percent occur on the hard or soft palate (Fig. 11.80), with the upper lip and buccal mucosa being the next most common locations. It is most common in older adults, having peak prevalence in the sixth to eighth decades of life. Two-thirds of all cases occur in females.

The tumor most often appears as a painless mass that may have been present for a long time with slow growth. Occasionally, it is associated with bleeding or discomfort. Palatal tumors sometimes will exhibit a rough, pebbly surface due to papillary hyperplasia of the overlying epithelium. Tumor can erode or infiltrate the underlying bone.

In 1999, a rare, distinctive group of salivary gland tumors known as **cribriform adenocarcinoma** were identified in the posterior tongue. Debate currently exists as to whether these lesions represent a unique tumor or simply a variant of polymorphous adenocarcinoma (*polymorphous adenocarcinoma, cribriform type*). Such tumors have been associated with *PRKD1, PRKD2,* or *PRKD3* gene fusions. Since its initial description, this tumor also has been identified in other minor salivary gland sites, as well as rare examples in the parotid gland.

Histopathologic Features

The tumor cells of polymorphous adenocarcinoma have a deceptively uniform appearance. They are round to polygonal in shape, with indistinct cell borders and pale to eosinophilic cytoplasm. The nuclei may be round, ovoid, or spindled; these nuclei usually are pale staining, although they can be more basophilic in some areas. The cells can exhibit different growth patterns, hence, the *polymorphous* term. The cells may grow in a solid pattern or form cords, ducts, or larger cystic spaces. In some tumors, a cribriform "Swiss cheese" pattern can be produced that mimics adenoid cystic carcinoma (Fig. 11.81). Mitotic figures are uncommon.

At low power, the tumor sometimes appears well circumscribed. However, the peripheral cells are usually infiltrative, invading the adjacent tissue in a single-file fashion (Fig. 11.82). Extension into underlying bone or skeletal muscle may be observed. The stroma is often mucoid in nature, or it may demonstrate hyalinization. Perineural invasion is common—another feature that may cause the tumor to be mistaken for adenoid cystic carcinoma (Fig. 11.83).

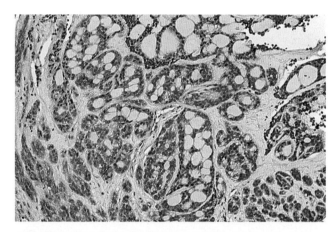

• **Fig. 11.81 Polymorphous Adenocarcinoma.** This medium-power view shows a cribriform arrangement of uniform tumor cells with pale-staining nuclei.

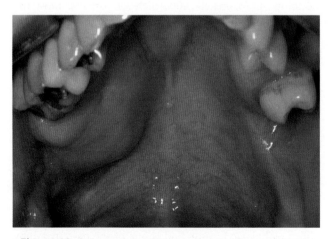

• **Fig. 11.80 Polymorphous Adenocarcinoma.** Slow-growing, firm mass of the right posterior lateral hard palate. (Courtesy of Dr. Kevin Riker.)

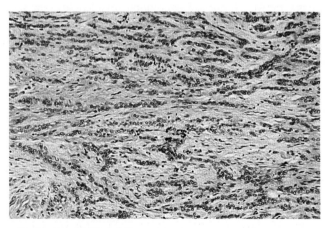

• **Fig. 11.82 Polymorphous Adenocarcinoma.** Pale-staining cells that infiltrate as single-file cords.

However, a distinction between these two tumors is important because of their vastly different prognoses.

Immunohistochemical staining can be helpful in distinguishing polymorphous adenocarcinoma from other salivary gland tumors that it may mimic. Lack of staining for glial fibrillary acidic protein (GFAP) can help to differentiate this tumor from pleomorphic adenoma, which is almost always strongly positive for GFAP. Immunostains for p40 and p63 can be valuable in distinguishing polymorphous adenocarcinoma from adenoid cystic carcinoma. Polymorphous adenocarcinoma will almost always be positive for p63 but negative for p40, whereas adenoid cystic carcinoma will be positive for both markers in almost 90% of cases. When compared with adenoid cystic carcinoma, polymorphous adenocarcinoma exhibits significantly weaker expression of CD43 and c-kit (CD117). However, other authors have questioned the usefulness of c-kit immunostaining.

Cribriform adenocarcinomas are characterized by a uniform population of basaloid cells that can form solid, microcystic, cribriform, and glomeruloid structures. The cells characteristically exhibit vesicular to optically clear nuclei resembling the pattern found in papillary thyroid carcinoma.

Treatment and Prognosis

The polymorphous adenocarcinoma is best treated by wide surgical excision, sometimes including resection of the underlying bone. Metastasis to regional lymph nodes is relatively uncommon, occurring in 9%–17% of patients. Therefore, neck dissection seems unwarranted in most cases unless there is clinical evidence of cervical metastases. Distant metastases are rare, occurring in only 2%–4% of patients.

The overall prognosis is good. Recurrent disease has been reported in 9%–32.5% of all patients, but this usually can be controlled with reexcision. Death from tumor is rare but may occur secondary to direct extension into vital structures. Microscopic identification of perineural invasion does not appear to affect the prognosis.

Cribriform adenocarcinoma is associated with a high rate of regional lymph metastasis, which can occur in up to 72% of cases. Therefore, neck dissection seems appropriate in

most cases, as well as possible radiation therapy. However, distant metastases are uncommon, and the overall survival rate is still relatively good.

◆ SALIVARY ADENOCARCINOMA, NOT OTHERWISE SPECIFIED

In spite of the wide variety of salivary gland malignancies that have been specifically identified and categorized, some tumors still defy the existing classification schemes. These tumors usually are designated as **salivary adenocarcinomas, not otherwise specified (NOS)**.

Clinical and Histopathologic Features

Because these adenocarcinomas represent such a diverse group of neoplasms, it is difficult to generalize about their clinical and microscopic features. Like most salivary tumors, they appear to be most common in the parotid gland, followed by the minor glands and the submandibular gland (Figs. 11.84 and 11.85). They may present as asymptomatic masses or cause pain or facial nerve paralysis. The microscopic appearance is highly variable but demonstrates features of a glandular malignancy with evidence of cellular pleomorphism, an infiltrative growth pattern, or both. These tumors exhibit a wide spectrum of differentiation, ranging from well-differentiated, low-grade neoplasms to poorly differentiated, high-grade malignancies.

As these tumors are studied more, it should be possible to classify some of them into separate, specific categories and allow more definitive analyses of their clinical and microscopic features.

Treatment and Prognosis

Because of their diversity, it is difficult to predict the prognosis for salivary adenocarcinoma (NOS), but patients with early-stage, well-differentiated tumors appear to have a better outcome. The survival rate is better for tumors of the oral

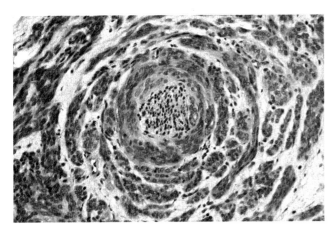

• **Fig. 11.83 Polymorphous Adenocarcinoma.** Perineural invasion.

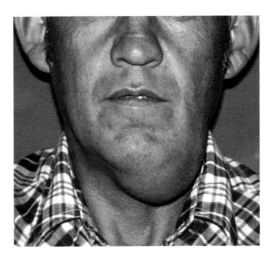

• **Fig. 11.84 Salivary Adenocarcinoma.** Large mass of the submandibular gland.

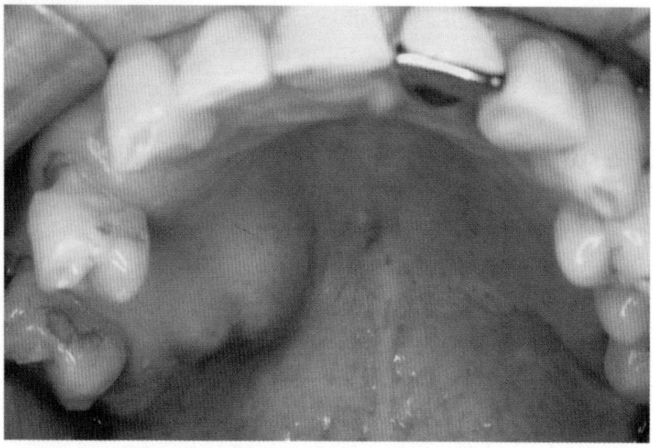

• **Fig. 11.85 Salivary Adenocarcinoma.** Mass of the posterior lateral hard palate.

cavity than for those in the major salivary glands. The reported 10-year survival rate for parotid tumors ranges from 26% to 55%; in contrast, one study reported a 10-year survival rate of 76% for intraoral tumors.

Bibliography

Salivary Gland Aplasia

Brotto D, Manara R, Vio S, et al.: Salivary glands abnormalities in oculo-auriculo-vertebral spectrum, *Clin Oral Invest* 22:395–400, 2018.

Chadi MJ, Georges GS, Albert F, et al.: Major salivary gland aplasia and hypoplasia in Down syndrome: review of the literature and report of a case, *Clin Case Rep* 5:939–944, 2017.

Hajianpour MJ, Bombei H, Lieberman SM, et al.: Dental issues in lacrimo-auriculo-dento-digital syndrome. An autosomal dominant condition with clinical and genetic variability, *J Am Dent Assoc* 148:157–163, 2017.

Seymen F, Koruyucu M, Toptanci IR, et al.: Novel *FGF10* mutation in autosomal dominant aplasia of lacrimal and salivary glands, *Clin Oral Invest* 21:167–172, 2017.

Taji SS, Savage N, Holcombe T, et al.: Congenital aplasia of the major salivary glands: literature review and case report, *Pediatr Dent* 33:113–118, 2011.

Togni L., Mascitti M., Santarelli A., et al: Unusual conditions impairing saliva secretion: developmental anomalies of salivary glands, Front Physiol 10:855. https://doi.org/10.3389/fphys.2019.00855.

Mucocele

Baurmash HD: Mucoceles and ranulas, *J Oral Maxillofac Surg* 61:369–378, 2003.

Campana F, Sibaud V, Chauvel A, et al.: Recurrent superficial mucoceles associated with lichenoid disorders, *J Oral Maxillofac Surg* 64:1830–1833, 2006.

Chi AC, Lambert PR 3rd, Richardson MS, et al.: Oral mucoceles: a clinicopathologic review of 1,824 cases, including unusual variants, *J Oral Maxillofac Surg* 69:1086–1093, 2011.

Choi YJ, Byun JS, Choi JK, et al.: Identification of predictive variables for the recurrence of oral mucocele, *Med Oral Patol Oral Cir Bucal* 24:e231–e235, 2019.

Eveson JW: Superficial mucoceles: pitfall in clinical and microscopic diagnosis, *Oral Surg Oral Med Oral Pathol* 66:318–322, 1988.

Jinbu Y, Kusama M, Itoh H, et al.: Mucocele of the glands of Blandin-Nuhn: clinical and histopathologic analysis of 26 cases, *Oral Surg Oral Med Oral Pathol Oral Radiol Endod* 95:467–470, 2003.

Joshi SR, Pendyala GS, Choudhari S, et al.: Mucocele of the glands of Blandin-Nuhn in children: a clinical, histopathologic, and retrospective study, *N Am J Med Sci* 4:379–383, 2012.

Ranula

Baurmash HD: Mucoceles and ranulas, *J Oral Maxillofac Surg* 61:369–378, 2003.

Chung YS, Cho Y, Kim BH: Comparison of outcomes of treatment for ranula: a proportion meta-analysis, *Br J Oral Maxillofac Surg* 57:620–626, 2019.

Harrison JD: Modern management and pathophysiology of ranula: literature review, *Head Neck* 32:1310–1320, 2010.

Jain P: Plunging ranulas and prevalence of the "tail sign" in 126 consecutive cases, *J Ultrasound Med* 39:273–278, 2020.

Kurabayashi T, Ida M, Yasumoto M, et al.: MRI of ranulas, *Neuroradiology* 42:917–922, 2000.

McGurk M, Eyeson J, Thomas B, et al.: Conservative treatment of oral ranula by excision with minimal excision of the sublingual gland: histological support for a traumatic etiology, *J Oral Maxillofac Surg* 66:2050–2057, 2008.

Zhao Y-F, Jia Y, Chen X-M, et al.: Clinical review of 580 ranulas, *Oral Surg Oral Med Oral Pathol Oral Radiol Endod* 98:281–287, 2004.

Salivary Duct Cyst

Eversole LR: Oral sialocysts, *Arch Otolaryngol* 113:51–56, 1987.

Takeda Y, Yamamoto H: Salivary duct cyst: its frequency in a certain Japanese population group (Tohoku districts), with special reference to adenomatous proliferation of the epithelial lining, *J Oral Sci* 43:9–13, 2001.

Stojanov IJ, Malik UA, Woo SB: Intraoral salivary duct cyst: clinical and histopathologic features of 177 cases, *Head Neck Pathol* 11:469–476, 2017.

Sialolithiasis

Fabie JE, Kompelli AR, Naylor TM, et al.: Gland-preserving surgery for salivary stones and the utility of sialendoscopes, *Head Neck* 41:1320–1327, 2019.

Guenzel T, Hoch S, Heinze N, et al.: Sialendoscopy plus laser lithotripsy in sialolithiasis of the submandibular gland in 64 patients: a simple and safe procedure, *Auris Nasus Larynx* 46:797–802, 2019.

Huoh KC, Eisele DW: Etiologic factors in sialolithiasis, *Otolaryngol Head Neck Surg* 145:935–939, 2011.

Jensen JL, Howell FV, Rick GM, et al.: Minor salivary gland calculi: a clinicopathologic study of forty-seven new cases, *Oral Surg Oral Med Oral Pathol* 47:44–50, 1979.

Sigismund PE, Zenk J, Koch M, et al.: Nearly 3,000 salivary stones: some clinical and epidemiologic aspects, *Laryngoscope* 125:1879–1882, 2015.

Sproll C, Naujoks C, Holtmann H, et al.: Removal of stones from the superficial lobe of the submandibular gland (SMG) via an intraoral endoscopy-assisted sialolithotomy, *Clin Oral Invest* 23:4145–4156, 2019.

Zenk J, Bozzato A, Winter M, et al.: Extracorporeal shock wave lithotripsy of submandibular stones: evaluation after 10 years, *Ann Otol Rhinol Laryngol* 113:378–383, 2004.

Zenk J, Koch M, Klintworth N, et al.: Sialendoscopy in the diagnosis and treatment of sialolithiasis: a study on more than 1000 patients, *Otolaryngol Head Neck Surg* 147:858–863, 2012.

Sialadenitis

Carlson ER: Diagnosis and management of salivary gland infections, *Oral Maxillofac Surg Clin N Am* 21:293–312, 2009.

Cung TD, Lai W, Svider PF, et al.: Sialendoscopy in the management of radioiodine induced sialadenitis: a systematic review, *Ann Otol Rhinol Laryngol* 126:768–773, 2017.

Fattahi TT, Lyu PE, Van Sickels JE: Management of acute suppurative parotitis, *J Oral Maxillofac Surg* 60:446–448, 2002.

Fowler CB, Brannon RB: Subacute necrotizing sialadenitis: report of 7 cases and a review of the literature, *Oral Surg Oral Med Oral Pathol Oral Radiol Endod* 89:600–609, 2000.

Gillespie MB, Intaphan J, Nguyen SA: Endoscopic-assisted management of chronic sialadenitis, *Head Neck* 33:1346–1351, 2011.

Hernandez S, Busso C, Walvekar RR: Parotitis and sialendoscopy of the parotid gland, *Otolaryngol Clin N Am* 49:381–393, 2016.

Ko YC, Philipone E, Florin W, et al.: Subacute necrotizing sialadenitis: a series of three cases and literature review, *Head Neck Pathol* 10:425–428, 2016.

Patel A, Karlis V: Diagnosis and management of pediatric salivary gland infections, *Oral Maxillofac Surg Clin N Am* 21:345–352, 2009.

Suresh L, Aguirre A: Subacute necrotizing sialadenitis: a clinicopathological study, *Oral Surg Oral Med Oral Pathol Oral Radiol Endod* 104:385–390, 2007.

Cheilitis Glandularis

Carrington PR, Horn TD: Cheilitis glandularis: a clinical marker for both malignancy and/or severe inflammatory disease of the oral cavity, *J Am Acad Dermatol* 54:336–337, 2006.

Nico MMS, Nakano de Melo J, Lourenço SV: Cheilitis glandularis: a clinicopathological study in 22 patients, *J Am Acad Dermatol* 62:233–238, 2010.

Reiter S, Vered M, Yarom N, et al.: Cheilitis glandularis: clinico-histopathological diagnostic criteria, *Oral Dis* 17:335–339, 2011.

Stoopler ET, Carrasco L, Stanton DC, et al.: Cheilitis glandularis: an unusual histopathologic presentation, *Oral Surg Oral Med Oral Pathol Oral Radiol Endod* 95:312–317, 2003.

Sialorrhea

Begley KA, Braswell LE, Noritz GH, et al.: Salivary gland ablation: introducing an interventional radiology treatment alternative in the management of sialorrhea, *Pediatr Radiol* 50:869–876, 2020.

Bronshtein M, Gover A, Beloosesky R, et al.: Characteristics and outcomes of ptyalism gravidarum, *Isr Med Assoc J* 20:573–575, 2018.

Calim OF, Hassouna HN, Yildirim YS: Pediatric sialorrhea: submandibular duct rerouting and intraparotid botulinum toxin A injection with literature review, *Ann Otol Rhinol Laryngol* 128:104–112, 2019.

Freudenreich O: Drug-induced sialorrhea, *Drugs Today* 41:411–418, 2005.

Jost WH, Bäumer T, Laskawi R, et al.: Therapy of sialorrhea with botulinum neurotoxin, *Neurol Ther* 8:273–288, 2019.

Lamey P-J, Clifford TJ, El-Karim IA, et al.: Personality analysis of patients complaining of sialorrhoea, *J Oral Pathol Med* 35:307–310, 2006.

Merello M: Sialorrhoea and drooling in patients with Parkinson's disease: epidemiology and management, *Drugs Aging* 25:1007–1019, 2008.

Petracca M, Guidubaldi A, Ricciardi L, et al.: Botulinum toxin A and B in sialorrhea: long-term data and literature overview, *Toxicon* 107:129–140, 2015.

Shirley WP, Hill JS, Woolley AL, et al.: Success and complications of four-duct ligation for sialorrhea, *Int J Pediatr Otorhinolaryngol* 67:1–6, 2003.

Xerostomia

Alajbeg I, Falcão DP, Tran SD, et al.: Intraoral electrostimulator for xerostomia relief: a long-term multicenter, open-label, uncontrolled, clinical study, *Oral Surg Oral Med Oral Pathol Oral Radiol* 113:773–781, 2012.

Cheng CQ, Xu H, Liu L, et al.: Efficacy and safety of pilocarpine for radiation-induced xerostomia in patients with head and neck cancer: a systematic review and meta-analysis, *J Am Dent Assoc* 147:236–243, 2016.

Fox PC: Salivary enhancement therapies, *Caries Res* 38:241–246, 2004.

Jensen SB, Pedersen AML, Vissink A, et al.: A systematic review of salivary gland hypofunction and xerostomia induced by cancer therapies: management strategies and economic impact, *Support Care Cancer* 18:1061–1079, 2010.

Mercadante V, Al Hamad A, Lodi G, et al.: Interventions for the management of radiotherapy-induced xerostomia and hyposalivation: a systematic review and meta-analysis, *Oral Oncol* 66:64–74, 2017.

Jose A, Siddiqi M, Cronin M, et al.: A randomized clinical trial in subjects with dry mouth evaluating subjective perceptions of an experimental oral gel, and oral rinse and a mouth spray compared to water, *Am J Dent* 29:58–64, 2016.

Porter SR, Scully C, Hegarty AM: An update of the etiology and management of xerostomia, *Oral Surg Oral Med Oral Pathol Oral Radiol Endod* 97:28–46, 2004.

Rao RS, Akula R, Satyanarayana TS, et al.: Recent advances of pacemakers in treatment of xerostomia: a systematic review, *J Int Soc Prev Community Dent* 9:311–315, 2019.

Scully C: Drug effects on salivary glands: dry mouth, *Oral Dis* 9:165–176, 2003.

Wolff A, Joshi RK, Ekström J, et al.: A guide to medications inducing salivary gland dysfunction, xerostomia, and subjective sialorrhea: a systemic review sponsored by the World Workshop on Oral Medicine VI, *Drugs R D* 17:1–28, 2017.

IgG4-Related Disease

Bhatti RM, Stelow EB: IgG4-related disease of the head and neck, *Adv Anat Pathol* 20:10–16, 2013.

Deshpande V, Zen Y, Chan JKC, et al.: Consensus statement on the pathology of IgG4-related disease, *Mod Pathol* 25:1181–1192, 2012.

Fragoulis GE, Zampeli E, Moutsopoulos HM: IgG4-related sialadenitis and Sjögren syndrome, *Oral Dis* 23:152–156, 2017.

Johnston J, Allen JE: IgG4-related disease in the head and neck, *Curr Opin Otolaryngol Head Neck Surg* 26:403–408, 2018.

Penfold CN: Mikulicz syndrome, *J Oral Maxillofac Surg* 43:900–905, 1985.

Stone JH, Zen Y, Deshpande V: IgG4-related disease, *N Engl J Med* 366:539–551, 2012.

Takano K, Yamamoto M, Takahashi H, et al.: Recent advances in knowledge regarding head and neck manifestations of IgG4-related disease, *Auris Nasus Larynx* 44:7–17, 2017.

Sjögren Syndrome

Baer AN, Walitt B: Sjögren syndrome and other causes of sicca in older adults, *Rheum Dis Clin North Am* 44:419–436, 2018.

Daniels TE: Labial salivary gland biopsy in Sjögren's syndrome: assessment as a diagnostic criterion in 362 suspected cases, *Arthritis Rheum* 27:147–156, 1984.

Daniels TE, Cox D, Shiboski CH, et al.: Associations between salivary gland histopathologic diagnoses and phenotypic features of Sjögren's syndrome (SS) among 1726 registry participants, *Arthritis Rheum* 63:2021–2030, 2011.

Fisher BA, Jonsson R, Daniels T, et al.: Standardisation of labial salivary gland histopathology in clinical trials in primary Sjögren's syndrome, *Ann Rheum Dis* 76:1161–1168, 2017.

Fox RI: Sjögren's syndrome, *Lancet* 366:321–331, 2005.

Jonsson MV, Theander E, Jonsson R: Predictors for the development of non-Hodgkin lymphoma in primary Sjögren's syndrome, *Presse Med* 41:e511–e516, 2012.

Jordan R, Diss TC, Lench NJ, et al.: Immunoglobulin gene rearrangements in lymphoplasmacytic infiltrates of labial salivary glands in Sjögren's syndrome. A possible predictor of lymphoma development, *Oral Surg Oral Med Oral Pathol Oral Radiol Endod* 79:723–729, 1995.

Kroese FGM, Haacke EA, Bombardieri M: The role of salivary gland histopathology in primary Sjögren's syndrome: promises and pitfalls, *Clin Exp Rheumatol* 36:s222–s233, 2018.

Manthorpe R, Benoni C, Jacobsson L, et al.: Lower frequency of focal lip sialadenitis (focus score) in smoking patients. Can tobacco diminish the salivary gland involvement as judged by histological examination and anti-SSA/Ro and anti-SSB/La antibodies in Sjögren's syndrome, *Ann Rheum Dis* 59:54–60, 2000.

Mariette X, Criswell LA: Primary Sjögren's syndrome, *N Engl J Med* 378:931–939, 2018.

Navazesh M, Kumar SKS: Measuring salivary flow. Challenges and opportunities, *JADA* 139:35S–40S, 2008.

Ramos-Casals M, Tzioufas AG, Stone JH, et al.: Treatment of primary Sjögren syndrome: a systematic review, *JAMA* 304:452–460, 2010.

Routsias JG, Goules JD, Charalampakis G, et al.: Malignant lymphoma in primary Sjögren's syndrome: an update on the pathogenesis and treatment, *Semin Arthritis Rheum* 43:178–186, 2013.

Shiboski CH, Shiboski SC, Seror R, et al.: 2016 American College of Rheumatology/European League Against Rheumatism classification criteria for primary Sjögren's syndrome. A consensus and data-driven methodology involving three international patient cohorts, *Ann Rheum Dis* 76:9–16, 2017.

Spijkervet FKL, Haacke E, Kroese FGM, et al.: Parotid gland biopsy, the alternative way to diagnose Sjögren syndrome, *Rheum Dis Clin N Am* 42:485–499, 2016.

Vivino FB, Bunya VY, Massaro-Giodorno G, et al.: Sjögren's syndrome: an update on disease pathogenesis, clinical manifestations and treatment, *Clin Immunol* 203:81–121, 2019.

Vivino FB, Gala I, Hermann GA: Change in final diagnosis on second evaluation of labial minor salivary gland biopsies, *J Rheumatol* 29:938–944, 2002.

Whitcher JP, Shiboski CH, Shiboski SC, et al.: A simplified quantitative method for assessing keratoconjunctivitis sicca from the Sjögren's Syndrome International Registry, *Am J Ophthalmol* 149:405–415, 2010.

Sialadenosis

Garcia BG, Ferrer AD, Jimenez ND, et al.: Bilateral parotid sialadenosis associated with long-standing bulimia: a case report and literature review, *J Maxillofac Oral Surg* 17:117–121, 2018.

Guggenheimer J, Close JM, Eghtesad B: Sialadenosis in patients with advanced liver disease, *Head Neck Pathol* 3:100–105, 2009.

Ihrler S, Rath C, Zengel P, et al.: Pathogenesis of sialadenosis: possible role of functionally deficient myoepithelial cells, *Oral Surg Oral Med Oral Pathol Oral Radiol Endod* 110:218–223, 2010.

Mignogna MD, Fedele S, Lo Russo L: Anorexia/bulimia-related sialadenosis of palatal minor salivary glands, *J Oral Pathol Med* 33:441–442, 2004.

Scully C, Bagán JV, Eveson JW, et al.: Sialosis: 35 cases of persistent parotid swelling from two countries, *Br J Oral Maxillofac Surg* 46:468–472, 2008.

Adenomatoid Hyperplasia

Arafat A, Brannon RB, Ellis GL: Adenomatoid hyperplasia of mucous salivary glands, *Oral Surg Oral Med Oral Pathol* 52:51–55, 1981.

Barrett AW, Speight PM: Adenomatoid hyperplasia of oral minor salivary glands, *Oral Surg Oral Med Oral Pathol Oral Radiol Endod* 79:482–487, 1995.

Buchner A, Merrell PW, Carpenter WM, et al.: Adenomatoid hyperplasia of minor salivary glands, *Oral Surg Oral Med Oral Pathol* 71:583–587, 1991.

Giansanti JS, Baker GO, Waldron CA: Intraoral, mucinous, minor salivary gland lesions presenting clinically as tumors, *Oral Surg Oral Med Oral Pathol* 32:918–922, 1971.

Necrotizing Sialometaplasia

Abrams AM, Melrose RJ, Howell FV: Necrotizing sialometaplasia: a disease simulating malignancy, *Cancer* 32:130–135, 1973.

Brannon RB, Fowler CB, Hartman KS: Necrotizing sialometaplasia: a clinicopathologic study of sixty-nine cases and review of the literature, *Oral Surg Oral Med Oral Pathol* 72:317–325, 1991.

Kaplan I, Alterman M, Kleinman S, et al.: The clinical, histologic, and treatment spectrum in necrotizing sialometaplasia, *Oral Surg Oral Med Oral Pathol Oral Radiol* 114:577–585, 2012.

Schöning H, Emshoff R, Kreczy A: Necrotizing sialometaplasia in two patients with bulimia and chronic vomiting, *Int J Oral Maxillofac Surg* 27:463–465, 1998.

Zhurakivska K, Maiorano E, Nocini R, et al.: Necrotizing sialometaplasia can hide the presence of salivary gland tumors: a case series, *Oral Dis* 25:1084–1090, 2019.

Salivary Gland Tumors: General Considerations

Andreasen S, Bjørndal K, Agander TK, et al.: Tumors of the sublingual gland: a national clinicopathologic study of 29 cases, *Eur Arch Otorhinolaryngol* 273:3847–3856, 2016.

Bishop JA, Thompson LDR, Wakely PE Jr, et al.: *Tumors of the salivary glands*, Arlington, 2021, American Registry of Pathology.

Buchner A, Merrell PW, Carpenter WM: Relative frequency of intraoral minor salivary gland tumors: a study of 380 cases from northern California and comparison to reports from other parts of the world, *J Oral Pathol Med* 36:207–214, 2007.

da Silva LP, Serpa MS, Viveiros SK, et al.: Salivary gland tumors in a Brazilian population: a 20-year retrospective and multicentric study of 2292 cases, *J Craniomaxillofac Surg* 46:2227–2233, 2018.

Ellies M, Schaffranietz F, Arglebe C, et al.: Tumor of the salivary glands in childhood and adolescence, *J Oral Maxillofac Surg* 64:1049–1058, 2006.

Ellis GL, Auclair PL: *Tumors of the salivary glands, AFIP atlas of tumor pathology, 4th series*, Silver Spring MD, 2008, ARP Press.

Ellis GL, Auclair PL, Gnepp DR: *Surgical pathology of the salivary glands*, Philadelphia, 1991, WB Saunders.

Eveson JW, Cawson RA: Salivary gland tumours: a review of 2410 cases with particular reference to histological types, site, age, and sex distribution, *J Pathol* 146:51–58, 1985a.

Eveson JW, Cawson RA: Tumours of the minor (oropharyngeal) salivary glands: a demographic study of 336 cases, *J Oral Pathol* 14:500–509, 1985b.

Gao M, Hao Y, Huang MX, et al.: Salivary gland tumours in a northern Chinese population: a 50-year retrospective study of 7190 cases, *Int J Oral Maxillofac Surg* 46:343–349, 2017.

Gnepp DR, Skalova A, Di Palma S, et al.: Salivary glands, In Gnepp DR, Bishop JA, editors: *Gnepp's diagnostic surgical pathology of the head and neck*, ed 3, 2021, Elsevier, pp 432–605.

Hay AJ, Migliacci J, Zanoni DK, et al.: Minor salivary gland tumors of the head and neck – Memorial Sloan Kettering experience:

incidence and outcomes by site and histological type, *Cancer* 125:3354–3366, 2019.

Jones AV, Craig GT, Speight PM, et al.: The range and demographics of salivary gland tumours diagnosed in a UK population, *Oral Oncol* 44:407–417, 2008.

Neville BW, Damm DD, Weir JC, et al.: Labial salivary gland tumors: an analysis of 103 cases, *Cancer* 61:2113–2116, 1988.

Pires FR, Pringle GA, de Almeida OP, et al.: Intra-oral minor salivary gland tumors: a clinicopathological study of 546 cases, *Oral Oncol* 43:463–470, 2007.

Seifert G, Miehlke A, Haubrich J, et al.: *Diseases of the salivary glands. Pathology—diagnosis—treatment—facial nerve surgery*, New York, 1986, George Thieme Verlag.

Sentani K, Ogawa I, Ozasa K, et al.: Characteristics of 5015 salivary gland neoplasms registered in the Hiroshima Tumor Tissue Registry over a period of 39 years, *J Clin Med* 8:566, 2019.

Spiro RH: Salivary neoplasms: overview of a 35-year experience with 2,807 patients, *Head Neck Surg* 8:177–184, 1986.

Tian Z, Li L, Wang L, et al.: Salivary gland neoplasms in oral and maxillofacial regions: a 23-year retrospective study of 6982 cases in an eastern Chinese population, *Int J Oral Maxillofac Surg* 39:235–242, 2010.

Waldron CA, EI-Mofty SK, Gnepp DR: Tumors of the intraoral minor salivary glands: a demographic and histologic study of 426 cases, *Oral Surg Oral Med Oral Pathol* 66:323–333, 1988.

Yih W-Y, Kratochvil FJ, Stewart JCB: Intraoral minor salivary gland neoplasms: review of 213 cases, *J Oral Maxillofac Surg* 63:805–810, 2005.

Pleomorphic Adenoma

Carlson ER, McCoy JM: Margins for benign salivary gland neoplasms of the head and neck, *Oral Maxillofac Surg Clin N Am* 29:325–340, 2017.

Dombrowski ND, Wolter NE, Irace AL, et al.: Pleomorphic adenoma of the head and neck in children: presentation and management, *Laryngoscope* 129:2603–2609, 2019.

Manor E, Joshua BZ, Brennan PA, et al.: Chromosomal aberrations in minor salivary gland pleomorphic adenoma, *J Oral Maxillofac Surg* 70:2798–2801, 2012.

Mendenhall WM, Mendenhall CM, Werning JW, et al.: Salivary gland pleomorphic adenoma, *Am J Clin Oncol* 31:95–99, 2008.

Sciubba JJ, Brannon R: Myoepithelioma of salivary glands: report of 23 cases, *Cancer* 47:562–572, 1982.

Silva SJ, Costa GT, Brant Filho AC, et al.: Metachronous bilateral pleomorphic adenoma of the parotid gland, *Oral Surg Oral Med Oral Pathol Oral Radiol Endod* 101:333–338, 2006.

Stennert E, Guntinas-Lichius O, Klussman JP, et al.: Histopathology of pleomorphic adenoma in the parotid gland: a prospective unselected series of 100 cases, *Laryngoscope* 111:2195–2200, 2001.

Triantafyllou A, Thompson LDR, Devaney KO, et al.: Functional histology of salivary gland pleomorphic adenoma: an appraisal, *Head Neck Pathol* 9:387–404, 2015.

Oncocytoma and Oncocytosis

Brandwein MS, Huvos AG: Oncocytic tumors of major salivary glands: a study of 68 cases with follow-up of 44 patients, *Am J Surg Pathol* 15:514–528, 1991.

Capone RB, Ha PK, Westra WH, et al.: Oncocytic neoplasms of the parotid gland: a 16-year institutional review, *Otolaryngol Head Neck Surg* 126:657–662, 2002.

Damm DD, White DK, Geissler RH Jr, et al.: Benign solid oncocytoma of intraoral minor salivary glands, *Oral Surg Oral Med Oral Pathol* 67:84–86, 1989.

Goode RK, Corio RL: Oncocytic adenocarcinoma of salivary glands, *Oral Surg Oral Med Oral Pathol* 65:61–66, 1988.

Rooper LM, Onenerk M, Siddiqui MT, et al.: Nodular oncocytic hyperplasia: can cytomorphology allow for preoperative diagnosis of a nonneoplastic salivary disease? *Cancer Cytopathol* 125:627–634, 2017.

Thompson LD, Wenig BM, Ellis GL: Oncocytomas of the submandibular gland: a series of 22 cases and a review of the literature, *Cancer* 78:2281–2287, 1996.

Zhan KY, Lentsch EJ: Oncocytic carcinoma of the major salivary glands: a population-based study of 278 cases, *Head Neck* 38: E1984–E1989, 2016.

Zhou C-X, Gao Y: Oncocytoma of the salivary glands: a clinicopathologic and immunohistochemical study, *Oral Oncol* 45:e232–e238, 2009.

Zhou C-X, Shi D-Y, Ma D-Q, et al.: Primary oncocytic carcinoma of the salivary glands: a clinicopathologic and immunohistochemical study of 12 cases, *Oral Oncol* 46:773–778, 2010.

Warthin Tumor

Fantasia JE, Miller AS: Papillary cystadenoma lymphomatosum arising in minor salivary glands, *Oral Surg Oral Med Oral Pathol* 52:411–416, 1981.

Franzen AM, Franzen CK, Guenzel T, et al.: Increased incidence of Warthin tumours of the parotid gland: a 42-year evaluation, *Eur Arch Otorhinolaryngol* 275:2593–2598, 2018.

Honda K, Kashima K, Daa T, et al.: Clonal analysis of the epithelial component of Warthin's tumor, *Hum Pathol* 31:1377–1380, 2000.

Kadletz L, Grasl S, Perisanidis C, et al.: Rising incidences of Warthin's tumors may be linked to obesity: a single-institution experience, *Eur Arch Otorhinolaryngol* 276:1191–1196, 2019.

Klussmann JP, Wittekindt C, Preuss SF, et al.: High risk for bilateral Warthin tumor in heavy smokers—review of 185 cases, *Acta Otolaryngol* 126:1213–1217, 2006.

Martins C, Fonseca I, Roque L, et al.: Cytogenetic characterisation of Warthin's tumour, *Oral Oncol* 33:344–347, 1997.

Psychogios G, Vlastos I, Thölken R, et al.: Warthin's tumor seems to be the most common benign neoplasm of the parotid gland in Germany, *Eur Arch Otorhinolaryngol* 277:2081–2084, 2020.

Takezawa K, Jackson C, Gnepp DR, et al.: Molecular characterization of Warthin tumor, *Oral Surg Oral Med Oral Pathol Oral Radiol Endod* 85:569–575, 1998.

Teymoortash A, Werner JA: Tissue that has lost its track: warthin's tumour, *Virchows Arch* 446:585–588, 2005.

Thangarajah T, Reddy VM, Castellanos-Arango F, et al.: Current controversies in the management of Warthin tumour, *Postgrad Med J* 85:3–8, 2009.

van der Wal JE, Davids JJ, van der Waal I: Extraparotid Warthin's tumours—report of 10 cases, *Br J Oral Maxillofac Surg* 31:43–44, 1993.

Veder LL, Kerrebijn JDF, Smedts FM, et al.: Diagnostic accuracy of fine-needle aspiration cytology in Warthin tumors, *Head Neck* 32:1635–1640, 2010.

Xu W, Lu H, Zhu Y, et al.: Warthin's tumour in oral and maxillofacial regions: an 18-year retrospective study of 1084 cases in an eastern-Chinese population, *Int J Oral Maxillofac Surg* 47:913–917, 2018.

Canalicular Adenoma

Daley TD, Gardner DG, Smout MS: Canalicular adenoma: not a basal cell adenoma, *Oral Surg Oral Med Oral Pathol* 57:181–188, 1984.

Gardner DG, Daley TD: The use of the terms monomorphic adenoma, basal cell adenoma, and canalicular adenoma as applied to salivary gland tumors, *Oral Surg Oral Med Oral Pathol* 56:608–615, 1983.

Neville BW, Damm DD, Weir JC, et al.: Labial salivary gland tumors: an analysis of 103 cases, *Cancer* 61:2113–2116, 1988.

Peraza AJ, Wright J, Gómez R: Canalicular adenoma: a systemic review, *J Craniomaxillofac Surg* 45:1754–1758, 2017.

Rousseau A, Mock D, Dover DG, et al.: Multiple canalicular adenomas: a case report and review of the literature, *Oral Surg Oral Med Oral Pathol Oral Radiol Endod* 87:346–350, 1999.

Suarez P, Hammond HL, Luna MA, et al.: Palatal canalicular adenoma: report of 12 cases and review of the literature, *Ann Diagn Pathol* 2:224–228, 1998.

Thompson LDR, Bauer JL, Chiosea S, et al.: Canalicular adenoma: a clinicopathologic and immunohistochemical analysis of 67 cases with a review of the literature, *Head Neck Pathol* 9:181–195, 2015.

Yoon AJ, Beller DE, Woo VL, et al.: Bilateral canalicular adenomas of the upper lip, *Oral Surg Oral Med Oral Pathol Oral Radiol Endod* 102:341–343, 2006.

Basal Cell Adenoma

Batsakis JG, Brannon RB: Dermal analogue tumours of major salivary glands, *J Laryngol* 95:155–164, 1981.

Ellis GL, Wiscovitch JG: Basal cell adenocarcinomas of the major salivary glands, *Oral Surg Oral Med Oral Pathol* 69:461–469, 1990.

Lee YH, Huang WC, Hsieh MS: *CTNNB1* mutations in basal cell adenoma of the salivary gland, *J Formos Med Assoc* 117:894–901, 2018.

Li BB, Zhou CX, Jia SN: Basal cell adenoma of salivary glands with a focal cribriform pattern: clinicopathologic and immunohistochemical study of 19 cases of a potential pitfall for diagnosis, *Ann Diagn Pathol* 18:5–9, 2014.

Machado de Sousa SO, Soares de Araújo N, Corrêa L, et al.: Immunohistochemical aspects of basal cell adenoma and canalicular adenoma of salivary glands, *Oral Oncol* 37:365–368, 2001.

Muller S, Barnes L: Basal cell adenocarcinoma of the salivary glands: report of seven cases and review of the literature, *Cancer* 78:2471–2477, 1996.

Tian Z, Hu Y, Wang L, et al.: An unusual cribriform variant of salivary basal cell tumours: a clinicopathological study of 22 cases, *Histopathology* 61:921–929, 2012.

Wilson TC, Robinson RA: Basal cell adenocarcinoma and basal cell adenoma of the salivary glands: a clinicopathologic review of seventy tumors with comparison of morphologic features and growth control indices, *Head Neck Pathol* 9:205–213, 2015.

Salivary Papillomas

Abrams AM, Finck FM: Sialadenoma papilliferum: a previously unreported salivary gland tumor, *Cancer* 24:1057–1063, 1969.

Brannon RB, Sciubba JJ, Giulani M: Ductal papillomas of salivary gland origin: a report of 19 cases and a review of the literature, *Oral Surg Oral Med Oral Pathol Oral Radiol Endod* 92:68–77, 2001.

Fowler CB, Damm DD: Sialadenoma papilliferum: analysis of seven new cases and review of the literature, *Head Neck Pathol* 12:193–201, 2018.

Gomes APN, Sobral APV, Loducca SVL, et al.: Sialadenoma papilliferum: immunohistochemical study, *Int J Oral Maxillofac Surg* 33:621–624, 2004.

Haberland-Carrodeguas C, Fornatora ML, Reich RF, et al.: Detection of human papillomavirus DNA in oral inverted ductal papillomas, *J Clin Pathol* 56:910–913, 2003.

Hsieh MS, Bishop JA, Wang YP, et al.: Salivary sialadenoma papilliferum consists of two morphologically, immunophenotypically, and genetically distinct subtypes, *Head Neck Pathol* 14:489–496, 2020.

Kubota N, Suzuki K, Kawai Y, et al.: Inverted ductal papilloma of minor salivary gland: case report with immunohistochemical study and literature review, *Pathol Int* 56:457–461, 2006.

Nakaguro M, Urano M, Ogawa I, et al.: Histopathologic evaluation of minor salivary gland papillary-cystic tumours: focus on genetic alterations in sialadenoma papilliferum and intraductal papillary mucinous neoplasm, *Histopathol* 76:411–422, 2020.

Sala-Pérez S, España-Tost A, Vidal-Bel A, et al.: Inverted ductal papilloma of the oral cavity secondary to lower lip trauma. A case report and literature review, *J Clin Exp Dent* 5:e112–e116, 2013.

de Sousa SO, Sesso A, de Araújo NS, et al.: Inverted ductal papilloma of minor salivary gland origin: morphological aspects and cytokeratin expression, *Eur Arch Otorhinolaryngol* 252:370–373, 1995.

Tomonao A, Kishino M, Masuda T, et al.: Intraductal papilloma arising from sublingual minor salivary gland: case report and immunohistochemical study, *Oral Surg Oral Med Oral Pathol Oral Radiol Endod* 107:e34–e37, 2009.

White DK, Miller AS, McDaniel RK, et al.: Inverted ductal papilloma: a distinctive lesion of minor salivary gland, *Cancer* 49:519–524, 1982.

Mucoepidermoid Carcinoma

Auclair PL, Goode RK, Ellis GL: Mucoepidermoid carcinoma of intraoral salivary glands, *Cancer* 69:2021–2030, 1992.

Birkeland AC, Foltin SK, Michmerhuizen NL, et al.: Correlation of *CRTC1/3-MAML2* fusion status, grade and survival in mucoepidermoid carcinoma, *Oral Oncol* 68:5–8, 2017.

Brandwein MS, Ivanov K, Wallace DI, et al.: Mucoepidermoid carcinoma: a clinicopathologic study of 80 patients with special reference to histological grading, *Am J Surg Pathol* 25:835–845, 2001.

Cipriani NA, Lusardi JJ, McElherne J, et al.: Mucoepidermoid carcinoma: a comparison of histologic grading systems and relationship to MAML2 rearrangement and prognosis, *Am J Surg Pathol* 43:885–897, 2019.

Dombrowski ND, Wolter NE, Irace AL, et al.: Mucoepidermoid carcinoma of the head and neck in children, *Int J Pediatr Otorhinolaryngol* 120:93–99, 2019.

Goode RK, Auclair PL, Ellis GL: Mucoepidermoid carcinoma of the major salivary glands: clinical and histopathologic analysis of 234 cases with evaluation of grading criteria, *Cancer* 82:1217–1224, 1998.

Hicks J, Flaitz C: Mucoepidermoid carcinoma of salivary glands in children and adolescents: assessment of proliferation markers, *Oral Oncol* 36:454–460, 2000.

Kolokythas A, Connor S, Kimgsoo D, et al.: Low-grade mucoepidermoid carcinoma of the intraoral minor salivary glands with cervical metastasis: report of 2 cases and review of the literature, *J Oral Maxillofac Surg* 68:1396–1399, 2010.

McHugh CH, Roberts DB, El-Naggar AK, et al.: Prognostic factors in mucoepidermoid carcinoma of the salivary glands, *Cancer* 118:3928–3936, 2012.

Navale P, Rooper LM, Bishop JA, et al.: Mucoepidermoid carcinoma of the oropharynx: a tumor type with a propensity for regional metastasis unrelated to histologic grade, *Human Pathol* 93:1–5, 2019.

Schwarz S, Stiegler C, Müller M, et al.: Salivary gland mucoepidermoid carcinoma is a clinically, morphologically and genetically heterogeneous entity: a clinicopathological study of 40 cases with emphasis on grading, histological variants and presence of the t(11;19) translocation, *Histopathology* 58:557–570, 2011.

Shafique K, Zhang PJ, Montone KT, et al.: Pathologic grading of mucoepidermoid carcinomas of the salivary gland and its effect on clinicopathologic follow-up: an institutional experience, *Human Pathol* 98:89–97, 2020.

Terauchi M, Michi Y, Hirai H, et al.: Prognostic factors in mucoepidermoid carcinoma of the minor salivary glands: a single-center retrospective study, *Oral Surg Oral Med Oral Pathol Oral Radiol* 131:209–216, 2021.

Védrine PO, Coffinet L, Temam S, et al.: Mucoepidermoid carcinoma of salivary glands in the pediatric age group: 18 clinical cases, including 11 second malignant neoplasms, *Head Neck* 28:827–833, 2006.

Intraosseous Mucoepidermoid Carcinoma

Bell D, Lewis C, El-Naggar AK, et al.: Primary intraosseous mucoepidermoid carcinoma of the jaw: reappraisal of the MD Anderson Cancer Center experience, *Head Neck* 38:E1312–E1317, 2016.

Brookstone MS, Huvos AG: Central salivary gland tumors of the maxilla and mandible: a clinicopathologic study of 11 cases with an analysis of the literature, *J Oral Maxillofac Surg* 50:229–236, 1992.

Browand BC, Waldron CA: Central mucoepidermoid tumors of the jaws, *Oral Surg Oral Med Oral Pathol* 40:631–643, 1975.

Li Y, Li LJ, Huang J, et al.: Central malignant salivary gland tumors of the jaw: retrospective clinical analysis of 22 cases, *J Oral Maxillofac Surg* 66:2247–2253, 2008.

Pires FR, Paes de Almeida O, Lopes MA, et al.: Central mucoepidermoid carcinoma of the mandible: report of four cases with long-term follow-up, *Int J Oral Maxillofac Surg* 32:378–382, 2003.

Waldron CA, Koh ML: Central mucoepidermoid carcinoma of the jaws: report of four cases with analysis of the literature and discussion of the relationship to mucoepidermoid, sialodontogenic, and glandular odontogenic cysts, *J Oral Maxillofac Surg* 48:871–877, 1990.

Zhou CX, Chen XM, Li TJ: Central mucoepidermoid carcinoma: a clinicopathologic and immunohistochemical study of 39 Chinese patients, *Am J Surg Pathol* 36:18–26, 2012.

Acinic Cell Carcinoma

Biron VL, Lentsch EJ, Gerry DR, et al.: Factors influencing survival in acinic cell carcinoma: a retrospective analysis of 2061 patients, *Head Neck* 37:870–877, 2015.

Bishop JA, Yonescu R, Batista D, et al.: Most nonparotid "acinic cell carcinomas" represent mammary analog secretory carcinomas, *Am J Surg Pathol* 37:1053–1057, 2013.

Chintakuntlawar AV, Shon W, Erickson-Johnson M, et al.: High-grade transformation of acinic cell carcinoma: an inadequately treated entity? *Oral Surg Oral Med Oral Pathol Oral Radiol* 121:542–549, 2016.

Chiosea SI, Griffith C, Assaad A, et al.: The profile of acinic cell carcinoma after recognition of mammary analog secretory carcinoma, *Am J Surg Pathol* 36:343–350, 2012.

Ellis GL, Corio RL: Acinic cell adenocarcinoma: a clinicopathologic analysis of 294 cases, *Cancer* 52:542–549, 1983.

Haller F, Skálová A, Ihrler S, et al.: Nuclear NR4A3 immunostaining is a specific and sensitive novel marker for acinic cell carcinoma of the salivary glands, *Am J Surg Pathol* 43:1264–1272, 2019.

Lei Y, Chiosea SI: Re-evaluating historic cohort of salivary acinic cell carcinoma with new diagnostic tools, *Head Neck Pathol* 6:166–170, 2012.

Michal M, Skálová A, Simpson RHW, et al.: Well-differentiated acinic cell carcinoma of salivary glands associated with lymphoid stroma, *Hum Pathol* 28:595–600, 1997.

Omlie JE, Koutlas IG: Acinic cell carcinoma of minor salivary glands: a clinicopathologic study of 21 cases, *J Oral Maxillofac Surg* 68:2053–2057, 2010.

Scherl C, Kato MG, Erkul E, et al.: Outcomes and prognostic factors for parotid acinic cell carcinoma: a National Cancer Database study of 2362 cases, *Oral Oncol* 82:53–60, 2018.

Schwarz S, Zenk J, Müller M, et al.: The many faces of acinic cell carcinomas of the salivary glands: a study of 40 cases relating histological and immunohistochemical subtypes to clinical parameters and prognosis, *Histopathology* 61:395–408, 2012.

Thompson LD, Aslam MN, Stall JN, et al.: Clinicopathologic and immunophenotypic characterization of 25 cases of acinic cell carcinoma with high-grade transformation, *Head Neck Pathol* 10:152–160, 2016.

Secretory Carcinoma

Bell D, Ferrarotto R, Liang L, et al.: Pan-Trk immunohistochemistry reliably identifies *ETV6-NTRK3* fusion in secretory carcinoma of the salivary gland, *Virchows Archiv* 476:295–305, 2020.

Bishop JA: Unmasking MASC: bringing to light the unique morphologic, immunohistochemical and genetic features of the newly recognized mammary analogue secretory carcinoma of salivary glands, *Head Neck Pathol* 7:35–39, 2013.

Boon E, Valstar MH, van der Graaf WTA, et al.: Clinicopathological characteristics and outcome of 31 patients with *ETV6-NTRK3* fusion gene confirmed (mammary analogue) secretory carcinoma of salivary glands, *Oral Oncol* 82:29–33, 2018.

Guilmette J, Dias-Santagata D, Nosé V, et al.: Novel gene fusions in secretory carcinoma of the salivary glands: enlarging the *ETV6* family, *Human Pathol* 83:50–58, 2019.

Kratochvil FJ III, Stewart JCB, Moore SR: Mammary analog secretory carcinoma of salivary glands: a report of 2 cases in the lips, *Oral Surg Oral Med Oral Pathol Oral Radiol* 114:630–635, 2012.

Skálová A: Mammary analogue secretory carcinoma of salivary gland origin: an update and expanded morphologic and immunohistochemical spectrum of recently described entity, *Head Neck Pathol* 7:S30–S36, 2013.

Skálová A, Vanecek T, Martinek P, et al.: Molecular profiling of mammary analog secretory carcinoma revealed a subset of tumors harboring a novel *ETV6-RET* translocation: report of 10 cases, *Am J Surg Pathol* 42:234–246, 2018.

Skálová A, Vanecek T, Sima R, et al.: Mammary analogue secretory carcinoma of salivary glands, containing the ETV6-NTRK3 fusion gene: a hitherto undescribed salivary gland tumor entity, *Am J Surg Pathol* 34:599–608, 2010.

Xu B, Haroon Al Rasheed MR, Antonescu CR, et al.: Pan-Trk immunohistochemistry is a sensitive and specific ancillary tool for diagnosing secretory carcinoma of the salivary gland and detecting *ETV6-NTRK3* fusion, *Histopathol* 76:375–382, 2020.

Malignant Mixed Tumors

Antony J, Gopalan V, Smith RA, et al.: Carcinoma ex pleomorphic adenoma: a comprehensive review of clinical, pathological and molecular data, *Head Neck Pathol* 6:1–9, 2012.

Auclair PL, Ellis GL: Atypical features in salivary gland mixed tumors: their relationship to malignant transformation, *Mod Pathol* 9:652–657, 1996.

Brandwein M, Huvos AG, Dardick I, et al.: Noninvasive and minimally invasive carcinoma ex mixed tumor: a clinicopathologic and ploidy study of 12 patients with major salivary tumors of low (or no?) malignant potential, *Oral Surg Oral Med Oral Pathol Oral Radiol Endod* 81:655–664, 1996.

Gnepp DR: Malignant mixed tumors of the salivary glands: a review, *Pathol Annu* 28(Pt 1):279–328, 1993.

Gupta A, Koochakzadeh S, Neskey DM, et al.: Salivary carcinosarcoma: an extremely rare and highly aggressive malignancy, *Laryngoscope* 130:E335–E339, 2020.

Hu YH, Zhang CY, Xia RH, et al.: Prognostic factors of carcinoma ex pleomorphic adenoma of the salivary glands, with emphasis on the widely invasive carcinoma: a clinicopathologic analysis of 361 cases in a Chinese population, *Oral Surg Oral Med Oral Pathol Oral Radiol* 122:598–608, 2016.

Katabi N, Gomez D, Klimstra DS, et al.: Prognostic factors of recurrence in salivary carcinoma ex pleomorphic adenoma, with emphasis on the carcinoma histologic subtype: a clinicopathologic study of 43 cases, *Hum Pathol* 41:927–934, 2010.

Knight J, Ratnasingham K: Metastasising pleomorphic adenoma: systematic review, *Int J Surg* 19:137–145, 2015.

Lewis JE, Olsen KD, Sebo TJ: Carcinoma ex pleomorphic adenoma: pathologic analysis of 73 cases, *Hum Pathol* 32:596–604, 2001.

LiVolsi VA, Perzin KH: Malignant mixed tumors arising in salivary glands. I. Carcinomas arising in benign mixed tumor: a clinicopathologic study, *Cancer* 39:2209–2230, 1977.

Nouraei SAR, Ferguson MS, Clarke PM, et al.: Metastasizing pleomorphic salivary adenoma, *Arch Otolaryngol Head Neck Surg* 132:788–793, 2006.

Spiro RH, Huvos AG, Strong EW: Malignant mixed tumor of salivary origin: a clinicopathologic study of 146 cases, *Cancer* 39:388–396, 1977.

Tortoledo ME, Luna MA, Batsakis JG: Carcinomas ex pleomorphic adenoma and malignant mixed tumors, *Arch Otolaryngol* 110:172–176, 1984.

Ye P, Gao Y, Mao C, et al.: Carcinoma ex pleomorphic adenoma: is it a high-grade malignancy? *J Oral Maxillofac Surg* 74:2093–2104, 2016.

Adenoid Cystic Carcinoma

Araújo VC, Loducca SVL, Sousa SOM, et al.: The cribriform features of adenoid cystic carcinoma and polymorphous low-grade adenocarcinoma: cytokeratin and integrin expression, *Ann Diagn Pathol* 5:330–334, 2001.

Atallah S, Casiraghi O, Fakhry N, et al.: A prospective multicentre REFCOR study of 470 cases of head and neck adenoid cystic carcinoma: epidemiology and prognostic factors, *Eur J Cancer* 130:241–249, 2020.

Bhayani MK, Yener M, El-Naggar A, et al.: Prognosis and risk factors for early-stage adenoid cystic carcinoma of the major salivary glands, *Cancer* 118:2872–2878, 2012.

Coca-Pelaz A, Rodrigo JP, Bradley PJ, et al.: Adenoid cystic carcinoma of the head and neck – an update, *Oral Oncol* 51:652–661, 2015.

Darling MR, Schneider JW, Phillips VM: Polymorphous low-grade adenocarcinoma and adenoid cystic carcinoma: a review and comparison of immunohistochemical markers, *Oral Oncol* 38:641–645, 2002.

Ellington CL, Goodman M, Kono SA, et al.: Adenoid cystic carcinoma of the head and neck: incidence and survival trends based on the 1973–2007 Surveillance, *Epidemiology, and End Results data, Cancer* 118:4444–4451, 2012.

Enamorado I, Lakhani R, Korkmaz H, et al.: Correlation of histopathological variants, cellular DNA content, and clinical outcome in adenoid cystic carcinoma of the salivary glands, *Otolaryngol Head Neck Surg* 131:646–650, 2004.

Han J, Gu T, Yang X, et al.: Primary intraosseous adenoid cystic carcinoma of the mandible: a comprehensive review and analysis of four new cases with emphasis on morphologic, immunophenotypic, and molecular characteristics, *Oral Surg Oral Med Oral Pathol Oral Radiol* 123:365–373, 2017.

Ju J, Li Y, Chai J, et al.: The role of perineural invasion on head and neck adenoid cystic carcinoma prognosis: a systematic review and meta-analysis, *Oral Surg Oral Med Oral Pathol Oral Radiol* 122:691–701, 2016.

Lloyd S, Yu JB, Wilson LD, et al.: Determinants and patterns of survival in adenoid cystic carcinoma of the head and neck, including an analysis of adjuvant radiation therapy, *Am J Clin Oncol* 34:76–81, 2011.

Penner CR, Folpe AL, Budnick SD: C-kit expression distinguishes salivary gland adenoid cystic carcinoma from polymorphous low-grade adenocarcinoma, *Mod Pathol* 15:687–691, 2002.

Rettig EM, Tan M, Ling S, et al.: MYB rearrangement and clinicopathologic characteristics in head and neck adenoid cystic carcinoma, *Laryngoscope* 125:E292–E299, 2015.

Skálová A, Simpson RH, Lehtonen H, et al.: Assessment of proliferative activity using the MIB1 antibody help to distinguish polymorphous low grade adenocarcinoma from adenoid cystic carcinoma of salivary glands, *Pathol Res Pract* 193:695–703, 1997.

Suárez C, Barnes L, Silver CE, et al.: Cervical lymph node metastasis in adenoid cystic carcinoma of oral cavity and oropharynx, *Auris Nasus Larynx* 43:477–484, 2016.

Woo VL, Bhuiya T, Kelsch R: Assessment of CD43 expression in adenoid cystic carcinomas, polymorphous low-grade adenocarcinomas, and monomorphic adenomas, *Oral Surg Oral Med Oral Pathol Oral Radiol Endod* 102:495–500, 2006.

Xiao R, Sethi RKV, Feng AL, et al.: The role of elective neck dissection in patients with adenoid cystic carcinoma of the head and neck, *Laryngoscope* 129:2094–2104, 2019.

Polymorphous Adenocarcinoma

Araújo VC, Loducca SVL, Sousa SOM, et al.: The cribriform features of adenoid cystic carcinoma and polymorphous low-grade adenocarcinoma: cytokeratin and integrin expression, *Ann Diagn Pathol* 5:330–334, 2001.

Batsakis JG, Pinkston GR, Luna MA, et al.: Adenocarcinomas of the oral cavity: a clinicopathologic study of terminal duct carcinomas, *J Laryngol Otol* 97:825–835, 1983.

Castle JT, Thompson LDR, Frommelt RA, et al.: Polymorphous low grade adenocarcinoma: a clinicopathologic study of 164 cases, *Cancer* 86:207–219, 1999.

Chi AC, Neville BW: Surface papillary epithelial hyperplasia (rough mucosa) is a helpful clue for identification of polymorphous low-grade adenocarcinoma, *Head Neck Pathol* 9:244–252, 2015.

Curran AE, White DK, Damm DD, et al.: Polymorphous low-grade adenocarcinoma versus pleomorphic adenoma of minor salivary glands: resolution of a diagnostic dilemma by immunohistochemical analysis with glial fibrillary acidic protein, *Oral Surg Oral Med Oral Pathol Oral Radiol Endod* 91:194–199, 2001.

Evans HL, Luna MA: Polymorphous low-grade adenocarcinoma: a study of 40 cases with long-term follow up and an evaluation of the importance of papillary areas, *Am J Surg Pathol* 24:1319–1328, 2000.

Freedman PD, Lumerman H: Lobular carcinoma of intraoral minor salivary glands, *Oral Surg Oral Med Oral Pathol* 56:157–165, 1983.

Mimica X, Katabi N, McGill MR, et al.: Polymorphous adenocarcinoma of salivary glands, *Oral Oncol* 95:52–58, 2019.

Penner CR, Folpe AL, Budnick SD: C-kit expression distinguishes salivary gland adenoid cystic carcinoma from polymorphous low-grade adenocarcinoma, *Mod Pathol* 15:687–691, 2002.

Sebastiao APM, Pareja F, Kumar R, et al.: Genomic analysis of recurrences and high-grade forms of polymorphous adenocarcinoma, *Histopathol* 75:193–201, 2019.

Sebastiao APM, Xu B, Lozada JR, et al.: Histologic spectrum of polymorphous adenocarcinoma of the salivary gland harbor genetic alterations affecting *PRKD* genes, *Mod Pathol* 33:65–73, 2020.

Seethala RR, Johnson JT, Barnes EL, et al.: Polymorphous low-grade adenocarcinoma: the University of Pittsburgh experience, *Arch Otolaryngol Head Neck Surg* 136:385–392, 2010.

Vander Poorten V, Triantafyllou A, Skálová A, et al.: Polymorphous adenocarcinoma of the salivary glands: reappraisal and update, *Eur Arch Otorhinolaryngol* 275:1681–1695, 2018.

Woo VL, Bhuiya T, Kelsch R: Assessment of CD43 expression in adenoid cystic carcinomas, polymorphous low-grade adenocarcinomas, and monomorphic adenomas, *Oral Surg Oral Med Oral Pathol Oral Radiol Endod* 102:495–500, 2006.

Xu B, Aneja A, Ghossein R, et al.: Predictors of outcome in the phenotypic spectrum of polymorphous low grade adenocarcinoma (PLGA) and cribriform adenocarcinoma of salivary gland (CASG): retrospective study of 69 patients, *Am J Surg Pathol* 40:1526–1537, 2016.

Xu B, Barbieri AL, Bishop JA, et al.: Histologic classification and molecular signature of polymorphous adenocarcinoma (PAC) and cribriform adencarcinoma of salivary gland (CASG). An international interobserver study, *Am J Surg Pathol* 44:545–552, 2020.

Salivary Adenocarcinoma, Not Otherwise Specified

Li J, Wang BY, Nelson M, et al.: Salivary adenocarcinoma, not otherwise specified: a collection of orphans, *Arch Pathol Lab Med* 128:1385–1394, 2004.

Matsuba HM, Mauney M, Simpson JR, et al.: Adenocarcinomas of major and minor salivary gland origin: a histopathologic review of treatment failure patterns, *Laryngoscope* 98:784–788, 1988.

Spiro RH, Huvos AG, Strong EW: Adenocarcinoma of salivary origin: clinicopathologic study of 204 patients, *Am J Surg* 144:423–431, 1982.

Stene T, Koppang HS: Intraoral adenocarcinomas, *J Oral Pathol* 10:216–225, 1981.

Wahlberg P, Anderson H, Biörklund A, et al.: Carcinoma of the parotid and submandibular glands—a study of survival in 2465 patients, *Oral Oncol* 38:706–713, 2002.

12

Soft Tissue Tumors

Mesenchymal soft tissue growths of the oral and maxillofacial region include both reactive tumor-like proliferations as well as true neoplasms. Virtually every different type of connective tissue has a number of both benign and malignant tumors, reflecting mutations that drive differentiation toward various tissue types, which results in a complex classification for these lesions. In addition, our knowledge of these tumors is rapidly and continuously expanding, especially as we learn more about the molecular/genetic changes that underlie many of these lesions (see Table 12.1). The discussion in this chapter will emphasize a number of the more common or more important tumors that may occur in the oral, head, and neck region.

◆ FIBROMA (IRRITATION FIBROMA; TRAUMATIC FIBROMA; FOCAL FIBROUS HYPERPLASIA; FIBROUS NODULE)

he **fibroma** is the most common "tumor" of the oral cavity. However, it is doubtful that it represents a true neoplasm in most instances; rather, it is a reactive hyperplasia of fibrous connective tissue in response to local irritation or trauma.

Clinical Features

Although the irritation fibroma can occur anywhere in the mouth, the most common location is the buccal mucosa along the bite line. Presumably, this is a consequence of trauma from biting the cheek (Figs. 12.1 and 12.2). The labial mucosa, tongue, and gingiva also are common sites (Figs. 12.3 and 12.4). It is likely that many gingival fibromas represent fibrous maturation of a preexisting pyogenic granuloma. The lesion typically appears as a smooth-surfaced pink nodule that is similar in color to the surrounding mucosa. In black patients, the mass may demonstrate gray-brown pigmentation. In some cases the surface may appear white as a result of hyperkeratosis from continued irritation. Most fibromas are sessile, although some are pedunculated. They range in size from tiny lesions that are only a couple of millimeters in diameter to large masses that are several centimeters across; however, most fibromas are 1.5 cm or less in diameter. The lesion usually produces no symptoms, unless secondary traumatic ulceration of the surface

has occurred. Irritation fibromas are most common in the fourth to sixth decades of life, and the male-to-female ratio is almost 1:2 for cases submitted for biopsy.

The **frenal tag** is a commonly observed type of fibrous hyperplasia, which most frequently occurs on the maxillary labial frenum. Such lesions present as small, asymptomatic, exophytic growths attached to the thin frenum surface (Fig. 12.5). One study of 5- to 13-year-old children found the prevalence of frenal tags to be 17.1%.

Histopathologic Features

Microscopic examination of the irritation fibroma shows a nodular mass of fibrous connective tissue covered by stratified squamous epithelium (Figs. 12.6 and 12.7). This connective tissue is usually dense and collagenized, although in some cases it is looser in nature. The lesion is not encapsulated; the fibrous tissue instead blends gradually into the surrounding connective tissues. The collagen bundles may be arranged in a radiating, circular, or haphazard fashion. The covering epithelium often demonstrates atrophy of the rete ridges because of the underlying fibrous mass. However, the surface may exhibit hyperkeratosis from secondary trauma. Scattered inflammation may be seen, most often beneath the epithelial surface. Usually this inflammation is chronic and consists mostly of lymphocytes and plasma cells.

Treatment and Prognosis

The irritation fibroma is treated by conservative surgical excision; recurrence is extremely rare. However, it is important to submit the excised tissue for microscopic examination because other benign or malignant tumors may mimic the clinical appearance of a fibroma.

Because frenal tags are small, innocuous growths that are easily diagnosed clinically, no treatment is usually necessary.

◆ GIANT CELL FIBROMA

The **giant cell fibroma** is a fibrous tumor with distinctive clinicopathologic features. Unlike the traumatic fibroma, it does not appear to be associated with chronic irritation. The giant cell fibroma represents approximately 2%–5% of all oral fibrous proliferations submitted for biopsy.

TABLE 12.1	Genetic Abnormalities of Various Soft Tissue Tumors	
Tumor	**Associated Gene Mutation/Translocation/ Rearrangement**
Solitary fibrous tumor	*NAB2::STAT6* gene fusion
Sinonasal-type hemangiopericytoma	*CTNNB1* mutation
Desmoid-type fibromatosis	*CTNNB1* mutation
Congenital hemangioma	*GNAQ* or *GNA11* mutation
Capillary vascular malformation	*GNAQ* or *PI3KCA* mutation
Venous malformation	*TIE2 (TEK)*, *PIK3CA*, or *MAP3K3* mutation
Arteriovenous malformation	*MAP2K1* mutation
Lymphatic malformation	*PIK3CA* mutation
Ectomesenchymal chondromyxoid tumor	*RREB1::MKL2* gene fusion
Embryonal rhabdomyosarcoma	Loss of heterozygosity of chromosome 11p15.5
Alveolar rhabdomyosarcoma	*PAX3::FOXO1* or *PAX7::FOXO1* gene fusion
Spindle cell/sclerosing rhabdomyosarcoma (congenital/infantile)	Gene fusions involving *VGLL2*, *SRF*, and *TEAD1*
Spindle cell/sclerosing rhabdomyosarcoma (adults)	*MYOD1* mutation
Monophasic synovial sarcoma	*SS18::SSX2* gene fusion
Biphasic synovial sarcoma	*SS18::SSX1* gene fusion
Alveolar soft part sarcoma	*ASPSCR1::TFE3* gene fusion

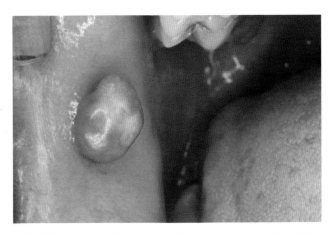

• **Fig. 12.2 Fibroma.** Black patient with a smooth-surfaced pigmented nodule on the buccal mucosa near the commissure.

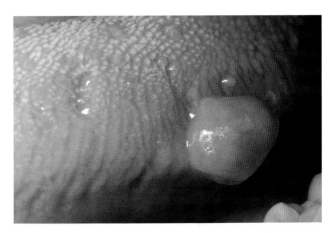

• **Fig. 12.3 Fibroma.** Lesion on the lateral border of the tongue.

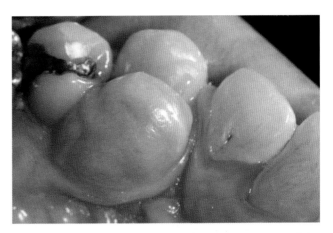

• **Fig. 12.4 Fibroma.** Smooth-surfaced, pink nodular mass of the palatal gingiva between the cuspid and first bicuspid.

Clinical Features

The giant cell fibroma is typically an asymptomatic sessile or pedunculated nodule, usually less than 1 cm in size (Fig. 12.8). The surface of the mass often appears papillary; therefore, the lesion may be clinically mistaken for a papilloma (Fig. 12.9). Compared with the common irritation

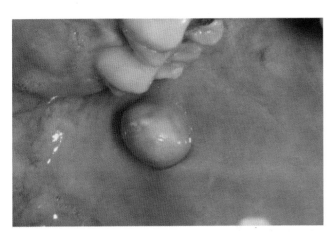

• **Fig. 12.1 Fibroma.** Pink nodule of the posterior buccal mucosa near the level of the occlusal plane.

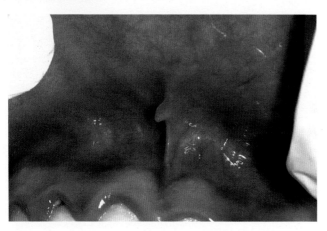

• **Fig. 12.5 Frenal Tag.** A small fingerlike projection of tissue attached to the maxillary labial frenum.

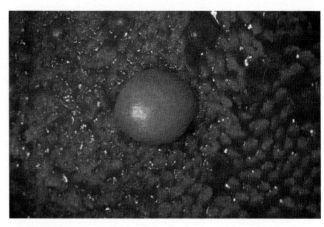

• **Fig. 12.8 Giant Cell Fibroma.** Exophytic nodule on the dorsum of the tongue.

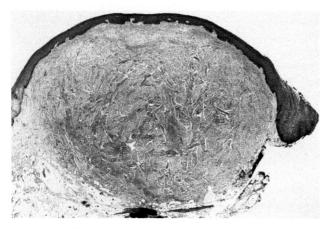

• **Fig. 12.6 Fibroma.** Low-power view showing an exophytic nodular mass of dense fibrous connective tissue.

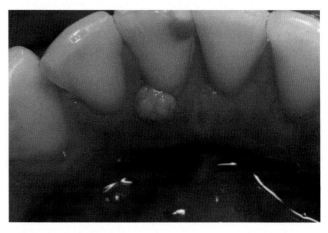

• **Fig. 12.9 Giant Cell Fibroma.** Papillary growth on the lingual mandibular gingiva. Because of the rough surface, this lesion would be easily mistaken for a papilloma.

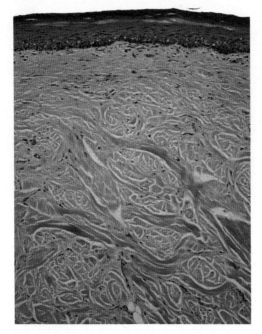

• **Fig. 12.7 Fibroma.** Higher-power view demonstrating dense collagen beneath the epithelial surface.

fibroma, the lesion usually occurs at a younger age. In about 60% of cases, the lesion is diagnosed during the first three decades of life. Some studies have suggested a slight female predilection. Approximately 50% of all cases occur on the gingiva. The mandibular gingiva is affected twice as often as the maxillary gingiva. The tongue and palate also are common sites.

The **retrocuspid papilla** is a microscopically similar developmental lesion that occurs on the gingiva lingual to the mandibular cuspid. It is frequently bilateral and typically appears as a small, pink papule that measures less than 5 mm in diameter (Fig. 12.10). Retrocuspid papillae are quite common, having been reported in 25%–99% of children and young adults. The prevalence in older adults drops to 6%–19%, suggesting that the retrocuspid papilla represents a normal anatomic variation that disappears with age.

Histopathologic Features

Microscopic examination of the giant cell fibroma reveals a mass of vascular fibrous connective tissue, which is usually loosely arranged (Fig. 12.11). The hallmark is the presence

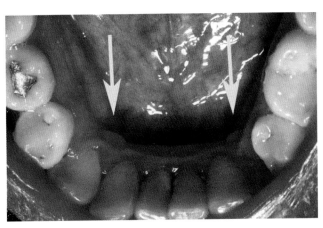

• **Fig. 12.10 Retrocuspid Papilla.** Bilateral papular lesions on the gingiva lingual to the mandibular canines (*arrows*).

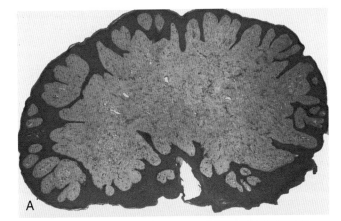

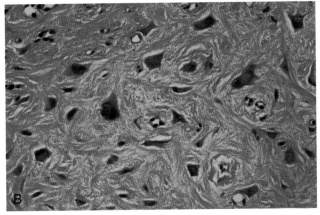

• **Fig. 12.11 Giant Cell Fibroma. A,** Low-power view showing a nodular mass of fibrous connective tissue covered by stratified squamous epithelium. Note the elongation of the rete ridges. **B,** High-power view showing multiple large stellate-shaped and multinucleated fibroblasts.

of numerous large, stellate fibroblasts within the superficial connective tissue. These cells may contain several nuclei. Frequently, the surface of the lesion is pebbly. The covering epithelium often is thin and atrophic, although the rete ridges may appear narrow and elongated.

Treatment and Prognosis

The giant cell fibroma is treated by conservative surgical excision. Recurrence is rare. Because of their characteristic appearance, retrocuspid papillae should be recognized clinically and do not need to be excised.

◆ EPULIS FISSURATUM (INFLAMMATORY FIBROUS HYPERPLASIA; DENTURE INJURY TUMOR; DENTURE EPULIS)

The **epulis fissuratum** is a tumor-like hyperplasia of fibrous connective tissue that develops in association with the flange of an ill-fitting complete or partial denture. Although the simple term *epulis* sometimes is used synonymously for epulis fissuratum, *epulis* is actually a generic term that can be applied to any tumor of the gingiva or alveolar mucosa. Therefore, some authors have advocated not using this term, preferring to call these lesions *inflammatory fibrous hyperplasia* or other descriptive names. However, the term *epulis fissuratum* is still widely used today and is well understood by virtually all clinicians. Other examples of epulides include the **giant cell epulis (peripheral giant cell granuloma)** (see page 527), **ossifying fibroid epulis (peripheral ossifying fibroma)** (see page 529), and **congenital epulis** (see page 546).

Clinical Features

The epulis fissuratum typically appears as a single or multiple fold or folds of hyperplastic tissue in the alveolar vestibule (Figs. 12.12 and 12.13). Most often, there are two folds of tissue, and the flange of the associated denture fits conveniently into the fissure between the folds. The redundant tissue is usually firm and fibrous, although some lesions appear erythematous and ulcerated, similar to the appearance of a pyogenic granuloma. Occasional examples of epulis fissuratum demonstrate surface areas of inflammatory papillary hyperplasia (see page 519). The size of the lesion can vary from localized hyperplasias less than 1 cm in size to massive lesions that involve most of the length of the vestibule. The epulis fissuratum usually develops on the facial aspect of the alveolar ridge, although occasional lesions are seen lingual to the mandibular alveolar ridge (Fig. 12.14).

The epulis fissuratum most often occurs in middle-aged and older adults, as would be expected with a denture-related lesion. It may occur on either the maxilla or mandible. The anterior portion of the jaws is affected much more often than the posterior areas. There is a pronounced female predilection; most studies show that two-thirds to three-fourths of all cases submitted for biopsy occur in women.

Another similar but less common fibrous hyperplasia, often called a **fibroepithelial polyp** or **leaflike denture fibroma,** occurs on the hard palate beneath a maxillary denture. This characteristic lesion is a flattened pink mass that is attached to the palate by a narrow stalk (Fig. 12.15). Usually, the flattened mass is closely applied to the palate and sits in a

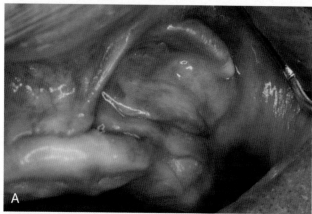

• **Fig. 12.12 Epulis Fissuratum.** Hyperplastic folds of tissue in the anterior maxillary vestibule.

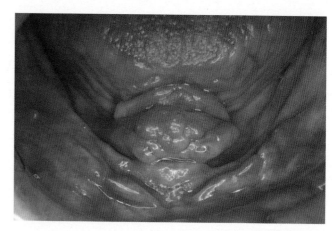

• **Fig. 12.14 Epulis Fissuratum.** Redundant folds of tissue arising in the floor of the mouth in association with a mandibular denture.

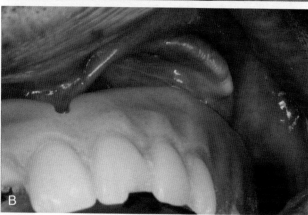
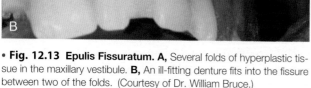

• **Fig. 12.13 Epulis Fissuratum. A,** Several folds of hyperplastic tissue in the maxillary vestibule. **B,** An ill-fitting denture fits into the fissure between two of the folds. (Courtesy of Dr. William Bruce.)

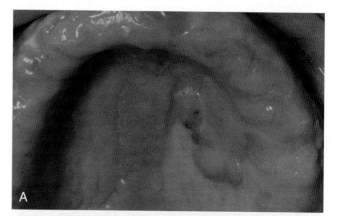
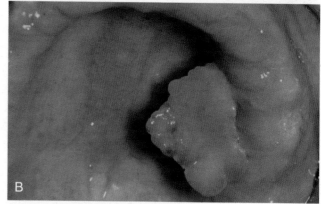

• **Fig. 12.15 Fibroepithelial Polyp.** Flattened mass of tissue arising on the hard palate beneath a maxillary denture; note its pedunculated nature. Because of its serrated edge, this lesion also is known as a *leaf-like denture fibroma.* Associated inflammatory papillary hyperplasia is visible in the palatal midline.

slightly cupped-out depression. However, it is easily lifted up with a probe, which demonstrates its pedunculated nature. The edge of the lesion often is serrated and resembles a leaf.

Histopathologic Features

Microscopic examination of the epulis fissuratum reveals hyperplasia of the fibrous connective tissue. Often multiple folds and grooves occur where the denture impinges on the

tissue (Fig. 12.16). The overlying epithelium is frequently hyperparakeratotic and demonstrates irregular hyperplasia of the rete ridges. In some instances, the epithelium shows inflammatory papillary hyperplasia (see page 519) or pseudoepitheliomatous (pseudocarcinomatous) hyperplasia. Focal areas of ulceration are not unusual, especially at the base of the grooves between the folds. A variable chronic inflammatory infiltrate is present; sometimes, it may include

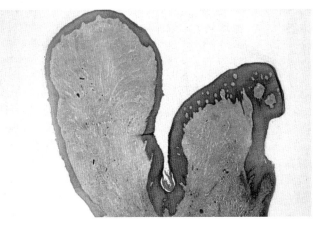

• **Fig. 12.16 Epulis Fissuratum.** Low-power photomicrograph demonstrating folds of hyperplastic fibrovascular connective tissue covered by stratified squamous epithelium.

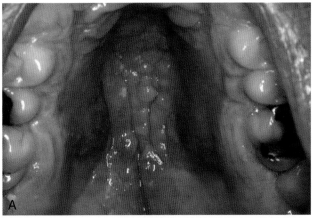

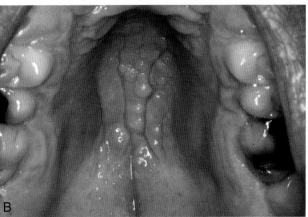

• **Fig. 12.17 Inflammatory Papillary Hyperplasia With Secondary Candidiasis. A,** Erythematous, pebbly appearance of the palatal vault. **B,** Resolution of the erythema following antifungal therapy.

eosinophils or show lymphoid follicles. If minor salivary glands are included in the specimen, then they usually show chronic sialadenitis.

In rare instances, the formation of osteoid or chondroid is observed. This unusual-appearing product, known as **osseous and chondromatous metaplasia,** is a reactive phenomenon caused by chronic irritation by the ill-fitting denture (see page 309). The irregular nature of this bone or cartilage can be microscopically disturbing, and the pathologist should not mistake it for a sarcoma.

The denture-related fibroepithelial polyp has a narrow core of dense fibrous connective tissue covered by stratified squamous epithelium. Like the epulis fissuratum, the overlying epithelium may be hyperplastic.

Treatment and Prognosis

The treatment of the epulis fissuratum or fibroepithelial polyp consists of surgical removal, with microscopic examination of the excised tissue. The ill-fitting denture should be remade or relined to prevent a recurrence of the lesion.

◆ INFLAMMATORY PAPILLARY HYPERPLASIA (DENTURE PAPILLOMATOSIS)

Inflammatory papillary hyperplasia is a reactive tissue growth that usually, although not always, develops beneath a denture. Some investigators classify this lesion as part of the spectrum of denture stomatitis (see page 205). Although the exact pathogenesis is unknown, the condition most often appears to be related to the following:
• An ill-fitting denture
• Poor denture hygiene
• Wearing the denture 24 hours a day

Approximately 20% of patients who wear their dentures 24 hours a day have inflammatory papillary hyperplasia. *Candida* organisms also have been suggested as a cause, but any possible role appears uncertain.

Clinical Features

Inflammatory papillary hyperplasia usually occurs on the hard palate beneath a denture base (Figs. 12.17 and 12.18). Early lesions may involve only the palatal vault, although advanced cases cover most of the palate. Less frequently, this hyperplasia develops on the edentulous mandibular alveolar ridge or on the surface of an epulis fissuratum. On rare occasions, the condition occurs on the palate of a patient without a denture, especially in people who habitually breathe through their mouth or have a high palatal vault. *Candida*-associated palatal papillary hyperplasia also has been reported in dentate patients with human immunodeficiency virus (HIV) infection.

Inflammatory papillary hyperplasia is usually asymptomatic. The mucosa is erythematous and has a pebbly or papillary surface. Many cases are associated with denture stomatitis.

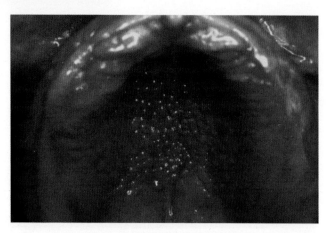

• **Fig. 12.18 Inflammatory Papillary Hyperplasia.** An advanced case exhibiting more pronounced papular lesions of the hard palate.

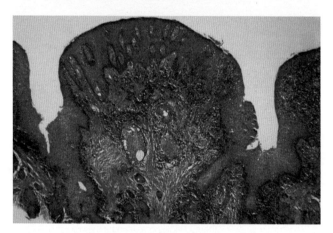

• **Fig. 12.19 Inflammatory Papillary Hyperplasia.** Medium-power view showing fibrous and epithelial hyperplasia resulting in papillary surface projections. Heavy chronic inflammation is present.

Histopathologic Features

The mucosa in inflammatory papillary hyperplasia exhibits numerous papillary growths on the surface that are covered by hyperplastic, stratified squamous epithelium (Fig. 12.19). In advanced cases, this hyperplasia is pseudoepitheliomatous in appearance, and the pathologist should not mistake it for carcinoma (Fig. 12.20). The connective tissue can vary from loose and edematous to densely collagenized. A chronic inflammatory cell infiltrate is usually seen, which consists of lymphocytes and plasma cells. Less frequently, polymorphonuclear leukocytes are also present. If underlying salivary glands are present, then they often show sclerosing sialadenitis.

Treatment and Prognosis

For very early lesions of inflammatory papillary hyperplasia, removal of the denture may allow the erythema and edema to subside, and the tissues may resume a more normal appearance. The condition also may show improvement after topical or systemic antifungal therapy. For more advanced and collagenized lesions, many clinicians prefer to excise the hyperplastic tissue before fabricating a new denture. Various surgical methods have been used, including the following:

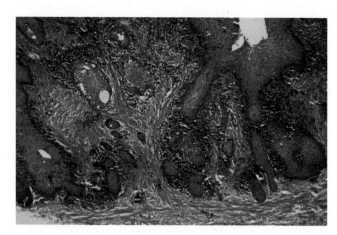

• **Fig. 12.20 Inflammatory Papillary Hyperplasia.** Higher-power view showing pseudoepitheliomatous hyperplasia of the epithelium. This epithelium has a bland appearance that should not be mistaken for carcinoma.

- Partial-thickness or full-thickness surgical blade excision
- Curettage
- Electrosurgery
- Cryosurgery
- Laser surgery

After surgery, the existing denture can be lined with a temporary tissue conditioner that acts as a palatal dressing and promotes greater comfort. After healing, the patient should be encouraged to leave the new denture out at night and to keep it clean.

◆ FIBROUS HISTIOCYTOMA

Fibrous histiocytomas are a diverse group of tumors that exhibit fibroblastic and histiocytic differentiation, although the cell of origin is uncertain. Because of the variable nature of these lesions, an array of terms has been used for them, including **dermatofibroma, sclerosing hemangioma, fibroxanthoma,** and **nodular subepidermal fibrosis.** Unlike other fibrous growths discussed previously in this chapter, the fibrous histiocytoma is generally considered to represent a true neoplasm.

Clinical Features

The fibrous histiocytoma can develop almost anywhere in the body. The most common site is the skin of the extremities, where the lesion is called a *dermatofibroma.* Tumors of the oral and perioral region are rare, and it is likely that many previously reported examples would be reclassified today as *solitary fibrous tumors* (see next topic). Rare intrabony lesions of the jaws also have been reported. Oral fibrous histiocytomas tend to occur in middle-aged and older adults; cutaneous examples are most frequent in young adults. The tumor is usually a painless nodular mass and can vary in size from a few millimeters to several centimeters in diameter (Fig. 12.21). Deeper tumors tend to be larger.

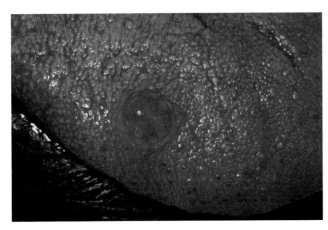

• **Fig. 12.21 Fibrous Histiocytoma.** Nodular mass on the dorsum of the tongue.

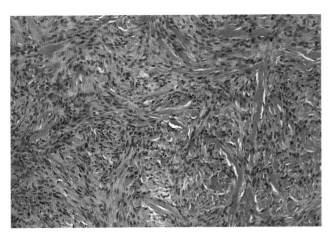

• **Fig. 12.22 Fibrous Histiocytoma.** Medium-power view of a skin tumor (*dermatofibroma*) showing spindle-shaped cells arranged in a storiform pattern.

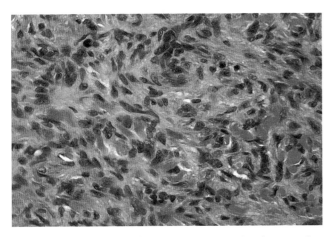

• **Fig. 12.23 Fibrous Histiocytoma.** High-power view demonstrating spindle-shaped cells with vesicular nuclei.

Histopathologic Features

Microscopically, the fibrous histiocytoma is characterized by a cellular proliferation of spindle-shaped fibroblastic cells with vesicular nuclei (Figs. 12.22 and 12.23). The margins of the tumor often are not sharply defined. The tumor cells are arranged in short, intersecting fascicles, known as a *storiform* pattern because of its resemblance to the irregular, whorled appearance of a straw mat. Rounded histiocyte-like cells, lipid-containing xanthoma cells, or multinucleated giant cells can be seen occasionally, as may scattered lymphocytes. The stroma may demonstrate areas of myxoid change or focal hyalinization.

Treatment and Prognosis

Local surgical excision is the treatment of choice. Recurrence is uncommon, especially for superficial tumors. Larger lesions of the deeper soft tissues have a greater potential to recur.

◆ SOLITARY FIBROUS TUMOR

The **solitary fibrous tumor** was initially described as a pleural neoplasm that was believed to arise from either mesothelial cells or submesothelial fibroblasts. However, examples of this tumor were later identified in a number of other anatomic sites, including the head and neck region. The term **hemangiopericytoma** originally was used for a rare soft tissue neoplasm that presumably was derived from pericytes (i.e., cells with processes that encircled endothelial cells of capillaries). However, a pericytic origin appears doubtful, and there is now general agreement that most so-called hemangiopericytomas represent cellular variants within the spectrum of solitary fibrous tumor. On the molecular level, solitary fibrous tumors have been shown to harbor a recurrent chromosomal translocation resulting in the fusion of the *NAB2* and *STAT6* genes.

In addition, a neoplasm microscopically similar to the hemangiopericytoma-like pattern of solitary fibrous tumor has been recognized in the sinonasal tract. This tumor does show myoid, pericyte-like differentiation and is thought to represent a separate entity known as a **sinonasal-type hemangiopericytoma (glomangiopericytoma; myopericytoma).** Recent studies have shown that this tumor harbors mutations of the *CTNNB1* gene that encodes for β-catenin.

Clinical Features

Solitary fibrous tumors have been reported primarily in adults and are rare in children. The tumor often is described as a slow-growing, painless, submucosal, or deep soft tissue mass that is easily removed from the surrounding tissues (Fig. 12.24). Solitary fibrous tumors of the oral cavity are most common in the buccal mucosa, which accounts for approximately 45% of such cases. Other common sites in the head and neck region include the sinonasal tract and the orbit.

Sinonasal-type hemangiopericytoma occurs primarily in middle-aged and older adults. Common presenting symptoms include nasal obstruction and epistaxis.

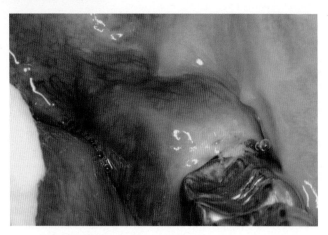

• **Fig. 12.24 Solitary Fibrous Tumor.** Nodular mass of the left retro-molar pad. (Courtesy of Dr. Caroline Bissonnette.)

Histopathologic Features

Solitary fibrous tumors are usually well-circumscribed lesions that exhibit a variable microscopic appearance. At one end of the spectrum, the lesional cells appear as tightly packed cells and surround endothelium-lined vascular channels—hence the concept of hemangiopericytoma. The cells are haphazardly arranged and demonstrate round to ovoid nuclei and indistinct cytoplasmic borders. The blood vessels often show irregular branching, which results in a characteristic "staghorn" and "antlerlike" appearance (Fig. 12.25, *A*).

At the other end of the spectrum, the cells are more spindled and arranged in either short fascicles or in a disorganized fashion ("patternless pattern") (see Fig. 12.25, *B*). The tumor often demonstrates alternating hypercellular and hypocellular zones with a variable degree of myxoid background change. Prominent hyalinized collagen bundles are characteristically observed in the hypocellular areas. Immunohistochemical studies show the lesional cells to be positive for CD34, bcl-2, and STAT6 in nearly all cases (see Fig. 12.25, *C*).

The identification of 4 or more mitoses per 10 high-power fields suggests a rapidly growing tumor that is capable of metastasis. The presence of necrosis also suggests malignancy. However, it is difficult to predict microscopically whether a particular tumor will act in a benign or malignant fashion.

Sinonasal-type hemangiopericytomas have a more prominent spindle cell pattern, with the cells arranged in a more orderly fashion. Mitotic figures are rare or absent. The vascular component is less intricate, and less interstitial collagen is found among the tumor cells. Most examples will express smooth muscle actin and nuclear β-catenin, but, in contrast to solitary fibrous tumor, the cells are usually negative for STAT6, CD34, and bcl-2.

Treatment and Prognosis

For solitary fibrous tumors with a benign histopathologic appearance, local excision is the treatment of choice. More extensive surgery is required for tumors with malignant

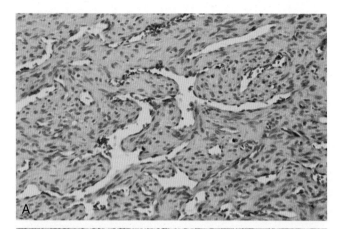

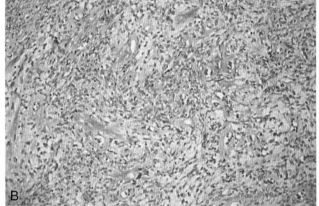

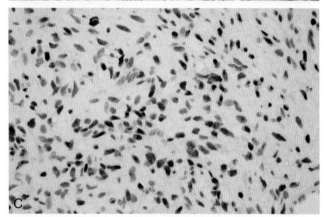

• **Fig. 12.25 Solitary Fibrous Tumor. A,** "Staghorn" blood vessels surrounded by haphazardly arranged cells. **B,** Moderately cellular fibrous proliferation ("patternless pattern") with prominent vascularity, slightly myxoid areas, and scattered dense collagen bundles. **C,** Immunohistochemistry showing strong nuclear positivity for STAT6.

characteristics. Oral examples usually behave in a benign fashion, although as many as 10% of extrapleural solitary fibrous tumors have been reported to show malignant behavior. Therefore, long-term follow-up of patients with this tumor is recommended.

The sinonasal-type hemangiopericytoma usually has a favorable prognosis with a recurrence rate of approximately 17%. Rare examples of locally aggressive or metastatic tumors have been reported.

◆ FIBROMATOSIS (DESMOID-TYPE FIBROMATOSIS)

The **fibromatoses** are a broad group of fibrous proliferations that have a biologic behavior and histopathologic pattern that is intermediate between those of benign fibrous lesions and fibrosarcoma. A number of different forms of fibromatosis are recognized throughout the body, and they often are named based on their particular clinicopathologic features. In the soft tissues of the head and neck, these lesions are frequently called **juvenile aggressive fibromatoses**, **desmoid-type fibromatoses**, or **extraabdominal desmoids.** Similar lesions within the bone have been called **desmoplastic fibromas** (see page 663). Individuals with familial adenomatous polyposis and Gardner syndrome (see page 656) have a greatly increased risk for developing desmoid-type fibromatosis. Activating *CTNNB1* gene mutations (located at chromosome 3p21) are detected in approximately 85% of cases.

Clinical and Radiographic Features

Soft tissue fibromatosis of the head and neck is a firm, painless mass, which may exhibit rapid or insidious growth (Fig. 12.26). The lesion most frequently occurs in children or young adults; hence, the term **juvenile fibromatosis.** However, cases also have been seen in middle-aged adults. The most common head and neck sites are the maxillary sinus and paramandibular soft tissue region, although the lesion can occur almost anywhere. The tumor can grow to considerable size, resulting in significant facial disfigurement. Destruction of adjacent bone may be observed on radiographs and other imaging studies.

Histopathologic Features

Soft tissue fibromatosis is characterized by a cellular proliferation of spindle-shaped cells that are arranged in streaming fascicles and are associated with a variable amount of collagen (Fig. 12.27). The lesion is usually poorly circumscribed and infiltrates the adjacent tissues. Hyperchromatism and pleomorphism of the cells should not be observed. Immunohistochemistry for smooth muscle actin (SMA) may be positive, which could be confused with other lesions showing myofibroblastic differentiation. However, desmoid-type fibromatoses typically show strong positivity for β-catenin in the cell nuclei.

Treatment and Prognosis

Because of its locally aggressive nature, the preferred treatment for soft tissue fibromatosis is wide excision that includes a generous margin of adjacent normal tissues. Adjuvant chemotherapy or radiation therapy sometimes has been used for incompletely resected or recurrent tumors. A 30% recurrence rate has been reported for aggressive fibromatosis of the head and neck. Metastasis does not occur.

◆ MYOFIBROMA (MYOFIBROMATOSIS)

Myofibroma is a rare spindle cell neoplasm that consists of myofibroblasts (i.e., cells with both smooth muscle and fibroblastic features). Such cells are not specific for this lesion, however, because they also can be identified in other fibrous proliferations. Most myofibromas occur as solitary lesions, but some patients develop a multicentric tumor process known as **myofibromatosis.**

Clinical and Radiographic Features

Although myofibromas are rare neoplasms, they demonstrate a predilection for the head and neck region. Solitary tumors develop most frequently in the first four decades of life, with a mean age of 23 years. The most common oral location is the mandible, followed by the alveolar mucosa/gingiva, buccal mucosa, and tongue. The tumor is typically a painless mass that sometimes exhibits rapid enlargement (Fig. 12.28). Intrabony tumors create radiolucent defects that usually tend to be poorly defined, although some may be well defined or multilocular (Fig. 12.29). Multicentric

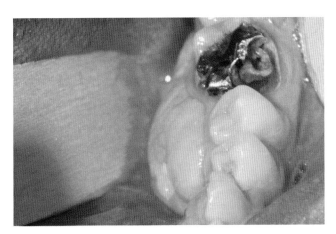

• **Fig. 12.26 Fibromatosis.** Locally aggressive proliferation of fibrous connective tissue of the lingual mandibular gingival mucosa.

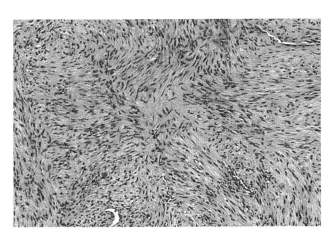

• **Fig. 12.27 Fibromatosis.** Streaming fascicles of fibroblastic cells that demonstrate little pleomorphism.

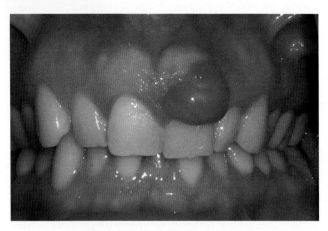

• **Fig. 12.28 Myofibroma.** Smooth-surfaced, nodular mass of the maxillary facial gingiva. (Courtesy of Dr. John Duckworth.)

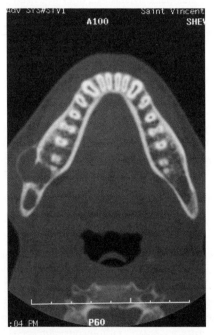

• **Fig. 12.29 Myofibroma.** Computed tomography (CT) scan showing an expansile lytic mass of the posterior mandible on the left side of the illustration. (Courtesy of Dr. Timothy Armanini.)

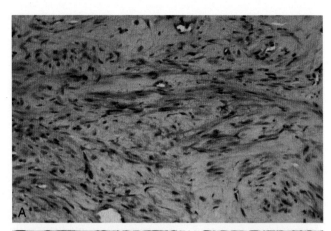

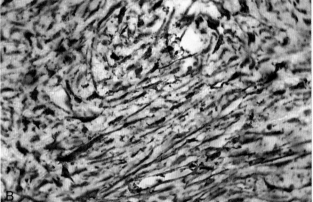

• **Fig. 12.30 Myofibroma. A,** Proliferation of spindle-shaped cells with both fibroblastic and smooth muscle features. **B,** Immunohistochemistry showing strong positivity for smooth muscle actin.

myofibromatosis primarily affects neonates and infants who may have tumors of the skin, subcutaneous tissue, muscle, bone, and viscera. The number of tumors can vary from several to more than 100.

Histopathologic Features

Myofibromas are composed of interlacing bundles of spindle cells with tapered or blunt-ended nuclei and eosinophilic cytoplasm (Fig. 12.30, *A*). Nodular fascicles may alternate with more cellular zones, imparting a biphasic appearance to the tumor. Scattered mitoses are not uncommon. Centrally, the lesion is often more vascular with a hemangiopericytoma-like appearance. The tumor cells are positive for smooth muscle actin and muscle-specific actin with immunohistochemistry (see Fig. 12.30, *B*), but they are negative for desmin and β-catenin.

Treatment and Prognosis

Solitary myofibromas are usually treated by surgical excision. A small percentage of tumors will recur after treatment, but typically these can be controlled with reexcision. Multifocal tumors arising in soft tissues and bone rarely recur after surgical removal. Spontaneous regression may occur in some cases. However, myofibromatosis involving the viscera or vital organs in infants can act more aggressively and sometimes proves to be fatal within a few days after birth.

◆ ORAL FOCAL MUCINOSIS

Oral focal mucinosis is an uncommon tumor-like mass that is believed to represent the oral counterpart of cutaneous focal mucinosis or a cutaneous myxoid cyst. The cause is unknown, although the lesion may result from overproduction of hyaluronic acid by fibroblasts.

Clinical Features

Oral focal mucinosis is most common in young adults and shows a 2:1 female-to-male predilection. The gingiva is the most common site, accounting for over half of all cases. The hard palate is the second most common location. The

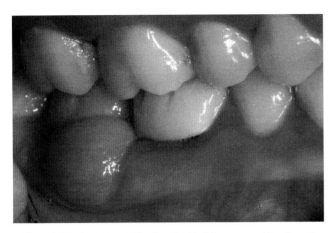

• **Fig. 12.31 Oral Focal Mucinosis.** Nodular mass arising from the gingiva between the mandibular first and second molars.

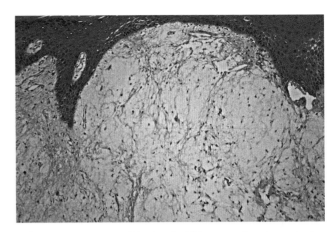

• **Fig. 12.33 Oral Focal Mucinosis.** High-power view demonstrating the myxomatous change.

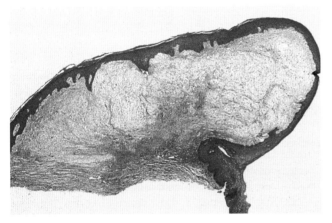

• **Fig. 12.32 Oral Focal Mucinosis.** Low-power view showing a nodular mass of loose, myxomatous connective tissue.

lesion usually presents as a sessile or pedunculated, painless nodular mass that is the same color as the surrounding mucosa (Fig. 12.31). The surface is typically smooth and nonulcerated, although occasional cases exhibit a lobulated appearance. The size varies from a few millimeters up to 2 cm in diameter. The patient often has been aware of the mass for many months or years before the diagnosis is made.

Histopathologic Features

Microscopic examination of oral focal mucinosis shows a well-localized but nonencapsulated area of loose, myxomatous connective tissue surrounded by denser, normal collagenous connective tissue (Figs. 12.32 and 12.33). The lesion is usually found just beneath the surface epithelium and often causes flattening of the rete ridges. The fibroblasts within the mucinous area can be ovoid, fusiform, or stellate, and they may demonstrate delicate, fibrillar processes. Few capillaries are seen within the lesion, especially compared with the surrounding denser collagen. Similarly, no significant inflammation is observed, although a perivascular lymphocytic infiltrate often is noted within the surrounding collagenous connective tissue. No appreciable reticulin is

evident within the lesion, and special stains suggest that the mucinous product is hyaluronic acid.

Treatment and Prognosis

Oral focal mucinosis is treated by surgical excision and does not tend to recur.

◆ PYOGENIC GRANULOMA (LOBULAR CAPILLARY HEMANGIOMA)

The **pyogenic granuloma** is a common tumor-like growth of the oral cavity that traditionally has been considered to be nonneoplastic in nature.* However, some pyogenic granulomas with a lobular endothelial growth pattern (known as *lobular capillary hemangiomas*) currently are categorized as *vascular tumors* under the classification scheme of the International Society for the Study of Vascular Anomalies (see Box 12.2, page 547).

Although originally theorized to be caused by pyogenic organisms, the pyogenic granuloma is now believed to be unrelated to infection. Instead, this lesion is thought to represent an exuberant tissue response related to local irritation, poor hygiene, or hormonal factors. In spite of its name, it is not a true granuloma.

Clinical Features

The pyogenic granuloma is a smooth or lobulated mass that is usually pedunculated, although some lesions are sessile (Figs. 12.34–12.36). The surface is characteristically ulcerated and ranges from pink to red to purple, depending on the age of the lesion. Young pyogenic granulomas are highly vascular in appearance; older lesions tend to become more

*However, some pyogenic granulomas (also known as *lobular capillary hemangiomas*) currently are categorized as *vascular tumors* under the classification scheme of the International Society for the Study of Vascular Anomalies (see Box 12.2, page 547).

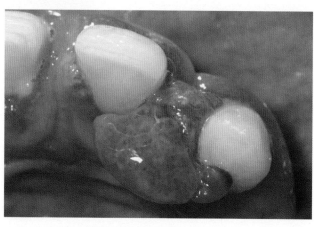

• **Fig. 12.34 Pyogenic Granuloma.** Erythematous, hemorrhagic mass arising from the maxillary anterior gingiva.

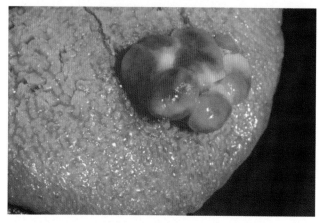

• **Fig. 12.35 Pyogenic Granuloma.** Ulcerated and lobulated mass on the dorsum of the tongue.

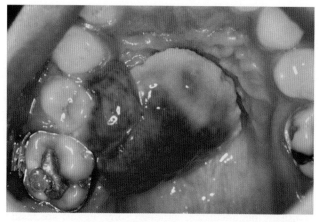

• **Fig. 12.36 Pyogenic Granuloma.** Unusually large lesion arising from the palatal gingiva in association with an orthodontic band. The patient was pregnant.

collagenized and pink. They vary from small growths only a few millimeters in size to larger lesions that may measure several centimeters in diameter. Typically, the mass is painless, although it often bleeds easily because of its extreme vascularity. Pyogenic granulomas may exhibit rapid growth, which

may create alarm for both the patient and the clinician, who may fear that the lesion might be malignant.

Oral pyogenic granulomas show a striking predilection for the gingiva, which accounts for approximately 75%–85% of all cases. Gingival irritation and inflammation that result from poor oral hygiene may be a precipitating factor in many patients. However, the lobular microscopic variant (lobular capillary hemangioma) tends to occur more frequently on the lips, tongue, and buccal mucosa. A history of trauma before the development of the lesion is not unusual, especially for extragingival pyogenic granulomas. Lesions are slightly more common on the maxillary gingiva than the mandibular gingiva; anterior areas are more frequently affected than posterior areas. These lesions are much more common on the facial aspect of the gingiva than the lingual aspect; some extend between the teeth and involve both the facial and the lingual gingiva.

Although the pyogenic granuloma can develop at any age, it is most common in children and young adults. Most studies also demonstrate a female predilection, possibly because of the vascular effects of female hormones. Pyogenic granulomas of the gingiva frequently develop in pregnant women, so much so that the terms *pregnancy tumor* or *granuloma gravidarum* often are used. Such lesions may begin to develop during the first trimester, and their prevalence increases up through the seventh month of pregnancy. The gradual rise in development of these lesions throughout pregnancy may be related to the increasing levels of estrogen and progesterone as the pregnancy progresses. After pregnancy and the return of normal hormone levels, some of these pyogenic granulomas resolve without treatment or undergo fibrous maturation and resemble a fibroma (Fig. 12.37).

Epulis granulomatosa is a term used to describe hyperplastic growths of granulation tissue that sometimes arise in healing extraction sockets (Fig. 12.38). These lesions resemble pyogenic granulomas and usually represent a granulation tissue reaction to bony sequestra in the socket.

Histopathologic Features

Microscopic examination of pyogenic granulomas shows a highly vascular proliferation that resembles granulation tissue (Figs. 12.39 and 12.40). Numerous small and larger endothelium-lined channels are formed that are engorged with red blood cells. In some examples, the vessels are organized in lobular aggregates—hence, the term *lobular capillary hemangioma.* The surface is usually ulcerated and replaced by a thick fibrinopurulent membrane. A mixed inflammatory cell infiltrate of neutrophils, plasma cells, and lymphocytes is evident. Neutrophils are most prevalent near the ulcerated surface; chronic inflammatory cells are found deeper in the specimen. Older lesions may have areas with a more fibrous appearance. In fact, many gingival fibromas probably represent pyogenic granulomas that have undergone fibrous maturation.

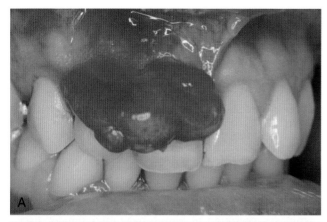

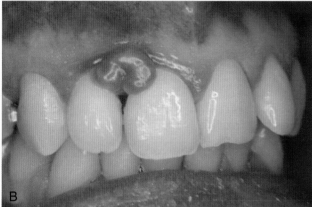

• **Fig. 12.37 Pyogenic Granuloma. A,** Large gingival mass in a pregnant woman just before childbirth. **B,** The mass has decreased in size and undergone fibrous maturation 3 months after childbirth. (Courtesy of Dr. George Blozis.)

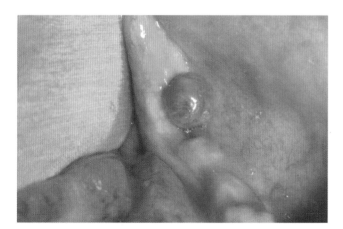

• **Fig. 12.38 Epulis Granulomatosa.** Nodular mass of granulation tissue that developed in a recent extraction site.

Treatment and Prognosis

The treatment of patients with pyogenic granuloma consists of conservative surgical excision, which is usually curative. The specimen should be submitted for microscopic examination to rule out other more serious diagnoses. For gingival lesions, the excision should extend down to periosteum

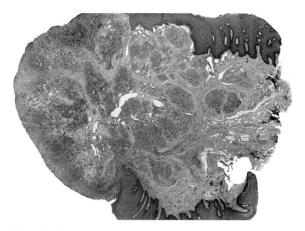

• **Fig. 12.39 Pyogenic Granuloma.** Low-power view showing an exophytic mass of granulation-like tissue with an ulcerated surface. Note the lobular endothelial proliferation in the deeper connective tissue.

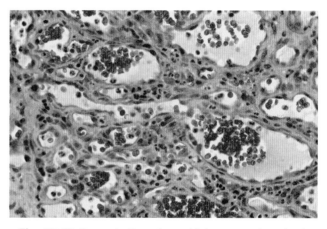

• **Fig. 12.40 Pyogenic Granuloma.** Higher-power view showing capillary blood vessels and scattered inflammation.

and the adjacent teeth should be thoroughly scaled to remove any source of continuing irritation. A recurrence rate of 3%–15% has been reported in most studies. In rare instances, multiple recurrences have been noted.

For lesions that develop during pregnancy, usually treatment should be deferred unless significant functional or aesthetic problems develop. The recurrence rate is higher for pyogenic granulomas removed during pregnancy, and some lesions will resolve spontaneously after parturition.

◆ PERIPHERAL GIANT CELL GRANULOMA

The **peripheral giant cell granuloma** is a relatively common tumor-like growth of the oral cavity. It probably does not represent a true neoplasm but rather is a reactive lesion caused by local irritation or trauma. In the past, it often was called a *peripheral giant cell reparative granuloma,* but any reparative nature appears doubtful. Some investigators believe that the giant cells show immunohistochemical features of osteoclasts, whereas other authors have suggested that the lesion is formed by cells from the mononuclear phagocyte system. The peripheral giant cell granuloma bears a close microscopic resemblance to the **central giant cell granuloma** (see page 631), and some pathologists believe that it may represent a soft tissue counterpart of this intraosseous lesion.

Clinical and Radiographic Features

The peripheral giant cell granuloma occurs exclusively on the gingiva or edentulous alveolar ridge, presenting as a red or red-blue nodular mass (Figs. 12.41 and 12.42). Examples also have been reported to arise adjacent to dental implants. Most lesions are smaller than 2 cm in diameter, although larger ones are seen occasionally. The lesion can be sessile or pedunculated and may or may not be ulcerated. The clinical appearance is similar to the more common pyogenic granuloma of the gingiva (see page 525), although the peripheral giant cell granuloma often is more blue-purple compared with the bright red of a typical pyogenic granuloma.

Peripheral giant cell granulomas can develop at almost any age, especially during the first through sixth decades of life. The mean age in several large series ranges from 31 to 46 years. Approximately 55% of cases occur in females. It may develop in either the anterior or posterior regions of the gingiva or alveolar mucosa, and the mandible is affected more often than the maxilla (ratio = 3:2). Although the peripheral giant cell granuloma develops within soft tissue, "cupping" resorption of the underlying alveolar bone sometimes is seen. On occasion, it may be difficult to determine whether the mass arose as a peripheral lesion or as a central giant cell granuloma that eroded through the cortical plate into the gingival soft tissues.

Histopathologic Features

Microscopic examination of a peripheral giant cell granuloma shows a proliferation of multinucleated giant cells within a background of plump ovoid and spindle-shaped mesenchymal cells (Figs. 12.43 and 12.44). The giant cells may contain only a few nuclei or up to several dozen. Some of these cells may have large, vesicular nuclei; others demonstrate small, pyknotic nuclei. Mitotic figures are fairly common in the background mesenchymal cells. Abundant hemorrhage is characteristically found throughout the mass, which often results in deposits of hemosiderin pigment, especially at the periphery of the lesion.

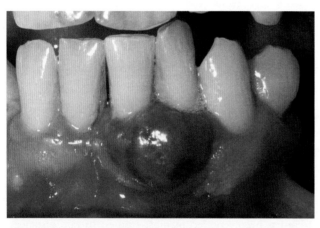

• **Fig. 12.41 Peripheral Giant Cell Granuloma.** Nodular blue-purple mass of the mandibular gingiva.

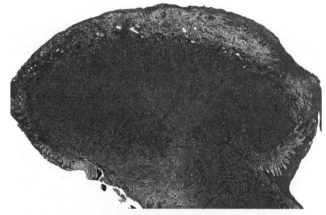

• **Fig. 12.43 Peripheral Giant Cell Granuloma.** Low-power view showing a nodular proliferation of multinucleated giant cells within the gingiva.

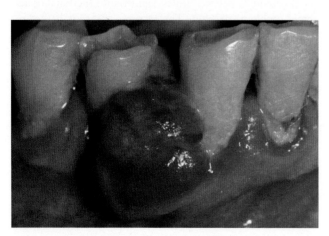

• **Fig. 12.42 Peripheral Giant Cell Granuloma.** Ulcerated mass of the mandibular gingiva.

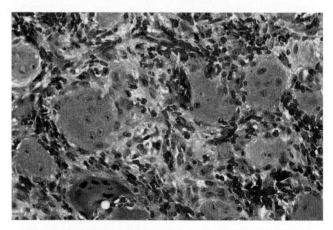

• **Fig. 12.44 Peripheral Giant Cell Granuloma.** High-power view showing scattered multinucleated giant cells within a hemorrhagic background of ovoid and spindle-shaped mesenchymal cells.

The overlying mucosal surface is ulcerated in about 50% of cases. A zone of dense fibrous connective tissue usually separates the giant cell proliferation from the mucosal surface. Adjacent acute and chronic inflammatory cells are frequently present. Areas of reactive bone formation or dystrophic calcifications are not unusual.

Treatment and Prognosis

The treatment of the peripheral giant cell granuloma consists of local surgical excision down to the underlying bone. The adjacent teeth should be carefully scaled to remove any source of irritation and to minimize the risk of recurrence. Approximately 10%–18% of lesions are reported to recur, and reexcision must be performed.

On rare occasions, lesions indistinguishable from peripheral giant cell granulomas have been seen in patients with hyperparathyroidism (see page 840). They apparently represent the so-called osteoclastic brown tumors associated with this endocrine disorder. Although brown tumors of hyperparathyroidism are more likely to be intraosseous in location and mimic a central giant cell granuloma, this endocrine disease also needs to be considered in patients with peripheral giant cell lesions.

◆ PERIPHERAL OSSIFYING FIBROMA (OSSIFYING FIBROID EPULIS; PERIPHERAL FIBROMA WITH CALCIFICATION)

The **peripheral ossifying fibroma** is a relatively common gingival growth that is considered to be reactive rather than neoplastic in nature. The pathogenesis of this lesion is uncertain. Because of their clinical and histopathologic similarities, researchers believe that some peripheral ossifying fibromas develop initially as pyogenic granulomas that undergo fibrous maturation and subsequent calcification. However, not all peripheral ossifying fibromas may develop in this manner. The mineralized product probably has its origin from cells of the periosteum or periodontal ligament.

Considerable confusion has existed over the nomenclature of this lesion, and several terms have been used to describe its variable histopathologic features. In the past, the terms *peripheral odontogenic fibroma* (see page 733) and *peripheral ossifying fibroma* often were used synonymously, but the peripheral odontogenic fibroma is now considered to be a distinct and separate entity. In addition, in spite of the similarity in names, the peripheral ossifying fibroma does not represent the soft tissue counterpart of the central ossifying fibroma (see page 652).

Clinical Features

The peripheral ossifying fibroma occurs exclusively on the gingiva. It appears as a nodular mass, either pedunculated or sessile, that usually emanates from the interdental papilla (Figs. 12.45 and 12.46). The color ranges from red to pink, and the surface is frequently, but not always, ulcerated. The growth probably begins as an ulcerated lesion; older ones are

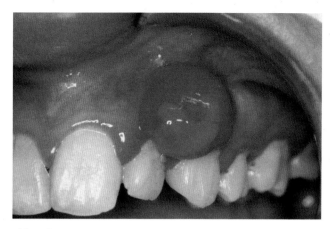

• **Fig. 12.45 Peripheral Ossifying Fibroma.** This red, ulcerated mass of the maxillary gingiva has recurred twice. Such ulcerated lesions are easily mistaken for a pyogenic granuloma.

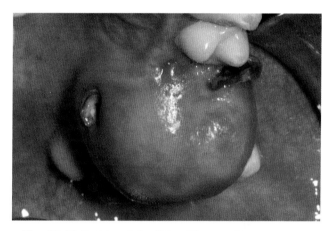

• **Fig. 12.46 Peripheral Ossifying Fibroma.** Pink, nonulcerated mass arising from the maxillary gingiva. The remaining roots of the first molar are present.

more likely to demonstrate healing of the ulcer and an intact surface. Red, ulcerated lesions often are mistaken for pyogenic granulomas; the pink, nonulcerated ones are clinically similar to irritation fibromas. Most lesions are less than 2 cm in size, although larger ones occasionally occur. The lesion often has been present for many weeks or months before the diagnosis is made.

The peripheral ossifying fibroma is predominantly a lesion of teenagers and young adults, with peak prevalence between the ages of 10 and 19. Almost two-thirds of all cases occur in females. There is a slight predilection for the maxillary arch, and more than 50% of all cases occur in the incisor-cuspid region. Usually, the teeth are unaffected; rarely, there can be migration and loosening of adjacent teeth.

Histopathologic Features

The basic microscopic pattern of the peripheral ossifying fibroma is one of a fibrous proliferation associated with the formation of a mineralized product (Figs. 12.47 and 12.48). If the epithelium is ulcerated, then the surface is

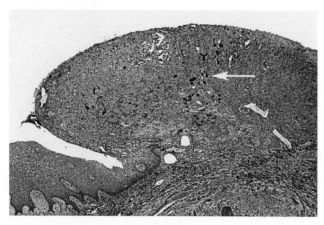

• **Fig. 12.47 Peripheral Ossifying Fibroma.** Ulcerated gingival mass demonstrating focal early mineralization (*arrow*).

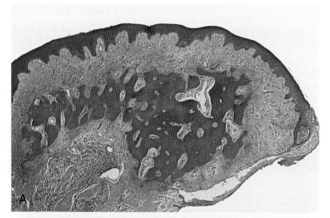

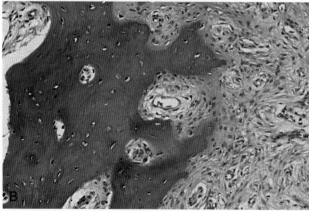

• **Fig. 12.48 Peripheral Ossifying Fibroma. A,** Nonulcerated fibrous mass of the gingiva showing central bone formation. **B,** Higher-power view showing trabeculae of bone with adjacent fibrous connective tissue.

covered by a fibrinopurulent membrane with a subjacent zone of granulation tissue. The deeper fibroblastic component often is cellular, especially in areas of mineralization. In some cases, the fibroblastic proliferation and associated mineralization is only a small component of a larger mass that resembles a fibroma or pyogenic granuloma.

The type of mineralized component is variable and may consist of bone, cementum-like material, or dystrophic calcifications. Frequently, a combination of products is formed. Usually, the bone is woven and trabecular in type, although older lesions may demonstrate mature lamellar bone. Trabeculae of unmineralized osteoid are not unusual. Less frequently, ovoid droplets of basophilic cementum-like material are formed. Dystrophic calcifications are characterized by multiple granules, tiny globules, or large, irregular masses of basophilic mineralized material. Such dystrophic calcifications are more common in early, ulcerated lesions; older, nonulcerated examples are more likely to demonstrate well-formed bone or cementum. In some cases, multinucleated giant cells may be found, usually in association with the mineralized product.

Treatment and Prognosis

The treatment of choice for the peripheral ossifying fibroma is local surgical excision with submission of the specimen for histopathologic examination. The mass should be excised down to periosteum because recurrence is more likely if the base of the lesion is allowed to remain. In addition, the adjacent teeth should be thoroughly scaled to eliminate any possible irritants. Periodontal surgical techniques, such as repositioned flaps or connective tissue grafts, may be necessary to repair the gingival defect in an aesthetic manner, particularly in the anterior maxillary region. Although excision is usually curative, a recurrence rate of 8%–16% has been reported.

◆ LIPOMA

The **lipoma** is a benign tumor of fat. Although it represents by far the most common mesenchymal neoplasm, most examples occur on the trunk and proximal portions of the extremities. Lipomas of the oral and maxillofacial region are much less frequent, accounting for only 1%–4% of all such tumors. The pathogenesis of lipomas is uncertain, but they appear to be more common in obese people. However, the metabolism of lipomas is completely independent of the normal body fat. If the caloric intake is reduced, then lipomas do not decrease in size, although normal body fat may be lost.

Clinical Features

Oral lipomas are usually soft, smooth-surfaced nodular masses that can be sessile or pedunculated (Figs. 12.49 and 12.50). Typically, the tumor is asymptomatic and often has been noted for many months or years before diagnosis. Most are less than 3 cm in size, but occasional lesions can become much larger. Although a subtle or more obvious yellow hue often is detected clinically, deeper examples may appear pink. The buccal mucosa and buccal vestibule are the most common intraoral sites and account for nearly 50% of all cases. Some buccal cases may not represent true tumors, but rather herniation of the buccal fat pad through the buccinator muscle, which may occur after local trauma in young children or subsequent to surgical removal of third molars in older patients. Less common sites include the tongue, lips, and floor of the mouth. Most patients are 40 years

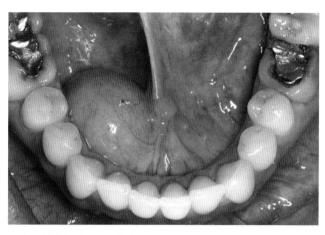

• **Fig. 12.49 Lipoma.** Soft, yellow nodular mass in the floor of the mouth. (Courtesy of Dr. Michael Tabor.)

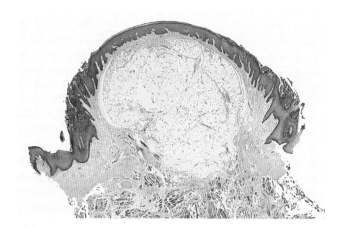

• **Fig. 12.51 Lipoma.** Low-power view of a tumor of the tongue demonstrating a mass of mature adipose tissue.

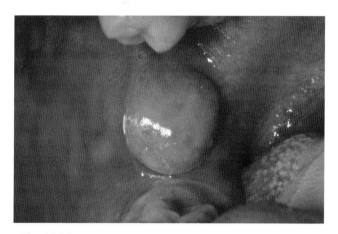

• **Fig. 12.50 Lipoma.** Nodular mass of the posterior buccal mucosa.

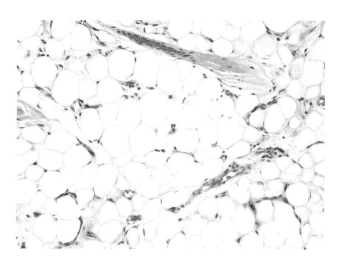

• **Fig. 12.52 Lipoma.** High-power view showing the similarity of the tumor cells to normal fat.

of age or older; lipomas are uncommon in children. Lipomas of the oral and maxillofacial region have shown a fairly balanced sex distribution in most studies.

Histopathologic Features

Most oral lipomas are composed of mature fat cells that differ little in microscopic appearance from the surrounding normal fat (Figs. 12.51 and 12.52). The tumor is usually well circumscribed and may demonstrate a thin fibrous capsule. A distinct lobular arrangement of the cells often is seen. On rare occasions, central cartilaginous or osseous metaplasia may occur within an otherwise typical lipoma.

A number of microscopic variants have been described. The most common of these is the **fibrolipoma,** which is characterized by a significant fibrous component intermixed with the lobules of fat cells. The remaining variants are rare.

The **angiolipoma** consists of an admixture of mature fat and numerous small blood vessels. The **spindle cell lipoma** demonstrates variable amounts of uniform-appearing spindle cells in conjunction with a more typical lipomatous component. These spindle cells are positive for CD34 with immunohistochemistry. Some spindle cell lipomas exhibit a

mucoid background *(myxoid lipoma)* and may be confused with myxoid liposarcomas. **Pleomorphic lipomas** are characterized by the presence of spindle cells plus bizarre, hyperchromatic giant cells; they can be difficult to distinguish from a pleomorphic liposarcoma. **Intramuscular (infiltrating) lipomas** often are more deeply situated and have an infiltrative growth pattern that extends between skeletal muscle bundles. The term **sialolipoma** was coined to describe tumors that secondarily entrap salivary gland tissue.

Traumatized oral lipomas can show degenerative cellular changes that can be mistaken for a form of well-differentiated liposarcoma known as *atypical lipomatous tumor*. Negative immunohistochemical expression for MDM2 and CDK4 can help to avoid overdiagnosis of such tumors as low-grade malignancies.

Treatment and Prognosis

Lipomas are treated by conservative local excision, and recurrence is rare. Most microscopic variants do not affect the prognosis. Intramuscular lipomas have a higher recurrence rate because of their infiltrative growth pattern, but this variant is rare in the oral and maxillofacial region.

◆ TRAUMATIC NEUROMA (AMPUTATION NEUROMA)

The **traumatic neuroma** is not a true neoplasm but a reactive proliferation of neural tissue after transection or other damage of a nerve bundle. After a nerve has been damaged or severed, the proximal portion attempts to regenerate and reestablish innervation of the distal segment by the growth of axons through tubes of proliferating Schwann cells. If these regenerating elements encounter scar tissue or otherwise cannot reestablish innervation, then a tumorlike mass may develop at the site of injury.

Clinical and Radiographic Features

Traumatic neuromas of the oral mucosa are typically smooth-surfaced, nonulcerated nodules. They can develop at any location but are most common in the mental foramen area, tongue, and lower lip (Figs. 12.53 and 12.54). A history

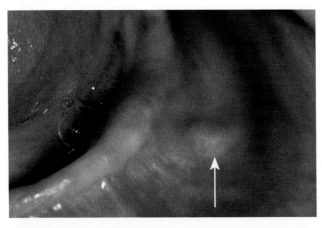

• **Fig. 12.53 Traumatic Neuroma.** Painful nodule of the mental nerve as it exits the mental foramen *(arrow)*.

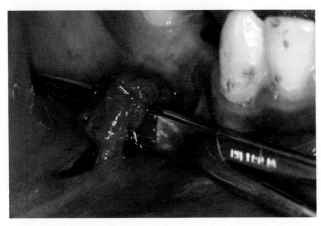

• **Fig. 12.54 Traumatic Neuroma.** Note the irregular nodular proliferation along the mental nerve that is being exposed at the time of surgery.

of trauma often can be elicited; some lesions arise subsequent to tooth extraction or other surgical procedures. Intraosseous traumatic neuromas may demonstrate a radiolucent defect on oral radiographs. Examples also may occur at other head and neck sites; it has been estimated that traumatic neuromas of the greater auricular nerve develop in 5%–10% of patients undergoing surgery for pleomorphic adenomas of the parotid gland.

Traumatic neuromas can occur at any age, but they are diagnosed most often in middle-aged adults. They appear to be slightly more common in women. Many traumatic neuromas are associated with altered nerve sensations that can range from anesthesia to dysesthesia to overt pain. Although pain has been traditionally considered a hallmark of this lesion, studies indicate that only one-fourth to one-third of oral traumatic neuromas are painful. This pain can be intermittent or constant and ranges from mild tenderness or burning to severe radiating pain. Neuromas of the mental nerve are frequently painful, especially when impinged on by a denture or palpated.

Histopathologic Features

Microscopic examination of traumatic neuromas shows a haphazard proliferation of mature, myelinated and unmyelinated nerve bundles within a fibrous connective tissue stroma that ranges from densely collagenized to myxomatous in nature (Figs. 12.55 and 12.56). An associated mild chronic inflammatory cell infiltrate may be present. Traumatic neuromas with inflammation are more likely to be painful than those without significant inflammation.

Treatment and Prognosis

The treatment of choice for the patient with a traumatic neuroma is surgical excision, including a small portion of the involved proximal nerve bundle. Most lesions do not recur; in some cases, however, the pain persists or returns at a later date.

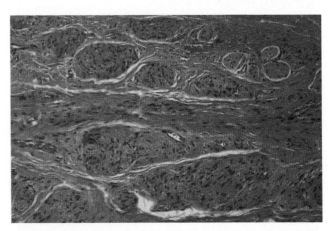

• **Fig. 12.55 Traumatic Neuroma.** Low-power view showing the haphazard arrangement of nerve bundles within the background fibrous connective tissue.

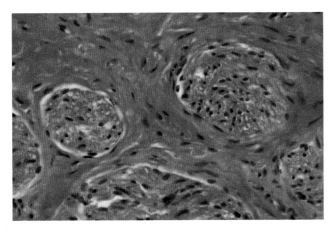

• **Fig. 12.56 Traumatic Neuroma.** High-power view showing cross-sectioned nerve bundles within dense fibrous connective tissue.

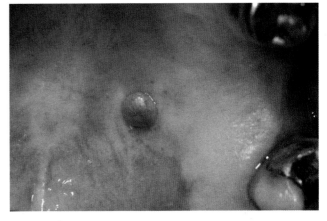

• **Fig. 12.57 Palisaded Encapsulated Neuroma.** Small, painless nodule of the lateral hard palate.

◆ PALISADED ENCAPSULATED NEUROMA (SOLITARY CIRCUMSCRIBED NEUROMA)

The **palisaded encapsulated neuroma** is a benign neural tumor with distinctive clinical and histopathologic features. It represents one of the more common superficial nerve tumors, especially in the head and neck region. The cause is uncertain, but some authors have speculated that trauma may play an etiologic role; the tumor is generally considered to represent a reactive lesion rather than a true neoplasm.

Clinical Features

The palisaded encapsulated neuroma shows a striking predilection for the face, which accounts for approximately 90% of reported cases. The nose and cheek are the most common specific sites. The lesion is most frequently diagnosed between the fifth and seventh decades of life, although the tumor often has been present for many months or years. It is a smooth-surfaced, painless, dome-shaped papule or nodule that is usually less than 1 cm in diameter.

Oral palisaded encapsulated neuromas are not uncommon, although many are probably diagnosed microscopically as neurofibromas or schwannomas. The lesion appears most frequently on the hard palate (Fig. 12.57), gingiva, and labial mucosa, although it also may occur in other oral locations.

Histopathologic Features

Palisaded encapsulated neuromas appear well circumscribed and often encapsulated (Fig. 12.58), although this capsule may be incomplete, especially along the superficial aspect of the tumor. Some lesions have a lobulated appearance. The tumor consists of moderately cellular interlacing fascicles of spindle cells that are consistent with Schwann cells. The nuclei are characteristically wavy and pointed, with no significant pleomorphism or mitotic activity. Although the nuclei show a similar parallel orientation within the fascicles, the more definite palisading and Verocay bodies

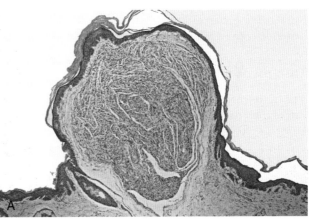

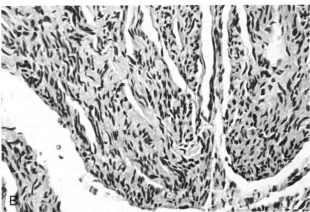

• **Fig. 12.58 Palisaded Encapsulated Neuroma. A,** Low-power view showing a well-circumscribed, nodular proliferation of neural tissue. **B,** Higher-power view demonstrating spindle cells with wavy nuclei.

typical of the Antoni A tissue of a schwannoma are usually not seen. Special stains reveal the presence of numerous axons within the tumor (a feature not seen in schwannoma) and the cells show a positive immunohistochemical reaction for S-100 protein (Fig. 12.59). Negative immunoreactivity for glial fibrillary acidic protein (GFAP) may be helpful in distinguishing the palisaded encapsulated neuroma from other neural tumors. Because the tumor is not always encapsulated and the cells are usually not truly palisaded, some

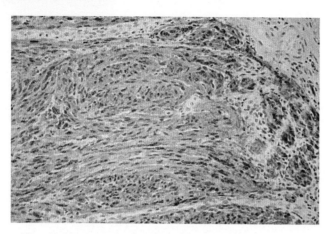

• **Fig. 12.59 Palisaded Encapsulated Neuroma.** Immunohisto-chemical reaction demonstrating spindle-shaped cells that are strongly positive for S-100 protein.

pathologists prefer **solitary circumscribed neuroma** as a better descriptive term for this lesion.

Treatment and Prognosis

The treatment for the palisaded encapsulated neuroma consists of conservative local surgical excision. Recurrence is rare. However, specific recognition of this lesion is important because it is not associated with neurofibromatosis or multiple endocrine neoplasia (MEN) type 2B.

◆ SCHWANNOMA (NEURILEMOMA)

The **schwannoma** is a benign neural neoplasm of Schwann cell origin. It is relatively uncommon, although 25%–48% of all cases occur in the head and neck region. Bilateral schwannomas of the auditory-vestibular nerve are a characteristic feature of the hereditary condition, **neurofibromatosis type II (NF2)**. Multiple schwannomas also occur in another genetic disorder known as **schwannomatosis** (Table 12.2).

Clinical and Radiographic Features

The solitary schwannoma is a slow-growing, encapsulated tumor that typically arises in association with a nerve trunk. As it grows, it pushes the nerve aside. Usually, the mass is asymptomatic, although tenderness or pain may occur in some instances. The lesion is most common in young and middle-aged adults and can range from a few millimeters to several centimeters in size.

The tongue and lips are the most common locations for oral schwannomas, although the tumor can occur almost anywhere in the mouth (Fig. 12.60). On occasion, the tumor arises centrally within bone and may produce bony expansion. Intraosseous examples are most common in the posterior mandible and usually appear as either unilocular or multilocular radiolucencies on radiographs. Pain and paresthesia are not unusual for intrabony tumors.

NF2 is an autosomal dominant condition caused by a mutation of a tumor suppressor gene (*NF2*) on chromosome 22,

which codes for a protein known as *merlin*. In addition to bilateral schwannomas ("acoustic neuromas") of the vestibular nerve, patients also develop schwannomas of peripheral nerves, plus meningiomas and gliomas of the central nervous system (CNS). On occasion, neurofibromas and *café au lait* skin pigmentation may be observed. Characteristic symptoms include progressive sensorineural deafness, dizziness, and tinnitus.

Schwannomatosis is related to mutations of the *SMARCB1* and *LZTR1* genes on chromosome 22. Patients develop multiple painful schwannomas at various sites but without involvement of the auditory-vestibular nerve.

Histopathologic Features

The schwannoma is usually an encapsulated tumor that demonstrates two microscopic patterns in varying amounts: (1) **Antoni A** and (2) **Antoni B**. Streaming fascicles of spindle-shaped Schwann cells characterize Antoni A tissue. These cells often form a palisaded arrangement around central acellular, eosinophilic areas known as **Verocay bodies** (Fig. 12.61). These Verocay bodies consist of reduplicated basement membrane and cytoplasmic processes. Antoni B tissue is less cellular and less organized; the spindle cells are randomly arranged within a loose, myxomatous stroma. Typically, neurites cannot be demonstrated within the tumor mass. The tumor cells will show a diffuse, positive immunohistochemical reaction for S-100 protein.

Degenerative changes can be seen in some older tumors **(ancient schwannomas)**. These changes consist of hemorrhage, hemosiderin deposits, inflammation, fibrosis, and nuclear atypia. However, these tumors are still benign, and the pathologist must be careful not to mistake these alterations for evidence of a sarcoma. Another rare variant is the **plexiform schwannoma,** which is characterized grossly and microscopically by a multinodular, plexiform growth pattern. Such tumors occasionally are associated with NF2 or schwannomatosis.

Treatment and Prognosis

The solitary schwannoma is treated by surgical excision, and the lesion should not recur. Malignant transformation does not occur or is extremely rare.

Vestibular schwannomas in patients with NF2 are difficult to manage. Surgical removal is indicated for large symptomatic tumors, but this often results in deafness and risks facial nerve damage. Stereotactic radiosurgery may be considered for older adult or frail patients, as well as for individuals who decline traditional surgery. Bevacizumab, a monoclonal antibody directed against vascular endothelial growth factor (VEGF)-A, may help to induce tumor shrinkage and improve hearing in up to half of affected patients.

◆ NEUROFIBROMA

The **neurofibroma** is the most common type of peripheral nerve neoplasm. It arises from a mixture of cell types, including Schwann cells and perineural fibroblasts.

TABLE 12.2 **Hereditary Neural and Neuroendocrine Syndromes**

Syndrome	Inheritance Pattern	Gene Mutation	Frequency	Common or Significant Clinical Features
Neurofibromatosis type I (NF1)	Autosomal dominant	*NF1* gene (chromosome 17q11.2)	1 in 2,500–3,000 births	Neurofibromas (especially plexiform type) *Café au lait* pigmentation Axillary and groin freckling Lisch nodules of the iris Optic glioma Epilepsy Hypertension Malignant peripheral nerve sheath tumor (8%–13% of patients)
Neurofibromatosis type II (NF2)	Autosomal dominant	*NF2* gene (chromosome 22q12.2)	1 in 25,000–87,000 births	Bilateral schwannomas ("acoustic neuromas") of the vestibular nerve (cranial nerve VIII) Cranial and spinal meningiomas Other cranial nerve and spinal schwannomas Cutaneous schwannomas Subcapsular cataracts *Café au lait* pigmentation (less common than in NF1) Cutaneous neurofibromas (uncommon)
Schwannomatosis	Autosomal dominant (although most cases have been sporadic)	*SMARCB1* gene or *LZTR1* gene (chromosome 22q11)	1 in 40,000 births	Multiple noncutaneous schwannomas (without involvement of cranial nerve VIII) Chronic pain associated with schwannomas
Multiple endocrine neoplasia type 1 (MEN 1)	Autosomal dominant	*MEN1* gene (chromosome 11q13)	1 in 20,000–40,000 births	Parathyroid tumors Pancreatic islet tumors Anterior pituitary tumors Adrenocortical tumors
Multiple endocrine neoplasia type 2A (MEN 2A)	Autosomal dominant	*RET* proto-oncogene (chromosome 10q11.2)	1 in 36,000–125,000 births	
Classical MEN 2A		95% of examples caused by mutations in codons 609, 611, 618, 620, and 634		MTC (90%) Pheochromocytoma (30%) Primary hyperparathyroidism (10%)
MEN 2A with cutaneous lichen amyloidosis		Most frequently caused by mutation in codon 634; occasionally associated with variants of codons 611 and 804		MTC (95%) Pheochromocytoma (50%) Primary hyperparathyroidism (15%)
MEN 2A with Hirschsprung disease		Caused by mutations in codons 609, 611, 618, and 620		MTC (80%) Pheochromocytoma (20%) Primary hyperparathyroidism (5%)
Familial medullary thyroid carcinoma		Associated with mutations in various codons (e.g., 533, 768, 804)		Patients develop only MTC Rarely develop other neuroendocrine tumors
Multiple endocrine neoplasia type 2B (MEN 2B)	Autosomal dominant	*RET* proto-oncogene (chromosome 10q.11.2; most frequently codon M918T [95%]; 5% at codon A883F)	1 in 400,000–4,000,000 births	MTC (100%) Pheochromocytoma (50%) Oral mucosal neuromas (88%) Intestinal ganglioneuromatosis (67%) Marfanoid habitus (73%) Corneal nerve hypertrophy (45%) Alacrima ("tearless crying") (40%)

MTC, medullary thyroid carcinoma.

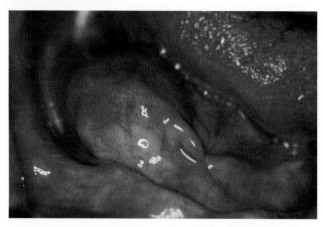

• **Fig. 12.60 Schwannoma.** Nodular mass in the floor of the mouth. (Courtesy of Dr. Art A. Gonty.)

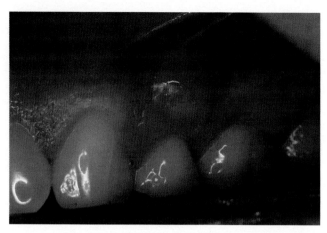

• **Fig. 12.62 Neurofibroma.** Smooth-surfaced, nodular mass of the maxillary gingiva and alveolar mucosa. (Courtesy of Dr. Neal Lemmerman.)

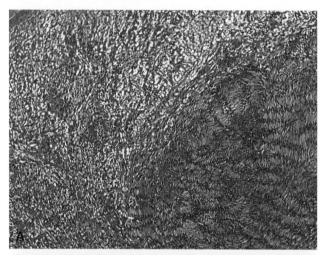

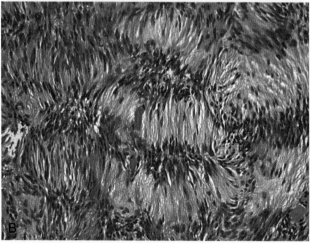

• **Fig. 12.61 Schwannoma. A,** Low-power view showing well-organized Antoni A tissue (*right*) with adjacent myxoid and less organized Antoni B tissue (*left*). **B,** The Schwann cells of the Antoni A tissue form a palisaded arrangement around acellular zones known as *Verocay bodies.*

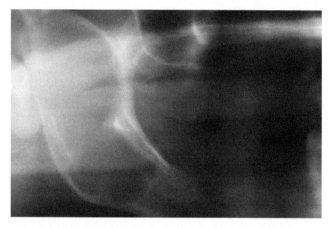

• **Fig. 12.63 Neurofibroma.** Intraosseous tumor filling the right mandibular ramus. (Courtesy of Dr. Paul Allen.)

slow-growing, soft, painless lesions that vary in size from small nodules to larger masses. The skin is the most frequent location for neurofibromas, but lesions of the oral cavity are not uncommon (Fig. 12.62). The tongue, palate, and gingiva are the most common intraoral sites. On rare occasions, the tumor can arise centrally within bone, where it may produce a well-demarcated or poorly defined unilocular or multilocular radiolucency (Fig. 12.63).

Histopathologic Features

The solitary neurofibroma often is well circumscribed, especially when the proliferation occurs within the perineurium of the involved nerve. Tumors that proliferate outside the perineurium may not appear well demarcated and tend to blend with the adjacent connective tissues.

The tumor is composed of interlacing bundles of spindle-shaped cells that often exhibit wavy nuclei (Figs. 12.64 and 12.65). These cells are associated with delicate collagen bundles and variable amounts of myxoid matrix. Mast cells tend to be numerous and can be a helpful diagnostic feature. Sparsely distributed small axons usually can be demonstrated within the tumor tissue by using silver stains. Immunohistochemically,

Clinical and Radiographic Features

Neurofibromas can arise as solitary tumors or be a component of neurofibromatosis (see page 537). Solitary tumors are most common in young adults and present as

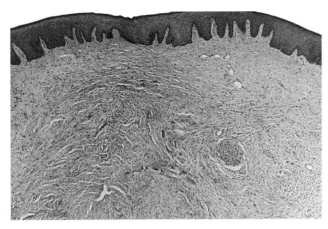

• **Fig. 12.64 Neurofibroma.** Low-power view showing a cellular tumor mass below the epithelial surface.

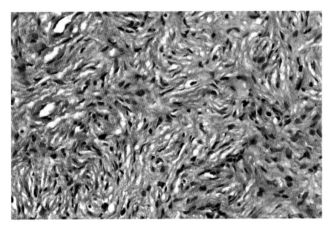

• **Fig. 12.65 Neurofibroma.** High-power view showing spindle-shaped cells with wavy nuclei.

the tumor cells show a scattered, positive reaction for S-100 protein.

Treatment and Prognosis

The treatment for solitary neurofibromas is local surgical excision, and recurrence is rare. Any patient with a lesion that is diagnosed as a neurofibroma should be evaluated clinically for the possibility of **neurofibromatosis** (see next topic). Malignant transformation of solitary neurofibromas can occur, although the risk appears to be remote, especially compared with that in patients with neurofibromatosis.

◆ NEUROFIBROMATOSIS TYPE I (VON RECKLINGHAUSEN DISEASE OF THE SKIN)

Neurofibromatosis type I is a relatively common hereditary condition that is estimated to occur in one of every 2,500–3,000 births (see Table 12.2, page 535). Several forms of neurofibromatosis have been recognized, but the most common type is **neurofibromatosis type I (NF1)**, which is discussed here. This form of the disease, also known

as **von Recklinghausen disease of the skin,** accounts for 85%–97% of neurofibromatosis cases and is inherited as an autosomal dominant trait (although 50% of all patients have no family history and apparently represent new mutations). It is caused by a wide variety of germline mutations of the *NF1* gene, which is located on chromosome region 17q11.2 and is responsible for a tumor suppressor protein product known as *neurofibromin*. The type and severity of the clinical manifestations are highly dependent on the specific mutational site in the *NF1* gene. *NF1* gene microdeletions and mutations of certain *NF1* codons are associated with more severe clinical features, whereas other *NF1* mutations confer a much milder clinical phenotype. Therefore, genetic testing is important to determine the specific mutation that is present.

Clinical and Radiographic Features

The current diagnostic criteria for NF1 are summarized in Box 12.1. Patients have multiple neurofibromas that can occur anywhere in the body but are most common on the skin. Cutaneous neurofibromas can vary from small papules to larger soft nodules, which often demonstrate the "buttonhole" sign (the ability to be invaginated into the subcutis by the tip of the index finger and then reappear when

---

• **BOX 12.1   Diagnostic Criteria for Neurofibromatosis Type I (NF1)***

A. The diagnostic criteria for NF1 are met in an individual who does not have a parent diagnosed with NF1 if two or more of the following are present:
   1. Six or more *café au lait* macules more than 5 mm in greatest diameter in prepubertal individuals and more than 15 mm in greatest diameter in postpubertal individuals[†]
   2. Freckling in the axillary or inguinal region[†]
   3. Two or more neurofibromas of any type *or* one plexiform neurofibroma
   4. Optic pathway glioma
   5. Two or more iris Lisch nodules identified by slit lamp examination or two or more choroidal abnormalities— defined as bright, patchy nodules imaged by optical coherence tomography/near-infrared reflectance imaging
   6. A distinctive osseous lesion such as sphenoid dysplasia,[‡] anterolateral bowing of the tibia, or pseudoarthrosis of a long bone
   7. A heterozygous pathogenic *NF1* variant with a variant allele fraction of 50% in apparently normal tissue such as white blood cells
B. A child of a parent who meets the diagnostic criteria specified in A merits diagnosis of NF1 if one or more of the criteria in A are present

*From Legius E, Messiaen L, Wolkenstein P, et al: Revised diagnostic criteria for neurofibromatosis type 1 and Legius syndrome: an international consensus recommendation, Genet Med 23:1506–1513, 2021.
[†]If only *café au lait* macules and freckling are present, the diagnosis is most likely NF1 but exceptionally the person might have another diagnosis such as Legius syndrome. At least one of the two pigmentary findings (*café au lait* macules or freckling) should be bilateral.
[‡]Sphenoid wing dysplasia is not a separate criterion in case of an ipsilateral orbital plexiform neurofibroma.

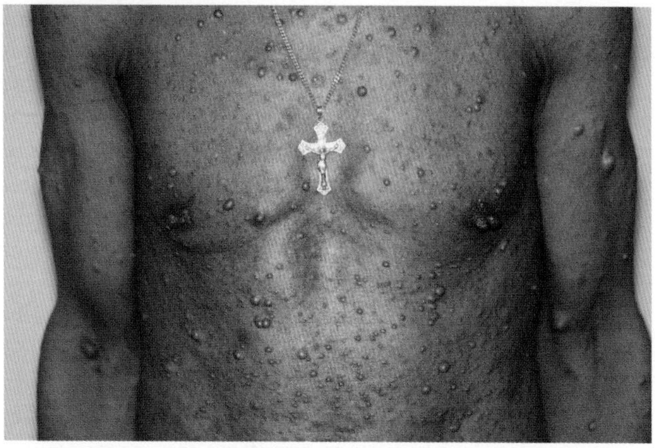

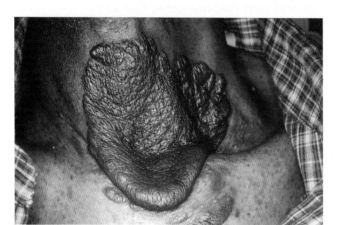

• **Fig. 12.66 Neurofibromatosis Type I.** Multiple tumors of the trunk and arms.

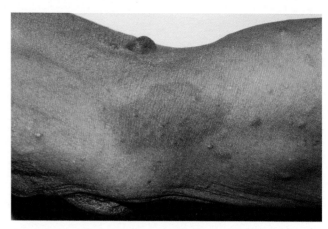

• **Fig. 12.68 Neurofibromatosis Type I.** Same patient as depicted in Fig. 12.66. Note the *café au lait* pigmentation on the arm.

• **Fig. 12.67 Neurofibromatosis Type I.** Baggy, pendulous neurofibroma of the lower neck.

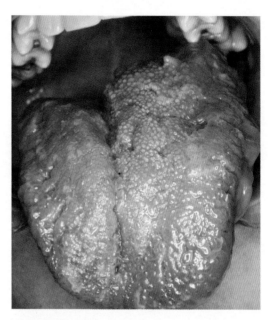

• **Fig. 12.69 Neurofibromatosis Type I.** Diffuse neurofibroma resulting in unilateral enlargement of the tongue.

pressure is released) (Fig. 12.66). The plexiform variant of neurofibroma, which feels like a "bag of worms," is considered pathognomonic for NF1. Some plexiform neurofibromas may evolve into massive baggy, pendulous masses (**elephantiasis neuromatosa**), which can exhibit increased pigmentation and hypertrichosis (Fig. 12.67).

The tumors may be present at birth, but they often begin to appear during puberty and may continue to develop slowly throughout adulthood. Accelerated growth may be seen during pregnancy. There is a wide variability in the expression of the disease. Some patients have only a few neurofibromas; others have literally hundreds or thousands of tumors. However, two-thirds of patients have relatively mild disease.

Another highly characteristic feature is the presence of *café au lait* (coffee with milk) pigmentation on the skin (Fig. 12.68). These spots occur as yellow-tan to dark-brown macules that vary in diameter from 1 to 2 mm to several centimeters. In NF1, this pigmentation typically has a smooth edge ("coast of California"), in contrast to the irregular border ("coast of Maine") of the *café au lait* spots that may occur with polyostotic fibrous dysplasia (see page 643). The pigmentation usually is present at birth or it may

develop during the first year of life. Freckling of the axilla (**Crowe sign**) or of other intertriginous zones is also a highly suggestive sign.

Lisch nodules, translucent brown-pigmented spots on the iris, are found in nearly all affected individuals. The most common general medical problem is hypertension, which may develop secondary to coarctation of the aorta, pheochromocytoma, or renal artery stenosis. Other possible abnormalities include CNS tumors, macrocephaly, mental deficiency, seizures, short stature, and scoliosis.

Studies indicate that oral manifestations may occur in as many as 72%–92% of cases, especially if a detailed clinical and radiographic examination is performed. The most commonly described finding is enlargement of the fungiform papillae, which has been reported in up to 50% of patients; however, the specificity of this finding for neurofibromatosis is unknown. Only about 25%–37% of patients will develop actual intraoral neurofibromas (Fig. 12.69). Radiographic findings may include enlargement of the mandibular foramen, enlargement or branching of the mandibular canal, increased bone density, concavity of the medial surface of the ramus, and increase in dimension of the coronoid notch. Cephalometric analysis often shows a short length of the mandible, maxilla, and cranial base.

Several unusual clinical variants of NF1 have been described. On occasion, the condition can present with unilateral involvement that, in the head and neck, may mimic hemifacial hyperplasia (see page 37). Such examples could represent *mosaic NF1*, being caused by a postzygotic somatic mutation later in embryonic development (rather than a germline mutation), which results in more limited areas of involvement. In patients with mosaic NF1, the risk for transmission to offspring can vary from 0% to 50%, depending on the degree to which the gonads may be affected by the mutation.

Several patients with NF1 have been described with central giant cell granulomas of the jaw. In addition, Legius syndrome and Noonan syndrome can show overlapping clinical features with NF1.

Treatment and Prognosis

There is no specific therapy for NF1, and treatment often is directed toward prevention or management of complications. Facial neurofibromas can be removed for cosmetic purposes. Carbon dioxide (CO_2) laser and dermabrasion have been used successfully for extensive lesions. NF1 patients with prominent hemifacial enlargement may require more significant cosmetic remodeling surgery.

One of the most feared complications is the development of cancer, most often a **malignant peripheral nerve sheath tumor (neurofibrosarcoma; malignant schwannoma),** which has been reported to occur in 8%–13% of cases. These tumors are most common on the trunk and extremities, although head and neck involvement is occasionally seen (Figs. 12.70–12.72). The 5-year survival rate for malignant peripheral nerve sheath tumors associated with NF1 is 15%–50%. Other malignancies also have been associated with NF1, including CNS tumors, pheochromocytoma, leukemia, rhabdomyosarcoma, and Wilms tumor. The average lifespan of individuals with NF1 is 8–15 years less than the general population, mostly related to vascular disease and malignant neoplasms.

In recent years, there has been considerable interest in Joseph (not John) Merrick, the so-called Elephant Man. Although Merrick once was mistakenly considered to have NF1, it is now generally accepted that his horribly disfigured appearance was not because of neurofibromatosis, but that he most likely had a rare condition known as **Proteus syndrome.** Because patients with NF1 may fear acquiring a similar clinical appearance,

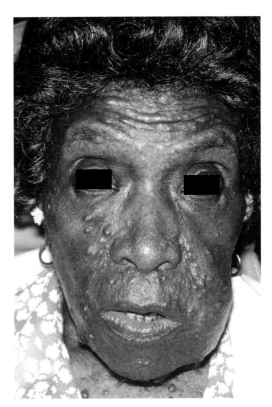

• **Fig. 12.70 Neurofibromatosis Type I.** Malignant peripheral nerve sheath tumor of the left cheek in a patient with type I neurofibromatosis. (From Neville BW, Hann J, Narang R, et al: Oral neurofibrosarcoma associated with neurofibromatosis type I, *Oral Surg Oral Med Oral Pathol* 72:456–461, 1991.)

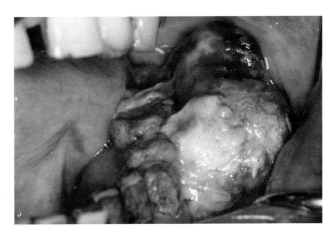

• **Fig. 12.71 Neurofibromatosis Type I.** Same patient as depicted in Fig. 12.70. Note the intraoral appearance of malignant peripheral nerve sheath tumor of the mandibular buccal vestibule. The patient eventually died of this tumor. (From Neville BW, Hann J, Narang R, et al: Oral neurofibrosarcoma associated with neurofibromatosis type I, *Oral Surg Oral Med Oral Pathol* 72:456–461, 1991.)

they should be reassured that they have a different condition. The phrase "Elephant Man disease" is incorrect and misleading, and it should be avoided. Genetic counseling is extremely important for all patients with neurofibromatosis.

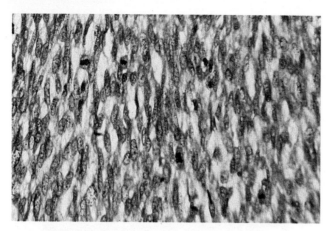

• **Fig. 12.72 Malignant Peripheral Nerve Sheath Tumor.** High-power view of an intraoral tumor that developed in a patient with neurofibromatosis type I. There is a cellular spindle cell proliferation with numerous mitotic figures.

◆ MULTIPLE ENDOCRINE NEOPLASIA TYPE 2B

The **multiple endocrine neoplasia (MEN) syndromes** are a group of rare autosomal dominant conditions characterized by tumors or hyperplasias of the neuroendocrine tissues (see Table 12.2, page 535). MEN type 1 is caused by mutations of the *MEN1* gene located on chromosome 11. Affected individuals can develop a variety of tumors of the parathyroid glands, pancreatic islets, anterior pituitary gland, and adrenal cortex. MEN2 is caused by mutations at various sites of the RET (*RE*arranged during *T*ransfection) proto-oncogene on chromosome 10, which predispose patients to the development of medullary thyroid carcinoma (MTC). Two distinct subtypes are recognized: MEN2A and MEN2B.

MEN type 2A encompasses a family of disorders with four phenotypes (classical MEN2A; MEN2A with cutaneous lichen amyloidosis; MEN2A with Hirschsprung disease; and familial MTC syndrome). Patients with classical MEN2A are at increased risk for MTC (over 90% of patients), adrenal pheochromocytomas, and primary hyperparathyroidism. MEN2A with cutaneous lichen amyloidosis is characterized by the same triad of neuroendocrine tumors, plus the presence of pruritic lesions in the scapular region that show amyloid deposition. Patients with MEN2A with Hirschsprung disease also have congenital absence of neural ganglion cells in the wall of the colon, which results in severe constipation and the risk of developing abnormal dilatation of the colon (megacolon). Individuals with familial MTC syndrome should develop only MTC with little to no risk for other neuroendocrine tumors. However, because long-term follow-up of these patients sometimes reveals eventual development of pheochromocytomas and primary hyperparathyroidism, the relevance of this fourth category of MEN2A recently has been questioned.

Over 95% of cases of MEN type 2B are caused by a germline mutation at codon 918 (M918T) of the RET

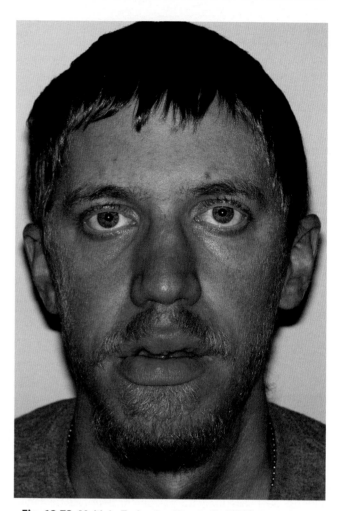

• **Fig. 12.73 Multiple Endocrine Neoplasia (MEN) Type 2B.** Note the narrow face and thick, protuberant lips.

proto-oncogene, although a few examples have been described with a mutation at codon 883 (A883F). In addition to MTC and pheochromocytomas, patients develop mucosal neuromas that especially involve the oral mucous membranes. Because oral manifestations are prominent only in MEN type 2B, the remainder of the discussion is limited to this condition.

Clinical Features

Patients with MEN type 2B usually have a marfanoid body build characterized by thin, elongated limbs with muscle wasting. The face is narrow, but the lips are characteristically thick and protuberant because of the diffuse proliferation of nerve bundles (Fig. 12.73). The upper eyelid sometimes is everted because of thickening of the tarsal plate. Small, pedunculated neuromas may be observable on the conjunctiva, eyelid margin, or cornea.

Oral mucosal neuromas are usually the first sign of the condition and may be detectable during infancy. These neuromas appear as soft, painless papules or nodules that principally affect the lips and anterior tongue but also may be seen on the buccal mucosa, gingiva, and palate (Fig. 12.74). Bilateral neuromas of the commissural mucosa are highly characteristic.

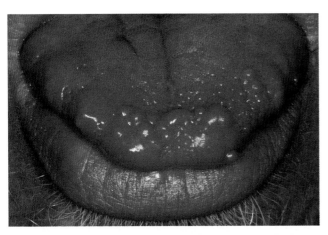

• Fig. 12.74 Multiple Endocrine Neoplasia (MEN) Type 2B. Multiple neuromas along the anterior margin of the tongue.

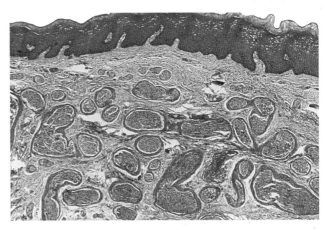

• Fig. 12.75 Multiple Endocrine Neoplasia (MEN) Type 2B. Low-power view of an oral mucosal neuroma showing marked hyperplasia of nerve bundles.

Pheochromocytomas of the adrenal glands develop in at least 50% of all patients and become more prevalent with increasing age. These neuroendocrine tumors are frequently bilateral or multifocal. The tumor cells secrete catecholamines, which result in symptoms such as profuse sweating, intractable diarrhea, headaches, flushing, heart palpitations, and hypertension. Also, approximately 67% of patients with MEN type 2B will develop ganglioneuromatosis of the gastrointestinal tract, which can result in abdominal distention, megacolon, constipation, and diarrhea. Corneal nerve hypertrophy and alacrima ("tearless crying") also may be observed.

The most significant aspect of this condition is the development of MTC, which occurs in virtually all cases. This aggressive tumor arises from the parafollicular cells (C cells) of the thyroid gland, which are responsible for calcitonin production. MTC silently develops early in life and, without prophylactic thyroidectomy before 1 year of age, most patients will develop metastatic tumor during childhood or adolescence.

Laboratory Values

If MTC is present, then serum or urinary levels of calcitonin are elevated. An increase in calcitonin levels may herald the onset of the tumor, and calcitonin also can be monitored to detect local recurrences or metastases after treatment. Pheochromocytomas may result in increased levels of urinary vanillylmandelic acid (VMA) and increased epinephrine-to-norepinephrine ratios.

Histopathologic Features

The mucosal neuromas are characterized by marked hyperplasia of nerve bundles in an otherwise normal or loose connective tissue background (Figs. 12.75 and 12.76). Prominent thickening of the perineurium is typically seen.

Treatment and Prognosis

The prognosis for patients with MEN type 2B centers on early recognition of the oral features. Because of the poor prognosis for MTC, the thyroid gland should be removed as soon as possible—preferably within the first year of life. The

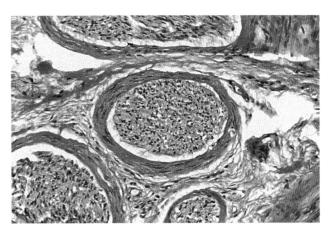

• Fig. 12.76 Multiple Endocrine Neoplasia (MEN) Type 2B. High-power view of the same neuroma as depicted in Fig. 12.75. Note the prominent thickening of the perineurium.

10-year survival rate after diagnosis for patients with MEN type 2B is 75% (compared to 97% for patients with MEN type 2A). It has been suggested that patients with the A883F mutation of the RET proto-oncogene may develop a less aggressive form of MTC than patients with the M918T mutation. Multikinase inhibitors with anti-*RET* activity (e.g., vandetanib, cabozantinib) recently have shown some promise in the management of MTC patients who are ineligible for surgery, but have symptomatic or progressive disease. Patients also should be observed for the development of pheochromocytomas because they may result in a life-threatening hypertensive crisis, especially if surgery with general anesthesia is performed.

◆ MELANOTIC NEUROECTODERMAL TUMOR OF INFANCY

The **melanotic neuroectodermal tumor of infancy** is a rare pigmented neoplasm that usually occurs during the first year of life. It is generally accepted that this lesion is of neural crest origin. In the past, however, a number of tissues were suggested as possible sources of this tumor. These included odontogenic epithelium and retina, which resulted in various older terms for this entity, such as **pigmented ameloblastoma, retinal anlage tumor,** and **melanotic progonoma.** Because these names are inaccurate, however, they should no longer be used.

Clinical and Radiographic Features

Melanotic neuroectodermal tumor of infancy almost always develops in young children during the first year of life; only 9% of cases are diagnosed after the age of 12 months. There is a striking predilection for the maxilla, which accounts for 62% of reported cases. Less frequently reported sites include the skull (16%), mandible (8%) epididymis and testis (5%), and brain (4%). (However, the percentages for sites other than the maxilla may be artificially high, because tumors occurring at less common locations probably are more likely to be submitted and accepted for publication.) A slight male predilection has been noted.

The lesion is most common in the anterior region of the maxilla, where it classically appears as a rapidly expanding mass that is frequently blue or black (Fig. 12.77). The tumor often destroys the underlying bone and may be associated with displacement of the developing teeth (Fig. 12.78). In some instances, there may be an associated osteogenic reaction, which exhibits a "sun ray" radiographic pattern that can be mistaken for osteosarcoma.

Laboratory Values

High urinary levels of vanillylmandelic acid (VMA) often are found in patients with melanotic neuroectodermal tumor of infancy. These levels may return to normal once the tumor has been resected. This finding supports the hypothesis of neural crest origin because other tumors from this tissue (e.g., pheochromocytoma and neuroblastoma) often secrete norepinephrine-like hormones that are metabolized to VMA and excreted in the urine.

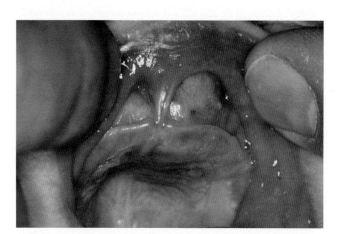

• **Fig. 12.77 Melanotic Neuroectodermal Tumor of Infancy.** Infant with an expansile mass of the anterior maxilla. (From Steinberg B, Shuler C, Wilson S: Melanotic neuroectodermal tumor of infancy: evidence for multicentricity, *Oral Surg Oral Med Oral Pathol* 66:666–669, 1988.)

Histopathologic Features

The tumor consists of a biphasic population of cells that form nests, tubules, or alveolar structures within a dense, collagenous stroma (Figs. 12.79 and 12.80). The alveolar and

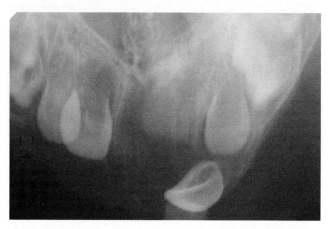

• **Fig. 12.78 Melanotic Neuroectodermal Tumor of Infancy.** Radiolucent destruction of the anterior maxilla associated with displacement of the developing teeth. (Courtesy of Dr. Len Morrow.)

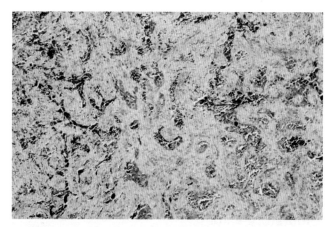

• **Fig. 12.79 Melanotic Neuroectodermal Tumor of Infancy.** Low-power view showing nests of epithelioid cells within a fibrous stroma.

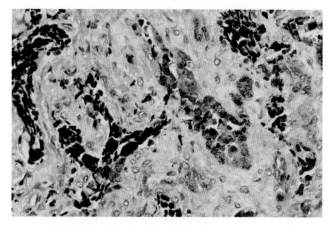

• **Fig. 12.80 Melanotic Neuroectodermal Tumor of Infancy.** High-power view of a tumor nest demonstrating two cell types: (1) small, hyperchromatic round cells and (2) larger epithelioid cells with vesicular nuclei. Some stippled melanin pigment is also present.

tubular structures are lined by cuboidal epithelioid cells that demonstrate vesicular nuclei and granules of dark-brown melanin pigment. The second cell type is neuroblastic in appearance and consists of small, round cells with hyperchromatic nuclei and little cytoplasm. These cells grow in loose nests and are frequently surrounded by the larger pigment-producing cells. Mitotic figures are rare.

Because of the tumor's characteristic microscopic features, immunohistochemistry usually is not essential to establish the diagnosis. However, the larger epithelioid cells typically are positive for cytokeratin, HMB-45, and neuron-specific enolase. In addition, the smaller cells usually are positive for neuron-specific enolase and synaptophysin.

Treatment and Prognosis

Despite their rapid growth and potential to destroy bone, most melanotic neuroectodermal tumors of infancy are benign. The lesion is best treated by surgical removal. Some clinicians prefer simple curettage, although others advocate that a 5-mm margin of normal tissue be included with the specimen. Recurrence of the tumor has been reported in about 20% of cases. Age at diagnosis is an important factor in predicting the risk of recurrence; infants diagnosed during the first 2 months of life have a significantly higher recurrence rate than children diagnosed after 4.5 months of age. In addition, about 7% of reported cases, mostly from the brain or skull, have acted in a malignant fashion, resulting in metastasis and death. Although this estimation of 7% is probably high (because unusual malignant cases are more likely to be reported), it underscores the potentially serious nature of this tumor and the need for careful clinical evaluation and follow-up of affected patients.

◆ PARAGANGLIOMA (CAROTID BODY TUMOR; CHEMODECTOMA; GLOMUS JUGULARE TUMOR; GLOMUS TYMPANICUM TUMOR)

The paraganglia are specialized tissues of neural crest origin that are associated with the autonomic nerves and ganglia throughout the body. Some of these cells act as chemoreceptors, such as the carotid body (located at the carotid bifurcation), which can detect changes in blood pH or oxygen tension and subsequently cause changes in respiration and heart rate. Tumors that arise from these structures are collectively known as **paragangliomas,** with the term preferably preceded by the anatomic site at which they are located. Therefore, tumors of the carotid body are appropriately known as **carotid body paragangliomas (carotid body tumors).** Other examples in the head and neck include **middle ear paragangliomas (glomus jugulare tumors; glomus tympanicum tumors), vagal paragangliomas,** and **laryngeal paragangliomas.**

Most head and neck paragangliomas occur as sporadic tumors, although 30%–40% of cases are associated with

heritable germline mutations of genes that encode for subunits or cofactors of the succinate dehydrogenase enzyme. Five hereditary paraganglioma syndromes (PGL1-5) have been recognized, all of which show an autosomal dominant inheritance pattern. However, PGL1 and PGL2 exhibit an unusual "parent-of-origin—dependent effect" consistent with maternal imprinting of the disease gene. Although the gene can be inherited from either the father or mother, only paternal transmission will result in development of tumors in the offspring. Therefore, the trait may appear to skip generations within a family. Development of head and neck paragangliomas also has been described rarely in several other genetic conditions, such as neurofibromatosis type 1, multiple endocrine neoplasia type 2, and von Hippel-Lindau syndrome.

Clinical and Radiographic Features

Although paragangliomas are rare, the head and neck area is the most common site for these lesions. Isolated, mutation-negative tumors show a 4:1 female:male ratio, whereas mutation-positive examples have an equal sex distribution. The tumor usually occurs in middle-aged adults (mean age of 41–47 years), although inherited cases tend to develop in patients over a decade younger. Hereditary cases have a greater chance of being multicentric; about 37% of such patients will develop more than one tumor.

The most common type is the carotid body paraganglioma, which develops at the bifurcation of the internal and external carotid arteries (Figs. 12.81 and 12.82). Most often it is a slowly enlarging, painless mass of the upper lateral neck below the angle of the jaw. It is seen more frequently in patients who live at high altitudes, indicating that some cases may arise from chronic hyperplasia of the carotid body in response to lower oxygen levels. Angiography can help to localize the tumor and demonstrate its characteristic vascular nature.

Middle ear paragangliomas are the next most common types of these tumors. The most common symptoms include

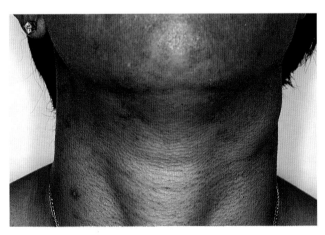

• **Fig. 12.81 Carotid Body Paraganglioma.** Large tumor in the left neck producing a visible external swelling. (Courtesy of Dr. Terry Day.)

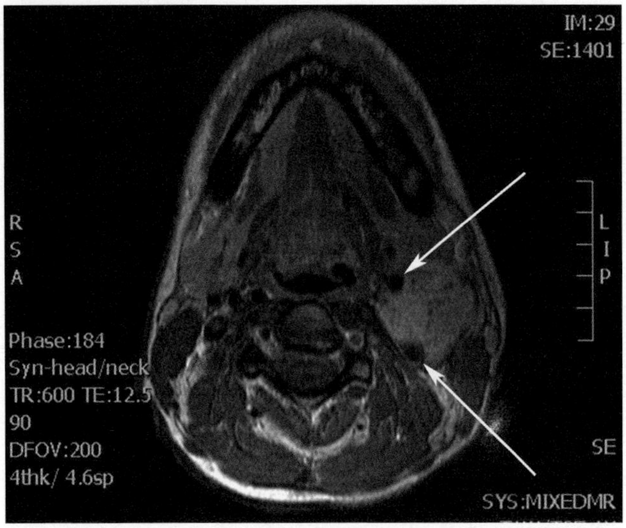

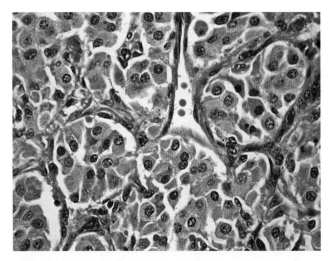

• **Fig. 12.82 Carotid Body Paraganglioma.** Same patient as depicted in Fig. 12.81. The magnetic resonance image (MRI) shows a tumor mass at the carotid bifurcation. *Arrows* indicate the external and internal branches of the carotid artery. (Courtesy of Dr. Terry Day.)

• **Fig. 12.83 Carotid Body Paraganglioma.** Nested arrangement of tumor cells.

dizziness, tinnitus (a ringing or other noise in the ear), hearing loss, and cranial nerve palsies.

Histopathologic Features

The paraganglioma is characterized by round or polygonal epithelioid cells that are organized into nests or *zellballen* (Fig. 12.83). The overall architecture is similar to that of the normal paraganglia, except the *zellballen* are usually larger and more irregular in shape. These nests consist primarily of chief cells, which demonstrate centrally located, vesicular nuclei and somewhat granular, eosinophilic cytoplasm. These cells are positive for neuroendocrine markers, such as chromogranin and synaptophysin. Loss of SDHB expression is indicative of an hereditary type of paraganglioma. The chief cells are surrounded by a flattened layer of sustentacular

cells that are immunoreactive for S-100 protein. The tumor is typically vascular and may be surrounded by a thin fibrous capsule.

Treatment and Prognosis

The treatment of paragangliomas may include surgery, radiation therapy, or both, depending on the extent and location of the tumor. Localized carotid body paragangliomas often can be treated by surgical excision with maintenance of the vascular tree. If the carotid artery is encased by tumor, it also may need to be resected, followed by vascular grafting. Although most carotid body paragangliomas can be controlled with surgery, vascular complications can lead to considerable surgical morbidity, such as intraoperative hemorrhage, stroke, and blood pressure instability. Radiation therapy may be used for unresectable tumors or as adjunctive treatment.

Because of their location near the base of the brain, middle ear paragangliomas are more difficult to manage. Hearing loss and other cranial nerve deficits are common postsurgical complications of jugular paragangliomas. Therefore, radiation therapy should be considered for primary management of such lesions. Stereotactic radiosurgery (gamma knife treatment) has shown promise in the management of primary or recurrent middle ear paragangliomas in patients who are poor surgical candidates. Stable tumors may require only active surveillance.

Approximately 6% of paragangliomas will metastasize, either to regional lymph nodes or distant sites. The risk varies from 2% for both middle ear and laryngeal tumors, to 4%–6% for carotid body tumors, and up to 16% for vagal tumors. Unfortunately, it is difficult to predict which tumors will act in a malignant fashion based on their microscopic features. However, the risk is much greater for patients with SDHB mutations (paraganglioma syndrome 4), where the rate of malignancy ranges from 30% to 50%.

◆ GRANULAR CELL TUMOR

The **granular cell tumor** is an uncommon benign soft tissue neoplasm that shows a predilection for the oral cavity. Originally, this lesion was believed to be of skeletal muscle origin and was called the *granular cell myoblastoma*. However, today most investigators believe that this tumor is derived from Schwann cells, sometimes calling it a **granular cell schwannoma/neurofibroma**. However, this tumor has characteristic clinicopathologic features, and **granular cell tumor** is the preferred designation.

Clinical Features

Granular cell tumors are most common in the oral cavity and on the skin. The single most common site is the tongue, which accounts for one-third to half of all reported cases. Tongue lesions most often occur on the dorsal surface. The lips and buccal mucosa are the next most common intraoral locations. The tumor most frequently occurs in the fourth to sixth decades of life and is rare in children. There is a 3:1 female predilection.

The granular cell tumor is typically an asymptomatic sessile nodule that is usually 2 cm or less in size (Figs. 12.84 and 12.85). The lesion often has been noted for many months or years, although sometimes the patient is unaware of its presence. The mass is typically pink, but some granular cell tumors appear yellow. The granular cell tumor is usually solitary, although multiple, separate tumors sometimes occur, especially in black patients.

Histopathologic Features

The granular cell tumor is composed of large, polygonal cells with abundant pale eosinophilic, granular cytoplasm and either dark or vesicular nuclei (Fig. 12.86). The cells are usually arranged in sheets, but they also may be found in cords and nests. The cell borders often are indistinct, which results in a syncytial appearance. The lesion is not encapsulated and often intermingles with the adjacent connective tissues. Often, there appears to be a transition from normal adjacent skeletal muscle fibers to granular tumor cells; this finding led

earlier investigators to suggest a muscle origin for this tumor. Less frequently, one may see groups of granular cells that envelop small nerve bundles. Immunohistochemical analysis reveals positivity for S-100 protein within the cells—a finding that is supportive, but not diagnostic, of neural origin. The lesional cells also are positive for CD-68, calretinin, and neuron-specific enolase.

An unusual and significant microscopic finding is the presence of acanthosis or pseudoepitheliomatous (pseudocarcinomatous) hyperplasia of the overlying epithelium, which has been reported in up to 50% of all cases (Fig. 12.87). Although this hyperplasia is usually minor in degree, in some cases it may be so striking that it results in a mistaken diagnosis of squamous cell carcinoma and subsequent unnecessary cancer surgery. The pathologist must be aware of this possibility, especially when dealing with a superficial biopsy sample or a specimen from the dorsum of the tongue—an unusual location for oral cancer.

Rare examples of S-100 negative granular cell tumors have been described. However, such lesions may represent a distinctly separate non-neural neoplasm.

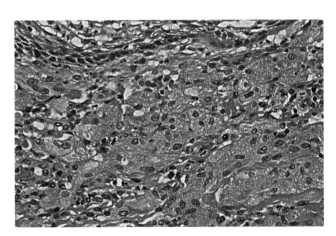

• **Fig. 12.86 Granular Cell Tumor.** Medium-high–power view showing polygonal cells with abundant granular cytoplasm.

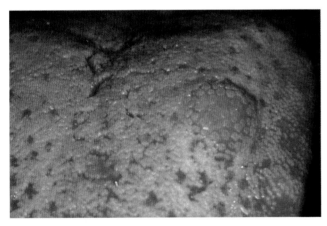

• **Fig. 12.84 Granular Cell Tumor.** Submucosal nodule on the dorsum of the tongue.

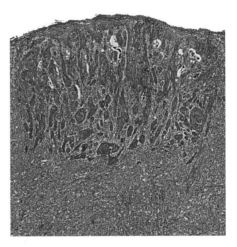

• **Fig. 12.87 Granular Cell Tumor.** Marked pseudoepitheliomatous hyperplasia overlying a granular cell tumor. Such cases may easily be mistaken for squamous cell carcinoma.

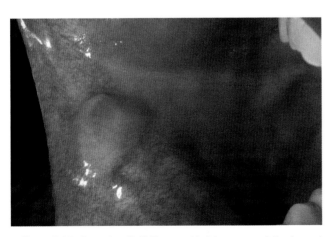

• **Fig. 12.85 Granular Cell Tumor.** Nodular mass of the buccal mucosa near the commissure.

Treatment and Prognosis

The granular cell tumor is best treated by conservative local excision, and recurrence is uncommon, even when the lesion is not entirely removed. Extremely rare examples of malignant granular cell tumor have been reported.

◆ CONGENITAL EPULIS (CONGENITAL EPULIS OF THE NEWBORN; CONGENITAL GRANULAR CELL LESION)

The **congenital epulis** is an uncommon soft tissue tumor that occurs almost exclusively on the alveolar ridges of newborns. It is often known by the redundant term, **congenital epulis of the newborn.** Rare examples also have been described on the tongue; therefore, some authors prefer using the term **congenital granular cell lesion,** because not all cases present as an *epulis* on the alveolar ridge. It also has been called **gingival granular cell tumor of the newborn,** but this term should be avoided. Although it bears a slight microscopic resemblance to the granular cell tumor (discussed previously), it exhibits ultrastructural and immunohistochemical differences that warrant its classification as a distinct and separate entity. However, the histogenesis of this tumor is still uncertain.

Clinical Features

The congenital epulis typically appears as a pink-to-red, smooth-surfaced, polypoid mass on the alveolar ridge of a newborn (Fig. 12.88). Most examples are 2 cm or less in size, although lesions as large as 7.5 cm have been reported. On occasion, the tumor has been detected *in utero* via ultrasound examination or magnetic resonance imaging (MRI). Multiple tumors develop in 10% of cases. A few rare examples on the tongue have been described in infants who also had alveolar tumors.

The tumor is two to three times more common on the maxillary ridge than on the mandibular ridge. It most frequently occurs lateral to the midline in the area of the developing lateral incisor and canine teeth. The congenital epulis shows a striking predilection for females, which suggests a hormonal influence in its development, although estrogen and progesterone receptors have not been detected. Nearly 90% of cases occur in females.

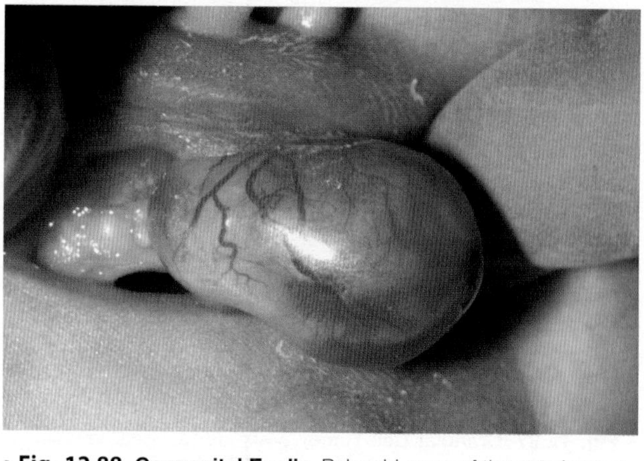

Histopathologic Features

The congenital epulis is characterized by large, rounded cells with abundant granular, eosinophilic cytoplasm and round to oval, lightly basophilic nuclei (Figs. 12.89 and 12.90). In older tumors, these cells may become elongated and separated by fibrous connective tissue. In contrast to the granular cell tumor, the overlying epithelium never shows pseudoepitheliomatous hyperplasia but typically demonstrates atrophy of the rete ridges. In addition, in contradistinction to the granular cell tumor, immunohistochemical analysis shows the tumor cells to be negative for S-100 protein.

Treatment and Prognosis

The congenital epulis is usually treated by surgical excision. The lesion never has been reported to recur, even with incomplete removal.

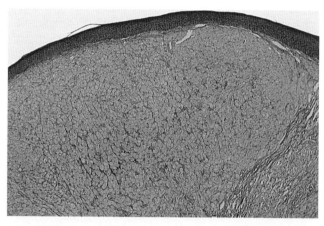

• **Fig. 12.89 Congenital Epulis.** Low-power photomicrograph showing a nodular tumor mass. Note the atrophy of the rete ridges.

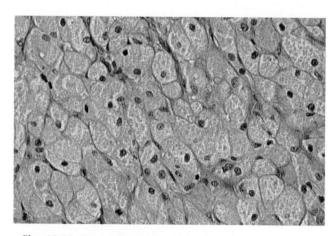

• **Fig. 12.90 Congenital Epulis.** High-power view of rounded cells with abundant granular cytoplasm.

• **Fig. 12.88 Congenital Epulis.** Polypoid mass of the anterior maxillary alveolar ridge in a newborn.

After birth, the tumor appears to stop growing and may even diminish in size. Eventual complete regression has been reported in a few patients, even without treatment (Fig. 12.91).

◆ HEMANGIOMA AND VASCULAR MALFORMATIONS

In recent years, great progress has been made in the classification and understanding of tumors and tumor-like proliferations of vascular origin. A modified classification scheme for these vascular anomalies is presented in Box 12.2.

The term **hemangioma** historically was used to describe a variety of developmental vascular anomalies. Currently, however, this term is reserved for benign vascular tumors characterized by proliferating endothelium, whereas the term **vascular malformation** is used for structural anomalies of blood vessels with normal endothelial cell turnover. Two major types of hemangioma are recognized: **infantile hemangiomas** and **congenital hemangiomas**. Infantile hemangiomas are the most common benign tumors of infancy, occurring in 4%–5% of children. They display a rapid growth phase with endothelial cell proliferation, followed by gradual involution. Most infantile hemangiomas cannot be recognized at birth but arise subsequently during the first several weeks of life. On the other hand, congenital hemangiomas are much rarer tumors that are present from birth; they may or may not undergo involution and are subclassified as *rapidly involuting congenital hemangioma [RICH], noninvoluting congenital hemangioma [NICH],* and *partially involuting congenital hemangioma [PICH]).* Molecular studies have shown that all three subtypes of congenital hemangioma may harbor point mutations in *GNAQ* or *GNA11*.

In comparison, vascular malformations usually are present at birth but persist throughout life. They can be categorized according to the type of vessel involved (capillary, venous, or arteriovenous) and according to hemodynamic features (low flow or high flow). Vascular malformations have been associated with a wide variety of gene mutations, including

GNAQ, PI3KCA, TIE2 (TEK), MAP3K3, and *MAP2K1* (see Table 12.1).

Clinical and Radiographic Features
Hemangiomas

Infantile hemangiomas are much more common in females than in males (ratio of 3:1 to 5:1), and they occur more frequently in whites than in other racial groups. The most common location is the head and neck, which accounts for 60% of all cases. Eighty percent of hemangiomas occur as single lesions, but 20% of affected patients will have multiple tumors.

Infantile hemangiomas are rarely present at birth, although a pale macule with threadlike telangiectasias may be noted on the skin. During the first few weeks of life, the tumor will demonstrate rapid development that occurs at a faster pace than the infant's overall growth. Superficial tumors of the skin appear raised and bosselated with a bright-red color ("strawberry" hemangioma) (Figs. 12.92

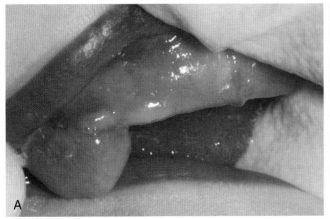
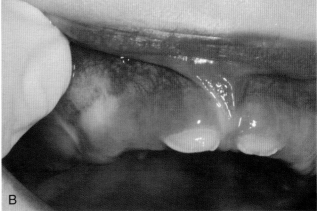

• **Fig. 12.91 Congenital Epulis. A,** Nodular mass on the maxillary alveolar ridge. Instead of being excised, the lesion was monitored clinically. **B,** Clinical appearance of the child at 1 year of age. The mass has disappeared without treatment. (Courtesy of Dr. Erwin Turner.)

and 12.93). They are firm and rubbery to palpation, and the blood cannot be evacuated by applying pressure. Deeper tumors may appear only slightly raised with a bluish hue.

The initial proliferative phase usually lasts for 6–12 months, after which the tumor grows proportionally with the child, followed by slow involution. The color gradually changes to a dull-purple hue, and the lesion feels less firm to palpation. By age 5, most of the red color is usually gone. About half of all hemangiomas will show complete resolution by 5 years of age, with 90% resolving by age 9. After tumor regression is complete, normal skin will be restored in about 50% of patients; however, up to 40% of affected individuals will show permanent changes such as atrophy, scarring, wrinkling, or telangiectasias.

Congenital hemangiomas, which are fully developed at birth, are equally divided between both sexes. Rapidly involuting congenital hemangiomas show early regression, with full involution by 9–14 months of age. Noninvoluting congenital hemangiomas grow proportionally with the child and do not undergo involution.

Complications occur in about 20% of hemangiomas. The most common problem is ulceration, which may occur with or without secondary infection. Although hemorrhage may be noted, significant blood loss does not usually occur.

Hemangiomas that occur in crucial areas can be associated with significant morbidity. Periocular tumors often result in amblyopia (dimness of vision), strabismus, or astigmatism. Patients with multiple cutaneous hemangiomas or large facial hemangiomas are at increased risk for concomitant visceral hemangiomas. Tumors in the neck and laryngeal region can lead to airway obstruction.

Large, segmental cervicofacial hemangioma can be a component of a well-recognized hemangioma syndrome—**PHACE (S) syndrome.** This acronym stands for the following:
- **P**osterior fossa brain anomalies (usually Dandy-Walker malformation)
- **H**emangioma (usually cervical segmental hemangioma)
- **A**rterial anomalies
- **C**ardiac defects and **C**oarctation of the aorta
- **E**ye anomalies
- **S**ternal cleft or **S**upraumbilical raphe

Kasabach-Merritt phenomenon is a serious coagulopathy that has been associated with two rare and potentially aggressive vascular tumors known as *tufted hemangioma* and *kaposiform hemangioendothelioma.* This disorder is characterized by severe thrombocytopenia and hemorrhage because of platelet trapping within the tumor. The mortality rate is as high as 20%–30%.

Vascular Malformations

Vascular malformations are present at birth and persist throughout life. Port wine stains are relatively common capillary malformations that occur in 0.3% of newborns.. They are most common on the face, particularly along the distribution of the trigeminal nerve. In Sturge-Weber syndrome, associated intracranial lesions are present (see page 551). Port wine stains are typically pink or purple macular lesions that grow commensurately with the patient. As the patient gets older, the lesion often darkens and becomes nodular because of vascular ectasia.

Low-flow **venous malformations** encompass a wide spectrum of lesions, from small isolated ectasias to complex growths that involve multiple tissues and organs. They are present at birth, although they may not always be immediately apparent. Typically, venous malformations are blue and are easily compressible (Fig. 12.94). They often grow

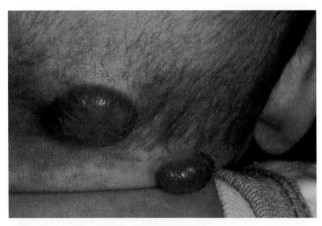

• **Fig. 12.92 Hemangioma.** Infant with two red, nodular masses on the posterior scalp and neck ("strawberry" hemangioma).

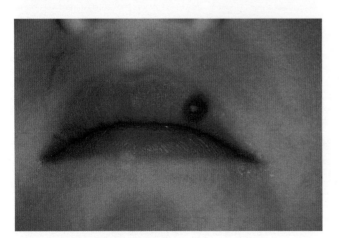

• **Fig. 12.93 Hemangioma.** Nodular, red mass on the upper lip vermilion in a 4-year-old child. (Courtesy of Dr. Lynn Wallace.)

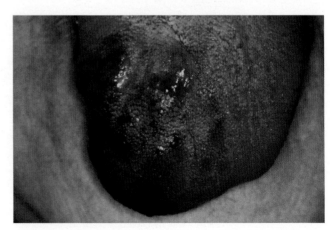

• **Fig. 12.94 Venous Malformation.** Blue-purple mass of the anterior tongue.

proportionately with the patient, but they may swell when dependent or with increased venous pressure. Secondary thrombosis and phlebolith formation can occur.

Arteriovenous malformations are high-flow lesions that result from persistent direct arterial and venous communication. Although they are present from birth, they may not become noticeable until later in childhood or adulthood. Because of the fast vascular flow through these lesions, a palpable thrill or bruit often is noticeable. The overlying skin typically feels warmer to touch. Presenting symptoms may include pain, bleeding, and skin ulceration.

Intrabony Vascular Malformations

Intrabony "hemangiomas" also may occur and usually represent either venous or arteriovenous malformations. In the jaws, such lesions are detected most often during the first three decades of life. They are slightly more common in females than in males and occur three times more often in the mandible than the maxilla. The lesion may be completely asymptomatic, although some examples are associated with pain and swelling. Mobility of teeth or bleeding from the gingival sulcus may occur. A bruit or pulsation may be apparent on auscultation and palpation.

The radiographic appearance of intrabony vascular malformations is variable. Most commonly, the lesion shows a multilocular radiolucent defect. The individual loculations may be small (honeycomb appearance) or large (soap bubble appearance). In other cases the lesion may present as an ill-defined radiolucent area or a well-defined, cystlike radiolucency (Fig. 12.95). Large malformations may cause cortical expansion, and occasionally a "sunburst" radiographic pattern is produced (Fig. 12.96). Angiography can be helpful in demonstrating the vascular nature of the lesion (Fig. 12.97).

Histopathologic Features

Early infantile hemangiomas are characterized by numerous plump endothelial cells and often-indistinct vascular lumina (Figs. 12.98 and 12.99). At this stage, such lesions often are known microscopically as *juvenile* or *cellular* hemangiomas. Because of their cellular nature, these lesions also have been called **juvenile hemangioendothelioma,** although this term should be avoided because hemangioendothelioma also is used to designate other vascular tumors of intermediate malignant potential. As the lesion matures, the endothelial cells become flattened, and the small, capillary-sized vascular spaces become more evident (Fig. 12.100). As the hemangioma undergoes involution, the vascular spaces become less prominent and are replaced by fibrofatty connective tissue.

Vascular malformations do not show active endothelial cell proliferation, and the channels resemble the vessels of origin. Therefore, capillary malformations may be similar to the capillary stage of hemangioma, whereas venous malformations may show more dilated vessels (Fig. 12.101). Because of their similar features, many vascular malformations are incorrectly categorized as *hemangiomas.* Arteriovenous malformations demonstrate a mixture of thick-walled arteries and veins, along with capillary vessels.

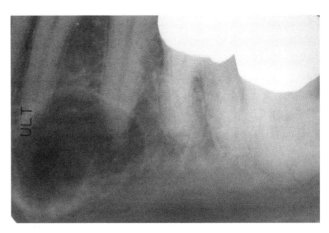

• **Fig. 12.95 Intrabony Venous Malformation.** Well-circumscribed radiolucency that contains fine trabeculations.

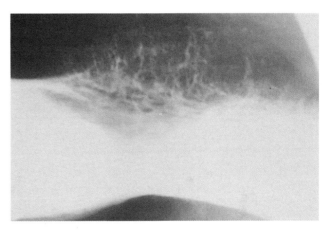

• **Fig. 12.96 Intrabony Venous Malformation.** Occlusal radiograph demonstrating cortical destruction and a "sunburst" periosteal reaction resembling osteosarcoma.

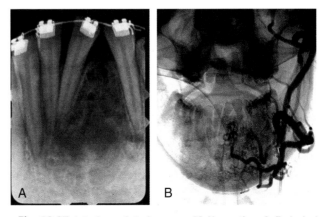

• **Fig. 12.97 Intrabony Arteriovenous Malformation. A,** Periapical radiograph showing an expansile, mottled radiolucency in the mandibular incisor region. Pulsatile hemorrhage was encountered when a biopsy of this lesion was attempted. **B,** Angiogram demonstrating a vascular proliferation between the mandibular incisors. (Courtesy of Dr. Larry Cunningham and Dr. Jason Ford.)

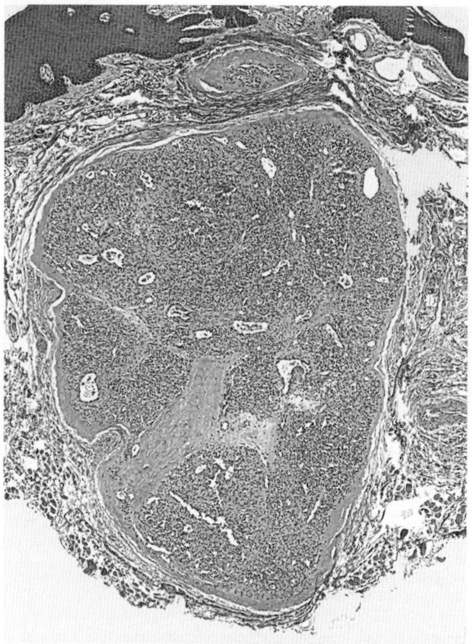

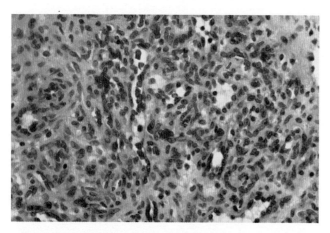

• **Fig. 12.98 Juvenile (Cellular) Hemangioma.** Low-power photomicrograph showing a circumscribed cellular mass of vascular endothelial cells arranged in lobular aggregates.

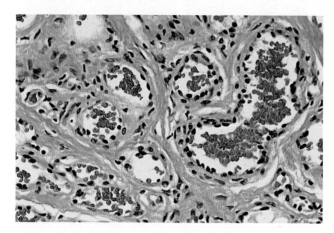

• **Fig. 12.99 Juvenile (Cellular) Hemangioma.** High-power view showing a highly cellular endothelial proliferation forming occasional indistinct vascular lumina.

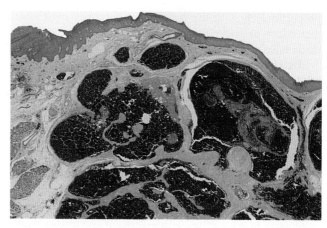

• **Fig. 12.100 Capillary Hemangioma.** High-power photomicrograph demonstrating well-formed capillary-sized vessels.

• **Fig. 12.101 Venous Malformation.** Low-power photomicrograph showing multiple large, dilated blood vessels.

GLUT1 is an immunohistochemical marker that is consistently positive in infantile hemangiomas. In contrast, this marker is negative in other developmental vascular tumors and anomalies listed in Box 12.2 (RICH, NICH, PICH, tufted angioma, kaposiform hemangioendothelioma, pyogenic granuloma, and vascular malformations).

Treatment and Prognosis

Because most hemangiomas of infancy undergo involution, management often consists of "watchful neglect." It is important to educate parents that although rapid growth may be seen, regression will occur. For problematic or life-threatening hemangiomas, pharmacologic therapy with the beta blocker propranolol has become the first-line treatment in recent years. Systemic corticosteroids also may help to reduce the size of the lesion, but this approach is associated with a greater risk potential than propranolol therapy. Intralesional and topical corticosteroids sometimes have been used for smaller localized, problematic lesions. Topical timolol maleate may be effective for thin or superficial infantile hemangiomas.

Surgical removal rarely is warranted for infantile hemangiomas, although excision may be effective for localized, pedunculated tumors that demonstrate ulceration or recurrent bleeding. Surgical management early in childhood also might be a consideration in situations where eventual surgical repair would be required anyway and the scar can be easily hidden. Upper eyelid tumors that can affect vision also may be candidates for surgery.

Flashlamp pulsed dye lasers can be effective in the treatment of port wine stains. The management of venous malformations depends on the size, location, and associated complications of the lesion. Small, stable malformations may not require treatment. Larger, problematic lesions may be treated with a combination of sclerotherapy and surgical excision. Sclerotherapy involves the injection of sclerosing agents, such as 95% ethanol, sodium tetradecyl sulfate, or ethanolamine oleate, directly into the lesion to induce fibrosis. Sclerotherapy alone may be sufficient for smaller lesions; for larger lesions, subsequent surgical resection can be accomplished with less risk of bleeding after sclerotherapy.

The treatment of arteriovenous malformations is more challenging and also depends on the size of the lesion and degree of involvement of vital structures. For cases that require resection, radiographic embolization often is performed 24–48 hours before surgery to minimize blood loss.

Vascular malformations of the jaws are potentially dangerous lesions because of the risk of severe bleeding, which may occur spontaneously or during surgical manipulation. Needle aspiration of any undiagnosed intrabony lesion before biopsy is a wise precaution to rule out the possibility of a vascular malformation. Severe and even fatal hemorrhages have occurred after incisional biopsy or extraction of teeth in the area of such lesions.

◆ STURGE-WEBER SYNDROME (ENCEPHALOTRIGEMINAL ANGIOMATOSIS; STURGE-WEBER ANGIOMATOSIS)

Sturge-Weber syndrome is a rare, nonhereditary developmental condition that is characterized by a hamartomatous vascular proliferation involving the tissues of the brain and face. The capillary malformation associated with this syndrome has been shown to be related to somatic mutations of the *GNAQ* and *PI3K* genes, resulting in aberrant activation of MAPK and/or PI3K.. It has been suggested that these embryologic mutations result in failure of the primitive cephalic venous plexus to regress and mature properly during the first trimester of pregnancy. The incidence of Sturge-Weber syndrome is estimated to be 1 in every 20,000 – 50,000 live births.

Clinical and Radiographic Features

Patients with Sturge-Weber syndrome are born with a dermal capillary vascular malformation of the face known as a **port wine stain** or **nevus flammeus** because of its deep-purple color. This port wine stain usually has a unilateral distribution along one or more segments of the trigeminal nerve. Occasionally, patients have bilateral involvement or additional port wine lesions elsewhere on the body. Risk for the condition occurs primarily in patients with involvement along the distribution of the ophthalmic branch of the trigeminal nerve (V1) (Figs. 12.102 and 12.103). Approximately 15%–20% of children with port-wine stains involving the distribution of V1 will have Sturge-Weber syndrome.

In addition to the facial port wine nevus, individuals with Sturge-Weber syndrome have leptomeningeal angiomas that overlie the ipsilateral cerebral cortex. This meningeal angiomatosis usually is associated with a convulsive disorder and often results in intellectual disability or contralateral hemiplegia. Other potential problems include migraine headaches, stroke-like episodes, growth hormone deficiency, and central hypothyroidism. Imaging studies of the brain may reveal gyriform "tramline" calcifications on the affected side (Fig. 12.104). Ocular involvement may be manifested

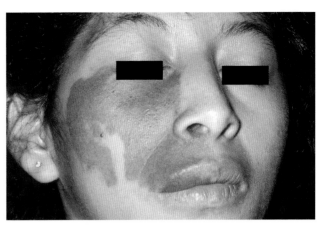

• **Fig. 12.102 Port Wine Stain.** Nevus flammeus of the malar area in a patient without Sturge-Weber syndrome. Unless the vascular lesion includes the region innervated by the ophthalmic branch of the trigeminal nerve, usually the patient does not have central nervous system (CNS) involvement.

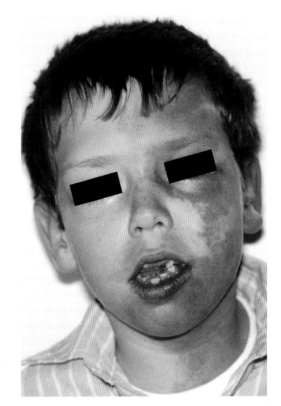

• **Fig. 12.103 Sturge-Weber Syndrome.** Port wine stain of the left face, including involvement along the ophthalmic branch of the trigeminal nerve. The patient also was intellectually disabled and had a seizure disorder.

by glaucoma and vascular malformations of the conjunctiva, episclera, choroid, and retina.

Intraoral involvement in Sturge-Weber syndrome is common, resulting in hypervascular changes to the ipsilateral mucosa (Fig. 12.105). The gingiva may exhibit slight vascular hyperplasia or a more massive hemangiomatous proliferation that can resemble a pyogenic granuloma. Such gingival

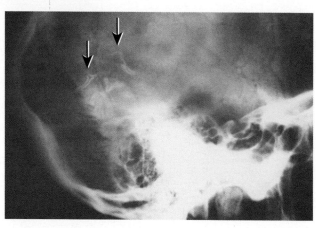

• **Fig. 12.104 Sturge-Weber Syndrome.** Skull film showing "tramline" calcifications (*arrows*). (Courtesy of Dr. Reg Munden.)

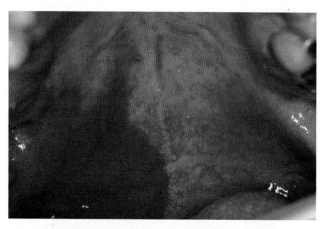

• **Fig. 12.105 Sturge-Weber Syndrome.** Unilateral vascular involvement of the soft palate.

hyperplasia may be attributable to the increased vascular component, anticonvulsant therapy used to control the epileptic seizures, or both. Destruction of the underlying alveolar bone has been reported in rare instances.

Histopathologic Features

The port wine nevus is characterized by excessive numbers of dilated blood vessels in the middle and deep dermis. The intraoral lesions show a similar vascular dilatation. Proliferative gingival lesions may resemble a pyogenic granuloma.

Treatment and Prognosis

The treatment and prognosis of Sturge-Weber syndrome depend on the nature and severity of the possible clinical features. Usually, facial port wine nevi can be improved by using flashlamp pulsed dye lasers. Cortical excision of angiomatous meningeal lesions may be necessary in some cases. Patients with intractable epilepsy and progressive intellectual disability eventually may require more extensive neurosurgical treatment, including lobectomy or hemispherectomy.

Port wine nevi that affect the gingiva can make flossing and dental prophylaxis difficult. Great care must be taken when performing surgical procedures in affected areas of the mouth because significant hemorrhage may be encountered. Lasers also may be helpful in the removal of hyperplastic oral lesions.

◆ NASOPHARYNGEAL ANGIOFIBROMA

The **nasopharyngeal angiofibroma** is a rare vascular and fibrous tumor-like lesion that occurs only in the nasopharynx. Although microscopically benign, it frequently exhibits locally destructive and aggressive behavior. It may represent a vascular malformation rather than a true neoplasm.

Clinical and Radiographic Features

Nasopharyngeal angiofibromas occur almost exclusively in males. The tumor is exceedingly rare in females—so much so that the diagnosis in a female patient should be viewed with skepticism and closely scrutinized. The lesion also shows a striking predilection for adolescents between the ages of 10 and 17 and often has been called the *juvenile nasopharyngeal angiofibroma.* However, rare examples also have been reported in slightly younger and older patients. Because of its almost exclusive occurrence in adolescent boys, a hormonal influence seems likely, although no definite endocrine abnormalities have been detected. Occasional examples of nasopharyngeal angiofibroma have been described in patients with familial adenomatous polyposis.

Unilateral nasal obstruction (80%) and epistaxis (60%) are common early symptoms. The lesion appears to arise in the pterygopalatine fossa and expands medially into the nasal cavity via the sphenopalatine foramen. Some cases show extension into the paranasal sinuses, orbits, cavernous sinus, or middle cranial fossa. Invasion into the oral cavity or cheek rarely has been reported. Computed tomography (CT) scans and magnetic resonance imaging (MRI) studies are helpful adjuncts in visualizing the extent of the lesion and degree of adjacent tissue destruction. Anterior bowing of the posterior wall of the maxillary sinus (Holman-Miller sign) is a characteristic feature (Fig. 12.106). Angiograms can be used to confirm the vascular nature of the lesion (Fig. 12.107).

Histopathologic Features

The nasopharyngeal angiofibroma consists of dense fibrous connective tissue that contains numerous dilated, thin-walled blood vessels of variable size (Fig. 12.108). Typically, the vascular component is more prominent at the periphery of the tumor, especially in lesions from younger patients.

Treatment and Prognosis

The primary treatment of nasopharyngeal angiofibroma usually consists of surgical excision. Depending on the extent of the lesion, this may be accomplished via endoscopic surgery,

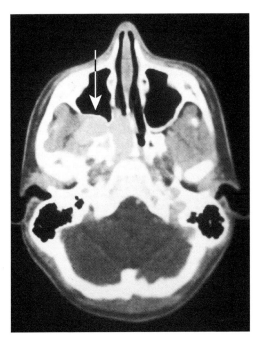

• **Fig. 12.106 Nasopharyngeal Angiofibroma.** A contrasted computed tomography (CT) scan showing a tumor of the nasopharynx and pterygopalatine fossa, with characteristic anterior bowing of the posterior wall of the right maxillary sinus *(arrow)*. (Courtesy of Dr. Pamela Van Tassel.)

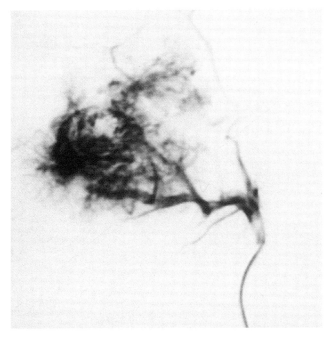

• **Fig. 12.107 Nasopharyngeal Angiofibroma.** A digital subtraction angiogram of the external carotid artery showing the intense vascular blush of the tumor. (Courtesy of Dr. Pamela Van Tassel.)

lateral rhinotomy, midfacial degloving procedure, infratemporal fossa approach, or combined craniofacial resection. Preoperative embolization of the tumor is helpful in controlling blood loss. Radiation therapy usually is reserved for recurrent lesions and extensive tumors with unusual vascular supplies or intracranial extension.

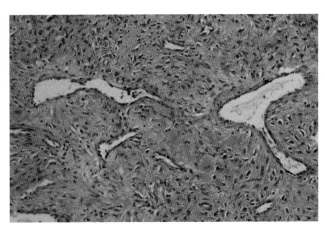

• **Fig. 12.108 Nasopharyngeal Angiofibroma.** Moderately cellular fibrous connective tissue with prominent blood vessels.

The recurrence rate varies from 20% to 40% in most studies. Such recurrences usually are retreated with further surgery or radiation therapy. Malignant transformation into fibrosarcoma rarely has been reported and probably is associated with prior radiation therapy.

◆ LYMPHATIC MALFORMATIONS (LYMPHANGIOMA; CYSTIC HYGROMA)

Lymphatic malformations are benign, hamartomatous tumor-like growths of lymphatic vessels. Like other vascular malformations, it is doubtful that they are true neoplasms; instead, they most likely represent developmental anomalies that arise from sequestrations of lymphatic tissue that do not communicate normally with the rest of the lymphatic system.

Lymphatic malformations can be classified into three types:
1. **Macrocystic**—composed of cystlike spaces measuring 2 cm or greater in diameter
2. **Microcystic**—composed of smaller vascular channels measuring less than 2 cm in diameter
3. **Mixed**—composed of a combination of macrocystic and microcystic spaces

The subtypes are probably variants of the same pathologic process, and the size of the vessels may depend on the nature of the surrounding tissues. Macrocystic lymphatic malformations ("cystic hygroma") often occur in the neck, where the loose adjacent connective tissues allow for more expansion of the vessels. Microcystic lesions are more frequent in the mouth, where the denser surrounding connective tissue and skeletal muscle limit vessel expansion.

Clinical Features

Lymphatic malformations have a marked predilection for the head and neck, which accounts for 50%–75% of all cases (Fig. 12.109). About half of all lesions are noted at birth, and around 90% develop by 2 years of age.

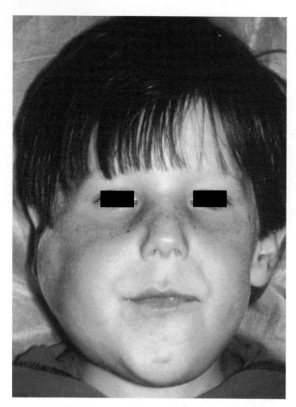

• **Fig. 12.109 Lymphatic Malformation.** Young boy with a cystic hygroma primarily involving the right side of the face. (Courtesy of Dr. Frank Kendrick.)

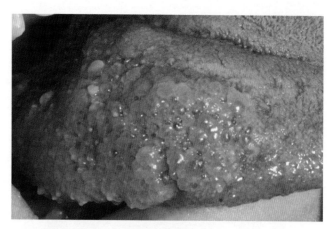

• **Fig. 12.110 Lymphatic Malformation.** Pebbly, vesicle-like appearance of a tumor of the right lateral tongue.

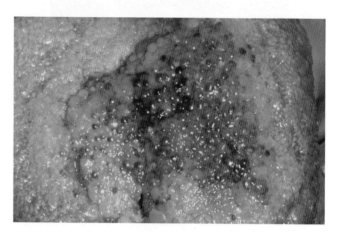

• **Fig. 12.111 Lymphatic Malformation.** Dorsal tongue lesion demonstrating a purple color, which can be caused by secondary hemorrhage or an associated hemangiomatous component.

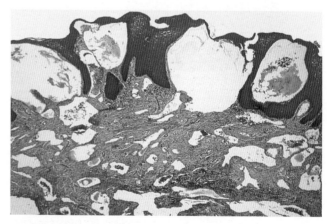

• **Fig. 12.112 Microcystic Lymphatic Malformation.** Lesion of the tongue showing dilated lymphatic vessels beneath the epithelium and in the deeper connective tissues.

Cervical lymphatic malformations are more common in the posterior triangle and are typically soft, fluctuant masses. They occur less frequently in the anterior triangle, although lesions in this location are more likely to result in respiratory difficulties or dysphagia if they grow large. Occasionally, cervical lesions will extend into the mediastinum or upward into the oral cavity. Such growths can become massive and can measure 15 cm or greater in size. Rapid enlargement may occur secondary to an upper respiratory tract infection, presumably because of increased lymph production, blocked lymphatic drainage, or secondary infection of the tumor.

Oral lymphatic malformations may occur at various sites but are most frequent on the anterior two-thirds of the tongue, where they often result in macroglossia (Figs. 12.110 and 12.111). Usually, the lesion is superficial in location and demonstrates a pebbly surface that resembles a cluster of translucent vesicles. The surface has been likened to the appearance of frog eggs or tapioca pudding. Secondary hemorrhage into the lymphatic spaces may cause some of these "vesicles" to become purple. Deeper tumors present as soft, ill-defined masses.

Small lymphatic anomalies less than 1 cm in size occur on the alveolar ridge in around 4% of black neonates. These lesions often occur bilaterally on the mandibular ridge and show a 2:1 male-to-female distribution. Most of these alveolar lymphangiomas apparently resolve spontaneously because they are not observed in older people.

Histopathologic Features

Lymphatic malformations are composed of lymphatic vessels that may show mild dilatation (microcystic) (Figs. 12.112 and 12.113) or macroscopic cystlike structures (macrocystic)

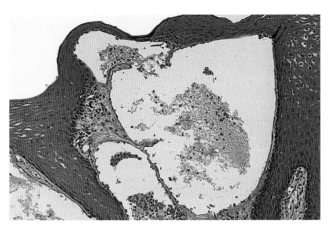

• **Fig. 12.113 Microcystic Lymphatic Malformation.** High-power photomicrograph showing dilated, lymph-filled vessels immediately below the atrophic surface epithelium.

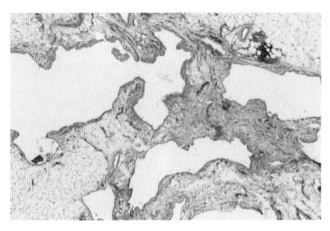

• **Fig. 12.114 Macrocystic Lymphatic Malformation.** Lesion from the neck showing markedly dilated lymphatic vessels.

(Fig. 12.114). The vessels often diffusely infiltrate the adjacent soft tissues and may demonstrate lymphoid aggregates in their walls. The lining endothelium is typically thin, and the spaces contain proteinaceous fluid and occasional lymphocytes. Some channels also may contain red blood cells, which creates uncertainty as to whether they are lymphatic or blood vessels. Although many of these likely represent secondary hemorrhage into a lymphatic vessel, some actually may be examples of mixed vascular malformations composed of both lymphatic and blood vessels.

In intraoral tumors, the lymphatic vessels are characteristically located just beneath the epithelial surface and often replace the connective tissue papillae. This superficial location results in the translucent, vesicle-like clinical appearance. However, extension of these vessels into the deeper connective tissue and skeletal muscle also may be seen.

Treatment and Prognosis

The treatment of lymphatic malformations of the head and neck depends on the size, location, and subtype of the anomaly. Smaller lesions not associated with significant functional or cosmetic problems may be managed best by observation alone. For example, some clinicians do not recommend treatment for nonenlarging lesions of the tongue because of the difficulty in removal and high recurrence rate. Spontaneous regression of lymphatic malformations is rare but has been reported in about 3% of cases.

When required, treatment usually consists of surgical excision, percutaneous sclerotherapy, or a combination of both. Total surgical removal may not be possible in all cases because of large size or involvement of vital structures. Recurrence after surgery is common, especially for microcystic lymphatic malformations of the oral cavity, because of their infiltrative nature. Macrocystic lesions of the cervical region are often well circumscribed and have a lower rate of recurrence.

In recent years, percutaneous sclerotherapy has proven to be a successful alternative to surgery for many lymphatic malformations. The most widely used sclerosants include doxycycline, OK-432, and bleomycin. Sclerotherapy is most successful in the management of macrocystic lesions, with over 80% of patients showing complete resolution or substantial response. A lower success rate is achieved in mixed and microcystic subtypes.

The prognosis is good for most patients, although large tumors of the neck or tongue may result in airway obstruction and death.

◆ LEIOMYOMA

Leiomyomas are benign tumors of smooth muscle that most commonly occur in the uterus, gastrointestinal tract, and skin. Leiomyomas of the oral cavity are rare. Most of these probably have their origin from vascular smooth muscle.

The three types are as follows:
1. Solid leiomyomas
2. Vascular leiomyomas (angiomyomas or angioleiomyomas)
3. Epithelioid leiomyomas (leiomyoblastomas)

Almost all oral leiomyomas are either solid or vascular in type; angiomyomas account for nearly 75% of all oral cases. Rare examples of developmental hamartomas composed primarily of smooth muscle (leiomyomatous hamartoma) also have been described in the oral cavity.

Clinical and Radiographic Features

The oral leiomyoma can occur at any age and is usually a slow-growing, firm, mucosal nodule (Fig. 12.115). Most lesions are asymptomatic, although occasional tumors can be painful. Solid leiomyomas are typically normal in color, although angiomyomas may exhibit a bluish hue. The most common sites are the lips, tongue, palate, and cheek, which together account for 80% of cases. Extremely rare intraosseous examples may present as unilocular radiolucencies of the jaws.

Oral leiomyomatous hamartomas occur most frequently on the anterior palatal gingiva in the incisive papilla region or on the midline dorsal tongue (Fig. 12.116). If the lesion is present at birth, then it may be mistaken for a congenital epulis (see page 546). Most other examples are discovered

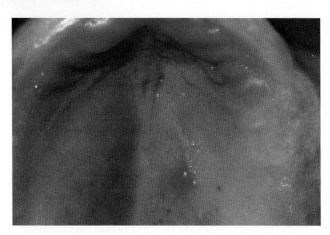

• **Fig. 12.115 Leiomyoma.** Small, pink-red nodule on the posterior hard palate lateral to the midline.

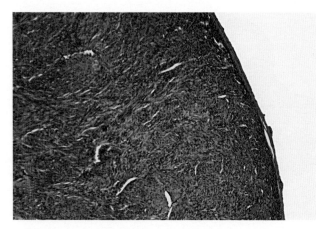

• **Fig. 12.117 Leiomyoma.** Low-power view showing a well-circumscribed cellular mass of spindle-shaped smooth muscle cells.

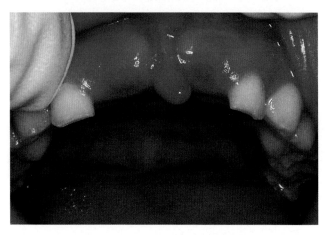

• **Fig. 12.116 Oral Leiomyomatous Hamartoma.** Small, papular growth on midline anterior maxillary alveolar ridge in a 7-year-old male. (Courtesy of Dr. Lon Doles.)

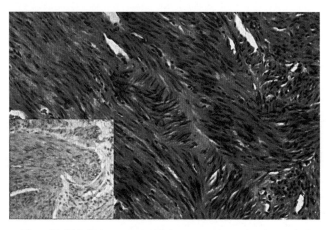

• **Fig. 12.118 Leiomyoma.** High-power view showing spindle-shaped cells with blunt-ended nuclei. Immunohistochemical analysis shows strong positivity for smooth muscle actin (*inset*).

during early childhood or adolescence. The lesion appears as a smooth, sessile or pedunculated nodule that usually is less than 1 cm in diameter.

Histopathologic Features

Solid leiomyomas are well-circumscribed tumors that consist of interlacing bundles of spindle-shaped smooth muscle cells (Figs. 12.117 and 12.118). The nuclei are elongated, pale staining, and blunt ended. Mitotic figures are uncommon. Rare examples with extensive ossification have been reported.

Angiomyomas also are well-circumscribed lesions that demonstrate multiple tortuous blood vessels with thickened walls caused by hyperplasia of their smooth muscle coats (Fig. 12.119). Intertwining bundles of smooth muscle may be found between the vessels, sometimes with inter-mixed adipose tissue. As its name implies, the epithelioid leiomyoma is composed primarily of epithelioid cells rather than spindle cells. Leiomyomatous hamartomas consist of interlacing fascicles sof eosinophilic spindle cells that may blend into the surrounding collagen.

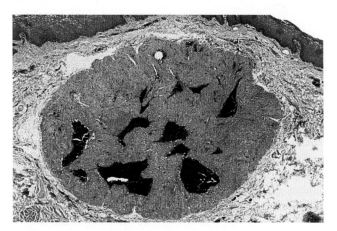

• **Fig. 12.119 Angiomyoma.** Well-circumscribed tumor exhibiting prominent blood vessels surrounded by smooth muscle.

Special stains and immunohistochemistry may be helpful to confirm the smooth muscle differentiation if the diagnosis is in doubt. The smooth muscle stains bright red with the Masson trichrome stain (Fig. 12.120). Immunohistochemi-cal analysis usually reveals the tumor cells to be positive for

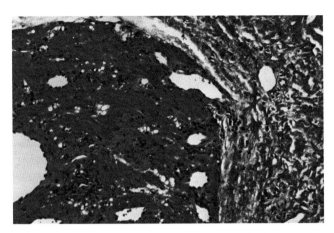

• **Fig. 12.120　Angiomyoma.** Masson trichrome stain demonstrating bundles of smooth muscle (*red*) with adjacent normal collagen (*blue*).

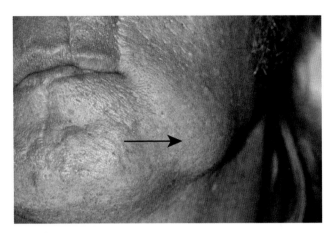

• **Fig. 12.121　Adult Rhabdomyoma.** Nodular mass (*arrow*) in the left cheek. (Courtesy of Dr. Craig Little.)

vimentin, smooth muscle actin, and muscle-specific actin; desmin positivity also may be seen.

Treatment and Prognosis

Oral leiomyomas are treated by local surgical excision. The lesion should not recur.

◆ RHABDOMYOMA

Benign neoplasms of skeletal muscle are called **rhabdomyomas.** The term *rhabdomyoma* also is used to describe a hamartomatous lesion of the heart that often is associated with tuberous sclerosis (see page 762). Despite the great amount of skeletal muscle throughout the body, benign skeletal muscle tumors are extremely rare. However, these extra-cardiac rhabdomyomas show a striking predilection for the head and neck. Rhabdomyomas of the head and neck can be subclassified into two major categories: (1) adult rhabdomyomas and (2) fetal rhabdomyomas.

Clinical Features
Adult Rhabdomyomas

Adult rhabdomyomas of the head and neck occur primarily in middle-aged and older patients, with about 80% of cases found in men. The most frequent sites are the pharynx, oral cavity, and larynx; intraoral lesions are most common in the floor of the mouth, soft palate, and base of tongue. The tumor appears as a nodule or mass that can grow many centimeters before discovery (Figs. 12.121 and 12.122). Laryngeal and pharyngeal lesions often lead to airway obstruction. Sometimes, the tumor is multinodular in nature, with two or more discrete nodules found in the same anatomic location. From 3% to 15% of adult rhabdomyomas are multicentric, with separate, distinct tumors at different sites.

Fetal Rhabdomyomas

Fetal rhabdomyomas usually occur in young children, although some also develop in adults. A similar male predilection is noted. The most common locations are the face and periauricular region.

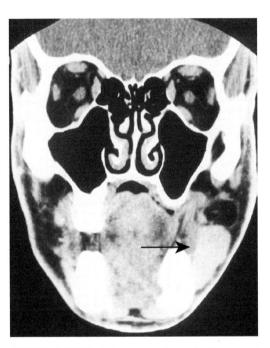

• **Fig. 12.122　Adult Rhabdomyoma.** Computed tomography (CT) scan of the same tumor depicted in Fig. 12.121. Note the mass (*arrow*) lateral to the left body of the mandible. (Courtesy of Dr. Craig Little.)

Histopathologic Features
Adult Rhabdomyomas

The adult rhabdomyoma is composed of well-circumscribed lobules of large, polygonal cells, which exhibit abundant granular, eosinophilic cytoplasm (Fig. 12.123). These cells often demonstrate peripheral vacuolization that results in a "spider web" appearance of the cytoplasm. Focal cells with cross striations can be identified in most cases (Fig. 12.124). Although rarely necessary for the diagnosis, immunohistochemical examination will show the tumor cells to be positive for myoglobin, desmin, and muscle-specific actin.

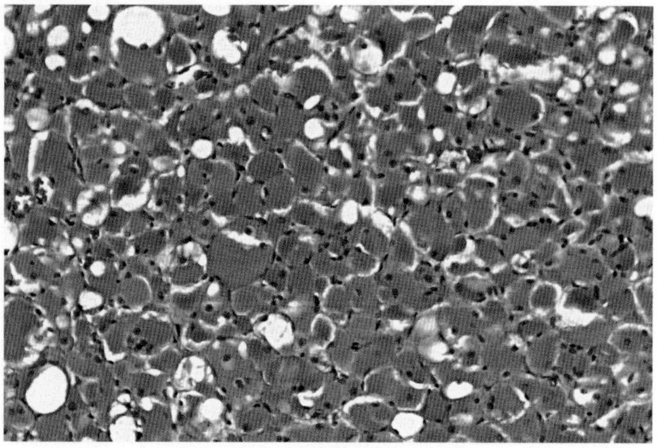

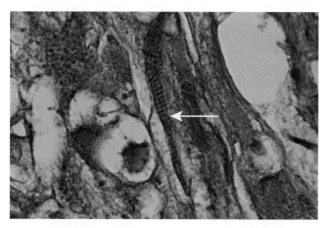

• **Fig. 12.123 Adult Rhabdomyoma.** Medium-power view showing a uniform tumor composed of rounded and polygonal cells with focal vacuolization.

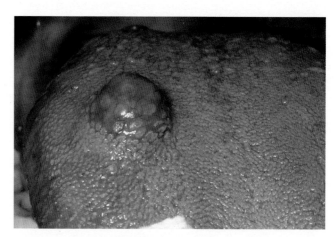

• **Fig. 12.125 Ectomesenchymal Chondromyxoid Tumor.** Nodular mass on the right dorsal tongue. (From Kannan R, Damm DD, White DK, et al: Ectomesenchymal chondromyxoid tumor of the anterior tongue: a report of three cases, *Oral Surg Oral Med Oral Pathol Oral Radiol Endod* 82:417–422, 1996.)

• **Fig. 12.124 Adult Rhabdomyoma.** Phosphotungstic acid hematoxylin (PTAH) stain that demonstrates focal cross striations in some cells (*arrow*).

Fetal Rhabdomyomas

The fetal rhabdomyoma has a less mature appearance and consists of a haphazard arrangement of spindle-shaped muscle cells that sometimes are found within a myxoid stroma. Some tumors may show considerable cellularity and mild pleomorphism, which makes them easily mistaken for rhabdomyosarcomas.

Treatment and Prognosis

The treatment of both variants of rhabdomyoma consists of local surgical excision. Recurrence has been reported in 10%–42% of cases, but this largely may be due to incomplete removal.

◆ ECTOMESENCHYMAL CHONDROMYXOID TUMOR

The **ectomesenchymal chondromyxoid tumor** is a rare benign intraoral neoplasm that was first identified in 1995. The histogenesis of this tumor is uncertain, although it has been suggested that it may arise from an uncommitted

ectomesenchymal cell of neural crest origin or from a soft tissue myoepithelial cell. The vast majority of these lesions have been related to *RREB1::MKL2* fusion genes; a much smaller subset have shown *EWSR1* gene rearrangements.

Clinical Features

Over 90% of ectomesenchymal chondromyxoid tumors occur on the anterior dorsal tongue, although rare examples also have been reported at the base of tongue, other oral soft tissue sites, and the mandible. The tumor shows a wide age range, most commonly being diagnosed in the third through the sixth decades of life. No sex predilection has been identified. The lesion usually presents at a painless nodular mass that may measure from less than 1 cm to several cm in diameter (Fig. 12.125).

Histopathologic Features

The ectomesenchymal chondromyxoid tumor can show a highly variable microscopic appearance. At low power, the tumor typically demonstrates a circumscribed, lobular growth pattern, although some cases may demonstrate focal infiltration into adjacent skeletal muscle. The cells can be polygonal to spindled or stellate in shape, with ovoid nuclei and pale eosinophilic to lightly basophilic cytoplasm. Varying degrees of cellularity are noted, including dense sheets of cells intermixed with zones of loosely arranged cells showing a myxoid appearance (Fig. 12.126). Focal hyalinized or chondroid stromal changes may be found. Immunohistochemistry usually shows the tumor cells to be positive for glial fibrillary acid protein (GFAP) and S100 protein.

Treatment and Prognosis

Treatment should consist of conservative surgical excision. Recurrence rarely has been reported.

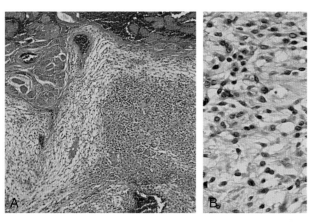

• **Fig. 12.126 Ectomesenchymal Chondromyxoid Tumor. A,** Low-power view showing a circumscribed tumor with both cellular areas (*right*) and less cellular myxoid zones (*left*). **B,** High-power view demonstrating spindle/stellate cells within a myxoid background.

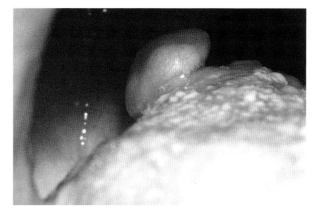

• **Fig. 12.127 Osseous Choristoma.** Hard pedunculated nodule on the posterior dorsum of the tongue. (Courtesy of Dr. Michael Meyrowitz.)

◆ OSSEOUS AND CARTILAGINOUS CHORISTOMAS

A **choristoma** is a tumor-like growth of microscopically normal tissue in an abnormal location. Several different tissue types may occur in the mouth as choristomas. These include gastric mucosa, glial tissue, and tumor-like masses of sebaceous glands. However, the most frequently observed choristomas of the oral cavity are those that consist of bone, cartilage, or both. These lesions sometimes have been called **soft tissue osteomas** or **soft tissue chondromas,** but *choristoma* is a better term because they do not appear to be true neoplasms.

Clinical Features

Osseous and cartilaginous choristomas show a striking predilection for the tongue, which accounts for 85% of cases. The most common location is the posterior tongue near the foramen cecum, although rare examples also have been reported elsewhere on the tongue and at other oral locations. The lesion is usually a firm, smooth-surfaced, sessile or pedunculated nodule between 0.5 and 2.0 cm in diameter (Fig. 12.127). Many patients are unaware of the lesion, although some complain of gagging or dysphagia.

Histopathologic Features

Microscopic examination of choristomas shows a well-circumscribed mass of dense lamellar bone or mature cartilage that is surrounded by dense fibrous connective tissue (Fig. 12.128). Sometimes a combination of bone and cartilage is formed. The bone has a well-developed Haversian canal system and occasionally demonstrates central fatty or hematopoietic marrow.

Treatment and Prognosis

Osseous and cartilaginous choristomas are best treated by local surgical excision. Recurrence has not been reported.

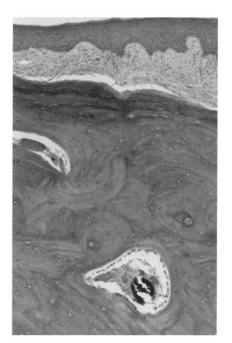

• **Fig. 12.128 Osseous Choristoma.** Mass of dense lamellar bone beneath the surface epithelium.

Soft Tissue Sarcomas

Fortunately, soft tissue sarcomas are rare in the oral and maxillofacial region and account for less than 1% of the cancers in this area. Because of their relative rarity, it is beyond the scope of this book to give a complete, detailed discussion of each of these tumors. However, a review of these entities is included in the following section.

◆ FIBROSARCOMA

The **fibrosarcoma** is a malignant tumor of fibroblasts. At one time, it was considered one of the most common soft tissue sarcomas. However, the diagnosis of fibrosarcoma rarely is made today because many spindle cell tumors with similar microscopic features have now been reclassified into separate, distinct categories. Fibrosarcomas are most common in the extremities; only 10%–19% occur in the head and neck region.

Clinical Features

Fibrosarcomas most often present as slow-growing masses that may reach considerable size before they produce pain (Fig. 12.129). They can develop at any age and occur anywhere in the head and neck region. A number of cases have been reported in the nose and paranasal sinuses, where they often result in obstructive symptoms. Development of fibrosarcoma following radiation therapy to the head and neck also has been described.

Histopathologic Features

Adult-type fibrosarcoma is often a diagnosis of exclusion, being used for spindle cell sarcomas that do not fit microscopically into other recognized categories. Well-differentiated examples consist of fascicles of spindle-shaped cells that classically form a "herringbone" pattern (Fig. 12.130). The cells often show little variation in size and shape, although variable numbers of

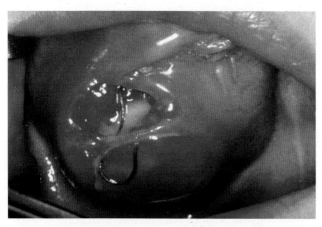

• **Fig. 12.129 Fibrosarcoma.** Child with a large mass of the hard palate and maxillary alveolar ridge. (Courtesy of Dr. John McDonald.)

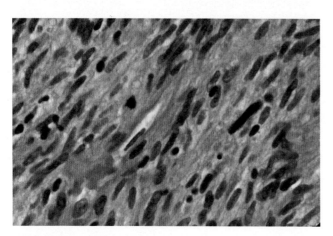

• **Fig. 12.130 Fibrosarcoma.** Cellular mass of spindle-shaped cells demonstrating mild pleomorphism.

mitotic figures usually can be identified. In more poorly differentiated tumors, the cells are less organized and may appear rounder or ovoid. Mild pleomorphism along with more frequent mitotic activity may be seen. Higher grade tumors tend to produce less collagen than do well-differentiated tumors. Immunohistochemical markers should be negative except for vimentin and minimal smooth muscle actin.

In addition to classic adult-type tumors, the classification of "fibrosarcoma" includes a number of variants, including *myxofibrosarcoma*, *low-grade fibromyxoid sarcoma*, *sclerosing epithelioid fibrosarcoma*, and *juvenile/infantile fibrosarcoma*.

Treatment and Prognosis

The treatment of choice is usually surgical excision, including a wide margin of adjacent normal tissue. Recurrence is noted in about half of cases, and 5-year survival rates range from 40% to 70%.

◆ UNDIFFERENTIATED PLEOMORPHIC SARCOMA (MALIGNANT FIBROUS HISTIOCYTOMA)

The term **malignant fibrous histiocytoma** was introduced in the 1960s to describe a group of sarcomas that were considered to show both fibroblastic and histiocytic features. This concept rapidly gained acceptance and malignant fibrous histiocytoma soon became the most commonly diagnosed soft tissue sarcoma in adults. However, experts today have questioned this concept because, with the help of immunohistochemistry and molecular studies, most tumors formerly diagnosed as malignant fibrous histiocytoma can now be reclassified into other categories, such as liposarcoma, leiomyosarcoma, rhabdomyosarcoma, myxofibrosarcoma, melanoma, and anaplastic carcinoma. However, there still remains a heterogeneous group of tumors from this former family, whose line of differentiation cannot be determined. The term **undifferentiated pleomorphic sarcoma** is now recommended for these lesions.

Clinical Features

Undifferentiated pleomorphic sarcomas occur primarily in older age groups. The most common complaint is an expanding mass that may or may not be painful or ulcerated. The extremities and deep tissues of the trunk are the most frequent locations. Tumors of the nasal cavity and paranasal sinuses produce obstructive symptoms.

Histopathologic Features

Several histopathologic patterns have been described. The most classic variety is the storiform-pleomorphic type, which is characterized by short fascicles of plump spindle cells arranged in a storiform pattern, admixed with areas of pleomorphic giant cells (Fig. 12.131).

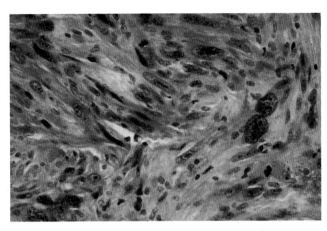

• **Fig. 12.131 Undifferentiated Pleomorphic Sarcoma.** Spindle cell neoplasm demonstrating marked pleomorphism and scattered mitoses.

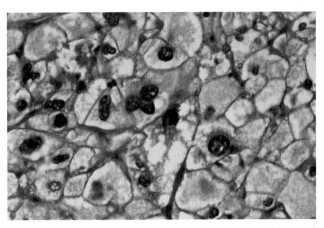

• **Fig. 12.132 Liposarcoma.** High-power view showing vacuolated lipoblasts with pleomorphic nuclei.

Treatment and Prognosis

Undifferentiated pleomorphic sarcoma is considered to be an aggressive tumor that is usually treated by radical surgical resection. Approximately 40% of patients with head and neck tumors will have local recurrence, and almost 30% will develop metastases. The overall 5-year survival rate is 52%–55%.

◆ LIPOSARCOMA

The **liposarcoma** is a malignant neoplasm of fatty origin. It currently is considered to be the most common soft tissue sarcoma and accounts for 15%–25% of all soft tissue malignancies in adults. The most common sites are the thigh, retroperitoneum, and inguinal region. Liposarcomas of the head and neck are rare, comprising only 3% of all such tumors.

Clinical Features

Liposarcomas are seen primarily in adults; the mean age for head and neck tumors is 57 years. The tumor is typically a soft, slow-growing, ill-defined mass that may appear normal in color or yellow. Pain or tenderness is uncommon; when present, it is usually a late feature. The neck is the most common site for liposarcomas of the head and neck region. The most frequent intraoral locations are the tongue and cheek.

Histopathologic Features

Most liposarcomas can be divided into several major categories:
1. Well-differentiated liposarcoma/atypical lipomatous tumor
2. Myxoid/round cell liposarcoma
3. Pleomorphic liposarcoma
4. Dedifferentiated liposarcoma

The most common of these variants in the oral cavity is the **well-differentiated liposarcoma,** which accounts for 67% of all cases. These tumors resemble benign lipomas but demonstrate scattered lipoblasts and atypical, hyperchromatic stromal cells (Fig. 12.132). Because well-differentiated liposarcoma in superficial soft tissue exhibits such low-grade behavior, these lesions often are referred to as *atypical lipomatous tumors*. Positive immunostaining for CDK4 and MDM2 can help to distinguish well-differentiated liposarcoma/atypical lipomatous tumor from benign lipomatous lesions. In more difficult cases, demonstration of *MDM2* gene amplification by fluorescence *in situ* hybridization (FISH) can help to confirm the diagnosis.

Myxoid liposarcomas demonstrate proliferating lipoblasts within a myxoid stroma that contains a rich capillary network. The **round cell liposarcoma** is a more aggressive form of myxoid liposarcoma with less differentiated, rounded cells.

Pleomorphic liposarcomas exhibit extreme cellular pleomorphism and bizarre giant cells. **Dedifferentiated liposarcomas** are characterized by the combination of well-differentiated liposarcoma with poorly differentiated, nonlipogenic sarcomatous changes. These features may coexist in the same neoplasm, or the dedifferentiated changes may develop in a recurrent tumor or metastasis.

Treatment and Prognosis

Radical excision is the treatment of choice for most liposarcomas throughout the body. In spite of this, at least 50% of all tumors recur. The overall 5-year survival rate ranges from 59% to 70%. There is a 10-year survival rate of approximately 50%. The histopathologic subtype is extremely important in predicting the prognosis; the outlook for pleomorphic liposarcomas is much worse than for myxoid and well-differentiated tumors.

In contrast, the prognosis for oral liposarcoma is more favorable because of the predominance of well-differentiated subtypes and because most tumors are small when diagnosed. Local recurrence has been reported in 15%–20% of cases, but metastasis and death as a result of tumor is rare.

◆ MALIGNANT PERIPHERAL NERVE SHEATH TUMOR (MALIGNANT SCHWANNOMA; NEUROFIBROSARCOMA; NEUROGENIC SARCOMA)

The principal malignancy of peripheral nerve origin is preferably called a **malignant peripheral nerve sheath tumor.** These tumors account for approximately 5%–10% of all soft tissue sarcomas, with one-fourth to one-half of such cases occurring in patients with neurofibromatosis type I (see page 537). The lesion is most common on the proximal portions of the extremities and the trunk; about 15% of cases occur in the head and neck region.

Clinical and Radiographic Features

Malignant peripheral nerve sheath tumors are most common in young adults. The mean age in patients with neurofibromatosis (29–36 years) is about one decade younger than in those without this condition (40–46 years). The tumor is an enlarging mass that sometimes exhibits rapid growth. Associated pain or a nerve deficit is common.

Oral tumors may occur anywhere, but the most common sites are the jaws, lips, and buccal mucosa (see Figs. 12.70 and 12.71, page 539). Radiographic examination of intraosseous tumors of the mandible may reveal widening of the mandibular canal or the mental foramen, with or without irregular destruction of the surrounding bone.

Histopathologic Features

The malignant peripheral nerve sheath tumor shows fascicles of atypical spindle-shaped cells, which often resemble the cells of adult-type fibrosarcoma (see Fig. 12.72, page 540). However, these cells frequently are more irregular in shape with wavy or comma-shaped nuclei. In addition to streaming fascicles, less cellular myxoid areas also may be present. With some tumors, there can be heterologous elements, which include skeletal muscle differentiation (**malignant Triton tumor**), cartilage, bone, or glandular structures.

A definitive diagnosis of neural origin often is difficult, especially in the absence of neurofibromatosis. Positive immunostaining for S-100 protein or SOX10 can be a helpful clue, but these are found in only about 50%–60% of all cases and may be focal. Also, these markers are not specific for neural origin, and sometimes they can be demonstrated in other spindle cell malignancies.

Treatment and Prognosis

The treatment of malignant peripheral nerve sheath tumors consists primarily of radical surgical excision, possibly along with adjuvant radiation therapy and chemotherapy. The prognosis is generally poor, with disease-specific survival ranging from 39% to 60% at 5 years, and 26% to 45% at 10 years. Some studies have suggested that patients with neurofibromatosis type I have a worse prognosis than sporadic cases, although other studies have shown no significant difference between these two groups. Tumors that are negative for S-100 protein have been reported to have a significantly worse prognosis.

◆ OLFACTORY NEUROBLASTOMA (ESTHESIONEUROBLASTOMA)

The **olfactory neuroblastoma** is a rare neuroectodermal neoplasm of the upper nasal vault that shows some similarities to neuroblastomas seen elsewhere in the body. It is believed to arise from sensory olfactory neuroepithelial cells.

Clinical and Radiographic Features

Unlike the usual neuroblastoma, the olfactory neuroblastoma is rare in patients younger than the age of 10 years. Instead, it is more common in adults, with a mean age at diagnosis of 45–56 years. The tumor arises high in the nasal cavity close to the cribriform plate. From there it may extend into the adjacent paranasal sinuses (especially the ethmoid sinus), the orbit, and the anterior cranial fossa (Fig. 12.133). The most common symptoms are nasal obstruction, epistaxis, pain, and anosmia.

Histopathologic Features

Olfactory neuroblastomas consist of small, round to ovoid basophilic cells that are arranged in sheets and lobules (Fig. 12.134). Rosette and pseudorosette formation and

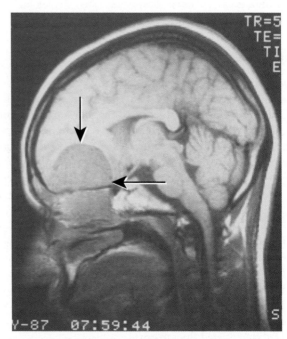

• **Fig. 12.133 Olfactory Neuroblastoma.** A T1-weighted sagittal magnetic resonance image (MRI) showing a tumor filling the superior nasal cavity and ethmoid sinus, with extension into the anterior cranial fossa (*arrows*). (Courtesy of Dr. Pamela Van Tassel.)

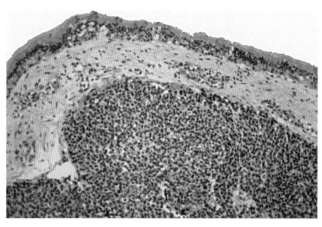

• **Fig. 12.134 Olfactory Neuroblastoma.** Sheet of small, basophilic cells adjacent to the sinonasal epithelium (*top*).

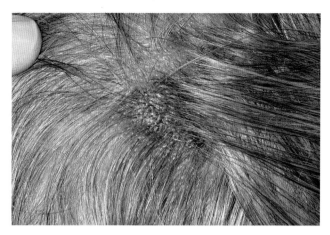

• **Fig. 12.135 Angiosarcoma.** Slightly elevated, bluish purple lesion on the scalp. (Courtesy of Dr. Terry Day.)

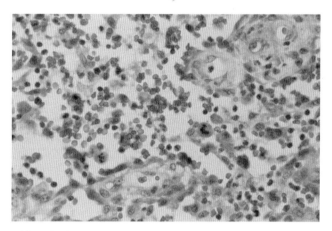

• **Fig. 12.136 Angiosarcoma.** Sinusoidal vascular spaces lined by pleomorphic endothelial cells.

areas of delicate neurofibrillary material may be seen. The tumor cells typically will express neuroendocrine markers, such as chromogranin, synaptophysin, and CD56.

Treatment and Prognosis

The treatment of olfactory neuroblastoma consists of surgical excision, often with adjuvant radiation therapy. A combined craniofacial surgical approach frequently is used. Adjuvant chemotherapy also has been shown to improve survival.

The prognosis depends on the histopathologic grade and clinical stage of the tumor. The overall 5-year survival is approximately 75%, and disease-free survival is 60%. At 10 years, these survival rates decrease to 60% and 40% respectively. Death is usually a result of local recurrence; metastasis occurs in approximately 20% of cases and is associated with an extremely poor prognosis.

◆ ANGIOSARCOMA

Angiosarcoma is a rare malignancy of vascular endothelium, which may arise from either blood or lymphatic vessels. Although it accounts for only 1% of all sarcomas, about half of all cases occur in the head and neck region, with the scalp and forehead being the most common sites. However, intraoral examples are exceedingly rare.

The term **hemangioendothelioma** is used to describe vascular tumors with microscopic features intermediate between those of hemangiomas and angiosarcomas. Such tumors also are rare and are considered to be of intermediate malignancy.

Clinical Features

Cutaneous angiosarcomas of the head and neck are most common in older adult patients. Early lesions often resemble a simple bruise, which may lead to a delay in diagnosis. However, the lesion continues to enlarge, which results in an elevated, nodular, or ulcerated surface (Fig. 12.135). Many examples appear multifocal in nature. Oral angiosarcomas

have been reported in various locations; the gingiva and tongue are the most common sites.

Histopathologic Features

Angiosarcoma is characterized by an infiltrative proliferation of endothelium-lined blood vessels that form an anastomosing network (Fig. 12.136). The endothelial cells appear hyperchromatic and atypical; they often tend to pile up within the vascular lumina. Increased mitotic activity may be seen. Immunohistochemical studies show the tumor cells to be positive for CD31 and ERG in most cases, whereas CD34 positivity is observed less consistently.

Treatment and Prognosis

Treatment usually consists of radical surgical excision, radiation therapy, or both. The prognosis for angiosarcoma of the head and neck is poor, with reported 5- and 10-year overall survival rates of only 26.5% and 16.9%, respectively. However, angiosarcomas of the oral cavity and salivary glands may have a somewhat better outcome. One recent review showed that 50% of patients with intraoral angiosarcoma died from their disease.

◆ KAPOSI SARCOMA

Kaposi sarcoma is an unusual vascular neoplasm that was first described in 1872 by Moritz Kaposi, a Hungarian dermatologist. Before the advent of the acquired immunodeficiency syndrome (AIDS) epidemic, it was a rare tumor; however, beginning in the early 1980s, Kaposi sarcoma became quite common because of its propensity to develop in individuals infected by HIV. Since the introduction of combination antiretroviral therapy (ART) in the mid- to late 1990s, the prevalence of AIDS-related Kaposi sarcoma in the Western world has declined.

Kaposi sarcoma is caused by infection with human herpesvirus 8 (HHV-8; Kaposi sarcoma-associated herpesvirus [KSHV]). The lesion most likely arises from endothelial cells, which may express markers for both lymphatic and blood vessel differentiation. Four clinical presentations are recognized:

1. Classic
2. Endemic (African)
3. Iatrogenic (transplant-associated)
4. AIDS-related

The first three forms are discussed here; AIDS-related Kaposi sarcoma is covered in the section on HIV disease (see page 254).

Clinical Features

Classic Type

Classic Kaposi sarcoma is primarily a disease of late adult life, and 90% of cases occur in men. Because HHV-8 exposure occurs with much greater frequency in some areas of the world, the prevalence of Kaposi sarcoma also is much higher in these regions, such as the Mediterranean, eastern Europe, and central equatorial Africa. Multiple blue-purple macules and plaques are present on the skin of the lower extremities (Fig. 12.137). These lesions grow slowly over many years and develop into painless tumor nodules. Oral lesions are rare and most frequently involve the palate. Some studies have

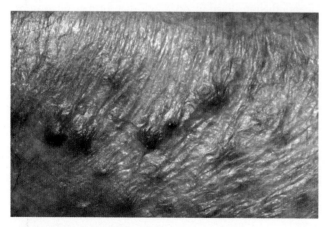

• **Fig. 12.137 Kaposi Sarcoma.** Classic Kaposi sarcoma in an older man presenting as multiple purple macules and plaques on the lower leg.

suggested that patients with classic Kaposi sarcoma have an increased prevalence of lymphoreticular malignancies, but other reports have questioned any significant association.

Endemic Type

Prior to the advent of HIV/AIDS, endemic Kaposi sarcoma was already recognized as a relatively common neoplasm of younger adults and children in sub-Saharan Africa. The course of the disease can vary widely; some patients develop indolent skin lesions similar to the pattern observed in classic Kaposi sarcoma, whereas others exhibit more aggressive tumors that involve deeper tissues, bone, and viscera. A particularly aggressive lymphadenopathic form also is recognized in young children, which is characterized by rapidly growing tumors of the lymph nodes, occasional visceral organ lesions, and sparse skin involvement. Although endemic Kaposi sarcoma used to be the most common form of the disease seen in Africa, AIDS-related Kaposi sarcoma is seen more frequently now.

Iatrogenic Type

Iatrogenic (transplant-associated) Kaposi sarcoma occurs in recipients of solid organ transplants. It affects 0.5% of renal transplant patients, usually several months to a few years after the transplant. It is probably related to the loss of cellular immunity from immunosuppressive therapy given to prevent organ rejection. Like classic Kaposi sarcoma, iatrogenic cases are more common in individuals of Mediterranean and eastern European ancestry; however, the disease may run a more aggressive course.

Histopathologic Features

Kaposi sarcoma typically evolves through three stages:

1. Patch (macular)
2. Plaque
3. Nodular

A proliferation of miniature vessels characterizes the **patch stage.** This results in an irregular, jagged vascular network that surrounds preexisting vessels. Sometimes normal structures, such as hair follicles or preexisting blood vessels, may appear to protrude into these new vessels (promontory sign). The lesional endothelial cells have a bland appearance and may be associated with scattered lymphocytes and plasma cells.

The **plaque stage** demonstrates further proliferation of these vascular channels along with the development of a significant spindle cell component. Tiny hyaline globules may be observed within or adjacent to the tumor cells.

In the **nodular stage,** the spindle cells increase to form a nodular tumor-like mass that may resemble a fibrosarcoma or other spindle cell sarcomas (Figs. 12.138 and 12.139). However, numerous extravasated erythrocytes are present, and slitlike vascular spaces may be discerned.

Other microscopic variants of Kaposi sarcoma include lymphangioma-like, telangiectatic, desmoplastic, lymphangiectatic, ecchymotic, and anaplastic subtypes.

Treatment and Prognosis

The treatment of Kaposi sarcoma depends on the clinical subtype and stage of the disease. For skin lesions in the classic form of the disease, radiation therapy (such as electron beam) may be used. Radiation therapy for oral lesions must be approached with caution, because an unusually severe mucositis can develop. Surgical excision can be performed for the control of individual lesions of the skin or mucosa. Systemic chemotherapy also may be helpful. Intralesional injection of vinblastine is used to control individual lesions.

The prognosis is variable, depending on the form of the disease and the patient's immune status. The classic form of the disease is slowly progressive; only 10%–20% of patients develop disseminated lesions. The mean survival time is 10–15 years, and patients often die from unrelated causes. Some patients with the endemic form of the disease develop indolent lesions similar in behavior to classic non-African Kaposi sarcoma. However, the other endemic African forms are more aggressive and the prognosis is poorer. The lymphadenopathic form runs a particularly fulminant course, usually resulting in the death of the patient within 2–3 years. In transplant patients, the disease also may be somewhat more aggressive; however, the tumors may regress if the patient's immunosuppressive therapy can be switched from cyclosporine to rapamycin, which is thought to have antitumor activity.

◆ LEIOMYOSARCOMA

The **leiomyosarcoma** is a malignant neoplasm of smooth muscle differentiation, which accounts for 5%–10% of all soft tissue sarcomas. The most common sites are the uterine wall and gastrointestinal tract. Leiomyosarcomas of the oral cavity are rare.

Clinical Features

In general, leiomyosarcomas are most common in middle-aged and older adults. However, tumors in the oral and maxillofacial region occur over a wide age range without a predilection for any age group. They have been reported at various sites, but about one-third of all oral cases arise in the mandible. The clinical appearance is nonspecific; there is usually an enlarging mass that may or may not be painful (Fig. 12.140). Secondary ulceration of the mucosal surface may occur.

Histopathologic Features

The microscopic examination of a leiomyosarcoma shows fascicles of spindle-shaped cells with abundant eosinophilic cytoplasm and blunt-ended, cigar-shaped nuclei (Fig. 12.141). Some tumors may be composed primarily of rounded epithelioid cells that have either eosinophilic or clear cytoplasm (epithelioid leiomyosarcoma). The degree of pleomorphism varies from one tumor to the next, but smooth muscle tumors with the presence of five or more mitoses per ten high-power fields should be considered potentially malignant. Glycogen usually can be demonstrated within the cells with a periodic acid-Schiff (PAS) stain, and the cell cytoplasm appears bright red with a Masson trichrome stain. Immunohistochemical analysis usually reveals the presence of one or more of the following

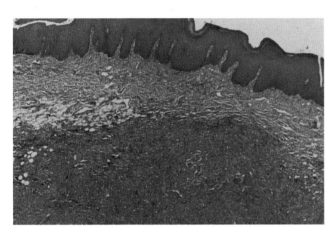

• **Fig. 12.138 Kaposi Sarcoma.** Low-power photomicrograph showing a cellular spindle cell tumor within the connective tissue.

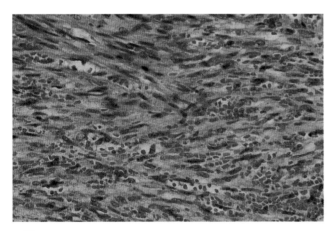

• **Fig. 12.139 Kaposi Sarcoma.** High-power photomicrograph showing spindle cells and poorly defined vascular slits.

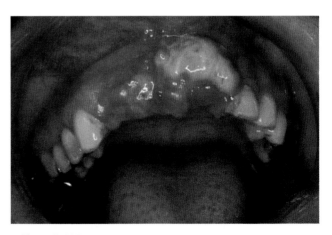

• **Fig. 12.140 Leiomyosarcoma.** Ulcerated mass of the anterior maxillary alveolar ridge. (Courtesy of Dr. Jim Weir.)

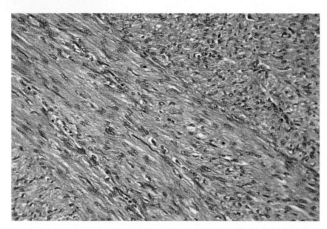

• **Fig. 12.141 Leiomyosarcoma.** Medium-high–power view of a pleomorphic spindle cell proliferation.

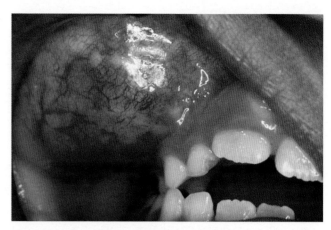

• **Fig. 12.142 Embryonal Rhabdomyosarcoma.** Young child with a mass of the right maxilla. (Courtesy of Dr. Robert Achterberg.)

myogenic markers: smooth muscle actin, muscle-specific actin (HHF 35), desmin, smooth muscle myosin (SMMS), and h-caldesmon.

Treatment and Prognosis

The treatment of leiomyosarcoma primarily consists of radical surgical excision, sometimes with adjunctive chemotherapy or radiation therapy. The prognosis for head and neck tumors depends on the degree of differentiation, with the potential for local recurrence and distant metastasis. A review of the Surveillance, Epidemiology, and End Results (SEER) database showed a 5-year disease-specific survival rate of 87.6% for patients with well-differentiated tumors, compared to 52.7% for patients with poorly differentiated tumors.

◆ RHABDOMYOSARCOMA

Rhabdomyosarcoma is a malignant neoplasm that is characterized by skeletal muscle differentiation. These tumors are much more common in young children, accounting for 50% of soft tissue sarcomas in childhood. In contrast, rhabdomyosarcoma comprises only 2%–5% of soft tissue sarcomas in adults. The most frequent site is the head and neck, which accounts for 26% of all cases. The genitourinary tract is the second most common location.

Four major subtypes of rhabdomyosarcoma are recognized:
• Embryonal
• Alveolar
• Pleomorphic
• Spindle/sclerosing

The discussion here will be limited primarily to the embryonal and alveolar subtypes, which comprise the vast majority of cases.

Clinical Features

Rhabdomyosarcoma primarily occurs during the first decade of life but also may occur in teenagers and young adults. It is rare in people older than 45 years, and approximately 60% of

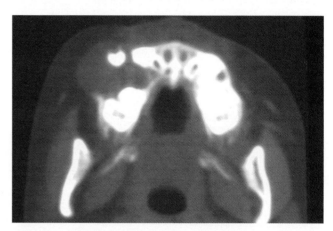

• **Fig. 12.143 Embryonal Rhabdomyosarcoma.** Computed tomography (CT) scan of patient from Fig. 12.142 showing expansile lytic lesion of the maxilla. (Courtesy of Dr. Robert Achterberg.)

all cases occur in males. Embryonal rhabdomyosarcomas are most common in the first 10 years of life and account for about 60% of all cases. Alveolar rhabdomyosarcomas occur most often in persons between 10 and 25 years of age; they account for approximately 30% of all tumors. Pleomorphic rhabdomyosarcomas represent less than 5% of all cases and show peak prevalence in patients older than 40 years of age. Spindle cell and sclerosing rhabdomyosarcomas formerly were classified as separate, distinct lesions. However, their overlapping microscopic and molecular features suggest that they are related entities. They represent 5%–10% of rhabdomyosarcomas.

Most head and neck lesions are embryonal or alveolar types; pleomorphic rhabdomyosarcomas primarily occur on the extremities. Spindle/sclerosing rhabdomyosarcomas in children are seen at a variety of sites, but adult cases show a predilection for the head and neck region.

The tumor is most often a painless, infiltrative mass that may grow rapidly (Figs. 12.142 and 12.143). In the head and neck region, the face and orbit are the most frequent locations, followed by the nasal cavity. The palate is the most frequent intraoral site, and some lesions may appear to arise in the maxillary sinus and break through into the oral cavity. Some embryonal rhabdomyosarcomas that arise within a cavity, such as the vagina or oropharynx, demonstrate an exophytic, polypoid growth pattern that resembles a cluster of grapes. The term *botryoid* (grapelike) *rhabdomyosarcoma* has been used for these lesions.

Histopathologic Features
Embryonal Type

The embryonal rhabdomyosarcoma resembles various stages in the embryogenesis of skeletal muscle. Poorly differentiated examples may be difficult to diagnose and consist of small round or oval cells with hyperchromatic nuclei and indistinct cytoplasm (Fig. 12.144). Alternating hypercellular and myxoid zones may be seen. Better-differentiated lesions show round to ovoid rhabdomyoblasts with distinctly eosinophilic cytoplasm and fibrillar material around the nucleus. Some tumors contain elongated, strap-shaped rhabdomyoblasts, but cross striations rarely are found (Fig. 12.145).

The **botryoid** subtype of embryonal rhabdomyosarcoma is sparsely cellular and has a pronounced myxoid stroma.

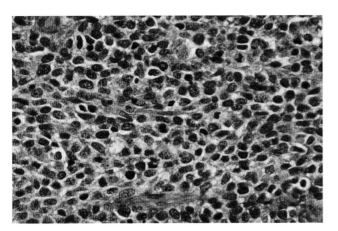

• **Fig. 12.144 Embryonal Rhabdomyosarcoma.** Medium-power view showing a sheet of small, round cells with hyperchromatic nuclei.

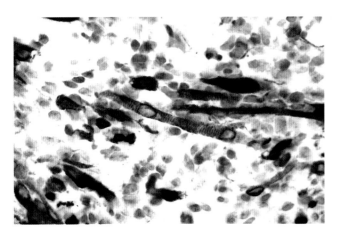

• **Fig. 12.145 Embryonal Rhabdomyosarcoma.** This tumor shows strap-shaped rhabdomyoblasts that are positive for desmin with immunohistochemical staining. Note the cross striations.

Increased cellularity, or a so-called *cambium layer,* is usually seen just beneath the mucosal surface.

Immunohistochemical analysis for the presence of desmin, myogenin, MyoD1, and muscle-specific actin can be helpful in supporting the muscular nature of the tumor. However, the intensity of the immunostaining can vary depending on the degree of rhabdomyoblastic differentiation.

Alveolar Type

Both classic and solid variants of alveolar rhabdomyosarcoma are recognized. The classic pattern is characterized by aggregates of poorly differentiated round to oval cells separated by fibrous septa. These cells demonstrate a central loss of cohesiveness, which results in an alveolar pattern. The peripheral cells of these aggregates adhere to the septal walls in a single layer. The central cells appear to float freely within the alveolar spaces. Mitoses are common, and multinucleated giant cells also may be seen. In contrast, solid alveolar rhabdomyosarcoma demonstrates cellular fields of small round basophilic cells without fibrovascular septa.

Cytogenetic and molecular studies play an important role in the diagnosis of rhabdomyosarcoma. Two distinct chromosomal translocations have been identified in alveolar rhabdomyosarcoma: *PAX3::FOXO1* and *PAX7::FOXO1.* Embryonal rhabdomyosarcoma frequently shows loss of heterozygosity at loci of chromosome 11p15.5. Congenital/infantile forms of spindle cell/sclerosing rhabdomyosarcoma are characterized by gene fusions involving *VGLL2, SRF,* and *TEAD1,* whereas "sclerosing rhabdomyosarcoma" in adults often shows *MYOD1* mutations.

Treatment and Prognosis

Before 1960 the prognosis for a patient with rhabdomyosarcoma was extremely poor, with more than 90% of patients dying. With the advent of multimodal therapy, the prognosis has improved dramatically.

Treatment typically consists of local surgical excision combined with multiagent chemotherapy (vincristine, actinomycin D, and cyclophosphamide). Postoperative radiation therapy also is used, except for localized tumors that have been completely resected at initial surgery. The 5-year overall survival rate for embryonal rhabdomyosarcoma of the head and neck is 63%, although the figure for botryoid variants (95%) is much better. The 5-year overall survival rate for alveolar rhabdomyosarcoma of the head and neck is only 35%. Congenital/infantile forms of spindle/sclerosing rhabdomyosarcoma have 5-year overall survival rate of 75%; however, this survival figure falls to 30% for those with *MYOD1* mutations.

◆ SYNOVIAL SARCOMA

Synovial sarcoma is an uncommon malignancy that represents 5%–10% of all soft tissue sarcomas. The tumor occurs primarily near large joints and bursae, especially in the extremities, but authorities now agree that this lesion probably does not arise from the synovium. Although it is often para-articular in location, the tumor rarely occurs within the joint capsule. In some instances, it arises in areas without any obvious relationship to synovial structures. Synovial sarcomas of the head and neck are rare (only 1.9%–3.7% of all cases), and many of these are unrelated to joint areas.

Over 90% of synovial sarcomas exhibit a balanced reciprocal translocation involving fusion of the *SS18* gene on chromosome 18 with either the *SSX1* or *SSX2* gene (or, rarely, *SSX4*) on the X chromosome. Detection of this translocation can be helpful in making the diagnosis and confirming the presence of metastatic disease.

Clinical Features

Synovial sarcomas most frequently occur in teenagers and young adults (mean age = 33.5 years), and there is a slight male predilection. The most common presentation is a gradually enlarging mass that often is associated with pain or tenderness. Tumors in the head and neck region are most common in the paravertebral and parapharyngeal areas. Often, they produce symptoms of dysphagia, dyspnea, or hoarseness. Rare intraoral examples have been reported in the tongue, cheek, and other sites.

Histopathologic Features

Two major patterns of synovial sarcoma are recognized: biphasic and monophasic. Biphasic synovial sarcomas usually are associated with *SS18::SSX1* gene fusions and are characterized by a combination of spindle cells and epithelial cells. The spindle cells usually predominate and produce a pattern that is similar to fibrosarcoma. Within this spindle cell background are groups of cuboidal to columnar epithelial cells that surround glandlike spaces or form nests, cords, or whorls (Fig. 12.146). Calcifications are seen in around 30% of cases.

Monophasic synovial sarcomas typically show *SS18::SSX2* gene fusions and are more common than biphasic

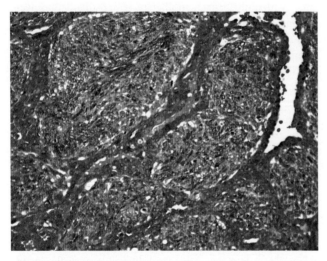

• **Fig. 12.146 Synovial Sarcoma.** Biphasic tumor consisting of spindle cells intermixed with cuboidal to columnar epithelial cells that line glandlike spaces.

forms of the tumor. Microscopically, they consist primarily or entirely of spindle cells, which can make distinction from other spindle cell malignancies difficult. However, many examples will demonstrate focal cells with epithelioid features and/or positive immunostaining for cytokeratin and epithelial membrane antigen. Nuclear immunoreactivity for TLE1 is also a useful screening marker. However, molecular genetic testing for the *SS18::SSX2* fusion gene transcript often is necessary to confirm the diagnosis. Rare examples of monophasic epithelial-predominant synovial sarcomas also have been reported.

Treatment and Prognosis

Treatment of synovial sarcoma usually consists of radical surgical excision, often with adjunctive radiation therapy or chemotherapy. The prognosis is guarded because the tumor has a high rate of recurrence and metastasis. The reported 5-year overall survival rates range from 56% to 76%. One recent series of head and neck synovial sarcomas showed 5- and 10-year disease specific survival rates of 79% and 68%, respectively.

◆ ALVEOLAR SOFT-PART SARCOMA

The **alveolar soft-part sarcoma** is a rare neoplasm of uncertain histogenesis, which accounts for 0.5%–1% of all soft tissue sarcomas. Molecular analysis of this tumor shows a characteristic genetic translocation, der(17)t(X;17)(p11.2q25), which results in an *ASPSCR1::TFE3* fusion gene.

Clinical Features

The alveolar soft-part sarcoma is usually a slow-growing, painless mass that is most common in adolescents and young adults between 15 and 35 years of age. The lower extremity is the most frequent location, especially the anterior thigh. However, examples that develop in infants and young children are most common in the head and neck region; the orbit and tongue are the most common head and neck sites. During the first two decades of life, the tumor shows nearly a 2:1 female predilection. However, cases that develop after the age of 30 are more common in men.

Histopathologic Features

Alveolar soft-part sarcomas are composed of groups of large, polygonal cells that are arranged around central alveolar spaces (Fig. 12.147, *A*). These cells have abundant granular, eosinophilic cytoplasm and one to several vesicular nuclei. Mitoses are rare. Special stains will reveal PAS-positive, diastase-resistant crystals that are highly characteristic for this tumor. Under the electron microscope, these crystals appear as rhomboid, polygonal, or rod-shaped structures with a regular latticework pattern.

Immunohistochemical analysis will demonstrate strong positivity for TFE3 transcription factor in the tumor nuclei (see Fig. 12.147, *B*). The diagnosis can be confirmed by

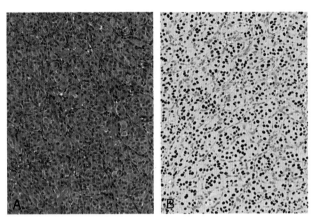

• **Fig. 12.147 Alveolar Soft-Part Sarcoma. A,** Alveolar collections of large, polygonal cells containing granular cytoplasm. **B,** Immunohisto-chemistry showing strong nuclear positivity for TFE3. (Courtesy of Dr. Mark Lingen.)

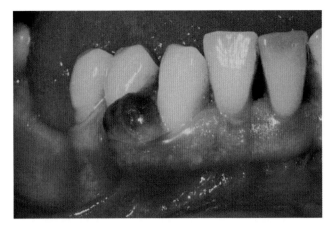

• **Fig. 12.148 Metastatic Melanoma.** Pigmented nodule of the man-dibular gingiva.

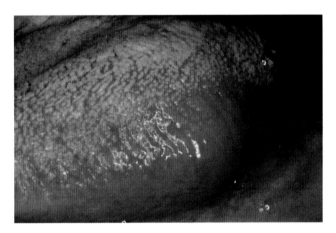

• **Fig. 12.149 Metastatic Renal Carcinoma.** Nodular mass of the left lateral border of the tongue. (Courtesy of Dr. Mark Bowden.)

identification of the *ASPSCR1::TFE3* fusion gene with reverse-transcription polymerase chain reaction (RT-PCR) or fluorescence *in situ* hybridization (FISH).

Treatment and Prognosis

Most patients with alveolar soft-part sarcomas are treated by radical surgical excision, often in conjunction with radiation therapy and chemotherapy. The prognosis is generally poor, often as a result of late metastasis. One study reported a 5-year survival rate of 60%, but the 20-year survival rate dropped to only 15%. Another series showed a 5-year disease-free survival of 71% for patients with localized dis-ease, compared with only 20% for patients who presented with metastatic disease. However, the prognosis for children appears to be better than for adults. Lingual and orbital tumors have much higher survival rates, possibly because of smaller tumor size at diagnosis and younger patient age.

◆ METASTASES TO THE ORAL SOFT TISSUES

Metastatic tumors to the oral cavity are uncommon and represent approximately 1% of all oral malignancies. Such metastases can occur to bone (see page 673) or to the oral soft tissues. The mechanism by which tumors can spread to the oral cavity is poorly understood. Primary malignancies from immediately adjacent tissues might be able to spread by a lymphatic route; however, such a mechanism cannot explain metastases from tumors from lower parts of the body, which are almost certainly blood-borne and should be filtered out by the lungs. One possible explanation for blood-borne metastases to the head and neck, especially in the absence of pulmonary metastases, is **Batson plexus,** a valveless vertebral venous plexus that might allow retrograde spread of tumor cells, bypassing filtration through the lungs.

Clinical Features

The most common site for oral soft tissue metastases is the gingiva, which accounts for 54% of all cases. The next most common site is the tongue, which accounts for 22.5% of cases. The lesion usually appears as a nodular mass that often resembles a hyperplastic or reactive growth, such as a pyo-genic granuloma (Figs. 12.148–12.150). Occasionally, the lesion appears as a surface ulceration. Adjacent teeth may become loosened by destruction of the underlying alveolar bone. The presence of teeth may play an important role in the preference of metastases for the gingiva. Once malignant cells reach the oral cavity, the rich vascular network of inflamed gingival tissues or an extraction site may serve as a fertile location for further growth.

Oral soft tissue metastases are more common in males and are seen most frequently in middle-aged and older adults. Almost any malignancy from any body site is capable of metastasis to the oral cavity, and a wide variety of tumors have been reported to spread to the mouth. (However, there is probably a bias in the literature toward reporting more unusual cases.) In the cases reported, lung cancer is respon-sible for nearly one-third of all oral soft tissue metastases in

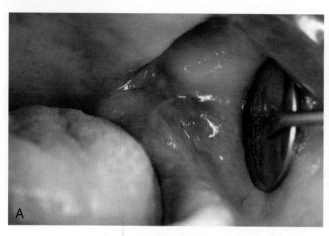
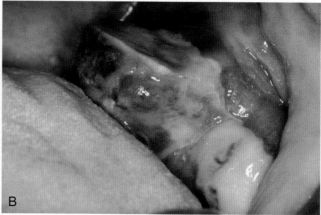

• **Fig. 12.150 Metastatic Adenocarcinoma of the Colon. A,** Focal swelling of the left retromolar pad area. **B,** Same patient 4 weeks later. Note the marked enlargement of the lesion.

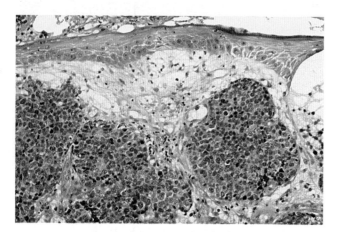

• **Fig. 12.151 Metastatic Carcinoma of the Lung.** Aggregates of malignant epithelial cells below the surface epithelium.

men, followed by renal carcinoma and melanoma. Although prostate cancer is common in men, metastases from these tumors have an affinity for bone and rarely occur in soft tissues. For women, breast cancer accounts for almost 25% of all cases, followed by malignancies of the genital organs, kidney, lung, and bone.

In most cases the primary tumor already is known when the metastatic lesion is discovered. In 25% of patients, however, the oral lesion is the first sign of the malignant disease.

Histopathologic Features

The microscopic appearance of the metastatic neoplasm should resemble the tumor of origin (Fig. 12.151). Most cases represent carcinomas; metastatic sarcomas to the oral region are rare.

Treatment and Prognosis

The prognosis for patients with metastatic tumors is generally poor because other metastatic sites also are frequently present. Management of the oral lesion is usually palliative and should be coordinated with the patient's overall treatment.

Bibliography

Fibroma and Giant Cell Fibroma

Brannon RB, Pousson RR: The retrocuspid papillae: a clinical evaluation of 51 cases, *J Dent Hyg* 77:180–184, 2003.

Gonsalves WC, Chi AC, Neville BW: Common oral lesions: part II. Masses and neoplasia, *Am Fam Physician* 75:509–512, 2007.

Houston GD: The giant cell fibroma: a review of 464 cases, *Oral Surg Oral Med Oral Pathol* 53:582–587, 1982.

Kuo RC, Wang YP, Chen HM, et al.: Clinicopathological study of oral giant cell fibromas, *J Formos Med Assoc* 108:725–729, 2009.

Magnusson BC, Rasmusson LG: The giant cell fibroma: a review of 103 cases with immunohistochemical findings, *Acta Odontol Scand* 53:293–296, 1995.

Safadi RA, Shaweesh AI, Hamasha AA, et al.: The significance of age group, gender and skin complexion in relation to the clinical distribution of developmental oral mucosal alterations in 5-13 year-old children, *J Stomatol Oral Maxillofac Surg* 119:122–128, 2018.

Savage NW, Monsour PA: Oral fibrous hyperplasias and the giant cell fibroma, *Aust Dent J* 30:405–409, 1985.

Souza LB, Andrade ES, Miguel MC, et al.: Origin of stellate giant cells in oral fibrous lesions determined by immunohistochemical expression of vimentin, HHF-35, CD68 and factor XIIIa, *Pathology* 36:316–320, 2004.

Weathers DR, Callihan MD: Giant cell fibroma, *Oral Surg Oral Med Oral Pathol* 37:374–384, 1974.

Epulis Fissuratum

Buchner A, Begleiter A, Hansen LS: The predominance of epulis fissuratum in females, *Quintessence Int* 15:699–702, 1984.

Canger EM, Celenk P, Kayipmaz S: Denture-related hyperplasia: a clinical study of a Turkish population group, *Braz Dent J* 20:243–248, 2009.

Coelho CMP, Zucoloto S, Lopes RA: Denture-induced fibrous inflammatory hyperplasia: a retrospective study in a school of dentistry, *Int J Prosthodont* 13:148–151, 2000.

Cutright DE: Osseous and chondromatous metaplasia caused by dentures, *Oral Surg Oral Med Oral Pathol* 34:625–633, 1972.

Cutright DE: The histopathologic findings in 583 cases of epulis fissuratum, *Oral Surg Oral Med Oral Pathol* 37:401–411, 1974.

Inflammatory Papillary Hyperplasia

Antonelli JR, Panno FV, Witko A: Inflammatory papillary hyperplasia: supraperiosteal excision by the blade-loop technique, *Gen Dent* 46:390–397, 1998.

Bhaskar SN, Beasley JD III, Cutright DE: Inflammatory papillary hyperplasia of the oral mucosa: report of 341 cases, *J Am Dent Assoc* 81:949–952, 1970.

Budtz-Jørgensen E: Oral mucosal lesions associated with the wearing of removable dentures, *J Oral Pathol* 10:65–80, 1981.

Cutright DE: Morphogenesis of inflammatory papillary hyperplasia, *J Prosthet Dent* 33:380–385, 1975.

Reichart PA, Schmidt-Westhausen A, Samaranayake LP, et al.: *Candida*-associated palatal papillary hyperplasia in HIV infection, *J Oral Pathol Med* 23:403–405, 1994.

Salonen MAM, Raustia AM, Oikarinen KS: Effect of treatment of palatal inflammatory papillary hyperplasia with local and systemic antifungal agents accompanied by renewal of complete dentures, *Acta Odontol Scand* 54:87–91, 1996.

Vaz Goulart MC, Lara VS: Inflammatory papillary hyperplasia of the palate: quantitative analysis of Candida albicans and its negative correlation with microscopic and demographic aspects, *Int J Prosthodont* 24:235–237, 2011.

Fibrous Histiocytoma
Gleason BC, Fletcher CDM: Deep "benign" fibrous histiocytoma: clinicopathologic analysis of 69 cases of a rare tumor indicating occasional metastatic potential, *Am J Surg Pathol* 32:354–362, 2008.

Gray PB, Miller AS, Loftus MJ: Benign fibrous histiocytoma of the oral/perioral regions: report of a case and review of 17 additional cases, *J Oral Maxillofac Surg* 50:1239–1242, 1992.

Heo M-S, Cho H-J, Kwon K-J, et al.: Benign fibrous histiocytoma in the mandible, *Oral Surg Oral Med Oral Pathol Oral Radiol Endod* 97:276–280, 2004.

Kirschnick LB, Schuch LF, Silveira FM, et al.: Benign fibrous histiocytoma of the oral and maxillofacial region: a systematic review, *Oral Surg Oral Med Oral Pathol Oral Radiol* 133:e43–e56, 2022.

Thompson SH, Shear M: Fibrous histiocytomas of the oral and maxillofacial regions, *J Oral Pathol* 13:282–294, 1984.

Solitary Fibrous Tumor
Bauer JL, Miklos AZ, Thompson LDR: Parotid gland solitary fibrous tumor: a case report and clinicopathologic review of 22 cases from the literature, *Head Neck Pathol* 6:21–31, 2012.

Cox DP, Daniels T, Jordan RCK: Solitary fibrous tumor of the head and neck, *Oral Surg Oral Med Oral Pathol Oral Radiol Endod* 110:79–84, 2010.

Goldblum JR, Folpe AL, Weiss SW: Solitary fibrous tumor (hemangiopericytoma), In Goldblum JR, Folpe AL, Weiss SW, editors: *Enzinger and Weiss's soft tissue tumors*, ed 7, Philadelphia, 2020, Elsevier, pp 1133–1147.

Nunes FB, Sant'Ana MSP, Silva AMB, et al.: Solitary fibrous tumour of the oral cavity: an update, *J Oral Pathol Med* 49:14–20, 2020.

O'Regan EM, Vanguri V, Allen CM, et al.: Solitary fibrous tumor of the oral cavity: clinicopathologic and immunohistochemical study of 21 cases, *Head Neck Pathol* 3:106–115, 2009.

Smith MH, Islam NM, Bhattacharyya I, et al.: STAT6 reliably distinguishes solitary fibrous tumors from myofibromas, *Head Neck Pathol* 12:110–117, 2018.

Smith SC, Gooding WE, Elkins M, et al.: Solitary fibrous tumors of the head and neck. A multi-institutional clinicopathologic study, *Am J Surg Pathol* 41:1642–1656, 2017.

Thompson LDR, Miettinen M, Wenig BM: Sinonasal-type hemangiopericytoma: a clinicopathologic and immunophenotypic analysis of 104 cases showing perivascular myoid differentiation, *Am J Surg Pathol* 27:737–749, 2003.

Yang XJ, Zheng JW, Ye WM, et al.: Malignant solitary fibrous tumors of the head and neck: a clinicopathological study of nine consecutive patients, *Oral Oncol* 45:678–682, 2009.

Fibromatosis
Al-Saraf A, Yassan L, Cipriani NA, et al.: Desmoid-type fibromatosis of the tongue, *Head Neck Pathol* 10:527–529, 2016.

Flucke U, Tops BBJ, van Diest PJ, et al.: Desmoid-type fibromatosis of the head and neck region in the paediatric population: a clinicopathological and genetic study of seven cases, *Histopathology* 64:769–776, 2014.

Fowler CB, Hartman KS, Brannon RB: Fibromatosis of the oral and paraoral region, *Oral Surg Oral Med Oral Pathol* 77:373–386, 1994.

Gnepp DR, Henley J, Weiss S, et al.: Desmoid fibromatosis of the sinonasal tract and nasopharynx: a clinicopathologic study of 25 cases, *Cancer* 78:2572–2579, 1996.

Kruse AL, Luebbers HT, Grätz KW, et al.: Aggressive fibromatosis of the head and neck: a new classification based on a literature review over 40 years (1968-2008), *Oral Maxillofac Surg* 14:227–232, 2010.

Wang W, Koirala U, Ma S, et al.: Age-based treatment of aggressive fibromatosis in the head and neck region, *J Oral Maxillofac Surg* 72:311–321, 2014.

Wilks DJ, Mowatt DJ, Merchant W, et al.: Facial paediatric desmoid fibromatosis: a case series, literature review and management algorithm, *J Plast Reconstr Aesthet Surg* 65:564–571, 2012.

Myofibroma (Myofibromatosis)
Abramowicz S, Simon LE, Kozakewich HP, et al.: Myofibromas of the jaws in children, *J Oral Maxillofac Surg* 70:1880–1884, 2012.

Foss RD, Ellis GL: Myofibromas and myofibromatosis of the oral region: a clinicopathologic analysis of 79 cases, *Oral Surg Oral Med Oral Pathol Oral Radiol Endod* 89:57–65, 2000.

Jones AC, Freedman PD, Kerpel SM: Oral myofibromas: a report of 13 cases and review of the literature, *J Oral Maxillofac Surg* 52:870–875, 1994.

Lingen MW, Mostofi RS, Solt DB: Myofibromas of the oral cavity, *Oral Surg Oral Med Oral Pathol Oral Radiol Endod* 80:297–302, 1995.

Sedghizadeh PP, Allen CM, Kalmar JR, et al.: Solitary central myofibroma presenting in the gnathic region, *Ann Diagn Pathol* 8:284–289, 2004.

Smith MH, Reith JD, Cohen DM, et al.: An update on myofibromas and myofibromatosis affecting the oral regions with report of 24 new cases, *Oral Surg Oral Med Oral Pathol Oral Radiol* 124:62–75, 2017.

Vered M, Allon I, Buchner A, et al.: Clinico-pathologic correlations of myofibroblastic tumor of the oral cavity. II. Myofibroma and myofibromatosis of the oral soft tissues, *J Oral Pathol Med* 36:304–314, 2007.

Oral Focal Mucinosis
Aldred MJ, Talacko AA, Ruljancich K, et al.: Oral focal mucinosis: report of 15 cases and review of the literature, *Pathology* 35:393–396, 2003.

Buchner A, Merrell PW, Leider AS, et al.: Oral focal mucinosis, *Int J Oral Maxillofac Surg* 19:337–340, 1990.

Soda G, Baiocchini A, Bosco D, et al.: Oral focal mucinosis of the tongue, *Pathol Oncol Res* 4:304–307, 1998.

Silva Cunha JL, Leite AA, de Castro AT, et al.: Oral focal mucinosis: a multi-institutional study and literature review, *J Cutan Pathol* 48:24–33, 2021.

Tomich CE: Oral focal mucinosis: a clinicopathologic and histochemical study of eight cases, *Oral Surg Oral Med Oral Pathol* 38:714–724, 1974.

Pyogenic Granuloma
Cardoso JA, Spanemberg JC, Cherubini K, et al.: Oral granuloma gravidarum: a retrospective study of 41 cases in southern Brazil, *J Appl Oral Sci* 21:215–218, 2013.

Epivatianos A, Antoniades D, Zaraboukas T, et al.: Pyogenic granuloma of the oral cavity: comparative study of its clinicopathological and immunohistochemical features, *Pathol Int* 55:391–397, 2005.

Gordón-Núñez MA, de Vasconcelos CM, Benevenuto TG, et al.: Oral pyogenic granuloma: a retrospective analysis of 293 cases in a Brazilian population, *J Oral Maxillofac Surg* 68:2185–2188, 2010.

Kerr DA: Granuloma pyogenicum, *Oral Surg Oral Med Oral Pathol* 4:158–176, 1951.

Mills SE, Cooper PH, Fechner RE: Lobular capillary hemangioma: the underlying lesion of pyogenic granuloma: a study of 73 cases from the oral and nasal mucous membranes, *Am J Surg Pathol* 4:471–479, 1980.

Ribeiro JL, Moraes RM, Carvalho BFC, et al.: Oral pyogenic granuloma: an 18-year retrospective clinicopathological and immunohistochemical study, *J Cutan Pathol* 48:863–869, 2021.

Toida M, Hasegawa T, Watanabe F, et al.: Lobular capillary hemangioma of the oral mucosa: clinicopathological study of 43 cases with a special reference to immunohistochemical characterization of the vascular elements, *Pathol Int* 53:1–7, 2003.

Zain RB, Khoo SP, Yeo JF: Oral pyogenic granuloma (excluding pregnancy tumor)—a clinical analysis of 304 cases, *Singap Dent J* 20:8–10, 1995.

Peripheral Giant Cell Granuloma

Chrcanovic BR, Gomes CC, Gomez RS: Peripheral giant cell granuloma: an updated analysis of 2824 cases reported in the literature, *J Oral Pathol Med* 47:454–459, 2018.

Giansanti JS, Waldron CA: Peripheral giant cell granuloma: review of 720 cases, *J Oral Surg* 17:787–791, 1969.

Katsikeris N, Kakarantza-Angelopoulou E, Angelopoulos AP: Peripheral giant cell granuloma: clinicopathologic study of 224 new cases and review of 956 reported cases, *Int J Oral Maxillofac Surg* 17:94–99, 1988.

Lester SR, Cordell KG, Rosebush MS, et al.: Peripheral giant cell granulomas: a series of 279 cases, *Oral Surg Oral Med Oral Pathol Oral Radiol* 118:475–482, 2014.

Limongelli L, Tempesta A, Lauritano D, et al.: Peripheral giant cell granuloma of the jaws as first sign of primary hyperparathyroidism: a case series, *J Clin Med* 9:4042, 2020.

Morais TM, Soares CD, Aguirre-Urizar JM, et al.: Peri-implant peripheral giant cell lesions: report of 13 new cases and comparative histological and immunohistochemical analysis with peripheral and central giant cell lesions, *Med Oral Patol Oral Cir Bucal* 24:e739–e745, 2019.

Smith BR, Fowler CB, Svane TJ: Primary hyperparathyroidism presenting as a "peripheral" giant cell granuloma, *J Oral Maxillofac Surg* 46:65–69, 1988.

Peripheral Ossifying Fibroma

Buchner A, Hansen LS: The histomorphologic spectrum of peripheral ossifying fibroma, *Oral Surg Oral Med Oral Pathol* 63:452–461, 1987.

Childers ELB, Morton I, Fryer CE, et al.: Giant peripheral ossifying fibroma: a case report and clinicopathologic review of 10 cases from the literature, *Head Neck Pathol* 7:356–360, 2013.

Cuisia ZE, Brannon RB: Peripheral ossifying fibroma—a clinical evaluation of 134 pediatric cases, *Pediatr Dent* 23:245–248, 2001.

Kenney JN, Kaugars GE, Abbey LM: Comparison between the peripheral ossifying fibroma and peripheral odontogenic fibroma, *J Oral Maxillofac Surg* 47:378–382, 1989.

Lázare H, Peteiro A, Pérez Sayáns M, et al.: Clinicopathological features of peripheral ossifying fibroma in a series of 41 patients, *Br J Oral Maxillofac Surg* 57:1081–1085, 2019.

Walters JD, Will JK, Hatfield RD, et al.: Excision and repair of the peripheral ossifying fibroma: a report of 3 cases, *J Periodontol* 72:939–944, 2001.

Zain RB, Fei YJ: Fibrous lesions of the gingiva: a histopathologic analysis of 204 cases, *Oral Surg Oral Med Oral Pathol* 70:466–470, 1990.

Lipoma

Cunha JLS, de Sousa SF, Mota CP, et al.: Sialolipomas of minor salivary glands: a multi-institutional study and literature review, *J Oral Pathol Med* 50:210–219, 2021.

Darling MR, Daley TD: Intraoral chondroid lipoma: a case report and immunohistochemical investigation, *Oral Surg Oral Med Oral Pathol Oral Radiol Endod* 99:331–333, 2005.

Furlong MA, Fanburg-Smith JC, Childers ELB: Lipoma of the oral and maxillofacial region: site and subclassification of 125 cases, *Oral Surg Oral Med Oral Pathol Oral Radiol Endod* 98:441–450, 2004.

Garavaglia J, Gnepp DR: Intramuscular (infiltrating) lipoma of the tongue, *Oral Surg Oral Med Oral Pathol* 63:348–350, 1987.

Horie N, Shimoyama T, Kaneko T, et al.: Traumatic herniation of the buccal fat pad, *Pediatr Dent* 23:249–252, 2001.

Lau SK, Bishop JA, Thompson LDR: Spindle cell lipoma of the tongue: a clinicopathologic study of 8 cases and review of the literature, *Head Neck Pathol* 9:253–259, 2015.

Perez-Sayáns M, Blanco-Carrión A, Oliveira-Alves MG, et al.: Multicentre retrospective study of 97 cases of intraoral lipoma, *J Oral Pathol Med* 48:499–504, 2019.

Pires FR, Souza L, Arruda R, et al.: Intraoral soft tissue lipomas: clinicopathological features from 91 cases diagnosed in a single oral pathology service, *Med Oral Patol Oral Cir Bucal* 26:e90–e96, 2021.

Starkman SJ, Olsen SM, Lewis JE, et al.: Lipomatous lesions of the parotid gland: analysis of 70 cases, *Laryngoscope* 123:651–656, 2013.

Stojanov IJ, Mariño-Enriquez A, Bahri N, et al.: Lipomas of the oral cavity: utility of MDM2 and CDK4 in avoiding overdiagnosis as atypical lipomatous tumor, *Head Neck Pathol* 13:169–176, 2019.

Studart-Soares EC, Costa FWG, Sousa FB, et al.: Oral lipomas in a Brazilian population: a 10-year study and analysis of 450 cases reported in the literature, *Med Oral Patol Oral Cir Bucal* 15:e691–e696, 2010.

Traumatic Neuroma

Lee EJ, Calcaterra TC, Zuckerbraun L: Traumatic neuromas of the head and neck, *Ear Nose Throat J* 77:670–676, 1998.

Peszkowski MJ, Larsson Å: Extraosseous and intraosseous oral traumatic neuromas and their association with tooth extraction, *J Oral Maxillofac Surg* 48:963–967, 1990.

Sist TC Jr, Greene GW: Traumatic neuroma of the oral cavity: report of thirty-one new cases and review of the literature, *Oral Surg Oral Med Oral Pathol* 51:394–402, 1981.

Tamiolakis P, Chrysomali E, Sklavounou-Andrikopoulou A, et al.: Oral neural tumors: clinicopathologic analysis of 157 cases and review of the literature, *J Clin Exp Dent* 11:e721–e731, 2019.

Vora AR, Loescher AR, Craig GT, et al.: A light microscopical study on the structure of traumatic neuromas of the human lingual nerve, *Oral Surg Oral Med Oral Pathol Oral Radiol Endod* 99:395–403, 2005.

Palisaded Encapsulated Neuroma

Chauvin PJ, Wysocki GP, Daley TD, et al.: Palisaded encapsulated neuroma of oral mucosa, *Oral Surg Oral Med Oral Pathol* 73:71–74, 1992.

Koutlas IG, Scheithauer BW: Palisaded encapsulated ("solitary circumscribed") neuroma of the oral cavity: a review of 55 cases, *Head Neck Pathol* 4:15–26, 2010.

Leblebici C, Savli TC, Yeni B, et al.: Palisaded encapsulated (solitary circumscribed) neuroma: a review of 30 cases, *Int J Surg Pathol* 27:506–514, 2019.

Magnusson B: Palisaded encapsulated neuroma (solitary circumscribed neuroma) of the oral mucosa, *Oral Surg Oral Med Oral Pathol Oral Radiol Endod* 82:302–304, 1996.

Schwannoma and Neurofibroma

Alotaiby FM, Fitzpatrick S, Upadhyaya J, et al.: Demographic, clinical and histopathological features of oral neural neoplasms: a retrospective study, *Head Neck Pathol* 13:208–214, 2019.

Butler RT, Patel RM, McHugh JB: Head and neck schwannomas: 20-year experience of a single institution excluding cutaneous and acoustic sites, *Head Neck Pathol* 10:286–291, 2016.

Campos MS, Fontes A, Marocchio LS, et al.: Clinicopathologic and immunohistochemical features of oral neurofibroma, *Acta Odontol Scand* 70:577–582, 2012.

Chi AC, Carey J, Muller S: Intraosseous schwannoma of the mandible: a case report and review of the literature, *Oral Surg Oral Med Oral Pathol Oral Radiol Endod* 96:54–65, 2003.

Chi AC, Neville BW, Cheng L: Plexiform schwannoma of the oral cavity: report of eight cases and a review of the literature, *Head Neck Pathol* 15:288–297, 2021.

Ellis GL, Abrams AM, Melrose RJ: Intraosseous benign neural sheath neoplasms of the jaws: report of seven new cases and review of the literature, *Oral Surg Oral Med Oral Pathol* 44:731–743, 1977.

Ferner RE: Neurofibromatosis 1 and neurofibromatosis 2: a twenty-first century perspective, *Lancet Neurol* 6:340–351, 2007.

Hoa M, Slattery WH 3rd: Neurofibromatosis 2, *Otolaryngol Clin N Am* 45:315–332, 2012.

Liu HL, Yu SY, Li GKH, et al.: Extracranial head and neck schwannomas: a study of the nerve of origin, *Eur Arch Otorhinolaryngol* 268:1343–1347, 2011.

Marocchio LS, Oliveira DT, Pereira MC, et al.: Sporadic and multiple neurofibromas in the head and neck region: a retrospective study of 33 years, *Clin Oral Investig* 11:165–169, 2007.

Merker VL, Esparza S, Smith MJ, et al.: Clinical features of schwannomatosis: a retrospective analysis of 87 patients, *Oncologist* 17:1317–1322, 2012.

Tamiolakis P, Chrysomali E, Sklavounou-Andrikopoulou A, et al.: Oral neural tumors: clinicopathologic analysis of 157 cases and review of the literature, *J Clin Exp Dent* 11:e721–e731, 2019.

Tamura R: Current understanding of neurofibromatosis type 1, 2, and schwannomatosis, *Int J Mol Sci* 22:5850, 2021. https://doi.org/10.3390/ijms22115850.

Thompson LDR, Koh SS, Lau SK: Tongue schwannoma: a clinicopathologic study of 19 cases, *Head Neck Pathol* 14:571–576, 2020.

Neurofibromatosis Type I

D'Ambrosio JA, Langlais RP, Young RS: Jaw and skull changes in neurofibromatosis, *Oral Surg Oral Med Oral Pathol* 66:391–396, 1988.

Edwards PC, Fantasia JE, Saini T, et al.: Clinically aggressive central giant cell granulomas in two patients with neurofibromatosis 1, *Oral Surg Oral Med Oral Pathol Oral Radiol Endod* 102:765–772, 2006.

Heervä E, Peltonen S, Pirttiniemi P, et al.: Short mandible, maxilla and cranial base are common in patients with neurofibromatosis 1, *Eur J Oral Sci* 119:121–127, 2011.

Hivelin M, Wolkenstein P, Lepage C, et al.: Facial aesthetic unit remodeling procedure for neurofibromatosis type 1 hemifacial hypertrophy: report on 33 consecutive adult patients, *Plast Reconstr Surg* 125:1197–1207, 2010.

Ingham S, Huson SM, Moran A, et al.: Malignant peripheral nerve sheath tumours in NF1: improved survival in women and in recent years, *Eur J Cancer* 47:2723–2728, 2011.

Jouhilahti EM, Visnapuu V, Soukka T, et al.: Oral soft tissue alterations in patients with neurofibromatosis, *Clin Oral Investig* 16:551–558, 2012.

Lee L, Yan Y-H, Pharoah MJ: Radiographic features of the mandible in neurofibromatosis: a report of 10 cases and review of the literature, *Oral Surg Oral Med Oral Pathol Oral Radiol Endod* 81:361–367, 1996.

Legius E, Messiaen L, Wolkenstein P, et al.: Revised diagnostic criteria for neurofibromatosis type I and Legius syndrome: an international consensus recommendation, *Genet Med* 23:1506–1513, 2021.

Ly KI, Blakeley JO: The diagnosis and management of neurofibromatosis type 1, *Med Clin N Am* 103:1035–1054, 2019.

Neville BW, Hann J, Narang R, et al.: Oral neurofibrosarcoma associated with neurofibromatosis type I, *Oral Surg Oral Med Oral Pathol* 72:456–461, 1991.

Shapiro SD, Abramovitch K, Van Dis ML, et al.: Neurofibromatosis: oral and radiographic manifestations, *Oral Surg Oral Med Oral Pathol* 58:493–498, 1984.

Visnapuu V, Peltonen S, Ellilä T, et al.: Periapical cemental dysplasia is common in women with NF1, *Eur J Med Genet* 50:274–280, 2007.

Visnapuu V, Peltonen S, Tammisalo T, et al.: Radiographic findings in the jaws of patients with neurofibromatosis 1, *J Oral Maxillofac Surg* 70:1351–1357, 2012.

Wilson BN, John AM, Handler MZ, et al.: Neurofibromatosis type 1: new developments in genetics and treatment, *J Am Acad Dermatol* 84:1667–1676, 2021.

Multiple Endocrine Neoplasia Type 2B

Carney JA: Familial multiple endocrine neoplasia: the first 100 years, *Am J Surg Pathol* 29:254–274, 2005.

Castinetti F, Moley J, Mulligan L, et al.: A comprehensive review on MEN2B, *Endocr Relat Cancer* 25:T29–T39, 2018.

Coyle D, Friedmacher F, Puri P: The association between Hirschsprung's disease and multiple endocrine neoplasia type 2a: a systematic review, *Pediatr Surg Int* 30:751–756, 2014.

Jasim S, Ying AK, Waguespack SG, et al.: Multiple endocrine neoplasia type 2B with a RET proto-oncogene A883F mutation displays a more indolent form of medullary thyroid carcinoma compared with a RET M918T mutation, *Thyroid* 21:189–192, 2011.

Mathiesen JS, Effraimidis G, Rossing M, et al.: Multiple endocrine neoplasia type 2: a review, *Semin Cancer Biol* 79:163–179, 2022.

Moline J, Eng C: Multiple endocrine neoplasia type 2: an overview, *Genet Med* 13:755–764, 2011.

Melanotic Neuroectodermal Tumor of Infancy

Barrett AW, Morgan M, Ramsay AD, et al.: A clinicopathologic and immunohistochemical analysis of melanotic neuroectodermal tumor of infancy, *Oral Surg Oral Med Oral Pathol Oral Radiol Endod* 93:688–698, 2002.

Chaudhary A, Wakhlu A, Mittal N, et al.: Melanotic neuroectodermal tumor of infancy: 2 decades of clinical experience with 18 patients, *J Oral Maxillofac Surg* 67:47–51, 2009.

Kruse-Lösler B, Gaertner C, Bürger H, et al.: Melanotic neuroectodermal tumor of infancy: systematic review of the literature and presentation of a case, *Oral Surg Oral Med Oral Pathol Oral Radiol Endod* 102:204–216, 2006.

Rachidi S, Sood AJ, Patel KG, et al.: Melanotic neuroectodermal tumor of infancy: a systematic review, *J Oral Maxillofac Surg* 73:1946–1956, 2015.

Paraganglioma

Boedeker CC, Hensen EF, Neumann HPH, et al.: Genetics of hereditary head and neck paragangliomas, *Head Neck* 36:907–916, 2014.

Capatina C, Ntali G, Karavitaki N, et al.: The management of head-and-neck paragangliomas, *Endocr Relat Cancer* 20:R291–R305, 2013.

Gandía-González ML, Kusak ME, Moreno NM, et al.: Jugulotympanic paragangliomas treated with Gamma Knife radiosurgery: a single-center review of 58 cases, *J Neurosurg* 121:1158–1165, 2014.

Offergeld C, Brase C, Yaremchuk S, et al.: Head and neck paragangliomas: clinical and molecular genetic classification, *Clinics* 67:19–28, 2012.

Valero C, Ganly I: Paragangliomas of the head and neck, *J Oral Pathol Med* 18, 2022. https://doi.org/10.1111/jop.13286.

Williams MD: Paragangliomas of the head and neck: an overview from diagnosis to genetics, *Head Neck Pathol* 11:278–287, 2017.

Granular Cell Tumor

Brannon RB, Anand PM: Oral granular cell tumors: an analysis of 10 new pediatric and adolescent cases and a review of the literature, *J Clin Pediatr Dent* 29:69–74, 2004.

Collins BM, Jones AC: Multiple granular cell tumors of the oral cavity: report of a case and review of the literature, *J Oral Maxillofac Surg* 53:707–711, 1995.

Ibáñez L, de Mendoza I, López Ortega K, et al.: Oral granular cell tumour: a multicentric study of 56 cases and a systematic review, *Oral Dis* 26:573–589, 2020.

Rawal YB, Dodson TB: S-100 negative granular cell tumor (so-called primitive polypoid non-neural granular cell tumor) of the oral cavity, *Head Neck Pathol* 11:404–412, 2017.

Rejas RA, Campos MS, Cortes AR, et al.: The neural histogenetic origin of the oral granular cell tumor: an immunohistochemical evidence, *Med Oral Patol Oral Cir Bucal* 16:e6–e10, 2011.

Vered M, Carpenter WM, Buchner A: Granular cell tumor of the oral cavity: updated immunohistochemical profile, *J Oral Pathol Med* 38:150–159, 2009.

Congenital Epulis

Bhatia SK, Goyal A, Ritwik P, et al.: Spontaneous regression of a congenital epulis in a newborn, *J Clin Pediatr Dent* 37:297–299, 2013.

Childers ELB, Fanburg-Smith JC: Congenital epulis of the newborn: 10 new cases of a rare oral tumor, *Ann Diagn Pathol* 15:157–161, 2011.

Damm DD, Cibull ML, Geissler RH, et al.: Investigation into the histogenesis of congenital epulis of the newborn, *Oral Surg Oral Med Oral Pathol* 76:205–212, 1993.

Kumar P, Kim HHS, Zahtz GD, et al.: Obstructive congenital epulis: prenatal diagnosis and perinatal management, *Laryngoscope* 112:1935–1939, 2002.

Lack EE, Worsham GF, Callihan MD, et al.: Gingival granular cell tumors of the newborn (congenital "epulis"): a clinical and pathologic study of 21 patients, *Am J Surg Pathol* 5:37–46, 1981.

Vered M, Dobriyan A, Buchner A: Congenital granular cell epulis presents an immunohistochemical profile that distinguishes it from the granular cell tumor of the adult, *Virchows Arch* 454:303–310, 2009.

Ye Y, Tang R, Liu B, et al.: Prenatal diagnosis and multidisciplinary management: a case report of congenital granular cell epulis and literature review, *J Int Med Res* 49:1–9, 2021.

Hemangioma and Vascular Malformations

Adams DM, Lucky AW: Cervicofacial vascular anomalies. I. Hemangiomas and other benign vascular tumors, *Semin Pediatr Surg* 15:124–132, 2006.

Du Z, Liu J-L, You Y-H, et al.: Genetic landscape of common venous malformations in the head and neck, *J Vasc Surg Venous Lymphat Disord* 9:1007–1016, 2021.

Fernandes D-T, Elias RA, Santos-Silva A-R, et al.: Benign oral vascular lesions treated by sclerotherapy with ethanolamine oleate: a retrospective study of 43 patients, *Med Oral Patol Oral Cir Bucal* 23:e180–e187, 2018.

Greene AK: Management of hemangiomas and other vascular tumors, *Clin Plast Surg* 38:45–63, 2011.

Greene AK, Goss JA: Vascular anomalies: from a clinicopathologic to a genetic framework, *Plast Reconstr Surg* 141:709e–717e, 2018.

Hogeling M: Propanolol for infantile hemangiomas: a review, *Curr Derm Rep* 1:179–185, 2012.

Huoh KC, Rosbe KW: Infantile hemangiomas of the head and neck, *Pediatr Clin N Am* 60:937–949, 2013.

Krowchuk DP, Frieden IJ, Mancini AJ, et al.: Clinical practice guideline for the management of infantile hemangiomas, *Pediatrics* 143:e20183475, 2019.

Kwon EKM, Seefeldt M, Drolet BA: Infantile hemangiomas: an update, *Am J Clin Dermatol* 14:111–123, 2013.

Lee A: Patel: Systematic review of pediatric mandibular arteriovenous malformations, *Int J Pediatr Otorhinolaryngol* 150:110942, 2021. https://doi.org/10.1016/j.ijporl.2021.110942.

Olsen GM, Nackers A, Drolet BA: Infantile and congenital hemangiomas, *Semin Pediatr Surg* 29(5):150969, 2020. https://doi.org/10.1016/j.sempedsurg.2020.150969.

Rudnick EF, Chen EY, Manning SC, et al.: PHACES syndrome: otolaryngic considerations in recognition and management, *Int J Pediatr Otorhinolaryngol* 73:281–288, 2009.

Taleb R, Koutlas IG, Argyris PP: Immunohistochemical and histochemical characterization of intraosseous arteriovenous malformations of the jaws: analysis of 16 cases with emphasis on GLUT-1 immunophenotype, *Oral Surg Oral Med Oral Pathol Oral Radiol* 124:165–174, 2017.

Zlotogorski A, Buchner A, Kaffe I, et al.: Radiological features of central haemangioma of the jaws, *Dentomaxillofac Radiol* 34:292–296, 2005.

Sturge-Weber Syndrome

Dowling MB, Zhao Y, Darrow DH: Orodental manifestations of facial port-wine stains, *J Am Acad Dermatol* 67:687–693, 2012.

Lo W, Marchuk DA, Ball KL, et al.: Updates and future horizons on the understanding, diagnosis, and treatment of Sturge-Weber syndrome brain involvement, *Dev Med Child Neurol* 54:214–223, 2012.

Nguyen V, Hochman M, Mihm MC Jr, et al.: The pathogenesis of port wine stain and Sturge Weber syndrome: complex interactions between genetic alterations and aberrant MAPK and PI3K activation, *Int J Mol Sci* 20:2243, 2019. https://doi.org/10.3390/ijms20092243.

Sabeti S, Ball KL, Burkhart C, et al.: Consensus statement for the management and treatment of port-wine birthmarks in Sturge-Weber syndrome, *JAMA Dermatol* 157:98–104, 2021.

Shirley MD, Tang H, Gallione CJ, et al.: Sturge-Weber syndrome and port-wine stains caused by somatic mutation in *GNAQ*, *N Engl J Med* 368:1971–1979, 2013.

Sudarsanam A, Ardern-Holmes SL: Sturge-Weber syndrome: from the past to the present, *Eur J Paediatr Neurol* 18:257–266, 2014.

Nasopharyngeal Angiofibroma

Bales C, Kotapka M, Loevner LA, et al.: Craniofacial resection of advanced juvenile nasopharyngeal angiofibroma, *Arch Otolaryngol Head Neck Surg* 128:1071–1078, 2002.

Boghani Z, Husain Q, Kanumuri VV, et al.: Juvenile nasopharyngeal angiofibroma: a systematic review and comparison of endoscopic, endoscopic-assisted, and open resection in 1047 cases, *Laryngoscope* 123:859–869, 2013.

Lee JT, Chen P, Safa A, et al.: The role of radiation in the treatment of advanced juvenile angiofibroma, *Laryngoscope* 112:1213–1220, 2002.

Leong SC: A systematic review of surgical outcomes for advanced juvenile nasopharyngeal angiofibroma with intracranial involvement, *Laryngoscope* 123:1125–1131, 2013.

Lloyd G, Howard D, Phelps P, et al.: Juvenile angiofibroma: the lessons of 20 years of modern imaging, *J Laryngol Otol* 113:127–134, 1999.

López F, Triantafyllou A, Snyderman CH, et al.: Nasal juvenile angiofibroma: current perspectives with emphasis on management, *Head Neck* 39:1033–1045, 2017.

Marshall AH, Bradley PJ: Management dilemmas in the treatment and follow-up of advanced juvenile nasopharyngeal angiofibroma, *ORL J Otorhinolaryngol Relat Spec* 68:273–278, 2006.

Lymphatic Malformations

Cahill AM, Nijs E, Ballah D, et al.: Percutaneous sclerotherapy in neonatal and infant head and neck lymphatic malformations: a single center experience, *J Pediatr Surg* 46:2083–2095, 2011.

Cheng J: Doxycycline sclerotherapy in children with head and neck lymphatic malformations, *J Pediatr Surg* 50:2143–2146, 2015.

Jian X-C: Surgical management of lymphangiomatous or lymphangiohemangiomatous macroglossia, *J Oral Maxillofac Surg* 63:15–19, 2005.

Levin LS, Jorgenson RJ, Jarvey BA: Lymphangiomas of the alveolar ridges in neonates, *Pediatrics* 58:881–884, 1976.

Okazaki T, Iwatani S, Yanai T, et al.: Treatment of lymphangioma in children: our experience of 128 cases, *J Pediatr Surg* 42:386–389, 2007.

Okazaki T, Iwatani S, Yanai T, et al.: Treatment of lymphangioma in children: our experience of 128 cases, *J Pediatr Surg* 42:386–389, 2007.

Tiwari P, Pandey V, Bera RN, et al.: Bleomycin sclerotherapy in lymphangiomas of the head and neck region: a prospective study, *Int J Oral Maxillofac Surg* 50:619–626, 2021.

Waner M: O TM: Multidisciplinary approach to the management of lymphatic malformations of the head and neck, *Otolaryngol Clin N Am* 51:159–172, 2018.

Wiegand S, Elvazi B, Zimmermann AP, et al.: Sclerotherapy of lymphangiomas of the head and neck, *Head Neck* 33:1649–1655, 2011.

Leiomyoma

de Araújo GR, Costa SFDS, Mesquita RA, et al.: Leiomyoma and leiomyosarcoma (primary and metastatic) of the oral and maxillofacial region: a clinicopathological and immunohistochemical study of 27 cases, *Head Neck Pathol* 16:294–303, 2022.

Damm DD, Neville BW: Oral leiomyomas, *Oral Surg Oral Med Oral Pathol* 47:343–348, 1979.

Frietas da Silva DM, Fernandes IA, Wu A, et al.: Oral leiomyomatous hamartoma of the anterior maxillary gingiva, *Clin Adv Periodontics* 6:190–194, 2016.

Gueiros LA, Romañach MJ, Pires-Soubhia AM, et al.: Angioleiomyoma affecting the lips: report of 3 cases and review of the literature, *Med Oral Patol Oral Cir Bucal* 16:e482–e487, 2011.

Koutlas IG, Manivel JC: Epithelioid leiomyoma of the oral mucosa, *Oral Surg Oral Med Oral Pathol Oral Radiol Endod* 82:670–673, 1996.

Liang H, Frederiksen NL, Binnie WH, et al.: Intraosseous leiomyoma: systematic review and report of one case, *Dentomaxillofac Radiol* 32:285–290, 2003.

Montague LJ, Fitzpatrick SG, Islam NM, et al.: Extensively ossifying oral leiomyoma: a rare histologic finding, *Head Neck Pathol* 8:311–316, 2014.

Rhabdomyoma

Cai Z, Thomas J, Alava I 3rd, et al.: Fetal type rhabdomyoma of the soft palate in an adult patient: report of one case and review of the literature, *Head Neck Pathol* 13:182–187, 2019.

Cleveland DB, Chen SY, Allen CM, et al.: Adult rhabdomyoma: a light microscopic, ultrastructural, virologic, and immunologic analysis, *Oral Surg Oral Med Oral Pathol* 77:147–153, 1994.

Kapadia SB, Meis JM, Frisman DM, et al.: Adult rhabdomyoma of the head and neck: a clinicopathologic and immunophenotypic study, *Hum Pathol* 24:608–617, 1993.

Kapadia SB, Meis JM, Frisman DM, et al.: Fetal rhabdomyoma of the head and neck: a clinicopathologic and immunophenotypic study of 24 cases, *Hum Pathol* 24:754–765, 1993.

Khalaf MG, Haddad R, Akiki M, et al.: Multifocal adult rhabdomyoma of the head and neck: case report and systematic review of the literature, *Int J Oral Maxillofac Surg* 50:327–334, 2021.

Ectomesenchymal Chondromyxoid Tumor

Allen CM: The ectomesenchymal chondromyxoid tumor: a review, *Oral Dis* 14:390–395, 2008.

Argyris PP, Bilodeau EA, Yancoskie AE, et al.: A subset of ectomesenchymal chondromyxoid tumours of the tongue show *EWSR1* rearrangements and are genetically linked to soft tissue myoepithelial neoplasms: a study of 11 cases, *Histopathology* 69:607–613, 2016.

Bubola J, Hagen K, Blanas N, et al.: Expanding awareness of the distribution and biologic potential of ectomesenchymal chondromyxoid tumor, *Head Neck Pathol* 15:319–322, 2021.

Dickson BC, Antonescu CR, Argyris PP, et al.: Ectomesenchymal chondromyxoid tumor: a neoplasm characterized by recurrent *RREB1-MKL2* fusions, *Am J Surg Pathol* 42:1297–1305, 2018.

Smith BC, Ellis GL, Meis-Kindblom JM, et al.: Ectomesenchymal chondromyxoid tumor of the anterior tongue: nineteen cases of a new clinicopathologic entity, *Am J Surg Pathol* 19:519–530, 1995.

Osseous and Cartilaginous Choristomas

Abdelsayed RA, Wetherington RW, Bent JP III, et al.: Glial choristoma of the tongue: a case report and review of the literature, *Oral Surg Oral Med Oral Pathol Oral Radiol Endod* 87:215–222, 1999.

Chou L, Hansen LS, Daniels TE: Choristomas of the oral cavity: a review, *Oral Surg Oral Med Oral Pathol* 72:584–593, 1991.

Norris O, Mehra P: Chondroma (cartilaginous choristoma) of the tongue: report of a case, *J Oral Maxillofac Surg* 70:643–646, 2012.

Supiyaphun P, Sampatanakul P, Kerekhanjanarong V, et al.: Lingual osseous choristoma: a study of eight cases and review of the literature, *Ear Nose Throat J* 77:316–318, 320, 325, 1998.

Soft Tissue Sarcomas

Goldblum JR, Folpe AL, Weiss SW: *Enzinger and Weiss's soft tissue tumors*, ed 7, Philadelphia, 2020, Elsevier.

Huh WW, Fitzgerald N, Mahajan A, et al.: Pediatric sarcomas and related tumors of the head and neck, *Cancer Treat Rev* 37:431–439, 2011.

Mendenhall WM, Mendenhall CM, Werning JW, et al.: Adult head and neck soft tissue sarcomas, *Head Neck* 27:916–922, 2005.

Moreira DGL, da Silva LP, de Morais EF, et al.: The occurrence and pattern of head and neck sarcomas: a comprehensive cancer center experience, *Eur Arch Otorhinolaryngol* 277:1473–1480, 2020.

Shellenberger TD, Sturgis EM: Sarcomas of the head and neck region, *Curr Oncol Rep* 11:135–142, 2009.

Fibrosarcoma

Bahrami A, Folpe AL: Adult-type fibrosarcoma: a reevaluation of 163 putative cases diagnosed at a single institution over a 48-year period, *Am J Surg Pathol* 34:1504–1513, 2010.

Baranov E, Hornick JL: Soft tissue special issue: fibroblastic and myofibroblastic neoplasms of the head and neck, *Head Neck Pathol* 14:43–58, 2020.

Mark RJ, Sercarz JA, Tran L, et al.: Fibrosarcoma of the head and neck: the UCLA experience, *Arch Otolaryngol Head Neck Surg* 117:396–401, 1991.

Zhu W, Hu F, Zhao T, et al.: Clinical characteristics of radiation-induced sarcoma of the head and neck: review of 15 cases and 323 cases in the literature, *J Oral Maxillofac Surg* 74:283–291, 2016.

Undifferentiated Pleomorphic Sarcoma

Clark DW, Moore BA, Patel SR, et al.: Malignant fibrous histiocytoma of the head and neck region, *Head Neck* 33:303–308, 2011.

Hardison SA, Davis PL 3rd, Browne JD: Malignant fibrous histiocytoma of the head and neck: a case series, *Am J Otolaryngol* 34:10–15, 2013.

Matushansky I, Charytonowicz E, Mills J, et al.: MFH classification: differentiating undifferentiated pleomorphic sarcoma in the 21st century, *Expert Rev Anticancer Ther* 9:1135–1144, 2009.

Nascimento AF, Raut CP: Diagnosis and management of pleomorphic sarcomas (so-called "MFH") in adults, *J Surg Oncol* 97:330–339, 2008.

Nguyen A, Vaudreuil A, Haun P, et al.: Clinical features and treatment of fibrous histiocytomas of the tongue: a systematic review, *Int Arch Otorhinolaryngol* 22:94–102, 2018.

Liposarcoma

Cheng J, Yu H, Wang L, et al.: Primary oral and maxillofacial liposarcoma: a clinicopathological and immunohistochemical study of eleven cases, *Arch Med Sci* 8:316–323, 2012.

Fanburg-Smith JC, Furlong MA, Childers ELB: Liposarcoma of the oral and salivary gland region: a clinicopathologic study of 18 cases with emphasis on specific sites, morphologic subtypes, and clinical outcome, *Mod Pathol* 15:1020–1031, 2002.

Gerry D, Fox NF, Spruill LS, et al.: Liposarcoma of the head and neck: analysis of 318 cases with comparison to non-head and neck sites, *Head Neck* 36:393–400, 2014.

Nascimento AF, McMenamin ME, Fletcher CDM: Liposarcomas/atypical lipomatous tumors of the oral cavity: a clinicopathologic study of 23 cases, *Ann Diagn Pathol* 6:83–93, 2002.

Pontes FSC, de Souza LL, Vulcão ENC: Liposarcoma of oral cavity: systematic review of cases reported to date and analysis of prognostic factors, *Head Neck* 42:2626–2634, 2020.

Malignant Peripheral Nerve Sheath Tumor

Ma C, Ow A, Shan OH, et al.: Malignant peripheral nerve sheath tumours in the head and neck region: retrospective analysis of clinicopathological features and treatment outcomes, *Int J Oral Maxillofac Surg* 43:924–932, 2014.

Martinez Devesa P, Mitchell TE, Scott I, et al.: Malignant peripheral nerve sheath tumors of the head and neck: two cases and a review of the literature, *Ear Nose Throat J* 85:392–396, 2006.

Minovi A, Basten O, Hunter B, et al.: Malignant peripheral nerve sheath tumors of the head and neck: management of 10 cases and literature review, *Head Neck* 29:439–445, 2007.

Stucky CCH, Johnson KN, Gray RJ, et al.: Malignant peripheral nerve sheath tumors (MPNST): the Mayo Clinic experience, *Ann Surg Oncol* 19:878–885, 2012.

Zou C, Smith KD, Liu J, et al.: Clinical, pathological, and molecular variables predictive of malignant peripheral nerve sheath tumor outcome, *Ann Surg* 249:1014–1022, 2009.

Olfactory Neuroblastoma

Bak M, Wein RO: Esthesioneuroblastoma: a contemporary review of diagnosis and management, *Hematol Oncol Clin North Am* 26:1185–1207, 2012.

Bell D, Saade R, Roberts D, et al.: Prognostic utility of Hyams histological grading and Kadish-Morita staging systems for esthesioneuroblastoma outcomes, *Head Neck Pathol* 9:51–59, 2015.

Faragalla H, Weinreb I: Olfactory neuroblastoma: a review and update, *Adv Anat Pathol* 16:322–331, 2009.

Fiani B, Quadri SA, Cathel A, et al.: Esthesioneuroblastoma: a comprehensive review of diagnosis, management, and current treatment options, *World Neurosurg* 126:194–211, 2019.

Ow TJ, Bell D, Kupferman ME, et al.: Esthesioneuroblastoma, *Neurosurg Clin N Am* 24:51–65, 2013.

Angiosarcoma

Albores-Saavedra J, Schwartz AM, Henson DE, et al.: Cutaneous angiosarcoma: analysis of 434 cases from the Surveillance, Epidemiology, and End Results Program, 1973-2007, *Ann Diagn Pathol* 15:93–97, 2011.

Chi AC, Weathers DR, Folpe AL, et al.: Epithelioid hemangioendothelioma of the oral cavity: report of two cases and review of the literature, *Oral Surg Oral Med Oral Pathol Oral Radiol Endod* 100:717–724, 2005.

Di Battista M, Darling MR, Scrivener E, et al.: Histologic and immunopathologic variability in primary intraoral angiosarcoma: a case report and review of the literature, *Head Neck Pathol* 14:1139–1148, 2020.

Fanburg-Smith JC, Furlong MA, Childers ELB: Oral and salivary gland angiosarcoma: a clinicopathologic study of 29 cases, *Mod Pathol* 16:263–271, 2003.

Favia G, Lo Muzio L, Serpico R, et al.: Angiosarcoma of the head and neck with intra-oral presentation: a clinico-pathological study of four cases, *Oral Oncol* 38:757–762, 2002.

Lee KC, Chuang S-K, Philipone EM, et al.: Characteristics and prognosis of primary head and neck angiosarcomas: a surveillance, epidemiology, and end results program (SEER) analysis of 1250 cases, *Head Neck Pathol* 13:378–385, 2019.

Perez MC, Padhya TA, Messina JL, et al.: Cutaneous angiosarcoma: a single-institution experience, *Ann Surg Oncol* 20:3391–3397, 2013.

Kaposi Sarcoma

Agaimy A, Mueller SK, Harrer T, et al.: Head and neck Kaposi sarcoma: clinicopathological analysis of 11 cases, *Head Neck Pathol* 12:511–516, 2018.

Brenner B, Weissmann-Brenner A, Rakowsky E, et al.: Classical Kaposi sarcoma: prognostic factor analysis of 248 patients, *Cancer* 95:1982–1987, 2002.

Bunn BK, Carvalho Mde V, Louw M, et al.: Microscopic diversity in oral Kaposi sarcoma, *Oral Surg Oral Med Oral Pathol Oral Radiol* 115:241–248, 2013.

Fatahzadeh M: Kaposi sarcoma: review and medical management update, *Oral Surg Oral Med Oral Pathol Oral Radiol* 113:2–16, 2012.

Flaitz CM, Jin Y-T, Hicks MJ, et al.: Kaposi's sarcoma-associated herpesvirus-like DNA sequences (KSHV/HHV-8) in oral AIDS-Kaposi's sarcoma: a PCR and clinicopathologic study, *Oral Surg Oral Med Oral Pathol Oral Radiol Endod* 83:259–264, 1997.

Guedes P.T.L, Pontes FSC, Prado-Ribeiro AC, et al.: HIV-positive patients with oral Kaposi's sarcoma: an overall survival analysis of 31 patients, *Oral Surg Oral Med Oral Pathol Oral Radiol* 131:702–710, 2021.

Hosseini-Moghaddam SM, Soleimanirahbar A, Mazzulli T, et al.: Post renal transplantation Kaposi's sarcoma: a review of its epidemiology, pathogenesis, diagnosis, clinical aspects, and therapy, *Transpl Infect Dis* 14:338–345, 2012.

Leiomyosarcoma

de Araújo GR, Costa SFDS, Mesquita RA, et al.: Leiomyoma and leiomyosarcoma (primary and metastatic) of the oral and maxillofacial region: a clinicopathological and immunohistochemical study of 27 cases, *Head Neck Pathol* 16:294–303, 2022.

Eppsteiner RW, DeYoung BR, Milhem MM, et al.: Leiomyosarcoma of the head and neck: a population-based analysis, *Arch Otolaryngol Head Neck Surg* 137:921–924, 2011.

Ko E: Primary oral leiomyosarcoma: a systemic review and update, *J Oral Pathol Med* 48:780–787, 2019.

Schütz A, Smeets R, Driemel O, et al.: Primary and secondary leiomyosarcoma of the oral and perioral region—clinicopathological and immunohistochemical analysis of a rare entity with a review of the literature, *J Oral Maxillofac Surg* 71:1132–1142, 2013.

Sedghizadeh PP, Angiero F, Allen CM, et al.: Post-irradiation leiomyosarcoma of the maxilla: report of a case in a patient with prior radiation treatment for retinoblastoma, *Oral Surg Oral Med Oral Pathol Oral Radiol Endod* 97:726–731, 2004.

Vilos GA, Rapidis AD, Lagogiannis GD, et al.: Leiomyosarcomas of the oral tissues: clinicopathologic analysis of 50 cases, *J Oral Maxillofac Surg* 63:1461–1477, 2005.

Rhabdomyosarcoma

Hicks J, Flaitz C: Rhabdomyosarcoma of the head and neck in children, *Oral Oncol* 38:450–459, 2002.

Iatrou I, Theologie-Lygidakis N, Schoinohoriti O, et al.: Rhabdomyosarcoma of the maxillofacial region in children and adolescents: report of 9 cases and literature review, *J Craniomaxillofac Surg* 45:831–838, 2017.

Kaste SC, Hopkins KP, Bowman LC: Dental abnormalities in long-term survivors of head and neck rhabdomyosarcoma, *Med Pediatr Oncol* 25:96–101, 1995.

Lee RJ, Lee KK, Lin T, et al.: Rhabdomyosarcoma of the head and neck: impact of demographic and clinicopathologic factors on survival, *Oral Surg Oral Med Oral Pathol Oral Radiol* 124:271–279, 2017.

Parham DM, Barr FG: Classification of rhabdomyosarcoma and its molecular basis, *Adv Anat Pathol* 20:387–397, 2013.

Pontes FSC, de Oliveira JI, de Souza LL, et al.: Clinicopathological analysis of head and neck rhabdomyosarcoma: a series of 10 cases and literature review, *Med Oral Patol Oral Cir Bucal* 23: e188–e197, 2018.

Turner JH, Richmon JD: Head and neck rhabdomyosarcoma: a critical analysis of population-based incidence and survival data, *Otolaryngol Head Neck Surg* 145:967–973, 2011.

Synovial Sarcoma

Al-Daraji W, Lasota J, Foss R, et al.: Synovial sarcoma involving the head: analysis of 36 cases with predilection to the parotid and temporal regions, *Am J Surg Pathol* 33:1494–1503, 2009.

Ferrari A, Gronchi A, Casanova M, et al.: Synovial sarcoma: a retrospective analysis of 271 patients of all ages treated at a single institution, *Cancer* 101:627–634, 2004.

Owosho AA, Estilo CL, Rosen EB, et al.: A clinicopathological study on SS18 fusion positive head and neck synovial sarcomas, *Oral Oncol* 66:46–51, 2017.

Salcedo-Hernández RA, Lino-Silva LS, Luna-Ortiz K: Synovial sarcoma of the head and neck: comparative analysis with synovial sarcoma of the extremities, *Auris Nasus Larynx* 40:476–480, 2013.

Stanbouly D, Litman E, Lee KC, et al.: Synovial sarcoma of the head & neck: a review of reported cases in the literature, *J Stomatol Oral Maxillofac Surg* 122:505–510, 2021.

Alveolar Soft-Part Sarcoma

Argyris PP, Reed RC, Manivel JC, et al.: Oral alveolar soft part sarcoma in childhood and adolescence: report of two cases and review of literature, *Head Neck Pathol* 7:40–49, 2013.

Fanburg-Smith JC, Miettinen M, Folpe AL, et al.: Lingual alveolar soft part sarcoma; 14 cases: novel clinical and morphological observations, *Histopathology* 45:526–537, 2004.

Folpe AL, Deyrup AT: Alveolar soft-part sarcoma: a review and update, *J Clin Pathol* 59:1127–1132, 2006.

Portera CA Jr, Ho V, Patel SR, et al.: Alveolar soft part sarcoma: clinical course and patterns of metastasis in 70 patients treated at a single institution, *Cancer* 91:585–591, 2001.

Wang HW, Qin XJ, Yang WJ, et al.: Alveolar soft part sarcoma of the oral and maxillofacial region: clinical analysis in a series of 18 patients, *Oral Surg Oral Med Oral Pathol Oral Radiol* 119:396–401, 2015.

Metastases to the Oral Soft Tissues

Allon I, Pessing A, Kaplan I, et al.: Metastatic tumors to the gingiva and the presence of teeth as a contributing factor: a literature analysis, *J Periodontol* 85:132–139, 2014.

Hirshberg A, Shnaiderman-Shapiro A, Kaplan I, et al.: Metastatic tumours to the oral cavity—pathogenesis and analysis of 673 cases, *Oral Oncol* 44:743–752, 2008.

Irani S: Metastasis to the oral soft tissues: a review of 412 cases, *J Int Soc Prevent Community Dent* 6:393–401, 2016.

Lim S-Y, Kim S-A, Ahn S-G, et al.: Metastatic tumours to the jaws and oral soft tissues: a retrospective analysis of 41 Korean patients, *Int J Oral Maxillofac Surg* 35:412–415, 2006.

13
Hematologic Disorders

◆ LYMPHOID HYPERPLASIA

The lymphoid tissue of the body plays an important role in the recognition and processing of foreign antigens, such as viruses, fungi, and bacteria. In addition, the lymphoid tissue has a protective function through a variety of direct and indirect mechanisms. In responding to antigenic challenges, lymphoid cells proliferate, thus increasing their numbers, to combat the offending agent more effectively. This proliferation results in enlargement of the lymphoid tissue, which is seen clinically as **lymphoid hyperplasia.**

Clinical Features

Lymphoid hyperplasia may affect the lymph nodes, the lymphoid tissue of Waldeyer ring, or the aggregates of lymphoid tissue that are normally scattered throughout the oral cavity, particularly in the oropharynx, the soft palate, the lateral tongue, and the floor of the mouth. When lymphoid hyperplasia affects the lymph nodes, usually the site that the lymph node drains can be identified as a source of active or recent infection. In the head and neck region, the anterior cervical chain of lymph nodes is most commonly involved, although any lymph node in the area may be affected.

With acute infections, the lymphadenopathy appears as enlarged, tender, relatively soft, freely movable nodules. Chronic inflammatory conditions produce enlarged, rubbery firm, nontender, freely movable nodes. Sometimes these chronic hyperplastic lymph nodes may be difficult to distinguish clinically from lymphoma, and a history of a preceding inflammatory process and lack of progressive enlargement are helpful clues that are consistent with a reactive process. Another condition, however, that should be considered in the differential diagnosis of multiple, persistently enlarged, nontender lymph nodes is human immunodeficiency virus (HIV) infection (see page 256).

Tonsillar size is variable from one person to the next, but lymphoid tissue is normally more prominent in younger individuals, usually reaching its peak early during the second decade of life and gradually diminishing thereafter. Some patients have such large tonsils that it seems as if they would occlude the airway (so-called kissing tonsils). Often, however, these patients have no symptoms and are unaware of a problem. As long as the large tonsils are symmetrical and asymptomatic (Fig. 13.1), it is likely that they are normal for that particular patient. Tonsillar asymmetry is a potentially serious sign that should be evaluated further to rule out the presence of a metastatic tumor or lymphoma.

Hyperplastic intraoral lymphoid aggregates appear as discrete, nontender, submucosal swellings, usually less than 1 cm in diameter, which may appear normal or dark pink in color if the aggregate is deeper; they may have a creamy yellow-orange to amber hue if the collection of lymphocytes is closer to the surface (Figs. 13.2 and 13.3). Lymphoid hyperplasia commonly involves the posterior lateral tongue, where it may appear somewhat ominous. The enlargement is usually bilaterally symmetrical, however, which helps to distinguish the condition from a malignancy. The buccal lymph node may also become hyperplastic and appear as a nontender, solitary, freely movable nodule, usually less than 1 cm in diameter, within the substance of the cheek. Infrequently, a more diffuse lymphoid hyperplasia involves the posterior hard palate, producing a slowly growing, nontender, boggy swelling with an intact mucosal surface and little color change. These palatal lesions may be clinically impossible to distinguish from extranodal lymphoma and would, therefore, necessitate biopsy.

Histopathologic Features

The microscopic features of lymphoid hyperplasia include sheets of small, well-differentiated lymphocytes with numerous interspersed, sharply demarcated collections of reactive lymphoblasts called **germinal centers.** The cells that comprise the germinal centers are primarily transformed B lymphocytes that may demonstrate numerous mitoses. Macrophages can also be identified by the presence of phagocytized material (**tingible bodies**) in their cytoplasm as they engulf nuclear debris from the proliferating lymphocytes. In some instances, immunohistochemical studies and clonality assays must be performed to rule out the possibility of follicular lymphoma.

Treatment and Prognosis

Once the diagnosis of lymphoid hyperplasia is confirmed, no treatment is usually required because it is a completely benign process. For those patients with palatal lymphoid hyperplasia that may interfere with a dental prosthesis, complete excision of the lesion is recommended.

◆ HEMOPHILIA

Hemophilia (*hemo* = blood; *philia* = loving) represents a variety of bleeding disorders associated with a genetic deficiency of any one of the clotting factors of the blood (Table 13.1). This condition was common in certain European royal families, with the initial mutation of the gene for factor IX affecting Queen Victoria of England, who then passed it on to her descendants. DNA analysis of the remains of the Russian royal family (Tsarina Alexandra was a granddaughter of Queen Victoria) confirmed a factor IX gene mutation that resulted in hemophilia B. Because this is an X-linked hereditary condition, a significant proportion of the male members of these families had hemophilia.

In the days before blood transfusions and clotting factor replacement therapy, many of these patients died as a direct result of, or from the complications of, uncontrolled hemorrhage. Because **hemophilia A** (factor VIII deficiency) is the most significant and widely recognized form of hemophilia and accounts for 80%–85% of the bleeding diatheses associated with a specific clotting factor deficiency, most of this discussion centers on that entity. Its estimated prevalence in the United States is 1 in 10,000 persons (or 1 in 5000 males).

As previously mentioned, a deficiency of factor IX or **hemophilia B (Christmas disease)** also may be encountered. Hemophilia B is similar to hemophilia A in its presentation, being transmitted in an X-linked fashion. Hemophilia B is much less common than hemophilia A, occurring with a prevalence of 1 in 60,000 (or 1 in 30,000 males). The term *Christmas disease* was obtained from the surname of the first person, a Canadian boy, who was identified as having hemophilia B in 1952.

Another clotting disorder that is sometimes seen, **von Willebrand disease**, is the result of a genetic deficiency of a plasma glycoprotein called **von Willebrand factor**. This glycoprotein aids in the adhesion of platelets at a site of bleeding, and it also binds to factor VIII, acting as a transport molecule. von Willebrand disease is a genetically heterogeneous condition, with

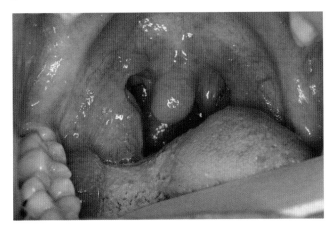

• **Fig. 13.1 Lymphoid Hyperplasia.** The large tonsil observed in this patient represents a benign hyperplasia of the lymphoid cells. If significant asymmetry is observed, further investigation may be warranted to rule out the possibility of lymphoma.

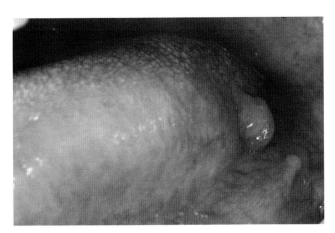

• **Fig. 13.2 Lymphoid Hyperplasia.** The smooth-surfaced papule of the posterior lateral tongue represents an enlarged lymphoid aggregate. The lesion exhibits a lighter color as a result of the accumulation of lymphocytes, which are white blood cells. (Courtesy of Dr. Dean White.)

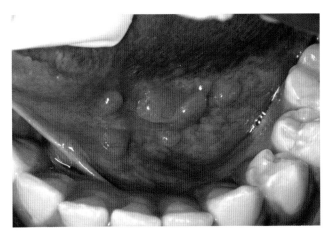

• **Fig. 13.3 Lymphoid Hyperplasia.** Multiple prominent lymphoid aggregates in the floor of the mouth.

TABLE 13.1	Comparison of the Most Commonly Encountered Inherited Bleeding Disorders		
Type	**Defect**	**Inheritance**	**Findings**
Hemophilia A (classic hemophilia)	Factor VIII deficiency	X-linked recessive	Abnormal PTT
Hemophilia B (Christmas disease)	Factor IX deficiency	X-linked recessive	Abnormal PTT
von Willebrand disease	Abnormal von Willebrand factor, abnormal platelets	Autosomal dominant	Abnormal PFA, abnormal PTT

PFA, platelet function assay (replaces bleeding time test); *PTT*, partial thromboplastin time.

several subtypes currently identified, and it may be transmitted in an autosomal dominant or recessive pattern. It is the most common of the inherited bleeding disorders, affecting an estimated 1 in 800–1000 persons. However, many cases of von Willebrand disease are mild and may be clinically insignificant.

Clinical Features

Hemophilia A is an X-linked disorder. Females typically carry the trait, but it is expressed primarily in males. Approximately 1 in 5000 males is born with this genetic disease, with about 30% of the cases representing new mutations. Failure of normal hemostasis after circumcision is typically one of the first signs that a bleeding disorder is present.

The severity of the bleeding disorder depends on the extent of the clotting factor deficiency. Hemophilia A is a heterogeneous disorder that is caused by any one of a variety of mutations associated with the gene for factor VIII. Because the mutations occur at different sites in the factor VIII gene (more than 2000 different mutations have been identified), a clinical spectrum of deficiency of factor VIII is seen. This results in varying degrees of disease expression, with those mutations affecting more significant or larger portions of the factor VIII gene causing more severe clinical disease. Not all patients have an absolute lack of the particular clotting factor; rather, the deficiency may be a percentage of the normal value in a given patient. For example, a patient with only 25% of normal factor VIII levels may be able to function normally under most circumstances; one with less than 5% commonly manifests a marked tendency to bruise with only minor trauma.

In infants, oral lacerations and ecchymoses that involve the lips and tongue are a frequent occurrence as a result of the common falls and bumps experienced by this age group. If not treated appropriately, then such lacerations may result in significant blood loss in more severely affected patients. Sometimes deep hemorrhage occurs during normal activity and may involve the muscles, soft tissues, and weight-bearing joints **(hemarthrosis),** especially the knees (Fig. 13.4). The

result of such uncontrolled bleeding is the formation of scar tissue as the body removes the extravasated blood. This often causes a crippling deformity of the knee joints secondary to arthritis and ankylosis. Sometimes the tissue hemorrhage results in the formation of a tumorlike mass, which has been called **pseudotumor of hemophilia.** Such lesions have been reported in the oral regions. In most instances, pseudotumors of hemophilia occur in patients affected with hemophilia A, but these lesions also have been described rarely in hemophilia B and von Willebrand disease.

An increased coagulation time (delay in blood clotting), of course, is the hallmark feature of this group of conditions. Uncontrollable or delayed hemorrhage may result from any laceration; this includes surgical incisions, dental extractions, and periodontal curettage (Fig. 13.5). Measurements of the platelet count, platelet function assay (PFA—an *in vitro* test of platelet function that has replaced the bleeding time test), prothrombin time (PT), and partial thromboplastin time (PTT) should be ordered as screening tests for any patient with a possible bleeding disorder.

Treatment and Prognosis

The treatment of clotting factor deficiencies essentially consists of replacement therapy with the appropriate clotting factor. Whether treatment is instituted depends on the severity of the clotting factor deficiency.

Patients who have greater than 25% of normal values of factor VIII may function normally. For patients with mild hemophilia (5%–40% of normal levels of factor VIII), no special treatment is typically required for normal activities. If surgery is to be performed, then clotting factor replacement therapy may be indicated.

For patients with severe deficiencies (less than 1% of normal levels of factor VIII), injections with the clotting factor must be performed as soon as a hemorrhagic episode occurs to prevent such complications as the crippling joint deformities of the knees.

The use of aspirin is strictly contraindicated because of its adverse effect on blood platelet function. Severe hemorrhage

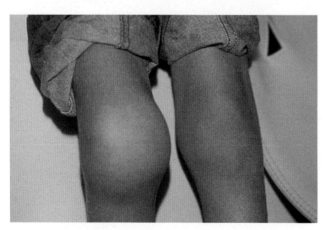

• **Fig. 13.4 Hemophilia.** The enlargement of the knees of this patient with factor VIII deficiency is due to repeated episodes of bleeding into the joints (hemarthrosis). Inflammation and scarring have resulted.

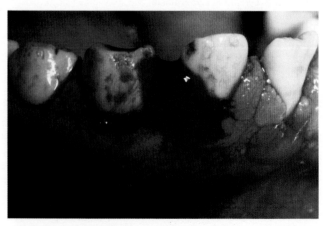

• **Fig. 13.5 Hemophilia.** Hemorrhage in a patient with factor IX deficiency occurred after routine periodontal curettage.

may result if these patients use aspirin-containing medications.

Genetic counseling should be provided to these patients and their families to help them understand the mechanism of inheritance. Using molecular techniques, women who are carriers can be confirmed. In addition, affected male fetuses can now be identified, and the severity of the factor VIII mutation can be assessed.

Optimal dental care is strongly encouraged for these patients to prevent oral problems that might require surgery. If oral or periodontal surgery is necessary, then consultation with the patient's physician is mandatory. The patient is usually prepared for the procedure by the administration of clotting factor just before the surgery. With an extensive surgical procedure, additional doses of clotting factor may be needed subsequently. In addition, epsilon-aminocaproic acid (EACA), an antifibrinolytic agent that inhibits clot degradation, should be given 1 day before the surgery and continued for 7–10 days afterward. Alternative therapy for patients who have levels of factor VIII greater than 5% of normal is desmopressin (1-deamino-8-D-arginine; DDAVP), which can be given just before surgery, either intravenously, subcutaneously, or intranasally. This drug causes the release of bound factor VIII, producing a temporary increase in the plasma levels of the clotting factor. Desmopressin may also be used to manage most patients affected by type 1 von Willebrand disease, which represents approximately 70%–80% of the cases of that disorder.

Although it saved many lives, clotting factor replacement therapy has also resulted in a tragic complication for many of these patients. Cryoprecipitation, the traditional method of concentrating clotting factors from the plasma, also resulted in the concentration of several viruses, including the hepatitis viruses and HIV. More than 40% of hemophilia A and B patients in the United States were estimated to be infected with hepatitis C virus. In addition, as many as 80%–90% of hemophiliac patients treated with multiple doses of factor VIII cryoprecipitate were infected with HIV, and many of these patients eventually developed acquired immunodeficiency syndrome (AIDS). The methods of preparing the clotting factors from pooled human plasma have been modified to eliminate or inactivate HIV; hepatitis A, B, and C; and parvovirus. Recombinant DNA technology also now provides a source of factor VIII that is manufactured by inserting the human factor VIII gene into bacteria that then synthesize the protein. Therefore, this product can now be manufactured without contamination by any viral organisms. Young people affected by hemophilia currently have minimal risk of contracting these infections as a result of their clotting factor replacement therapy.

Other problems must occasionally be confronted, however. Approximately 25%–30% of patients with severe hemophilia A may develop antibodies directed against factor VIII, and this is a very serious complication. Because the antibodies react with the factor VIII molecule, the result is an inhibition of the activity of the clotting factor, and these patients are once more faced with the prospect of uncontrolled bleeding. Patients with factor IX deficiency can develop similar inhibitory antibodies to factor IX, but this appears to occur much less frequently. Attempts to induce immune tolerance may help some individuals, although more immediate care has generally centered on bypassing the factor VIII–related portion of the clotting cascade by administration of recombinant factor VIIa or activated prothrombin complex. More recently, a bispecific monoclonal antibody, emicizumab, has been developed. Emicizumab essentially acts as a substitute for active factor VIII by forming a link between active factor IX and factor X, resulting in activation of factor X, which allows the clotting process to proceed. These methods that are necessary to bypass the inhibitory antibodies are expensive however. Hemophilia research centers are currently focused on developing gene therapy that will correct the condition at the molecular level.

◆ PLASMINOGEN DEFICIENCY (LIGNEOUS CONJUNCTIVITIS; HYPOPLASMINOGENEMIA)

Plasminogen deficiency is a rare autosomal recessive condition that is caused by any one of several mutations of the gene responsible for the production of plasminogen, the precursor to plasmin. In the clotting cascade, factors are activated that lead to the development of a clot; however, simultaneously serum proteins such as plasminogen are converted to plasmin, which is responsible for degrading the clot. Without the formation of plasmin, the clot tends to grow and persist despite having performed its original hemostatic function. The result of plasminogen deficiency is a buildup of fibrin, deposited as irregular plaques and nodules that primarily affect mucosal surfaces. Involvement of the conjunctival mucosa is characterized by the formation of thick, firm plaques, for which the term *ligneous conjunctivitis* has been used (*ligneous* means "woodlike"). Even though this condition was initially described in the 19th century, it was during the late 1990s that an explanation for the majority of these cases was provided. Similar lesions have been produced in mice that have been genetically manipulated to create knock-out mutations of the plasminogen gene.

Clinical Features

The most striking aspect of plasminogen deficiency is the development of thick, creamy yellow to erythematous, firm plaques and nodules involving primarily the conjunctival mucosa of the upper eyelid. Typically the condition is detected during the first decade of life, but lesions can develop later as well. Even though this is an autosomal recessive condition, there is a tendency for the disease to present more often in women, although the reason for this is unknown.

In addition to the conjunctival lesions, other mucosal surfaces can be affected, including the oral mucosa, laryngeal mucosa, and vaginal mucosa. In a recent series of 50 patients with this condition, ocular lesions were documented in 80%, gingival lesions in 34%, respiratory tract lesions in 16%, and vaginal lesions in 8%. Laryngeal mucosal involvement often includes the vocal cords, which typically results in a raspy,

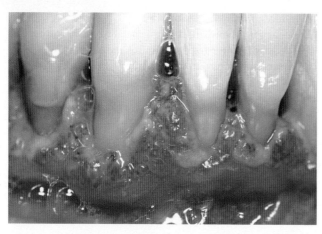

• **Fig. 13.6 Plasminogen Deficiency.** The ulcerated plaques and papules seen on the gingiva of this patient with plasminogen deficiency represent accumulations of fibrin. (Courtesy of Dr. Kenneth Rasenberger.)

hoarse voice. Occlusion of the airway by a fibrin mass has been described rarely.

Oral lesions of plasminogen deficiency primarily involve the gingivae, presenting as patchy ulcerated papules and nodules with a very irregular surface (Fig. 13.6). These lesions may be few in number or distributed diffusely in all quadrants, and they tend to wax and wane in severity.

Histopathologic Features

The microscopic features of the lesions associated with this condition can be very confusing for the pathologist who is not familiar with the disease. The accumulation of fibrin appears as diffuse sheets of acellular eosinophilic material that bears a close resemblance to amyloid (Fig. 13.7). Special stains for amyloid (such as Congo red) are negative, however, because this material represents fibrin. Confirmation that the eosinophilic material is fibrin can be done using the Fraser-Lendrum histochemical staining method. Variable numbers of inflammatory cells are seen, and granulation tissue is usually seen adjacent to the fibrin deposits.

Treatment and Prognosis

Treatment of plasminogen deficiency remains a problem. Damage to the mucosal tissues, including surgical trauma, should be minimized to reduce the likelihood of fibrin accumulation. Careful, thorough oral hygiene practices should be encouraged to diminish the effect of local inflammation. Sporadic reports describe resolution of the conjunctival lesions with either topical or systemic plasminogen; however, this agent is not available commercially. Some patients have experienced spontaneous regression of their lesions over time. Topical heparin combined with prednisone has helped control the gingival lesions in some patients. Alternatively, surgical excision of the gingival nodules, followed by low-dose systemic doxycycline, topical chlorhexidine mouth rinse, and systemic warfarin has also reportedly been effective in managing the lesions. Currently, these may be the two most

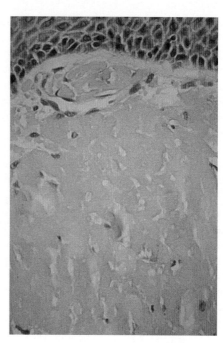

• **Fig. 13.7 Plasminogen Deficiency.** This high-power photomicrograph shows attenuated surface epithelium and a collection of relatively acellular eosinophilic material that superficially resembles amyloid, but is actually fibrin.

reasonable approaches for treating the oral lesions, although successful human trials using replacement plasminogen have been published, and this treatment awaits approval by the U.S. Food and Drug Administration. In the future, gene therapy may be feasible. Interestingly, these patients do not have any unusual problems with intravascular thrombus formation, and their lifespan does not appear to be shortened.

◆ ANEMIA

Anemia is a general term for either a decrease in the volume of red blood cells (hematocrit) or in the concentration of hemoglobin. This problem can result from a number of factors, including a decreased production of erythrocytes or an increased destruction or loss of erythrocytes. Laboratory studies, such as the red blood cell (RBC) count, hematocrit, hemoglobin concentration, mean corpuscular volume (MCV), mean corpuscular hemoglobin (MCH), and mean corpuscular hemoglobin concentration (MCHC), can help indicate the probable cause of the anemia.

Rather than being a disease itself, anemia is often a sign of an underlying disease, such as renal failure, liver disease, chronic inflammatory conditions, malignancies, or vitamin or mineral deficiencies. The diverse causes and complexity of the problem of anemia are presented in Box 13.1.

Clinical Features

The symptoms of anemia are typically related to the reduced oxygen-carrying capacity of the blood, which is a result of the reduced numbers of erythrocytes. Symptoms such as tiredness, headache, shortness of breath, or lightheadedness are often present.

• BOX 13.1 Causes of Anemia

Anemias With Disturbed Iron Metabolism
- Iron deficiency anemia
- Sideroblastic anemias

Megaloblastic Anemias
- Cobalamin (B_{12}) deficiency (pernicious anemia)
- Folic acid deficiency

Anemia Associated With Chronic Disorders
- Anemia of chronic infection (infective endocarditis, tuberculosis, osteomyelitis, lung abscess, and pyelonephritis)
- Anemia of inflammatory connective tissue disorders (rheumatoid arthritis, lupus erythematosus, sarcoidosis, temporal arteritis, and regional enteritis)
- Anemia associated with malignancy
  - Secondary to chronic bleeding
  - Myelophthisic anemia
- Anemia of uremia
- Anemia of endocrine failure
- Anemia of liver disease

Hemolytic Anemias
- Extrinsic causes
  - Splenomegaly
  - Red cell antibodies
  - Trauma in the circulation
  - Direct toxic effects (various microorganisms, copper salts, and venom of certain snakes)
- Membrane abnormalities
  - Spur cell anemia
  - Paroxysmal nocturnal hemoglobinuria
  - Hereditary spherocytosis
  - Hereditary elliptocytosis
- Disorders of the interior of the red cell
  - Defects in the Embden-Meyerhof pathway
  - Defects in the hexose monophosphate shunt

Disorders of Hemoglobin
- Sickle cell anemia
- Thalassemias

Pallor of the mucous membranes may be observed in severe cases of anemia. The palpebral conjunctiva is often the site where this paleness is most easily appreciated, but the oral mucosa may show similar signs.

Treatment and Prognosis

The treatment of anemia depends on determining the underlying cause of the anemia and correcting that problem, if possible.

◆ SICKLE CELL ANEMIA

Sickle cell anemia is one of the more severe genetic disorders of hemoglobin synthesis (**hemoglobinopathies**). Because of the mutational substitution of a thymine molecule for an adenine in DNA, the codon is altered to code for the amino acid valine rather than glutamic acid in the β-globin chain of hemoglobin. This results in a hemoglobin molecule that, in the deoxygenated state, is prone to molecular aggregation and polymerization. Consequently, the red blood cells (RBCs) of patients with sickle cell anemia have a marked tendency to undergo deformation from the normal biconcave disk shape to a rigid-and-curved (sickle) shape. Because the genes for hemoglobin synthesis are codominant, if only one allele is affected, then only 40%–50% of that patient's hemoglobin will be abnormal. Such a patient is simply a carrier and is said to have **sickle cell trait,** a condition that has no significant clinical manifestations in most everyday circumstances. Some sickling may be precipitated under certain conditions, such as dehydration or low-oxygen tensions related to either exercise or high altitudes.

This abnormal gene has persisted in the human race perhaps because it confers a degree of resistance to the malarial organism. As a result, the gene is seen most frequently in populations, such as African, Mediterranean, and Asian, who reside in areas where malaria is endemic. In the United States, nearly 2.5 million people (approximately 8% of the black population) carry this trait.

Unfortunately, in patients who inherit two alleles that code for sickle hemoglobin, the RBCs contain primarily sickle hemoglobin, which results in the condition called **sickle cell disease.** In the United States, about 1 of every 350–400 blacks is born with this disease. Such patients are often susceptible to the problems associated with abnormal RBC morphology. The sickled erythrocytes are more fragile than normal, lasting only 12–16 days in the circulation (about one-tenth of the lifespan of a normal RBC), and they tend to block the capillaries because of their shape and adherence properties. As a result, these patients have a chronic hemolytic anemia and many difficulties related to reduced blood flow to organs and tissues, which produces ischemia, infarction, and tissue death.

Clinical and Radiographic Features

Virtually any tissue or organ may be affected in sickle cell disease. The clinical spectrum of involvement can vary tremendously, with approximately one-third of patients exhibiting severe manifestations. Perhaps the most dramatic sign of this disease is the **sickle cell crisis,** a situation in which the sickling of the erythrocytes becomes severe. Hypoxia, infection, hypothermia, or dehydration may precipitate a crisis; however, for most crises there is no identifiable predisposing factor. Patients who experience a crisis suffer extreme pain from ischemia and infarction of the affected tissue. The long bones, lungs, and abdomen are among the most commonly affected sites, and each episode lasts 3–10 days. Pulmonary involvement, known as **acute chest syndrome,** is particularly serious, and one large study indicated that this is frequently precipitated by fat embolism or community-acquired pneumonia. Some patients may experience such crises monthly; others may go for 1 year or longer without problems. Often fever accompanies the crisis; therefore, infection must be considered in the differential diagnosis.

Patients with sickle cell disease are susceptible to infections, especially those caused by *Streptococcus pneumoniae*, probably because of the destruction of the spleen at an early age by repeated infarctions. Such infections are the most common cause of death among children affected by sickle cell disease in the United States.

Other problems include delayed growth and development in most patients. Impaired kidney function and ocular abnormalities develop secondary to the damage caused by vaso-occlusive episodes in the capillary networks of those organs. If the patient lives long enough, then renal failure may eventually develop. In addition, approximately 5%–8% of these patients will experience central nervous system (CNS) damage in the form of a stroke, which occurs at an average age of about 8 years.

The oral radiographic features of sickle cell disease are relatively nonspecific. They consist of a reduced trabecular pattern of the mandible because of increased hematopoiesis occurring in the marrow spaces. Occasionally, a "hair-on-end" appearance is seen on the skull radiograph, although this is less prominent than that seen in thalassemia (Fig. 13.8). Other oral problems that have been reported include an increased prevalence of osteomyelitis of the mandible, mandibular bone infarction, prolonged paresthesia of the mandibular nerve, and asymptomatic pulpal necrosis.

Histopathologic Features

In homozygous sickle cell disease, a peripheral blood smear shows a peculiar curved distortion of the erythrocytes, resembling a sickle or boomerang shape.

Treatment and Prognosis

The patient experiencing a sickle cell crisis should be managed with supportive care, including fluids, rest, and appropriate analgesic therapy (usually narcotic preparations). It is important, but often difficult, to rule out the possibility of

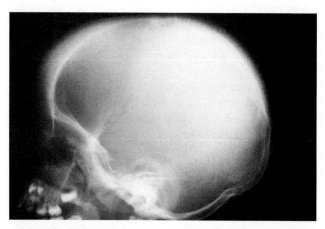

• **Fig. 13.8 Sickle Cell Anemia.** Lateral skull radiograph reveals an altered trabecular pattern, including a slight degree of "hair-on-end" appearance of the cranial bones. (Courtesy of Dr. Reg Munden.)

infection. Acute chest syndrome or cerebral infarct may require treatment with RBC transfusions.

All 50 states now screen for this hemoglobin disorder as part of their newborn infant health care system to identify affected individuals as soon as possible so that appropriate therapy can be instituted. For children with a diagnosis of sickle cell disease, continuous prophylactic penicillin therapy is indicated until at least 5 years of age. In addition, the child should be given polyvalent pneumococcal vaccinations. Situations that might precipitate a crisis, such as strenuous exercise, dehydration, or exposure to cold, should be avoided.

For nearly two decades, hydroxyurea that had been approved for treatment of adults with relatively severe disease. This drug increases the fetal form of hemoglobin (hemoglobin F), which may inhibit polymerization of hemoglobin S and may also reduce the adherence of erythrocytes to the vessel walls. Unfortunately, hydroxyurea has a number of potential side effects and should be used judiciously. In recent years, three new agents have been approved by the U.S. Food and Drug Administration for reduction of the number of crisis episodes in sickle cell disease patients. Each of these drugs has a different mechanism of action, and each is quite costly. Available in 2017, L-glutamine oral powder has to be mixed with water and taken twice daily by patients who are over 5 years of age. The mechanism of action is uncertain, but the medication may cause a decrease in oxidative damage in the sickled erythrocytes. Crizanlizumab-tmca and voxelotor were both approved in 2019. Crizanlizumab-tmca is a monoclonal antibody that is directed against P-selectin, a protein that is associated with the pathophysiologic mechanisms of the sickle cell crisis. This medication is given to patients over 15 years of age as a monthly intravenous infusion. Voxelotor can be given as a daily tablet to patients over 11 years of age, and it reduces sickling of the erythrocyte by inhibiting hemoglobin-S polymerization. Hemoglobin levels also increase in patients taking this medication.

Bone marrow transplantation is curative, but this is a procedure with multiple potential complications and is used primarily for severely affected patients having a histocompatibility antigen (HLA)-matched donor sibling. Only about 18% of sickle cell anemia patients currently meet these criteria. Gene therapy is another potential approach to curing sickle cell anemia, and several clinical trials are currently ongoing. To date, only one patient has been reported to have undergone successful lentivirus-mediated insertion of the corrected β-globin gene into the genome of his hematopoietic stem cells, resulting in resolution of the sickle cell disease. This treatment is not without risks, however, as illustrated by a recent report describing the development of acute myeloid leukemia in a woman who had undergone the same procedure. Although the insertion of the corrected gene itself was not thought to be responsible for the development of malignancy, other factors related to sickle cell anemia itself and the transplantation protocol could have played a role.

When surgery is necessary, local anesthesia, if possible, is usually preferred. If general anesthesia is indicated, then precautions should be taken to avoid conditions that might induce a crisis, such as hypoxia, vascular stasis, acidosis, infection, reduced body temperature, or dehydration.

For patients who have the sickle cell trait or the disease, genetic counseling is appropriate. DNA diagnostic techniques have been used for several years to assess whether a fetus is affected by sickle cell disease, permitting consideration of termination of the pregnancy. Molecular evaluation of the DNA from a single cell obtained from an embryo that was fertilized *in vitro* has allowed selection of a nonaffected embryo for uterine implantation. For parents who are carriers of the sickle cell trait, this is one method to ensure that their offspring do not have sickle cell disease.

Although the mortality rate for sickle cell disease in developed countries has improved dramatically over the past few years, the prognosis is variable because of the wide spectrum of disease activity. Those who are severely affected, however, often are quite disabled because of the many complications of the disease and have a decreased lifespan.

◆ THALASSEMIA

Thalassemia represents a group of disorders of hemoglobin synthesis that are characterized by reduced synthesis of either the α-globin or β-globin chains of the hemoglobin molecule. As in those with sickle cell trait, people who carry the trait for one of the forms of thalassemia seem to be more resistant to infection by the malarial organism; an increased frequency of these genes is seen in Mediterranean, African, Indian, and Southeast Asian populations. Because the original cases were reported from the region of the Mediterranean Sea, the name *thalassemia* was given, derived from the Greek word *thalassa,* meaning "sea." The thalassemias are considered to be among the most common inherited conditions that affect humans.

An understanding of the structure and synthesis of hemoglobin is helpful in explaining the pathophysiology of these conditions. The hemoglobin molecule is a tetramer that is composed of two α chains and two β chains; if one of the chains is not being made in adequate quantities, then the normal amount of hemoglobin cannot be made. Furthermore, the excess globin chains accumulate within the erythrocyte, further compromising the structure and function of the cell.

These abnormal erythrocytes are recognized by the spleen and selected for destruction **(hemolysis).** In addition, there is evidence of ineffective erythropoiesis caused by premature cell death of erythrocyte precursors in the bone marrow because of activation of apoptotic mechanisms. The net result is that the patient has hypochromic, microcytic anemia.

Because two genes code for the β chain and four genes code for the α chain, the degree of clinical severity in these conditions can vary considerably. The severity depends on which specific genetic alteration is present and whether it is heterozygous or homozygous. In the heterozygous state, an adequate amount of normal hemoglobin can be made and the affected patient experiences few signs or symptoms. In the homozygous state, however, the problems are often severe or even fatal. In addition, variations in the severity of the clinical presentation may be a reflection of the specific alteration in the genetic code, because more than 200 different mutations have been documented for β-thalassemia alone.

Clinical and Radiographic Features
β-Thalassemia

If only one defective gene for the β-globin molecule is inherited **(thalassemia minor)**, no significant clinical manifestations are usually present.

When two defective genes for the β-globin molecule are inherited, the patient typically is affected with **thalassemia major**, also called **Cooley anemia** or **Mediterranean anemia.** The disease is usually detected during the first year of life because a severe microcytic, hypochromic anemia develops when fetal hemoglobin synthesis ceases after 3–4 months of age. The red blood cells (RBCs) that are produced are extremely fragile and survive for only a few days in the peripheral circulation.

In an attempt to maintain adequate oxygenation, the rate of hematopoiesis (despite being ineffective) is greatly increased (up to 30 times normal), resulting in massive bone marrow hyperplasia, as well as hepatosplenomegaly and lymphadenopathy because of extramedullary hematopoiesis. The bone marrow hyperplasia may affect the jaws especially, producing an altered trabecular pattern and marked, painless enlargement of the mandible and maxilla (Fig. 13.9). This results in a characteristic "chipmunk" facies and causes

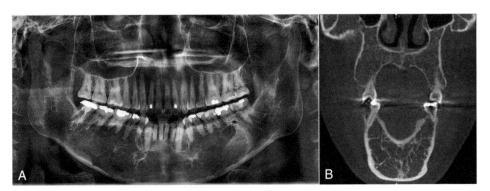

• **Fig. 13.9 Thalassemia. A,** Panoramic radiograph of a 42-year-old male with β-thalassemia shows mandibular enlargement, marked radiolucent change, and wispy trabeculae. **B,** Coronal CT image shows similar changes in the jaws. (Panel A: Courtesy of Dr. Nicole S. Pheifer. Panel B: Courtesy of Dr. Andrew P. Wightman.)

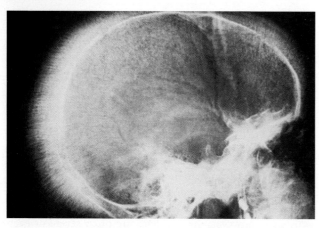

• **Fig. 13.10 Thalassemia.** Lateral skull radiograph depicting the characteristic "hair-on-end" appearance in a patient with thalassemia.

reduced size or obliteration of the paranasal sinuses. Frontal bossing is also present, and a skull radiograph may show a prominent "hair-on-end" appearance of the calvaria (Fig. 13.10). Generalized maturational delay of the patient is typically seen. Delayed development of the dentition also has been described, with the teeth showing a mean delay of approximately 1 year compared with a matched population.

Without therapy, tissue hypoxia worsens and serious bacterial infections with pneumococcal organisms often develop. Eventually, high-output cardiac failure occurs; many patients die by 1 year of age as a result of infection or heart problems.

α-Thalassemia

Because four α-globin genes may be affected, **α-thalassemia** has a broader spectrum of involvement than does β-thalassemia. The condition is caused by deletion at the α-globin gene locus.

When only one deleted gene is inherited, no disease can be detected. With the inheritance of two deleted genes, the condition is known as **α-thalassemia trait**. These patients have a mild degree of anemia and microcytosis that is usually not clinically significant. With three deleted genes, the term **hemoglobin H (HbH) disease** is applied. Patients have problems with hemolytic anemia and splenomegaly. For patients with severe hemolysis, splenectomy may be indicated.

The homozygous state, in which all four genes are deleted, causes severe generalized fetal edema, a condition that has been termed **hydrops fetalis.** Hydrops fetalis is not specific for α-thalassemia and can be seen as a manifestation of other diseases, such as severe Rh incompatibility. Infants with α-thalassemia who are affected by this problem typically die within a few hours of birth.

Treatment and Prognosis

Thalassemia major is treated today primarily by means of blood transfusions. These should be administered every 2–3 weeks to simulate the normal hematologic state. Unfortunately, with repeated blood transfusions, iron overload inevitably develops because of the constant infusion of exogenous RBCs. This is a serious problem, and often death is

due to **hemochromatosis,** an abnormal deposition of iron throughout the tissues of the body. The heart, liver, and endocrine glands are particularly affected by the toxic accumulation of iron. To combat this problem, an iron-chelating agent, deferoxamine (also known as *desferrioxamine*), must be given. If such therapy is used steadfastly, patients with β-thalassemia may have a relatively normal life span; however, problems may arise with patient compliance because this medication must be infused, either parenterally or subcutaneously, over several hours for at least 250 nights each year. If adequate control of iron levels is not obtained, the addition of an orally administered iron chelator, either deferiprone or deferasirox, is often considered. Deferiprone used alone is not as effective as deferoxamine, but the number of weekly infusions of the latter drug can be reduced when combined with deferiprone. Hematologic studies are done weekly due to agranulocytosis developing in 1% of patients taking deferiprone. Deferasirox does not seem to have significant side effects. All of these iron chelators are expensive, although the oral medications used in combination are more cost effective because patient compliance is better and infusion-related costs are eliminated. Hematopoietic stem cell transplantation has also been used with considerable success for individuals who are relatively young, have little organ damage, and have an HLA-matched donor.

Clinicians can now identify α-thalassemia, with its attendant hydrops fetalis (historically considered a fatal condition), *in utero* by molecular testing, and the fetus can be given intrauterine umbilical vein transfusions. An 80% survival rate has been reported for these infants, although they will require either lifelong transfusion therapy or hematopoietic stem cell transplantation. Prenatal diagnosis is also available for β-thalassemia.

For patients who have developed an abnormal facial appearance caused by thalassemia, surgical correction can be performed in many cases. Prevention of thalassemia also is desirable, either by screening for carriers of the genetic trait and providing genetic counseling, or by prenatal diagnosis.

◆ APLASTIC ANEMIA

Aplastic anemia is a rare, life-threatening hematologic disorder that is characterized by failure of the hematopoietic precursor cells in the bone marrow to produce adequate numbers of all types of blood cells (pancytopenia). A significant amount of evidence supports the concept that most cases of aplastic anemia represent an immune-mediated disease caused by cytotoxic T lymphocytes that target differentiating hematopoietic cells in the marrow. As a result, the hematopoietic stem cells do not seem to undergo normal maturation despite normal or increased levels of cytokines, such as granulocyte-macrophage colony-stimulating factor (GM-CSF), which normally induce the production and maturation of several types of white blood cells.

Although the underlying trigger for the immune-mediated destruction of the hematopoietic cells is unknown, some cases of aplastic anemia are associated with exposure to certain environmental toxins (e.g., benzene), treatment with certain drugs (especially the antibiotic chloramphenicol), or infection with certain viruses (particularly non-A, non-B, non-C, or non-G hepatitis). It is possible that the abnormal immune response is perhaps initiated by such exogenous stimuli in certain instances. A few genetic disorders, such as **Fanconi anemia** and **dyskeratosis congenita** (see page 752), also are associated with an increased frequency of aplastic anemia.

Clinical Features

Because all of the formed elements of the blood are decreased in patients with aplastic anemia, the initial symptoms may be related to any one or several of the deficiencies. The erythrocyte deficiency produces signs and symptoms related to a decreased oxygen-carrying capacity of the blood; therefore, patients may experience fatigue, lightheadedness, tachycardia, or weakness. The platelet deficiency (thrombocytopenia) is seen as a marked tendency for bruising and bleeding, which affects a variety of sites. Retinal and cerebral hemorrhages are some of the more devastating manifestations of this bleeding tendency. Deficiency of white blood cells (neutropenia, leukopenia, or granulocytopenia) is the most significant complication of this disease, predisposing the patient to bacterial and fungal infections that often are the cause of death.

The oral findings related to thrombocytopenia include gingival hemorrhage (Fig. 13.11), oral mucosal petechiae, purpura, and ecchymoses. The oral mucosa may appear pale because of the decreased numbers of red blood cells (RBCs). Oral ulcerations associated with infection due to neutropenia, particularly those that involve the gingival tissues, may be present. Minimal erythema is usually associated with the periphery of the ulcers. Gingival hyperplasia has also been reported in association with aplastic anemia.

Histopathologic Features

A bone marrow biopsy specimen usually demonstrates a relatively acellular marrow with extensive fatty infiltration. The histopathologic features of an oral ulceration in a patient with aplastic anemia show numerous microorganisms in addition to a remarkable lack of inflammatory cells in the ulcer bed.

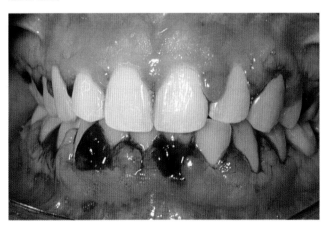

• **Fig. 13.11 Aplastic Anemia.** Diffuse gingival hyperplasia with sulcular hemorrhage.

Diagnosis

The diagnosis of aplastic anemia is usually established by laboratory studies. A pancytopenia is characterized by at least two of the following findings:
- Fewer than 500 granulocytes/µL
- Fewer than 20,000 platelets/µL
- Fewer than 20,000 reticulocytes/µL

Treatment and Prognosis

The course for patients with aplastic anemia is unpredictable. For the milder forms of the disease, spontaneous recovery of the marrow may occur in some instances; progression to severe aplastic anemia may be seen in others. Generally, in severe cases, the chances of spontaneous recovery are slim. If a particular environmental toxin or drug is associated with the process, then withdrawal of the offending agent may sometimes result in recovery.

The treatment is initially supportive. Appropriate antibiotics are given for the infections that develop, and transfusions of packed RBCs or platelets are administered for symptomatic treatment of anemia and bleeding problems, respectively.

Definitive therapy for aplastic anemia is to replace the defective marrow with normal marrow, either by bone marrow transplantation or peripheral blood stem cell transplantation from a matched donor. Patients must be carefully selected; patients younger than 50 years of age and those with an HLA-matched donor (usually a sibling) have the best prognosis, but unfortunately only about 30% of patients meet these criteria.

For those patients who would not be a good prospect for bone marrow transplantation because of their advanced age or no matched donor, immunosuppressive therapy is recommended. Antithymocyte globulin combined with cyclosporine produces a response in the majority of these patients. Compared with treatment results from only 35 years ago, the prognosis for this condition has markedly improved. In the past, for patients with severe aplastic anemia treated with only antibiotics and transfusions, the mortality rate was greater than 80% in the first year after the diagnosis. Currently, an overall long-term survival of 85% of these patients can be achieved with either bone marrow transplant or immunosuppressive therapy. However, even if the disease is controlled, then these patients remain at risk for recurrent marrow aplasia and are at increased risk for acute leukemia.

◆ NEUTROPENIA

Neutropenia refers to a decrease in the number of the circulating neutrophils below 1.5×10^9/L in an adult. It is often associated with an increased susceptibility of the patient to bacterial infections. Clinicians must be aware of this disorder because infection of the oral mucosa may be the initial sign of the disease. Interestingly, several ethnic groups, including patients of African and Middle Eastern background, will consistently have neutrophil counts that would qualify as neutropenia (as low as 1.2×10^9/L), yet these individuals are otherwise healthy. This finding has been termed **benign ethnic neutropenia,** and it appears to have no effect on the health of the patient because neutrophil counts respond to bacterial challenge.

A decrease in neutrophils may be precipitated by several mechanisms, most of which involve decreased production or increased destruction of these important inflammatory cells. When infections are noted in infancy and neutropenia is detected, the problem is usually the result of a congenital or genetic abnormality, such as **Schwachman-Diamond syndrome, dyskeratosis congenita** (see page 752), **cartilage-hair syndrome,** or **severe congenital neutropenia.** If the neutropenia is detected later in life, it usually represents one of the acquired forms. Many acquired neutropenia conditions have an unknown cause; however, others are clearly associated with various causes. A decreased production of neutrophils and the other formed elements of the blood may result from the destruction of the bone marrow by malignancies, such as leukemia (see page 593), or by metabolic diseases, such as Gaucher disease (see page 821), and osteopetrosis (see page 620). Several different types of malignancy, including Hodgkin and non-Hodgkin lymphoma, melanoma, renal cell carcinoma, and T-cell large granular lymphocyte leukemia (Fig. 13.12), have been reported to trigger destruction of neutrophils by various autoimmune mechanisms.

Many drugs may affect neutrophil production, either through direct toxic effects on the bone marrow progenitor cells or by triggering autoimmune mechanisms that destroy neutrophils. These drugs include the following:

- Anticancer chemotherapeutic agents (e.g., nitrogen mustard, busulfan, chlorambucil, and cyclophosphamide)
- Antibiotics (e.g., penicillins and sulfonamides)
- Phenothiazines
- Tranquilizers
- Diuretics

Neutropenia can also be a late manifestation of rituximab therapy, occurring 4–5 weeks after treatment on average. Nutritional deficiencies of vitamin B_{12} or folate, which may be a consequence of malabsorption syndromes, can inhibit neutrophil production as well.

A variety of viral and bacterial infections not only may reduce production of neutrophils but also seem to increase their destruction, typically at the sites of infection. Autoimmune mechanisms of neutrophil destruction may also be induced by viral or bacterial infections. Viral infections that have been implicated include the following:

- Hepatitis A and B
- Rubella
- Measles
- Respiratory syncytial virus
- Varicella
- HIV

Numerous bacterial infections, such as typhoid, tuberculosis, brucellosis, and tularemia, may also cause neutropenia. The increased destruction of neutrophils by an autoimmune mechanism also occurs in such disorders as systemic lupus erythematosus (SLE), in which autoantibodies directed against the neutrophil are produced.

Clinical Features

Most patients with neutropenia have some form of bacterial infection rather than a viral or fungal infection, particularly if the other elements of the immune system (lymphocytes, plasma cells, and monocytes) are still intact. *Staphylococcus aureus* and gram-negative organisms seem to cause the most problems for patients with neutropenia. The suppuration and abscess formation normally associated with such infections may be markedly reduced because of the lack of neutrophils. The most common sites of infection include the middle ear, the oral cavity, and the perirectal area. When neutrophil counts drop below 0.5×10^9/L, however, pulmonary infections often develop.

The oral lesions of neutropenia consist of ulcerations that usually involve the gingival mucosa, probably because of the heavy bacterial colonization of this area and the chronic trauma that it receives. These ulcers characteristically lack an erythematous periphery (Fig. 13.12), although this finding has been variable. Premature periodontal bone loss with exfoliation of the deciduous dentition has been described.

Histopathologic Features

A biopsy specimen of neutropenic ulceration usually shows a reduced number or the absence of neutrophils. Bacterial invasion of the host tissue may be apparent in some instances.

Treatment and Prognosis

Infections related to neutropenia are managed with appropriate antibiotic therapy. The patient should be encouraged to maintain optimal oral hygiene to decrease the bacterial load in the oral cavity. Studies using recombinant human granulocyte colony-stimulating factor (G-CSF; filgrastim; pegfilgrastim), a cytokine that promotes the growth and differentiation of neutrophils, have shown remarkable

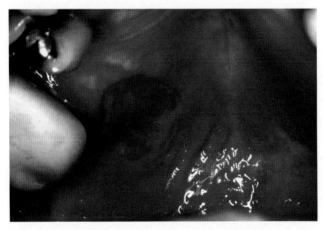

• **Fig. 13.12 Neutropenia.** Palatal neutropenic ulceration that was seen in a patient with large granular lymphocyte leukemia, a rare form of leukemia that induces a severe decrease in neutrophils.

results. Patients with severe neutropenia have a significant increase in neutrophil counts and resolution of infections after treatment with this agent. Prophylactic use of filgrastim or pegfilgrastim reduces the risk of febrile neutropenia in patients who are receiving certain antineoplastic chemotherapeutic regimens. Patients who do not respond to G-CSF may have to be considered for hematopoietic stem cell transplantation, depending on the severity of the neutropenia and subsequent infections.

◆ AGRANULOCYTOSIS

Agranulocytosis is a condition in which the cells of the granulocytic series, particularly neutrophils, are absent. As in other disorders of the formed elements of the blood, agranulocytosis may occur as a result of decreased production or increased destruction or use of these cells. Although some cases are idiopathic, most are induced by exposure to one of several drugs. Some drugs, such as the anticancer chemotherapeutic agents, induce agranulocytosis by inhibiting the normal mitotic division and maturation of the hematopoietic stem cells. In other instances, the drugs trigger an immunologic reaction that results in the destruction of granulocytes. Rarely, agranulocytosis may be a congenital syndrome (**congenital agranulocytosis, Kostmann syndrome**) that results from a decreased level of the cytokine granulocyte colony-stimulating factor (G-CSF).

Clinical Features

Agranulocytosis typically develops within a few days after a person ingests the offending drug. Because of the lack of granulocytes (especially neutrophils), bacterial infections often develop and patients may show signs and symptoms of malaise, sore throat, swelling, fever, chills, bone pain, pneumonia, and shock. The erythrocyte and platelet counts are usually normal or only slightly depressed.

Oral lesions are common and include necrotizing, deep, punched-out ulcerations of the buccal mucosa, tongue, and palate. The gingivae are especially susceptible to infection, often resembling the pattern of necrotizing ulcerative gingivitis (NUG) (see page 151).

Histopathologic Features

Microscopic examination of a biopsy specimen from one of the oral ulcerations in agranulocytosis characteristically shows abundant bacterial organisms, both on the surface and within the tissue. The host inflammatory response is relatively sparse, with few granulocytes, particularly neutrophils, seen in the ulcer bed.

Treatment and Prognosis

If the clinician believes that a particular drug has caused the agranulocytosis, the medication should be discontinued as soon as is reasonably possible. In many instances, the granulocyte count returns to normal within 10–14 days after cessation of the offending agent. For patients who have agranulocytosis secondary to cancer chemotherapy, oral hygiene should be meticulous to foster an immaculate oral environment. In addition, the use of chlorhexidine-containing mouth rinses seems to reduce the severity of the oral lesions. Active infections are treated with appropriate antibiotic medications.

If the agranulocytosis is related to cancer treatment, the white blood cell count usually returns to normal after a period of weeks. For patients whose granulocyte counts do not recover, administration of G-CSF or granulocyte-macrophage colony-stimulating factor (GM-CSF) may be beneficial. The overall mortality rate for this condition in the past was 20%–30%, although cytokine therapy and the newer broad-spectrum antibiotics have improved the outlook for these patients.

◆ CYCLIC NEUTROPENIA (CYCLIC HEMATOPOIESIS)

Cyclic neutropenia is a rare idiopathic hematologic disorder that is characterized by regular periodic reductions in the neutrophil population of the affected patient. The underlying cause seems to be a mutation of the neutrophil elastase *(ELA-2* or *ELANE)* gene, resulting in arrested development of neutrophils at the promyelocyte stage within the marrow. This mutation is also associated with premature apoptosis of these myeloid precursor cells. The best estimated frequency of this disease in the population is about 1 in 1 million. Although an autosomal dominant pattern of inheritance has been described in a few cases, most examples of cyclic neutropenia are isolated.

Symptoms usually begin in childhood and tend to correlate with the neutrophil counts. When the neutrophil count is at its nadir (i.e., lowest point), the patient experiences problems with infection. As the neutrophil count rises toward normal, the signs and symptoms abate. Very low neutrophil counts usually are present for 3–6 days, and blood monocyte and eosinophil levels are typically increased when the neutrophil count is depressed. Even when the neutrophil count is at its peak, the levels are often less than normal.

Clinical and Radiographic Features

The signs and symptoms of cyclic neutropenia occur in rather uniformly spaced episodes, which usually have a 21-day cycle. Patients typically complain of recurrent episodes of fever, anorexia, cervical lymphadenopathy, malaise, pharyngitis, and oral mucosal ulcerations. Other gastrointestinal mucosal areas, including the colon, rectum, and anus, may be affected by recurrent ulcerations.

The oral ulcerations develop on any oral mucosal surface that is exposed to even minor trauma, particularly the lips, tongue, buccal mucosa, and oropharynx (Fig. 13.13). An erythematous halo is variably present at the periphery of the ulcers. The gingiva is the most severely affected region of the oral cavity. Severe periodontal bone loss with marked

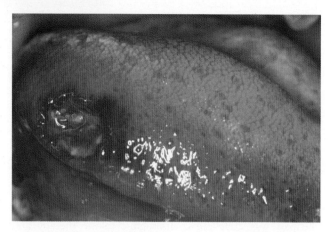

• **Fig. 13.13 Cyclic Neutropenia.** Ulceration of the lateral tongue is typical of the lesions associated with cyclic neutropenia. (From Allen CM, Camisa C: Diseases of the mouth and lips. In Sams WM, Lynch P, editors: *Principles and practice of dermatology*, ed 2, New York, 1996, Churchill Livingstone.)

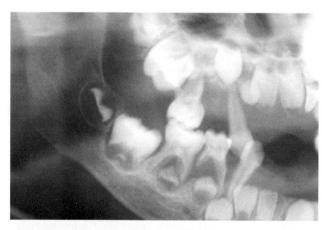

• **Fig. 13.14 Cyclic Neutropenia.** Cyclic neutropenia is one of several conditions that may produce premature bone loss, as shown in the interradicular regions of the mandibular deciduous molar teeth.

gingival recession and tooth mobility also is characteristic (Fig. 13.14).

Diagnosis

The diagnosis of cyclic neutropenia should be established by sequential complete blood counts (typically three times per week for 6–8 weeks) to determine whether cycling of the neutrophil levels occurs. The neutrophil count should be less than $500/mm^3$ for 3–5 days during each of at least three successive cycles to make this diagnosis.

Histopathologic Features

The histopathologic features of cyclic neutropenia are similar to those of the other neutropenic and granulocytopenic ulcerations if the biopsy is performed during the nadir of the neutrophil count.

Treatment and Prognosis

Supportive care for the patient with cyclic neutropenia includes antibiotic therapy for significant infections that might occur while the neutrophil count is at its lowest. Unfortunately, this approach cannot be considered a permanent treatment. Other methods that have been used with marginal success include splenectomy, corticosteroid therapy, and nutritional supplementation. Administration of the cytokine granulocyte colony-stimulating factor (G-CSF) several times weekly seems to correct the lack of production of neutrophils. This treatment results in a decrease in the time of neutropenia from 5 days to 1 day, which improves the clinical course of the disease. The cycles are reduced from 18 to 21 days to 11 to 13 days, and the severity of mucositis and infection are reduced.

Supportive care in the form of optimal oral hygiene should be maintained to reduce the number and severity of oral infections and improve the prognosis of the periodontal structures. Fortunately, for many of these patients, the severity of symptoms related to cyclic neutropenia seems to diminish after the second decade of life, despite the fact that the cycling of the neutrophils continues.

◆ THROMBOCYTOPENIA

Thrombocytopenia is a hematologic disorder that is characterized by a markedly decreased number of circulating blood platelets (formed elements derived from megakaryocyte precursors in the bone marrow). Platelets are necessary for hemostasis and clot formation. A platelet count of $200,000–400,000/mm^3$ is considered normal. The decrease in platelets may be the result of the following:
• Reduced production
• Increased destruction
• Sequestration in the spleen

REDUCED PLATELET PRODUCTION

Reduced production of platelets may be the result of various causes, such as infiltration of the bone marrow by malignant cells or the toxic effects of cancer chemotherapeutic drugs. In such instances, decreases in the other formed elements of the blood are also seen.

INCREASED PLATELET DESTRUCTION

Increased destruction of platelets may be caused by an immunologic reaction, which is often precipitated by any one of more than 100 different drugs; heparin is one of the most common offending agents. This type of reaction is typically idiosyncratic and, therefore, not related to the dose of the drug. Similarly, autoantibodies directed against platelets, specifically certain surface glycoproteins, may on rare occasions be induced by viral infection or vaccination. In addition, certain systemic diseases may have thrombocytopenia as a component, such as systemic lupus erythematosus (SLE) and HIV infection. Increased destruction may also occur because of increased consumption of platelets associated with abnormal blood clot formation. This occurs in patients with conditions, such as **thrombotic thrombocytopenic purpura (TTP).** This serious disorder of coagulation is caused by a deficiency of a von Willebrand factor-cleaving metalloprotease (ADAMTS13), which triggers the formation of numerous thrombi within the small blood vessels of the body. The condition is usually caused by antibodies directed against ADAMTS13, but TTP can also rarely be inherited as an autosomal recessive condition when mutations of the ADAMTS13 gene are present.

SEQUESTRATION IN THE SPLEEN

Under normal conditions, one-third of the platelet population is sequestered in the spleen. Consequently, conditions that cause splenomegaly (e.g., portal hypertension secondary to liver disease, splenic enlargement secondary to tumor infiltration, and splenomegaly associated with Gaucher disease) also cause larger numbers of platelets to be taken out of circulation. Regardless of the cause, the result for the patient is a bleeding problem because normal numbers of platelets are not available for proper hemostasis.

Clinical Features

Clinical evidence of thrombocytopenia is not usually seen until the platelet levels drop below 100,000/mm^3. The severity of involvement is directly related to the extent of platelet reduction. The condition often is initially detected because of the presence of oral lesions. Minor traumatic events are continuously inflicted on the oral mucosa during chewing and swallowing of food. The small capillaries that are damaged during this process are normally sealed off with microscopic thrombi. In a patient with thrombocytopenia, however, the thrombi do not form properly. This results in a leakage of blood from the small vessels. Clinically, this usually produces pinpoint hemorrhagic lesions known as **petechiae.** If a larger quantity of blood is extravasated, then an **ecchymosis** or bruise results (Fig. 13.15). With even larger amounts of extravasated blood, a **hematoma** (*hemat* = blood; *oma* = tumor) will develop (Fig. 13.16). Spontaneous gingival hemorrhage often occurs in these patients, as does bleeding from sites of minor trauma.

Similar hemorrhagic events occur throughout the body. With severe thrombocytopenia (<10,000 platelets/mm^3), massive bleeding from the gastrointestinal or urinary tract may be fatal. Epistaxis is often present in these patients, and hemoptysis indicates significant pulmonary hemorrhage. Intracranial hemorrhage is also a potentially fatal complication of severe thrombocytopenia.

Immune thrombocytopenic purpura (ITP) or **immune thrombocytopenia,** which used to be known as idiopathic thrombocytopenic purpura or idiopathic thrombocytopenia, can present as either an acute or chronic process. Acute ITP usually occurs during childhood, classically after a nonspecific viral infection. The symptoms of thrombocytopenia appear quickly and may be severe. Most cases, however, resolve

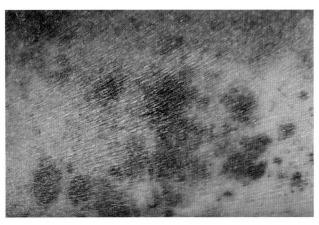

• **Fig. 13.15 Thrombocytopenia.** The bruising (purpura) seen on this patient's forearm is a result of reduced platelet count secondary to myelodysplasia, a preleukemic bone marrow disorder.

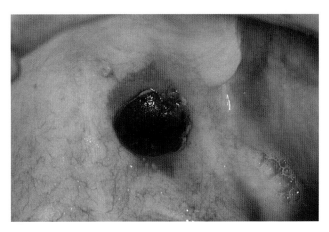

• **Fig. 13.16 Thrombocytopenia.** This dark palatal lesion represents a hematoma caused by a lack of normal coagulation, characteristic of thrombocytopenia.

spontaneously within 4–6 weeks, and 90% of patients recover by 3–6 months. Chronic ITP most frequently affects women between 20 and 40 years. Autoantibodies directed against antigens on the platelet surface result in sequestration and destruction of the platelets in the spleen. Consequently many of these patients may respond to splenectomy.

Histopathologic Features

Gingival biopsy may be performed for diagnostic purposes in patients with suspected TTP. Approximately 30%–40% of such biopsy specimens show the presence of fibrin deposits in the small vessels. These deposits are more readily appreciated after staining the tissue section using the periodic acid-Schiff (PAS) method.

Treatment and Prognosis

If the clinician believes the thrombocytopenia to be drug-related, the drug should be discontinued immediately. In most instances, the platelet count returns to normal after several days. Platelet transfusions and corticosteroid therapy may be necessary if life-threatening hemorrhage occurs. As mentioned earlier, ITP often resolves spontaneously, but those cases that are more severe may require corticosteroid therapy or intravenous immunoglobulin (IVIG) therapy. Good success has been documented with rituximab (which targets B lymphocytes) or thrombopoietin-receptor agonists (which stimulate megakaryocytes to produce more platelets). Splenectomy is generally reserved for those cases of ITP that are refractory to medical treatment. For some forms of thrombocytopenia, such as TTP, the patient's prognosis is relatively guarded. In the past, the condition was almost uniformly fatal, although the outlook has greatly improved since therapy with plasma exchange transfusions, combined with corticosteroids or rituximab, became available. More than 70% of these patients now survive with proper treatment.

◆ POLYCYTHEMIA VERA (PRIMARY POLYCYTHEMIA; POLYCYTHEMIA RUBRA VERA; PRIMARY ACQUIRED ERYTHROCYTOSIS)

Polycythemia vera is a rare idiopathic hematologic disorder that is best thought of as an increase in the mass of the red blood cells (RBCs). Uncontrolled production of platelets and granulocytes, however, is often seen concurrently, and most authorities feel that this condition represents a relatively non-aggressive myeloproliferative disorder. Researchers believe the over-production is related to the abnormal behavior of a single progenitor marrow stem cell, which begins multiplying without regard to the normal regulatory hormones, such as erythropoietin. This gives rise to a group or clone of unregulated cells that then produce the excess numbers of these formed elements of the blood at two to three times the normal rate. These cells generally function in a normal fashion.

Clinical Features

Polycythemia vera typically affects older adults. The median age at diagnosis is 60 years. Only 5% of cases are diagnosed before the age of 40 years. No sex predilection is seen, and the annual incidence in the United States is estimated to be approximately 20 cases per million population. An acquired mutation of one of the tyrosine kinase genes, Janus kinase 2 (*JAK2*), plays a significant role in the development of this disorder, and more than 95% of patients with polycythemia vera have been shown to have this mutation.

The initial symptoms of the disease are nonspecific and include the following:
- Headache
- Weakness
- Dizziness
- Drowsiness
- Visual disturbances
- Sweating
- Weight loss
- Dyspnea
- Epigastric pain

A ruddy complexion may be evident on physical examination. One relatively characteristic complaint, described in about 40% of affected patients, is that of generalized pruritus (itching), particularly after bathing, without evidence of a rash.

The problems caused by thrombus formation, which would be expected with the increased viscosity of the blood and the increased platelet numbers, include transient ischemic attacks, cerebrovascular accidents, and myocardial infarctions. Hypertension and splenomegaly are also common.

A peculiar peripheral vascular event called **erythromelalgia** affects the hands and feet. Patients experience a painful burning sensation accompanied by erythema and warmth. This may eventually lead to thrombotic occlusion of the vessels that supply the digits. Digital gangrene and necrosis may result. Erythromelalgia is probably caused by excessive platelets, and its onset seems to be precipitated by exercise, standing, or warm temperatures.

Strangely enough, these patients may also have problems with excess hemorrhage. Epistaxis and ecchymoses are sometimes a problem, and gingival hemorrhage has been described.

Treatment and Prognosis

With the initial diagnosis of polycythemia vera, an immediate attempt is made to reduce the RBC mass. The first treatment is usually phlebotomy, with as much as 500 mL of blood removed every other day until a hematocrit of less than 45% is achieved. If thrombotic events are an immediate problem, then treatment with low-dose aspirin should be started. If difficulty in controlling the platelet levels is encountered, anagrelide hydrochloride, a selective inhibitor of megakaryocyte maturation and platelet production, may be prescribed. Antihistamines are used to help control the symptoms of pruritus.

Long-term management may include intermittent phlebotomy, as well as the relatively mild chemotherapeutic drug, hydroxyurea. Hydroxyurea is one chemotherapeutic agent that may not pose an increased risk of leukemia, however, because it acts as an antimetabolite and does not appear to have any mutagenic properties. If the patient cannot tolerate hydroxyurea, or if an inadequate response is seen, then treatment with recently developed medications that target the JAK2 pathway, such as pegylated interferon and ruxolitinib, may be appropriate. For resistant cases, myelosuppressive therapy has also been advocated, although an increased risk of leukemia is associated with some chemotherapeutic drugs. Nevertheless, in 2%–10% of patients with polycythemia vera, acute leukemia ultimately develops.

Overall, the prognosis is fair; patients with polycythemia vera survive an average of 10–12 years after the diagnosis, if treated. Given the fact that the median age at diagnosis is 60 years, the majority of affected patients do not seem to have a markedly higher death rate compared with their unaffected peers.

◆ LEUKEMIA

Leukemia represents several types of malignancies of hematopoietic stem cell derivation. The disease begins with the malignant transformation of one of the stem cells, which initially proliferates in the bone marrow and eventually overflows into the peripheral blood of the affected patient. Problems arise when the leukemic cells crowd out the normal defense cell and erythrocyte precursors. In the United States, approximately 3.4% of all cancers are leukemia, and 3.8% of deaths from cancer can be attributed to this disease.

Leukemias are usually classified according to their histogenesis and clinical behavior. Therefore, the broad categories would be **acute** or **chronic** (referring to the clinical course) and **myeloid** or **lymphocytic/lymphoblastic** (referring to the histogenetic origin). Myeloid leukemias can differentiate along several different pathways; thus they produce malignant cells that usually show features of granulocytes or monocytes, and less frequently, erythrocytes or megakaryocytes.

Acute leukemias, if untreated, run an aggressive course and often result in the death of the patient within a few months. Chronic leukemias tend to follow a more indolent course, although the end result is the same. One of the greatest successes in cancer treatment has been achieved in acute lymphoblastic leukemia of childhood, a condition that used to be uniformly fatal but now is often capable of being controlled.

Leukemias are probably the result of a combination of environmental and genetic factors. Certain syndromes are associated with an increased risk. These genetic disorders include the following:

- Down syndrome
- Bloom syndrome
- Neurofibromatosis type I
- Schwachman syndrome
- Ataxia-telangiectasia syndrome
- Klinefelter syndrome
- Fanconi anemia
- Wiskott-Aldrich syndrome

In addition, certain types of leukemia show specific chromosomal abnormalities. The first chromosomal abnormality to be detected was found in patients with **chronic myeloid leukemia,** and this malignancy was characterized by a genetic alteration called the **Philadelphia chromosome.** This abnormality represents a translocation of the chromosomal material between the long arms of chromosomes 22 and 9. This rearrangement of the genetic material occurs in such a fashion as to fuse the breakpoint cluster region *(BCR)* gene with the Abelson *(ABL)* oncogene, producing an entirely new gene: *BCR-ABL.* This gene is continuously transcribed, and the resulting protein product, a tyrosine kinase, causes the uncontrolled proliferation of the leukemic cells. Identifying such pathogenetic mechanisms has opened up an entirely new field of chemotherapy that targets specific molecular mechanisms of carcinogenesis. A variety of other genetic alterations in the bone marrow stem cells has been associated with the **myelodysplasia syndromes,** a group of disorders that appear to represent early stages in the evolution of **acute myeloid leukemia.** As the genetic alterations accumulate in the stem cells, the chances of the patient developing leukemia increase.

Some environmental agents are associated with an increased risk of leukemia, but their overall contribution to the leukemia problem is thought to be less than 5%. Exposure to pesticides, benzene, and benzene-like chemicals has been associated with an increased risk of developing leukemia. Ionizing radiation has also been implicated; this was documented by the increased frequency of chronic myeloid leukemia in the survivors of the atomic bomb blasts at Hiroshima and Nagasaki during World War II. Viruses have also been shown to produce leukemia, although this is not a common finding. The most thoroughly studied is the retrovirus known as *human T-cell leukemia/lymphoma virus type 1 (HTLV-1),* which is transmitted by contaminated blood from infected to uninfected individuals. This virus can cause a relatively rare form of malignancy of T lymphocytes, which may present as a leukemia or non-Hodgkin lymphoma (see page 600). Most cases have been identified in parts of the Caribbean, central Africa, and southwestern Japan.

As knowledge about this group of diseases increases, the fact that the leukemias are diverse and complex cannot be overlooked. For example, at least 11 distinct subtypes of acute myeloid leukemia have now been identified, and each subtype has a different treatment approach and prognosis. Because of the complexity of this area, the discussion is limited to those aspects of leukemia that are more directly related to the oral or head and neck region.

Clinical Features

If all types of leukemia are considered, this condition occurs at a rate of 13 cases per 100,000 population annually. Slightly more males than females are affected. The myeloid leukemias generally affect an adult population; **acute myeloid leukemia** affects a broader age range, which includes children. The median age of patients diagnosed with **chronic myeloid leukemia** is approximately 59 years. **Acute lymphoblastic leukemia,** in contrast, occurs predominantly in children and represents one of the more common childhood malignancies. **Chronic lymphocytic leukemia,** the most common type of leukemia, primarily affects older adults.

Many of the clinical signs and symptoms of leukemia are related to the marked reduction in the numbers of normal white and red blood cells, a phenomenon that results from the crowding out of the normal hematopoietic stem cells by the malignant proliferation **(myelophthisic anemia).** Because of the reduced red blood cell (RBC) count and subsequent reduction in oxygen-carrying capacity of the blood, patients complain of fatigue, easy tiring, and dyspnea on mild exertion. The malignant cells may also infiltrate other organs and often cause splenomegaly, hepatomegaly, and lymphadenopathy.

Leukemic patients may also complain of easy bruising and bleeding, problems that are caused by a lack of blood platelets

(thrombocytopenia), the result of megakaryocytes being crowded out of the marrow. Petechial hemorrhages of the posterior hard palate and the soft palate may be observed, and these may be accompanied by spontaneous gingival hemorrhage, especially with platelet counts less than 10,000–20,000/mm³. Because disturbances in stem cell differentiation accompany the myelodysplasia syndromes, thrombocytopenia is often present in these patients, and gingival hemorrhage has been reported in this setting. Serious hemorrhagic complications may result from bleeding into the CNS or the lungs.

A fever associated with infection may be the initial sign of the leukemic process. Perirectal infections, pneumonia, urinary tract infections, and septicemia are common infectious complications. The microorganisms that are typically involved include gram-negative bacteria, gram-positive cocci, and certain *Candida* species.

Ulceration of the oral mucosa is often present as a result of the impaired ability of the host to combat the normal microbial flora. Usually, the gingival mucosa is the most severely affected because of the abundant bacteria normally present around the teeth. The neutropenic ulcers that are produced are typically deep, punched-out lesions with a gray-white necrotic base. Oral candidiasis is often a complication of leukemia, involving the oral mucosa diffusely. Herpetic infections are the most common viral lesions, and these may involve any area of the oral mucosa rather than being confined to the keratinized mucosa, as in immunocompetent patients.

Occasionally, the leukemic cells infiltrate the oral soft tissues and produce a diffuse, boggy, nontender swelling that may or may not be ulcerated. This occurs most frequently with the myelomonocytic types of leukemia, and it may result in diffuse gingival enlargement (Figs. 13.17 and 13.18) or a prominent tumorlike growth (Fig. 13.19). The tumorlike collection of leukemic cells is known as **myeloid sarcoma,** a designation that has replaced the older terms, **granulocytic sarcoma** and **extramedullary myeloid tumor.** Historically the proliferation of leukemic cells was called

chloroma because it is often greenish (*chlor* = green; *oma* = tumor) on fresh-cut sections. Other oral manifestations include infiltration of the periapical tissues, simulating periapical inflammatory disease both clinically and radiographically.

Histopathologic Features

Microscopic examination of leukemia-affected tissue shows diffuse infiltration and destruction of the normal host tissue by sheets of poorly differentiated cells with either myelomonocytic characteristics or lymphoid features.

Diagnosis

The diagnosis is usually established by confirming the presence of poorly differentiated leukemic cells in the peripheral blood and bone marrow. Bone marrow biopsy is normally performed in conjunction with the peripheral blood studies because some patients may go through an aleukemic phase in which the atypical cells are absent from

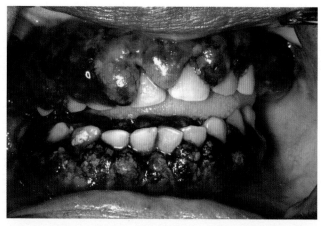

• **Fig. 13.18 Leukemia.** Extensive hemorrhagic enlargement of the maxillary and mandibular gingivae. (Courtesy of Dr. Michael Tabor.)

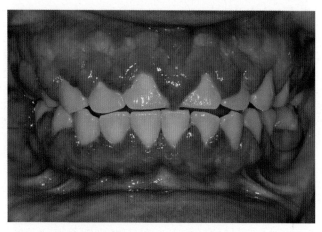

• **Fig. 13.17 Leukemia.** Diffuse gingival enlargement, as depicted in this photograph, may occur in leukemic patients, particularly in those with monocytic leukemia. (Courtesy of Dr. Spencer Shoff.)

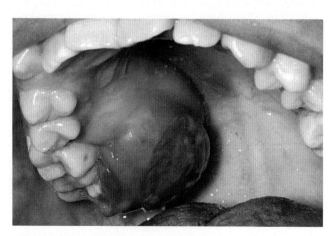

• **Fig. 13.19 Leukemia.** The ulcerated soft tissue nodule of the hard palate represents leukemic cells that have proliferated in this area.

the circulation. Classifying the type of leukemia requires establishing the immunophenotype by using immunohistochemical markers to identify cell surface antigens expressed by the tumor cells. Immunohistochemical confirmation of certain characteristic enzymes (e.g., myeloperoxidase and lysozyme) is necessary to identify and classify the myeloid leukemias. In addition, cytogenetic and molecular characterization of the lesional cells is typically necessary. In many cases, the results of these various studies will be significant because both the patient's treatment and the patient's prognosis are directly affected.

Treatment and Prognosis

Although a detailed discussion is beyond the scope of this text, the treatment of a patient with leukemia typically consists of various forms of chemotherapy; the type of leukemia dictates the chemotherapeutic regimen. In most cases the purpose of chemotherapy is to destroy as many of the atypical cells as possible in a short time, thus inducing a remission. For this reason, this technique has been termed **induction chemotherapy.** Usually, this phase of chemotherapy requires high doses of toxic chemotherapeutic agents; often, the patient experiences a number of unpleasant side effects during treatment. Once remission has been induced, this state must be maintained. This is the purpose of **maintenance chemotherapy,** which typically requires lower doses of chemotherapeutic drugs given over a longer period.

If the *BCR-ABL* fusion is identified in the leukemic cells of a patient with chronic myeloid leukemia, then treatment with a tyrosine kinase inhibitor is appropriate. The first tyrosine kinase inhibitor to be developed and marketed was imatinib mesylate, and at least half of these patients will respond dramatically to this therapy. Imatinib must be taken continuously, because relapses develop quickly if the drug is stopped. Unfortunately over 100 different mutations have been identified in this fused gene; consequently, 33% of chronic myelogenous leukemia patients will be resistant to imatinib. Additional BCR-ABL tyrosine kinase inhibitors, such as dasatinib, nilotinib, and bosutinib, have been developed and can be used as first-, second-, or third-line therapy. Chronic lymphocytic leukemia is considered curable only by treatment with allogeneic hematopoietic stem cell transplantation, a procedure that has its own risks and can be considered in patients less than 60 years of age. Most patients achieve a significant response when treated with traditional chemotherapeutic agents that are combined with monoclonal antibodies directed against one of the B-lymphocyte cell surface antigens. Rituximab, which is a CD20 antibody, has been effective in managing this disease; however, other monoclonal B-cell surface antibodies are being investigated. Drug therapy may be combined with radiation therapy to the CNS because the chemotherapeutic drugs often do not cross the blood-brain barrier effectively. Therefore, the leukemic cells may survive in this site and cause a relapse of the leukemia. Direct intrathecal infusion of the chemotherapeutic agent may be performed to circumvent the problem of the blood-brain barrier. If this strategy succeeds in inducing a remission, then a bone marrow transplant may be considered as a therapeutic option, particularly for the types of leukemia that tend to relapse. This option often is reserved for patients younger than 45 years of age because the success rate is less favorable in older patients.

Supportive care is often necessary if these patients are to survive their leukemia. For patients with bleeding problems, transfusions with platelets may be necessary. If severe anemia is present, packed RBCs may be required. Infections, of course, should be evaluated with respect to the causative organism, and appropriate antibiotics must be prescribed. Support must be maintained from an oral perspective because many of these patients experience infections of the oral mucosa during the course of their disease. Optimal oral hygiene should be encouraged, and aggressive investigation of any oral complaint should be performed as soon as possible to prevent potentially serious oral infectious complications.

The prognosis of a particular patient depends on a number of variables, including the type of leukemia, the age of the patient, and the cytogenetic alterations associated with the disease. In children with **acute lymphoblastic leukemia,** nearly 90% of these patients are now considered to be cured after appropriate treatment. In an adult with the same diagnosis, even though the rate of initial remission induction is 80%, the 5-year survival rate is generally much lower in most reported series.

Patients younger than 60 years of age with **acute myeloid leukemia** have a 5-year survival rate of approximately 40% today. This form of leukemia in a patient older than 60 years, however, has a much poorer prognosis, with less than a 10% chance of survival seen in that population. Similarly, patients with a previous history of myelodysplasia have an unfavorable prognosis.

Even though an indolent period is experienced with **chronic myeloid leukemia,** eventually the neoplastic cells undergo a process known as **blast transformation,** in which they become less differentiated, proliferate wildly, and cause the patient's death within 3–6 months. In the past, the 5-year survival rate for chronic myeloid leukemia was in the 20% range. Today, most centers are reporting 5-year survival rates of approximately 80%, a dramatic improvement presumably because of the effect of tyrosine kinase inhibitor therapy. Additional factors that may play a role in improved survival include diagnosis of the disease at an earlier stage and the availability of better supportive care. Attempts to control chronic myeloid leukemia by bone marrow transplantation from an HLA-matched donor have resulted in 5-year survival rates of 60%–70% in younger patients with this disease. This may be an option for those patients who do not respond to tyrosine kinase inhibitor therapy.

Chronic lymphocytic leukemia is considered to be incurable, but its course is highly variable and depends on the stage of the disease. Patients with limited disease have an average survival time of more than 10 years. Those with more advanced disease survive an average of only 2 years.

◆ LANGERHANS CELL HISTIOCYTOSIS (HISTIOCYTOSIS X; LANGERHANS CELL DISEASE; IDIOPATHIC HISTIOCYTOSIS; EOSINOPHILIC GRANULOMA; LANGERHANS CELL GRANULOMA; LANGERHANS CELL GRANULOMATOSIS)

The term *histiocytosis X* was introduced as a collective designation for a spectrum of rare clinicopathologic disorders characterized by proliferation of histiocyte-like cells that are accompanied by varying numbers of eosinophils, lymphocytes, plasma cells, and multinucleated giant cells. The distinctive histiocytic cells present in this lesion have been identified as Langerhans cells, and the condition is now designated as **Langerhans cell histiocytosis.** In persons under 15 years of age, approximately 5 cases per million are diagnosed annually, however in adults the incidence drops to 1 in a million.

Langerhans cells are dendritic mononuclear cells normally found in the epidermis, mucosa, lymph nodes, and bone marrow. These cells process and present antigens to T lymphocytes. For many years, researchers have debated whether Langerhans cell histiocytosis represents a nonneoplastic condition or a true neoplasm. Studies examining the clonality of the lesional cells of this condition have shown this to be a monoclonal proliferation, a finding that is more consistent with a neoplastic process. *BRAF* or *MAP2K1* mutations have been identified in 40%–60% of Langerhans cell histiocytosis lesions, and these molecular alterations have been implicated in uncontrolled cell division related to several other neoplasms. Investigators have suggested that the varied clinical presentations of this condition may be related to the stage in the development of the Langerhans cell in which the *BRAF* or *MAP2K1* mutation occurs. When the mutation occurs early in the maturation process, a more aggressive, disseminated disease results; if the mutation happens in the later stages of maturation, a more localized, benign lesion develops.

Clinical and Radiographic Features

The clinicopathologic spectrum traditionally considered under the designation of Langerhans cell histiocytosis includes the following:

- Monostotic or polyostotic eosinophilic granuloma of bone—solitary or multiple bone lesions without visceral involvement
- Chronic disseminated histiocytosis—a disease involving bone, skin, and viscera (**Hand-Schüller-Christian disease)**
- Acute disseminated histiocytosis—a disease with prominent cutaneous, visceral, and bone marrow involvement occurring mainly in infants (**Letterer-Siwe disease)**

It is difficult to categorize many patients into one of these classic designations because of overlapping clinical features.

The often-cited Hand-Schüller-Christian triad—bone lesions, exophthalmos, and diabetes insipidus—is present in only a few patients with chronic disseminated disease. It is widely believed that the traditional designations of Hand-Schüller-Christian and Letterer-Siwe disease serve no useful purpose and should be discontinued. Many cases reported as Letterer-Siwe disease in the older literature probably included obscure infections, immunodeficiency syndromes, and malignant histiocytic lesions. Pulmonary Langerhans cell histiocytosis has also been described, but this probably is unrelated to the condition that affects the jaws. Patients who develop pulmonary Langerhans cell histiocytosis are usually adults with a history of smoking, and clonality studies suggest that this is probably a reactive process. The Histiocyte Society, in order to better define prognostic categories of Langerhans cell histiocytosis, has proposed the following classification:

- Single organ involvement—typically bone or skin
  - Unifocal disease
  - Multifocal disease
- Multiorgan involvement
  - No organ dysfunction
  - Organ dysfunction
    - Low-risk (skin, bone, lymph nodes, and/or pituitary gland)
    - High-risk (lung, liver, spleen, and/or bone marrow)

Although Langerhans cell histiocytosis may be encountered in patients over a wide age range, more than 50% of all cases are seen in patients younger than age 15. Although some series have reported a male predilection, overall the sexes appear to be equally affected. Bone lesions, either solitary or multiple, are the most common clinical presentation. Lesions may be found in almost any bone, but the skull, ribs, vertebrae, and mandible are among the most frequent sites. Children younger than age 10 most often have skull and femoral lesions; patients older than age 20 more often have lesions in the ribs, shoulder girdle, and mandible. Adult patients with solitary or multiple bone lesions may have lymphadenopathy but usually do not have significant visceral involvement.

The jaws are affected in 10%–20% of all cases. Dull pain and tenderness often accompany bone lesions. Radiographically, the lesions often appear as sharply punched-out radiolucencies without a corticated rim, but occasionally an ill-defined radiolucency is seen. Bone involvement in the mandible usually occurs in the posterior areas, and a characteristic "scooped out" appearance may be evident when the superficial alveolar bone is destroyed. The resulting bone destruction and loosening of the teeth clinically may resemble severe periodontitis (Fig. 13.20). Extensive alveolar involvement causes the teeth to appear as if they are "floating in air" (Fig. 13.21).

Ulcerative or proliferative mucosal lesions or a proliferative gingival mass may develop if the disease breaks out of bone (Fig. 13.22). Occasionally, this process may involve only the oral soft tissues. Lesions also can occur within the body of the mandible or maxilla, where they may simulate a periapical inflammatory condition.

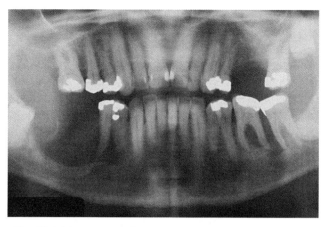

• **Fig. 13.20 Langerhans Cell Histiocytosis.** Severe bone loss in the mandibular molar regions that resembles advanced periodontitis. (Courtesy of Dr. James White.)

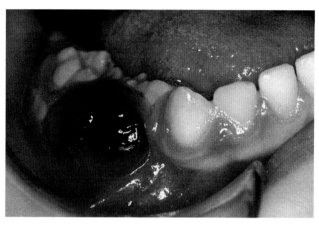

• **Fig. 13.22 Langerhans Cell Histiocytosis**. Clinical photograph of the same patient shown in Fig. 13.21. The lesion has broken out of bone and produced this soft tissue mass.

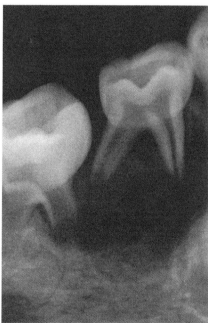

• **Fig. 13.21 Langerhans Cell Histiocytosis.** Periapical radiograph showing marked bone loss involving the mandibular teeth in a young girl, resulting in a "floating-in-air" appearance of the teeth.

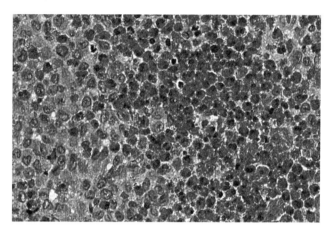

• **Fig. 13.23 Langerhans Cell Histiocytosis.** There is a diffuse infiltrate of pale-staining Langerhans cells intermixed with numerous red granular eosinophils.

Histopathologic Features

The bone lesions of patients with Langerhans cell histiocytosis show a diffuse infiltration of large, pale-staining mononuclear cells that resemble histiocytes. These cells have indistinct cytoplasmic borders and rounded or indented vesicular nuclei. Varying numbers of eosinophils are typically interspersed among the histiocyte-like cells (Fig. 13.23). Plasma cells, lymphocytes, and multinucleated giant cells are often seen, and areas of necrosis and hemorrhage may be present.

The identification of lesional Langerhans cells is necessary to confirm the diagnosis. Because Langerhans cells cannot be differentiated from other histiocytes by routine histologic staining, additional diagnostic methods are required. Electron microscopic evaluation of lesional tissue was the gold standard for many years because, ultrastructurally, Langerhans cells contain rod-shaped cytoplasmic structures known as **Birbeck granules,** which differentiate them from other mononuclear phagocytes (Fig. 13.24). Immunohistochemical procedures are now used to identify the lesional Langerhans cells because of their immunoreactivity with antibodies directed against either CD-1a or CD-207 (langerin), and both markers are specific for Langerhans cell histiocytosis when seen in the correct clinical setting.

Treatment and Prognosis

Because this condition is relatively rare, treatment recommendations are often based on anecdotal experience, rather than randomized controlled trials. Most patients with oral involvement have single organ disease affecting the jaws, although other skeletal lesions may be present. Accessible bone lesions, such as those in the maxilla and mandible, are usually treated by curettage. Low doses of radiation

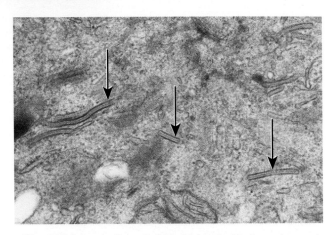

• **Fig. 13.24 Langerhans Cell Histiocytosis.** Electron micrograph showing rod-shaped Birbeck bodies *(black arrows)* in the cytoplasm of a Langerhans cell. (Courtesy of Richard Geissler.)

may be used for less accessible bone lesions, although the potential for induction of malignancy secondary to this treatment is a concern in younger patients. Intralesional injection with corticosteroid agents has also been reported to be effective in some patients with localized bone lesions. Infrequently, the apparent spontaneous regression of localized Langerhans cell histiocytosis has been reported. The prognosis for bone lesions in the absence of significant visceral involvement is generally good; however, progression or dissemination of the disease may occur, particularly for patients who have three or more bones affected.

When multiple organs are involved, the low-risk pattern is often associated with considerable morbidity, but the mortality is much less than that of patients with high-risk organ involvement. Because of the relative rarity of disseminated cases, treatment protocols continue to be refined. Single-agent chemotherapy using prednisolone, etoposide, vincristine, or cyclosporine has produced a good response in a significant percentage of such patients, although recurrence is typically seen in over half of the cases. A combination of vincristine and prednisone, given over the period of a year, seems to reduce this risk of recurrence, particularly in children. Lesions in adults, however, respond much better to low-dose cytarabine (ara-C). Multiple high-risk organ involvement seen in infants and young children may not respond to these more conservative approaches, and multiple chemotherapeutic agents are given in that situation. In addition, hematopoietic stem cell transplantation may be an option. Patients who improve significantly with induction chemotherapy during the first 6 weeks have a much better prognosis (nearly 90% survival) compared to those who do not respond. In that group, only 20%–35% have survived historically. Drugs that specifically target the *BRAF* pathway, such as vemurafenib and dabrafenib, have shown promising initial results in experimental treatment trials examining their impact on multifocal high-risk Langerhans cell histiocytosis. In general, the prognosis is poorer for patients in whom the first sign of the disease develops at a very young age and somewhat better for patients who are older at the time of onset.

◆ HODGKIN LYMPHOMA (HODGKIN DISEASE)

Hodgkin lymphoma represents a malignant lymphoproliferative disorder, although for many years the exact nature of the process was poorly understood. The difficulty in comprehending the character of the condition is reflected in the relatively noncommittal term *Hodgkin disease*, which was used for decades and still may be heard today. Perhaps one reason why Hodgkin lymphoma was not easily understood is that, unlike most malignancies, the neoplastic cells **(Reed-Sternberg cells)** make up only about 0.1%–2% of the cells in the enlarged lymph nodes that characterize this condition. Current evidence regarding the histogenesis of the Reed-Sternberg cell points to a B-lymphocyte origin. Certainly, the disease can cause death if appropriate therapy is not instituted, although the treatment of this malignancy is one of the few major success stories in cancer therapy during the past 30 years. In the United States, Hodgkin lymphoma is about one-tenth as common as non-Hodgkin lymphoma; approximately 8500 cases are diagnosed annually. Although the cause of this disease is unknown, epidemiologic and molecular studies have linked Epstein-Barr virus (EBV) infection to a significant percentage of these lesions.

Clinical Features

Hodgkin lymphoma almost always begins in the lymph nodes, and any lymph node group is susceptible. The most common sites of initial presentation are the cervical and supraclavicular nodes (70%–75%) or the axillary and mediastinal nodes (5%–10% each). The disease initially appears less than 5% of the time in the abdominal and inguinal lymph nodes.

Overall, a male predilection is observed, and a bimodal pattern is noted with respect to the patient's age at diagnosis. One peak is observed between 15 and 35 years of age; another peak is seen after the age of 50.

The usual presenting sign is the identification by the patient of a persistently enlarging, nontender, discrete mass or masses in one lymph node region (Fig. 13.25). In the early stages, the involved lymph nodes are often rather movable; as the condition progresses, the nodes become more matted and fixed to the surrounding tissues. If it is untreated, then the condition spreads to other lymph node groups and eventually involves the spleen and other extralymphatic tissues, such as bone, liver, and lung. Oral involvement has been reported, but it is rare. In about 30%–40% of patients with Hodgkin disease, other systemic signs and symptoms may be present, such as weight loss, fever, night sweats, and generalized pruritus (itching). The absence of these systemic signs and symptoms is considered to be better in terms of the patient's prognosis, and this information is used in staging the disease. Patients who have no systemic signs are assigned to category A and those with systemic signs to category B.

The staging of Hodgkin lymphoma is important for planning treatment and estimating the prognosis for a given

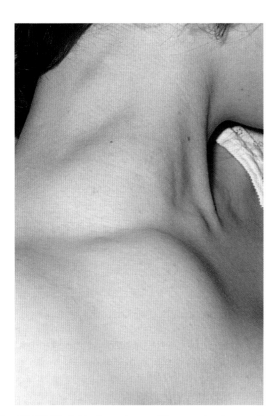

• **Fig. 13.25 Hodgkin Lymphoma.** The prominent supraclavicular and cervical masses represent Hodgkin lymphoma.

TABLE 13.2	Ann Arbor System for Classification of Hodgkin Lymphoma
Stage	Defining Features
I	Involvement of a single lymph node region (I) or a single extralymphatic organ or site (I_E)
II	Involvement of two or more lymph node regions on the same side of the diaphragm (II) or one or more lymph node regions with an extralymphatic site (II_E)
III	Involvement of lymph node regions on both sides of the diaphragm (III), possibly with an extralymphatic organ or site (III_E), the spleen (III_S), or both (III_{SE})
IV	Diffuse or disseminated involvement of one or more extralymphatic organs (identified by symbols), with or without associated lymph node involvement
	A: Absence of systemic signs B: Presence of fever, night sweats, and/or unexplained loss of 10% or more of body weight during the 6-month period before diagnosis

Adapted from Gobbi PG, Ferreri AJM, Ponzoni M, et al: Hodgkin lymphoma, *Crit Rev Oncol Hematol* 85:216–237, 2013.

patient. The staging procedure typically includes confirmation of the pathologic diagnosis, careful history and physical examination, abdominal and thoracic computed tomography (CT) scans or magnetic resonance imaging (MRI) studies, chest radiographs, and routine hematologic studies (e.g., complete blood count, serum chemistries, and erythrocyte sedimentation rate). Evaluation of the extent of disease involvement using (^{18}F)-fluorodeoxyglucose positron emission tomography (FDG PET/CT) scans is now part of the standard protocol, particularly at large institutions. The radiolabeled glucose is given intravenously, and the Hodgkin lymphoma cells metabolize this compound to a much greater extent than the normal tissues, thus identifying sites where tumor is present. Staging procedures that were used in the past, such as lymphangiography, gallium scan, bone marrow biopsy, exploratory laparotomy, and splenectomy, are often not necessary today. A summary of the staging system for Hodgkin lymphoma is presented in Table 13.2.

Histopathologic Features

Hodgkin lymphoma is recognized to comprise two main forms, (1) nodular lymphocyte–predominant Hodgkin lymphoma and (2) classical Hodgkin lymphoma, the latter of which is divided into five subtypes. Although this group of diseases has certain features in common, current immunohistochemical and molecular biologic techniques have allowed distinctions to be made among the various types. The common features include effacement of the normal nodal

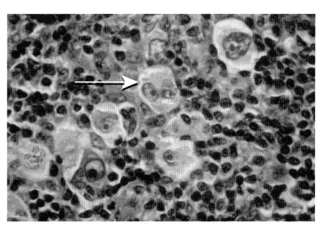

• **Fig. 13.26 Hodgkin Lymphoma.** This high-power photomicrograph shows the characteristic Reed-Sternberg cell *(arrow)* of Hodgkin lymphoma, identified by its "owl-eye" nucleus.

architecture by a diffuse, often mixed, infiltrate of inflammatory cells that is interspersed with large, atypical neoplastic lymphoid cells. In the case of classical Hodgkin lymphoma, this atypical cell is known as a **Reed-Sternberg cell** (Fig. 13.26). The Reed-Sternberg cell is typically binucleated ("owl-eye" nuclei), although it may be multinucleated ("pennies on a plate"), with prominent nucleoli. The malignant cell in nodular lymphocyte–predominant Hodgkin lymphoma is the "popcorn cell," which is so-named because of the resemblance of the nucleus to a kernel of popped corn. The pathologist must see one of these types of distinctive atypical cells to make a diagnosis of Hodgkin lymphoma, although their presence does not automatically imply that diagnosis, because similar cells may be seen in certain viral infections, especially infectious mononucleosis. To summarize, Hodgkin lymphoma is currently classified in the following manner:

- Nodular lymphocyte–predominant Hodgkin lymphoma, or
- Classical Hodgkin lymphoma (comprising five histopathologic subtypes):
  1. Lymphocyte rich
  2. Nodular sclerosis
  3. Mixed cellularity
  4. Lymphocyte depletion
  5. Unclassifiable

These names describe the most prominent histopathologic feature of each type, and specific epidemiologic and prognostic characteristics are associated with each type.

Nodular lymphocyte–predominant Hodgkin lymphoma constitutes 4%–5% of all cases of Hodgkin lymphoma in the United States. In the past, this form was probably combined with the lymphocyte-rich subtype, but the presence of the characteristic popcorn cells is a significant clue to the diagnosis.

Lymphocyte-rich classical Hodgkin lymphoma represents about 6% of all cases. Sheets of small lymphocytes with few Reed-Sternberg cells characterize this form.

The **nodular sclerosis** subtype makes up 60%–80% of cases and occurs more frequently in females during the second decade of life. This type gets its name from the broad fibrotic bands that extend from the lymph node capsule into the lesional tissue. Reed-Sternberg cells in the nodular sclerosis form appear to reside in clear spaces and, therefore, are referred to as *lacunar cells.*

The **mixed cellularity** form accounts for about 15%–30% of the cases and is characterized by a mixture of small lymphocytes, plasma cells, eosinophils, and histiocytes with abundant Reed-Sternberg cells.

The **lymphocyte depletion** subtype, the most aggressive type, makes up less than 1% of the cases in recent reports. Before modern immunohistochemical techniques, many examples of large cell lymphoma or anaplastic T-cell lymphoma were undoubtedly included in this category. In this form of Hodgkin lymphoma, numerous bizarre giant Reed-Sternberg cells are present, with few lymphocytes.

Occasionally, examples of Hodgkin lymphoma are encountered that really do not fit the criteria for any of the known subtypes, and these are designated as **unclassifiable.**

Treatment and Prognosis

The treatment of Hodgkin lymphoma depends on the stage of involvement. In the past, patients who had limited disease (stages I and II) often were managed by local radiation therapy alone. Recent treatment trends, however, combine less extensive radiotherapy fields with milder multiagent chemotherapy regimens to maximize disease control and minimize long-term complications of therapy. Patients with stage III or IV disease require chemotherapy; radiation therapy is used conjointly if significant mediastinal involvement or residual disease is

detected. For many years a regimen known as **MOPP** (mechlorethamine, Oncovin, procarbazine, prednisone) was widely used to treat Hodgkin lymphoma. Because significant long-term side effects can be associated with this chemotherapy, other regimens, known as **ABVD** (Adriamycin, bleomycin, vinblastine, dacarbazine [DTIC]) and **BEACOPP** (bleomycin, etoposide, Adriamycin, cyclophosphamide, vincristine [Oncovin], procarbazine, prednisone), are now used most often because they have fewer complications.

Before modern cancer therapy was developed for Hodgkin lymphoma, the 5-year survival rate was only 5%. The prognosis for this disease is fairly good today; the best treatment results occur in those who present in the early stages. Patients with stage I and II disease often have an 80%–90% relapse-free 10-year survival rate; those with stage III and IV disease have a 55%–75% 10-year survival rate.

The histopathologic subtype of Hodgkin lymphoma appears to have minimal impact on the response to therapy. In the past, researchers believed that the lymphocyte depletion form had a poorer prognosis than the other subtypes. However, with newer immunohistochemical studies, clinicians now realize that many of these cases were misdiagnosed. In most instances, the stage of disease now plays a more important role in determining the patient's prognosis than does the histopathologic subtype.

After 15 years posttreatment, patient mortality is due more often to the complications of therapy: either secondary malignancy or cardiovascular disease. Currently, research is focused on the development of treatment regimens that continue to have a superior cure rate, while simultaneously decreasing the risk of treatment-related complications.

◆ NON-HODGKIN LYMPHOMA

The **non-Hodgkin lymphomas** include a diverse and complex group of malignancies of lymphoreticular histogenesis and differentiation. In most instances, they initially arise within lymph nodes and tend to grow as solid masses. This is in contrast to lymphocytic leukemias (see page 593), which begin in the bone marrow and are characterized by a large proportion of malignant cells that circulate in the peripheral blood. The non-Hodgkin lymphomas most commonly originate from cells of the B-lymphocyte series, with an estimated 85% of European and American lymphoid neoplasms having this derivation. Tumors with a T-lymphocyte derivation are less common, whereas true histiocyte-derived lymphomas are even rarer.

The microscopic appearance of the lesional cells was used in the past to classify the tumors as either *lymphocytic* or *histiocytic.* With the development of modern immunologic techniques, however, it is now known that many of the lesions that had been classified as *histiocytic* were in fact neoplasms composed of transformed B lymphocytes. In the early 1980s, a group of American pathologists devised a classification scheme, known as the *Working Formulation for Clinical Use,* which may still be referred to in the United States. Based on this classification, lymphomas were broadly grouped into three categories:

1. Low grade
2. Intermediate grade
3. High grade

Unfortunately, the Working Formulation has been shown to be somewhat limited in its utility and accuracy. Many lesions that have been recently defined are not included in this classification. For these reasons, an international study group in the early 1990s devised a new method of categorizing the lymphomas, known as the *REAL (revised European-American lymphoma) classification.* With this system, a combination of histopathologic features, immunologic cell surface markers, and gene rearrangement studies are used to organize this group of neoplasms. Further revisions to the World Health Organization (WHO) lymphoma classification system appear periodically as knowledge about this challenging area of pathology accumulates (Box 13.2).

• BOX 13.2 Classification of Hematopoietic and Lymphoid Neoplasms, Modified From the Revised European-American Lymphoma (REAL)/World Health Organization (WHO) Classification

B-Cell Neoplasms

I. Precursor B-cell neoplasm: Precursor B-acute lymphoblastic leukemia/LBL
II. Peripheral (mature) B-cell neoplasms
  A. B-cell chronic lymphocytic leukemia/small lymphocytic lymphoma
  B. B-cell prolymphocytic leukemia
  C. Lymphoplasmacytic lymphoma/immunocytoma
  D. Mantle cell lymphoma
  E. Follicular lymphoma
  F. Extranodal marginal zone B-cell lymphoma of MALT type
  G. Nodal marginal zone B-cell lymphoma (± monocytoid B-cells)
  H. Splenic marginal zone lymphoma (± villous lymphocytes)
  I. Hairy cell leukemia
  J. Plasmacytoma/plasma cell myeloma
  K. Diffuse large B-cell lymphoma
  L. Burkitt lymphoma

T-Cell and Putative NK-Cell Neoplasms

I. Precursor T-cell neoplasm: Precursor T-acute lymphoblastic leukemia/LBL
II. Peripheral (mature) T-cell and NK-cell neoplasms
  A. T-cell chronic lymphocytic leukemia/prolymphocytic leukemia
  B. T-cell granular lymphocytic leukemia
  C. Mycosis fungoides/Sézary syndrome
  D. Peripheral T-cell lymphoma, not otherwise characterized
  E. Hepatosplenic gamma/delta T-cell lymphoma
  F. Subcutaneous panniculitis-like T-cell lymphoma
  G. Angioimmunoblastic T-cell lymphoma
  H. Extranodal T-/NK-cell lymphoma, nasal-type
  I. Enteropathy-type intestinal T-cell lymphoma
  J. Adult T-cell lymphoma/leukemia (HTLV 1+)
  K. Anaplastic large cell lymphoma, primary systemic type
  L. Anaplastic large cell lymphoma, primary cutaneous type
  M. Aggressive NK-cell leukemia

HTLV, human T-lymphotropic virus; *LBL,* lymphoblastic lymphoma; *MALT,* mucosa-associated lymphoid tissue; *NK,* natural killer.

This classification is more precise than the Working Formulation, and currently most pathologists in the United States categorize lymphomas according to the modified REAL system, although some of the more sophisticated molecular studies may not be available at smaller laboratories.

Approximately 77,000 cases of non-Hodgkin lymphoma are diagnosed in the United States annually; slightly more than one-fourth of this number will die of the disease each year. The incidence of this malignancy has been declining slightly in the United States over the past decade. The prevalence of lymphoma is increased in patients who have immunologic problems, such as congenital immunodeficiencies (e.g., Bloom syndrome, Wiskott-Aldrich syndrome, and common variable immunodeficiency), AIDS, organ transplantation, and autoimmune disease (e.g., Sjögren syndrome, systemic lupus erythematosus (SLE), and rheumatoid arthritis).

Viruses may play a role in the pathogenesis of at least some of these lesions. For example, Epstein-Barr virus (EBV) has been implicated, but not proven, to be an etiopathogenic agent in Burkitt lymphoma (see page 606), a type of high-grade, small, noncleaved B-cell lymphoma. EBV is more convincingly related to the development of various lymphoproliferative conditions (known as **EBV-associated lymphoproliferative disorders**) that range from benign, reactive processes through overt malignancies. Some of these occur in the setting of immune senescence (decreased function of the immune system with aging), whereas others are related to immunosuppressive medications (Fig. 13.27), immunosuppression after solid organ or bone marrow transplant, or in association with AIDS (see page 256). Human herpesvirus 8 (HHV-8) has not only been associated with Kaposi sarcoma but also with primary body cavity lymphoma and some cases of plasmablastic lymphoma. The blood-borne human retrovirus, human T-cell leukemia/lymphoma virus type I (HTLV-1), has been shown to cause an aggressive form of peripheral T-cell lymphoma among certain populations in the Caribbean, central Africa, and southwest Japan.

Even bacteria have been shown to induce the formation of so-called **mucosa-associated lymphoid tissue (MALT) lymphoma** of the stomach. Antibiotic treatment of *Helicobacter pylori* infection of the stomach lining often results in complete regression of this low-grade lymphoma.

Clinical and Radiographic Features

Non-Hodgkin lymphoma occurs primarily in adults, although children may be affected, particularly by the more aggressive intermediate- and high-grade lymphomas. The condition most commonly develops in the lymph nodes, but so-called extranodal lymphomas are also found. In the United States, approximately 20%–40% of lymphomas develop in an extranodal site, but in Asian countries such as Korea and Japan, nearly half of all lymphomas are extranodal.

With a nodal presentation, the patient usually is aware of a nontender mass that has been slowly enlarging for months. The lesion typically involves a local lymph node collection, such as the cervical, axillary, or inguinal nodes; one or two freely movable nodules are noticed initially. As the

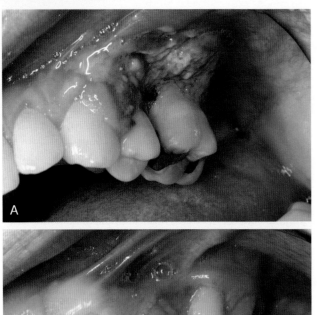

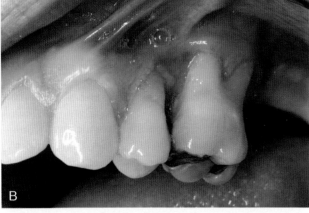

• **Fig. 13.27 Epstein-Barr Virus (EBV)-Associated Lymphoproliferative Disorder. A,** This 42-year-old woman, treated for autoimmune hepatitis with mycophenolate mofetil, developed painful gingival ulcers. **B,** Resolution of the lesion after immune suppression was stopped and rituximab therapy was initiated.

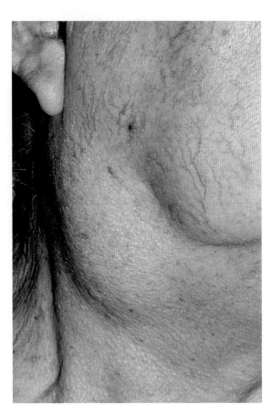

• **Fig. 13.28 Non-Hodgkin Lymphoma.** The matted, nontender lymph node enlargement in the lateral cervical region represents a common presentation of lymphoma.

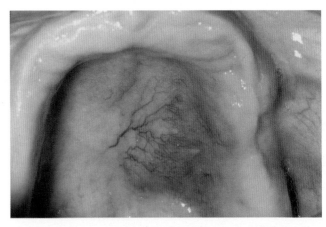

• **Fig. 13.29 Non-Hodgkin Lymphoma.** One of the frequent locations of extranodal lymphoma in the head and neck area is the palate, where the tumor appears as a nontender, boggy swelling. Note the overlying telangiectatic blood vessels, a feature often seen with malignancy.

malignancy progresses, the nodes become more numerous and are fixed to adjacent structures or matted together (Fig. 13.28). Gradually, the process involves other lymph node groups, and invasion of adjoining normal tissues occurs.

In the oral cavity, lymphoma usually appears as extranodal disease. Although the oral lesions of lymphoma are often a component of more widely disseminated disease, at times the lymphoma begins in the oral tissues and has not spread to other sites. The malignancy may develop in the oral soft tissues or centrally within the jaws. Soft tissue lesions appear as nontender, diffuse swellings; they most commonly affect the buccal vestibule, posterior hard palate, or gingiva (Figs. 13.29 and 13.30). Such swellings characteristically have a boggy consistency. The lesion may appear erythematous or purplish, and it may or may not be ulcerated. Patients who wear a denture that contacts the lesional site often complain that their denture does not fit because it feels too tight.

Lymphoma of bone may cause vague pain or discomfort, which might be mistaken for a toothache. The patient may complain of paresthesia, particularly with a mandibular lesion (so-called numb chin syndrome). Radiographs usually show an ill-defined or ragged radiolucency, although in the early stages, the radiographic changes may be subtle or non-existent. If untreated, then the process typically causes

expansion of the bone, eventually perforating the cortical plate and producing a soft tissue swelling. Such lesions have been mistaken for a dental abscess, although a significant amount of pain is not present in most cases.

Clinical staging to determine the extent to which the disease has spread is an important factor in assessing the prognosis for a particular patient. The staging evaluation should include a history, physical examination, complete blood

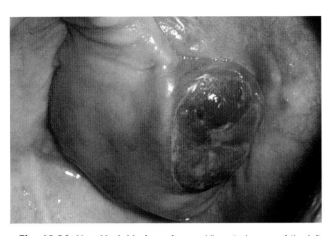

• **Fig. 13.30 Non-Hodgkin Lymphoma.** Ulcerated mass of the left posterior maxilla.

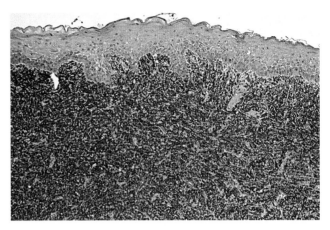

• **Fig. 13.31 Non-Hodgkin Lymphoma.** This low-power photomicrograph shows a diffuse infiltration of the subepithelial connective tissue by lymphoma.

count, liver function studies, CT scans of the thoracic, pelvic and abdominal regions, and bone marrow biopsy. PET/CT scans are also very useful in staging, but this technique often is available only at larger medical centers. PET/CT is also employed to assess response to treatment, in addition to staging. Because of the information obtained with CT or PET/CT imaging, studies such as chest radiographs, lymphangiography, and staging laparotomy are not routinely performed today. The staging system for Hodgkin lymphoma (see Table 13.2) has been widely adopted for use with the non-Hodgkin lymphomas.

Histopathologic Features

Non-Hodgkin lymphomas are histopathologically characterized by a proliferation of lymphocytic-appearing cells that may show varying degrees of differentiation, depending on the type of lymphoma. Low-grade lesions consist of well-differentiated small lymphocytes. High-grade lesions tend to be composed of less differentiated cells. All lymphomas grow as infiltrative, broad sheets of relatively uniform neoplastic cells that usually show little or no evidence of lesional tissue necrosis (Figs. 13.31 and 13.32). In some lesions, particularly those of B-lymphocyte origin, a vague semblance of germinal center formation may be seen (i.e., a *nodular* or *follicular* pattern). Other lymphomas show no evidence of such differentiation, and this pattern is termed *diffuse.* If the lymphoma arises in a lymph node, then the tumor destroys the normal architecture of the node. An extranodal lymphoma destroys the normal adjacent host tissue by infiltrating throughout the area. In the oral cavity, diffuse large B-cell lymphoma, which is considered to be a high-grade lymphoma, is the most common diagnosis, comprising approximately 60% of the cases.

Standard of care demands that appropriate immunohistochemical and cytogenetic studies be performed for a tumor diagnosed as lymphoma. In general, these studies can become quite involved and, therefore, are beyond the scope of this text.

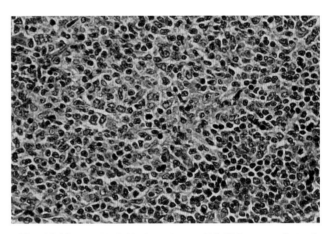

• **Fig. 13.32 Non-Hodgkin Lymphoma.** This high-power photomicrograph shows lesional cells of lymphoma, consisting of a population of poorly differentiated cells of the lymphocytic series with minimal cytoplasm.

Treatment and Prognosis

The treatment of a patient with non-Hodgkin lymphoma is based on several factors, including the type of lymphoma, the stage and grade of the lymphoma, the overall health of the patient, and the patient's pertinent past medical history. The patient's health must be considered because many of the chemotherapeutic regimens are quite debilitating. Surgical management is not usually indicated.

Because most non-Hodgkin lymphomas are of B-cell differentiation, many treatment strategies now incorporate monoclonal antibodies directed against CD20, a B-cell surface antigen, as part of the chemotherapeutic regimen for both low-grade and high-grade lymphomas. Rituximab is one of the more commonly used agents (see Fig. 13.27), although several others are now available. Novel monoclonal antibodies to CD20 and other lymphoid cell surface antigens are continually being developed and examined in clinical trials.

Low-grade (indolent) lymphomas are perhaps the most controversial in terms of treatment. Some authorities recommend no particular treatment because these tumors are slow growing and tend to recur despite chemotherapy. Given the fact that low-grade lymphomas arise in older adults and the median survival without treatment is 8–10 years, many oncologists in the past would opt for a "watch and wait" strategy, treating the patient only if symptoms develop. With the development of rituximab therapy, however, median survival in these patients is now 15 years. Unfortunately, approximately 40% of low-grade lymphomas eventually transform to a high-grade lymphoma, leading to the patient's demise. Because these low-grade lymphomas have been considered "incurable," new treatments are being investigated.

For **high-grade** (aggressive) lymphomas, the treatment of localized disease may consist of radiation plus chemotherapy. With more advanced and disseminated disease, chemotherapy alone usually is implemented. Multiagent chemotherapy is used routinely, and new combinations that include recently developed drugs, such as proteasome inhibitors and thalidomide analogues, are being evaluated continuously. Autologous hematopoietic stem transplantation or allogeneic bone marrow transplantation may also be used in some situations. In recent years, the response rate of many high-grade lymphomas has shown much improvement, although the cure rate generally is not high. Patients with some high-grade lymphomas may have a 60% survival rate at 5 years after diagnosis and treatment.

◆ MYCOSIS FUNGOIDES (CUTANEOUS T-CELL LYMPHOMA)

From its name, one might think that **mycosis fungoides** is a fungal infection. The early dermatologists who first recognized mycosis fungoides knew that this was not the case; however, they still thought the disease resembled a fungal condition. Thus this term has persisted. This condition, in fact, represents a lymphoma that is derived from T lymphocytes, specifically the T-helper (CD4+) lymphocyte. With modern diagnostic techniques, clinicians now know that there are several types of cutaneous lymphomas, each having specific T-lymphocyte or B-lymphocyte differentiation patterns. Even though mycosis fungoides is the most common of these cutaneous lymphomas, it is still a relatively rare malignancy; only about 1300 new cases are diagnosed in the United States annually. This condition exhibits a peculiar property called **epidermotropism** (i.e., a propensity to invade the epidermis of the skin). Oral involvement, although infrequent, may also be present.

Clinical Features

Mycosis fungoides is a condition that usually affects middle-aged adult men; there is a 2:1 male-to-female ratio and a mean age at diagnosis of 55–60 years. African-Americans appear to be affected approximately 1.5 times more frequently than other ethnic groups. The disease progresses through three stages, usually over the course of several years.

The first stage, known as the **eczematous (erythematous) stage,** is often mistaken for psoriasis of the skin because

of the well-demarcated, scaly, erythematous patches that characterize these lesions. Patients may complain of pruritus. With time, the erythematous patches evolve into slightly elevated, red lesions **(plaque stage).** These plaques tend to grow and become distinct papules and nodules. At this time, the disease has entered the **tumor stage** (Fig. 13.33). Visceral involvement is also seen at this point.

Approximately 60 cases of mycosis fungoides with oral involvement have been reported. The most commonly affected sites are the tongue, palate, and gingiva (Fig. 13.34). The buccal mucosa, tonsils, lips, sinuses, and nasopharynx may also be affected. The oral lesions present as erythematous, indurated plaques or nodules that are typically ulcerated. Generally, these lesions appear late in the course of the disease and develop after the cutaneous lesions.

Sézary syndrome is an aggressive expression of mycosis fungoides that essentially represents a dermatopathic T-cell leukemia. The patient has a generalized exfoliative erythroderma, as well as lymphadenopathy, hepatomegaly, and splenomegaly.

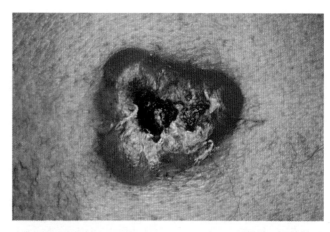

• **Fig. 13.33 Mycosis Fungoides.** In the tumor stage of the disease, patients with mycosis fungoides have ulcerated nodules of the skin. (From Damm DD, White DK, Cibull ML, et al: Mycosis fungoides: initial diagnosis via palatal biopsy with discussion of diagnostic advantages of plastic embedding, *Oral Surg Oral Med Oral Pathol* 58:413–419, 1984.)

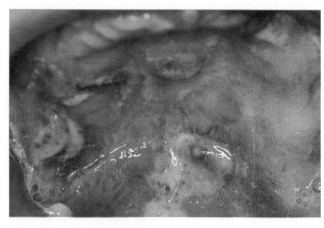

• **Fig. 13.34 Mycosis Fungoides.** The ulcerated palatal lesions represent a rare example of oral mucosal involvement by mycosis fungoides.

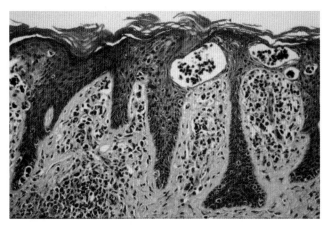

• **Fig. 13.35 Mycosis Fungoides.** This medium-power photomicrograph of a cutaneous lesion of mycosis fungoides shows infiltration of the epithelium by the malignant infiltrate that forms Pautrier microabscesses.

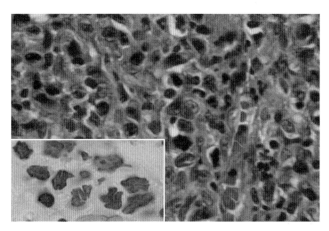

• **Fig. 13.36 Mycosis Fungoides.** This high-power photomicrograph of an oral biopsy specimen reveals the atypical, malignant lymphoid cells of mycosis fungoides that exhibit cerebriform morphology *(inset)*.

The lung, kidneys, and CNS can also be involved. This condition follows a fulminant course and typically results in the patient's death within a short period of time; the median survival for this form of the disease is 2–3 years.

Histopathologic Features

Eczematous Stage

The early stages of mycosis fungoides may be difficult to diagnose histopathologically because of the subtle changes that characterize the initial lesions. A psoriasiform pattern of epithelial alteration is seen, with parakeratin production and elongation of the epithelial rete ridges. Scattered, slightly atypical lymphocytic cells may be seen in the connective tissue papillae, but such features are often mistaken for an inflammatory process.

Plaque Stage

With the development of the plaque stage, a more readily identifiable microscopic pattern emerges. Examination of the surface epithelium reveals infiltration by atypical lymphocytic cells, which are sometimes referred to as *mycosis cells* or *Sézary cells.* These atypical lymphocytes classically form small intraepithelial aggregates termed *Pautrier microabscesses* (Fig. 13.35). The lesional cells have an extremely unusual nucleus because of the marked infolding of the nuclear membrane, which results in what is termed a *cerebriform nucleus.* This feature can best be appreciated when viewed in special semithin, plastic-embedded microscopic sections (Fig. 13.36). The diagnosis of mycosis fungoides can be confirmed by demonstrating positivity for CD4 (a cell surface marker for T-helper cells) in the lesional cell population. In addition, T-cell receptor gene rearrangement analysis should identify a monoclonal population of T lymphocytes. A mixed infiltrate of eosinophils, histiocytes, and plasma cells may be observed in the subepithelial connective tissue.

Tumor Stage

As the condition progresses to the tumor stage, the diffuse infiltration of the dermis and epidermis by atypical lymphocytic cells makes it easier to identify as a malignant process.

Other types of lymphoma would enter into the histopathologic differential diagnosis.

Immunohistochemical studies demonstrating a T-helper phenotype, combined with the T-cell receptor gene rearrangement studies, would help to distinguish the malignant infiltrate from other lymphomas and establish the diagnosis of mycosis fungoides. Examination of the peripheral blood of a patient with Sézary syndrome shows circulating atypical lymphoid cells.

Treatment and Prognosis

Topical nitrogen mustard, topical carmustine, superpotent topical corticosteroids, topical bexarotene (a synthetic retinoid), imiquimod, electron beam therapy, or photochemotherapy (**PUVA** [8-methoxy-**p**soralen + **u**ltra**v**iolet **A**]) are effective in controlling mycosis fungoides during the early stages. Ultimately, the topical forms of therapy fail, and aggressive chemotherapy is necessary, particularly if there is visceral involvement. Newer agents that may be added to the chemotherapy regimen include monoclonal antibodies (alemtuzumab; mogamulizumab), so-called HDAC-inhibitors (vorinostat and romidepsin), certain retinoid compounds (including systemic bexarotene), and specific interferon compounds. If Sézary syndrome develops, then extracorporeal photopheresis or chemotherapy is used as a treatment modality. Extracorporeal photopheresis involves removing of a small amount of the patient's blood and separating the red and white blood cells. The red blood cells are returned to the patient immediately. The white blood cells are mixed with the photoactive drug 8-methoxypsoralen, and are irradiated outside the body (extracorporeal) with ultraviolet A. These altered white cells are then infused back into the patient. Many of the altered white cells undergo apoptosis, but the procedure also may help generate an immunologic response to the patient's own abnormal lymphocytes. Allogeneic stem cell transplantation may also be an option for patients with advanced disease that has failed other treatments.

Although mycosis fungoides is not considered to be curable, the disease is usually slowly progressive. If the condition is identified in an early stage, the median overall survival can range from 20 to 35 years, and patients may die of causes unrelated to their lymphoma. Once the disease progresses beyond the cutaneous involvement, the course becomes much worse. In its later stages, the median overall survival rate typically ranges from 2 to 5 years, with the patient usually dying of organ failure or sepsis.

◆ BURKITT LYMPHOMA

Burkitt lymphoma is a malignancy of B-lymphocyte origin that represents an undifferentiated lymphoma. It was named after the missionary doctor, Denis Burkitt, who first documented the process. In the original report, this type of lymphoma was described in young African children, and it seemed to have a predilection for the jaws. Because it was seen frequently in sub-Saharan Africa, the term **African Burkitt lymphoma** has been applied to the disease. It is now known to have increased prevalence in areas of the world where malaria is also seen, such as northeastern Brazil and New Guinea, and some investigators now refer to such tumors arising in these areas of increased prevalence as **endemic Burkitt lymphoma.** Examination of tumor tissue from the African cases led to the discovery of Epstein-Barr virus (EBV) by virologists in 1964. Although the mechanism is unknown, the pathogenesis of endemic Burkitt lymphoma is undoubtedly related to EBV because more than 90% of the tumor cells show expression of EBV nuclear antigen, and affected patients have elevated antibody titers to EBV. Malarial infection somehow plays a role in endemic Burkitt lymphoma as well, because patients with the highest antibody titers to *Plasmodium falciparum,* the causative organism of malaria, are most likely to develop the malignancy. Tumors with a similar histomorphology, commonly referred to as **sporadic** or **American Burkitt lymphoma,** have been observed in other countries, where the neoplasm is usually first detected as an abdominal mass. EBV is much less frequently identified in the sporadic tumors, however. Some HIV-related lymphomas may also have the microscopic features of Burkitt lymphoma, and these lesions have been designated **immunodeficiency-associated Burkitt lymphoma.** Similar tumors have been reported in other immunodeficiency settings, such as in patients who have received allografts or have a congenital immunodeficiency syndrome. Characteristic cytogenetic chromosomal translocations, which may also be responsible for neoplastic transformation, have been described in all three forms of Burkitt lymphoma.

Clinical and Radiographic Features

As many as 50%–70% of the cases of endemic Burkitt lymphoma present in the jaws. The malignancy usually affects children (peak prevalence, about 7 years of age) who live in Central Africa, and a male predilection is usually reported. The posterior segments of the jaws are more commonly affected, and the maxilla is involved more often than the

mandible (a 2:1 ratio). Sometimes all four quadrants of the jaws show tumor involvement.

The tendency for jaw involvement seems to be age related; nearly 90% of 3-year-old patients have jaw lesions, in contrast to only 25% of patients older than age 15. Sporadic Burkitt lymphoma tends to affect patients over a greater age range than is noted for the African tumor. Although the abdominal region is typically affected, jaw lesions have been reported in sporadic Burkitt lymphoma (Fig. 13.37).

The growth of the tumor mass may produce facial swelling and proptosis. Pain, tenderness, and paresthesia are usually minimal, although marked tooth mobility may be present because of the aggressive destruction of the alveolar bone. Premature exfoliation of deciduous teeth and enlargement of the gingiva or alveolar process may also be seen.

The radiographic features are consistent with a malignant process and include a radiolucent destruction of the bone with ragged, ill-defined margins (Fig. 13.38). This process may begin as several smaller sites, which eventually enlarge and coalesce. Patchy loss of the lamina dura has been mentioned as an early sign of Burkitt lymphoma.

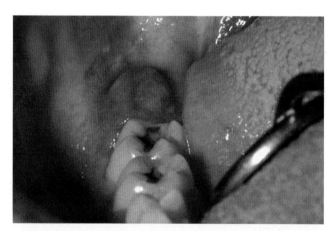

• **Fig. 13.37 Burkitt Lymphoma.** This patient had documented American Burkitt lymphoma involving the abdominal region. The retromolar swelling represents oral involvement with the malignancy.

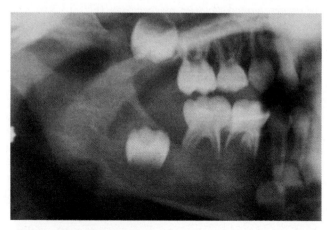

• **Fig. 13.38 Burkitt Lymphoma.** This 4-year-old child had evidence of bone destruction with tooth mobility in all four quadrants of his jaws. Note the patchy, ill-defined loss of bone. (Courtesy of Dr. Gregory Anderson.)

Histopathologic Features

Burkitt lymphoma histopathologically represents an undifferentiated, small, noncleaved B-cell lymphoma. The lesion invades as broad sheets of tumor cells that exhibit round nuclei with minimal cytoplasm. Each tumor nucleus often has several prominent nucleoli, and numerous mitoses are seen. Immunohistochemical studies using markers that identify proliferating cells (e.g., Ki-67) typically indicate that almost 100% of the tumor cells are in the process of replicating. On viewing the lesion on low-power magnification, a classic "starry-sky" pattern is often appreciated—a phenomenon that is caused by the presence of macrophages within the tumor tissue (Fig. 13.39). These macrophages have abundant cytoplasm, which microscopically appears less intensely stained in comparison with the surrounding process. Thus these cells tend to stand out as "stars" set against the "night sky" of deeply hyperchromatic neoplastic lymphoid cells (Fig. 13.40).

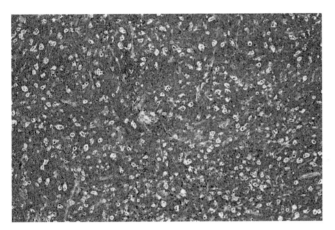

• **Fig. 13.39 Burkitt Lymphoma.** This low-power photomicrograph shows the classic "starry-sky" appearance, a pattern caused by interspersed histiocytic cells with abundant cytoplasm ("stars") set against a background of malignant, darkly staining lymphoma cells ("night sky").

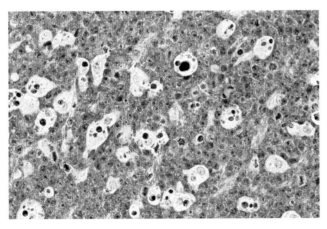

• **Fig. 13.40 Burkitt Lymphoma.** This high-power photomicrograph demonstrates the undifferentiated, small, dark lesional cells with numerous histiocytes.

Because the histopathologic features of Burkitt lymphoma can appear similar to some cases of diffuse large B-cell lymphoma, standard of care now dictates that, in addition to immunohistochemical studies, molecular genetic analysis of the tumor tissue should be performed. This distinction is important because these two malignancies are treated differently. Burkitt lymphoma is characterized by one of several specific translocations, the most common being t(8;14)(q24; q32), that results in overexpression of the oncogene *c-myc,* an event that presumably drives the neoplastic proliferation.

Treatment and Prognosis

Burkitt lymphoma is an aggressive malignancy that usually results in the death of the patient within 4–6 months after diagnosis if it is not treated. In the past, even with treatment, the prognosis for Burkitt lymphoma was poor, with a median survival time of only 10.5 months.

More recently, intensive, multiagent chemotherapeutic protocols, which emphasize the use of high doses of cyclophosphamide, have shown an 85%–95% event-free (no evidence of recurrence) survival rate 3–5 years after treatment for younger patients, particularly those with relatively early, stage I or II, disease. Adults tend to be less tolerant of intensive multiagent chemotherapy; however, a large controlled study has shown that the addition of the monoclonal antibody, rituximab, to a less aggressive multiagent chemotherapeutic regimen can improve the 3-year, event-free survival rate in adults with Burkitt lymphoma to 75%, compared to 62% for those patients who received chemotherapy without rituximab. Relapsed Burkitt lymphoma has a very poor prognosis unfortunately.

◆ EXTRANODAL NK/T-CELL LYMPHOMA, NASAL-TYPE (ANGIOCENTRIC T-CELL LYMPHOMA; MIDLINE LETHAL GRANULOMA; IDIOPATHIC MIDLINE DESTRUCTIVE DISEASE; POLYMORPHIC RETICULOSIS; MIDLINE MALIGNANT RETICULOSIS; ANGIOCENTRIC IMMUNOPROLIFERATIVE LESION)

Extranodal NK/T-cell lymphoma, nasal-type is a rare malignancy that is characterized clinically by aggressive, nonrelenting destruction of the midline structures of the palate and nasal fossa. For many decades, the nature of this process was controversial, a fact that can readily be appreciated by the wide variety of terms by which it has been called. In actuality, many of the cases reported as "midline lethal granuloma" in the past represented a wide variety of immunologic (e.g., Wegener granulomatosis) and infectious (e.g., tertiary syphilis) diseases. The term **midline lethal granuloma** should be used only as a descriptive designation of a destructive midline condition, and thorough diagnostic evaluation, including biopsy and culture, is necessary to make a definitive diagnosis. Once the other causes of midline destruction have been eliminated, in most cases this disorder can be identified as a *natural killer (NK)/T-cell lymphoma,* based on modern cytogenetic, immunologic, and molecular studies. Epstein-Barr virus (EBV) is thought to play a significant role in the pathogenesis of this malignancy, and by the WHO criteria, *in situ* evidence of EBV in the lesional cells is necessary to make this diagnosis. The difficulty in distinguishing among these destructive disorders can be appreciated by the fact that **lymphomatoid granulomatosis,** which had been considered part of this T-cell lymphoma spectrum, is now known to be an EBV-driven proliferation of B lymphocytes.

Even though extranodal NK/T-cell lymphoma often does not have the classic histopathologic features of lymphoma microscopically, it behaves in a malignant fashion and responds to the same treatments to which lymphomas respond. For reasons that are unclear, this condition is seen with greater frequency in Asian, Guatemalan, and Peruvian populations.

Clinical Features

Extranodal NK/T-cell lymphoma is typically observed in adults, and a male predilection is noted in most case series. The initial signs and symptoms are often localized to the nasal region and include nasal stuffiness or epistaxis. Pain may accompany the nasal symptoms. Swelling of the soft palate or posterior hard palate may precede the formation of a deep, necrotic ulceration, which usually occupies a midline position. This ulceration enlarges and destroys the palatal tissues, which typically creates an oronasal fistula (Fig. 13.41). Secondary infection may complicate the course of the disease, and life-threatening hemorrhage is a potential problem in some instances.

Histopathologic Features

Histopathologic examination of one of these lesions shows a mixed infiltrate of a variety of inflammatory cells, often arranged around blood vessels (angiocentric) (Fig. 13.42).

The lesional process appears to invade and destroy the normal tissue in the area. Necrosis is often present in some areas of the lesion, presumably secondary to infiltration of the blood vessels by the tumor cells. Medium to large, angular, lymphocytic cells with an atypical appearance are usually identified as a component of the cellular infiltrate. Immunohistochemical evaluation of this infiltrate shows that the atypical cells mark with antibodies directed against either NK-cell antigens (such as CD56) or T-lymphocyte antigens (such as CD3). Probes for EBV-encoded RNA (EBER) should label nearly all of the tumor cells as well. Molecular genetic studies may show monoclonal gene rearrangements of the T-lymphocyte receptor, consistent with a lymphoreticular malignancy, in those tumors that have T-cell, rather than NK-cell, differentiation.

Treatment and Prognosis

Without treatment, extranodal NK/T-cell lymphoma is a relentlessly progressive, highly destructive process that ultimately leads to the patient's death by secondary infection,

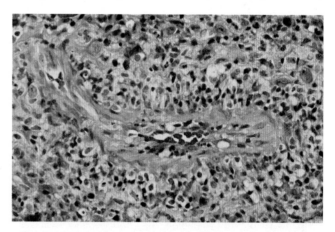

• **Fig. 13.42 Extranodal NK/T-Cell Lymphoma, Nasal-Type.** This medium-power photomicrograph shows atypical lymphoid cells infiltrating the wall and filling the lumen of a blood vessel. Such a pattern is termed *angiocentric* (i.e., around blood vessels).

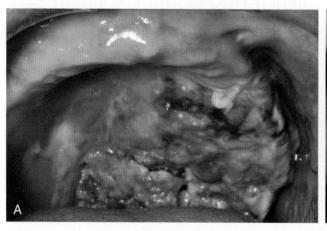

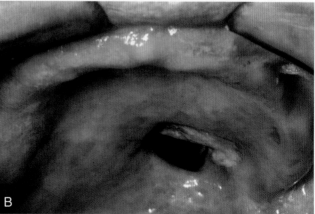

• **Fig. 13.41 Extranodal NK/T-Cell Lymphoma, Nasal-Type. A,** This 62-year-old man had a destructive palatal lesion that proved to be a T-cell lymphoma, and evaluation showed cervical lymph node involvement as well. **B,** Resolution of the lesion 1 month later, after multiagent chemotherapy.

massive hemorrhage, or infiltration of vital structures in the area. Lesions that are localized usually respond to radiation therapy, a feature that is similar to that of T-cell lymphomas of other sites. Treatment with 40–50 Gy will appear to control the disease, although dissemination of the lesion develops in approximately 30% of these patients. Similarly, multiagent chemotherapy that includes anthracyclines results in relapse. Concurrent or sequential radiation therapy, in conjunction with a multidrug chemotherapeutic regimen that includes a platinum compound or pegylated asparaginase, is now recommended. Five-year survival rates are usually reported to be in the range of 65%–85%. For patients with more disseminated disease, combination chemotherapy is indicated, and a less favorable prognosis can be expected, with 30%–50% 5-year survival generally reported.

◆ MULTIPLE MYELOMA

Multiple myeloma is a relatively uncommon malignancy of plasma cell origin that often appears to have a multicentric origin within bone. The cause of the condition is unknown, although sometimes a plasmacytoma (see page 611) may evolve into multiple myeloma. This disease makes up about 1% of all malignancies and 10%–15% of hematologic malignancies. If metastatic disease is excluded, then multiple myeloma accounts for nearly 50% of all malignancies that involve the bone. Over 32,000 cases are diagnosed annually in the United States.

The abnormal plasma cells that compose this tumor are typically monoclonal. The abnormal cells probably arise from a single malignant precursor that has undergone uncontrolled mitotic division and has spread throughout the body. Because the neoplasm develops from a single cell, all of the daughter cells that comprise the lesional tissue have the same genetic makeup and produce the same proteins. These proteins are the immunoglobulin components that the plasma cell would normally produce, although in the case of this malignant tumor the immunoglobulins are not normal or functional. The signs and symptoms of this disease result from the uncontrolled proliferation of the tumor cells and the uncontrolled manufacture of their protein products.

Clinical and Radiographic Features

Multiple myeloma is typically a disease of adults, with men being affected slightly more often than women. The median age at diagnosis is between 60 and 70 years, and it is rarely diagnosed before age 40. For reasons that are not understood, the disease occurs twice as frequently in blacks as whites, making this the most common hematologic malignancy among black persons in the United States.

Bone pain, particularly in the lumbar spine, is the most characteristic presenting symptom. Some patients experience pathologic fractures caused by tumor destruction of bone. They may also complain of fatigue as a consequence of myelophthisic anemia. Petechial hemorrhages of the skin and oral mucosa may be seen if platelet production has been affected. Fever may be present as a result of neutropenia with increased susceptibility to infection. Metastatic calcifications may involve the soft tissues and are thought to be caused by hypercalcemia secondary to tumor-related osteolysis.

Radiographically, multiple well-defined, punched-out radiolucencies or ragged radiolucent lesions may be seen in multiple myeloma (Fig. 13.43). These may be especially evident on a skull film. Although any bone may be affected, the jaws have been reported to be involved in as many as 30% of cases. The radiolucent areas of the bone contain the abnormal plasma cell proliferations that characterize multiple myeloma.

Renal failure may be a presenting sign in these patients because the kidneys become overburdened with the excess circulating light chain proteins of the tumor cells. These light chain products, which are found in the urine of 30%–50% of patients with multiple myeloma, are called **Bence Jones proteins,** after the British physician who first described them in detail.

Approximately 10%–15% of patients with multiple myeloma show deposition of amyloid (see page 824) in various soft tissues of the body, and this may be the initial manifestation of the disease. Amyloid deposits are due to the accumulation of the abnormal light chain proteins. A recent study found that approximately 3% of newly diagnosed multiple myeloma patients presented with oral mucosal amyloid deposition. The tongue is the oral site that is most common affected, typically showing diffuse enlargement and firmness. A nodular pattern may also involve tongue, and sometimes the nodules are ulcerated. Another area that is commonly

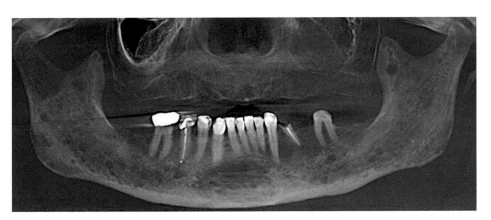

• **Fig. 13.43 Multiple Myeloma.** Multiple myeloma affecting the mandible. The disease produced multiple, small, "punch-out" radiolucencies. (Courtesy of Dr. Matthew D'Addario.)

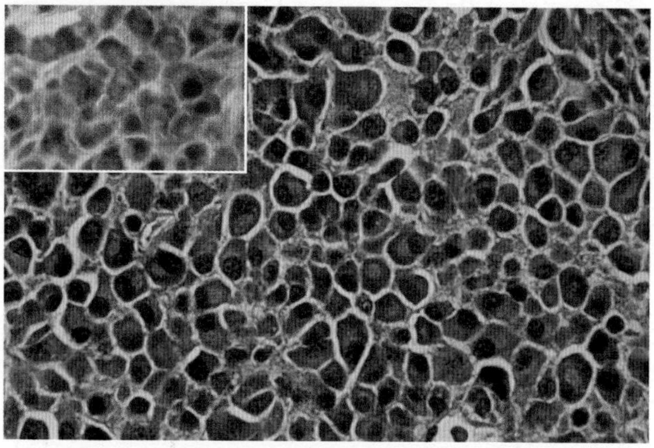

• **Fig. 13.44 Multiple Myeloma.** This high-power photomicrograph reveals sheets of malignant plasma cells with eccentric nuclei and stippled nuclear chromatin. Immunohistochemical studies *(inset)* show a uniform reaction of the lesional cells for antibodies directed against kappa light chains, indicating a monoclonal neoplastic proliferation.

affected is the periorbital skin, with the amyloid deposits appearing as waxy, firm, plaquelike lesions (see Fig. 17.7 on page 825).

Histopathologic Features

Histopathologic examination of the lesional tissue in multiple myeloma shows diffuse, monotonous sheets of neoplastic, variably differentiated, plasmacytoid cells that invade and replace the normal host tissue (Fig. 13.44). Mitotic activity may be seen with some frequency. The monoclonality of the plasma cell population can be demonstrated using antibodies directed against the lambda and kappa light chain components of the immunoglobulin molecule. In a neoplastic proliferation of plasma cells, virtually all of the lesional cells will mark with only one of these antibodies. In contrast, a reactive plasma cell infiltrate will show a mixture of lambda- and kappa-producing plasma cells. Occasionally, deposition of amyloid may be observed in association with the neoplastic cells. Like other types of amyloid, this material appears homogeneous, eosinophilic, and relatively acellular. It stains metachromatically with crystal violet and shows an affinity for Congo red, demonstrating apple-green birefringence on viewing with polarized light. A biopsy specimen of bone marrow from a patient with multiple myeloma should show at least 10% atypical plasma cells making up the marrow cell population.

Diagnosis

Although the histopathologic and radiographic findings may strongly suggest a diagnosis of multiple myeloma, screening of the serum or urine by protein electrophoresis should be performed. If an abnormality is detected, then this should be confirmed by protein immunoelectrophoresis, which is a more sensitive test, as an additional parameter to establish the diagnosis. The serum and urine protein immunoelectrophoresis should show the presence of myeloma protein (M-protein). This represents the massive over-production of one abnormal immunoglobulin by the neoplastic clone of plasma cells, thus this feature is termed **monoclonal gammopathy.**

This monoclonal protein consists of two heavy chain polypeptides of the same immunoglobulin (Ig) class (IgA, IgG, IgM, IgD, or IgE) and one of two light chain polypeptides of the same class (kappa or lambda). Occasionally, the neoplastic cells produce only the light chain component.

Treatment and Prognosis

The goals of treatment related to multiple myeloma include not only controlling the malignancy but also making the patient comfortable and prolonging the patient's survival. Initial attempts to control multiple myeloma generally consist of chemotherapy. Several combinations of chemotherapeutic agents are available, and the choice of which regimen to use in a particular patient often depends on the cytogenetic profile of their myeloma cells. The cytogenetic profile identifies the presence or absence of any of several chromosomal translocations, deletions, or trisomies of patient's tumor, which predicts a low-, standard-, intermediate- or high-risk of progression of the malignancy. Detailed discussion of the treatment of multiple myeloma is beyond the scope of this text, however the drugs that are used to treat this disease typically include a corticosteroid (usually dexamethasone or prednisone) in addition to one or more other drugs, such as an alkylating agent (melphalan or cyclophosphamide), an immune-modulating agent (thalidomide, lenalidomide, or pomalidomide), a proteasome inhibitor (bortezomib, carfilzomib, or ixazomib), or a monoclonal antibody (elotuzumab, daratumumab, or isatuximab). Usually the malignancy responds to the multidrug therapy, however relapse is common, and autologous stem cell transplantation is then performed. More aggressive chemotherapeutic regimens, as well as allogeneic bone marrow transplantation, may be considered in otherwise healthy patients under the age of 55–65 years, but these individuals comprise a minority of multiple myeloma patients. Radiation therapy is useful only as palliative treatment for painful bone lesions. Any one of several bisphosphonate medications (clodronate, pamidronate, or zoledronic acid) can be prescribed to reduce the possibility of myeloma-related fracture with its attendant pain, but these medications do not increase survival. A small percentage of these patients may experience the complication of medication-related osteonecrosis of the jaws (see page 286), and many oncology centers insist that myeloma patients receive a complete oral examination in order to identify and resolve any potential conditions that could predispose to jaw infection.

While it is unlikely that multiple myeloma can be cured, the prognosis varies considerably among affected individuals. A variety of factors play a role in predicting prognosis, with younger patients tending to do better than older ones. Patients with other systemic diseases have a worse prognosis, as do patients who present with more widespread lesions, and patients who do not respond well to initial therapy. As mentioned earlier, the prognosis is also dependent on certain chromosomal and molecular genetic features, with hyperdiploid lesions being more aggressive, as well as those with certain chromosomal translocations.

Patients who fall in the standard-risk category can expect to have a median survival rate of 6–7 years following diagnosis, whereas those who are high-risk can expect a median survival of 2–3 years. These figures, while not encouraging at first glance, are much improved compared to just two to three decades ago, when a 10% 5-year survival was typical.

◆ PLASMACYTOMA

The **plasmacytoma** is a unifocal, monoclonal, neoplastic proliferation of plasma cells that usually arises within bone. Infrequently, it is seen in soft tissue, in which case, the term **extramedullary plasmacytoma** is used. Some investigators believe that this lesion represents the least aggressive part of a spectrum of plasma cell neoplasms that extends to **multiple myeloma.** Therefore, the plasmacytoma is important because it may ultimately give rise to the more serious problem of multiple myeloma.

Clinical and Radiographic Features

The plasmacytoma usually is detected in an adult male, with an average age at diagnosis of 55 years. The male-to-female ratio is approximately 2:1. Most of the lesions present centrally within a single bone, and the spine is the most commonly involved site. About one-third of the cases are reported in that location. The initial symptoms often relate to swelling or bone pain; occasionally, however, this lesion is detected on routine radiographic examination. The extramedullary plasmacytoma appears as a relatively nondescript, well-circumscribed, nontender soft tissue mass. A slightly stronger male predilection is seen with this lesion, approaching a 3:1 male-to-female ratio. Approximately 25% of extramedullary plasmacytomas develop in the head and neck region, and such lesions have been reported in the tonsils, the nasopharynx, the paranasal sinuses, the nose, and the parotid gland.

Radiographically, the lesion may be seen as a well-defined, unilocular radiolucency with no evidence of sclerotic borders or as a ragged radiolucency similar to the appearance of multiple myeloma (Fig. 13.45). No other lesions should be identifiable by a skeletal survey using MRI, PET/CT, and careful physical examination, however.

Histopathologic Features

The histopathologic features of the plasmacytoma are identical to those of multiple myeloma. Sheets of plasma cells show varying degrees of differentiation. Immunohistochemical studies demonstrate that these plasma cells are monoclonal. As many as 25%–50% of these patients also show a monoclonal gammopathy on evaluation by serum protein immunoelectrophoresis, although the amount of abnormal protein is much less than that seen with multiple myeloma. Solitary plasmacytoma also differs from multiple myeloma in that no evidence of plasma cell infiltration should be seen by a random bone marrow biopsy, and the patient should not show signs of anemia, hypercalcemia, or renal failure.

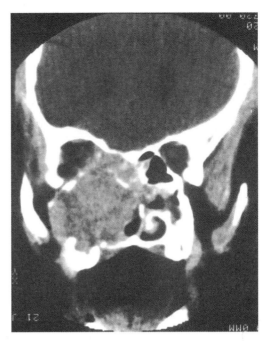

• **Fig. 13.45 Plasmacytoma.** This computed tomography (CT) scan depicts a solitary plasmacytoma involving the left maxillary sinus and nasal cavity.

Immunohistochemically, extramedullary plasmacytoma appears to differ from its intrabony counterparts in that it shows a marked decrease or lack of immunoreactivity for antibodies directed against cyclin D1 and CD56.

Treatment and Prognosis

Plasmacytomas are usually treated with radiation therapy, and typically a dose of at least 40 Gy is delivered to the tumor site. A few lesions have been surgically excised with good results, although this is not the preferred treatment in most instances. PET/CT is typically used to determine the efficacy of therapy, based on the marked reduction in metabolic activity at the tumor site. Unfortunately, when patients with plasmacytoma of bone are observed on a long-term basis, most will eventually develop multiple myeloma. From 65%–85% show evidence of disseminated disease by 10 years after their initial diagnosis. However, virtually all of these patients will develop multiple myeloma by 15 years following their diagnosis. Extramedullary plasmacytoma seems to have a much better prognosis, with less than 30% of these patients showing progression to multiple myeloma and 70% having a 10-year disease-free period after treatment.

Bibliography

Lymphoid Hyperplasia

Jham BC, Binmadi NO, Scheper MA, et al.: Follicular hyperplasia of the palate: case report and literature review, *J Craniomaxillofac Surg* 37:79–82, 2009.

Kolokotronis A, Dimitrakopoulos I, Asimaki A: Follicular lymphoid hyperplasia of the palate: report of a case and review of the literature, *Oral Surg Oral Med Oral Pathol Oral Radiol Endod* 96:172–175, 2003.

Menasce LP, Shanks JH, Banerjee SS, et al.: Follicular lymphoid hyperplasia of the hard palate and oral mucosa: report of three cases and a review of the literature, *Histopathology* 39:353–358, 2001.

Wright J, Dunsworth A: Follicular lymphoid hyperplasia of the hard palate: a benign lymphoproliferative process, *Oral Surg Oral Med Oral Pathol* 55:162–168, 1983.

Hemophilia

Almazrooa S, Binmadi N, Khalifa H, et al.: A progressively enlarging swelling in the mandible, *Oral Surg Oral Med Oral Pathol Oral Radiol* 123:283–287, 2017.

Argyris PP, Anim SO, Koutlas IG: Maxillary pseudotumor as initial manifestation of von Willebrand disease, type 2: report of a rare case and literature review, *Oral Surg Oral Med Oral Pathol Oral Radiol* 121:e27–e31, 2016.

Ben-Ami T, Revel-Vilk S: The use of DDAVP in children with bleeding disorders, *Pediatr Blood Cancer* 60:S42–S43, 2013.

Berntorp E, Shapiro AD: Modern haemophilia care, *Lancet* 379:1447–1456, 2012.

Bhat R, Cabey W: Evaluation and management of congenital bleeding disorders, *Hematol Oncol Clin North Am* 31:1105–1122, 2017.

Blanco-Carrion J, Liñares-Gonzalez A, Batalla-Vazquez P, et al.: Morbidity and economic complications following mucogingival surgery in a hemophiliac HIV-infected patient: a case report, *J Periodontol* 75:1413–1416, 2004.

Chattopadhyay PK, Nagori SA, Menon RP, et al.: Hemophilic pseudotumor of the mandible in a patient with hemophilia B, *Oral Maxillofac Surg* 21:467–469, 2017.

Cox DP, Solar A, Huang J, et al.: Pseudotumor of the mandible as first presentation of hemophilia in a 2-year-old male: a case report and review of jaw pseudotumors of hemophilia, *Head Neck Pathol* 5:226–232, 2011.

Croteau SE: Evolving complexity in hemophilia management, *Pediatr Clin North Am* 65:407–425, 2018.

Doyle AJ, Back DL, Austin S: Characteristics and management of the haemophilia-associated pseudotumours, *Haemophilia* 26:33–40, 2020.

Escobar MA, Brewer A, Caviglia H, et al.: Recommendations on multidisciplinary management of elective surgery in people with haemophilia, *Haemophilia* 24:693–702, 2018.

Evatt BL: The AIDS epidemic in haemophilia patients II: pursuing absolute viral safety of clotting factor concentrates 1985-1988, *Haemophilia* 18:649–654, 2012.

Federici AB, Berntorp E, Lee CA: The 80th anniversary of von Willebrand's disease: history, management and research, *Haemophilia* 12:563–572, 2006.

Fijnvandraat K, Cnossen MH, Leebeek FWG, et al.: Diagnosis and management of haemophilia, *Br Med J* 344, 2012, e2707.

Gröner A: Pathogen safety of plasma-derived products—Haemate/Humate-P, *Haemophilia* 14(Suppl 5):54–71, 2008.

Heiland M, Weber M, Schmelzle R: Life-threatening bleeding after dental extraction in a hemophilia A patient with inhibitors to factor VIII: a case report, *J Oral Maxillofac Surg* 61:1350–1353, 2003.

Izumi Y, Taniguchi T, Maruyama Y, et al.: Effective periodontal treatment in a patient with type IIA von Willebrand's disease: report of a case, *J Periodontol* 70:548–553, 1999.

Kizilocak H, Young G: Diagnosis and treatment of hemophilia, *Clin Adv Hematol Oncol* 17:344–351, 2019.

Laguna P, Klukowska A: Management of oral bleedings with recombinant factor VIIa in children with haemophilia A and inhibitor, *Haemophilia* 11:2–4, 2005.

Lofqvist T, Nilsson IM, Berntorp E, et al.: Haemophilia prophylaxis in young patients—a long-term follow-up, *J Intern Med* 241:395–400, 1997.

Mahlangu J: Emicizumab for the prevention of bleeds in hemophilia A, *Expert Opin Biol Ther* 19:753–761, 2019.

Mannucci PM: Treatment of von Willebrand's disease, *N Engl J Med* 351:683–694, 2004.

O'Brien SH, Saini S: von Willebrand disease in pediatrics: evaluation and management, *Hematol Oncol Clin North Am* 33:425–438, 2019.

Perrin GQ, Herzog RW, Markusic DM: Update on clinical gene therapy for hemophilia, *Blood* 133:407–414, 2019.

Pruthi RK: Hemophilia: a practical approach to genetic testing, *Mayo Clin Proc* 80:1485–1499, 2005.

Rogaev EI, Grigorenko AP, Faskhutdinova G, et al.: Genotype analysis identifies the cause of the "Royal Disease", *Science* 326:817, 2009.

Smith JA: Hemophilia: what the oral and maxillofacial surgeon needs to know, *Oral Maxillofac Surg Clin North Am* 28:481–489, 2016.

Swystun LL, James PD: Genetic diagnosis in hemophilia and von Willebrand disease, *Blood Rev* 31:47–56, 2017.

van Galen KPM, Engelen ET, Mauser-Bunschoten EP, et al.: Antifibrinolytic therapy for preventing oral bleeding in patients with haemophilia or Von Willebrand disease undergoing minor oral surgery or dental extractions, *Cochrane Database Syst Rev* (12):CD011385, 2015. https://doi.org/10.1002/14651858.CD011385.pub2.

Plasminogen Deficiency

Celkan T: Plasminogen deficiency, *J Thromb Thrombolysis* 43:132–138, 2017.

Chi AC, Prichard E, Richardson MS, et al.: Pseudomembranous disease (ligneous inflammation) of the female genital tract, peritoneum, gingiva, and paranasal sinuses associated with plasminogen deficiency, *Ann Diagn Pathol* 13:132–139, 2009.

Cohen J, Cohen S, Cymberknoh MC, et al.: Laryngeal obstruction in congenital plasminogen deficiency, *Pediatr Pulmonol* 47:923–925, 2012.

Fine G, Bauer K, Al-Mohaya M, et al.: Successful treatment of ligneous gingivitis with warfarin, *Oral Surg Oral Med Oral Pathol Oral Radiol Endod* 107:77–80, 2009.

Gokbuget AY, Mutlu S, Scully C, et al.: Amyloidaceous ulcerated gingival hyperplasia: a newly described entity related to ligneous conjunctivitis, *J Oral Pathol Med* 26:100–104, 1997.

Mehta R, Shapiro AD: Plasminogen deficiency, *Haemophilia* 14:1261–1268, 2008.

Sadasivan A, Ramesh R, Mathew DG: Ligneous periodontitis in a patient with type 1 plasminogen deficiency: a case report and review of the literature, *Case Rep Dent*, 2020, 5680535. https://doi.org/10.1155/2020/5680535.

Schuster V, Seregard S: Ligneous conjunctivitis, *Surv Ophthalmol* 48:369–388, 2003.

Scully C, Gokbuget AY, Allen C, et al.: Oral lesions indicative of plasminogen deficiency (hypoplasminogenemia), *Oral Surg Oral Med Oral Pathol Oral Radiol Endod* 91:334–337, 2001.

Shapiro AD, Nakar C, Parker JM, et al.: Plasminogen replacement therapy for the treatment of children and adults with congenital plasminogen deficiency, *Blood* 131:1301–1310, 2018.

Shapiro AD, Menegatti M, Palla R, et al.: An international registry of patients with plasminogen deficiency (HISTORY), *Haematologica* 105:554–561, 2020.

Sivolella S, De Biagi M, Sartori MT, et al.: Destructive membranous periodontal disease (ligneous gingivitis): a literature review, *J Periodontol* 83:465–476, 2012.

Tefs K, Gueorguieva M, Klammt J, et al.: Molecular and clinical spectrum of type I plasminogen deficiency: a series of 50 patients, *Blood* 108:3021–3026, 2006.

Tu Y, Gonzalez-Gronow M, Kolomeyer AM, et al.: Adult-onset ligneous conjunctivitis with detection of a novel plasminogen gene mutation and anti-plasminogen IgA antibody: a clinicopathologic study and review of literature, *Semin Ophthalmol* 31:526–531, 2016.

Watts P, Suresh P, Mezer E, et al.: Effective treatment of ligneous conjunctivitis with topical plasminogen, *Am J Ophthalmol* 133:451–455, 2002.

Anemia

Cullis JO: Diagnosis and management of anaemia of chronic disease: current status, *Br J Haematol* 154:289–300, 2011.

Green R: Anemias beyond B12 and iron deficiency: the buzz about other B's, elementary, and nonelementary problems, *Hematology Am Soc Hematol Educ Program* 2012:492–498, 2012.

Groopman JE, Itri LM: Chemotherapy-induced anemia in adults: incidence and treatment, *J Natl Cancer Inst* 91:1616–1634, 1999.

Halwachs-Baumann G: Diagnosis of anaemia: old things rearranged, *Wien Med Wochenschr* 162:478–488, 2012.

Koury MJ, Rhodes M: How to approach chronic anemia, *Hematology Am Soc Hematol Educ Program* 2012:183–190, 2012.

Powell DJ, Achebe MO: Anemia for the primary care physician, *Prim Care* 43:527–542, 2016.

Remuzzi G, Ingelfinger JR: Correction of anemia—payoffs and problems, *N Engl J Med* 355:2144–2146, 2006.

Richards T: Anaemia in hospital practice, *Br J Hosp Med* 73:571–575, 2012.

Tefferi A: Anemia in adults: a contemporary approach to diagnosis, *Mayo Clin Proc* 78:1274–1280, 2003.

Vieth JT, Lane DR: Anemia, *Hematol Oncol Clin North Am* 31:1045–1060, 2017.

Sickle Cell Anemia

Blair HA: Crizanlizumab: first approval, *Drugs* 80:79–84, 2020.

Carden MA, Little J: Emerging disease-modifying therapies for sickle cell disease, *Haematologica* 104:1710–1719, 2019.

Goyal S, Tisdale J, Schmidt M, et al.: Acute myeloid leukemia case after gene therapy for sickle cell disease, *N Engl J Med* 386:138–147, 2022.

Hamdoun E, Davis L, McCrary SJ, et al.: Bilateral mental nerve neuropathy in an adolescent during sickle cell crises, *J Child Neurol* 27:1028–1041, 2012.

Hoppe C, Neumayr L: Sickle cell disease: monitoring, current treatment, and therapeutics under development, *Hematol Oncol Clin North Am* 33:355–371, 2019.

Houwing ME, de Pagter PJ, van Beers EJ, et al.: Sickle cell disease: clinical presentation and management of a global health challenge, *Blood Rev* 37, 2019, 100580.

Meier ER: Treatment options for sickle cell disease, *Pediatr Clin North Am* 65:427–443, 2018.

Pecker LH, Lanzkron S: Sickle cell disease, *Ann Intern Med* 174:ITC1–ITC16, 2021.

Piel FB, Steinberg MH, Rees DC: Sickle cell disease, *N Engl J Med* 376:1561–1573, 2017.

Ribeil J-A, Hacein-Bey-Abina S, Payen E, et al.: Gene therapy in a patient with sickle cell disease, *N Engl J Med* 376:848–855, 2017.

Souza SFC, de Carvalho HLCC, Costa CPS, et al.: Association of sickle cell haemoglobinopathies with dental and jaw bone abnormalities, *Oral Dis* 24:393–403, 2018.

Sundd P, Gladwin MT, Novelli EM: Pathophysiology of sickle cell disease, *Annu Rev Pathol* 14:263–292, 2019.

Vanderhave KL, Perkins CA, Scannell B, et al.: Orthopaedic manifestations of sickle cell disease, *J Am Acad Orthop Surg* 26:94–101, 2018.

Vichinsky E, Hoppe CC, Ataga KI, et al.: A phase 3 randomized trial of voxelotor in sickle cell disease, *N Engl J Med* 381:509–519, 2019.

Watanabe M, Saito N, Nadgir RN, et al.: Craniofacial bone infarcts in sickle cell disease: clinical and radiological manifestations, *J Comput Assist Tomogr* 37:91–97, 2013.

Thalassemia

Akcalıa A, Yıldıza MS, Akcalıc Z, et al.: Periodontal condition of patients with Thalassemia Major: a systematic review and meta-analysis, *Arch Oral Biol* 102:113–121, 2019.

Bollig C, Schell LK, Rücker G, et al.: Deferasirox for managing iron overload in people with thalassaemia, *Cochrane Database Syst Rev* (8):CD007476, 2017. https://doi.org/10.1002/14651858.CD007476.pub3.

Cannell H: The development of oral and facial signs in beta-thalassaemia major, *Br Dent J* 164:50–51, 1988.

Hazza'a AM, Al-Jamal G: Radiographic features of the jaws and teeth in thalassemia major, *Dentomaxillofac Radiol* 35:283–288, 2006.

Higgs DR, Engel JD, Stamatoyannopoulos G: Thalassaemia, *Lancet* 379:373–383, 2012.

Javid B, Said-Al-Naief N: Craniofacial manifestations of β-thalassemia major, *Oral Surg Oral Med Oral Pathol Oral Radiol* 119:e33–e40, 2015.

Khandros E, Kwiatkowski JL: Beta thalassemia: monitoring and new treatment approaches, *Hematol Oncol Clin North Am* 33:339–353, 2019.

Taher AT, Weatherall DJ, Cappellini MD: Thalassaemia, *Lancet* 391:155–167, 2018.

Taher AT, Musallam KM, Cappellini MD: Thalassaemia, *N Engl J Med* 384:727–743, 2021.

Tyler PA, Madani G, Chaudhuri R, et al.: The radiological appearances of thalassaemia, *Clin Radiol* 61:40–52, 2006.

Viprakasit V, Ekwattanakit S: Clinical classification, screening and diagnosis for thalassemia, *Hematol Oncol Clin North Am* 32:193–211, 2018.

Aplastic Anemia

Agnihotri R, Bhat KM, Bhat GS, et al.: Periodontal management of a patient with severe aplastic anemia: a case report, *Spec Care Dentist* 29:141–144, 2009.

Clucas DB, Fox LC, Wood EM, et al.: Revisiting acquired aplastic anaemia: current concepts in diagnosis and management, *Intern Med J* 49:152–159, 2019.

Comito RR, Badu LA, Forcello N: Nivolumab-induced aplastic anemia: a case report and literature review, *J Oncol Pharm Pract* 25:221–225, 2019.

Luker J, Scully C, Oakhill A: Gingival swelling as a manifestation of aplastic anemia, *Oral Surg Oral Med Oral Pathol* 71:55–56, 1991.

Sepúlveda E, Brethauer U, Rojas J, et al.: Oral manifestations of aplastic anemia in children, *J Am Dent Assoc* 137:474–478, 2006.

Scheinberg P: Recent advances and long-term results of medical treatment of acquired aplastic anemia: are patients cured? *Hematol Oncol Clin North Am* 32:609–618, 2018.

Wang L, Liu H: Pathogenesis of aplastic anemia, *Hematology* 24:559–566, 2019.

Young NS: Aplastic anemia, *N Engl J Med* 379:1643–1656, 2018.

Neutropenia

Afzal W, Owlia MB, Hasni S, et al.: Autoimmune neutropenia updates: etiology, pathology, and treatment, *South Med J* 110:300–307, 2017.

Antonio AG, Alcantara PCC, Ramos MEB, et al.: The importance of dental care for a child with severe congenital neutropenia: a case report, *Spec Care Dentist* 30:261–265, 2010.

Atallah-Yunes SA, Ready A, Newburger PE: Benign ethnic neutropenia, *Blood Rev* 37:100586, 2019. https://doi.org/10.1016/j.blre.2019.06.003.

Barilà G, Calabretto G, Teramo A, et al.: T cell large granular lymphocyte leukemia and chronic NK lymphocytosis, *Best Pract Res Clin Haematol* 32:207–216, 2019.

Mehta HM, Malandra M, Corey SJ: G-CSF and GM-CSF in neutropenia, *J Immunol* 195:1341–1349, 2015. https://doi.org/10.4049/jimmunol.1500861.

Palmblad J, Nilsson CC, Höglund P, et al.: How we diagnose and treat neutropenia in adults, *Expert Rev Hematol* 9:479–487, 2016.

Palmblad J, Siersma V, Lind B, et al.: Age-related prevalence and clinical significance of neutropenia—isolated or combined with other cytopenias: real world data from 373,820 primary care individuals, *Am J Hematol* 95:521–528, 2020.

White L, Ybarra M: Neutropenic fever, *Hematol Oncol Clin North Am* 31:981–993, 2017.

Ye Y, Carlsson G, Wondimu B, et al.: Mutations in the *ELANE* gene are associated with development of periodontitis in patients with severe congenital neutropenia, *J Clin Immunol* 31:936–945, 2011.

Zaromb A, Chamberlain D, Schoor R, et al.: Periodontitis as a manifestation of chronic benign neutropenia, *J Periodontol* 77:1921–1926, 2006.

Zecha JAEM, Raber-Durlacher JE, Laheij AMGA, et al.: The impact of the oral cavity in febrile neutropenia and infectious complications in patients treated with myelosuppressive chemotherapy, *Support Care Cancer* 27:3667–3679, 2019.

Agranulocytosis

Carey PJ: Drug-induced myelosuppression: diagnosis and management, *Drug Saf* 26:691–706, 2003.

di Fonzo H, Villegas Gutsh M, Castroagudin A, et al.: Agranulocytosis induced by vancomycin. Case report and literature review, *Am J Case Rep* 19:1053–1056, 2018.

Johnston A, Uetrecht J: Current understanding of the mechanisms of idiosyncratic drug-induced agranulocytosis, *Expert Opin Drug Metab Toxicol* 11:243–257, 2015.

Kurago ZB, Kerr AR, Narayana N: Clinical pathologic conference case 5: agranulocytosis, *Head Neck Pathol* 5:286–291, 2011.

Tewari S, Tewari S, Sharma RK, et al.: Necrotizing stomatitis: a possible periodontal manifestation of deferiprone-induced agranulocytosis, *Oral Surg Oral Med Oral Pathol Oral Radiol Endod* 108:e13–e19, 2009.

Vicente N, Cardoso L, Barros L, et al.: Antithyroid drug-induced agranulocytosis: state of the art on diagnosis and management, *Drugs R D* 17:91–96, 2017.

Cyclic Neutropenia

Aota K, Kani K, Yamanoi T, et al.: Management of tooth extraction in a patient with ELANE gene mutation-induced cyclic neutropenia. A case report, *Medicine* 98(39):e17372, 2019.

Aprikyan AAG, Liles WC, Boxer LA, et al.: Mutant elastase in pathogenesis of cyclic and severe congenital neutropenia, *J Pediatr Hematol Oncol* 24:784–786, 2002.

Baer PN, Iacono VJ: Cyclic neutropenia: report of a case with a 15-year follow-up, *Periodontal Clin Investig* 16:14–19, 1994.

Chen X, Peng W, Zhang Z, et al.: ELANE gene mutation-induced cyclic neutropenia manifesting as recurrent fever with oral mucosal ulcer. A case report, *Medicine* 97(10):e0031, 2018.

Jung S, Gies V, Korganow A-S, et al.: Primary immunodeficiencies with defects in innate immunity: focus on orofacial manifestations, *Front Immunol* 11:1065, 2020.

Nakai Y, Ishihara C, Ogata S, et al.: Oral manifestations of cyclic neutropenia in a Japanese child: case report with a 5-year follow-up, *Pediatr Dent* 25:383–388, 2003.

Pernu HE, Pajari UH, Lanning M: The importance of regular dental treatment in patients with cyclic neutropenia: follow-up of 2 cases, *J Periodontol* 67:454–459, 1996.

Thrombocytopenia

Cooper N, Ghanima W: Immune thrombocytopenia, *N Engl J Med* 381:945–955, 2019.

Dou X, Yang R: Current and emerging treatments for immune thrombocytopenia, *Expert Rev Hematol* 12(9):723–732, 2019. https://doi.org/10.1080/17474086.2019.1636644.

Hong X, Wang X, Wang Z: A rare case report of acyclovir-induced immune thrombocytopenia with tongue hematomas as the first sign, and a literature review, *BMC Pharmacol Toxicol* 18:12, 2017.

Kappler S, Ronan-Bentle S, Graham A: Thrombotic microangiopathies (TTP, HUS, HELLP), *Hematol Oncol Clin North Am* 31:1081–1103, 2017.

Kim TO, Despotovic JM: Primary and secondary immune cytopenias: evaluation and treatment approach in children, *Hematol Oncol Clin North Am* 33:489–506, 2019.

Loirat C, Coppo P, Veyradier A: Thrombotic thrombocytopenic purpura in children, *Curr Opin Pediatr* 25:216–224, 2013.

Pandy M, Yarlagadda L: Drug-induced thrombocytopenia: a less known interaction, *Blood Coagul Fibrinolysis* 23:778–780, 2012.

Thompson CC, Tacke RB, Woolley LH, et al.: Purpuric oral and cutaneous lesions in a case of drug-induced thrombocytopenia, *J Am Dent Assoc* 105:465–467, 1982.

Polycythemia Vera

Marchioli R, Ginazzi G, Specchia G, et al.: Cardiovascular events and intensity of treatment in polycythemia vera, *N Engl J Med* 368:22–33, 2013.

McMullin MF, Harrison CN, Ali S, et al.: A guideline for the diagnosis and management of polycythaemia vera. A British Society for Haematology Guideline, *Br J Haematol* 184:176–191, 2019.

Rumi E, Baratè C, Benevolo G, et al.: Myeloproliferative and lymphoproliferative disorders: state of the art, *Hematol Oncol* 38:121–128, 2020.

Spivak JL: How I treat polycythemia vera, *Blood* 134:341–352, 2019.

Leukemia

Boras VV, Juras DV, Aurer I, et al.: Gingival ulcerations in a patient with acute myeloid leukemia: a case report and literature review, *Acta Clin Croat* 58:556–560, 2019.

Chapple ILC, Saxby MS, Murray JA: Gingival hemorrhage, myelodysplastic syndromes, and acute myeloid leukemia: a case report, *J Periodontol* 70:1247–1253, 1999.

Coltro G, Patnaik MM: Chronic myelomonocytic leukemia: insights into biology, prognostic factors, and treatment, *Curr Oncol Rep* 21:101, 2019. https://doi.org/10.1007/s11912-019-0855-6.

Foran JM, Shammo JM: Clinical presentation, diagnosis, and prognosis of myelodysplastic syndromes, *Am J Med* 125:S6–S13, 2012.

Francisconi CF, Caldas RJ, Martins LJO, et al.: Leukemic oral manifestations and their management, *Asian Pac J Cancer Prev* 17:911–915, 2016.

Hallek M, Shanafelt TD, Eichhorst B: Chronic lymphocytic leukaemia, *Lancet* 391:1524–1537, 2018.

Hollsberg P, Hailer DA: Pathogenesis of diseases induced by human lymphotropic virus type I infection, *N Engl J Med* 328:1173–1182, 1993.

Ishikawa S, Kato Y, Kabasawa T, et al.: A case of myeloid sarcoma of the mandibular gingiva as extramedullary relapse of acute myeloid leukemia, *Oral Maxillofac Surg* 24:121–126, 2020.

Kaplan JA: Leukemia in children, *Pediatr Rev* 40:319–331, 2019. https://doi.org/10.1542/pir.2018-0192.

Menasce LP, Banerjee SS, Beckett E, et al.: Extra-medullary myeloid tumour (granulocytic sarcoma) is often misdiagnosed: a study of 26 cases, *Histopathology* 34:391–398, 1999.

Papamanthos MK, Kolokotronis AD, Skulakis HE, et al.: Acute myeloid leukaemia diagnosed by intra-oral myeloid sarcoma, *Head Neck Pathol* 4:132–135, 2010.

Peters SM, Han C, Yoon AJ, et al.: Chronic lymphocytic leukemia in association with a ranula: a report and review of the literature, *Oral Surg Oral Med Oral Pathol Oral Radiol* 123:e160–e163, 2017.

Peterson DE, Gerad H, Williams LT: An unusual instance of leukemic infiltrate: diagnosis and management of periapical tooth involvement, *Cancer* 51:1716–1719, 1983.

Rhee D, Myssiorek D, Zahtz G, et al.: Recurrent attacks of facial nerve palsy as the presenting sign of leukemic relapse, *Laryngoscope* 112:235–237, 2002.

Rose-Inman H, Kuehl D: Acute leukemia, *Hematol Oncol Clin North Am* 31:1011–1028, 2017.

Shallisa RM, Wang R, Davidoff A, et al.: Epidemiology of the classical myeloproliferative neoplasms: the four corners of an expansive and complex map, *Blood Rev* 42:100706, 2020. https://doi.org/10.1016/j.blre.2020.100706.

Short NJ, Rytting ME, Cortes JE: Acute myeloid leukaemia, *Lancet* 392:593–606, 2018.

Sollecito TP, Draznin J, Parisi E, et al.: Leukemic gingival infiltrate as an indicator of chemotherapeutic failure following monoclonal antibody therapy: a case report, *Spec Care Dentist* 23:108–110, 2003.

Soverini S, Bassan R, Lion T: Treatment and monitoring of Philadelphia chromosome-positive leukemia patients: recent advances and remaining challenges, *J Hematol Oncol* 12:39, 2019. https://doi.org/10.1186/s13045-019-0729-2.

Stoopler ET, Pinto A, Alawi F, et al.: Granulocytic sarcoma: an atypical presentation in the oral cavity, *Spec Care Dentist* 24:65–69, 2004.

Vibhute P, Carneiro E, Genden E, et al.: Palatal enlargement in chronic lymphocytic leukemia, *AJNR Am J Neuroradiol* 27:1649–1650, 2006.

Vural F, Ozcan MA, Ozsan GH, et al.: Gingival involvement in a patient with CD56+ chronic myelomonocytic leukemia, *Leuk Lymphoma* 45:415–418, 2004.

Langerhans Cell Histiocytosis

Abla O, Rollins B, Ladisch S: Langerhans cell histiocytosis: progress and controversies, *Br J Haematol* 187:559–562, 2019.

Allen CE, Merad M, McClain KL: Langerhans-cell histiocytosis, *N Engl J Med* 379:856–868, 2018.

Annibali S, Cristalli MP, Solidani M, et al.: Langerhans cell histiocytosis: oral/periodontal involvement in adult patients, *Oral Dis* 15:596–601, 2009.

Bedran NR, Carlos R, Benevenuto de Andrade BA, et al.: Clinicopathological and immunohistochemical study of head and neck Langerhans cell histiocytosis from Latin America, *Head Neck Pathol* 12:431–439, 2018.

Cantu MA, Lupo PJ, Bilgi M, et al.: Optimal therapy for adults with Langerhans cell histiocytosis bone lesions, *PLoS One* 7:e43257, 2012.

Cleveland DB, Goldberg KM, Greenspan JS, et al.: Langerhans' cell histiocytosis. Report of three cases with unusual oral soft tissue involvement, *Oral Surg Oral Med Oral Pathol Oral Radiol Endod* 82:541–548, 1996.

Dagenais M, Pharoah MJ, Sikorski PA: The radiographic characteristics of histiocytosis X: a study of 29 cases that involve the jaws, *Oral Surg Oral Med Oral Pathol* 74:230–236, 1992.

Donadieu J, Larabi IA, Tardieu M, et al.: Vemurafenib for refractory multisystem Langerhans cell histiocytosis in children: an international observational study, *J Clin Oncol* 37:2857–2865, 2019.

Hartman KH: A review of 114 cases of histiocytosis X, *Oral Surg Oral Med Oral Pathol* 49:38–54, 1980.

Hicks J, Flaitz CM: Langerhans cell histiocytosis: current insights in a molecular age with emphasis on clinical oral and maxillofacial pathology practice, *Oral Surg Oral Med Oral Pathol Oral Radiol Endod* 100:S42–S66, 2005.

Key SJ, O'Brien CJ, Silvester KC, et al.: Eosinophilic granuloma: resolution of maxillofacial bony lesions following minimal intervention. Report of three cases and a review of the literature, *J Craniomaxillofac Surg* 32:170–175, 2004.

Krooks J, Minkov M, Weatherall AG: Langerhans cell histiocytosis in children. History, classification, pathobiology, clinical manifestations, and prognosis, *J Am Acad Dermatol* 78:1035–1044, 2018.

Krooks J, Minkov M, Weatherall AG: Langerhans cell histiocytosis in children. Diagnosis, differential diagnosis, treatment, sequelae, and standardized follow-up, *J Am Acad Dermatol* 78:1047–1056, 2018.

Murray M, Dean J, Slater L: Multifocal oral Langerhans cell histiocytosis, *J Oral Maxillofac Surg* 69:2585–2591, 2011.

Postini AM, Andreacchio A, Boffano M, et al.: Langerhans cell histiocytosis of bone in children: a long-term retrospective study, *J Pediatr Orthop B* 21:457–462, 2012.

Putters TF, de Visscher JGAM, van Veen A, et al.: Intralesional infiltration of corticosteroids in the treatment of localized Langerhans' cell histiocytosis of the mandible. Report of known cases and three new cases, *Int J Oral Maxillofac Surg* 34:571–575, 2005.

Sahm F, Capper D, Preusser M, et al.: BRAFV600E mutant protein is expressed in cells of variable maturation in Langerhans cell histiocytosis, *Blood* 120:e28–e34, 2012.

Tran G, Huynh TN, Paller AS: Langerhans cell histiocytosis: a neoplastic disorder driven by Ras-ERK pathway mutations, *J Am Acad Dermatol* 78:579–590, 2018.

Yousem SA, Colby TV, Chen Y-Y, et al.: Pulmonary Langerhans' cell histiocytosis. Molecular analysis of clonality, *Am J Surg Pathol* 25:630–636, 2001.

Hodgkin Lymphoma

Ansell SM: Hodgkin lymphoma: 2018 update on diagnosis, risk-stratification, and management, *Am J Hematol* 93:704–715, 2018.

Bröckelmann PJ, Sasse S, Engert A: Balancing risk and benefit in early-stage classical Hodgkin lymphoma, *Blood* 131:1666–1678, 2018.

Darling MR, Cuddy KK, Rizkalla K: Hodgkin lymphoma of the oral mucosa, *Head Neck Pathol* 6:507–510, 2012.

Depaus J, Delcourt A, André M: Therapeutic recommendations for early stage Hodgkin lymphomas, *Br J Haematol* 184:9–16, 2019.

Gómez-Almaguer D, González-Llano O, Jiménez-Antolinez V, et al.: Treatment of classical Hodgkin's lymphoma in children and adolescents, *Expert Opin Pharmacother* 20(10):1227–1234, 2019. https://doi.org/10.1080/14656566.2019.1606212.

Herrin HK: The oral implications of Hodgkin's disease, *Gen Dent* 47:572–575, 1999.

Hodgson DC: Late effects of modern therapy for Hodgkin lymphoma, *Hematology Am Soc Hematol Educ Program* 2011:323–329, 2011.

Iyengar P, Mazloom A, Shihadeh F, et al.: Hodgkin lymphoma involving extranodal and nodal head and neck sites, *Cancer* 116:3825–3829, 2010.

Küppers R, Hansmann M-L: The Hodgkin and Reed/Sternberg cell, *Int J Biochem Cell Biol* 37:511–517, 2005.

Levinea I, Kaliszb K, Smith DA, et al.: Update on Hodgkin lymphoma from a radiologist's perspective, *Clin Imaging* 65:65–77, 2020.

van Leeuwen FE, Ng AK: Late sequelae in Hodgkin lymphoma survivors, *Hematol Oncol* 35:S60–S66, 2017.

Yencha MW: Primary parotid gland Hodgkin's lymphoma, *Ann Otol Rhinol Laryngol* 111:338–342, 2002.

Non-Hodgkin Lymphoma

Amorim Pellicioli AC, Alves Luciano A, Carrinho Ayroza Rangel AL, et al.: Epstein-Barr virus (EBV)-associated post-transplant lymphoproliferative disorder appearing as mandibular gingival ulcers, *Oral Surg Oral Med Oral Pathol Oral Radiol* 121:e80–e86, 2016.

Ando M, Matsuzaki M, Murofushi T: Mucosa-associated lymphoid tissue lymphoma presented as diffuse swelling of the parotid gland, *Am J Otolaryngol* 26:285–288, 2005.

Armitage JO, Gascoyne JD, Lunning MA, et al.: Non-Hodgkin lymphoma, *Lancet* 390:298–310, 2017.

Bhattacharyya S, Bains APS, Sykes DL, et al.: Lymphoid neoplasms of the oral cavity with plasmablastic morphology—a case series and review of the literature, *Oral Surg Oral Med Oral Pathol Oral Radiol* 128:651–659, 2019.

Broadwater DR, Peker D: Systemic non-Hodgkin T cell lymphomas presenting in the head and neck region: an institutional experience of a rare entity, *Head Neck Pathol* 12:481–487, 2018.

Dojcinov SD, Venkataraman G, Pittaluga S, et al.: Age-related EBV-associated lymphoproliferative disorders in the Western population: a spectrum of reactive lymphoid hyperplasia and lymphoma, *Blood* 117:4726–4735, 2011.

Folk GS, Abbondanzo SL, Childers EL, et al.: Plasmablastic lymphoma: a clinicopathologic correlation, *Ann Diagn Pathol* 10:8–12, 2006.

Guerard EJ, Bishop MR: Overview of non-Hodgkin's lymphoma, *Dis Mon* 58:208–218, 2012.

Guggisberg K, Jordan RCK: Mantle cell lymphoma of the oral cavity: case series and comprehensive review of the literature, *Oral Surg Oral Med Oral Pathol Oral Radiol Endod* 109:98–104, 2010.

Hashimoto K, Nagao T, Saito T, et al.: Methotrexate-associated lymphoproliferative disorders of the tongue developing in patients with rheumatoid arthritis: a report of 2 cases and a review, *Oral Surg Oral Med Oral Pathol Oral Radiol* 119:e1–e5, 2015.

Hussein MRA: Non-Hodgkin's lymphoma of the oral cavity and maxillofacial region: a pathologist viewpoint, *Expert Rev Hematol* 11:737–748, 2018.

Kolokotronis A, Konstantinou N, Christakis I, et al.: Localized B-cell non-Hodgkin's lymphoma of the oral cavity and maxillofacial region: a clinical study, *Oral Surg Oral Med Oral Pathol Oral Radiol Endod* 99:303–310, 2005.

Mealey BL, Tunder GS, Pemble CW: Primary extranodal malignant lymphoma affecting the periodontium, *J Periodontol* 73:937–941, 2002.

Rizvi MA, Evens AM, Tallman MS, et al.: T-cell non-Hodgkin lymphoma, *Blood* 107:1255–1264, 2006.

Rodrigues-Fernandes CI, Lacerda de Souza L, Ferreira dos Santos-Costa S, et al.: Clinicopathological analysis of oral diffuse large B-cell lymphoma, NOS: a systematic review, *J Oral Pathol Med* 48:185–191, 2019.

Sánchez-Romero C, Rebelo Pontes HA, Sirotheau Corrêa Pontes F, et al.: Acute lymphoblastic leukemia/lymphoma of the oral and maxillofacial region, *Oral Surg Oral Med Oral Pathol Oral Radiol* 126:152–164, 2018.

Scherfler S, Freier K, Seeberger R, et al.: Cranio-maxillofacial non-Hodgkin's lymphoma: clinical and histological presentation, *J Craniomaxillofac Surg* 40:e211–e213, 2012.

Thaker R, Lee KC, Peters S, et al.: Asymptomatic nodule in the right cheek in a 65-year-old female, *Oral Surg Oral Med Oral Pathol Oral Radiol* 128:567–571, 2019.

Theander E, Vasaitis L, Baecklund E, et al.: Lymphoid organisation in labial salivary gland biopsies is a possible predictor for the development of malignant lymphoma in primary Sjögren's syndrome, *Ann Rheum Dis* 70:1363–1368, 2011.

Tomich CE, Shafer WG: Lymphoproliferative disease of the hard palate: a clinicopathologic entity, *Oral Surg Oral Med Oral Pathol* 39:754–768, 1975.

Triantafillidou K, Dimitrakopoulos J, Iordanidis F, et al.: Extranodal non-Hodgkin lymphomas of the oral cavity and maxillofacial region: a clinical study of 58 cases and review of the literature, *J Oral Maxillofac Surg* 70:2776–2785, 2012.

Van der Waal RIF, Huijgens PC, van der Valk P, et al.: Characteristics of 40 primary extranodal non-Hodgkin lymphomas of the oral cavity in perspective of the new WHO classification and the International Prognostic Index, *Int J Oral Maxillofac Surg* 34:391–395, 2005.

Zapater E, Bagán JV, Carbonell F, et al.: Malignant lymphoma of the head and neck, *Oral Dis* 16:119–128, 2010.

Mycosis Fungoides

Chua MS-T, Veness MJ: Mycosis fungoides involving the oral cavity, *Australas Radiol* 46:336–339, 2002.

Damm DD, White DK, Cibull ML, et al.: Mycosis fungoides: initial diagnosis via palatal biopsy with discussion of diagnostic advantages of plastic embedding, *Oral Surg Oral Med Oral Pathol* 58:413–419, 1984.

Hata T, Aikoh T, Hirokawa M, et al.: Mycosis fungoides with involvement of the oral mucosa, *Int J Oral Maxillofac Surg* 27:127–128, 1998.

Hristov AC, Tejasvi T, Wilcox RA: Mycosis fungoides and Sézary syndrome: 2019 update on diagnosis, risk-stratification, and management, *Am J Hematol* 94:1027–1041, 2019.

Larocca C, Kupper T: Mycosis fungoides and Sézary syndrome: an update, *Hematol Oncol Clin North Am* 33:103–120, 2019.

Larocca CA, LeBoeuf NR: Overview of cutaneous T-cell lymphomas, *Hematol Oncol Clin North Am* 33:669–686, 2019.

Lovgren M-L, Scarisbrick JJ: Update on skin directed therapies in mycosis fungoides, *Chin Clin Oncol* 8(1):7, 2019. https://doi.org/10.21037/cco.2018.11.03.

May SA, Jones D, Medeiros LJ, et al.: Oral-cutaneous CD4-positive T-cell lymphoma: a study of two patients, *Am J Dermatopathol* 29:62–67, 2007.

Rosebush MS, Allen CM, Accurso BT, et al.: Oral mycosis fungoides: a report of three cases and review of the literature, *Head Neck Pathol* 13:492–499, 2019.

Sirois DA, Miller AS, Harwick RD, et al.: Oral manifestations of cutaneous T-cell lymphoma: a report of eight cases, *Oral Surg Oral Med Oral Pathol* 75:700–705, 1993.

Sultan AS, Mostoufi B, Papadimitriou JC, et al.: Large cell transformation of oral mycosis fungoides, *Head Neck Pathol* 12:247–251, 2018.

Wright JM, Balciunas BA, Muus JH: Mycosis fungoides with oral manifestations: report of a case and review of the literature, *Oral Surg Oral Med Oral Pathol* 51:24–31, 1981.

Burkitt Lymphoma

Atallah-Yunes SA, Murphy DJ, Noy A: HIV-associated Burkitt lymphoma, *Lancet Haematol* 7:e594–e600, 2020.

Casulo C, Friedberg JW: Burkitt lymphoma—a rare but challenging lymphoma, *Best Pract Res Clin Haematol* 31:279–284, 2018.

Dave SS, Fu K, Wright GW, et al.: Molecular diagnosis of Burkitt's lymphoma, *N Engl J Med* 354:2431–2442, 2006.

Draz A, Elias W, El-Sissi A, et al.: Pediatric unilateral facial swelling, *Oral Surg Oral Med Oral Pathol Oral Radiol* 123:519–523, 2017.

Dunleavy K, Little RF, Wilson WH: Update on Burkitt lymphoma, *Hematol Oncol Clin North Am* 30:1333–1343, 2016.

Hussein MRA: Non-Hodgkin's lymphoma of the oral cavity and maxillofacial region: a pathologist viewpoint, *Expert Rev Hematol* 11:737–748, 2018.

Kikuchi K, Inoue H, Miyazaki Y, et al.: Adult sporadic Burkitt lymphoma of the oral cavity: a case report and literature review, *J Oral Maxillofac Surg* 70:2936–2943, 2012.

Molyneux EM, Rochford R, Griffen B, et al.: Burkitt's lymphoma, *Lancet* 379:1234–1244, 2012.

Ribrag V, Koscielny S, Bosq J, et al.: Rituximab and dose-dense chemotherapy for adults with Burkitt's lymphoma: a randomised, controlled, open-label, phase 3 trial, *Lancet* 387:2402–2411, 2016.

Uğar DA, Bozkaya S, Karaca I, et al.: Childhood craniofacial Burkitt's lymphoma presenting as maxillary swelling: report of a case and review of literature, *J Dent Child* 73:45–50, 2006.

Walusansa V, Okuku F, Orem J: Burkitt lymphoma in UGANDA, the legacy of Denis Burkitt and an update on the disease status, *Br J Haematol* 156:757–760, 2012.

Extranodal NK/T-Cell Lymphoma, Nasal-Type

Al-Hakeem DA, Fedele S, Carlos R, et al.: Extranodal NK/T-cell lymphoma, nasal type, *Oral Oncol* 43:4–14, 2007.

Allen PB, Lechowicz MJ: Management of NK/T-cell lymphoma, nasal type, *J Oncol Pract* 15:513–520, 2019.

Kim SJ, Kim WS: Treatment of localized extranodal NK/T cell lymphoma, nasal type, *Int J Hematol* 92:690–696, 2010.

Lanzel E, Syrbu SI, Hellstein JW, et al.: Destructive soft tissue mass in the maxilla/maxillary sinus, *Oral Surg Oral Med Oral Pathol Oral Radiol* 125:510–515, 2018.

Li S, Feng X, Li T, et al.: Extranodal NK/T-cell lymphoma, nasal type. A report of 73 cases at MD Anderson Cancer Center, *Am J Surg Pathol* 37:14–23, 2013.

Meng W, Zhou Y, Zhang H, et al.: Nasal-type NK/T-cell lymphoma with palatal ulcer as the earliest clinical manifestation: a case report with literature review, *Pathol Oncol Res* 16:133–137, 2010.

Mosqueda-Taylor A, Meneses-Garcia A, Zarate-Osorno A, et al.: Angiocentric lymphomas of the palate: clinico-pathological considerations in 12 cases, *J Oral Pathol Med* 26:93–97, 1997.

Sánchez-Romero C, Paes de Almeida O, Rendón Henao J, et al.: Extranodal NK/T-cell lymphoma, nasal type in Guatemala: an 86-case series emphasizing clinical presentation and microscopic characteristics, *Head Neck Pathol* 13:624–634, 2019.

Sokolowska-Wojdylo M, Florek A, Barańska-Rybak W, et al.: Natural killer/T-cell lymphoma, nasal type, masquerading as recalcitrant periodontitis in a patient with a diagnosis of Wegener's granulomatosis, *Am J Med Sci* 345:163–167, 2013.

Tse E, Kwong Y-L: The diagnosis and management of NK/T-cell lymphomas, *J Hematol Oncol* 10:85, 2017. https://doi.org/10.1186/s13045-017-0452-9.

Tse E, Kwong Y-L: NK/T-cell lymphomas, *Best Pract Res Clin Haematol* 32:253–261, 2019.

Yamaguchi M, Suzuki R, Oguchi M: Advances in the treatment of extranodal NK/T-cell lymphoma, nasal type, *Blood* 131:2528–2540, 2018.

Multiple Myeloma

Elias HG, Scott J, Metheny L, et al.: Multiple myeloma presenting as mandibular ill-defined radiolucent lesion with numb chin syndrome: a case report, *J Oral Maxillofac Surg* 67:1991–1996, 2009.

Ferreira L, Efebera Y, Allen CM: Clinical pathologic conference case 2: a diffuse swelling of the neck, *Oral Surg Oral Med Oral Pathol Oral Radiol* 115:e36–e40, 2013.

Gandolfi S, Laubach JP, Hideshima T, et al.: The proteasome and proteasome inhibitors in multiple myeloma, *Cancer Metastasis Rev* 36:561–584, 2017.

Gerecke C, Fuhrmann S, Strifler S, et al.: The diagnosis and treatment of multiple myeloma, *Dtsch Arztebl Int* 113:470–476, 2016.

Gouvêa AF, Ribeiro ACP, León JE, et al.: Head and neck amyloidosis: clinicopathological features and immunohistochemical analysis of 14 cases, *J Oral Pathol Med* 41:178–185, 2012.

Leiba M, Jarjoura S, Abboud W, et al.: Role of oral examination in newly diagnosed multiple myeloma patients: a safe and simple way to detect light chain amyloidosis, *Oral Dis* 24:1343–1348, 2018.

Mateos M-V, San Miguel JF: Management of multiple myeloma in the newly diagnosed patient, *Hematology Am Soc Hematol Educ Program* 2017(1):498–507, 2017.

Mhaskar R, Redzepovic J, Wheatley K, et al.: Bisphosphonates in multiple myeloma: a network meta-analysis, *Cochrane Database Syst Rev* (5):CD003188, 2012.

Rajkumar SV: Multiple myeloma: 2020 update on diagnosis, risk-stratification, and management, *Am J Hematol* 95:548–567, 2020.

Rajkumar SV: Multiple myeloma: every year a new standard? *Hematol Oncol* 37(Suppl 1):62–65, 2019.

Smith D, Yong K: Multiple myeloma, *Br Med J* 346, 2013, f3863.

Tsang RW, Campbell BA, Goda JS, et al.: Radiation therapy for solitary plasmacytoma and multiple myeloma: guidelines from the International Lymphoma Radiation Oncology Group, *Int J Radiat Oncol Biol Phys* 101:794–808, 2018.

Plasmacytoma

Alwan H, Moor JW, Wright D, et al.: Extramedullary plasmacytoma of the tongue base: a case report and clinical review of head and neck plasmacytoma, *Ear Nose Throat J* 89:369–373, 2010.

Fotiou D, Dimopoulos MA, Kastritis E: How we manage patients with plasmacytomas, *Curr Hematol Malig Rep* 13:227–235, 2018.

Kremer M, Ott G, Nathrath M, et al.: Primary extramedullary plasmacytoma and multiple myeloma: phenotypic differences revealed by immunohistochemical analysis, *J Pathol* 205:92–101, 2005.

Lesmes D, Laster Z: Plasmacytoma in the temporomandibular joint: a case report, *Br J Oral Maxillofac Surg* 46:322–324, 2008.

Madruga Lombardoa E, Dal Moro Maitob FL, Heitza C, et al.: Solitary plasmacytoma of the jaws: therapeutical considerations and prognosis based on a case reports systematic survey, *Braz J Otorhinolaryngol* 84:790–798, 2018.

Majumdar S, Raghavan U, Jones NS: Solitary plasmacytoma and extramedullary plasmacytoma of the paranasal sinuses and soft palate, *J Laryngol Otol* 116:962–965, 2002.

Pham A, Mahindra A: Solitary plasmacytoma: a review of diagnosis and management, *Curr Hematol Malig Rep* 14:63–69, 2019.

Rodríguez-Caballero B, Sanchez-Santolino S, Garciá-Montesinos-Perea B: Mandibular solitary plasmacytoma of the jaw: a case report, *Med Oral Pathol Oral Cir Bucal* 16:e647–e650, 2011.

Rothfield RE, Johnson JT, Slavrides A: Extramedullary plasmacytoma of the parotid, *Head Neck* 12:352–354, 1990.

Venkatesulu B, Mallick S, Giridhar P, et al.: Pattern of care and impact of prognostic factors on the outcome of head and neck extramedullary plasmacytoma: a systematic review and individual patient data analysis of 315 cases, *Eur Arch Otorhinolaryngol* 275:595–606, 2018.

14

Bone Pathology

◆ OSTEOGENESIS IMPERFECTA ("BRITTLE BONE DISEASE")

Osteogenesis imperfecta comprises a heterogeneous group of heritable disorders characterized by osteopenia (low bone density) and bone fragility. This condition represents one of the most common heritable bone diseases and is estimated to affect 1 in 10,000 to 15,000 live births.

Approximately 90% of cases exhibit an autosomal dominant inheritance pattern with mutations in one of two type I collagen genes: *COL1A1* and *COL1A2*. In addition, there are numerous other variants (mainly autosomal recessive) caused by recently discovered mutations in genes related to type I collagen post-translational modification, processing, and cross-linking; bone mineralization; osteoblast differentiation; and other functions. Sporadic cases are possible as well.

Type I collagen is a major constituent of bone, dentin, sclerae, ligaments, and skin; osteogenesis imperfecta may affect any of these tissue types. Type I collagen is a triple helical molecule composed of peptide chains encoded by *COL1A1* and *COL1A2*. Defects in the complex process of synthesis, post-translational modification (including hydroxylation, crosslinking, and terminal propeptide cleavage), and chaperone-guided protein folding result in abnormal type I collagen with low tensile strength. Consequently, the bone is brittle; upon fracture, healing will occur but may be associated with exuberant callus formation.

Classification of the various forms of osteogenesis imperfecta continues to evolve as molecular genetic discoveries are made. Based on clinical and genetic findings, at least 18 types are recognized by the Online Mendelian Inheritance in Man (OMIM) database. Other authorities prefer to delineate disease types based on a functional genetic approach. In clinical practice, classification based on phenotype alone is used most widely. Table 14.1 summarizes the International Skeletal Dysplasia Society (ISDS) Nosology Committee's clinical classification scheme (which represents an adaptation of the original Sillence classification) along with corresponding genetic mutations and OMIM disease types.

Clinical and Radiographic Features

Severity varies widely by disease type, and mutations in even a single gene locus may produce extensive phenotypic variation. Disease characterization as mild, moderate, or severe generally is based on the number of bone fractures, degree of long bone and spine deformity, degree of growth impairment, and age at which abnormalities initially become evident. For example, osteogenesis imperfecta type 1—the mildest and most common form—is characterized by a variable number of bone fractures, no significant bone deformity, and essentially normal growth. Typically, fractures first occur when the patient begins to walk and decrease in frequency after puberty. In contrast, osteogenesis imperfecta type 2 is the most severe form, characterized by extreme bone fragility and deformity. Most patients with this disease type die *in utero* or shortly after birth; death often results from respiratory distress due to multiple rib fractures and a small thorax.

Additional clinical findings may include blue sclerae (Fig. 14.1), hearing loss, and joint hyperextensibility or contractures. Infrequently, patients may develop muscle weakness and cardiopulmonary complications. The radiographic hallmarks include osteopenia, bowing deformity of the long bones, multiple fractures, and an increased number of Wormian bones in the skull. Wormian bones are small sutural bones arranged in a mosaic pattern; they also can be seen in other processes, such as cleidocranial dysplasia (see page 623).

Dental alterations that appear clinically and radiographically identical to dentinogenesis imperfecta (see page 104) may be evident as well. Both dentitions demonstrate blue, yellow, or brown translucence (Fig. 14.2, *A*); however, this finding may be less prominent in the permanent teeth. The underlying dentinal defects often lead to severe attrition, resulting in loss of vertical dimension and potential tooth loss. Radiographs typically reveal premature pulpal obliteration (Fig. 14.2, *B*), although shell teeth rarely may be seen. The teeth often exhibit bulbous crowns, cervical constriction, and narrow or corncob-shaped roots. Other possible dental findings include pulp stones, taurodontism, radicular dilaceration, hypodontia, and microdontia. Despite exhibiting similar tooth alterations, osteogenesis imperfecta and dentinogenesis imperfecta are distinct diseases resulting from different mutations. Therefore, the dental defects associated with the systemic disorder osteogenesis imperfecta should be designated **opalescent teeth**, whereas the term *dentinogenesis imperfecta* should be reserved for patients with alterations isolated to the teeth.

Craniofacial findings in osteogenesis imperfecta may include triangular facies, frontal bossing, relative macrocephaly, a flattened vertex and skull base, and a prominent

TABLE 14.1 Osteogenesis Imperfecta Classification Scheme

ISDS Classification	Phenotype	Inheritance Pattern(s)	Gene(s) Mutated	OMIM Disease Type(s)
OI type 1	Mild, nondeforming disease with persistently blue sclerae	AD	COL1A1, COL1A2	I
OI type 2	Severe, perinatal lethal disease	AD, AR	COL1A1, COL1A2, CRTAP, LEPRE1, PPIB	II, VII, VIII, IX
OI type 3	Moderate to severe, progressively deforming disease	AD, AR	COL1A1, COL1A2, IFITM5, SERPINF1, CRTAP, LEPRE1, PPIB, SERPINH1, FKBP10, TMEM38B, BMP1, WNT1, CREB3L1, SPARC, TENT5A	III, V, VI, VII, VIII, IX, X, XI, XIII, XIV, XVI, XVII, XVIII
OI type 4	Moderate disease, normal sclera in adults	AD, AR	COL1A1, COL1A2, WNT1, IFITM5, CRTAP, PPIB, FKBP10, SP7	IV, V, VII, IX, XI, XII, XV
OI type 5	Moderate disease with calcification of interosseous membranes and/or hypertrophic callus formation	AD	IFITM5	

AD, Autosomal dominant; *AR*, autosomal recessive; *BMP1*, bone morphogenetic protein 1 gene; *COL1A1*, collagen, type 1, alpha 1 gene; *COL1A2*, collagen, type 1, alpha 2 gene; *CREB3L1*, cAMP response element-binding protein 3-like 1 gene; *CRTAP*, cartilage-associated protein gene; *FKBP10*, FK506 binding protein 10 gene; *IFITM5*, interferon-induced transmembrane protein 5 gene; *ISDS*, International Skeletal Dysplasia Society; *LEPRE1*, leucine- and proline-enriched proteoglycan 1 gene; *OI*, osteogenesis imperfecta; *OMIM*, Online Mendelian Inheritance in Man; *PPIB*, peptidylprolyl isomerase B gene; *SERPINF1*, serpin peptidase inhibitor, clade F, member 1 gene; *SERPINH1*, serpin peptidase inhibitor gene; *SPARC*, secreted protein, acidic, cysteine-rich; *SP7*, transcription factor Sp7 gene; *TENT5A*, terminal nucleotidyltransferase 5A gene; *TMEM38*, transmembrane protein 38B gene; *WNT1*, wingless-type MMTV integration site family, member 1 gene.

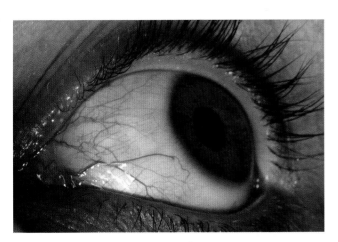

• **Fig. 14.1 Osteogenesis Imperfecta.** Blue sclera in a patient with osteogenesis imperfecta.

occiput. Craniocervical junction anomalies may result in brainstem compression, central apnea, and decreased muscle tone. In addition, there is an increased prevalence of Class III malocclusion (caused by maxillary hypoplasia, with or without mandibular hyperplasia), crossbite, open bite, and deviated nasal septum (Fig. 14.2, *A*). Individuals with osteogenesis imperfecta type 5 may exhibit bimaxillary retrusive malocclusion with reduced lower face height. Furthermore, a few investigators have noted somewhat accelerated tooth development and eruption among pediatric patients with osteogenesis imperfecta and no history of bisphosphonate therapy.

There are a few reported probands with osteogenesis imperfecta occurring in association with other heritable conditions, such as Ehlers-Danlos syndrome (see page 760), Stickler syndrome, and *gnathodiaphyseal dysplasia*. The latter condition previously was thought to represent a variation of osteogenesis imperfecta but currently is considered a distinct condition, characterized by *ANO5* mutations, autosomal dominant inheritance, generalized bone fragility, bowing and cortical sclerosis of tubular bones, and fibro-osseous lesions of the jaws (similar to florid cemento-osseous dysplasia or familial gigantiform cementoma).

Diagnosis

Diagnosis requires correlation of the clinical features, radiographic and/or prenatal ultrasound findings, and family history. For diagnostic confirmation, genetic testing is more sensitive than electrophoresis for type I collagen secreted by cultured dermal fibroblasts. Bone biopsy may be helpful in select cases. Serum concentrations of vitamin D, calcium, phosphorus, and alkaline phosphatase usually are normal, although occasionally the latter may be slightly elevated.

Treatment and Prognosis

Management of bone fractures and deformity may be difficult. The mainstays of treatment are physiotherapy, rehabilitation, and orthopedic surgery. In addition, intravenous

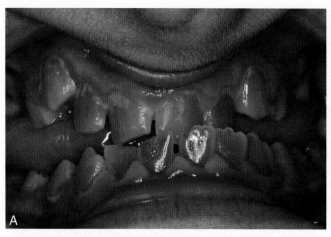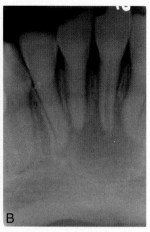

• **Fig. 14.2 Osteogenesis Imperfecta. A,** Opalescent teeth, class III malocclusion, and posterior open bite in a patient with osteogenesis imperfecta. **B,** Periapical radiograph of the same patient showing several teeth with pulpal obliteration. (Courtesy of Dr. Taylor Cox.)

bisphosphonates typically are administered to children with moderate to severe disease. Such therapy may decrease pain, induce reshaping of vertebrae after compression fractures, improve growth, and increase mobility. However, there is conflicting data regarding whether this treatment reduces fracture rates. The benefits of bisphosphonate therapy for adult or mild childhood disease and the long-term safety of bisphosphonate therapy require further study. Investigational treatments for osteogenesis imperfecta include denosumab (a monoclonal antibody targeting receptor activator of nuclear factor-kappa B ligand [RANKL]), growth hormone, recombinant human parathyroid hormone (teriparatide), transforming growth factor-beta (TGF-β) inhibitors, sclerostin inhibitors, and stem cell therapy.

Dental treatment is similar to that for dentinogenesis imperfecta (see page 104). Successful implant placement has been reported in a few cases, although the impact of the altered bone on osseointegration is not well studied. In patients with significant malocclusion, orthognathic surgery and orthodontic treatment may be performed. Alternatively, osteodistraction may be considered to reduce the risk of atypical fractures from conventional orthognathic procedures (e.g., Le Fort I osteotomy). Presurgical planning should take into account an increased risk for bleeding disorders, cardiac malformations, and hyperthermia. Intubation may be difficult because of a short neck, kyphoscoliosis, and fragility of the mandible and cervical vertebrae. Also, patients previously treated with bisphosphonates may exhibit delayed healing after osteotomy. Although there is concern regarding the potential for bisphosphonates to induce osteonecrosis of the jaws, this complication has not been reported thus far among children and young adults who have been administered these medications for the management of osteogenesis imperfecta. In addition, some studies suggest that patients receiving intravenous bisphosphonate therapy for osteogenesis imperfecta are at increased risk for tooth impaction, ectopic teeth, pulp stones, and pulpal obliteration.

The prognosis varies by disease type. Patients with mild disease exhibit a normal life span, whereas those with especially severe disease die *in utero* or in the perinatal period.

◆ OSTEOPETROSIS (ALBERS-SCHÖNBERG DISEASE; MARBLE BONE DISEASE)

Osteopetrosis is a group of rare hereditary skeletal disorders characterized by markedly increased bone density. The name of this disease is derived from the Greek words for "bone" (*osteo*) and "stone" (*petros*). The condition is characterized by a failure of osteoclast function or differentiation. Decreased osteoclastic bone resorption results in sclerotic yet fragile bone.

The underlying genetic abnormality is unknown in about 25% of patients. Mutations discovered thus far primarily cause defects in osteoclastic proteins necessary for formation and acidification of resorption lacunae. In particular, such defects may interfere with intracellular lysosomal/vesicular trafficking, fusion of acidified vesicles with the "ruffled border" (folded osteoclast cell membrane in areas of bone resorption), and regulation of ionic charge across the cell membrane. In addition, some patients have mutations that interfere with the RANK (receptor activator of nuclear factor-kappa B)/RANK ligand pathway, which is important for osteoclastogenesis.

Although several disease subtypes have been identified, there are three major clinical patterns:
1. **Autosomal recessive infantile ("malignant") type**
2. **Intermediate autosomal recessive type**
3. **Autosomal dominant adult ("benign") type**

The estimated frequency is 1 in 250,000 live births for the recessive types and 1 in 20,000 live births for the autosomal dominant type. A very rare X-linked recessive type has been described as well.

Table 14.2 summarizes a classification system based on phenotype and corresponding genetic defects. Disease

TABLE 14.2 Classification Scheme for Major Forms of Osteopetrosis

Form	Mutated Gene(s)	Gene Product and/or Affected Osteoclast Function(s)	Clinical Phenotype
Autosomal recessive infantile	*TCIRG1*	Proton pump subunit, acid secretion, vesicular trafficking	Severe, osteopetrorickets
	CLCN7	Chloride channel, lysosomal trafficking, acidification	Severe, possible neurodegeneration
	OSTM1	Chloride channel function, lysosomal trafficking, acidification	Severe, neurodegeneration
	RANK (TNFRSF11A)	Cell surface receptor, osteoclast differentiation	Severe
	RANKL (TNFSF11)	Ligand that binds RANK receptor, osteoclast differentiation	Severe
	SNX10	Endolysosomal trafficking/fusion	Severe, osteopetrorickets
Intermediate autosomal recessive	*PLEKHMI*	Vesicle trafficking and acidification	Intermediate
	CAII	Acidification	Intermediate, renal tubular acidosis, cerebral calcifications
Autosomal dominant	*CLCN7*	Chloride channel, lysosomal trafficking, acidification	Mild to severe, rarely lethal
X-linked recessive	*IKBKG (NEMO)*	Osteoclast differentiation and activation	Severe, immunodeficiency, ectodermal dysplasia

CAII, carbonic anhydrase II gene; *CLCN7,* chloride channel 7 gene; *IKBKG,* inhibitor of nuclear factor kappa B kinase subunit gamma gene; *NEMO,* nuclear factor-kappa B essential modulator gene; *OSTM1,* osteopetrosis-associated transmembrane protein 1 gene; *PLEKHM1,* pleckstrin homology domain gene; *RANK,* receptor activator of nuclear factor-kappa B gene; *RANKL,* receptor activator of nuclear factor-kappa B ligand gene; *SNX10,* sorting nexin 10 gene; *TCIRG1,* T-cell immune regulator 1 gene; *TNFRSF11A,* tumor necrosis factor receptor superfamily, member 11A gene (also known as *RANK*); *TNFSF11,* tumor necrosis factor ligand superfamily member 11 gene (also known as *RANKL*).

severity varies widely, potentially even among patients with the same disease subtype.

Clinical and Radiographic Features

Autosomal Recessive Infantile Osteopetrosis

This severe form usually is diagnosed at birth or in early infancy. Typical findings include a diffusely sclerotic skeleton, bone marrow failure, frequent fractures with defective healing, cranial nerve compression, and growth impairment.

The initial signs often are normocytic anemia with hepatosplenomegaly resulting from compensatory extramedullary hematopoiesis. Granulocytopenia causes increased susceptibility to infection. The bone is dense but prone to pathologic fracture. A paradoxical condition termed *osteopetrorickets* often develops; the altered bone is unable to mobilize its overly abundant mineral stores, which results in hypocalcemia, hypophosphatemia, and impaired mineralization of newly formed bone. Individuals with autosomal recessive infantile osteopetrosis typically exhibit a broad face, hypertelorism, snub nose, frontal bossing, and macrocephaly. Cognitive function is usually normal, although neurodegeneration may develop in some disease subtypes. Failure of resorption and remodeling of the skull produces hydrocephalus and narrow skull foramina; cranial nerve compression

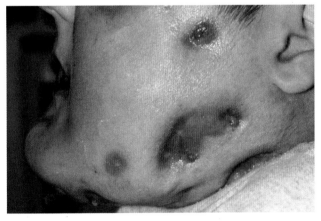

• **Fig. 14.3 Osteopetrosis.** This 24-year-old white man has the infantile form of osteopetrosis. He has mandibular osteomyelitis, and multiple draining fistulae are present on his face. (Courtesy of Dr. Dan Sarasin.)

may result in blindness, deafness, and facial paralysis. Osteomyelitis of the jaws is a frequent complication of tooth extraction (Fig. 14.3).

Radiographically, there is a widespread increase in skeletal density with defects in metaphyseal remodeling. The radiographic distinction between cortical and cancellous bone is

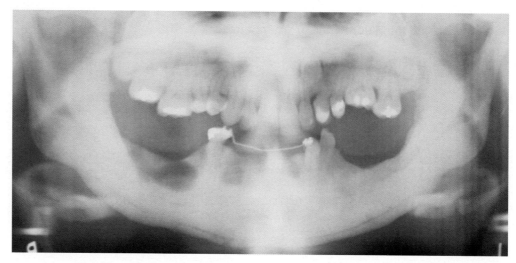

• **Fig. 14.4 Osteopetrosis.** Extensive mandibular involvement is apparent in this radiograph of a 31-year-old woman. She received a diagnosis of osteopetrosis as a child. There is a history of multiple fractures and osteomyelitis of the jaws. (Courtesy of Dr. Dan Sarasin.)

lost (Fig. 14.4). There is often marked thickening of the calvarium and skull base, and there may be poor sinus development. Tooth roots often are difficult to visualize radiographically because of the density of the surrounding bone. In addition, failure of tooth eruption is common. Other possible dental findings include tooth agenesis, malformed crowns and roots, and enamel hypoplasia.

Intermediate Autosomal Recessive Osteopetrosis

Affected patients often are asymptomatic at birth but exhibit fractures by the end of the first decade. Mild to moderate anemia and extramedullary hematopoiesis are common, but bone marrow failure is rare. Short stature, mandibular prognathism, unerupted teeth, and osteomyelitis also have been reported. Individuals with intermediate disease caused by carbonic anhydrase II deficiency typically exhibit renal tubular acidosis and cerebral calcifications.

Autosomal Dominant Adult Osteopetrosis

This most common type usually is discovered in adolescence or adulthood and exhibits less severe manifestations. Sclerosis mainly affects the axial skeleton, with relative sparing of the long bones. Marrow failure is infrequent, and approximately 40% of affected patients are asymptomatic. Among symptomatic patients, findings may include bone pain, frequent fractures, and cranial nerve compression.

Occasionally, the diagnosis is discovered initially on review of dental radiographs that reveal diffusely increased radiopacity of the medullary bone. Mandibular involvement may be associated with an increased risk for fracture and osteomyelitis following tooth extraction.

Other rare conditions causing widespread osteosclerosis should be considered in the differential diagnosis. Such diseases include autosomal dominant endosteal hyperostosis (autosomal dominant osteosclerosis), sclerosteosis, and van Buchem disease.

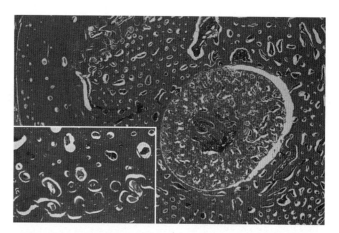

• **Fig. 14.5 Osteopetrosis.** Low-power photomicrograph showing sclerotic bone that is replacing the normal cancellous bone. The *inset* shows a nodular pattern of the dense bone obliterating the marrow spaces.

Histopathologic Features

Several patterns of abnormal endosteal bone formation have been described. These include the following:
• Tortuous lamellar trabeculae replacing the cancellous portion of the bone
• Globular amorphous bone deposition in the marrow spaces (Fig. 14.5)
• Osteophytic bone formation

Osteoclasts may be increased, decreased, or normal in number; however, they do not appear to be functional because Howship lacunae are absent or minimal. In osteoclast-rich disease forms, the scant remaining hematopoetic marrow is fibrotic, and there may be a concurrent increase in the number of activated osteoblasts. In osteoclast-poor disease, the scant residual marrow does not exhibit fibrosis.

Treatment and Prognosis

Treatment is guided by the disease subtype and underlying genetic defect. Because a variety of complications are possible, management may require a multidisciplinary team, including specialists in orthopedics, hematology, developmental pediatrics, endocrinology, infectious disease, neurology, neurosurgery, otolaryngology, and ophthalmology. In addition, dental evaluation is recommended for all patients regardless of disease severity. Preventive oral health care is essential for avoiding extractions or other surgical procedures that may increase the risk for developing osteomyelitis.

For autosomal dominant adult osteopetrosis, no specific treatment is available other than management of disease complications. Although the prognosis varies, most patients exhibit long-term survival.

In contrast, the prognosis for untreated autosomal recessive infantile osteopetrosis is poor, with most patients dying during the first decade of life. For patients with certain disease subtypes, allogeneic hematopoietic stem cell transplantation (HSCT) potentially may be curative. The rationale for this procedure is based on the hematopoietic origin of osteoclasts. HSCT should be performed as soon as possible (before the age of 10 months) in order improve the likelihood of a favorable outcome. However, finding an appropriate donor can be difficult, and the procedure is associated with considerable risk. Alternative treatments include interferon gamma-1b and corticosteroids.

Supportive measures include blood transfusions, analgesics for bone pain, and bone fracture stabilization. Osteomyelitis of the jaws requires rapid intervention to minimize osseous destruction; management typically includes drainage and surgical débridement, bacterial culture with sensitivity testing, and prolonged IV antibiotic therapy. Hyperbaric oxygen may be a useful adjunct in recalcitrant cases, and surgical reconstruction may be necessary.

◆ CLEIDOCRANIAL DYSPLASIA (CLEIDOCRANIAL DYSOSTOSIS; SCHEUTHAUER-MARIE-SAINTON SYNDROME; MARIE-SAINTON DISEASE)

Best known for its dental and clavicular abnormalities, **cleidocranial dysplasia** is a generalized bone disorder caused by mutations in the *RUNX2* (or *CBFA1*) gene on chromosome 6p21. This gene encodes a key transcription factor for osteoblastic differentiation and skeletal morphogenesis. This condition initially was thought to involve only membranous bones (e.g., clavicles, skull, and flat bones), but it is now known to affect endochondral ossification as well. Studies suggest that *RUNX2* additionally plays an important role in odontogenesis via participation in odontoblast differentiation, osteoclastogenesis (in association with the dental follicle and periodontal ligament), enamel organ formation, and dental lamina proliferation. Disruption of these functions might explain the distinct dental anomalies associated

with this disorder. The estimated worldwide prevalence is 1:1,000,000. There is an autosomal dominant inheritance pattern, although as many as 40% of cases may represent spontaneous mutations. In addition, investigators have proposed that an autosomal recessive form and germline mosaicism are possible.

Clinical and Radiographic Features

The bone defects chiefly involve the clavicles and skull, although various other skeletal anomalies may be present (Table 14.3). The clavicles typically are hypoplastic or discontinuous, either unilaterally or bilaterally; in about 10% of cases, the clavicles are completely absent. The patient's neck appears long, and the shoulders are narrow with marked drooping. The clavicular abnormalities result in unusual

TABLE 14.3	Major Clinical and Radiographic Features of Cleidocranial Dysplasia
Anatomic Region	**Features**
Craniofacial/ oral region	• Large skull • Frontal and parietal bossing • Brachycephaly • Ocular hypertelorism • Nose with depressed bridge and broad base • Delayed closure of sutures and fontanels • Wormian bones • Small or absent paranasal sinuses • Narrow, high-arched palate; cleft palate • Numerous unerupted/variably misshapen permanent and supernumerary teeth • Retention of primary dentition; delayed eruption of permanent dentition • Mandible: Prognathism, coarse trabeculation, narrow and parallel-sided rami, slender and pointed coronoid processes with distal curvature, patent symphysis • Hypoplastic maxilla
Thorax	• Hypoplastic, discontinuous, or absent clavicles • Hypoplastic scapulae • Narrow upper thorax • Absent ribs
Pelvis	• Hypoplastic iliac wings • Widening of the pubic symphysis and sacroiliac joints • Delayed ossification of the pubic bone
Extremities	• Genus valgus (knock knees) • Pes planus (flat feet) • Brachydactyly • Tapered fingers and short, broad thumbs • Short terminal phalanges • Long second metacarpals • Short and deformed middle phalanges
Other	• Short stature • Scoliosis

hypermobility, and many patients can approximate their shoulders anteriorly (Fig. 14.6).

Additional features include short stature, narrow chest, wide pubic symphysis, short arms, genu valgu (knock knee deformity), flat feet, and scoliosis. Craniofacial findings include enlarged skull, brachycephaly, and pronounced frontal and parietal bossing. Ocular hypertelorism and a broad-based nose with a depressed bridge often are noted as well. On skull radiographs, the sutures and fontanels show delayed closure or may remain open throughout life. Secondary centers of ossification appear in the suture lines, and many

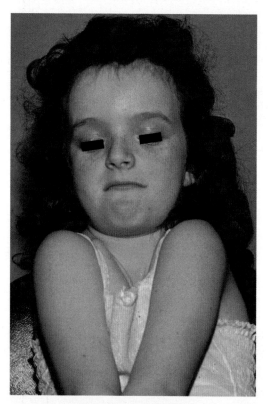

• **Fig. 14.6 Cleidocranial Dysplasia.** Patient can almost approximate her shoulders in front of her chest. (Courtesy of Dr. William Bruce.)

Wormian bones may be seen. Abnormal development of the temporal bone and eustachian tube may lead to conductive or sensorineural hearing loss and recurrent ear infections.

The gnathic and dental manifestations are distinctive and may lead to the initial diagnosis. Patients often have a narrow, high-arched palate, and there is an increased prevalence of cleft palate. Over-retained deciduous teeth and delay or complete failure of permanent tooth eruption are characteristic features. There may be abnormal spacing in the mandibular incisor area because of widening of the alveolar bone. On dental radiographs, the most dramatic finding is the presence of numerous unerupted permanent and supernumerary teeth, often exhibiting distorted crown and root shapes (Fig. 14.7). Dentigerous cysts occasionally may arise in association with these unerupted teeth. The number of supernumerary teeth can be impressive, with some patients demonstrating more than 60 such teeth. In addition, the mandible often demonstrates coarse trabeculation with areas of increased density; narrow rami with nearly parallel anterior and posterior borders; and slender, pointed coronoid processes with a distal curvature. In some cases, the mandibular symphysis remains patent. There may be a thin zygomatic arch with a downward bend and small or absent maxillary sinuses. Generalized hypoplasia of the paranasal sinuses may predispose the patient to recurrent sinus infections.

As the patient ages, a short lower face height, acute gonial angle, anterior inclination of the mandible, and mandibular prognathism develop. These changes may result from inadequate vertical growth of the maxilla and hypoplastic alveolar ridge development caused by delay or lack of permanent tooth eruption.

Histopathologic Features

The reason for failure of permanent tooth eruption in cleidocranial dysplasia is poorly understood. Some microscopic studies have reported a lack of secondary cementum in unerupted teeth, although other studies have disputed this finding. Additional proposed hypotheses include increased

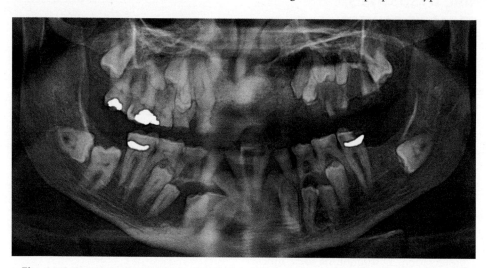

• **Fig. 14.7 Cleidocranial Dysplasia.** Panoramic radiograph showing multiple unerupted and supernumerary teeth. (Courtesy of Dr. Samer Joudeh.)

jawbone density, abnormally coarse trabecular pattern of the jaws, and insufficient alveolar bone resorption—possibly resulting from altered periodontal ligament cells with reduced capacity to induce osteoclastogenesis. The development of supernumerary teeth has been theorized to result from hyperactive or persistent dental lamina.

Treatment and Prognosis

Most patients function well. An affected individual may be unaware of the disease until a professional calls it to his or her attention.

The dental problems may be difficult to address, and early intervention is recommended. Treatment typically involves removal of primary and supernumerary teeth followed by exposure and orthodontic extrusion of permanent teeth. The extractions may be conducted in stages (according to the extent of root development of the unerupted permanent dentition) or in a single procedure. If completed before adulthood, then such treatment may prevent short lower face height and mandibular prognathism. Orthognathic surgery also may be considered after growth completion. Additional treatment options include full-mouth extractions or autotransplantation of selected impacted teeth followed by fabrication of an appropriate prosthesis. In several reported cases, dental implants have been placed successfully; however, further studies are needed to assess whether the altered bone might compromise osseointegration.

◆ FOCAL OSTEOPOROTIC MARROW DEFECT

The **focal osteoporotic marrow defect** is an area of hematopoietic marrow that is sufficient in size to produce a radiolucency. This entity does not represent a pathologic process, but its radiographic features may be confused with an intraosseous neoplasm or other pathosis. The pathogenesis is unknown, although the following theories have been proposed:

- Aberrant bone regeneration after tooth extraction or dental implant placement
- Persistence of fetal marrow
- Marrow hyperplasia in response to increased demand for erythrocytes

Clinical and Radiographic Features

Approximately 75% of cases occur in adult females, and about 70% involve the posterior mandible, most often in edentulous areas. The defect is typically asymptomatic and nonexpansile. Most cases are detected incidentally during radiographic examination, which shows a radiolucency ranging from several millimeters to several centimeters in diameter. The borders typically appear well-circumscribed on panoramic radiographs; however, more detailed periapical radiographs may exhibit ill-defined borders and fine central trabeculation (Fig. 14.8). There is usually an isolated defect, although multifocal involvement is possible.

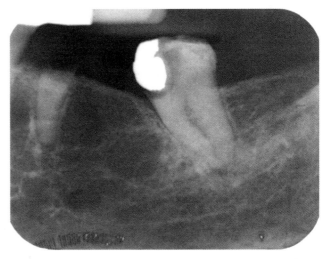

• **Fig. 14.8 Focal Osteoporotic Marrow Defect.** Fairly well-circumscribed radiolucency with fine central trabeculation in the extraction site of a mandibular molar. (Courtesy of Dr. R. Sidney Jones.)

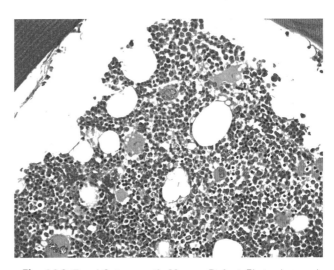

• **Fig. 14.9 Focal Osteoporotic Marrow Defect.** Photomicrograph showing normal hematopoietic bone marrow.

Histopathologic Features

Microscopically, the defect contains cellular hematopoietic and/or fatty marrow (Fig. 14.9). The associated bony trabeculae show no evidence of abnormal osteoblastic or osteoclastic activity.

Treatment and Prognosis

The radiographic findings are often suggestive of the diagnosis but are nonspecific. Incisional biopsy, therefore, often is necessary to establish the diagnosis. Once the diagnosis is made, no further treatment is needed. The prognosis is excellent, and there appears to be no significant association with anemia or other hematologic disorders.

◆ IDIOPATHIC OSTEOSCLEROSIS

Idiopathic osteosclerosis represents focally increased bone density of unknown cause. It cannot be attributed to any inflammatory, dysplastic, neoplastic, or systemic disorder. Some authorities consider this condition to represent a developmental variation of normal bony architecture. Idiopathic osteosclerosis also has been termed *dense bone island, bone eburnation, bone whorl, bone scar, enostosis,* and *focal periapical osteopetrosis.* The following discussion focuses on jaw involvement, although similar sclerotic areas may occur in other bones.

In addition, similar radiopaque foci may develop in the periapical areas of teeth with nonvital or inflamed pulps; these lesions most likely represent a response to inflammation. Such reactive foci are termed **condensing osteitis** or **focal chronic sclerosing osteomyelitis** (see page 141) and should not be designated *idiopathic osteosclerosis.* Because past studies did not distinguish between idiopathic and inflammatory lesions, confusion in terminology has resulted.

Clinical and Radiographic Features

The estimated prevalence is 6%, with some investigators suggesting a slightly increased frequency in blacks and Asians. Most authors report either a female predilection or no significant sex predilection. According to several long-term studies, most examples of idiopathic osteosclerosis arise in the late first or early second decade. The sclerotic area may slowly increase in size, with peak diameter usually attained once the patient reaches full maturity. The peak prevalence is in the third decade, with peak bone mass in the fourth decade. Later in adulthood, the sclerosis typically remains stable, decreases in size, or undergoes complete regression.

Idiopathic osteosclerosis is invariably asymptomatic and nonexpansile. The condition typically is detected incidentally during routine radiographic examination. About 90%

of cases occur in the mandible, most often in the molar and premolar regions. In most patients, only one sclerotic focus is present, although some patients have two to four foci. For patients with multifocal involvement, the possibility of multiple osteomas within the setting of Gardner syndrome (see page 656) should be excluded.

Radiographically, idiopathic osteosclerosis typically appears as a well-defined radiopacity, ranging from 0.2 to 2.0 cm in diameter. However, ill-defined borders, diameter as large as 7.0 cm, or a mixed radiolucent-radiopaque appearance have been described infrequently. The radiopacity may be round, oval, square, elongated, triangular, or irregular. There is no radiolucent rim, with the exception of unusual cases involving the mandibular canal. Most examples are uniformly radiopaque, although a nonhomogeneous core sometimes may be evident. The condition often is associated with tooth roots—the opacity may obscure a portion of the root, contact the lamina dura, or arise in close proximity to the root. Many examples are associated with a root apex or occur between the roots of teeth, but cases unrelated to teeth also are possible (Fig. 14.10). Rarely, the sclerotic bone may surround an impacted tooth. Root resorption and tooth movement have been noted infrequently.

Histopathologic Features

Microscopic examination shows dense lamellar bone with scant fibrofatty marrow. Inflammatory cells are inconspicuous or absent.

Diagnosis

Usually a diagnosis of idiopathic osteosclerosis may be made with confidence, based on history, clinical features, and radiographic findings. Biopsy is warranted if there are symptoms or significant cortical expansion. Although idiopathic osteosclerosis demonstrates radiographic and histopathologic

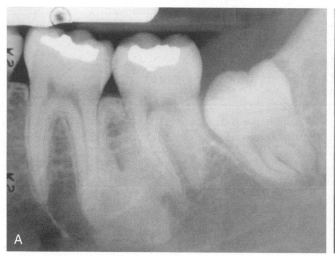
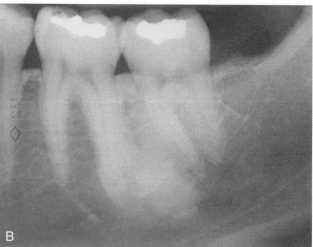

• **Fig. 14.10** **Idiopathic Osteosclerosis. A,** An asymptomatic area of bone sclerosis is seen between and apical to the roots of the first and second mandibular molars. **B,** No appreciable change can be seen on this radiograph taken 10 years later. (Courtesy of Dr. Michael Quinn.)

similarities with a compact osteoma (see page 655), lack of cortical expansion and failure of continued growth rule against a neoplastic process. Tooth vitality and the absence of a deep restoration or caries help to distinguish idiopathic osteosclerosis from condensing osteitis.

Treatment and Prognosis

If the lesion is discovered during adolescence, periodic radiographs appear prudent until the area stabilizes. After that point, no treatment is indicated, because there is little or no tendency for the lesions to progress in adulthood.

◆ MASSIVE OSTEOLYSIS (GORHAM DISEASE; GORHAM-STOUT SYNDROME; VANISHING BONE DISEASE; PHANTOM BONE DISEASE; IDIOPATHIC OSTEOLYSIS)

Massive osteolysis is a rare disease characterized by spontaneous and usually progressive destruction of one or more bones. The destroyed bone is replaced by a vascular proliferation and, ultimately, dense fibrous tissue without bone regeneration.

The etiopathogenesis is unknown. There is no evidence of underlying metabolic or endocrine imbalance. Proposed pathogenetic mechanisms include the following:
* Trauma-induced proliferation of vascular granulation tissue
* Trauma-induced activation of a previously silent hamartoma
* Slow blood flow through dilated lesional vessels, resulting in local hypoxia, reduced pH, and activation of hydrolytic enzymes
* Increased osteoclastic activity (mediated by interleukin-6) and increased sensitivity of osteoclast precursors to humoral factors (such as receptor activator of nuclear factor kappa B ligand [RANKL] and macrophage colony-stimulating factor [M-CSF])
* Lymphangiogenesis mediated by vascular endothelial growth factor (VEGF) and platelet-derived growth factor (PDGF)
* Agenesis or dysfunction of thyroid C cells

In addition, based on molecular genetic studies in a limited number of cases, some investigators have suggested a potential pathogenetic role for *TNFRSF11A*, *TREM2*, and *PTEN* mutations.

Clinical and Radiographic Features

The disease occurs over a broad age range (1 month to 76 years), with a predilection for children and young adults. Among patients with jaw involvement, the mean age is approximately 32 years, and the male-to-female ratio is 1.7:1. Although any bone can be affected, commonly reported sites include the pelvic bones, shoulder bones, craniomaxillofacial skeleton, ribs, sternum, and spine.

Multicentric involvement and extension into soft tissue may be evident.

Gnathic lesions most often involve the mandible. Simultaneous involvement of both jaws and extension to adjacent extragnathic sites are possible. About half of patients are symptomatic. Signs and symptoms include mobile teeth, pain, malocclusion, deviation of the mandible, and clinically obvious deformity. Potential sequelae include pathologic fracture and obstructive sleep apnea; the latter may occur secondary to posterior mandibular displacement after extensive osteolysis. Temporomandibular joint (TMJ) involvement may be confused with other conditions that can cause TMJ dysfunction. Elevated serum alkaline phosphatase has been noted in about a fourth of reported gnathic cases.

Radiographically, the earliest changes consist of intramedullary radiolucent foci of varying size with indistinct margins (Fig. 14.11). Loss of the lamina dura and thinning of the cortical plates may precede development of obvious radiolucency. In some cases, the bone destruction may mimic periodontitis or periapical inflammatory disease. With progression, the radiolucent foci coalesce, enlarge, and extend to the cortical bone. Eventually, large portions of bone disappear (Fig. 14.12).

Histopathologic Features

Microscopically, early lesions exhibit a nonspecific vascular proliferation intermixed with fibrous connective tissue and chronic inflammatory cells (Fig. 14.13). Blood vessels and/or lymphatic vessels may be present, although current evidence suggests the latter predominate. Immunohistochemistry with the D2-40 antibody may be performed to highlight lymphatic endothelium. The vascular channels are thin-walled and may vary in size. Within the adjacent bone, the osteocyte lacunae may be enlarged without significant alteration in the number of osteoclasts present. In later stages, there is fibrosis without bone regeneration.

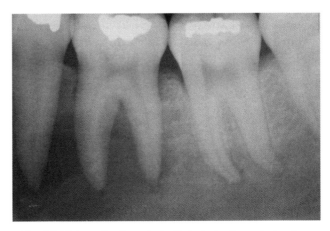

• **Fig. 14.11 Massive Osteolysis.** Periapical radiograph showing an ill-defined radiolucency associated with vital mandibular teeth. Note the loss of lamina dura. (Courtesy of Dr. John R. Cramer.)

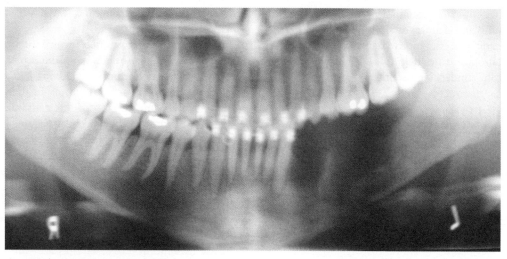

• **Fig. 14.12 Massive Osteolysis.** Panoramic radiograph of the same patient shown in Fig. 14.11, showing extensive bone loss and a pathologic fracture of the left mandible. This destruction occurred over an 8-month period. (Courtesy of Dr. John R. Cramer.)

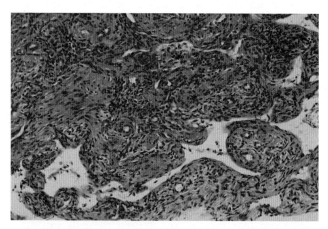

• **Fig. 14.13 Massive Osteolysis.** Biopsy specimen from the same patient shown in Figs. 14.11 and 14.12. The loose, highly vascular connective tissue shows a diffuse chronic inflammatory cell infiltrate.

Treatment and Prognosis

The clinical course of massive osteolysis is variable and unpredictable. In most cases, bone destruction progresses over months to a few years and results in complete loss of the affected bone or bones. Some patients, however, experience spontaneous arrest of the process without complete loss of the affected bone. Uncommonly, death results from respiratory compromise due to severe thoracic involvement or from spinal cord compression due to vertebral destruction.

There is no standardized therapy, and treatment is not particularly satisfactory. Maxillofacial lesions most commonly are managed by observation or surgical resection. Surgical reconstruction may be complicated by bone graft resorption and inadequate bone for fixation; therefore, it is advisable to delay reconstruction until arrest of the osteolytic disease phase. Alternative treatment options includes radiation therapy or medications, which at times may be combined with surgery. However, particularly in young patients, there are concerns regarding the potential for post-irradiation sarcoma and radiation-induced developmental defects. Medical treatments include bisphosphonates, interferon alpha-2b, sirolimus, anti-VEGF antibodies, corticosteroids, calcitonin, vitamin D, and calcium-containing compounds. However, the effectiveness of any therapeutic intervention is difficult to evaluate because the disease is so rare and the condition may arrest spontaneously in some patients. Therefore, further studies are needed.

◆ PAGET DISEASE OF BONE (OSTEITIS DEFORMANS)

Paget disease of bone is characterized by abnormal, anarchic resorption and deposition of bone, resulting in skeletal distortion and weakening. It represents the second most common metabolic bone disorder after osteoporosis and primarily affects older adults of Anglo-Saxon ancestry. There is marked variation in reported prevalence by geographic region, with the highest rates in the United Kingdom. The disease also frequently occurs in Australia, New Zealand, Western and Southern Europe, and North America. In the United States, the disease affects approximately 1%–2% of the general population. For reasons unclear, significant declines in disease incidence and severity have been observed in recent decades in many high-prevalence regions.

The etiology is unknown, but both genetic and environmental factors have been proposed. Approximately one-third of patients have a first-degree relative with the disease, and an autosomal dominant inheritance pattern with incomplete penetrance has been observed. In about 40% of familial cases and 5% of sporadic cases, germline mutations in the sequestosome 1 gene *(SQSTM1)* (which encodes the p62 protein) have been identified. Patients with *SQSTM1* mutations tend to have more severe disease than those without such mutations. *SQSTM1* mutations result in activation of the nuclear factor-kappa B (NF-κB) signaling pathway and increased osteoclastic activity. In addition, rare mutations in other genes affecting this pathway have been detected in some patients with familial Paget disease or Paget-like disorders. Furthermore, genome-wide association studies have identified polymorphisms in various genes that appear to confer increased susceptibility to Paget disease.

The possibility that Paget disease results from a slow virus infection has received considerable attention but remains controversial. Inclusion bodies resembling nucleocapsids from a paramyxovirus have been detected in osteoclasts from affected individuals; however, attempts to demonstrate mRNA and proteins from paramyxoviruses in patient tissue samples have yielded variable results. In animal models, interactions between measles virus infection and *SQSTM1* mutations can produce Paget-like bone lesions. Additional circumstantial evidence is provided by epidemiologic studies that have noted an association with rural living, thereby suggesting possible transmission of an infectious agent via contact with farm animals.

The primary underlying abnormality in Paget disease appears to be in the osteoclasts, which are increased in size, number, and activity. *In vitro* studies suggest that increased osteoclastogenesis may result from hyperresponsiveness of osteoclast precursors to receptor activator of nuclear factor kappa B ligand (RANKL), tumor necrosis factor-alpha (TNF-α), and 1, 25-dihydroxyvitamin D3. In response to increased bone resorption by osteoclasts, there is accelerated but haphazard bone formation by osteoblasts.

Clinical and Radiographic Features

Paget disease of bone primarily affects older patients. Disease frequency increases with age, and the mean age at diagnosis has been increasing in many populations. The condition is rare in patients younger than 50 years. Most studies report a male predilection.

At diagnosis many patients present with bone pain, although at least 25% are asymptomatic. Asymptomatic disease may be discovered incidentally when radiographic examination or serum alkaline phosphatase measurement is performed for unrelated reasons. Bone pain may result from either increased bone turnover or secondary complications (e.g., osteoarthritis, spinal stenosis, pathologic fracture, and pseudofracture). Pagetic bone pain typically is mild to moderate, with worsening at rest and improvement during movement. In contrast, secondary osteoarthritic pain tends to be severe and excerbated by movement.

The disease arises in one or more bones simultaneously, and involvement typically remains restricted to these original sites throughout the disease course. The pelvis, vertebrae, femur, tibia, and skull are involved most commonly. Affected bones become thickened, enlarged, and weakened, with an increased risk for fracture. Involvement of weight-bearing bones often leads to bowing deformity, resulting in a "simian (monkeylike) stance." Skull involvement generally causes a progressive increase in head circumference. Deafness and visual impairment may result from nerve compression or other mechanisms. Cardiovascular complications,

including arterial calcifications and high-output congestive heart failure, also are possible.

Jaw involvement is present in about 17% of patients, with a predilection for the maxilla (approximate 2:1 maxilla-to-mandible ratio). Maxillary disease produces enlargement of the middle third of the face and may result in nasal obstruction, enlarged turbinates, obliterated sinuses, and deviated septum. In extreme cases, there is a lion-like facial deformity **(leontiasis ossea).** The alveolar ridges tend to remain symmetrical but become grossly enlarged. Alveolar enlargement may cause spacing between teeth, and edentulous patients may complain that their dentures feel too tight.

Radiographically, in early disease stages, the affected bone exhibits decreased radiodensity and a coarse trabecular pattern. Particularly in the skull, large circumscribed radiolucencies may be present **(osteoporosis circumscripta).** In later disease stages, patchy areas of bone sclerosis form and tend to become confluent. The patchy sclerotic areas characteristically exhibit a "cotton wool" appearance, and marked bony expansion is evident (Figs. 14.14 and 14.15). In addition, the teeth may demonstrate generalized hypercementosis.

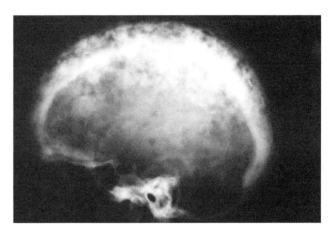

• **Fig. 14.14 Paget Disease.** Lateral skull film shows marked enlargement of the cranium with new bone formation above the outer table of the skull and a patchy, dense, "cotton wool" appearance. (Courtesy of Dr. Reg Munden.)

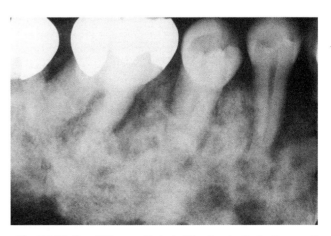

• **Fig. 14.15 Paget Disease.** Periapical film showing the "cotton wool" appearance of the bone.

Radiographic findings of Paget disease may resemble those of cemento-osseous dysplasia (see page 645). Patients with presumed cemento-osseous dysplasia who develop significant jaw expansion should be evaluated further to rule out Paget disease.

Histopathologic Features

Microscopic examination shows uncontrolled resorption and formation of bone. In the resorptive phase, numerous hyperactive osteoclasts surround the bone trabeculae; these osteoclasts tend to be enlarged with an increased number of nuclei. In addition, highly vascular fibrous connective tissue replaces the marrow. Behind the "leading edge" of osteoclastic activity, there is a gradual conversion from predominantly osteoclastic to osteoblastic activity. The osteoblasts form osteoid rims around the bone trabeculae, and the bone lacks an organized lamellar pattern. Basophilic reversal lines, which indicate the junction between alternating bone resorption and formation, result in a characteristic "jigsaw puzzle" or "mosaic" appearance (Fig. 14.16). In the sclerotic phase, there are large masses of dense bone with prominent reversal lines.

Diagnosis

Diagnosis typically requires correlation of the clinical and radiographic findings with laboratory test results. In addition, bone scintigraphy may help to determine the extent of involvement. Histopathologic examination can be confirmatory but often is unnecessary for diagnosis.

Laboratory testing typically shows elevated serum alkaline phosphatase levels with normal blood calcium and phosphorus levels. Although serum bone-specific alkaline phosphatase is considered the most sensitive marker of bone formation, total serum alkaline phosphatase is more widely available and, thus, typically used in routine clinical practice. When measuring total serum alkaline phosphatase, liver enzymes also should be assessed in order to exclude elevated alkaline phosphatase of hepatic origin.

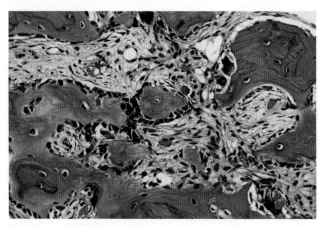

• **Fig. 14.16 Paget Disease.** Prominent osteoblastic and osteoclastic activity surround the bone trabeculae. Note the resting and reversal lines.

In patients with limited disease extent, total serum alkaline phosphatase may be within normal range. In such cases, it may be helpful to assess specialized markers of bone formation (e.g., serum procollagen type 1 N-terminal propeptide) or resorption (e.g., urinary N-terminal telopeptide of type 1 collagen).

Treatment and Prognosis

Paget disease is chronic and slowly progressive but seldom fatal. Asymptomatic patients with limited disease do not require treatment. Patients with symptomatic or extensive disease typically receive bisphosphonate therapy (i.e., single infusion of zoledronic acid; oral risedronate or alendronate administered daily for several months). Studies have demonstrated that such treatment can reduce bone turnover, induce normalization of alkaline phosphatase levels, and decrease bone pain. In particular, single-infusion therapy with zoledronic acid is highly effective in achieving sustained disease remission. However, there is currently insufficient evidence regarding whether bisphosphonates may reduce the risk for long-term complications, such as osteoarthritis, bone deformity, and deafness. Analgesics and nonsteroidal anti-inflammatory drugs (NSAIDs) may be useful for controlling pain caused by secondary osteoarthritis. Management of Paget disease also may include orthotics, canes or other mobility devices, and orthopedic surgery (e.g., hip or joint replacement). Prior to orthopedic surgery involving an active disease site, bisphosphonates may be administered in order to reduce the risk for excessive blood loss.

Potential dental complications include difficulties in extracting teeth with hypercementosis and/or ankylosis; extensive hemorrhage from oral surgical procedures performed during the vascular lytic phase; and poor wound healing with increased susceptibility to osteomyelitis during the avascular sclerotic phase. Edentulous patients may require new dentures periodically to compensate for progressive alveolar enlargement. Pagetic bone and a history of bisphosphonate therapy generally are considered unfavorable factors for osseointegration of dental implants, although successful implant placement has been reported in a few cases.

Malignant transformation of pagetic bone into osteosarcoma or other sarcomas is a rare disease complication, with an estimated lifetime risk of less than 1%. A sudden increase in bone pain or swelling should raise suspicion of possible underlying malignancy. Osteosarcoma in adults older than 40 years is quite uncommon in individuals who do not have Paget disease. Most Paget-related osteosarcomas develop in the pelvis and long bones of the extremities—the skull and jaws are affected only rarely. Osteosarcoma in Paget disease is very aggressive and associated with a poor prognosis.

Another rare complication of Paget disease is the development of benign and malignant giant cell tumors (see page 633), most often involving the craniofacial skeleton. Heritable mutations in the *ZNF687* gene recently have been identified in an unusual subset of patients with early-onset Paget disease, subsequent development of giant cell tumors, and often Italian descent.

◆ CENTRAL GIANT CELL GRANULOMA (GIANT CELL LESION; GIANT CELL TUMOR)

The **central giant cell granuloma** is an intraosseous lesion of unknown etiology. There has been much debate regarding whether this entity represents a reactive process or a benign neoplasm, with mounting evidence favoring the latter. In the past, it was hypothesized to represent a reparative response to trauma-induced hemorrhage—hence, its former designation *giant cell reparative granuloma*. However, there is little evidence to support a reparative response; therefore, most oral and maxillofacial pathologists today prefer the term *giant cell granuloma* or the more noncommittal term *giant cell lesion*. In fact, some examples demonstrate locally aggressive behavior similar to that of a benign neoplasm, and the recent identification of pathogenic mutations supports a monoclonal proliferation. In particular, genetic studies have demonstrated recurrent somatic mutations in *TRPV4, KRAS,* or *FGFR1* in approximately 70% of cases examined. These mutations activate the Ras-MAPK (mitogen-activated protein kinase) pathway and appear to be important drivers in disease development. Interestingly, similar mutations stimulating this pathway have been identified in a host of other conditions that produce giant cell proliferations in the oral cavity (Table 14.4). Furthermore, the nonossifying fibroma—a lesion often occurring in the metaphysis of long bones in young individuals—frequently harbors activating mutations in *KRAS, FGFR1,* and *NF1*. This observation has prompted some investigators to suggest that the nonossifying fibroma of long bones and the central giant cell granuloma of the jaws may represent variants of the same entity.

Clinical and Radiographic Features

Central giant cell granulomas of the jaws occur over a broad age range (0–86 years), although about 70% of cases occur before age 30. There is a female predilection, and approximately 70% of cases arise in the mandible. Lesions are more common in the anterior portions of the jaws, and mandibular lesions frequently cross the midline. Although central giant cell granulomas also have been reported in various extragnathic sites, it is uncertain whether such cases actually represent true **giant cell tumors** (see next topic).

Based on the clinical and radiographic features, central giant cell granulomas of the jaws may be divided into two categories:

1. **Nonaggressive lesions** comprise most cases. They are relatively small, exhibit few or no symptoms, grow slowly, and do not cause cortical perforation or root resorption. Such lesions typically are discovered during routine radiographic examination or as a result of painless jaw expansion.

2. **Aggressive lesions** are characterized by pain, rapid growth, cortical perforation, root resorption, tooth displacement, and/or paresthesia. Extension into soft tissue and ulceration of the overlying mucosal surface also are possible (Fig. 14.17). Compared to nonaggressive lesions, aggressive lesions tend to be larger at diagnosis, develop in somewhat younger patients, and exhibit a greater recurrence potential.

Radiographically, the central giant cell granuloma appears as a unilocular or multilocular radiolucency, with well-delineated but generally noncorticated borders (Fig. 14.18). The lesion may vary from a 5 mm incidental radiographic

TABLE 14.4	Lesions or Conditions with Oral Giant Cell Proliferation and Mutations Activating the Ras-MAPK Pathway
Lesion or Condition	**Comment**
Central giant cell granuloma	Recent studies have demonstrated recurrent somatic activating mutations in *TRPV4, KRAS,* or *FGFR1* in approximately 70% of cases examined.
Peripheral giant cell granuloma (see page 527)	This gingival lesion may be considered the soft tissue counterpart of the central giant cell granuloma. In one study, activating mutations in *KRAS* and *FGFR1* were detected in about 70% and 10% of examined cases, respectively. Implant-associated peripheral giant cell granulomas also may exhibit *KRAS* mutations.
Brown tumor of hyperparathyroidism (see page 840)	In one study, about half of examined cases from the jaws exhibited activating *KRAS* mutations.
"RASopathies" (disorders of the Ras-MAPK pathway)	These disorders are caused by germline mutations in genes encoding Ras-MAPK signaling pathway components. Multifocal giant cell lesions of the jaws can occur in association with various heritable syndromes within this category, including Noonan syndrome, neurofibromatosis type 1 (see page 537), cardio-facio-cutaneous syndrome, and Noonan syndrome with multiple lentigines (LEOPARD syndrome).
Osteoglophonic dysplasia	This rare heritable disorder is caused by FGFR1 mutations. Giant cell lesions of the gingiva and nonossifying fibromas of long bones may develop. Other features include craniosynostosis, rhizomelic dwarfism, hypertelorism, depressed nasal bridge, midface hypoplasia, frontal bossing, macroglossia, prognathism, oligodontia or anodontia, and impacted teeth.

FGFR1, fibroblast growth factor receptor 1 gene; *KRAS*, Kirsten rat sarcoma viral oncogene; LEOPARD, multiple lentigines, electrocardiographic conduction abnormalities, ocular hypertelorism, pulmonic stenosis, abnormal genitalia, retardation of growth, and sensorineural deafness; MAPK, mitogen-activated protein kinase; *TRPV4*, transient receptor potential cation channel subfamily V member 4 gene.

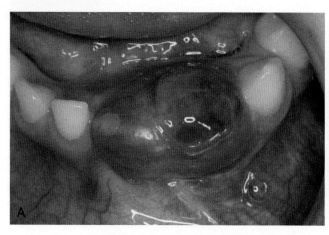 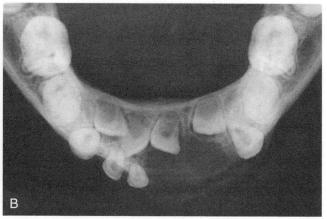

• **Fig. 14.17 Central Giant Cell Granuloma. A,** A blue-purple, ulcerated mass is present on the anterior alveolar ridge of this 4-year-old white boy. **B,** The occlusal radiograph shows a radiolucent lesion with cortical expansion.

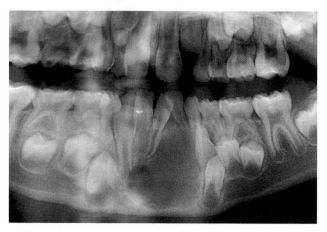

• **Fig. 14.18 Central Giant Cell Granuloma.** Panoramic radiograph showing a well-delineated radiolucent lesion in the anterior mandible.

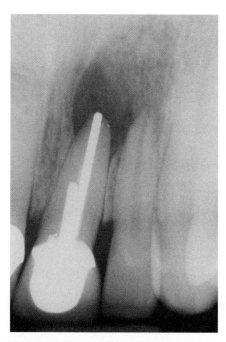

• **Fig. 14.19 Central Giant Cell Granuloma.** The periapical radiograph shows a radiolucent area involving the apex of an endodontically treated tooth. This was considered preoperatively to represent a periapical granuloma or periapical cyst.

finding to a destructive lesion greater than 10 cm. Small unilocular lesions may be confused with periapical granulomas or cysts (Fig. 14.19), and multilocular lesions may appear similar to ameloblastomas. On CBCT examination, the bone at the periphery of the lesion may demonstrate a subtle, granular pattern, and multilocular examples may exhibit a mixture of wispy and coarse septa.

Histopathologic Features

Microscopically, giant cell lesions of the jaws exhibit few to many multinucleated giant cells in a background of ovoid to spindle-shaped mononuclear stromal cells (Fig. 14.20). Investigators have proposed that the spindle cell component is the proliferating cell population and recruits monocyte-macrophage precursors, inducing them to differentiate into osteoclastic giant cells by activation of the RANK/RANKL signaling pathway. The giant cells may be aggregated focally in the lesional tissue or may be present diffusely throughout the lesion. These cells vary considerably in size and shape from case to case. Some are small and irregular in shape with

only a few nuclei, whereas others are large and round with 20 or more nuclei.

The stroma may be loosely arranged and edematous or more cellular. Older lesions may show considerable stromal fibrosis. Erythrocyte extravasation and hemosiderin deposition are often prominent. Focal bone or osteoid formation may be present.

Correlation of the histopathologic features with clinical behavior remains debatable. There are conflicting reports regarding whether more aggressive giant cell lesions of the jaws may be associated with an increased number of giant cells, larger giant cells, a greater fractional surface area occupied by giant cells, and a higher mitotic index. A few studies

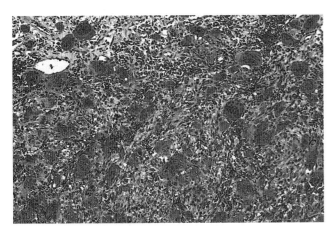

• **Fig. 14.20 Central Giant Cell Granuloma.** Numerous multinucleated giant cells within a background of plump proliferating mesenchymal cells. Note extensive red blood cell extravasation.

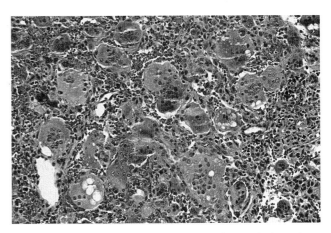

• **Fig. 14.21 Giant Cell Tumor.** This photomicrograph shows large giant cells that are distributed in a cellular mesenchymal tissue. This specimen was from an aggressive lesion that had destroyed most of the maxilla.

suggest that increased vascular density, increased expression of markers of angiogenesis, and increased expression of matrix metalloproteinases might correlate with aggressive clinical behavior.

The microscopic differential diagnosis includes numerous other entities. Because giant cell granulomas are histopathologically identical to brown tumors, hyperparathyroidism (see page 840) should be ruled out in all instances. In addition, areas microscopically identical to central giant cell granuloma have been noted in aneurysmal bone cysts (see page 638) and intermixed with central odontogenic fibromas (see page 731). Associations with benign fibro-osseous lesions and, more rarely, melorheostosis (an unusual bone disease characterized by cortical hyperostosis with a radiographic pattern likened to dripping candle wax and recently found to harbor somatic mutations in *MAP2K1* or other genes) have been noted as well. Furthermore, multifocal giant cell lesions of the jaws may occur infrequently as an isolated finding or in association with certain heritable conditions, including cherubism (see page 634), Ramon syndrome, Jaffe-Campanacci syndrome, and so-called "RASopathies" (see Table 14.4).

Treatment and Prognosis

Central giant cell granulomas of the jaws usually are treated by thorough curettage. Recurrent lesions may require further curettage (at times combined with peripheral ostectomy) or *en bloc* resection. Alternative treatments include intralesional corticosteroid injections, subcutaneous or nasal calcitonin, subcutaneous interferon alpha-2a, imatinib, denosumab, and bisphosphonates. Although further studies are needed, nonsurgical approaches may be desirable when surgical removal of a large tumor would result in significant deformity.

Among reported cases, the overall recurrence rate is approximately 18%. Lesions with aggressive clinicoradiographic features exhibit increased recurrence potential. In spite of the potential for recurrence, the long-term prognosis is good.

◆ GIANT CELL TUMOR ("TRUE GIANT CELL TUMOR")

The relationship between **giant cell tumors** of the extragnathic skeleton and giant cell lesions of the jaws is uncertain and controversial. Many authorities regard these two groups of lesions as distinct entities, based on differences in clinicopathologic features and biologic behavior. Extragnathic giant cell tumors have been found to exhibit somatic mutations in *H3F3A* (which encodes a histone protein) and, less often, *IDH1 or IDH2* (which encode isocitrate dehydrogenase 1 and 2, respectively), whereas giant cell lesions of the jaws have not been found to harbor such alterations. Instead, recent studies suggest that somatic *TRPV4*, *KRAS*, and *FGFR1* mutations are important drivers in the etiopathogenesis of the jaw lesions. Clinically, extragnathic giant cell tumors most often occur in the epiphyses of long bones. Compared to giant cell lesions of the jaws, extragnathic tumors are more likely to cause pain and tend to be diagnosed in patients who are 1 to 2 decades older on average. Some microscopic studies suggest that extragnathic giant cell tumors tend to exhibit more stromal cellularity and larger, more uniformly distributed giant cells, with a greater number of nuclei. Nonetheless, jaw lesions occasionally may exhibit microscopic features that are indistinguishable from typical extragnathic giant cell tumors (Fig. 14.21). In terms of biologic behavior, compared to jaw lesions, extragnathic lesions tend to be more aggressive, with higher recurrence rates after curettage. Pulmonary metastases ("benign pulmonary implants") and malignant transformation have been noted in approximately 2% of extragnathic giant cell tumors.

On the other hand, some researchers have found that giant cell granulomas of the jaws and giant cell tumors of the extragnathic skeleton are similar in many respects when substratification by clinical behavior is taken into account. These investigators hypothesize that giant cell lesions tend to be diagnosed earlier in the jaws compared to other sites simply because of frequent routine dental examinations and readily apparent changes in facial appearance.

◆ CHERUBISM

Cherubism is a rare developmental jaw condition that can be inherited as an autosomal dominant trait with variable expressivity. However, some cases appear to represent *de novo* mutations. A few investigators have reported a higher penetrance in males than in females, but others have questioned this finding.

Most cases are caused by gain-of-function mutations in the *SH3BP2* gene on chromosome 4p16. These mutations lead to enhanced stability of the 3BP2 adaptor protein and consequent upregulation of various signal transduction pathways. As a result, enhanced osteoclastogenesis and hyperactive osteoclasts produce lytic bone lesions. In addition, mouse model studies demonstrating increased production of tumor necrosis factor-alpha (TNF-α) by macrophages suggest a role for inflammation in this disorder. However, it is unclear why the lesions in cherubism primarily affect the jaws. Investigators hypothesize that rapid bone remodeling during childhood tooth eruption and oral commensal bacteria may play a role.

The name *cherubism* was applied to this condition because the facial appearance is similar to that of the plump-cheeked little angels (cherubs) depicted in Renaissance paintings. Although cherubism also has been called *familial fibrous dysplasia,* this term should be avoided because cherubism has no relationship to fibrous dysplasia of bone (see page 641).

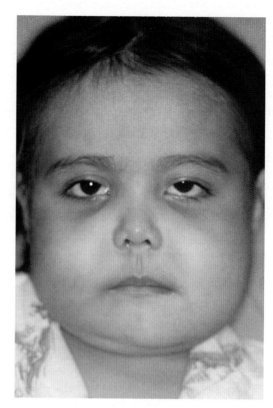

• **Fig. 14.22 Cherubism.** This young girl shows the typical cherubic facies resulting from bilateral expansile mandibular and maxillary lesions. (Courtesy of Dr. Román Carlos.)

Clinical and Radiographic Features

The condition usually first becomes evident at around 2–9 years of age, although in mild cases the diagnosis may not be made until 10–12 years. The clinical alterations typically progress until puberty and stabilize during adolescence. Some patients exhibit slow regression of lesions during adulthood, but others continue to experience marked bony changes and deformity.

The plump, cherub-like cheeks result from painless, bilaterally symmetric expansion of the posterior mandible (Fig. 14.22). In early disease, cervical lymphadenopathy also may contribute to the apparent fullness. In severe cases, involvement of the inferior and/or lateral orbital walls may tilt the eyeballs upward and retract the lower eyelid, thereby exposing the sclera below the iris to produce an "eyes upturned to heaven" appearance. Rare reports of unilateral cherubism are difficult to accept as true examples of this disease unless there is a strong family history or genetic confirmation.

In the mandible, lesions frequently develop in the angles, ascending rami, and coronoid processes, but the condyles usually are spared. In severe cases, most of the mandible is affected. Involvement of the maxillary tuberosities or entire maxilla also is possible, and there may be a V-shaped palatal arch. Extensive jaw involvement causes marked widening and distortion of the alveolar ridges. In addition to aesthetic compromise, the condition may cause tooth displacement, tooth mobility, premature loss of deciduous teeth, impacted or missing permanent teeth (especially molars), impaired

mastication, speech difficulties, upper airway obstruction, and vision or hearing loss.

Radiographic examination typically shows bilateral, multilocular, expansile radiolucencies (Fig. 14.23, *A*). This radiographic presentation is virtually diagnostic. Less commonly, the lesions may appear unilocular. Additional findings may include resorption of adjacent tooth roots and thinning or perforation of the cortical bone. Although cherubism primarily is limited to the craniofacial region, rib involvement also has been reported in a few cases.

Biochemical findings (including serum calcium and phosphorus) typically are normal in patients with cherubism, although serum alkaline phosphatase and other markers of bone remodeling may be elevated in patients with active disease. If laboratory results do not suggest hyperparathyroidism, then most children with bilaterally symmetric giant cell lesions of the jaws represent examples of cherubism. However, multiple giant cell lesions may be seen in association with other conditions, including Ramon syndrome, Jaffe-Campanacci syndrome, and so-called "RASopathies" (e.g., Noonan syndrome, neurofibromatosis type 1) (see Table 14.4).

Histopathologic Features

Because the microscopic findings of cherubism are similar to those of isolated giant cell granulomas, correlation with the clinical and radiographic findings is essential for diagnosis. Microscopic examination shows vascular fibrous tissue with

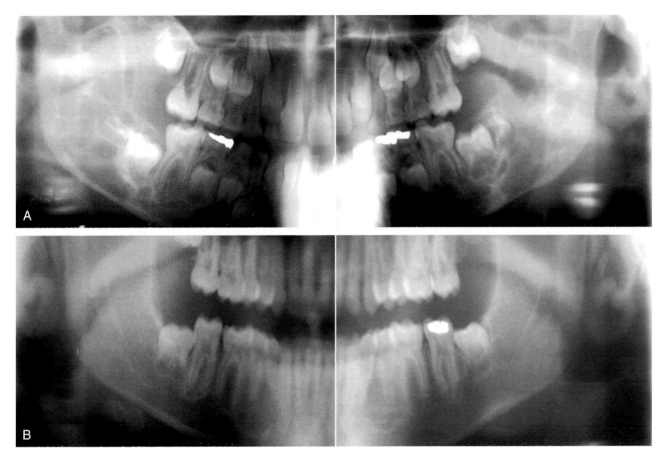

• **Fig. 14.23 Cherubism. A,** Panoramic radiograph of a 7-year-old white boy. Bilateral multilocular radiolucencies can be seen in the posterior mandible. **B,** Same patient 6 years later. The lesions in the mandibular rami demonstrate significant resolution, but areas of involvement are still present in the body of the mandible. (Courtesy of Dr. John R. Cramer.)

variable numbers of multinucleated giant cells and scattered hemorrhage. The giant cells tend to be small and aggregated focally (Fig. 14.24). Like the giant cells in central giant cell granulomas, the giant cells in cherubism express markers suggestive of osteoclastic origin. The stroma in cherubism tends to be more loosely arranged than that in giant cell granulomas. In some cases, cherubism reveals eosinophilic, cuff-like deposits surrounding small blood vessels. This eosinophilic cuffing appears to be specific for cherubism but has been described in only about 28% of reported cases. In older, resolving lesions of cherubism, the tissue becomes more fibrous, the number of giant cells decreases, and new bone formation is seen.

Treatment and Prognosis

In most instances, lesion progression spontaneously ceases after puberty. According to a recent systematic review of the literature, lesion growth after 21 years of age has been noted in only about 5% of reported and genetically confirmed cases. Over time some patients exhibit lesion regression, with facial features approaching normalcy (Fig. 14.23). Nevertheless, the prognosis in any given case is difficult to predict, and persistent facial deformity or continued disease progression is possible.

A conservative treatment approach generally is preferred. Mild cases may require only observation. However, treatment typically is indicated for patients with aggressive lesions, severe functional impairment, or marked facial deformity. Surgical intervention may consist of curettage, recontouring, partial resection, or complete resection. The surgical defects may be filled with autogenous cancellous bone and bone marrow grafts. Outcomes of surgery performed during the active disease phase are variable, with some investigators reporting excellent results and others reporting aggressive regrowth. Generally, it is preferable to delay surgery until the disease has become quiescent, although severe aesthetic and functional compromise may demand earlier intervention. Alternative treatment with calcitonin, interferon, imatinib, denosumab, or tacrolimus has been reported anecdotally but requires further study. Attempts to treat cherubism with adalimumab (a TNF-α antagonist)—alone or in combination with bisphosphonates—have yielded disappointing results thus far. Radiation therapy is contraindicated because of the risk for post-irradiation sarcoma.

Dental management may include extraction or orthodontic extrusion of impacted teeth; orthodontics for malocclusion; and prostheses for missing teeth. Placement of dental implants and autotransplantation of teeth also have been reported in a few cases.

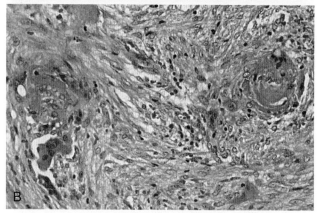

• **Fig. 14.24 Cherubism. A,** Photomicrograph showing scattered giant cells within a background of cellular, hemorrhagic mesenchymal tissue. **B,** High-power view showing perivascular eosinophilic cuffing.

◆ SIMPLE BONE CYST (TRAUMATIC BONE CYST; HEMORRHAGIC BONE CYST; SOLITARY BONE CYST; IDIOPATHIC BONE CAVITY; UNICAMERAL BONE CYST)

The **simple bone cyst** is an empty or fluid-containing bone cavity. Because this lesion lacks an epithelial lining, it represents a pseudocyst rather than a true cyst.

The etiopathogenesis is uncertain, and several theories have been proposed. In particular, the **trauma-hemorrhage theory** has many advocates, as evidenced by the widely used designation **traumatic bone cyst.** According to this theory, trauma that is insufficient to cause a bone fracture results in an intraosseous hematoma. If the hematoma does not undergo organization and repair, it may liquefy and result in a pseudocystic defect. However, a history of trauma to the affected area and the presence of blood within the cavity have been inconsistent findings. Other proposed theories include venous obstruction, interstitial fluid blockage, local disturbance in bone growth, altered calcium metabolism, ischemic marrow necrosis, aberrant synovial development, low-grade infection, and degeneration of a bone tumor or cyst. In addition, investigators recently have identified

FUS::NFATC2 or *EWSR1::NFATC2* fusions in a subset of extragnathic cases.

Clinical and Radiographic Features

Simple bone cysts have been reported in almost every bone of the body. Most cases involve the metaphyses of long bones, with a predilection for the proximal humerus and proximal femur. In addition, solitary bone cysts may arise in the jaws, with a marked mandibular predominance. Although any area of the mandible may be involved, the premolar, molar, and symphyseal regions are affected most commonly. Maxillary lesions tend to occur in the anterior region. Most solitary bone cysts are diagnosed in young patients, with a peak in the second decade. Jaw lesions exhibit no significant gender bias, whereas extragnathic lesions exhibit a male predilection. Unlike extragnathic lesions, jaw lesions tend to lack clinical signs or symptoms; thus, the true frequency of jaw lesions is undoubtedly greater than the literature would suggest. About 20% of patients, however, have a painless jaw swelling. Pain and paresthesia are noted infrequently.

Simple bone cysts of the jaws often are discovered incidentally during radiographic examination for some other reason. The lesion typically appears as a well-delineated, unilocular radiolucency. However, ill-defined and multilocular lesions also are possible. The defect may range from 1 to 10 cm in diameter. Occasionally, the radiolucent defect shows domelike projections that scallop upward between the roots of adjacent teeth. This feature is highly suggestive but not diagnostic of a simple bone cyst (Figs. 14.25 and 14.26). In many cases, a cone-shaped outline (pointed at one or both ends in the anterior-posterior direction) may be noted, particularly when the lesion is large. Oval, irregular, or rounded borders are possible as well. The adjacent teeth are generally vital and not displaced. Root resorption, loss of lamina dura, cortical expansion, cortical thinning or perforation, and displacement of the mandibular canal are evident in a minority of cases. Most lesions are solitary, but multifocal involvement has been reported occasionally. Extensive lesions involving a substantial portion of the mandibular body and ascending ramus also are possible.

Simple bone cysts at times may arise in association with cemento-osseous dysplasia (see page 645) (Fig. 14.27) and other fibro-osseous proliferations. Such cases tend to occur in older females.

Histopathologic Features

There is never an epithelial lining. Instead, the walls of the defect are lined by a thin band of vascular fibrous connective tissue (Fig. 14.28) or a thickened myxofibromatous proliferation with reactive bone. In addition, there may be fibrin, scattered erythrocytes, occasional giant cells, and lacelike dystrophic calcifications (Fig. 14.29). Some authors also have noted amorphous, cementum-like material, which may represent osteoid. The bony surface next to the cavity may show resorptive areas (Howship lacunae) indicative of past osteoclastic activity.

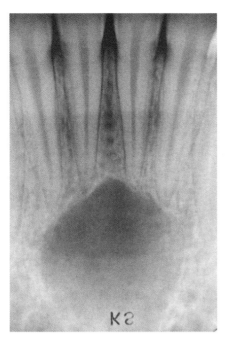

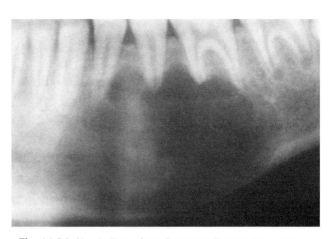

• **Fig. 14.26 Simple Bone Cyst.** Panoramic film showing a large simple bone cyst of the mandible in a 12-year-old girl. The scalloping superior aspect of the cyst between the roots of the teeth is highly suggestive of, but not diagnostic for, a simple bone cyst. (Courtesy of Dr. Lon Doles.)

• **Fig. 14.25 Simple Bone Cyst.** Periapical radiograph showing a radiolucent area in the apical region of the anterior mandible. The incisor teeth responded normally to vitality testing, and no restorations are present.

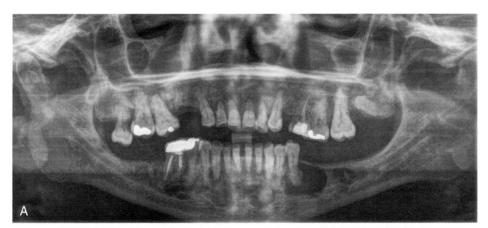

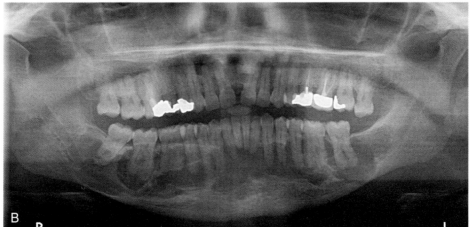

• **Fig. 14.27 Simple Bone Cyst and Cemento-Osseous Dysplasia. A,** Panoramic radiograph showing florid cemento-osseous dysplasia with secondary formation of a simple bone cyst in the left mandibular premolar region. **B,** Panoramic radiograph showing florid cemento-osseous dysplasia with secondary formation of a large simple bone cyst extending from the left to right molar regions of the mandible. (**A,** Courtesy of Fallon Berger. **B,** Courtesy of Dr. Hal Levine.)

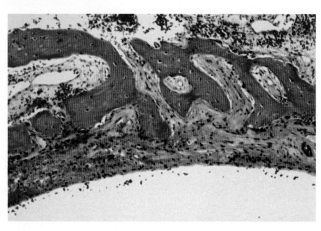

• **Fig. 14.28 Simple Bone Cyst.** Photomicrograph of the bony wall of a simple bone cyst. A thin, vascular connective tissue membrane is adjacent to the bone, and no epithelial lining is identified.

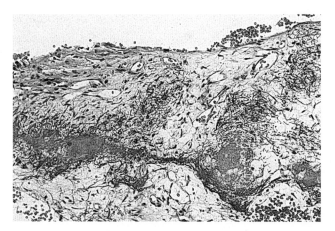

• **Fig. 14.29 Simple Bone Cyst.** Loose vascular connective tissue exhibiting areas of basophilic lacelike calcification in the wall of a simple bone cyst.

Diagnosis

The radiographic features of the simple bone cyst are not entirely specific and may be confused with a wide variety of odontogenic and non-odontogenic radiolucent jaw lesions. Surgical exploration is necessary to establish the diagnosis.

Typically, little to no tissue is obtained at the time of surgery; therefore, the diagnosis is based primarily on the clinical, radiographic, and intraoperative findings. In about one-third of cases, there is an empty cavity with smooth, shiny bony walls. In about two-thirds of cases, the cavity contains small amounts of serosanguineous fluid. The mandibular neurovascular bundle may be seen lying free in the cavity.

Treatment and Prognosis

Simple bone cysts of the long bones often are treated aggressively, with various combinations of curettage, cryosurgery, decompression, intralesional steroid injections, bone substitute or autologous bone marrow injection, and bone grafting. Reported recurrence rates are relatively high (mean 29%, range 12%–48%).

In contrast, simple bone cysts of the jaws typically are managed by surgical exploration and curettage. Intraoperatively, the bony walls of the cavity usually appear smooth and shiny, although it is wise to curette them and submit the small amount of tissue obtained for microscopic examination to rule out more serious diseases. Surgical exploration with or without curettage usually induces bone regeneration; normal radiographic findings typically are evident 12–17 months after surgery. Periodic radiographic examination should be performed until complete resolution has been confirmed. There are also anecdotal reports of favorable results with bone grafting, plasma-rich protein, or packing materials. Most studies report very low recurrence rates (approximately 1%–2%), although some report recurrence rates as high as 26%. There is an increased potential for recurrence when there are multiple lesions or with lesions arising in association with cemento-osseous dysplasia. In addition, one study reported an increased recurrence potential among jaw lesions exhibiting scalloped margins, resorption of the lamina dura, nodular bone expansion, and multiple cavities. Overall, the prognosis is excellent.

◆ ANEURYSMAL BONE CYST

The **aneurysmal bone cyst** is an intraosseous accumulation of variable-sized, blood-filled spaces surrounded by cellular fibrous connective tissue and reactive bone. Because the lesion lacks an epithelial lining, it represents a pseudocyst rather than a true cyst. Aneurysmal bone cysts may be classified as *primary* (i.e., arising *de novo*) or *secondary* (i.e., arising in association with another bone lesion). In extremely rare cases, the lesion may arise in soft tissue as well.

The etiopathogenesis is poorly understood. Traditionally, the aneurysmal bone cyst has been thought to result from a reactive process and/or altered hemodynamics. Many authors have theorized that a traumatic event, vascular malformation, neoplasm, or other pathologic condition may disrupt normal osseous hemodynamics, resulting in an enlarging area of hemorrhage and osteolysis. Consistent with this hypothesis is the observation that approximately 30% of aneurysmal bone cysts overall and 15% of gnathic examples form in association with other lesions. In contrast, cytogenetic evidence suggests that primary aneurysmal bone cysts may be neoplastic in nature. The majority of primary lesions analyzed exhibit recurrent translocations and consequent transcriptional upregulation of the ubiquitin-specific protease 6 *(USP6)* (also known as *Tre-2* or *TRE17*) oncogene on chromosome 17p13. The most commonly observed translocation is t(16;17)(q22;p13), which results in fusion of *USP6* with the cadherin 11 gene *(CDH11)*. Other possible *USP6* fusion partners include the zinc-finger 9 gene *(ZNF9)*, collagen 1A1 gene *(COL1A1)*, thyroid receptor-associated protein gene *(TRAP150)*, and osteomodulin gene *(OMD)*. However, *USP6* translocations have been detected in very few craniofacial lesions thus far. The underlying mechanisms by which *USP6* upregulation leads to tumor formation remain poorly understood. Some studies suggest there may be downstream dysregulation of bone morphogenetic protein resulting in disrupted osteoblastic maturation, and others have noted nuclear factor-kappa B (NF-κB)-mediated induction of matrix metalloproteinases that play an important role in angiogenesis and inflammatory processes.

Clinical and Radiographic Features

Aneurysmal bone cysts arise primarily in the long bones or vertebrae of patients younger than 30 years. Only about 2% of cases involve the jaws. Gnathic lesions mainly affect young patients (peak in the second decade) but may occur over a broad age range. Most authors report either no significant sex predilection or a slight female predilection. The lesions arise more often in the mandible than the maxilla, and the vast majority arises in the posterior segments of the jaws. Within the mandible, involvement of the ascending ramus and posterior body is common, whereas involvement of the condylar and coronoid processes is infrequent.

The most common clinical manifestation is a rapidly enlarging swelling. Pain is a variable finding; paresthesia and crepitus have been noted rarely. Malocclusion, mobility, migration, or resorption of involved teeth may be present. Maxillary lesions often bulge into the adjacent sinus and occasionally cause nasal obstruction, nasal bleeding, proptosis, and diplopia.

Radiographic examination shows a unilocular or multilocular radiolucency, often with marked cortical expansion and thinning (Fig. 14.30). The radiographic borders may be well defined or poorly defined. There is frequently a ballooning or "blow-out" distention of the affected bone. Uncommonly, small radiopaque foci, thought to be small trabeculae of reactive bone, are noted within the radiolucency.

Intraoperatively, intact periosteum and a thin shell of bone typically are evident overlying the lesion, although cortical perforation is possible. When the periosteum and bony shell are removed, the lesion exhibits dark venous-like bleeding with a "blood-soaked sponge" appearance.

Histopathologic Features

Microscopically, the aneurysmal bone cyst is characterized by blood-filled spaces of varying size. These blood-filled spaces lack an endothelial or epithelial lining (Fig. 14.31). The surrounding septa exhibit a proliferation of fibroblastic or myofibroblastic spindle cells with associated multinucleated giant cells, osteoid, and woven bone. The spindle cells harbor *USP6* and *CDH11* rearrangement and, thus, appear to represent the neoplastic component in primary lesions. Similar to the multinucleated giant cells in giant cell granulomas, the multinucleated giant cells in aneurysmal bone cysts exhibit an osteoclastic phenotype, as evidenced by immunohistochemical and *in situ* hybridization studies. Osteoid deposits may appear linear, nodular, or lacelike. Mitotic figures may be evident but should not be atypical. As noted earlier, aneurysmal bone cysts may be associated with other pathoses, such as cemento-ossifying fibromas, fibrous dysplasia, or central giant cell granulomas.

Treatment and Prognosis

Aneurysmal bone cysts of the jaws usually are treated by curettage or enucleation, sometimes supplemented with cryosurgery. *En bloc* resection is reserved for extensive or recurrent lesions. Preoperative embolization may be considered to control bleeding but often is unnecessary, because most gnathic lesions exhibit low-flow vascularity. Typically, the surgical defect heals within 6 months to 1 year and does not necessitate bone grafting. Alternative treatments reported anecdotally in the literature include denosumab and intralesional injection of various agents (e.g., aqueous calcium sulfate, calcitonin with methyprednisolone, Ethibloc). Irradiation generally is contraindicated.

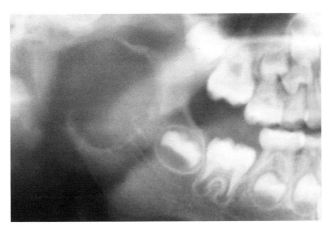

• **Fig. 14.30 Aneurysmal Bone Cyst.** A large radiolucent lesion involves most of the ascending ramus in a 5-year-old white boy. (Courtesy of Dr. Samuel McKenna.)

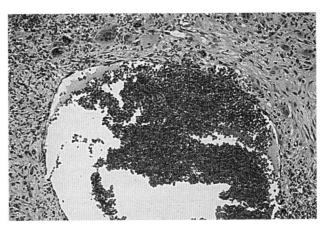

• **Fig. 14.31 Aneurysmal Bone Cyst.** Photomicrograph showing a blood-filled space surrounded by fibroblastic connective tissue. Scattered multinucleated giant cells are seen adjacent to the vascular space.

Recent reviews of the literature have noted recurrence rates of 3%–23% among reported jaw lesions. The risk for recurrence may be greater among secondary lesions compared to primary lesions. In addition, some reported recurrences actually may represent persistence after incomplete removal. Occasionally, recurrence also may be related to incomplete removal of a coexisting lesion, such as an ossifying fibroma or osteoblastoma. Overall, despite recurrences, the long-term prognosis is favorable.

◆ CENTRAL XANTHOMA OF THE JAWS (PRIMARY XANTHOMA OF BONE; PRIMARY INTRAOSSEOUS XANTHOMA; FIBROUS XANTHOMA OF BONE; FIBROXANTHOMA OF BONE)

The central xanthoma of the jaws is a rare lesion characterized by the presence of lipid-laden macrophages (termed *xanthoma cells* or *foam cells*). Its etiopathogenesis is unclear, although it is believed to represent either a reactive process or a benign neoplasm. Some investigators have proposed that this lesion results from phagocytosis of lipids leaked from blood vessels after local trauma or hemorrhage. Unlike xanthomas involving soft tissue or extragnathic bones, central xanthomas of the jaws are not closely associated with metabolic or endocrine disorders, such as hyperlipidemia or diabetes mellitus.

Some authors consider xanthomas of the jaws to belong to a spectrum of conditions that also includes the nonossifying fibroma (fibrous cortical defect) and benign fibrous histiocytoma. The nonossifying fibroma is a lesion commonly arising in the metaphysis of the long bones in children and adolescents; it frequently undergoes spontaneous resolution, unlike the more slowly progressive central xanthoma of the mandible. The benign fibrous histiocytoma only rarely develops intraosseously, with a predilection for the pelvis and long bones; it typically exhibits more progressive growth compared to xanthomas of the jaws. Based on differences in clinicopathologic presentation and behavior, it seems more appropriate to regard the central xanthoma of the jaws as a distinct entity.

Clinical and Radiographic Features

The central xanthoma of the jaws has been reported over a broad age range, with a peak in the second and third decades of life and no significant gender predilection. The mandible is affected much more often than the maxilla. Mandibular lesions tend to occur in the posterior region. Most patients are asymptomatic, although swelling and pain are possible. Some cases have been discovered incidentally during radiographic examination performed for other reasons. Infrequent findings include tooth mobility and lower lip numbness.

Radiographic examination typically shows a solitary, unilocular radiolucency, although some examples appear as a multilocular radiolucency (Fig. 14.32), a mixed radiolucency-radiopacity, or a "ground-glass" radiopacity. Reported lesion size varies from 1 to 11 cm (median 2 cm). The borders may be either well- or ill-defined and may appear punched out or sclerotic. Larger tumors may exhibit cortical expansion. Infrequent findings include a scalloped border, resorption or splaying of adjacent tooth roots, cortical resorption or perforation, displacement of the inferior alveolar canal, and elevation of the maxillary sinus floor.

Histopathologic Features

Grossly, the tumor typically presents as a soft, yellow mass or yellow granules. Microscopic examination shows a sheet-like proliferation of ovoid cells with abundant, foamy or granular cytoplasm and small, round nuclei (Fig. 14.33). Unlike the nonossifying fibroma and benign fibrous histiocytoma, the

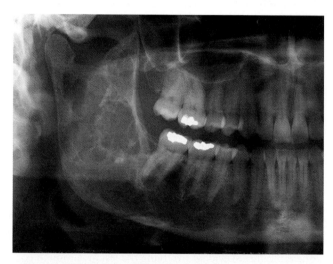

• **Fig. 14.32 Central Xanthoma of the Jaws.** Large multilocular radiolucency in the right posterior body and ramus of the mandible. (Courtesy of Dr. Patrick Morris.)

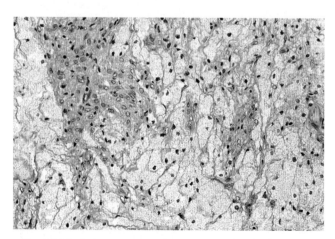

• **Fig. 14.33 Central Xanthoma of the Jaws.** Proliferation of ovoid cells with abundant foamy cytoplasm and small, round nuclei. There is only a minor fibrous connective tissue component.

central xanthoma of the jaws include a variable fibrous connective tissue component, lacks a storiform growth pattern, and rarely exhibits multinucleated giant cells. Lymphocytes and plasma cells occasionally may be present within the background; however, the lack of a prominent mixed inflammatory background aids in avoiding confusion with periapical inflammatory disease. Small bony trabeculae and metaplastic ossification around bone spicules may be noted as well.

The foam cells exhibit strong immunoreactivity for CD68. Negative expression of S-100 protein, CD1a, and CD207 aids in distinction from Langerhans cell histiocytosis (see page 596). The microscopic differential diagnosis also includes Erdheim-Chester disease and lipid reticuloendothelioses (see page 821), although these entities can be ruled out readily by clinical correlation.

Treatment and Prognosis

Most cases are treated by curettage, enucleation, or partial excision. Recurrence after complete removal has been reported rarely.

FIBRO-OSSEOUS LESIONS OF THE JAWS

Fibro-osseous lesions are a diverse group of processes that are characterized by replacement of normal bone by fibrous tissue containing a newly formed mineralized product. The term *fibro-osseous lesion* is descriptive and does not constitute a specific diagnosis. Lesions belonging to this category may be developmental (hamartomatous), reactive, dysplastic, or neoplastic.

The major types of fibro-osseous lesions of the jaws are listed in Box 14.1. Although these conditions differ in etiology, they may exhibit very similar histopathologic features. Therefore, correlation of the histopathologic findings with

• BOX 14.1 Major Types of Fibro-Osseous Lesions of the Jaws

Fibrous dysplasia
- Monostotic fibrous dysplasia
- Polyostotic fibrous dysplasia
  - Isolated
  - Syndrome-related (i.e., McCune-Albright syndrome, Mazabraud syndrome)
- Cemento-osseous dysplasia
  - Focal cemento-osseous dysplasia
  - Periapical cemento-osseous dysplasia
  - Florid cemento-osseous dysplasia
- Ossifying fibroma
  - Cemento-ossifying fibroma
  - Juvenile ossifying fibroma
    - Trabecular variant
    - Psammomatoid variant

the clinical and radiographic features typically is essential for establishing a specific diagnosis. (However, in some cases of cemento-osseous dysplasia, a presumptive diagnosis may be made based on the clinical and radiographic findings.) A specific diagnosis is critical because the treatment, biologic behavior, and prognosis of these pathoses vary greatly. Some fibro-osseous lesions only require monitoring, whereas others necessitate surgical recontouring or complete removal.

FIBROUS DYSPLASIA

Fibrous dysplasia is a developmental tumorlike condition, characterized by replacement of normal bone by a proliferation of cellular fibrous connective tissue with irregular bony trabeculae. This sporadic condition results from postzygotic, activating mutations in the *GNAS* gene, which encodes the alpha subunit of a stimulatory G protein. Such mutations have not been detected in ossifying fibroma or cemento-osseous dysplasia.

Clinically, fibrous dysplasia may involve one bone or multiple bones; in some cases, involvement of multiple bones may occur in conjunction with cutaneous and endocrine abnormalities. The extent of disease depends on when the *GNAS* mutation occurs. During early embryonic development, mutation of a pluripotent stem cell can cause abnormalities in multiple cell types, including osteoblasts, melanocytes, and endocrine cells. In contrast, if the mutation occurs in a skeletal progenitor cell in a later stage of embryonic development, then only osteoblasts will be affected. Alternatively, if the mutation occurs during postnatal life, then osteoblasts in only a single bone will be affected. Furthermore, the parental origin of the mutated *GNAS* allele may affect the phenotype, because in certain cell types (such as pituitary somatotrophs) genomic imprinting results in expression of only the maternal allele.

Constitutive activation of G-protein signaling impairs differentiation of skeletal progenitor cells into mature osteoblasts and osteocytes, induces an abnormal fibroblastic phenotype among bone marrow stromal cells, stimulates melanin production in melanocytes, and causes hyperplasia and hyperfunction of various endocrine cell types. In addition, mutated osteoblasts, osteocytes, and stromal cells overexpress interleukin (IL)-6 and receptor activator of nuclear factor-kappa B ligand (RANKL), which stimulate osteoclastogenesis and may contribute to bone lesion expansion.

Clinical and Radiographic Features
Monostotic Fibrous Dysplasia

About 80% of patients with fibrous dysplasia have disease limited to a single bone (**monostotic fibrous dysplasia**). Commonly involved sites include the craniofacial bones, ribs, femur, and tibia. Males and females are affected with about equal frequency. The condition is diagnosed most often during the second and third decades of life. The mean age at diagnosis for cases involving the jaws is approximately 24–37 years; some studies suggest that gnathic lesions may be diagnosed in a somewhat older age group compared to extragnathic lesions.

Among jaw cases, the maxilla is affected more often than the mandible. There is a predilection for the posterior region. Although mandibular lesions are truly monostotic, maxillary lesions often extend to involve adjacent bones (e.g., zygoma, sphenoid, ethmoid, frontal bone, temporal bone, occiput)—in which case the term **craniofacial fibrous dysplasia** is appropriate. Painless, unilateral swelling is the most common clinical finding (Fig. 14.34). Growth is generally slow, and many cases are discovered incidentally during radiographic examination. Occasionally, however, the growth may be fairly rapid. Adjacent teeth may be displaced by the bony mass but usually remain firm.

The classic radiographic finding is a fine "ground-glass" opacification with poorly defined margins (Figs. 14.35 through 14.37). However, some examples may appear radiolucent or mixed radiolucent-radiopaque. Sometimes there is "ground-glass" opacification surrounding a central radiolucency. As the patient ages, there may be increased lesion heterogeneity or sclerosis. Mottled, diffusely sclerotic, "rind" sign (thick sclerotic margin), cotton wool, chalky, soap bubble, and fingerprint patterns (Fig. 14.38) are possible. There is often buccolingual expansion with cortical thinning, which may be appreciated best by CT; the outer cortical contour typically remains smooth, although endosteal scalloping may be noted. Mandibular lesions may cause displacement of the inferior alveolar canal and bulging of the inferior border. Periapical radiographs may demonstrate narrowing of the periodontal ligament space and an ill-defined lamina dura that blends with the abnormal bone. Infrequent findings include tooth impaction and root resorption. Maxillary lesions often cause superior displacement of the sinus floor and obliteration of the antrum. In addition, extensive skull involvement may be evident (Fig. 14.39). CT is superior to conventional radiographs for visualizing the characteristic bony changes and determining the extent of disease. In addition, skeletal scintigraphy may aid in detecting metabolically active lesions and ruling out polyostotic disease.

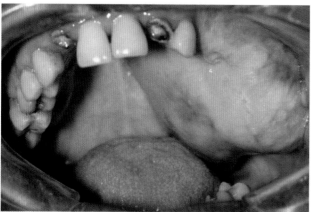

• **Fig. 14.34 Fibrous Dysplasia.** Expansile mass of the left maxilla in a 45-year-old woman. This lesion was known to have been present for at least 20 years.

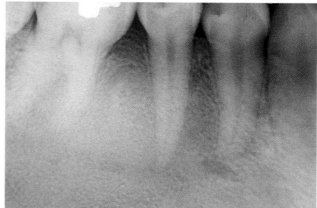

• **Fig. 14.36 Fibrous Dysplasia.** Periapical radiograph showing a diffuse "ground-glass" radiographic appearance.

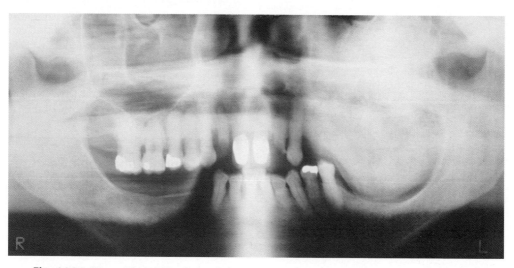

• **Fig. 14.35 Fibrous Dysplasia.** Panoramic radiograph of the patient shown in Fig. 14.34. A diffuse "ground-glass" radiopacity is evident. (Courtesy of Dr. Richard Brock.)

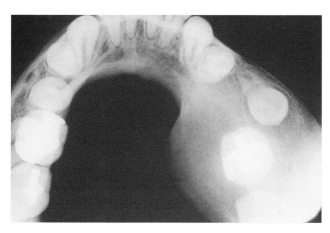

• **Fig. 14.37 Fibrous Dysplasia.** Occlusal radiograph showing localized expansion of the mandible and the "ground-glass" radiographic appearance. The margins of the lesion are not well defined and blend into the adjacent bone. (From Waldron CA, Giansanti JS: Benign fibro-osseous lesions of the jaws: a clinical-radiologic-histologic review of 65 cases. I. Fibrous dysplasia of the jaws, *Oral Surg Oral Med Oral Pathol* 35:190–201, 1973.)

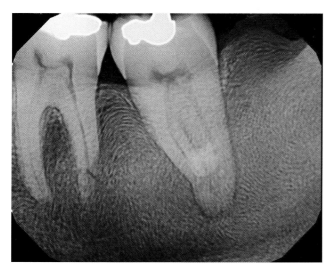

• **Fig. 14.38 Fibrous Dysplasia.** Radiograph showing a "fingerprint" pattern.

Polyostotic Fibrous Dysplasia; McCune-Albright Syndrome

A minority of patients with fibrous dysplasia exhibits involvement of two or more bones (**polyostotic fibrous dysplasia**). Most patients with polyostotic disease are diagnosed before 10 years of age, and there is a female predilection. The number of involved bones varies from a few to 75% of the entire skeleton. Commonly involved sites include the craniofacial region, pelvic bones, and femur.

Presenting signs and symptoms related to long bone involvement may include pain, pathologic fracture, limping, leg length discrepancy, and bowing deformity. Radiographic examination may reveal malformation of the proximal femur (known as *coxa vara, shepherd's crook deformity,* or *hockey stick deformity*). Craniofacial involvement is present in as many as 87% of patients with polyostotic disease and may result in facial asymmetry (Fig. 14.40), malocclusion, vision changes,

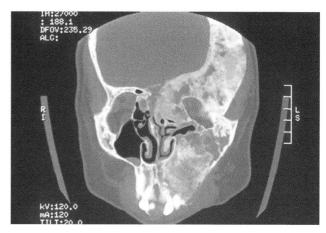

• **Fig. 14.39 Fibrous Dysplasia.** Computed tomography (CT) image showing extensive involvement of the maxilla and skull.

hearing impairment, sinonasal congestion, and airway obstruction. Hypophosphatemia caused by renal phosphate wasting is a fairly common finding, which appears to be related to the release of fibroblast growth factor 23 *(FGF23)* by the affected bones.

A small subset of patients may exhibit polyostotic fibrous dysplasia in association with the following syndromes:
- **McCune-Albright syndrome**, characterized by two or more of the following features: polyostotic fibrous dysplasia, *café au lait* (coffee with milk) pigmentation, and hyperfunctioning endocrinopathies (In the past, some authors used the term *Jaffe-Lichtenstein syndrome* for cases of polyostotic fibrous dysplasia with café au lait pigmentation but no endocrinopathy; however, according to current convention, such cases are regarded as a variation of McCune-Albright syndrome.)
- **Mazabraud syndrome**, characterized by fibrous dysplasia and intramuscular myxomas

The *café au lait* pigmentation typically is seen on the skin at or shortly after birth. It consists of well-defined, tan macules with very irregular, jagged margins, resembling a map of the coastline of Maine (Fig. 14.41). In contrast, the *café au lait* spots of neurofibromatosis (see page 537) usually exhibit smooth borders (like the coast of California). The cutaneous lesions in McCune-Albright syndrome tend to be unilateral and more or less respect the midline. In addition, similar pigmentation of the lips and intraoral mucosa may be noted; however, unlike the skin lesions, the oral lesions tend to develop in adulthood and may progress with age.

In McCune-Albright syndrome, the most common endocrine abnormality is sexual precocity, particularly in females. Menstrual bleeding, breast development, and pubic hair may be apparent within the first few months or years of life. Other possible endocrinopathies include hyperthyroidism, hyperparathyroidism, neonatal hypercortisolism, and excess growth hormone. In addition, in one study of craniofacial fibrous dysplasia mainly occurring in McCune-Albright syndrome, investigators reported various dental anomalies, including tooth displacement, oligodontia, enamel hypoplasia, enamel hypomineralization, taurodontism, and retained deciduous teeth.

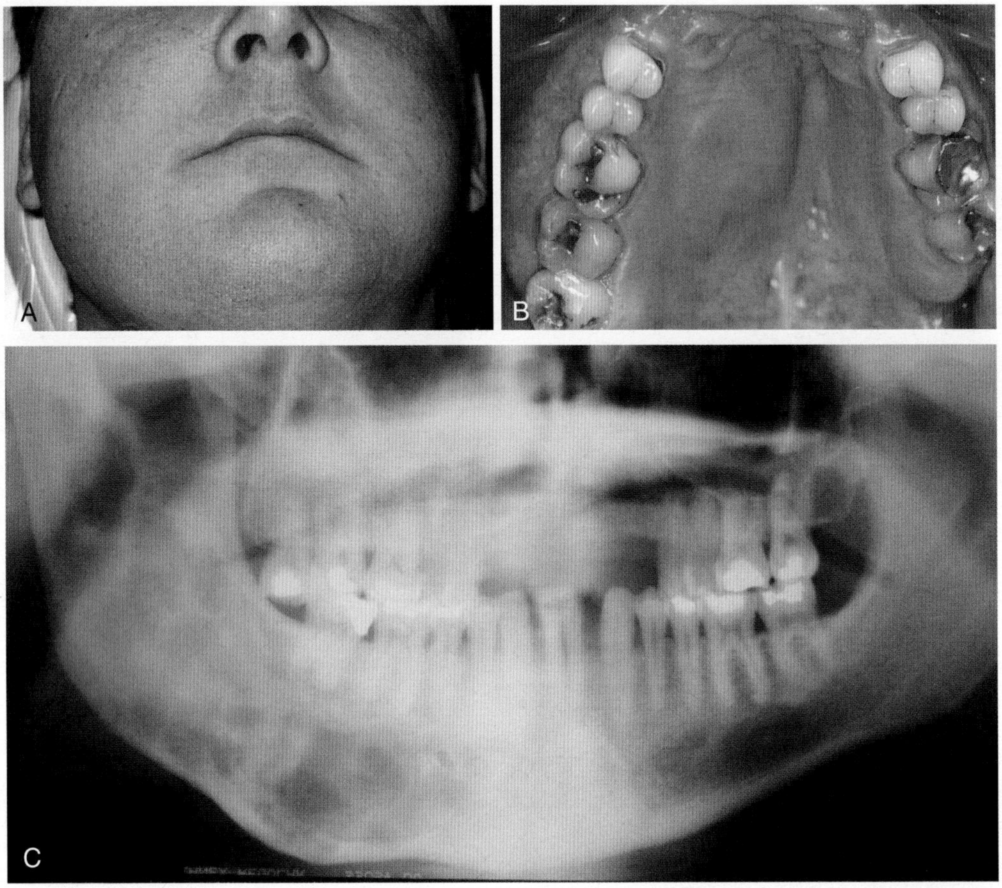

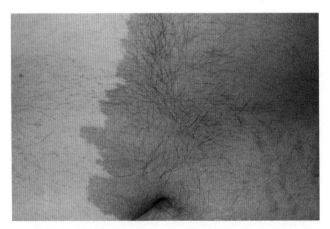

• **Fig. 14.40 Polyostotic Fibrous Dysplasia.** McCune-Albright syndrome. **A,** Young man exhibiting enlargement of the right maxilla and mandible. **B,** Intraoral photograph showing unilateral maxillary expansion. **C,** Panoramic radiograph showing ill-defined lesions of the right side of both jaws.

• **Fig. 14.41 Polyostotic Fibrous Dysplasia.** McCune-Albright syndrome. *Café au lait* pigmentation of the abdomen. This is the same patient as shown in Fig. 14.40.

Histopathologic Features

Microscopic examination typically shows irregularly shaped trabeculae of immature (woven) bone in a cellular fibrous stroma (Fig. 14.42). At the periphery, the lesional bone fuses with normal bone, without a capsule or line of demarcation.

The abnormal bony trabeculae tend to be thin and disconnected, with elongated, curvilinear shapes likened to Chinese characters or alphabet soup (often forming the letters "C," "Y," and "U"). Osteoblastic rimming is usually absent or minimal, and peritrabecular clefting (artifactual retraction of the stroma from the bony trabeculae) is common. In addition, tiny calcified spherules rarely may be seen but are never numerous. In later stages, the woven bone is replaced by lamellar bone with roughly parallel trabeculae (Fig. 14.43). The rather monotonous pattern of calcification in fibrous dysplasia differs from the more haphazard mixture of woven bone, lamellar bone, and spheroid particles characteristic of ossifying fibroma and cemento-osseous dysplasia.

Fibrous dysplasia may appear more sclerotic in the jaw and skull than other sites. Microscopic variations include a pagetoid pattern (characterized by thick, interconnected bone trabeculae) and a hypercellular pattern (characterized by parallel bone trabeculae with numerous osteocytes and polarized osteoblastic rimming). Secondary aneurysmal bone cyst formation has been reported as well.

Genetic testing for *GNAS* mutations can be performed on lesional tissue or, possibly, peripheral blood samples. Such testing may be helpful when there is diagnostic uncertainty, but it exhibits low sensitivity and is not performed routinely.

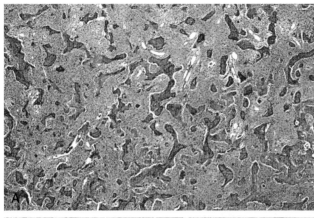

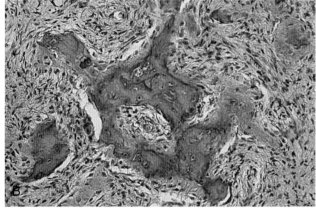

• **Fig. 14.42 Fibrous Dysplasia. A,** Irregularly shaped trabeculae of woven bone in a fibrous stroma. **B,** Medium-power view showing peripheral osteoid without osteoblastic rimming.

• **Fig. 14.43 Mature Fibrous Dysplasia. A,** This long-standing lesion shows separate, broad trabeculae of bone within fibrous connective tissue. **B,** Note the lamellar maturation of the bone.

Treatment and Prognosis

Fibrous dysplasia tends to stabilize upon skeletal maturation, and spontaneous regression even has been reported in a few cases. Therefore, conservative management is preferred. Some lesions, nevertheless, exhibit continued growth into adulthood. The risk for severe deformity and complications is particularly elevated among patients with widespread polyostotic fibrous dysplasia—especially in the setting of McCune-Albright syndrome with uncontrolled growth hormone excess.

Patients with minimal cosmetic and functional disturbances may not require surgical treatment. For young patients with significant problems due to large or extensive lesions, surgical contouring, shaving, or other debulking procedures may be performed. However, subsequent regrowth may require additional surgery. Approximately 20%–50% of patients show some regrowth after surgical debulking, and the risk for regrowth is greater among younger than older patients. Therefore, if possible, many authorities prefer to delay surgery until the disease is quiescent.

Alternatively, complete surgical removal may be considered in some cases, such as small monostotic lesions, very aggressive lesions, or lesions refractory to repeated debulking. Combined orthodontic treatment and orthognathic surgery may be performed to correct malocclusion. Successful placement of dental implants has been reported in a few cases, but additional studies are needed. Investigational treatments include bisphosphonates and denosumab; these agents may help to relieve bone pain in fibrous dysplasia. Radiation therapy is contraindicated because of the risk for post-irradiation bone sarcoma.

Transformation into malignancy, usually an osteosarcoma, is estimated to occur in less than 1% of patients with fibrous dysplasia. The risk for sarcomatous transformation is greatest among those with a history of radiation therapy, McCune-Albright syndrome, or Mazabraud syndrome. Rapid lesion growth, sudden onset of pain, neurosensory changes, or marked changes in radiographic appearance should alert the clinician to rule out malignant transformation.

◆ CEMENTO-OSSEOUS DYSPLASIAS (OSSEOUS DYSPLASIA)

Cemento-osseous dysplasia occurs in the tooth-bearing areas of the jaws and is probably the most common fibro-osseous lesion encountered in clinical practice. Because the histopathologic features share many similarities with fibrous dysplasia and ossifying fibroma, correct diagnosis can be problematic but is critical for appropriate management.

Some investigators have suggested that cemento-osseous dysplasia originates from the periodontal ligament, because of microscopic similarity and lesion proximity to this structure. Others believe this condition represents a defect in extra-ligamentary bone remodeling that may be triggered by local injury or, possibly, an underlying hormonal imbalance.

Occasionally, simple bone cysts (see page 636) may arise in association with cemento-osseous dysplasia (Fig. 14.27) or other fibro-osseous proliferations. Investigators have suggested that these simple bone cysts may result from interstitial fluid obstruction by the fibro-osseous proliferation.

Clinical and Radiographic Features

Based on clinical and radiographic features, cemento-osseous dysplasia includes the following variants: (1) **focal,** (2) **periapical,** and (3) **florid.**

Focal Cemento-Osseous Dysplasia

Focal cemento-osseous dysplasia involves a single site. Before the concept of focal cemento-osseous dysplasia was clarified in the mid-1990s, most cases were misdiagnosed as a variant of ossifying fibroma.

About 90% of cases of focal cemento-osseous dysplasia occur in females, with an approximate mean age of 41 years and a predilection for the third to sixth decades. The lesion has been reported across ethnic groups—most often blacks followed by East Asians and whites. In contrast to the peri-apical and florid variants, the focal variant seems to affect a greater proportion of whites, although this finding may be due to study population bias.

Focal cemento-osseous dysplasia most commonly involves the posterior mandible. The disease typically is asymptomatic and is detected incidentally by radiographic examination. Most lesions are smaller than 1.5 cm in diameter.

Radiographically, the lesion varies from completely radiolucent to densely radiopaque with a thin peripheral radiolucent rim. Most commonly, however, there is a mixed radiolucent and radiopaque pattern (Fig. 14.44). The borders

tend to be well defined but slightly irregular, and a sclerotic margin occasionally may be noted. The condition typically occurs around tooth apices or in extraction sites. Thinning or perforation of the cortex and resorption of adjacent tooth roots may be evident in some cases on CBCT examination. Most examples are not expansile, although mild expansion is possible. A focal lesion occasionally may represent an early stage in the transition to multifocal involvement, especially in black females.

Periapical Cemento-Osseous Dysplasia (Osseous Dysplasia; Periapical Cemental Dysplasia; Periapical Cementoma; Anterior Mandibular Osseous Dysplasia)

Periapical cemento-osseous dysplasia predominantly involves the periapical region of the anterior mandible. Solitary lesions may occur, but multiple foci typically are present. There is a marked female predilection (female-to-male ratio ranging from about 10:1 to 14:1), and approximately 70% of cases arise in blacks. East Asians often are affected as well. Most patients are diagnosed initially between 30 and 50 years of age, with the diagnosis almost never made in individuals younger than 20 years. The associated teeth are usually vital and seldom have restorations.

Periapical cemento-osseous dysplasia is an asymptomatic condition that often is discovered when radiographs are taken for other purposes. Early lesions appear as circumscribed periapical radiolucencies, similar to periapical granulomas or periapical cysts (Fig. 14.45). However, unlike periapical inflammatory disease, periapical cemento-osseous dysplasia may produce lesions that are not exactly centered on the anatomic root apices, as evidenced by CBCT examination. In some cases, adjacent lesions fuse to form a linear radiolucency that envelops the apices of several teeth (Fig. 14.46). Over time, the lesions tend to "mature" and become mixed radiolucent-radiopaque (Fig. 14.47). The radiopaque component may appear round, ovoid, or irregular. In the end stage, the lesions appear as circumscribed, dense radiopacities with narrow radiolucent rims. The radiolucent rims may be

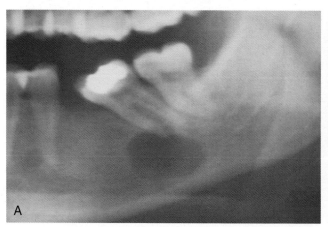
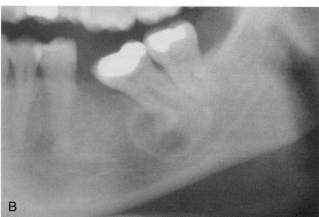

• **Fig. 14.44 Focal Cemento-Osseous Dysplasia. A,** A radiolucent area involves the edentulous first molar area and the apical area of the second molar. **B,** Radiograph of the same patient taken 9 years later showing a mixed radiolucent and radiopaque pattern.

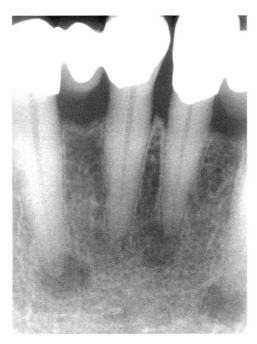

• **Fig. 14.45 Periapical Cemento-Osseous Dysplasia.** Periapical radiograph showing multiple radiolucent lesions at the apices of the anterior mandibular teeth. (Courtesy of Dr. Aaron Carner.)

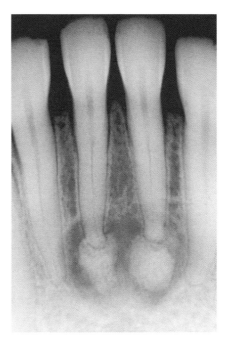

• **Fig. 14.47 Periapical Cemento-Osseous Dysplasia.** Later-stage lesions exhibiting significant mineralization.

Florid Cemento-Osseous Dysplasia

Florid cemento-osseous dysplasia exhibits multifocal involvement not limited to the anterior mandible. Although many cases affect only the posterior portions of the jaws, synchronous involvement of the anterior mandible may be observed as well (Fig. 14.48). Like the periapical pattern, this form predominantly affects black females (in some series, more than 90% of patients), with a marked predilection for middle-aged to older adults. An intermediate frequency among East Asian populations also has been described.

The lesions show a tendency for bilateral and fairly symmetrical involvement of the mandible (Fig. 14.49), and occasionally there may be extensive involvement in all four quadrants. At times the disease may be asymptomatic and discovered only when radiographs are taken for unrelated reasons. In other cases, patients may have dull pain, alveolar sinus tracts, and exposure of yellowish, avascular bone to the oral cavity (Fig. 14.50). Although rarely prominent, some jaw expansion may be evident.

Radiographically, the lesions demonstrate a maturation pattern similar to that noted in the other forms of cemento-osseous dysplasia. Initially, the lesions are predominantly radiolucent but with time become mixed, then predominantly radiopaque with only a thin radiolucent rim (see Fig. 14.49). On occasion, a lesion can become almost totally radiopaque and blend with the adjacent normal-appearing bone. Both dentulous and edentulous areas may be affected. Typically, the radiopacities remain separated from adjacent teeth with an intervening, intact periodontal ligament space. However, in some end-stage lesions, the cemento-osseous material may fuse with the tooth root surface to produce thickened root apices surrounded by radiolucency (or a "hypercementosis-like"

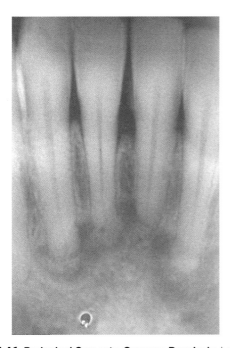

• **Fig. 14.46 Periapical Cemento-Osseous Dysplasia.** Later-stage lesions exhibiting significant mineralization.

surrounded by sclerotic margins. The periodontal ligament space usually appears intact, and fusion to the tooth is rare. Most lesions exhibit self-limiting growth, with individual lesions seldom exceeding 1.0 cm in diameter. The lesions are typically nonexpansile; however, mild expansion and thinning or perforation of the cortical plates at times may be appreciated with CBCT. In some cases, resorption of adjacent tooth roots also may be demonstrated by 3-dimensional imaging.

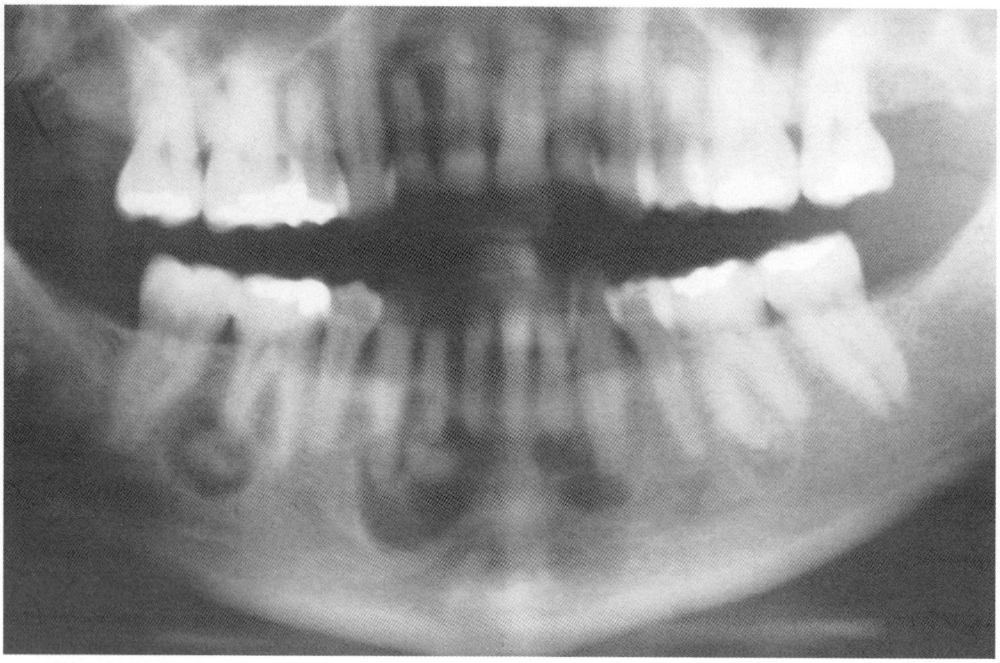

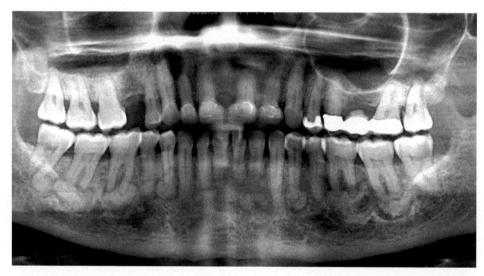

• **Fig. 14.48 Florid Cemento-Osseous Dysplasia.** Multiple mixed radiolucent and radiopaque lesions involving the anterior and posterior regions of the mandible.

• **Fig. 14.49 Florid Cemento-Osseous Dysplasia.** Multiple mixed radiolucent and radiopaque lesions throughout the mandible. (Courtesy of Dr. Haitham Hadeed.)

appearance). Cortical thinning or perforation, mild expansion, and adjacent tooth root resorption occasionally may be noted with CBCT examination.

Histopathologic Features

All three patterns of cemento-osseous dysplasia demonstrate similar histopathologic features. There are typically fragments of cellular fibrovascular connective tissue with scattered hemorrhage and a variable mixture of woven bone, lamellar bone, and cementum-like particles (Figs. 14.51 and 14.52). As the lesions mature, the ratio of fibrous connective tissue to mineralized material decreases. Over time, the bony trabeculae become thick and curvilinear, with

shapes likened to ginger roots. In the final radiopaque stage, the individual trabeculae fuse to form sheetlike or globular masses of sclerotic, disorganized cemento-osseous material (Fig. 14.53).

Diagnosis

In most instances of florid or periapical cemento-osseous dysplasia, the distinctive clinical and radiographic findings (e.g., a black female patient with multiquadrant involvement or multiple lesions involving vital lower incisor teeth) allow a strong presumptive diagnosis. In contrast, the features of focal cemento-osseous dysplasia tend to be less specific, and biopsy often is needed for diagnosis.

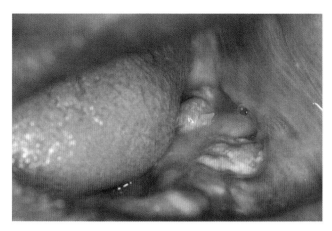

• **Fig. 14.50 Florid Cemento-Osseous Dysplasia.** Yellowish, avascular cementum-like material is beginning to exfoliate through the oral mucosa.

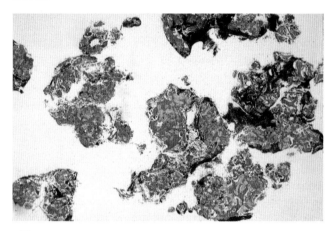

• **Fig. 14.51 Cemento-Osseous Dysplasia.** Low-power photomicrograph showing fragments of cellular fibrous connective tissue containing scattered trabeculae of bone.

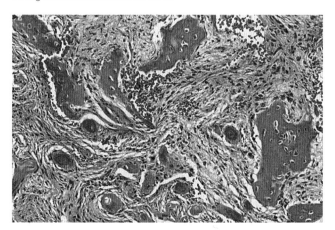

• **Fig. 14.52 Cemento-Osseous Dysplasia.** High-power photomicrograph showing spicules of bone and cementum-like hard tissue within moderately cellular fibrous connective tissue. Note the hemorrhage around the bony trabeculae.

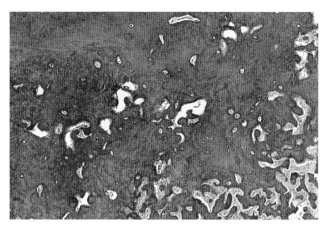

• **Fig. 14.53 Cemento-Osseous Dysplasia.** Late-stage lesion showing a sclerotic mass of cemento-osseous material.

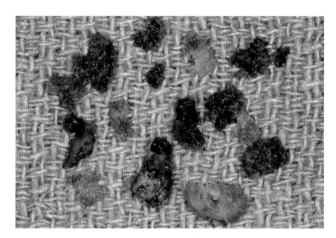

• **Fig. 14.54 Cemento-Osseous Dysplasia.** Gross specimen comprised of small, gritty tissue fragments.

surgeon typically curettes into small fragments during biopsy (Fig. 14.54). In contrast, ossifying fibromas tend to separate cleanly and are removed in one or several large masses. Microscopically, both lesion types demonstrate a mixture of bone and cementum-like particles, although subtle histopathologic differences may be appreciated. The bony trabeculae in ossifying fibroma tend to be more delicate and show more prominent osteoblastic rimming compared to those in cemento-osseous dysplasia. Also, the cementum-like particles in cemento-osseous dysplasia are irregularly shaped and often exhibit retraction from the adjacent stroma, whereas those in ossifying fibroma are more ovoid and often demonstrate brush borders in intimate association with the adjacent stroma. Although ossifying fibroma can exhibit peripheral hemorrhage, cemento-osseous dysplasia typically reveals hemorrhage throughout the lesion and sinusoidal vascularity in close association with the bony trabeculae.

Treatment and Prognosis

Cemento-osseous dysplasia does not appear to be neoplastic and, therefore, generally does not require removal. During the predominantly radiolucent phase, the lesions cause few problems. However, in the sclerotic phase, the lesions tend

In particular, distinguishing focal cemento-osseous dysplasia from ossifying fibroma can be difficult. However, the findings at surgery may be helpful in discriminating between these two lesions. Before the final sclerotic stage, cemento-osseous dysplasia consists of gritty tissue that the to be hypovascular and prone to necrosis and secondary infection with minimal provocation. For the asymptomatic patient, the best management consists of regular recall examinations with prophylaxis and oral hygiene reinforcement to control periodontal disease and prevent tooth loss.

Because the onset of symptoms usually is associated with exposure of the sclerotic masses to the oral cavity, surgical procedures (e.g., biopsy, elective tooth extraction) should be avoided. In some instances, symptoms begin after lesion exposure resulting from progressive alveolar atrophy under a denture. Therefore, affected patients should be encouraged to retain their teeth. Dental implant placement in an area of cemento-osseous generally is not recommended, although there are anecdotal reports of successful implant placement. Management of the symptomatic patient who has developed secondary osteomyelitis is more difficult. Antibiotics may be indicated but often are not effective. Sequestration of the sclerotic cementum-like masses occurs slowly and is followed by healing. Saucerization of dead bone may speed healing. When simple bone cysts arise within foci of cemento-osseous dysplasia, surgical exploration is necessary to establish the diagnosis. These simple bone cysts often do not heal as rapidly as those noted in younger patients without cemento-osseous dysplasia. In some cases the cysts persist or enlarge after surgical intervention; when they fill in, the bone retains an abnormal radiographic appearance. Thorough curettage of the cyst and the surrounding fibro-osseous proliferation may assist healing.

Some investigators have noted a rare subset of cases (termed *expansive osseous dysplasia*) that exhibit progressive growth but otherwise typical clinicopathologic features of cemento-osseous dysplasia (Fig. 14.55). Such lesions have been reported most often in the anterior mandible of African black females, with a somewhat younger age at onset compared to conventional cemento-osseous dysplasia. Tooth displacement, cortical perforation, and limited extension into soft tissue are possible. Such lesions typically require surgical removal.

Overall, the prognosis is good. Development of a sarcoma within an area of cemento-osseous dysplasia has been reported but is extremely rare.

◆ FAMILIAL GIGANTIFORM CEMENTOMA (FAMILIAL EXPANSIVE OSSEOUS DYSPLASIA)

Although the term *gigantiform cementoma* has been used in the past as a synonym for florid cemento-osseous dysplasia, most authorities now restrict use of this term to a rare hereditary disorder known as **familial gigantiform cementoma.** This extremely rare disorder exhibits an autosomal dominant pattern of transmission with high penetrance and variable expressivity. It is characterized by a cemento-osseous proliferation involving multiple quadrants of the jaws with early onset and often massive expansion.

Based on microscopic similarities, some authors consider familial gigantiform cementoma to be a variant of cemento-osseous dysplasia (*familial expansive osseous dysplasia, familial florid cemento-osseous dysplasia*). Comparable to cemento-osseous dysplasia, familial gigantiform cementoma progresses through an early radiolucent stage, an intermediate mixed radiolucent-radiopaque stage, and a mature radiopaque stage with lesion stabilization. However, a tendency for early onset, gross bony expansion, and an extended growth phase prior to maturation distinguish this condition from cemento-osseous dysplasia. Alternatively, based on a tendency for marked lesion growth, other authors prefer to regard familial gigantiform cementoma as a distinct neoplasm or a subtype of ossifying fibroma.

Sporadic cases with clinical and radiographic features similar to those of familial gigantiform cementoma also have been reported using various terms, including *(nonfamilial) gigantiform cementoma, (nonfamilial) expansive osseous dysplasia, multiple (cemento-) ossifying fibromas,* and *bilateral ossifying fibromas.* Such sporadic examples appear to be more common than familial ones. Whether these sporadic cases represent an expansive form of cemento-osseous dysplasia, spontaneous mutations, or a variant of ossifying fibroma remains uncertain. Molecular genetic studies are needed to improve the understanding and appropriate classification of this problematic disease spectrum.

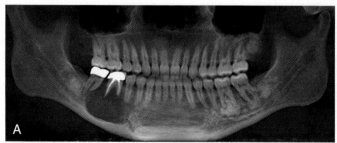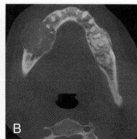

• **Fig. 14.55 Expansive Osseous Dysplasia. A,** Black female with bilateral mandibular cemento-osseous dysplasia, including an expansile lesion on the patient's right side. **B,** The computed tomography (CT) scan demonstrates both buccal and lingual expansion. (Courtesy of Dr. Peter Franco.)

Clinical and Radiographic Findings

Unlike florid cemento-osseous dysplasia, familial gigantiform cementoma exhibits neither a predilection for blacks nor a significant gender predilection. Although blacks may be affected, most reported families are Asian or white. Radiographic alterations may begin to develop during the first decade of life. By adolescence, most patients exhibit clinically obvious expansion of the jaws (Fig. 14.56). The lesions affect multiple quadrants, often with simultaneous involvement of the maxilla and mandible. Lesion growth may be rapid or slow. In a few reported cases, especially rapid growth has been noted during pregnancy. Although the course is variable, many patients develop significant facial deformity, as well as impaction, malposition, and malocclusion of the involved dentition. If not treated, then the osseous enlargement typically ceases by the fifth decade.

Radiographically, the lesions initially may appear as multiple periapical radiolucencies, resembling cemento-osseous dysplasia. With progression, the affected sites expand to replace much of the normal bone within the involved quadrant and develop a mixed radiolucent and radiopaque pattern. With further maturation, the lesions become predominantly radiopaque but often maintain a thin radiolucent rim. As noted in cemento-osseous dysplasia, the affected bone during the final radiopaque stage is very sensitive to inflammatory stimuli and becomes necrotic with minimal provocation.

Some investigators have reported elevated serum alkaline phosphatase that subsequently declines after surgical removal of the osseous proliferations. Anemia also has been reported in a number of affected females in different kindreds. In one family, two affected females demonstrated multifocal polypoid adenomas of the uterus that were associated with chronic hemorrhage and apparently caused anemia.

Furthermore, in a few kindreds diagnosed with familial gigantiform cementoma, bone fragility and a tendency for long bone fractures have been noted. However, such cases actually may represent examples of another entity known as *gnathodiaphyseal dysplasia* (a heritable autosomal dominant condition characterized by *GDD1* [or anoctamin 5 gene (*ANO5*)] mutations, diffuse fibro-osseous lesions of the jaws often with a prominent psammomatoid body component, bone fragility, and bowing/cortical sclerosis of tubular bones).

Histopathologic Features

Histopathologically, familial gigantiform cementoma shows features similar to cemento-ossifying fibroma and florid cemento-osseous dysplasia.

Treatment and Prognosis

Before the final sclerotic stage, shave-down surgical procedures typically are unsuccessful because the dysplastic tissue rapidly regrows. Once the lesions are predominantly radiopaque, partial removal may lead to sequestration of the remaining affected bone. Therefore, if feasible, complete resection and reconstruction are recommended. Because familial gigantiform cementoma might be associated with polypoid adenomas of the uterus, gynecologic evaluation is prudent for female patients—especially those with anemia.

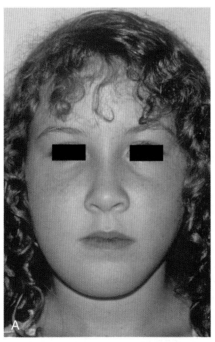
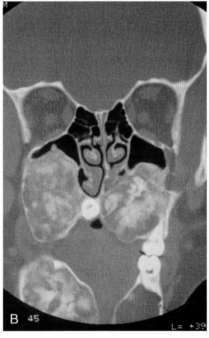

• **Fig. 14.56 Familial Gigantiform Cementoma.** Young woman with massive lesions involving all four quadrants of the jaws. (**A,** From Abdelsayed RA, Eversole LR, Singh BS, et al: Gigantiform cementoma: clinicopathologic presentation of 3 cases, *Oral Surg Oral Med Oral Pathol Oral Radiol Endod* 91:438–444, 2001; **B,** Courtesy of Dr. Rafik Abdelsayed.)

◆ CEMENTO-OSSIFYING FIBROMA (CONVENTIONAL OSSIFYING FIBROMA; OSSIFYING FIBROMA; CEMENTIFYING FIBROMA)

Although it can resemble focal cemento-osseous dysplasia radiographically and histopathologically, **cemento-ossifying fibroma** is a true neoplasm with significant growth potential. This neoplasm is relatively rare, and many examples reported in the older literature actually represent cases of focal cemento-osseous dysplasia.

The origin of cemento-ossifying fibroma is somewhat controversial. Based upon its predilection for tooth-bearing areas of the jaws and ability to produce a variable mixture of bony trabeculae and cementum-like spherules, investigators have suggested that the origin is odontogenic or from periodontal ligament progenitor cells. However, microscopically identical neoplasms with cementum-like differentiation also have been reported in the orbital, frontal, ethmoid, sphenoid, and temporal bones or non-tooth-bearing areas of the jaws, and many authorities regard the cementum-like material in cemento-ossifying fibromas as a variation of bone. Indeed, some contend that bone and cementum are essentially the same mineralized product and only can be distinguished based on anatomic location (i.e., presence of cementum along root surfaces). Therefore, a non-odontogenic origin also has been proposed.

In this section, we use the term *cemento-ossifying fibroma*. However, various alternative terms (including *ossifying fibroma, conventional ossifying fibroma—odontogenic and non-odontogenic types,* and *cementifying fibroma*) have been applied to this tumor as well. Furthermore, some authors prefer the term *conventional ossifying fibroma* in order to distinguish this lesion from juvenile ossifying fibroma (see page 653).

Mutations in the tumor suppressor gene *HRPT2* (or *CDC73*) (which encodes the parafibromin protein) have been identified in patients with *hyperparathyroidism-jaw tumor syndrome.* This rare autosomal dominant disorder is characterized by parathyroid adenoma or carcinoma, cemento-ossifying fibromas of the jaws, renal cysts, Wilms tumors, and uterine tumors. In addition, investigators have found *HRPT2* mutations in a few sporadic cases of cemento-ossifying fibroma of the jaws. However, the potential pathogenetic role of such mutations in cemento-ossifying fibroma remains poorly understood. Also of interest, a recent study detected frequent copy number alterations—especially involving chromosomes 7 and 12—in cemento-ossifying fibromas but not fibrous dysplasia of the jaws.

Clinical and Radiographic Features

Cemento-ossifying fibromas occur over a broad age range, with a peak in the third and fourth decades of life. There is a female predilection, with the mandible involved far more often than the maxilla. The mandibular premolar and molar area is the most common site. Maxillary lesions tend to involve the antrum and canine fossa.

Small lesions are often asymptomatic and may be detected only by radiographic examination. Larger tumors may produce painless jaw swelling (Fig. 14.57) and obvious facial asymmetry. Some lesions may become massive and cause considerable deformity. Pain and tooth mobility are infrequent, and paresthesia is rare. Most examples are solitary; however, multiple synchronous lesions have been reported very rarely—either as an isolated finding or as a component of hyperparathyroidism-jaw tumor syndrome.

Depending on the amount of calcification, radiographic examination shows a well-defined lesion that is radiolucent, mixed radiolucent and radiopaque, or mostly radiopaque. Some examples exhibit a sclerotic border. Most radiolucent lesions are unilocular. Multilocular lesions at times may represent concurrent aneurysmal bone cyst (see page 638) formation. True ossifying fibromas that appear largely radiopaque with only a thin radiolucent periphery are

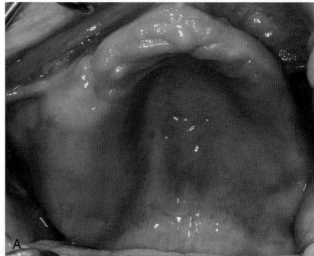

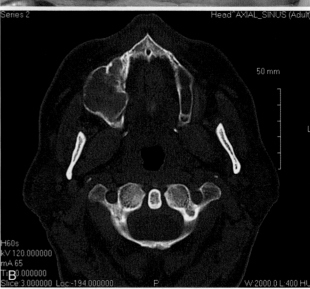

• **Fig. 14.57 Cemento-ossifying Fibroma.** Clinical image **(A)** and computed tomography (CT) scan **(B)** showing a large, expansile lesion of the posterior maxilla. (Courtesy of Dr. Greg Cobetto.)

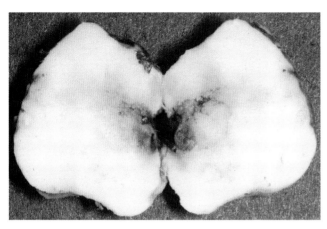

• **Fig. 14.58 Cemento-ossifying Fibroma.** Gross specimen showing a well-circumscribed tumor that shelled out in one piece and subsequently was hemisected.

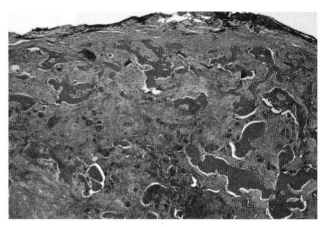

• **Fig. 14.59 Cemento-ossifying Fibroma.** This low-magnification photomicrograph shows a well-circumscribed solid tumor mass. Trabeculae of bone and droplets of cementum-like material can be seen forming within a background of cellular fibrous connective tissue.

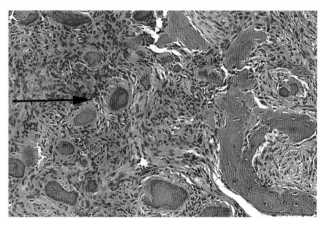

• **Fig. 14.60 Cemento-ossifying Fibroma.** High-power photomicrograph showing a mixture of woven bone and cementum-like material. Note the spherules demonstrating peripheral brush borders (arrow).

infrequent; many reported examples with this radiographic pattern likely represent end-stage focal cemento-osseous dysplasia. Buccolingual bony expansion is common; in addition, large mandibular lesions often demonstrate a characteristic downward bowing of the inferior cortex, and inferior displacement of the mandibular canal is possible. The adjacent teeth may exhibit root divergence or root resorption. Maxillary lesions may displace the sinus floor.

Histopathologic Features

At surgery, the lesion tends to separate easily from the surrounding bone; thus, the tumor usually is submitted as one mass or a few large pieces (Fig. 14.58). Grossly and microscopically, most lesions are well demarcated but unencapsulated. However, a fibrous capsule may be present in some cases.

Microscopic examination shows cellular fibrous tissue with mineralized product (Fig. 14.59). The mineralized component may include a variable admixture of osteoid, bone, and basophilic acellular (or "cementum-like") spherules. The bony trabeculae vary in size and frequently demonstrate both woven and lamellar patterns. Peripheral osteoid and osteoblastic rimming are usually present. The cementum-like spherules often demonstrate brush borders that blend into the adjacent connective tissue (Fig. 14.60). These spherules may be surrounded by radiating collagen fibers reminiscent of Sharpey fibers within the periodontal ligament. Under polarized light, this cementum-like material may exhibit a quilted pattern. Significant intralesional hemorrhage is unusual. The heterogeneous mineralized product characteristic of cemento-ossifying fibroma differs from the more uniform osseous pattern of fibrous dysplasia. Rarely, a lesion may exhibit combined features of cemento-ossifying fibroma and central giant cell granuloma.

Treatment and Prognosis

The circumscribed nature of the cemento-ossifying fibroma generally permits enucleation or curettage of the tumor with relative ease. Large lesions that have caused considerable

bone destruction may necessitate surgical resection and bone grafting. Recurrence after complete removal is uncommon, with an average recurrence rate of approximately 10% among various reported case series. Overall, the prognosis is very good, and there is no apparent potential for malignant transformation.

◆ JUVENILE OSSIFYING FIBROMA (JUVENILE ACTIVE OSSIFYING FIBROMA; JUVENILE AGGRESSIVE OSSIFYING FIBROMA; AGGRESSIVE OSSIFYING FIBROMA)

The **juvenile ossifying fibroma** is a controversial lesion that has been distinguished from cemento-ossifying fibroma on the basis of patient age, site predilection, and clinical behavior. The term includes two distinct clinicopathologic variants: (1) **trabecular** and (2) **psammomatoid**. Among lesions involving the craniofacial skeleton, the psammomatoid variant has been reported more frequently than the trabecular variant.

The etiopathogenesis is poorly understood. In a small number of orbital psammomatoid ossifying fibromas, investigators have demonstrated nonrandom chromosomal breakpoints at Xq26 and 2q33 resulting in (X;2) translocation. Researchers also have identified *MDM2* (E3 ubiquitin-protein ligase gene) and *RASAL1* (RAS protein activator like 1 gene) amplification in juvenile ossifying fibromas; these changes may be associated with locally aggressive behavior and have been detected at a significantly higher frequency in this tumor type compared to cemento-ossifying fibroma and craniofacial fibrous dysplasia. Among studies conducted thus far, failure to detect *GNAS* or *HRPT2* mutations in juvenile ossifying fibromas suggests that these lesions are distinct from fibrous dysplasia and cemento-ossifying fibromas.

Clinical and Radiographic Features

Juvenile ossifying fibromas most often arise in children, adolescents, and young adults; however, a broader age range has been reported for the psammomatoid variant (3 months to 72 years) than the trabecular variant (1–33 years). The average age at diagnosis is somewhat younger for the trabecular variant than the psammomatoid variant (approximately 12 years versus 19 years, respectively). Most authors report either a slight male predilection or no significant gender predilection. The trabecular variant arises primarily in the jaws, whereas the psammomatoid variant often involves the paranasal sinuses and orbital region. In both variants, gnathic involvement slightly favors the maxilla.

Although some cases exhibit slow, progressive enlargement, others exhibit rapid, aggressive growth. Small lesions may be discovered incidentally during routine radiographic examination, whereas larger lesions tend to cause painless swelling and obvious facial enlargement. Pain and paresthesia are infrequent findings. Tumors arising in the paranasal sinuses may penetrate the orbital, nasal, and cranial cavities. Nasal obstruction, epistaxis, sinusitis, headaches, proptosis, diplopia, and blindness may result. Rarely, intracranial extension may cause encephalitis and meningitis.

Radiographic examination typically shows a well-circumscribed radiolucency or mixed radiolucency and radiopacity (Fig. 14.61). A sclerotic border may be evident in some cases. Homogeneous "ground-glass" opacification, "ground-glass" opacification with central radiolucency, discrete calcifications, or a multilocular "honeycomb" pattern also may be observed. Aggressive lesions often cause expansion and cortical thinning or perforation. Similar to cemento-ossifying fibromas, juvenile ossifying fibromas may produce downward bowing of the inferior cortex of the mandible and inferior displacement of the mandibular canal. Jaw lesions also can cause tooth displacement, root resorption, and failure of tooth development. Sinus involvement may appear radiographically as cloudy opacification mimicking sinusitis.

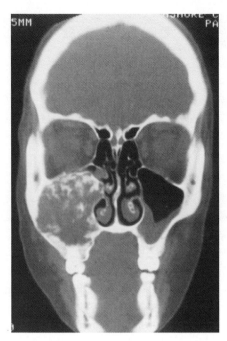

• **Fig. 14.61 Juvenile Ossifying Fibroma.** Computed tomography (CT) scan showing a large tumor involving the left maxilla and maxillary sinus of a 12-year-old girl. Clinically, the tumor was growing rapidly.

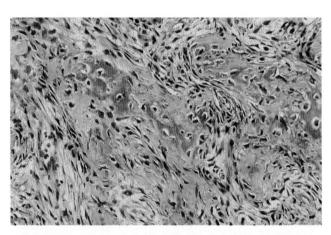

• **Fig. 14.62 Juvenile Ossifying Fibroma, Trabecular Variant.** Trabeculae of cellular woven bone are present in a cellular fibrous stroma.

Histopathologic Features

Both patterns are typically well demarcated but unencapsulated. However, the mineralized component differs between the two variants. The trabecular variant shows irregular strands of highly cellular osteoid encasing plump and irregular osteocytes (Fig. 14.62). These strands often are lined by plump osteoblasts and multinucleated osteoclasts. In contrast, the psammomatoid variant exhibits concentric lamellated ossicles that vary in size and may be round, ovoid, or crescentic in shape. The ossicles typically appear basophilic with peripheral eosinophilic osteoid rims and brush borders that blend into the surrounding stroma (Fig. 14.63).

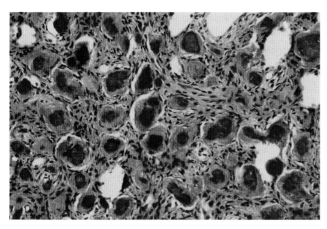

• **Fig. 14.63 Juvenile Ossifying Fibroma, Psammomatoid Variant.** Cellular fibrous connective tissue containing spherical ossicles with basophilic centers and peripheral eosinophilic rims.

In both variants, the mineralized product is set within the background of a fibrous stroma. The stroma is often hypercellular, although cellularity may vary. Mitotic figures may be noted but are neither numerous nor atypical. Scattered aggregates of osteoclastic giant cells are often evident in the trabecular variant, whereas giant cells are an infrequent finding in the psammomatoid variant. In the trabecular variant, the newly formed osteoid often blends imperceptibly with the surrounding fibrous stroma. Zones of hemorrhage, giant cells, edema, and pseudocystic degeneration may correlate with grossly evident brown, curvilinear strands on the tumor's cut surface. In both variants, hemorrhagic cystic degeneration may resemble aneurysmal bone cyst formation.

Treatment and Prognosis

For small lesions, complete local excision or thorough curettage appears adequate. Combining enucleation with curettage or peripheral ostectomy may decrease the risk for recurrence. For large or aggressive lesions, wider resection may be required.

In contrast to the negligible recurrence rate for cemento-ossifying fibromas, an overall recurrence rate of 21% has been reported for juvenile ossifying fibromas. Many reported recurrences actually may represent tumor persistence after incomplete surgical removal. Malignant transformation has not been documented. Tumor-related deaths are extremely rare and primarily result from complications caused by direct intracranial extension.

◆ OSTEOMA

Osteomas are benign tumors composed of mature compact or cancellous bone. Osteomas primarily involve the craniofacial skeleton and rarely, if ever, are diagnosed in other bones. They may arise on the bone surface (**periosteal, peripheral,** or **exophytic osteomas**) or within medullary bone (**endosteal** or **central osteomas**). **Extraskeletal osteomas,** typically located within muscle or the dermis of the skin (**osteoma cutis**), also are possible.

There is some question whether osteomas represent true neoplasms, and not all lesions designated as osteomas may represent a single entity. Some likely result from injury, an inflammatory process, or a hamartomatous process. Because some osteomas arise in areas where muscle attaches to bone, investigators have hypothesized that muscle traction may be a contributory factor. Common palatal tori, mandibular tori, and buccal exostoses (see page 19) are not considered to be osteomas, although they are histopathologically identical. Because many osteomas are small and asymptomatic, there is little reliable information regarding their frequency and demographic distribution.

Clinical and Radiographic Features

Osteomas of the jaws most often are detected in adults, with a predilection for the mandibular body and condyle. Lesions involving the mandibular body frequently are found on the lingual surface adjacent to the premolars or molars. Less common mandibular locations include the angle (particularly at the inferior border), ramus, and coronoid process.

Most examples are solitary and asymptomatic with very slow growth. Pain, tooth displacement, and tooth impaction have been reported in a minority of cases. Rarely, a lesion may become especially large and produce marked facial deformity. Periosteal osteomas appear as polypoid or sessile masses on the bone surface, whereas endosteal osteomas may not be evident clinically unless they are large enough to cause expansion. Multifocal lesions may arise in association with Gardner syndrome (see page 656). In addition, unilateral osteomas of the jaws have been reported in association with encephalocraniocutaneous lipomatosis (Haberland syndrome).

Osteomas involving the mandibular condyle may limit mouth opening or cause malocclusion, with deviation of the dental midline and chin toward the unaffected side. Pain and swelling also are possible. Some authorities consider condylar osteomas to be true neoplasms, whereas others designate them as *hyperostoses*. Distinguishing this process from condylar hyperplasia can be difficult; however, a condylar osteoma typically is lobulated, whereas a hyperplastic condyle usually retains its original shape.

Osteomas of the sinonasal and orbital region (*sino-orbital osteomas*) are even more common than gnathic lesions. Among the paranasal sinuses, the frontal sinus is most often involved, followed by the ethmoid and maxillary sinuses. Sinus lesions are usually asymptomatic, although pain, swelling, sinusitis, and nasal discharge are possible. Orbital osteomas may cause proptosis, diplopia, and decreased visual acuity. Infrequently, intracranial extension may result in meningitis, cerebral abscesses, and intracranial mucoceles.

Radiographically, osteomas typically appear as circumscribed sclerotic masses, although early lesions may appear radiolucent or mixed radiolucent-radiopaque. Periosteal osteomas may show a uniformly sclerotic pattern or may demonstrate a sclerotic periphery with central trabeculation (Fig. 14.64). Smaller endosteal osteomas are difficult, if not impossible, to differentiate radiographically from condensing osteitis, focal chronic sclerosing osteomyelitis, or idiopathic osteosclerosis. The true nature of these osteomas can be confirmed only by documentation of continued growth.

Histopathologic Features

Compact (or **"ivory"**) osteomas are composed of normal-appearing, dense bone with minimal marrow (Fig. 14.65). **Cancellous** osteomas are composed of bony trabeculae and fibrofatty marrow. Osteoblastic activity may be fairly prominent. Some sino-orbital osteomas exhibit so-called "osteoblastoma-like features," characterized by enlarged osteoblasts, woven bone, and loosely arranged fibrovascular stroma.

Treatment and Prognosis

Small, asymptomatic osteomas may not require treatment but should be observed periodically. Conservative excision is appropriate for large or symptomatic osteomas of the mandibular body. Because they are frequently symptomatic, condylar osteomas usually are removed by local resection or

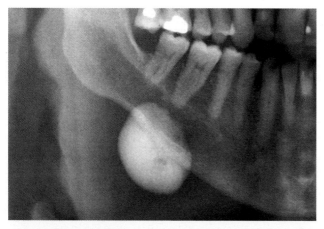

• **Fig. 14.64 Osteoma.** Panoramic radiograph showing a uniformly sclerotic mass arising from the surface of the posterior mandible. (Courtesy of Dr. James Lemon.)

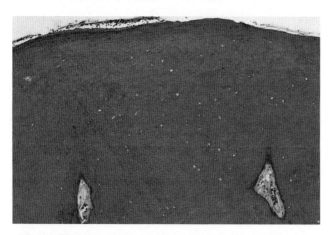

• **Fig. 14.65 Osteoma.** This compact osteoma is composed of dense bone, with only minimal marrow elements.

condylectomy. Symptomatic paranasal sinus osteomas may be removed endoscopically or via an open surgical approach. Recurrence after excision is extremely rare, and there are no reports of malignant transformation.

◆ GARDNER SYNDROME

Gardner syndrome is a rare disorder, characterized by intestinal polyps as well as various abnormalities of bone, teeth, skin, soft tissue, and other sites. This syndrome represents a variant of *familial adenomatous polyposis*—an autosomal dominant disorder characterized by mutations in the adenomatous polyposis coli *(APC)* tumor suppressor gene on chromosome 5q21 and a markedly increased risk for colorectal cancer. The specific position of mutations within the *APC* gene determines the severity of gastrointestinal disease and the nature of the extraintestinal findings. In both classical familial adenomatous polyposis and the Gardner syndrome variant, patients develop hundreds to thousands of colorectal adenomatous polyps, with nearly 100% progression to colorectal cancer if left untreated. The term *Gardner syndrome* generally refers to cases in which the extraintestinal manifestations are especially prominent. Another disease variant, *attenuated familial adenomatous polyposis*, is characterized by similar extraintestinal findings but a smaller number (a few to a hundred) of colorectal polyps. The estimated frequency of familial adenomatous polyposis coli ranges from about 1 in 7,000 to 1 in 31,000 live births, although it is difficult to determinate the exact proportion of cases represented by Gardner syndrome or other disease variants.

Clinical and Radiographic Features

In patients with Gardner syndrome, colorectal polyps typically develop by the second decade of life (Fig. 14.66). The lesions often are asymptomatic but may cause diarrhea, constipation, rectal bleeding, anemia, and abdominal pain. The colorectal polyps are adenomatous (i.e., precancerous with varying degrees of dysplasia) and, if untreated, ultimately transform into adenocarcinoma. In addition, polyps

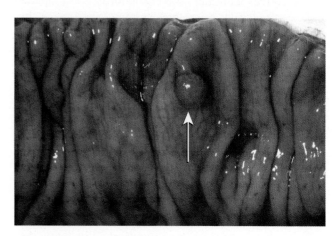

• **Fig. 14.66 Gardner Syndrome.** A segment of resected large bowel showing polyp formation *(arrow)*.

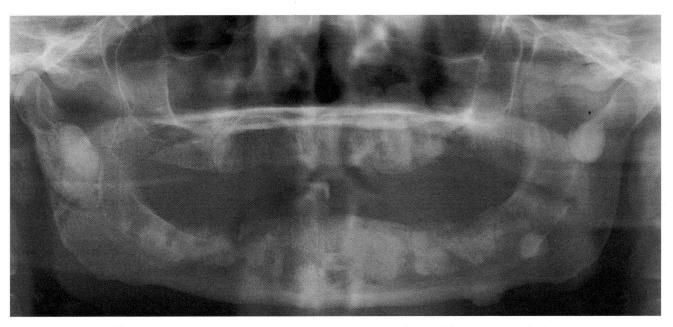

• **Fig. 14.67 Gardner Syndrome.** Panoramic radiograph showing multiple osteomas of the jaws. (Courtesy of Dr. Terry Day.)

often arise in the duodenum or gastric fundus, although only a small percentage of polyps in these sites undergo carcinomatous transformation.

Up to 90% of patients with Gardner syndrome demonstrate skeletal abnormalities, the most common of which are osteomas. The osteomas usually are noted around puberty and often become evident before the intestinal polyps; indeed, the presence of multiple osteomas may lead to an early diagnosis of Gardner syndrome. Although the osteomas may affect any part of the skeleton, they most commonly involve the skull, paranasal sinuses, and mandible. Mandibular lesions often occur at the angle and may cause marked facial deformity. Occasionally, osteomas of the condyle may limit mouth opening. Most patients demonstrate between three and six osseous lesions. The osteomas appear as radiopacities that vary from a few millimeters to several centimeters in diameter (Fig. 14.67).

Dental abnormalities occur in about 22%–30% of patients and include odontomas, supernumerary teeth, and impacted teeth. The frequency of supernumerary teeth in Gardner syndrome is not nearly as high as that noted in cleidocranial dysplasia. Hypercementosis, fused or unusually long tooth roots, and congenitally missing teeth also have been reported in some individuals with Gardner syndrome.

Most patients show one or several epidermoid cysts of the skin (Fig. 14.68). Other cutaneous findings may include lipomas, fibromas, neurofibromas, and leiomyomas. Desmoid tumors (locally aggressive fibrous neoplasms of soft tissue) arise in approximately 10% of patients. These lesions are more frequent in females than males and often develop in the abdominal scar that forms after colectomy. Other possible extraintestinal neoplasms include thyroid carcinoma, adrenal adenoma or adenocarcinoma, hepatoblastoma, pancreatic adenocarcinoma, nasopharyngeal angiofibroma, and brain

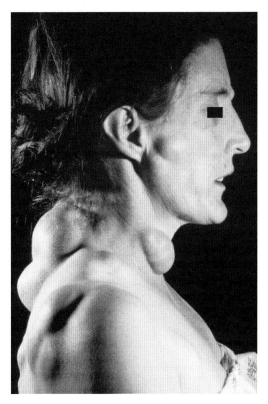

• **Fig. 14.68 Gardner Syndrome.** This patient has multiple, large epidermoid cysts. (Courtesy of Dr. William Welton.)

tumors. Furthermore, pigmented lesions of the ocular fundus (also known as *congenital hypertrophy of the retinal pigment epithelium*) are evident in about 75% of patients with familial adenomatous polyposis. This ocular abnormality correlates with specific mutated loci within the *APC* gene.

Histopathologic Features

Histopathologically, the osteomas are generally of the compact type. An individual lesion cannot be differentiated microscopically from a solitary osteoma.

Treatment and Prognosis

The major problem for patients with Gardner syndrome is the high risk for transformation of colorectal polyps into adenocarcinoma. Without treatment, approximately 50% of patients will develop colorectal cancer by 30 years of age, and the frequency of malignant change approaches 100% by the fifth decade. Therefore, prophylactic colectomy usually is recommended. Clinical trials have shown some regression of polyps with cyclooxygenase-2 (COX-2) inhibitors, such as sulindac, but further studies are needed.

Patients also should be monitored for development of extracolonic malignancies or desmoid tumors. Genetic counseling is indicated as well. Osteomas and epidermoid cysts may be removed if they cause functional or cosmetic problems. Dental management typically involves surgical extraction of impacted teeth, removal of odontomas, and prosthodontic treatment. Orthodontic tooth movement may be difficult due to increased bone density from the osteomas.

◆ OSTEOBLASTOMA (GIANT OSTEOID OSTEOMA) AND OSTEOID OSTEOMA

Osteoblastoma and **osteoid osteoma** are closely related benign bone tumors that arise from osteoblasts. They exhibit very similar histopathologic features but differ somewhat in clinical presentation. The osteoid osteoma exhibits more limited growth potential than osteoblastoma; traditionally, the lesions are distinguished based on lesion size, with osteoid osteomas measuring less than 1.5 or 2 cm in diameter and osteoblastomas measuring at or above this threshold. In addition, although both lesion types often cause pain, the osteoid osteoma is associated more specifically with nocturnal pain relieved by nonsteroidal anti-inflammatory drugs (NSAIDs). This characteristic feature may be explained by the presence of a tumor nidus with a high concentration of peripheral nerves and prostaglandins.

Most investigators consider these lesions to be true neoplasms, although some have proposed that the limited growth of osteoid osteoma suggests an inflammatory or unusual healing process. In support of a neoplastic nature, recurrent *FOS* and *FOSB* rearrangements recently have been identified in both osteoblastoma and osteoid osteoma. These shared genetic alterations suggest that these entities may represent variants of the same lesion.

Clinical and Radiographic Features

Osteoblastoma

Osteoblastomas are rare and represent approximately 1% of all primary bone tumors. The most frequently affected sites are the vertebral column, long bones, pelvis, talus, facial bones, and small bones of the hands and feet. Among gnathic lesions, there is a mandibular predilection, with most examples involving the posterior regions. Approximately 85% of gnathic osteoblastomas occur before 30 years of age, and there is a slight female predominance.

Most osteoblastomas are between 2 and 4 cm, but they may be as large as 10 cm. Dull pain, tenderness, and swelling are common presenting features. Unlike the pain associated with osteoid osteoma, the pain associated with osteoblastoma usually is not relieved by NSAIDs. Painful jaw lesions may be misinterpreted as odontogenic infections. Gnathic tumors also may cause tooth mobility, root resorption, or tooth displacement.

Radiographically, the osteoblastoma typically appears as a well- or ill-defined, round to oval radiolucency with patchy areas of mineralization (Fig. 14.69). Some examples demonstrate considerable mineralization. Surrounding reactive sclerosis is less prominent in osteoblastoma than osteoid osteoma. Most osteoblastomas arise within medullary bone, although a periosteal or intracortical origin also is possible.

A small subset of osteoblastomas (**aggressive osteoblastomas**) is characterized by atypical histopathologic features and locally aggressive behavior. These tumors usually occur in patients older than 30 years. A variety of bones, including the mandible, may be involved. Pain is common and may be severe. Aggressive osteoblastomas exhibit radiographic findings similar to those of conventional osteoblastoma but tend to be larger (typically greater than 4 cm in diameter).

Osteoid Osteoma

Osteoid osteoma comprises about 3% of all primary bone tumors. The lesion occurs most often in the femur and tibia but is very rare in the jaws. Gnathic tumors tend to occur in the posterior regions, with a slight mandibular predominance and a peak in the second and third decades of life. Although

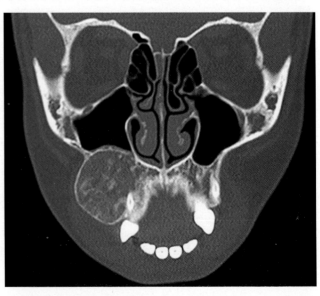

• **Fig. 14.69 Osteoblastoma.** Computed tomography (CT) image showing an expansile, mixed radiolucent and radiopaque lesion of the maxilla. (Courtesy of Dr. Michael Zetz.)

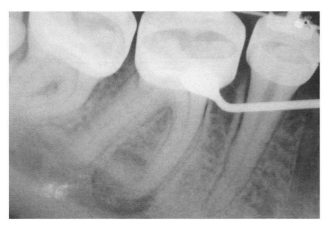

• **Fig. 14.70 Osteoid Osteoma.** A circumscribed, mixed radiolucent and radiopaque lesion near the apex of mesial root of mandibular first molar. The patient had dull, nocturnal pain that was relieved by aspirin. (Courtesy of Dr. Ellen Eisenberg.)

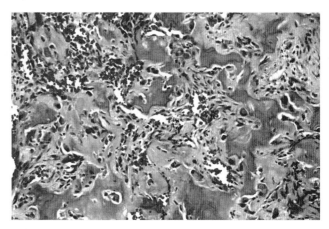

• **Fig. 14.71 Osteoblastoma.** High-power photomicrograph showing irregular bony trabeculae with prominent osteoblastic rimming and osteoclasts.

extragnathic lesions demonstrate a male predilection, jaw lesions exhibit no significant gender predilection. The most prominent clinical symptom is pain that is most severe at night and alleviated by NSAIDs. However, nocturnal pain relieved by NSAIDs has been documented more often among extragnathic lesions than jaw lesions.

Radiographically, the osteoid osteoma typically appears as a well-circumscribed, round to ovoid radiolucency (or "nidus") with a variable degree of surrounding reactive sclerosis. The radiolucent nidus may contain a small, central radiopacity, resulting in a target-like appearance (Fig. 14.70). The nidus typically measures less than 1.5 cm in diameter and most commonly arises within cortical bone, although a medullary or periosteal origin also is possible. A periosteal reaction occasionally may be seen.

Histopathologic Features

Microscopically, both osteoid osteoma and osteoblastoma centrally exhibit irregular trabeculae of osteoid or woven bone, which are surrounded by numerous osteoblasts and scattered osteoclasts. The osteoblasts have ample cytoplasm and hyperchromatic nuclei (Fig. 14.71). The loose fibrous stroma includes dilated vessels and occasional hemorrhage. The vascularity tends to be more prominent in osteoblastoma than osteoid osteoma. At the periphery, there is typically a more prominent zone of dense, sclerotic bone in osteoid osteoma than osteoblastoma.

Aggressive osteoblastomas typically demonstrate sheets or single layers of large (epithelioid) osteoblasts with occasional mitotic activity, lacelike osteoid ("blue bone matrix"), and irregular bony trabeculae. However, epithelioid morphology does not always correlate with aggressive clinical behavior. Differentiation between aggressive osteoblastoma and low-grade osteosarcoma may be very difficult, although infiltrative growth, marked cytologic atypia, and atypical mitotic figures favor the latter. Another rare osteoblastoma variant is the *epithelioid multinodular osteoblastoma*, characterized

by a multinodular proliferation of epithelioid osteoblasts with or without bone matrix.

Fluorescence *in situ* hybridization (FISH) may be performed to detect *FOS* or *FOSB* rearrangements in osteoblastomas and osteoid osteomas. In addition, FOS overexpression may be demonstrated by immunohistochemistry, although specimen decalcification may decrease immunoreactivity.

Treatment and Prognosis

Most osteoid osteomas and osteoblastomas of the jaws are treated by local excision or curettage. Some osteoid osteomas may regress spontaneously; however, most clinicians prefer surgical removal over long-term observation and pain management with NSAIDs. For extragnathic lesions, minimally invasive techniques (e.g., computed tomography [CT]-guided excision and radiofrequency ablation) have gained popularity recently.

Recurrence after complete removal is uncommon; many reported recurrences may be attributed to incomplete excision. Osteoid osteoma exhibits no potential for malignant transformation, and osteoblastoma only rarely transforms into osteosarcoma. Whether aggressive osteoblastoma exhibits a greater recurrence potential than conventional osteoblastoma is controversial, although metastasis or death from aggressive osteoblastoma has not been reported.

◆ CEMENTOBLASTOMA (TRUE CEMENTOMA)

Cementoblastoma is a benign neoplasm of cementoblasts and represents less than 1% of all odontogenic tumors. Many authorities believe this lesion represents the only true neoplasm of cementum. Alternatively, because cementoblastoma bears a close histopathologic resemblance to osteoblastoma (see previous section), others consider cementoblastoma to be a variant of osteoblastoma. The primary distinguishing

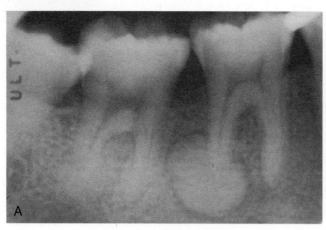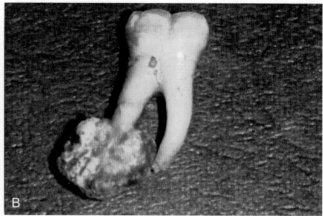

• **Fig. 14.72 Cementoblastoma. A,** A densely mineralized mass is seen at the apex of the distal root of the first molar. The root is partially resorbed. **B,** The surgical specimen shows that the mass is attached to the root. (Courtesy of Dr. John Wright.)

factor is whether or not the lesion is fused to a tooth root. Because of its similarity to osteoblastoma, cementoblastoma is discussed here rather than in Chapter 15.

Clinical and Radiographic Features

Nearly 80% of cases arise in the mandible, primarily in the molar and premolar region. In particular, almost 50% of cases involve the mandibular first permanent molar. Impacted, unerupted, or deciduous teeth rarely may be affected as well. There is no sex predilection. The neoplasm predominantly affects young patients, with a mean age of 24 years and a peak in the second and third decades of life. The mean lesion size is about 2 cm (range 0.5 to 8 cm). Pain and swelling are present in approximately 70% of reported cases. The associated tooth usually responds normally to vitality tests, although a loss of vitality is noted in about 20% of cases. Most investigators consider this lesion rather innocuous; however, signs of locally aggressive behavior may be observed, including bony expansion, cortical perforation, displacement of adjacent teeth, envelopment of multiple teeth, maxillary sinus involvement, and infiltration into the pulp chamber and root canals.

Radiographically, the tumor typically appears as a radiopaque mass that is fused to one or more tooth roots and is surrounded by a thin radiolucent rim (Fig. 14.72). In rare instances, the lesion may appear entirely radiolucent. The outline of the root or roots of the involved tooth usually is obscured by root resorption and fusion of the tumor with the tooth. Inferior displacement of the mandibular canal may be evident in about one-fourth of cases.

Histopathologic Features

The histopathologic features of cementoblastoma closely resemble those of osteoblastoma. However, the primary distinguishing feature of cementoblastoma is fusion with the involved tooth (Fig. 14.73). Microscopic examination shows sheets and thick trabeculae of mineralized material with irregularly placed lacunae and prominent basophilic reversal

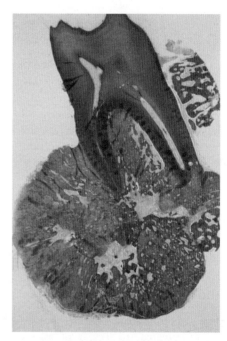

• **Fig. 14.73 Cementoblastoma.** Low-power photomicrograph showing the tumor attached to the roots of the tooth.

lines. The background stroma is comprised of cellular fibrovascular tissue. Multinucleated giant cells often are present, and prominent blast-like cells frequently line the mineralized trabeculae (Fig. 14.74). Radiating columns of uncalcified matrix typically are seen at the periphery, corresponding to the radiolucent rim seen radiographically. In few instances, the lesion may infiltrate the pulp chamber and root canals of the involved tooth.

Treatment and Prognosis

Treatment usually consists of surgical extraction of the tooth and the attached calcified mass. A potential alternative is excision of the mass with root amputation followed by endodontic treatment of the remaining tooth. Some

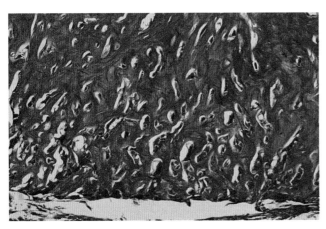

• **Fig. 14.74 Cementoblastoma.** Mineralized tissue containing numerous plump cementoblasts.

investigators suggest that supplementing extraction or excision with osseous curettage may decrease the risk for recurrence. Unusually large lesions may require surgical resection. The overall recurrence rate is approximately 12%. An increased risk for recurrence has been noted among cases exhibiting bony expansion or cortical perforation.

◆ CHONDROMA

Chondromas are benign tumors of mature hyaline cartilage. They comprise about 16% of benign bone tumors and most often arise in the small bones of the hands and feet. In the craniofacial bones, a diagnosis of chondroma should be viewed with great skepticism because many purported cases have recurred and exhibited malignant behavior. There are only a few individual reports and small series of gnathic chondromas, with most examples thought to arise from cartilage or cartilaginous rests in the condyle, anterior maxilla, mandibular symphysis, and coronoid process.

Chondromas predominantly arise within medullary bone (*enchondromas*), but some may develop just beneath the periosteum (*periosteal chondromas*). Most chondromas are solitary, although multiple lesions (*enchondromatosis*) may develop in the following nonheritable disorders:
- **Ollier disease** (enchondromatosis with predominantly unilateral involvement of the appendicular skeleton)
- **Maffucci syndrome** (enchondromatosis with extraskeletal angiomas)

Enchondromatosis differs from solitary chondroma in that it appears to represent a developmental disorder of endochondral ossification (or "cartilage dysplasia") rather than a true neoplasm.

Chondromas frequently harbor somatic mutations in *IDH1* and *IDH2* (isocitrate dehydrogenase 1 and 2 genes). They also may exhibit mutations or structural alterations of *COL2A1* and *YEATS2*. Such genetic abnormalities may be found in chondrosarcomas as well; however, additional alterations (such as *CDKN2A* amplification) may aid in distinguishing chondrosarcomas from chondromas.

Clinical and Radiographic Features

More than 60% of chondromas are diagnosed in the second, third, and fourth decades of life, and there is no significant sex predilection. Most gnathic examples occur in the condyle or anterior maxilla of adult patients. Usually, the lesions are painless and grow slowly. However, condylar tumors may cause pain, limited mouth opening, and deviation of the mandible from the midline. Lesions arising adjacent to teeth may cause tooth mobility and root resorption. Radiographically, the chondroma typically appears as a well-defined radiolucency with central opacification.

Histopathologic Features

Histopathologically, a chondroma appears as a well-circumscribed, lobular mass of mature hyaline cartilage. The cartilage typically demonstrates well-formed lacunae containing small chondrocytes with pale cytoplasm and small, round nuclei. Microscopic distinction between a chondroma and a low-grade chondrosarcoma of the jaws may be difficult (see page 669).

Treatment and Prognosis

It is wise to consider any jaw lesion diagnosed as a chondroma to represent a potential chondrosarcoma. Treatment typically consists of complete surgical removal.

◆ CHONDROMYXOID FIBROMA

The **chondromyxoid fibroma** is a rare, benign cartilaginous neoplasm that represents less than 1% of all primary bone tumors. Cytogenetic studies have detected frequent abnormalities in chromosome 6, and upregulation of the glutamate receptor metabotropic-1 gene (*GRM1*) located on chromosome 6q24.3 appears to be an important event in tumor development.

Clinical and Radiographic Features

Chondromyxoid fibromas exhibit a predilection for young adults and most commonly involve the metaphyseal region of long bones, especially the proximal tibia and distal femur. Only about 2% of cases arise in the craniofacial bones, where possible sites of involvement include the sinonasal region, occipital bone, temporal bone, orbital region, and jaws. Depending on tumor location, symptoms may include sinonasal congestion, headache, hearing loss, tinnitus, vertigo, cranial nerve palsy, and visual disturbance.

Among reported jaw lesions, the average age at diagnosis is approximately 28 years (range 9–67 years), with a peak in the second and third decades. There is no significant sex predilection. The lesion occurs more often in the mandible than the maxilla. Initial signs and symptoms often include swelling and pain. However, some cases are asymptomatic and detected incidentally by radiographic examination.

Radiographically, chondromyxoid fibromas of the jaws typically appear as well-circumscribed radiolucencies with sclerotic margins. The lesion borders may appear scalloped, lobulated, or oval. The maximum diameter may range from 1.0 to 6.5 cm (average 3.3 cm). Cortical thinning or destruction (often with a "bite-like" hemispherical pattern) is common, but the periosteum usually remains intact. Internal trabeculation may be evident, and central radiopacities are noted in about 10% of cases.

Histopathologic Features

Microscopic examination shows lobules of spindle-shaped or stellate cells with abundant myxoid or chondroid intercellular substance. The lobules characteristically exhibit increased cellularity at the periphery. Between the lobules there is cellular fibrous tissue with spindle-shaped or round cells and varying numbers of multinucleated giant cells (Fig. 14.75). Coarse, irregular calcifications and residual bone spicules also may be present. Focal hyaline cartilage formation is rare. Occasionally, large pleomorphic cells may cause confusion with chondrosarcoma; however, chondrosarcoma typically shows hypercellularity throughout the tumor lobules and lacks a benign radiographic appearance.

Treatment and Prognosis

There is controversy regarding the most appropriate treatment for chondromyxoid fibroma. Many authors advocate conservative surgical removal, whereas others prefer wide resection. In general, relatively small lesions of the jaws are treated by local enucleation or curettage, but larger lesions often necessitate resection. In addition, some investigators have reported that filling the surgical defect with bone graft material following curettage results in a lower recurrence rate than curettage alone. Radiation therapy is contraindicated because of the risk for inducing malignant transformation or osteoradionecrosis.

Although the chondromyxoid fibroma is a benign tumor, approximately 25% of cases in the long bones recur after

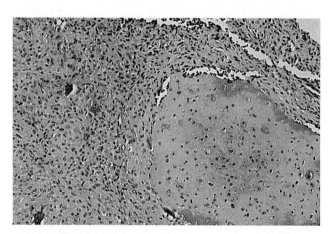

• **Fig. 14.75 Chondromyxoid Fibroma.** Myxoid connective tissue with scattered giant cells and foci of cartilaginous differentiation.

curettage alone. Among reported jaw tumors, recurrence has been noted in less than 10% of cases.

◆ SYNOVIAL CHONDROMATOSIS (SYNOVIAL CHONDROMETAPLASIA; SYNOVIAL OSTEOCHONDROMATOSIS)

Synovial chondromatosis is a rare, benign arthropathy characterized by development of cartilaginous nodules within the synovial membrane. The etiopathogenesis is poorly understood. Traditionally, synovial chondromatosis has been regarded as a reactive, metaplastic process. However, recent studies demonstrating *FN1* (fibronectin 1) and/or *ACVRA2* (activin receptor 2A) gene rearrangement in more than half of examined cases suggest that it may represent a true, benign neoplasm. Examples may be subclassified as *primary synovial chondromatosis* (i.e., cases with no identifiable etiologic factors) or *secondary synovial chondromatosis* (i.e., cases associated with trauma, joint overuse, inflammatory joint disease, or non-inflammatory arthropathy).

The condition typically proceeds through three stages. In the first stage, cartilaginous or osteocartilaginous nodules develop in the synovial lining. Subsequently, these nodules begin to detach, with some lying free in the joint space and others remaining in the synovial membrane. In the final stage, the nodules are found only in the joint space. The detached particles are called **loose bodies** (or "joint mice").

Clinical and Radiographic Features

The disease most commonly affects large joints, such as the knee, elbow, hip, and shoulder. Temporomandibular joint (TMJ) involvement is uncommon, although in recent years there has been an increase in reported cases, possibly because of improved imaging techniques and increased disease awareness.

Synovial chondromatosis of the TMJ occurs over a broad age range (12–82 years), with a mean age at diagnosis of approximately 40–50 years. In contrast to the findings in other joints, there is a predilection for females. The clinical presentation is nonspecific and, thus, delay in diagnosis is common. Typical findings include periarticular swelling, pain, crepitus, limited mouth opening, and deviation of the mandible from the midline. Headache, sensory disturbances, and facial nerve paralysis are infrequent. In rare instances, the disease may produce no symptoms.

The process usually is confined to a single joint. However, bilateral involvement and extra-articular extension (e.g., TMJ lesions with erosion of the condylar head, skull base, or intracranial structures) have been reported in a few cases. Within the TMJ, the disease primarily involves the superior compartment, although involvement of the inferior compartment also is possible.

Radiographically, the loose bodies in the joint may appear as round to irregular, radiopaque structures of variable size (Fig. 14.76). Other findings may include

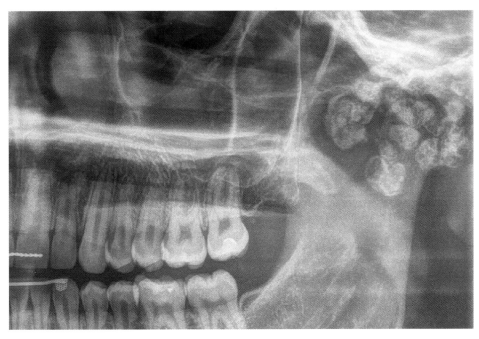

• **Fig. 14.76 Synovial Chondromatosis.** Computed tomography (CT) scan showing opacities of variable size within the temporomandibular joint (TMJ) region. (Courtesy of Dr. Ankur Johri.)

irregularity of the joint surface, widening of the joint space, and sclerosis or hyperostosis of the glenoid fossa or condyle. Similar features, however, may be seen in other degenerative joint diseases. Likewise, failure to detect loose bodies on imaging studies does not preclude a diagnosis of synovial chondromatosis. CT and magnetic resonance imaging (MRI) are more sensitive than plain radiography for demonstrating many of the characteristic features of synovial chondromatosis.

Histopathologic Features

Nodules of hyaline cartilage are present within the synovium and lie loose in the joint space. There may be anywhere from 1 to more than 200 loose bodies. The cartilaginous nodules often become calcified or ossified. Particularly in primary lesions, the chondrocytes may appear atypical with enlarged, hyperchromatic nuclei and binucleation (Fig. 14.77). However, correlation with the clinical and radiographic findings may aid in distinguishing synovial chondromatosis from chondrosarcoma.

Treatment and Prognosis

Synovial chondromatosis of the TMJ typically is treated by partial or complete synovectomy and removal of all loose bodies, at times combined with meniscectomy. Condylectomy is reserved for unusual cases with severe condylar destruction. Surgery is performed most commonly via open arthrotomy, although arthroscopy or arthrocentesis may be used for biopsy and, in select cases, for treatment. A wider approach is typically necessary for rare cases with extensive extra-articular involvement.

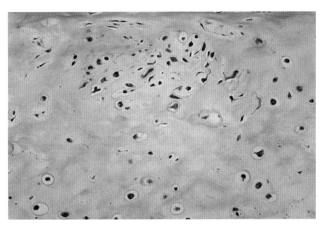

• **Fig. 14.77 Synovial Chondromatosis.** Photomicrograph from one of many nodules removed at the time of synovectomy. The cartilage shows some degree of atypia, and in a different clinical setting this histopathology could be interpreted to represent a low-grade chondrosarcoma.

The prognosis is good, with an overall low frequency of recurrence after surgical excision. However, some investigators have noted more aggressive behavior and a higher recurrence rate among primary lesions compared to secondary lesions. Thus periodic follow-up examinations would appear to be prudent. Malignant transformation of synovial chondromatosis of the TMJ is extremely rare.

◆ DESMOPLASTIC FIBROMA

The **desmoplastic fibroma** of bone is a benign, locally aggressive, fibroblastic neoplasm that comprises less than 1% of primary bone tumors. Clinicopathologic and ultrastructural findings suggest that this tumor represents the osseous counterpart of soft tissue fibromatosis (desmoid tumor) (see page 523). Thus far, however, there are only limited genetic studies of desmoplastic fibromas of bone for identification of *CTTNB1* and *APC* mutations; these genes are involved in the Wnt/beta-catenin pathway and have been implicated in the pathogenesis of soft tissue fibromatosis. In addition, immunohistochemical studies for nuclear expression of beta-catenin in desmoplastic fibromas have yielded variable results. In a few cases, desmoplastic fibroma-like lesions of the jaws have been reported in association with tuberous sclerosis.

Clinical and Radiographic Features

Most desmoplastic fibromas of bone arise in patients younger than 30 years old. The most common locations are the mandible, femur, pelvis, tibia, and radius.

Among jaw lesions reported in the English literature, the age range is 6 months to 70 years, with a mean of approximately 14 years. There is no significant sex predilection. More than 80% of cases affect the mandible—most often the posterior body, the angle, and the ramus. Most patients exhibit a painless swelling with slow to rapid growth, although pain has been reported in some examples. Limited opening, malocclusion, tooth mobility, tooth displacement, root resorption, delayed tooth eruption, temporomandibular joint dysfunction, pathologic fracture, proptosis, nasal obstruction, concurrent infection, and dysesthesia also are possible.

Radiographically, the lesion appears as a multilocular or unilocular radiolucency with well- or ill-defined margins (Fig. 14.78). The bone is expanded, and the cortex is thinned; cortical reaction mimicking the appearance of an osteosarcoma is rare. Erosion through the cortex and extension into soft tissue may be evident. In such cases, it may be difficult to determine whether the lesion is a desmoplastic fibroma of bone with soft tissue extension or a soft tissue fibromatosis with extension into bone.

Histopathologic Findings

The tumor is composed of small, elongated fibroblasts and abundant collagen fibers (Fig. 14.79). The degree of cellularity may vary within a given lesion, and the cellular areas may show plump fibroblasts. However, the fibroblasts are not atypical, and mitoses are absent or sparse. Bone spicules may be present at the interface between the tumor and adjacent bone but are never an integral part of the lesion. This reactive bone at the periphery may be mistaken for osteoid production, which may lead to a misdiagnosis of a benign fibro-osseous lesion or low-grade osteosarcoma. Therefore, diagnostic biopsies should be sampled generously from the center rather than the periphery of the lesion. Immunohistochemistry often shows reactivity among the tumor cells for smooth muscle actin and muscle specific actin, and nuclear expression of beta catenin is variable. The Ki-67 proliferation index is less than 5%.

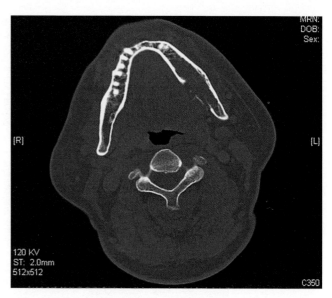

• **Fig. 14.78 Desmoplastic Fibroma.** Ill-defined, destructive radiolucency of the left mandible.

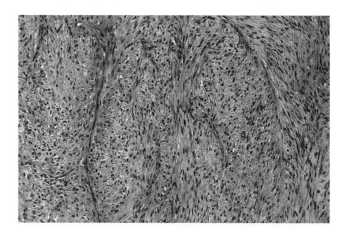

• **Fig. 14.79 Desmoplastic Fibroma.** The tumor consists of a cellular proliferation of fibroblasts arranged in interlacing fascicles.

Treatment and Prognosis

Although the desmoplastic fibroma is a benign tumor, it often behaves in a locally aggressive fashion, with extensive bone destruction and soft tissue extension; thus, radical surgery may be required to control the disease. Most cases are treated by resection, although enucleation or curettage may be adequate for localized lesions without cortical perforation or soft tissue extension. Anecdotal reports of patients treated with chemotherapy (e.g., vincristine, doxorubicin, dacarazine, actinomycin D, cyclophosphamide) have noted variable results.

The recurrence rate is approximately 5% following resection, 30% following enucleation, and as high as 70% following curettage. Given the potential for recurrence, patients should be monitored postoperatively for at least 3 years. The long-term prognosis is good, but there may be considerable morbidity. Malignant transformation is rare.

It may be very difficult to distinguish desmoplastic fibroma of bone from well-differentiated fibrosarcoma. Some authorities suggest that all desmoplastic fibromas of bone be considered potentially malignant.

◆ OSTEOSARCOMA (OSTEOGENIC SARCOMA)

Osteosarcoma is a malignancy characterized by the production of osteoid or immature bone. Excluding hematopoietic neoplasms, osteosarcoma is the most common malignancy to originate within bone. In the United States, approximately 1000 new cases are diagnosed per year, with about half occurring in children and adolescents.

The etiopathogenesis of osteosarcoma is not completely understood. The tumor generally is thought to originate from mesenchymal stem cells or committed osteoblast precursors. A strong association with the adolescent growth spurt and the metaphyses of long bones suggests that rapid bone growth and hormonal factors may play a role. Additional risk factors include radiation exposure, alkylating agents, Paget disease of bone (see page 628), and certain rare heritable syndromes (e.g., Li-Fraumeni syndrome, hereditary retinoblastoma, Rothmund-Thompson syndrome, Bloom syndrome, Werner syndrome, Diamond-Blackfan anemia). Studies have demonstrated a complex genetic profile in most osteosarcomas, with alterations detected in *TP53, RB1, MDM2, CDKN2A, ATRX, DLG2,* and other genes. In addition, some investigators have detected co-amplification of *RASAL1* and *MDM2* in a subtype of high-grade mandibular ostesarcomas; this finding has been noted in the juvenile ossifying fibroma (see page 653) as well.

Osteosarcomas may be classified as *central* (arising within the medullary cavity), *surface* (arising in the juxtacortical region), or, vary rarely, *extraskeletal* (arising within soft tissue) (Table 14.5). The vast majority of cases are central. Surface osteosarcomas are discussed in the next section (see page 668). In addition, some authors regard gnathic osteosarcomas as a separate entity, because these lesions exhibit somewhat distinctive clinical features and biologic behavior.

Clinical and Radiographic Features

Extragnathic osteosarcoma demonstrates a bimodal age distribution, with a major peak during adolescence and a lesser peak among adults older than 60 years. The initial peak occurs during the period of greatest bone growth, with most cases arising in the distal femoral and proximal tibial metaphyses. Among tumors involving the extremities, there is a slight male predilection. In older patients, osteosarcoma often is attributed to Paget disease of bone or previous irradiation, and the axial skeleton and flat bones are involved most frequently. In both the axial and appendicular skeleton, the age-adjusted incidence for osteosarcoma in the United States is somewhat greater among blacks compared to Hispanics and whites.

TABLE 14.5	Osteosarcoma Types	
Type		**Grade**
Central (intramedullary)	Conventional: • Osteoblastic • Chondroblastic • Fibroblastic	High
	Other rare variants (e.g., telangiectatic, small cell, epithelioid, giant cell-rich, osteoblastoma-like, and chondroblastoma-like)	High
	Low-grade central	Low
Surface (juxtacortical)	Parosteal	Low
	Periosteal	Intermediate
	High-grade surface	High
Extraskeletal		Low to high

About 6% of all osteosarcomas arise in the jaws. Jaw lesions exhibit no significant gender predilection and occur over a broad age range, with a peak in the third through fifth decades of life. The mean age is approximately 35–41 years, which is about 2 decades older than the mean age for osteosarcomas of the long bones.

Most studies report either a fairly even distribution between the mandible and maxilla or a mandibular predilection. Mandibular tumors arise most frequently in the body, followed by the angle, symphysis, and ramus. Maxillary lesions develop more often in the inferior portion (alveolar ridge, sinus floor, and/or palate) than the superior aspect (zygoma and orbital rim).

Swelling and pain are the most common clinical findings (Figs. 14.80 and 14.81). Tooth mobility, paresthesia, and nasal obstruction (in the case of maxillary tumors) also may be noted. Some patients report symptoms for relatively long periods before diagnosis, which suggests that some osteosarcomas of the jaws grow rather slowly.

Radiographic examination may show a radiopaque, mixed radiolucent-radiopaque, or entirely radiolucent lesion with ill-defined borders (Figs. 14.80, *B,* 14.81, *B,* and 14.82). Cortical destruction, cortical expansion, and a periosteal reaction also may be evident. The latter may appear as a "classic" sunburst pattern (present in about 25% of jaw osteosarcomas) or a triangular elevation of the periosteum (*Codman triangle*). Occasionally, the adjacent teeth exhibit "spiking" root resorption (with tapered narrowing of the root). Symmetrical widening of the periodontal ligament space (*Garrington sign*) (Fig. 14.83) may be an important clue for diagnosis of early osteosarcoma, although this feature also

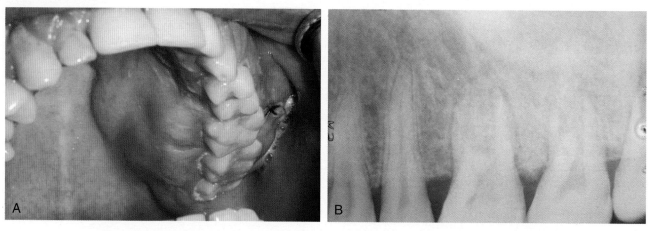

• **Fig. 14.80 Osteosarcoma. A,** This patient shows a firm, painful swelling of the left maxilla of recent onset. **B,** The periapical radiograph shows a dense sclerotic change in the bone pattern. (Courtesy of Dr. Len Morrow.)

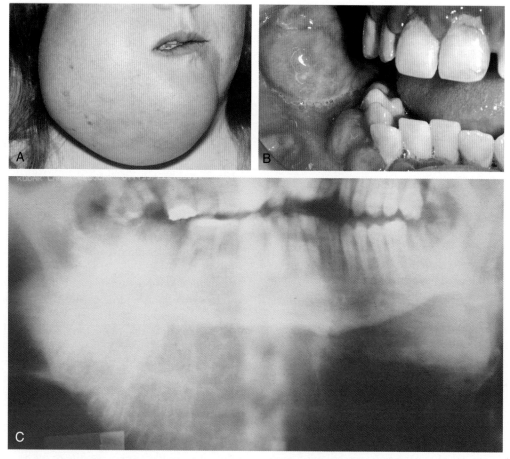

• **Fig. 14.81 Osteosarcoma. A,** This massive tumor had been present for many months before the patient sought treatment. **B,** Intraoral photograph of the tumor mass. **C,** The panoramic radiograph shows a "sunburst" pattern of trabeculation.

may be seen in other malignancies. At times an extensive osteosarcoma may show only subtle variation in the trabecular pattern. Plain radiography and CT often are used for initial evaluation. However, MRI is superior for assessment of primary tumor extent.

Histopathologic Features

Although osteosarcomas exhibit considerable histopathologic variation, the essential microscopic criterion is direct production of osteoid by malignant mesenchymal cells (Fig. 14.84). In addition to osteoid, the tumor cells may

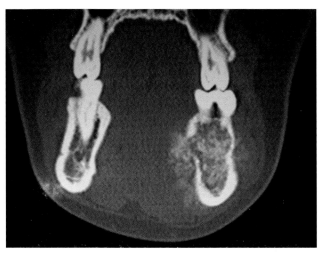

• **Fig. 14.82 Osteosarcoma.** Computed tomography (CT) scan showing a mottled radiopacity of the mandible with cortical destruction and a focal "sunburst" periosteal reaction. (Courtesy of Dr. Steve Anderson.)

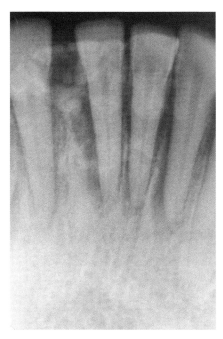

• **Fig. 14.83 Osteosarcoma.** This 26-year-old woman had a 6-cm painful tumor of the anterior mandible. The periapical radiograph shows widening of the periodontal ligament spaces and a mottled radiopacity superimposed on the teeth. (Courtesy of Dr. Charles Ferguson.)

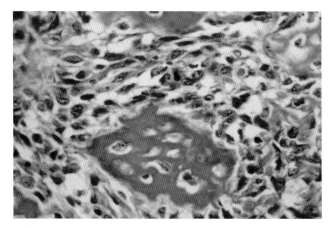

• **Fig. 14.84 Osteosarcoma.** Anaplastic tumor cells forming cellular disorganized bone.

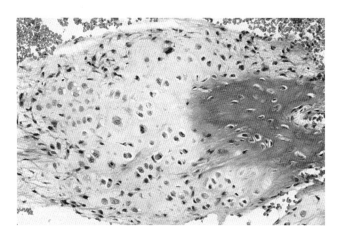

• **Fig. 14.85 Osteosarcoma.** This tumor produced a combination of malignant cartilage and bone.

produce chondroid and fibrous connective tissue. Histopathologic findings may range from relatively uniform, round or spindle-shaped cells in low-grade tumors to markedly pleomorphic cells with bizarre nuclear and cytoplasmic shapes in high-grade tumors. The amount of matrix produced by the tumor may vary considerably. In some instances, osteoid production may be very minimal and difficult to demonstrate.

Greater than 90% of ostesarcomas are classified as the conventional type. Depending on whether there is a predominance of osteoid, cartilage, or collagen produced, such tumors can be subclassified as osteoblastic, chondroblastic, or fibroblastic. Less common variants are listed in Table 14.5.

Chondroblastic osteosarcomas constitute a substantial proportion of all osteosarcomas of the jaws. Some examples may be composed almost entirely of malignant cartilage growing in lobules with only small foci of direct osteoid production by tumor cells (Fig. 14.85). Such lesions, however, should be classified as osteosarcomas rather than chondrosarcomas. Some investigators have reported that chondroblastic osteosarcomas lack isocitrate dehydrogenase 1 *(IDH1)* gene and isocitrate dehydrogenase 2 *(IDH2)* gene mutations, whereas such mutations are frequent among chondrosarcomas and chondromas.

Low-grade osteosarcomas show minimal cellular atypia and may be difficult to differentiate from benign bone lesions, such as fibrous dysplasia or ossifying fibroma. Correlation with imaging studies is essential for accurate diagnosis. Immunohistochemical expression of MDM2 and CDK4 or demonstration of *MDM2* amplification by fluorescence *in situ* hybridization (FISH) also may help to distinguish low-grade osteosarcoma from benign fibro-osseous lesions and other benign bone tumors.

Treatment and Prognosis

The treatment of choice for osteosarcoma of the jaws is wide surgical resection. The additional use of chemotherapy and/or radiotherapy for gnathic osteosarcomas is controversial but may be considered in some cases (e.g., tumors of questionable resectability, surgical margins positive for tumor, and recurrent tumors). For high-grade osteosarcomas of the long bones, management usually consists of neoadjuvant (preoperative) chemotherapy followed by radical surgery and adjuvant (postoperative) chemotherapy. Among patients with localized disease at diagnosis, such treatment has resulted in 5-year survival rates of approximately 60%–80%, compared to less than 20% with surgery alone. However, for patients with gnathic osteosarcomas, such protocols have yielded variable outcomes, and further studies are needed.

The most important prognostic factor is the ability to achieve initial complete surgical removal. Compared to mandibular lesions, maxillary lesions often are more difficult to resect and exhibit a worse prognosis. Additional adverse factors include prior radiation exposure, advanced age, and underlying Paget disease of bone. Interestingly, some investigators have reported a better prognosis for osteosarcoma of the jaws than osteosarcoma of the long bones. This observation may be related to a tendency for gnathic osteosarcomas to exhibit a low rate of metastasis despite often high-grade histopathologic features. However, other studies have shown no significant survival advantage among patients with gnathic osteosarcoma.

For patients with osteosarcoma of the jaws, death results more often from uncontrolled local disease than from distant metastases. Most deaths from uncontrolled local disease occur within 2 years of initial treatment. Metastases most often affect the lungs. According to Surveillance, Epidemiology, and End Results (SEER) data in the United States, the 5-year overall and disease-specific survival rates for osteosarcoma of the jaws from 1973 to 2011 were approximately 53% and 62%, respectively. However, some centers have reported greater than 80% long-term survival.

SURFACE (JUXTACORTICAL) OSTEOSARCOMAS

Although most osteosarcomas arise within the medullary cavity of bone, some cases originate in the periosteal or cortical region with little or no medullary involvement. Such surface lesions typically involve the long bones, although gnathic cases rarely have been reported. Surface osteosarcoma includes the following subtypes:

• Parosteal osteosarcoma
• Periosteal osteosarcoma
• High-grade surface osteosarcoma

Parosteal osteosarcoma appears as a lobulated, exophytic nodule attached to the cortex by a short, broad stalk

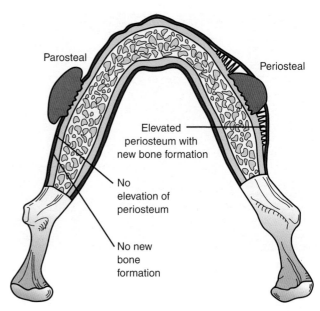

• **Fig. 14.86 Peripheral (Juxtacortical) Osteosarcoma.** Illustration comparing different types of peripheral osteosarcoma. Parosteal osteosarcoma presents as a lobulated nodule without a peripheral periosteal reaction. Periosteal osteosarcoma presents as a sessile mass associated with significant periosteal new bone formation.

(Fig. 14.86). There is no elevation of the periosteum and no peripheral periosteal reaction. Radiographs may demonstrate a radiolucent line ("string sign") that corresponds to the periosteum between the sclerotic tumor and the underlying cortex. Histopathologic examination shows a spindle cell fibroblast-like proliferation with well-developed, elongated bony trabeculae, often arranged in a parallel streaming or "pulled steel wool" pattern. A cartilaginous component also may be evident in some examples. Amplification of *CDK4* and *MDM2* has been reported in about 79% of cases. Parosteal osteosarcomas are low-grade tumors, with a low risk for recurrence and metastasis following wide excision. However, long-standing or inadequately excised tumors may become higher grade osteosarcomas.

Periosteal osteosarcoma appears as a sessile lesion that arises between the cortex and the inner (or cambium) layer of the periosteum (see Fig. 14.86). Thus, a periosteal reaction often is evident radiographically. The tumor frequently perforates the periosteum and extends into the surrounding soft tissue. Histopathologically, the tumor demonstrates primitive sarcomatous cells with chondroblastic differentiation. Close inspection reveals focal osteoid or immature bone formation. Treatment typically consists of wide resection alone or combined with chemotherapy. Periosteal osteosarcoma is an intermediate-grade tumor, with a prognosis better than conventional intramedullary osteosarcoma but worse than parosteal osteosarcoma.

High-grade surface osteosarcoma is extremely rare. This variant is similar to conventional intramedullary osteosarcoma in terms of microscopic features and biologic behavior.

POST-IRRADIATION BONE SARCOMA

Sarcoma arising in bone previously subjected to radiation therapy is an uncommon but well-recognized phenomenon. Bone sarcomas have been reported to develop 3–55 years after radiation exposure, with a mean latency period of about 4–17 years. Studies estimate that 0.03%–0.2% of irradiated patients develop post-irradiation bone or soft tissue sarcomas. Within the head and neck region, nasopharyngeal cancer represents the most common primary tumor type associated with post-irradiation sarcoma development, and the most frequent locations for such sarcomas include the sinonasal region and mandible.

Some studies indicate that the risk for post-irradiation bone sarcomas increases with cumulative radiation dose. Reported mean and median radiation doses vary from 43 to 64 Gy. However, the radiation dose applied to the primary tumor may be greater than the dose delivered to the area where a sarcoma later arises. Thus, medium- to low-dose radiation may be sufficient and, possibly, even more effective than high-dose radiation for inducing sarcoma development.

Osteosarcoma is the most common post-irradiation bone sarcoma type, accounting for 49%–85% of cases. Other reported types include undifferentiated pleomorphic sarcoma (malignant fibrous histiocytoma), fibrosarcoma, and chondrosarcoma. The lesions tend to be poorly differentiated, and the prognosis is generally poor. According to a systematic review of radiation-induced sarcomas of the head and neck, about 41% of patients died of disease after a mean interval of 14 months. Another review limited to radiation-induced sarcomas of the oral cavity reported a 5-year survival rate of 15%.

◆ CHONDROSARCOMA

Chondrosarcoma is a malignant neoplasm in which the tumor cells form cartilage but not bone. Chondrosarcoma is about half as common as osteosarcoma and twice as common as Ewing sarcoma. Chondrosarcomas comprise about 11% of all primary malignant bone tumors but involve the jaws only rarely. Approximately 1%–12% of all chondrosarcomas arise in the head and neck, and such lesions comprise only 0.1% of all head and neck malignancies.

Chondrosarcoma may develop *de novo (primary chondrosarcoma)* or from a preexisting benign cartilaginous tumor *(secondary chondrosarcoma)*. The histogenesis is controversial; investigators have hypothesized that the tumor may originate from chondrocytes, embryonal chondroid, or pluripotential mesenchymal stem cells. Interestingly, there is an increased risk for chondrosarcoma among patients with Ollier disease and Maffucci syndrome (see page 661). These forms of chondromatosis are associated with somatic mutations in the isocitrate dehydrogenase 1 *(IDH1)* gene and isocitrate dehydrogenase 2 *(IDH2)* gene; likewise, chondromas and chondrosarcomas of bone frequently exhibit mutations in these genes.

Clinical and Radiographic Findings

Although chondrosarcoma develops over a broad age range, most affected patients are older. In the United States, the median age at diagnosis is approximately 53 years, and the male-to-female ratio is 1.3:1. The most frequently involved sites are the ilium, femur, and humerus.

Gnathic chondrosarcomas exhibit a predilection for the anterior maxilla. In contrast, mandibular tumors tend to favor the posterior region. Other possible sites of involvement in the head and neck include the paranasal sinuses, nasal septum, skull base, and cervical vertebrae. Most head and neck chondrosarcomas develop within the bones or joints, but approximately one-third of cases originate in either laryngotracheal cartilage or soft tissue. According to a systematic review of the literature, chondrosarcomas of the jaws occur over a broad age range (2–82 years), with a peak in the third decade and a mean age at diagnosis of approximately 33 years. The male-to-female ratio is approximately 1.2:1. At presentation, the most commonly reported signs or symptoms include swelling, pain, and facial asymmetry. Separation or loosening of teeth also is possible. Infrequent findings include regional lymphadenopathy and paresthesia. Lesions involving the temporomandibular joint can cause trismus. Patients with maxillary tumors may develop nasal obstruction, congestion, epistaxis, photophobia, or visual loss as well.

Radiographically, chondrosarcoma usually appears as an ill-defined radiolucency with radiopaque foci (Fig. 14.87). These radiopaque foci correspond to calcification or ossification of the cartilage matrix. Some cases show extensive calcification and primarily appear radiopaque. Infrequently, there is lobular growth with minimal or no calcification; such lesions may appear as multilocular radiolucencies that mimic a benign process. Penetration of the cortex can result in a sunburst pattern similar to that seen in some osteosarcomas. Jaw tumors may cause root resorption or symmetrical widening of the periodontal ligament space of adjacent teeth.

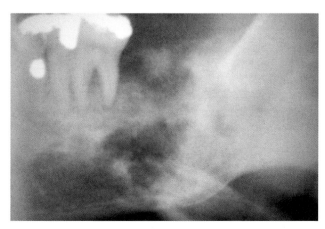

• **Fig. 14.87 Chondrosarcoma.** Ill-defined radiolucent lesion of posterior mandible containing radiopaque foci. (Courtesy of Dr. Ben B. Henry.)

Chondrosarcomas tend to be highly infiltrative. Although plain radiography typically is used for initial evaluation, MRI is the best method for assessing tumor extent. In addition, CT may help to demonstrate calcifications.

Histopathologic Features

Chondrosarcomas are composed of cartilage showing varying degrees of maturation and cellularity. In most cases, lacunar formation within the chondroid matrix is evident, although this feature may be scarce in poorly differentiated tumors. The tumor often shows a lobular growth pattern. The central areas of the lobules demonstrate the greatest degree of maturation, whereas the peripheral areas tend to exhibit immature cartilage and mesenchymal tissue consisting of round or spindle-shaped cells. Calcification or ossification may occur within the chondroid matrix. Neoplastic cartilage may be replaced by bone in a manner similar to normal endochondral ossification. Distinction between metaplastic bone formation and malignant osteoid production is important for differentiating chondrosarcoma from chondroblastic osteosarcoma.

Chondrosarcomas may be assigned a histopathologic grade of I through III. Low-grade tumors closely resemble normal cartilage and may be very difficult to distinguish from chondromas or synovial chondromatosis. With increasing tumor grade, there is a decreased amount of cartilaginous matrix but increased cellularity, nuclear size, nuclear pleomorphism, binucleated or multinucleated chondrocytes, cellular spindling, mitotic activity, and necrosis. Most chondrosarcomas of the jaws are grade I or II (Fig. 14.88). In general, chondrosarcomas of the head and neck tend to exhibit a lower grade and often are diagnosed at an earlier stage compared to those arising in other regions.

Variants

Uncommon microscopic variants of chondrosarcoma include the following:

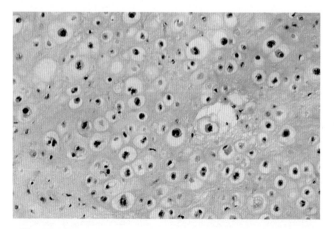

• **Fig. 14.88 Chondrosarcoma.** This grade II chondrosarcoma shows a variation in size of chondrocyte nuclei. Occasional double nuclei are seen in the lacunae.

- **Clear cell chondrosarcoma** is a low-grade variant exhibiting cells with abundant clear cytoplasm. This variant may be difficult to differentiate from metastatic clear cell carcinoma.
- **Dedifferentiated chondrosarcoma** is a high-grade variant that shows an admixture of well-differentiated chondrosarcoma and a high-grade sarcoma. This variant is exceedingly rare in the jaws.
- **Myxoid chondrosarcoma** classically is described as a soft tissue tumor, although intraosseous lesions are possible. This variant is characterized by a proliferation of cells with clear, vacuolated, or eosinophilic cytoplasm within a background of mucoid material.
- **Mesenchymal chondrosarcoma** is discussed in the next section.

Treatment and Prognosis

Surgical resection is the mainstay of treatment for chondrosarcoma. Curettage followed by cryosurgery may be an alternative for grade I chondrosarcomas confined within bone, although this technique mainly is used for long bone tumors. Radiation and chemotherapy are less effective for chondrosarcoma than osteosarcoma. However, radiation may be considered for unresectable disease. In addition, for high-grade, clear cell, or extracompartmental (i.e., extending beyond bone) chondrosarcomas, radiation therapy may be administered either preoperatively for tumors deemed borderline resectable or postoperatively for residual disease. Systemic agents typically are reserved for select cases of chondrosarcoma (e.g., dasatinib or pazopanib for widespread metastasis, ivosidenib for *IDH1*-mutant conventional/dedifferentiated tumors).

Major prognostic factors for chondrosarcoma include clinical stage, histopathologic grade, and adequacy of resection. In the United States, the overall relative 5-year survival rate is approximately 78%. The relative 5-year survival rates for patients with localized disease, regional metastasis, and distant metastasis are 91%, 75%, and 22%, respectively. Because recurrence often is a late sequela, patients must be followed for their lifetime.

Head and neck chondrosarcomas typically are locally aggressive with low metastatic potential. Metastasis mainly is seen among rare high-grade tumors. Nevertheless, death may occur by direct extension into vital structures. In particular, maxillary tumors often are large at diagnosis, occur adjacent to the central nervous system, and are difficult to resect; therefore, they are difficult to cure. According to Surveillance, Epidemiology, and End Results (SEER) registry data, 5-year disease-specific and overall survival rates for head and neck chondrosarcomas are 90% and 81%, respectively.

MESENCHYMAL CHONDROSARCOMA

Mesenchymal chondrosarcoma is an aggressive variant of chondrosarcoma with a distinctive biphasic histopathologic pattern. It is considered high-grade based on clinical behavior rather than histopathologic features. This variant represents only about 2%–9% of all chondrosarcomas. *HEY1-NCOA2* fusion has been identified in approximately 90% of cases; *IRF2BP2-CDX1* fusion also is possible. Unlike conventional chondrosarcomas, mesenchymal chondrosarcomas do not harbor *IDH1* mutations.

Clinical and Radiographic Features

In contrast to other chondrosarcoma types, the mesenchymal variant is unusual in that it most frequently affects individuals in the second and third decades of life and most often arises in the jaws (22%–27% of cases). Other commonly affected sites are the ribs, shoulder, pelvic girdle, and vertebrae. In addition, approximately 30%–60% of cases arise in soft tissue rather than bone.

Swelling and pain, often of fairly short duration, are the most common symptoms. Radiographically, the tumor typically appears as an ill-defined radiolucency with or without stippled calcification (Fig. 14.89). However, some examples may appear predominantly radiopaque, particularly within the maxilla.

Histopathologic Features

Microscopic examination shows two distinct elements: well-differentiated cartilaginous nodules and sheets of small, undifferentiated, spindled or round cells (Fig. 14.90). The degree of cellularity and atypia within the cartilaginous component may vary from that of a benign chondroma to a low-grade chondrosarcoma. The undifferentiated component may exhibit a branching vascular pattern that mimics solitary fibrous tumor ("hemangiopericytoma"). In addition, the undifferentiated component may appear similar to rhabdomyosarcoma, Ewing sarcoma, lymphoma, or metastatic small cell carcinoma. The undifferentiated cells may exhibit immunohistochemical expression of CD99, SOX9, and NKX3.1, whereas the cartilaginous component expresses S-100 protein.

Treatment and Prognosis

Surgical excision with wide margins is the mainstay of therapy. Some studies have suggested that supplemental radiation therapy and/or chemotherapy may be beneficial, although further investigation is needed. Some individuals are treated with regimens similar to those used for patients with Ewing sarcoma (see next section). Close long-term follow-up is recommended, because local recurrence and metastasis are common and may be discovered more than 20 years after initial therapy. Metastasis most frequently develops in the lungs. According to Surveillance, Epidemiology, and End Results (SEER) registry data, 5- and 10-year overall survival rates are 51% and 43%, respectively; cases arising in the head and neck exhibit better survival compared to those developing in other sites (median survival 95.7 months versus 67.4 months, respectively).

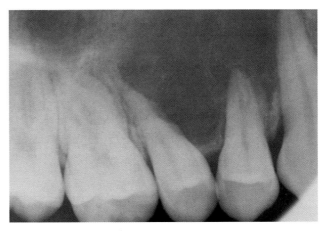

• **Fig. 14.89 Mesenchymal Chondrosarcoma.** Periapical radiograph showing an ill-defined radiolucency with associated root resorption. (Courtesy of Dr. Michael Robinson.)

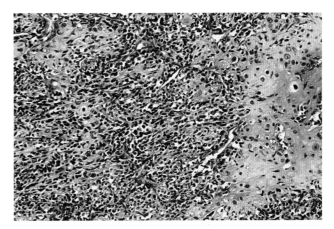

• **Fig. 14.90 Mesenchymal Chondrosarcoma.** Medium-power photomicrograph showing sheets of small basophilic cells with focal areas of cartilaginous differentiation *(right)*.

◆ EWING SARCOMA

Ewing sarcoma is a malignant neoplasm composed of small, undifferentiated round cells. In the United States, the annual incidence is approximately 1 per million population. Although rare, Ewing sarcoma is the second most common primary malignant bone tumor in pediatric patients after osteosarcoma. The term *Ewing sarcoma* (or the *Ewing sarcoma family of tumors*) includes classical Ewing sarcoma of bone, extraosseous Ewing sarcoma, primitive neuroectodermal tumor (Ewing sarcoma with neuronal differentiation), and Askin tumor (small round cell tumor of the chest wall). Based on shared histologic, immunohistochemical, and genetic characteristics, authorities currently consider these entities to represent the same tumor type.

The histogenesis of Ewing sarcoma is unknown. Investigators previously have hypothesized that the tumor originates from the neural crest. However, current evidence favors an origin from mesenchymal stem cells with potential for limited neural differentiation. At the molecular level, Ewing sarcoma is defined by balanced chromosomal translocations that result in fusion of the RNA-binding protein

EWS (or the closely related FUS protein) with ETS family transcription factors (e.g., FLI1, ERG, ETV1, ETV4, and FEV). In particular, more than 85% of cases demonstrate the translocation t(11;22) (q24;q12), which encodes the EWS::FLI1 fusion protein.

Recent molecular studies have identified additional rare types of undifferentiated small round cell sarcomas of bone and soft tissue, including round cell sarcoma with *EWSR1–non-ETS* fusions, *CIC*-rearranged sarcoma, and sarcoma with *BCOR* genetic alterations. Such tumors formerly were considered subtypes of Ewing sarcoma (or "Ewing-like sarcoma") but currently are recognized as distinct entities.

Clinical and Radiographic Features

Most patients with Ewing sarcoma are adolescents, and the median age at diagnosis is 15 years. However, advances in molecular diagnosis have led to an increase in the number of cases diagnosed in young adults. There is a slight male predominance, and the majority of patients are white. Osseous lesions most frequently involve the long bones, pelvis, and ribs. Only 1%–2% of cases arise in the gnathic or craniofacial bones. Primary extraosseous lesions are also possible but very rare.

The most common clinical findings are pain and swelling. Fever, leukocytosis, and an elevated erythrocyte sedimentation rate also may be present in advanced disease. The tumor often penetrates the cortex, resulting in a soft tissue mass overlying the affected area of the bone (Fig. 14.91). Jaw involvement is more common in the mandible than the maxilla and may result in tooth displacement, tooth mobility, root resorption, and paresthesia. Cervical lymphadenopathy may be evident as well. The nonspecific clinicoradiographic presentation may lead to a misdiagnosis of odontogenic infection or osteomyelitis.

Radiographically, most osseous lesions appear as ill-defined radiolucencies, although a mixed radiolucent and radiopaque pattern also is possible. Cortical destruction or expansion may or may not be present. The characteristic "onionskin" periosteal reaction, commonly observed in

Ewing sarcoma of long bones, seldom is seen in jaw lesions. Although plain radiography often is used for initial evaluation, CT and MRI are superior for assessing lesion extent.

Histopathologic Features

Ewing sarcoma typically is composed of broad sheets of small, monotonous, round cells with well-delineated nuclear outlines and ill-defined cellular borders (Fig. 14.92). In some cases, variable-sized nests of tumor cells are separated by fibrovascular septa, creating a lobular pattern. Extensive necrosis and hemorrhage are common. Cytoplasmic clearing and rosette formation are variable findings.

Diagnosis may be difficult. Ewing sarcoma must be differentiated from other pediatric small round cell tumors, such as metastatic neuroblastoma, malignant lymphoma, small cell osteosarcoma, and alveolar rhabdomyosarcoma. Metastatic small cell carcinoma also may be considered in the differential diagnosis of a suspected Ewing sarcoma in an older patient.

Ewing sarcomas typically exhibit cytoplasmic periodic acid-Schiff (PAS)-positive glycogen granules. Membranous reactivity for CD99 (MIC2) and nuclear reactivity for NKX2.2 usually can be demonstrated by immunohistochemistry. In addition, immunohistochemical expression of FLI1 or ERG may be noted in cases harboring *EWSR1::FLI1* or *EWSR1::ERG* mutations, respectively. Identification of characteristic chromosomal translocations by reverse transcription polymerase chain reaction (RT-PCR) or fluorescence *in situ* hybridization (FISH) may aid in confirming the diagnosis.

Treatment and Prognosis

Treatment usually consists of multidrug chemotherapy with surgery and/or radiotherapy. Systemic chemotherapy typically is indicated, because seemingly localized disease often is associated with occult micrometastases.

With the development of modern multimodal therapy, the prognosis for patients with Ewing sarcoma has improved dramatically in recent decades. In the United States, overall

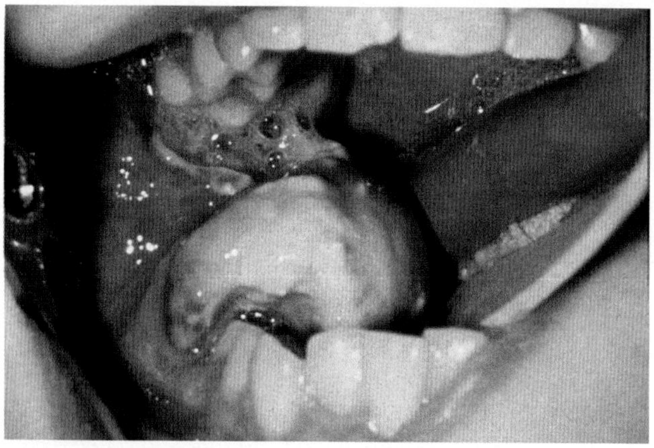

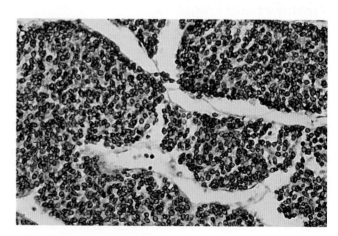

• **Fig. 14.91 Ewing Sarcoma.** A rapidly growing, ulcerated tumor of the right posterior mandible. (Courtesy of Dr. George Blozis.)

• **Fig. 14.92 Ewing Sarcoma.** Broad sheets of small round cells with well-defined nuclear outlines and ill-defined cytoplasmic borders.

5-year relative survival is approximately 61%, and 5-year survival rates for patients with localized disease, regional metastasis, and distant metastasis at presentation are approximately 81%, 67%, and 38%, respectively. The presence of metastasis is the most important prognostic factor, and metastasis is evident at initial diagnosis in about 25% of patients. The most common sites of metastasis are the lungs and bones; for reasons unknown, patients with extrapulmonary metastasis tend to fare worse than those with metastasis confined to the lungs. There is limited data regarding gnathic Ewing sarcoma, although lesions arising in the jaws appear to exhibit a more favorable prognosis compared to those arising in the long bones and pelvis.

◆ METASTATIC TUMORS TO THE JAWS

Metastatic carcinoma is the most common form of cancer involving bone. The most common primary sites for carcinomas that metastasize to bone are the breast, lung, thyroid, prostate, and kidney. The bones that most frequently exhibit metastasis include the vertebrae, ribs, pelvis, and skull.

Jaw metastasis is rare but may occur more often than generally appreciated. In an autopsy study of mandibles from patients with various extraoral primary carcinomas, microscopic examination revealed metastasis in 16% of cases, with most of these metastases found to be clinically, radiographically, and grossly undetectable. Metastatic spread of a carcinoma to the jaws usually occurs by the hematogenous route. Sarcomas arising in soft tissues or other bones metastasize to the jaws only very rarely.

Clinical and Radiographic Features

Jaw metastases have been reported over a broad age range but most often affect older adults; the mean age is approximately 43–52 years, with no significant gender bias. There is a marked predilection for the mandible, especially the molar region.

Clinical signs and symptoms of jaw metastasis may include pain, swelling, tooth mobility, trismus, and paresthesia. In particular, mandibular metastasis with involvement of the mental nerve may produce paresthesia in the lower lip and chin (**numb-chin syndrome**). The rarity of jaw metastases and the nonspecific clinical presentation may lead to a mistaken impression of an inflammatory process. Sometimes an osseous metastasis is discovered in a nonhealing extraction site from which a tooth was removed because of local pain or significant mobility. In other instances, the patient may be completely asymptomatic, and the lesion is discovered incidentally by radiographic examination.

Occasionally, diagnosis of a jaw metastasis is the first indication that the patient has a primary malignancy at some other anatomic site. Location of the occult primary tumor may be difficult and may require extensive evaluation.

Most radiographically evident jaw metastases appear as ill-defined or "moth-eaten" radiolucencies (Fig. 14.93). However, some examples—particularly metastatic prostate

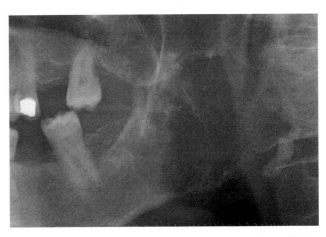

• **Fig. 14.93 Thyroid Carcinoma Metastatic to the Jaws.** Radiograph showing an ill-defined, destructive radiolucency with irregular borders at the angle of the mandible. (Courtesy of Dr. Terry Day.)

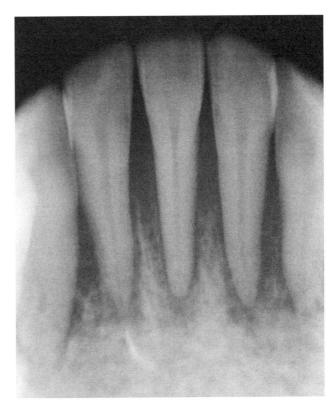

• **Fig. 14.94 Carcinoma Metastatic to the Jaws.** Periapical radiograph showing widening of the periodontal ligament spaces.

and breast carcinomas—may appear radiopaque or mixed radiolucent-radiopaque. *Osteolytic* (bone-resorbing) and/or *osteoblastic* (bone-forming) activity may result from various growth factors and other substances produced by tumor cells. Some lesions may mimic periapical inflammatory disease or periodontal disease. Cortical erosion, pathologic fracture, and widening of the periodontal ligament space may be noted as well (Fig. 14.94). Compared to plain radiography,

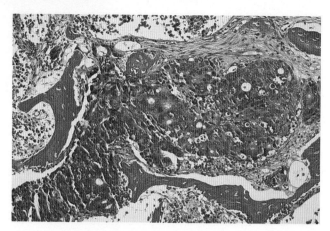

• **Fig. 14.95 Carcinoma Metastatic to the Jaws.** Islands of malignant cells can be seen filling the marrow spaces.

bone scintigraphy is more sensitive for detecting osseous metastases.

Histopathologic Features

The microscopic appearance of metastatic carcinoma in bone varies. In some instances, the metastasis exhibits well-differentiated features that suggest an origin from a specific site, such as the kidney, colon, or thyroid. More often, however, metastatic carcinomas are poorly differentiated, and the tumor origin is not readily apparent (Fig. 14.95). Poorly differentiated metastatic carcinoma may be difficult to differentiate from lymphoma, melanoma, or anaplastic sarcoma. In such cases, immunohistochemistry may aid in diagnosis. Definitive diagnosis requires correlation of laboratory studies with a thorough medical history, complete physical examination, and imaging studies.

Treatment and Prognosis

Although a solitary metastatic focus may be treated by excision or radiation therapy, jaw metastasis almost always is associated with widely disseminated disease. Management depends on the specific underlying tumor type and often is palliative in nature. Administration of bisphosphonates may help to slow progression of bone metastases, decrease bone pain, and reduce the risk for pathologic fracture. By definition, osseous metastasis constitutes stage IV disease. Accordingly, the prognosis for metastatic carcinoma to the jaws is poor, and most patients survive less than 1 year.

Bibliography

Osteogenesis Imperfecta
Binger T, Rücker M, Spitzer WJ: Dentofacial rehabilitation by osteo-distraction, augmentation and implantation despite osteogenesis imperfecta, *Int J Oral Maxillofac Surg* 35:559–562, 2006.

Forlino A, Marini JC: Osteogenesis imperfecta, *Lancet* 387: 1657–1671, 2016.

Dwan K, Phillipi CA, Steiner RD, et al.: Bisphosphonate therapy for osteogenesis imperfecta, *Cochrane Database Syst Rev* 10: CD005088, 2016.

López-Arcas JM, Chamorro M, Del Castillo JL, et al.: Osteogenesis imperfecta and orthognathic surgery: case report and literature review, *J Oral Maxillofac Surg* 67:1128–1132, 2009.

Madhuri V, Selina A, Loganathan L, et al.: Osteogenesis imperfecta: novel genetic variants and clinical observations from a clinical exome study of 54 Indian patients, *Ann Hum Genet* 85:37–46, 2021.

Marçal FF, Ribeiro EM, Costa FWG, et al.: Dental alterations on panoramic radiographs of patients with osteogenesis imperfecta in relation to clinical diagnosis, severity, and bisphosphonate regimen aspects: a STROBE-compliant case-control study, *Oral Surg Oral Med Oral Pathol Oral Radiol* 128:621–630, 2019.

Marom R, Rabenhorst BM, Morello R: Osteogenesis imperfecta: an update on clinical features and therapies, *Eur J Endocrinol* 183: R95–R106, 2020.

Mortier GR, Cohn DH, Cormier-Daire V, et al.: Nosology and classification of genetic skeletal disorders: 2019 revision, *Am J Med Genet Part A* 179A:2393–2419, 2019.

O'Connell AC, Marini JC: Evaluation of oral problems in an osteogenesis imperfecta population, *Oral Surg Oral Med Oral Pathol Oral Radiol Endod* 87:189–196, 1999.

Palomo T, Vilaça T, Lazaretti-Castro M: Osteogenesis imperfecta: diagnosis and treatment, *Curr Opin Endocrinol Diabetes Obes* 24:381–388, 2017.

Prabhu N, Duckmanton N, Stevenson AR: The placement of osseointegrated dental implants in a patient with type IVB osteogenesis imperfecta: a 9-year follow-up, *Oral Surg Oral Med Oral Pathol Oral Radiol Endod* 103:349–354, 2007.

Reznikov N, Dagdeviren D, Tamimi F, et al.: Cone-beam computed tomography of osteogenesis imperfecta types III and IV: three-dimensional evaluation of craniofacial features and upper airways, *JBMR Plus* 3:e10124, 2019.

Rizkallah J, Schwartz S, Rauch F, et al.: Evaluation of the severity of malocclusions in children affected by osteogenesis imperfecta with the peer assessment rating and discrepancy indexes, *Am J Orthod Dentofacial Orthop* 143:336–341, 2013.

Rosén A, Modig M, Larson O: Orthognathic bimaxillary surgery in two patients with osteogenesis imperfecta and a review of the literature, *Int J Oral Maxillofac Surg* 40:866–886, 2011.

Rossi V, Lee B, Marom R: Osteogenesis imperfecta: advancements in genetics and treatment, *Curr Opin Pediatr* 31:708–715, 2019.

Sillence DO, Senn A, Danks PM: Genetic heterogeneity in osteogenesis imperfecta, *J Med Genet* 16:101–116, 1979.

Tashima H, Wattanawong K, Ho CT, et al.: Orthognathic surgery considerations for patients with undiagnosed type I osteogenesis imperfecta, *J Oral Maxillofac Surg* 69:2233–2241, 2011.

Thomas IH, DiMeglio LA: Advances in the classification and treatment of osteogenesis imperfecta, *Curr Osteoporos Rep* 14:1–9, 2016.

Thuesen KJ, Gjørup H, Hald JD, et al.: The dental perspective on osteogenesis imperfecta in a Danish adult population, *BMC Oral Health* 18:175, 2018.

Vuorimies I, Arponen H, Valta H, et al.: Timing of dental development in osteogenesis imperfecta patients with and without bisphosphonate treatment, *Bone* 94:29–33, 2017.

Wannfors K, Johansson C, Donath K: Augmentation of the mandible via a "tent-pole" procedure and implant treatment in a patient with type III osteogenesis imperfecta: clinical and histologic considerations, *Int J Oral Maxillofac Implants* 24:1144–1148, 2009.

Osteopetrosis

Hennekam RCM, Krantz ID, Allanson JE: Osteopetrosis, In *Gorlin's syndromes of the head and neck*, ed 5, New York, 2010, Oxford University Press, pp 245–250.

Mikami T, Miake Y, Bologna-Molina R, et al.: Ultrastructural analyses of alveolar bone in a patient with osteomyelitis secondary to osteopetrosis: a review of the literature, *J Oral Maxillofac Surg* 74:1584–1595, 2016.

Oğütcen-Toller M, Tek M, Sener I, et al.: Intractable bimaxillary osteomyelitis in osteopetrosis: review of the literature and current therapy, *J Oral Maxillofac Surg* 68:167–175, 2010.

Palagano E, Menale C, Sobacchi C, et al.: Genetics of osteopetrosis, *Curr Osteoporos Rep* 16:13–25, 2018.

Penna S, Capo V, Palagano E, et al.: One disease, many genes: implications for the treatment of osteopetrosis, *Front Endocrinol (Lausanne)* 10:85, 2019.

Rikhotso E, Reyneke JP, Ferretti C: Osteopetrosis: literature review and report of three cases, *SADJ* 63:302–307, 2008.

Satomura K, Kon M, Tokuyama R, et al.: Osteopetrosis complicated by osteomyelitis of the mandible: a case report including characterization of the osteopetrotic bone, *Int J Oral Maxillofac Surg* 36:86–93, 2007.

Teti A, Econs MJ: Osteopetroses, emphasizing potential approaches to treatment, *Bone* 102:50–59, 2017.

Younai F, Eisenbud L, Sciubba JJ: Osteopetrosis: a case report including gross and microscopic findings in the mandible at autopsy, *Oral Surg Oral Med Oral Pathol* 65:214–221, 1988.

Wu CC, Econs MJ, DiMeglio LA, et al.: Diagnosis and management of osteopetrosis: consensus guidelines from the osteopetrosis working group, *J Clin Endocrinol Metab* 102:3111–3123, 2017.

Cleidocranial Dysplasia

Atil F, Culhaoglu A, Kocyigit ID, et al.: Oral rehabilitation with implant-supported fixed dental prostheses of a patient with cleidocranial dysplasia, *J Prosthet Dent* 119:12–16, 2018.

Bufalino A, Paranaíba LMR, Gouvêa AF, et al.: Cleidocranial dysplasia: oral features and genetic analysis of 11 patients, *Oral Dis* 18:184–190, 2012.

D'Alessandro G, Tagariello T, Piana G: Cleidocranial dysplasia: etiology and stomatognathic and craniofacial abnormalities, *Minerva Stomatol* 59:117–127, 2010.

Farrow E, Nicot R, Wiss A, et al.: Cleidocranial dysplasia: a review of clinical, radiological, genetic implications and a guidelines proposal, *J Craniofac Surg* 29:382–389, 2018.

Kreiborg S, Jensen BL: Tooth formation and eruption - lessons learnt from cleidocranial dysplasia, *Eur J Oral Sci* 126(Suppl 1):72–80, 2018.

Pan CY, Tseng YC, Lan TH, et al.: Craniofacial features of cleidocranial dysplasia, *J Dent Sci* 12:313–318, 2017.

Roberts T, Stephen L, Beighton P: Cleidocranial dysplasia: a review of the dental, historical, and practical implications with an overview of the South African experience, *Oral Surg Oral Med Oral Pathol Oral Radiol* 115:46–55, 2013.

Sberna MT, De Angelis D, Laruffa R, et al.: Oral manifestation of cleido cranial displasia, *Minerva Stomatol* 61:421–429, 2012.

Zhu Y, Zou Y, Yu Q, et al.: Combined surgical-orthodontic treatment of patients with cleidocranial dysplasia: case report and review of the literature, *Orphanet J Rare Dis* 13:271, 2018.

Focal Osteoporotic Marrow Defect

Barker BF, Jensen JL, Howell FV: Focal osteoporotic marrow defects of the jaws, *Oral Surg Oral Med Oral Pathol* 38:404–413, 1974.

Crawford BE, Weathers DR: Osteoporotic marrow defects of the jaws, *J Oral Surg* 28:600–603, 1970.

Garcia NG, Barros FB, Carvalho MM, et al.: Focal osteoporotic bone marrow defect involving dental implant: a case report, *Int J Implant Dent* 1:18, 2015.

Makek M, Lello GE: Focal osteoporotic bone marrow defects of the jaws, *J Oral Maxillofac Surg* 44:268–273, 1986.

Schneider LC, Mesa ML, Fraenkel D: Osteoporotic bone marrow defect: radiographic features and pathogenic factors, *Oral Surg Oral Med Oral Pathol* 65:127–129, 1988.

Standish SM, Shafer WG: Focal osteoporotic bone marrow defects of the jaws, *J Oral Surg* 20:123–128, 1962.

Idiopathic Osteosclerosis

Gamba TO, Maciel NAP, Rados PV, et al.: The imaging role for diagnosis of idiopathic osteosclerosis: a retrospective approach based on records of 33,550 cases, *Clin Oral Investig* 25:1755–1765, 2021.

Geist JR, Katz JO: The frequency and distribution of idiopathic osteosclerosis, *Oral Surg Oral Med Oral Pathol* 69:388–393, 1990.

Halse A, Molven O: Idiopathic osteosclerosis of the jaws followed through a period of 20–27 years, *Int Endod J* 35:747–751, 2002.

Ledesma-Montes C, Jiménez-Farfán MD, Hernández-Guerrero JC: Idiopathic osteosclerosis in the maxillomandibular area, *Radiol Med* 124:27–33, 2019.

MacDonald D, Yu W: Incidental findings in a consecutive series of digital panoramic radiographs, *Imaging Sci Dent* 50:53–64, 2020.

MacDonald-Jankowski DS: Idiopathic osteosclerosis in the jaws of Britons and of the Hong Kong Chinese: radiology and systematic review, *Dentomaxillofac Radiol* 28:357–363, 1999.

Petrikowski CG, Peters E: Longitudinal radiographic assessment of dense bone islands of the jaws, *Oral Surg Oral Med Oral Pathol Oral Radiol Endod* 83:627–634, 1997.

Sisman Y, Ertas ET, Ertas H, et al.: The frequency and distribution of idiopathic osteosclerosis of the jaw, *Eur J Dent* 5:409–414, 2011.

Williams TP, Brooks SL: A longitudinal study of idiopathic osteosclerosis and condensing osteitis, *Dentomaxillofac Radiol* 27:275–278, 1998.

Yonetsu K, Yuasa K, Kanda S: Idiopathic osteosclerosis of the jaws: panoramic radiographic and computed tomographic findings, *Oral Surg Oral Med Oral Pathol Oral Radiol Endod* 83:517–521, 1997.

Massive Osteolysis

Al-Jamali J, Glaum R, Kassem A, et al.: Gorham-Stout syndrome of the facial bones: a review of pathogenesis and treatment modalities and report of a case with a rare cutaneous manifestations, *Oral Surg Oral Med Oral Pathol Oral Radiol* 114:e23–e29, 2012.

Chrcanovic BR, Gomez RS: Gorham-Stout disease with involvement of the jaws: a systematic review, *Int J Oral Maxillofac Surg* 48:1015–1021, 2019.

Escande C, Schouman T, Françoise G, et al.: Histological features and management of a mandibular Gorham disease: a case report and review of maxillofacial cases in the literature, *Oral Surg Oral Med Oral Pathol Oral Radiol Endod* 106:e30–e37, 2008.

Gondivkar SM, Gadbail AR: Gorham-Stout syndrome: a rare clinical entity and review of literature, *Oral Surg Oral Med Oral Pathol Oral Radiol Endod* 109:e41–e48, 2010.

Heyd R, Micke O, Surholt C, et al.: Radiation therapy for Gorham-Stout syndrome: results of a national patterns-of-care study and literature review, *Int J Radiation Oncol* 8:e179–e185, 2011.

Kayada Y, Yoshiga K, Takada K, et al.: Massive osteolysis of the mandible with subsequent obstructive sleep apnea syndrome: a case report, *J Oral Maxillofac Surg* 53:1463–1465, 1995.

Mignogna MD, Fedele S, Lo Russo L, et al.: Gorham's disease of the mandible mimicking periodontal disease on radiograph, *J Clin Periodontol* 32:1022–1025, 2005.

Rossi M, Buonuomo PS, Battafarano G, et al.: Dissecting the mechanisms of bone loss in Gorham-Stout disease, *Bone* 130:115068, 2020.

Sansare K, Saalim M, Jogdand M, et al.: Radiographic extent of maxillofacial Gorham's disease and its impact on recurrence: a systematic review, *Oral Surg Oral Med Oral Pathol Oral Radiol* 132:80–92, 2021.

Zhang S, Wu D, Shi L: Gorham disease of the mandible: a report of two cases and a literature review, *Oral Surg Oral Med Oral Pathol Oral Radiol* 127:e71–e76, 2019.

Paget Disease of Bone

Carrillo R, Morales A, Rodriguez-Peralto JL, et al.: Benign fibro-osseous lesions in Paget's disease of the jaws, *Oral Surg Oral Med Oral Pathol* 71:588–592, 1991.

Cheng YSL, Wright JM, Walstad WR, et al.: Osteosarcoma arising in Paget's disease of the mandible, *Oral Oncol* 38:785–792, 2002.

Corral-Gudino L, Borao-Cengotita-Bengoa M, del Pino-Montes J, et al.: Epidemiology of Paget's disease of bone: a systematic review and meta-analysis of secular changes, *Bone* 55:347–352, 2013.

Cundy T: Paget's disease of bone, *Metabolism* 80:5–14, 2018.

Friedrich RE, Luebke AM, Amling M, et al.: Clinical and microstructural findings in Paget disease of the entire mandible, *J Oral Maxillofac Surg* 76:336–346, 2018.

Ralston SH, Corral-Gudino L, Cooper C, et al.: Diagnosis and management of Paget's disease of bone in adults: a clinical guideline, *J Bone Miner Res* 34:579–604, 2019.

Singer FR: The evaluation and treatment of Paget's disease of bone, *Best Pract Res Clin Rheumatol* 34:101506, 2020.

Tillman H: Paget's disease of bone: a clinical, radiographic and histopathologic study of 24 cases involving the jaws, *Oral Surg Oral Med Oral Pathol* 15:1225–1234, 1962.

Torres T, Tamimi F, Garcia I, et al.: Dental implants in a patient with Paget disease under bisphosphonate treatment: a case report, *Oral Surg Oral Med Oral Pathol Oral Radiol Endod* 107:387–392, 2009.

Central Giant Cell Granuloma

Alsufyani NA, Aldosary RM, Alrasheed RS, et al.: A systematic review of the clinical and radiographic features of hybrid central giant cell granuloma lesions of the jaws, *Acta Odontol Scand* 79:124–131, 2021.

Amary F, Berisha F, Ye H, et al.: H3F3A (histone 3.3) G34W immunohistochemistry: a reliable marker defining benign and malignant giant cell tumor of bone, *Am J Surg Pathol* 41:1059–1068, 2017.

Auclair PL, Cuenin P, Kratochvil FJ, et al.: A clinical and histomorphologic comparison of the central giant cell granuloma and the giant cell tumor, *Oral Surg Oral Med Oral Pathol* 66:197–208, 1988.

Bredell M, Rordorf T, Kroiss S, et al.: Denosumab as a treatment alternative for central giant cell granuloma: a long-term retrospective cohort sudy, *J Oral Maxillofac Surg* 76:775–784, 2018.

Camarini C, de Souza Tolentino E: Non-surgical treatment as an alternative for the management of central giant cell granuloma: a systematic review, *Clin Oral Investig* 26:2111–2132, 2022.

Chrcanovic BR, Gomes CC, Dos Santos TR, et al.: Clinical factors associated with the recurrence of central giant cell lesions, *J Oral Pathol Med* 48:799–802, 2019.

Chrcanovic BR, Gomes CC, Gomez RS: Central giant cell lesion of the jaws: an updated analysis of 2270 cases reported in the literature, *J Oral Pathol Med* 47:731–739, 2018.

Czerniak B: Chapter 10, Giant cell lesions, In *Dorfman and Czerniak's Bone Tumors*, ed 2, Philadelphia, 2016, Elsevier Saunders, pp 692–759.

DeLange J, van den Akker HP: Clinical and radiological features of central giant-cell lesions of the jaw, *Oral Surg Oral Med Oral Pathol Oral Radiol Endod* 99:464–470, 2005.

DeLange J, van der Akker HP, van Zanten GOV, et al.: Calcitonin therapy in central giant cell granuloma of the jaw: a randomized double-blind placebo-controlled study, *Int J Oral Maxillofac Surg* 35:791–795, 2006.

Ferretti C, Muthray E: Management of central giant cell granuloma of mandible using intralesional corticosteroids: case report and review of literature, *J Oral Maxillofac Surg* 69:2824–2829, 2011.

Gomes CC, Diniz MG, Amaral FR, et al.: The highly prevalent H3F3A mutation in giant cell tumours of bone is not shared by sporadic central giant cell lesion of the jaws, *Oral Surg Oral Med Oral Pathol Oral Radiol* 118:583–585, 2014.

Gomes CC, Diniz MG, Bastos VC, et al.: Making sense of giant cell lesions of the jaws (GCLJ): lessons learned from next-generation sequencing, *J Pathol* 250:126–133, 2020.

Gomes CC, Gayden T, Bajic A, et al.: *TRPV4* and *KRAS* and *FGFR1* gain-of-function mutations drive giant cell lesions of the jaw, *Nat Commun* 9:4572, 2018.

Guimarães LM, Gomes IP, Pereira TDSF, et al.: *KRAS* mutations in brown tumor of the jaws in hyperparathyroidism, *J Oral Pathol Med* 49:796–802, 2021.

Jadu FM, Pharoah MJ, Lee L, et al.: Central giant cell granuloma of the mandibular condyle: a case report and review of the literature, *Dentomaxillofac Radiol* 40:60–64, 2011.

Kang H, Jha S, Deng Z, et al.: Somatic activating mutations in *MAP2K1* cause melorheostosis, *Nat Commun* 9:1390, 2018.

Kato Kaneko M, Liu X, Oki H, et al.: Isocitrate dehydrogenase mutation is frequently observed in giant cell tumor of bone, *Cancer Sci* 105:744–748, 2014.

Kruse-Lösler B, Diallo R, Gaertner C, et al.: Central giant cell granuloma of the jaws: a clinical, radiologic, and histopathologic study of 26 cases, *Oral Surg Oral Med Oral Pathol Oral Radiol Endod* 101:346–354, 2006.

Martins-Chaves RR, Guimarães LM, Pereira TDSF, et al.: KRAS mutations in implant-associated peripheral giant cell granuloma, *Oral Dis* 26:334–340, 2020.

Palmerini E, Picci P, Reichardt P, et al.: Malignancy in giant cell tumor of bone: a review of the literature, *Technol Cancer Res Treat* 18, 2019. 1533033819840000.

Peacock ZS, Resnick CM, Susarla SM, et al.: Do histologic criteria predict biologic behavior of giant cell lesions? *J Oral Maxillofac Surg* 70:2573–2580, 2012.

Reddy V, Saxena S, Aggarwal P, et al.: Incidence of central giant cell granuloma of the jaws with clinical and histological confirmation: an archival study in Northern India, *Br J Oral Maxillofac Surg* 50:668–672, 2012.

Resnick CM, Margolis J, Susarla SM, et al.: Maxillofacial and axial/appendicular giant cell lesions: unique tumor or variants of the same disease?—a comparison of phenotypic, clinical, and radiographic characteristics, *J Oral Maxillofac Surg* 68:130–137, 2010.

Richardson J, Stanbouly D, Litman E, et al.: Central giant cell granuloma of the head & neck: a case report and systematic review, *J Stomatol Oral Maxillofac Surg*, 2021. S2468-7855(21)00164-6.

Stavropoulos F, Katz J: Central giant cell granulomas: a systematic review of the radiographic characteristics with the addition of 20 new cases, *Dentomaxillofac Radiol* 31:213–217, 2002.

Schreuder WH, van den Berg H, Westermann AM, et al.: Pharmacological and surgical therapy for the central giant cell granuloma: a long-term retrospective cohort study, *J Craniomaxillofac Surg* 45:232–243, 2017.

Suárez-Roa Mde L, Reveiz L, Ruíz-Godoy Rivera LM, et al.: Interventions for central giant cell granuloma (CGCG) of the jaws, *Cochrane Database Syst Rev* 4):CD007404, 2009.

Triantafillidou K, Venetis G, Karakinaris G, et al.: Central giant cell granuloma of the jaws: a clinical study of 17 cases and a review of the literature, *Ann Otol Rhinol Laryngol* 120:167–174, 2011.

Whitaker SB, Waldron CA: Central giant cell lesions of the jaws: a clinical, radiologic and histopathologic study, *Oral Surg Oral Med Oral Pathol* 75:199–208, 1993.

Cherubism

Bar Droma E, Beck-Rosen G, Ilgiyaev A, et al.: Positive outcomes of denosumab treatment in 2 patients with cherubism, *J Oral Maxillofac Surg* 78:2226–2234, 2020.

Chrcanovic BR, Guimarães LM, Gomes CC, et al.: Cherubism: a systematic literature review of clinical and molecular aspects, *Int J Oral Maxillofac Surg* 50:43–53, 2021.

Miranda Galvis M, Faustino ISP, Ferraz FC, et al.: Orthodontic treatment in a patient with cherubism: benefits and limitations, *Spec Care Dentist* 40:291–297, 2020.

Kadlub N, Vazquez MP, Galmiche L, et al.: The calcineurin inhibitor tacrolimus as a new therapy in severe cherubism, *J Bone Miner Res* 30:878–885, 2015.

Kueper J, Tsimbal C, Olsen BR, et al.: *SH3BP2*-related fibro-osseous disorders of the maxilla and mandible: a systematic review, *Int J Oral Maxillofac Surg* 51:54–61, 2022.

Meng XM, Yu SF, Yu GY: Clinicopathologic study of 24 cases of cherubism, *Int J Oral Maxillofac Surg* 34:350–356, 2005.

Papadaki ME, Lietman SA, Levine MA, et al.: Cherubism: best clinical practice, *Orphanet J Rare Dis* 7(Suppl 1):S6, 2012.

Reichenberger EJ, Levine MA, Olsen BR, et al.: The role of SH3BP2 in the pathophysiology of cherubism, *Orphanet J Rare Dis* 7(Suppl 1):S5, 2012.

Roginsky VV, Ivanov AL, Ovtchinnikov IA: Familial cherubism: the experience of the Moscow Central Institute for Stomatology and Maxillo-facial Surgery, *Int J Oral Maxillofac Surg* 38:218–223, 2009.

Stoor P, Suomalainen A, Kemola W, et al.: Craniofacial and dental features in six children with cherubism, *J Craniofac Surg* 28:1806–1811, 2017.

Ueki Y, Tiziani V, Santanna C, et al.: Mutations in the gene encoding c-Abl-binding protein SH3BP2 cause cherubism, *Nat Genet* 125–126, 2001.

Simple Bone Cyst

An SY, Lee JS, Benavides E, et al.: Multiple simple bone cysts of the jaws: review of the literature and report of three cases, *Oral Surg Oral Med Oral Pathol Oral Radiol* 117:e458–e469, 2014.

Chadwick JW, Alsufyani NA, Lam EWN: Clinical and radiographic features of solitary and cemento-osseous dysplasia-associated simple bone cysts, *Dentomaxillofac Radiol* 40:230–235, 2011.

Copete MA, Kawamata A, Langlais RP: Solitary bone cyst of the jaws: radiographic review of 44 cases, *Oral Surg Oral Med Oral Pathol Oral Radiol Endod* 85:221–225, 1998.

Hung YP, Fisch AS, Diaz-Perez JA, et al.: Identification of *EWSR1-NFATC2* fusion in simple bone cysts, *Histopathology* 78:849–856, 2021.

Kaugars GE, Cale AE: Traumatic bone cyst, *Oral Surg Oral Med Oral Pathol* 63:318–324, 1987.

Lima LB, de Freitas Filho SA, Barbosa de Paulo LF, et al.: Simple bone cyst: description of 60 cases seen at a Brazilian School of Dentistry and review of international literature, *Med Oral Patol Oral Cir Bucal* 25:e616–e625, 2020.

Martins-Filho PR, Santos Tde S, Araújo VL, et al.: Traumatic bone cyst of the mandible: a review of 26 cases, *Braz J Otorhinolaryngol* 78:16–21, 2012.

Perdigão PF, Silva EC, Sakurai E, et al.: Idiopathic bone cavity: a clinical, radiographic, and histological study, *Br J Oral Maxillofac Surg* 41:407–409, 2003.

Pižem J, Šekoranja D, Zupan A, et al.: *FUS-NFATC2* or *EWSR1-NFATC2* fusions are present in a large proportion of simple bone cysts, *Am J Surg Pathol* 44:1623–1634, 2020.

Suei Y, Taguchi A, Nagasaki T, et al.: Radiographic findings and prognosis of simple bone cyst of the jaws, *Dentomaxillofac Radiol* 39:65–71, 2012.

Suei Y, Taguchi A, Tanimoto K: A comparative study of simple bone cysts of the jaw and extracranial bones, *Dentomaxillofac Radiol* 36:125–129, 2007.

Suei Y, Taguchi A, Tanimoto K: Simple bone cyst of the jaws: evaluation of treatment outcome by review of 132 cases, *J Oral Maxillofac Surg* 65:918–923, 2007.

Tariq MU, Din NU, Ahmad Z, et al.: Cementum-like matrix in solitary bone cysts: a unique and characteristic but yet underrecognized feature of promising diagnostic utility, *Ann Diagn Pathol* 18:1–4, 2014.

Aneurysmal Bone Cyst

Alhumaid I, Abu-Zaid A: Denosumab therapy in the management of aneurysmal bone cysts: a comprehensive literature review, *Cureus* 11:e3989, 2019.

Arora SS, Paul S, Arora S, et al.: Secondary jaw aneurysmal bone cyst (JABC)—a possible misnomer? A review of literature on secondary JABCs, their pathogenesis and oncogenesis, *J Oral Pathol Med* 43:647–651, 2014.

Henriques AC, Carvalho Mde V, Miguel MC, et al.: Clinical pathological analysis of nine cases of aneurysmal bone cyst of the jaws in a Brazilian population, *Eur Arch Otorhinolaryngol* 269:971–976, 2012.

Liu Y, Zhou J, Shi J: Clinicopathology and recurrence analysis of 44 jaw aneurysmal bone cyst cases: a literature review, *Front Surg* 8:678696, 2021.

Mankin HJ, Hornicek FJ, Ortiz-Cruz E, et al.: Aneurysmal bone cyst: a review of 150 patients, *J Clin Oncol* 23:6756–6762, 2005.

McMullen PD, Bridge JA, Blair EA, et al.: Aneurysmal bone cyst of the maxillary sinus with *USP6* rearrangement: case report of a rare entity and review of the literature, *Head Neck Pathol* 13:281–285, 2019.

Motamedi MH, Navi F, Eshkevari PS, et al.: Variable presentations of aneurysmal bone cysts of the jaws: 51 cases treated during a 30-year period, *J Oral Maxillofac Surg* 66:2098–2103, 2008.

Ogle OE, Santosh AB: Medication management of jaw lesions for dental patients, *Dent Clin N Am* 60:483–495, 2016.

Oliveira AM, Chou MM: The TRE17/USP6 oncogene: a riddle wrapped in a mystery inside an enigma, *Front Biosci (Schol Ed)* 4:321–334, 2012.

Rehman R, Dekhou A, Osto M, et al.: Aneurysmal bone cysts of the craniofacial origin: a systematic review, *OTO Open* 5, 2021. 2473974X211052950.

Struthers PJ, Shear M: Aneurysmal bone cyst of the jaws. I. Clinicopathologic features, *Int J Oral Surg* 13:85–91, 1984.

Struthers PJ, Shear M: Aneurysmal bone cyst of the jaws. II. Pathogenesis, *Int J Oral Surg* 13:92–100, 1984.

Sun ZJ, Sun HL, Yang RL, et al.: Aneurysmal bone cysts of the jaws, *Int J Surg Pathol* 17:311–322, 2009.

Sun ZJ, Zhao YF, Yang RL, et al.: Aneurysmal bone cysts of the jaws: analysis of 17 cases, *J Oral Maxillofac Surg* 68:2122–2128, 2010.

Central Xanthoma of the Jaws

Bowers LM, Cohen DM, Bhattacharyya I, et al.: The non-ossifying fibroma: a case report and review of the literature, *Head Neck Pathol* 7:203–210, 2013.

de Arruda JAA, Almeida TFA, Abreu LG, et al.: Intraosseous xanthoma of the mandible: A multi-institutional case series with a literature review, *J Oral Pathol Med* 48:935–942, 2019.

Daley T, Dunn G, Darling MR: Central xanthoma of the jaws: a clinicopathologic entity? *Oral Surg Oral Med Oral Pathol Oral Radiol* 119:92–100, 2015.

Harsanyi BB, Larsson A: Xanthomatous lesions of the mandible: osseous expression of non-X histiocytosis and benign fibrous histiocytoma, *Oral Surg Oral Med Oral Pathol* 65:551–566, 1988.

Morel D, Kelsch RD, Nolan PJ: Primary xanthoma of the mandible: report of a rare case, *Head Neck Pathol* 10:245–251, 2016.

Olson NJ, Addante RR, de Abreu FB, et al.: Central xanthoma of the jaw in association with Noonan syndrome, *Hum Pathol* 82:202–205, 2018.

Rawal YB, Chandra SR, Hall JM: Central xanthoma of the jaw bones: a benign tumor, *Head Neck Pathol* 11:192–202, 2017.

Whitehouse L, Bobinskas A, Chengot P, et al.: Intraosseous mandibular xanthomas – an interesting diagnostic dilemma? *Oral Surg* 11:213–223, 2018.

Fibro-Osseous Lesions—General Aspects and Classification

Abramovitch K, Rice DD: Benign fibro-osseous lesions of the jaws, *Dent Clin N Am* 60:167–193, 2016.

Ahmad M, Gaalaas L: Fibro-osseous and other lesions of bone in the jaws, *Radiol Clin North Am* 56:91–104, 2018.

de Noronha Santos Netto J, Machado Cerri J, Miranda AM, et al.: Benign fibro-osseous lesions: clinicopathologic features from 143 cases diagnosed in an oral diagnosis setting, *Oral Surg Oral Med Oral Pathol Oral Radiol* 115:e56–e65, 2013.

El-Mofty SK: Fibro-osseous lesions of the craniofacial skeleton: an update, *Head Neck Pathol* 8:432–444, 2014.

Eversole R, Su L, El-Mofty S: Benign fibro-osseous lesions of the craniofacial complex: a review, *Head Neck Pathol* 2:177–202, 2008.

Hameed M, Horvai AE, Jordan RCK: Soft tissue special issue: gnathic fibro-osseous lesions and osteosarcoma, *Head Neck Pathol* 14:70–82, 2020.

MacDonald-Jankowski DS: Fibro-osseous lesions of the face and jaws, *Clin Radiol* 59:11–25, 2004.

Mainville GN, Turgeon DP, Kauzman A: Diagnosis and management of benign fibro-osseous lesions of the jaws: a current review for the dental clinician, *Oral Dis* 23:440–450, 2017.

Nelson BL, Phillips BJ: Benign fibro-osseous lesions of the head and neck, *Head Neck Pathol* 13:466–475, 2019.

Noffke CE, Raubenheimer EJ, MacDonald D: Fibro-osseous disease: harmonizing terminology with biology, *Oral Surg Oral Med Oral Pathol Oral Radiol* 114:388–392, 2012.

Waldron CA: Fibro-osseous lesions of the jaws, *J Oral Maxillofac Surg* 51:828–835, 1993.

Soluk-Tekkesin M, Sinanoglu A, Selvi F, et al.: The importance of clinical and radiological findings for the definitive histopathologic diagnosis of benign fibro-osseous lesions of the jaws: study of 276 cases, *J Stomatol Oral Maxillofac Surg*, 2021. S2468-7855(21)00084-7.

Fibrous Dysplasia

Akintoye SO, Boyce AM, Collins MT: Dental perspectives in fibrous dysplasia and McCune-Albright syndrome, *Oral Surg Oral Med Oral Pathol Oral Radiol* 116:e149–e155, 2013.

Akintoye SO, Lee JS, Feimster T, et al.: Dental characteristics of fibrous dysplasia and McCune-Albright syndrome, *Oral Surg Oral Med Oral Pathol Oral Radiol Endod* 96:275–282, 2003.

Burke AB, Collins MT, Boyce AM: Fibrous dysplasia of bone: craniofacial and dental implications, *Oral Dis* 23:697–708, 2017.

Cheng J, Wang Y, Yu H, et al.: An epidemiological and clinical analysis of craniomaxillofacial fibrous dysplasia in a Chinese population, *Orphanet J Rare Dis* 7:80, 2012.

Cheng J, Yu H, Wang D, et al.: Spontaneous malignant transformation in craniomaxillofacial fibrous dysplasia, *J Craniofac Surg* 24:141–145, 2013.

Davidova LA, Bhattacharyya I, Islam MN, et al.: An analysis of clinical and histopathologic features of fibrous dysplasia of the jaws: a series of 40 cases and review of literature, *Head Neck Pathol* 14:353–361, 2020.

de Castro LF, Ovejero D, Boyce AM: Diagnosis of endocrine disease: mosaic disorders of FGF23 excess: fibrous dysplasia/McCune-Albright syndrome and cutaneous skeletal hypophosphatemia syndrome, *Eur J Endocrinol* 182:R83–R99, 2020.

Hartley I, Zhadina M, Collins MT, et al.: Fibrous dysplasia of bone and McCune-Albright syndrome: a bench to bedside review, *Calcif Tissue Int* 104:517–529, 2019.

Javaid MK, Boyce A, Appelman-Dijkstra N, et al.: Best practice management guidelines for fibrous dysplasia/McCune-Albright syndrome: a consensus statement from the FD/MAS international consortium, *Orphanet J Rare Dis* 14:139, 2019.

Kushchayeva YS, Kushchayev SV, Glushko TY, et al.: Fibrous dysplasia for radiologists: beyond ground glass bone matrix, *Insights Imaging* 9:1035–1056, 2018.

Lee JS, FitzGibbon EJ, Chen YR, et al.: Clinical guidelines for the management of craniofacial fibrous dysplasia, *Orphanet J Rare Dis* 7(Suppl 1):S2, 2012.

MacDonald-Jankowski D: Fibrous dysplasia: a systematic review, *Dentomaxillofac Radiol* 38:196–215, 2009.

Pereira TDSF, Gomes CC, Brennan PA, et al.: Fibrous dysplasia of the jaws: integrating molecular pathogenesis with clinical, radiological, and histopathological features, *J Oral Pathol Med* 48:3–9, 2019.

Prado Ribeiro AC, Carlos R, Speight PM, et al.: Peritrabecular clefting in fibrous dysplasia of the jaws: an important histopathologic feature for differentiating fibrous dysplasia from central ossifying fibroma, *Oral Surg Oral Med Oral Pathol Oral Radiol* 114:503–508, 2012.

Ricalde P, Magliocca KR, Lee JS: Craniofacial fibrous dysplasia, *Oral Maxillofac Surg Clin N Am* 24:427–441, 2012.

Waldron CA, Giansanti JS: Benign fibro-osseous lesions of the jaws. I. Fibrous dysplasia of the jaws, *Oral Surg Oral Med Oral Pathol* 35:190–201, 1973.

Cemento-Osseous Dysplasias

Alsufyani NA, Lam EWN: Osseous (cemento-osseous) dysplasia of the jaws: clinical and radiographic analysis, *J Can Dent Assoc* 77:b70, 2011.

Alsufyani NA, Lam EWN: Cemento-osseous dysplasia of the jaw bones: key radiographic features, *Dentomaxillofac Radiol* 40:141–146, 2011.

Esfahanizadeh N, Yousefi H: Successful implant placement in a case of florid cemento-osseous dysplasia: a case report and literature review, *J Oral Implantol* 44:275–279, 2018.

Groot RH, van Merkesteyn JPR, Bras J: Diffuse sclerosing osteomyelitis and florid osseous dysplasia, *Oral Surg Oral Med Oral Pathol Oral Radiol Endod* 81:333–342, 1996.

Gumru B, Akkitap MP, Deveci S, et al.: A retrospective cone beam computed tomography analysis of cemento-osseous dysplasia, *J Dent Sci* 16:1154–1161, 2021.

Kawai T, Hiranuma H, Kishino M, et al.: Cemento-osseous dysplasia of the jaws in 54 patients: a radiographic study, *Oral Surg Oral Med Oral Pathol Oral Radiol Endod* 87:107–114, 1999.

MacDonald-Jankowski DS: Florid cemento-osseous dysplasia: a systematic review, *Dentomaxillofac Radiol* 32:141–149, 2003.

MacDonald-Jankowski DS: Focal cemento-osseous dysplasia: a systematic review, *Dentomaxillofac Radiol* 37:350–360, 2008.

Mahomed F, Altini M, Meer S, et al.: Cemento-osseous dysplasia with associated simple bone cysts, *J Oral Maxillofac Surg* 63:1549–1554, 2005.

Melrose RJ: The clinico-pathologic spectrum of cemento-osseous dysplasia, *Oral Maxillofac Clin North Am* 9:643–653, 1997.

Olgac V, Sinanoglu A, Selvi F, et al.: A clinicopathologic analysis of 135 cases of cemento-osseous dysplasia: to operate or not to operate? *J Stomatol Oral Maxillofac Surg* 122:278–282, 2021.

Raubenheimer EJ, Noffke CE, Boy SC: Osseous dysplasia with gross jaw expansion: a review of 18 lesions, *Head Neck Pathol* 10:437–443, 2016.

Schneider LC, Dolinsky HB, Grodjesk JE, et al.: Malignant spindle cell tumor arising in the mandible of a patient with florid osseous dysplasia, *Oral Surg Oral Med Oral Pathol Oral Radiol Endod* 88:69–73, 1999.

Schneider LC, Mesa ML: Differences between florid osseous dysplasia and diffuse sclerosing osteomyelitis, *Oral Surg Oral Med Oral Pathol* 70:308–312, 1990.

Su L, Weathers DR, Waldron CA: Distinguishing features of focal cemento-osseous dysplasias and cemento-ossifying fibromas. I. A pathologic spectrum of 316 cases, *Oral Surg Oral Med Oral Pathol Oral Radiol Endod* 84:301–309, 1997.

Summerlin DJ, Tomich CE: Focal cemento-osseous dysplasia: a clinicopathologic study of 221 cases, *Oral Surg Oral Med Oral Pathol* 78:611–620, 1994.

Waldron CA: Fibro-osseous lesions of the jaws, *J Oral Maxillofac Surg* 43:249–262, 1985.

Zillo Martini M, Caroli Rocha A, Lemos CA Jr, et al.: Fibro-osseous lesions associated with simple bone cysts: three case reports and review of the literature, *Minerva Stomatol* 59:671–676, 2010.

Familial Gigantiform Cementoma

Abdelsayed RA, Eversole LR, Singh BS, et al.: Gigantiform cementoma: clinicopathologic presentation of 3 cases, *Oral Surg Oral Med Oral Pathol Oral Radiol Endod* 91:438–444, 2001.

Cannon JS, Keller EE, Dahlin DC: Gigantiform cementoma: report of two cases (mother and son), *J Oral Surg* 38:65–70, 1980.

Chi AC, Collins LHC: Familial gigantiform cementoma, In WHO classification of tumours editorial board, editor: *World Health Organization Classification of Head and Neck Tumours*, ed 5, Lyon, France, 2022, International Agency for Research on Cancer. Available at: https://tumourclassification.iarc.who.int/chaptercontent/52/180. (Internet; beta version ahead of print).

Coleman H, Altini M, Kieser J, et al.: Familial florid cemento-osseous dysplasia—a case report and review of the literature, *J Dent Assoc S Afr* 51:766–770, 1996.

Finical SJ, Kane WJ, Clay RP, et al.: Familial gigantiform cementoma, *Plast Reconstr Surg* 103:949–954, 1999.

Kumar VV, Ebenezer S, Narayan TV, et al.: Clinicopathologic conference: multiquadrant expansile fibro-osseous lesion in a juvenile, *Oral Surg Oral Med Oral Pathol Oral Radiol* 113:286–292, 2012.

Ma C, Wang H, He G, et al.: Familial gigantiform cementoma: case report of an unusual clinical manifestation and possible mechanism related to "calcium steal disorder,", *Medicine (Baltimore)* 95:e2956, 2016.

Moshref M, Khojasteh A, Kazemi B, et al.: Autosomal dominant gigantiform cementoma associated with bone fractures, *Am J Med Genet A* 146A:644–648, 2008.

Nel C, Yakoob Z, Schouwstra CM, et al.: Familial florid cemento-osseous dysplasia: a report of three cases and review of the literature, *Dentomaxillofac Radiol* 50:20190486, 2021.

Noffke CE, Raubenheimer EJ: Expansive osseous dysplasia: report of 9 lesions in an African population sample and review of the literature, *Oral Surg Oral Med Oral Pathol Oral Radiol Endod* 111:e35–e41, 2011.

Otaify GA, Whyte MP, Gottesman GS, et al.: Gnathodiaphyseal dysplasia: Severe atypical presentation with novel heterozygous mutation of the anoctamin gene (ANO5), *Bone* 107:161–171, 2018.

Raubenheimer EJ, Noffke CE: Regarding the use of the term "cementum" in pathologic proliferations, *Head Neck Pathol* 12:629–630, 2018.

Rossbach HC, Letson D, Lacson A, et al.: Familial gigantiform cementoma with brittle bone disease, pathologic fractures, and osteosarcoma: a possible explanation of an ancient mystery, *Pediatr Blood Cancer* 44:390–396, 2005.

Shah S, Huh KH, Yi WJ, et al.: Follow-up CT findings of recurrent familial gigantiform cementoma of a female child, *Skeletal Radiol* 41:341–346, 2012.

Toffanin A, Benetti R, Manconi R: Familial florid cemento-osseous dysplasia: a case report, *J Oral Maxillofac Surg* 58:1440–1446, 2000.

Wang HW, Yu M, Qin XJ, et al.: Familial gigantiform cementoma: distinctive clinical features of a large Chinese pedigree, *Br J Oral Maxillofac Surg* 53:83–85, 2015.

Young SK, Markowitz NR, Sullivan S, et al.: Familial gigantiform cementoma: classification and presentation of a large pedigree, *Oral Surg Oral Med Oral Pathol* 68:740–747, 1989.

Cemento-Ossifying Fibroma

Akcam T, Altug HA, Karakoc O, et al.: Synchronous ossifying fibromas of the jaws: a review, *Oral Surg Oral Med Oral Pathol Oral Radiol* 114(Suppl 5):S120–S125, 2012.

Baumhoer D, Haefliger S, Ameline B, et al.: Ossifying fibroma of non-odontogenic origin: a fibro-osseous lesion in the craniofacial skeleton to be (re-)considered, *Head Neck Pathol*, 2021 (Epub ahead of print June 26, 2021.).

Chi AC, Collins LHC: Cemento-ossifying fibroma, In WHO Classification of Tumours Editorial Board, editor: *World Health Organization Classification of Head and Neck Tumours*, ed 5, Lyon, France, 2022, International Agency for Research on Cancer. Available at: https://tumourclassification.iarc.who.int/chaptercontent/52/162. (Internet; beta version ahead of print).

de Mesquita Netto AC, Gomez RS, Diniz MG, et al.: Assessing the contribution of HRPT2 to the pathogenesis of jaw fibrous dysplasia, ossifying fibroma, and osteosarcoma, *Oral Surg Oral Med Oral Pathol Oral Radiol* 115:359–367, 2013.

Eversole LR, Leider AS, Nelson K: Ossifying fibroma: a clinicopathologic study of 64 cases, *Oral Surg Oral Med Oral Pathol* 60:505–511, 1985.

Kaplan I, Manor I, Yahalom R, et al.: Central giant cell granuloma associated with central ossifying fibroma of the jaws: a clinicopathologic study, *Oral Surg Oral Med Oral Pathol Oral Radiol Endod* 103:e35–e41, 2007.

Kaur T, Dhawan A, Bhullar RS, et al.: Cemento-ossifying fibroma in maxillofacial region: a series of 16 cases, *J Maxillofac Oral Surg* 20:240–245, 2021.

Ma M, Liu L, Shi R, et al.: Copy number alteration profiling facilitates differential diagnosis between ossifying fibroma and fibrous dysplasia of the jaws, *Int J Oral Sci* 13:21, 2021.

MacDonald-Jankowski DS: Ossifying fibroma: a systematic review, *Dentomaxillofac Radiol* 38:495–513, 2009.

MacDonald-Jankowski DS, Li TK: Ossifying fibromas in a Hong Kong community: the clinical and radiological features and outcomes of treatment, *Dentomaxillofac Radiol* 38:514–523, 2009.

Su L, Weathers DR, Waldron CA: Distinguishing features of focal cemento-osseous dysplasias and cemento-ossifying fibromas. I. A pathologic spectrum of 316 cases, *Oral Surg Oral Med Oral Pathol Oral Radiol Endod* 84:301–309, 1997.

Titinchi F, Morkel J: Ossifying fibroma: analysis of treatment methods and recurrence patterns, *J Oral Maxillofac Surg* 74:2409–2419, 2016.

Torresan F, Iacobone M: Clinical features, treatment, and surveillance of hyperparathyroidism-jaw tumor syndrome: an up-to-date and review of the literature, *Int J Endocrinol* 2019:1761030, 2019.

Triantafillidou K, Venetis G, Karakinaris G, et al.: Ossifying fibroma of the jaws: a clinical study of 14 cases and review of the literature, *Oral Surg Oral Med Oral Pathol Oral Radiol* 114:193–199, 2012.

Waldron CA, Giansanti JS: Benign fibro-osseous lesions of the jaws. II. Benign fibro-osseous lesions of periodontal ligament origin, *Oral Surg Oral Med Oral Pathol* 35:340–350, 1973.

Woo SB: Central cemento-ossifying fibroma: primary odontogenic or osseous neoplasm? *J Oral Maxillofac Surg* 73(12 Suppl):S87–S93, 2015.

Juvenile Ossifying Fibroma

Chi AC, Collins LHC: Juvenile trabecular ossifying fibroma, In WHO Classification of Tumours Editorial Board, editor: *World Health Organization Classification of Head and Neck Tumours*, ed 5, Lyon, France, 2022, International Agency for Research on Cancer. Available at: https://tumourclassification.iarc.who.int/chaptercontent/52/164. (Internet; beta version ahead of print).

Chi AC, Collins LHC: Psammomatoid ossifying fibroma, In WHO Classification of Tumours Editorial Board, editor: *World Health Organization Classification of Head and Neck Tumours*, ed 5, Lyon, France, 2022, International Agency for Research on Cancer. Available at: https://tumourclassification.iarc.who.int/chaptercontent/52/163. (Internet; beta version ahead of print).

Chrcanovic BR, Gomez RS: Juvenile ossifying fibroma of the jaws and paranasal sinuses: a systematic review of the cases reported in the literature, *Int J Oral Maxillofac Surg* 49:28–37, 2020.

El-Mofty S: Psammomatoid and trabecular juvenile ossifying fibroma of the craniofacial skeleton: two distinct clinico-pathologic entities, *Oral Surg Oral Med Oral Pathol Oral Radiol Endod* 93:296–304, 2002.

Han J, Hu L, Zhang C, et al.: Juvenile ossifying fibroma of the jaw: a retrospective study of 15 cases, *Int J Oral Maxillofac Surg* 45:368–376, 2016.

Owosho AA, Hughes MA, Prasad JL, et al.: Psammomatoid and trabecular juvenile ossifying fibroma: two distinct radiologic entities, *Oral Surg Oral Med Oral Pathol Oral Radiol* 118:732–738, 2014.

Sarode SC, Sarode GS, Waknis P, et al.: Juvenile psammomatoid ossifying fibroma: a review, *Oral Oncol* 47:1110–1116, 2011.

Slootweg PJ: Juvenile trabecular ossifying fibroma: an update, *Virchows Arch* 461:699–703, 2012.

Sultan AS, Schwartz MK, Caccamese JF, et al.: Juvenile trabecular ossifying fibroma, *Head Neck Pathol* 12:567–571, 2018.

Tabareau-Delalande F, Collin C, Gomez-Brouchet A, et al.: Chromosome 12 long arm rearrangement covering *MDM2* and *RASAL1* is associated with aggressive craniofacial juvenile ossifying fibroma and extracranial psammomatoid fibro-osseous lesions, *Mod Pathol* 28:48–56, 2015.

Titinchi F: Juvenile ossifying fibroma of the maxillofacial region: analysis of clinico-pathological features and management, *Med Oral Patol Oral Cir Bucal* 26:e590–e597, 2021.

Urs AB, Kumar P, Arora S, et al.: Clinicopathologic and radiologic correlation of ossifying fibroma and juvenile ossifying fibroma—an institutional study of 22 cases, *Ann Diagn Pathol* 17:198–203, 2013.

Osteoma

Arslan HH, Tasli H, Cebeci S, Gerek M: The management of the paranasal sinus osteomas, *J Craniofac Surg* 28:741–745, 2017.

Bhatt G, Gupta S, Ghosh S, et al.: Central osteoma of maxilla associated with an impacted tooth: report of a rare case with literature review, *Head Neck Pathol* 13:554–561, 2019.

Dell'Aversana Orabona G, Salzano G, Iaconetta G, et al.: Facial osteomas: fourteen cases and a review of literature, *Eur Rev Med Pharmacol Sci* 19:1796–1802, 2015.

Ghita I, Brooks JK, Bordener SL, et al.: Central compact osteoma of the mandible: case report featuring unusual radiographic and computed tomographic presentations and brief literature review, *J Stomatol Oral Maxillofac Surg*, 2020. S2468-7855(20)30226-3.

Halawi AM, Maley JE, Robinson RA, et al.: Craniofacial osteoma: clinical presentation and patterns of growth, *Am J Rhinol Allergy* 27:128–133, 2013.

Herford AS, Stoffella E, Tandon R: Osteomas involving the facial skeleton: a report of 2 cases and review of the literature, *Oral Surg Oral Med Oral Pathol Oral Radiol* 115:e1–e6, 2013.

Larrea-Oyarbide N, Valmaseda-Castellón E, Berini-Aytés L, et al.: Osteomas of the craniofacial region. Review of 106 cases, *J Oral Pathol Med* 37:38–42, 2008.

McHugh JB, Mukherji SK, Lucas DR: Sino-orbital osteoma: a clinicopathologic study of 45 surgically treated cases with emphasis on tumors with osteoblastoma-like features, *Arch Pathol Lab Med* 133:1587–1593, 2009.

Ostrofsky M, Morkel JA, Titinchi F: Osteoma of the mandibular condyle: a rare case report and review of the literature, *J Stomatol Oral Maxillofac Surg* 120:584–587, 2019.

Sayan BN, Ucok C, Karasu HA, et al.: Peripheral osteoma of the oral and maxillofacial region: a study of 35 new cases, *J Oral Maxillofac Surg* 60:1299–1301, 2002.

Woldenberg Y, Nash M, Bodner L: Peripheral osteoma of the maxillofacial region. Diagnosis and management: a study of 14 cases, *Med Oral Patol Oral Cir Bucal* 10(Suppl 2):E139–E142, 2005.

Gardner Syndrome

Boffano P, Bosco GF, Gerbino G: The surgical management of oral and maxillofacial manifestations of Gardner syndrome, *J Oral Maxillofac Surg* 68:2549–2554, 2010.

Cristofaro MG, Giudice A, Amantea A, et al.: Gardner's syndrome: a clinical and genetic study of a family, *Oral Surg Oral Med Oral Pathol Oral Radiol* 115:e1–e6, 2013.

Pereira DL, Carvalho PA, Achatz MI, et al.: Oral and maxillofacial considerations in Gardner's syndrome: a report of two cases, *Ecancermedicalscience* 10:623, 2016.

Galiatsatos P, Foulkes WD: Familial adenomatous polyposis, *Am J Gastroenterol* 101:385–398, 2006.

Gorlin RJ, Cohen MM Jr: Hennekam RCM: Gardner syndrome, In *Gorlin's syndromes of the head and neck*, ed 5, New York, 2010, Oxford University Press, pp 526–532.

Half E, Bercovich D, Rozen P: Familial adenomatous polyposis, *Orphanet J Rare Dis* 4:22, 2009.

Jasperson KW, Patel SG, Ahnen DJ: APC-associated polyposis conditions, In Adam MP, Ardinger HH, Pagon RA, et al., editors: *GeneReviews® [Internet]*, Seattle, 2022, University of Washington, pp 1993–2022. https://www.ncbi.nlm.nih.gov/books/NBK1345/. Accessed February 15, 2022.

Lagha NB, Galeazzi JM, Chapireau D, et al.: Surgical management of osteoma associated with a familial Gardner's syndrome, *J Oral Maxilofac Surg* 65:1234–1240, 2007.

National Cancer Institute: *Genetics of Colorectal Cancer (PDQ) (website)*, https://www.cancer.gov/types/colorectal/hp/colorectal-genetics-pdq. Accessed December 26, 2020.

Wijn MA, Keller JJ, Giardiello FM, et al.: Oral and maxillofacial manifestations of familial adenomatous polyposis, *Oral Dis* 13:360–365, 2007.

Osteoblastoma and Osteoid Osteoma

Alvares Capelozza AL, Gião Dezotti MS, Casati Alvares L, et al.: Osteoblastoma of the mandible: systematic review of the literature and report of a case, *Dentomaxillofac Radiol* 34:1–8, 2005.

Amary F, Markert E, Berisha F, et al.: FOS expression in osteoid osteoma and osteoblastoma: a valuable ancillary diagnostic tool, *Am J Surg Pathol* 43:1661–1667, 2019.

An SY, Shin HI, Choi KS, et al.: Unusual osteoid osteoma of the mandible: report of case and review of the literature, *Oral Surg Oral Med Oral Pathol Oral Radiol* 116:e134–e140, 2013.

Capodiferro S, Maiorano E, Giardina C, et al.: Osteoblastoma of the mandible: clinicopathologic study of four cases and literature review, *Head Neck* 27:616–625, 2005.

Fittall MW, Mifsud W, Pillay N, et al.: Recurrent rearrangements of *FOS* and *FOSB* define osteoblastoma, *Nat Commun* 9:2150, 2018.

Harrington C, Accurso BT, Kalmar JR, et al.: Aggressive osteoblastoma of the maxilla: a case report and review of the literature, *Head Neck Pathol* 5:165–170, 2011.

Jones AC, Prihoda TJ, Kacher JE, et al.: Osteoblastoma of the maxilla and mandible: a report of 24 cases, review of the literature, and discussion of its relationship to osteoid osteoma of the jaws, *Oral Surg Oral Med Oral Pathol Oral Radiol Endod* 102:639–650, 2006.

Kashikar S, Steinle M, Reich R, et al.: Epithelioid multinodular osteoblastoma of the mandible: a case report and review of literature, *Head Neck Pathol* 10(2):182–187, 2016.

Lam SW, Cleven AHG, Kroon HM, et al.: Utility of FOS as diagnostic marker for osteoid osteoma and osteoblastoma, *Virchows Arch* 476:455–463, 2020.

Pereira TDSF, Andrade BAB, Romañach MJ, et al.: Clinicopathologic study of 6 cases of epithelioid osteoblastoma of the jaws with immunoexpression analysis of FOS and FOSB, *Oral Surg Oral Med Oral Pathol Oral Radiol* 130:191–199, 2020.

Rawal YB, Angiero F, Allen CM, et al.: Gnathic osteoblastoma: clinicopathologic review of seven cases with long-term follow-up, *Oral Oncol* 42:123–130, 2006.

Singh A, Solomon MC: Osteoid osteoma of the mandible: a case report with review of the literature, *J Dent Sci* 12:185–189, 2017.

Cementoblastoma

Brannon RB, Fowler CB, Carpenter WM, et al.: Cementoblastoma: an innocuous neoplasm? A clinicopathologic study of 44 cases and review of the literature with special emphasis on recurrence, *Oral Surg Oral Med Oral Pathol Oral Radiol Endod* 93:311–320, 2002.

Chrcanovic BR, Gomez RS: Cementoblastoma: an updated analysis of 258 cases reported in the literature, *J Craniomaxillofac Surg* 45:1759–1766, 2017.

Jelic JS, Loftus MJ, Miller AS, et al.: Benign cementoblastoma: report of an unusual case and analysis of 14 additional cases, *J Oral Maxillofac Surg* 51:1033–1037, 1993.

Ohki K, Kumamoto H, Nitta Y, et al.: Benign cementoblastoma involving multiple maxillary teeth: report of a case with a review of the literature, *Oral Surg Oral Med Oral Pathol Oral Radiol Endod* 97:53–58, 2004.

Slootweg PJ: Cementoblastoma and osteoblastoma: a comparison of histologic features, *J Oral Pathol Med* 21:385–389, 1992.

Chondroma

Czerniak B: Enchondroma.: *In Dorfman and Czerniak's bone tumors*, Philadelphia, 2016, Elsevier Saunders, pp 356–386.

Czerniak B: Enchondromatosis, In *Dorfman and Czerniak's bone tumors*, Philadelphia, 2016, Elsevier Saunders, pp 386–400.

Heitz C, Vogt BF, Bergoli RD, et al.: Chondroma in the temporomandibular region—case report and therapeutic considerations, *Oral Maxillofac Surg* 16:75–78, 2012.

Joseph NM, McGill KC, Horvai AE: Genomic profiling of low-grade intramedullary cartilage tumors can distinguish enchondroma from chondrosarcoma, *Am J Surg Pathol* 45:812–819, 2021.

Marchetti C, Mazzoni S, Bertoni F: Chondroma of the mandibular condyle—relapse of a rare benign chondroid tumor after 5 years' follow-up: case report, *Br J Oral Maxillofac Surg* 50:e69–e71, 2012.

Unni KK: *Dahlin's bone tumors: general aspects and data on 10,165 cases*, ed 6, Philadelphia, 2009, Lippincott-Raven, pp 22–40.

Chondromyxoid Fibroma

De La Peña NM, Yekzaman BR, Patra DP, et al.: Craniofacial chondromyxoid fibromas: a systematic review and analysis based on anatomic locations, *World Neurosurg*, 2021. S1878-8750(21)01637-5.

Hammad HM, Hammond HL, Kurago ZB, et al.: Chondromyxoid fibroma of the jaws: case report and review of the literature, *Oral Surg Oral Med Oral Pathol Oral Radiol Endod* 85:293–300, 1998.

Khatana S, Singh V, Gupta A: Unilocular anterior mandibular swelling, *Int J Pediatr Otorhinolaryngol* 77:964–971, 2013.

Meredith DM, Fletcher CDM, Jo VY: Chondromyxoid fibroma arising in craniofacial sites: a clinicopathologic analysis of 25 cases, *Am J Surg Pathol* 42:392–400, 2018.

Müller S, Whitaker SB, Weathers DR: Chondromyxoid fibroma of the mandible: diagnostic image cytometry findings and review of the literature, *Oral Surg Oral Med Oral Pathol* 73:465–468, 1992.

Nord KH, Lilljebjörn H, Vezzi F, et al.: *GRM1* is upregulated through gene fusion and promoter swapping in chondromyxoid fibroma, *Nat Genet* 46:474–477, 2014.

Romeo S, Duim RAJ, Bridge JA, et al.: Heterogeneous and complex rearrangements of chromosome arm 6q in chondromyxoid fibroma, *Am J Pathol* 177:1365–1376, 2010.

Vuletić M, Sušić M, Gabrić D: Chondromyxoid fibroma of the mandible in an older adult: a case report, *J Oral Maxillofac Surg Med Pathol* 30:523–527, 2018.

Wu CT, Inwards CY, O'Laughlin S, et al.: Chondromyxoid fibroma of bone: a clinicopathologic review of 278 cases, *Hum Pathol* 29:438–446, 1998.

Synovial Chondromatosis

Amary F, Perez-Casanova L, Ye H, et al.: Synovial chondromatosis and soft tissue chondroma: extraosseous cartilaginous tumor defined by *FN1* gene rearrangement, *Mod Pathol* 32:1762–1771, 2019.

Cai XY, Yang C, Chen MJ, et al.: Arthroscopic management for synovial chondromatosis of the temporomandibular joint: a retrospective review of 33 cases, *J Oral Maxillofac Surg* 70:2106–2113, 2012.

Coleman H, Chandraratnam E, Morgan G, et al.: Synovial chondrosarcoma arising in synovial chondromatosis of the temporomandibular joint, *Head Neck Pathol* 7:304–309, 2013.

Gross AJ, Houston KR, Hudson JW, et al.: A multidisciplinary approach to synovial chondromatosis of the temporomandibular joint with cranial base involvement: a brief review of the literature and case report, *J Oral Maxillofac Surg* 78:1759–1765, 2020.

Guarda-Nardini L, Piccotti F, Ferronato G, et al.: Synovial chondromatosis of the temporomandibular joint: a case description with systematic literature review, *Int J Oral Maxillofac Surg* 39:745–755, 2010.

Lee LM, Zhu YM, Zhang DD, et al.: Synovial chondromatosis of the temporomandibular joint: a clinical and arthroscopic study of 16 cases, *J Craniomaxillofac Surg* 47:607–610, 2019.

Liu X, Huang Z, Zhu W, et al.: Clinical and imaging findings of temporomandibular joint synovial chondromatosis: an analysis of 10 cases and literature review, *J Oral Maxillofac Surg* 74:2159–2168, 2016.

Meng J, Guo C, Yi B, et al.: Clinical and radiographic findings of synovial chondromatosis affecting the temporomandibular joint, *Oral Surg Oral Med Oral Pathol Oral Radiol Endod* 109:441–448, 2010.

Nishiyama M, Nozawa M, Ogi N, et al.: Computed tomographic features of synovial chondromatosis of the temporomandibular joint with a few small calcified loose bodies, *Oral Radiol* 37:236–244, 2021.

Shah SB, Ramanojam S, Gadre PK, et al.: Synovial chondromatosis of temporomandibular joint: journey through 25 decades and a case report, *J Oral Maxillofac Surg* 69:2795–2814, 2011.

Sink J, Bell B, Mesa H: Synovial chondromatosis of the temporomandibular joint: clinical, cytologic, histologic, radiologic, therapeutic aspects, and differential diagnosis of an uncommon lesion, *Oral Surg Oral Med Oral Pathol Oral Radiol* 117:e269–e274, 2014.

Von Lindern JJ, Theuerkauf I, Niederhagen B, et al.: Synovial chondromatosis of the temporomandibular joint: clinical, diagnostic, and histomorphologic findings, *Oral Surg Oral Med Oral Pathol Oral Radiol Endod* 94:31–38, 2002.

Desmoplastic Fibroma

Horvai AE, Jordan RC: Fibro-osseous lesions of the craniofacial bones: β-catenin immunohistochemical analysis and *CTNNB1* and *APC* mutation analysis, *Head Neck Pathol* 8:291–297, 2014.

Kadowaki H, Oyama Y, Nishida H, et al.: A case of desmoplastic fibroma of bone with *CTNNB1* point mutation, *Oral Surg Oral Med Oral Pathol Oral Radiol* 129:e230–e233, 2020.

Khatib B, Pogrel MA: Desmoplastic fibroma of the mandible in young children-a case series, *Int J Oral Maxillofac Surg* 46:173–180, 2017.

Madakshira MG, Bal A, Verma RK: Desmoplastic fibroma of the mandible: a rare gnathic bone tumor with a review of the literature, *Autops Case Rep* 27(9):e2019091, 2019.

Said-Al-Naief N, Fernandes R, Louis P, et al.: Desmoplastic fibroma of the jaw: a case report and review of literature, *Oral Surg Oral Med Oral Pathol Oral Radiol Endod* 101:82–94, 2006.

Shekhar MG, Reddy RS, Ravikanth M, et al.: Desmoplastic fibroma of the mandible: case report and review of literature, *Prim Dent Care* 18:115–118, 2011.

Suurmeijer AJH, Cleton-Jansen AM: Desmoplastic fibroma of bone, In WHO Classification Editorial Board, editor: *WHO classification of tumours: soft tissue and bone tumours*, ed 5, Lyon, France, 2020, IARC Press, pp 422–423.

Tandon S, Garg RK: Intraoral desmoplastic fibroma: a manifestation of tuberous sclerosis, *Fetal Pediatr Pathol* 31:195–201, 2012.

Woods TR, Cohen DM, Islam MN, et al.: Desmoplastic fibroma of the mandible: a series of three cases and review of literature, *Head Neck Pathol* 9:196–204, 2015.

Osteosarcoma

Amary MF, Bacsi K, Maggiani F, et al.: *IDH*1 and *IDH2* mutations are frequent events in central chondrosarcoma and central and periosteal chondromas but not in other mesenchymal tumours, *J Pathol* 224:334–343, 2011.

American Cancer Society: *Osteosarcoma*, https://www.cancer.org/cancer/osteosarcoma.html. Accessed March 3, 2021.

Baumhoer D, Brunner P, Eppenberger-Castori S, et al.: Osteosarcomas of the jaws differ from their peripheral counterparts and require a distinct treatment approach. Experiences from the DOESAK Registry, *Oral Oncol* 50:147–153, 2014.

Bennett JH, Thomas G, Evans AW, et al.: Osteosarcoma of the jaws: a 30-year retrospective review, *Oral Surg Oral Med Oral Pathol Oral Radiol Endod* 90:323–333, 2000.

Bertin H, Gomez-Brouchet A, Rédini F: Osteosarcoma of the jaws: an overview of the pathophysiological mechanisms, *Crit Rev Oncol Hematol* 156, 2020, 103126.

Canadian Society of Otolaryngology—Head and Neck Surgery Oncology Study Group: Osteogenic sarcoma of the mandible and maxilla: a Canadian review (1980–2000), *J Otolaryngol* 33:139–144, 2004.

Chaudhary M, Chaudhary SD: Osteosarcoma of jaws, *J Oral Maxillofac Pathol* 16:233–236, 2012.

Chen YM, Shen QC, Gokavarapu S, et al.: Osteosarcoma of the mandible: a site-specific study on survival and prognostic factors, *J Craniofac Surg* 27:1929–1933, 2016.

Duong LM, Richardson LC: Descriptive epidemiology of malignant primary osteosarcoma using population-based registries, United States, 1999–2008, *J Registry Manag* 40:59–64, 2013.

Granowski-LeCornu M, Chuang SK, Kaban LB, et al.: Osteosarcoma of the jaws: factors influencing prognosis, *J Oral Maxillofac Surg* 69:2368–2375, 2011.

Guadagnolo BA, Zagars GK, Raymond AK, et al.: Osteosarcoma of the jaw/craniofacial region. Outcomes after multimodality treatment, *Cancer* 115:3252–3270, 2009.

Guérin M, Thariat J, Ouali M, et al.: A new subtype of high-grade mandibular osteosarcoma with *RASAL1/MDM2* amplification, *Hum Pathol* 50:70–78, 2016.

Jafari F, Javdansirat S, Sanaie S, et al.: Osteosarcoma: a comprehensive review of management and treatment strategies, *Ann Diagn Pathol* 49:151654, 2020.

Jaffe N, Bruland OS, Bielack SS, editors: *Pediatric and adolescent osteosarcoma*, New York, 2009, Springer.

Kerr DA, Lopez HU, Deshpande V, et al.: Molecular distinction of chondrosarcoma from chondroblastic osteosarcoma through IDH1/2 mutations, *Am J Surg Pathol* 37:787–795, 2013.

Lee RJ, Arshi A, Schwartz HC, et al.: Characteristics and prognostic factors of osteosarcoma of the jaws: a retrospective cohort study, *JAMA Otolaryngol Head Neck Surg* 141:470–477, 2015.

Limbach AL, Lingen MW, McElherne J, et al.: The utility of MDM2 and CDK4 immunohistochemistry and *MDM2* FISH in craniofacial osteosarcoma, *Head Neck Pathol* 14:889–898, 2020.

Luo Z, Chen W, Shen X, et al.: Head and neck osteosarcoma: CT and MR imaging features, *Dentomaxillofac Radiol* 49:20190202, 2020.

Malik F, Gleysteen JP, Agarwal S: Osteosarcoma of the jaw: report of 3 cases (including the rare epithelioid variant) with review of literature, *Oral Surg Oral Med Oral Pathol Oral Radiol* 131:e71–e80, 2021.

Mirabello L, Troisi RJ, Savage SA: Osteosarcoma incidence and survival rates from 1973 to 2004: data from the Surveillance, Epidemiology, and End Results Program, *Cancer* 115:1531–1543, 2009.

Mirabello L, Zhu B, Koster R, et al.: Frequency of pathogenic germline variants in cancer-susceptibility genes in patients with osteosarcoma, *JAMA Oncol* 6:724–734, 2020.

Paparella ML, Olvi LG, Brandizzi D, et al.: Osteosarcoma of the jaw: an analysis of a series of 74 cases, *Histopathology* 63:551–557, 2013.

Patel SG, Meyers P, Huvos AG, et al.: Improved outcomes in patients with osteogenic sarcoma of the head and neck, *Cancer* 95:1495–1503, 2002.

PDQ Pediatric Treatment Editorial Board: Osteosarcoma and undifferentiated pleomorphic sarcoma of bone treatment (PDQ®): health professional version, In *PDQ Cancer Information Summaries*, Bethesda, 2021, National Cancer Institute. https://www.ncbi.nlm.nih.gov/books/NBK65942/#_NBK65942_pubdet_. Accessed March 3, 2021.

Smeele LE, Kostense PJ, van der Waal I, et al.: Effect of chemotherapy on survival of craniofacial osteosarcoma: a systematic review of 201 patients, *J Clin Oncol* 15:363–367, 1997.

Thariat J, Julieron M, Brouchet A, et al.: Osteosarcomas of the mandible: are they different from other tumor sites? *Crit Rev Oncol Hematol* 82:280–295, 2012.

Thariat J, Schouman T, Brouchet A, et al.: Osteosarcomas of the mandible: multidisciplinary management of a rare tumor of the young adult a cooperative study of the GSF-GETO, Rare Cancer Network, GETTEC/REFCOR and SFCE, *Ann Oncol* 24:824–831, 2013.

Wang S, Shi H, Yu Q: Osteosarcoma of the jaws: demographic and CT imaging features, *Dentomaxillofac Radiol* 41:37–42, 2012.

Post-irradiation Bone Sarcoma

Coca-Pelaz A, Mäkitie AA, Strojan P, et al.: Radiation-induced sarcomas of the head and neck: a systematic review, *Adv Ther* 38:90–108, 2021.

de Souza LL, Pontes HAR, Santos-Silva AR, et al.: Oral radiation-induced sarcomas: systematic review, *Head Neck* 42:2660–2668, 2020.

Liao LQ, Yan HH, Mai JH, et al.: Radiation-induced osteosarcoma of the maxilla and mandible after radiotherapy for nasopharyngeal carcinoma, *Chin J Cancer* 35:89, 2016.

Mavrogenis AF, Pala E, Guerra G, et al.: Post-radiation sarcomas: clinical outcome of 52 patients, *J Surg Oncol* 150:570–576, 2012.

Samartzis D, Nishi N, Hayashi M, et al.: Exposure to ionizing radiation and development of bone sarcoma: new insights based on atomic-bomb survivors of Hiroshima and Nagasaki, *J Bone Joint Surg Am* 93:1008–1015, 2011.

Sheppard DG, Libshitz HI: Post-radiation sarcomas: a review of the clinical and imaging features in 63 cases, *Clin Radiol* 56:22–29, 2001.

Chondrosarcoma

Almansoori AA, Kim HY, Kim B, et al.: Chondrosarcoma of the jaw: a retrospective series, *Oral Surg Oral Med Oral Pathol Oral Radiol* 128:106–111, 2019.

American Cancer Society: *Bone cancer early detection, diagnosis, and staging*, https://www.cancer.org/cancer/bone-cancer/detection-diagnosis-staging/survival-statistics.html. Accessed June 29, 2021.

Asioli S, Ruengwanichayakun P, Zoli M, et al.: Association of clinicopathological features with outcome in chondrosarcomas of the head and neck, *Otolaryngol Head Neck Surg* 164:807–814, 2021.

Coca-Pelaz A, Rodrigo JP, Triantafyllou A, et al.: Chondrosarcomas of the head and neck, *Eur Arch Otorhinolaryngol* 271:2601–2609, 2014.

de Souza LL, Pontes FSC, Fonseca FP, et al.: Chondrosarcoma of the jaw bones: a review of 224 cases reported to date and an analysis of prognostic factors, *Int J Oral Maxillofac Surg* 48:452–460, 2019.

Ellis MA, Gerry DR, Byrd JK: Head and neck chondrosarcomas: analysis of the Surveillance, *Epidemiology, and End Results database, Head Neck* 38:1359–1366, 2016.

Faro TF, Martins-de-Barros AV, Lima GTWF, et al.: Chondrosarcoma of the temporomandibular joint: systematic review and survival analysis of cases reported to date, *Head Neck Pathol* 15:923–934, 2021.

Garrington GE, Collett WK: Chondrosarcoma. I.: A selected literature review, *J Oral Pathol* 17:1–11, 1988.

Garrington GE, Collett WK: Chondrosarcoma. II. Chondrosarcoma of the jaws: analysis of 37 cases, *J Oral Pathol* 17:12–20, 1988.

Giuffrida AY, Burgueno JE, Koniaris LG, et al.: Chondrosarcoma in the United States (1973 to 2003): an analysis of 2890 cases from the SEER database, *J Bone Joint Surg Am* 9:1063–1072, 2009.

Hong P, Taylor SM, Trites JR, et al.: Chondrosarcoma of the head and neck: report of 11 cases and literature review, *J Otolaryngol Head Neck Surg* 38:279–285, 2009.

Nakashima Y, Unni KK, Shives TC, et al.: Mesenchymal chondrosarcoma of bone and soft tissue: a review of 111 cases, *Cancer* 57:2444–2453, 1985.

National Comprehensive Care Network: NCCN Clinical Practice Guidelines in Oncology, Bone Cancer (Version 1.2021). https://www.nccn.org/professionals/physician_gls/pdf/bone.pdf. Accessed March 12, 2021.

Pelliteri PK, Ferlito A, Fagan JJ, et al.: Mesenchymal chondrosarcoma of the head and neck, *Oral Oncol* 43:970–975, 2007.

Pontes HAR, Pontes FSC, de Abreu MC, et al.: Clinicopathological analysis of head and neck chondrosarcoma: three case reports and literature review, *Int J Oral Maxillofac Surg* 41:203–210, 2012.

Prado FO, Nishimoto IN, Perez DE, et al.: Head and neck chondrosarcoma: analysis of 16 cases, *Br J Oral Maxillofac Surg* 47:555–557, 2009.

Saito K, Unni KK, Wollan PC, et al.: Chondrosarcoma of the jaw and facial bones, *Cancer* 76:1550–1558, 1995.

Schneiderman BA, Kliethermes SA, Nystrom LM: Survival in mesenchymal chondrosarcoma varies based on age and tumor location: a survival analysis of the SEER database, *Clin Orthop Relat Res* 475:799–805, 2017.

Tien N, Chaisuparat R, Fernandes R, et al.: Mesenchymal chondrosarcoma of the maxilla: case report and literature review, *J Oral Maxillofac Surg* 65:1260–1266, 2007.

Vencio EF, Reeve CM, Unni KK, et al.: Mesenchymal chondrosarcoma of the jaw bones. Clinicopathologic study of 19 cases, *Cancer* 82:2350–2355, 1998.

Wang L, Motoi T, Khanin R, et al.: Identification of a novel, recurrent *HEY1-NCOA2* fusion in mesenchymal chondrosarcoma based on a genome-wide screen of exon-level expression data, *Genes Chromosomes Cancer* 51:127–139, 2012.

Ewing Sarcoma

Bornstein MM, von Arx T, Altermatt HJ: Loss of pulp sensitivity and pain as the first symptoms of Ewing's sarcoma in the right maxillary sinus and alveolar process: report of a case, *J Endod* 34:1549–1553, 2009.

Bosma SE, Ayu O, Fiocco M, et al.: Prognostic factors for survival in Ewing sarcoma: a systematic review, *Surg Oncol* 27:603–610, 2018.

Casaroto AR, DA Silva Sampieri MB, Soares CT, et al.: Ewing's sarcoma family tumors in the jaws: case report, immunohistochemical analysis and literature review, *In Vivo* 31:481–491, 2017.

Grünewald TGP, Cidre-Aranaz F, Surdez D, et al.: Ewing sarcoma, *Nat Rev Dis Primers* 4:5, 2018.

Hafezi S, Seethala RR, Stelow EB, et al.: Ewing's family of tumors of the sinonasal tract and maxillary bone, *Head Neck Pathol* 5:8–16, 2011.

Karimi A, Shirinbak I, Beshkar M, et al.: Ewing sarcoma of the jaws, *J Craniofac Surg* 22:1657–1660, 2011.

Ko E, Brouns EREA, Korones DN, et al.: Primary Ewing sarcoma of the anterior mandible localized to the midline, *Oral Surg Oral Med Oral Pathol Oral Radiol* 115:e46–e50, 2013.

Margaix-Muñoz M, Bagán J, Poveda-Roda R: Ewing sarcoma of the oral cavity. A review, *J Clin Exp Dent* 9:e294–e301, 2017.

National Cancer Institute: *Ewing Sarcoma Treatment (PDQ) (website)*, https://www.cancer.gov/types/bone/hp/ewing-treatment-pdq. Accessed June 29, 2021.

Rehman R, Osto M, Parry N, et al.: Ewing sarcoma of the craniofacial bones: a qualitative systematic review, *Otolaryngol Head Neck Surg*, 2021b. 1945998211022228, 2021.

Sbaraglia M, Righi A, Gambarotti M, et al.: Ewing sarcoma and Ewing-like tumors, *Virchows Arch* 476:109–119, 2020.

Whaley JT, Indelicato DJ, Morris CG, et al.: Ewing sarcoma of the head and neck, *Am J Clin Oncol* 33:321–326, 2010.

Metastatic Tumors to the Jaws

Akinbami BO: Metastatic carcinoma of the jaws: a review of literature, *Niger J Med* 18:139–142, 2009.

D'Silva NJ, Summerlin DJ, Cordell KG, et al.: Metastatic tumors in the jaws: a retrospective study of 114 cases, *J Am Dent Assoc* 137:1667–1672, 2006.

Hashimoto N, Kurihara K, Yamasaki H, et al.: Pathologic characteristics of metastatic carcinoma in the human mandible, *J Oral Pathol* 16:362–367, 1987.

Hirshberg A, Shnaiderman-Shapiro A, Kaplan I, et al.: Metastatic tumors to the oral cavity—pathogenesis and analysis of 673 cases, *Oral Oncol* 44:743–752, 2008.

Irani S: Metastasis to the jawbones: a review of 453 cases, *J Int Soc Prev Community Dent* 7:71–81, 2017.

Kumar GS, Manjunatha BS: Metastatic tumors to the jaws and oral cavity, *J Oral Maxillofac Pathol* 17:71–75, 2013.

15

Odontogenic Cysts and Tumors

Odontogenic cysts and tumors constitute an important aspect of oral and maxillofacial pathology. Odontogenic cysts are encountered relatively commonly in dental practice. Odontogenic tumors, by contrast, are uncommon lesions. Even in the specialized oral and maxillofacial pathology laboratory, less than 1% of all specimens received are odontogenic tumors.

ODONTOGENIC CYSTS

With rare exceptions, epithelium-lined cysts in bone are seen only in the jaws. Other than a few cysts that may result from the inclusion of epithelium along embryonic lines of fusion, most jaw cysts are lined by epithelium that is derived from odontogenic epithelium. These are referred to as **odontogenic cysts.** (Non-odontogenic jaw cysts are discussed in Chapter 1.)

Odontogenic cysts are subclassified as developmental or inflammatory in origin. The inciting factors that initiate the formation of **developmental cysts** are unknown, but these lesions do not appear to be the result of an inflammatory reaction. **Inflammatory cysts** are the result of inflammation. Box 15.1 presents categories of odontogenic cysts modified from the 2022 World Health Organization (WHO) classification. (The periapical cyst is discussed in Chapter 3.)

◆ DENTIGEROUS CYST (FOLLICULAR CYST)

The **dentigerous cyst** is defined as a cyst that originates by the separation of the follicle from around the crown of an unerupted tooth. This is the most common type of developmental odontogenic cyst, making up about 20% of all epithelium-lined cysts of the jaws. The dentigerous cyst encloses the crown of an unerupted tooth and is attached to the tooth at the cementoenamel junction (Fig. 15.1). The pathogenesis of this cyst is uncertain, but apparently it develops by accumulation of fluid between the reduced enamel epithelium and the tooth crown.

Although most dentigerous cysts are considered to be developmental in origin, there are some examples that appear to have an inflammatory pathogenesis. For example, it has been suggested that, on occasion, a dentigerous cyst may develop around the crown of an unerupted permanent tooth as a result of periapical inflammation from an overlying primary tooth (Fig. 15.2). Another scenario involves a partially erupted mandibular third molar that develops an inflamed cystlike lesion along the distal or buccal aspect. Although many such lesions probably are due to inflammation associated with recurrent pericoronitis, these lesions are usually diagnosed as examples of dentigerous cyst, especially because it is impossible to determine histopathologically whether the inflammatory component is primary or secondary in nature. The term **paradental cyst** sometimes has been applied to these lesions, but the use of this term in the literature is confusing because it also has been used to describe examples of what is known as the *buccal bifurcation cyst* (see page 704).

Clinical and Radiographic Features

Although dentigerous cysts may occur in association with any unerupted tooth, most often they involve mandibular third molars, accounting for approximately 65% of all cases. Other relatively frequent sites include maxillary canines, maxillary third molars, and mandibular second premolars. Dentigerous cysts rarely involve unerupted deciduous teeth. Occasionally, they are associated with supernumerary teeth or odontomas. Multiple dentigerous cysts have been reported, although this is an infrequent finding.

Although dentigerous cysts may be encountered in patients across a wide age range, they are discovered most frequently in patients between 10 and 30 years of age. There is a slight male predilection, and the prevalence is higher for whites than for blacks. Small dentigerous cysts are usually completely asymptomatic and are discovered only on a routine radiographic examination or when films are taken to determine the reason for the failure of a tooth to erupt. Dentigerous cysts can grow to a considerable size, and large cysts may be associated with a painless expansion of the bone in the involved area. Extensive lesions may result in facial asymmetry. Large dentigerous cysts are uncommon, and most lesions that are considered to be large dentigerous cysts on radiographic examination prove to be odontogenic keratocysts (OKCs) or ameloblastomas. Dentigerous cysts may become infected and be associated with pain and swelling. Such infections may arise in a dentigerous cyst that is associated with a partially erupted tooth or by extension from a periapical or periodontal lesion that affects an adjacent tooth.

• BOX 15.1 Classification of Odontogenic Cysts

Developmental

- Dentigerous cyst
- Eruption cyst
- Odontogenic keratocyst (OKC)*
- Orthokeratinized odontogenic cyst
- Gingival (alveolar) cyst of the newborn
- Gingival cyst of the adult
- Lateral periodontal cyst
- Calcifying odontogenic cyst†
- Glandular odontogenic cyst

Inflammatory

- Periapical (radicular) cyst
- Residual periapical (radicular) cyst
- Buccal bifurcation cyst

*The OKC currently is included with the odontogenic cysts in the 2022 World Health Organization (WHO) classification; however, some authors and clinicians favor classifying it in the odontogenic tumor category ("keratocystic odontogenic tumor").

†Some odontogenic "ghost cell" lesions occur as solid, neoplastic growths that should be classified as odontogenic tumors ("dentinogenic ghost cell tumor" and "ghost cell odontogenic carcinoma").

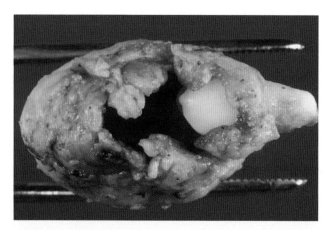

• **Fig. 15.1 Dentigerous Cyst.** Gross specimen of a dentigerous cyst involving a maxillary canine tooth. The cyst has been cut open to show the cyst-to-crown relationship.

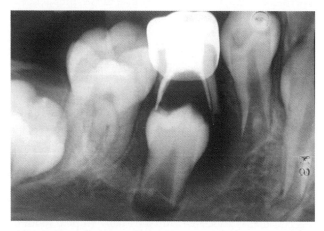

• **Fig. 15.2 Dentigerous Cyst.** Well-circumscribed radiolucency surrounding the crown of the mandibular second molar. The overlying primary molar previously had root canal therapy.

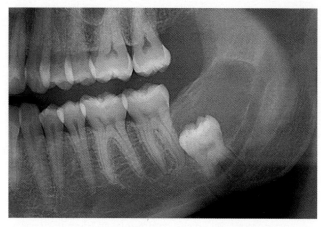

• **Fig. 15.3 Dentigerous Cyst.** Unilocular radiolucency surrounding the crown of an impacted mandibular third molar. (Courtesy of Dr. William Dunlap.)

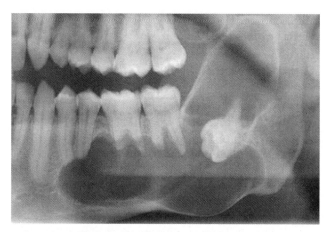

• **Fig. 15.4 Dentigerous Cyst.** This unusually large dentigerous cyst shows a somewhat multilocular radiographic pattern. Note the root resorption of the adjacent molars and bicuspids. (Courtesy of Dr. John Werther.)

Radiographically, the dentigerous cyst typically shows a unilocular radiolucent area that is associated with the crown of an unerupted tooth (Fig. 15.3). The radiolucency usually has a well-defined and often corticated border, but an infected cyst may show ill-defined borders. A large dentigerous cyst may give the impression of a multilocular process because of the persistence of bone trabeculae within the radiolucency (Fig. 15.4). The cyst-to-crown relationship shows several radiographic variations. In the **central** variety, which is the most common, the cyst surrounds the crown of the tooth and the crown projects into the cyst (Fig. 15.5). The **lateral** variety is usually associated with mesioangular impacted mandibular third molars that are partially erupted. The cyst grows laterally along the root surface and partially surrounds the crown (Fig. 15.6). In the **circumferential** variant, the cyst surrounds the crown and extends for some distance along the root so that a significant portion of the root appears to lie within the cyst (Fig. 15.7). Rarely, a third molar may be displaced to the

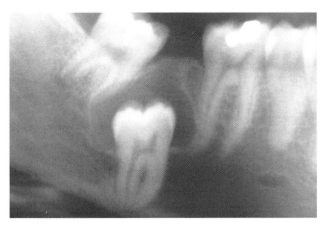

• **Fig. 15.5 Dentigerous Cyst.** Central type showing the crown projecting into the cystic cavity. (Courtesy of Dr. Stephen E. Irwin.)

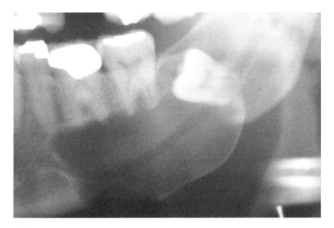

• **Fig. 15.6 Dentigerous Cyst.** Lateral variety showing a large cyst along the mesial root of the unerupted molar. This cyst exhibited mucous cell prosoplasia. (Courtesy of Dr. John R. Cramer.)

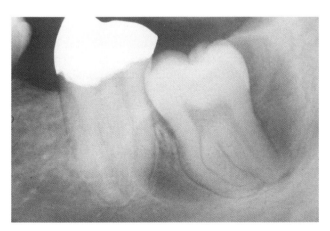

• **Fig. 15.7 Dentigerous Cyst.** Circumferential variety showing cyst extension along the mesial and distal roots of the unerupted tooth. (Courtesy of Dr. Richard Marks.)

lower border of the mandible or higher up into the ascending ramus. Maxillary anterior teeth may be displaced into the floor of the nose, and other maxillary teeth may be moved through the maxillary sinus to the floor of the orbit. Dentigerous cysts may displace the involved tooth for a

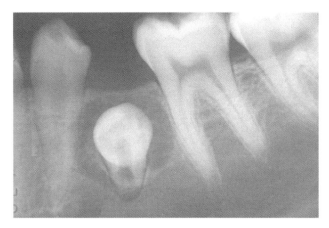

• **Fig. 15.8 Dentigerous Cyst or Enlarged Follicle.** Radiolucent lesion involving the crown of an unerupted mandibular premolar. Distinction between a dentigerous cyst and an enlarged follicle for a lesion of this size by radiographic and even histopathologic means is difficult, if not impossible. (Courtesy of Dr. Wally Austelle.)

considerable distance. Root resorption of adjacent erupted teeth can occur (see Fig. 15.4).

Radiographic distinction between a small dentigerous cyst and an enlarged follicle about the crown of an unerupted tooth is difficult and may be largely an academic exercise (Fig. 15.8). For the lesion to be considered a dentigerous cyst, some investigators believe that the radiolucent space surrounding the tooth crown should be at least 3–4 mm in diameter. Radiographic findings are not diagnostic for a dentigerous cyst, however, because OKCs, unilocular ameloblastomas, and many other odontogenic and nonodontogenic tumors may have radiographic features that are essentially identical to those of a dentigerous cyst.

Histopathologic Features

The histopathologic features of dentigerous cysts vary, depending on whether the cyst is inflamed or not inflamed. In the **noninflamed dentigerous cyst,** the fibrous connective tissue wall is loosely arranged and contains considerable glycosaminoglycan ground substance. Small islands or cords of inactive-appearing odontogenic epithelial rests may be present in the fibrous wall. Occasionally these rests may be numerous, and at times pathologists who are not familiar with oral lesions have misinterpreted this finding as ameloblastoma. The epithelial lining consists of two to four layers of flattened nonkeratinizing cells, and the epithelium and connective tissue interface is flat (Fig. 15.9).

In the fairly common **inflamed dentigerous cyst,** the fibrous wall is more collagenized, with a variable infiltration of chronic inflammatory cells. The epithelial lining may show varying amounts of hyperplasia with the development of rete ridges and more definite squamous features (Fig. 15.10). A keratinized surface is sometimes seen, but these changes must be differentiated from those observed in the OKC. Focal areas of mucous cells may be found in the epithelial lining of dentigerous cysts (Fig. 15.11). Rarely,

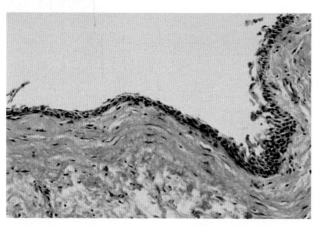

• **Fig. 15.9 Dentigerous Cyst.** This noninflamed dentigerous cyst shows a thin, nonkeratinized epithelial lining.

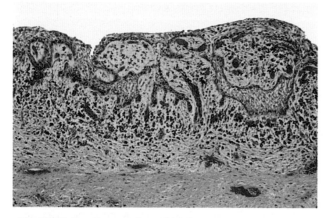

• **Fig. 15.10 Dentigerous Cyst.** This inflamed dentigerous cyst shows a thicker epithelial lining with hyperplastic rete ridges. The fibrous cyst capsule shows a diffuse chronic inflammatory infiltrate.

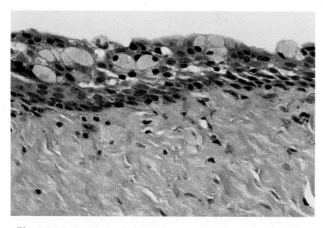

• **Fig. 15.11 Dentigerous Cyst.** Scattered mucous cells can be seen within the epithelial lining.

ciliated columnar cells are present. Small nests of sebaceous cells rarely may be noted within the fibrous cyst wall. These mucous, ciliated, and sebaceous elements are believed to represent the multipotentiality of the odontogenic epithelial lining in a dentigerous cyst.

Gross examination of the wall of a dentigerous cyst may reveal one or several areas of nodular thickening on the luminal surface. These areas must be examined microscopically to rule out the presence of early neoplastic change.

Because a thin layer of reduced enamel epithelium normally lines the dental follicle surrounding the crown of an unerupted tooth, it can be difficult to distinguish a small dentigerous cyst from simply a normal or enlarged dental follicle based on microscopic features alone. Again, this distinction often represents largely an academic exercise; the most important consideration is ensuring that the lesion does not represent a more significant pathologic process (e.g., OKC or ameloblastoma).

Treatment and Prognosis

The usual treatment for a dentigerous cyst is careful enucleation of the cyst together with removal of the unerupted tooth. If eruption of the involved tooth is considered feasible, then the tooth may be left in place after partial removal of the cyst wall. Patients may need orthodontic treatment to assist eruption. Large dentigerous cysts also may be treated by marsupialization. This permits decompression of the cyst, with a resulting reduction in the size of the bone defect. The cyst can then be excised at a later date, with a less extensive surgical procedure. In situations where the tooth roots are in close proximity to the inferior alveolar nerve, coronectomy and cyst removal can be performed. This procedure allows the roots to remain in place, thereby reducing the risk of damage to the neurovascular bundle.

The prognosis for most dentigerous cysts is excellent, and recurrence seldom is noted after complete removal of the cyst. However, several potential complications must be considered. Much has been written about the possibility that the lining of a dentigerous cyst might undergo neoplastic transformation to an **ameloblastoma.** Although undoubtedly this can occur, the frequency of such neoplastic transformation is low. Rarely, a **squamous cell carcinoma** may arise in the lining of a dentigerous cyst (see page 705). It is likely that some **intraosseous mucoepidermoid carcinomas** (see page 496) develop from mucous cells in the lining of a dentigerous cyst.

◆ ERUPTION CYST (ERUPTION HEMATOMA)

The **eruption cyst** is the soft tissue analogue of the dentigerous cyst. The cyst develops as a result of separation of the dental follicle from around the crown of an erupting tooth that is within the soft tissues overlying the alveolar bone.

Clinical Features

The eruption cyst appears as a soft, often translucent swelling in the gingival mucosa overlying the crown of an erupting deciduous or permanent tooth. Most examples are seen in children younger than age 10. Although the cyst can occur around any tooth, the lesion most commonly has been associated with the central incisors and first molars in both dentitions. On occasion, bilateral cysts may be observed. Surface trauma may result in a considerable amount of blood in the cystic fluid, which imparts a blue to purple-brown color. Such lesions sometimes are referred to as **eruption hematomas** (Fig. 15.12).

Histopathologic Features

Intact eruption cysts seldom are submitted to the oral and maxillofacial pathology laboratory, and most examples consist of the excised roof of the cyst, which has been removed to facilitate tooth eruption. These show surface oral epithelium on the superior aspect. The underlying lamina propria shows a variable inflammatory cell infiltrate. The deep portion of the specimen, which represents the roof of the cyst, shows a thin layer of nonkeratinizing squamous epithelium (Fig. 15.13).

Treatment and Prognosis

Treatment may not be required because the cyst usually ruptures spontaneously, permitting the tooth to erupt. If this does not occur, then simple excision of the roof of the cyst generally permits speedy eruption of the tooth.

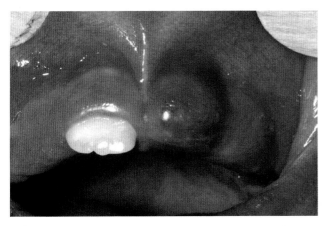

• **Fig. 15.12 Eruption Cyst.** This soft gingival swelling contains considerable blood and can also be designated as an eruption hematoma.

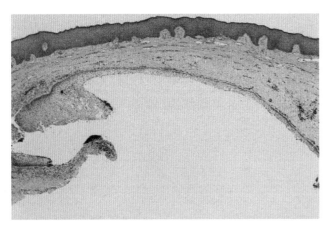

• **Fig. 15.13 Eruption Cyst.** A cystic epithelial cavity can be seen below the mucosal surface.

◆ PRIMORDIAL CYST

The concept and meaning of the term **primordial cyst** often have been controversial and confusing. In the older classification of cysts used in the United States, the primordial cyst was considered to originate from cystic degeneration of the enamel organ epithelium before the development of dental hard tissue. Therefore, the primordial cyst would occur in place of a tooth.

In the mid-1950s, oral and maxillofacial pathologists in Europe introduced the term **odontogenic keratocyst (OKC)** to denote a cyst with specific histopathologic features and clinical behavior, which was believed to arise from the dental lamina (i.e., the dental primordium). Subsequently, this concept was widely accepted, and the terms *odontogenic keratocyst* and *primordial cyst* were used synonymously. The 1972 WHO classification used the designation *primordial cyst* as the preferred term for this lesion. The 1992 WHO classification, however, listed *odontogenic keratocyst* as the preferred designation.

Almost all examples of so-called primordial cysts (i.e., a cyst that develops in the place of a tooth) microscopically will be OKCs (Fig. 15.14). Whether there could be such a radiographic presentation that is not microscopically an OKC is still unsettled. If such a lesion exists, then it must be exceedingly rare.

◆ ODONTOGENIC KERATOCYST (KERATOCYSTIC ODONTOGENIC TUMOR)

The **odontogenic keratocyst (OKC)** is a distinctive form of developmental odontogenic cyst that deserves special consideration because of its specific histopathologic features and potentially aggressive clinical behavior. There is general agreement that the OKC arises from cell rests of the dental lamina. This cyst shows a different growth mechanism and biologic behavior from the more common dentigerous cyst and radicular cyst.

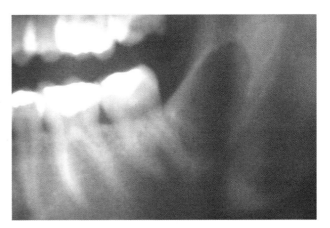

• **Fig. 15.14 Primordial Cyst.** This patient gave no history of extraction of the third molar. A cyst is located in the third molar area. The cyst was excised, and histopathologic examination revealed an odontogenic keratocyst (OKC).

Some investigators have suggested that the OKC be regarded as a benign cystic neoplasm rather than a cyst. Indeed, in the 2005 WHO monograph on head and neck tumors, this lesion was reclassified under the name **keratocystic odontogenic tumor (KCOT)**. However, subsequent editions of the WHO classification reverted to using OKC as the preferred designation. The arguments to support classification as a tumor largely rely on studies that have shown certain molecular genetic alterations that are also present in some neoplasms. Recent studies have reported that 93% of sporadic OKCs, as well as 90% of OKCs associated with the nevoid basal cell carcinoma syndrome, show inactivating mutations of the *PTCH1* gene, an important component of the Hedgehog signaling pathway. When compared to other odontogenic cysts, the OKC shows significantly greater expression of proliferating cell nuclear antigen (PCNA) and Ki-67, especially in the suprabasilar layer. Also, genetic analyses have demonstrated loss of heterozygosity for various other tumor suppressor genes (*p16, p53, MCC, TSLC1, LATS2,* and *FHIT*) in many OKCs.

Whether such molecular findings warrant reclassification of the OKC as a neoplasm (KCOT) remains a hotly debated topic in oral and maxillofacial pathology circles. The authors currently favor retaining "odontogenic keratocyst" as the primary term for this lesion, although both terms are acceptable and should be considered synonymous. Regardless of which term is preferred, these lesions are significant for three reasons:

1. Greater growth potential than most other odontogenic cysts
2. Higher recurrence rate
3. Possible association with the nevoid basal cell carcinoma syndrome

Although there are wide variations in the reported frequency of OKCs compared with that of other types of odontogenic cysts, most studies indicate that OKCs make up 3%–11% of all odontogenic cysts.

Clinical and Radiographic Features

OKCs may be found in patients who range in age from infancy to old age, but about 60% of all cases are diagnosed in people between 10 and 40 years of age. There is a slight male predilection. The mandible is involved in 60%–80% of cases, with a marked tendency to involve the posterior body and ramus (Fig. 15.15).

Small OKCs are usually asymptomatic and discovered only during the course of a radiographic examination. Larger OKCs may be associated with pain, swelling, or drainage. Some extremely large cysts, however, may cause no symptoms.

OKCs tend to grow in an anteroposterior direction within the medullary cavity of the bone without causing obvious bone expansion. This feature may be useful in differential clinical and radiographic diagnosis because dentigerous and radicular cysts of comparable size are usually associated with bony expansion. Multiple OKCs may be present, and

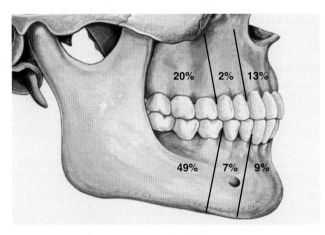

• **Fig. 15.15 Odontogenic Keratocyst (OKC).** Relative distribution of OKCs in the jaws.

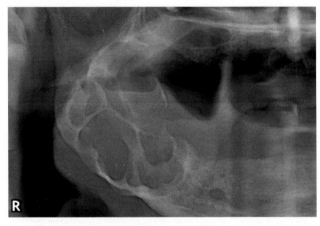

• **Fig. 15.16 Odontogenic Keratocyst (OKC).** Large, multilocular cyst involving most of the angle and ramus of the right mandible. (Courtesy of Dr. Dan Cook.)

such patients should be evaluated for other manifestations of the **nevoid basal cell carcinoma (Gorlin) syndrome** (see page 694).

OKCs demonstrate a well-defined radiolucent area with smooth and often corticated margins. Large lesions, particularly in the posterior body and ramus of the mandible, may appear multilocular (Fig. 15.16). An unerupted tooth is involved in the lesion in 25%–40% of cases; in such instances, the radiographic features suggest the diagnosis of dentigerous cyst (Figs. 15.17 and 15.18). In these cases, the cyst has presumably arisen from dental lamina rests near an unerupted tooth and has grown to envelop the unerupted tooth. Resorption of the roots of erupted teeth adjacent to OKCs is less common than that noted with dentigerous and radicular cysts.

The diagnosis of OKC is based on the histopathologic features. The radiographic findings, although often highly suggestive, are not diagnostic. The radiographic findings in an OKC may simulate those of a dentigerous cyst, a radicular cyst, a residual cyst, a lateral periodontal cyst (Fig. 15.19), or the so-called globulomaxillary cyst (which is no longer considered to be a true entity). OKCs of the anterior midline

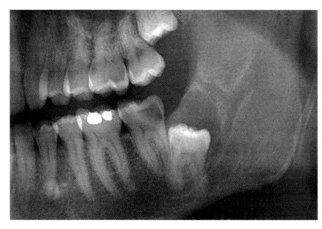

• **Fig. 15.17 Odontogenic Keratocyst (OKC).** Small radiolucency surrounding the crown of the mandibular third molar. Such lesions underscore the importance of microscopic examination of even small pericoronal radiolucencies. (Courtesy of Dr. Chad Seubert.)

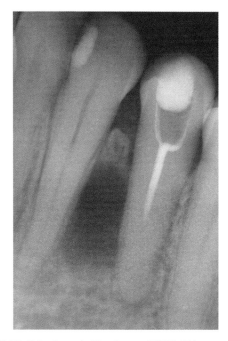

• **Fig. 15.19 Odontogenic Keratocyst (OKC).** This cyst cannot be radiographically differentiated from a lateral periodontal cyst. (Courtesy of Dr. Keith Lemmerman.)

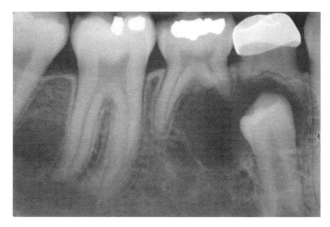

• **Fig. 15.18 Odontogenic Keratocyst (OKC).** This cyst involves the crown of an unerupted premolar. Radiographically, this lesion cannot be differentiated from a dentigerous cyst.

maxillary region can mimic nasopalatine duct cysts (Fig. 15.20). For unknown reasons, this particular subset of keratocyst usually occurs in older individuals with a mean age of nearly 70 years. Rare examples of peripheral OKCs within the gingival soft tissues have been reported.

Histopathologic Features

The OKC typically shows a thin, friable wall, which is often difficult to enucleate from the bone in one piece. The cystic lumen may contain a clear liquid that is similar to a transudate of serum, or it may be filled with a cheesy material that, on microscopic examination, consists of keratinaceous debris. Microscopically, the thin fibrous wall is usually devoid of significant inflammation. The epithelial lining is composed of a uniform layer of stratified squamous epithelium, usually four to eight cells in thickness. The epithelium and connective tissue interface is usually flat, and rete ridge formation is inconspicuous. Detachment of portions of the cyst-lining epithelium from the fibrous wall is commonly

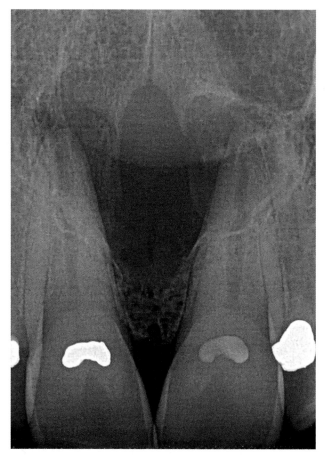

• **Fig. 15.20 Odontogenic Keratocyst (OKC).** This radiolucency in the anterior midline maxillary region mimics a nasopalatine duct cyst. (Courtesy of Dr. Trent Tucker.)

observed. The luminal surface shows flattened parakeratotic epithelial cells, which exhibit a wavy or corrugated appearance (Fig. 15.21). On occasion, isolated foci of orthokeratin production may be found in addition to the parakeratin. The basal epithelial layer is composed of a palisaded layer of cuboidal or columnar epithelial cells, which are often hyperchromatic. Small satellite cysts, cords, or islands of odontogenic epithelium may be seen within the fibrous wall. Rare examples of a so-called solid variant of odontogenic keratocyst have been described, which are characterized by a combination of both solid islands of odontogenic epithelium and keratin-filled cystic spaces. In rare instances, cartilage has been observed in the wall of an OKC.

In the presence of inflammatory changes, the typical features of the OKC may be altered. The parakeratinized luminal surface may disappear, and the epithelium may proliferate to form rete ridges with the loss of the characteristic palisaded basal layer (Fig. 15.22). When these changes involve most of the cyst lining, the diagnosis of OKC cannot be confirmed unless other sections show the typical features described earlier.

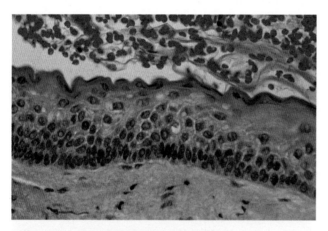

• **Fig. 15.21 Odontogenic Keratocyst (OKC).** The epithelial lining is 6–8 cells thick, with a hyperchromatic and palisaded basal cell layer. Note the corrugated parakeratotic surface.

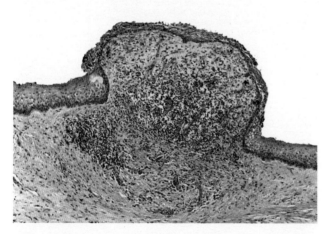

• **Fig. 15.22 Odontogenic Keratocyst (OKC).** The characteristic microscopic features have been lost in the central area of this portion of the cystic lining because of the heavy chronic inflammatory cell infiltrate.

In the past, some investigators recognized a purely orthokeratotic variant of the OKC. However, these cysts do not demonstrate a hyperchromatic and palisaded basal cell layer, which is so characteristic of true OKCs. In addition, the clinical behavior of these orthokeratinized cysts differs markedly from that of the typical parakeratinized cysts described in this section. Therefore, these orthokeratinizing cysts should be classified as a separate entity (see following section).

Treatment and Prognosis

Although the presence of an OKC may be suspected on clinical or radiographic grounds, histopathologic confirmation is required for the diagnosis. Consequently, most OKCs are treated similarly to other odontogenic cysts—i.e., by enucleation and curettage. Complete removal of the cyst in one piece is often difficult because of the thin, friable nature of the cyst wall. In contrast to other odontogenic cysts, OKCs often tend to recur after treatment. Whether this is due to fragments of the original cyst that were not removed at the time of the operation or a "new" cyst that has developed from dental lamina rests in the general area of the original cyst cannot be determined with certainty.

The reported frequency of recurrence in various studies ranges from 5% to 62%. This wide variation may be related to the total number of cases studied, the length of follow-up periods, and the inclusion or exclusion of orthokeratinized cysts in the study group. Several reports that include large numbers of cases indicate a recurrence rate of approximately 21%–30%. Recurrence is encountered more often in mandibular OKCs, particularly those in the posterior body and ramus. Multiple recurrences are not unusual. Although many OKCs recur within 5 years of the original surgery, a significant number of recurrences may not be manifested until 10 or more years after the original surgical procedure. Long-term clinical and radiographic follow-up, therefore, is necessary.

Many surgeons recommend peripheral ostectomy of the bony cavity with a bone bur to reduce the frequency of recurrence. Others advocate chemical cauterization of the bony cavity with Carnoy's solution after cyst removal (although use of Carnoy's solution may not be permitted by many hospitals). Intraluminal injection of Carnoy's solution also has been used to free the cyst from the bony wall, thereby allowing easier removal with a lower recurrence rate. After cystotomy and incisional biopsy, some surgeons have treated large OKCs by insertion of a polyethylene drainage tube to allow decompression and subsequent reduction in size of the cystic cavity (Fig. 15.23). Such decompression treatment results in thickening of the cyst lining, allowing easier removal with an apparently lower recurrence rate.

Other than the tendency for recurrences, the overall prognosis for most OKCs is good. Occasionally, a locally aggressive OKC cannot be controlled without local resection and bone grafting. In extremely rare instances, keratocysts have been seen to extend up into the skull base region. A few examples of carcinoma arising in an OKC have been

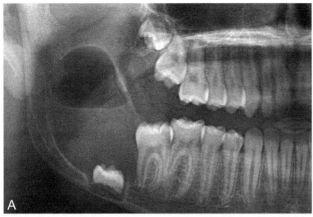

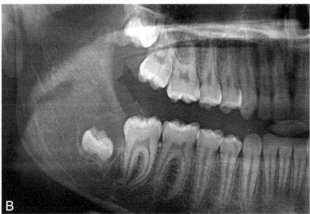

• **Fig. 15.23 Decompression of an Odontogenic Keratocyst (OKC). A,** Large unilocular radiolucency associated with the right mandibular third molar. **B,** Six months after insertion of a polyethylene drainage tube to allow decompression, the cyst has shrunk and the third molar has migrated upward. (Courtesy of Dr. Brad Gregory.)

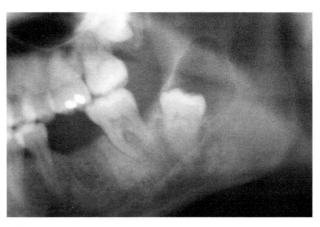

• **Fig. 15.24 Orthokeratinized Odontogenic Cyst.** Small unilocular radiolucency associated with the impacted mandibular left third molar. (Courtesy of Dr. Tom McDonald.)

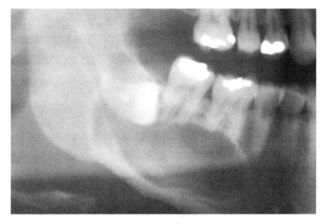

• **Fig. 15.25 Orthokeratinized Odontogenic Cyst.** A large cyst involving a horizontally impacted lower third molar. (Courtesy of Dr. Carroll Gallagher.)

reported, but the propensity for an OKC to undergo malignant alteration is no greater and is possibly less than that for other types of odontogenic cysts. Patients with OKCs should be evaluated for manifestations of the nevoid basal cell carcinoma syndrome (see page 694), particularly if the patient is in the first or second decade of life or if multiple keratocysts are identified.

♦ ORTHOKERATINIZED ODONTOGENIC CYST

The designation **orthokeratinized odontogenic cyst** does not denote a specific clinical type of odontogenic cyst but refers only to an odontogenic cyst that microscopically has an orthokeratinized epithelial lining. Although such lesions were originally called the *orthokeratinized variant of odontogenic keratocyst,* it is generally accepted that they are clinicopathologically different from the more common parakeratinized odontogenic keratocyst (OKC) and should be placed into a different category. Orthokeratinized odontogenic cysts represent 7%–17% of all keratinizing jaw cysts.

Clinical and Radiographic Features

Orthokeratinized odontogenic cysts occur predominantly in young adults and show a 2.6:1 male-to-female ratio. The lesion occurs more frequently in the mandible than the maxilla (3:1 ratio), with a tendency to involve the posterior areas of the jaws. They have no clinical or radiographic features that differentiate them from other inflammatory or developmental odontogenic cysts. The lesion usually appears as a unilocular radiolucency, but occasional examples have been multilocular. About two-thirds of orthokeratinized odontogenic cysts are encountered in a lesion that appears clinically and radiographically to represent a dentigerous cyst; they most often involve an unerupted mandibular third molar tooth (Figs. 15.24 and 15.25). The size can vary from less than 1 cm to large lesions greater than 7 cm in diameter. Occasional examples of multiple orthokeratinized odontogenic cysts have been described.

Histopathologic Features

The cyst lining is composed of stratified squamous epithelium, which shows an orthokeratotic surface of varying thickness. Keratohyaline granules may be prominent in the superficial

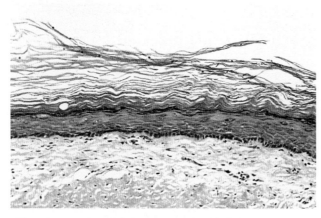

• **Fig. 15.26 Orthokeratinized Odontogenic Cyst.** Microscopic features showing a thin epithelial lining. The basal epithelial layer does not demonstrate palisading. Keratohyaline granules are present, and a thick layer of orthokeratin is seen on the luminal surface.

epithelial layer subjacent to the orthokeratin. In rare instances, focal sebaceous differentiation has been reported. The epithelial lining may be relatively thin, and a prominent palisaded basal layer, characteristic of the OKC, is not present (Fig. 15.26).

Treatment and Prognosis

Enucleation with curettage is the usual treatment for orthokeratinized odontogenic cysts. Recurrence has rarely been noted, and the reported frequency is around 2%, which is in marked contrast with the 30% or higher recurrence rate associated with OKCs. It has been suggested that cysts with an orthokeratinized surface may be at slightly greater risk for malignant transformation, but evidence for this is scant. Orthokeratinized odontogenic cysts typically are not associated with nevoid basal cell carcinoma syndrome, even in rare situations when multiple cysts are identified.

◆ NEVOID BASAL CELL CARCINOMA SYNDROME (GORLIN SYNDROME)

Nevoid basal cell carcinoma syndrome (Gorlin syndrome; NBCCS) is an autosomal dominant inherited condition that exhibits high penetrance and variable expressivity. The syndrome usually is caused by mutations in **patched** *(PTCH),* a tumor suppressor gene mapped to chromosome 9q22.3-q31, which plays an important role in the sonic hedgehog (SHH) signaling pathway. A much smaller percentage of cases have been related to germline mutations of *SUFU,* another member of the SHH pathway. Approximately 20%–30% of affected patients represent new mutations. One of the most common clinical features is development of OKCs, which can lead to early diagnosis. The prevalence of Gorlin syndrome is estimated to be anywhere from 1 in 19,000 to 1 in 164,000, depending on the population studied.

Clinical and Radiographic Features

There is great variability in the expressivity of NBCCS, and no single component is present in all patients. The most

• **BOX 15.2** **Major Clinical Features of the Nevoid Basal Cell Carcinoma Syndrome**

50% or Greater Frequency
• Multiple basal cell carcinomas
• Odontogenic keratocysts (OKCs)
• Epidermal cysts of the skin
• Palmar/plantar pits
• Calcified falx cerebri
• Enlarged head circumference
• Rib anomalies (splayed, fused, partially missing, and/or bifid)
• Mild ocular hypertelorism
• Spina bifida occulta of cervical or thoracic vertebrae

15%–49% Frequency
• Calcified ovarian fibromas
• Short fourth metacarpals
• Kyphoscoliosis or other vertebral anomalies
• Pectus excavatum or carinatum
• Strabismus (exotropia)

Less Than 15% Frequency (But Not Random)
• Medulloblastoma
• Meningioma
• Lymphomesenteric cysts
• Cardiac fibroma
• Fetal rhabdomyoma
• Marfanoid build
• Cleft lip and/or palate
• Hypogonadism in males
• Intellectual disability

From Gorlin RJ: Nevoid basal-cell carcinoma syndrome, *Medicine* 66:98–113, 1987.

common and significant features are summarized in Box 15.2. The patient often has a characteristic facies, with frontal and temporoparietal bossing, which results in an increased cranial circumference (more than 60 cm in adults). The eyes may appear widely separated, and many patients have true mild ocular hypertelorism. Mild mandibular prognathism is also commonly present (Fig. 15.27).

Basal cell carcinomas of the skin are a major component of the syndrome. These tumors usually begin to appear at puberty or in the second and third decades of life, although they can develop in young children. The lesions may vary from flesh-colored papules to ulcerating plaques. They often appear on skin that is not exposed to sunlight, but they are most commonly located in the midface area (Fig. 15.28). Tumors on the neck and eyelids often are pedunculated and can be mistaken for skin tags (acrochordons). The number of skin tumors may vary from only a few to many hundreds. Blacks with the syndrome tend to develop basal cell carcinomas less frequently than whites (40% versus 90%), and they have fewer of these lesions, probably because of protective skin pigmentation. Less than 15% of dark-skinned patients develop more than two basal cell carcinomas.

Palmar and plantar pits are present in about 65%–85% of patients (Fig. 15.29). These punctate lesions represent a localized impairment of the maturation of basal epithelial cells, resulting in a focally depressed area as the result of a

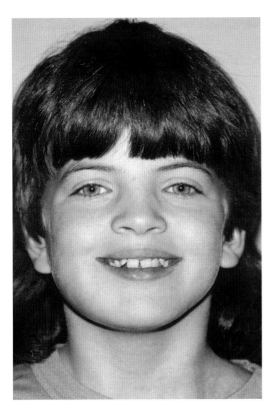

• **Fig. 15.27 Nevoid Basal Cell Carcinoma Syndrome.** This 11-year-old girl shows hypertelorism and mandibular swelling. (Courtesy of Dr. Richard DeChamplain.)

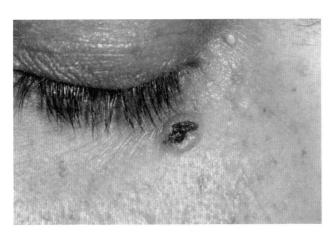

• **Fig. 15.28 Nevoid Basal Cell Carcinoma Syndrome.** An ulcerating basal cell carcinoma is present on the upper face.

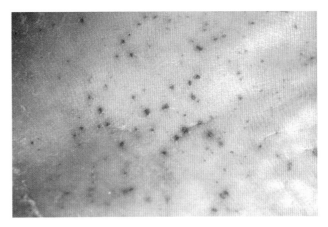

• **Fig. 15.29 Nevoid Basal Cell Carcinoma Syndrome.** Plantar pits.

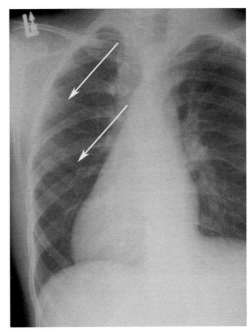

• **Fig. 15.30 Nevoid Basal Cell Carcinoma Syndrome.** Chest film showing presence of bifid ribs *(arrows)*.

markedly thinned keratin layer. Basal cell carcinomas rarely may develop at the base of the pits.

Ovarian cysts and fibromas have been reported in 25%–50% of women with this syndrome. A number of other tumors also have been reported to occur with lesser frequency. These include desmoplastic medulloblastoma within the first 4 years of life, meningioma, cardiac fibroma, and fetal rhabdomyoma. The risk for medulloblastoma is approximately 2%–5% for patients with *PTCH* mutations, but this risk can be as high as 33% for those with *SUFU* mutations.

Skeletal anomalies are present in 60%–75% of patients with this syndrome. The most common anomaly is a bifid rib or splayed ribs (Fig. 15.30). This anomaly may involve several ribs and may be bilateral. Kyphoscoliosis has been observed in about 30%–40% of patients, and a number of other anomalies, such as spina bifida occulta and shortened metacarpals, seem to occur with unusual frequency. A distinctive lamellar calcification of the falx cerebri, noted on an anteroposterior skull radiograph or computed tomography (CT) image, is a common finding and is present in most affected patients (Fig. 15.31).

Jaw cysts are one of the most constant features of the syndrome and are present in 90% of the patients. The cysts are OKCs, although there are some differences between the cysts in patients with NBCCS and in those with isolated OKCs. The cysts are frequently multiple; some patients have had as many as ten separate cysts. The patient's age when the first

OKC is removed is significantly younger in those affected by this syndrome than in those with isolated OKCs. For most patients with this syndrome, their first OKC is removed before age 19. About one-third of patients with NBCCS have only a solitary cyst at the time of the initial presentation, but in most cases additional cysts will develop over periods ranging from 1 to 20 years. Interestingly, OKCs may not occur in individuals with *SUFU*-related NBCCS.

Radiographically, the cysts in patients with NBCCS do not differ significantly from isolated OKCs. The cysts in patients with this syndrome are often associated with the crowns of unerupted teeth; on radiographs they may mimic dentigerous cysts (Fig. 15.32).

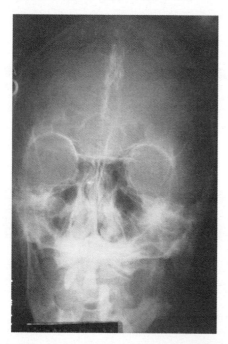

• **Fig. 15.31 Nevoid Basal Cell Carcinoma Syndrome.** Anteroposterior skull film showing calcification of the falx cerebri. (Courtesy of Dr. Ramesh Narang.)

Diagnostic criteria for NBCCS are provided in Box 15.3.

Histopathologic Features

The cysts in NBCCS histopathologically are invariably OKCs. The keratocysts in patients with this syndrome tend to have more satellite cysts, solid islands of epithelial proliferation, and odontogenic epithelial rests within the fibrous capsule than do isolated keratocysts (Fig. 15.33). Foci of calcification also appear to be more common. These features, however, are not diagnostic for NBCCS because they may be seen in isolated keratocysts.

The basal cell tumors of the skin cannot be distinguished from ordinary basal cell carcinomas. They exhibit a wide spectrum of histopathologic findings, from superficial basal cell lesions to aggressive, noduloulcerative basal cell carcinomas.

Treatment and Prognosis

Most of the anomalies in NBCCS are minor and usually not life threatening. The prognosis generally depends on the behavior of the skin tumors. In a few cases, aggressive basal cell carcinomas have caused the death of the patient as a result of tumor invasion of the brain or other vital structures (Figs. 15.34 and 15.35). Because the development of the basal cell carcinomas seems to be triggered by ultraviolet (UV) light exposure, patients should take appropriate precautions to avoid sunlight. For the same reason, radiation therapy should be avoided if at all possible. The jaw cysts are treated in the same manner as isolated OKCs, but in many patients additional cysts will continue to develop. Varying degrees of jaw deformity may result from the operations for multiple cysts. Infection of the cysts in patients with this syndrome is also relatively common.

The recent development of SHH pathway inhibitors, such as vismodegib, has shown promise in the management of basal cell carcinomas in patients with NBCCS. In

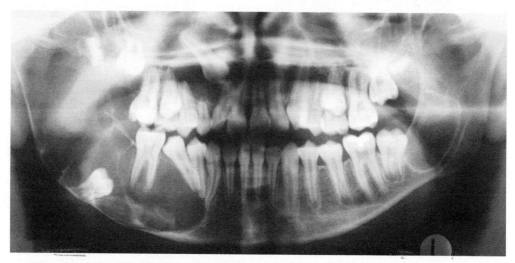

• **Fig. 15.32 Nevoid Basal Cell Carcinoma Syndrome.** Large cysts are present in the right and left mandibular molar regions, together with a smaller cyst involving the right maxillary canine in the same patient shown in Fig. 15.27. (Courtesy of Dr. Richard DeChamplain.)

• BOX 15.3 Diagnostic Criteria for the Nevoid Basal Cell Carcinoma Syndrome

A diagnosis can be made if the patient has:
1. Two major criteria
2. One major and two minor criteria
3. One major criterion and genetic confirmation

Major Criteria

1. Lamellar (sheet-like) calcification of the falx cerebri
2. Odontogenic keratocyst (OKC)
3. Two or more palmar or plantar pits
4. Five or more basal cell carcinomas *or* one before the age of 30 years
5. First degree relative with the nevoid basal cell carcinoma syndrome

Minor Criteria

1. Childhood medulloblastoma
2. Lymphomesenteric or pleural cysts
3. Macrocephaly
4. Cleft lip or palate
5. Rib or vertebral anomalies: bifid, splayed, or extra ribs; bifid vertebrae
6. Preaxial or postaxial polydactyly
7. Ovarian or cardiac fibromas
8. Ocular anomalies (e.g., cataracts, developmental defects, and pigmentary changes of the retinal epithelium)

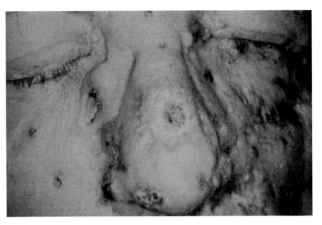

• **Fig. 15.34 Nevoid Basal Cell Carcinoma Syndrome.** This 52-year-old man had more than 100 basal cell carcinomas removed from his face over a 30-year period. Several basal cell carcinomas are present in this photograph. The lesion at the inner canthus of the left eye was deeply invasive and was eventually fatal as a result of brain invasion.

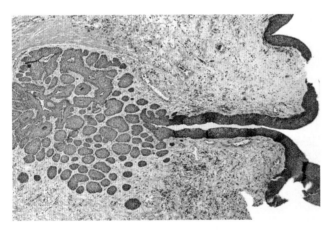

• **Fig. 15.33 Nevoid Basal Cell Carcinoma Syndrome.** Odontogenic keratocyst (OKC) showing numerous odontogenic epithelial rests in the cyst wall.

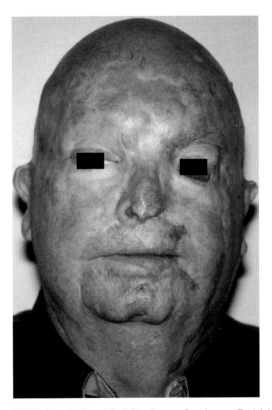

• **Fig. 15.35 Nevoid Basal Cell Carcinoma Syndrome.** Facial deformity secondary to multiple surgical procedures to remove basal cell carcinomas.

addition, vismodegib has been shown to be effective in inducing shrinkage of odontogenic keratocysts in some syndrome patients. Unfortunately, this medication often is associated with intolerable side effects that can cause patients to discontinue therapy. However, continuing research into this class of SHH pathway inhibitors may result in better medications for the treatment of these lesions.

Some investigators have suggested that affected children should have magnetic resonance imaging (MRI) studies every 6 months until 7 years of age to monitor for the development of medulloblastoma. Fortunately, this malignancy appears to have a better prognosis in syndrome patients than

in patients without the syndrome. Genetic counseling is appropriate for affected individuals.

◆ GINGIVAL (ALVEOLAR) CYST OF THE NEWBORN

Gingival cysts of the newborn are small, superficial, keratin-filled cysts that are found on the alveolar mucosa of infants. These cysts arise from remnants of the dental

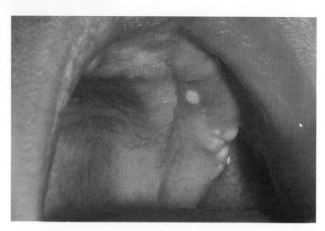

• **Fig. 15.36** **Gingival Cyst of the Newborn.** Multiple whitish papules on the alveolar ridge of a newborn infant.

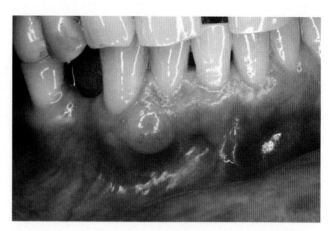

• **Fig. 15.37** **Gingival Cyst of the Adult.** Tense, fluid-filled swelling on the facial gingiva.

lamina. They are common lesions, having been reported in 25%–53% of all newborns. However, because they disappear spontaneously by rupture into the oral cavity, the lesions seldom are noticed or sampled for biopsy. Similar inclusion cysts (e.g., **Epstein's pearls** and **Bohn's nodules**) are also found in the midline of the palate or laterally on the hard and soft palate (see page 25).

Clinical Features

Gingival cysts of the newborn appear as small, usually multiple whitish papules on the mucosa overlying the alveolar processes of neonates (Fig. 15.36). The individual cysts are usually no more than 2–3 mm in diameter. The maxillary alveolus is more commonly involved than the mandibular.

Histopathologic Features

Examination of an intact gingival cyst of the newborn shows a thin, flattened epithelial lining with a parakeratotic luminal surface. The lumen contains keratinaceous debris.

Treatment and Prognosis

No treatment is indicated for gingival cysts of the newborn because the lesions spontaneously involute as a result of the rupture of the cysts and resultant contact with the oral mucosal surface. The lesions are rarely seen after 3 months of age.

◆ GINGIVAL CYST OF THE ADULT

The **gingival cyst of the adult** is an uncommon lesion. It is considered to represent the soft tissue counterpart of the **lateral periodontal cyst** (see next topic), being derived from rests of the dental lamina (rests of Serres). The diagnosis of gingival cyst of the adult should be restricted to lesions with the same histopathologic features as those of the lateral periodontal cyst. On rare occasions, a cyst may develop in the gingiva at the site of a gingival graft; however, such lesions

probably represent *epithelial inclusion cysts* that are a result of the surgical procedure.

Clinical Features

Like the lateral periodontal cyst, the gingival cyst of the adult shows a striking predilection to occur in the mandibular canine and premolar area (60%–75% of cases). Gingival cysts of the adult are most commonly found in patients in the fifth through the seventh decades of life. They are almost invariably located on the facial gingiva or alveolar mucosa. Maxillary gingival cysts are usually found in the incisor, canine, and premolar areas.

Clinically, the cysts appear as painless, domelike swellings, usually less than 0.5 cm in diameter, although rarely they may be somewhat larger (Fig. 15.37). They are often bluish or blue-gray. In some instances, the cyst may cause a superficial "cupping out" of the alveolar bone, which is usually not detected on a radiograph but is apparent when the cyst is excised. If more bone is missing, one could argue that the lesion may be a lateral periodontal cyst that has eroded the cortical bone rather than a gingival cyst that originated in the mucosa.

Histopathologic Features

The histopathologic features of the gingival cyst of the adult are similar to those of the lateral periodontal cyst, consisting of a thin, flattened epithelial lining with or without focal plaques that contain clear cells (Figs. 15.38 and 15.39). Small nests of these glycogen-rich clear cells, which represent rests of the dental lamina, also may be seen in the surrounding connective tissue. Sometimes the cystic lining is so thin that it is easily mistaken for the endothelial lining of a dilated blood vessel.

Treatment and Prognosis

The gingival cyst of the adult responds well to simple surgical excision. The prognosis is excellent.

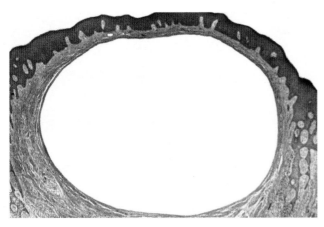

• **Fig. 15.38 Gingival Cyst of the Adult.** Low-power photomicrograph showing a thin-walled cyst in the gingival soft tissue.

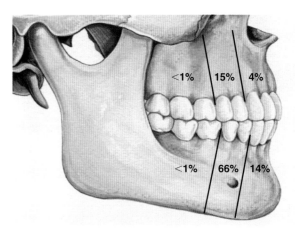

• **Fig. 15.40 Lateral Periodontal Cyst.** Relative distribution of lateral periodontal cysts in the jaws.

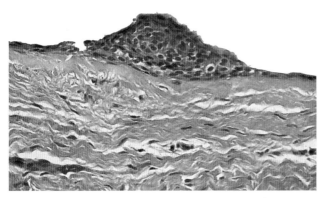

• **Fig. 15.39 Gingival Cyst of the Adult.** High-power photomicrograph showing a plaquelike thickening of the epithelial lining.

◆ LATERAL PERIODONTAL CYST (BOTRYOID ODONTOGENIC CYST)

The **lateral periodontal cyst** is an uncommon type of developmental odontogenic cyst that typically occurs along the lateral root surface of a tooth. It is believed to arise from rests of the dental lamina, and it represents the intrabony counterpart of the gingival cyst of the adult. The lateral periodontal cyst accounts for less than 2% of all epithelium-lined jaw cysts.

In the past, the term *lateral periodontal cyst* was used to describe any cyst that developed along the lateral root surface, including lateral radicular cysts (see page 126) and OKCs (see page 689). However, the lateral periodontal cyst has distinctive clinical and microscopic features that distinguish it from other lesions that sometimes develop in the same location.

Clinical and Radiographic Features

The lateral periodontal cyst is most often an asymptomatic lesion that is detected only during a radiographic examination. It most frequently occurs in patients in the fifth

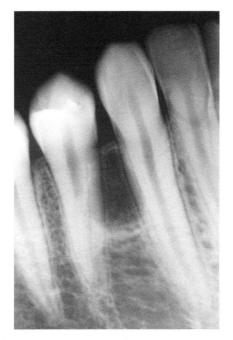

• **Fig. 15.41 Lateral Periodontal Cyst.** Radiolucent lesion between the roots of a vital mandibular canine and first premolar.

through the seventh decades of life; rarely does it occur in someone younger than age 30. Around 75%–80% of cases occur in the mandibular premolar-canine-lateral incisor area. Maxillary examples also usually involve this same tooth region (Fig. 15.40).

Radiographically, the cyst usually appears as a well-circumscribed radiolucent area located laterally to the root or roots of vital teeth. Most such cysts are less than 1.0 cm in greatest diameter (Figs. 15.41 and 15.42). In rare instances, multifocal lateral periodontal cysts have been described. In addition, some examples can develop in edentulous sites.

Occasionally, the lesion may have a polycystic appearance; such examples have been termed **botryoid odontogenic cysts.** Grossly and microscopically, they show a grapelike cluster of small individual cysts (Fig. 15.43). These

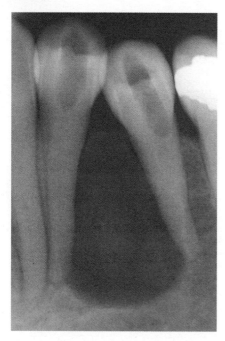

• **Fig. 15.42 Lateral Periodontal Cyst.** A larger lesion causing root divergence.

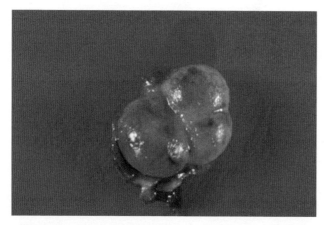

• **Fig. 15.43 Lateral Periodontal Cyst.** Gross specimen of a botryoid variant. Microscopically, this grapelike cluster revealed three separate cavities.

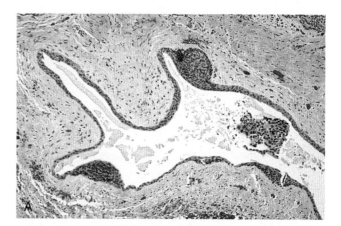

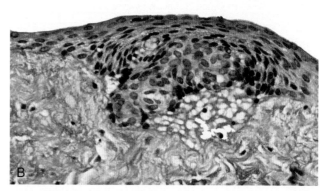

• **Fig. 15.44 Lateral Periodontal Cyst. A,** This photomicrograph shows a thin epithelial lining with focal nodular thickenings. **B,** These thickenings often show a swirling appearance of the cells.

lesions are generally considered to represent a variant of the lateral periodontal cyst, possibly the result of cystic degeneration and subsequent fusion of adjacent foci of dental lamina rests. The botryoid variant often shows a multilocular radiographic appearance, but it also may appear unilocular.

The radiographic features of the lateral periodontal cyst are not diagnostic; an OKC that develops between the roots of adjacent teeth may show identical radiographic findings. An inflammatory radicular cyst that occurs laterally to a root in relation to an accessory foramen or a cyst that arises from periodontal inflammation also may simulate a lateral periodontal cyst radiographically (see page 126). In one study of 46 cases of cystic lesions in the lateral periodontal region, only 13 met the histopathologic criteria for the lateral periodontal cyst; eight were OKCs, 20 were inflammatory cysts, and five were of undetermined origin.

Histopathologic Features

The lateral periodontal cyst has a thin, generally noninflamed, fibrous wall, with an epithelial lining that is only one to three cells thick in most areas. This epithelium usually consists of flattened squamous cells, but sometimes the cells are cuboidal in shape. Foci of glycogen-rich clear cells may be interspersed among the lining epithelial cells. Some cysts show focal nodular thickenings of the lining epithelium, which are composed chiefly of clear cells (Fig. 15.44). Clear cell epithelial rests sometimes are seen within the fibrous wall. Rarely, lateral periodontal cysts exhibit focal areas that histopathologically are suggestive of the glandular odontogenic cyst (see page 703).

Treatment and Prognosis

Conservative enucleation of the lateral periodontal cyst is the treatment of choice. Usually, this can be accomplished without damage to the adjacent teeth. Recurrence is unusual, although it has been reported with the botryoid variant, presumably because of its polycystic nature. An exceedingly rare case of squamous cell carcinoma, which apparently originated in a lateral periodontal cyst, also has been reported.

♦ CALCIFYING ODONTOGENIC CYST (CALCIFYING CYSTIC ODONTOGENIC TUMOR; GORLIN CYST; DENTINOGENIC GHOST CELL TUMOR; GHOST CELL ODONTOGENIC CARCINOMA)

First described in 1962 by Gorlin and associates, the **calcifying odontogenic cyst** is part of a spectrum of lesions characterized by odontogenic epithelium containing "ghost cells," which then may undergo calcification. Most examples grow in a cystic fashion, although some lesions occur as solid tumorlike growths. Therefore, in the 2022 WHO classification system, ghost cell lesions have been categorized under three separate headings (based on the cystic, solid, or malignant nature of the lesion):

1. Calcifying odontogenic cyst
2. Dentinogenic ghost cell tumor
3. Ghost cell odontogenic carcinoma

At this point, it is uncertain whether these categories are variations of the same pathologic process or represent distinct, separate lesions. Molecular studies have shown that calcifying odontogenic cysts harbor mutations of *CTNNB1*, which encodes for β-catenin. Similar mutations also have been described in the dentinogenic ghost cell tumor and ghost cell odontogenic carcinoma.

The overwhelming majority of intraosseous ghost cell odontogenic lesions grow as cystic lesions, and less than 5% of cases can be classified as solid dentinogenic ghost cell tumors or ghost cell odontogenic carcinomas. Approximately one-third of peripheral lesions will be solid in nature, although these peripheral examples are not as aggressive as their intraosseous counterparts.

The calcifying odontogenic cyst may be associated with other recognized odontogenic tumors, most commonly **odontomas.** However, **adenomatoid odontogenic tumors** and **ameloblastomas** also have been associated with calcifying odontogenic cysts.

Clinical and Radiographic Features

Intraosseous calcifying odontogenic cysts occur with about equal frequency in the maxilla and mandible. About 65% of cases are found in the incisor and canine areas (Fig. 15.45). The mean age is 30 years, and most cases are diagnosed in the second to fourth decades of life. Calcifying odontogenic cysts that are associated with odontomas tend to occur in younger patients, with a mean age of 17 years.

The central calcifying odontogenic cyst is usually a unilocular, well-defined radiolucency, although the lesion occasionally may appear multilocular. Radiopaque structures within the lesion, either irregular calcifications or toothlike

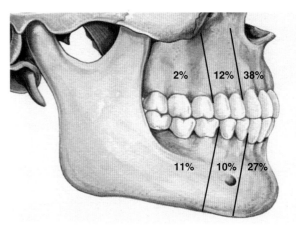

• **Fig. 15.45 Calcifying Odontogenic Cyst.** Relative distribution of calcifying odontogenic cysts in the jaws.

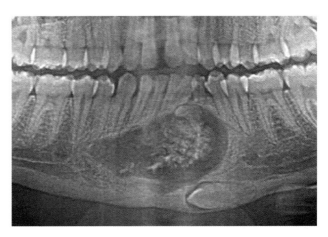

• **Fig. 15.46 Calcifying Odontogenic Cyst.** Well-circumscribed mixed radiolucent/radiopaque lesion in the anterior mandible. This cyst was associated with an odontoma. (Courtesy of Dr. Michael Border).

densities, are present in about one-third to one-half of cases (Fig. 15.46). In approximately one-third of cases, the radiolucent lesion is associated with an unerupted tooth, most often a canine. Most calcifying odontogenic cysts are between 2.0 and 4.0 cm in greatest diameter, but lesions as large as 12.0 cm have been noted. Root resorption or divergence of adjacent teeth is seen with some frequency (Fig. 15.47).

Intraosseous dentinogenic ghost cell tumors are most common in the third through the fifth decades of life, occurring most often in the posterior areas of both jaws. These solid tumors are capable of acting more aggressively than their cystic counterparts, sometimes resulting in root resorption, perforation of the cortical plate, or sinus destruction.

Extraosseous odontogenic ghost cell lesions comprise from 5% to 17% of all cases, appearing as localized sessile or pedunculated gingival masses with no distinctive clinical features (Fig. 15.48). They can resemble common gingival fibromas, gingival cysts, or peripheral giant cell granulomas. Peripheral examples tend to occur later in life, with peak prevalence during the sixth to eighth decades.

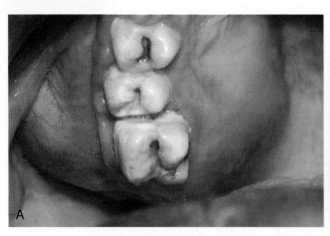

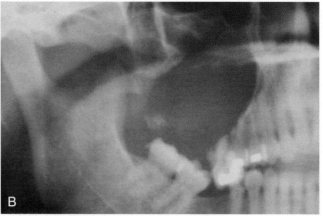

• **Fig. 15.47 Calcifying Odontogenic Cyst. A,** Expansion of the posterior maxillary alveolus caused by a large calcifying odontogenic cyst. **B,** Panoramic radiograph of the same patient showing a large radiolucency in the posterior maxilla. A small calcified structure is seen in the lower portion of the cyst. (Courtesy of Dr. Tom Brock.)

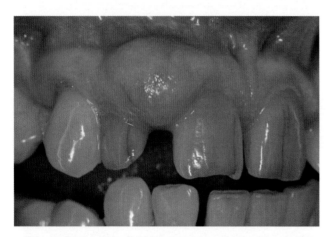

• **Fig. 15.48 Peripheral Calcifying Odontogenic Cyst.** Nodular mass of the maxillary facial gingiva. (Courtesy of Dr. Kenneth Rasenberger.)

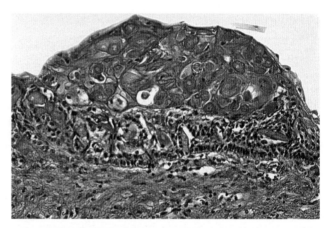

• **Fig. 15.49 Calcifying Odontogenic Cyst.** The cyst lining shows ameloblastoma-like epithelial cells, with a columnar basal layer. Large eosinophilic ghost cells are present within the epithelial lining.

Ghost cell odontogenic carcinomas are extremely rare, aggressive neoplasms that may arise *de novo* or from malignant degeneration of calcifying odontogenic cyst or dentinogenic ghost cell tumor. Such tumors have been reported more often in the maxilla than in the mandible.

Histopathologic Features

The calcifying odontogenic cyst most commonly occurs as a well-defined cystic lesion with a fibrous capsule and a lining of odontogenic epithelium of four to ten cells in thickness. The basal cells of the epithelial lining may be cuboidal or columnar and are similar to ameloblasts. The overlying layer of loosely arranged epithelium may resemble the stellate reticulum of an ameloblastoma.

The most characteristic histopathologic feature of the calcifying odontogenic cyst is the presence of variable numbers of "ghost cells" within the epithelial component. These eosinophilic ghost cells are altered epithelial cells that are

characterized by the loss of nuclei with preservation of the basic cell outline (Fig. 15.49).

The nature of the ghost cell change is controversial. Some believe that this change represents coagulative necrosis or accumulation of enamel protein; others contend it is a form of normal or aberrant keratinization of odontogenic epithelium. Masses of ghost cells may fuse to form large sheets of amorphous, acellular material. Calcification within the ghost cells is common. This first appears as fine basophilic granules that may increase in size and number to form extensive masses of calcified material. Areas of an eosinophilic matrix material that are considered by some authors to represent dysplastic dentin (dentinoid) also may be present adjacent to the epithelial component. This is believed to be the result of an inductive effect by the odontogenic epithelium on the adjacent mesenchymal tissue (Fig. 15.50).

Several variants of the cystic type of calcifying odontogenic cyst are seen. In some cases, the epithelial lining proliferates into the lumen so that the lumen is largely filled with

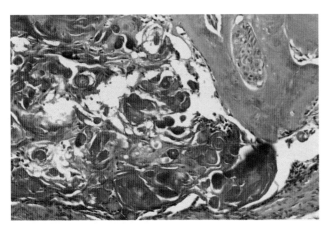

• **Fig. 15.50 Calcifying Odontogenic Cyst.** Eosinophilic dentinoid material is present adjacent to a sheet of ghost cells.

masses of ghost cells and dystrophic calcifications. Multiple daughter cysts may be present within the fibrous wall, and a foreign body reaction to herniated ghost cells may be conspicuous.

In another variant, unifocal or multifocal epithelial proliferation of the cyst lining into the lumen may resemble ameloblastoma. These proliferations are intermixed with varying numbers of ghost cells. These epithelial proliferations superficially resemble, but do not meet, the strict histopathologic criteria for ameloblastoma.

About 20% of calcifying odontogenic cysts are associated with odontomas. This variant is usually a unicystic lesion that shows the features of a calcifying odontogenic cyst together with those of a small complex or compound odontoma.

Solid dentinogenic ghost cell tumors may occur intraosseously or extraosseously. The **extraosseous** forms appear to be more common. These show varying-sized islands of odontogenic epithelium in a fibrous stroma. The epithelial islands show peripheral palisaded columnar cells and central stellate reticulum, which resemble ameloblastoma. Nests of ghost cells, however, are present within the epithelium, and juxtaepithelial dentinoid is commonly present. These features differentiate this lesion from the peripheral ameloblastoma.

The rare **intraosseous** dentinogenic ghost cell tumor is a solid neoplasm that consists of ameloblastoma-like strands and islands of odontogenic epithelium in a mature fibrous connective tissue stroma. Variable numbers of ghost cells and juxtaepithelial dentinoid are present.

Ghost cell odontogenic carcinomas grow as solid tumors but also exhibit malignant features, such as cellular pleomorphism, increased mitotic activity, necrosis, and invasion of the surrounding tissues.

Treatment and Prognosis

The prognosis for a patient with a calcifying odontogenic cyst is good; only a few recurrences after simple enucleation have been reported. Peripheral examples appear to have the same prognosis as a peripheral ameloblastoma, with a minimal chance of recurrence after simple surgical excision.

However, intraosseous dentinogenic ghost cell tumors are potentially aggressive neoplasms. One study reported a recurrence rate of 73% for lesions treated in a conservative fashion (enucleation or curettage), whereas the recurrence rate was 33% for lesions treated more aggressively (marginal or segmental resection). Although few cases of ghost cell odontogenic carcinoma have been reported, such tumors have an unpredictable behavior. Recurrences are common, and a few patients have died from either uncontrolled local disease or metastases. An overall 5-year survival rate of 73% has been calculated for reported cases.

◆ GLANDULAR ODONTOGENIC CYST (SIALO-ODONTOGENIC CYST)

The **glandular odontogenic cyst** is a rare type of developmental odontogenic cyst that can show aggressive behavior. Although it is generally accepted as being of odontogenic origin, it also shows glandular or salivary features that presumably are an indication of the pluripotentiality of odontogenic epithelium.

Clinical and Radiographic Features

The glandular odontogenic cyst occurs most commonly in middle-aged adults, with a mean age of 46–48 years at the time of diagnosis; rarely does it occur before the age of 20. Approximately 68%–75% of reported cases have occurred in the mandible. The cyst has a strong predilection for the anterior region of the jaws, and many mandibular lesions will cross the midline.

The size of the cyst can vary from small lesions less than 1 cm in diameter to large destructive lesions that may involve most of the jaw. Small cysts may be asymptomatic; however, large cysts often produce clinical expansion, which sometimes can be associated with pain or paresthesia (Fig. 15.51).

Radiographically, the lesion presents as either a unilocular or multilocular radiolucency. The margins of the radiolucency are usually well defined with a corticated rim.

Histopathologic Features

The glandular odontogenic cyst is lined by squamous epithelium of varying thickness. The interface between the epithelium and the fibrous connective tissue wall is generally flat. The fibrous cyst wall is usually devoid of any inflammatory cell infiltrate. The superficial epithelial cells that line the cyst cavity tend to be cuboidal to columnar, resulting in an uneven hobnail and sometimes papillary surface (Fig. 15.52). The surface layer often includes mucin-producing goblet cells, occasionally with the presence of cilia. Glandular, ductlike spaces within the epithelial lining are another characteristic finding. These spaces are lined by cuboidal cells and often contain mucicarmine-positive fluid. In focal areas,

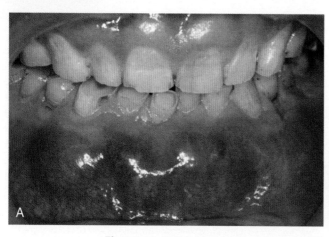
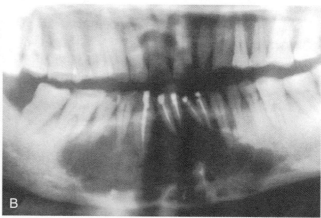

• **Fig. 15.51 Glandular Odontogenic Cyst. A,** Expansile lesion of the anterior mandible. **B,** The panoramic radiograph shows a large multilocular radiolucency. (Courtesy of Dr. Cheng-Chung Lin.)

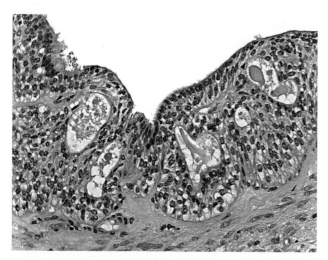

• **Fig. 15.52 Glandular Odontogenic Cyst.** The cyst is lined by stratified squamous epithelium that exhibits surface columnar cells with cilia. Numerous microcysts containing mucinous material are present.

the epithelial lining cells may form spherical nodules, similar to those seen in lateral periodontal cysts.

There is some histopathologic overlap between the features of the glandular odontogenic cyst and those of some intraosseous, low-grade, predominantly cystic mucoepidermoid carcinomas (see page 496). In selected microscopic fields, the microscopic features may be identical. Examination of multiple sections, however, usually permits the differentiation of these lesions. Also, glandular odontogenic cysts will not show *MAML2* gene rearrangements, which often are found in central mucoepidermoid carcinomas.

Treatment and Prognosis

Most cases of glandular odontogenic cyst have been treated by enucleation or curettage. However, this cyst shows a propensity for recurrence, which is observed in approximately 22%–30% of all cases. Recurrence appears to be more common among the lesions that present in a multilocular fashion. Because of its potentially aggressive nature and tendency for

recurrence, some authors have advocated *en bloc* resection, particularly for multilocular lesions. Marsupialization and decompression may be attempted for larger lesions to promote shrinkage prior to surgery. One example of central mucoepidermoid carcinoma apparently arising from a recurrent glandular odontogenic cyst has been reported.

◆ BUCCAL BIFURCATION CYST (INFLAMMATORY COLLATERAL CYST)

The **buccal bifurcation cyst** is an uncommon inflammatory odontogenic cyst that characteristically develops on the buccal aspect of the mandibular first permanent molar, although some cases have involved the second molar. The pathogenesis of this cyst is uncertain. One theory suggests that early tooth eruption may be associated with inflammation of the buccal sulcular or junctional epithelium, resulting in epithelial proliferation and cyst formation. In addition, a few of these lesions have been associated with teeth that demonstrate cervical enamel extensions into the bifurcation area (see page 90). Such extensions may predispose these teeth to buccal pocket formation, which could then enlarge to form a cyst in response to pericoronitis.

The term **paradental cyst** sometimes has been used synonymously for the buccal bifurcation cyst. Such lesions typically occur distal or buccal of partially erupted mandibular third molars with a history of pericoronitis. The pathogenesis of the so-called paradental cyst also is uncertain. However, the distinction of paradental cysts from secondarily inflamed dentigerous cysts is difficult, if not impossible, in many instances (see page 685).

Clinical and Radiographic Features

The buccal bifurcation cyst typically occurs in children from 5 to 13 years of age. The patient has slight-to-moderate tenderness on the buccal aspect of the mandibular first or second molar, which may be in the process of erupting. The patient often notes associated clinical swelling and a foul-tasting discharge. Periodontal probing usually reveals pocket formation

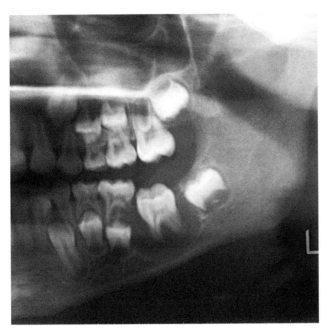

• Fig. 15.53 Buccal Bifurcation Cyst. Well-circumscribed unilocular radiolucency superimposed on the roots of the mandibular first permanent molar. (Courtesy of Dr. Michael Pharoah.)

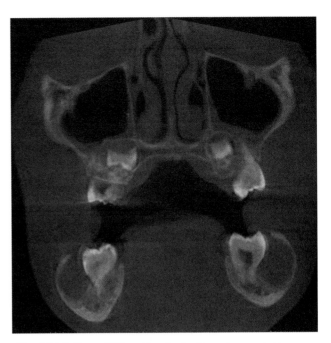

• Fig. 15.54 Buccal Bifurcation Cysts. Coronal computed tomography (CT) image showing bilateral cysts buccal to the roots of the mandibular first molars. (Courtesy of Dr. Brent Newby.)

on the buccal aspect of the involved tooth. Around one-third of patients have been reported to have bilateral involvement of the first molars.

Radiographs typically show a well-circumscribed unilocular radiolucency involving the buccal bifurcation and root area of the involved tooth (Fig. 15.53). The average size of the lucent defect is 1.2 cm, but the lesion may be as large as 2.5 cm in diameter. An occlusal radiograph or cone-beam computed tomography (CBCT) can be helpful in demonstrating the buccal location of the lesion. The root apices of the molar are characteristically tipped toward the lingual mandibular cortex (Fig. 15.54). Many cases are associated with proliferative periostitis (see page 141) of the overlying buccal cortex, which is characterized by a single or multiple layers of reactive bone formation.

Histopathologic Features

The microscopic features are nonspecific and show a cyst that is lined by nonkeratinizing stratified squamous epithelium with areas of hyperplasia. A prominent chronic inflammatory cell infiltrate is present in the surrounding connective tissue wall.

Treatment and Prognosis

The buccal bifurcation cyst is usually treated by enucleation; extraction of the associated tooth is unnecessary. Within 1 year of surgery, there is usually complete healing with normalization of periodontal probing depths and radiographic evidence of bone fill. Several reports have described cases that resolved without surgery—either with no treatment at all or by daily irrigation of the buccal pocket with saline and hydrogen peroxide.

◆ CARCINOMA ARISING IN ODONTOGENIC CYSTS

Carcinoma arising within bone is a rare lesion that is essentially limited to the jaws. Because the putative source of the epithelium giving rise to the carcinoma is odontogenic, these intraosseous jaw carcinomas are collectively known as **odontogenic carcinomas.** Odontogenic carcinomas may arise in an ameloblastoma, rarely from other odontogenic tumors, *de novo* (without evidence of a preexisting lesion), or from the epithelial lining of odontogenic cysts. Some intraosseous mucoepidermoid carcinomas (see page 496) also may arise from mucous cells lining a dentigerous cyst.

Most intraosseous carcinomas apparently arise in odontogenic cysts. Although infrequently documented in the literature, carcinomatous transformation of the lining of an odontogenic cyst may be more common than is generally appreciated. Several studies have shown that 1%–2% of all oral cavity carcinomas seen in some oral and maxillofacial pathology services may originate from odontogenic cysts. The pathogenesis of carcinomas arising in odontogenic cysts is unknown. Occasionally, areas within the lining of odontogenic cysts histopathologically demonstrate varying degrees of epithelial dysplasia, and such changes likely give rise to the carcinoma.

Clinical and Radiographic Features

Although carcinomas arising in cysts may be seen in patients across a wide age range, they are encountered most often in older patients. The mean reported age is 60 years. This lesion is over twice as common in men as in women. Pain and swelling are the most common complaints. However, many

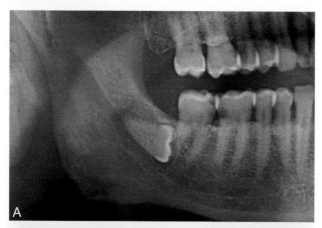

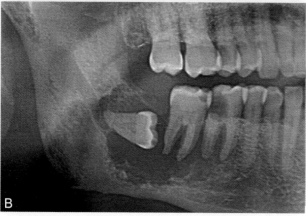

• **Fig. 15.55   Carcinoma Arising in a Dentigerous Cyst. A,** Impacted mandibular third molar surrounded by a narrow radiolucent rim. **B,** Radiographic appearance 5 years later, which shows a large destructive radiolucency with ragged borders. (Courtesy of Dr. Matthew Lee.)

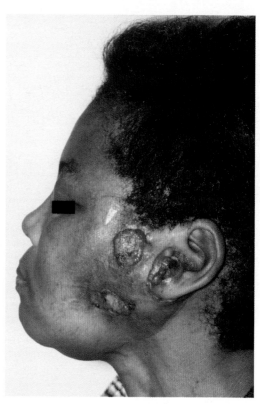

• **Fig. 15.56   Carcinoma Arising in a Cyst.** There is a massive carcinoma of the mandible, with extension into the parotid gland, the face, and the base of the brain. Nineteen years previously, a large odontogenic keratocyst (OKC) with areas of epithelial dysplasia had been removed from the ascending ramus. The patient had suffered multiple recurrences, with eventual change into invasive carcinoma.

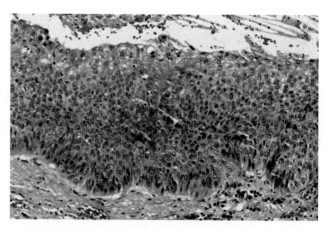

• **Fig. 15.57   Carcinoma Arising in a Cyst.** High-power view of a dentigerous cyst from a 53-year-old man. The lining demonstrates full-thickness epithelial dysplasia.

patients have no symptoms, and the diagnosis of carcinoma is made only after microscopic examination of a presumed odontogenic cyst.

Radiographic findings may mimic those of any odontogenic cyst, although the margins of the radiolucent defect are usually irregular and ragged. CT scans of the lesion may demonstrate a destructive pattern that is not appreciated on viewing plain radiographs. A lesion considered to be a **residual periapical cyst** is apparently the most common type associated with carcinomatous transformation, although routine periapical cysts can also exhibit malignant change. These account for 60% of reported cases. In about 16% of cases, the carcinoma appeared to have arisen in a **dentigerous cyst** (Fig. 15.55). Examples of malignant transformation of calcifying odontogenic cysts also have been reported. In one patient, the carcinoma was thought to originate from a **lateral periodontal cyst.**

A number of examples of carcinoma arising in an OKC also have been documented (Fig. 15.56). However, some reported examples do not appear to have arisen in true parakeratinized OKCs, but rather in **orthokeratinized odontogenic cysts.**

Histopathologic Features

Most carcinomas arising in cysts histopathologically have been **well-differentiated** or **moderately well-differentiated squamous cell carcinomas.** Sometimes it is possible to identify a transition from a normal-appearing cyst lining to invasive squamous cell carcinoma (Figs. 15.57 and 15.58).

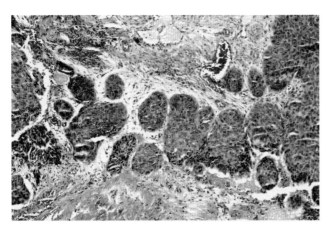

• **Fig. 15.58 Carcinoma Arising in a Cyst.** Same case as Fig. 15.57 showing islands of invasive epithelial cells in the cyst wall.

Treatment and Prognosis

The treatment of patients with carcinomas arising in cysts has varied from local block excision to radical resection, with or without radiation or adjunctive chemotherapy. The prognosis is difficult to evaluate because most reports consist of isolated cases. Metastases to regional lymph nodes have been demonstrated in a few cases. One review showed an overall 2-year survival rate of 62%, but the 5-year survival rate dropped to 38%.

Before a given lesion can be accepted as an example of primary intraosseous carcinoma, the possibility that the tumor represents metastatic spread from an intraoral or extraoral site must be ruled out by appropriate studies.

ODONTOGENIC TUMORS

Odontogenic tumors comprise a complex group of lesions of diverse histopathologic types and clinical behavior. Some of these lesions are true neoplasms and may rarely exhibit malignant behavior. Others may represent tumorlike malformations (hamartomas).

Odontogenic tumors, like normal odontogenesis, demonstrate varying inductive interactions between odontogenic epithelium and odontogenic ectomesenchyme. This ectomesenchyme was formerly referred to as *mesenchyme* because it was thought to be derived from the mesodermal layer of the embryo. It is now accepted that this tissue differentiates from the ectodermal layer in the cephalic portion of the embryo. **Tumors of odontogenic epithelium** are composed only of odontogenic epithelium without any participation of odontogenic ectomesenchyme.

Other odontogenic neoplasms, sometimes referred to as **mixed odontogenic tumors,** are composed of odontogenic epithelium and ectomesenchymal elements. Dental hard tissue may or may not be formed in these lesions.

A third group, **tumors of odontogenic ectomesenchyme,** is composed principally of ectomesenchymal elements. Although odontogenic epithelium may be included within these lesions, it does not appear to play any essential role in their pathogenesis.

Box 15.4 presents categories of odontogenic tumors, listing the most common and important odontogenic tumors that are discussed in this textbook.

Because many of these lesions are quite rare, it is sometimes difficult to assess certain epidemiologic features accurately, as well as recommendations regarding treatment. It should be kept in mind that reports in the literature may be biased due to geopolitical/economic variations in submission of biopsies or the tendency of journal editors to publish reports of lesions that are unusual or aggressive.

TUMORS OF ODONTOGENIC EPITHELIUM

Epithelial odontogenic tumors are composed of odontogenic epithelium without participation of odontogenic ectomesenchyme. Several distinctly different tumors are included in the group; ameloblastoma is the most important and common of them.

◆ AMELOBLASTOMA

The **ameloblastoma** is the most common clinically significant odontogenic tumor. Its relative frequency equals the combined frequency of all other odontogenic tumors, excluding odontomas. Ameloblastomas are tumors of odontogenic epithelial origin. Theoretically, they may arise from rests of dental lamina, from a developing enamel organ, from the epithelial lining of an odontogenic cyst, or from the basal cells of the oral mucosa. As many as 80% of ameloblastomas will show mutations in *BRAF* p.V600E, a gene involved in the mitogen-activated protein kinase (MAP kinase) cell signaling pathway.

Ameloblastomas are slow-growing, locally invasive tumors that run a benign course in most cases. They typically have been described as having three different clinicoradiographic presentations, which deserve separate consideration because of potentially differing therapeutic considerations and prognosis:

1. Conventional solid or multicystic (about 75%–86% of all cases)
2. Unicystic (about 13%–21% of all cases)
3. Peripheral (extraosseous) (about 1%–4% of all cases)

CONVENTIONAL SOLID OR MULTICYSTIC INTRAOSSEOUS AMELOBLASTOMA

Clinical and Radiographic Features

Conventional solid or **multicystic intraosseous ameloblastoma** is encountered in patients across a wide age range. It is rare in children younger than age 10 and relatively uncommon in the 10- to 19-year-old group. The tumor shows an approximately equal prevalence in the third to seventh decades of life. There is no significant sex predilection. Some studies indicate a greater frequency in blacks; others show no racial predilection. About 80%–85% of conventional ameloblastomas occur in the mandible, most often in the molar-ascending ramus area. About 15%–20% of ameloblastomas occur in the maxilla, usually in the posterior regions (Fig. 15.59). The tumor is often asymptomatic, and smaller lesions are detected only during a radiographic examination. A painless swelling or expansion of the jaw is the usual clinical presentation (Figs. 15.60 and 15.61). If untreated, then the lesion may grow slowly to massive or grotesque proportions (Fig. 15.62). Pain and paresthesia are uncommon, even with large tumors.

The most typical radiographic feature is that of a multilocular radiolucent lesion, although one large international study suggested that a unilocular presentation was just as likely. Multilocular lesions are described as having a "soap bubble" appearance (when the radiolucent loculations are large) or as being "honeycombed" (when the loculations are small) (Figs. 15.63–15.65). Buccal and lingual cortical expansion is frequently present. Resorption of the roots of

teeth adjacent to the tumor is common. In many cases an unerupted tooth, most often a mandibular third molar, is associated with the radiolucent defect (Fig. 15.66). Solid ameloblastomas may radiographically appear as unilocular radiolucent defects, which may resemble almost any type of cystic lesion (Fig. 15.67). The margins of these radiolucent lesions, however, often show irregular scalloping. Although the radiographic features, particularly of the typical multilocular defect, may be highly suggestive of ameloblastoma, a variety of odontogenic and non-odontogenic lesions may show similar radiographic features (see Appendix).

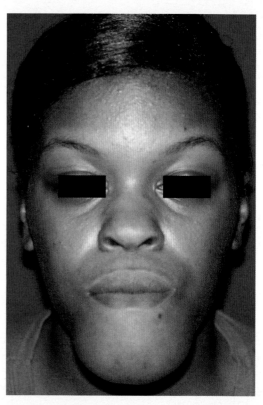

• **Fig. 15.60 Ameloblastoma.** Large expansile mass of the anterior mandible. (Courtesy of Dr. Michael Tabor.)

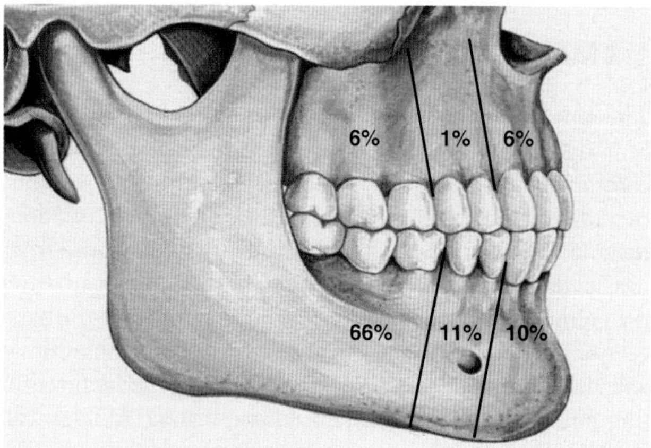

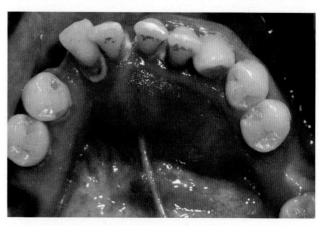

• **Fig. 15.61 Ameloblastoma.** Prominent expansion of the lingual alveolus caused by a large ameloblastoma of the mandibular symphysis.

• **Fig. 15.59 Ameloblastoma.** Relative distribution of ameloblastomas in the jaws.

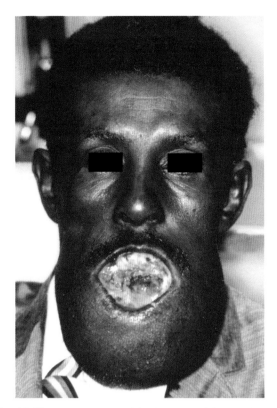

• **Fig. 15.62 Ameloblastoma.** Massive tumor of the anterior mandible. (Courtesy of Dr. Ronald Baughman.)

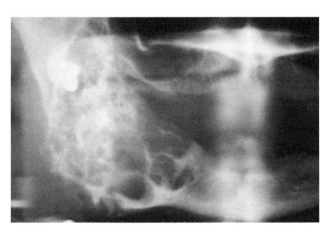

• **Fig. 15.63 Ameloblastoma.** Large multilocular lesion involving the mandibular angle and ascending ramus. The large loculations show the "soap bubble" appearance. An unerupted third molar has been displaced high into the ramus.

One histopathologic form of ameloblastoma that does not have these characteristic features is the desmoplastic ameloblastoma, a variant that Eversole and colleagues documented initially in the literature in 1984. The desmoplastic ameloblastoma has a marked predilection to occur in the anterior regions of the jaws, with equal distribution between the mandible and the maxilla. Radiographically, this type may not suggest the diagnosis of ameloblastoma; the majority of these tumors resemble a fibro-osseous lesion because of their mixed radiolucent and radiopaque appearance (Fig. 15.68).

This mixed radiographic appearance is due to osseous metaplasia within the dense fibrous septa that characterize the lesion, not because the tumor itself is producing a mineralized product.

Histopathologic Features

Conventional solid or multicystic intraosseous ameloblastomas show a remarkable tendency to undergo cystic change; grossly, most tumors have varying combinations of cystic and solid features. The cysts may be seen only at the microscopic level or may be present as multiple large cysts that include most of the tumor. Several microscopic subtypes of conventional ameloblastoma are recognized, but these microscopic patterns generally have little bearing on the behavior of the tumor. Large tumors often show a combination of microscopic patterns.

The **follicular** and **plexiform** patterns are the most common. Less common histopathologic patterns include the **acanthomatous, granular cell, desmoplastic,** and **basal cell** types.

Follicular Pattern

The follicular histopathologic pattern is the most common and recognizable. Islands of epithelium resemble enamel organ epithelium in a mature fibrous connective tissue stroma. The epithelial nests consist of a core of loosely arranged angular cells resembling the stellate reticulum of an enamel organ. A single layer of tall columnar ameloblast-like cells surrounds this central core. The nuclei of these cells are located at the opposite pole to the basement membrane (**reversed polarity**). In other areas, the peripheral cells may be more cuboidal and resemble basal cells. Cyst formation is common and may vary from microcysts, which form within the epithelial islands, to large macroscopic cysts, which may be several centimeters in diameter (Figs. 15.69 and 15.70). If an incisional biopsy is taken from the latter area, an inappropriate diagnosis of "unicystic ameloblastoma" may be rendered by the pathologist.

Plexiform Pattern

The plexiform type of ameloblastoma consists of long, anastomosing cords or larger sheets of odontogenic epithelium. The cords or sheets of epithelium are bounded by columnar or cuboidal ameloblast-like cells surrounding more loosely arranged epithelial cells. Occasionally the cuboidal cells may form structures resembling ducts, resulting in what has been termed an adenoid pattern. Such lesions may be misdiagnosed as adenomatoid odontogenic tumor or adenocarcinoma by the pathologist who is not familiar with this pattern. The supporting stroma in the plexiform pattern of ameloblastoma tends to be loosely arranged and vascular. Cyst formation is relatively uncommon in this variety. When it occurs, it is more often associated with stromal degeneration rather than cystic change within the epithelium (Fig. 15.71).

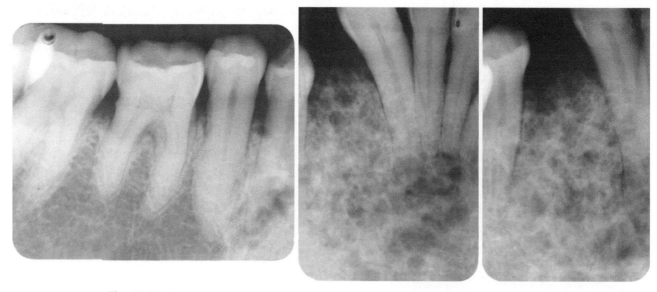

• **Fig. 15.64 Ameloblastoma.** Periapical films showing the "honeycombed" appearance. (Courtesy of Dr. John Hann.)

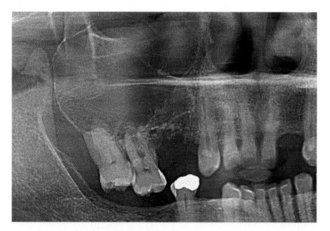

• **Fig. 15.65 Ameloblastoma.** Expansile, radiolucent mass of the right posterior maxilla, which fills the maxillary sinus. (Courtesy of Dr. Doug Oliver.)

If the duct-like structures are accompanied by dentinoid deposition, then the diagnosis of a rare, relatively recently described, ameloblastoma-like tumor called adenoid ameloblastoma may be appropriate. One report has suggested that the characteristic mutations of *BRAF* p.V600E gene are not present in this lesion.

Acanthomatous Pattern

When extensive squamous metaplasia, often associated with keratin formation, occurs in the central portions of the epithelial islands of a follicular ameloblastoma, the term **acanthomatous ameloblastoma** is sometimes applied. This change does not indicate a more aggressive course for the lesion; histopathologically, however, such a lesion may be confused with squamous cell carcinoma or squamous odontogenic tumor (Fig. 15.72).

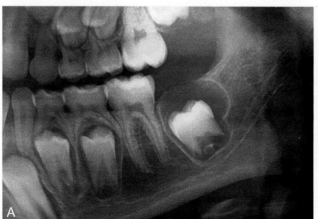
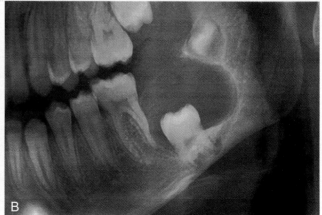

• **Fig. 15.66 Ameloblastoma. A,** Unilocular radiolucency surrounding the crown of the developing left mandibular second molar, which mimics a small dentigerous cyst. **B,** This radiograph from 3 years later shows enlargement of the lesion, including inferior displacement of the tooth. (Courtesy of Dr. Patrick Scioscia.)

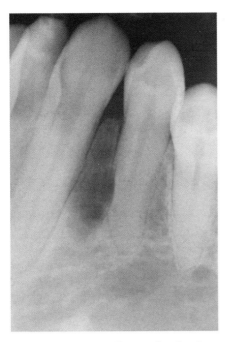

• **Fig. 15.67 Ameloblastoma.** This small unilocular radiolucency lesion could easily be mistaken for a lateral periodontal cyst. (Courtesy of Dr. Tony Traynham.)

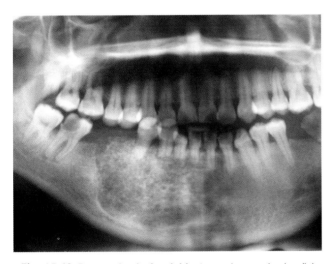

• **Fig. 15.68 Desmoplastic Ameloblastoma.** Large mixed radiolucent and radiopaque lesion of the anterior and right body of the mandible. (Courtesy of Dr. Román Carlos.)

Granular Cell Pattern

Ameloblastomas may sometimes show transformation of groups of lesional epithelial cells to granular cells. These cells have abundant cytoplasm filled with eosinophilic granules that resemble lysosomes ultrastructurally and histochemically. Although originally considered to represent an aging or degenerative change in long-standing lesions, this variant has been seen in young patients. When this granular cell change is extensive in an ameloblastoma, the designation of **granular cell ameloblastoma** is appropriate (Fig. 15.73).

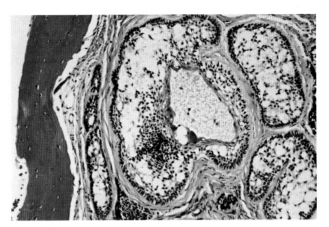

• **Fig. 15.69 Ameloblastoma (Follicular Pattern).** Multiple islands of odontogenic epithelium demonstrating peripheral columnar differentiation with reverse polarization. The central zones resemble stellate reticulum and exhibit foci of cystic degeneration.

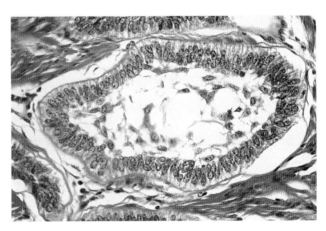

• **Fig. 15.70 Ameloblastoma (Follicular Pattern).** This high-power photomicrograph highlights the peripheral columnar cells exhibiting reverse polarization.

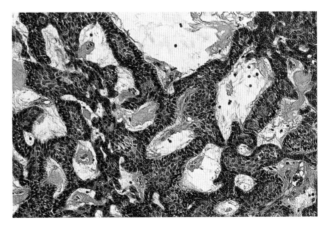

• **Fig. 15.71 Ameloblastoma (Plexiform Pattern).** Anastomosing cords of odontogenic epithelium.

Desmoplastic Pattern

This type of ameloblastoma contains small islands and cords of odontogenic epithelium in a densely collagenized stroma. Immunohistochemical studies have shown increased

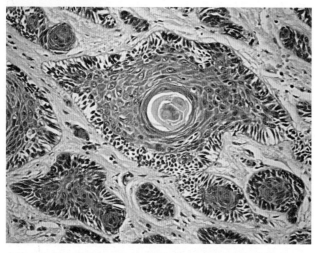

• **Fig. 15.72 Ameloblastoma (Acanthomatous Pattern).** Islands of ameloblastoma demonstrating central squamous differentiation.

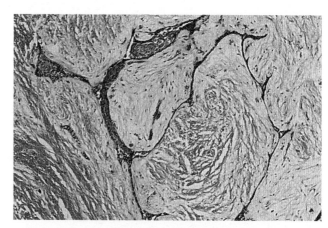

• **Fig. 15.74 Ameloblastoma (Desmoplastic Variant).** Thin cords of ameloblastic epithelium within a dense fibrous connective tissue stroma.

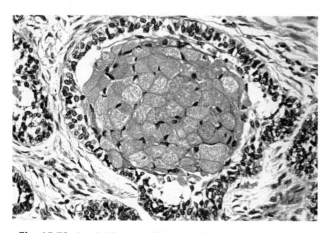

• **Fig. 15.73 Ameloblastoma (Granular Cell Variant).** Tumor island exhibiting central cells with prominent granular cytoplasm.

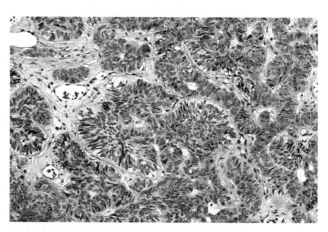

• **Fig. 15.75 Ameloblastoma (Basal Cell Variant).** Islands of hyperchromatic basaloid cells with peripheral palisading.

production of the cytokine known as *transforming growth factor-β (TGF-β)* in association with this lesion, suggesting that this may be responsible for the desmoplasia. Peripheral columnar ameloblast-like cells are inconspicuous about the epithelial islands (Fig. 15.74).

Basal Cell Pattern

The basal cell variant of ameloblastoma is the least common type. These lesions are composed of nests of uniform basaloid cells, and they histopathologically are very similar to basal cell carcinoma of the skin. No stellate reticulum is present in the central portions of the nests. The peripheral cells about the nests tend to be cuboidal rather than columnar (Fig. 15.75).

Treatment and Prognosis

Patients with conventional solid or multicystic intraosseous ameloblastomas have been treated by a variety of means. These range from simple enucleation and curettage to *en bloc* resection

(Fig. 15.76). The optimal method of treatment has been the subject of controversy for many years, primarily because this tumor is rather uncommon, and designing well-controlled, randomized clinical trials with sufficient follow-up periods is a logistical challenge. The conventional ameloblastoma tends to infiltrate between intact cancellous bone trabeculae at the periphery of the lesion before bone resorption becomes radiographically evident. Therefore, the actual margin of the tumor often extends beyond its apparent radiographic or clinical margin. Attempts to remove the tumor by curettage often leave small islands of tumor within the bone, which later manifest as recurrences. Recurrence rates of 50%–90% have been reported in various studies after curettage. Recurrence often takes many years to become clinically manifest, and 5-year disease-free periods do not indicate a cure.

Marginal resection is the most widely used treatment, but recurrence rates of up to 15% have been reported after marginal or block resection. Some surgeons advocate a more conservative approach to treatment by planning surgery after careful evaluation of CT scans of the tumor. Removal of

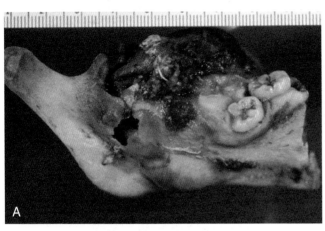 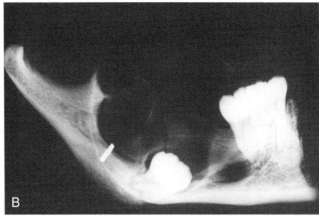

• **Fig. 15.76 Ameloblastoma. A,** Gross photograph of a mandibular resection specimen. **B,** The radiograph of the specimen shows a large radiolucent defect associated with an inferiorly displaced third molar. (Courtesy of Dr. Mary Richardson.)

the tumor, followed by peripheral ostectomy, often reduces the need for extensive reconstructive surgery. Some tumors may not be amenable to this approach because of their size or growth pattern.

Other surgeons advocate that the margin of the resection should be at least 1.0–2.0 cm past the radiographic limits of the tumor. Ameloblastomas of the posterior maxilla are particularly dangerous because of the difficulty of obtaining an adequate surgical margin around the tumor. Orbital invasion by maxillary ameloblastomas occasionally has been described. Although some studies suggest that the ameloblastoma may be radiosensitive, radiation therapy has seldom been used as a treatment modality because of the intraosseous location of the tumor and the potential for secondary radiation-induced malignancy developing in a relatively young patient population.

The conventional ameloblastoma is a persistent, infiltrative neoplasm that very seldom may kill the patient by progressive spread to involve vital structures. Most of these tumors, however, are not life-threatening lesions. Rarely, an ameloblastoma exhibits frank malignant behavior. These are discussed separately.

UNICYSTIC AMELOBLASTOMA

The **unicystic ameloblastoma** has for several decades been given separate consideration based on its clinical, radiographic, and pathologic features. Although its response to treatment in reports from the 1970s and 1980s suggested that this lesion might behave in a less aggressive fashion, recent reports have disputed this concept. Unicystic ameloblastomas account for 10%–46% of all intraosseous ameloblastomas in various studies. Whether the unicystic ameloblastoma originates *de novo* as a neoplasm or whether it is the result of neoplastic transformation of nonneoplastic cyst epithelium has been long debated. Both mechanisms probably occur, but proof of which is involved in an individual patient is virtually impossible to obtain.

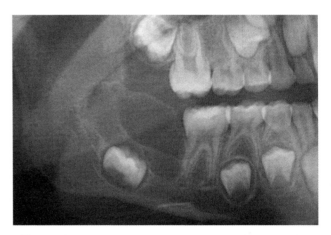

• **Fig. 15.77 Unicystic Ameloblastoma.** Radiolucency associated with the crown of the developing mandibular second molar. (Courtesy of Dr. Joseph Van Sickels.)

Clinical and Radiographic Features

Unicystic ameloblastomas are seen most often in younger patients, with about 50% of all such tumors diagnosed during the second decade of life. The average age in one large series was 23 years. More than 90% of unicystic ameloblastomas are found in the mandible, usually in the posterior regions. The lesion is often asymptomatic, although large lesions may cause a painless swelling of the jaws.

In many patients, this lesion typically appears as a circumscribed radiolucency that surrounds the crown of an unerupted mandibular third molar (Figs. 15.77 and 15.78), clinically resembling a dentigerous cyst. Other tumors simply appear as sharply defined radiolucent areas and are usually considered to be a primordial, radicular, or residual cyst, depending on the relationship of the lesion to teeth in the area. In some instances, the radiolucent area may have scalloped margins but is still a unicystic ameloblastoma. Whether a unicystic ameloblastoma can have a truly multilocular radiographic presentation is arguable.

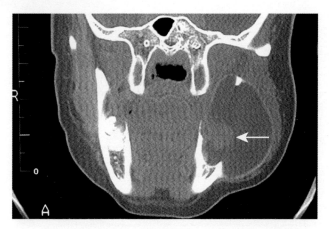

• **Fig. 15.78 Unicystic Ameloblastoma (Intraluminal Plexiform Type).** Coronal computed tomography (CT) image that shows a large cystic lesion with an intraluminal mass arising from the cyst wall (*arrow*).

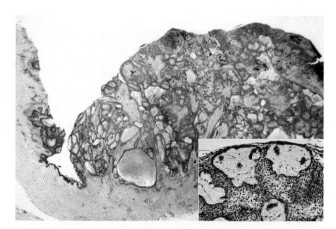

• **Fig. 15.80 Unicystic Ameloblastoma (Intraluminal Plexiform Type).** Photomicrograph of an intraluminal mass arising from the cyst wall. The *inset* shows the intraluminal mass at higher magnification.

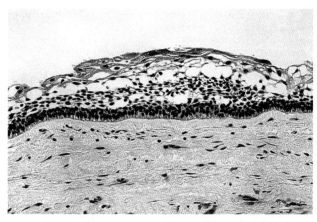

• **Fig. 15.79 Unicystic Ameloblastoma (Luminal Type).** The cyst is lined by ameloblastic epithelium showing a hyperchromatic, polarized basal layer. The overlying epithelial cells are loosely cohesive and resemble stellate reticulum.

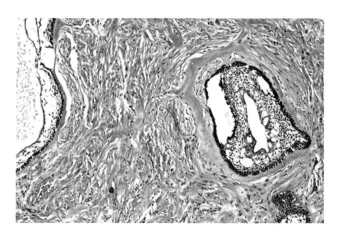

• **Fig. 15.81 Unicystic Ameloblastoma (Mural Type).** The epithelial lining of the cystic component can be seen on the left edge of the photomicrograph. Islands of follicular ameloblastoma are infiltrating into the fibrous connective tissue wall on the right.

The surgical findings may also suggest that the lesion in question is a cyst, and the diagnosis of ameloblastoma is made only after microscopic study of the specimen.

Histopathologic Features

Three histopathologic variants of unicystic ameloblastoma have been described. In the first type **(luminal unicystic ameloblastoma),** the tumor is confined to the luminal surface of the cyst. The lesion consists of a fibrous cyst wall with a lining composed totally or partially of ameloblastic epithelium. The lining demonstrates a basal layer of columnar or cuboidal cells with hyperchromatic nuclei that show reverse polarity and basilar cytoplasmic vacuolization (Fig. 15.79). The upper epithelial cells are loosely cohesive and resemble stellate reticulum. This finding does not seem to be related to inflammatory edema.

In the second microscopic variant, one or more nodules of ameloblastoma project from the cystic lining Tunto the lumen of the cyst. This type is called an **intraluminal unicystic**

ameloblastoma. These nodules may be relatively small or largely fill the cystic lumen. In some cases, the nodule of tumor that projects into the lumen demonstrates an edematous, plexiform pattern that resembles the plexiform pattern seen in conventional ameloblastomas (Fig. 15.80). These lesions are sometimes referred to as **plexiform unicystic ameloblastomas.** The intraluminal cellular proliferation does not always meet the strict histopathologic criteria for ameloblastoma, and this may be secondary to inflammation that nearly always accompanies this pattern. Typical ameloblastoma, however, may be found in other, less inflamed parts of the specimen.

In the third variant, known as **mural unicystic ameloblastoma,** the fibrous wall of the cyst is infiltrated by typical follicular or plexiform ameloblastoma. The extent and depth of the ameloblastic infiltration may vary considerably. With any presumed unicystic ameloblastoma, multiple sections through many levels of the specimen are necessary to rule out the possibility of mural invasion of tumor cells (Fig. 15.81).

Treatment and Prognosis

The clinical and radiographic findings in most cases of unicystic ameloblastoma suggest that the lesion is an odontogenic cyst. These tumors are usually treated as cysts by enucleation. The diagnosis of ameloblastoma is made only after microscopic examination of the presumed cyst. If the ameloblastic elements are confined to the lumen of the cyst with or without intraluminal tumor extension, then the cyst enucleation has probably been adequate treatment. The patient, however, should be kept under long-term follow-up. If the specimen shows extension of the tumor into the fibrous cyst wall for any appreciable distance, then subsequent management of the patient is more controversial. Some surgeons believe that local resection of the area is indicated as a prophylactic measure; others prefer to keep the patient under close radiographic observation and delay further treatment until there is evidence of recurrence.

Recurrence rates of 10%–20% were described after enucleation and curettage of unicystic ameloblastomas in many of the earlier series of cases. This range is considerably less than the 50%–90% recurrence rates noted after curettage of conventional solid and multicystic intraosseous ameloblastomas. A systematic review of the literature up to 2018 determined that 21% of these lesions recurred after enucleation, and only 3% recurred following radical resection. It is possible that some of those tumors that are designated as "unicystic" may, in fact, have a more characteristic invasive component that has not been detected histopathologically because it is essentially impossible to examine these lesions in every 360-degree plane of section.

PERIPHERAL (EXTRAOSSEOUS) AMELOBLASTOMA

The **peripheral ameloblastoma** is uncommon and accounts for about 1%–4% of all ameloblastomas. This tumor probably arises from rests of dental lamina beneath the oral mucosa or from the basal epithelial cells of the surface epithelium. Histopathologically, these lesions have the same features as the intraosseous form of the tumor.

Clinical Features

The peripheral ameloblastoma is usually a painless, nonulcerated sessile or pedunculated gingival or alveolar mucosal lesion. The clinical features are non-specific, and most lesions are clinically considered to represent a fibroma or pyogenic granuloma. Most examples are smaller than 1.5 cm, but larger lesions have been reported (Fig. 15.82). The tumor has been found in patients across a wide age range, but most are seen in middle-aged persons, with an average reported age of 52 years.

Peripheral ameloblastomas are most commonly found on the posterior gingival and alveolar mucosa, and they are somewhat more common in mandibular than in maxillary areas. In some cases, the superficial alveolar bone becomes

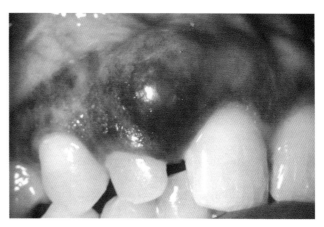

• **Fig. 15.82 Peripheral Ameloblastoma.** Sessile gingival mass. (Courtesy of Dr. Dean K. White.)

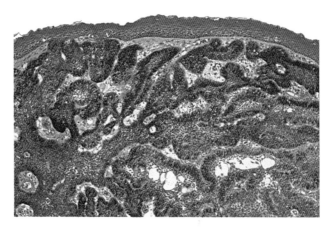

• **Fig. 15.83 Peripheral Ameloblastoma.** Interconnecting cords of ameloblastic epithelium filling the lamina propria.

slightly eroded, but significant bone involvement does not occur. A few examples of a microscopically identical lesion have been reported in the buccal mucosa at some distance from the alveolar or gingival soft tissues.

Histopathologic Features

Peripheral ameloblastomas have islands of ameloblastic epithelium that occupy the lamina propria underneath the surface epithelium (Fig. 15.83). The proliferating epithelium may show any of the features described for the intraosseous ameloblastoma; plexiform or follicular patterns are the most common. Connection of the tumor with the basal layer of the surface epithelium is seen in about 50% of cases. This may represent origin of the tumor from the basal layer of the epithelium in some cases, but in other instances the tumor could develop in the gingival connective tissue and merge with the surface epithelium.

Basal cell carcinomas of the gingival mucosa have been reported, but most of these would be designated best as peripheral ameloblastomas. A **peripheral odontogenic fibroma** may be confused microscopically with a peripheral ameloblastoma, particularly if a prominent epithelial component is present in the former. The presence of dysplastic dentin or cementum-like elements in the peripheral odontogenic fibroma and the lack of peripheral columnar epithelial cells showing reverse polarity of their nuclei should serve to distinguish the two lesions.

Treatment and Prognosis

Unlike the intraosseous ameloblastoma, the peripheral ameloblastoma shows an innocuous clinical behavior. Patients respond well to local surgical excision. Although local recurrence has been noted in 15%–20% of cases, further local excision almost always results in a cure. Several examples of malignant change in a peripheral ameloblastoma have been reported, but this is rare.

◆ MALIGNANT AMELOBLASTOMA AND AMELOBLASTIC CARCINOMA

Rarely, an ameloblastoma exhibits frank malignant behavior with development of metastases. The frequency of malignant behavior in ameloblastomas is difficult to determine but probably occurs in far less than 1% of all ameloblastomas.

The terminology for these lesions is somewhat confusing, but should not be considered controversial. The term *malignant ameloblastoma*, also known as *metastasizing ameloblastoma*, is used for a tumor that shows the histopathologic features of ameloblastoma, both in the primary tumor and in the metastatic deposits. This is a very rare neoplasm, with fewer than 30 well-documented cases described in the literature. The term *ameloblastic carcinoma* should be reserved for an ameloblastoma that has cytologic features of malignancy in the primary tumor, in a recurrence, or in any metastatic deposit. This is also a rare condition, although approximately 200 cases have been reported. These lesions may follow a markedly aggressive local course, but metastases do not necessarily occur. Other malignancies of odontogenic

differentiation that are quite rare, but deserve mention, include sclerosing odontogenic carcinoma, primary intraosseous carcinoma, ghost cell odontogenic carcinoma, odontogenic carcinosarcoma, odontogenic carcinoma with dentinoid, and odontogenic sarcomas.

Clinical and Radiographic Features

Malignant ameloblastomas have been observed in patients who range in age from 6 to 61 years (mean age, 30 years), and no sex predilection is seen. For patients with documented metastases, the interval between the initial treatment of the ameloblastoma and first evidence of metastasis varies from 3 to 45 years. In nearly one-third of cases, metastases do not become apparent until 10 years after treatment of the primary tumor. Ameloblastic carcinomas, in contrast, tend to develop later in life, with the mean age at diagnosis typically being in the sixth decade of life. Men are affected twice as frequently as women.

Metastases from ameloblastomas are found most often in the lungs. These have sometimes been regarded as aspiration or implant metastases. However, the peripheral location of some of these lung metastases suggests that they must have occurred by blood or lymphatic routes rather than aspiration.

Cervical lymph nodes are the second most common site for metastasis of an ameloblastoma. Spread to vertebrae, other bones, and viscera has also occasionally been confirmed.

The radiographic findings of malignant ameloblastomas may be essentially the same as those in typical nonmetastasizing ameloblastomas. Ameloblastic carcinomas are often more aggressive lesions, with ill-defined margins and cortical destruction (Fig. 15.84).

Histopathologic Features

With malignant ameloblastomas, the primary jaw tumor and the metastatic deposits show no microscopic features that differ from those of ameloblastomas with a completely

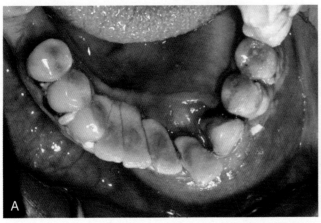
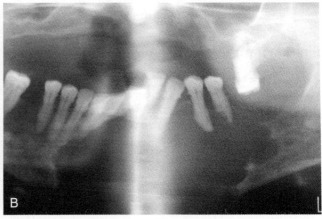

• **Fig. 15.84 Ameloblastic Carcinoma. A,** Rapidly growing tumor showing prominent labial expansion of the mandible in the incisor and premolar area. **B,** The panoramic radiograph shows irregular destruction of the mandible. (From Neville BW, Damm DD, White DK: *Color atlas of clinical oral pathology,* ed 2, Hamilton, 1999, BC Decker.)

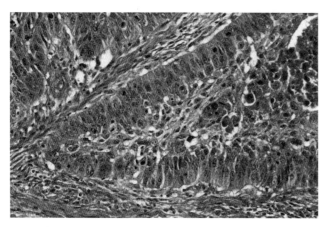

• **Fig. 15.85 Ameloblastic Carcinoma.** Ameloblastic epithelium demonstrating hyperchromatism, pleomorphism, and numerous mitotic figures.

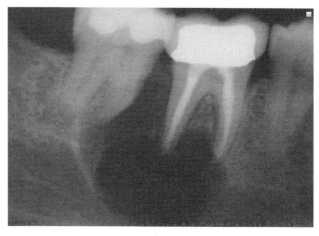

• **Fig. 15.86 Clear Cell Odontogenic Carcinoma.** A radiolucent defect at the apex of the mandibular first molar. (Courtesy of Dr. John Werther.)

benign local course. With ameloblastic carcinomas, the metastatic deposit or primary tumor shows the microscopic pattern of ameloblastoma in addition to cytologic features of malignancy. These include an increased nuclear-to-cytoplasmic ratio, nuclear hyperchromatism, and the presence of mitoses (Fig. 15.85). Necrosis in tumor islands and areas of dystrophic calcification may also be present.

Treatment and Prognosis

The prognosis of patients with malignant ameloblastomas appears to be poor, but the paucity of documented cases with long-term follow-up does not permit accurate assumptions to be made. About 50% of the patients with documented metastases and long-term follow-up have died of their disease. Lesions designated as *ameloblastic carcinoma* have demonstrated a uniformly aggressive clinical course, with perforation of the cortical plates of the jaw and extension of the tumor into adjacent soft tissues. One review of the literature identified a mean 5-year survival rate of nearly 70% when ameloblastic carcinoma was treated by surgical resection having disease-free margins. Radiation therapy has been used infrequently to treat this malignancy, although isolated reports indicate some benefit for those patients who are not candidates for extensive surgical procedures.

◆ CLEAR CELL ODONTOGENIC CARCINOMA (CLEAR CELL ODONTOGENIC TUMOR)

Clear cell odontogenic carcinoma is a rare jaw tumor that was first described in 1985. To date, approximately 120 examples have been documented. The tumor appears to be of odontogenic origin, but its histogenesis is uncertain. Histochemical and ultrastructural studies have suggested that the clear cells, which are the prominent feature of this neoplasm, may have similarities to glycogen-rich presecretory ameloblasts. Molecular studies of clear cell odontogenic carcinoma, however, have identified translocation of the

EWSR1 gene, which is often fused with the *ATF1* gene. This genetic alteration can be found in a variety of tumors, but it is often seen in hyalinizing clear cell carcinoma, a rare salivary gland malignancy.

Clinical and Radiographic Features

The clear cell odontogenic carcinoma exhibits a variable clinical pattern. A wide age range (from 17 to 89 years of age; mean age—55 years) has been described, and 65% of cases are diagnosed in females. Slightly more than 80% of the lesions develop in the mandible. Approximately 50% of patients complain of pain or lower lip paresthesia, and bony swelling has been described as a presenting sign in 80% of affected patients. Other patients are relatively symptom free. A significant number of patients will have evidence of soft tissue involvement by the tumor at the time of diagnosis because the lesion perforates bone.

Radiographically, the lesions appear as unilocular or multilocular radiolucencies. The margins of the radiolucency are often somewhat ill-defined or irregular (Fig. 15.86).

Histopathologic Features

Three histopathologic patterns have been described for clear cell odontogenic carcinoma. The biphasic pattern consists of varying-sized nests of epithelial cells, with a clear or faintly eosinophilic cytoplasm admixed with more eosinophilic polygonal epithelial cells (Fig. 15.87). The second pattern is more monophasic, characterized by only clear cells that are arranged in nests and cords. Thin strands of hyalinized connective tissue often separate the clear cell nests. The third pattern has a resemblance to ameloblastoma in that the peripheral cells of the clear cell islands may infrequently demonstrate palisading (Fig. 15.88). Often the lesional cells do not exhibit a significant degree of nuclear or cytologic pleomorphism. Furthermore, mitoses are generally sparse and necrosis is not a prominent feature. The clear cells contain small amounts of glycogen, but mucin stains are negative. In some cases, islands more typical of ameloblastoma are interspersed among the other tumor elements.

Hyalinizing clear cell carcinoma resembles clear cell odontogenic carcinoma, and although the salivary gland tumor develops in the soft tissues, for those lesions that have significant bone destruction, it may be difficult to identify the site of origin. Clear cell odontogenic carcinoma also may be difficult to distinguish from intraosseous mucoepidermoid carcinoma with a prominent clear cell component, although the negative mucin stains are consistent with the former. Amyloid stains would confirm the diagnosis of clear cell variant of the calcifying epithelial odontogenic tumor, because amyloid would not be present in clear cell odontogenic tumor. A metastatic clear cell neoplasm, such as a renal cell carcinoma, clear cell breast carcinoma, or clear cell melanoma, may also need to be ruled out before the diagnosis of clear cell odontogenic carcinoma can be established. If the diagnosis is unresolved using routine studies, molecular analysis can be employed to identify the characteristic translocation of the *EWSR1* gene and the fusion products that have been described in clear cell odontogenic carcinoma.

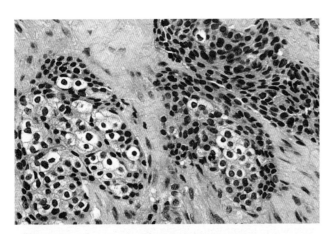

• **Fig. 15.87 Clear Cell Odontogenic Carcinoma.** Hyperchromatic epithelial nests including clusters of cells with abundant clear cytoplasm.

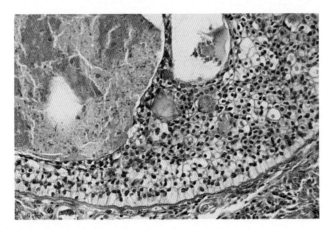

• **Fig. 15.88 Clear Cell Odontogenic Carcinoma.** Tumor island demonstrating cells with a clear cytoplasm. Note the peripheral columnar differentiation.

Treatment and Prognosis

Clear cell odontogenic carcinomas largely demonstrate an aggressive clinical course, with invasion of contiguous structures and a significant tendency to recur, particularly if the initial treatment is enucleation or curettage. Most patients require fairly radical surgery that may include hemimandibulectomy or hemimaxillectomy. Metastatic involvement of regional lymph nodes has been documented in about 9% of these patients, and pulmonary metastases have been identified in approximately 15%.

◆ ADENOMATOID ODONTOGENIC TUMOR

The **adenomatoid odontogenic tumor** represents 2%–7% of all odontogenic tumors, and more than 1,500 examples have been reported in the literature. Although this lesion was formerly considered to be a variant of the ameloblastoma and was designated as "adenoameloblastoma," its clinical features and biologic behavior indicate that it is a separate entity. Postulated histogenetic sources of the tumor cells have included enamel organ epithelium, reduced enamel epithelium, and rests of Malassez; however, some investigators have suggested that the lesion arises from remnants of dental lamina associated with the gubernacular cord. The lack of recurrence following enucleation, combined with the immunohistochemical profile of this lesion, have led some to the hypothesis that the adenomatoid odontogenic tumor is perhaps better thought of as a hamartoma, rather than a neoplasm.

Clinical and Radiographic Features

Adenomatoid odontogenic tumors are largely limited to younger patients, and two-thirds of all cases are diagnosed when patients are 10–19 years of age. This tumor is definitely uncommon in a patient older than age 30. It has a striking tendency to occur in the anterior portions of the jaws and is found twice as often in the maxilla as in the mandible (Fig. 15.89). Females are affected about twice as often as males.

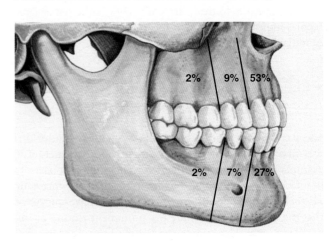

• **Fig. 15.89 Adenomatoid Odontogenic Tumor.** Relative distribution of adenomatoid odontogenic tumor in the jaws.

Most adenomatoid odontogenic tumors are relatively small. They seldom exceed 3 cm in greatest diameter, although a few large lesions have been reported. Peripheral (extraosseous) forms of the tumor are also encountered but are rare. These usually appear as small, sessile masses on the facial gingiva of the maxilla. Clinically, these lesions cannot be differentiated from the common gingival fibrous lesions.

Adenomatoid odontogenic tumors are frequently asymptomatic and are discovered during the course of a routine radiographic examination or when films are made to determine why a tooth has not erupted. Larger lesions cause a painless expansion of the bone.

In about 75% of cases, the tumor appears as a circumscribed, unilocular radiolucency that involves the crown of an unerupted tooth, most often a canine. This follicular type of adenomatoid odontogenic tumor may be impossible to differentiate radiographically from the more common dentigerous cyst. The radiolucency associated with the follicular type of adenomatoid odontogenic tumor sometimes extends apically along the root past the cementoenamel junction. This feature may help to distinguish an adenomatoid odontogenic tumor from a dentigerous cyst (Fig. 15.90). Rare examples of multiple adenomatoid odontogenic tumors associated with impacted teeth have been described in nevus sebaceus syndrome (Schimmelpenning syndrome).

The adenomatoid odontogenic tumor also may present as a well-delineated unilocular radiolucency that is not related to an unerupted tooth, but rather is located between the roots of erupted teeth (extrafollicular type) (Fig. 15.91), although this is less common than the follicular type.

The lesion may appear completely radiolucent; often, however, it contains fine (snowflake) calcifications (Fig. 15.92). This feature may be helpful in differentiating the adenomatoid odontogenic tumor from a dentigerous cyst.

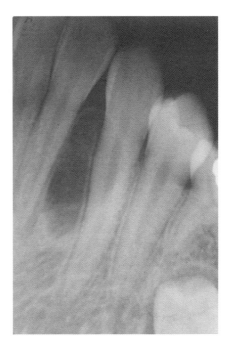

• **Fig. 15.91 Adenomatoid Odontogenic Tumor.** A small radiolucency is present between the roots of the lateral incisor and canine. (Courtesy of Dr. Ramesh Narang.)

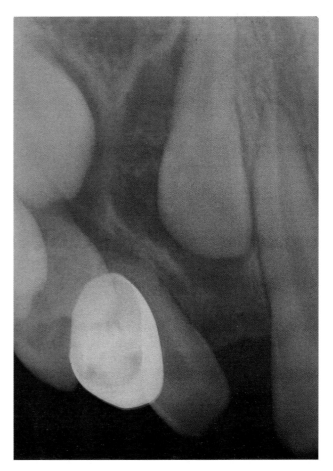

• **Fig. 15.92 Adenomatoid Odontogenic Tumor.** Well-defined pericoronal radiolucency enveloping the maxillary right lateral incisor in a 14-year-old male. Note the subtle snowflake-like calcifications within the lesion. (Courtesy of Dr. Jason Barker.)

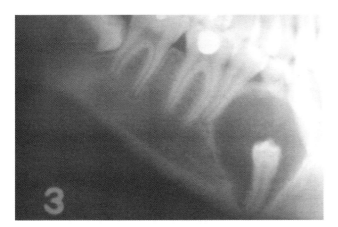

• **Fig. 15.90 Adenomatoid Odontogenic Tumor.** Radiolucent lesion involving an unerupted mandibular first premolar. In contrast to the usual dentigerous cyst, the radiolucency extends almost to the apex of the tooth. (Courtesy of Dr. Tony Traynham.)

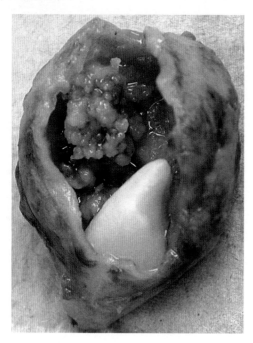

• **Fig. 15.93 Adenomatoid Odontogenic Tumor.** A well-circumscribed cystlike mass can be seen enveloping the crown of a maxillary cuspid. Note the intraluminal vegetations, which represent nodular tumor growth.

Histopathologic Features

The adenomatoid odontogenic tumor is a well-defined lesion that is usually surrounded by a thick, fibrous capsule. When the lesion is bisected, the central portion of the tumor may be essentially solid or may show varying degrees of cystic change (Fig. 15.93).

Microscopically, the tumor is composed of spindle-shaped epithelial cells that form sheets, strands, or whorled masses of cells in a scant fibrous stroma. The epithelial cells may form rosettelike structures about a central space, which may be empty or contain small amounts of eosinophilic material. This material may stain for amyloid.

The tubular or ductlike structures, which are the characteristic feature of the adenomatoid odontogenic tumor, may be prominent, scanty, or even absent in a given lesion. These consist of a central space surrounded by a layer of columnar or cuboidal epithelial cells. The nuclei of these cells tend to be polarized away from the central space. The mechanism of formation of these tubular structures is not entirely clear but is likely the result of the secretory activity of the tumor cells, which appear to be preameloblasts. In any event, these structures are not true ducts, and no glandular elements are present in the tumor (Fig. 15.94).

Small foci of calcification may also be scattered throughout the tumor. These have been interpreted as abortive enamel formation. Some adenomatoid odontogenic tumors contain larger areas of matrix material or calcification. This material has been interpreted as dentinoid or cementum. Some lesions also have another pattern, particularly at the periphery of the tumor adjacent to the capsule. This consists of narrow, often anastomosing cords of epithelium in an eosinophilic, loosely arranged matrix.

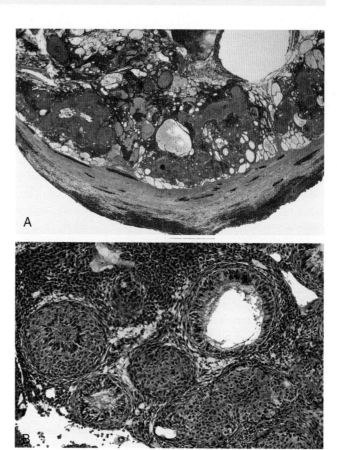

• **Fig. 15.94 Adenomatoid Odontogenic Tumor. A,** Low-power view demonstrating a thick capsule surrounding the tumor. **B,** Higher magnification showing the ductlike epithelial structures. The nuclei of the columnar cells are polarized away from the central spaces.

The histopathologic features of this lesion are distinctive and should not be confused with any other odontogenic tumor. Interestingly, some adenomatoid odontogenic tumors have been described with focal areas that resemble calcifying epithelial odontogenic tumor, odontoma, or calcifying odontogenic cyst. These lesions appear to behave as a routine adenomatoid odontogenic tumor, however. The chief problem relates to mistaking this tumor for an ameloblastoma by a pathologist who is not familiar with this lesion. This error can lead to unnecessary radical surgery.

Treatment and Prognosis

The adenomatoid odontogenic tumor is completely benign; because of its capsule, it enucleates easily from the bone. Aggressive behavior has not been documented, and recurrence after enucleation seldom, if ever, occurs.

◆ CALCIFYING EPITHELIAL ODONTOGENIC TUMOR (PINDBORG TUMOR)

The **calcifying epithelial odontogenic tumor,** also widely known as the **Pindborg tumor,** is an uncommon lesion that accounts for less than 1% of all odontogenic tumors.

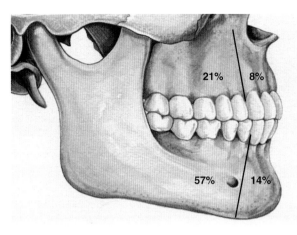

• **Fig. 15.95 Calcifying Epithelial Odontogenic Tumor.** Relative distribution of calcifying epithelial odontogenic tumor in the jaws.

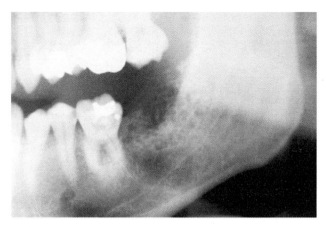

• **Fig. 15.96 Calcifying Epithelial Odontogenic Tumor.** Honeycombed multilocular radiolucency containing fine calcifications.

Approximately 360 cases have been reported to date. Although the tumor is clearly of odontogenic origin, its histogenesis is uncertain. The tumor cells bear a close morphologic resemblance to the cells of the stratum intermedium of the enamel organ; however, some investigators have recently suggested that the tumor arises from dental lamina remnants based on its anatomic distribution in the jaws. Mutations of the *PTCH1* gene have been identified in one small series of this neoplasm. This gene is characteristically associated with nevoid basal cell carcinoma syndrome (see page 694), but the calcifying epithelial odontogenic tumor is not a component of that condition.

Clinical and Radiographic Features

Although the calcifying epithelial odontogenic tumor has been found in patients across a wide age range and in many parts of the jaw, it is most often encountered in patients between 30 and 50 years of age. There is no sex predilection. About two-thirds of all reported cases have been found in the mandible, most often in the posterior areas (Fig. 15.95). A painless, slow-growing swelling is the most common presenting sign. Rare examples of multiple, synchronous calcifying epithelial odontogenic tumors also have been reported.

Radiographically, the tumor exhibits either a unilocular or a multilocular radiolucent defect (Fig. 15.96), with the unilocular pattern encountered more commonly in the maxilla. The margins of the lytic defect are often scalloped and usually relatively well defined. However, approximately 20% of cases have an ill-defined periphery, and an additional 20% exhibit a corticated border. The tumor is frequently associated with an impacted tooth, most often a mandibular molar. The lesion may be entirely radiolucent, but calcified structures of varying size and density are commonly seen. Although some authors have suggested that these are often most prominent around the crown of the impacted tooth (Fig. 15.97), a review of the literature identified this feature in only 12% of published cases with adequate radiographic documentation. Similarly, the description of a "driven-snow" pattern of the

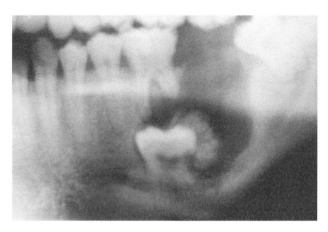

• **Fig. 15.97 Calcifying Epithelial Odontogenic Tumor.** Prominent calcification around the crown of an impacted second molar that is involved in the tumor. (Courtesy of Dr. Harold Peacock.)

calcifications appears to be much less common than previously believed.

A few cases of peripheral (extraosseous) calcifying epithelial odontogenic tumor have been reported. These appear as nonspecific, sessile gingival masses, most often on the anterior gingiva. Some of these have been associated with cupped-out erosion of the underlying bone.

Histopathologic Features

The calcifying epithelial odontogenic tumor has discrete islands, strands, or sheets of polyhedral epithelial cells in a fibrous stroma (Fig. 15.98). The cellular outlines of the epithelial cells are distinct, and intercellular bridges may be noted. The nuclei show considerable variation, and giant nuclei may be seen. Some tumors show considerable nuclear pleomorphism, but this feature is not considered to indicate malignancy. Large areas of amorphous, eosinophilic, hyalinized (amyloid-like) extracellular material are also often present. The tumor islands frequently enclose masses of this hyaline material, resulting in a cribriform appearance. Calcifications, which are a distinctive feature of the tumor,

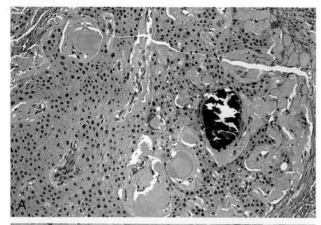

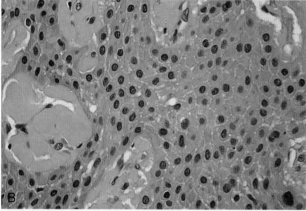

• **Fig. 15.98 Calcifying Epithelial Odontogenic Tumor. A,** Sheets of epithelial tumor cells that surround pools of amorphous, eosinophilic amyloid with focal calcification. **B,** Higher-power view showing polyhedral cells with eosinophilic cytoplasm and intercellular bridging. Adjacent amyloid deposits can be seen.

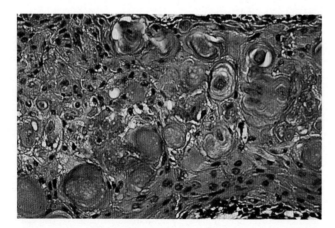

• **Fig. 15.99 Calcifying Epithelial Odontogenic Tumor.** Multiple concentric Liesegang ring calcifications.

develop within the amyloid-like material and form concentric rings *(Liesegang ring calcifications)* (Fig. 15.99). These tend to fuse and form large, complex masses.

Several microscopic variations may be encountered. Some tumors consist of large sheets of epithelial cells with minimal

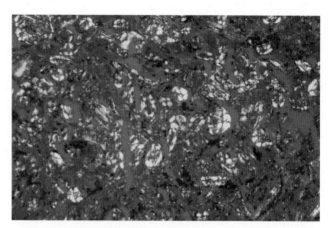

• **Fig. 15.100 Calcifying Epithelial Odontogenic Tumor.** With Congo red staining, the pools of amyloid exhibit an apple-green birefringence when viewed with polarized light.

production of amyloid-like material and calcifications. Others show large diffuse masses of amyloid-like material that contain only small nests or islands of epithelium. A clear cell variant has been described, in which clear cells constitute a significant portion of the epithelial component, and this tumor also has been reported to have a cystic growth pattern. A microcystic pattern has also been described in some Pindborg tumors.

The amyloid-like material in the Pindborg tumor has been extensively investigated by histochemical, immunohistochemical, and biochemical methods, as well as by electron microscopy. The material generally stains as amyloid (i.e., positive staining results with Congo red). After Congo red staining, the amyloid will exhibit apple-green birefringence when viewed with polarized light (Fig. 15.100). Investigators have identified this material as a unique protein that is produced by this tumor, as well as by the normal odontogenic apparatus and other odontogenic neoplasms. Both the protein structure and the DNA sequence of the responsible gene have been described, and this material has been designated as odontogenic ameloblast-associated protein (ODAM).

Treatment and Prognosis

Although it was originally believed that the calcifying epithelial odontogenic tumor had about the same biologic behavior as the ameloblastoma, accumulating experience indicates that it tends to be less aggressive. Conservative local resection to include a narrow rim of surrounding bone appears to be the treatment of choice, although lesions in the posterior maxilla should probably be treated more aggressively. A recurrence rate of about 15% has been reported; tumors treated by curettage have the highest frequency of recurrence. The overall prognosis appears good, although rare examples of malignant or borderline malignant calcifying epithelial odontogenic tumor have been reported, with documented metastasis to regional lymph nodes and lung.

◆ SQUAMOUS ODONTOGENIC TUMOR

Squamous odontogenic tumor is a rare benign odontogenic neoplasm that was first described in 1975 and is now recognized as a distinct entity. Approximately 110 examples have been reported to date, although a recent review of the literature suggested that some of these may have been misdiagnosed, based on accompanying photomicrographs, or had no microscopic documentation. Thus, a more accurate figure is likely closer to 50 cases. Most of these have been located within bone, although a few peripheral examples have been described. Before 1975, this lesion was probably believed to represent an atypical acanthomatous ameloblastoma or even a squamous cell carcinoma. The squamous odontogenic tumor may arise from neoplastic transformation of dental lamina rests or perhaps the epithelial rests of Malassez. In some cases, the tumor appears to originate within the periodontal ligament that is associated with the lateral root surface of an erupted tooth.

Clinical and Radiographic Features

Squamous odontogenic tumors have been found in patients whose ages ranged from 9 to 67 years (average age, 34). They are randomly distributed throughout the alveolar processes of the maxilla and mandible, with no site of predilection. A few patients have had multiple squamous odontogenic tumors that involved several quadrants of the mouth; one family with three affected siblings who each had multiple lesions has been reported. There is no apparent sex predilection. A painless or mildly painful gingival swelling, often associated with mobility of the associated teeth, is the most common complaint. About 10% of reported patients have had no symptoms, and their lesions were detected during a radiographic examination.

The radiographic findings are not specific or diagnostic and consist of a triangular radiolucent defect lateral to the root or roots of the teeth (Fig. 15.101). In some instances, this suggests vertical periodontal bone loss. The radiolucent area may be somewhat ill defined or may show a well-defined, corticated margin. Most examples are relatively small lesions that seldom exceed 1.5 cm in greatest diameter.

Histopathologic Features

The microscopic findings of squamous odontogenic tumor are distinctive and consist of varying-shaped islands of bland-appearing squamous epithelium in a mature fibrous connective tissue stroma. The peripheral cells of the epithelial islands do not show the characteristic polarization seen in ameloblastomas (Fig. 15.102). Vacuolization and individual cell keratinization within the epithelial islands are common features. Small microcysts are sometimes observed within the epithelial islands. Laminated calcified bodies and globular eosinophilic structures, which do not stain for amyloid, are present within the epithelium in some cases. The former probably represents dystrophic calcifications; the nature of the latter is unknown.

Islands of epithelium that closely resemble those of the squamous odontogenic tumor have been observed within the fibrous walls of dentigerous and radicular cysts. These have been designated as *squamous odontogenic tumorlike proliferations* in odontogenic cysts. These islands do not appear to have any significance relative to the behavior of the cyst,

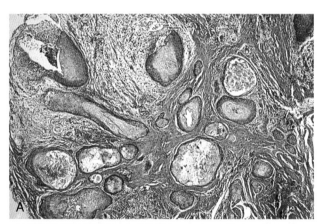
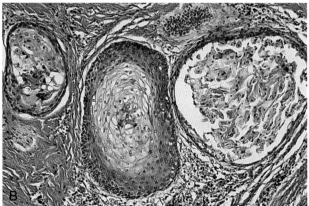

• **Fig. 15.102   Squamous Odontogenic Tumor. A,** Low-power photomicrograph showing islands of bland-appearing squamous epithelium in a fibrous stroma. **B,** Higher-power photomicrograph showing bland appearance of the epithelium with microcyst formation.

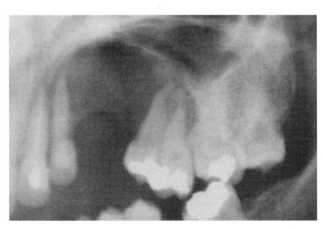

• **Fig. 15.101   Squamous Odontogenic Tumor.** Lucent defect extending along the roots of the lateral incisor and first premolar teeth. (Courtesy of Dr. Ed McGaha.)

and evaluation of the clinical, radiographic, and histopathologic features should permit differentiation from a squamous odontogenic tumor.

In published reports, some squamous odontogenic tumors have been misdiagnosed initially as ameloblastomas, resulting in unnecessary radical surgery.

Treatment and Prognosis

Conservative local excision or curettage appears to be effective for patients with squamous odontogenic tumors, and most reported cases have not recurred after local excision. A few instances of recurrence have been reported, but these have responded well to further local excision. The overall recurrence rate following conservative treatment is estimated to be approximately 19%. Maxillary squamous odontogenic tumors may be somewhat more aggressive than mandibular lesions, with a greater tendency to invade adjacent structures. This may be because of the porous, spongy nature of the maxillary bone. The multicentric lesions have typically exhibited a less aggressive, almost hamartomatous behavior when compared with solitary lesions. A well-documented example of apparent malignant transformation of squamous odontogenic tumor has been reported.

MIXED ODONTOGENIC TUMORS

The group of mixed odontogenic tumors, composed of proliferating odontogenic epithelium in a cellular ectomesenchyme resembling the dental papilla, poses problems in classification. Some of these lesions show varying degrees of inductive effect by the epithelium on the mesenchyme, leading to the formation of varying amounts of enamel and dentin. Some of these lesions (the common odontomas) are clearly nonneoplastic developmental anomalies; others appear to be true neoplasms. The nature of others is uncertain.

In some instances, the histopathologic findings alone cannot distinguish between the neoplastic lesions and the developmental anomalies. Clinical and radiographic features often are of considerable assistance in making this distinction.

◆ AMELOBLASTIC FIBROMA

The **ameloblastic fibroma** is considered to be a true mixed tumor in which the epithelial and mesenchymal tissues are both neoplastic. It is an uncommon tumor, but the data regarding its frequency are difficult to evaluate because (particularly in earlier reports) some lesions that were diagnosed as ameloblastic fibroma may actually have represented the early developing stage of an odontoma.

Clinical and Radiographic Features

Ameloblastic fibromas tend to occur in younger patients; most lesions are diagnosed in the first two decades of life, with an average age of 15 years. This lesion, however, is occasionally encountered in middle-aged patients. The tumor is

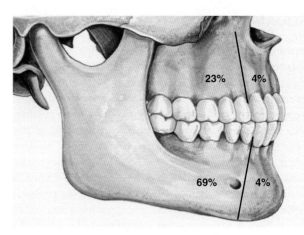

• **Fig. 15.103 Ameloblastic Fibroma.** Relative distribution of ameloblastic fibroma in the jaws.

slightly more common in males than in females. Small ameloblastic fibromas are asymptomatic; larger tumors are associated with swelling of the jaws. The posterior mandible is the most common site; about 70% of all cases are located in this area (Fig. 15.103). Convincing examples of this tumor arising within the gingival soft tissue have been described, but this appears to represent a rare phenomenon.

Radiographically, either a unilocular or multilocular radiolucent lesion is seen, with the smaller lesions tending to be unilocular. The radiographic margins tend to be well defined, and they may be corticated. An unerupted tooth is associated with the lesion in about 75% of cases. The ameloblastic fibroma may grow to a large size, and cases that involve a considerable portion of the body and ascending ramus of the mandible or the posterior maxilla have been reported (Fig. 15.104).

Histopathologic Features

The ameloblastic fibroma appears as a solid, soft tissue mass with a smooth outer surface. A definite capsule may or may not be present. Microscopically, the tumor is composed of a cell-rich mesenchymal tissue resembling the primitive dental papilla admixed with proliferating odontogenic epithelium. The latter may have one of two patterns, both of which are usually present in any given case. The most common epithelial pattern consists of long, narrow cords of odontogenic epithelium, often in an anastomosing arrangement. These cords are usually only two cells in thickness and are composed of cuboidal or columnar cells (Fig. 15.105). In the other pattern, the epithelial cells form small, discrete islands that resemble the follicular stage of the developing enamel organ. These show peripheral columnar cells, which surround a mass of loosely arranged epithelial cells that resemble stellate reticulum. In contrast to the follicular type of ameloblastoma, these follicular islands in the ameloblastic fibroma seldom demonstrate microcyst formation.

The mesenchymal portion of the ameloblastic fibroma consists of plump stellate and ovoid cells in a loose matrix, which closely resembles the developing dental papilla.

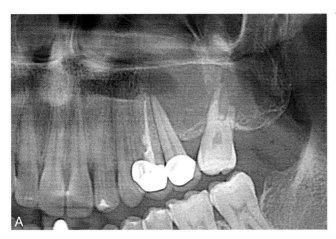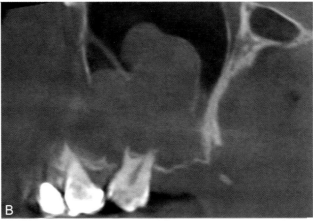

• **Fig. 15.104 Ameloblastic Fibroma. A,** Panoramic radiograph showing a destructive radiolucent lesion of the left posterior maxilla. **B,** Cone-beam computed tomography (CBCT) image demonstrating extension of the tumor into the maxillary sinus. (Courtesy of Dr. Michael Menis.)

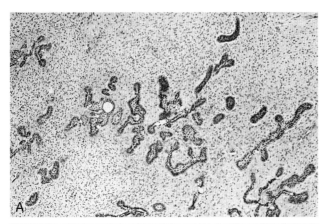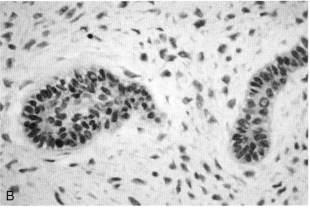

• **Fig. 15.105 Ameloblastic Fibroma. A,** Long, narrow cords of odontogenic epithelium supported by richly cellular, primitive connective tissue. **B,** Basophilic epithelial islands with peripheral nuclear palisading.

Collagen formation is generally inconspicuous. Juxtaepithelial hyalinization of the mesenchymal portion of the tumor is sometimes seen, and occasionally diffuse areas of hyalinized acellular lesional tissue are evident.

A few examples of ameloblastic fibroma occurring in conjunction with calcifying odontogenic cyst also have been reported.

Treatment and Prognosis

The proper management of ameloblastic fibroma has been an ongoing topic of debate. Although initially it was believed that the ameloblastic fibroma was an innocuous lesion that seldom recurred after simple local excision or curettage, subsequent reports seemed to indicate a substantial risk of recurrence after conservative therapy. The highest recurrence rate (43.5%) was recorded in a series of cases from the Armed Forces Institute of Pathology, and it could be argued that this was a biased sample of larger lesions that were inherently more difficult to manage. In analysis of cases reported in the literature, approximately 19% of ameloblastic fibromas were reported to recur after enucleation or marginal resection and an adequate follow-up period. Based on these data, recent recommendations have emphasized conservative initial therapy for ameloblastic fibroma, followed by long-term monitoring. More aggressive surgical excision should probably be reserved for recurrent lesions. Approximately 26% of the cases of the rare ameloblastic fibrosarcoma develop in the setting of a recurrent ameloblastic fibroma.

◆ AMELOBLASTIC FIBRO-ODONTOMA

The **ameloblastic fibro-odontoma** is defined as a tumor with the general features of an ameloblastic fibroma but that also contains enamel and dentin. Some investigators believe that the ameloblastic fibro-odontoma is only a stage in the development of an odontoma and do not consider it to be a separate entity. Certainly the histopathologic features of a developing odontoma may overlap somewhat with ameloblastic fibro-odontoma. There are well-documented examples, however, of this tumor exhibiting progressive growth and causing considerable deformity and bone destruction. Such lesions appear to be true neoplasms. However, distinguishing between a developing odontoma and an ameloblastic fibro-odontoma may be difficult based on histopathologic grounds alone, and it is quite likely that some examples of developing odontoma have been reported in the literature as ameloblastic fibro-odontoma. A recent publication that analyzed reported cases of odontoma and ameloblastic fibro-odontoma found that lesions that were 2.1 cm or greater in size and developed in patients younger than 13.5 years of age were more likely to have features consistent with a neoplasm. The latest World Health Organization has eliminated the ameloblastic fibro-odontoma from its classification of odontogenic tumors, an action with which the authors of this textbook disagree, for reasons noted above. Whether molecular genetic studies that might be performed at some time in the future will resolve this dilemma remains to be seen.

Clinical and Radiographic Features

The ameloblastic fibro-odontoma is usually seen in children with an average age of 10 years. It is rarely encountered in adults. Like the **ameloblastic fibroma,** ameloblastic fibro-odontomas occur more frequently in the posterior regions of the jaws, and the majority involves the mandible (Fig. 15.106). Males are affected somewhat more often than females, with a 3:2 ratio noted in the literature. The lesion is commonly asymptomatic and is discovered when radiographs are taken to determine the reason for failure of a tooth to erupt. Large examples may be associated with a painless swelling of the affected bone.

Radiographically, the tumor shows a well-circumscribed unilocular or, infrequently, multilocular radiolucent defect that contains a variable amount of calcified material with the radiodensity of tooth structure. The calcified material within the lesion may appear as multiple, small radiopacities or as a solid conglomerate mass (Fig. 15.107). In most instances, an unerupted tooth is present at the margin of the lesion, or the crown of the unerupted tooth may be included within the defect. Approximately 5% of ameloblastic fibro-odontomas contain only a minimal amount of calcifying enamel and dentin matrix and appear primarily as radiolucent lesions (Fig. 15.108). These cannot be

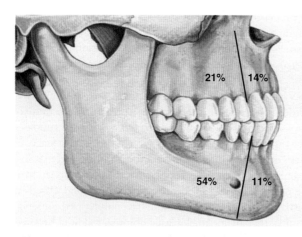

• **Fig. 15.106 Ameloblastic Fibro-Odontoma.** Relative distribution of ameloblastic fibro-odontoma in the jaws.

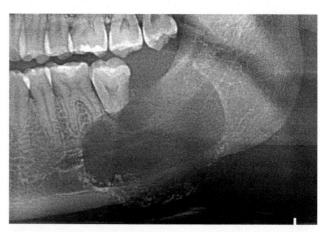

• **Fig. 15.108 Ameloblastic Fibro-Odontoma.** Large, expansile radiolucent defect that is associated with root resorption of the overlying molars. Flecks of mineralized material are present at the periphery. (Courtesy of Dr. Mark Spinazze.)

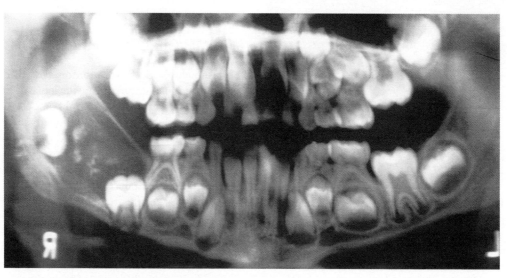

• **Fig. 15.107 Ameloblastic Fibro-Odontoma.** Radiolucent defect in the ramus containing small calcifications having the radiodensity of tooth structure.

differentiated from the wide variety of unilocular radiolucencies that may involve the jaws. At the other extreme, some ameloblastic fibro-odontomas appear as largely calcified masses with only a narrow rim of radiolucency about the periphery of the lesion, which would be a pattern that certainly suggests a maturing odontoma.

Histopathologic Features

The soft tissue component of the ameloblastic fibro-odontoma is microscopically identical to the **ameloblastic fibroma** and has narrow cords and small islands of odontogenic epithelium in a loose primitive-appearing connective tissue that resembles the dental papilla. The calcifying element consists of foci of enamel and dentin matrix formation in close relationship to the epithelial structures (Fig. 15.109). The more calcified lesions show mature dental structures in the form of rudimentary small teeth or conglomerate masses of enamel and dentin. Some researchers have designated a similar tumor in which the calcifying component consists only of dentin matrix and dentinoid material as **ameloblastic

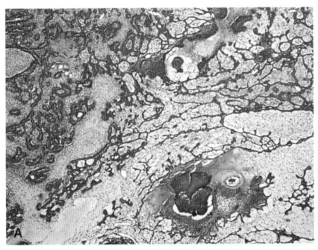

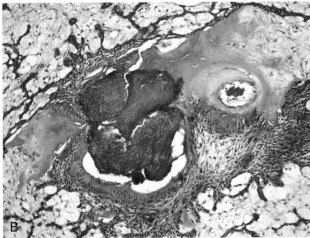

• **Fig. 15.109 Ameloblastic Fibro-Odontoma. A,** The soft tissue component of the tumor is indistinguishable from an ameloblastic fibroma. **B,** Formation of disorganized tooth structure can be seen.

fibro-dentinoma.** It is questionable whether this lesion represents a separate entity, and it is probably best considered as only a variant of the ameloblastic fibro-odontoma.

Treatment and Prognosis

A patient with an ameloblastic fibro-odontoma is generally treated by conservative curettage, and the lesion usually separates easily from its bony bed. The tumor is well circumscribed and does not invade the surrounding bone.

The prognosis is excellent, and the recurrence rate after conservative removal is estimated to be about 7%. Development of an ameloblastic fibrosarcoma after curettage of an ameloblastic fibro-odontoma has been reported, but this is exceedingly rare.

◆ AMELOBLASTIC FIBROSARCOMA (AMELOBLASTIC SARCOMA)

The rare **ameloblastic fibrosarcoma** is considered to be the malignant counterpart of the ameloblastic fibroma, and approximately 110 cases have been documented in the literature. Interestingly, in most cases, only the mesenchymal portion of the lesion shows features of malignancy; the epithelial component remains rather bland. These tumors may apparently arise *de novo;* however, in approximately one-quarter of known cases, the malignant lesion represents a recurrence of a tumor previously diagnosed as an ameloblastic fibroma or an ameloblastic fibro-odontoma. Recent molecular analysis of a small series of this tumor has identified mutations of *BRAF*, and less commonly, *NRAS*. Pharmacologic blocking agents for these genetic pathways are currently available, and evaluation of their efficacy in clinical treatment trials may determine their therapeutic benefit in the future.

Clinical and Radiographic Features

Ameloblastic fibrosarcomas occur slightly more often in males as in females, based on reported cases. The lesion tends to occur in younger patients (mean reported age, approximately 30 years). Although either the maxilla or the mandible may be involved, about 80% of cases have occurred in the mandible. Pain and swelling associated with rapid clinical growth are the common complaints.

Radiographically, the ameloblastic fibrosarcoma may show an ill-defined destructive radiolucent presentation, suggestive of a malignant process (Fig. 15.110).

Histopathologic Features

Ameloblastic fibrosarcomas contain an epithelial component similar to that seen in the ameloblastic fibroma, although it is frequently less prominent. The epithelial component appears histopathologically benign and does not demonstrate any cytologic atypia. The mesenchymal portion of the tumor,

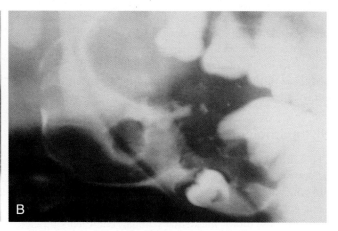

• **Fig. 15.110 Ameloblastic Fibrosarcoma. A,** A 21-year-old woman complained of facial asymmetry and recent increase in size of a mandibular mass that had been present for some years. **B,** Radiograph of the same patient. Note the lytic destruction of the posterior mandible. (Courtesy of Dr. Sam McKenna.)

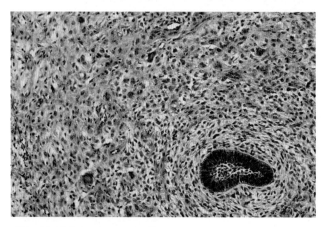

• **Fig. 15.111 Ameloblastic Fibrosarcoma.** The cellular mesenchymal tissue shows hyperchromatism and atypical cells. A small island of ameloblastic epithelium is present.

however, is highly cellular and shows hyperchromatic and often bizarre pleomorphic cells (Fig. 15.111). Mitoses are usually prominent. In some cases with multiple recurrences, the epithelial component becomes progressively less conspicuous so that the tumor eventually shows only a poorly differentiated fibrosarcoma.

In a few instances, dysplastic dentin or small amounts of enamel may be formed. Some have called such lesions **ameloblastic dentinosarcomas** or **ameloblastic fibro-odontosarcomas.** This additional subclassification, however, appears unnecessary. Another rare event that actually may be overrepresented in the literature is concurrent malignant transformation of both the epithelial and mesenchymal elements of an ameloblastic fibroma, resulting in an **ameloblastic** (or **odontogenic**) **carcinosarcoma.**

Treatment and Prognosis

Once the diagnosis of ameloblastic fibrosarcoma has been confirmed, radical surgical excision appears to be the treatment of choice. Curettage or local excision is usually followed by rapid local recurrence. The tumor is locally aggressive and infiltrates adjacent bone and soft tissues.

The long-term prognosis is difficult to ascertain because of the few reported cases with adequate follow-up, with the best estimates suggesting that 20% of these patients will succumb to their tumor. Most deaths have resulted from uncontrolled local disease, and metastatic tumor has been documented in only four of 54 evaluable cases.

◆ ODONTOAMELOBLASTOMA

The **odontoameloblastoma** is an extremely rare odontogenic tumor that contains an ameloblastomatous component and odontoma-like elements. Fewer than 20 cases have been reported with sufficient documentation to support this diagnosis, and odontoameloblastoma as an entity was formally eliminated from the World Health Organization Classification of Head and Neck Tumours as of 2017. This tumor was formerly called *ameloblastic odontoma* and was confused with the more common (though still relatively rare) lesion currently designated as **ameloblastic fibro-odontoma.** Because the clinical behavior of these two tumors is quite different, they should be distinguished from one another. This neoplasm is also frequently confused with an odontoma that is in its early stages of development. Some investigators believe that this lesion represents simply an ameloblastoma that has developed in conjunction with an odontoma, with the two lesions being otherwise unrelated.

Clinical and Radiographic Features

Because of the rarity of odontoameloblastomas, little reliable information is available. The lesion appears to occur more often in younger patients, and either jaw can be affected. Pain, delayed eruption of teeth, and expansion of the affected bone may be noted.

Radiographically, the tumor shows a radiolucent, destructive process that contains calcified structures. These have the radiodensity of tooth structure and may resemble miniature teeth or occur as larger masses of calcified material similar to a complex odontoma.

Histopathologic Features

The histopathologic features of the odontoameloblastoma are complex. The proliferating epithelial portion of the tumor has features of an **ameloblastoma,** most often of the plexiform or follicular pattern. The ameloblastic component is intermingled with immature or more mature dental tissue in the form of developing rudimentary teeth, which is similar to the appearance of a **compound odontoma,** or conglomerate masses of enamel, dentin, and cementum, as seen in a **complex odontoma.**

Treatment and Prognosis

Multiple recurrences of odontoameloblastomas have been reported after local curettage, and it appears that this tumor has the same biologic potential as the ameloblastoma. It is probably wise to treat a patient with this lesion in the same manner as one with an ameloblastoma. However, there are no valid data on the long-term prognosis.

◆ ODONTOMA

Odontomas are the most common types of odontogenic tumors. Their prevalence exceeds that of all other odontogenic tumors combined. Odontomas are considered to be developmental anomalies **(hamartomas),** rather than true neoplasms. When fully developed, odontomas consist chiefly of enamel and dentin, with variable amounts of pulp and cementum. In their earlier developmental stages, varying amounts of proliferating odontogenic epithelium and mesenchyme are present.

Odontomas are further subdivided into compound and complex types. The **compound odontoma** is composed of multiple, small toothlike structures. The **complex odontoma** consists of a conglomerate mass of enamel and dentin, which bears no anatomic resemblance to a tooth. In most series, compound odontomas are more frequently diagnosed than complex, and it is possible that some compound odontomas are not submitted for microscopic examination because the clinician is comfortable with the clinical and radiographic diagnosis. Occasionally, an odontoma may show both compound and complex features.

Clinical and Radiographic Features

Most odontomas are detected during the first two decades of life, and the mean age at the time of diagnosis is 14 years. The majority of these lesions are completely asymptomatic, being discovered on a routine radiographic examination or when films are taken to determine the reason for failure of a tooth to erupt. Odontomas are typically relatively small and seldom exceed the size of a tooth in the area where they are located. However, large odontomas up to 6 cm or more in

diameter are occasionally seen. These large odontomas can cause expansion of the jaw.

Odontomas occur somewhat more frequently in the maxilla than in the mandible. Although compound and complex odontomas may be found in any site, the compound type is more often seen in the anterior maxilla; complex odontomas occur more often in the molar regions of either jaw. Occasionally, an odontoma will develop completely within the gingival soft tissues.

Radiographically, the **compound odontoma** appears as a collection of toothlike structures of varying size and shape surrounded by a narrow radiolucent zone (Figs. 15.112 and 15.113). The **complex odontoma** appears as a calcified mass with the radiodensity of tooth structure, which is also surrounded by a narrow radiolucent rim. An unerupted

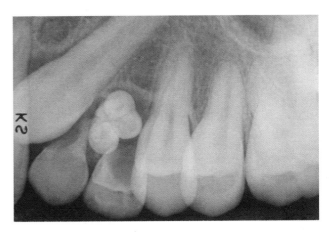

• **Fig. 15.112 Compound Odontoma.** A small cluster of toothlike structures is preventing the eruption of the maxillary canine. (Courtesy of Dr. Robert J. Powers.)

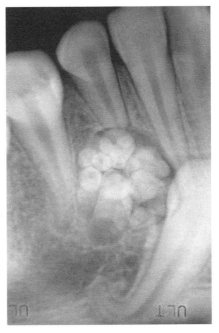

• **Fig. 15.113 Compound Odontoma.** Multiple toothlets preventing the eruption of the mandibular cuspid. (Courtesy of Dr. Brent Bernard.)

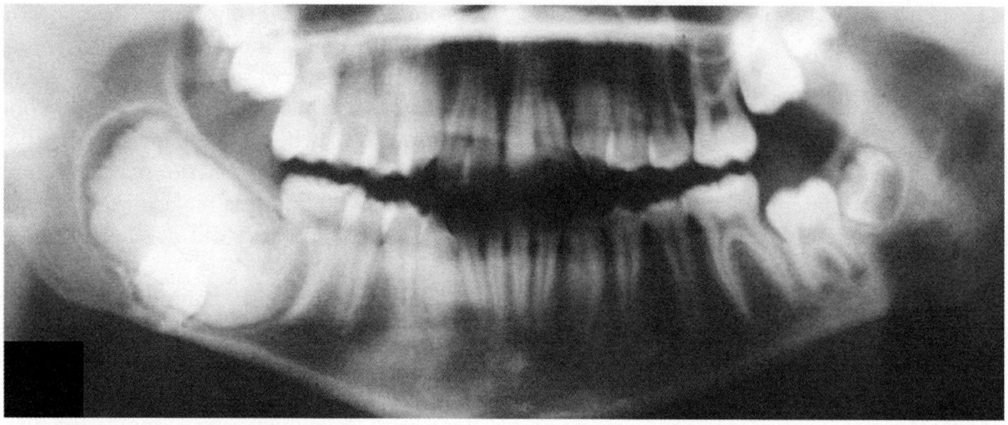

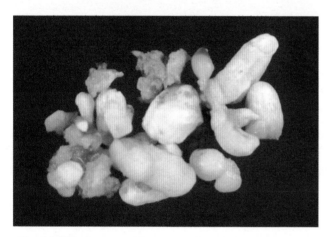

• **Fig. 15.114 Complex Odontoma.** A large radiopaque mass is overlying the crown of the mandibular right second molar, which has been displaced to the inferior border of the mandible.

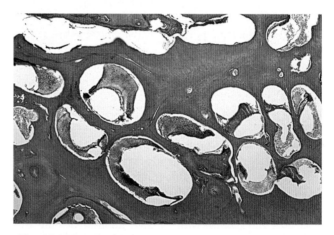

• **Fig. 15.115 Compound Odontoma.** Surgical specimen consisting of more than 20 malformed toothlike structures.

• **Fig. 15.116 Complex Odontoma.** This decalcified section shows a disorganized mass of dentin intermixed with small pools of enamel matrix.

tooth is frequently associated with the odontoma, and the odontoma prevents eruption of the tooth (Fig. 15.114). Some small odontomas are present between the roots of erupted teeth and are not associated with disturbance in eruption. The radiographic findings are usually diagnostic, and the compound odontoma is seldom confused with any other lesion. A developing odontoma may show little evidence of calcification and appear as a circumscribed radiolucent lesion. A complex odontoma, however, may be radiographically confused with an osteoma or some other highly calcified bone lesion.

Histopathologic Features

The compound odontoma consists of multiple structures resembling small, single-rooted teeth, contained in a loose fibrous matrix (Fig. 15.115). The mature enamel caps of the toothlike structures are lost during decalcification for preparation of the microscopic section, but varying amounts of enamel matrix are often present. Pulp tissue may be seen in the coronal and root portions of the toothlike structures. In patients with developing odontomas, structures that resemble tooth germs are present.

Complex odontomas consist largely of mature tubular dentin. This dentin encloses clefts or hollow circular structures that contained the mature enamel that was removed during decalcification. The spaces may contain small amounts of enamel matrix or immature enamel (Fig. 15.116). Small islands of eosinophilic-staining epithelial ghost cells are present in about 20% of complex odontomas. These may represent remnants of odontogenic epithelium that have undergone keratinization and cell death from the local anoxia. A thin layer of cementum is often present about the periphery of the mass. Occasionally, a dentigerous cyst may arise from the epithelial lining of the fibrous capsule of a complex odontoma.

Treatment and Prognosis

Odontomas are treated by simple local excision, and the prognosis is excellent.

◆ PRIMORDIAL ODONTOGENIC TUMOR

The primordial odontogenic tumor is the most recent addition to the spectrum of odontogenic neoplasms, being first identified as a distinct entity in 2014. Previously these rare lesions were categorized as an unusual example of ameloblastic fibroma, myxoma, or central odontogenic fibroma. As more cases were documented over the years, it became apparent that this tumor was unique and deserved to be recognized in its own right.

Clinical and Radiographic Features

The primordial odontogenic tumor typically affects patients in the first or second decade of life, presenting as a firm, painless swelling of the posterior mandible, or less commonly, maxilla. Radiographically, the lesion appears as an expansile, unilocular or bilocular, well-demarcated radiolucency that is associated with the crown of a posterior tooth (Fig. 15.117), although sometimes the tooth appears to be completely contained within the lesion. The 3rd molars and primary molars are affected most frequently. Some of these tumors attain significant size, with the greatest dimension ranging from 1.5 to 9.0 cm.

Histopathologic Features

Microscopically the primordial odontogenic tumor is usually encapsulated, and the bulk of the lesion consists of sheets of myxoid to cellular ectomesenchymal tissue that often has a lobulated or undulating periphery. The edge of the tumor is lined by a thin layer of cuboidal to columnar epithelium that resembles the inner enamel epithelium of a developing tooth (Fig. 15.118). Stellate reticulum-like differentiation adjacent to the columnar epithelium has been described in half of reported cases. In some instances, this epithelium may be somewhat more prominent, dipping between the ectomesenchymal lobules of the tumor. Occasionally eosinophilic mineralized tissue that has been described as "enameloid" in appearance is identified in the lesion, as well as basophilic calcifications that resemble enamel matrix.

Treatment and Prognosis

Enucleation or conservative excision, including the involved tooth, has been the preferred treatment, and this appears to be curative despite the relatively large size of some primordial odontogenic tumors. To date, of the 24 reported cases of this tumor, only one has recurred.

TUMORS OF ODONTOGENIC ECTOMESENCHYME

◆ CENTRAL ODONTOGENIC FIBROMA

The **central odontogenic fibroma** is an uncommon and somewhat controversial lesion. Approximately 235 examples have been reported. Formerly, some oral and maxillofacial pathologists designated solid fibrous masses that were almost always associated with the crown of an unerupted tooth as *odontogenic fibromas*. Most oral and maxillofacial pathologists today consider such lesions to represent only hyperplastic dental follicles, and these should not be considered to be neoplasms.

Clinical and Radiographic Features

Odontogenic fibromas have been reported in patients whose ages ranged from 3 to 77 years (mean age, 33 years). Of those cases reported in the literature, a 1.35:1.0 female-to-male ratio has been noted, indicating a strong female predilection. The maxilla and mandible are affected nearly equally, with most maxillary lesions located anterior to the first molar

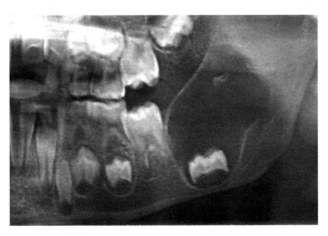

• **Fig. 15.117 Primordial Odontogenic Tumor.** Panoramic radiograph depicting a large demarcated radiolucency involving the left posterior mandible and ramus. The developing 2nd molar is displaced inferiorly, and a faint opacity represents the developing 3rd molar that is displaced superiorly. (Courtesy of Dr. Amy Bogardus.)

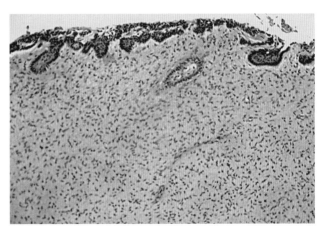

• **Fig. 15.118 Primordial Odontogenic Tumor.** Sheets of uniform spindle-shaped cells resembling dental papilla are covered by a thin layer of odontogenic epithelium that resembles the inner enamel epithelium. (Courtesy of Dr. Amy Bogardus.)

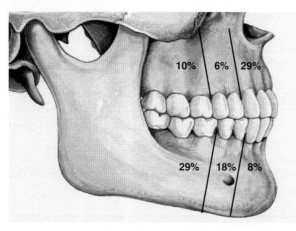

• **Fig. 15.119 Odontogenic Fibroma.** Relative distribution of odontogenic fibroma in the jaws.

tooth (Fig. 15.119). In the mandible, however, about half of the tumors are located posterior to the first molar. A systematic review of odontogenic fibromas reported in the literature found that approximately 5% are associated with an unerupted tooth. Smaller odontogenic fibromas are usually completely asymptomatic; larger lesions may be associated with localized bony expansion or loosening of teeth. Interestingly, the palatal mucosa that overlies the tumor occasionally may exhibit a defect or groove.

Radiographically, smaller odontogenic fibromas tend to be well-defined, unilocular, radiolucent lesions often associated with the periradicular area of erupted teeth (Fig. 15.120). Larger lesions tend to be multilocular radiolucencies. Many lesions have a corticated border. Root resorption of associated teeth is common, and lesions located between the teeth often cause root divergence. Approximately 12% of central odontogenic fibromas will exhibit radiopaque flecks within the lesion.

Histopathologic Features

Lesions reported as central odontogenic fibroma have shown considerable histopathologic diversity; in the past, this led some authors to describe two separate types, although this concept has been questioned. The simple type of odontogenic fibroma is rare, being composed of stellate fibroblasts, often arranged in a whorled pattern with fine collagen fibrils and considerable ground substance (Fig. 15.121). Small foci of odontogenic epithelial rests may be present. Spindle cell collagenous lesions that do not have epithelial rests may represent other entities, such as desmoplastic fibroma, myofibroma, or neurofibroma. Occasional foci of dystrophic calcification may be seen.

Epithelium-rich odontogenic fibromas (sometimes called WHO odontogenic fibromas) are more common and have a more complex pattern, which often consists of a fairly cellular fibrous connective tissue with collagen fibers arranged in interlacing bundles. Odontogenic epithelium in the form of long strands or isolated nests is present throughout the

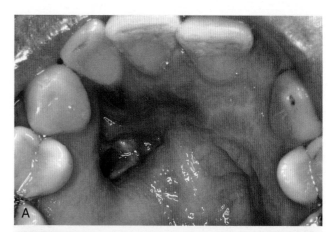

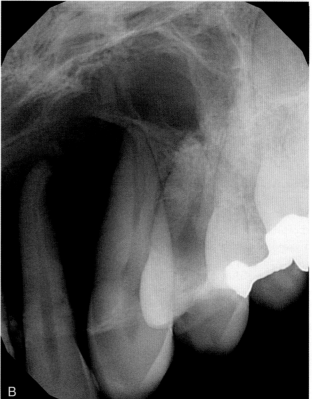

• **Fig. 15.120 Odontogenic Fibroma. A,** Clinical image showing a groove or defect in the palatal mucosa, a feature that has been described with maxillary lesions. **B,** Radiograph of this patient, depicting a multilocular radiolucency of the anterior maxilla. (Courtesy of Dr. Greg Adams.)

lesion and may be a prominent component (Fig. 15.122). The fibrous component may vary from myxoid to densely hyalinized.

Calcifications composed of cementum-like material or dentinoid are present in some cases. Focal deposits of odontogenic ameloblast-associated protein (ODAM), which represent a form of amyloid, have been described in a few central odontogenic fibromas, and Langerhans cells are often identified in these lesions as well. The possibility that some of these lesions may have been reported as non-calcifying Langerhans cell-rich calcifying epithelial odontogenic tumors cannot be

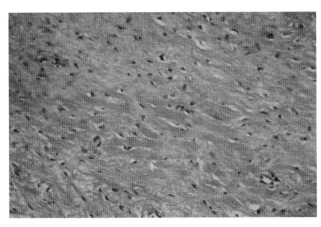

• **Fig. 15.121 Odontogenic Fibroma.** Simple type of odontogenic fibroma showing scattered fibroblasts within a collagenous background. No epithelial rests were found on multiple sections from this tumor.

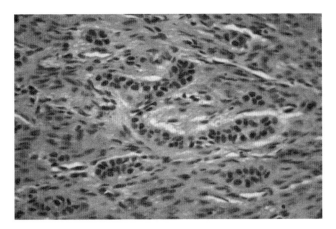

• **Fig. 15.122 Odontogenic Fibroma.** Epithelium-rich variant showing a cellular fibroblastic proliferation containing narrow cords of odontogenic epithelium.

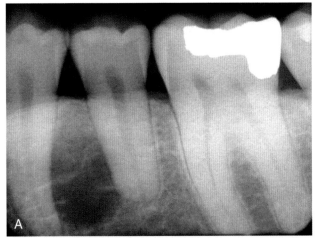

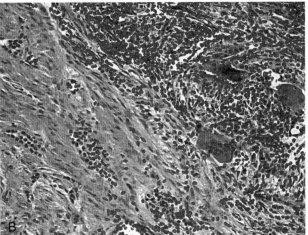

• **Fig. 15.123 Odontogenic Fibroma with Associated Giant Cell Granuloma. A,** Unilocular radiolucency between the left mandibular bicuspids. **B,** Microscopic examination reveals two distinct patterns. On the left, one can see cords of odontogenic epithelium within a fibrous background, consistent with odontogenic fibroma. Typical features of central giant cell granuloma are present on the right side of the field.

excluded. Approximately 40 examples of central odontogenic fibroma associated with a **giant cell granuloma**–like component have been reported since 1992 (Fig. 15.123). It seems unlikely that this process represents a "collision" tumor with synchronous occurrence of an odontogenic fibroma and a giant cell granuloma. Several of these lesions have recurred, and the recurrences typically exhibit both components. Whether the odontogenic fibroma somehow induced a giant cell response in these patients, a giant cell granuloma triggered formation of an odontogenic fibroma, or whether this is a distinct biphasic lesion remains to be clarified.

Treatment and Prognosis

Odontogenic fibromas are usually treated by enucleation and vigorous curettage. Although the tumor does not have a definite capsule, it appears to have a limited growth potential, particularly in the anterior regions of the jaws. A few recurrences have been documented, but the prognosis is very good.

◆ PERIPHERAL ODONTOGENIC FIBROMA

The relatively uncommon **peripheral odontogenic fibroma** is considered to represent the soft tissue counterpart of the **central (intraosseous) odontogenic fibroma.** In the past, some authors have designated clinically and histopathologically similar lesions as **odontogenic epithelial hamartoma** or as **peripheral fibroameloblastic dentinoma.** It is likely that all of these terms refer to the same lesion, and peripheral odontogenic fibroma seems to be the most appropriate designation. A few series of this lesion have been reported in the past three decades, bringing the total number of cases in the literature to over 420.

Clinical and Radiographic Features

The peripheral odontogenic fibroma appears as a firm, slow-growing, and usually sessile gingival mass covered by normal-appearing mucosa (Fig. 15.124). Rarely, multifocal or diffuse lesions have been described. Clinically, the peripheral odontogenic fibroma cannot be distinguished from the much more common fibrous gingival lesions (see Chapter 12). The lesion is most often encountered on the facial gingiva of the mandible. Most lesions are between 0.5 and 1.5 cm in diameter, and they infrequently cause displacement of the teeth. Peripheral odontogenic fibromas have been recorded in patients across a wide age range, with most identified from the second to the fourth decades of life.

Radiographic studies demonstrate a soft tissue mass, which in some cases has shown areas of calcification. The lesion typically does not involve the underlying bone, although occasionally a "cupped out" appearance has been noted. Rarely resorption caused by the tumor, affecting either the root or crown of the adjacent tooth, can be seen radiographically.

Histopathologic Features

The peripheral odontogenic fibroma shows similar histopathologic features to the central odontogenic fibroma (WHO type). The tumor consists of interwoven fascicles of cellular fibrous connective tissue, which may be interspersed with areas of less cellular, myxoid connective tissue. A granular cell change has been rarely identified in the connective tissue component, and giant cell granuloma–like areas have been described in a few lesions. Islands or strands of odontogenic epithelium are scattered throughout the connective tissue. These may be prominent or scarce. The epithelial cells may show vacuolization. Dysplastic dentin, amorphous ovoid cementum-like calcifications, and trabeculae of osteoid may also be present.

Treatment and Prognosis

The peripheral odontogenic fibroma is treated by local surgical excision, and the prognosis is good. Recurrence of this lesion has been documented, however, so the patient and clinician should be aware of this possibility.

◆ GRANULAR CELL ODONTOGENIC TUMOR (GRANULAR CELL ODONTOGENIC FIBROMA)

The rare **granular cell odontogenic tumor** was initially reported as "granular cell ameloblastic fibroma." Subsequently, it was designated as **granular cell odontogenic fibroma,** although the authors prefer the noncommittal term **granular cell odontogenic tumor.** Approximately 40 cases of this unusual neoplasm have been reported.

Clinical and Radiographic Features

Patients with granular cell odontogenic tumors have all been adults at the time of diagnosis, with more than half being older than 40 years of age. More than 70% of the cases have developed in women. The tumor occurs primarily in the mandible and most often in the premolar and molar region. Some lesions are completely asymptomatic; others present as a painless, localized expansion of the affected area. A few cases of granular cell odontogenic tumor have been described in the gingival soft tissues as well.

Radiographically, the lesion appears as a well-demarcated radiolucency, which may be unilocular or multilocular and occasionally shows small calcifications (Fig. 15.125).

Histopathologic Features

The granular cell odontogenic tumor is composed of large eosinophilic granular cells, which closely resemble the granular cells seen in the soft tissue granular cell tumor (see page 544) or the granular cells seen in the granular cell variant of the ameloblastoma (see page 711). Narrow cords or small islands of odontogenic epithelium are scattered among the granular cells (Fig. 15.126). Small cementum-like or dystrophic calcifications associated with the granular cells have been seen in some lesions.

The nature of the granular cells is controversial. Ultrastructural studies reveal the features of mesenchymal cells, and bodies consistent with lysosomal structures have been

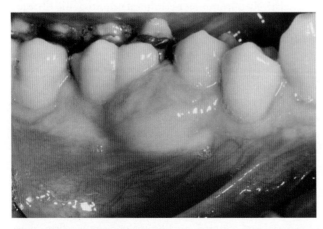

• **Fig. 15.124 Peripheral Odontogenic Fibroma.** This sessile gingival mass cannot be clinically distinguished from the common peripheral ossifying fibroma. (Courtesy of Dr. Jerry Stovall.)

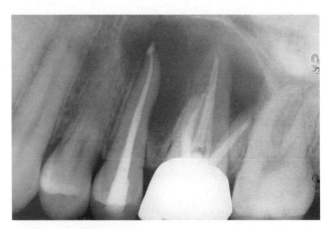

• **Fig. 15.125 Granular Cell Odontogenic Tumor.** Radiolucent lesion involving the apical area of endodontically treated maxillary teeth. (Courtesy of Dr. Steve Ferry.)

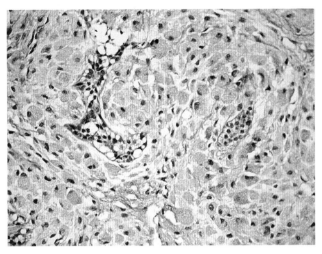

• **Fig. 15.126 Granular Cell Odontogenic Tumor.** Sheet of large granular mesenchymal cells with small nests of odontogenic epithelium.

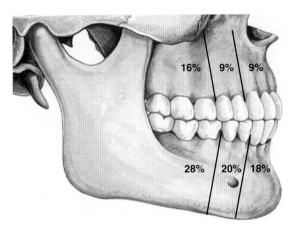

• **Fig. 15.127 Odontogenic Myxoma.** Relative distribution of odontogenic myxoma in the jaws.

identified within the lesional cell cytoplasm. Immunohistochemically, the granular cells in the granular cell odontogenic tumor do not react with antibodies directed against S-100 protein, in contrast to the positive S-100 reactivity of the granular cell tumor.

Treatment and Prognosis

The granular cell odontogenic fibroma appears to be completely benign in the overwhelming majority of instances and responds well to curettage. Only one recurrence has been documented, and a solitary example of a malignant central granular cell odontogenic fibroma has been reported.

◆ ODONTOGENIC MYXOMA

Myxomas of the jaws are believed to arise from odontogenic ectomesenchyme. They bear a close microscopic resemblance to the mesenchymal portion of a developing tooth. Formerly, some investigators made a distinction between **odontogenic myxomas** (derived from odontogenic mesenchyme) and **osteogenic myxomas** (presumably derived from primitive bone tissue). However, most authorities in orthopedic pathologic practice do not accept that myxomas occur in the extragnathic skeleton, and all myxomas of the jaws are currently considered to be of odontogenic origin.

Clinical and Radiographic Features

Myxomas are predominantly found in young adults but may occur across a wide age group. The average age for patients with myxomas is 25–30 years. Recent systematic reviews of the literature suggest a slight female sex predilection. The tumor may be found in almost any area of the jaws, and the mandible is involved more commonly than the maxilla (Fig. 15.127). Smaller lesions may be asymptomatic and are discovered only during a radiographic examination. Larger lesions are often associated with a painless expansion

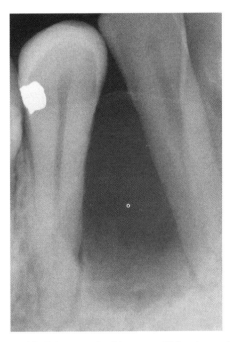

• **Fig. 15.128 Odontogenic Myxoma.** Unilocular radiolucency between the right mandibular lateral incisor and cuspid.

of the involved bone. In some instances, clinical growth of the tumor may be rapid; this is probably related to the accumulation of myxoid ground substance in the tumor.

Radiographically, the myxoma appears as a unilocular or multilocular radiolucency that may displace or cause resorption of teeth in the area of the tumor (Fig. 15.128). The margins of the radiolucency are often irregular or scalloped. The radiolucent defect may contain thin, wispy trabeculae of residual bone, which are often arranged at right angles to one another (Fig. 15.129). Large myxomas of the mandible may show a "soap bubble" radiolucent pattern, which is indistinguishable from that seen in ameloblastomas (Fig. 15.130). In addition, a few large odontogenic myxomas have been reported as having a "sun-burst" or "sun-ray"

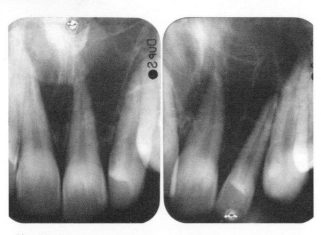

• **Fig. 15.129 Odontogenic Myxoma.** Radiolucent lesion of anterior maxilla showing fine residual bone trabeculae arranged at right angles to one another ("stepladder" pattern).

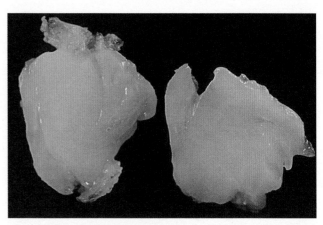

• **Fig. 15.131 Odontogenic Myxoma.** Gross specimen of case shown in Fig. 15.128, demonstrating a white gelatinous mass.

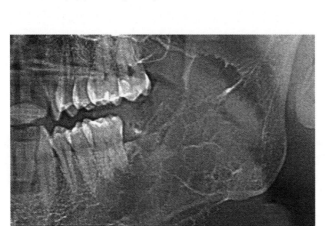

• **Fig. 15.130 Odontogenic Myxoma.** Multilocular expansile radiolucency of the posterior mandible. (Courtesy of Dr. Robert Pulliam.)

radiographic appearance that mimics osteosarcoma radiographically.

Histopathologic Features

At the time of surgery or gross examination of the specimen, the gelatinous, loose structure of the myxoma is obvious (Fig. 15.131). Microscopically, the tumor is composed of haphazardly arranged stellate, spindle-shaped, and round cells in an abundant, loose myxoid stroma that contains only a few collagen fibrils (Fig. 15.132). Histochemical study shows that the ground substance is composed of glycosaminoglycans, chiefly hyaluronic acid and chondroitin sulfate. Immunohistochemically, the myxoma cells show diffuse immunoreactivity with antibodies directed against vimentin, with some cases having focal reactivity for muscle-specific actin. Small islands of inactive-appearing odontogenic epithelial rests may be scattered throughout the myxoid ground substance. These epithelial rests are not required for the diagnosis and are not obvious in most cases. In some patients, the tumor may have a greater

tendency to form collagen fibers; such lesions are sometimes designated as **fibromyxomas** or **myxofibromas.** There is no evidence that the more collagenized variants deserve separate consideration, although some investigators have suggested that these may represent part of a spectrum that includes the central odontogenic fibroma at the other endpoint. Myxomas may rarely exhibit cementum-like calcifications.

A myxoma may be microscopically confused with other myxoid jaw neoplasms, such as the rare chondromyxoid fibroma (see page 661) or the myxoid neurofibroma (see page 534). Chondromyxoid fibroma should have areas of cartilaginous differentiation, whereas myxoid neurofibromas tend to have areas in which lesional cells are arranged in vague fascicles, as well as scattered cells that are positive for antibodies directed against S-100 protein. Myxoid change in an enlarged dental follicle or the dental papilla of a developing tooth may be microscopically similar to a myxoma. Evaluation of the clinical and radiographic features, however, prevents overdiagnosis of these lesions as myxomas.

Another tumor that should be considered in the histopathologic differential diagnosis is the sinonasal myxoma, a lesion that has been recognized only in the past two decades. This lesion typically develops in the first 2 years of life, presenting as a swelling of the maxilla. A unilocular or multilocular radiolucency is seen with imaging studies. Microscopically, the tumor appears very similar to odontogenic myxoma; however, a few sinonasal myxomas have been reported to show positivity for antibodies directed against β-catenin immunohistochemically, unlike odontogenic myxoma. It should also be noted that odontogenic myxomas are exceedingly rare in the first decade of life.

Treatment and Prognosis

Small myxomas are generally treated by curettage, but careful periodic reevaluation is necessary for at least 5 years. For larger lesions, more extensive resection may be required

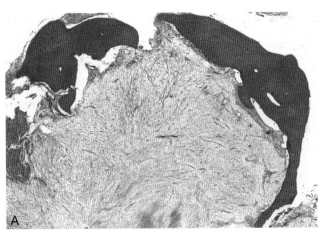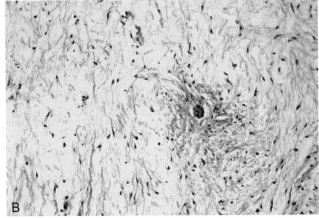

• **Fig. 15.132 Odontogenic Myxoma. A,** A loose, myxomatous tumor can be seen filling the marrow space between the bony trabeculae. **B,** Higher-power view showing loosely arranged spindle cells and fine collagen fibrils. A small odontogenic epithelial rest is seen in the center of the image.

because myxomas are not encapsulated and tend to infiltrate the surrounding bone. Complete removal of a large tumor by curettage is often difficult to accomplish, and lesions of the posterior maxilla, in particular, should be treated more aggressively in most instances. Recurrence rates from various studies average approximately 25%. In spite of local recurrences, the overall prognosis is good, and metastases do not occur.

In rare cases the myxoma microscopically shows marked cellularity and cellular atypism. Some have designated these lesions as *myxosarcomas* or *malignant odontogenic myxoma*. They appear to have a more aggressive local course than do the usual myxomas. Death because of involvement of vital structures by the tumor has been described, but distant metastases have not been reported.

◆ CEMENTOBLASTOMA ("TRUE CEMENTOMA")

Many oral and maxillofacial pathologists consider the **cementoblastoma** to represent an odontogenic tumor. However, other pathologists have pointed out that the histopathologic features of cementoblastomas of the jaws are identical to those of a bone tumor, osteoblastoma, seen both in the jaws and extragnathic skeleton. Cementoblastomas are discussed in Chapter 14 (see page 659).

Bibliography

Odontogenic Cysts and Tumors—General References and Classification

Barnes L, Eveson JW, Reichart P, et al., editors: *World Health Organization classification of tumours: pathology and genetics of head and neck tumours,* Lyon, France, 2005, IARC Press.

El-Naggar AK, Chan JKC, Grandis JR, et al.: *WHO classification of head and neck tumours,* ed 4, Lyon, 2017, IARC, pp 204–260. Chapter 8.

WHO Classification of Tumours Editorial Board: Head and neck tumours [Internet; beta version ahead of print], In *WHO classification of tumours series,* ed 5, vol. 9, Lyon (France), 2022, International Agency for Research on Cancer. Available from: https://tumourclassification.iarc.who.int/chapters/52.

Johnson NR, Gannon OM, Savage NW, et al.: Frequency of odontogenic cysts and tumors: a systematic review, *J Investig Clin Dent* 5:9–14, 2014.

Jones AV, Craig GT, Franklin CD: Range and demographics of odontogenic cysts diagnosed in a UK population over a 30-year period, *J Oral Pathol Med* 35:500–507, 2006.

Philipsen HP, Reichart PA: The development and fate of epithelial residues after completion of the human odontogenesis with special reference to the origins of epithelial odontogenic neoplasms, hamartomas and cysts, *Oral Biosci Med* 1:171–179, 2004.

Sharifian MJ, Khalili M: Odontogenic cysts: a retrospective study of 1227 cases in an Iranian population from 1987 to 2007, *J Oral Sci* 53:361–367, 2011.

Shear M: Developmental odontogenic cysts: an update, *J Oral Pathol Med* 23:1–11, 1994.

Shear M, Speight P: *Cysts of the oral and maxillofacial regions,* ed 4, Oxford, 2007, Blackwell.

Dentigerous Cyst

Ackermann G, Cohen MA, Altini M: The paradental cyst: a clinicopathologic study of 50 cases, *Oral Surg Oral Med Oral Pathol* 64:308–312, 1987.

Austin RP, Nelson BL: Sine qua non: dentigerous cyst, *Head Neck Pathol* 15:1261–1264, 2021.

Benn A, Altini M: Dentigerous cysts of inflammatory origin: a clinicopathologic study, *Oral Surg Oral Med Oral Pathol Oral Radiol Endod* 81:203–209, 1996.

Craig GT: The paradental cyst: A specific inflammatory odontogenic cyst, *Br Dent J* 141:9–14, 1976.

Curran AE, Damm DD, Drummond JF: Pathologically significant pericoronal lesions in adults: histopathologic evaluation, *J Oral Maxillofac Surg* 60:613–617, 2002.

Daley TD, Wysocki GP: The small dentigerous cyst: a diagnostic dilemma, *Oral Surg Oral Med Oral Pathol Oral Radiol Endod* 79:77–81, 1995.

Delbem AC, Cunha RF, Afonso RL, et al.: Dentigerous cysts in primary dentition: report of 2 cases, *Pediatr Dent* 28:269–272, 2006.

Gorlin RJ: Potentialities of oral epithelium manifest by mandibular dentigerous cysts, *Oral Surg Oral Med Oral Pathol* 10:271–284, 1957.

Henien M, Sproat C, Kwok J, et al.: Coronectomy and dentigerous cysts: a review of 68 patients, *Oral Surg Oral Med Oral Pathol Oral Radiol* 123:670–674, 2017.

Lin HP, Wang YP, Chen HM, et al.: A clinicopathologic study of 338 dentigerous cysts, *J Oral Pathol Med* 42:462–467, 2013.

Lustmann L, Bodner L: Dentigerous cysts associated with supernumerary teeth, *Int J Oral Maxillofac Surg* 17:100–102, 1988.

Motamedi MHK, Talesh KT: Management of extensive dentigerous cysts, *Br Dent J* 198:203–206, 2005.

Narang RS, Manchanda AS, Arora P, et al.: Dentigerous cyst of inflammatory origin—a diagnostic dilemma, *Ann Diagn Pathol* 16:119–123, 2012.

Qian WT, Ma ZG, Xie QY, et al.: Marsupialization facilitates eruption of dentigerous cyst-associated mandibular premolars in preadolescent patients, *J Oral Maxillofac Surg* 71:1825–1832, 2013.

Takeda Y, Oikawa Y, Furuya I, et al.: Mucous and ciliated cell metaplasia in epithelial linings of odontogenic inflammatory and developmental cysts, *J Oral Sci* 47:77–81, 2005.

Yao L, Xu X, Ren M, et al.: Inflammatory dentigerous cyst of mandibular first premolar associated with endodontically treated primary first molar: a rare case report, *Eur J Paediatr Dent* 16:201–204, 2015.

Zhang LL, Yang R, Zhang L, et al.: Dentigerous cyst: a retrospective clinicopathological analysis of 2082 dentigerous cysts in British Columbia, Canada, *Int J Oral Maxillofac Surg* 39:876–882, 2010.

Eruption Cyst

Aguiló L, Cibrián R, Bagán JV, et al.: Eruption cysts: retrospective clinical study of 36 cases, *ASDC J Dent Child* 65:102–106, 1998.

Bodner L, Goldstein J, Sarnat H: Eruption cysts: a clinical report of 24 new cases, *J Clin Pediatr Dent* 28:183–186, 2004.

Clark CA: A survey of eruption cysts in the newborn, *Oral Surg Oral Med Oral Pathol* 15:917, 1962.

Şen-Tunç E, Açikel H, Şaroğlu-Sönmez I, et al.: Eruption cysts: a series of 66 cases with clinical features, *Med Oral Patol Oral Cir Bucal* 22:e228–e232, 2017.

Seward MH: Eruption cyst: an analysis of its clinical features, *J Oral Surg* 31:31–35, 1973.

Primordial Cyst

Brannon RB: The odontogenic keratocyst—a clinicopathologic study of 312 cases, *Part I: clinical features, Oral Surg Oral Med Oral Pathol* 42:54–72, 1976.

Robinson HBG: Classification of cysts of the jaws, *Am J Orthod Oral Surg* 31:370–375, 1945.

Odontogenic Keratocyst

Ahlfors E, Larsson A, Sjögren S: The odontogenic keratocyst: a benign cystic tumor? *J Oral Maxillofac Surg* 42:10–19, 1984.

Agaram NP, Collins BM, Barnes L, et al.: Molecular analysis to demonstrate that odontogenic keratocysts are neoplastic, *Arch Pathol Lab Med* 128:313–317, 2004.

Barnes L, Eveson JW, Reichart P, et al., editors: *World Health Organization classification of tumours: pathology and genetics of head and neck tumours*, Lyon, France, 2005, IARC Press.

Brannon RB: The odontogenic keratocyst—a clinicopathologic study of 312 cases. Part I: clinical features, *Oral Surg Oral Med Oral Pathol* 42:54–72, 1976.

Brannon RB: The odontogenic keratocyst—a clinicopathologic study of 312 cases. Part II: histologic features, *Oral Surg Oral Med Oral Pathol* 43:233–255, 1977.

Brøndum N, Jensen VJ: Recurrence of keratocysts and decompression treatment: a long-term follow-up of forty-four cases, *Oral Surg Oral Med Oral Pathol* 72:265–269, 1991.

Chi AC, Owings JR, Muller S: Peripheral odontogenic keratocyst: report of two cases and review of the literature, *Oral Surg Oral Med Oral Pathol Oral Radiol Endod* 99:71–78, 2005.

Chrcanovic BR, Gomez RS: Recurrence probability for keratocystic odontogenic tumors: an analysis of 6247 cases, *J Craniomaxillofac Surg* 45:244–251, 2017.

Finkelstein MW, Hellstein JW, Lake KS, et al.: Keratocystic odontogenic tumor: a retrospective analysis of genetic, immunohistochemical and therapeutic features. Proposal of a multicenter clinical survey tool, *Oral Surg Oral Med Oral Pathol Oral Radiol* 116:75–83, 2013.

Fornatora ML, Reich RF, Chotkowski G, et al.: Odontogenic keratocyst with mural cartilaginous metaplasia: a case report and a review of the literature, *Oral Surg Oral Med Oral Pathol Oral Radiol Endod* 92:430–434, 2001.

Garlock JA, Pringle GA, Hicks ML: The odontogenic keratocyst: a potential endodontic misdiagnosis, *Oral Surg Oral Med Oral Pathol Oral Radiol Endod* 85:452–456, 1988.

Henley J, Summerlin D-J, Tomich C, et al.: Molecular evidence supporting the neoplastic nature of odontogenic keratocyst: a laser capture microdissection study of 15 cases, *Histopathology* 47:582–586, 2005.

Jackson IT, Potparic Z, Fasching M, et al.: Penetration of the skull base by dissecting keratocyst, *J Craniomaxillofac Surg* 21:319–325, 1993.

Kolokythas A, Fernandes RP, Pazoki A, et al.: Odontogenic keratocyst: to decompress or not to decompress? A comparative study of decompression and enucleation versus resection/peripheral ostectomy, *J Oral Maxillofac Surg* 65:640–644, 2007.

Kratochvil FJ, Brannon RB: Cartilage in the walls of odontogenic keratocysts, *J Oral Pathol Med* 22:282–285, 1993.

Kumchai H, Champion AF, Gates JC: Carcinomatous transformation of odontogenic keratocyst and primary intraosseous carcinoma: a systematic review and report of a case, *J Oral Maxillofac Surg* 79:1081.e1–1081.e9, 2021.

Li T-J: The odontogenic keratocyst: a cyst, or a cystic neoplasm? *J Dent Res* 90:133–142, 2011.

Meiselman F: Surgical management of the odontogenic keratocyst: conservative approach, *J Oral Maxillofac Surg* 52:960–963, 1994.

Morgan TA, Burton CC, Qian F: A retrospective review of treatment of the odontogenic keratocyst, *J Oral Maxillofac Surg* 63:635–639, 2005.

Neville BW, Damm DD, Brock TR: Odontogenic keratocysts of the midline maxillary region, *J Oral Maxillofac Surg* 55:340–344, 1997.

Pogrel MA, Jordan RCK: Marsupialization as a definitive treatment for the odontogenic keratocyst, *J Oral Maxillofac Surg* 62:651–655, 2004.

Preston RD, Narayana N: Peripheral odontogenic keratocyst, *J Periodontol* 76:2312–2315, 2005.

Rodu B, Tate AL, Martinez MG: The implications of inflammation in odontogenic keratocysts, *J Oral Pathol* 16:518–521, 1987.

Shear M: The aggressive nature of the odontogenic keratocyst: is it a benign cystic neoplasm? Part 1 Clinical and early experimental evidence of aggressive behavior, *Oral Oncol* 38:219–226, 2002.

Shear M: The aggressive nature of the odontogenic keratocyst: is it a benign cystic neoplasm? Part 2. Proliferation and genetic studies, *Oral Oncol* 38:323–331, 2002.

Shear M: The aggressive nature of the odontogenic keratocyst: is it a benign cystic neoplasm? Part 3. Immunocytochemistry of cytokeratin and other epithelial cell markers, *Oral Oncol* 38:407–415, 2002.

Slusarenko da Silva Y, Stoelinga PJW, Grillo R, et al.: Cyst or tumor? A systematic review and meta-analysis on the expression of p53 marker in odontogenic keratocysts, *J Craniomaxillofac Surg* 49:1101–1106, 2021.

Stojanov IJ, Schaefer IM, Menon RS, et al.: Biallelic *PTCH1* inactivation is a dominant genomic change in sporadic keratocystic odontogenic tumors, *Am J Surg Pathol* 44:553–560, 2020.

Williams TP, Connor FA Jr: Surgical management of the odontogenic keratocyst: aggressive approach, *J Oral Maxillofac Surg* 52:964–966, 1994.

Zhang R, Yang J, Zhang J, et al.: Should the solid variant of odontogenic keratocyst and keratoameloblastoma be classified as the same entity? A clinicopathological analysis of nine cases and a review of the literature, *Pathology* 53:478–486, 2021.

Orthokeratinized Odontogenic Cysts

Chi AC, Neville BW, McDonald TA, et al.: Jaw cysts with sebaceous differentiation: report of 5 cases and a review of the literature, *J Oral Maxillofac Surg* 65:2568–2574, 2007.

Crane H, Da Forno P, Kyriakidou E, et al.: Multiple orthokeratinized odontogenic cysts: a report of two cases and review of the literature, *Head Neck Pathol* 14:381–385, 2020.

Dong Q, Pan S, Sun LS, et al.: Orthokeratinized odontogenic cyst: a clinicopathologic study of 61 cases, *Arch Pathol Lab Med* 134:271–275, 2010.

Li T-J, Kitano M, Chen X-M, et al.: Orthokeratinized odontogenic cyst: a clinicopathological and immunocytochemical study of 15 cases, *Histopathology* 32:242–251, 1998.

MacDonald-Jankowski DS: Orthokeratinized odontogenic cyst: a systemic review, *Dentomaxillofac Radiol* 39:455–467, 2010.

Oh KY, Kim JE, Cho SD, et al.: Orthokeratinized odontogenic cyst: a large series and comprehensive literature review with emphasis on synchronous multiple occurrence and neoplastic transformation, *Oral Surg Oral Med Oral Pathol Oral Radiol* 133:e72–e82, 2022.

Wright JM: The odontogenic keratocyst: orthokeratinized variant, *Oral Surg Oral Med Oral Pathol* 51:609–618, 1981.

Nevoid Basal Cell Carcinoma Syndrome

Ally MS, Tang JY, Joseph T, et al.: The use of vismodegib to shrink keratocystic odontogenic tumors in patients with basal cell nevus syndrome, *JAMA Dermatol* 150:542–545, 2014.

Amlashi SFA, Riffaud L, Brassier G, et al.: Nevoid basal cell carcinoma syndrome: relation with desmoplastic medulloblastoma in infancy. A population-based study and review of the literature, *Cancer* 98:618–624, 2003.

Bree AF, Shah MR: BCNS Colloquium Group: consensus statement from the first international colloquium on basal cell nevus syndrome (BCNS), *Am J Med Genet A* 155:2091–2097, 2011.

Evans DG, Farndon PA, Adam MP, et al.: Nevoid basal cell carcinoma syndrome, In *GeneReview® [Internet]*, Seattle (WA), 2002, University of Washington, Seattle. June 20 [Updated 2018 Mar 29], 1993–2022.

Goldstein AM, Pastakia B, DeGiovanna JJ, et al.: Clinical findings in two African-American families with the nevoid basal cell carcinoma syndrome (NBCC), *Am J Med Genet* 50:272–281, 1994.

Gorlin RJ: Nevoid basal cell carcinoma (Gorlin) syndrome, *Genet Med* 6:530–539, 2004.

Gorlin RJ, Goltz R: Multiple nevoid basal cell epithelioma, jaw cysts and bifid rib syndrome, *N Engl J Med* 262:908–914, 1960.

Gururangan S, Robinson G, Ellison DW, et al.: Gorlin syndrome and desmoplastic medulloblastoma: report of 3 cases with unfavorable clinical course and novel mutations, *Pediatr Blood Cancer* 62:1855–1858, 2015.

Karhade DS, Afshar S, Padwa BL: What is the prevalence of undiagnosed nevoid basal cell carcinoma syndrome in children with an odontogenic keratocyst? *J Oral Maxillofac Surg* 77:1389–1391, 2019.

Kimonis VE, Goldstein AM, Pastakia B, et al.: Clinical manifestations in 105 persons with nevoid basal cell carcinoma syndrome, *Am J Med Genet* 69:299–308, 1997.

Lam C, Ou JC, Billingsley EM: PTCH-ing it together: a basal cell nevus syndrome review, *Dermatol Surg* 39:1557–1572, 2013.

Lin MJ, Dubin DP, Khorasani H, et al.: Basal cell nevus syndrome: From DNA to therapeutics, *Clin Dermatol* 38:467–476, 2020.

Lo Muzio L, Staibano S, Pannone G, et al.: Expression of cell cycle and apoptosis-related proteins in sporadic odontogenic keratocysts and odontogenic keratocysts associated with the nevoid basal cell carcinoma syndrome, *J Dent Res* 78:1345–1353, 1999.

Shanley S, Ratcliffe J, Hockey A, et al.: Nevoid basal cell carcinoma syndrome: review of 118 affected individuals, *Am J Med Genet* 50:282–290, 1994.

Woolgar JA, Rippin JW, Browne RM: A comparative histologic study of odontogenic keratocysts in basal cell nevus syndrome and non-syndrome patients, *J Oral Pathol* 16:75–80, 1987.

Woolgar JA, Rippin JW, Browne RM: The odontogenic keratocyst and its occurrence in the nevoid basal cell carcinoma syndrome, *Oral Surg Oral Med Oral Pathol* 64:727–730, 1987.

Gingival Cyst of the Newborn

Bilodeau EA, Hunter KD: Odontogenic and developmental oral lesions in pediatric patients, *Head Neck Pathol* 15:71–84, 2021.

Cataldo E, Berkman M: Cysts of the oral mucosa in newborns, *Am J Dis Child* 116:44–48, 1968.

Fromm A: Epstein's pearls, Bohn's nodules and inclusion cysts of the oral cavity, *J Dent Child* 34:275–287, 1967.

Jorgenson RJ, Shapiro SD, Salinas CF, et al.: Intraoral findings and anomalies in neonates, *Pediatrics* 69:577–582, 1982.

Monteagudo B, Labandeira J, Cabanillas M, et al.: Prevalence of milia and palatal and gingival cysts in Spanish newborns, *Pediatr Dermatol* 29:301–305, 2012.

Paula JDR, Dezan CC, Frossard WTG, et al.: Oral and facial inclusion cysts in newborns, *J Clin Pediatr Dent* 31:127–129, 2006.

Gingival Cyst of the Adult

Bell RC, Chauvin PJ, Tyler MT: Gingival cyst of the adult: a review and report of eight cases, *J Can Dent Assoc* 63:533–535, 1997.

Breault LG, Billman MA, Lewis DM: Report of a gingival "surgical cyst" developing secondarily to a subepithelial connective tissue graft, *J Periodontol* 68:392–395, 1997.

Buchner A, Hansen LS: The histomorphologic spectrum of the gingival cyst in the adult, *Oral Surg Oral Med Oral Pathol* 48:532–539, 1979.

Chrcanovic BR, Gomez RS: Gingival cyst of the adult, lateral periodontal cyst, and botryoid odontogenic cyst: an updated systematic review, *Oral Dis* 25:26–33, 2019.

Giunta JL: Gingival cysts in the adult, *J Periodontol* 73:827–831, 2002.

Viveiros SK, Pinho RFC, Custódio M, et al.: A rare odontogenic cyst: gingival cyst of the adult. A series of 20 new cases from a single center, *J Craniomaxillofac Surg* 47:647–650, 2019.

Lateral Periodontal Cyst

Baker RD, D'Onofrio ED, Corio RL: Squamous-cell carcinoma arising in a lateral periodontal cyst, *Oral Surg Oral Med Oral Pathol* 47:495–499, 1979.

Carter LC, Carney YL, Perez-Pudlewski D: Lateral periodontal cyst: multifactorial analysis of a previously unreported series, *Oral Surg Oral Med Oral Pathol Oral Radiol Endod* 81:210–216, 1996.

Chrcanovic BR, Gomez RS: Gingival cyst of the adult, lateral periodontal cyst, and botryoid odontogenic cyst: an updated systematic review, *Oral Dis* 25:26–33, 2019.

Cohen D, Neville B, Damm D, et al.: The lateral periodontal cyst: a report of 37 cases, *J Periodontol* 55:230–234, 1984.

Deeb JG, Deeb GR, Schafer DR: Odontogenic keratocyst is frequently misdiagnosed for a lateral periodontal cyst in premolar and anterior tooth-bearing areas, *J Endod* 48:337–344, 2022.

Fantasia JE: Lateral periodontal cyst: an analysis of forty-six cases, *Oral Surg Oral Med Oral Pathol* 48:237–243, 1979.

Gurol M, Burkes EJ Jr, Jacoway J: Botryoid odontogenic cyst: analysis of 33 cases, *J Periodontol* 66:1069–1073, 1995.

Ramer M, Valauri D: Multicystic lateral periodontal cyst and botryoid odontogenic cyst: multifactorial analysis of previously unreported series and review of literature, *N Y State Dent J* 71:47–51, 2005.

Santos PP, Freitas VS, Freitas Rde A, et al.: Botryoid odontogenic cyst: a clinicopathologic study of 10 cases, *Ann Diagn Pathol* 15:221–224, 2011.

Siponen M, Neville BW, Damm DD, et al.: Multifocal lateral periodontal cysts: a report of 4 cases and review of the literature, *Oral Surg Oral Med Oral Pathol Oral Radiol Endod* 111:225–233, 2011.

Wysocki GP, Brannon RB, Gardner DG, et al.: Histogenesis of the lateral periodontal cyst and the gingival cyst of the adult, *Oral Surg Oral Med Oral Pathol* 50:327–334, 1980.

Calcifying Odontogenic Cyst

de Arruda JAA, Monteiro JLGC, Abreu LG, et al.: Calcifying odontogenic cyst, dentinogenic ghost cell tumor, and ghost cell odontogenic carcinoma: a systematic review, *J Oral Pathol Med* 47:721–730, 2018.

de Arruda JAA, Schuch LF, Abreu LG, et al.: A multicentre study of 268 cases of calcifying odontogenic cyst and a literature review, *Oral Dis* 24:1282–1293, 2018.

Buchner A, Akrish SJ, Vered M: Central dentinogenic ghost cell tumor: an update on a rare aggressive odontogenic tumor, *J Oral Maxillofac Surg* 74:307–314, 2016.

Ellis GL: Odontogenic ghost cell tumor, *Semin Diagn Pathol* 16:288–292, 1999.

Ellis GL, Shmookler BM: Aggressive (malignant?) epithelial odontogenic ghost cell tumor, *Oral Surg Oral Med Oral Pathol* 61:471–478, 1986.

Gomes CC, de Sousa SF, Gomez RS: Craniopharyngiomas and odontogenic tumors mimic normal odontogenesis and share genetic mutations, histopathologic features, and molecular pathways activation, *Oral Surg Oral Med Oral Pathol Oral Radiol* 127:231–236, 2019.

Gorlin RJ, Pindborg JJ, Clausen FP, et al.: The calcifying odontogenic cyst—a possible analogue to the cutaneous calcifying epithelioma of Malherbe: an analysis of fifteen cases, *Oral Surg Oral Med Oral Pathol* 15:1235–1243, 1962.

Hong SP, Ellis GL, Hartman KS: Calcifying odontogenic cyst: a review of ninety-two cases with reevaluation of their nature as cysts or neoplasms, the nature of the ghost cells and subclassification, *Oral Surg Oral Med Oral Pathol* 72:56–64, 1991.

Johnson A III, Fletcher M, Gold L, et al.: Calcifying odontogenic cyst: a clinicopathologic study of 57 cases with immunohistochemical evaluation for cytokeratin, *J Oral Maxillofac Surg* 55:679–683, 1997.

Ledesma-Montes C, Gorlin RJ, Shear M, et al.: International collaborative study on ghost cell odontogenic tumours: calcifying cystic odontogenic tumour, dentinogenic ghost cell tumour and ghost cell odontogenic carcinoma, *J Oral Pathol Med* 37:302–308, 2008.

Li T-J, Yu S-F: Clinicopathologic spectrum of the so-called calcifying odontogenic cysts: a study of 21 intraosseous cases with reconsideration of the terminology and classification, *Am J Surg Pathol* 27:372–384, 2003.

Lu Y, Mock D, Takata T, et al.: Odontogenic ghost cell carcinoma: report of four new cases and review of the literature, *J Oral Pathol Med* 28:323–329, 1999.

Ohata Y, Kayamori K, Yukimori A, et al.: A lesion categorized between ghost cell odontogenic carcinoma and dentinogenic ghost cell tumor with CTNNB1 mutation, *Pathol Int* 68:307–312, 2018.

Praetorius F, Hjørting-Hansen E, Gorlin RJ, et al.: Calcifying odontogenic cyst: range, variations and neoplastic potential, *Acta Odontol Scand* 39:227–240, 1981.

Sekine S, Sato S, Takata T, et al.: β-catenin mutations are frequent in calcifying odontogenic cysts, but rare in ameloblastomas, *Am J Surg Pathol* 163:1707–1712, 2003.

de Souza VG, de Pinho MP, Rozza-de-Menezes RE, et al.: Comparative analysis between dentinogenic ghost cell tumor and ghost cell odontogenic carcinoma: a systematic review, *Head Neck Pathol* 15:1265–1283, 2021.

Yoshida M, Kumamoto H, Ooya K, et al.: Histopathological and immunohistochemical analysis of calcifying odontogenic cysts, *J Oral Pathol Med* 30:582–588, 2001.

Glandular Odontogenic Cyst

Bishop JA, Yonescu R, Batista D, et al.: Glandular odontogenic cysts (GOCs) lack MAML2 rearrangements: a finding to discredit the putative nature of GOC as a precursor to central mucoepidermoid carcinoma, *Head Neck Pathol* 8:287–290, 2014.

Chrcanovic BR, Gomez RS: Glandular odontogenic cyst: an updated analysis of 169 cases reported in the literature, *Oral Dis* 24:717–724, 2018.

Fowler CB, Brannon RB, Kessler HP, et al.: Glandular odontogenic cyst: analysis of 46 cases with special emphasis on microscopic criteria for diagnosis, *Head Neck Pathol* 5:364–375, 2011.

Gardner DG, Kessler HP, Morency R, et al.: The glandular odontogenic cyst: an apparent entity, *J Oral Pathol* 17:359–366, 1988.

Kaplan I, Anavi Y, Hirshberg A: Glandular odontogenic cyst: a challenge in diagnosis and treatment, *Oral Dis* 14:575–581, 2008.

Kaplan I, Gal G, Anavi Y, et al.: Glandular odontogenic cyst: treatment and recurrence, *J Oral Maxillofac Surg* 63:435–441, 2005.

Nagasaki A, Ogawa I, Sato Y, et al.: Central mucoepidermoid carcinoma arising from glandular odontogenic cyst confirmed by analysis of *MAML2* rearrangement: a case report, *Pathol Int* 68:31–35, 2018.

Nel C, Robinson L, Roza ALOC, et al.: Clinical and radiologic spectrum of glandular odontogenic cysts: a multicenter study of 92 cases, *Oral Surg Oral Med Oral Pathol Oral Radiol* 133:593–603, 2022.

Shen J, Fan M, Chen X, et al.: Glandular odontogenic cyst in China: report of 12 cases and immunohistochemical study, *J Oral Pathol Med* 35:175–182, 2006.

Buccal Bifurcation Cyst

Ackermann G, Cohen MA, Altini M: The paradental cyst: a clinicopathologic study of 50 cases, *Oral Surg Oral Med Oral Pathol* 64:308–312, 1987.

David LA, Sàndor GKB, Stoneman DW: The buccal bifurcation cyst: is non-surgical treatment an option? *J Can Dent Assoc* 64:712–716, 1998.

Fowler CB, Brannon RB: The paradental cyst: a clinicopathologic study of six new cases and review of the literature, *J Oral Maxillofac Surg* 47:243–248, 1989.

Philipsen HP, Reichart PA, Ogawa I, et al.: The inflammatory paradental cyst: a critical review of 342 cases from a literature survey, including 17 new cases from the author's files, *J Oral Pathol Med* 33:147–155, 2004.

Pompura JR, Sàndor GKB, Stoneman DW: The buccal bifurcation cyst: a prospective study of treatment outcomes in 44 sites, *Oral Surg Oral Med Oral Pathol Oral Radiol Endod* 83:215–221, 1997.

Ruddocks LA, Fitzpatrick SG, Bhattacharyya I, et al.: Buccal bifurcation cyst: a case series and review of the literature, *JADA* 153:421–428, 2022.

Shohat I, Buchner A, Taicher S: Mandibular buccal bifurcation cyst: enucleation without extraction, *Int J Oral Maxillofac Surg* 32:610–613, 2003.

Stoneman DW, Worth HM: The mandibular infected buccal cyst-molar area, *Dent Radiogr Photogr* 56:1–14, 1983.

Carcinoma Arising in Odontogenic Cysts

Bodner L, Manor E, Shear M, et al.: Primary intraosseous squamous cell carcinoma arising in an odontogenic cyst—a clinicopathologic analysis of 116 reported cases, *J Oral Pathol Med* 40:733–738, 2011.

Chaisuparat R, Coletti D, Kolokythas A, et al.: Primary intraosseous odontogenic carcinoma arising in an odontogenic cyst or de novo: a clinicopathologic study of six new cases, *Oral Surg Oral Med Oral Pathol Oral Radiol Endod* 101:196–202, 2006.

Ghita I, Nagai MY, Lubek JE, et al.: Ghost cell odontogenic carcinoma arising in a previous calcifying odontogenic cyst: a case report and review of the literature, *Head Neck Pathol* 16:828–835, 2022. https://doi.org/10.1007/s12105-022-01445-6.

Hennis HL, Stewart WC, Neville B, et al.: Carcinoma arising in an odontogenic keratocyst with orbital invasion, *Doc Ophthalmol* 77:73–79, 1991.

Nel C, Robinson L, van Heerden WFP: Ghost cell odontogenic carcinoma arising in the background of a calcifying odontogenic cyst, *Oral Radiol* 37:537–542, 2021.

Stoelinga PJ, Bronkhorst FB: The incidence, multiple presentation and recurrence of aggressive cysts of the jaws, *J Craniomaxillofac Surg* 16:184–195, 1988.

van der Waal I, Rauhamaa R, van der Kwast WAM, et al.: Squamous cell carcinoma arising in the lining of odontogenic cysts: report of 5 cases, *Int J Oral Surg* 14:146–152, 1985.

Waldron CA, Mustoe TA: Primary intraosseous carcinoma of the mandible with probable origin in an odontogenic cyst, *Oral Surg Oral Med Oral Pathol* 67:716–724, 1989.

Ye P, Wei T, Gao Y, et al.: Primary intraosseous squamous cell carcinoma arising from an odontogenic keratocyst: case series and literature review, *Med Oral Patol Oral Cir Bucal* 26:e49–e55, 2021.

Ameloblastoma

Anand R, Sarode GS, Sarode SC, et al.: Clinicopathological characteristics of desmoplastic ameloblastoma: a systematic review, *J Investig Clin Dent* 9(1), 2018. https://doi.org/10.1111/jicd.12282.

Anpalagan A, Tzortzis A, Twigg J, et al.: Current practice in the management of peripheral ameloblastoma: a structured review, *Br J Oral Maxillofac Surg* 59:e1–e8, 2021.

Bilodeau EA, Seethala RR: Update on odontogenic tumors: proceedings of the North American Head and Neck Pathology Society, *Head Neck Pathol* 13:457–465, 2019.

Buchner A, Merrell PW, Carpenter WM: Relative frequency of central odontogenic tumors: a study of 1,088 cases from northern California and comparison to studies from other parts of the world, *J Oral Maxillofac Surg* 64:1343–1352, 2006.

de Arruda JAA, Noronha MS, Abreu LG, et al.: Adenoid ameloblastoma in the posterior maxilla: a case report and review of the literature, *Oral Maxillofac Surg* 24:243–249, 2020.

De Silva I, Rozen WM, Ramakrishnan A, et al.: Achieving adequate margins in ameloblastoma resection: the role for intra-operative specimen imaging. Clinical report and systematic review, *PLoS One* 7:e47897, 2012.

Eversole LR, Leider AS, Hansen LS: Ameloblastomas with pronounced desmoplasia, *J Oral Maxillofac Surg* 42:735–740, 1984.

Hendra FN, Natsir Kalla DS, Van Cann EM, et al.: Radical vs conservative treatment of intraosseous ameloblastoma: Systematic review and meta-analysis, *Oral Dis* 25:1683–1696, 2019.

Hong J, Yun P-Y, Chung I-H, et al.: Long-term follow up on recurrence of 305 ameloblastoma cases, *Int J Oral Maxillofac Surg* 36:283–288, 2007.

Jayasooriya PR, Abeyasinghe WAMUL, Liyanage REPR, et al.: Diagnostic enigma of adenoid ameloblastoma: literature review based evidence to consider it as a new sub type of ameloblastoma, *Head Neck Pathol* 16:344–352, 2022.

Kishino M, Murakami S, Fukuda Y, et al.: Pathology of the desmoplastic ameloblastoma, *J Oral Pathol Med* 30:35–40, 2001.

Kurppa KJ, Catón J, Morgan PR, et al.: High frequency of BRAF V600E mutations in ameloblastoma, *J Pathol* 232:492–498, 2014.

Leibovitch I, Schwarcz RM, Modjtahedi S, et al.: Orbital invasion by recurrent maxillary ameloblastoma, *Ophthalmology* 113:1227–1230, 2006.

Philipsen HP, Reichart PA: Classification of odontogenic tumours: a historical review, *J Oral Pathol Med* 35:525–529, 2006.

Philipsen HP, Reichart PA, Takata T: Desmoplastic ameloblastoma (including "hybrid" lesion of ameloblastoma): biological profile based on 100 cases from the literature and own files, *Oral Oncol* 37:455–460, 2001.

Pizziolo-Coura B, Nunes-Dos Santos J, Paiva-Fonseca F, et al.: Adenoid ameloblastoma with dentinoid is molecularly different from ameloblastomas and adenomatoid odontogenic tumors, *J Oral Pathol Med* 50:1067–1071, 2021.

Pogrel MA, Montes DM: Is there a role for enucleation in the management of ameloblastoma? *Int J Oral Maxillofac Surg* 38:807–812, 2009.

Raubenheimer EJ, van Heerden WFP, Noffke CEE: Infrequent clinicopathological findings in 108 ameloblastomas, *J Oral Pathol Med* 24:227–232, 1995.

Richard BM, Thyveetil M, Sharif H, et al.: Ameloblastoma with stromal multinucleated giant cells, *Histopathology* 25:497–499, 1994.

SantAna MSP, Dos Santos Costa SF, da Silva MP, et al.: BRAF p. V600E status in epithelial areas of ameloblastoma with different histological aspects: implications to the clinical practice, *J Oral Pathol Med* 50:478–484, 2021.

Sharma A, Ingole S, Deshpande M, et al.: Retrospective analysis of desmoplastic ameloblastoma: clinical review, *Med Oral Patol Oral Cir Bucal* 26:e246–e255, 2021.

Siriwardena BSMS, Crane H, O'Neill N, et al.: Odontogenic tumors and lesions treated in a single specialist oral and maxillofacial pathology unit in the United Kingdom in 1992-2016, *Oral Surg Oral Med Oral Pathol Oral Radiol* 127:151–166, 2019.

Small IA, Waldron CA: Ameloblastoma of the jaws, *Oral Surg Oral Med Oral Pathol* 8:281–297, 1955.

Sun Z-J, Wu Y-R, Cheng N, et al.: Desmoplastic ameloblastoma—a review, *Oral Oncol* 45:752–759, 2009.

Takata T, Miyauchi M, Ogawa I, et al.: Immunoexpression of transforming growth factor b in desmoplastic ameloblastoma, *Virchows Arch* 436:319–323, 2000.

Troiano G, Dioguardi M, Cocco A, et al.: Conservative vs radical approach for the treatment of solid/multicystic ameloblastoma: a systematic review and meta-analysis of the last decade, *Oral Health Prev Dent* 15:421–426, 2017.

Waldron CA, El-Mofty S: A histopathologic study of 116 ameloblastomas with special reference to the desmoplastic variant, *Oral Surg Oral Med Oral Pathol* 63:441–451, 1987.

Zhang J, Gu Z, Jiang L, et al.: Ameloblastoma in children and adolescents, *Br J Oral Maxillofac Surg* 48:549–554, 2010.

Unicystic Ameloblastoma

Ackerman GL, Altini M, Shear M: The unicystic ameloblastoma: a clinicopathologic study of 57 cases, *J Oral Pathol* 17:541–546, 1988.

Antonoglou GN, Sándor GK: Recurrence rates of intraosseous ameloblastomas of the jaws: a systematic review of conservative versus aggressive treatment approaches and meta-analysis of non-randomized studies, *J Craniomaxillofac Surg* 43:149–157, 2015.

Peacock ZS: Controversies in oral and maxillofacial pathology, *Oral Maxillofacial Surg Clin N Am* 29:475–486, 2017.

Philipsen HP, Reichart PA: Unicystic ameloblastoma: a review of 193 cases from the literature, *Oral Oncol* 34:317–325, 1998.

Robinson L, Martinez MG: Unicystic ameloblastoma: a prognostically distinct entity, *Cancer* 40:2278–2285, 1977.

Siriwardena BSMS, Tennakoon TMPB, Hunter KD, et al.: Unicystic ameloblastoma: analysis of 370 cases in a single center in Sri Lanka, *J Oral Pathol Med* 47:706–709, 2018.

Vickers RA, Gorlin RJ: Ameloblastoma: delineation of early histopathologic features of neoplasia, *Cancer* 26:699–710, 1970.

Peripheral (Extraosseous) Ameloblastoma

Anpalagan A, Tzortzis A, Twigg J, et al.: Current practice in the management of peripheral ameloblastoma: a structured review, *Br J Oral Maxillofac Surg* 59:e1–e8, 2021.

Baden E, Doyle JL, Petriella V: Malignant transformation of peripheral ameloblastoma, *Oral Surg Oral Med Oral Pathol* 75:214–219, 1993.

Bologna-Molina R, Mosqueda-Taylor A, de Almeida-Oslei P, et al.: Peripheral desmoplastic ameloblastoma: histopathological and immunohistochemical profile of a case, *Med Oral Patol Oral Cir Bucal* 15:e846–e849, 2010.

Gardner DG: Peripheral ameloblastoma: a study of 21 cases including 5 reported as basal cell carcinoma of the gingiva, *Cancer* 39:1625–1633, 1977.

Ide F, Kusama K, Tanaka A, et al.: Peripheral ameloblastoma is not a hamartoma but rather more of a neoplasm, *Oral Oncol* 38:318–320, 2002.

Ide F, Mishima K, Miyazaki Y, et al.: Peripheral ameloblastoma in-situ: an evidential fact of surface epithelium origin, *Oral Surg Oral Med Oral Pathol Oral Radiol Endod* 108:763–767, 2009.

Philipsen HP, Reichart PA, Nikai H, et al.: Peripheral ameloblastoma: biological profile based on 160 cases from the literature, *Oral Oncol* 37:17–27, 2001.

Yamanishi T, Ando S, Aikawa T, et al.: A case of extragingival peripheral ameloblastoma in the buccal mucosa, *J Oral Pathol Med* 36:184–186, 2007.

Malignant Ameloblastoma and Ameloblastic Carcinoma

Aoki T, Akiba T, Kondo Y, et al.: The use of radiation therapy in the definitive management of ameloblastic carcinoma: a case report, *Oral Surg Oral Med Oral Pathol Oral Radiol* 127:e56–e60, 2019.

Corio RL, Goldblatt LI, Edwards PA, et al.: Ameloblastic carcinoma: a clinicopathologic assessment of eight cases, *Oral Surg Oral Med Oral Pathol* 64:570–576, 1987.

Dissanayake RKG, Jayasooriya PR, Siriwardena DJL, et al.: Review of metastasizing (malignant) ameloblastoma (METAM): pattern of metastasis and treatment, *Oral Surg Oral Med Oral Pathol Oral Radiol Endod* 111:734–741, 2011.

Dos Santos JN, Servato JPS, Cardoso SV, et al.: Odontogenic carcinosarcoma: morphologic and immunohistochemical description of a case, *Oral Surg Oral Med Oral Pathol Oral Radiol* 126:e264–e270, 2018.

Giridhar P, Mallick S, Upadhyay AD, et al.: Pattern of care and impact of prognostic factors in the outcome of ameloblastic carcinoma: a systematic review and individual patient data analysis of 199 cases, *Eur Arch Otorhinolaryngol* 274:3803–3810, 2017.

Hall JM, Weathers DR, Unni KK: Ameloblastic carcinoma: an analysis of 14 cases, *Oral Surg Oral Med Oral Pathol Oral Radiol Endod* 103:799–807, 2007.

Huang J-W, Luo H-Y, Li Q, et al.: Primary intraosseous squamous cell carcinoma of the jaws. Clinicopathologic presentation and prognostic factors, *Arch Pathol Lab Med* 133:1834–1840, 2009.

Matsushita Y, Fujita S, Yanamoto S, et al.: Spindle cell variant of ameloblastic carcinoma: a case report and literature review, *Oral Surg Oral Med Oral Pathol Oral Radiol* 121:e54–e61, 2016.

McLean-Holden AC, Bishop JA, Kessler HP, et al.: Spindle-cell variant of ameloblastic carcinoma: a report of 3 cases and demonstration of epithelial-mesenchymal transition in tumor progression, *Oral Surg Oral Med Oral Pathol Oral Radiol* 128:e113–e121, 2019.

Sakuranaka H, Sekine A, Miyamoto I, et al.: Pulmonary malignant ameloblastoma without local recurrence 31 years after primary resection: a case report and literature review, *Intern Med* 59:1423–1426, 2020.

Van Dam S, Unni KK, Keller EE: Metastasizing (malignant) ameloblastoma: review of a unique histopathologic entity and report of Mayo Clinic experience, *J Oral Maxillofac Surg* 68:2962–2974, 2010.

Clear Cell Odontogenic Tumor

Bilodeau EA, Weinreb I, Antonescu CR, et al.: Clear cell odontogenic carcinomas show EWSR1 rearrangements. A novel finding and a biological link to salivary clear cell carcinoma, *Am J Surg Pathol* 37:1001–1005, 2013.

Ebert CS, Dubin MG, Hart CF, et al.: Clear cell odontogenic carcinoma: a comprehensive analysis of treatment strategies, *Head Neck* 27:536–542, 2005.

Ginat DT, Villaflor V, Cipriani NA: Oral cavity clear cell odontogenic carcinoma, *Head Neck Pathol* 10:217–220, 2016.

Guastaldi FPS, Faquin WC, Gootkind F, et al.: Clear cell odontogenic carcinoma: a rare jaw tumor. A summary of 107 reported cases, *Int J Oral Maxillofac Surg* 48:1405–1410, 2019.

Hansen LS, Eversole LR, Green TL, et al.: Clear cell odontogenic tumor—a new histologic variant with aggressive potential, *Head Neck Surg* 8:115–123, 1985.

Labrador AJP, Marin NRG, Valdez LHM, et al.: Clear cell odontogenic carcinoma a systematic review, *Head Neck Pathol*, 2021. https://doi.org/10.1007/s12105-021-01383-9.

Santana T, de Andrade FL, de Sousa Melo MC, et al.: Clear cell odontogenic carcinoma harboring the EWSR1-ATF1 fusion gene: report of a rare case, *Head Neck Pathol* 14:847–851, 2020.

Vogels R, Baumhoer D, van Gorp J, et al.: Clear cell odontogenic carcinoma: occurrence of EWSR1-CREB1 as alternative fusion gene to EWSR1-ATF1, *Head Neck Pathol* 13:225–230, 2019.

Waldron CA, Small IA, Silverman H: Clear cell ameloblastoma—an odontogenic carcinoma, *J Oral Maxillofac Surg* 43:709–717, 1985.

Adenomatoid Odontogenic Tumor

Chaves RRM, Júnior AACP, Gomes CC, et al.: Multiple adenomatoid odontogenic tumors in a patient with Schimmelpenning syndrome, *Oral Surg Oral Med Oral Pathol Oral Radiol* 129:e12–e17, 2020.

Chrcanovic BR, Gomez RS: Adenomatoid odontogenic tumor: an updated analysis of the cases reported in the literature, *J Oral Pathol Med* 48:10–16, 2019.

Damm DD, White DK, Drummond JF, et al.: Combined epithelial odontogenic tumor: adenomatoid odontogenic tumor and calcifying epithelial odontogenic tumor, *Oral Surg Oral Med Oral Pathol* 55:487–496, 1983.

Ide F, Mishima K, Kikuchi K, et al.: Development and growth of adenomatoid odontogenic tumor related to formation and eruption of teeth, *Head Neck Pathol* 5:123–132, 2011.

Ide F, Matsumoto N, Miyazaki Y, et al.: Recurrence of adenomatoid odontogenic tumor, *J Oral Pathol Med* 48:96–97, 2019.

Martínez A, Mosqueda-Taylor A, Marchesani FJ, et al.: Adenomatoid odontogenic tumor concomitant with cystic complex odontoma: case report, *Oral Surg Oral Med Oral Pathol Oral Radiol Endod* 108:e25–e29, 2009.

Naidu A, Slater LJ, Hamao-Sakamoto A, et al.: Adenomatoid odontogenic tumor with peripheral cemento-osseous reactive proliferation: report of 2 cases and review of the literature, *Oral Surg Oral Med Oral Pathol Oral Radiol* 122:e86–e92, 2016.

Nel C, Uys A, Robinson L, et al.: Multiple adenomatoid odontogenic tumours associated with eight impacted teeth, *Oral Radiol* 37:321–327, 2021.

Reichart PA, Philipsen HP, Khongkhunthian P, et al.: Immunoprofile of the adenomatoid odontogenic tumor, *Oral Dis* 23:731–736, 2017.

Roza ALOC, Carlos R, van Heerden WFP, et al.: An international collaborative study of 105 new cases of adenomatoid odontogenic tumors, *Oral Surg Oral Med Oral Pathol Oral Radiol* 132:327–338, 2021.

Calcifying Epithelial Odontogenic Tumor

Cheng Y-SL, Wright JM, Walstad WR, et al.: Calcifying epithelial odontogenic tumor showing microscopic features of potential malignant behavior, *Oral Surg Oral Med Oral Pathol Oral Radiol Endod* 93:287–295, 2002.

Chrcanovic BR, Gomez RS: Calcifying epithelial odontogenic tumor: an updated analysis of 339 cases reported in the literature, *J Craniomaxillofac Surg* 45:1117–1123, 2017.

de Arruda JAA, Abreu LG, Silva LVO, et al.: Calcifying epithelial odontogenic tumours: Collaborative study of 32 cases and review of literature, *Oral Dis* 25:192–205, 2019.

Demian N, Harris RJ, Abramovitch K, et al.: Malignant transformation of calcifying epithelial odontogenic tumor is associated with the loss of p53 transcriptional activity: a case report with review of the literature, *J Oral Maxillofac Surg* 68:1964–1973, 2010.

Franklin CD, Pindborg JJ: The calcifying epithelial odontogenic tumor: a review and analysis of 113 cases, *Oral Surg Oral Med Oral Pathol* 42:753–765, 1976.

Gaiger de Oliveira M, Moraes Chaves AC, Visioli F, et al.: Peripheral clear cell variant of calcifying epithelial odontogenic tumor affecting 2 sites: report of a case, *Oral Surg Oral Med Oral Pathol Oral Radiol Endod* 107:407–411, 2009.

Germanier Y, Bornstein MM, Stauffer E, et al.: Calcifying epithelial odontogenic (Pindborg) tumor of the mandible with clear cell component treated by conservative surgery: report of a case, *J Oral Maxillofac Surg* 63:1377–1382, 2005.

Gopalakrishnan R, Simonton S, Rohrer MD, et al.: Cystic variant of calcifying epithelial odontogenic tumor, *Oral Surg Oral Med Oral Pathol Oral Radiol Endod* 102:773–777, 2006.

Ide F, Matsumoto N, Miyazaki Y, et al.: What is the non-calcifying Langerhans cell-rich variant of calcifying epithelial odontogenic tumor? *Head Neck Pathol* 13:489–491, 2019.

Kaplan I, Buchner A, Calderon S, et al.: Radiological and clinical features of calcifying epithelial odontogenic tumour, *Dentomaxillofac Radiol* 30:22–28, 2001.

Kawano K, Ono K, Yada N, et al.: Malignant calcifying epithelial odontogenic tumor of the mandible: report of a case with pulmonary metastasis showing remarkable response to platinum derivatives, *Oral Surg Oral Med Oral Pathol Oral Radiol Endod* 104:76–81, 2007.

Kestler DP, Foster JS, Macy SD, et al.: Expression of odontogenic ameloblast-associated protein (ODAM) in dental and other epithelial neoplasms, *Mol Med* 14:318–326, 2008.

McCloy R, Bacaj P, Bouquot JE, et al.: Thirteen synchronous multifocal calcifying epithelial odontogenic tumors (CEOT): case report and review of the literature, *J Oral Maxillofac Surg* 79:2078–2085, 2021.

Murphy CL, Kestler DP, Foster JS, et al.: Odontogenic ameloblast-associated protein nature of the amyloid found in calcifying epithelial odontogenic tumors and unerupted tooth follicles, *Amyloid* 15:89–95, 2008.

Peacock ZS, Cox D, Schmidt BL: Involvement of *PTCH1* mutations in the calcifying epithelial odontogenic tumor, *Oral Oncol* 46:387–392, 2010.

Philipsen HP, Reichart PA: Calcifying epithelial odontogenic tumour: biological profile based on 181 cases from the literature, *Oral Oncol* 36:17–26, 2000.

Pindborg JJ: A calcifying epithelial odontogenic tumor, *Cancer* 11:838–843, 1958.

Ruddocks LA, Fitzpatrick SG, Bhattacharyya I, et al.: Calcifying epithelial odontogenic tumor: a case series spanning 25 years and review of the literature, *Oral Surg Oral Med Oral Pathol Oral Radiol* 131:684–693, 2021.

Rydin K, Sjöström M, Warfvinge G: Clear cell variant of intraosseous calcifying epithelial odontogenic tumor: a case report and review of the literature, *Oral Surg Oral Med Oral Pathol Oral Radiol* 122: e125–e130, 2016.

Sánchez-Romero C, Carlos R, de Almeida OP, et al.: Microcystic calcifying epithelial odontogenic tumor, *Head Neck Pathol* 12:598–603, 2018.

Santosh N, McNamara KK, Kalmar JR, et al.: Non-calcifying Langerhans cell-rich variant of calcifying epithelial odontogenic tumor: a distinct entity with predilection for anterior maxilla, *Head Neck Pathol* 13:718–721, 2019.

Sedghizadeh PP, Wong D, Shuler CF, et al.: Multifocal calcifying epithelial odontogenic tumor, *Oral Surg Oral Med Oral Pathol Oral Radiol Endod* 104:e30–e34, 2007.

Seim P, Regezi JA, O'Ryan F: Hybrid ameloblastoma and calcifying epithelial odontogenic tumor: case report, *J Oral Maxillofac Surg* 63:852–855, 2005.

Shetty SJ, Pereira T, Desai RS: Peripheral clear cell variant of calcifying epithelial odontogenic tumor: case report and review of the literature, *Head Neck Pathol* 10:481–485, 2016.

Só BB, Carrard VC, Hildebrand LC, et al.: Synchronous calcifying epithelial odontogenic tumor: case report and analysis of the 5 cases in the literature, *Head Neck Pathol* 14:435–441, 2020.

Squamous Odontogenic Tumor

Baden E, Doyle J, Mesa M, et al.: Squamous odontogenic tumor: report of three cases including the first extraosseous case, *Oral Surg Oral Med Oral Pathol* 75:733–738, 1993.

Chrcanovic BR, Gomez RS: Squamous odontogenic tumor and squamous odontogenic tumor-like proliferations in odontogenic cysts: an updated analysis of 170 cases reported in the literature, *J Craniomaxillofac Surg* 46:504–510, 2018.

Elmuradi S, Mair Y, Suresh L, et al.: Multicentric squamous odontogenic tumor: a case report and review of the literature, *Head Neck Pathol* 11:168–174, 2017.

Goldblatt LI, Brannon RB, Ellis GL: Squamous odontogenic tumor: report of five cases and review of the literature, *Oral Surg Oral Med Oral Pathol* 54:187–196, 1982.

Ide F, Shimoyama T, Horie N, et al.: Intraosseous squamous cell carcinoma arising in association with a squamous odontogenic tumour of the mandible, *Oral Oncol* 35:431–434, 1999.

Leider AS, Jonker A, Cook HE: Multicentric familial squamous odontogenic tumor, *Oral Surg Oral Med Oral Pathol* 68:175–181, 1989.

Mills WP, Davilla MA, Beattenmuller EA, et al.: Squamous odontogenic tumor: report of a case with lesions in three quadrants, *Oral Surg Oral Med Oral Pathol* 61:557–563, 1986.

Parmar RM, Brannon RB, Fowler CB: Squamous odontogenic tumor-like proliferations in radicular cysts: a clinicopathologic study of forty-two cases, *J Endod* 37:623–626, 2011.

Philipsen HP, Reichart PA: Squamous odontogenic tumor (SOT): a benign neoplasm of the periodontium. A review of 36 reported cases, *J Clin Periodontol* 23:922–926, 1996.

Pullon PA, Shafer WG, Elzay RP, et al.: Squamous odontogenic tumor: report of six cases of a previously undescribed lesion, *Oral Surg Oral Med Oral Pathol* 40:616–630, 1975.

Upadhyaya JD, Banasser A, Cohen DM, et al.: Squamous odontogenic tumor: review of the literature and report of a new case, *J Oral Maxillofac Surg* 79:164–176, 2021.

Wright JM: Squamous odontogenic tumor-like proliferations in odontogenic cysts, *Oral Surg Oral Med Oral Pathol* 47:354–358, 1979.

Mixed Odontogenic Tumors

Bilodeau EA, Collins BM: Odontogenic cysts and neoplasms, *Surg Pathol Clin* 10:177–222, 2017.

Bilodeau EA, Seethala RR: Update on odontogenic tumors: proceedings of the North American Head and Neck Pathology Society, *Head Neck Pathol* 13:457–465, 2019.

Hansen LS, Ficarra G: Mixed odontogenic tumors: an analysis of 23 new cases, *Head Neck Surg* 10:330–343, 1988.

Philipsen HP, Reichart PA: Classification of odontogenic tumors: a historical review, *J Oral Pathol Med* 35:525–529, 2006.

Philipsen HP, Reichart PA: Praetorius F: Mixed odontogenic tumours and odontomas. Considerations on interrelationship. Review of the literature and presentation of 134 new cases of odontomas, *Oral Oncol* 33:86–99, 1997.

Tomich CE: Benign mixed odontogenic tumors, *Semin Diagn Pathol* 16:308–316, 1999.

Ameloblastic Fibroma

Chrcanovic BR, Brennan PA, Rahimi S, et al.: Ameloblastic fibroma and ameloblastic fibrosarcoma: a systematic review, *J Oral Pathol Med* 47:315–325, 2018.

Cohen DM, Bhattacharyya I: Ameloblastic fibroma, ameloblastic fibro-odontoma, and odontoma, *Oral Maxillofac Surg Clin North Am* 16:375–384, 2004.

Dallera P, Bertoni F, Marchetti C, et al.: Ameloblastic fibroma: a follow-up of six cases, *Int J Oral Maxillofac Surg* 25:199–202, 1996.

Darling MR, Daley TD: Peripheral ameloblastic fibroma, *J Oral Pathol Med* 35:190–192, 2006.

Lin C-C, Chen C-H, Lin L-M, et al.: Calcifying odontogenic cyst with ameloblastic fibroma: report of three cases, *Oral Surg Oral Med Oral Pathol Oral Radiol Endod* 98:451–460, 2004.

Mosby EL, Russell D, Noren S, et al.: Ameloblastic fibroma in a 7-week-old infant: a case report and review of the literature, *J Oral Maxillofac Surg* 56:368–372, 1998.

Nelson BL, Folk GS: Ameloblastic fibroma, *Head Neck Pathol* 3:51–53, 2009.

Pereira da Costa DO, Novellino Alves ATN, Calasans-Maia MD, et al.: Maxillary ameloblastic fibroma: a case report, *Braz Dent J* 22:171–174, 2011.

Trodahl JN: Ameloblastic fibroma: a survey of cases from the Armed Forces Institute of Pathology, *Oral Surg Oral Med Oral Pathol* 33:547–558, 1972.

Ameloblastic Fibro-Odontoma

Boxberger NR, Brannon RB, Fowler CB: Ameloblastic fibro-odontoma: a clinicopathologic study of 12 cases, *J Clin Pediatr Dent* 35:397–404, 2011.

Buchner A, Kaffe I, Vered M: Clinical and radiological profile of ameloblastic fibro-odontoma: an update on an uncommon odontogenic tumor based on a critical analysis of 114 cases, *Head Neck Pathol* 7:54–63, 2013.

Chrcanovic BR, Gomez RS: Ameloblastic fibrodentinoma and ameloblastic fibro-odontoma: an updated systematic review of cases reported in the literature, *J Oral Maxillofac Surg* 75:1425–1437, 2017.

Furst I, Pharoah M, Phillips J: Recurrence of an ameloblastic fibro-odontoma in a 9-year-old boy, *J Oral Maxillofac Surg* 57:620–623, 1999.

Howell RM, Burkes EJ: Malignant transformation of ameloblastic fibro-odontoma to ameloblastic fibrosarcoma, *Oral Surg Oral Med Oral Pathol* 43:391–401, 1977.

Miller AS, Lopez CF, Pullon PA, et al.: Ameloblastic fibro-odontoma, *Oral Surg Oral Med Oral Pathol* 41:354–365, 1976.

Peters SM, Bergen MS, Philipone EM, et al.: Ameloblastic fibro-odontoma in an adolescent: a case report and review of literature, *J Clin Pediatr Dent* 42:458–460, 2018.

Soluk-Tekkesin M, Vered M: Ameloblastic fibro-odontoma: at the crossroad between "developing odontoma" and true odontogenic tumour, *Head Neck Pathol* 15:1202–1211, 2021.

Speight PM, Takata T: New tumour entities in the 4th edition of the World Health Organization Classification of Head and Neck tumours: odontogenic and maxillofacial bone tumours, *Virchows Arch* 472:331–339, 2018.

Van Wyk CW, Van der Vyver PC: Ameloblastic fibroma with dentinoid formation/immature dentinoma: a microscopic and ultrastructural study of the epithelial-connective tissue interface, *J Oral Pathol* 12:37–46, 1983.

Ameloblastic Fibrosarcoma

Agaimy A, Skalova A, Franchi A, et al.: Ameloblastic fibrosarcoma: clinicopathological and molecular analysis of seven cases highlighting frequent BRAF and occasional NRAS mutations, *Histopathology* 76:814–821, 2020.

Al Shetawi H, Alpert EH, Buchbinder D, et al.: Ameloblastic fibrosarcoma of the mandible: a case report and a review of the literature, *J Oral Maxillofac Surg* 73:1661.e1–1661.e7, 2015.

Bertoni F, Del Corso G, Bacchini P, et al.: Ameloblastic fibrosarcoma of the mandible evolving from a prior ameloblastic fibroma after two years: an unusual finding, *Int J Surg Pathol* 24:656–659, 2016.

Carlos-Bregni R, Mosqueda-Taylor A, Meneses-Garcia A: Ameloblastic fibrosarcoma of the mandible: report of two cases and review of the literature, *J Oral Pathol Med* 30:316–320, 2001.

Chrcanovic BR, Brennan PA, Rahimi S, et al.: Ameloblastic fibroma and ameloblastic fibrosarcoma: a systematic review, *J Oral Pathol Med* 47:315–325, 2018.

DeLair D, Bejarano PA, Peleg M, et al.: Ameloblastic carcinosarcoma of the mandible arising in ameloblastic fibroma: a case report and review of the literature, *Oral Surg Oral Med Oral Pathol Oral Radiol Endod* 103:516–520, 2007.

Kobayashi K, Murakami R, Fujii T, et al.: Malignant transformation of ameloblastic fibroma to ameloblastic fibrosarcoma: case report and review of the literature, *J Craniomaxillofac Surg* 33:352–355, 2005.

Kousar A, Hosein MM, Ahmed Z, et al.: Rapid sarcomatous transformation of an ameloblastic fibroma of the mandible: case report and literature review, *Oral Surg Oral Med Oral Pathol Oral Radiol Endod* 108:e80–e85, 2009.

Lai J, Blanas N, Higgins K, et al.: Ameloblastic fibrosarcoma: report of a case, study of immunophenotype, and comprehensive review of the literature, *J Oral Maxillofac Surg* 70:2007–2012, 2012.

Servato JPS, Faria PR, Ribeiro CV, et al.: Ameloblastic fibrosarcoma: a case report and literature review, *Braz Dent J* 28:262–272, 2017.

Odontoameloblastoma

El-Naggar AK, Chan JKC, Grandis JR, et al.: *WHO classification of head and neck tumours*, ed 4, Lyon, 2017, IARC, pp 204–260. Chapter 8.

Kaugars GE: Ameloblastic odontoma (odonto-ameloblastoma), *Oral Surg Oral Med Oral Pathol* 71:371–373, 1991.

Mosca RC, Marques MM, Barbosa SC, et al.: Odontoameloblastoma: report of two cases, *Indian J Dent Res* 20:230–234, 2009.

Mosqueda-Taylor A, Carlos-Bregni R, Ramírez-Amador V, et al.: Odontoameloblastoma. Clinico-pathologic study of three cases and critical review of the literature, *Oral Oncol* 38:800–805, 2002.

Speight PM, Takata T: New tumour entities in the 4th edition of the World Health Organization Classification of Head and Neck tumours: odontogenic and maxillofacial bone tumours, *Virchows Arch* 472:331–339, 2018.

Odontoma

Ashkenazi M, Greenberg BP, Chodik G, et al.: Postoperative prognosis of unerupted teeth after removal of supernumerary teeth or odontomas, *Am J Orthod Dentofac Orthop* 131:614–619, 2007.

Bilodeau EA, Collins BM: Odontogenic cysts and neoplasms, *Surg Pathol Clin* 10:177–222, 2017.

Cohen DM, Bhattacharyya I: Ameloblastic fibroma, ameloblastic fibro-odontoma, and odontoma, *Oral Maxillofac Surg Clin North Am* 16:375–384, 2004.

da Silva Rocha OKM, da Silva Barros CC, da Silva LAB, et al.: Peripheral compound odontoma: a rare case report and literature review, *J Cutan Pathol* 47:720–724, 2020.

Ide F, Shimoyama T, Horie N: Gingival peripheral odontoma in an adult: case report, *J Periodontol* 71:830–832, 2000.

Maltagliati A, Ugolini A, Crippa R, et al.: Complex odontoma at the upper right maxilla: Surgical management and histomorphological profile, *Eur J Paediatr Dent* 21:199–202, 2020.

Sedano HO, Pindborg JJ: Ghost cell epithelium in odontomas, *J Oral Pathol* 4:27–30, 1975.

Servato JPS, de Souza MCR, Horta DC, et al.: Odontogenic tumours in children and adolescents: a collaborative study of 431 cases, *Int J Oral Maxillofac Surg* 41:768–773, 2012.

Tekkesin MS, Pehlivan S, Olgac V, et al.: Clinical and histopathological investigation of odontomas: review of the literature and presentation of 160 cases, *J Oral Maxillofac Surg* 70:1358–1361, 2012.

Tomizawa M, Otsuka Y, Noda T: Clinical observations of odontomas in Japanese children: 39 cases including one recurrent case, *Int J Paediatr Dent* 15:37–43, 2005.

Primordial Odontogenic Tumor

Almazyad A, Li C-C, Tapia ROC, et al.: Primordial odontogenic tumour: report of two cases, *Histopathology* 72:1221–1227, 2018.

Almazyad A, Collette D, Zhang D, et al.: Recurrent primordial odontogenic tumor: epithelium-rich variant, *Head Neck Pathol*, 2022. https://doi.org/10.1007/s12105-021-01354-0.

Ando T, Shrestha M, Nakamoto T, et al.: A case of primordial odontogenic tumor: a new entity in the latest WHO classification (2017), *Pathol Int* 67:365–369, 2017.

Azzi L, Tettamanti L, Di Francesco A, et al.: Primordial odontogenic tumour: a systematic review of the common but also unusual features of this novel entity, *J Stomatol Oral Maxillofac Surg* 121:408–417, 2020.

Bologna-Molina R, Mikami T, Pereira-Prado V, et al.: Primordial odontogenic tumor: an immunohistochemical profile, *Med Oral Patol Oral Cir Bucal* 22:e314–e323, 2017.

Bomfim BB, Prado R, Sampaio RK, et al.: Primordial odontogenic tumor: report of a new case and literature review, *Head Neck Pathol* 13:125–130, 2019.

Kayamori K, Tsuchiya M, Michi Y, et al.: Primordial odontogenic tumor occurred in the maxilla with unique calcifications and its crucial points for differential diagnosis, *Pathol Int* 71:80–87, 2021.

Mikami T, Ohashi Y, Bologna-Molina R, et al.: Primordial odontogenic tumor: a case report with histopathological analyses, *Pathol Int* 67:638–643, 2017.

Mikami T, Bologna-Molina R, Mosqueda-Taylor A, et al.: Pathogenesis of primordial odontogenic tumour based on tumourigenesis and odontogenesis, *Oral Dis* 24:1226–1234, 2018.

Mosqueda-Taylor A, Pires FR, Aguirre-Urízar JM, et al.: Primordial odontogenic tumour: clinicopathological analysis of six cases of a previously undescribed entity, *Histopathology* 65:606–612, 2014.

Slater LJ, Eftimie LF, Herford AS: Primordial odontogenic tumor: report of a case, *J Oral Maxillofac Surg* 74:547–551, 2016.

Central Odontogenic Fibroma

Allen CM, Hammond HL, Stimson PG: Central odontogenic fibroma WHO type: a report of 3 cases with an unusual associated giant cell reaction, *Oral Surg Oral Med Oral Pathol* 73:62–66, 1992.

Bilodeau EA, Collins BM: Odontogenic cysts and neoplasms, *Surg Pathol Clin* 10:177–222, 2017.

Correa Pontes FS, Lacerda de Souza L, Paula de Paula L, et al.: Central odontogenic fibroma: an updated systematic review of cases reported in the literature with emphasis on recurrence influencing factors, *J Craniomaxillofac Surg* 46:1753–1757, 2018.

Eversole LR: Odontogenic fibroma, including amyloid and ossifying variants, *Head Neck Pathol* 5:335–343, 2011.

Handlers JP, Abrams AM, Melrose RJ, et al.: Central odontogenic fibroma: clinicopathologic features of 19 cases and review of the literature, *J Oral Maxillofac Surg* 49:46–54, 1991.

Ide F, Sakashita H, Kusama K: Ameloblastomatoid, central odontogenic fibroma: an epithelium-rich variant, *J Oral Pathol Med* 31:612–614, 2002.

Kakuguchi W, Nakamichi Y, Kitamura T: Amyloid variant of central odontogenic fibroma in the mandible: a case report and literature review, *Am J Case Rep* 21:e925165, 2020.

Mosqueda-Taylor A, Martínez-Mata G, Carlos-Bregni R, et al.: Central odontogenic fibroma: new findings and report of a multicentric collaborative study, *Oral Surg Oral Med Oral Pathol Oral Radiol Endod* 112:349–358, 2011.

Odell EW, Lombardi T, Barrett AW, et al.: Hybrid central giant cell granuloma and central odontogenic fibroma-like lesions of the jaws, *Histopathology* 30:165–171, 1997.

Roza ALOC, Sousa EM, Leite AA, et al.: Central odontogenic fibroma: an international multicentric study of 62 cases, *Oral Surg Oral Med Oral Pathol Oral Radiol* 131:549–557, 2021.

Tosios KI, Gopalakrishnan R, Koutlas IG: So-called hybrid central odontogenic fibroma/central giant cell lesion of the jaws. A report on seven additional cases, including an example in a patient with cherubism, and hypotheses on the pathogenesis, *Head Neck Pathol* 2:333–338, 2008.

Upadhyaya JD, Cohen DM, Islam MN, et al.: Hybrid central odontogenic fibroma with giant cell granuloma like lesion: a report of three additional cases and review of the literature, *Head Neck Pathol* 12:166–174, 2018.

Zhou CX, Li TJ: A clinicopathologic study on central odontogenic fibroma: with special reference to amyloid variant, *Oral Surg Oral Med Oral Pathol Oral Radiol* 126:513–520, 2018.

Peripheral Odontogenic Fibroma

Alaeddini M, Salehizadeh S, Baghaii F, et al.: A retrospective analysis of peripheral odontogenic fibroma in an Iranian population, *J Oral Maxillofac Surg* 68:2099–2103, 2010.

Baden E, Moskow BS, Moskow R: Odontogenic epithelial hamartoma, *J Oral Surg* 26:702–714, 1968.

Buchner A, Merrell PW, Carpenter WM: Relative frequency of peripheral odontogenic tumors: a study of 45 new cases and comparison with studies from the literature, *J Oral Pathol Med* 35:385–391, 2006.

Ficarra G, Sapp JP, Eversole LR: Multiple peripheral odontogenic fibroma, World Health Organization type, and central giant cell granuloma: a case report of an unusual association, *J Oral Maxillofac Surg* 51:325–328, 1993.

Heithersay GS, Musu D, Cotti E: External tooth resorption associated with a peripheral odontogenic fibroma: review and case report, *Aust Dent J* 62:516–522, 2017.

Ide F, Obara K, Mishima K, et al.: Peripheral odontogenic tumor: a clinicopathologic study of 30 cases. General features and hamartomatous lesions, *J Oral Pathol Med* 34:552–557, 2005.

Martelli-Junior H, Mesquita RA, de Paula AM, et al.: Peripheral odontogenic fibroma (WHO type) of the newborn: a case report, *Int J Paediatr Dent* 16:376–379, 2006.

Ritwik P, Brannon RB: Peripheral odontogenic fibroma: a clinicopathologic study of 151 cases and review of the literature with special emphasis on recurrence, *Oral Surg Oral Med Oral Pathol Oral Radiol Endod* 110:357–363, 2010.

Siar CH, Ng KH: Clinicopathological study of peripheral odontogenic fibromas (WHO-type) in Malaysians (1967-95), *Br J Oral Maxillofac Surg* 38:19–22, 2000.

Weber A, van Heerden WF, Ligthelm AJ, et al.: Diffuse peripheral odontogenic fibroma: report of 3 cases, *J Oral Pathol Med* 21:82–84, 1992.

Granular Cell Odontogenic Tumor

Brannon RB, Goode RK, Eversole LR, et al.: The central granular cell odontogenic tumor: report of 5 new cases, *Oral Surg Oral Med Oral Pathol Oral Radiol Endod* 94:614–621, 2002.

Chiang C-T, Hu K-Y, Tsai C-C: Central granular cell odontogenic tumor: the first reported case in Oriental people and literature review, *J Formos Med Assoc* 113:321–325, 2014.

Mesquita AT, Santos CR, Gomez RS, et al.: Central granular cell odontogenic tumor: a histopathologic and immunohistochemical study, *Ann Diagn Pathol* 13:405–412, 2009.

Piattelli A, Rubini C, Goteri G, et al.: Central granular cell odontogenic tumour: report of the first malignant case and review of the literature, *Oral Oncol* 39:78–82, 2003.

Rinaggio J, Cleveland D, Koshy R, et al.: Peripheral granular cell odontogenic fibroma, *Oral Surg Oral Med Oral Pathol Oral Radiol Endod* 104:676–679, 2007.

Roza ALOC, Sousa EM, Leite AA, et al.: Central odontogenic fibroma: an international multicentric study of 62 cases, *Oral Surg Oral Med Oral Pathol Oral Radiol* 131:549–557, 2021.

Sarode SC, Sarode GS, Vaidya K: Central granular cell odontogenic tumor: a systematic review, *J Oral Pathol Med* 43:167–176, 2014.

Vincent SD, Hammond HL, Ellis GL, et al.: Central granular cell odontogenic fibroma, *Oral Surg Oral Med Oral Pathol* 63:715–721, 1987.

Waldron CA, Thompson CW, Conner WA: Granular cell ameloblastic fibroma, *Oral Surg Oral Med Oral Pathol* 16:1202–1213, 1963.

Myxoma

Alhousami T, Sabharwal A, Gupta S, et al.: Fibromyxoma of the jaw: case report and review of the literature, *Head Neck Pathol* 12:44–51, 2018.

Barker BF: Odontogenic myxoma, *Semin Diagn Pathol* 16:297–301, 1999.

Chrcanovic BR, Gomez RS: Odontogenic myxoma: an updated analysis of 1,692 cases reported in the literature, *Oral Dis* 25:676–683, 2019.

Dotta JH, Miotto LN, Spin-Neto R, et al.: Odontogenic myxoma: systematic review and bias analysis, *Eur J Clin Investig* 50:e13214, 2020.

Friedrich RE, Scheuer HA, Fuhrmann A, et al.: Radiographic findings of odontogenic myxomas on conventional radiographs, *Anticancer Res* 32:2173–2178, 2012.

Hammad HM, Hasen YM, Odat AA, et al.: Odontogenic myxoma with diffuse calcifications: a case report and review of a rare histologic feature, *Oral Surg Oral Med Oral Pathol Oral Radiol* 122:e116–e124, 2016.

Lahey E, Woo S-B, Park H-K: Odontogenic myxoma with diffuse calcifications: a case report and review of the literature, *Head Neck Pathol* 7:97–102, 2013.

Mewar P, González-Torres KE, Jacks TM, et al.: Sinonasal myxoma: a distinct lesion of infants, *Head Neck Pathol* 14:212–219, 2020.

Pahl S, Henn W, Binger T, et al.: Malignant odontogenic myxoma of the maxilla: case with cytogenetic confirmation, *J Laryngol Otol* 114:533–535, 2000.

Titinchi F, Hassan BA, Morkel JA, et al.: Odontogenic myxoma: a clinicopathological study in a South African population, *J Oral Pathol Med* 45:599–604, 2016.

Vasconcelos ACU, Silveira FM, Gomes APN, et al.: Odontogenic myxoma: a 63-year retrospective multicenter study of 85 cases in a Brazil population and a review of 999 cases from literature, *J Oral Pathol Med* 47:71–77, 2018.

White JA, Ramer N, Wentland TR, et al.: The rare radiographic sunburst appearance of odontogenic myxomas: a case report and review of the literature, *Head Neck Pathol* 14:1105–1110, 2020.

16
Dermatologic Diseases

◆ ECTODERMAL DYSPLASIA

Ectodermal dysplasia represents a group of inherited conditions in which two or more ectodermally derived anatomic structures fail to develop. Thus depending on the type of ectodermal dysplasia, hypoplasia or aplasia of tissues (e.g., skin, hair, nails, teeth, and sweat glands) may be seen. The various types of this disorder may be inherited in any one of several genetic patterns, including autosomal dominant, autosomal recessive, and X-linked patterns. Even though by some accounts almost 200 different subtypes of ectodermal dysplasia can be defined, these disorders are considered to be relatively rare, with an estimated frequency of seven cases occurring in every 10,000 births. For fewer than 50% of these conditions, the specific genetic mutations and their chromosomal locations have been identified. Systematically classifying these conditions can be challenging because of their wide-ranging clinical features; however, some investigators have suggested that a classification scheme based on the molecular genetic alteration associated with each type might be appropriate. Thus groups of ectodermal dysplasia syndromes could be categorized as being caused by mutations in genes encoding cell-cell signals, genes encoding adhesion molecules, or genes regulating transcription.

Clinical Features

Perhaps the best known of the ectodermal dysplasia syndromes is **hypohidrotic ectodermal dysplasia**. In most instances, this disorder seems to show an X-linked inheritance pattern, with the gene mapping to Xq12-q13.1; therefore, a male predominance is usually seen. However, a few families have been identified that show autosomal recessive or autosomal dominant patterns of inheritance.

Affected individuals typically display heat intolerance because of a reduced number of eccrine sweat glands. Sometimes the diagnosis is made during infancy because the baby appears to have a fever of undetermined origin; however, the infant simply cannot regulate body temperature appropriately because of the decreased number of sweat glands. Uncommonly, death results from the markedly elevated body temperature, although this generally happens only when the condition is not identified. Sometimes, as a diagnostic aid, a special impression can be made of the patient's fingertips and then examined microscopically to count the density of the sweat glands. Such findings should be interpreted in conjunction with appropriate age-matched controls.

Other signs of this disorder include fine, sparse hair, including a reduced density of eyebrow and eyelash hair (Fig. 16.1). The periocular skin may show a fine wrinkling with hyperpigmentation (Fig. 16.2), and midface hypoplasia is frequently observed, often resulting in protuberant lips. Because the salivary glands are ectodermally derived, these glands may be hypoplastic or absent, and patients may exhibit varying degrees of xerostomia. The nails may also appear dystrophic and brittle.

The teeth are usually markedly reduced in number (**oligodontia** or **hypodontia**), and their crown shapes are characteristically abnormal (Fig. 16.3). The incisor crowns usually appear tapered, conical, or pointed, and the molar crowns are reduced in diameter. Complete lack of tooth development (**anodontia**) has also been reported, but this appears to be uncommon.

Female patients may show partial expression of the abnormal gene; that is, their teeth may be reduced in number or may have mild structural changes. This incomplete presentation can be explained by the **Lyon hypothesis,** with half of the female patient's X chromosomes expressing the normal gene, and the other half expressing the defective gene.

Histopathologic Features

Histopathologic examination of the skin from a patient with hypohidrotic ectodermal dysplasia shows a decreased number of sweat glands and hair follicles. The adnexal structures that are present are hypoplastic and malformed.

Treatment and Prognosis

Management of hypohidrotic ectodermal dysplasia warrants genetic counseling for the parents and the patient. The dental problems are best managed by a team of dental specialists, including prosthodontists, orthodontists, and oral and maxillofacial surgeons. Treatment options include prosthetic replacement of the dentition with complete dentures, overdentures, or fixed appliances, depending on the number and location of the remaining teeth. With careful site selection, endosseous dental implants may be considered for facilitating prosthetic management of patients older than 6 years of age. Orthognathic surgery may be necessary to correct skeletal

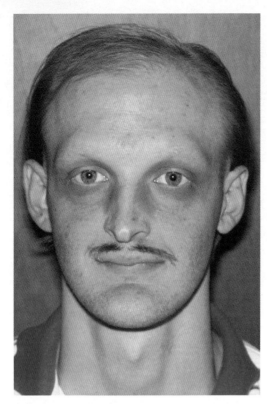

• **Fig. 16.1 Ectodermal Dysplasia.** The sparse hair, periocular hyperpigmentation, and mild midfacial hypoplasia are characteristic features evident in this affected patient.

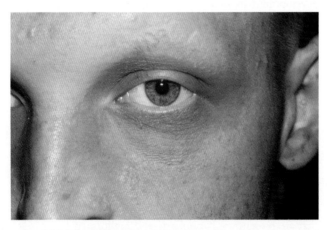

• **Fig. 16.2 Ectodermal Dysplasia.** Closer view of the same patient depicted in Fig. 16.1. Fine periocular wrinkling, as well as sparse eyelash and eyebrow hair, can be observed.

discrepancies of the jaws, and orthodontic movement of the existing teeth may benefit the placement and function of fixed or removable prostheses.

◆ WHITE SPONGE NEVUS (CANNON DISEASE)

White sponge nevus is a relatively rare genodermatosis (a genetically determined skin disorder) that is inherited as an autosomal dominant trait displaying a high degree of

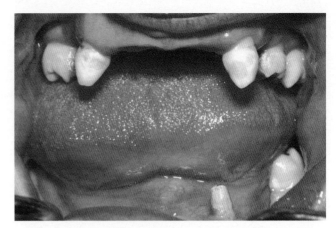

• **Fig. 16.3 Ectodermal Dysplasia.** Oligodontia and conical crown forms are typical oral manifestations. (Courtesy of Dr. Charles Hook and Dr. Bob Gellin.)

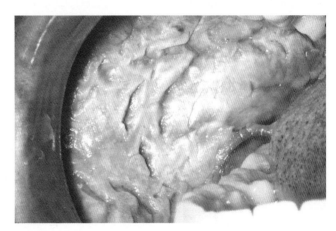

• **Fig. 16.4 White Sponge Nevus.** Diffuse, thickened white plaques of the buccal mucosa.

penetrance and variable expressivity. This condition is due to a defect in the normal keratinization of the oral mucosa. In the 30-member family of keratin filaments, the pair of keratins known as *keratin 4* and *keratin 13* is specifically expressed in the spinous cell layer of mucosal epithelium. Mutations in either of these keratin genes have been shown to be responsible for the clinical manifestations of white sponge nevus.

Clinical Features

The lesions of white sponge nevus usually appear at birth or in early childhood, but sometimes the condition develops during adolescence. Symmetrical, thickened, white, corrugated or velvety, diffuse plaques affect the buccal mucosa bilaterally in most instances (Fig. 16.4). Other common intraoral sites of involvement include the ventral tongue, labial mucosa, soft palate, alveolar mucosa, and floor of the mouth, although the extent of involvement can vary from patient to patient. Extraoral mucosal sites, such as the nasal, esophageal, laryngeal, and anogenital mucosa, appear to be less commonly affected. Patients are usually asymptomatic.

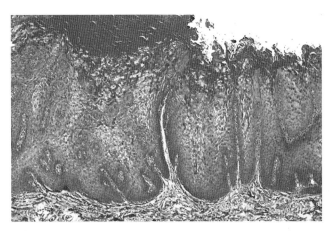

• **Fig. 16.5 White Sponge Nevus.** This low-power photomicrograph shows prominent hyperparakeratosis, marked thickening (acanthosis), and vacuolation of the spinous cell layer.

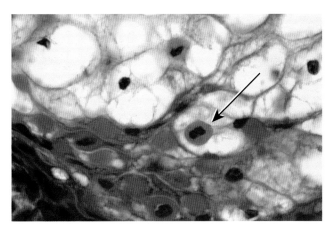

• **Fig. 16.6 White Sponge Nevus.** This high-power photomicrograph shows vacuolation of the cytoplasm of the cells of the spinous layer, with no evidence of epithelial atypia. Perinuclear condensation of keratin tonofilaments can also be observed in some cells.

Histopathologic Features

The microscopic features of white sponge nevus are characteristic but not necessarily pathognomonic. Prominent hyperparakeratosis and marked acanthosis with clearing of the cytoplasm of the cells in the spinous layer are common features (Figs. 16.5 and 16.6); however, similar microscopic findings may be associated with leukoedema and hereditary benign intraepithelial dyskeratosis (HBID). In some instances, an eosinophilic condensation is noted in the perinuclear region of the cells in the superficial layers of the epithelium, a feature that is unique to white sponge nevus. Ultrastructurally, this condensed material can be identified as tangled masses of keratin tonofilaments.

Exfoliative cytologic studies may provide more definitive diagnostic information. A cytologic preparation stained with the Papanicolaou method often shows the eosinophilic perinuclear condensation of the epithelial cell cytoplasm to a greater extent than does the histopathologic section (Fig. 16.7).

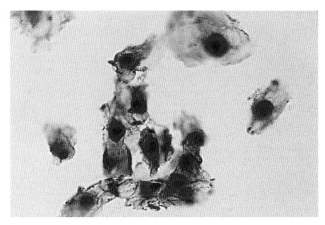

• **Fig. 16.7 White Sponge Nevus.** This high-power photomicrograph of a Papanicolaou-stained cytologic preparation shows the pathognomonic perinuclear condensation of keratin tonofilaments.

Treatment and Prognosis

Because this is a benign condition, no treatment is necessary. The prognosis is good.

◆ HEREDITARY BENIGN INTRAEPITHELIAL DYSKERATOSIS (WITKOP-VON SALLMANN SYNDROME)

Hereditary benign intraepithelial dyskeratosis (HBID) is a rare autosomal dominant genodermatosis primarily affecting descendants of a triracial isolate (Native American, black, and white) of people who originally lived in North Carolina. Examples of HBID have sporadically been reported from other areas of the United States because of migration of affected individuals, and descriptions of affected patients with no apparent connection to North Carolina have also appeared in the literature.

Clinical Features

The lesions of HBID usually develop during childhood, in most instances affecting the oral and conjunctival mucosa. The oral lesions are similar to those of white sponge nevus, with both conditions showing thick, corrugated white plaques involving the buccal and labial mucosa (Fig. 16.8). Milder cases may exhibit the opalescent appearance of leukoedema. Other oral mucosal sites, such as the floor of the mouth and lateral tongue, may also be affected. These oral lesions may exhibit a superimposed candidal infection as well.

The most interesting feature of HBID is the ocular lesions, which begin to develop very early in life. These appear as thick, opaque, gelatinous plaques affecting the bulbar conjunctiva adjacent to the cornea (Fig. 16.9) and sometimes involving the cornea itself. When the lesions are active, patients may experience tearing, photophobia, and itching of the eyes. In many patients, the plaques are most prominent in the spring and tend to regress during the summer or

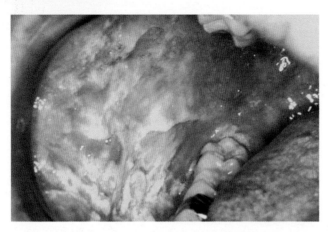

• **Fig. 16.8 Hereditary Benign Intraepithelial Dyskeratosis (HBID).** Oral lesions appear as corrugated white plaques of the buccal mucosa. (Courtesy of Dr. John McDonald.)

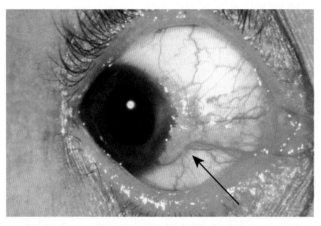

• **Fig. 16.9 Hereditary Benign Intraepithelial Dyskeratosis (HBID).** Ocular lesions appear as gelatinous plaques *(arrow)* of the bulbar conjunctivae. (Courtesy of Dr. Carl Witkop.)

autumn. Sometimes blindness may result from the induction of vascularity of the cornea secondary to the shedding process.

Histopathologic Features

The histopathologic features of HBID include prominent parakeratin production in addition to marked acanthosis. A peculiar dyskeratotic process, similar to that of Darier disease, is scattered throughout the upper spinous layer of the surface oral epithelium (Fig. 16.10). With this dyskeratotic process, an epithelial cell appears to be surrounded or engulfed by an adjacent epithelial cell, resulting in the so-called *cell-within-a-cell* phenomenon.

Treatment and Prognosis

Because HBID is a benign condition, no treatment is generally required or indicated for the oral lesions. If superimposed candidiasis develops, then an antifungal medication can be used. Patients with symptomatic ocular lesions should be

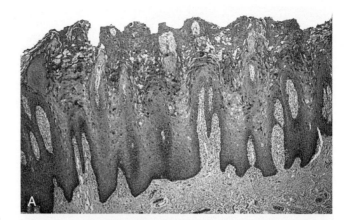

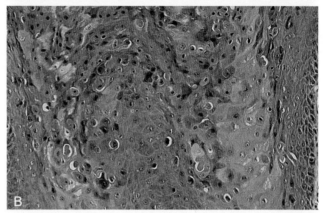

• **Fig. 16.10 Hereditary Benign Intraepithelial Dyskeratosis (HBID). A,** Medium-power photomicrograph exhibiting hyperparakeratosis, acanthosis, and dyskeratosis. **B,** Higher magnification showing dyskeratotic cells.

referred to an ophthalmologist. Typically, the plaques that obscure vision must be surgically excised. This procedure, however, is recognized as a temporary measure because the lesions often recur.

◆ PACHYONYCHIA CONGENITA (JADASSOHN-LEWANDOWSKY TYPE; JACKSON-LAWLER TYPE)

Pachyonychia congenita is a group of rare genodermatoses that are usually inherited as an autosomal dominant trait, although a *de novo* mutation is seen in approximately 45% of affected patients. Mutations of genes that encode for keratin 6a, 6b, 6c, 16, or 17 are responsible for this condition, with different phenotypic expressions depending on the particular mutation. The nails, especially the toenails, are dramatically affected in most patients. Oral lesions are seen most frequently in patients who have mutation of the keratin 6a (*KRT6A*) gene, but can be found in a reduced percentage of the other keratin mutations. Throughout the world, approximately 5000–10,000 people are thought to have this condition. Historically, pachyonychia congenita has been divided into the Jadassohn-Lewandowsky type

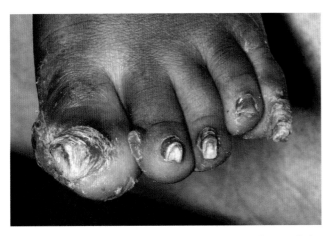

• **Fig. 16.11 Pachyonychia Congenita.** The nails often have a tubular configuration due to keratin accumulation beneath the nailbed.

(pachyonychia congenita, type 1) and the Jackson-Lawler type (pachyonychia congenita, type 2). It may be more appropriate, however, to categorize this group of disorders based on the specific keratin mutation that affects a particular patient.

Clinical Features

Virtually all patients with pachyonychia congenita exhibit characteristic nail changes, either at birth or in the early neonatal period. The free margins of the nails are lifted up because of an accumulation of keratinaceous material in the nail beds. This results in a pinched, tubular configuration (Fig. 16.11). Ultimately, nail loss may occur.

Other skin changes that may occur include marked hyperkeratosis of the palmar and plantar surfaces, producing thick, callous-like lesions (Fig. 16.12). Hyperhidrosis of the palms and soles is also commonly present. The rest of the skin shows punctate papules, representing an abnormal accumulation of keratin in the hair follicles. One disabling feature of the syndrome is severe pain with walking, which is believed to be due to the formation of blisters beneath the thick calluses on the soles of the feet, although recent studies have suggested that neuropathic pain may be a contributing factor. Fissuring of the thickened plantar calluses can also occur and cause pain upon walking.

The oral lesions seen in pachyonychia congenita consist of thickened white plaques that involve the lateral margins and dorsal surface of the tongue. Other oral mucosal regions that are frequently exposed to mild trauma, such as the palate, buccal mucosa, and alveolar mucosa, may also be affected (Fig. 16.13). Neonatal teeth are seen in a majority of patients with mutations of the keratin 17 gene, but only one-third of these individuals have oral white lesions. The increased incidence in dental caries that is identified in these patients may be related to the impact that abnormal keratin proteins have on enamel structure. Hoarseness and dyspnea have been described in some patients as a result of laryngeal mucosal involvement.

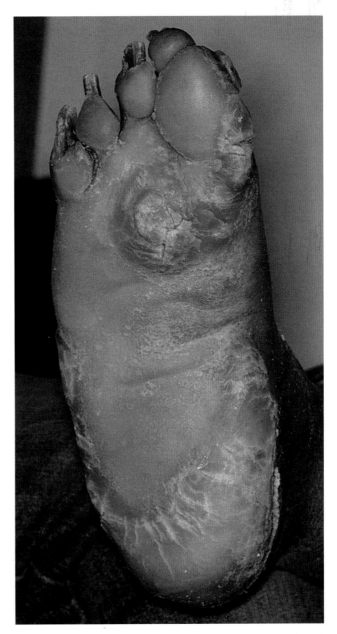

• **Fig. 16.12 Pachyonychia Congenita.** The soles of the feet of affected patients typically show marked callus-like thickenings.

Histopathologic Features

Microscopic examination of lesional oral mucosa shows marked hyperparakeratosis and acanthosis with perinuclear clearing of the epithelial cells.

Treatment and Prognosis

Because the oral lesions of pachyonychia congenita show no apparent tendency for malignant transformation, no treatment is required. The nails are often lost or may need to be surgically removed because of the deformity. In addition, the keratin accumulation on the palms and soles can be quite uncomfortable and distressing to many of the affected individuals. Most patients have to pay continuous attention to

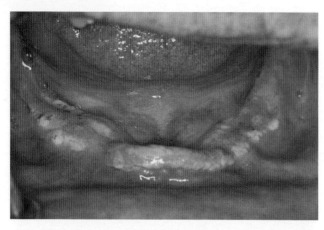

• **Fig. 16.13 Pachyonychia Congenita.** Although tongue lesions are more common in patients with pachyonychia congenita, other oral mucosal sites exposed to minor trauma, such as the alveolar mucosa, may develop thickened white patches. (Courtesy of Dr. John Lenox.)

removal of the excess keratin, and issues related to quality of life often arise. If laryngeal involvement results in dyspnea, laser debulking may improve airway function. Oral retinoids may be of some benefit for select patients, but the dosage has to be carefully monitored in order to minimize medication side effects. Patients should receive genetic counseling, as an aid in family planning. Chorionic villus sampling can be used to identify the various keratin mutations associated with these disorders, thereby allowing prenatal diagnosis.

◆ DYSKERATOSIS CONGENITA (COLE-ENGMAN SYNDROME; ZINSSER-COLE-ENGMAN SYNDROME)

Dyskeratosis congenita is a rare genodermatosis that is usually inherited as an X-linked recessive trait, resulting in a striking male predilection. Autosomal dominant and autosomal recessive forms, although less common, have been reported. Mutations in the *DKC1* gene initially were determined to cause the X-linked form of dyskeratosis congenita. The mutated gene appears to disrupt the normal maintenance of telomerase, an enzyme that is critical in determining normal cellular longevity. Subsequently, mutations of 14 other genes responsible for telomere maintenance have been identified for the other inheritance patterns of dyskeratosis congenital, and the condition is now considered part of a spectrum of telomere biology disorders. The clinician should be aware of the condition because the oral lesions may undergo malignant transformation, and patients are susceptible to aplastic anemia.

Clinical Features

Dyskeratosis congenita usually becomes evident during the first 10 years of life. A reticular pattern of skin hyperpigmentation develops, affecting the face, neck, and upper chest. In addition, abnormal, dysplastic changes of the nails are evident at this time (Fig. 16.14).

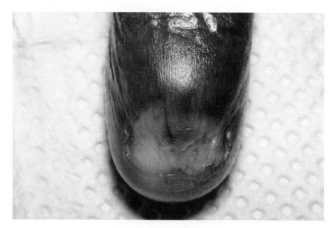

• **Fig. 16.14 Dyskeratosis Congenita.** Dysplastic nail changes.

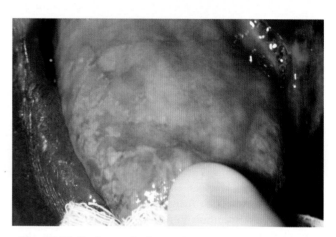

• **Fig. 16.15 Dyskeratosis Congenita.** Atrophy and hyperkeratosis of the dorsal tongue mucosa are visible.

Intraorally, the tongue and buccal mucosa develop bullae; these are followed by erosions and, eventually, leukoplakic lesions (Fig. 16.15). The leukoplakic lesions are considered to be premalignant, and approximately one-third of them become malignant in a 10- to 30-year period. The actual rate of transformation may be higher, but this may not be appreciated because of the shortened life span of these patients. Rapidly progressive periodontal disease has been reported sporadically.

Thrombocytopenia is usually the first hematologic problem that develops, typically during the second decade of life, followed by anemia. Ultimately, aplastic anemia develops in approximately 80% of these patients (see page 586). Mild to moderate intellectual disability may also be present. Generally, the autosomal recessive and X-linked recessive forms show a more severe pattern of disease expression.

Histopathologic Features

Biopsy specimens of the early oral mucosal lesions show hyperorthokeratosis with epithelial atrophy. As the lesions progress, epithelial dysplasia develops until frank squamous cell carcinoma evolves.

Treatment and Prognosis

The discomfort of the oral lesions is managed symptomatically, and careful periodic oral mucosal examinations are performed to check for evidence of malignant transformation. Routine medical evaluation is warranted to monitor the patient for the development of aplastic anemia. Certain anabolic steroids have been shown to increase telomerase activity, and treatment with these drugs may result in temporary improvement in the hematologic status. Bone marrow failure ultimately ensues, however. Selected patients may be considered for allogeneic hematopoietic stem cell transplantation once the aplastic anemia is identified.

As a result of these potentially life-threatening complications, the prognosis is guarded. The average life span for the more severely affected patients is 32 years of age. The parents and the patient should receive genetic counseling.

◆ XERODERMA PIGMENTOSUM

Xeroderma pigmentosum is a rare genodermatosis in which numerous cutaneous malignancies develop at a very early age. The prevalence of the condition in the United States is estimated to be 1 in 250,000–500,000. The condition is inherited as an autosomal recessive trait and is caused by one of several defects in the excision repair and/or postreplication repair mechanism of DNA. As a result of the inability of the epithelial cells to repair ultraviolet (UV) light–induced damage, mutations in the epithelial cells occur, leading to the development of nonmelanoma skin cancer at a rate 10,000 times what would normally be expected in people younger than 20 years of age.

Clinical Features

During the first few years of life, patients affected by xeroderma pigmentosum show a markedly increased tendency to sunburn. Skin changes, such as atrophy, freckled pigmentation, and patchy depigmentation, soon follow (Fig. 16.16). In early childhood, **actinic keratoses** begin developing, a process that normally does not take place before 40 years of age. These lesions quickly progress to **squamous cell carcinoma,** with **basal cell carcinoma** also appearing; consequently, in most patients a nonmelanoma skin cancer develops during the first decade of life. Melanoma develops in about 5% of patients with xeroderma pigmentosum, but it evolves at a slightly later time. As a consequence of sun exposure, the head and neck region is the site most frequently affected by these cutaneous malignancies. Neurologic degenerative changes occur in 20% to 30% of affected patients and include subnormal intelligence, ataxia, sensorineural deafness, and impaired eyesight. The precise cause for the neurologic problems is currently unclear.

Oral manifestations, which often occur before 20 years of age, include development of **squamous cell carcinoma** of the lower lip and the tip of the tongue. This latter site is most unusual for oral cancer, and its involvement is again

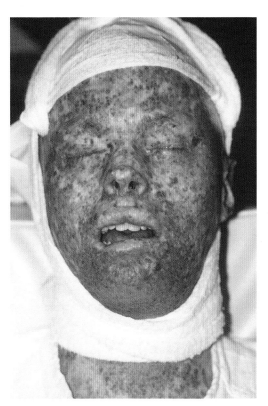

• **Fig. 16.16 Xeroderma Pigmentosum.** The atrophic changes and pigmentation disturbances shown are characteristic of xeroderma pigmentosum.

undoubtedly related to the increased sun exposure, however minimal, which this area receives in contrast to the rest of the oral mucosa.

The diagnosis of xeroderma pigmentosum is usually made when the patient is evaluated for the cutaneous lesions, because it is highly unusual for a very young person to have skin cancer. Because xeroderma pigmentosum is an autosomal recessive trait, a family history of the disorder is not likely to be present, but the possibility of a consanguineous relationship of the affected child's parents should be investigated.

Histopathologic Features

The histopathologic features of xeroderma pigmentosum are relatively nonspecific, in that the cutaneous premalignant lesions and malignancies that occur are microscopically indistinguishable from those observed in unaffected patients.

Treatment and Prognosis

Treatment of xeroderma pigmentosum is challenging because in most instances significant sun damage has already occurred by the time of diagnosis. Patients are advised to avoid sunlight and unfiltered fluorescent light and to wear appropriate protective clothing and sunscreens if they cannot avoid sun exposure. Because sunlight exposure is reduced, these patients often require vitamin D supplementation. Before receiving dental treatment, a calibrated UV light meter should be used to evaluate the amount of UV light being emitted from various sources in the dental office, such as the examination light, the radiograph view box, computer screens in the area, fiber-optic lights, or lights that are used for curing composite restorations. Some authors have suggested that any reading greater than 0 nm/cm² would be unacceptable. A dermatologist should evaluate the patient every 3 months to monitor the development of cutaneous lesions.

Topical chemotherapeutic agents (e.g., 5-fluorouracil or imiquimod) may be used to treat actinic keratoses. Nonmelanoma skin cancers should be excised conservatively, preferably with microscopically controlled excision (Mohs surgery) to preserve as much normal tissue as possible. Patients should also receive genetic counseling, because a high number of consanguineous marriages have been reported in some series.

The prognosis is still poor. Most patients die 30 years earlier than the normal population, either directly from cutaneous malignancy or from complications associated with the treatment of the cancer. The outlook is much better if patients adhere to a strict program of life-long UV light avoidance, but this can be difficult to achieve.

◆ HEREDITARY MUCOEPITHELIAL DYSPLASIA

Hereditary mucoepithelial dysplasia is a rare disorder that may occur sporadically or may be inherited as an autosomal dominant trait; however, the precise genetic alteration is currently unknown. Approximately 60 cases have been reported, although affected patients may not be recognized due to the rarity of condition. For reasons that are not entirely understood, the mucosal epithelial cells do not develop in a normal fashion, and for this reason the designation of *dysplasia* has been given. However, in this situation, no increased risk of malignant transformation is seen. When a cervical exfoliative cytologic preparation (Pap smear) is done, the epithelial cells that are harvested may be interpreted as appearing cytologically unusual or atypical; in the past, some female patients have been advised to undergo hysterectomy because of this misinterpretation. Consequently, accurate identification of this disorder is extremely important for these patients.

Clinical Features

Hereditary mucoepithelial dysplasia is characterized by both cutaneous and mucosal abnormalities. Patients typically have sparse, coarse hair with nonscarring alopecia. Eyelashes and eyebrows are generally affected (Fig. 16.17). Severe photophobia develops at an early age, and most of these patients will have evidence of cataracts beginning in childhood or early adult life. Corneal vascularization, keratitis secondary to corneal erosions, cataracts, and nystagmus are also commonly described. As would be expected, vision is usually markedly impaired for these patients. Other skin

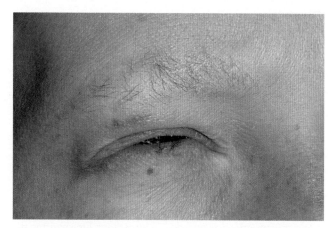

• **Fig. 16.17 Hereditary Mucoepithelial Dysplasia.** Sparse hair is noted on the eyebrows and eyelashes.

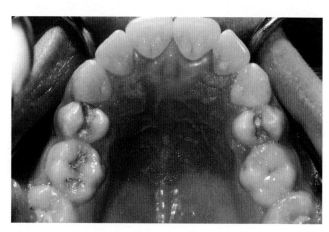

• **Fig. 16.18 Hereditary Mucoepithelial Dysplasia.** Marked erythema of the anterior hard palate.

manifestations include a prominent perineal rash that appears during infancy, as well as a widespread rough, dry texture because of follicular keratosis.

Pulmonary complications related to mucoepithelial dysplasia can range in severity, presumably because of the degree of gene expression. In one family, cavitary bullae were reported to form within the lung parenchyma, and these led to recurrent bouts of pneumonia, often resulting in life-threatening complications.

The oral manifestations of hereditary mucoepithelial dysplasia are usually quite striking, appearing as demarcated fiery-red erythema of the hard palate (Fig. 16.18), with generally less involvement of the attached gingivae and tongue mucosa. These mucosal alterations are typically asymptomatic, despite their remarkable clinical appearance. The nasal, conjunctival, vaginal, cervical, urethral, and bladder mucosa may have the same unusual erythematous features.

Histopathologic Features

Biopsies of the mucosal lesions of hereditary mucoepithelial dysplasia show epithelium with minimal keratinization and a disorganized maturation pattern. The squamous epithelial

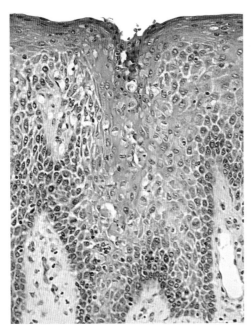

• **Fig. 16.19 Hereditary Mucoepithelial Dysplasia.** Disorganized epithelium exhibiting scattered intracytoplasmic vacuoles.

cells may have a relatively high nuclear/cytoplasmic ratio, but significant nuclear or cellular pleomorphism is not observed. Cytoplasmic vacuoles have been described and may appear as grayish inclusions (Fig. 16.19). These vacuoles also may be observed in exfoliative cytology samples. Ultrastructurally, the lesional cells have been described as having reduced numbers of desmosomes and internalized gap junctions.

Treatment and Prognosis

Given the genetic nature of this disease, supportive care and genetic counseling are typically offered. Affected patients should be monitored for development of pulmonary disease.

◆ INCONTINENTIA PIGMENTI (BLOCH-SULZBERGER SYNDROME)

Incontinentia pigmenti is a relatively rare inherited disorder, with approximately 800 cases reported worldwide. It typically evolves in several stages, primarily affecting the skin, eyes, and central nervous system (CNS), as well as oral structures. There is a marked female predilection, with a 37:1 female-to-male ratio reported. The condition is inherited as an X-linked dominant trait, with the single unpaired gene on the X chromosome being lethal for most males. The mutated gene responsible for producing the phenotypic features of incontinentia pigmenti maps to the Xq28 locus, where the *IKBKG* gene (*inhibitor of kappa B kinase gamma*, formerly known as *NEMO*) is found. This gene is active in early embryogenesis, and acts to protect the developing tissues of the embryo from apoptosis. Mutation of this gene in females has less of an impact, due to the presence of two X chromosomes. If this mutated gene is present in a male

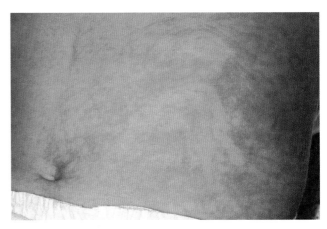

• **Fig. 16.20 Incontinentia Pigmenti.** Swirling pattern of pigmentation on the abdomen of an infant.

embryo, that embryo will not remain viable. Of the few males who survive, a small percentage have Klinefelter syndrome (XXY karyotype), whereas the rest usually show mosaicism for the *IKBKG* gene, suggesting a postzygotic mutation.

Clinical Features

The clinical manifestations of incontinentia pigmenti usually begin in the first few weeks of infancy. There are four classic stages associated with the cutaneous lesions:
1. Vesicular stage: Vesiculobullous lesions appear on the skin of the trunk and limbs. Spontaneous resolution usually occurs within 4 months.
2. Verrucous stage: Verrucous cutaneous plaques develop, affecting the limbs. These clear by 6 months of age, evolving into the third stage.
3. Hyperpigmentation stage: Macular, brown skin lesions appear, characterized by a strange swirling pattern (Fig. 16.20), although these tend to fade around the time of puberty.
4. Atrophy and depigmentation stage: Atrophy and depigmentation of the skin ultimately occur. Considerable overlap among these stages can occur at times, however.

CNS abnormalities occur in approximately 30% of affected patients. The most common problems are intellectual disability, seizure disorders, and motor difficulties. Ocular problems (e.g., strabismus, nystagmus, cataracts, retinal vascular abnormalities, and optic nerve atrophy) may also be identified in nearly 35% of these patients.

The oral manifestations of incontinentia pigmenti, noted in 70%–95% of the cases, include **oligodontia (hypodontia),** delayed eruption, high-arched palate, and hypoplasia or malformed crowns of the teeth (Fig. 16.21). The teeth are often small and cone shaped; both the primary and permanent dentitions are affected.

Histopathologic Features

The microscopic findings in incontinentia pigmenti vary, depending on when a biopsy of the skin lesions is performed.

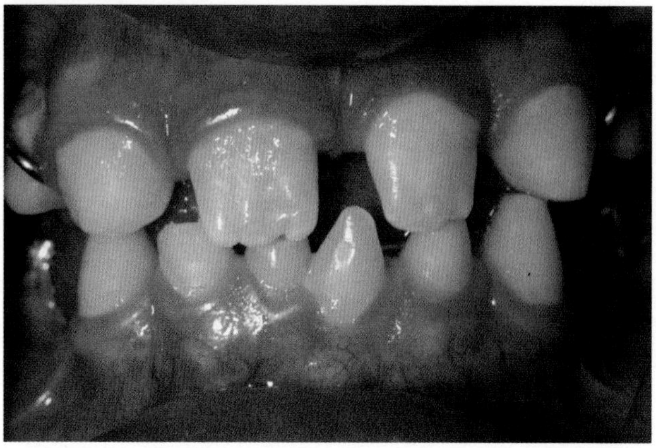

• **Fig. 16.21 Incontinentia Pigmenti.** Hypodontia and conical teeth.

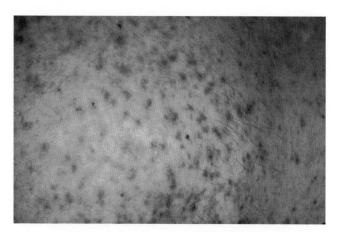

• **Fig. 16.22 Darier Disease.** Erythematous cutaneous papules on the chest.

In the initial vesicular stage, intraepithelial clefts filled with eosinophils are observed. During the verrucous stage, hyper-keratosis, acanthosis, and papillomatosis are noted. The hyperpigmentation stage shows numerous melanin-containing macrophages (melanin incontinence) in the sube-pithelial connective tissue, the feature from which the disorder derives its name.

Treatment and Prognosis

Treatment of incontinentia pigmenti is directed toward the various abnormalities. Dental management includes appropriate prosthodontic and restorative care, although this is sometimes difficult if CNS problems are severe. Prenatal genetic testing can be performed, but currently this is not widely available.

◆ DARIER DISEASE (KERATOSIS FOLLICULARIS; DYSKERATOSIS FOLLICULARIS; DARIER-WHITE DISEASE)

Darier disease is an uncommon genodermatosis with rather striking skin involvement and relatively subtle oral mucosal lesions. The condition is generally inherited as an autosomal dominant trait, having a high degree of penetrance and variable expressivity, although as much as 40-50% of cases may represent new mutations. A lack of cohesion among the surface epithelial cells characterizes this disease, and mutation of a gene (identified as *ATP2A2*) that encodes an intracellular calcium pump (SERCA2—sarco/endoplasmic reticulum Ca^{2+}-ATPase isoform 2) has been identified as the cause for abnormal desmosomal organization in the affected epithelial cells. Estimates of the prevalence of Darier disease in Northern European populations range from 1 in 36,000–1 in 100,000.

Clinical Features

Patients with Darier disease have numerous erythematous, often pruritic, papules on the skin of the trunk and the scalp that develop during the first or second decade of life

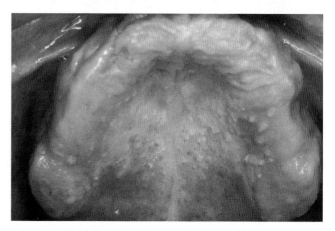

• **Fig. 16.23 Darier Disease.** The oral mucosa may show multiple white papules. (Courtesy of Dr. George Blozis.)

(Fig. 16.22). An accumulation of keratin, producing a rough texture, may be seen in association with the lesions, and a foul odor may be present as a result of bacterial degradation of the keratin. The process generally becomes worse during the summer months, either because of sensitivity of some patients to UV light or because increased heat results in sweating, which induces more epithelial clefting. The palms and soles often exhibit pits and keratoses. The nails show longitudinal lines, ridges, or painful splits.

The oral lesions are typically asymptomatic and are discovered on routine examination. The frequency of occurrence of oral lesions ranges from 15% to 50%. They consist of multiple, normal-colored or white, flat-topped papules that, if numerous enough to be confluent, result in a cobblestone mucosal appearance (Fig. 16.23). These lesions affect the hard palate and alveolar mucosa primarily, although the buccal mucosa or tongue may be occasionally involved. If the palatal lesions are prominent, then the condition may resemble inflammatory papillary hyperplasia or nicotine stomatitis. Some patients with this condition also experience recurrent obstructive parotid swelling secondary to duct abnormalities.

Histopathologic Features

Microscopic examination of the cutaneous or mucosal lesions shows a dyskeratotic process characterized by a central keratin plug that overlies epithelium exhibiting a suprabasilar cleft (Fig. 16.24). This intraepithelial clefting phenomenon, also known as **acantholysis,** is not unique to Darier disease and may be seen in conditions, such as pemphigus vulgaris (see page 769). In addition, the epithelial rete ridges associated with the lesions appear narrow, elongated, and "test tube"–shaped. Closer inspection of the epithelium reveals varying numbers of two types of dyskeratotic cells, called *corps ronds* (round bodies) or **grains** (because they resemble cereal grains).

Treatment and Prognosis

Treatment of Darier disease depends on the severity of involvement. Photosensitive patients should use a sunscreen, and all patients should minimize unnecessary exposure to hot environments. For relatively mild cases, keratolytic agents or emollients may be the only treatment required. For more severely affected patients, systemic retinoids are often beneficial, but the side effects of such medications are often quite bothersome to the patient and can be significant; therefore, the physician should carefully monitor their use. Although the condition is not premalignant or otherwise life threatening, genetic counseling is appropriate.

◆ WARTY DYSKERATOMA (ISOLATED DARIER DISEASE; ISOLATED DYSKERATOSIS FOLLICULARIS; FOCAL ACANTHOLYTIC DYSKERATOSIS; FOLLICULAR DYSKERATOMA)

The **warty dyskeratoma** is a distinctly uncommon solitary lesion that can occur on skin or oral mucosa. It is histopathologically identical to Darier disease. For this reason the lesion has been termed **isolated Darier disease.** The lesion is not otherwise related to Darier disease, however, and its cause remains unknown.

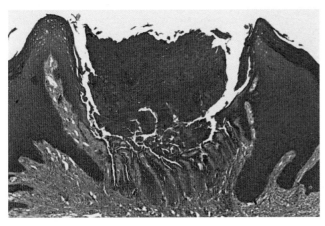

• **Fig. 16.24 Darier Disease.** Low-power photomicrograph showing a thick keratin plug, intraepithelial clefting, and elongated rete ridges.

Clinical Features

The cutaneous warty dyskeratoma typically appears as a solitary, asymptomatic, umbilicated papule on the skin of the head or neck of an older adult, although multiple cutaneous lesions have been reported. The intraoral lesion also develops in patients older than age 40, and a slight male predilection has been identified. The intraoral warty dyskeratoma appears as a pink or white, umbilicated papule located on the keratinized mucosa, especially the hard palate and the alveolar ridge (Fig. 16.25). A warty or roughened surface is noted in some lesions. Most warty dyskeratomas are smaller than 0.5 cm in diameter.

Histopathologic Features

Histopathologically, the warty dyskeratoma appears very similar to **keratosis follicularis.** Both conditions display dyskeratosis, basilar hyperplasia, and a suprabasilar cleft (Fig. 16.26). The warty dyskeratoma is a solitary lesion, however, and the formation of *corps ronds* and grains is not a prominent feature.

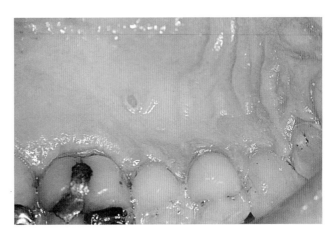

• **Fig. 16.25 Warty Dyskeratoma.** Umbilicated papule on the hard palate. (Courtesy of Dr. Greg Adams.)

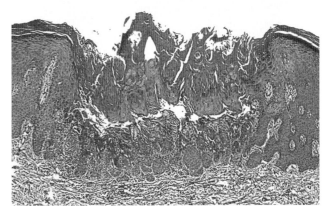

• **Fig. 16.26 Warty Dyskeratoma.** Well-circumscribed invagination filled with a thick parakeratin plug. There is hyperplasia of the basilar cells with a suprabasilar cleft.

Treatment and Prognosis

Treatment of the warty dyskeratoma consists of conservative excision. The prognosis is excellent; these lesions have not been reported to recur, and they have no apparent malignant potential. Careful histopathologic evaluation of the tissue should be performed, because some epithelial dysplasias may show a marked lack of cellular cohesiveness, resulting in a similar acantholytic appearance microscopically.

◆ PEUTZ-JEGHERS SYNDROME

Peutz-Jeghers syndrome is a relatively rare but well-recognized condition, having a prevalence of approximately 1 in 50,000–200,000 births. It is characterized by freckle-like lesions of the hands, perioral skin, and oral mucosa, in conjunction with intestinal polyposis and predisposition for affected patients to develop cancer. The syndrome is generally inherited as an autosomal dominant trait, although as many as 35% of cases represent new mutations. Mutation of the tumor suppressor gene, *STK11* (also known as *LKB1*) is responsible for most cases of Peutz-Jeghers syndrome. This gene, which encodes for a serine/threonine kinase, is located on chromosome 19p13.3.

Clinical Features

The skin lesions of Peutz-Jeghers syndrome usually develop early in childhood and involve the periorificial areas (e.g., mouth, nose, anus, and genital region). The skin of the extremities is affected in about 50% of patients (Fig. 16.27). The lesions resemble freckles, but they do not wax and wane with sun exposure, as do true freckles.

The intestinal polyps, generally considered to be hamartomatous growths, are scattered throughout the mucus-producing areas of the gastrointestinal tract. The jejunum and ileum are most commonly affected. Patients often have problems with intestinal obstruction because of intussusception ("telescoping" of a proximal segment of the bowel into a distal portion), a problem that usually becomes evident during the third decade of life. Most of these episodes are self-correcting, but surgical intervention is sometimes necessary to prevent ischemic necrosis of the bowel, with subsequent peritonitis. Gastrointestinal adenocarcinoma develops in a significant percentage of affected patients, although the polyps themselves do not appear to be premalignant. In one large series of cases, 9% of the patients had developed gastrointestinal malignancy by 40 years of age and 33% by 60 years of age. This compares to 0.1% and 1.0%, respectively, in the general population. Other tumors affecting the pancreas, male and female genital tract, breast, and ovary may also develop. In women, the risk of developing breast cancer approaches 50% by 60 years of age. The increased frequency of malignancy in these patients overall is estimated to be approximately 10–18 times greater than normal.

The oral lesions essentially represent an extension of the perioral freckling. These 1- to 4-mm brown to blue-gray macules primarily affect the vermilion zone, the labial and buccal mucosa, and the tongue; they are seen in more than 90% of these patients (Fig. 16.28). The number of lesions and the extent of involvement can vary markedly from patient to patient. Some degree of fading of the pigmented lesions may be noted during adolescence.

Histopathologic Features

The gastrointestinal polyps of Peutz-Jeghers syndrome histopathologically represent benign overgrowths of intestinal glandular epithelium supported by a core of smooth muscle. Epithelial atypia is not usually a prominent feature, unlike the polyps of Gardner syndrome (see page 656).

Microscopic evaluation of the pigmented cutaneous lesions shows slight acanthosis of the epithelium with elongation of the rete ridges. No apparent increase in melanocyte number is detected by electron microscopy, but the dendritic processes of the melanocytes are elongated. Furthermore, the melanin pigment appears to be retained in the melanocytes rather than being transferred to adjacent keratinocytes.

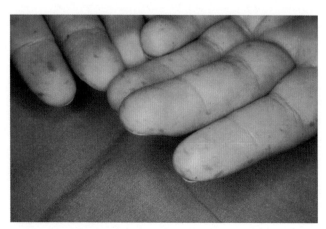

• **Fig. 16.27 Peutz-Jeghers Syndrome.** Cutaneous lesions appear as brown, macular, freckle-like areas, often concentrated around the mouth or on the hands. (Courtesy of Dr. Ahmed Uthman.)

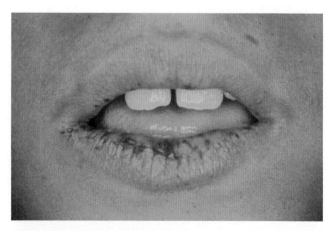

• **Fig. 16.28 Peutz-Jeghers Syndrome.** Oral manifestations include multiple, dark, freckle-like lesions of the lips. (Courtesy of Dr. Ahmed Uthman.)

Treatment and Prognosis

Patients with Peutz-Jeghers syndrome should be monitored for development of intussusception or tumor formation. Genetic counseling is also appropriate; moreover, prenatal or preimplantation genetic testing may now be available at some tertiary care centers.

◆ HEREDITARY HEMORRHAGIC TELANGIECTASIA (OSLER-WEBER-RENDU SYNDROME)

Hereditary hemorrhagic telangiectasia (HHT) is an uncommon mucocutaneous disorder that is inherited as an autosomal dominant trait, and epidemiologic studies suggest a prevalence that ranges from 1 in 5000 to 18,000 people, depending on the geographic region. Mutation of either one of two different genes at two separate loci is responsible for the condition. HHT1 is caused by a mutation of the *endoglin (ENG)* gene on chromosome 9, whereas mutation of *activin receptor-like kinase-1 (ALK1; ACVRL1)*, a gene located on chromosome 12, produces HHT2. The proteins produced by these genes may play a role in blood vessel wall integrity. With both types of HHT, numerous vascular hamartomas develop, affecting the skin and mucosa; however, other vascular problems, such as arteriovenous fistulas, may also be seen. Patients affected with HHT1 tend to have more pulmonary and cerebral involvement, whereas those with HHT2 generally have a later onset of their telangiectasias and a greater degree of hepatic involvement. A much less common mutation, involving the *MADH4* gene, has also been identified, and these patients exhibit an overlap syndrome characterized by HHT and juvenile polyposis. The polyps involve both the upper and lower gastrointestinal tract, and these patients have an increased risk for developing colorectal carcinoma at an early age. The clinician should be familiar with HHT because the oral lesions are often the most dramatic and most easily identified component of this syndrome.

Clinical Features

Patients with HHT are often diagnosed initially because of frequent episodes of epistaxis. On further examination, the nasal and oropharyngeal mucosae exhibit numerous scattered red papules, 1–2 mm in size, which blanch when diascopy is used. This blanching indicates that the red color is due to blood contained within blood vessels (in this case, small collections of dilated capillaries [**telangiectasias**] that are close to the surface of the mucosa). These telangiectatic vessels are most frequently found on the vermilion zone of the lips, tongue, and buccal mucosa, although any oral mucosal site may be affected (Figs. 16.29 and 16.30). With aging, the telangiectasias tend to become more numerous and slightly larger.

In many patients, telangiectasias are seen on the hands and feet. The lesions are often distributed throughout the

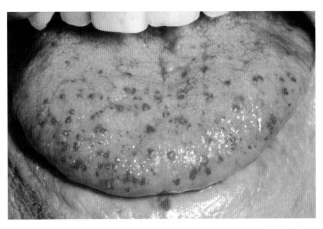

• **Fig. 16.29** Hereditary Hemorrhagic Telangiectasia (HHT). The tongue of this patient shows multiple red papules, which represent superficial collections of dilated capillary spaces.

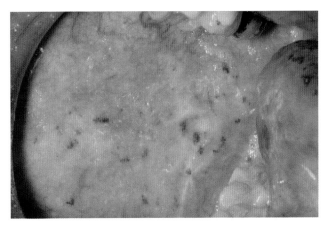

• **Fig. 16.30** Hereditary Hemorrhagic Telangiectasia (HHT). Red macules similar to the tongue lesions are observed on the buccal mucosa.

gastrointestinal mucosa, the genitourinary mucosa, and the conjunctival mucosa. The gastrointestinal telangiectasias have a tendency to rupture, which may cause significant blood loss. Chronic iron-deficiency anemia is often a problem for such individuals. Significantly, arteriovenous fistulas may develop in the lungs (15%–45% of HHT patients), liver (30%), or brain (10%–20%). The pulmonary arteriovenous malformations seem to predispose these patients to the development of brain abscesses due to right-to-left shunting of bacteria that might be introduced into the bloodstream. In at least one instance, periodontal vascular malformations were felt to be the cause of septic pulmonary emboli that resolved only after several teeth with periodontal abscesses were extracted.

A diagnosis of HHT can be made if a patient has three of the following four criteria:
1. Recurrent spontaneous epistaxis
2. Telangiectasias of the mucosa and skin
3. Arteriovenous malformation involving the lungs, liver, or CNS
4. Family history of HHT

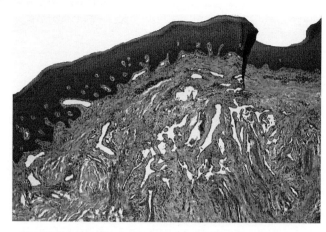

• **Fig. 16.31** **Hereditary Hemorrhagic Telangiectasia (HHT).** This low-power photomicrograph shows multiple dilated vascular spaces located immediately subjacent to the epithelium.

In some instances, CREST syndrome (**C**alcinosis cutis, **R**aynaud phenomenon, **E**sophageal dysfunction, **S**clerodactyly, and **T**elangiectasia) (see page 805) must be considered in the differential diagnosis. In these cases, serologic studies for anticentromere autoantibodies often help to distinguish between the two conditions because these antibodies typically would be present only in CREST syndrome.

Histopathologic Features

If one of the telangiectasias is submitted for biopsy, the microscopic features essentially show a superficially located collection of thin-walled vascular spaces that contain erythrocytes (Fig. 16.31).

Treatment and Prognosis

For mild cases of HHT, no treatment may be required. Moderate cases may be managed by selective cryosurgery or electrocautery of the most bothersome of the telangiectatic vessels. Laser ablation of the telangiectatic lesions has also been used, although this approach appears to be most successful for patients with mild to moderate disease. More severely affected patients, particularly those troubled by repeated episodes of epistaxis, may require a surgical procedure of the nasal septum (septal dermoplasty). The involved nasal mucosa is removed and replaced by a skin graft; however, some long-term follow-up studies suggest that the grafts eventually become revascularized, resulting in recurrence of the problem. Nasal closure is another surgical technique that has been performed for patients with severe epistaxis in whom other methods have failed.

Combined progesterone and estrogen therapy may benefit some patients, but because of the potentially serious side effects, this should be limited to the most severely affected individuals. Bevacizumab, an antibody directed against vascular endothelial growth factor, has shown some promise in controlling epistaxis, but this is a costly medication. Iron replacement therapy is indicated for the iron-deficient

patient, and occasionally blood transfusions may be necessary to compensate for blood loss.

From a dental standpoint, the use of prophylactic antibiotics is indicated before dental procedures that might cause bacteremia in patients with HHT and a history of either a treated or untreated pulmonary arteriovenous malformation. For patients with a history of HHT, such antibiotics are advocated until a pulmonary arteriovenous malformation is ruled out because of the 1% prevalence of brain abscesses in affected individuals. Researchers believe that antibiotic coverage, similar to that for endocarditis prophylaxis, may prevent this serious complication. Patients with a history of HHT should be screened for arteriovenous malformations, which can be eliminated by embolization or other vasodestructive techniques using interventional radiologic methods. The decision to treat such a lesion often depends on the anatomic site and the severity of the malformation. For patients who have been treated for a pulmonary arteriovenous malformation, monitoring for recurrence of the condition and for development of additional arteriovenous malformations in other pulmonary sites is recommended.

The prognosis is generally good, although studies indicate a reduced lifespan, which can range from 7 to 14 years shorter than average. Patients with milder disease expression may have a more modest decrease in longevity. A 1%–2% mortality rate is reported from complications related to blood loss. For patients with brain abscesses, the mortality rate can range up to 40%, even with early diagnosis and appropriate therapy.

◆ EHLERS-DANLOS SYNDROMES

The **Ehlers-Danlos syndromes,** a group of inherited connective tissue disorders, are relatively heterogeneous. At least thirteen types have been described over the years, and these are typically distinguished based on clinical and molecular features. The affected patient exhibits problems that are usually attributed to the production of abnormal collagen, the protein that is the main structural component of the connective tissue. Because the production of collagen necessitates many biochemical steps that are controlled by several genes, the potential exists for any one of these genes to mutate, producing selective defects in collagen synthesis. The various forms of abnormal collagen result in many overlapping clinical features for each of the types of the Ehlers-Danlos syndrome (Table 16.1). This discussion concentrates on the three most common and significant forms of this group of conditions.

Typical clinical findings include hypermobility of the joints, easy bruisability, and marked elasticity of the skin. In the past, some affected individuals worked in circus sideshows as the "rubber" man and the "contortionist" as a result of their pronounced joint mobility and ability to stretch the skin.

Clinical Features

The pattern of inheritance and the clinical manifestations vary with the type of Ehlers-Danlos syndrome being examined. About 80% of patients have the **classical type** in either

TABLE 16.1 Ehlers-Danlos Syndromes

Common Types	Clinical Features	Inheritance	Defect
Classical (severe)	Hyperextensible skin, easy bruising, hypermobile joints, papyraceous scarring of skin	AD	Collagen type V mutations
Classical (mild)	Less severe classical manifestations	AD	Collagen type V mutations
Hypermobility	Soft skin, no scarring, marked joint hyperextensibility	AD	Not known
Vascular	Severe bruising; risk for arterial, bowel, and uterine rupture	AD	Collagen type III mutations

Rare Types	Clinical Features	Inheritance	Defect
Kyphoscoliotic EDS	Ocular globe fragility, hyperextensible skin, hypermobile joints, scoliosis	AR	Lysyl hydroxylase point mutations
Arthrochalasia EDS	Congenital hip dislocation, joint hypermobility, normal scarring, mandibular hypoplasia	AD	Collagen type I mutations
Dermatosparaxis EDS	Severe skin fragility, sagging skin	AR	Procollagen peptidase deficiency
Classical-like	Hyperextensible skin, easy and severe bruising, hypermobile joints, no abnormal scarring of skin	AR	Tenascin X glycoprotein deficiency
Periodontal EDS	Considerable range of features related to skin and joints; early onset of periodontitis	AR	Mutations in C1R and C1S
Brittle cornea syndrome	Thin cornea (microcornea); predisposition to corneal rupture; early onset keratoconus and keratoglobus; joint hypermobility	AR	Mutations of ZNF469 and PRDM5
Musculo-contractural EDS	Kyphoscoliosis; adducted thumbs, congenital talipes, arachnodactyly; joint hypermobility, hyperextensible, fragile skin; poor wound healing	AR	Mutations of CHST14 and DSE genes, with CHST14 more severe
Myopathic	Muscle hypotonia; proximal joint contractures; hypermobile distal joints	AD or AR	Mutation of COL12A1 causing Type XII collagen abnormalities
Spondylo-dysplastic	Short stature; muscle hypotonia; bowing of limbs; skin hyperextensibility	AR	Mutation of B4GALT7, B3GALT6, and SLC39A13

AD, Autosomal dominant; *AR,* autosomal recessive; *XLR,* X-linked recessive.

the **mild** or **severe** form. Classical Ehlers-Danlos syndrome is inherited as an autosomal dominant trait, and mutations of genes responsible for type V collagen (*COL5A1* or *COL5A2*) have been identified in these patients. Hyperelasticity of the skin (Fig. 16.32) and cutaneous fragility can be observed as a result. An unusual healing response that often occurs with relatively minor injury to the skin is termed **papyraceous scarring** because it resembles crumpled cigarette paper (Fig. 16.33).

Patients with the **hypermobility type** of Ehlers-Danlos syndrome exhibit remarkable joint hypermobility but no evidence of unusual scarring. Chronic musculo-skeletal pain is often present to a greater degree than is seen with other types of Ehlers-Danlos syndrome.

The **vascular type** of Ehlers-Danlos used to be known as the **ecchymotic** type because of the extensive bruising that occurs with everyday trauma. Defects in type III collagen have been identified in this disorder. This form is inherited

in an autosomal dominant pattern, and a young patient may be mistaken for a victim of child abuse. The life expectancy of these patients is often greatly reduced because of the tendency for aortic aneurysm formation and rupture.

Periodontal Ehlers-Danlos syndrome is a rare variant that has dental manifestations as a hallmark feature, with patients showing marked periodontal disease activity at a relatively early age, as well as reduced or no attached gingiva. Although these patients may have overlapping features with either the classical or vascular forms of the disease, genetic analysis of this form of Ehlers-Danlos syndrome has found specific mutations of two genes, *C1R* and *C1S.*

The oral manifestations of Ehlers-Danlos syndrome include the ability of 50% of these patients to touch the tip of their nose with their tongue **(Gorlin sign)** (Fig. 16.34), a feat that can be achieved by less than 10% of the general population. Some authors have noted easy bruising and bleeding during minor manipulations of the

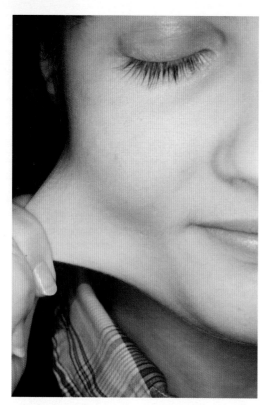

• **Fig. 16.32 Ehlers-Danlos Syndrome.** The hyperelasticity of the skin is evident in this patient affected by the mild form of classical Ehlers-Danlos syndrome.

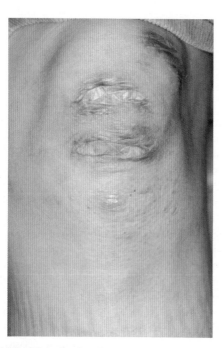

• **Fig. 16.33 Ehlers-Danlos Syndrome.** Scarring that resembles crumpled cigarette paper (papyraceous scarring) is associated with minimal trauma in patients with Ehlers-Danlos syndromes. These lesions involve the skin of the knee.

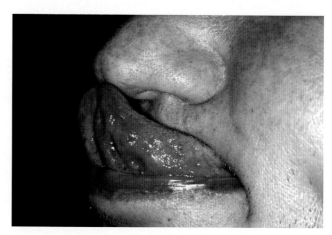

• **Fig. 16.34 Ehlers-Danlos Syndrome.** Patient demonstrating the Gorlin sign by touching the tip of the nose with their tongue.

oral mucosa; others state that oral mucosal friability is present. A tendency for recurrent subluxation of the temporomandibular joint (TMJ) and the development of other TMJ disorders has also been reported.

Most patients with Ehlers-Danlos syndrome have relatively normal teeth, although high cusps and deep developmental fissures in the posterior teeth have been described. A variety of dental abnormalities have been described, however, including malformed, stunted tooth roots, large pulp stones, and hypoplastic enamel. Although most of these findings have not been consistently correlated with any particular type of the syndrome, pulp stones seem to occur more commonly in patients affected by classical Ehlers-Danlos syndrome.

Treatment and Prognosis

The prognosis for the patient with Ehlers-Danlos syndrome depends on the type. Some forms, such as the vascular type, can be very serious, with sudden death occurring from rupture of the aorta secondary to the weakened, abnormal collagen that constitutes the vessel wall. The mild classical type is generally compatible with a normal life span, although affected women may have problems with placental tearing and hemorrhage during gestation. Pain management for patients with Ehlers-Danlos syndrome often requires physical therapy and pharmacologic treatment.

Accurate diagnosis is important because it affects the prognosis heavily. Similarly, because the various types of this syndrome show a variety of inheritance patterns, an accurate diagnosis is required so that appropriate genetic counseling can be provided.

◆ TUBEROUS SCLEROSIS (EPILOIA; BOURNEVILLE-PRINGLE SYNDROME)

Tuberous sclerosis is an uncommon syndrome that is classically characterized by intellectual disability, seizure disorders, and angiofibromas of the skin. The condition is often inherited as an autosomal dominant trait, but two-thirds of the cases are sporadic and appear to represent new mutations. These mutations involve either one of two tumor suppressor genes: *TSC1* (found on chromosome 9) or, more commonly, *TSC2* (found on chromosome 16). Both of these gene products are components of the same intracellular biochemical pathway known as mechanistic (formerly "mammalian") Target of Rapamycin (mTOR) that is one of the regulators of cell growth. The multiple hamartomatous growths that are seen in this disorder are thought to arise from disruption of the normal regulatory function of these genes. Tuberous sclerosis has a wide range of clinical severity, although two-thirds of these patients have the *TSC2* mutation, and these patients have a more severe expression of the disease than those who have the *TSC1* mutation. Milder forms of tuberous sclerosis may be difficult to diagnose.

The prevalence is approximately 1 in 10,000 in the general population, although in some long-term care facilities tuberous sclerosis accounts for as high as 1% of the intellectually disabled patients. Nevertheless, average intelligence is present in over half of tuberous sclerosis patients.

Clinical Features

Several clinical features characterize tuberous sclerosis. The first of these, **facial angiofibromas,** used to be called *adenoma sebaceum.* Because these lesions are neither adenomas nor sebaceous, the use of that term should be discontinued. Facial angiofibromas appear as multiple, smooth-surfaced papules and occur primarily in the nasolabial fold area (Fig. 16.35). Similar lesions, called *ungual* or *periungual fibromas,* are seen around or under the margins of the nails (Fig. 16.36).

Two other characteristic skin lesions are connective tissue hamartomas called **shagreen patches** and ovoid areas of hypopigmentation called **ash-leaf spots.** Even though approximately 5% of the general population may have an ash-leaf spot, studies have reported that 90%–98% of children with tuberous sclerosis display these lesions. The shagreen patches, so named because of their resemblance to sharkskin-derived shagreen cloth, affect the skin of the trunk. The ash-leaf spots may appear on any cutaneous surface and

may be best visualized using UV (Wood's lamp) illumination. "Confetti" spots also may be seen in tuberous sclerosis patients, appearing as 1–3 mm, pale macules that are symmetrically distributed on the trunk or extremities, somewhat resembling confetti that was tossed onto the skin.

CNS manifestations include seizure disorders in 80%–85% of affected patients and intellectual disability in approximately 30%. In addition, hamartomatous proliferations in the CNS develop into the potato-like growths ("tubers") seen at autopsy, from which the term *tuberous sclerosis* is derived (Fig. 16.37). The tuberous hamartomas can best be visualized using T2-weighted magnetic resonance imaging (MRI) and are present in 80%–95% of these patients. Also, approximately 10% of tuberous sclerosis patients will develop a type of benign brain tumor known as *subependymal giant cell astrocytoma.*

A relatively rare tumor of the heart muscle, called **cardiac rhabdomyoma,** is also typically associated with this syndrome. This lesion, which probably represents a hamartoma rather than a true neoplasm, occurs in approximately 30% to 50% of affected patients and is typically identified in early

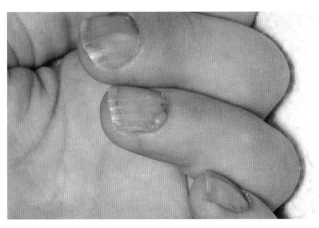

• **Fig. 16.36 Tuberous Sclerosis.** Examination of the fingers often shows periungual fibromas.

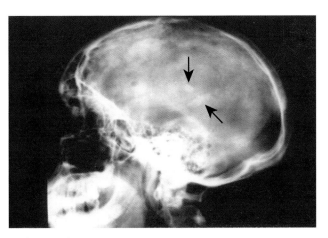

• **Fig. 16.37 Tuberous Sclerosis.** Patchy calcifications *(arrows)* associated with intracranial hamartoma formation are seen on this lateral skull radiograph. (Courtesy of Dr. Reg Munden.)

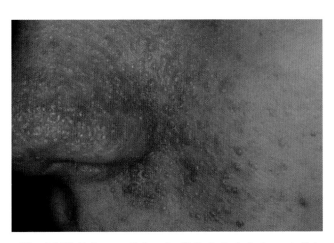

• **Fig. 16.35 Tuberous Sclerosis.** Patients typically have multiple papular facial lesions that microscopically are angiofibromas.

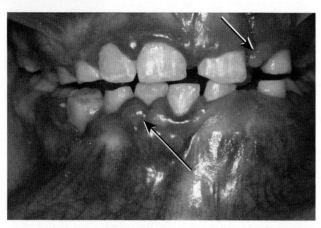

• **Fig. 16.38 Tuberous Sclerosis.** Patients often exhibit gingival hyperplasia, which may be secondary to phenytoin medications used to control seizures in some cases. Fibrous papules of the gingiva *(arrows)* may also be present.

childhood. Problems with myocardial function may develop as a result of this process, but many of these tumors undergo spontaneous regression.

Another hamartomatous type of growth related to this disorder is the **angiomyolipoma.** This is a benign neoplasm composed of vascular smooth muscle and adipose tissue and occurs primarily in the kidney, typically bilaterally. Even though the angiomyolipoma is benign, the tumors are often associated with large dilated blood vessels, and significant clinical problems can arise if these vessels rupture spontaneously.

Oral manifestations of tuberous sclerosis include developmental enamel pitting on the facial aspect of the anterior permanent dentition in 50% to 100% of patients. These pits are more readily appreciated after applying a dental plaque–disclosing solution to the teeth. Multiple fibrous papules affect 11% to 56% of patients. The fibrous papules are seen predominantly on the anterior gingival mucosa (Fig. 16.38), although the lips, buccal mucosa, palate, and tongue may be involved. Diffuse fibrous gingival enlargement is reported in affected patients—even those who are not taking phenytoin; however, most cases of gingival hyperplasia in these individuals are probably related to medication taken to control seizures. Some patients with tuberous sclerosis may also exhibit radiolucencies of the jaws that represent dense fibrous connective tissue proliferations (Fig. 16.39).

The diagnosis of tuberous sclerosis can be based on finding at least two of the following major features:
• Facial angiofibromas
• Ungual or periungual fibromas
• Hypomelanotic macules (three or more)
• Shagreen patch
• CNS hamartomas
• Subependymal nodules
• Subependymal giant cell astrocytoma
• Cardiac rhabdomyoma
• Renal angiomyolipoma
• Multiple retinal nodular hamartomas
• Lymphangioleiomyomatosis of the lung

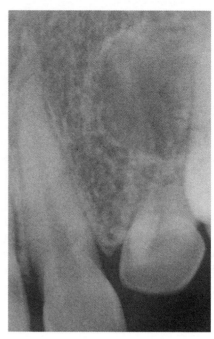

• **Fig. 16.39 Tuberous Sclerosis.** Periapical radiograph exhibiting a well-defined radiolucency apical to the maxillary left lateral incisor. Biopsy revealed an intraosseous fibrous proliferation.

The presence of one major and two minor features may also confirm the diagnosis. The minor features include the following:
• Multiple, randomly distributed enamel pits
• Gingival fibromas
• Bone "cysts" (actually fibrous proliferations)
• "Confetti" skin lesions
• Multiple renal cysts
• Non-renal hamartomas

Histopathologic Features

Microscopic examination of the fibrous papules of the oral mucosa or the enlarged gingivae shows a nonspecific fibrous hyperplasia. Similarly, the radiolucent jaw lesions consist of dense fibrous connective tissue that resembles desmoplastic fibroma or the simple type of central odontogenic fibroma. The angiofibroma of the skin is a benign aggregation of delicate fibrous connective tissue characterized by plump, uniformly spaced fibroblasts with numerous interspersed thin-walled vascular channels.

Treatment and Prognosis

For patients with tuberous sclerosis, most of the treatment is directed toward the management of the seizure disorder with anticonvulsant agents. Periodic MRI of the head may be done to screen for intracranial lesions, whereas ultrasound evaluation is performed for evaluation of kidney involvement. Intellectually disabled patients may have problems with oral hygiene procedures, and poor oral hygiene contributes to phenytoin-induced gingival hyperplasia. Studies examining medications (such as, sirolimus and everolimus) that block the mTOR pathway that causes tuberous sclerosis have shown significant shrinkage of several tumor types associated with this disorder, including renal angiomyolipoma, facial angiofibroma, and subependymal giant cell astrocytoma. A decrease in tuberous sclerosis-related seizures has also been noted with this treatment. Patients affected by tuberous sclerosis have a slightly reduced life span compared with the general population, with death usually related to CNS or kidney disease.

Genetic counseling is also appropriate for affected patients, and careful clinical evaluation of the patient's parents is recommended in order to rule out overlooked mild expression of tuberous sclerosis affecting one of them. Genetic testing is available for both *TSC1* and *TSC2* mutations if prenatal or preimplantation family planning is desired.

♦ MULTIPLE HAMARTOMA SYNDROME (COWDEN SYNDROME; *PTEN* HAMARTOMA-TUMOR SYNDROME)

Multiple hamartoma syndrome is a rare condition that has important implications for the affected patient, because malignancies, in addition to the benign hamartomatous growths, develop in a high percentage of these individuals. Usually, the syndrome is inherited as an autosomal dominant trait showing a high degree of penetrance and a range of expressivity, although new mutations may account for as many as 45% of cases. The gene responsible for this disorder has been mapped to chromosome 10, and a mutation of the *phosphatase and tensin homolog deleted on chromosome 10 (PTEN)* gene has been implicated in its pathogenesis. The estimated prevalence of this condition is approximately 1 in 200,000, and more than 300 affected patients have been described in the literature. In recent years, overlapping clinical features of multiple hamartoma syndrome with **Lhermitte-Duclos disease, Bannayan-Riley-Ruvalcaba syndrome,** and **Proteus-like syndrome** have been noted, and all of these disorders have demonstrated mutations of the *PTEN* gene.

Clinical Features

Cutaneous manifestations are present in almost all patients with multiple hamartoma syndrome, usually developing during the second decade of life. The majority of the skin lesions appear as multiple, small (less than 1 mm) papules, primarily on the facial skin, especially around the mouth, nose, and ears (Fig. 16.40). Microscopically, most of these papules represent hair follicle hamartomas called **trichilemmomas.** Other commonly noted skin lesions are **acral keratosis,** a warty-appearing growth that develops on the dorsal surface of the hand, and **palmoplantar keratosis,** a prominent callus-like lesion on the palms or soles. Cutaneous **hemangiomas, sclerotic fibromas, neuromas, xanthomas,** and **lipomas** have also been described.

Other problems can appear in these patients as well. Thyroid disease usually presents as either a goiter or a thyroid adenoma, but papillary or follicular adenocarcinoma may develop. In one large series, thyroid malignancy was identified in 14% of patients with this condition. In women, fibrocystic disease of the breast is frequently observed. Unfortunately, breast cancer occurs with a relatively high frequency (25%–50%) in these patients. The mean age at diagnosis of breast malignancy is 40 years, which is much younger than usual. In the gastrointestinal tract, multiple benign hamartomatous polyps may be present. In addition, several types of benign and malignant tumors of the female genitourinary tract occur more often than in the normal population.

The oral lesions vary in severity from patient to patient and usually consist of multiple papules affecting the gingivae, dorsal tongue, and buccal mucosa (Figs. 16.41 and 16.42). These lesions have been reported in more than 80% of affected patients and generally produce no symptoms. Other possible oral findings include a high-arched palate, periodontitis, and extensive dental caries, although it is unclear whether the latter two conditions are significantly related to the syndrome.

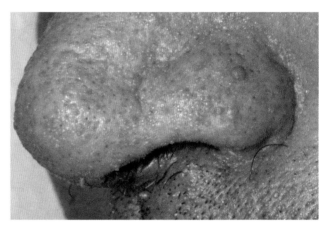

• **Fig. 16.40 Multiple Hamartoma Syndrome.** These tiny cutaneous facial papules represent hair follicle hamartomas (trichilemmomas).

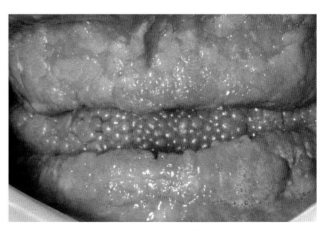

• **Fig. 16.41 Multiple Hamartoma Syndrome.** Multiple, irregular fibroepithelial papules involve the tongue *(center)* and alveolar ridge mucosa.

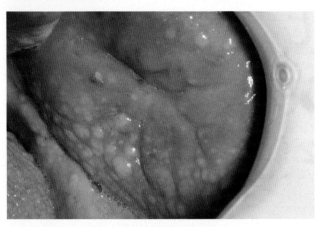

• **Fig. 16.42 Multiple Hamartoma Syndrome.** Multiple papules on the left buccal mucosa.

Histopathologic Features

The histopathologic features of the oral lesions are rather nonspecific, essentially representing fibroepithelial hyperplasia. Other lesions associated with this syndrome have their own characteristic histopathologic findings, depending on the hamartomatous or neoplastic tissue origin.

Diagnosis

The diagnosis can be based on the finding of two of the following three pathognomonic signs:
1. Multiple facial trichilemmomas
2. Multiple oral papules
3. Acral keratoses

A variety of other major and minor diagnostic criteria, as well as a positive family history, are also helpful in confirming the diagnosis. Genetic testing for mutations of the *PTEN* gene are clinically available, but 20% of patients who otherwise have characteristic multiple hamartoma syndrome will not demonstrate a genetic abnormality; therefore, a negative test does not necessarily preclude the diagnosis of multiple hamartoma syndrome.

Treatment and Prognosis

Treatment of multiple hamartoma syndrome is controversial. Although most of the tumors that develop are benign, the prevalence of malignancy is higher than in the general population; therefore, annual physical examinations should be performed that focus specifically on anatomic sites of increased tumor prevalence, particularly breast, uterus, and thyroid. Because longitudinal studies have found that 85% of women with multiple hamartoma syndrome will develop breast cancer, some investigators have recommended bilateral prophylactic mastectomies as early as the third decade of life for female patients.

◆ EPIDERMOLYSIS BULLOSA

The term **epidermolysis bullosa** describes a heterogeneous group of inherited blistering mucocutaneous disorders. Each has a specific defect in the attachment mechanisms of the epithelial cells, either to each other or to the underlying connective tissue. Recent advances in the understanding of the clinical features, epidemiology, immunofluorescence mapping, and molecular genetic abnormalities of these conditions have led to the identification of more than 30 different forms. Depending on the defective mechanism of cellular cohesion, there are four broad categories:
1. Simplex
2. Junctional
3. Dystrophic
4. Kindler syndrome

Each category consists of several forms of the disorder. A variety of inheritance patterns may be seen, depending on the particular form. The degree of severity can range from relatively mild, annoying forms, such as the **simplex** types, through a spectrum that includes severe, fatal disease. For example, many cases of **junctional** epidermolysis bullosa result in death at birth because of the significant sloughing of the skin during passage through the birth canal. Specific mutations in the genes encoding keratin 5 and keratin 14 have been identified as being responsible for most of the **simplex** types, whereas mutations in the genetic codes of laminin-332, type XVII collagen, or α6β4 integrin have been documented for the **junctional** types. Most of the **dystrophic** types are caused by mutations in the genes responsible for type VII collagen production, with over 300 distinctly different mutations identified to date. **Kindler syndrome** is the most recently characterized pattern of this group of disorders, and mutations of the gene that encodes for a hemidesmosomal attachment protein, kindlin-1, are responsible for this rare condition.

A few representative examples of the types of epidermolysis bullosa are summarized in Table 16.2. Because oral lesions are most commonly observed in the dystrophic forms, this discussion centers on these forms. Dental abnormalities, such as anodontia, enamel hypoplasia, pitting of the enamel, neonatal teeth, severe periodontitis, and severe dental caries, have been variably associated with several of the different types of epidermolysis bullosa, although studies have suggested that the prevalence of dental abnormalities is significantly increased only with the **junctional** type. A disorder termed **epidermolysis bullosa acquisita** is mentioned because of the similarity of its name; however, this is an unrelated condition, having an autoimmune (rather than a genetic) origin (see page 778).

Clinical Features
Dominant Dystrophic Types

The **dystrophic** forms of epidermolysis bullosa that are inherited in an autosomal dominant fashion are not usually life threatening, although they may certainly be disfiguring and pose many problems. The initial lesions are vesicles or bullae, which are seen early in life and develop on areas exposed to low-grade, chronic trauma, such as the knuckles or knees (Fig. 16.43). The bullae rupture, resulting in erosions or ulcerations that ultimately heal with scarring. In the process, appendages such as fingernails may be lost.

The oral manifestations are typically mild, with some gingival erythema and tenderness. Gingival recession and

TABLE 16.2	**Examples of Epidermolysis Bullosa**			

Form	Inheritance	Clinical Features	Defect
EB simplex	AD	Blistering of the hands and feet; mucosal involvement uncommon; blisters heal without scarring; prognosis usually good	Keratin gene defects
Junctional EB, generalized gravis variant	AR	Severe blistering at birth; granulation tissue around the mouth; oral erosions common; pitted enamel hypoplasia; often fatal (previously called *EB letalis*)	Defects of hemidesmosomes
Dominant, dystrophic EB, Pasini type	AD	Generalized blistering, white papules	Defect in type VII collagen
Dominant, dystrophic EB, Cockayne-Touraine type	AD	Extremities primarily affected	Defect in type VII collagen
Recessive, dystrophic EB, generalized gravis type	AR	Severe mucosal involvement; mittenlike scarring; deformities of hands and feet; patients usually do not survive past early adulthood	Defect in type VII collagen
Recessive, dystrophic EB, inverse type	AR	Involvement of groin and axilla; severe oral and esophageal lesions	Defect in type VII collagen

EB, Epidermolysis bullosa; *AD*, autosomal dominant; *AR*, autosomal recessive.

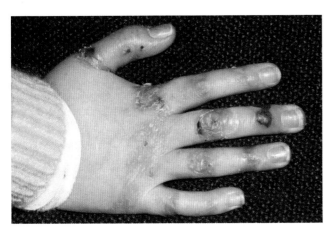

• **Fig. 16.43 Epidermolysis Bullosa.** A young girl, affected by the dominant dystrophic form of epidermolysis bullosa, shows the characteristic hemorrhagic bullae, scarring, and erosion associated with minimal trauma to the hands.

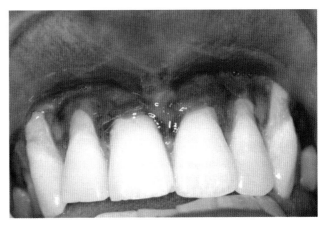

• **Fig. 16.44 Epidermolysis Bullosa.** A teenaged boy, affected by dominant dystrophic epidermolysis bullosa, shows a reduced depth of the labial vestibule caused by repeated mucosal tearing and healing with scarring.

reduction in the depth of the buccal vestibule may be observed (Fig. 16.44).

Recessive Dystrophic Types

Generalized recessive dystrophic epidermolysis bullosa represents one of the more debilitating forms of the disease. Vesicles and bullae form with even minor trauma. Secondary infections are often a problem because of the large surface areas that may be involved. If the patient manages to survive into the second decade, then hand function is often greatly diminished because of the repeated episodes of cutaneous breakdown and healing with scarring, resulting in fusion of the fingers into a mittenlike deformity (Fig. 16.45).

The oral problems are no less severe. Bulla and vesicle formation is induced by virtually any food having some degree of texture. Even with a soft diet, the repeated cycles of scarring often result in microstomia (Fig. 16.46) and

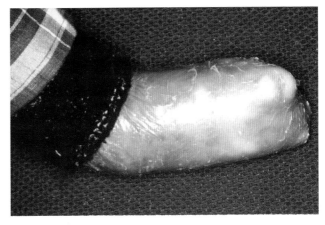

• **Fig. 16.45 Epidermolysis Bullosa.** A 19-year-old man, affected by recessive dystrophic epidermolysis bullosa, shows the typical mitten-like deformity of the hand caused by scarring of the tissue after damage associated with normal activity.

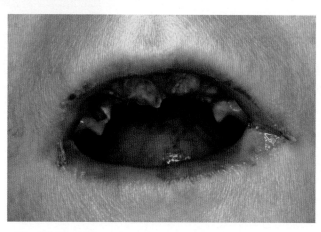

• **Fig. 16.46 Epidermolysis Bullosa.** Same patient as depicted in Fig. 16.45. Microstomia has been caused by repeated trauma and healing with scarring. Note the severe dental caries activity associated with a soft cariogenic diet.

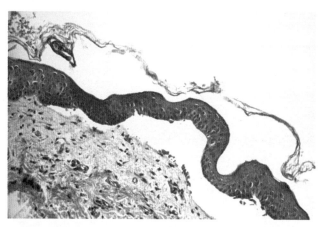

• **Fig. 16.47 Epidermolysis Bullosa.** Complete separation of the epithelium from the connective tissue is seen in this photomicrograph of a tissue section obtained from a patient affected by a junctional form of epidermolysis bullosa.

ankyloglossia. Similar mucosal injury and scarring may cause severe stricture of the esophagus. Because a soft diet is usually highly cariogenic, carious destruction of the dentition at an early age is common.

Histopathologic Features

The histopathologic features of epidermolysis bullosa vary with the type being examined. The **simplex** form shows intraepithelial clefting by light microscopy. **Junctional, dystrophic,** and **Kindler** forms show subepithelial clefting (Fig. 16.47). Electron microscopic examination reveals clefting at the level of the lamina lucida of the basement membrane in the **junctional** forms and below the lamina densa of the basement membrane in the **dystrophic** forms. In contrast, the **Kindler** form shows clefting just below the basal cell layer, at its interface with the lamina lucida. Immunohistochemical evaluation of perilesional tissue is now typically used to identify specific defects to classify and subtype the condition further. Molecular genetic analysis may also be helpful for confirming the diagnosis in some instances.

Treatment and Prognosis

Treatment of epidermolysis bullosa varies with the type. For milder cases, no treatment other than local wound care may be needed. Sterile drainage of larger blisters and the use of topical antibiotics are often indicated in these situations. For the more severe cases, intensive management with oral antibiotics may be necessary if cellulitis develops; despite intensive medical care, some patients die as a result of infectious complications.

The "mitten" deformity of the hands, seen in recessive dystrophic epidermolysis bullosa, can be corrected with plastic surgery, but the problem usually recurs after a period of time, and surgical intervention is required every 2 years on average. With esophageal involvement, dysphagia may be a significant problem, resulting in malnutrition and weight loss. Placement of a gastrostomy tube may be necessary at times. Patients with the recessive dystrophic forms are also predisposed to development of **cutaneous squamous cell carcinoma.** This malignancy often develops in areas of chronic ulceration during the second through third decades of life and represents a significant cause of death for these patients. Infrequently, the lingual mucosa of affected patients has been reported to undergo malignant transformation as well.

Management of the oral manifestations also depends on the type of the disease. For patients who are susceptible to mucosal bulla formation, dental manipulation should be kept to a minimum. To achieve this, topical 1% neutral sodium fluoride solution should be administered daily to prevent dental caries. Occlusal sealants are also recommended. A soft diet that is as noncariogenic as possible, as well as atraumatic oral hygiene procedures, should be encouraged. Maintaining adequate nutrition for affected patients is critical to ensure optimal wound healing. Endosseous dental implants, followed by fixed dental prostheses, have been successfully placed in some patients with recessive dystrophic epidermolysis bullosa.

If dental restorative care is required, the lips should be lubricated to minimize trauma. Injections for local anesthesia can usually be accomplished by depositing the anesthetic slowly and deeply within the tissues. For extensive dental care, including extractions, endotracheal anesthesia may be performed without significant problems in most cases.

Unfortunately, because of the genetic nature of these diseases, no cure exists. Genetic counseling of affected families is indicated. Both prenatal diagnosis and preimplantation diagnosis are available as adjuncts to family planning.

IMMUNE-MEDIATED DISEASES AND THEIR EVALUATION

Several conditions discussed in this chapter are the result of inappropriate production of antibodies by the patient (autoantibodies). These autoantibodies are directed against various constituents of the molecular apparatus that hold epithelial cells together or that bind the surface epithelium to the underlying connective tissue. The ensuing damage

Direct immunofluorescence

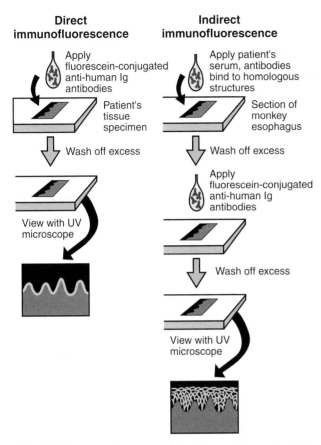

Apply fluorescein-conjugated anti-human Ig antibodies

Patient's tissue specimen

Wash off excess

View with UV microscope

Indirect immunofluorescence

Apply patient's serum, antibodies bind to homologous structures

Section of monkey esophagus

Wash off excess

Apply fluorescein-conjugated anti-human Ig antibodies

Wash off excess

View with UV microscope

• **Fig. 16.48 Immunofluorescence Techniques.** Comparison of the techniques for direct and indirect immunofluorescence. The left side depicts the direct immunofluorescent findings in mucous membrane pemphigoid, a disease that has autoantibodies directed toward the basement zone. The right side shows the indirect immunofluorescent findings for pemphigus vulgaris, a disease that has autoantibodies directed toward the intercellular areas between the spinous cells of the epithelium. *Ig,* Immunoglobulin; *UV,* ultraviolet.

produced by the interaction of these autoantibodies with the host tissue is seen clinically as a disease process, often termed an **immunobullous** disease. Because each disease is characterized by production of specific types of autoantibodies, identification of the antibodies and the tissues against which they are targeted is important diagnostically. The two techniques that are widely used to investigate the immunobullous diseases are (1) direct immunofluorescence and (2) indirect immunofluorescence studies. Following is a brief overview of how they work.

Direct immunofluorescence is used to detect autoantibodies that are bound to the patient's tissue. Before testing can take place, several procedures must occur. Inoculating human immunoglobulins into a goat creates antibodies directed against these human immunoglobulins. The antibodies raised in response to the human immunoglobulins are harvested from the animal and tagged with fluorescein, a dye that glows when viewed with UV light. As illustrated on the left side of Fig. 16.48, a frozen section of the patient's tissue is placed on a slide, and this is incubated with fluorescein-conjugated goat antihuman antibodies. These

antibodies bind to the tissue at any site where human immunoglobulin is present. The excess antibody suspension is washed off, and the section is then viewed with a microscope having a UV light source.

With indirect immunofluorescence studies, the patient is being evaluated for presence of antibodies that are circulating in the blood. As shown on the right side of Fig. 16.48, a frozen section of tissue that is similar to human oral mucosa (e.g., Old World monkey esophagus) is placed on a slide and incubated with the patient's serum. If there are autoantibodies directed against epithelial attachment structures in the patient's serum, then they will attach to the homologous structures on the monkey esophagus. The excess serum is washed off, and fluorescein-conjugated goat antihuman antibody is incubated with the section. The excess is washed off, and the section is examined with UV light to detect the presence of autoantibodies that might have been in the serum.

Examples of the molecular sites of attack of the autoantibodies are seen diagrammatically in Fig. 16.49. Each site is distinctive for a particular disease; however, the complexities of the epithelial attachment mechanisms are still being elucidated, and more precise mapping may be possible in the future. A summary of the clinical, microscopic, and immunopathologic features of the more important immunemediated mucocutaneous diseases is found in Table 16.3.

◆ PEMPHIGUS

The condition known as **pemphigus** represents four related diseases of an autoimmune origin:
1. Pemphigus vulgaris
2. Pemphigus vegetans
3. Pemphigus erythematosus
4. Pemphigus foliaceus

Only the first two of these affect the oral mucosa, and the discussion is limited to **pemphigus vulgaris. Pemphigus vegetans** is rare; most authorities now feel it represents simply a variant of pemphigus vulgaris.

Pemphigus vulgaris is the most common of these disorders (*vulgaris* is Latin for *common*). Even so, it is not seen very often. The estimated incidence is one to five cases per million people diagnosed each year in the general population. Nevertheless, pemphigus vulgaris is an important condition because, if untreated, it often results in the patient's death. Furthermore, the oral lesions are often the first sign of the disease, and they are the most difficult to resolve with therapy. This has prompted the description of the oral lesions as "the first to show, and the last to go."

The blistering that typifies this disease is due to an abnormal production, for unknown reasons, of autoantibodies that are directed against the epidermal cell surface glycoproteins, desmoglein 3 and desmoglein 1. These desmogleins are components of **desmosomes** (structures that bond epithelial cells to each other), and the autoantibodies attach to these desmosomal components, effectively inhibiting the molecular interaction that is responsible for adherence. As a result of this immunologic attack on the desmosomes, a split develops

Normal structures

Targeted structures for immune-mediated diseases

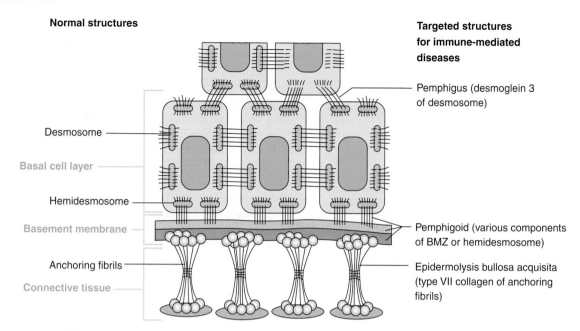

Desmosome

Basal cell layer

Hemidesmosome

Basement membrane

Anchoring fibrils

Connective tissue

Pemphigus (desmoglein 3 of desmosome)

Pemphigoid (various components of BMZ or hemidesmosome)

Epidermolysis bullosa acquisita (type VII collagen of anchoring fibrils)

• **Fig. 16.49 Epithelial Attachment Apparatus.** Schematic diagram demonstrating targeted structures in several immune-mediated diseases. *BMZ,* Basement membrane zone.

within the epithelium, causing a blister to form. Desmoglein 3 is preferentially expressed in the parabasal region of the epidermis and oral epithelium, whereas desmoglein 1 is found primarily in the superficial portion of the epidermis, with minimal expression in oral epithelium. Patients who have developed autoantibodies directed against desmoglein 3, with or without desmoglein 1, will histopathologically show intraepithelial clefting just above the basal layer, and clinically oral mucosal blisters of pemphigus vulgaris will form. Patients who develop autoantibodies directed against only desmoglein 1 will histopathologically show superficial intraepithelial clefting of the epidermis, but oral mucosa will not be affected. Clinically, the fine scaly red lesions of pemphigus foliaceus or pemphigus erythematosus will be evident.

Occasionally, a pemphigus-like oral and cutaneous eruption may occur in patients taking certain medications (e.g., penicillamine, angiotensin-converting enzyme [ACE] inhibitors, nonsteroidal anti-inflammatory drugs [NSAIDs]) (see page 337) or in patients with malignancy, especially lymphoreticular malignancies (so-called **paraneoplastic pemphigus**) (see page 774). Similarly, a variety of other conditions may produce chronic vesiculoulcerative or erosive lesions of the oral mucosa, and these often need to be considered in the differential diagnosis (see Table 16.3). In addition, a rare genetic condition termed **chronic benign familial pemphigus** or **Hailey-Hailey disease** may have erosive cutaneous lesions, but oral involvement in that process appears to be uncommon.

Clinical Features

The initial manifestations of pemphigus vulgaris often involve the oral mucosa, typically in adults. The average age at diagnosis is 50 years, although rare cases may be seen in childhood.

A slight female predilection is observed in some reports, and the condition seems to be more common in persons of Mediterranean, South Asian, or Jewish heritage.

Patients usually complain of oral soreness, and examination shows superficial, ragged erosions and ulcerations distributed haphazardly on the oral mucosa (Figs. 16.50–16.53). Such lesions may affect virtually any oral mucosal location, although the palate, labial mucosa, buccal mucosa, ventral tongue, and gingivae are often involved. Patients rarely report vesicle or bulla formation intraorally, and such lesions can seldom be identified by the examining clinician, probably because of early rupture of the thin, friable roof of the blisters. More than 50% of the patients have oral mucosal lesions before the onset of cutaneous lesions, sometimes by as much as 1 year or more. Eventually, however, nearly all patients have intraoral involvement. The skin lesions appear as flaccid vesicles and bullae (Fig. 16.54) that rupture quickly, usually within hours to a few days, leaving an erythematous, denuded surface. Infrequently ocular involvement may be seen, usually appearing as bilateral conjunctivitis. Unlike mucous membrane pemphigoid, the ocular lesions of pemphigus typically do not cause scarring and symblepharon formation (see page 776).

Without proper treatment, the oral and cutaneous lesions tend to persist and progressively involve more surface area. A characteristic feature of pemphigus vulgaris is that a bulla can be induced on normal-appearing skin if firm lateral pressure is exerted. This is called a **positive Nikolsky sign.**

Histopathologic Features

Biopsy specimens of perilesional tissue show characteristic intraepithelial separation, which occurs just above the basal cell layer of the epithelium (Fig. 16.55). Sometimes the entire superficial layers of the epithelium are stripped away,

TABLE 16.3 Chronic Vesiculoulcerative Diseases

Condition	Mean Age	Sex Predilection	Clinical Features	Histopathologic Features	Direct Immunofluorescence	Indirect Immunofluorescence
Pemphigus vulgaris	Fourth to sixth decade	Equal	Vesicles, erosions, and ulcerations on any oral mucosal or skin surface	Intraepithelial clefting	Positive intercellular	Positive
Paraneoplastic pemphigus	Sixth to seventh decade	Equal	Vesicles, erosions, and ulcerations on any mucosal or skin surface	Subepithelial and intraepithelial clefting	Positive, intercellular and basement membrane zone	Positive (rat bladder)
Mucous membrane pemphigoid	Sixth to seventh decade	Female	Primarily mucosal lesions	Subepithelial clefting	Positive, basement membrane zone	Negative
Bullous pemphigoid	Seventh to eighth decade	Equal	Primarily skin lesions	Subepithelial clefting	Positive, basement membrane zone	Positive
Erythema multiforme	Third to fourth decade	Male	Skin and mucosa involved; target lesions on skin	Subepithelial edema and perivascular inflammations	Nondiagnostic	Negative
Lichen planus	Fifth to sixth decade	Female	Oral and/or skin lesions; may or may not be erosive	Hyperkeratosis, saw-toothed rete ridges, bandlike infiltrate of lymphocytes	Fibrinogen, basement membrane zone (characteristic, but not specific for lichen planus)	Negative

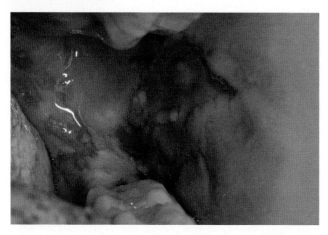

• **Fig. 16.50 Pemphigus Vulgaris.** Multiple erosions of the left buccal mucosa and soft palate.

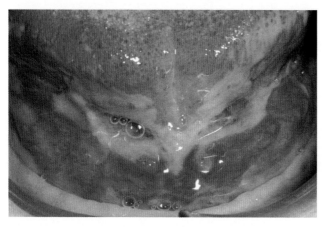

• **Fig. 16.51 Pemphigus Vulgaris.** Large, irregularly shaped ulcerations involving the floor of the mouth and ventral tongue.

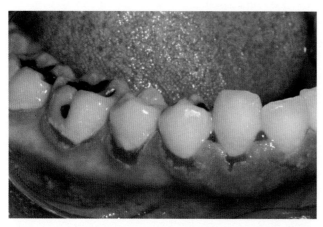

• **Fig. 16.52 Pemphigus Vulgaris.** Multiple erosions affecting the marginal gingiva.

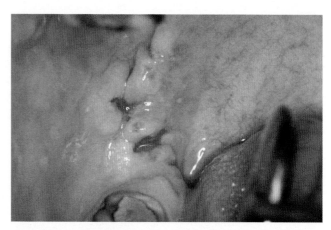

• **Fig. 16.53 Pemphigus Vulgaris.** The patient, with a known diagnosis of pemphigus vulgaris, had been treated with immunosuppressive therapy. The oral erosions shown here were the only persistent manifestation of her disease.

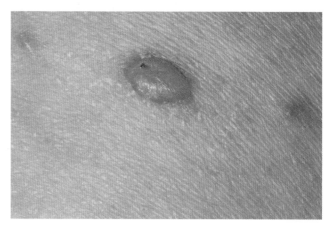

• **Fig. 16.54 Pemphigus Vulgaris.** This flaccid cutaneous bulla is characteristic of skin involvement.

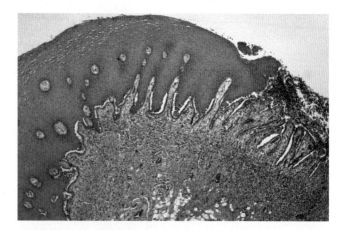

• **Fig. 16.55 Pemphigus Vulgaris.** Low-power photomicrograph of perilesional mucosa affected by pemphigus vulgaris. An intraepithelial cleft is located just above the basal cell layer.

leaving only the basal cells, which have been described as resembling a "row of tombstones." The cells of the spinous layer of the surface epithelium typically appear to fall apart, a feature that has been termed **acantholysis,** and the loose cells tend to assume a rounded shape (Fig. 16.56). This feature of pemphigus vulgaris can be used in making a diagnosis based on the identification of these rounded cells (**Tzanck cells**) in an exfoliative cytologic preparation. A mild-to-moderate chronic inflammatory cell infiltrate is usually seen in the underlying connective tissue.

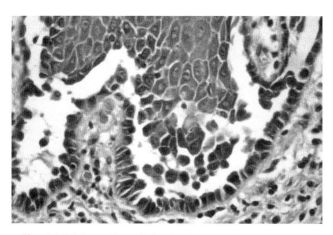

• **Fig. 16.56 Pemphigus Vulgaris.** High-power photomicrograph showing rounded, acantholytic epithelial cells sitting within the intraepithelial cleft.

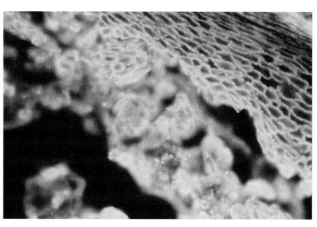

• **Fig. 16.57 Pemphigus Vulgaris.** Photomicrograph depicting the direct immunofluorescence pattern of pemphigus vulgaris. Immunoreactants are deposited in the intercellular areas between the surface epithelial cells, resulting in a "chicken wire" pattern.

The diagnosis of pemphigus vulgaris should be confirmed by direct immunofluorescence examination of fresh perilesional tissue or tissue submitted in Michel's solution. With this procedure, antibodies (usually IgG or IgM) and complement components (usually C3) can be demonstrated in the intercellular spaces between the epithelial cells (Fig. 16.57) in almost all patients with this disease. Indirect immunofluorescence is also typically positive in 80% to 90% of cases, demonstrating the presence of circulating autoantibodies in the patient's serum. Enzyme-linked immunosorbent assays (ELISAs) have been developed to detect circulating autoantibodies as well.

It is critical that perilesional tissue be obtained for both light microscopy and direct immunofluorescence to maximize the probability of a diagnostic sample. If ulcerated mucosa is submitted for testing, then the results are often inconclusive because of either a lack of an intact interface between the epithelium and connective tissue or a great deal of nonspecific inflammation.

Treatment and Prognosis

A diagnosis of pemphigus vulgaris should be made as early in its course as possible because control is generally easier to achieve. Pemphigus is a systemic disease; therefore, treatment requires a systemic approach. In the recent past, treatment consisted primarily of systemic corticosteroids (usually prednisone or prednisolone), often in combination with other immunosuppressive drugs (so-called steroid-sparing agents), such as mycophenolate mofetil or azathioprine. Currently the use of rituximab, a monoclonal antibody that targets B-lymphocytes, is often mentioned as a first-line approach to managing this disease, as it targets the cells responsible for producing the autoantibodies that cause pemphigus. Usually rituximab is used in conjunction with a lower dose of systemic corticosteroids, resulting in a more rapid clearing of the lesions, as well as faster and more prolonged remission of the disease. Newer anti-B-cell monoclonal antibodies that are more effective are now being tested to determine their impact on treatment of pemphigus vulgaris. There is interest in these new therapeutic approaches because the potential side effects associated with the long-term use of systemic corticosteroids are significant and include the following:

• Diabetes mellitus
• Adrenal suppression
• Weight gain
• Osteoporosis
• Peptic ulcers
• Severe mood swings
• Increased susceptibility to a wide range of infections

Ideally, a physician with expertise in immunosuppressive therapy should manage the patient. Often the clinician can monitor the success of therapy by measuring the titers of circulating autoantibodies using indirect immunofluorescence, because disease activity frequently correlates with the abnormal antibody levels. Although some clinicians have advocated the use of topical corticosteroids in the management of oral lesions, the observed improvement is undoubtedly because of the absorption of the topical agents, resulting in a greater systemic dose.

Pemphigus may undergo complete resolution, although remissions and exacerbations are common. One study suggested that up to 75% of patients will have disease resolution after 10 years of treatment, although most centers have historically reported a remission rate of approximately 30%.

Before the development of corticosteroid therapy, as many as 60% to 90% of these patients died, primarily as a result of infections and electrolyte imbalances. Currently the mortality rate associated with pemphigus vulgaris is in the range of 5% to 10%, usually because of the complications of long-term systemic corticosteroid use. The mortality rate may improve in the future as anti-B-cell therapeutic approaches become more widely used.

◆ PARANEOPLASTIC PEMPHIGUS (NEOPLASIA-INDUCED PEMPHIGUS; PARANEOPLASTIC AUTOIMMUNE MULTIORGAN SYNDROME)

Paraneoplastic pemphigus is a rare vesiculobullous disorder that affects patients who have a neoplasm, usually **lymphoma** or **chronic lymphocytic leukemia.** Approximately 500 cases have been documented. Although the precise pathogenetic mechanisms are unknown, some evidence suggests abnormal levels of the cytokine, interleukin-6 (IL-6), could be produced by host lymphocytes in response to the patient's tumor. IL-6 may then be responsible for stimulating the abnormal production of antibodies directed against antigens associated with the desmosomal complex and the basement membrane zone of the epithelium. In addition to a variety of different antibodies that attack these epithelial adherence structures, some investigators have described cutaneous and mucosal damage that appears to be mediated by cytotoxic T lymphocytes in some cases of paraneoplastic pemphigus. As a result of this multifaceted immunologic attack, the disease manifests in an array of clinical features, histopathologic findings, and immunopathologic findings that may be perplexing if the clinician is unfamiliar with this condition. Some investigators prefer the term *paraneoplastic autoimmune multiorgan syndrome (PAMS)* because of the much greater array of tissues that are targeted by a variety of immunologic assaults.

Clinical Features

Patients typically have a history of a malignant lymphoreticular neoplasm, or less commonly, a benign lymphoproliferative disorder such as angiofollicular lymph node hyperplasia (Castleman disease). In approximately one-third of reported cases, paraneoplastic pemphigus developed before a neoplasm was identified, thus signaling the presence of a tumor. The neoplastic disease may or may not be under control at the time of onset of the paraneoplastic condition. Signs and symptoms of paraneoplastic pemphigus usually begin suddenly and may appear polymorphous. In some instances, multiple vesiculobullous lesions affect the skin (Fig. 16.58) and oral mucosa. Palmar or plantar bullae may be evident, a feature that is uncommon in pemphigus vulgaris. For other patients, skin lesions can appear more papular and pruritic, similar to cutaneous lichen planus. The lips often show hemorrhagic crusting similar to that of erythema multiforme (Fig. 16.59). Oral mucosal involvement is an early, consistent feature of paraneoplastic pemphigus, and patients develop multiple areas of erythema and diffuse, irregular ulceration (Fig. 16.60), affecting virtually any oral mucosal surface. If the lesions remain untreated, then they persist and worsen. Some patients may develop only oropharyngeal lesions, without cutaneous involvement.

Other mucosal surfaces are also commonly affected, with 70% of patients having involvement of the conjunctival mucosa. In this area, a cicatrizing (scarring) conjunctivitis

develops, similar to that seen with mucous membrane pemphigoid (Fig. 16.61). The anogenital, nasopharyngeal, esophageal, and respiratory tract mucosa may also be involved. Involvement of the bronchiolar mucosa is particularly significant because the lining epithelium sloughs and

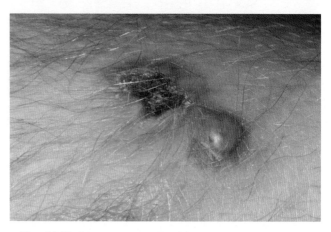

• **Fig. 16.58 Paraneoplastic Pemphigus.** The bulla and crusted ulcerations on this patient's arm are representative of the polymorphous cutaneous lesions.

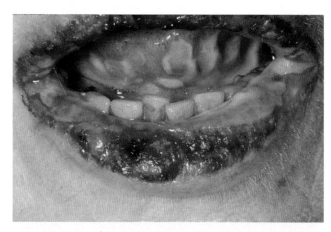

• **Fig. 16.59 Paraneoplastic Pemphigus.** Crusted, hemorrhagic lip lesions may be mistaken for erythema multiforme or herpes simplex infection.

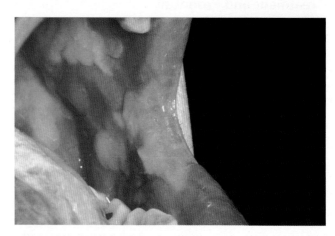

• **Fig. 16.60 Paraneoplastic Pemphigus.** These diffuse oral ulcerations are quite painful.

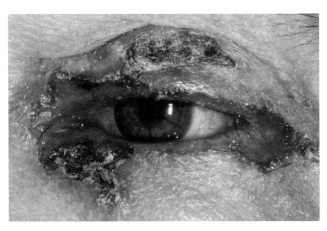

• **Fig. 16.61 Paraneoplastic Pemphigus.** Ocular involvement.

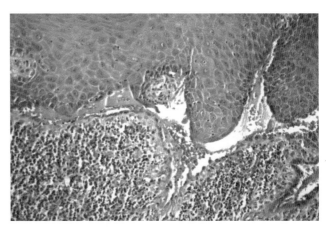

• **Fig. 16.62 Paraneoplastic Pemphigus.** This medium-power photomicrograph shows both intraepithelial and subepithelial clefting.

occludes the bronchiolar lumina and the alveoli of the lung, resulting in a condition known as **bronchiolitis obliterans.**

Histopathologic Features

The features of paraneoplastic pemphigus on light microscopic examination may be as diverse as the clinical features. In most cases, a lichenoid mucositis is seen, usually with subepithelial clefting (like pemphigoid) or intraepithelial clefting (like pemphigus) (Fig. 16.62).

Direct immunofluorescence studies may show a weakly positive deposition of immunoreactants (IgG and complement) in the intercellular zones of the epithelium and/or a linear deposition of immunoreactants at the basement membrane zone. Although antibodies directed against desmoglein 1 and 3, as well as the bullous pemphigoid antigens are often produced, antibodies directed against the plakin family of desmosomal components are more commonly identified and are more specific for paraneoplastic pemphigus. ELISA or immunoblotting techniques are used to confirm the presence of antibodies directed against periplakin or envoplakin specifically. If these tests are not available, then indirect immunofluorescence can be conducted using a transitional type of epithelium (e.g., rat urinary bladder mucosa) as the substrate due to its rich expression of plakins. This technique shows a fairly specific pattern of antibody localization to the intercellular areas of the epithelium. Examples of paraneoplastic pemphigus that show only a lichenoid reaction with no demonstrable autoantibody production have infrequently been described.

Treatment and Prognosis

Paraneoplastic pemphigus is often a very serious condition with a high morbidity and mortality rate, with cases documented in the literature having an overall mortality rate of 60%, although some series have reported a mortality rate of 90%. For the infrequent cases associated with a benign lymphoproliferative condition, surgical removal of the tumor may result in regression of the paraneoplastic pemphigus. For those cases associated with malignancy, treatment usually consists of systemic prednisone combined with cyclosporine. Cyclophosphamide, another immunosuppressive agent, may be added to this regimen, although other immunosuppressive and immune-modulating drugs are also being evaluated. Rituximab, the anti-B-cell monoclonal antibody that has shown very promising results as a treatment for pemphigus vulgaris does not appear to have a significant impact on the course of paraneoplastic pemphigus. As with pemphigus vulgaris, the skin lesions of paraneoplastic pemphigus usually respond more quickly to treatment than the oral lesions. Unfortunately, although the immunosuppressive therapy often manages to control the autoimmune disease, this immunosuppression often seems to trigger a reactivation of the malignant neoplasm. Thus a high mortality rate is seen, with patients succumbing to complications of the vesiculobullous lesions, complications of immune suppressive therapy, respiratory failure due to bronchiolitis obliterans, or progression of malignant disease. Occasionally, long-term survivors are reported, but these seem to be in the minority. As more of these patients are identified, therapeutic strategies can be better evaluated and modified for optimal care in the future.

◆ MUCOUS MEMBRANE PEMPHIGOID (CICATRICIAL PEMPHIGOID; BENIGN MUCOUS MEMBRANE PEMPHIGOID)

Evidence has accumulated to suggest that **mucous membrane pemphigoid** represents a group of chronic, blistering, mucocutaneous autoimmune diseases in which tissue-bound autoantibodies are directed against one or more components of the basement membrane. As such, this condition has a heterogeneous origin, with autoantibodies being produced against any one of a variety of basement membrane components, all of which produce similar clinical manifestations. The precise prevalence is unknown, but most authors believe that it is at least twice as common as pemphigus vulgaris.

The term **pemphigoid** is used because clinically it often appears similar (the meaning of the *-oid* suffix) to **pemphigus.** The prognosis and microscopic features of pemphigoid, however, are very different.

Although a variety of terms have been used over the decades to designate this condition, a group of experts from both medicine and dentistry met in 1999 and came to an agreement that **mucous membrane pemphigoid** would be the most appropriate name for the disease. **Cicatricial pemphigoid,** another commonly used name for this process, is derived from the word **cicatrix,** meaning *scar.* When the conjunctival mucosa is affected, the scarring that results is the most significant aspect of this disorder because it invariably results in blindness unless the condition is recognized and treated. Interestingly, the oral lesions seldom exhibit this tendency for scar formation.

Clinical Features

Mucous membrane pemphigoid usually affects older adults, with an average age of 50–60 years at the onset of disease. Females are affected more frequently than males by a 2:1 ratio. Oral lesions are seen in most patients, but other sites, such as conjunctival, nasal, esophageal, laryngeal, and vaginal mucosa, as well as the skin (Fig. 16.63), may be involved.

The oral lesions of pemphigoid begin as either vesicles or bullae that may occasionally be identified clinically (Fig. 16.64). In contrast, patients with pemphigus rarely display such blisters. The most likely explanation for this difference is that the pemphigoid blister forms in a subepithelial location, producing a thicker, stronger roof than the intraepithelial, acantholytic pemphigus blister. Eventually, the oral blisters rupture, leaving large, superficial, ulcerated, and denuded areas of mucosa (Fig. 16.65). The ulcerated lesions are usually painful and persist for weeks to months if untreated.

Often this process is seen diffusely throughout the mouth, but it may be limited to certain areas, especially the gingiva (Fig. 16.66). Gingival involvement produces a clinical reaction pattern termed **desquamative gingivitis** (see page 155).

This pattern may also be seen in other conditions, such as **erosive lichen planus** or, much less frequently, **pemphigus vulgaris.**

The most significant complication of mucous membrane pemphigoid, however, is ocular involvement. Although exact figures are not available, up to 25% of patients with oral lesions may eventually develop ocular disease. One eye may be affected before the other. The earliest change is subconjunctival fibrosis, which usually can be detected by an ophthalmologist using slit-lamp microscopic examination. As the disease progresses, the conjunctiva becomes inflamed and eroded. Attempts at healing lead to scarring between the bulbar (lining the globe of the eye) and palpebral (lining the inner surface of the eyelid) conjunctivae. Adhesions called **symblepharons** result (Fig. 16.67). Without treatment the inflammatory changes become more severe, although conjunctival vesicle formation is rarely seen. Scarring can ultimately cause the eyelids to turn inward **(entropion).** This causes the eyelashes to rub against the cornea and globe **(trichiasis)** (Fig. 16.68). The scarring closes off the openings of

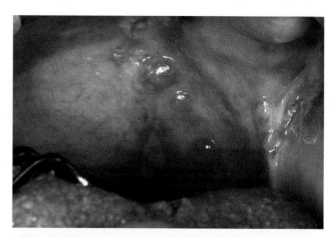

• **Fig. 16.64 Mucous Membrane Pemphigoid.** One or more intraoral vesicles, as seen on the soft palate, may be detected in patients with mucous membrane pemphigoid. Usually, shallow ulcerations of the oral mucosa are also present, as seen in the midline posterior soft palate, where one of the vesicles has ruptured.

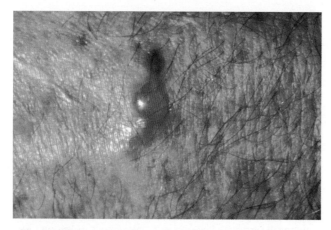

• **Fig. 16.63 Mucous Membrane Pemphigoid.** Although cutaneous lesions are not common, tense bullae such as these may develop on the skin of 20% of affected patients. (Courtesy of Dr. Charles Camisa.)

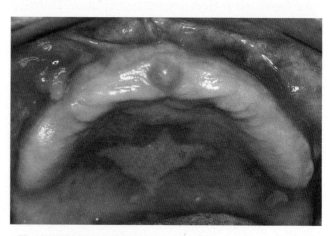

• **Fig. 16.65 Mucous Membrane Pemphigoid.** Large, irregular oral ulcerations characterize the lesions after the initial bullae rupture.

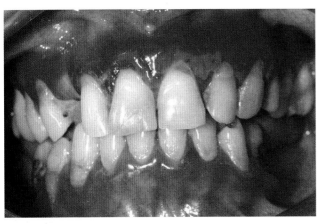

• **Fig. 16.66 Mucous Membrane Pemphigoid.** Often the gingival tissues are the only affected site, resulting in a clinical pattern known as *desquamative gingivitis*. Such a pattern may also be seen with lichen planus and pemphigus vulgaris.

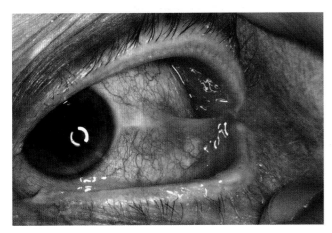

• **Fig. 16.67 Mucous Membrane Pemphigoid.** Although the earliest ocular changes are difficult to identify, patients with ocular involvement may show adhesions (symblepharons) between the bulbar and palpebral conjunctivae before severe ocular damage occurs.

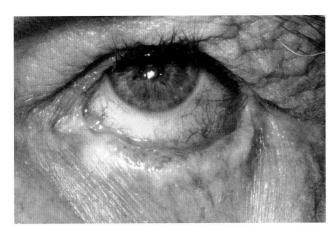

• **Fig. 16.68 Mucous Membrane Pemphigoid.** The disease has caused the upper eyelid of this patient to turn inward (entropion), resulting in the eyelashes rubbing against the eye itself (trichiasis). Also note the obliteration of the lower fornix of the eye.

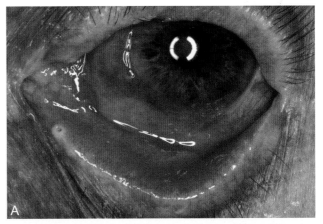

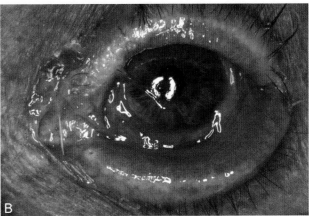

• **Fig. 16.69 Mucous Membrane Pemphigoid. A,** This patient with ocular involvement shows severe conjunctival inflammation. **B,** Four months later, the progression of his conjunctival involvement is striking, with adhesions and scarring involving the cornea.

the lacrimal glands as well, and with the loss of tears, the eye becomes extremely dry. The cornea then produces keratin as a protective mechanism; however, keratin is an opaque material, and blindness ensues (Fig. 16.69, A and B). End-stage ocular involvement may also be characterized by adhesions between the upper and lower eyelids themselves.

Other mucosal sites may also be involved and cause considerable difficulty for the patient. In females, the vaginal mucosal lesions may cause considerable pain during attempts at intercourse (**dyspareunia**).

Laryngeal lesions, which are fairly uncommon, may be especially significant because of the possibility of airway obstruction by the bullae that are formed. Patients who experience a sudden change in vocalization or who have difficulty breathing should undergo examination with laryngoscopy.

Histopathologic Features

Biopsy of perilesional mucosa shows a split between the surface epithelium and the underlying connective tissue in the region of the basement membrane (Fig. 16.70). A mild chronic inflammatory cell infiltrate is present in the superficial submucosa.

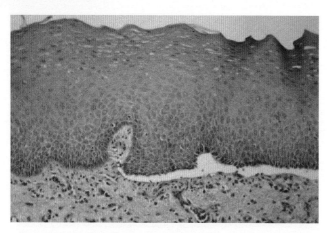

• **Fig. 16.70 Mucous Membrane Pemphigoid.** Medium-power photomicrograph of perilesional tissue shows characteristic subepithelial clefting.

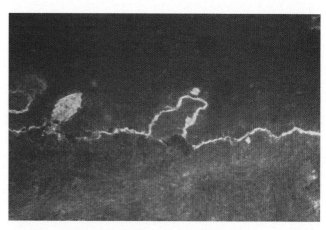

• **Fig. 16.71 Mucous Membrane Pemphigoid.** Direct immunofluorescence studies show a deposition of immunoreactants at the basement membrane zone of the epithelium. (Courtesy of Dr. Ronald Grimwood.)

Direct immunofluorescence studies of perilesional mucosa show a continuous linear band of immunoreactants at the basement membrane zone in nearly 90% of affected patients (Fig. 16.71). The immune deposits consist primarily of IgG and C3, although IgA and IgM may also be identified. One study has suggested that, when IgG and IgA deposits are found in the same patient, the disease may be more severe. All of these immunoreactants may play a role in the pathogenesis of the subepithelial vesicle formation by weakening the attachment of the basement membrane through a variety of mechanisms, including complement activation with recruitment of inflammatory cells, particularly neutrophils.

Indirect immunofluorescence is positive in only 5%–25% of these patients, indicating a relatively consistent lack of readily detectable circulating autoantibodies. One type of mucous membrane pemphigoid produces low levels of circulating autoantibodies to epiligrin (laminin-5), a component of the basement membrane. Approximately 30% of patients with this variant of mucous membrane pemphigoid have been shown to have a solid malignancy, and the pemphigoid may be the initial sign that the patient has cancer. Antiepiligrin mucous membrane pemphigoid seems to have more widespread involvement, affecting oral, nasal, ocular, and laryngeal mucosa, compared with other forms of mucous membrane pemphigoid. In contrast, another group of investigators has shown that pemphigoid patients with only oral mucosal involvement have circulating autoantibodies to α6 integrin, a component of the hemidesmosome.

For an accurate diagnosis, perilesional tissue—rather than the ulcerated lesion itself—should be obtained. Often the epithelium in the area of the lesion is so loosely attached that it strips off as the clinician attempts to perform the biopsy. Such tissue is not usually adequate for diagnostic purposes because the interface between the epithelium and connective tissue is no longer intact (although some investigators have shown positive immunofluorescence with this tissue).

Other relatively rare conditions can mimic pemphigoid histopathologically. These include pemphigoid-like reactions to various medications (see page 337), **linear IgA**

bullous dermatosis, angina bullosa hemorrhagica, and **epidermolysis bullosa acquisita.**

Linear IgA Bullous Dermatosis

Linear IgA bullous dermatosis, as the name indicates, is characterized by the linear deposition of only IgA along the basement membrane zone. Even though some cases of mucous membrane pemphigoid may have IgA antibodies, linear IgA bullous dermatosis predominantly affects the skin and, therefore, can usually be distinguished from mucous membrane pemphigoid on a clinical basis.

Angina Bullosa Hemorrhagica

Angina bullosa hemorrhagica is a rare, poorly characterized oral mucosal disorder that exhibits variably painful, blood-filled vesicles or bullae, usually affecting the soft palate of middle-aged or older adults (Fig. 16.72). The blisters typically rupture spontaneously and heal without scarring. A subepithelial cleft is noted microscopically. No hematologic or immunopathologic abnormalities have been detected, and although the cause is unknown, many patients have a history of trauma or corticosteroid inhaler use.

Epidermolysis Bullosa Acquisita

Epidermolysis bullosa acquisita is an immunologically mediated condition characterized by autoantibodies directed against type VII collagen, the principal component of the anchoring fibrils. The anchoring fibrils play an important role in bonding the epithelium to the underlying connective tissue. As a result, their immunologic destruction leads to the formation of bullous lesions of the skin and mucosa with minimal trauma. The disease was named epidermolysis bullosa acquisita ("acquisita" means "acquired") because of its clinical resemblance to the inherited condition, dystrophic epidermolysis bullosa. Unlike the inherited disorder, epidermolysis bullosa acquisita typically affects middle-aged or older adults.

Oral lesions are present in up to 50% of the cases, although such lesions are uncommon in the absence of

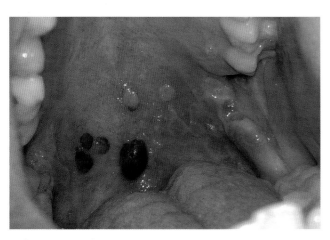

• **Fig. 16.72 Angina Bullosa Hemorrhagica.** Hemorrhagic blisters on the soft palate in a patient who regularly used a corticosteroid inhaler. (Courtesy of Dr. Peter Lyu.)

cutaneous lesions. To distinguish epidermolysis bullosa acquisita from other immunobullous diseases with subepithelial clefting, a special technique is performed. A sample of the patient's perilesional skin is incubated in a concentrated salt solution; this causes the epithelium to separate from the connective tissue, forming an artificially induced bulla. Immunohistochemical evaluation shows deposition of IgG autoantibodies on the floor (connective tissue side) of the bulla where type VII collagen resides. This finding is in contrast to that of most forms of mucous membrane pemphigoid, in which the autoantibodies are usually localized to the roof of the induced blister.

Treatment and Prognosis

Once the diagnosis of mucous membrane pemphigoid has been established by light microscopy and direct immunofluorescence, the patient should be referred to an ophthalmologist who is familiar with the ocular lesions of this condition for a baseline examination of the conjunctivae. This should be done whether or not the patient is experiencing ocular complaints. In addition, if the patient is experiencing symptoms at other anatomic sites, then the appropriate specialist should be consulted.

Because this condition is characterized by heterogeneous pathogenetic mechanisms, it is not surprising that treatments advocated over the years have been varied. In fact, there is no single good therapy for every patient; treatment must be individualized, depending on lesional distribution, disease activity, and therapeutic response. Perhaps as the various forms of pemphigoid are better defined immunopathologically, more specific, directed therapy can be devised. In addition, most of the therapies are based on empirical recommendations, primarily because mucous membrane pemphigoid is relatively rare, and being able to acquire sufficient numbers of patients for randomized, placebo-controlled treatment studies is quite challenging.

Topical Agents

If only oral lesions are present, sometimes the disease can be controlled with application of one of the more potent topical corticosteroid gel preparations to the lesions several times each day. Once control is achieved, the applications can be discontinued, although the lesions are certain to flare up again. Sometimes alternate-day application prevents such exacerbations of disease activity.

Patients with only gingival lesions often benefit from good oral hygiene measures, which can help to decrease the severity of the lesions and reduce the amount of topical corticosteroids required. As an additional aid in treating gingival lesions, a flexible mouth guard may be fabricated to use as a carrier for the corticosteroid medication.

Systemic Agents

If topical corticosteroids are unsuccessful, systemic treatments are available. Dapsone, which is a sulfa drug derivative, can be used to treat patients with mild-to-moderate involvement by mucous membrane pemphigoid. Systemic treatment with dapsone typically has fewer serious side effects when compared to systemic corticosteroid therapy, for example.

Some centers report good results with dapsone, but others observe that a minority of patients respond adequately. Contraindications to its use include glucose-6-phosphate dehydrogenase deficiency or allergy to sulfa drugs.

Another alternative systemic therapy that may be used for patients with less severe disease is tetracycline or minocycline and niacinamide (nicotinamide). Systemic daily divided doses of 0.5–2.0 g of each drug have been reported (in open-label trials) to be effective in controlling mucous membrane pemphigoid. Double-blind, placebo-controlled studies on larger groups of patients should be done to confirm this form of therapy, however.

For more severely affected patients with mucous membrane pemphigoid, corticosteroids plus other immunosuppressive/immune modulating agents, (such as, rituximab, mycophenolate mofetil, or cyclophosphamide) may be used. This type of aggressive treatment is often indicated in the presence of advancing ocular disease, but it must be realized that many of these patients are older and may have preexisting medical conditions that may preclude aggressive immune suppression. Some studies have suggested that treatment with intravenous (IV) human immunoglobulin (which is very expensive) may be more effective in managing ocular lesions of pemphigoid than systemic corticosteroid therapy. Attempts at surgical correction of any symblepharons that might have formed must be done when the disease is under control or quiescent; otherwise, the manipulation often induces an acute flare of the ocular lesions.

◆ BULLOUS PEMPHIGOID

Bullous pemphigoid is the most common of the autoimmune blistering conditions, occurring at an estimated rate of ten cases per million population per year, although the

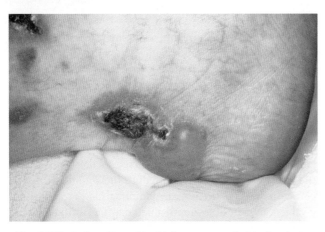

• **Fig. 16.73 Bullous Pemphigoid.** Cutaneous vesiculobullous lesions of the heel. The bullae eventually rupture, leaving hemorrhagic crusted areas.

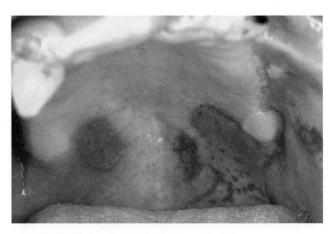

• **Fig. 16.74 Bullous Pemphigoid.** These oral lesions appear as large, shallow ulcerations involving the soft palate.

incidence is much greater in patients over 60 years of age. The disease is characterized by the production of autoantibodies directed against components of the basement membrane. In many respects, bullous pemphigoid resembles **mucous membrane pemphigoid,** but most investigators note that there are enough differences to consider these diseases as distinct but related entities. One significant difference is that the clinical course in patients with bullous pemphigoid is usually characterized by periods of remission followed by relapse, whereas the course in patients with mucous membrane pemphigoid is usually protracted and progressive.

Clinical Features

Bullous pemphigoid typically develops in older people; most patients are between 75 and 80 years of age. No sex or racial predilection is generally reported, although one group of investigators noted that men are overrepresented in this disease by a 2:1 margin when one corrects for the skewing of the aging population toward the female gender. Pruritus is often an early symptom. This is followed by the development of multiple, tense bullae on either normal or erythematous skin (Fig. 16.73). These lesions eventually rupture after several days, causing a superficial crust to form. Eventually, healing takes place without scarring.

Oral mucosal involvement is uncommon, with approximately 10%–20% of patients being affected. The oral lesions, like the skin lesions, begin as bullae, but they tend to rupture sooner, probably as a result of the constant low-grade trauma to which the oral mucosa is subjected. Large, shallow ulcerations with smooth, distinct margins are present after the bullae rupture (Fig. 16.74).

Histopathologic Features

Microscopic examination of tissue obtained from the perilesional margin of a bulla shows separation of the epithelium from the connective tissue at the basement membrane zone, resulting in a subepithelial separation. Modest numbers of

both acute and chronic inflammatory cells are typically seen in the lesional area, and the presence of eosinophils within the bulla itself is characteristic.

Direct immunofluorescence studies show a continuous linear band of immunoreactants, usually IgG and C3, localized to the basement membrane zone in 90%–100% of affected patients. These antibodies bind to proteins associated with **hemidesmosomes,** structures that bind the basal cell layer of the epithelium to the basement membrane and the underlying connective tissue. These proteins have been designated as **bullous pemphigoid antigens (BP180 and BP230),** and immunoelectron microscopy has demonstrated the localization of BP180 to the upper portion of the lamina lucida of the basement membrane.

In addition to the tissue-bound autoantibodies, 50%–90% of the patients also have circulating autoantibodies in the serum, producing an indirect immunofluorescent pattern that is identical to that of the direct immunofluorescence. Unlike pemphigus vulgaris, the antibody titers seen in bullous pemphigoid do not appear to correlate with disease activity. The antibodies alone do not appear to be capable of inducing bullae in this disease. Instead, binding of the antibodies to the basement membrane initiates the complement cascade, which in turn results in degranulation of mast cells, with recruitment of neutrophils and eosinophils to the area. The damage to the basement membrane is thought to be mediated by elastases and matrix metalloproteinases released by these inflammatory cells.

Treatment and Prognosis

Treatment of patients with mild or localized bullous pemphigoid consists of application of one of the stronger topical corticosteroid preparations. Management of the patient with moderate-to-severe, widespread bullous pemphigoid consists of systemic immunosuppressive therapy. Moderate daily doses of systemic prednisone usually control the condition, after which alternate-day therapy may be given to reduce the risk of corticosteroid complications. If the lesions do not respond to prednisone alone, then another immunosuppressive, corticosteroid-sparing agent may be added to the regimen, including azathioprine, methotrexate, mycophenolate mofetil, or an anti-CD20 monoclonal antibody, such as rituximab. Dapsone, a sulfa derivative, may be used as an alternative therapeutic agent, and tetracycline and niacinamide therapy is reported to be effective for some patients. The more severe, resistant cases require prednisone combined with cyclophosphamide; however, this regimen has the potential for significant side effects.

The prognosis is generally good with respect to control of the skin lesions, with many patients experiencing remission. Recent reports based on a relatively large series of bullous pemphigoid patients have suggested that problems frequently develop due to the immunosuppressive therapy used in this older adult population. Mortality rates that are three times that of an age- and sex-matched control population may be seen, with approximately 20% of patients expiring 1 year after diagnosis.

◆ ERYTHEMA MULTIFORME

Erythema multiforme is a blistering, ulcerative mucocutaneous condition of uncertain etiopathogenesis. A cell-mediated (rather than humoral) immunologic attack on the oral mucosa and/or epidermis is thought to play a significant role, although the precise cause is poorly understood. In about 50%–60% of the cases, the clinician can identify an apparent precipitating cause, usually a preceding infection, such as **herpes simplex** or *Mycoplasma pneumoniae*, or less commonly, exposure to any one of a variety of drugs and medications, particularly antibiotics or analgesics. These agents may trigger the immunologic derangement that produces the disease. Sophisticated techniques in molecular biology have demonstrated the presence of herpes simplex DNA in patients with recurrent erythema multiforme, thus supporting the concept of an immunologic precipitating event. Interestingly, direct and indirect immunofluorescence studies are nonspecific and are not really very useful diagnostically except to rule out other vesiculobullous diseases.

For many years it was thought that erythema multiforme exhibited a spectrum of severity, ranging from **erythema multiforme minor** through **erythema multiforme major** (traditionally thought to be synonymous with **Stevens-Johnson syndrome**) and **toxic epidermal necrolysis (Lyell disease).** Most authorities currently feel that erythema multiforme minor and major may represent a distinctly different process from the latter two conditions. Therefore, Stevens-Johnson syndrome and toxic epidermal necrolysis will be discussed separately in the next section.

Clinical Features

Erythema multiforme typically has an acute onset and usually affects young adults in their 20s or 30s, with no striking sex predilection. Prodromal symptoms are often present and include fever, malaise, headache, cough, and sore throat, occurring approximately 1 week before onset. The condition may show varying degrees of severity in affected patients. Milder cases, known as **erythema multiforme minor,** usually begin with the development of slightly elevated, round, dusky-red patches on the skin of the extremities. These lesions may have a variety of appearances, however *(multiforme* means *many forms).* Some of these skin lesions develop features that are highly characteristic for the disease. These lesions appear as concentric circular erythematous rings resembling a target or bull's-eye **(target lesions)** (Fig. 16.75). In more severe cases, these may evolve into bullae with necrotic centers.

The oral cavity is the most frequently involved mucosal site, although the conjunctival, genitourinary, and respiratory mucosa also may be affected. Involvement of extraoral mucosal areas is usually associated with the more severe form of this condition, erythema multiforme major.

The frequency of oral involvement is difficult to determine and is reported to range from 25% to 70%. Discrepancies in the prevalence may be due to referral patterns or degree of scrutiny of the oral mucosa. The oral lesions begin as erythematous patches that undergo epithelial necrosis and evolve into large, shallow erosions and ulcerations with irregular borders (Fig. 16.76). Hemorrhagic crusting of the vermilion zone of the lips is common (Fig. 16.77). These oral lesions, like the skin lesions, emerge quickly and are uncomfortable. Sometimes patients are dehydrated because they are unable to ingest liquids as a result of mouth pain. The ulcerations often have a diffuse distribution. The lips, labial mucosa, buccal mucosa, tongue, floor of the mouth, and soft palate are the most common sites of involvement. Usually, the gingivae and hard palate are relatively spared.

Erythema Multiforme Major

A diagnosis of *erythema multiforme major* can be made if two or more mucosal sites are affected in conjunction with widespread skin lesions. In most cases the oral mucosa is involved in addition to either the ocular (Fig. 16.78) or genital mucosae. With severe ocular involvement, scarring (symblepharon formation) may occur, similar to that in mucous membrane pemphigoid (see page 776).

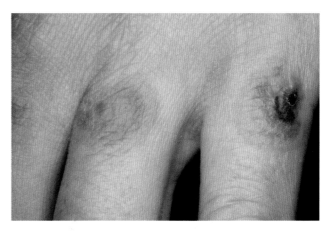

• **Fig. 16.75 Erythema Multiforme.** The concentric erythematous pattern of the cutaneous lesions on the fingers resembles a target or bull's-eye.

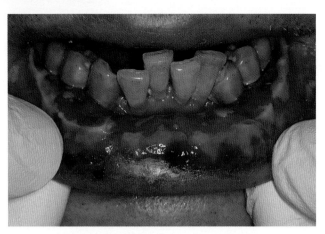

• **Fig. 16.76 Erythema Multiforme.** Focal hemorrhagic crusting of the lips is seen in conjunction with diffuse shallow ulcerations and erosions involving this patient's mandibular labial mucosa.

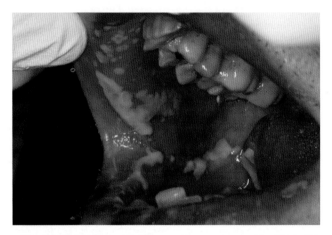

• **Fig. 16.77 Erythema Multiforme.** Same patient as Fig. 16.76. Diffuse shallow ulcerations of varying sizes are noted on the right buccal mucosa. The patient had finished a course of sulfamethoxazole and trimethoprim for a urinary tract infection a few days before the onset of the lesions.

Histopathologic Features

Histopathologic examination of the perilesional mucosa in erythema multiforme reveals a pattern that is characteristic but not pathognomonic. Subepithelial or intraepithelial vesiculation may be seen in association with necrotic basal keratinocytes (Fig. 16.79). A mixed inflammatory infiltrate is present, consisting of lymphocytes, neutrophils, and often eosinophils. Sometimes these cells are arranged in a perivascular orientation (Fig. 16.80). Because the immunopathologic features are also nonspecific, the diagnosis is often based on the clinical presentation and the exclusion of other vesiculobullous disorders.

Treatment and Prognosis

Management of erythema multiforme, in many respects, remains controversial. In the past, the use of systemic or topical corticosteroids was often advocated, especially in the

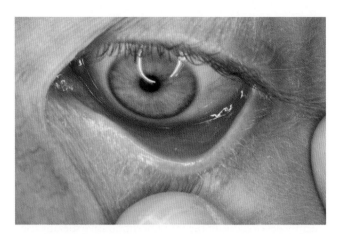

• **Fig. 16.78 Erythema Multiforme Major.** While involvement of other mucosal surfaces is more frequently seen with Stevens-Johnson syndrome, this patient's condition was preceded by oral herpetic infection. This finding, combined with his cutaneous manifestations, resulted in a diagnosis of erythema multiforme major, in this case causing the severe conjunctivitis depicted in this photograph.

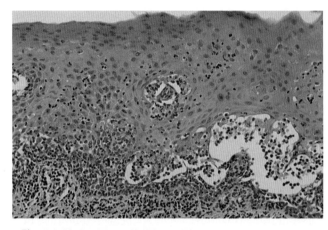

• **Fig. 16.79 Erythema Multiforme.** This medium-power photomicrograph shows inflammation and intraepithelial vesicle formation in the basilar portion of the epithelium. Numerous necrotic and apoptotic eosinophilic keratinocytes are present in the blister area.

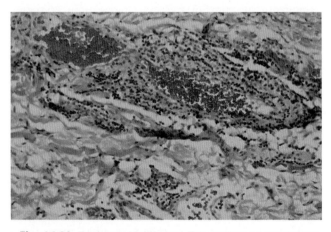

• **Fig. 16.80 Erythema Multiforme.** This medium-power photomicrograph shows the perivascular inflammatory infiltrate, typically seen in erythema multiforme.

early stages of the disease. Although there is little good clinical evidence from controlled trials that such treatment is beneficial, this treatment is typically used at most centers. If a causative drug is identified or suspected, then it should be discontinued immediately.

If the patient is dehydrated as a result of an inability to eat because of oral pain, then IV rehydration may be necessary along with topical anesthetic agents to decrease discomfort.

Even though the disease is self-limiting, usually lasting 2–6 weeks, about 20% of patients experience recurrent episodes, usually in the spring and autumn. If recurrent episodes of erythema multiforme are a problem, then an initiating factor, such as recurrent herpesvirus infection or drug exposure, should be sought. If disease is triggered by herpes simplex, then continuous oral acyclovir or valacyclovir therapy can prevent recurrences. Very infrequently patients may have continuous lesions of erythema multiforme. In most cases erythema multiforme is not life-threatening except in its most severe form.

◆ STEVENS-JOHNSON SYNDROME AND TOXIC EPIDERMAL NECROLYSIS

In the past, many dermatologists considered Stevens-Johnson syndrome and toxic epidermal necrolysis to represent the most severe end of the erythema multiforme spectrum. As careful documentation of the clinical features of these uncommon diseases was compiled, it became evident that there were subtle, but distinct, differences between erythema multiforme and Stevens-Johnson/toxic epidermal necrolysis. Although the inciting event in erythema multiforme is usually a herpesvirus infection, Stevens-Johnson syndrome and toxic epidermal necrolysis are almost always triggered by drug exposure, with more than 200 different medications having been implicated. Recent studies have shown that the damage to the epithelium is due to increased apoptosis of the epithelial cells, and several mechanisms have been postulated to account for this phenomenon.

Clinical Features

The difference between Stevens-Johnson syndrome and toxic epidermal necrolysis is the degree of skin involvement, with Stevens-Johnson syndrome having less than 10% of the body surface affected by lesions, and toxic epidermal necrolysis having more than 30% involvement. These severe blistering diseases are rare. Stevens-Johnson syndrome occurs at an average rate of one to seven cases per million population per year, whereas toxic epidermal necrolysis occurs at a rate of about one case per million per year. In contrast to Stevens-Johnson syndrome, which is usually seen in younger patients, toxic epidermal necrolysis tends to occur in people over 60 years of age. A female predilection is observed.

These patients usually have flu-like prodromal signs and symptoms, including fever, malaise, sore throat, headache, and loss of appetite. Within a few days, skin lesions begin

to develop, but unlike erythema multiforme, the cutaneous lesions of Stevens-Johnson syndrome and toxic epidermal necrolysis initially appear on the trunk, presenting as erythematous macules (completely flat). Within 1–14 days, however, sloughing of the skin and flaccid bullae develop. Virtually all of these patients will have mucosal sites of involvement (Fig. 16.81), particularly the oral mucosa. Diffuse sloughing of a significant proportion of the skin and mucosal surfaces makes it appear as if the patient had been badly scalded (Figs. 16.82 and 16.83). If the patient survives, then the cutaneous process resolves in 3–5 weeks; however, oral lesions may take longer to heal, and significant residual ocular damage is evident in half of the patients.

Histopathologic Features

Biopsy of a developing bulla of Stevens-Johnson syndrome or toxic epidermal necrolysis typically shows a subepithelial blister that is characterized by degenerating, necrotic basal keratinocytes. The underlying connective tissue usually supports a rather sparse population of chronic inflammatory cells.

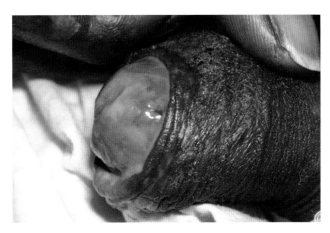

• **Fig. 16.81 Stevens-Johnson Syndrome.** Genital ulcerations, demonstrated in this patient by the involvement of the glans penis, may be a component of Stevens-Johnson syndrome, which tends to be more severe than erythema multiforme major.

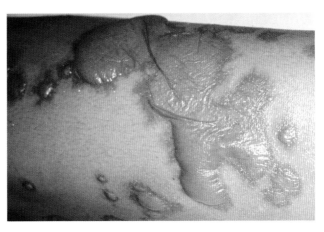

• **Fig. 16.82 Toxic Epidermal Necrolysis.** This serious mucocutaneous disorder is characterized by diffuse bullous skin lesions. (Courtesy of Dr. Peter Larsen.)

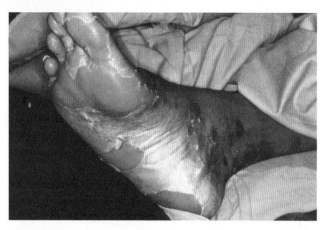

• **Fig. 16.83 Toxic Epidermal Necrolysis.** The desquamation of the skin of the foot is characteristic of the diffuse sloughing cutaneous lesions. (Courtesy of Dr. Peter Larsen.)

Treatment and Prognosis

One of the most important aspects in managing patients with Stevens-Johnson syndrome and toxic epidermal necrolysis is identifying and immediately discontinuing any drug that might be initiating the condition. Because the lesions of toxic epidermal necrolysis are analogous to those suffered by burn patients, management of these patients in the burn unit of the hospital is recommended. Corticosteroids should be avoided in the management of toxic epidermal necrolysis because some investigators have found that such drugs may be detrimental. IV administration of pooled human immunoglobulins has been shown in several open-label trials to produce remarkable resolution of toxic epidermal necrolysis, presumably because of blockade of Fas ligand, which is believed to play a role in inducing epithelial cell apoptosis. The mortality rate in patients with toxic epidermal necrolysis historically has been approximately 25%–30%; the rate in those with Stevens-Johnson syndrome is 1%–5%.

◆ ERYTHEMA MIGRANS (GEOGRAPHIC TONGUE; BENIGN MIGRATORY GLOSSITIS; WANDERING RASH OF THE TONGUE; ERYTHEMA AREATA MIGRANS; STOMATITIS AREATA MIGRANS)

Erythema migrans is a common benign condition that primarily affects the tongue. It is often detected on routine examination of the oral mucosa. The lesion occurs in 1%–3% of the population. Some epidemiologic studies have shown that females are affected more frequently than males by a 2:1 ratio, whereas other series do not identify a gender predilection. Patients occasionally may consult a health care professional if they happen to notice the unusual appearance of their tongue or if the lingual mucosa becomes sensitive to hot or spicy foods as a result of the process.

Even though erythema migrans has been documented for many years, the etiopathogenesis is still unknown. Some

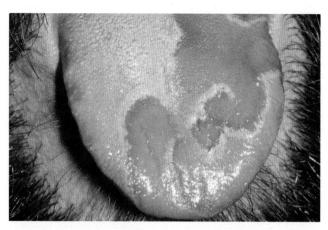

• **Fig. 16.84 Erythema Migrans.** The erythematous, well-demarcated areas of papillary atrophy are characteristic of erythema migrans affecting the tongue (benign migratory glossitis). Note the asymmetrical distribution and the tendency to involve the lateral aspects of the tongue.

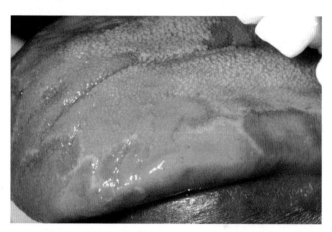

• **Fig. 16.85 Erythema Migrans.** Lingual mucosa of a different patient than the one in Fig. 16.84. The lateral distribution of the lesions is shown.

investigators have suggested that erythema migrans occurs with increased frequency in atopic individuals; however, one large epidemiologic study in the United States found no statistically significant association between erythema migrans and a variety of conditions that had previously been postulated either to cause or influence this process. Erythema migrans was not seen as frequently in cigarette smokers, while there seemed to be no significant differences in frequency related to age, sex, oral contraceptive use, presence of allergies, diabetes mellitus, or psychological or dermatologic conditions. A similar study in Turkey essentially agreed with these findings, with the exception of an association with a history of allergy or atopy.

Clinical Features

The characteristic lesions of erythema migrans are seen on the anterior two-thirds of the dorsal tongue mucosa. They appear as multiple, well-demarcated zones of erythema (Figs. 16.84 and 16.85), concentrated at the tip and lateral borders of the tongue. This erythema is due to atrophy of the filiform papillae, and these atrophic areas are typically surrounded at least partially by a slightly elevated, yellow-white, serpentine or scalloped border (Fig. 16.86). The patient who is aware of the process is often able to describe the lesions as appearing quickly in one area, healing within a few days or weeks, and then developing in a very different area. Frequently, the lesion begins as a small white patch, which then develops a central erythematous atrophic zone and enlarges centrifugally. Approximately one-third of patients with **fissured tongue** (see page 11) are affected with erythema migrans as well. Some patients may have only a solitary lesion, but this is uncommon. The lesions are usually asymptomatic, although a burning sensation or sensitivity to hot or spicy foods may be noted when the lesions are active. Only rarely is the burning sensation more constant and severe.

Very infrequently, erythema migrans may occur on oral mucosal sites other than the tongue. In these instances, the tongue is almost always affected; however, other lesions develop on the buccal mucosa, on the labial mucosa, and (less frequently) on the soft palate or floor of the mouth (Figs. 16.87 and 16.88). These lesions typically produce no symptoms and can be identified by a yellow-white serpentine or scalloped border that surrounds an erythematous zone. These features should prevent confusion with such conditions as candidiasis or erythroplakia.

Histopathologic Features

If a biopsy specimen of the peripheral region of erythema migrans is examined, a characteristic histopathologic pattern is observed. Hyperparakeratosis, spongiosis, acanthosis, and elongation of the epithelial rete ridges are seen (Fig. 16.89). In addition, collections of neutrophils **(Munro abscesses)** are observed within the epithelium (Fig. 16.90); lymphocytes and neutrophils involve the lamina propria. The intense neutrophilic infiltrate may be responsible for the destruction of the superficial portion of the epithelium, thus producing an atrophic, reddened mucosa as the lesion progresses. Because these histopathologic features are reminiscent of **psoriasis,** this is called a **psoriasiform mucositis.** Despite the apparent lack of association between dermatologic conditions and erythema migrans in some reports, at least one case-control study of psoriatic patients showed that erythema migrans occurred at a rate of about 10%; only 2.5% of an age-matched and sex-matched population were affected. A Brazilian study determined that both patients with psoriasis and those with benign migratory glossitis were more likely to have the same human

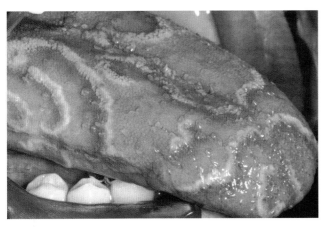
• **Fig. 16.86 Erythema Migrans.** Striking involvement of the dorsal and lateral surfaces of the tongue.

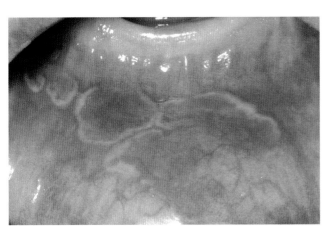
• **Fig. 16.87 Erythema Migrans.** Lesions of the lower labial mucosa.

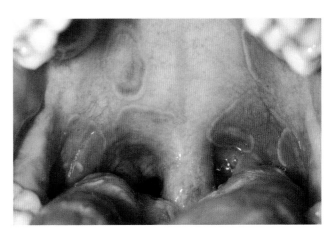
• **Fig. 16.88 Erythema Migrans.** These palatal lesions show well-demarcated erythematous areas surrounded by a white border, similar to the process involving the tongue.

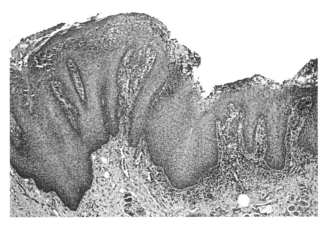
• **Fig. 16.89 Erythema Migrans.** This low-power photomicrograph shows the elongation of the rete ridges with parakeratosis and neutrophilic infiltration. Such features are also common in psoriasis, which explains why this is known as a *psoriasiform mucositis.*

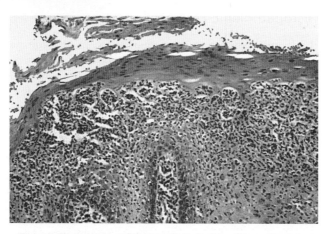

• **Fig. 16.90 Erythema Migrans.** This medium-power photomicrograph shows collections of neutrophils in the superficial spinous layer of the epithelium.

leukocyte antigen (HLA) group, namely HLA-Cw6. In addition, a Croatian study found that patients with erythema migrans, compared to a control group with no oral lesions, were statistically more likely to have celiac disease, a gluten-sensitive enteropathy. Whether these findings mean that erythema migrans represents oral psoriasis or oral celiac disease is debatable. It may simply reflect an immunologic milieu that predisposes patients to be more susceptible to developing erythema migrans.

Treatment and Prognosis

Generally no treatment is indicated for patients with erythema migrans. Reassuring the patient that the condition is completely benign is often all that is necessary. Infrequently, patients may complain of tenderness or a burning sensation that is so severe that it disrupts their lifestyle. In such cases, topical corticosteroids, such as fluocinonide or betamethasone gel, may provide relief when applied as a thin film several times a day to the lesional areas.

◆ REACTIVE ARTHRITIS (REITER SYNDROME)

Reactive arthritis represents a group of uncommon diseases that most likely have an immunologically mediated cause. Current evidence suggests that these disorders may be triggered by any one of several infectious agents in a genetically susceptible person. In some instances, the arthritis will be accompanied by mucocutaneous findings, including oral lesions. A classic triad of signs has been described:
1. Nongonococcal urethritis
2. Arthritis
3. Conjunctivitis

However, most patients do not exhibit all three of these signs. Although reactive arthritis with a mucocutaneous component is also known as **Reiter syndrome,** some authors have advocated removing the *Reiter* eponym because of Hans Reiter's Nazi criminal activities during World War II, and he was not the first to describe this syndrome.

It is interesting that reactive arthritis has been reported with some frequency in patients infected with the human immunodeficiency virus (HIV).

Clinical Features

Reactive arthritis is particularly prevalent in young adult men. In some series, a male-to-female ratio of up to 9:1 has been reported. The majority (60%–80%) of these patients are positive for HLA-B27, a haplotype present in only 10% of the population. The syndrome usually develops 1–4 weeks after an episode of dysentery or venereal disease; in fact, two French physicians published a description of this entity affecting four postdysenteric soldiers 1 week before Reiter's paper appeared.

Urethritis is often the first sign and is seen in both affected males and females. Females may also have inflammation of the uterine cervix. Conjunctivitis usually appears concurrently with the urethritis, and after several days, arthritis ensues. The arthritis usually affects the joints of the lower extremities, although TMJ involvement has been identified in one-third of these patients, typically as erosion of the condylar head. Skin lesions often take the form of a characteristic lesion of the glans penis **(balanitis circinata).** These lesions develop in about 20%–30% of patients with reactive arthritis, and they appear as well-circumscribed erythematous erosions with a scalloped, whitish linear boundary.

The oral lesions, which occur in slightly less than 20% of patients with this disorder, are described in various ways. Some reports mention painless erythematous papules distributed on the buccal mucosa and palate; other reports describe shallow, painless ulcers that affect the tongue, buccal mucosa, palate, and gingiva. Some authors have even implied that **geographic tongue** may be a component of reactive arthritis, probably because geographic tongue bears a superficial resemblance to the lesions of balanitis circinata.

The American Rheumatism Association has defined reactive arthritis based on the clinical findings of a peripheral arthritis that lasts longer than 1 month in conjunction with urethritis, cervicitis, or both.

Histopathologic Features

The histopathologic findings of the cutaneous lesions in patients with reactive arthritis are frequently similar to those found in patients with **psoriasis,** particularly with respect to the presence of microabscesses within the superficial layers of the surface epithelium. Other features in common with psoriasis include hyperparakeratosis with elongated, thin rete ridges.

Treatment and Prognosis

Some patients with reactive arthritis experience spontaneous resolution of their disease after 3–12 months, but many others have chronic symptoms that may wax and wane. Treatment may not be necessary for the milder cases. NSAIDs are initially used for managing arthritis, and sulfasalazine may be helpful in resolving cases that do not respond. Immunosuppressive or immune modulating agents, including corticosteroids, azathioprine, etanercept, and methotrexate, are reserved for the most resistant cases if they are not associated with HIV infection.

Physical therapy probably helps to reduce joint fibrosis associated with arthritis. About 15%–20% of patients with this disorder have severe disability, usually from arthritis.

◆ LICHEN PLANUS

Lichen planus is a relatively common, chronic dermatologic disease that often affects the oral mucosa. The strange name of the condition was provided by the British physician Erasmus Wilson, who first described it in 1869. Lichens are primitive plants composed of symbiotic algae and fungi. The term *planus* is Latin for *flat*. Wilson probably thought that the skin lesions looked similar enough to the lichens growing on rocks to merit this designation. Even though the term *lichen planus* suggests a flat, fungal condition, current evidence indicates that this is an immunologically mediated mucocutaneous disorder.

A variety of medications may induce lesions that can appear clinically very similar to the idiopathic form of the condition; however, the term **lichenoid mucositis (or lichenoid dermatitis,** depending on the site involved) is probably a better name for the drug-related alterations (see page 337). Similarly, foreign material that becomes inadvertently embedded in the gingiva may elicit a host response that is termed **lichenoid foreign body gingivitis** (see page 154). Reports of hepatitis C infection associated with oral lichen planus occasionally have appeared in the literature, usually from the Mediterranean countries, but this does not appear to be a significant association in the United States or Great Britain. More recent, carefully controlled epidemiologic studies do not appear to support an association of oral lichen planus with hepatitis C. However, genetic influences presumably may have an effect on the expression of lichen planus in select populations.

The relationship of stress or anxiety to the development of lichen planus is controversial, and most cited cases appear to be anecdotal or lack appropriate controls. Those studies that have applied psychologic questionnaires often find increased levels of anxiety in these patients; however, many patients who have been told that they have lichen planus are aware that anxiety has been linked to the disorder. Whether this awareness may influence the manner in which they answer the psychologic questionnaires could be debated. In one study that used psychologic questionnaires to attempt to resolve this question, patients with oral lichen planus had no greater degree of stress in their lives than did age-matched and sex-matched control patients. It might be that stress has no bearing on the pathogenesis of lichen planus; however, an alternative explanation might be that those patients who have lichen planus simply respond in this fashion to levels of stress that do not induce lesions in other people.

Recently some investigators have identified a link between hypothyroidism and oral lichen planus, including the

association of thyroid medication and oral lichen planus. Autoantibodies directed against thyroid tissue may also play a role in the pathogenesis of oral lichen planus in some patients.

Clinical Features

Most patients with lichen planus are middle-aged adults. It is rare for children to be affected. Women predominate in most series of cases, usually by a 3:2 ratio over men. Approximately 1% of the population may have cutaneous lichen planus. The prevalence of oral lichen planus is between 0.1% and 2.2%.

The skin lesions of lichen planus have been classically described as purple, pruritic, polygonal papules (Fig. 16.91). These usually affect the flexor surfaces of the extremities. Excoriations may not be visible, despite the fact that the lesions itch, because it hurts the patient when he or she scratches them.

Careful examination of the surface of the skin papules reveals a fine, lacelike network of white lines **(Wickham striae)** (Fig. 16.92). Other sites of extraoral involvement include the glans penis, the vulvar mucosa, and the nails. Essentially there are two forms of oral lesions: reticular and erosive.

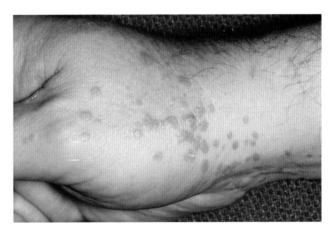

• **Fig. 16.91 Lichen Planus.** The cutaneous lesions on the wrist appear as purple, polygonal papules.

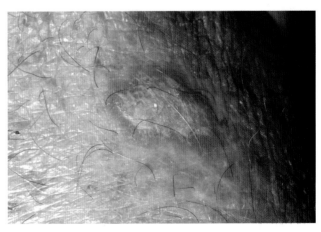

• **Fig. 16.92 Lichen Planus.** Closer view of a skin lesion of lichen planus. Careful examination shows a network of fine white lines (Wickham striae) on the surface of the papules.

Reticular Lichen Planus

Reticular lichen planus is much more common than the erosive form, but the erosive form predominates in several studies. This is probably because of referral bias (because the erosive form is symptomatic and, therefore, the patient is more likely to be referred to an academic center for evaluation). The reticular form usually causes no symptoms and involves the posterior buccal mucosa bilaterally (Fig. 16.93). Post-inflammatory melanosis occasionally accompanies the reticular striae, particularly in persons of color (Fig. 16.94). Other oral mucosal surfaces may also be involved concurrently, such as the lateral and dorsal tongue, the gingivae, the palate, and vermilion border (Fig. 16.95).

Reticular lichen planus is thus named because of its characteristic pattern of interlacing white lines (also referred to as *Wickham striae*); however, the white lesions may appear as papules in some instances. These lesions are typically not static but wax and wane over weeks or months (Fig. 16.96). The reticular pattern may not be as evident in some sites, such as the dorsal tongue, where the lesions appear more as

keratotic plaques with atrophy of the papillae (Fig. 16.97). In addition, superficial mucoceles may develop within, or adjacent to, mucosal areas that are involved by lichen planus.

Erosive Lichen Planus

Erosive lichen planus, although not as common as the reticular form, is more significant for the patient because the lesions are usually symptomatic. Clinically, there are atrophic, erythematous areas with central ulceration of varying degrees. The periphery of the atrophic regions is usually bordered by fine, white radiating striae (Figs. 16.98 and 16.99). Sometimes the atrophy and ulceration are confined to the gingival mucosa, producing the reaction pattern called **desquamative gingivitis** (see page 155) (Fig. 16.100). In such cases, biopsy specimens should be obtained for light microscopic and immunofluorescent studies of perilesional tissue, because mucous membrane pemphigoid (see page 775) and pemphigus vulgaris (see page 769) may appear in a similar fashion.

If the erosive component is severe, epithelial separation from the underlying connective tissue may occur. This results in the relatively rare presentation of **bullous lichen planus.**

Histopathologic Features

The histopathologic features of lichen planus are characteristic but may not be specific, because other conditions, such as **lichenoid drug reaction, lichenoid amalgam reaction, lichenoid foreign body gingivitis, oral graft-versus-host disease (GVHD), lupus erythematosus (LE), chronic ulcerative stomatitis, oral mucosal cinnamon reaction,** and the incipient phase of **proliferative verrucous leukoplakia** may also show a similar histopathologic pattern. Varying degrees of orthokeratosis and parakeratosis may be present on the surface of the epithelium, depending on whether the biopsy specimen is taken from an erosive or reticular lesion.

The thickness of the spinous layer can also vary. The rete ridges may be absent or hyperplastic, but they classically have a pointed or "saw-toothed" shape (Fig. 16.101).

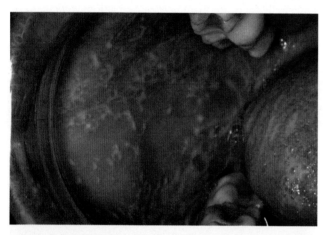

• **Fig. 16.93 Lichen Planus.** The interlacing white lines and papules are typical of reticular lichen planus involving the buccal mucosa, the most common site of oral involvement.

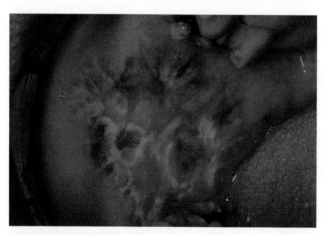

• **Fig. 16.94 Lichen Planus.** In persons of color who develop lichen planus, it is not unusual to see patchy areas of reactive (benign) melanosis develop in the lesions, presumably due to stimulation of the melanocytes in this area by the inflammatory cells that cause this condition.

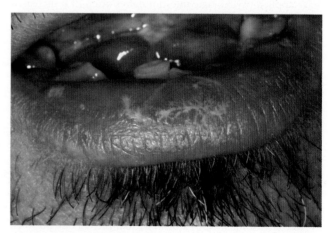

• **Fig. 16.95 Lichen Planus.** Reticular lesions of the lower lip vermilion.

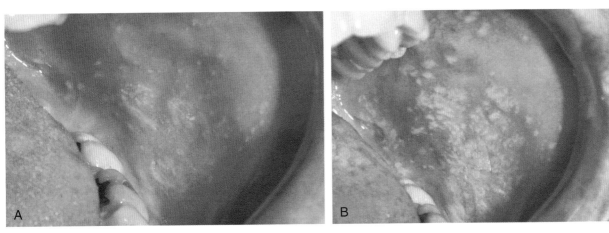

• **Fig. 16.96 Lichen Planus. A,** A middle-aged woman with mild reticular lichen planus of the left buccal mucosa. **B,** Same patient 2 weeks later, showing exacerbation of the lesions. Such waxing and waning is characteristic of lichen planus.

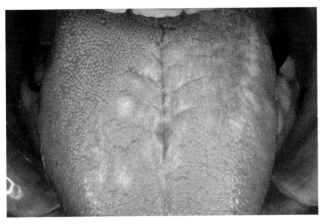

• **Fig. 16.97 Lichen Planus.** With involvement of the dorsal tongue by reticular lichen planus, the characteristic interlacing striae seen in the buccal mucosal lesions are usually not present. Instead, smooth white plaques are typically observed replacing the normal papillary surface of the tongue.

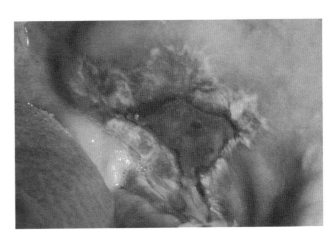

• **Fig. 16.98 Lichen Planus.** Ulceration of the buccal mucosa shows peripheral radiating keratotic striae, characteristic of oral erosive lichen planus.

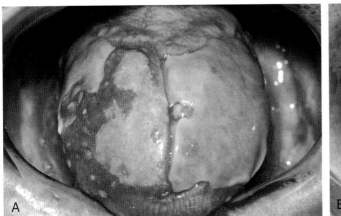

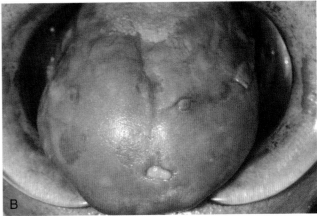

• **Fig. 16.99 Lichen Planus. A,** The dorsal surface of the tongue shows extensive ulceration caused by erosive lichen planus. Note the fine white streaks at the periphery of the ulcerations. **B,** Same patient after systemic corticosteroid therapy. Much of the mucosa has reepithelialized, with only focal ulcerations remaining.

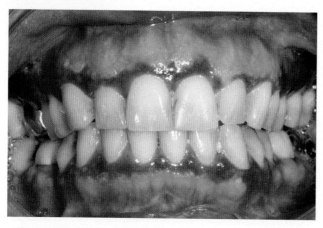

• **Fig. 16.100 Lichen Planus.** Erosive lichen planus often appears as a desquamative gingivitis, producing gingival erythema and tenderness.

Destruction of the basal cell layer of the epithelium **(hydropic degeneration)** is also evident. This is accompanied by an intense, bandlike infiltrate of predominantly T lymphocytes immediately subjacent to the epithelium (Fig. 16.102). Degenerating keratinocytes may be seen in the area of the epithelium and connective tissue interface and have been termed **colloid, cytoid, hyaline,** or **Civatte bodies.** No significant degree of epithelial atypia is expected in oral lichen planus, although lesions having a superimposed candidal infection may appear worrisome. These should be reevaluated histopathologically after the candidal infection is treated. On occasion, the chronic inflammatory host response to the atypical cells of **epithelial dysplasia** can appear virtually indistinguishable histopathologically from lichen planus, particularly in milder cases of epithelial dysplasia. Such ambiguity may contribute to the controversy related to the malignant transformation potential of lichen planus.

The immunopathologic features of lichen planus are nonspecific. Most lesions show the deposition of a shaggy band of fibrinogen at the basement membrane zone, however a similar pattern of fibrinogen deposition can be found with epithelial dysplasia.

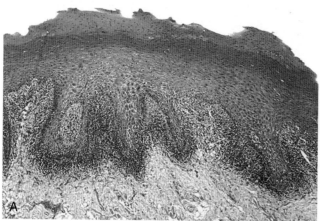
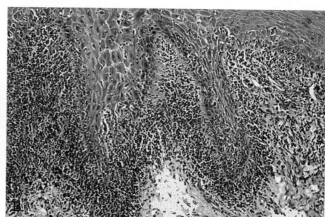

• **Fig. 16.101 Lichen Planus. A,** This low-power photomicrograph of an oral lesion shows hyperkeratosis, saw-toothed rete ridges, and a bandlike infiltrate of lymphocytes immediately subjacent to the epithelium. **B,** Higher-power view showing migration of lymphocytes into the lower epithelium with interface degeneration of the basal cell layer.

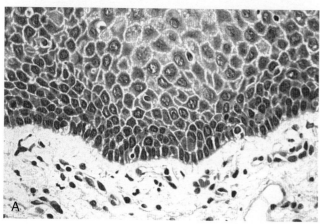
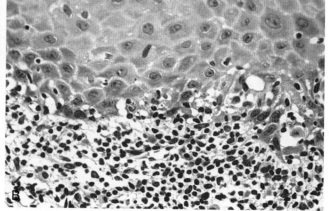

• **Fig. 16.102 Lichen Planus. A,** High-power photomicrograph of normal epithelium showing an intact basal cell layer and no inflammation. **B,** High-power photomicrograph of lichen planus showing degeneration of the basal epithelial layer and an intense lymphocytic infiltrate in the superficial lamina propria.

Diagnosis

The diagnosis of **reticular lichen planus** can often be made based on the clinical findings alone. The interlacing white striae appearing bilaterally on the posterior buccal mucosa are virtually pathognomonic, however if the clinical features are not completely characteristic, biopsy would be appropriate. In addition, difficulties in diagnosis may arise if candidiasis is superimposed on the lesions because the organism may alter the characteristic reticular pattern of the lichen planus (Fig. 16.103).

Erosive lichen planus is sometimes more challenging to diagnose (based on clinical features alone) than the reticular form. If the typical radiating white striae and erythematous, atrophic mucosa are present at the periphery of well-demarcated ulcerations on the posterior buccal mucosa bilaterally, then the clinician may certainly consider a diagnosis of erosive lichen planus. However, a biopsy may be necessary to rule out other ulcerative or erosive diseases, such as lupus erythematosus or chronic ulcerative stomatitis. If the diagnosis is still in question, then direct immunofluorescence studies sometimes prove helpful in distinguishing between these diseases.

Specimens of isolated erosive lichenoid lesions, particularly those of the soft palate, the lateral and ventral tongue, or the floor of the mouth, should be obtained for biopsy to rule out premalignant changes or malignancy. Another condition that may mimic an isolated lesion of lichen planus, both clinically and histopathologically, is a **lichenoid reaction to dental amalgam** (see page 346).

Treatment and Prognosis

Reticular lichen planus typically produces no symptoms, and no treatment is needed. Occasionally, affected patients may have superimposed candidiasis, in which case they may complain of a burning sensation of the oral mucosa at the site of the lesion. Antifungal therapy is necessary in such a case. Some investigators recommend annual reevaluation of the reticular lesions of oral lichen planus.

Erosive lichen planus is often bothersome because of the open sores in the mouth. Because it is an immunologically mediated condition, corticosteroids are recommended. The lesions respond to systemic corticosteroids, but such drastic therapy is usually not necessary. One of the stronger topical corticosteroids (e.g., fluocinonide, betamethasone, or clobetasol gel) applied as a thin film several times per day to the most symptomatic areas is usually sufficient to induce healing within 1 or 2 weeks. The patient should be warned that the condition will undoubtedly flare up again, in which case the corticosteroids should be reapplied. In addition, the possibility of iatrogenic candidiasis associated with corticosteroid use should be monitored (Fig. 16.104). Some investigators have recommended compounding corticosteroid ointments with an adhesive methylcellulose base, but patient compliance may be reduced because this material is difficult to apply. Although the use of other agents (such as, topical retinoids, tacrolimus, mycophenolate mofetil, or cyclosporine) has occasionally been advocated for recalcitrant cases of erosive lichen planus, reports of their efficacy have usually been limited to small series of cases or have been contradictory. Furthermore, their side effects can be significant, and in the case of tacrolimus or cyclosporine, the cost of the drug may be prohibitive. Some investigators suggest that patients with oral erosive lichen planus be evaluated every 3–6 months, particularly if the lesions are not typical.

The question of the malignant potential of lichen planus, particularly the erosive form, is yet to be resolved. Most cases of reported malignant transformation are rather poorly documented. Some of these reported cases may not have been true lichen planus, but rather they may have actually been dysplastic leukoplakias with a secondary lichenoid inflammatory infiltrate that mimicked lichen planus, such as proliferative verrucous leukoplakia. In addition, the argument can be made that because both lichen planus and squamous cell

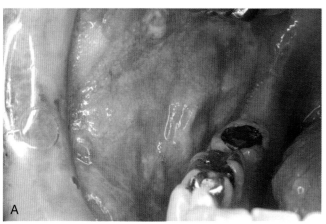 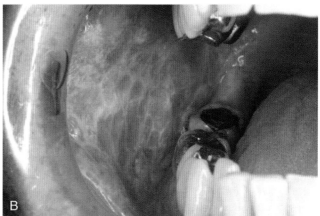

• **Fig. 16.103 Lichen Planus. A,** These relatively nondescript white lesions affected the buccal mucosa of a patient who had complained of a burning sensation. Histopathologic evaluation of the lesion showed a lichenoid mucositis with superimposed candidiasis. **B,** Same patient 2 weeks after antifungal therapy. Once the mucosal reaction to the candidal organism was eliminated, the characteristic white striae of reticular lichen planus were identified.

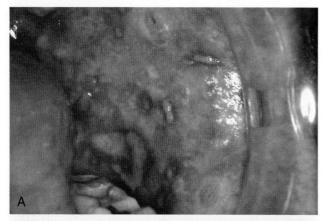

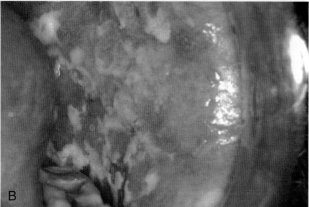

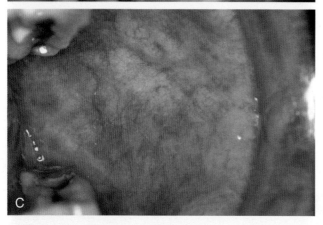

• **Fig. 16.104** Lichen Planus. **A,** This patient was diagnosed with erosive lichen planus affecting the buccal mucosa and was treated with topical corticosteroids. **B,** Same patient 2 weeks later. The creamy-white plaques of pseudomembranous candidiasis have developed as a result of the corticosteroid therapy. **C,** Same patient after antifungal therapy. At this point, he was asymptomatic.

of oral epithelial dysplasia, squamous cell carcinoma, normal oral mucosa, and oral reactive lesions. The molecular profile of oral lichen planus more closely resembled that of normal or reactive oral mucosa, a finding that provides less support for the concept of lichen planus being precancerous. Another study evaluated the malignant transformation rate of typical oral lichen planus compared with oral "lichenoid" lesions. The lichenoid lesions had some features of lichen planus, but were not completely representative, either clinically or histopathologically, of that disease. These investigators found that there was no transformation of characteristic lichen planus, although several of the "lichenoid" lesions developed into squamous cell carcinoma. Additional prospective clinical studies with strict clinical and histopathologic criteria for the definition of oral lichen planus will need to be performed to resolve this question. If the potential for malignant transformation exists, then it appears to be small. Most of the reported cases have been confined to patients with either the erosive or so-called plaque-type form of lichen planus.

◆ CHRONIC ULCERATIVE STOMATITIS

Chronic ulcerative stomatitis is another immune-mediated disorder that affects the oral mucosa. This condition was initially described in 1990, and slightly more than 70 cases have been reported. Although the precise pathogenetic mechanisms are unknown, these patients develop autoantibodies against a 70-kDa nuclear protein, $\Delta Np63\alpha$, an isoform of p63, and *in vitro* studies suggest that these antibodies play a role in development of this disease by interrupting the normal maintenance of the epithelium/connective tissue interface.

The prevalence of this disease may be more common than is realized. Because of its clinical similarity to erosive lichen planus, it is possible that only a clinical diagnosis is made when an affected patient is encountered, and a biopsy is not performed. Even if a biopsy is done, the tissue is often submitted for routine light microscopy alone, and the direct immunofluorescence studies that are required for its diagnosis are not ordered. Distinction from lichen planus should be made because chronic ulcerative stomatitis typically does not respond as well to corticosteroid therapy, and just as is the case with lupus erythematosus (LE), chronic ulcerative stomatitis has been reported to improve using antimalarial drugs.

Clinical Features

Chronic ulcerative stomatitis usually affects adult women, and the mean age at diagnosis is late in the sixth decade of life. The condition may appear as desquamative gingivitis, although ulcerations or erosions of the tongue or buccal mucosa are also quite common (Fig. 16.105). The ulcers are generally surrounded by patchy zones of erythema and streaky keratosis that somewhat resemble lichen planus, although classic striae formation usually is not evident. The ulcers heal without scarring and often migrate around

carcinoma are not rare, some people may have both problems simultaneously, and the two processes may be unrelated to one another. Conversely, some investigators say that the atrophic epithelium of lichen planus may be more susceptible to the action of carcinogens, resulting in an increased risk of malignant transformation. Two studies have examined the molecular characteristics of classic reticular lichen planus, comparing the loss of heterozygosity at purported tumor suppressor gene loci in these lesions with that of varying grades

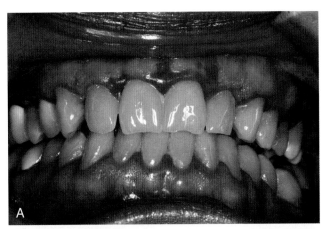

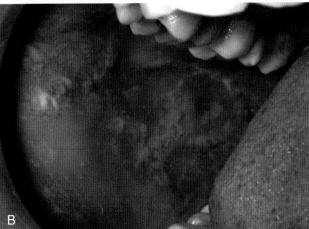

• **Fig. 16.105 Chronic Ulcerative Stomatitis. A,** Gingival lesions having a "desquamative gingivitis" presentation, requiring biopsy with direct immunofluorescence studies for diagnosis. **B,** Buccal mucosal involvement. The lesions appear somewhat lichenoid, although classic Wickham striae are not evident.

the oral mucosa. As is typical with most immune-mediated conditions, the severity of the oral lesions tends to wax and wane. Fewer than 20% of affected patients will develop concurrent lichenoid skin lesions.

Histopathologic Features

Although the histopathologic features of chronic ulcerative stomatitis are similar to those of lichen planus, the epithelium is generally more atrophic and the inflammatory infiltrate usually contains significant numbers of plasma cells in addition to lymphocytes (Fig. 16.106). Artifactual epithelial separation from the underlying connective tissue is not unusual.

Diagnosis

The diagnosis of chronic ulcerative stomatitis is essentially based on its characteristic immunopathologic pattern. Although it may not be economically feasible to do immunologic testing on every case of lichen planus, this procedure should be considered for erosive lichenoid lesions that do not have a characteristic appearance or distribution, as well as for erosive lesions that do not respond to topical corticosteroid therapy. With direct immunofluorescence studies, autoantibodies (usually IgG) that are directed against the nuclei of stratified squamous epithelial cells in the basal and parabasal regions of the epithelium are detected (Fig. 16.107). Indirect immunofluorescence studies are also positive for these stratified epithelium-specific antinuclear antibodies (ANAs), and some investigators believe that confirmation of the diagnosis is necessary using serum for indirect immunofluorescence evaluation. An ELISA test has been developed, and if it becomes commercially available, this should make screening for this condition much more cost-effective. Other immune-mediated conditions (e.g., systemic sclerosis and LE) may show ANA deposition with direct immunofluorescence; however, nuclei throughout the entire thickness of the epithelium are positive with those diseases.

Treatment and Prognosis

Unlike the lesions of erosive lichen planus, the lesions associated with chronic ulcerative stomatitis may not respond as well to topical or systemic corticosteroid therapy. If the

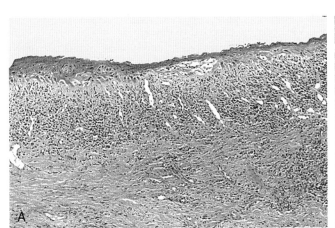

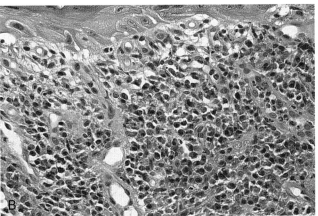

• **Fig. 16.106 Chronic Ulcerative Stomatitis. A,** Low-power photomicrograph showing epithelial atrophy with a heavy chronic inflammatory cell infiltrate in the superficial lamina propria. **B,** High-power photomicrograph showing interface degeneration of the basilar epithelium in association with the inflammation. Unlike lichen planus, this infiltrate includes numerous plasma cells, as well as lymphocytes.

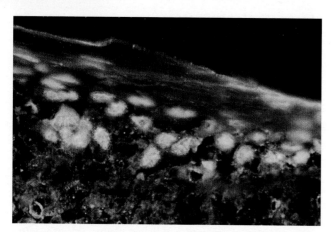

• **Fig. 16.107 Chronic Ulcerative Stomatitis.** Direct immunofluorescence studies show presence of IgG in the basal and parabasal epithelial nuclei.

lesions are not adequately controlled with corticosteroids, then management with hydroxychloroquine, an antimalarial drug, should be considered. Hydroxychloroquine therapy, however, requires both periodic ophthalmologic evaluation to monitor for drug-related retinopathy and periodic hematologic evaluation.

◆ GRAFT-VERSUS-HOST DISEASE

Graft-versus-host disease (GVHD) occurs mainly in recipients of allogeneic bone marrow transplantation, a procedure performed on approximately 8000 patients in the United States each year. Such transplants are performed at major medical centers to treat life-threatening diseases of the blood or bone marrow, such as leukemia, lymphoma, multiple myeloma, aplastic anemia, thalassemia, sickle cell anemia, or disseminated metastatic disease. Cytotoxic drugs, radiation, or both may be used to destroy the malignant cells, but in the process the normal hematopoietic cells of the patient are destroyed. To provide the patient with an immune system, an HLA-matched donor must be found. The donor supplies hematopoietic stem cells obtained from bone marrow, peripheral blood, or umbilical cord blood. These stem cells are transfused into the patient, whose own hematopoietic and immune cells have been destroyed. The transfused hematopoietic cells make their way to the recipient's bone marrow and begin to reestablish normal function.

Unfortunately, the HLA match is not always exact, and despite the use of immunomodulating and immunosuppressive drugs (such as, cyclosporine, methotrexate, and prednisone), the engrafted cells often recognize that they are not in their native environment. When this happens, these cells start attacking what they perceive as a foreign body. The result of this attack is GVHD, and it can be quite devastating to the patient.

In recent years, oncologists have taken advantage of this type of immunologic attack when treating leukemia patients, and often a beneficial "graft-versus-leukemia" effect is seen when the donor cells interpret the leukemic cells as being foreign. For older patients, who tend to have more significant side effects with traditional bone marrow transplantation, the concept of a "mini-allograft" has been developed. Not all of the patient's white blood cells (WBCs) are destroyed in this procedure, which is also known as *nonmyeloablative allogenic hematopoietic cell transplantation,* to allow the donor cells to mount a more aggressive assault on the patient's leukemic cells.

Autologous stem cell transplantation has also become an increasingly popular method of treatment for some of these life-threatening diseases. Because these cells are derived from the patient, there is no risk of GVHD in this setting.

Clinical Features

The systemic signs of GVHD are varied, depending on the organ system involved and whether the problem is acute or chronic. The severity of GVHD depends on several factors, with milder disease seen in patients who have a better histocompatibility match, are younger, have received cord blood, and are female. In addition, wide ranges in the percentage of patients who develop GVHD and its oral manifestations are to be expected, given the variety of disorders that are treated with bone marrow transplantation and the spectrum of conditioning regimens.

Acute GVHD is typically observed within the first few weeks after bone marrow transplantation. Although acute GVHD has arbitrarily been defined as occurring within 100 days after the procedure, most investigators make this diagnosis based on the clinical features rather than a specific time point. The disease affects about 50% of bone marrow transplant patients. The skin lesions that develop may range from a mild rash to a diffuse severe sloughing that resembles toxic epidermal necrolysis (see page 783). These signs may be accompanied by diarrhea, nausea, vomiting, abdominal pain, and liver dysfunction.

Chronic GVHD may represent a continuation of a previously diagnosed case of acute GVHD, or it may develop later than 100 days after bone marrow transplantation, sometimes not appearing for several years after the procedure. Chronic GVHD can be expected to develop in 30% to 70% of bone marrow transplant recipients, and it often mimics any one of a variety of autoimmune conditions, such as systemic lupus erythematosus (SLE), Sjögren syndrome, or primary biliary cirrhosis. Skin involvement, which is the most common manifestation, may resemble lichen planus or even systemic sclerosis.

The oral mucosal manifestations of GVHD can also vary, depending on the duration and severity of the attack and the targeted oral tissues. Of patients with acute GVHD, 33%–75% will have oral involvement; of patients with chronic GVHD, 80% or more will have oral lesions. Sometimes the oral lesions of GVHD are the only sign of the disorder. In most patients with oral GVHD, there is a fine, reticular network of white striae that resembles oral lichen planus, although a more diffuse pattern of pinpoint white papules has also been described (Figs. 16.108–16.110). The tongue, the gingivae, the labial mucosa, and the buccal mucosa are the oral mucosal sites most frequently involved. Patients often complain of a burning sensation of the oral mucosa, and care must be taken not to overlook possible candidiasis. Atrophy of the oral mucosa may be present, and this can contribute to the mucosal discomfort. Ulcerations that are

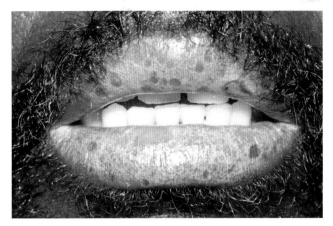

• Fig. 16.108 **Graft-Versus-Host Disease (GVHD).** Confluent, interlacing white linear lesions of the vermilion zone superficially resemble oral lichen planus.

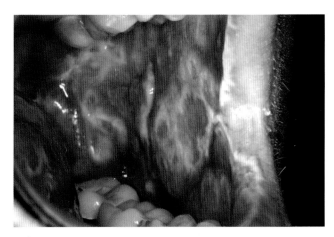

• Fig. 16.109 **Graft-Versus-Host Disease (GVHD).** Lichenoid and erosive lesions of the left buccal mucosa.

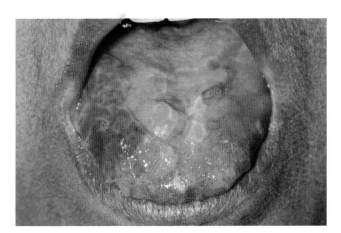

• Fig. 16.110 **Graft-Versus-Host Disease (GVHD).** Involvement of the tongue showing erosions and ulcerations that resemble erosive lichen planus.

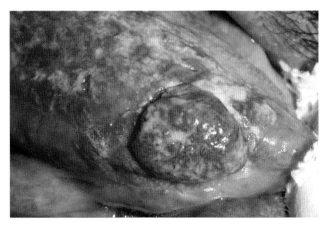

• Fig. 16.111 **Squamous Cell Carcinoma Arising in Graft-Versus-Host Disease (GVHD).** Erythematous, ulcerated mass arising on the lateral border of the tongue. Note the surrounding mucosal erosions, which represent GVHD.

related to the chemotherapeutic conditioning and neutropenic state of the patient often develop during the first 2 weeks after bone marrow transplantation. Ulcers that persist longer than 2 weeks may represent acute GVHD, and these should be differentiated from intraoral herpesvirus infection or bacterial infection. Bone marrow transplant patients have a small but increased risk for the development of both oral and cutaneous epithelial dysplasia and squamous cell carcinoma. Demarcated white or red plaques of the oral mucosa that do not have the characteristic lichenoid features should be biopsied to rule out preneoplastic or neoplastic changes (Fig. 16.111).

Xerostomia is also a common complaint. If the patient is not taking drugs that dry the mouth, it is likely that the immunologic response is destroying the salivary gland tissue. Other evidence of salivary gland involvement includes the development of small superficial mucoceles, particularly on the soft palate.

Histopathologic Features

The histopathologic features of GVHD resemble those of oral lichen planus to a certain degree. Both lesions display hyperorthokeratosis, short and pointed rete ridges, and degeneration of the basal cell layer. The inflammatory response in GVHD is usually not as intense as in lichen planus. With advanced cases, an abnormal deposition of collagen is present, similar to the pattern in systemic sclerosis. Minor salivary gland tissue usually shows periductal inflammation in the early stages, with gradual acinar destruction and extensive periductal fibrosis appearing later.

Diagnosis

The diagnosis of GVHD may be difficult because of the varied clinical manifestations. Such a diagnosis is of great clinical significance to the patient because complications of the condition and its treatment may be lethal. Although the diagnosis of GVHD is based on the clinical and histopathologic findings, each patient may have a different constellation of signs and symptoms. Oral lesions appear to have value as a highly predictive index of the presence of GVHD.

Treatment and Prognosis

The primary strategy for dealing with GVHD is to reduce or prevent its occurrence. Careful tissue histocompatibility matching is performed, and the patient is given prophylactic therapy with immunomodulatory and immunosuppressive agents, such as prednisone in combination with either cyclosporine or tacrolimus. If GVHD develops, then the doses of these drugs may be increased or similar pharmacologic agents may be added, although detailed description of the medical management of systemic GVHD is beyond the scope of this text. Suffice it to say that a wide range of treatment modalities are available and their selection and frequency of use varies among tertiary care centers. A partial list would include mycophenolate mofetil, azathioprine, extracorporeal photopheresis, mTOR inhibitors (sirolimus and everolimus), JAK inhibitors (ruxolitinib and tofacitinib), and anti-CD20 monoclonal antibody (rituximab) .

With respect to oral lesions, topical corticosteroids may facilitate the healing of focal oral ulcerations associated with GVHD, and some reports have suggested that topical tacrolimus may be useful in managing ulcers that are resistant to corticosteroids. Topical anesthetic agents are administered to provide patient comfort while the lesions are present, although narcotic analgesics may be required in some cases. The use of **p**soralen and **u**ltra**v**iolet **A** (PUVA) therapy also has been shown to improve the cutaneous and oral lesions of patients with the lichenoid form of GVHD. If significant xerostomia is present in a dentulous patient, then topical fluorides should be used daily to prevent xerostomia-related caries. If significant amounts of salivary acinar tissue remain, then treatment with pilocarpine hydrochloride or cevimeline hydrochloride may improve the salivary flow. Current recommendations are to evaluate the oral status of patients before bone marrow transplantation and eliminate any potential sources of infection. Interestingly, one study showed no differences in posttransplant infections or survival between a group of patients who received dental treatment before their transplant and a group who did not.

In general, some degree of GVHD is expected in most allogeneic bone marrow transplant recipients. The prognosis depends on the extent to which the condition progresses and whether or not it can be controlled. The significance of this complication is reflected in the survival of more than 70% of patients with relatively mild GVHD at 6 years posttransplant, compared with approximately 15% of patients with severe GVHD.

◆ PSORIASIS

Psoriasis is a common chronic skin disease affecting approximately 3% of people in the United States. According to some estimates, roughly 8 million people in this country have psoriasis, and more than 250,000 new cases are diagnosed each year.

Psoriasis is characterized by an increased proliferative activity of the cutaneous keratinocytes. Recent advances in cell kinetics, immunology, and molecular biology have increased the understanding of the etiopathogenesis of the keratinocyte proliferation in this disorder. Although the triggering agent has yet to be identified, activated T lymphocytes appear to orchestrate a complex scenario that includes abnormal production of cytokines, adhesion molecules, chemotactic polypeptides, and growth factors. Genetic factors also seem to play a role, because as many as one-third of these patients have affected relatives. Currently nine different genetic loci have been identified that may be related to the development of psoriasis. If one twin in a set of identical twins has psoriasis, there is a 35%–72% chance that the other twin will have it. This suggests that genetic factors are not entirely responsible for the condition, and that one or more unidentified environmental agents must influence its pathogenesis.

Clinical Features

Psoriasis often has its onset during the second or third decade of life and tends to persist for years, with periods of exacerbation and quiescence. Patients frequently report that the lesions improve during the summer and worsen during the winter, an observation that may be related to lesional exposure to UV light. The lesions are typically symmetrically distributed in certain favored locations, such as the scalp, elbows, and knees. The classic description is a well-demarcated, erythematous plaque with a silvery scale on its surface (Fig. 16.112). The lesions are often asymptomatic, but it is not unusual for a patient to complain of itching—in fact, the term *psoriasis* is

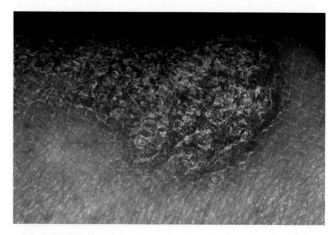

• **Fig. 16.112 Psoriasis.** Characteristic cutaneous lesion, characterized by an erythematous plaque surmounted by silvery keratotic scales.

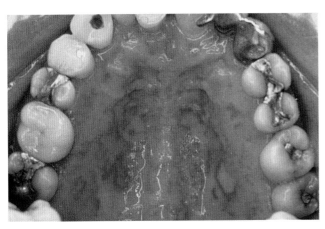

• **Fig. 16.113 Psoriasis.** This is an example of relatively rare involvement of the oral mucosa by psoriasis. The erythematous linear patches tended to flare with the patient's cutaneous lesions. (Courtesy of Dr. George Blozis.)

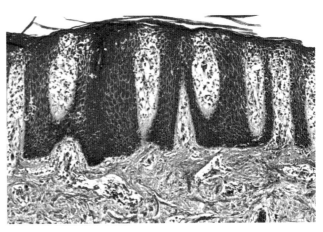

• **Fig. 16.114 Psoriasis.** Low-power photomicrograph showing elongation of the rete ridges, hyperkeratosis, and inflammation of the papillary dermis.

derived from the Greek word for itching. An unfortunate complication affecting approximately 25%–30% of these patients is **psoriatic arthritis,** which may involve the TMJ. Other co-morbidities that have been described in patients with psoriasis include inflammatory bowel disease, non-alcoholic liver disease, mood disorders, and cardiovascular disease. A recent study found that periodontitis is more prevalent among psoriatic patients as well.

Oral lesions may occur in patients with psoriasis, but they are distinctly uncommon. Because descriptions of these lesions have ranged from white plaques to red plaques to ulcerations, it is difficult to determine the true nature of intraoral psoriasis (Fig. 16.113). To render a diagnosis of intraoral psoriasis, some investigators say that the activity of the oral lesions should parallel that of the cutaneous lesions. Some authors refer to **erythema migrans** (see page 784) as *intraoral psoriasis,* and the prevalence of erythema migrans in psoriatic patients appears to be slightly greater than that seen in the rest of the population. It is difficult, however, to prove a direct correlation of that common mucosal alteration with psoriasis.

Histopathologic Features

Microscopically, psoriasis has a characteristic pattern. The surface epithelium shows marked parakeratin production, and the epithelial rete ridges are elongated (Fig. 16.114). The connective tissue papillae, which contain dilated capillaries, approach close to the epithelial surface, and a perivascular chronic inflammatory cell infiltrate is present. In addition, collections of neutrophils **(Munro abscesses),** are seen within the parakeratin layer.

With respect to oral lesions, good correlation with skin disease activity should be seen in addition to the characteristic histopathologic features, because other intraoral lesions, such as erythema migrans and oral mucosal cinnamon reaction (see page 344), exhibit a psoriasiform microscopic appearance.

Treatment and Prognosis

The treatment of psoriasis depends on the severity of the disease activity, as well as the presence or absence of psoriatic arthritis. For mild lesions, which generally means that no more than 3%–5% of the skin surface is affected, no treatment may be necessary.

For patients with moderate skin involvement (5%–10% skin surface involvement), or for mild lesions that are bothersome or cosmetically unacceptable, topical corticosteroids are commonly prescribed in the United States. Coal tar derivatives and keratolytic agents also may be used. Other topical drugs that have proven effective include vitamin D_3 analogues (calcipotriene, calcipotriol, and calcitriol), and tazarotene, a retinoid (vitamin A) compound. Newer topical biologic agents include the calcineurin inhibitors, tacrolimus and pimecrolimus, although these are usually reserved for recalcitrant lesions. Exposure to UV radiation may also be helpful for mild to moderate disease.

The treatment approach related to moderate or severe (greater than 10% skin surface involvement) psoriasis has changed dramatically over the past several years and is continuing to evolve due to development of newer systemic biologic agents that target specific disease-related components of the psoriatic pathophysiologic pathways. A relatively brief listing would include certolizumab, infliximab, adalimumab, and etanercept (directed against tumor necrosis factor-alpha [TNF-α]); alefacept (directed against T-cell receptors); guselkumab, tildrakizumab-asmn, risankizumab-rzaa, and mirikizumab (directed against IL-23); secukinumab, ixekizumab, brodalumab, and bimekizumab (directed against IL-17); or ustekinumab (directed against IL-12 and IL-23). For severe cases, psoralen and ultraviolet A (PUVA) therapy or ultraviolet B (UVB) therapy may be needed. Methotrexate or cyclosporine may also be used as systemic treatments for severe disease; however, these drugs have significant side effects.

Although the mortality rate is not increased in patients with psoriasis, the condition often persists for years despite therapy. A 30-year prospective study has shown a definite increase in the risk for cutaneous squamous cell carcinoma in psoriasis patients who have received over 350 life-time

PUVA treatments, but those who received fewer than 150 had a very modest increase. Interestingly, the risk for development of basal cell carcinoma did not seem to be significantly elevated. Broad-band UV-B treatment has much less carcinogenic potential compared to PUVA, and narrow-band UV-B treatment has the least of the three phototherapies.

◆ LUPUS ERYTHEMATOSUS

Lupus erythematosus (LE) is a classic example of an immunologically mediated condition, and is the most common of the so-called collagen vascular or connective tissue diseases in the United States, with more than 1.5 million people affected. It may exhibit any one of several clinicopathologic forms.

Systemic lupus erythematosus (SLE) is a serious multisystem disease with a variety of cutaneous and oral manifestations. There is an increase in the activity of the humoral limb (B lymphocytes) of the immune system in conjunction with abnormal function of the T lymphocytes. Although genetic factors probably play a role in the pathogenesis of SLE, the precise cause is unknown. Undoubtedly, interplay between genetic and environmental factors occurs, for if SLE develops in one monozygotic (identical) twin, then the other twin has a 24% chance of having SLE as well. In contrast, if one dizygotic (fraternal) twin has SLE, then the other twin has only a 2% chance of being affected.

Chronic cutaneous lupus erythematosus (CCLE) may represent a different, but related, process. It primarily affects the skin and oral mucosa, and the prognosis is good.

Subacute cutaneous lupus erythematosus (SCLE) is a third form of the disease, which has clinical features intermediate between those of SLE and CCLE.

Clinical Features

Systemic Lupus Erythematosus

SLE can be a very difficult disease to diagnose in its early stages because it often appears in a nonspecific, vague fashion, frequently with periods of remission or disease inactivity. Women are affected nearly 8–10 times more frequently than men. The average age at diagnosis is 31 years. Common findings include fever, weight loss, arthritis, fatigue, and general malaise. In 40% to 50% of affected patients, a characteristic rash, having the pattern of a butterfly, develops over the malar area and nose (Fig. 16.115), typically sparing the nasolabial folds. Sunlight often makes the lesions worse.

The kidneys are affected in approximately 40%–50% of SLE patients. This complication may ultimately lead to kidney failure; thus it is typically the most significant aspect of the disease.

Cardiac involvement is also common, with pericarditis being the most frequent complication. At autopsy nearly 50% of SLE patients display warty vegetations affecting the heart valves **(Libman-Sacks endocarditis).** Its significance is debatable, although some patients may develop superimposed subacute bacterial endocarditis on these otherwise sterile outgrowths of fibrinoid material and connective tissue cells.

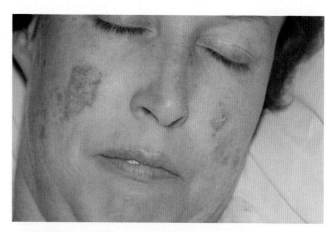

• **Fig. 16.115 Systemic Lupus Erythematosus (SLE).** The erythematous patches seen in the malar regions are a characteristic sign.

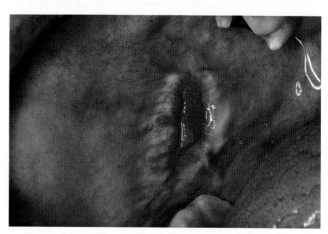

• **Fig. 16.116 Systemic Lupus Erythematosus (SLE).** This ulceration of the buccal mucosa exhibits fine radiating white striae at its periphery, clinically appearing similar to erosive lichen planus.

Oral lesions of SLE develop in 5%–25% of these patients, although some studies indicate prevalence as high as 40%. The lesions usually affect the palate, buccal mucosa, and gingivae. Sometimes they appear as lichenoid areas, but they may also look nonspecific or even somewhat granulomatous (Fig. 16.116). Involvement of the vermilion zone of the lower lip **(lupus cheilitis)** is sometimes seen. Varying degrees of ulceration, pain, erythema, and hyperkeratosis may be present. Other oral complaints such as xerostomia, stomatodynia, candidiasis, periodontal disease, and dysgeusia have been described, but the direct association of these problems with SLE remains to be proven. In some cases, the oral problems may be related directly or indirectly to medications that are used to treat SLE.

Confirming the diagnosis of SLE can often be difficult, particularly in the early stages. Criteria for making the diagnosis of SLE were established by the American College of Rheumatology in 1997, however the Systemic Lupus International Collaborating Clinic Criteria, published in 2012, have also been frequently applied diagnostically. Both of these diagnostic approaches to SLE have considerable overlap, with both requiring certain specific clinical and laboratory findings in order to confirm the diagnosis of SLE (Table 16.4).

TABLE 16.4	Prevalence of Clinical and Laboratory Manifestations of Systemic Lupus Erythematosus	
Findings		**Affected Patients (%)**
Systemic Signs and Symptoms: Fatigue, Malaise, Fever, Anorexia, Weight Loss		95%
MUSCULOSKELETAL SYMPTOMS		95%
Arthralgia/myalgia		95%
Nonerosive polyarthritis		60%
CUTANEOUS SIGNS		80%
Photosensitivity		70%
Malar rash		50%
Oral ulcers		40%
Discoid rash		20%
HEMATOLOGIC SIGNS		85%
Anemia (chronic disease)		70%
Leukopenia (<4000/μL)		65%
Lymphopenia (<1500/μL)		50%
Thrombocytopenia (<100,000/μL)		15%
Hemolytic anemia		10%
NEUROLOGIC SIGNS AND SYMPTOMS		60%
Cognitive disorder		50%
Headache		25%
Seizures		20%
CARDIOPULMONARY SIGNS		60%
Pleurisy, pericarditis, effusions		30%–50%
Myocarditis, endocarditis		10%
RENAL SIGNS		30%–50%
Proteinuria >500 mg/24 h, cellular casts		30%–50%
Nephrotic syndrome		25%
End-stage renal disease		5%–10%

Adapted from Hahn BH: Systemic lupus erythematosus. In Jameson JL, Fauci AS, Kasper DL, et al., editors: *Harrison's principles of internal medicine,* ed 20, New York, 2018, McGraw-Hill, pp 2515–2526. Reproduced with permission of The McGraw-Hill Companies.

Chronic Cutaneous Lupus Erythematosus

Patients with CCLE usually have few or no systemic signs or symptoms, with lesions being limited to skin or mucosal surfaces. The skin lesions of CCLE most commonly present as **discoid lupus erythematosus.** They begin as scaly, round ("discoid") erythematous patches that are frequently distributed on sun-exposed skin, especially in the head and neck area (Fig. 16.117). Patients may indicate that the lesions

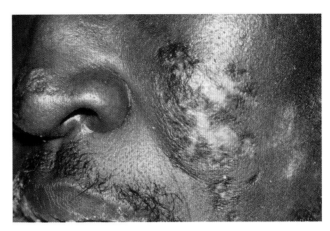

• **Fig. 16.117 Chronic Cutaneous Lupus Erythematosus (CCLE).** The skin lesions are characterized by scaling, atrophy, and pigmentary disturbances, which are most evident on sun-exposed skin.

are exacerbated by sun exposure. With time, the lesions may heal spontaneously in one area, only to appear in another area. The healing process usually results in cutaneous atrophy with scarring and hypopigmentation or hyperpigmentation of the resolving lesion. Conjunctival involvement by CCLE has rarely been reported to cause cicatrizing conjunctivitis, clinically similar to mucous membrane pemphigoid.

In most cases the oral manifestations of CCLE essentially appear clinically identical to the lesions of erosive lichen planus. Unlike the oral lesions of lichen planus, however, the oral lesions of CCLE seldom occur in the absence of skin lesions. An ulcerated or atrophic, erythematous central zone, surrounded by white, fine, radiating striae, characterizes the oral lesion of CCLE (Figs. 16.118 and 16.119). Sometimes the erythematous, atrophic central region of a lesion may show a fine stippling of white dots. As with erosive lichen planus, the ulcerative and atrophic oral lesions of CCLE may be painful, especially when exposed to acidic or salty foods.

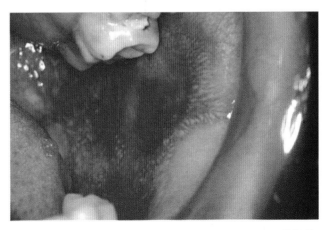

• **Fig. 16.118 Chronic Cutaneous Lupus Erythematosus (CCLE).** Radiating keratotic striae surround erythematous zones of the buccal mucosa. These features are similar to those of erosive lichen planus.

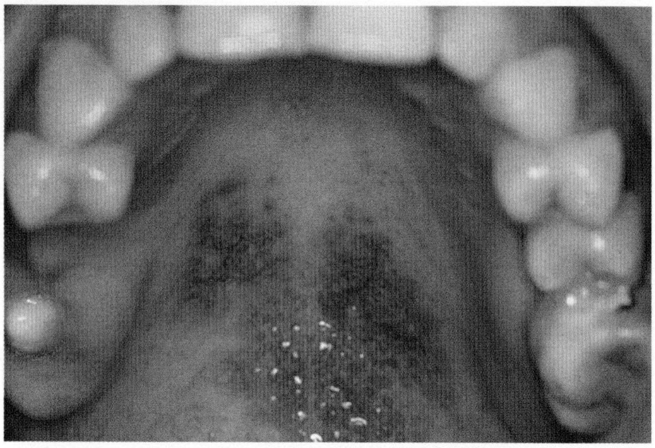

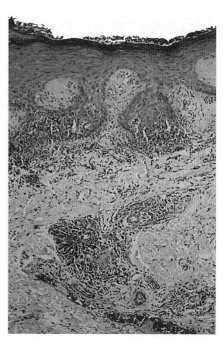

• **Fig. 16.119 Chronic Cutaneous Lupus Erythematosus (CCLE).** Oral involvement may also include relatively nondescript erythematous patches, such as this one in the palate.

Subacute Cutaneous Lupus Erythematosus

Patients with SCLE have clinical manifestations intermediate between those of SLE and CCLE. The skin lesions are the most prominent feature of this variation. They are characterized by photosensitivity and are, therefore, generally present in sun-exposed areas. These lesions do not show the induration and scarring seen with the skin lesions of CCLE. Oral lesions similar to those of CCLE have been described in this variant of lupus as well. Usually, the renal or neurologic abnormalities associated with SLE are not present, although most patients will have arthritis or musculoskeletal problems. SCLE may be triggered by any one of a variety of medications (see page 337).

Histopathologic Features

The histopathologic features of the skin and oral lesions of the various forms of LE show some features in common but are different enough to warrant separate discussions.

The skin lesions of CCLE are characterized by hyperkeratosis, often displaying keratin packed into the openings of hair follicles ("follicular plugging"). In all forms of LE, degeneration of the basal cell layer is frequently observed, and the underlying connective tissue supports patchy to dense aggregates of chronic inflammatory cells (Figs. 16.120 and 16.121). In the deeper connective tissue, the inflammatory infiltrate often surrounds the small blood vessels.

The oral lesions demonstrate hyperkeratosis, alternating atrophy and thickening of the spinous cell layer, degeneration of the basal cell layer, and subepithelial lymphocytic infiltration. These features may also be seen in oral lichen planus; however, the two conditions can usually be distinguished by the presence in LE of patchy deposits of a periodic acid-Schiff (PAS)-positive material in the basement membrane zone, subepithelial edema (sometimes to the point of vesicle formation), and a more diffuse, deep inflammatory infiltrate, often in a perivascular orientation. Some authorities, however, feel that differentiating lichen planus from LE is best done by direct immunofluorescence studies or histopathologic examination of the cutaneous lesions.

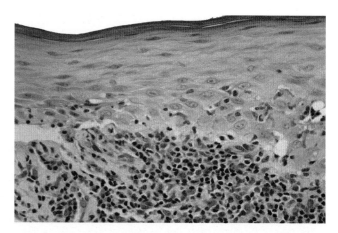

• **Fig. 16.120 Lupus Erythematosus (LE).** Low-power photomicrograph showing hyperparakeratosis with interface mucositis and perivascular inflammation.

• **Fig. 16.121 Lupus Erythematosus (LE).** High-power photomicrograph of the interface mucositis.

Diagnosis

In addition to the clinical and microscopic features, a number of additional immunologic studies may be helpful in making the diagnosis of LE.

Direct immunofluorescence testing of lesional tissue shows deposition of one or more immunoreactants (usually IgM, IgG, or C3) in a shaggy or granular band at the basement membrane zone. In addition, direct immunofluorescence testing of clinically normal skin of SLE patients often shows a similar deposition of IgG, IgM, or complement components. This finding is known as a **positive lupus band test.** Although a positive lupus band test is consistent with the diagnosis of LE, it is now known that other conditions, such as rheumatoid arthritis, Sjögren syndrome, and systemic sclerosis, may also have similar positive findings.

TABLE 16.5 Selected Abnormal Immunologic Findings in Lupus Erythematosus

Findings	Frequency	Significance
Direct immunofluorescence, lesional skin	CCLE: 90% SLE: 95%	May help distinguish among the various types of LE
Direct immunofluorescence, normal skin	CCLE: 0% SLE: 25%–60%	Lupus band test
Antinuclear antibodies (ANAs)	CCLE: 0%–10% SLE: 98%	Very sensitive for SLE, but not very specific; not useful for CCLE diagnosis
Anti-double-stranded DNA antibodies	CCLE: 0% SLE: 70%	Specific for SLE; may indicate disease activity or kidney involvement
Anti-Sm antibodies	CCLE: 0% SLE: 25%	Specific for SLE

CCLE, Chronic cutaneous lupus erythematosus; *SLE,* systemic lupus erythematosus; *LE,* lupus erythematosus.

Furthermore, some patients with LE may not have a positive lupus band test; therefore, this study must always be interpreted in the context of other clinical signs.

Evaluation of serum obtained from a patient with SLE shows various immunologic abnormalities. Approximately 95% of these patients have antibodies directed against multiple nuclear antigens (i.e., antinuclear antibodies [ANAs]). Although this is a nonspecific finding that may be seen in other autoimmune diseases, as well as in otherwise healthy older individuals, it is nevertheless useful as a screening study. Furthermore, if results are negative on multiple occasions, then the diagnosis of SLE should probably be doubted. Antibodies directed against double-stranded DNA are noted in 70% of patients with SLE, and these are more specific for the disease. Another 30% of patients show antibodies directed against Sm, a protein that is complexed with small nuclear RNA. This finding is very specific for SLE.

A summary of selected immunologic findings in LE is shown in Table 16.5.

Treatment and Prognosis

Patients with SLE should avoid excessive exposure to sunlight because UV light may precipitate disease activity. Mild active disease may be effectively managed using NSAIDs combined with antimalarial drugs, such as hydroxychloroquine. For more severe, acute episodes that involve arthritis, pericarditis, thrombocytopenia, or nephritis, systemic corticosteroids are generally indicated; these may be combined with other immunosuppressive and immunomodulating agents. If oral lesions are present, they typically respond to the systemic therapy.

As with SLE patients, patients with CCLE should avoid excessive sunlight exposure. Because most of the manifestations of CCLE are cutaneous, topical corticosteroids are often reasonably effective. Topical calcineurin inhibitors (tacrolimus or pimecrolimus) may also be used, although these medications are relatively expensive. For cases that are resistant to topical therapy, systemic antimalarial drugs, immunosuppressive drugs, immunomodulating drugs, or low-dose thalidomide may produce a response. Topical corticosteroids are also helpful in treating the oral lesions of CCLE.

The prognosis for the patient with SLE is variable. For patients undergoing treatment today, the 5-year survival rate is approximately 95%; however, by 20 years, the survival rate falls to 78%. Ultimately, the prognosis depends on which organs are affected and how frequently the disease is reactivated. The most common cause of death is renal failure; however, chronic immunosuppression also predisposes these patients to increased mortality because of infection and development of malignancy. For reasons that are poorly understood, the prognosis is worse for men than for women. In addition, blacks tend to fare more poorly than whites.

The prognosis for patients with CCLE is considerably better than that for patients with SLE, although transformation to SLE may be seen in approximately 5%–15% of CCLE patients. Usually, CCLE remains confined to the skin, but it may persist and be quite a nuisance. For about 50% of CCLE patients, the problem eventually resolves after several years.

◆ SYSTEMIC SCLEROSIS (PROGRESSIVE SYSTEMIC SCLEROSIS; SCLERODERMA; DIFFUSE CUTANEOUS SYSTEMIC SCLEROSIS; HIDE-BOUND DISEASE)

Systemic sclerosis is a relatively rare condition that probably has an immunologically mediated pathogenesis involving abnormal interactions among vascular tissue, connective tissue, and immune cells in genetically predisposed individuals. For reasons that are not understood, dense collagen is deposited in the tissues of the body in extraordinary amounts. Although its most dramatic effects are seen in association with the skin, the disease is often quite serious, with most organs of the body affected.

Clinical and Radiographic Features

Systemic sclerosis affects approximately 10–40 persons per million population each year. Women have the condition three to five times more frequently than do men. Most patients are adults. The onset of the disease is generally insidious, with the cutaneous changes often responsible for bringing the problem to the patient's attention.

Often one of the first signs of the disease is **Raynaud phenomenon**, a vasoconstrictive event triggered by emotional distress or exposure to cold. Raynaud phenomenon (see CREST syndrome, on page 805) is not specific for systemic sclerosis, however, because it may be present in other immunologically mediated diseases and in otherwise healthy people. Resorption of the terminal phalanges (**acro-osteolysis**) and flexion contractures produce shortened, clawlike fingers (Fig. 16.122). The vascular events and the abnormal collagen deposition contribute to the production of ulcerations on the fingertips (Fig. 16.123).

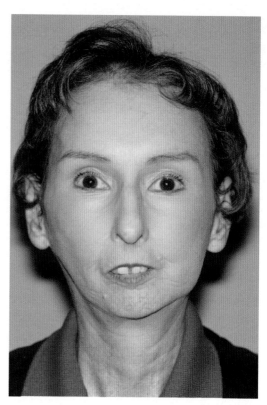

• **Fig. 16.124 Systemic Sclerosis.** The involvement of the facial skin with abnormal collagen deposition produces a mask-like facies. Note the loss of the alae of the nose.

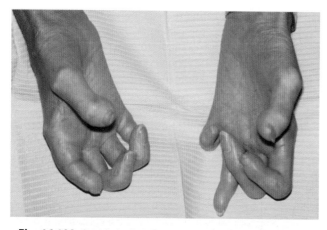

• **Fig. 16.122 Systemic Sclerosis.** The tense, shiny appearance of the skin is evident. Note that the fingers are fixed in a claw-like position, with some showing shortening as a result of acro-osteolysis.

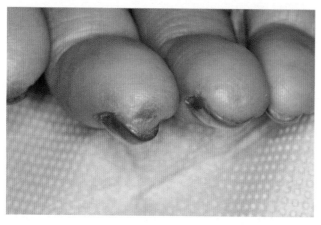

• **Fig. 16.123 Systemic Sclerosis.** Ulcerations of the fingertips.

The skin develops a diffuse, hard texture (*sclero* = hard; *derma* = skin), and its surface is usually smooth. Involvement of the facial skin by subcutaneous collagen deposition results in the characteristic smooth, taut, masklike facies (Fig. 16.124). Similarly, the nasal alae become atrophied, resulting in a pinched appearance to the nose, called a *mouse facies*. When the skin changes are confined to the hands, face, feet, and lower portions of the limbs, the designation of *limited cutaneous systemic sclerosis* is applied. If these changes progress rapidly to involve the skin of the trunk and the proximal limbs, or if the changes begin in these areas, then the process is termed *diffuse cutaneous systemic sclerosis*. These two presentations seem to have different prognoses.

Involvement of other organs may be subtle at first, but the results are more serious. Fibrosis of the lungs, heart, kidneys, and gastrointestinal tract are seen primarily in patients with diffuse cutaneous systemic sclerosis, and the abnormal collagen deposition leads to organ failure, typically within the first 3 years after the diagnosis is made. Pulmonary fibrosis is particularly significant, leading to pulmonary hypertension and heart failure, a primary cause of death for these patients. Patients with limited cutaneous systemic sclerosis tend to develop pulmonary hypertension later than those with a diffuse presentation.

The oral manifestations occur in varying degrees. **Microstomia** often develops as a result of collagen deposition in the perioral tissues. This causes a limitation of opening the mouth

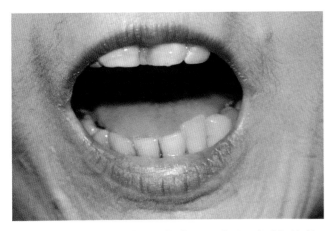

• **Fig. 16.125 Systemic Sclerosis.** Same patient as depicted in Fig. 16.124. Because of the associated microstomia, this is the patient's maximal opening.

in nearly 70% of these patients (Fig. 16.125). Characteristic furrows radiating from the mouth produce a "purse string" appearance. Loss of attached gingival mucosa and multiple areas of gingival recession may occur in some patients. Dysphagia often develops as a result of deposition of collagen in the lingual and esophageal submucosa, producing a firm, hypomobile (boardlike) tongue and an inelastic esophagus, thus hindering swallowing. Xerostomia is frequently identified in these patients, and the possibility of concurrent secondary Sjögren syndrome may require consideration.

On dental radiographs, diffuse widening of the periodontal ligament space is often present throughout the dentition. The extent of the widening may vary, with some examples being subtle and others quite dramatic (Fig. 16.126). Varying degrees of resorption of the posterior ramus of the mandible, the coronoid process, the chin, and the condyle may be detected on panoramic radiographs, affecting approximately 10%–20% of patients (Fig. 16.127). In theory, these areas are resorbed because of the increased pressure associated with the abnormal collagen production. Individual tooth resorption has also been reported to occur at a higher frequency in these patients.

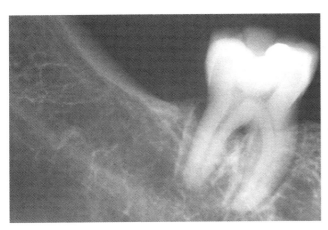

• **Fig. 16.126 Systemic Sclerosis.** Diffuse widening of the periodontal ligament space is often identified on evaluation of periapical radiographs.

A milder condition that resembles cutaneous systemic sclerosis has been called **localized scleroderma** or **morphea,** and it usually affects only a solitary patch of skin. Because these lesions often look like scars, the name *en coup de sabre* ("strike of the sword") is used to describe them (Fig. 16.128). This problem is primarily cosmetic and, unlike systemic sclerosis, it is rarely life threatening. For this reason, many authorities now feel that this disorder may be unrelated to systemic sclerosis.

Histopathologic Features

Microscopic examination of tissue involved by systemic sclerosis shows diffuse deposition of dense collagen within and around the normal structures (Fig. 16.129). This abnormal collagen replaces and destroys the normal tissue, causing the loss of normal tissue function.

Diagnosis

During the early phases, it may be difficult to make a diagnosis of systemic sclerosis. Generally, the clinical signs of stiffened skin texture along with the development of Raynaud phenomenon are suggestive of the diagnosis. A skin biopsy may be supportive of the diagnosis if abundant collagen deposition is observed microscopically.

Laboratory studies may be helpful to the diagnostic process if anticentromere antibodies, anti-RNA polymerase III, or anti-Scl 70 (topoisomerase I) is detected. Antitopoisomerase I and anti-RNA polymerase III antibodies are seen more often with diffuse cutaneous systemic sclerosis and development of pulmonary fibrosis; anticentromere antibodies are usually associated with limited cutaneous systemic sclerosis (including **CREST syndrome**—see next topic), as well as development of late-onset pulmonary hypertension.

Treatment and Prognosis

The management of systemic sclerosis is difficult. Unfortunately, many of the recommended treatments have not been examined in controlled trials, and the natural waxing and waning course of the disease makes it difficult to assess the effectiveness of a given treatment in an open-label trial. Systemic medications, such as penicillamine, are prescribed in an attempt to inhibit collagen production. One double-blind study, however, showed no difference in measured patient outcomes with high-dose versus low-dose penicillamine, suggesting that perhaps this medication has limited efficacy. Surprisingly, corticosteroids are of little benefit, and some studies have suggested that their use may increase the risk of renal disease. For patients in the early stages of diffuse cutaneous systemic sclerosis, treatment with relatively low doses of methotrexate has been shown to improve the skin changes. Extracorporeal photopheresis also has been shown to have some beneficial effect on the skin lesions.

Other management strategies are directed at controlling symptoms. Such techniques as esophageal dilation are used,

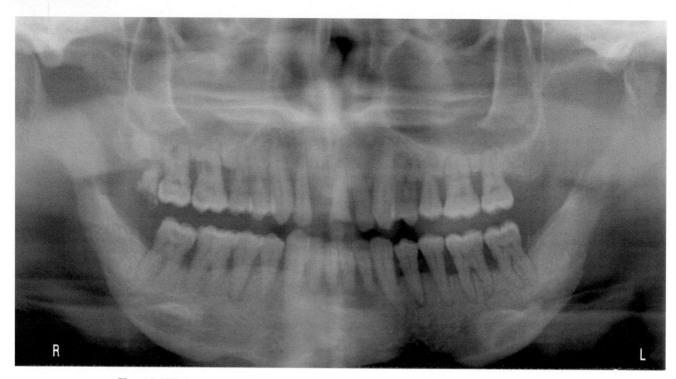

• **Fig. 16.127 Systemic Sclerosis.** Panoramic radiographic evaluation may show a characteristic resorption of the ramus, coronoid process, or condyle.

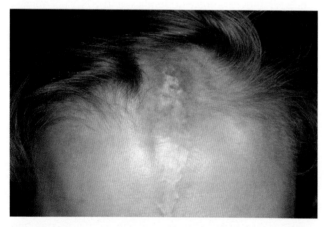

• **Fig. 16.128 Localized Scleroderma (Morphea).** The cutaneous alteration on the patient's forehead represents a limited form of sclero-derma called *en coup de sabre,* because the lesion resembles a scar that might result from a cut with a sword.

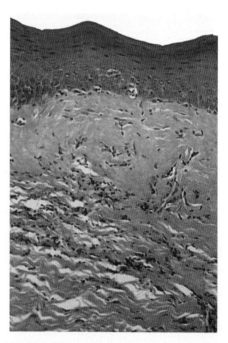

• **Fig. 16.129 Systemic Sclerosis.** Medium-power photomicrograph of an oral biopsy specimen. Diffuse deposition of collagen is apparent throughout the lamina propria.

for example, to temporarily correct esophageal strictures. Proton pump inhibitors can reduce gastric acid production and improve symptoms of gastroesophageal reflux disease. Calcium channel blocking agents or phosphodiesterase type 5 inhibitors help to increase peripheral blood flow and lessen the symptoms of Raynaud phenomenon, but many patients can reduce episodes by keeping warm (especially their hands and feet) or by stopping cigarette smoking. Angiotensin-converting enzyme (ACE) inhibitors often effectively control hypertension if kidney involvement is prominent.

From a dental standpoint, problems may develop for patients who wear prostheses because of the microstomia and inelasticity of the mouth. Collapsible dental appliances with special hinges have been made to facilitate the insertion and removal of dentures. Microstomia and inelastic soft tissue also hamper the maintenance of good oral hygiene, and affected patients have a decreased ability to manipulate a manual toothbrush as a result of sclerotic changes in the fingers and hands. In such situations, the use of an electric toothbrush should be considered in order to optimize dental plaque control. Reduced salivary flow is not uncommon in these patients, and daily application of a 1% neutral sodium fluoride gel will help prevent cervical dental caries. Surgical correction of open bite associated with condylar resorption has been described. Infrequently, the resorption of the mandible may become so great as to cause a pathologic fracture.

The prognosis is poor, although the outlook is better for patients with limited cutaneous involvement than for those with diffuse involvement. If the heart is affected, then the prognosis is particularly poor, but most patients die because of pulmonary involvement. Overall survival figures are difficult to calculate due to a variety of factors, including the rarity of the disease, the inherent variability of its natural course, and the variation in treatments provided at medical centers around the world. With current treatment regimens, it is estimated that 10-year survival rates for patients with limited cutaneous systemic sclerosis approach 75%–80%, whereas survival drops to 55%–60% for patients with diffuse cutaneous systemic sclerosis.

◆ CREST SYNDROME (ACROSCLEROSIS; LIMITED SCLERODERMA; LIMITED CUTANEOUS SYSTEMIC SCLEROSIS)

CREST syndrome is an uncommon condition that many authorities now believe represents a variant of limited cutaneous systemic sclerosis. The term *CREST* is an acronym for **C**alcinosis cutis, **R**aynaud phenomenon, **E**sophageal dysfunction, **S**clerodactyly, and **T**elangiectasia.

Clinical Features

As with all types of systemic sclerosis, most patients with CREST syndrome are women in the sixth or seventh decade of life. The characteristic signs may not appear synchronously but instead may develop sequentially over a period of months to years.

Calcinosis cutis occurs in the form of movable, nontender, subcutaneous nodules, 0.5–2.0 cm in size, which are usually multiple (Fig. 16.130). Larger, more numerous or superficial calcifications may occasionally become bothersome and require removal.

Raynaud phenomenon may be observed when a person's hands or feet are exposed to cold temperatures. The initial clinical sign is a dramatic blanching of the digits, which appear dead-white in color as a result of severe vasospasm. A few minutes later, the affected extremity takes on a bluish color because of venous stasis. After warming, increased blood flow results in a dusky-red hue with the return of hyperemic blood

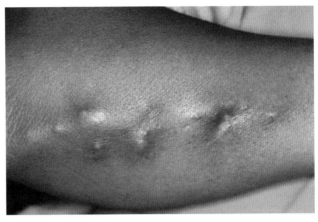

• **Fig. 16.130 CREST Syndrome.** The subcutaneous nodules on this patient's arm represent deposition of calcium salts (calcinosis cutis). (Courtesy of Dr. Román Carlos.)

flow. This may be accompanied by varying degrees of throbbing pain.

Esophageal dysfunction, caused by abnormal collagen deposition in the esophageal submucosa, may not be noticeable in the early phases of CREST syndrome. Often the subtle initial signs of this problem must be demonstrated by barium swallow radiologic studies.

The **sclerodactyly** of CREST syndrome is rather remarkable. The fingers become stiff, and the skin takes on a smooth, shiny appearance. Often the fingers undergo permanent flexure, resulting in a characteristic "claw" deformity (Fig. 16.131). As with other forms of cutaneous systemic sclerosis, this change is due to abnormal deposition of collagen within the dermis in these areas.

The **telangiectasias** in this syndrome are similar to those seen in hereditary hemorrhagic telangiectasia (HHT) (see page 759). As with that condition, significant bleeding from the superficial dilated capillaries may occur. The facial skin and the vermilion zone of the lips are commonly affected (Fig. 16.132).

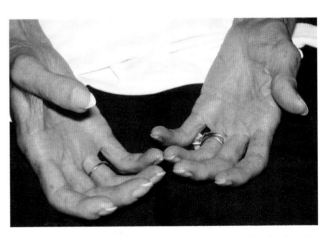

• **Fig. 16.131 CREST Syndrome.** Claw-like deformity affecting the hands (sclerodactyly).

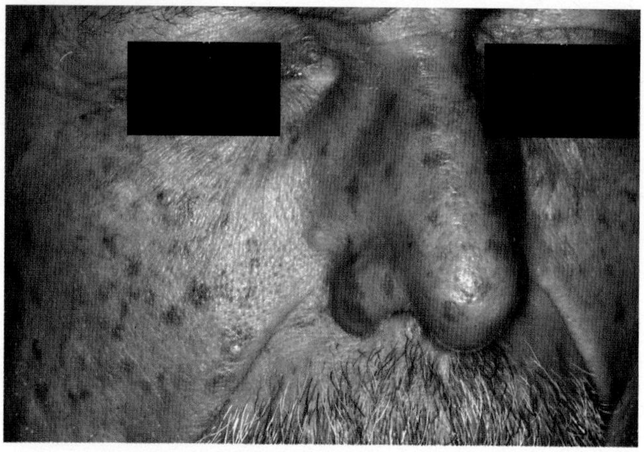

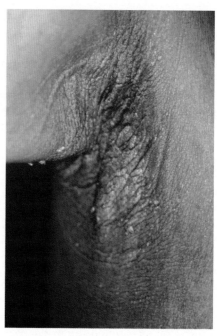

• **Fig. 16.132 CREST Syndrome.** The patient shows numerous red facial macules representing telangiectatic blood vessels.

Histopathologic Features

The histopathologic findings in CREST syndrome are similar, although milder, to those seen in systemic sclerosis. Superficial dilated capillaries are observed if a telangiectatic vessel is included in the biopsy specimen.

Diagnosis

Sometimes, HHT may be considered in the differential diagnosis if the history is unclear and the other signs of CREST syndrome are not yet evident. In these cases, laboratory studies directed at identifying anticentromere antibodies may be useful, because this test is relatively specific for CREST syndrome and other types of limited cutaneous systemic sclerosis.

Treatment and Prognosis

The treatment of patients with CREST syndrome is essentially the same as that of those with systemic sclerosis. Because CREST syndrome usually is not as severe, the treatment does not have to be as aggressive. Although the prognosis for this condition is much better than that for systemic sclerosis, patients should be monitored for an increased risk of developing pulmonary hypertension or primary biliary cirrhosis, generally more than 10 years after the initial diagnosis.

◆ ACANTHOSIS NIGRICANS

Acanthosis nigricans is an acquired dermatologic problem characterized by the development of a velvety, brownish alteration of the skin. In rare instances, this unusual condition develops in conjunction with a malignancy, usually gastrointestinal cancer, and is termed **malignant acanthosis nigricans.** The cutaneous lesion itself is benign, yet it is significant because it represents a cutaneous marker for internal malignancy. The cause of malignant acanthosis nigricans is unknown, although a cytokine-like peptide capable of affecting the epidermal cells may be produced by the malignancy.

Most cases, estimated to affect as many as 5% of adults, are not associated with a malignancy and are termed **benign**

• **Fig. 16.133 Acanthosis Nigricans.** The lesions are characterized by numerous fine, almost velvety, confluent papules. The lesions most often affect the flexural areas, such as the axilla depicted in this photograph. (From Hall JM, Moreland A, Cox GJ, et al: Oral acanthosis nigricans: report of a case and comparison of oral and cutaneous pathology, *Am J Dermatopathol* 10:68–73, 1988.)

acanthosis nigricans. A clinically similar form, **pseudoacanthosis nigricans,** may occur in some obese people. Some benign forms of acanthosis nigricans may be inherited or may occur in association with various endocrinopathies, such as diabetes mellitus, Addison disease, hypothyroidism, and acromegaly. Furthermore, benign acanthosis nigricans may occur with certain syndromes (e.g., Crouzon syndrome) or drug ingestion (e.g., oral contraceptives or corticosteroids). These forms of the condition are typically associated with resistance of the tissues to the effects of insulin, similar to the insulin resistance seen in non–insulin-dependent diabetes mellitus (NIDDM). Even though the affected individuals may not have overt diabetes mellitus, they often show increased levels of insulin or an abnormal response to exogenously administered insulin.

Clinical Features

The malignant form of acanthosis nigricans develops in association with an internal malignancy, particularly adenocarcinoma of the gastrointestinal tract. Approximately 20% of the cases of malignant acanthosis nigricans are identified before the malignancy is found, but most appear at about the same time as discovery of the gastrointestinal tumor or thereafter.

Both forms of acanthosis nigricans affect the intertriginous and flexural areas of the skin predominantly, appearing as finely papillary, hyperkeratotic, brownish patches that are usually asymptomatic (Fig. 16.133). The texture of the lesions has been variably described as either velvety or leathery.

Oral lesions of acanthosis nigricans have also been reported and may occur in 25% to 50% of affected patients, especially

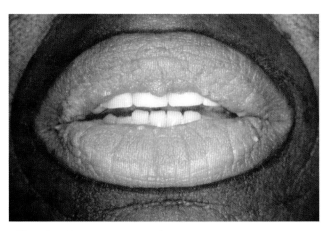

• **Fig. 16.134 Acanthosis Nigricans.** The vermilion zone of the lips is affected. (Courtesy of Dr. George Blozis.)

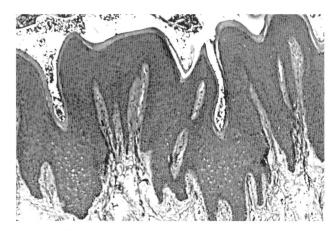

• **Fig. 16.136 Acanthosis Nigricans.** Medium-power photomicrograph of an oral lesion showing papillomatosis, mild hyperkeratosis, and acanthosis of the epithelium.

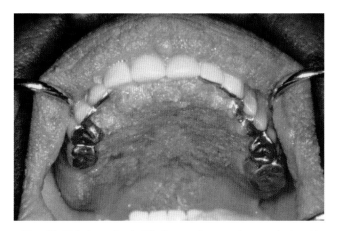

• **Fig. 16.135 Acanthosis Nigricans.** Same patient as depicted in Fig. 16.134. Note involvement of the palatal mucosa. (Courtesy of Dr. George Blozis.)

those with the malignant form. These lesions appear as diffuse, finely papillary areas of mucosal alteration that most often involve the tongue or lips, particularly the upper lip (Figs. 16.134 and 16.135). The buccal mucosa may also be affected. The brownish pigmentation associated with the cutaneous lesions is usually not seen in oral acanthosis nigricans.

Histopathologic Features

The histopathologic features of the various forms of acanthosis nigricans are essentially identical. The epidermis exhibits hyperorthokeratosis and papillomatosis. Usually, some degree of increased melanin deposition is noted, but the extent of acanthosis (thickening of the spinous layer) is really rather mild. The oral lesions have much more acanthosis, but show minimal increased melanin pigmentation (Fig. 16.136).

Treatment and Prognosis

Although acanthosis nigricans itself is a harmless process, the patient should be evaluated to ascertain which form of the disease is present. Abrupt onset of acanthosis nigricans in

an adult who has none of the benign predisposing factors related to this condition should trigger medical evaluation to rule out internal malignancy. Identification and treatment of the underlying malignancy obviously are important for patients with the malignant type; unfortunately, the prognosis for these individuals is very poor. Interestingly, malignant acanthosis nigricans may resolve when the cancer is treated. Keratolytic agents may improve the appearance of the benign forms.

Bibliography

Ectodermal Dysplasia

Anbouba GM, Carmany EP, Natoli JL: The characterization of hypodontia, hypohidrosis, and hypotrichosis associated with X-linked hypohidrotic ectodermal dysplasia: a systematic review, *Am J Med Genet* 182A:831–841, 2020.

Aswegan AL, Josephson KD, Mowbray R, et al.: Autosomal dominant hypohidrotic ectodermal dysplasia in a large family, *Am J Med Genet* 72:462–467, 1997.

Clauss F, Manière M-C, Obry F, et al.: Dento-craniofacial phenotypes and underlying molecular mechanisms in hypohidrotic ectodermal dysplasia (HED): a review, *J Dent Res* 87:1089–1099, 2008.

Ho L, Williams MS, Spritz RA: A gene for autosomal dominant hypohidrotic ectodermal dysplasia (EDA3) maps to chromosome 2q11-q13, *Am J Hum Genet* 62:1102–1106, 1998.

Itin PH, Fistarol SK: Ectodermal dysplasias, *Am J Med Genet* 131C:45–51, 2004.

Jorgenson RJ, Salinas CF, Dowben JS, et al.: A population study on the density of palmar sweat pores, *Birth Defects Orig Artic Ser* 24:51–63, 1988.

Kantaputra PN, Hamada T, Kumchai T, et al.: Heterozygous mutation in the SAM domain of p63 underlies Rapp-Hodgkin ectodermal dysplasia, *J Dent Res* 82:433–437, 2003.

Knaudt B, Volz T, Krug M, et al.: Skin symptoms in four ectodermal dysplasia syndromes including two case reports of Rapp-Hodgkin syndrome, *Eur J Dermatol* 22:605–613, 2012.

Knobloch LA, Larsen PE, Saponaro PC, et al.: Early implant placement for a patient with ectodermal dysplasia: thirteen years of clinical care, *J Prosthet Dent* 119:702–709, 2018.

Liu G, Wang X, Qin M, et al.: A novel splicing mutation of ectodysplasin A gene responsible for hypohidrotic ectodermal dysplasia, *Oral Dis* 24:1101–1106, 2018.

Munoz F, Lestringant G, Sybert V, et al.: Definitive evidence for an autosomal recessive form of hypohidrotic ectodermal dysplasia clinically indistinguishable from the more common X-linked disorder, *Am J Hum Genet* 61:94–100, 1997.

Reyes-Reali J, Mendoza-Ramos MI, Garrido-Guerrero E, et al.: Hypohidrotic ectodermal dysplasia: clinical and molecular review, *Int J Dermatol* 57:965–972, 2018.

Schnabl D, Grunert I, Schmuth M, et al.: Prosthetic rehabilitation of patients with hypohidrotic ectodermal dysplasia: A systematic review, *J Oral Rehabil* 45:555–570, 2018.

Singh P, Warnakulasuriya S: Aplasia of submandibular salivary glands associated with ectodermal dysplasia, *J Oral Pathol Med* 33:634–636, 2004.

Wohlfart S, Meiller R, Johanna Hammersen J, et al.: Natural history of X-linked hypohidrotic ectodermal dysplasia: a 5-year follow-up study, *Orphanet J Rare Dis* 15:7, 2020.

Wright T, Fete M, Schneider H, et al.: Ectodermal dysplasias: classification and organization by phenotype, genotype and molecular pathway, *Am J Med Genet A* 179:442–447, 2019.

White Sponge Nevus

Bezerra KT, Leite TC, Roza ALOC, et al.: White sponge nevus: a condition not always clinically suspected, *J Cutan Pathol* 47:22–26, 2020.

Cutlan JE, Saunders N, Olsen SH, et al.: White sponge nevus presenting as genital lesions in a 28-year-old female, *J Cutan Pathol* 37:386–389, 2010.

Kimura M, Nagao T, Machida J, et al.: Mutation of keratin 4 gene causing white sponge nevus in a Japanese family, *Int J Oral Maxillofac Surg* 42:615–618, 2013.

Kürklü E, Öztürk S, Cassidy AJ, et al.: Clinical features and molecular genetic analysis in a Turkish family with oral white sponge nevus, *Med Oral Patol Oral Cir Bucal* 23:e144–e150, 2018.

Martins-Filho PRS, Ferreira-Brasileiro B, Luciano-Trento C, et al.: Familial case of oral white sponge nevus—a rare hereditary condition, *An Bras Dermatol* 86(4 Suppl. 1):S39–S41, 2011.

Müller S: Frictional keratosis, contact keratosis and smokeless tobacco keratosis: features of reactive white lesions of the oral mucosa, *Head Neck Pathol* 13:16–24, 2019.

Pinna R, Cocco F, Campus G, et al.: Genetic and developmental disorders of the oral mucosa: epidemiology; molecular mechanisms; diagnostic criteria; management, *Periodontol* 2000(80):12–27, 2019.

Rugg EL, McLean WHI, Allison WE, et al.: A mutation in the mucosal keratin K4 is associated with oral white sponge nevus, *Nat Genet* 11:450–452, 1995.

Sobhan M, Alirezaei P, Farshchian M, et al.: White sponge nevus: report of a case and review of the literature, *Acta Medica Iranica* 55:533–535, 2017.

Westin M, Rekabdar E, Blomstrand L, et al.: Mutations in the genes for keratin-4 and keratin-13 in Swedish patients with white sponge nevus, *J Oral Pathol Med* 47:152–157, 2018.

Zhang JM, Yang ZW, Chen RY, et al.: Two new mutations in the keratin 4 gene causing oral white sponge nevus in Chinese family, *Oral Dis* 15:100–105, 2009.

Hereditary Benign Intraepithelial Dyskeratosis

Bui T, Young JW, Frausto RF, et al.: Hereditary benign intraepithelial dyskeratosis: report of a case and re-examination of the evidence for locus heterogeneity, *Ophthalmic Genet* 37:76–80, 2016.

Haisley-Royster CA, Allingham RR, Klintworth GK, et al.: Hereditary benign intraepithelial dyskeratosis: report of two cases with prominent oral lesions, *J Am Acad Dermatol* 45:634–636, 2001.

McLean IW, Riddle PJ, Scruggs JH, et al.: Hereditary benign intraepithelial dyskeratosis: a report of two cases from Texas, *J Ophthalmol* 88:164–168, 1981.

Sadeghi EM, Witkop CJ: The presence of *Candida albicans* in hereditary benign intraepithelial dyskeratosis: an ultrastructural observation, *Oral Surg Oral Med Oral Pathol* 48:342–346, 1979.

Shields CL, Shields JA, Eagle RC: Hereditary benign intraepithelial dyskeratosis, *Arch Ophthalmol* 105:422–423, 1987.

Pachyonychia Congenita

Brill S, Sprecher E, Smith FJD, et al.: Chronic pain in pachyonychia congenita: evidence for neuropathic origin, *Br J Dermatol* 179:154–162, 2018.

Dabbagh B, Cukier O, Yeganeh M, et al.: Pachyonychia congenita associated with a novel variant of KRT17 presenting unusual oral manifestations, *J Dent Child* 86:61–63, 2019.

Duverger O, Carlson JC, Karacz CM, et al.: Genetic variants in pachyonychia congenital-associated keratins increase susceptibility to tooth decay, *PLoS Genet* 14:e1007168, 2018.

Eliason MJ, Leachman SA, Feng B-J, et al.: A review of the clinical phenotype of 254 patients with genetically confirmed pachyonychia congenita, *J Am Acad Dermatol* 67:680–686, 2012.

Forrest CE, Casey G, Mordaunt DA, et al.: Pachyonychia congenita: a spectrum of KRT6a mutations in Australian patients, *Pediatr Dermatol* 33:337–342, 2016.

Gruber R, Edlinger M, Kaspar RL, et al.: An appraisal of oral retinoids in the treatment of pachyonychia congenita, *J Am Acad Dermatol* 66:e193–e199, 2012.

Liu J, Zhong W, Yu B, et al.: Generalized bullae in a young girl with KRT6A-related pachyonychia congenita, *Pediatr Dermatol* 37:974–976, 2020.

McLean WHI, Hansen CD, Eliason MJ, et al.: The phenotypic and molecular genetic features of pachyonychia congenita, *J Invest Dermatol* 131:1015–1017, 2011.

O'Kane AM, Jackson CP, Mahadevan M, et al.: Laryngeal manifestations of pachyonychia congenita: a clinical case and discussion on management for the otolaryngologist, *J Laryngol Otol* 131(Suppl. S2):S53–S56, 2017.

Wilson NJ, Leachman SA, Hansen CD, et al.: A large mutational study in pachyonychia congenita, *J Invest Dermatol* 131:1018–1024, 2011.

Zieman AG, Coulombe PA: Pathophysiology of pachyonychia congenita-associated palmoplantar keratoderma: new insight into skin epithelial homeostasis and avenues for treatment, *Br J Dermatol* 182:564–573, 2020.

Dyskeratosis Congenita

Abdel-Karim A, Frezzini C, Viggor S, et al.: Dyskeratosis congenita: a case report, *Oral Surg Oral Med Oral Pathol Oral Radiol Endod* 108:e20–e24, 2009.

Agarwal S: Evaluation and management of hematopoietic failure in dyskeratosis congenita, *Hematol Oncol Clin North Am* 32:669–685, 2018.

Bongiorno M, Rivard S, Hammer D, et al.: Malignant transformation of oral leukoplakia in a patient with dyskeratosis congenita, *Oral Surg Oral Med Oral Pathol Oral Radiol* 124:e239–e242, 2017.

Calado RT, Young NS: Telomere diseases, *N Engl J Med* 361:2353–2365, 2009.

Davidovitch E, Eimerl D, Aker M, et al.: Dyskeratosis congenita: dental management of a medically complex child, *Pediatr Dent* 27:244–248, 2005.

Elliot AM, Graham GE, Bernstein M, et al.: Dyskeratosis congenita: an autosomal recessive variant, *Am J Med Genet* 83:178–182, 1999.

Jyonouchi S, Forbes L, Ruchelli E, et al.: Dyskeratosis congenita: a combined immunodeficiency with broad clinical spectrum—a single-center pediatric experience, *Pediatr Allergy Immunol* 22:313–319, 2011.

Kanegane H, Kasahara Y, Okamura J, et al.: Identification of DKC1 gene mutations in Japanese patients with X-linked dyskeratosis congenita, *Br J Haematol* 129:432–434, 2005.

Knight SW, Heiss NS, Vulliamy TJ, et al.: X-linked dyskeratosis congenita is predominantly caused by missense mutations in the DKC1 gene, *Am J Hum Genet* 65:50–58, 1999.

Li F, Li W, Qiao X, et al.: Clinical features of dyskeratosis congenita in mainland China: case reports and literature review, *Int J Hematol* 109:328–335, 2019.

Lourenço SV, Boggio PA, Fezzi FA, et al.: Dyskeratosis congenita—report of a case with emphasis on gingival aspects, *Pediatr Dermatol* 26:176–179, 2009.

Niewisch MR, Savage SA: An update on the biology and management of dyskeratosis congenita and related telomere biology disorders, *Expert Rev Hematol* 12(12):1037–1052, 2019. https://doi.org/10.1080/17474086.2019.1662720.

Stoopler ET, Shanti RM: Dyskeratosis congenital, *Mayo Clin Proc* 94:1668–1669, 2019.

Trott KE, Briddell JW, Corao-Uribe D, et al.: Dyskeratosis congenita and oral cavity squamous cell carcinoma: report of a case and literature review, *J Pediatr Hematol Oncol* 41:501–503, 2019.

Xeroderma Pigmentosum

Alwatban L, Binamer Y: Xeroderma pigmentosum at a tertiary care center in Saudi Arabia, *Ann Saudi Med* 37:240–244, 2017.

Black JO: Xeroderma pigmentosum, *Head and Neck Pathol* 10:139–144, 2016.

Carneiro MC, de Carvalho KT, de Souza TE, et al.: Unusual intraoral cancer with unexpected outcome in a patient with xeroderma pigmentosum: an alert for antineoplastic treatment, *Oral Surg Oral Med Oral Pathol Oral Radiol* 129:e1–e11, 2020.

DiGiovanna JJ, Kraemer KH: Shining a light on xeroderma pigmentosum, *J Invest Dermatol* 132:785–796, 2012.

Kraemer KH, Lee MM, Scotto J: Xeroderma pigmentosum: cutaneous, ocular, and neurologic abnormalities in 830 published cases, *Arch Dermatol* 123:241–250, 1987.

Lehmann A, Seebode C, Martens MC, et al.: Xeroderma pigmentosum—facts and perspectives, *Anticancer Res* 38:1159–1164, 2018.

Park S, Dock M: Xeroderma pigmentosum: a case report, *Pediatr Dent* 25:397–400, 2003.

Zghal M, Fazaaa B, Abdelhak S, et al.: Xeroderma pigmentosum, *Ann Dermatol Venereol* 145:706–722, 2018.

Hereditary Mucoepithelial Dysplasia

Avadhanam VS, Khaw PT, Martin KR: Long-term ocular follow-up in a case with hereditary mucoepithelial dysplasia, *J Pediatr Ophthalmol Strabismus* 47:e1–e4, 2010.

Boralevi F, Haftek M, Vabres P, et al.: Hereditary mucoepithelial dysplasia: clinical, ultrastructural and genetic study of eight patients and literature review, *Br J Dermatol* 153:310–318, 2005.

Chacon-Camacho OF, Arce-Gonzalez R, Ordaz-Robles T, et al.: Exome sequencing identifies a SREBF1 recurrent ARG557CYS mutation as the cause of hereditary mucoepithelial dysplasia in a family with high clinical variability, *Am J Med Genet A* 182:2773–2777, 2020.

Hernández-Martin A, Colmenero I, Torrelo A: Hereditary mucoepithelial dysplasia: report of two sporadic cases, *Pediatr Dermatol* 29:311–315, 2012.

Kulkarni T, de Andrade J, Zhou Y, et al.: Alveolar epithelial disintegrity in pulmonary fibrosis, *Am J Physiol Lung Cell Mol Physiol* 311: L185–L191, 2016.

Leithauser LA, Mutasim DF: Hereditary mucoepithelial dysplasia: unique histopathological findings in skin lesions, *J Cutan Pathol* 39:431–439, 2012.

Scheman AJ, Ray DJ, Witkop CJ, et al.: Hereditary mucoepithelial dysplasia: case report and review of the literature, *J Am Acad Dermatol* 21:351–357, 1989.

Witkop CJ, White JG, Sauk JJ, et al.: Clinical, histologic, cytologic and ultrastructural characteristics of the oral lesions from hereditary mucoepithelial dysplasia, *Oral Surg Oral Med Oral Pathol* 46:645–657, 1978.

Incontinentia Pigmenti

Cammarata-Scalisi F, Fusco F, Ursini MV: Incontinentia pigmenti, *Actas Dermosifiliogr* 110:273–278, 2019.

Greene-Roethke C: Incontinentia pigmenti: a summary review of this rare ectodermal dysplasia with neurologic manifestations, including treatment protocols, *J Pediatr Health Care* 31: e45–e52, 2017.

Hsiao P-F, Lin S-P, Chiang S-S, et al.: *NEMO* gene mutations in Chinese patients with incontinentia pigmenti, *J Formos Med Assoc* 109:192–200, 2010.

O'Doherty M, McCreery K, Green AJ, et al.: Incontinentia pigmenti—ophthalmological observation of a series of cases and review of the literature, *Br J Ophthalmol* 95:11–16, 2011.

Phan TA, Wargon O, Turner AM: Incontinentia pigmenti case series: clinical spectrum of incontinentia pigmenti in 53 female patients and their relatives, *Clin Exp Dermatol* 30:474–480, 2005.

Rosser T: Neurocutaneous disorders, *Continuum (Minneap Minn)* 24(1):96–129, 2018. Child Neurology.

Santa-Maria FD, Monteavaro Mariath L, Poziomczyk CS, et al.: Dental anomalies in 14 patients with IP: clinical and radiological analysis and review, *Clin Oral Investig* 21:1845–1852, 2017.

Scheuerle AE: Incontinentia pigmenti in adults, *Am J Med Genet* 179A:1415–1419, 2019.

Sun S, Li F, Liu Y, et al.: A novel inhibitor of nuclear factor kappa-B kinase subunit gamma mutation identified in an incontinentia pigmenti patient with syndromic tooth agenesis, *Arch Oral Biol* 101:100–107, 2019.

Wang R, Lara-Corrales I, Kannu P, et al.: Unraveling incontinentia pigmenti: a comparison of phenotype and genotype variants, *J Am Acad Dermatol* 81:1142–1149, 2019.

Darier Disease

Adams AM, Macleod RI, Munro CS: Symptomatic and asymptomatic salivary duct abnormalities in Darier's disease: a sialographic study, *Dentomaxillofac Radiol* 23:25–28, 1994.

Burge SM, Wilkinson JD: Darier-White disease: a review of the clinical features in 163 patients, *J Am Acad Dermatol* 27:40–50, 1992.

Frezzini C, Cedro M, Leao JC, et al.: Darier disease affecting the gingival and oral mucosal surfaces, *Oral Surg Oral Med Oral Pathol Oral Radiol Endod* 102:e29–e33, 2006.

Letulé V, Herzinger T, Ruzicka T, et al.: Treatment of Darier disease with oral alitretinoin, *Clin Exp Dermatol* 38:523–525, 2013.

Macleod RI, Munro CS: The incidence and distribution of oral lesions in patients with Darier's disease, *Br Dent J* 171:133–136, 1991.

Nellen RGL, Steijlen PM, van Steensel MAM, et al.: Mendelian disorders of cornification caused by defects in intracellular calcium pumps: mutation update and database for variants in ATP2A2 and ATP2C1 associated with Darier disease and Hailey–Hailey disease, *Hum Mutat* 38:343–356, 2017.

Savignac M, Edir A, Simon M, et al.: Darier disease: a disease model of impaired calcium homeostasis in the skin, *Biochim Biophys Acta* 1813:1111–1117, 2011.

Schwartz JL, Clinton TS: Darier's disease misdiagnosed as severe seborrheic dermatitis, *Mil Med* 176:1457–1459, 2011.

Sehgal VN, Srivastava G: Darier's (Darier-White) disease/keratosis follicularis, *Int J Dermatol* 44:184–192, 2005.

Shi B-J, Xue M, Zhong G-S, et al.: The *ATP2A2* gene in patients with Darier's disease: one novel splicing mutation, *Int J Dermatol* 51:1074–1077, 2012.

Takagi A, Kamijo M, Ikeda S: Darier disease, *J Dermatol* 43:275–279, 2016.

Warty Dyskeratoma

Allon I, Buchner A: Warty dyskeratoma/focal acantholytic dyskeratosis—an update on a rare oral lesion, *J Oral Pathol Med* 41:261–267, 2012.

Chau MNY, Radden BG: Oral warty dyskeratoma, *J Oral Pathol* 13:546–556, 1984.

Kaddu S, Dong H, Mayer G, et al.: Warty dyskeratoma—"follicular dyskeratoma": analysis of clinicopathologic features of a distinctive follicular adnexal neoplasm, *J Am Acad Dermatol* 47:423–428, 2002.

Kaugars GE, Lieb RJ, Abbey LM: Focal oral warty dyskeratoma, *Int J Dermatol* 23:123–130, 1984.

Laskaris G, Sklavounou A: Warty dyskeratoma of the oral mucosa, *Br J Oral Maxillofac Surg* 23:371–375, 1985.

Xie Y, Zhang Q, Wang L: Multiple warty dyskeratomas with severe pruritus: a case report and literature review, *Am J Dermatopathol* 40:e44–e45, 2018.

Peutz-Jeghers Syndrome

Arber N, Moshkowitz M: Small bowel polyposis syndromes, *Curr Gastroenterol Rep* 13:435–441, 2011.

Beggs AD, Latchford AR, Vasen HFA, et al.: Peutz-Jeghers syndrome: a systematic review and recommendations for management, *Gut* 59:975–986, 2010.

Chen H-Y, Jin XW, Li B-R, et al.: Cancer risk in patients with Peutz–Jeghers syndrome: a retrospective cohort study of 336 cases, *Tumor Biol* 1–7, 2017.

Jelsig AM, Qvist N, Sunde L: Disease pattern in Danish patients with Peutz-Jeghers syndrome, *Int J Colorectal Dis* 31:997–1004, 2016.

Jenne DE, Reimann H, Nezu J-I, et al.: Peutz-Jeghers syndrome is caused by mutations in a novel serine threonine kinase, *Nat Genet* 18:38–43, 1998.

Korsse SE, van Leerdam ME, Dekker E: Gastrointestinal diseases and their oro-dental manifestations: Part 4: Peutz-Jeghers syndrome, *Br Dent J* 222:214–217, 2017.

Kumar S, Arora P, Goswami P: Recurrent intestinal obstruction in a patient of Peutz–Jeghers syndrome, *J Cancer Res Ther* 15:252–254, 2019.

Latchford A, Cohen S, Auth M, et al.: Management of Peutz-Jeghers syndrome in children and adolescents: a position paper from the ESPGHAN Polyposis Working Group, *J Pediatr Gastroenterol Nutr* 68:442–452, 2019.

Meserve EEK, Nucci MR: Peutz-Jeghers syndrome - pathobiology, pathologic manifestations, and suggestions for recommending genetic testing in pathology reports, *Surg Pathol* 9:243–268, 2016.

van Lier MGF, Westerman AM, Wagner A, et al.: High cancer risk and increased mortality in patients with Peutz-Jeghers syndrome, *Gut* 60:141–147, 2011.

Wang Z, Liu S, Liu S, et al.: Prenatal diagnosis in a hereditary Peutz-Jeghers syndrome family with high cancer, *BMC Med Genet* 19:66, 2018.

Westerman AM, Entius MM, de Baar E, et al.: Peutz-Jeghers syndrome: 78-year follow-up of the original family, *Lancet* 353:1211–1215, 1999.

Hereditary Hemorrhagic Telangiectasia

Bowers EMR, Lee S: Treatment of tongue telangiectasia in a patient with hereditary haemorrhagic telangiectasia, *BMJ Case Rep* 13:e238485, 2020.

Corre P, Perret C, Isidor B, et al.: A brain abscess following dental extractions in a patient with hereditary hemorrhagic telangiectasia, *Br J Oral Maxillofac Surg* 49:e9–e11, 2011.

Da Silva Santos PS, Fernandes KS, Magalhães MH: Osler-Weber-Rendu syndrome—dental implications, *J Can Dent Assoc* 75:527–530, 2009.

Droege F, Thangavelu K, Stuck BA, et al.: Life expectancy and comorbidities in patients with hereditary hemorrhagic telangiectasia, *Vasc Med* 23:377–383, 2018.

Faughnan ME, Mager JJ, Hetts SW, et al.: Second International Guidelines for the diagnosis and management of hereditary hemorrhagic telangiectasia, *Ann Intern Med* 173:989–1001, 2020.

Favia G, Tempesta A, Limongelli L, et al.: Diode laser treatment and clinical management of multiple oral lesions in patients with hereditary haemorrhagic telangiectasia, *Br J Oral Maxillofac Surg* 54:379–383, 2016.

Fiorella ML, Ross D, Henderson KJ, et al.: Outcome of septal dermoplasty in patients with hereditary hemorrhagic telangiectasia, *Laryngoscope* 115:301–305, 2005.

Kjeldsen AD, Vase P, Green A: Hereditary haemorrhagic telangiectasia: a population-based study of prevalence and mortality in Danish patients, *J Intern Med* 245:31–39, 1999.

Koubaa M, Lahiani D, Mâaloul I, et al.: Actinomycotic brain abscess as the first clinical manifestation of hereditary hemorrhagic telangiectasia—case report and review of the literature, *Ann Hematol* 92:1141–1143, 2013.

Kritharis A, Al-Samkari H, Kuter DJ: Hereditary hemorrhagic telangiectasia: diagnosis and management from the hematologist's perspective, *Haematologica* 103:1433–1443, 2018.

Kühnel T, Wirsching K, Wohlgemuth W, et al.: Hereditary hemorrhagic telangiectasia, *Otolaryngol Clin N Am* 51:237–254, 2018.

Russi EW, Dazzi H, Gäumann N: Septic pulmonary embolism due to periodontal disease in a patient with hereditary hemorrhagic telangiectasia, *Respiration* 63:117–119, 1996.

Schwenter F, Faughnen ME, Gradinger AB, et al.: Juvenile polyposis, hereditary hemorrhagic telangiectasia, and early onset colorectal cancer in patients with *SMAD4* mutation, *J Gastroenterol* 47:795–804, 2012.

Shovlin C, Bamford K, Carlo Sabbà C, et al.: Prevention of serious infections in hereditary hemorrhagic telangiectasia: roles for prophylactic antibiotics, the pulmonary capillaries—but not vaccination, *Haematologica* 104:e85, 2019.

Ehlers-Danlos Syndromes

Bowen JM, Sobey GJ, Burrows NP, et al.: Ehlers–Danlos syndrome, classical type, *Am J Med Genet Part C (Semin Med Genet)* 175C:27–39, 2017.

Byers PH, Belmont J, Black J, et al.: Diagnosis, natural history, and management in vascular Ehlers–Danlos syndrome, *Am J Med Genet Part C (Semin Med Genet)* 175C:40–47, 2017.

Chopra P, Tinkle B, Hamonet C, et al.: Pain management in the Ehlers–Danlos syndromes, *Am J Med Genet Part C (Semin Med Genet)* 175C:212–219, 2017.

De Coster PJ, Martens LC, De Paepe A: Oral health in prevalent types of Ehlers-Danlos syndromes, *J Oral Pathol Med* 34:298–307, 2005.

Fridrich KL, Fridrich HH, Kempf KK, et al.: Dental implications in Ehlers-Danlos syndrome: a case report, *Oral Surg Oral Med Oral Pathol* 69:431–435, 1990.

Ghali N, Sobey G, Burrows N: Ehlers-Danlos syndromes, *BMJ* 366: l4966, 2019.

Jesudas R, Chaudhury A, Laukaitis CM: An update on the new classification of Ehlers-Danlos syndrome and review of the causes of bleeding in this population, *Haemophilia* 25:558–566, 2019.

Kapferer-Seebacher I, Lundberg P, Malfait F, et al.: Periodontal manifestations of Ehlers–Danlos syndromes: a systematic review, *J Clin Periodontol* 44:1088–1100, 2017.

Kapferer-Seebacher I, Pepin M, Werner R, et al.: Periodontal Ehlers-Danlos syndrome is caused by mutations in *C1R* and *C1S*, which encode subcomponents C1r and C1s of complement, *Am J Hum Genet* 99:1005–1014, 2016.

Kapferer-Seebacher I, Schnabl D, Zschocke J, et al.: Dental manifestations of Ehlers-Danlos syndromes: a systematic review, *Acta Derm Venereol* 100:adv00092, 2020.

Malfait F, De Coster P, Hausser I, et al.: The natural history, including orofacial features of three patients with Ehlers-Danlos syndrome, dermatosparaxis type (EDS type VIIC), *Am J Med Genet* 131A:18–28, 2004.

Malfait F, Francomano C, Byers P, et al.: The 2017 international classification of the Ehlers–Danlos syndromes, *Am J Med Genet Part C (Semin Med Genet)* 175C:8–26, 2017.

Mitakides J, Tinkle BT: Oral and mandibular manifestations in the Ehlers–Danlos syndromes, *Am J Med Genet Part C (Semin Med Genet)* 175C:220–225, 2017.

Norton LA, Assael LA: Orthodontic and temporomandibular joint considerations in treatment of patients with Ehlers-Danlos syndrome, *Am J Orthod Dentofac Orthop* 111:75–84, 1997.

Riley B: The many facets of hypermobile Ehlers-Danlos syndrome, *J Am Osteopath Assoc* 120:30–32, 2020.

Tinkle B, Castori M, Berglund B, et al.: Hypermobile Ehlers–Danlos syndrome (a.k.a. Ehlers–Danlos syndrome type III and Ehlers–Danlos syndrome hypermobility type): clinical description and natural history, *Am J Med Genet Part C (Semin Med Genet)* 175C:48–69, 2017.

Yassin OM, Rihani FB: Multiple developmental dental anomalies and hypermobility type Ehlers-Danlos syndrome, *J Clin Pediatr Dent* 30:337–341, 2006.

Tuberous Sclerosis
de Araujo LJ, Lima LS, Alvarenga TM, et al.: Oral and neurocutaneous phenotypes of familial tuberous sclerosis, *Oral Surg Oral Med Oral Pathol Oral Radiol Endod* 111:87–94, 2011.

Cardis MA, DeKlotz CMC: Cutaneous manifestations of tuberous sclerosis complex and the paediatrician's role, *Arch Dis Child* 102:858–863, 2017.

Cross NJ, Fung DE: Tuberous sclerosis: a case report, *Spec Care Dentist* 30:157–159, 2010.

Damm DD, Tomich CE, White DK, et al.: Intraosseous fibrous lesions of the jaws: a manifestation of tuberous sclerosis, *Oral Surg Oral Med Oral Pathol Oral Radiol Endod* 87:334–340, 1999.

Ebrahimi-Fakhari D, Mann LL, Poryo M, et al.: Incidence of tuberous sclerosis and age at first diagnosis: new data and emerging trends from a national, prospective surveillance study, *Orphanet J Rare Dis* 13:117, 2018.

Fahmy MD, Gupta A, Padilla RJ, et al.: Desmoplastic fibroma associated with tuberous sclerosis: case report and literature review, *Oral Surg Oral Med Oral Pathol Oral Radiol* 128:e92–e99, 2019.

Franz DN, Belousova E, Sparagana S, et al.: Long-term use of everolimus in patients with tuberous sclerosis complex: final results from the EXIST-1 study, *PLoS One* 11(6):e0158476, 2016. https://doi.org/10.1371/journal.pone.0158476.

Li M, Zhou Y, Chen C-Y, et al.: Efficacy and safety of mTOR inhibitors (rapamycin and its analogues) for tuberous sclerosis complex: a meta-analysis, *Orphanet J Rare Dis* 14(1):39, 2019. https://doi.org/10.1186/s13023-019-1012-x.

Nguyen Q-BD, DarConte MD, Hebert AA: The cutaneous manifestations of tuberous sclerosis complex, *Am J Med Genet* 178C:321–325, 2018.

Peron A, Au KS, Northrup H: Genetics, genomics, and genotype–phenotype correlations of TSC: insights for clinical practice, *Am J Med Genet* 178C:281–290, 2018.

Peron A, Northrup H: Tuberous sclerosis complex, *Am J Med Genet* 178C:274–277, 2018.

Portocarrero LKL, Quental KN, Samorano LP, et al.: Tuberous sclerosis complex: review based on new diagnostic criteria, *An Bras Dermatol* 93:323–331, 2018.

Salussolia CL, Klonowska K, Kwiatkowski DJ, et al.: Genetic etiologies, diagnosis, and treatment of tuberous sclerosis complex, *Annu Rev Genomics Hum Genet* 20:217–240, 2019.

Sampson JR, Attwood D, Al Mughery AS, et al.: Pitted enamel hypoplasia in tuberous sclerosis, *Clin Genet* 42:50–52, 1992.

Thomas D, Rapley J, Strathman R, et al.: Tuberous sclerosis with gingival overgrowth, *J Periodontol* 63:713–717, 1992.

Multiple Hamartoma Syndrome
Alexander EK, Chan-Smutko G, Saksena MA: Case 19-2013: A 35-year-old woman with recurrent goiter and ductal carcinoma of the breast, *N Engl J Med* 368:2416–2424, 2013.

Assis Machado R, Ribeiro Parana LM, Martins L, et al.: Variable expressivity and novel PTEN mutations in Cowden syndrome, *Oral Surg Oral Med Oral Pathol Oral Radiol* 127:55–61, 2019.

Bagán JV, Penarrocha M, Vera-Sempere F: Cowden syndrome: clinical and pathological considerations in two new cases, *J Oral Maxillofac Surg* 47:291–294, 1989.

Elo JA, Sun H-H, Laudenbach JM, et al.: Multiple oral mucosal hamartomas in a 34-year old female, *Head Neck Pathol* 11:393–398, 2017.

Glavina A, Bradamante M, Durdov MG, et al.: Gingival papillomatosis as the oral sign of Cowden syndrome: a case report, *Acta Dermatovenerol Croat* 27:260–264, 2019.

Hammerschmidt M, Lourenc SV, Simonsen Nico MM: A clinicopathological study of the oral lesions of Cowden disease, *J Oral Pathol Med* 46:637–643, 2017.

Kieselova K, Santiago F, Henrique M, et al.: Multiple sclerotic fibromas of the skin: an important clue for the diagnosis of Cowden syndrome, *BMJ Case Rep*, 2017. https://doi.org/10.1136/bcr-2017-221695.

Lin SI, Mort JR, Hinchey PM, et al.: Clinical pathologic conference: diffuse papillomatous lesions of the gingiva with posterolateral neck skin tags, *Oral Surg Oral Med Oral Pathol Oral Radiol* 125:209–214, 2018.

Macken WL, Tischkowitz M, Lachlan KL: PTEN Hamartoma tumor syndrome in childhood: a review of the clinical literature, *Am J Med Genet* 181C:591–610, 2019.

Perića M, Tomab S, Lasserre JF, et al.: Cowden syndrome associated with severe periodontal disease: a short literature review and a case report, *Oral Health Prev Dent* 16:225–232, 2018.

Pilarski R, Eng C: Will the real Cowden syndrome please stand up (again)? Expanding mutational and clinical spectra of the PTEN hamartoma tumour syndrome, *J Med Genet* 41:323–326, 2004.

Porter S, Cawson R, Scully C, et al.: Multiple hamartoma syndrome presenting with oral lesions, *Oral Surg Oral Med Oral Pathol Oral Radiol Endod* 82:295–301, 1996.

Epidermolysis Bullosa

Azrak B, Kaevel K, Hofmann L, et al.: Dystrophic epidermolysis bullosa: oral findings and problems, *Spec Care Dentist* 26:111–115, 2006.

Bello YM, Falabella AF, Schachner LA: Management of epidermolysis bullosa in infants and children, *Clin Dermatol* 21:278–282, 2003.

Brain JH, Paul BF, Assad DA: Periodontal plastic surgery in a dystrophic epidermolysis bullosa patient: review and case report, *J Periodontol* 70:1392–1396, 1999.

Çagirankaya LB, Hatipoglu MG, Hatipoglu H: Localized epidermolysis bullosa simplex with generalized enamel hypoplasia in a child, *Pediatr Dermatol* 23:167–168, 2006.

De Benedittis M, Petruzzi M, Favia G, et al.: Oro-dental manifestations in Hallopeau-Siemens type recessive dystrophic epidermolysis bullosa, *Clin Exp Dermatol* 29:128–132, 2004.

Delebarre H, Chiaverini C, Vandersteen C, et al.: Orofacial management for epidermolysis bullosa during wisdom tooth removal surgery: a technical note, *J Stomatol Oral Maxillofac Surg* 120:467–470, 2019.

Has C, Nyströma A, Saeidian AH, et al.: Epidermolysis bullosa: molecular pathology of connective tissue components in the cutaneous basement membrane zone, *Matrix Biol* 71-72:313–329, 2018.

Has C, Liu L, Bolling MC, et al.: Clinical practice guidelines for laboratory diagnosis of epidermolysis bullosa, *Br J Dermatol* 182:574–592, 2020.

Has C, Bauer JW, Bodemer C, et al.: Consensus reclassification of inherited epidermolysis bullosa and other disorders with skin fragility, *Br J Dermatol* 183:614–627, 2020.

Krämer S, Lucas J, Gamboa F, et al.: Clinical practice guidelines: oral health care for children and adults living with epidermolysis bullosa, *Spec Care Dentist* 40:3–81, 2020.

Li AW, Prindaville B, Bateman ST, et al.: Inpatient management of children with recessive dystrophic epidermolysis bullosa: a review, *Pediatr Dermatol* 34:647–655, 2017.

McGrath JA, O'Grady A, Mayou BJ, et al.: Mitten deformity in severe generalized recessive dystrophic epidermolysis bullosa: histological, immunofluorescence, and ultrastructural study, *J Cutan Pathol* 19:385–389, 1992.

Momeni A, Pieper K: Junctional epidermolysis bullosa: a case report, *Int J Paediatr Dent* 15:146–150, 2005.

Pekiner FN, Yücelten D, Özbayrak S, et al.: Oral-clinical findings and management of epidermolysis bullosa, *J Clin Pediatr Dent* 30:59–66, 2005.

Peñarrocha-Oltra D, Aloy-Prósper A, Ata-Ali J, et al.: Implants placed simultaneously with particulated bone graft in patients diagnosed with recessive dystrophic epidermolysis bullosa, *J Oral Maxillofac Surg* 70:e51–e57, 2012.

Serrano-Martínez MC, Bagán JV, Silvestre FJ, et al.: Oral lesions in recessive dystrophic epidermolysis bullosa, *Oral Dis* 9:264–268, 2003.

Silva LC, Cruz RA, Abou-Id LR, et al.: Clinical evaluation of patients with epidermolysis bullosa: review of the literature and case reports, *Spec Care Dentist* 24:22–27, 2004.

Wright JT: Oral manifestations in the epidermolysis bullosa spectrum, *Dermatol Clin* 28:159–164, 2010.

Pemphigus

Arduino PG, Broccoletti R, Carbone M, et al.: The prompt use of rituximab could decrease adverse effects in patient with pemphigus vulgaris: a preliminary evaluation, *J Oral Pathol Med* 49:177–180, 2020.

Beissert S, Mimouni D, Kanwar A, et al.: Treating pemphigus vulgaris with prednisone and mycophenolate mofetil: a multicenter, randomized, placebo-controlled trial, *J Invest Dermatol* 130:2041–2048, 2010.

Black M, Mignogna MD, Scully C: Pemphigus vulgaris, *Oral Dis* 11:119–130, 2005.

Brenner S, Bialy-Golan A, Ruocco V: Drug-induced pemphigus, *Clin Dermatol* 16:393–397, 1998.

Eisenberg E, Ballow M, Wolfe SH, et al.: Pemphigus-like mucosal lesions: a side effect of penicillamine therapy, *Oral Surg Oral Med Oral Pathol* 51:409–414, 1981.

Fortuna G, Calabria E, Ruoppo E, et al.: The use of rituximab as an adjuvant in the treatment of oral pemphigus vulgaris, *J Oral Pathol Med* 49:91–95, 2020.

Harman KE, Seed PT, Gratian MJ, et al.: The severity of cutaneous and oral pemphigus is related to desmoglein 1 and 3 antibody levels, *Br J Dermatol* 144:775–780, 2001.

Kridin K, Ahn C, Huang WC, et al.: Treatment update of autoimmune blistering diseases, *Dermatol Clin* 37:215–228, 2019.

Laskaris G, Stoufi E: Oral pemphigus vulgaris in a 6-year-old girl, *Oral Surg Oral Med Oral Pathol* 69:609–613, 1990.

Leshem YA, Hodak E, David M, et al.: Successful treatment of pemphigus with biweekly 1-g infusions of rituximab: a retrospective study of 47 patients, *J Am Acad Dermatol* 68:404–411, 2013.

Mays JW, Carey BP, Posey R, et al.: World Workshop of Oral Medicine VII: a systematic review of immunobiologic therapy for oral manifestations of pemphigoid and pemphigus, *Oral Dis* 25(Suppl. 1):111–121, 2019.

Mignogna MD, Fortuna G, Leuci S, et al.: Oropharyngeal pemphigus vulgaris and clinical remission. A long-term, longitudinal study, *Am J Clin Dermatol* 11:137–145, 2010.

Mignogna MD, Lo Muzio L, Bucci E: Clinical features of gingival pemphigus vulgaris, *J Clin Periodontol* 28:489–493, 2001.

Rashid H, Lamberts A, Diercks GFH, et al.: Oral lesions in autoimmune bullous diseases: an overview of clinical characteristics and diagnostic algorithm, *Am J Clin Dermatol* 20:847–861, 2019.

Schmidt E, Kasperkiewicz M, Joly P: Pemphigus, *Lancet* 394:882–894, 2019.

Sultan AS, Villa A, Saavedra AP, et al.: Oral mucous membrane pemphigoid and pemphigus vulgaris—a retrospective two-center cohort study, *Oral Dis* 23:498–504, 2017.

Temel AB, Murrell DF: Pharmacological advances in pemphigus, *Curr Opin Pharmacol* 46:44–49, 2019.

Venugopal SS, Murrell DF: Diagnosis and clinical features of pemphigus vulgaris, *Immunol Allergy Clin N Am* 32:233–243, 2012.

Paraneoplastic Pemphigus

Allen CM, Camisa C: Paraneoplastic pemphigus: a review of the literature, *Oral Dis* 6:208–214, 2000.

Amber KT, Valdebrana M, Grando DA: Paraneoplastic autoimmune multiorgan syndrome (PAMS): beyond the single phenotype of paraneoplastic pemphigus, *Autoimmun Rev* 17:1002–1010, 2018.

Anhalt GJ, Kim SC, Stanley JR, et al.: Paraneoplastic pemphigus: an autoimmune mucocutaneous disease associated with neoplasia, *N Engl J Med* 323:1729–1735, 1990.

Cummins DL, Mimouni D, Tzu J, et al.: Lichenoid paraneoplastic pemphigus in the absence of detectable antibodies, *J Am Acad Dermatol* 56:153–159, 2007.

Didona D, Fania L, Didona B, et al.: Paraneoplastic dermatoses: a brief general review and an extensive analysis of paraneoplastic pemphigus and paraneoplastic dermatomyositis, *Int J Mol Sci* 21:2178, 2020. https://doi.org/10.3390/ijms21062178.

Frew JW, Murrell DF: Paraneoplastic pemphigus (paraneoplastic autoimmune multiorgan syndrome): clinical presentations and pathogenesis, *Dermatol Clin* 29:419–425, 2011.

Helm TN, Camisa C, Valenzuela R, et al.: Paraneoplastic pemphigus: a distinct autoimmune vesiculobullous disorder associated with neoplasia, *Oral Surg Oral Med Oral Pathol* 75:209–213, 1993.

Kim J-H, Kim S-C: Paraneoplastic pemphigus: paraneoplastic autoimmune disease of the skin and mucosa, *Front Immunol*, 2019. https://doi.org/10.3389/fimmu.2019.01259.

Maruta CW, Miyamoto D, Aoki V, et al.: Paraneoplastic pemphigus: a clinical, laboratorial, and therapeutic overview, *An Bras Dermatol* 94:388–398, 2019.

Mimouni D, Anhalt GJ, Lazarova Z, et al.: Paraneoplastic pemphigus in children and adolescents, *Br J Dermatol* 147:725–732, 2002.

Nousari HC, Deterding R, Wojtczack H, et al.: The mechanism of respiratory failure in paraneoplastic pemphigus, *N Engl J Med* 340:1406–1410, 1999.

Ouedraogo E, Gottlieb J, de Masson A, et al.: Risk factors for death and survival in paraneoplastic pemphigus associated with hematologic malignancies in adults, *J Am Acad Dermatol* 80:1544–1549, 2019.

Paolino G, Didona D, Magliulo G, et al.: Paraneoplastic pemphigus: insight into the autoimmune pathogenesis, clinical features and therapy, *Int J Mol Sci* 18:2532, 2017. https://doi.org/10.3390/ijms18122532.

Schmidt E, Kasperkiewicz M, Joly P: Pemphigus, *Lancet* 394:882–894, 2019.

Wang D, Chen Z: Paraneoplastic pemphigus associated with small lymphocytic lymphoma: a case report, *Medicine* 100(2):e24039, 2021.

Yokokura H, Demitsu T, Kakurai M, et al.: Paraneoplastic pemphigus mimicking erosive mucosal lichen planus associated with primary hepatocellular carcinoma, *J Dermatol* 33:842–845, 2006.

Mucous Membrane Pemphigoid

Bagan J, Muzio LL, Scully C: Mucous membrane pemphigoid, *Oral Dis* 11:197–218, 2005.

Bhol KC, Goss L, Kumari S, et al.: Autoantibodies to human α6 integrin in patients with oral pemphigoid, *J Dent Res* 80:1711–1715, 2001.

Carey B, Setterfield J: Mucous membrane pemphigoid and oral blistering diseases, *Clin Exp Dermatol* 44:732–739, 2019.

Chaidemenos G: Tetracycline and niacinamide in the treatment of blistering skin diseases, *Clin Dermatol* 19:781–785, 2001.

Chan LS: Ocular and oral mucous membrane pemphigoid (cicatricial pemphigoid), *Clin Dermatol* 30:34–37, 2012.

Daniel BS, Murrell DF: Review of autoimmune blistering diseases: the pemphigoid diseases, *J Eur Acad Dermatol Venereol* 33:1685–1694, 2019.

Egan CA, Lazarova Z, Darling TN, et al.: Anti-epiligrin cicatricial pemphigoid: clinical findings, immunopathogenesis and significant associations, *Medicine* 82:177–186, 2003.

Fatahzadeh M, Radfar L, Sirois DA: Dental care of patients with autoimmune vesiculobullous diseases: case reports and literature review, *Quintessence Int* 37:777–787, 2006.

Finn DJ, Graham C, Holt DJ, et al.: Management of mucous membrane pemphigoid in a joint oral medicine–dermatology clinic, *Clin Exp Dermatol* 45:685–690, 2020.

Fortuna G, Marinkovich MP: Linear immunoglobulin A bullous dermatosis, *Clin Dermatol* 30:38–50, 2012.

Guiliani M, Favia GF, Lajolo C, et al.: Angina bullosa haemorrhagica: presentation of eight new cases and review of the literature, *Oral Dis* 8:54–58, 2002.

Gupta R, Woodley DT, Chen M: Epidermolysis bullosa acquisita, *Clin Dermatol* 30:60–69, 2012.

Hansen MS, Klefter ON, Julian HO, et al.: Management of patients with ocular manifestations in vesiculobullous disorders affecting the mouth, *Oral Dis* 23:849–853, 2017.

Horie N, Kawano R, Inaba J, et al.: Angina bullosa hemorrhagica of the soft palate: a clinical study of 16 cases, *J Oral Sci* 50:33–36, 2008.

Jalil BA, Abdou YG, Rosen SA, et al.: Mucous membrane pemphigoid causing central airway obstruction, *J Bronchol Intervent Pulmonol* 24:334–338, 2017.

Kridina K, Kneiberb D, Kowalski EH, et al.: Epidermolysis bullosa acquisita: a comprehensive review, *Autoimmun Rev* 18:786–795, 2019.

Kulkarni R, Payne AS, Werth VP, et al.: Custom dental trays with topical corticosteroids for management of gingival lesions of mucous membrane pemphigoid, *Int J Dermatol* 59:e195–e224, 2020.

Lambiel S, Dulguerov P, Laffitte E, et al.: Paraneoplastic mucous membrane pemphigoid with ocular and laryngeal involvement, *BMJ Case Rep*, 2017. https://doi.org/10.1136/bcr-2017-220887.

Letko E, Miserocchi E, Daoud YJ, et al.: A nonrandomized comparison of the clinical outcome of ocular involvement in patients with mucous membrane (cicatricial) pemphigoid between conventional immunosuppressive and intravenous immunoglobulin therapies, *Clin Immunol* 111:303–310, 2004.

Mays JW, Carey BP, Posey R, et al.: WWOM VII: a systematic review of immunobiologic therapy for oral manifestations of pemphigoid and pemphigus, *Oral Dis* 25(Suppl 1):111–121, 2019.

O'Regan E, Bane A, Flint S, et al.: Linear IgA disease presenting as desquamative gingivitis, *Arch Otolaryngol Head Neck Surg* 130:469–472, 2004.

Rashid KA, Gürcan HM, Ahmed AR: Antigen specificity in subsets of mucous membrane pemphigoid, *J Invest Dermatol* 126:2631–2636, 2006.

Sami N, Bhol KC, Ahmed AR: Intravenous immunoglobulin therapy in patients with multiple mucosal involvement in mucous membrane pemphigoid, *Clin Immunol* 102:59–67, 2002.

Santi CG, Gripp AC, Roselino AM, et al.: Consensus on the treatment of autoimmune bullous dermatoses: bullous pemphigoid, mucous membrane pemphigoid and epidermolysis bullosa acquisita—Brazilian Society of Dermatology, *An Bras Dermatol* 94(2 Suppl 1):S33–S47, 2019.

Setterfield J, Shirlaw PJ, Kerr-Muir M, et al.: Mucous membrane pemphigoid: a dual circulating antibody response with IgG and IgA signifies a more severe and persistent disease, *Br J Dermatol* 138:602–610, 1998.

Staines K, Hampton PJ: Treatment of mucous membrane pemphigoid with the combination of mycophenolate mofetil, dapsone, and prednisolone: a case series, *Oral Surg Oral Med Oral Pathol Oral Radiol* 114:e49–e56, 2012.

Stephenson P, Lamey P-J, Scully C, et al.: Angina bullosa haemorrhagica: clinical and laboratory features in 30 patients, *Oral Surg Oral Med Oral Pathol* 63:560–565, 1987.

Sultan A, Stojanov IJ, Lerman MA, et al.: Oral lichen planus pemphigoides: a series of four cases, *Oral Surg Oral Med Oral Pathol Oral Radiol* 120:58–68, 2015.

Taylor J, McMillan R, Shephard M, et al.: World Workshop on Oral Medicine VI: a systematic review of the treatment of mucous membrane pemphigoid, *Oral Surg Oral Med Oral Pathol Oral Radiol* 120:161–171, 2015.

Walton R, Robinson M, Carrozzo M: A service evaluation of the diagnostic testing for mucous membrane pemphigoid in a UK oral medicine unit, *J Oral Pathol Med* 49:687–692, 2020.

Wang K, Seitzman G, Gonzales JA: Ocular cicatricial pemphigoid, *Curr Opin Ophthalmol* 29:543–551, 2018.

Yamamoto K, Fujimoto M, Inoue M, et al.: Angina bullosa hemorrhagica of the soft palate: report of 11 cases and literature review, *J Oral Maxillofac Surg* 64:1433–1436, 2006.

Bullous Pemphigoid

Bağcı IS, Horváth ON, Ruzicka T, et al.: Bullous pemphigoid, *Autoimmun Rev* 16:445–455, 2017.

Genovese G, Di Zenzo G, Cozzani E, et al.: New insights into the pathogenesis of bullous pemphigoid: 2019 update, *Front Immunol*, 2019. https://doi.org/10.3389/fimmu.2019.01506.

Kridin K, Ahn C, Huang WC, et al.: Treatment update of autoimmune blistering diseases, *Dermatol Clin* 37:215–228, 2019.

Kridin K, Bergman R: Assessment of the prevalence of mucosal involvement in bullous pemphigoid, *JAMA Dermatol* 155:166–171, 2019.

Maglie R, Hertl M: Pharmacological advances in pemphigoid, *Curr Opin Pharmacol* 46:34–43, 2019.

Miyamoto D, Santi CG, Aoki V, et al.: Bullous pemphigoid, *An Bras Dermatol* 94:133–146, 2019.

Santi CG, Gripp AC, Roselino AM, et al.: Consensus on the treatment of autoimmune bullous dermatoses: bullous pemphigoid, mucous membrane pemphigoid and epidermolysis bullosa acquisita—Brazilian Society of Dermatology, *An Bras Dermatol* 94(2 Suppl 1): S33–S47, 2019.

Thomas RM, Colon A, Motaparthi K: Rituximab in autoimmune pemphigoid diseases: indications, optimized regimens, and practice gaps, *Clin Dermatol* 38:384–396, 2020.

Erythema Multiforme

Celentano A, Tovaru S, Yap T, et al.: Oral erythema multiforme: trends and clinical findings of a large retrospective European case series, *Oral Surg Oral Med Oral Pathol Oral Radiol* 120:707–716, 2015.

Du Y, Wang F, Liu T, et al.: Recurrent oral erythema multiforme: a case series report and review of the literature, *Oral Surg Oral Med Oral Pathol Oral Radiol* 129:e224–e229, 2020.

Hao M, Zang P, Miller M, et al.: Herpes associated erythema multiforme: a retrospective study, *Am J Emerg Med* 38:2761.e1–2761.e3, 2020.

Langley A, Anooshiravani N, Kwan S, et al.: Erythema multiforme in children and *Mycoplasma pneumoniae* aetiology, *J Cutan Med Surg* 20:453–457, 2016.

Samim F, Auluck A, Zed C, et al.: Erythema multiforme: a review of the epidemiology, pathogenesis, clinical features, and treatment, *Dent Clin N Am* 57:583–596, 2013.

Sanchis JM, Bagán JV, Gavaldá C, et al.: Erythema multiforme: diagnosis, clinical manifestations and treatment in a retrospective study of 22 patients, *J Oral Pathol Med* 39:747–752, 2010.

Spencer S, Buhary T, Coulson I, et al.: Mucosal erosions as the presenting symptom in erythema multiforme: a case report, *Br J Gen Pract*, 2016. https://doi.org/10.3399/bjgp16X684205.

Trayes KP, Love G, Studdiford JS: Erythema multiforme: recognition and management, *Am Fam Physician* 100:82–88, 2019.

Williams PM, Conklin RJ: Erythema multiforme: a review and contrast from Stevens-Johnson syndrome/toxic epidermal necrolysis, *Dent Clin N Am* 49:67–76, 2005.

Zoghaib S, Kechichian E, Souaid K, et al.: Triggers, clinical manifestations, and management of pediatric erythema multiforme: a systematic review, *J Am Acad Dermatol* 81:813–822, 2019.

Stevens-Johnson Syndrome/Toxic Epidermal Necrolysis

Barea-Jiménez N, Calero J, Molina-Negrón D, et al.: Treatment for oral lesions in pediatric patients with Stevens-Johnson's syndrome: A case report and literature, *Int J Paediatr Dent* 30:489–496, 2020.

Coelho Mendes B, de Souza Santos AM, da Cunha Cervantes LC, et al.: Lip synechia resulting from toxic epidermal necrolysis: a rare condition, *J Craniofac Surg* 31:e593–e595, 2020.

Lee HY, Walsh SA, Creamer D: Long-term complications of Stevens–Johnson syndrome/toxic epidermal necrolysis (SJS/TEN): the spectrum of chronic problems in patients who survive an episode of SJS/TEN necessitates multidisciplinary follow-up, *Br J Dermatol* 177:924–935, 2017.

Lyell A: Toxic epidermal necrolysis: an eruption resembling scalding of the skin, *Br J Dermatol* 68:355–361, 1956.

Nowsheen S, Lehman JS, el-Azhary RA: Differences between Stevens-Johnson syndrome versus toxic epidermal necrolysis, *Int J Dermatol* 60:53–59, 2021.

Papp A, Sikora S, Evans M, et al.: Treatment of toxic epidermal necrolysis by a multidisciplinary team. A review of literature and treatment results, *Burns* 44:807–815, 2018.

Schwartz RA, McDonough PH, Lee BW: Toxic epidermal necrolysis. Part I. Introduction, history, classification, clinical features, systemic manifestations, etiology, and immunopathogenesis, *J Am Acad Dermatol* 69:173.e1–173.e13, 2013.

Schwartz RA, McDonough PH, Lee BW: Toxic epidermal necrolysis. Part II. Prognosis, sequelae, diagnosis, differential diagnosis, prevention, and treatment, *J Am Acad Dermatol* 69:187.e1–187.e16, 2013.

Seminario-Vidal L, Kroshinsky D, Malachowski SJ, et al.: Society of Dermatology Hospitalists supportive care guidelines for the management of Stevens-Johnson syndrome/toxic epidermal necrolysis in adults, *J Am Acad Dermatol* 82:1553–1567, 2020.

Sharma N, Venugopal R, Maharana PK, et al.: Multistep grading system for evaluation of chronic ocular sequelae in patients with Stevens-Johnson syndrome, *Am J Ophthalmol* 203:69–77, 2019.

Wang F, Ma Z, Wu X, et al.: Allopurinol-induced toxic epidermal necrolysis featuring almost 60% skin detachment, *Medicine* 98(25):e16078, 2019.

Wolf B, Sadoff R, Nannini V: Toxic epidermal necrolysis: a dermatologic emergency and the role of the oral and maxillofacial surgeon, *J Oral Maxillofac Surg* 76:1688–1694, 2018.

Erythema Migrans

Cigic L, Galic T, Kero D, et al.: The prevalence of celiac disease in patients with geographic tongue, *J Oral Pathol Med* 45:791–796, 2016.

Darling MR, Su N, Masen S, et al.: Geographic tongue: assessment of peripheral nerve status, Langerhans cell, and HLA-DR expression, Oral Surg Oral Med Oral Pathol, *Oral Radiol* 124:371–377, 2017.

Gonzaga HFS, Torres EA, Alchorne MMA, et al.: Both psoriasis and benign migratory glossitis are associated with HLA-Cw6, *Br J Dermatol* 135:368–370, 1996.

González-Álvarez L, García-Martín JM, García-Pola MJ: Association between geographic tongue and psoriasis: a systematic review and meta-analyses, *J Oral Pathol Med* 48:365–372, 2019.

McNamara KK, Kalmar JR: Erythematous and vascular oral mucosal lesions: a clinicopathologic review of red entities, *Head Neck Pathol* 13:4–15, 2019.

Miloğlu Ö, Göregen M, Akgül HM, et al.: The prevalence and risk factors associated with benign migratory glossitis lesions in 7619 Turkish dental outpatients, *Oral Surg Oral Med Oral Pathol Oral Radiol Endod* 107:e29–e33, 2009.

Morris LF, Phillips CM, Binnie WH, et al.: Oral lesions in patients with psoriasis: a controlled study, *Cutis* 49:339–344, 1992.

Ogueta IC, Ramírez MP, Jiménez CO, et al.: Geographic tongue: what a dermatologist should know, *Actas Dermosifiliogr* 110:341–346, 2019.

Picciani BLS, Domingos TA, Teixeira-Souza T, et al.: Geographic tongue and psoriasis: clinical, histopathological, immunohistochemical and genetic correlation—a literature review, *An Bras Dermatol* 91:410–421, 2016.

Shulman JD, Carpenter WM: Prevalence and risk factors associated with geographic tongue among US adults, *Oral Dis* 12:381–386, 2006.

Zagari O: The prevalence and significance of fissured tongue and geographical tongue in psoriatic patients, *Clin Exp Dermatol* 31:192–195, 2006.

Reactive Arthritis

García-Kutzbach A, Chacón-Súchite J, García-Ferrer H, et al.: Reactive arthritis: update 2018, *Clin Rheumatol* 37:869–874, 2018.

Kataria RK, Brent LH: Spondyloarthropathies, *Am Fam Physician* 69:2853–2860, 2004.

Könönen M, Kovero O, Wenneberg B, et al.: Radiographic signs in the temporomandibular joint in Reiter's disease, *J Orofac Pain* 16:143–147, 2002.

Panush RS, Wallace DJ, Dorff EN, et al.: Retraction of the suggestion to use the term "Reiter's syndrome" sixty-five years later: the legacy of Reiter, a war criminal, should not be eponymic honor but rather condemnation (letter), *Arthritis Rheum* 56:693–694, 2007.

Schempp CM, Schauer F, Huhn CK, et al.: Skin inflammation associated with arthritis, synovitis and enthesitis. Part 2: rheumatoid arthritis, reactive arthritis, Reiter's syndrome, Lyme borreliosis, dermatomyositis and lupus erythematosus, *J Dtsch Dermatol Ges*, 2019. https://doi.org/10.1111/ddg.13761.

Wu IB, Schwartz RA: Reiter's syndrome: the classic triad and more, *J Am Acad Dermatol* 59:113–121, 2008.

Lichen Planus

Accurso BT, Warner BM, Knobloch TJ, et al.: Allelic imbalance in oral lichen planus and assessment of its classification as a premalignant condition, *Oral Surg Oral Med Oral Pathol Oral Radiol Endod* 112:359–366, 2011.

Arduino PG, Campolongo MG, Sciannameo V, et al.: Randomized, placebo-controlled, double-blind trial of clobetasol propionate 0.05% in the treatment of oral lichen planus, *Oral Dis* 24:772–777, 2018.

Belfiore P, Di Fede O, Cabibi D, et al.: Prevalence of vulval lichen planus in a cohort of women with oral lichen planus: an interdisciplinary study, *Br J Dermatol* 155:994–998, 2006.

Campisi G, Di Fede O, Craxì A, et al.: Oral lichen planus, hepatitis C virus, and HIV: no association in a cohort study from an area of high hepatitis C virus endemicity, *J Am Acad Dermatol* 51:364–370, 2004.

Carrozzo M, Francia di Celle P, Gandolfo S, et al.: Increased frequency of HLA-DR6 allele in Italian patients with hepatitis C virus-associated oral lichen planus, *Br J Dermatol* 144:803–808, 2001.

Carrozzo M, Porter S, Mercadante V, et al.: Oral lichen planus: a disease or a spectrum of tissue reactions? Types, causes, diagnostic algorhythms, prognosis, management strategies, *Periodontology* 2000(80):105–125, 2019.

Cheng Y-S L, Gould A, Kurago Z, et al.: Diagnosis of oral lichen planus: a position paper of the American Academy of Oral and Maxillofacial Pathology, *Oral Surg Oral Med Oral Pathol Oral Radiol* 122:332–354, 2016.

Davidova LA, Fitzpatrick SG, Bhattacharyya I, et al.: Lichenoid characteristics in premalignant verrucous lesions and verrucous carcinoma of the oral cavity, *Head Neck Pathol* 13:573–579, 2019.

Eisenberg E: Oral lichen planus: a benign lesion, *J Oral Maxillofac Surg* 58:1278–1285, 2000.

Giuliani M, Troiano G, Cordaro M, et al.: Rate of malignant transformation of oral lichen planus: a systematic review, *Oral Dis* 25:693–709, 2019.

González-García A, Diniz-Freitas M, Gándara-Vila P, et al.: Triamcinolone acetonide mouth rinses for treatment of erosive oral lichen planus: efficacy and risk of fungal over-infection, *Oral Dis* 12:559–565, 2006.

Guan G, Mei L, Polonowita A, et al.: Malignant transformation in oral lichen planus and lichenoid lesions: a 14-year longitudinal retrospective cohort study of 829 patients in New Zealand, *Oral Surg Oral Med Oral Pathol Oral Radiol* 130:411–418, 2020.

Harden D, Skelton H, Smith KJ: Lichen planus associated with hepatitis C virus: no viral transcripts are found in the lichen planus, and effective therapy for hepatitis C virus does not clear lichen planus, *J Am Acad Dermatol* 49:847–852, 2003.

Ingafou M, Leao JC, Porter SR, et al.: Oral lichen planus: a retrospective study of 690 British patients, *Oral Dis* 12:463–468, 2006.

Jainkittivong A, Kuvatanasuchati J, Pipattanagovit P, et al.: *Candida* in oral lichen planus patients undergoing topical steroid therapy, *Oral Surg Oral Med Oral Pathol Oral Radiol Endod* 104:61–66, 2007.

Laeijendecker R, Tank B, Dekker SK, et al.: A comparison of treatment of oral lichen planus with topical tacrolimus and triamcinolone acetonide ointment, *Acta Derm Venereol* 86:227–229, 2006.

Le Cleach L, Chosidow O: Lichen planus, *N Engl J Med* 366:723–732, 2012.

Leao JC, Ingafou M, Khan A, et al.: Desquamative gingivitis: retrospective analysis of disease associations of a large cohort, *Oral Dis* 14:556–560, 2008.

Lv K, Liu J, Ye W, et al.: Multiple superficial mucoceles concomitant with oral lichen planus: a case series, *Oral Surg Oral Med Oral Pathol Oral Radiol* 127:e95–e101, 2019.

Mattsson U, Jontell M, Holmstrup P: Oral lichen planus and malignant transformation: is a recall of patients justified? *Crit Rev Oral Biol Med* 13:390–396, 2002.

Patel S, Yeoman CM, Murphy R: Oral lichen planus in childhood: a report of three cases, *Int J Paediatr Dent* 15:118–122, 2005.

Montague LJ, Bhattacharyya I, Islam MN, et al.: Direct immunofluorescence testing results in cases of premalignant and malignant oral lesions, *Oral Surg Oral Med Oral Pathol Oral Radiol* 119:675–683, 2015.

Robledo-Sierra J, Landin-Wilhelmsen K, Filipsson Nyström H, et al.: A mechanistic linkage between oral lichen planus and autoimmune thyroid disease, *Oral Dis* 24:1001–1011, 2018.

Roosaar A, Yin L, Sandborgh-Englund G, et al.: On the natural course of oral lichen lesions in a Swedish population-based sample, *J Oral Pathol Med* 35:257–261, 2006.

Setterfield JF, Neill S, Shirlaw PJ, et al.: The vulvovaginal gingival syndrome: a severe subgroup of lichen planus with characteristic clinical features and a novel association with the class II HLA DQB1*0201 allele, *J Am Acad Dermatol* 55:98–113, 2006.

Shearston K, Fateh B, Tai S, et al.: Oral lichenoid dysplasia and not oral lichen planus undergoes malignant transformation at high rates, *J Oral Pathol Med* 48:538–545, 2019.

Shen Z-Y, Liu W, Feng J-Q, et al.: Squamous cell carcinoma development in previously diagnosed oral lichen planus: de novo or transformation? *Oral Surg Oral Med Oral Pathol Oral Radiol Endod* 112:592–596, 2011.

Siponen M, Huuskonen L, Kallio-Pulkkinen S, et al.: Topical tacrolimus, triamcinolone acetonide, and placebo in oral lichen planus: a pilot randomized controlled trial, *Oral Dis* 23:660–668, 2017.

Thorne JE, Jabs DA, Nikolskaia OV, et al.: Lichen planus and cicatrizing conjunctivitis: characterization of five cases, *Am J Ophthalmol* 136:239–243, 2003.

Thornhill MH, Sankar V, Xu X-J, et al.: The role of histopathological characteristics in distinguishing amalgam-associated oral lichenoid reactions and oral lichen planus, *J Oral Pathol Med* 35:233–240, 2006.

Tucker SC, Coulson IH: Lichen planus is not associated with hepatitis C infection in patients from North West England, *Acta Derm Venereol* 79:378–379, 1999.

Van der Meij EH, Mast H, van der Waal I: The possible premalignant character of oral lichen planus and oral lichenoid lesions: a prospective follow-up study of 192 patients, *Oral Oncol* 43:742–748, 2007.

Van der Meij EH, Slootweg PJ, van der Wal JE, et al.: Interobserver and intraobserver variability in the histologic assessment of oral lichen planus, *J Oral Pathol Med* 28:274–277, 1999.

Van der Meij EH, van der Waal I: Lack of clinicopathologic correlation in the diagnosis of oral lichen planus based on the presently available diagnostic criteria and suggestions for modifications, *J Oral Pathol Med* 32:507–512, 2003.

Vilar-Villanueva M, Gándara-Vila P, Blanco-Aguilera E, et al.: Psychological disorders and quality of life in oral lichen planus patients and a control group, *Oral Dis* 25:1645–1651, 2019.

Voûte ABE, Schulten EAJM, Langendijk PNJ, et al.: Fluocinonide in an adhesive base for treatment of oral lichen planus: a double-blind, placebo-controlled clinical study, *Oral Surg Oral Med Oral Pathol* 75:181–185, 1993.

Wee JS, Shirlaw PJ, Challacombe SJ, et al.: Efficacy of mycophenolate mofetil in severe mucocutaneous lichen planus: a retrospective review of 10 patients, *Br J Dermatol* 167:36–43, 2012.

Zhang LW, Michelsen C, Cheng X, et al.: Molecular analysis of oral lichen planus: a premalignant lesion? *Am J Pathol* 151:323–327, 1997.

Chronic Ulcerative Stomatitis

Azzi L, Cerati M, Lombardo M, et al.: Chronic ulcerative stomatitis: a comprehensive review and proposal for diagnostic criteria, *Oral Dis* 25:1465–1491, 2019.

Carlson MW, Garlick JA, Solomon LW: Chronic ulcerative stomatitis: evidence of autoimmune pathogenesis, *Oral Surg Oral Med Oral Pathol Oral Radiol Endod* 111:742–748, 2011.

Jaremko WM, Beutner EH, Kumar V, et al.: Chronic ulcerative stomatitis associated with a specific immunologic marker, *J Am Acad Dermatol* 22:2115–2120, 1990.

Ko EM, Danciu TE, Fullen DR, et al.: Chronic ulcerative stomatitis: case series of an under-recognized entity, *J Cutan Pathol* 45:927–932, 2018.

Lee LA, Walsh P, Prater CA, et al.: Characterization of an autoantigen associated with chronic ulcerative stomatitis: the CUSP autoantigen is a member of the p53 family, *J Invest Dermatol* 113:146–151, 1999.

Qari H, Villasante C, Richert J, et al.: The diagnostic challenges of separating chronic ulcerative stomatitis from oral lichen planus, *Oral Surg Oral Med Oral Pathol Oral Radiol* 120:622–627, 2015.

Reddy R, Fitzpatrick SG, Bhattacharyya I, et al.: Seventeen new cases of chronic ulcerative stomatitis with literature review, *Head Neck Pathol* 13:386–396, 2019.

Solomon LW, Aguirre A, Neiders M, et al.: Chronic ulcerative stomatitis: clinical, histopathologic, and immunopathologic findings, *Oral Surg Oral Med Oral Pathol Oral Radiol Endod* 96:718–726, 2003.

Solomon LW, Stark PC, Winter L, et al.: ELISA test for p63 antibodies in chronic ulcerative stomatitis, *Oral Dis* 16:151–155, 2010.

Graft-Versus-Host Disease

Abdelsayed RA, Sumner T, Allen CM, et al.: Oral precancerous and malignant lesions associated with graft-versus-host disease: report of 2 cases, *Oral Surg Oral Med Oral Pathol Oral Radiol Endod* 93:75–80, 2002.

Brand HS, Bots CP, Raber-Durlacher JE: Xerostomia and chronic oral complications among patients treated with haematopoietic stem cell transplantation, *Br Dent J* 207(E17):1–4, 2009.

Brown RS, Edwards D, Walsh-Chocolaad T, et al.: Topical tacrolimus with custom trays in the treatment of severe oral chronic graft-versus-host disease refractory to a potent topical steroid therapy, *Oral Surg Oral Med Oral Pathol Oral Radiol* 115:e26–e30, 2013.

Csanadi M, Agh T, Tordai A, et al.: (2019) A systematic literature review of incidence, mortality, and relapse of patients diagnosed with chronic graft versus host disease, *Expert Rev Hematol* 12(5):311–323, 2019. https://doi.org/10.1080/17474086.2019.1605288.

Eckardt A, Starke O, Stadler M, et al.: Severe oral chronic graft-versus-host disease following allogeneic bone marrow transplantation: highly effective treatment with topical tacrolimus, *Oral Oncol* 40:811–814, 2004.

Fall-Dickson JM, Pavletic SZ, Mays JW, et al.: Oral complications of chronic graft-versus-host disease, *J Natl Cancer Inst Monogr* 2019 (53):54–62, 2019.

García-F-Villalta MJ, Pascual-López M, Elices M, et al.: Superficial mucoceles and lichenoid graft versus host disease: report of three cases, *Acta Derm Venereol* 82:453–455, 2002.

Haverman TM, Raber-Durlacher JE, Raghoebar II, et al.: Oral chronic graft-versus-host disease. What the general dental practitioner needs to know, *JADA* 151:846–856, 2020.

Imanguli MM, Atkinson JC, Mitchell SA, et al.: Salivary gland involvement in chronic graft-versus-host disease: prevalence, clinical significance, and recommendations for evaluation, *Biol Blood Marrow Transplant* 16:1362–1369, 2010.

Ion D, Stevenson K, Woo S-B, et al.: Characterization of oral involvement in acute graft-versus-host disease, *Biol Blood Marrow Transplant* 20:1717–1721, 2014.

Mawardi H, Hashmi SK, Elad S, et al.: Chronic graft-versus-host disease: current management paradigm and future perspectives, *Oral Dis* 25:931–948, 2019.

Melkos AB, Massenkeil G, Arnold R, et al.: Dental treatment prior to stem cell transplantation and its influence on the posttransplantation outcome, *Clin Oral Investig* 7:113–115, 2003.

Nygaard M, Wichert S, Berlin G, et al.: Extracorporeal photopheresis for graft-vs-host disease: a literature review and treatment guidelines proposed by the Nordic ECP Quality Group, *Eur J Haematol* 104:361–375, 2020.

Ramachandran V, Kolli SS, Strowd LC: Review of graft-versus-host disease, *Dermatol Clin* 37:569–582, 2019.

Rocha V, Wagner JE, Sobocinski KA, et al.: Graft-versus-host disease in children who have received a cord-blood or bone marrow transplant from an HLA-identical sibling, *N Engl J Med* 342:1846–1854, 2000.

Sánchez AR, Sheridan PJ, Rogers RS: Successful treatment of oral lichen planus-like chronic graft-versus-host disease with topical tacrolimus: a case report, *J Periodontol* 75:613–619, 2004.

Sarantopoulos S, Cardones AR, Sullivan KM: How I treat refractory chronic graft-versus-host disease, *Blood* 133:1191–1200, 2019.

Sedghizadeh PP, Allen CM, Anderson KE, et al.: Oral graft-versus-host disease and programmed cell death: pathogenetic and clinical correlates, *Oral Surg Oral Med Oral Pathol Oral Radiol Endod* 97:491–498, 2004.

Soares AB, Faria PR, Magna LA, et al.: Chronic GVHD in minor salivary glands and oral mucosa: histopathological and immunohistochemical evaluation of 25 patients, *J Oral Pathol Med* 34:368–373, 2005.

Treister N, Li S, Kim H, et al.: An open-label Phase II randomized trial of topical dexamethasone and tacrolimus solutions for the treatment of oral chronic graft-versus-host disease, *Biol Blood Marrow Transplant* 22:2084–2091, 2016.

Weng X, Xing Y, Cheng B: Multiple and recurrent squamous cell carcinoma of the oral cavity after graft-versus-host disease, *J Oral Maxillofac Surg* 75:1899–1905, 2017.

Woo S-B, Lee SJ, Schubert MM: Graft-vs-host disease, *Crit Rev Oral Biol Med* 8:201–216, 1997.

Psoriasis

Armstrong AW, Read C: Pathophysiology, clinical presentation, and treatment of psoriasis: a review, *JAMA* 323:1945–1960, 2020.

Brooks JK: Psoriasis: a review of systemic comorbidities and dental management considerations, *Quintessence Int* 49:209–217, 2018.

Bruce AJ, Rogers RS: Oral psoriasis, *Dermatol Clin* 21:99–104, 2003.

Costa SC, Hirota SK, Takahashi MDF, et al.: Oral lesions in 166 patients with cutaneous psoriasis: a controlled study, *Med Oral Patol Oral Cir Bucal* 14:e371–e375, 2009.

Doffy DL, Spelman LS, Martin NG: Psoriasis in Australian twins, *J Am Acad Dermatol* 29:428–434, 1993.

Mattsson U, Warfvinge G, Jontell M: Oral psoriasis - a diagnostic dilemma: a report of two cases and a review of the literature, *Oral Surg Oral Med Oral Pathol Oral Radiol* 120:e183–e189, 2015.

Mendes LS, Cota LOM, Costa AA, et al.: Periodontitis as another comorbidity associated with psoriasis: a case-control study, *J Periodontol* 90:358–366, 2019.

Myers WA, Gottlieb AB, Mease P: Psoriasis and psoriatic arthritis: clinical features and disease mechanisms, *Clin Dermatol* 24:438–447, 2006.

Picciani BLS, Domingos TA, Teixeira-Souza T, et al.: Geographic tongue and psoriasis: clinical, histopathological, immunohistochemical and genetic correlation—a literature review, *An Bras Dermatol* 91:410–421, 2016.

Pietrzak D, Pietrzak A, Krasowska D, et al.: Digestive system in psoriasis: an update, *Arch Dermatol Res* 309:679–693, 2017.

Reid C, Griffiths CEM: Psoriasis and treatment: past, present and future aspects, *Acta Derm Venereol* 100:adv00032, 2020.

Stern RS: The risk of squamous cell and basal cell cancer associated with psoralen and ultraviolet A therapy: a 30-year prospective study, *J Am Acad Dermatol* 66:553–562, 2012.

von Csiky-Sessoms S, Lebwohl M: What's new in psoriasis, *Dermatol Clin* 37:129–136, 2019.

Lupus Erythematosus

Aringer M, Johnson SR: Classifying and diagnosing systemic lupus erythematosus in the 21st century, *Rheumatology* 59:v4–v11, 2020.

Arvanitidou I-E, Nikitakis NG, Georgaki M, et al.: Multiple primary squamous cell carcinomas of the lower lip and tongue arising in discoid lupus erythematosus: a case report, *Oral Surg Oral Med Oral Pathol Oral Radiol* 125:e22–e30, 2018.

Benli N, Batool F, Stutz C, et al.: Orofacial manifestations and dental management of systemic lupus erythematosus: a review, *Oral Dis* 27:151–167, 2021.

Brennan MT, Valerin MA, Napeñas JJ, et al.: Oral manifestations of patients with lupus erythematosus, *Dent Clin N Am* 49:127–141, 2005.

Chang AY, Werth VP: Treatment of cutaneous lupus, *Curr Rheumatol Rep* 13:300–307, 2011.

Deapen D, Escalante A, Weinrib L, et al.: A revised estimate of twin concordance in systemic lupus erythematosus, *Arthritis Rheum* 35:311–318, 1992.

Del Barrio-Díaz P, Reyes-Vivanco C, Cifuentes-Mutinelli M, et al.: Association between oral lesions and disease activity in lupus erythematosus, *J Eur Acad Dermatol Venereol* 34:349–356, 2020.

Doria A, Iaccarino L, Ghirardello A, et al.: Long-term prognosis and causes of death in systemic lupus erythematosus, *Am J Med* 119:700–706, 2006.

Fava A, Petri M: Systemic lupus erythematosus: diagnosis and clinical management, *J Autoimmun* 96:1–13, 2019.

Filotico R, Mastrandrea V: Cutaneous lupus erythematosus: clinico-pathologic correlation, *G Ital Dermatol Venereol* 153:216–229, 2018.

Gagari E, De Villiers P, Antoniou C: Clinico-pathologic conference: case 5, *Head Neck Pathol* 3:295–298, 2009.

Hahn BH: Systemic lupus erythematosus, In Jameson JL, Fauci AS, Kasper DL, et al., editors: *Harrison's principles of internal medicine*, ed 20, New York, 2018, McGraw-Hill, pp 2515–2526.

Lam N-CV, Ghetu MV, Bieniek ML: Systemic lupus erythematosus: primary care approach to diagnosis and management, *Am Fam Physician* 94:284–294, 2016.

Menzies S, O'Shea F, Galvin S, et al.: Oral manifestations of lupus, *Ir J Med Sci* 187:91–93, 2018.

Nico MMS, Romiti R, Lourenço SV: Oral lesions in four cases of subacute cutaneous lupus erythematosus, *Acta Derm Venereol* 91:436–439, 2011.

Ribero S, Sciascia S, Borradori L, et al.: The cutaneous spectrum of lupus erythematosus, *Clinic Rev Allerg Immunol* 53:291–305, 2017.

Rhodus NL, Johnson DK: The prevalence of oral manifestations of systemic lupus erythematosus, *Quintessence Int* 21:461–465, 1990.

Rodsaward P, Prueksrisakul T, Deekajorndech T, et al.: Oral ulcers in juvenile-onset systemic lupus erythematosus: a review of the literature, *Am J Clin Dermatol* 18:755–762, 2017.

Stojan G, Petri M: Epidemiology of systemic lupus erythematosus: an update, *Curr Opin Rheumatol* 30:144–150, 2018.

Tanaka Y: State-of-the-art treatment of systemic lupus erythematosus, *Int J Rheum Dis* 23:465–471, 2020.

Thorne JE, Jabs DA, Nikolskaia O, et al.: Discoid lupus erythematosus and cicatrizing conjunctivitis: clinicopathologic study of two cases, *Ocul Immunol Inflamm* 10:287–292, 2002.

Systemic Sclerosis

Alhendi FJ, Werth VP, Sollecito TP, et al.: Systemic sclerosis: update for oral health care providers, *Spec Care Dentist* 40:418–430, 2020.

Anbiaee N, Tafakhori Z: Early diagnosis of progressive systemic sclerosis (scleroderma) from a panoramic view: report of three cases, *Dentomaxillofac Radiol* 40:457–462, 2011.

Burchfield C, Vorrasi J: Maxillofacial implications of scleroderma and systemic sclerosis: a case report and literature review, *J Oral Maxillofac Surg* 77:1203–1208, 2019.

Dagenais M, MacDonald D, Baron M, et al.: The Canadian Systemic Sclerosis Oral Health Study IV: oral radiographic manifestations in systemic sclerosis compared with the general population, *Oral Surg Oral Med Oral Pathol Oral Radiol* 120:104–111, 2015.

Demir Y, Karaaslan T, Aktepe F, et al.: Linear scleroderma "en coup de sabre" of the cheek, *J Oral Maxillofac Surg* 61:1091–1094, 2003.

Denton CP, Khanna D: Systemic sclerosis, *Lancet* 390:1685–1699, 2017.

Eversole LR, Jacobsen PL, Stone CE: Oral and gingival changes in systemic sclerosis (scleroderma), *J Periodontol* 55:175–178, 1984.

Gomes da Silva GS, Maymone de Melo ML, Leão JC, et al.: Oral features of systemic sclerosis: a case–control study, *Oral Dis* 25:1995–2002, 2019.

Haers PE, Sailer HF: Mandibular resorption due to systemic sclerosis: case report of surgical correction of a secondary open bite deformity, *Int J Oral Maxillofac Surg* 24:261–267, 1995.

Ioannidis JPA, Vlachoyiannopoulos PG, Haidich A-B, et al.: Mortality in systemic sclerosis: an international meta-analysis of individual patient data, *Am J Med* 118:2–10, 2005.

Isola G, Williams RC, Lo Gullo A, et al.: Risk association between scleroderma disease characteristics, periodontitis, and tooth loss, *Clin Rheumatol* 36:2733–2741, 2017.

Jung S, Martin T, Schmittbuhl M, et al.: The spectrum of orofacial manifestations in systemic sclerosis: a challenging management, *Oral Dis* 23:424–439, 2017.

Kirby DF, Chatterjee S: Evaluation and management of gastrointestinal manifestations in scleroderma, *Curr Opin Rheumatol* 26:621–629, 2014.

Knobler RM, French LE, Kim Y, et al.: A randomized, double-blind, placebo-controlled trial of photopheresis in systemic sclerosis, *J Am Acad Dermatol* 54:793–799, 2006.

Leung WK, Chu CH, Mok MY, et al.: Periodontal status of adults with systemic sclerosis: case-control study, *J Periodontol* 82:1140–1145, 2011.

Medsger TA: Natural history of systemic sclerosis and the assessment of disease activity, severity, functional status, and psychologic well-being, *Rheum Dis Clin N Am* 29:255–273, 2003.

Pearson DR, Werth VP, Pappas-Taffer L: Systemic sclerosis: current concepts of skin and systemic manifestations, *Clin Dermatol* 36:459–474, 2018.

Rout PGJ, Hamburger J, Potts AJC: Orofacial radiological manifestations of systemic sclerosis, *Dentomaxillofac Radiol* 25:193–196, 1996.

Sticherling M: Systemic sclerosis—dermatological aspects. Part 1: Pathogenesis, epidemiology, clinical findings, *J Dtsch Dermatol Ges* 10:705–716, 2012.

van den Hoogen F, Khanna D, Fransen J, et al.: 2013 Classification criteria for systemic sclerosis: an American college of rheumatology/European league against rheumatism collaborative initiative, *Ann Rheum Dis* 72:1747–1755, 2013.

Varga J: Systemic sclerosis (scleroderma) and related disorders, In Jameson JL, Fauci AS, Kasper DL, et al., editors: *Harrison's principles of internal medicine*, ed 20, New York, 2018, McGraw-Hill, pp 2546–2560.

Yenisey M, Külünk T, Kurt S, et al.: A prosthodontics management alternative for scleroderma patients, *J Oral Rehabil* 32:696–700, 2005.

CREST Syndrome

Chamberlain AJ, Walker NPJ: Successful palliation and significant remission of cutaneous calcinosis in CREST syndrome with carbon dioxide laser, *Dermatol Surg* 968–970, 2003.

Daoussis D, Antonopoulos I, Liossis S-NC, et al.: Treatment of systemic sclerosis-associated calcinosis: a case report of rituximab-induced regression of CREST-related calcinosis and review of the literature, *Semin Arthritis Rheum* 41:822–829, 2012.

Ferreli C, Gasparini G, Parodi A, et al.: Cutaneous manifestations of scleroderma and scleroderma-like disorders: a comprehensive review, *Clinic Rev Allerg Immunol* 53:306–336, 2017.

Frantza C, Huscherb D, Avouac J, et al.: Outcomes of limited cutaneous systemic sclerosis patients: results on more than 12,000 patients from the EUSTAR database, *Autoimmun Rev* 19:102452, 2020.

Pearson DR, Werth VP, Pappas-Taffer L: Systemic sclerosis: current concepts of skin and systemic manifestations, *Clin Dermatol* 36:459–474, 2018.

Sparsa A, Lesaux N, Kessler E, et al.: Treatment of cutaneous calcinosis in CREST syndrome by extracorporeal shock wave lithotripsy, *J Am Acad Dermatol* 53:S263–S265, 2005.

Acanthosis Nigricans

Abu-Safieh Y, Khelfa S: Acanthosis nigricans: a presentation of gastric adenocarcinoma, *Arab J Gastroenterol* 12:156–157, 2011.

Cairo F, Rubino I, Rotundo R, et al.: Oral acanthosis nigricans as a marker of internal malignancy, *A case report, J Periodontol* 72:1271–1275, 2001.

Hall JM, Moreland A, Cox GJ, et al.: Oral acanthosis nigricans: report of a case and comparison of oral and cutaneous pathology, *Am J Dermatopathol* 10:68–73, 1988.

Karadağ AS, You Y, Danarti R, et al.: Acanthosis nigricans and the metabolic syndrome, *Clin Dermatol* 36:48–53, 2018.

Mignogna MD, Fortuna G, Falleti J, et al.: Gastric diffuse large B-cell lymphoma (DLBCL) exhibiting oral acanthosis nigricans and tripe palms, *Dig Liver Dis* 41:766–768, 2009.

Mostofi RS, Hayden NP, Soltani K: Oral malignant acanthosis nigricans, *Oral Surg Oral Med Oral Pathol* 56:372–374, 1983.

Ramirez-Amador V, Esquivel-Pedraza L, Caballero-Mendoza E, et al.: Oral manifestations as a hallmark of malignant acanthosis nigricans, *J Oral Pathol Med* 28:278–281, 1999.

Rizwan M, Iftikhar N, Sarfraz T, et al.: Malignant acanthosis nigricans: an indicator of internal malignancy, *J Coll Physicians Surg Pak* 29:888–890, 2019.

Schwartz RA: Acanthosis nigricans, *J Am Acad Dermatol* 31:1–19, 1994.

Scully C, Barrett WA, Gilkes J, et al.: Oral acanthosis nigricans, the sign of Leser-Trélat and cholangiocarcinoma, *Br J Dermatol* 145:505–526, 2001.

Shah KR, Boland CR, Patel M, et al.: Cutaneous manifestations of gastrointestinal disease: part I, *J Am Acad Dermatol* 68:189e1–189e21, 2013.

Wick MR, Patterson JW: Cutaneous paraneoplastic syndromes, *Semin Diagn Pathol* 36:211–228, 2019.

Yu Q, Li X-L, Ji G, et al.: Malignant acanthosis nigricans: an early diagnostic clue for gastric adenocarcinoma, *World J Surg Oncol* 15:208, 2017.

17

Oral Manifestations of Systemic Diseases

◆ MUCOPOLYSACCHARIDOSIS

The **mucopolysaccharidoses** are a heterogeneous group of metabolic disorders that are usually inherited in an autosomal recessive fashion. These disorders are all characterized by the lack of any one of several normal enzymes needed to process the important intercellular substances known as *glycosaminoglycans*. These substances used to be known as *mucopolysaccharides,* thus the term *mucopolysaccharidosis.* Examples of glycosaminoglycans include the following:

- Heparan sulfate
- Dermatan sulfate
- Keratan sulfate
- Chondroitin sulfate

The type of mucopolysaccharidosis that is seen clinically depends on which of these substrates lacks its particular enzyme. The mucopolysaccharidoses as a group occur with a frequency of approximately 1 in 15,000 to 29,000 live births, although some types are much less common.

Clinical and Radiographic Features

The clinical features of the mucopolysaccharidoses vary, depending on the particular syndrome that is examined (Table 17.1). Furthermore, affected patients with a particular type of this disorder often exhibit a wide range of severity of involvement. Most types of mucopolysaccharidosis are associated with some degree of intellectual disability. Often the facial features of affected patients are somewhat coarse, with heavy brow ridges (Fig. 17.1), and there are other skeletal changes, such as stiff joints. Cloudy degeneration of the corneas, a problem that frequently leads to blindness, is seen in several forms of mucopolysaccharidosis.

The oral manifestations vary according to the particular type of mucopolysaccharidosis. Most types show some degree of macroglossia. Gingival hyperplasia may be present, particularly in the anterior regions, as a result of the drying and irritating effects of mouth breathing. The dental changes include thin enamel with pointed cusps on the posterior teeth, although this seems to be a feature unique to mucopolysaccharidosis type IVA. Other dental manifestations include numerous impacted teeth with prominent follicular spaces (Fig. 17.2), possibly caused by the accumulation of glycosaminoglycans in the follicular connective tissue. Some investigators have reported the occurrence of multiple impacted teeth that are congregated in a single large follicle, forming a rosette pattern radiographically. Taurodonts (see page 92) are seen with increased frequency in affected individuals, and deformities of the condylar head, described as flattening or distortion, have been identified in these patients.

Although the clinical findings may suggest that a patient is affected by one of the mucopolysaccharidoses, the diagnosis is confirmed by finding elevated levels of glycosaminoglycans in the urine, as well as deficiencies of the specific enzymes in the patient's leukocytes and fibroblasts.

Treatment and Prognosis

No satisfactory systemic treatment of the mucopolysaccharidoses exists at this time. Several forms of mucopolysaccharidosis are associated with a markedly reduced life span and with intellectual disability. Attempts to improve the survival and quality of life of these patients using hematopoietic stem cell transplantation have met with some success. Unfortunately, not all aspects of the disease are corrected, and the complications associated with transplantation must be addressed. Such complications are associated with a 15%–20% mortality rate. Enzyme replacement therapy currently is available for mucopolysaccharidosis types I, II, and VI. Initiation of the respective recombinant human enzymes—laronidase, idursulfase, and galsulfase—early in the patient's life appears to improve significantly many of the aspects of the disease, although complete resolution does not occur. Because of the rarity of these conditions and the expense of developing the treatments, the annual cost for such therapy can range from $176,000 for laronidase to $657,000 for idursulfase, which currently has the dubious distinction of being the most expensive prescription medication. Genetic counseling is indicated for the parents and siblings of a patient affected by one of the mucopolysaccharidosis syndromes. Prenatal diagnosis is available for family planning as well.

TABLE 17.1	Features of Selected Mucopolysaccharidosis Syndromes				
Type	Eponym	Inheritance	Enzyme Deficiency	Stored Substrate	Clinical Features
I-H	Hurler	AR	α-ʟ-Iduronidase	HS and DS	Appears in infancy; cloudy corneas, growth impairment, reduced intelligence, coronary artery disease; rarely live 10 years
I-S	Scheie	AR	α-ʟ-Iduronidase	HS and DS	Onset in late childhood; cloudy corneas, normal intelligence, aortic regurgitation; survive to adulthood
II	Hunter	X-linked R	Iduronate-2-sulfatase	HS and DS	Appears at 1–2 years of age; clear corneas, reduced intelligence, growth impairment, stiff joints
III-A	Sanfilippo-A	AR	Heparan N-sulphatase	HS	Appears at 4–6 years of age; clear corneas, reduced intelligence, mild skeletal changes; death in adolescence
III-B	Sanfilippo-B	AR	α-N-acetylglucosaminidase	HS	Generally same as Sanfilippo-A
IV-A	Morquio-A	AR	Galactose-6-sulfatase	KS and CS	Appears at 1–2 years of age; cloudy corneas, normal intelligence, lax joints; may survive to middle age
IV-B	Morquio-B	AR	β-Galactosidase	KS	Generally similar to Morquio-A
VI	Maroteaux-Lamy	AR	Arylsulphatase B	DS and CS	Appears at 2–6 years of age; cloudy corneas, normal intelligence, growth impairment, stiff joints; may survive to adulthood

AR, Autosomal recessive; *CS*, chondroitin sulfate; *DS*, dermatan sulfate; *HS*, heparan sulfate; *KS*, keratan sulfate; *R*, recessive.

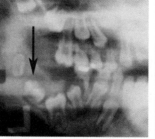 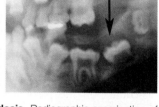

• **Fig. 17.2 Mucopolysaccharidosis.** Radiographic examination of the dentition of a child affected by Hunter syndrome typically shows radiolucencies (arrows) associated with the crowns of unerupted teeth.

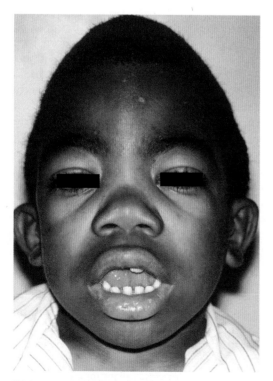

• **Fig. 17.1 Mucopolysaccharidosis.** This patient affected by Hunter syndrome exhibits the characteristic facial features of this disorder.

Management of the dental problems of these patients is essentially no different from that of other patients. However, several factors may have to be taken into account:

- Degree of intellectual disability (if any)
- Presence or absence of a seizure disorder
- Degree of joint stiffening
- Extent of other related medical problems

Depending on which of these factors is present and the extent of involvement, dental care may warrant sedation, hospitalization, or general anesthesia of the patient for optimal results. General anesthesia and sedation may be challenging, however, because of excess amounts of pharyngeal tissues that often produce a smaller than normal airway. In severely affected patients, general anesthesia probably should be considered only in life-threatening situations.

◆ LIPID RETICULOENDOTHELIOSES

The **lipid reticuloendothelioses** are a relatively rare group of inherited disorders. These include the following conditions:

- Gaucher disease
- Niemann-Pick disease
- Tay-Sachs disease

These conditions are seen with increased frequency in patients with Ashkenazi Jewish heritage. Affected patients lack certain enzymes necessary for processing specific lipids; this results in an accumulation of the lipids within a variety of cells. Because of this accumulation, it appeared that cells were attempting to store these substances; therefore, the term *storage disease* was commonly used for these disorders.

In **Gaucher disease** (the most common of the reticuloendothelioses), a lack of glucocerebrosidase results in the accumulation of glucosylceramide, particularly within the lysosomes of cells of the macrophage and monocyte lineage. Three types of Gaucher disease are now recognized: type 1 (nonneuronopathic) is seen primarily in the Ashkenazi Jewish population, and types 2 and 3 (neuronopathic) have a panethnic distribution.

Niemann-Pick disease is characterized by a deficiency of acid sphingomyelinase, resulting in the accumulation of sphingomyelin, also within the lysosomes of macrophages.

Tay-Sachs disease is caused by a lack of β-hexosaminidase A, which results in the accumulation of a ganglioside, principally within the lysosomes of neurons.

All these disorders are inherited as autosomal recessive traits. The genetic mutation known to cause Gaucher disease has been evaluated for the Ashkenazi Jewish population, and approximately 1 in 12–17 persons carry the defective gene. Most of the individuals identified as having the gene, however, were heterozygous and, therefore, asymptomatic.

Clinical and Radiographic Features
Gaucher Disease

The clinical features of Gaucher disease are generally the result of the effects of the abnormal storage of glucosylceramide. Macrophages laden with this glucocerebroside are typically rendered relatively nonfunctional, and they tend to accumulate within the liver, spleen, and bone marrow of the affected patient. Bone marrow accumulation displaces the normal hematopoietic cells and produces anemia and thrombocytopenia. In addition, these patients are susceptible to bone infarctions. The resulting bone pain is often the presenting complaint. Characteristic *Erlenmeyer flask* deformities of the long bones, particularly of the femur, are often identified. Accumulations of the macrophages in the spleen and liver result in visceral enlargement. Many affected patients show a significant degree of growth impairment. Neurologic deterioration occurs in patients with the less common types 2 and 3 Gaucher disease. Jaw lesions typically appear as ill-defined radiolucencies that usually affect the mandible, producing thinning of the cortical bone without causing devitalization of the teeth or significant resorption

of the lamina dura. The walls of the mandibular canal may also be obliterated by the disease process. Decreased salivary flow has been documented for patients with Gaucher disease compared with an age- and sex-matched population, although this decrease may not be clinically important.

Niemann-Pick Disease

Niemann-Pick disease occurs as three different types, each associated with a different clinical expression and prognosis. Types A and B are caused by a deficiency of acid sphingomyelinase, whereas type C is primarily the result of mutations of either *NPC-1* or *NPC-2,* genes involved with cholesterol processing. Types A and C have **neuronopathic** features, characterized by psychomotor impairment, dementia, spasticity, and hepatosplenomegaly, with death occurring during the first or second decade of life. Type B patients normally survive into adulthood and exhibit **visceral signs,** primarily hepatosplenomegaly, and sometimes pulmonary involvement.

Tay-Sachs Disease

Tay-Sachs disease may have a wide clinical range because the condition is genetically heterogeneous. Some forms are mild, with patients surviving into adulthood. In the severe infantile form, however, rapidly progressive neuronal degeneration develops shortly after birth. Signs and symptoms include blindness, developmental impairment, and intractable seizures. Death usually occurs by 3–5 years of age.

Histopathologic Features

Histopathologic examination of an osseous lesion of Gaucher disease shows sheets of lipid-engorged macrophages (Gaucher cells) exhibiting abundant bluish cytoplasm, which has a fine texture resembling wrinkled silk. In Niemann-Pick disease, the characteristic cell seen on examination of a bone marrow aspirate is the "sea blue" histiocyte.

Treatment and Prognosis
Gaucher Disease

For patients with a mild expression of Gaucher disease, no treatment may be necessary. For more severe forms of Gaucher disease, enzyme replacement therapy with one of the macrophage-targeted glucocerebrosidases, including imiglucerase, velaglucerase alfa, and taliglucerase alfa, is used. All of these medications require intravenous (IV) infusion and are quite expensive, often costing more than $150,000 per year for treatment. After 9–12 months of therapy, patients exhibit improvement in the status of their anemia, a decrease in plasma glucocerebroside levels, and a decrease in hepatosplenomegaly. Resolution of the radiographic bone changes takes place over a longer period. Children treated with this regimen may show significant gain in height. Unfortunately enzyme replacement therapy has shown minimal effect on the neuronopathic Gaucher disease types 2 and 3, primarily because the medication cannot cross the blood-brain barrier. Bone marrow transplantation has also been attempted;

however, the problems inherent in graft-versus-host disease (GVHD) are still present with that form of therapy, and thus it is not recommended. A case-control study showed that adults with Gaucher disease have an increased risk for hematologic malignancies, particularly lymphoma and multiple myeloma. Genetic counseling should be provided to all affected patients.

Niemann-Pick and Tay-Sachs Disease

The neuronopathic forms of Niemann-Pick disease and the infantile form of Tay-Sachs disease are associated with a poor prognosis. Genetic counseling should be provided for affected families. Molecular markers of these disorders have been developed to identify carriers. Such identification allows earlier intervention in terms of counseling, and targeted population screening for the gene that causes Tay-Sachs disease has resulted in a marked decrease in affected patients during the past three decades.

◆ LIPOID PROTEINOSIS (HYALINOSIS CUTIS ET MUCOSAE; URBACH-WIETHE SYNDROME)

A rare condition, **lipoid proteinosis** is inherited as an autosomal recessive trait. It is characterized by the deposition of a waxy material in the dermis and submucosal connective tissue of affected patients. The earliest thorough description of lipoid proteinosis was by Urbach and Wiethe in 1929, and more than 300 patients, most being of European background, have been reported to date. Mutations of the *ECM1* gene, which encodes a glycoprotein known as *extracellular matrix protein 1*, have been identified as the cause for this condition.

Clinical Features

The laryngeal mucosa and vocal cords are usually the sites that are initially affected by lipoid proteinosis. Therefore, the first sign of the disease may be one of the following:
- An inability of the infant to make a crying sound
- A hoarse cry in infancy
- The development of a hoarse voice during early childhood

The vocal cords become thickened as the accumulation of an amorphous material begins to affect the laryngeal mucosa. This infiltrative mucosal process may also involve the pharynx, esophagus, tonsils, vulva, and rectum. Skin lesions also develop early in life, appearing as thickened, yellowish, waxy papules; plaques; or nodules that often affect the face, particularly the lips and the margins of the eyelids (Fig. 17.3). Some lesions may begin as dark-crusted vesicles that heal as atrophic hyperpigmented patches.

Eventually, most patients exhibit a thickened, furrowed appearance of the skin. Other areas of the skin that may be involved include the neck, palms, axillae, elbows, scrotum, knees, and digits. In those areas subjected to chronic trauma, a hyperkeratotic, verrucous surface often develops. In addition

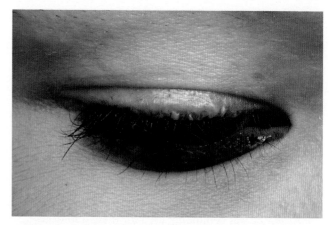

• **Fig. 17.3 Lipoid Proteinosis.** Thickened papules are present along the margin of the eyelid. (Courtesy of Dr. Maria Copete.)

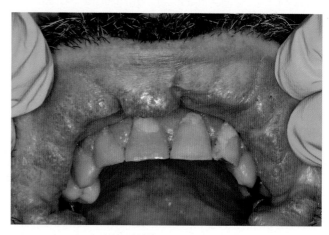

• **Fig. 17.4 Lipoid Proteinosis.** The vermilion zone of the upper lip exhibits yellow-white, nodular thickenings.

to the cutaneous manifestations, symmetrical intracranial calcifications of the medial temporal lobes have been identified in approximately 70% of affected patients. These lesions are usually asymptomatic, although a few patients with such calcifications have been reported to have a seizure disorder.

The oral mucosal abnormalities typically become evident in the second decade of life. The tongue, labial mucosa, and buccal mucosa become nodular, diffusely enlarged, and thickened because of infiltration with waxy, yellow-white plaques and nodules (Fig. 17.4). The dorsal tongue papillae are eventually destroyed, and the tongue develops a smooth surface. The accumulation of the amorphous material within the tongue may result in its being bound to the floor of the mouth. Therefore, the patient may not be able to protrude the tongue, and the lack of oral soft tissue mobility may hinder the delivery of optimal dental care in some instances. Gingival enlargement appears to be an infrequent finding.

Histopathologic Features

A biopsy specimen of an early lesion of lipoid proteinosis typically reveals the deposition of a lamellar material around the blood vessels, nerves, hair follicles, and sweat glands. This

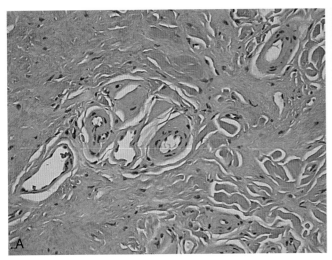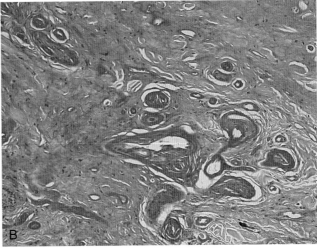

• **Fig. 17.5 Lipoid Proteinosis. A,** This medium-power photomicrograph shows perivascular deposition of a lamellar, acellular material. **B,** The periodic acid-Schiff (PAS) method is used to stain and highlight the perivascular deposits. (Courtesy of Dr. Maria Copete.)

material stains positively with the periodic acid-Schiff (PAS) method and is not digested by diastase. The location of this material, its staining properties, and the presence of increased laminin, type IV collagen, and type V collagen suggest a basement membrane origin.

A biopsy specimen of a lesion in its later stages usually shows not only the lamellar material but also deposition of an amorphous substance within the dermal connective tissue (Fig. 17.5).

Treatment and Prognosis

Generally, no specific treatment is available for lipoid proteinosis other than genetic counseling. In rare instances, the infiltration of the laryngeal mucosa may produce difficult breathing for some infants, in which case debulking of the mucosal lesions may be necessary. Most patients with lipoid proteinosis have a normal life span. Certainly, however, the vocal hoarseness and the appearance of the skin may influence the quality of life for affected patients. As is the case with several other hyperkeratotic genodermatoses, the rough, scaly skin lesions may respond to systemic retinoid therapy, but the deposits of abnormal material in the dermis and submucosa do not.

◆ JAUNDICE (ICTERUS)

Jaundice is a condition characterized by excess bilirubin in the bloodstream. The bilirubin accumulates in the tissues, which results in a yellowish discoloration of the skin and mucosa. To understand jaundice, it is important to know something about the metabolism of bilirubin. Most bilirubin is derived from the breakdown of hemoglobin, the oxygen-carrying pigment of erythrocytes. The average life span of an erythrocyte in the circulation is 120 days. After this time, it undergoes physiologic breakdown. The hemoglobin is degraded and processed by the cells of the reticuloendothelial system, and bilirubin is liberated into the bloodstream in an unconjugated state. In the liver, bilirubin is taken up by the hepatocytes and conjugated with glucuronic acid, which produces conjugated bilirubin, a soluble product that can be excreted in the bile.

There are numerous causes for increased serum levels of bilirubin; some are physiologic, and many are pathologic. Therefore, the presence of jaundice is not a specific sign and generally necessitates physical examination and laboratory studies to determine the precise cause. The basic disturbances associated with increased bilirubin levels include an increased production of bilirubin. This occurs when the red blood cells (RBCs) are being broken down at such a rapid rate that the liver cannot keep pace with processing. This breakdown is seen in such conditions as **autoimmune hemolytic anemia** or **sickle cell anemia.**

In addition, the liver may not be functioning correctly, resulting in decreased uptake of the bilirubin from the circulation or decreased conjugation of bilirubin in the liver cells. Jaundice is frequently present at birth as a result of the low level of activity of the enzyme system that conjugates bilirubin. Defects in this enzyme system may also be seen with certain inherited problems, one of the more common of which is **Gilbert syndrome.** This innocuous condition is often detected on routine examination, and it is estimated to affect up to 5% of people in the United States. Because most of these examples of jaundice occur with impaired processing of bilirubin, laboratory studies usually show unconjugated bilirubin in the serum.

The presence of conjugated bilirubinemia in jaundice can usually be explained by the reduced excretion of bilirubin into the bile ducts. This can be the result of swelling of the hepatocytes (resulting in an occlusion of the bile canaliculi) or hepatocyte necrosis, with disruption of the bile canaliculi and liberation of conjugated bilirubin. Thus liver function may be disturbed because of any one of a variety of infections (e.g., viruses) or toxins (e.g., alcohol).

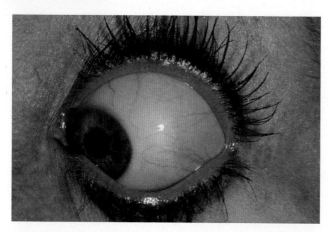

• **Fig. 17.6 Jaundice.** The yellow color of the sclera represents a common finding.

Occlusion of the bile duct from gallstones, stricture, or cancer can also force conjugated bilirubin into the bloodstream.

Clinical Features

The patient affected by jaundice exhibits a diffuse, uniform, yellowish discoloration of the skin and mucosa. The color varies in intensity, depending on the serum level of bilirubin and the anatomic site. Because elastin fibers have an affinity for bilirubin, tissues that have a high content of elastin, including the sclera, lingual frenum, and soft palate, are prominently affected. The sclera of the eye is often the first site at which the yellow color is noted (Fig. 17.6). The yellow discoloration caused by **hypercarotenemia** (resulting from excess ingestion of carotene, a vitamin-A precursor found in yellow vegetables and fruits) may be confused with jaundice, but the sclera is not involved in that condition.

Other signs and symptoms associated with jaundice vary with the underlying cause of the hyperbilirubinemia. For example, patients with viral hepatitis usually have a fever, abdominal pain, anorexia, and fatigue. The patient with jaundice typically requires a complete medical evaluation to determine the precise cause of the condition so that proper therapy can be instituted.

Treatment and Prognosis

The treatment and prognosis of the patient with jaundice vary with the cause. The jaundice that is commonly noted at birth often resolves spontaneously; however, if the infant is placed under special lights, then the clearing will occur more quickly because conjugation of the bilirubin molecule is triggered by exposure to blue light. If the episode of jaundice is due to significant liver damage, as may be seen with viral hepatitis B or hepatotoxic chemical injury, then the prognosis will vary, depending on the extent of liver damage. The prognosis for patients with jaundice secondary to liver damage associated with metastatic malignancy is poor.

♦ AMYLOIDOSIS

Amyloidosis represents a heterogeneous group of conditions characterized by the deposition of an extracellular proteinaceous substance called **amyloid.** Virchow coined the term *amyloid* in the middle of the nineteenth century because he believed it to be a starch-like material (*amyl* = starch; *oid* = resembling). We now understand that amyloid can be formed in a variety of settings, each with its own specific type of amyloid protein. Many of these amyloid proteins have been identified precisely with respect to their biochemical composition, and ideally an attempt should be made to categorize the type of amyloid specifically when this diagnosis is made. The various amyloid proteins are designated with an *A*, to indicate amyloid, followed by an abbreviation for the specific amyloid protein. For example, *AL* would identify amyloid composed of immunoglobulin light (L) chain molecules. Although amyloid may have several sources, all types of amyloid have the common feature of a β-pleated sheet molecular configuration, which can be seen with X-ray diffraction crystallographic analysis. Because of this similarity of molecular structure, the different types of amyloid have similar staining patterns with special stains.

Amyloidosis can produce a variety of effects, depending on the organ of involvement and the extent to which the amyloid is deposited. With limited cutaneous forms of amyloidosis, virtually no effect on survival is seen. With some forms of systemic amyloidosis, however, death may occur within a few years of the diagnosis as a result of cardiac or renal failure. Furthermore, the presence of amyloid may be associated with other problems, such as multiple myeloma or chronic infections.

Clinical Features

Several classifications of amyloidosis have been proposed in the past decade, each evolving as the knowledge of this unusual condition increases. None of the classifications is completely satisfactory, although in recent years, the biochemical makeup of these proteins has figured more prominently in most classifications. This discussion attempts to be as concise and direct as possible. Essentially, amyloidosis may be divided into **organ-limited** and **systemic** forms from a clinical standpoint.

Organ-Limited Amyloidosis

Although organ-limited amyloidosis may occur in a variety of organs, it has infrequently been reported in the oral soft tissues. An example of a limited form of amyloidosis is the amyloid nodule, which appears as a solitary, otherwise asymptomatic, submucosal deposit. Most of the organ-limited forms of amyloidosis consist of aggregates of immunoglobulin light chains, which in some cases are produced by a focal collection of monoclonal plasma cells. By definition, such amyloid deposits are not associated with any systemic alteration.

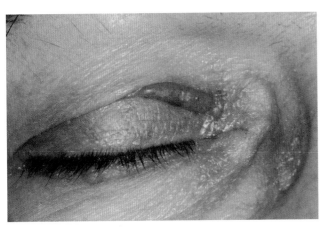

• **Fig. 17.7 Amyloidosis.** This patient exhibits a firm, waxy nodular lesion in the periocular region, a finding that is characteristic of this condition.

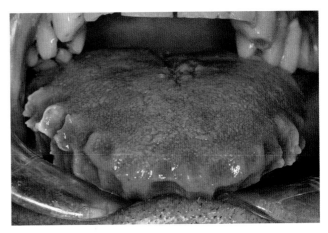

• **Fig. 17.8 Amyloidosis.** The patient exhibits an enlarged and crenated tongue. (Courtesy of Dr. Gregory Erena.)

Systemic Amyloidosis

Systemic amyloidosis may occur in several forms:

- Primary
- Myeloma associated
- Secondary
- Hemodialysis associated
- Heredofamilial

Primary and Myeloma-Associated Amyloidosis

The primary and myeloma-associated forms of amyloidosis usually affect older adults (average age, 65 years), and a slight male predilection is present. These types of amyloidosis are caused by deposition of light chain molecules (thus the designation *AL*), with most cases being idiopathic, although approximately 15%–20% are associated with multiple myeloma. The initial signs and symptoms may be nonspecific, often resulting in a delayed diagnosis. Fatigue, weight loss, paresthesia, hoarseness, edema, and orthostatic hypotension are among the first indications of this disease process. Eventually, carpal tunnel syndrome, mucocutaneous lesions, hepatomegaly, and macroglossia develop as a result of the deposition of the amyloid protein. The skin lesions appear as smooth-surfaced, firm, waxy papules and plaques. These most commonly affect the eyelid region (Fig. 17.7), the retroauricular region, the neck, and the lips. The lesions are often associated with petechiae and ecchymoses. Macroglossia has been reported in 10%–40% of these patients and may appear as diffuse or nodular enlargement of the tongue (Fig. 17.8). Sometimes oral amyloid nodules show ulceration and submucosal hemorrhage overlying the lesions. Infrequently, patients may complain of dry eyes or dry mouth, which is secondary to amyloid infiltration and destruction of the lacrimal and salivary glands. When significant blood vessel infiltration has occurred, claudication of the jaw musculature may be noticed.

Secondary Amyloidosis

Secondary amyloidosis is so named because it characteristically develops as a result of a chronic inflammatory process, such as long-standing osteomyelitis, tuberculosis, or sarcoidosis. Cleavage fragments of a circulating acute-phase reactant protein appear to comprise this type of amyloidosis, which is thus designated *AA*. The heart is usually not affected as in other forms of amyloidosis. Liver, kidney, spleen, and adrenal involvement are typical, however. With the advent of modern antibiotic therapy, this form of amyloidosis has become much less common in the United States.

Hemodialysis-Associated Amyloidosis

Patients who have undergone long-term renal dialysis also are susceptible to amyloidosis, although in this case the amyloid protein has been identified as β_2-microglobulin, and this type of amyloidosis is designated as $A\beta_2M$. β_2-Microglobulin is a normally occurring protein that usually is not removed by the dialysis procedure, and it accumulates in the plasma. Eventually, it forms deposits, particularly in the bones and joints. Often, carpal tunnel syndrome occurs, as well as cervical spine pain and dysfunction. Tongue involvement has been reported. This type of amyloidosis may become less of a problem in the future because of increased use of dialyzers with larger pores that permit removal of the large β_2-microglobulin molecule.

Heredofamilial Amyloidosis

Heredofamilial amyloidosis is an uncommon but significant form of the disease. Several kindred have been identified in Swedish, Portuguese, and Japanese populations, and most types are inherited as autosomal dominant traits. Hereditary transthyretin amyloidosis is one example of this type of amyloidosis, and this form of amyloid deposition is characterized by gradual onset of both sensory and motor nerve polyneuropathy. Affected patients develop a variety of signs and symptoms, including difficulty walking, bilateral carpel tunnel syndrome, paroxysmal intense pain affecting their extremities, cardiomyopathy, and gastrointestinal disturbances. An autosomal recessive form, known as *familial Mediterranean fever*, has also been described. Other inherited forms of amyloidosis may also present with polyneuropathies, and other manifestations, such as cardiac arrhythmias, congestive heart

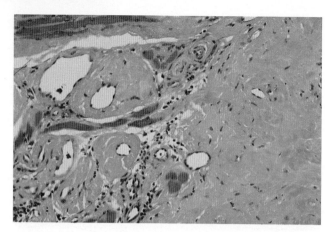

• **Fig. 17.9 Amyloidosis.** This medium-power photomicrograph shows the eosinophilic, acellular deposits that are characteristic of amyloid deposition.

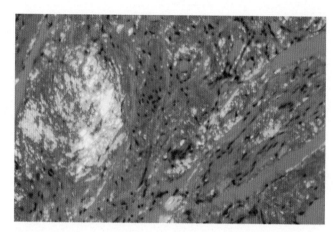

• **Fig. 17.10 Amyloidosis.** High-power photomicrograph of a Congo red–stained section, demonstrating characteristic apple-green birefringence when viewed with polarized light. (Courtesy of Dr. John Kalmar.)

failure, and renal failure, eventually develop as the amyloid deposition continues.

Histopathologic Features

Biopsy of rectal mucosa has classically been used to confirm a diagnosis of primary or myeloma-associated amyloidosis, with up to 80% of such biopsy specimens being positive. Aspiration biopsy of abdominal subcutaneous fat is a simpler procedure, however, and the sensitivity of this technique has been reported to range from 55% to 75%. Alternative tissue sources, however, are the gingiva and labial salivary glands. Histopathologic examination of gingival tissue that has been affected by amyloidosis shows extracellular deposition in the submucosal connective tissue of an amorphous, eosinophilic material, which may be arranged in a perivascular orientation or may be diffusely present throughout the tissue (Fig. 17.9). Relatively low sensitivity has been reported for gingival biopsies, whereas labial salivary gland tissue shows deposition of amyloid in a periductal or perivascular location in more than 80% of the cases.

If the amorphous eosinophilic material represents amyloid, it will be stained by the dye, Congo red, which has an affinity for the abnormal protein. In tissue sections stained with Congo red, the amyloid appears red. When the tissue that takes up the Congo red stain is viewed with polarized light, it exhibits an apple-green birefringence (Fig. 17.10). This Congo red staining method is considered to be the "gold standard" for identifying the presence of amyloid. Other techniques have been used, but these are less sensitive or specific. Microscopic sections stained with crystal violet reveal a characteristic metachromasia; this normally purple dye appears more reddish when it reacts with amyloid. Staining with thioflavine T, a fluorescent dye, also gives positive results if amyloid is present. Ultrastructurally, amyloid is seen as a collection of 7.5- to 10-nm diameter, nonbranching, linear fibrils.

Diagnosis

Once the histopathologic diagnosis of amyloidosis has been made, the patient must be evaluated medically to determine the type of amyloidosis that is present. This often entails a workup that includes serum immunoelectrophoresis to determine whether a monoclonal gammopathy exists so that multiple myeloma can be ruled out. Immunohistochemical studies are proving to be very useful in distinguishing the specific type of amyloid protein. Family history and physical examination findings are also important.

Treatment and Prognosis

In most instances, no effective therapy is available for amyloidosis. Surgical debulking of amyloid deposition in the tongue has met with limited success. Selected forms of amyloidosis may respond to treatment, or at least their progression may be slowed, depending on the underlying cause. In cases of secondary amyloidosis associated with an infectious agent, treatment of the infection and reduction of the inflammation often result in clinical improvement. Renal transplantation may arrest the progression of the bone lesions in hemodialysis-associated amyloidosis, but this procedure apparently does not reverse the process. Liver transplantation has been shown to improve the prognosis of several forms of inherited amyloidosis, particularly the transthyretin variant. Newly approved treatments for transthyretin amyloidosis include inotersen and patisiran, which disrupt the intracellular molecular synthesis of transthyretin amyloid, resulting in reduction in symptoms and markedly improving the prognosis of this condition. Familial Mediterranean fever may respond to systemic colchicine therapy. Genetic counseling is also appropriate for patients affected by the inherited forms of amyloidosis. Treatment of primary amyloidosis (AL) with colchicine, prednisone, and melphalan appears to improve the prognosis of patients who do not have cardiac or renal involvement, although the outlook is guarded to poor in most instances. Autologous stem cell transplantation has shown to improve survival rates, but unfortunately only 20%–25% of AL amyloid patients meet the criteria for undergoing this rigorous form of therapy. Most patients die of cardiac failure, arrhythmia, or renal disease within months to a few years after the diagnosis.

◆ XANTHELASMA (XANTHELASMA PALPEBRARUM)

Xanthelasma is the most common of the cutaneous xanthomas, occurring in approximately 4% of the adult population. The condition is mentioned because these lesions appear somewhat similar to cutaneous amyloid deposits. In addition, the presence of xanthelasma has been related to an increased risk of atherosclerosis as well as elevated serum lipids.

Clinical Features

Xanthelasma is typically identified in middle-aged or older adults, presenting as one or more soft, yellowish plaques associated with the periocular skin (Fig. 17.11). The lesions tend to develop on the medial aspect of the upper eyelid. Their soft consistency and yellow color clinically should help distinguish xanthelasma from amyloid deposits.

Histopathologic Features

Biopsy of xanthelasma shows a collection of lipid-laden histiocytes in the superficial to mid-dermal connective tissue.

Treatment and Prognosis

Treatment of xanthelasma itself is not necessary and is generally considered a cosmetic procedure. If the patient has not been evaluated recently with respect to their cholesterol levels, referral to a primary care physician for serum lipid assessment would be prudent. The lesions can be surgically removed, or they can be removed by laser ablation. Both techniques have similar acceptable cosmetic results, although recurrence is not unusual, even if serum lipids are controlled.

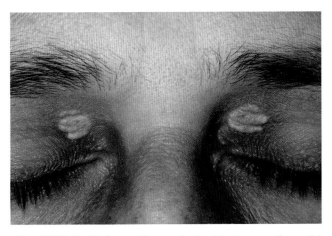

• **Fig. 17.11 Xanthelasma.** These soft yellowish plaques on the medial aspect of the skin of the upper eyelid are characteristic of xanthelasma.

◆ VITAMIN DEFICIENCY

In the United States today, significant vitamin deficiencies are not common. Patients with malabsorption syndromes or eating disorders, persons who follow "fad diets," and alcoholics are the groups most commonly affected.

Vitamin A (retinol) is essential for the maintenance of vision, and it also plays a role in growth and tissue differentiation. Vitamin A can be obtained directly from dietary sources, such as organ meats (particularly liver), or the body can synthesize it from β-carotene, which is abundant in dark green, red, or yellow vegetables.

Vitamin B_1 (thiamin) acts as a coenzyme for several metabolic reactions and is thought to maintain the proper functioning of neurons. Thiamin is found in many animal and vegetable food sources.

Vitamin B_2 (riboflavin) is necessary for cellular oxidation-reduction reactions. Foods that contain significant amounts of riboflavin include milk, green vegetables, lean meat, fish, legumes, and eggs.

Vitamin B_3 (niacin) acts as a coenzyme for oxidation-reduction reactions. Rich sources include food from animal sources, especially lean meat and liver, milk, eggs, whole grains, peanuts, yeast, and cereal bran or germ.

Vitamin B_6 (pyridoxine) serves as a cofactor associated with enzymes that participate in amino acid synthesis. It is found in many animal and vegetable food sources.

Vitamin C (ascorbic acid) is necessary for the proper synthesis of collagen. This vitamin is present in a wide variety of vegetables and fruits, although it is particularly abundant in citrus fruits.

Vitamin D, which is now considered to be a hormone, can be synthesized in adequate amounts within the epidermis if the skin is exposed to a moderate degree of sunlight. Most milk and processed cereal is fortified with vitamin D in the United States today, however. Appropriate levels of vitamin D and its active metabolites are necessary for calcium absorption from the gut.

Vitamin E (α-tocopherol) is a fat-soluble vitamin that is widely stored throughout the body. It probably functions as an antioxidant. Vegetable oils, meats, nuts, cereal grains, and fresh greens and vegetables are good sources of vitamin E.

Vitamin K is a fat-soluble vitamin found in a wide variety of green vegetables, as well as milk, butter, and liver; intestinal bacteria also produce it. This vitamin is necessary for the proper synthesis of various proteins, including the clotting factors II, VII, IX, and X.

Clinical Features

Vitamin A

A severe deficiency of vitamin A during infancy may result in blindness, and is considered one of the leading causes of childhood blindness in underdeveloped parts of the world. The early changes associated with a lack of this vitamin later in life include an inability of the eye to adapt to reduced light conditions (i.e., night blindness). With more severe, prolonged deficiency, dryness of the skin and conjunctiva develop, and the ocular changes may progress to ulceration of the cornea, leading to blindness.

Thiamin

A deficiency of thiamin results in a condition called **beriberi,** a problem that is relatively uncommon in the Western world except in alcoholics or other individuals who do not receive a balanced diet. Thiamin deficiency has also been documented in patients who have had gastric bypass surgery for weight control, presumably because an adequate amount of the vitamin is not obtained in the diet. The condition became prevalent in Southeast Asia when the practice of removing the outer husks of the rice grain by machine was introduced. Because these outer husks contained nearly all of the thiamin, people who subsisted on the "polished" rice became deficient in this vitamin. The disorder is manifested by cardiovascular problems (e.g., peripheral vasodilation, heart failure, and edema) and neurologic problems (including peripheral neuropathy and Wernicke encephalopathy). Patients with Wernicke encephalopathy experience vomiting, nystagmus, and progressive mental deterioration, which may lead to coma and death.

Riboflavin

A diet that is chronically deficient in riboflavin causes a number of oral alterations, including glossitis, angular cheilitis, sore throat, and swelling and erythema of the oral mucosa. A normocytic, normochromic anemia may be present, and seborrheic dermatitis may affect the skin.

Niacin

A deficiency of niacin causes a condition known as **pellagra,** a term derived from the Italian words *pelle agra,* meaning *rough skin.* This condition may occur in populations that use maize as a principal component of their diets, because corn is a poor source of niacin. Pellagra was once common in the southeastern United States and may still be seen in some parts of the world. The classic systemic signs and symptoms include the triad of dermatitis, dementia, and diarrhea. The dermatitis is distributed symmetrically; sun-exposed areas, such as the face, neck, and forearms, are affected most severely (Fig. 17.12). The oral manifestations have been described as stomatitis and glossitis, with the tongue appearing red, smooth, and raw. Without correction of the niacin deficiency, the disease may evolve and persist over a period of years, eventually leading to death.

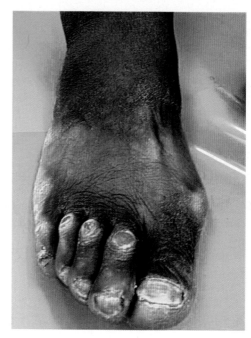

• **Fig. 17.12 Pellagra.** The skin on the foot is rough and hyperpigmented, except for a central band that was protected from sunlight by a sandal strap. (Courtesy of Dr. Sylvie Brener.)

Pyridoxine

A deficiency of pyridoxine is unusual because of its widespread occurrence in a variety of foods. A number of drugs, such as the antituberculosis drug isoniazid, act as pyridoxine antagonists; therefore, patients who receive these medications may have a deficiency state. Because the vitamin plays a role in neuronal function, patients may show weakness, dizziness, or seizure disorders. Cheilitis and glossitis, reported in people with pellagra, are also reported in patients with pyridoxine deficiency.

Vitamin C

A deficiency of vitamin C is known as **scurvy,** and its occurrence in the United States is usually limited to people whose diets lack fresh fruits and vegetables. Commonly affected groups include inner-city infants (whose diets often consist entirely of milk), children affected by autism or other neurodevelopmental disorders (due to limited diet that is chosen), bone marrow transplant recipients (due to oral mucositis related to graft-vs-host disease), children with iron overload related to multiple transfusions (due to sickle cell anemia and thalassemia), and older edentulous men, particularly those who live alone.

The clinical signs of scurvy are typically related to inadequate collagen synthesis. For example, weakened vascular walls may result in widespread petechial hemorrhage and ecchymosis. Similarly, wound healing is delayed, and recently healed wounds may break down. In childhood, painful subperiosteal hemorrhages may occur.

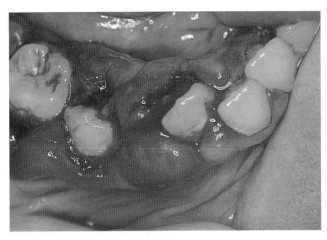

• **Fig. 17.13 Scurvy.** Hemorrhagic gingival enlargement (scorbutic gingivitis) because of capillary fragility. (Courtesy of Dr. James Hargan.)

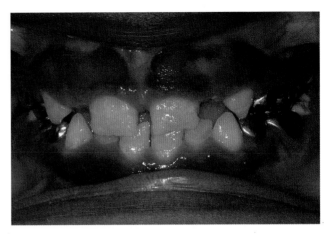

• **Fig. 17.14 Vitamin D Deficiency.** Hypocalcification of the teeth is seen in this child who had vitamin D deficiency related to a diet of breast milk exclusively and lack of adequate sunlight exposure. (Courtesy of Dr. Pamela McDonald.)

The oral manifestations are well documented and include generalized gingival swelling with spontaneous hemorrhage, ulceration, tooth mobility, and increased severity of periodontal infection and periodontal bone loss. The gingival lesions have been termed **scorbutic gingivitis** (Fig. 17.13). If untreated, scurvy may ultimately lead to death, often as a result of intracranial hemorrhage.

Vitamin D

A deficiency of vitamin D during infancy results in a condition called **rickets;** adults who are deficient in this vitamin develop **osteomalacia.** With the vitamin-D supplementation of milk and cereal, rickets is a relatively uncommon disease today in the United States. In past centuries, however, rickets was often seen, particularly in the temperate zones of the world, which often do not receive adequate sunlight to ensure physiologic levels of vitamin D. Even today in the United States, children who are dark-skinned and do not receive adequate sun exposure, as well as solely breast-fed infants, remain at risk for developing rickets. Nutritional rickets remains a problem in many developing countries, although the condition is thought to be associated more with calcium deficiency than vitamin-D deficiency.

Clinical manifestations of rickets include irritability, growth impairment, and prominence of the costochondral junctions (*rachitic rosary*). As the child ages and begins to put weight on the long bones of the legs, significant bowing results because of the poor mineralization of the skeleton. Vitamin-D deficiency occurring during the period of tooth development will result hypomineralization of the teeth (Fig. 17.14).

A similar pattern of poorly mineralized bone is seen in osteomalacia in adults. Bone normally undergoes continuous remodeling and turnover, and the osteoid that is produced during this process does not have sufficient calcium to mineralize completely. Thus a weak, fragile bone structure results. Patients affected by osteomalacia frequently complain of diffuse skeletal pain, and their bones are susceptible to fracture with relatively minor injury.

Vitamin E

A deficiency of vitamin E is rare and occurs primarily in children who suffer from chronic cholestatic liver disease. These patients have severe malabsorption of all fat-soluble vitamins, but particularly vitamin E. Multiple neurologic signs develop as a result of abnormalities in the central nervous system (CNS) and peripheral nervous system.

Vitamin K

A deficiency of vitamin K may be seen in patients with malabsorption syndromes or in those whose intestinal microflora has been eliminated by long-term broad-spectrum antibiotic use. Oral anticoagulants in the dicumarol family also inhibit the normal enzymatic activity of vitamin K. A deficiency or inhibition of synthesis of vitamin K leads to a coagulopathy because of the inadequate synthesis of prothrombin and other clotting factors. Intraorally, this coagulopathy is most often manifested by gingival bleeding. If the coagulopathy is not corrected, death may result from uncontrolled systemic hemorrhage.

Treatment and Prognosis

Replacement therapy is indicated for vitamin deficiencies. However, such deficiencies are uncommon in most developed countries, except for the situations described earlier. In fact, vitamin excess is perhaps more likely to be encountered in the United States today because so many people self-medicate with unnecessary and potentially harmful vitamin supplements. For example, excess vitamin A may cause abdominal pain, vomiting, headache, joint pain, and exostoses, whereas excess vitamin C may induce the formation of additional kidney stones in individuals with a history of nephrolithiasis. Similarly, an increased prevalence of kidney stones can be seen with excess oral intake of vitamin D.

◆ IRON-DEFICIENCY ANEMIA

Iron-deficiency anemia is the most common cause of anemia in the United States and throughout the world. This form of anemia develops when the amount of iron available to the body cannot keep pace with the need for iron in the production of red blood cells (RBCs). This type of anemia develops under four conditions:
1. Excessive blood loss
2. Increased demand for RBCs
3. Decreased intake of iron
4. Decreased absorption of iron

It is estimated up to 11% of women of childbearing age in the United States are iron deficient as a result of the chronic blood loss associated with excessive menstrual flow **(menorrhagia).** Similarly, 1%–2% of adult men are iron deficient because of chronic blood loss, usually associated with gastrointestinal disease, such as peptic ulcer disease, diverticulosis, hiatal hernia, or malignancy.

An increased demand for erythrocyte production occurs during childhood growth spurts and during pregnancy. A decreased intake of iron may be seen during infancy when the diet consists of relatively iron-poor foods, such as cereals and milk. Likewise, the diets of older people may be deficient if their dental condition prohibits them from eating the proper foods or if they cannot afford iron-rich foods, such as meats and vegetables. In the developing world, intestinal parasites (especially hookworms) are a common cause of iron deficiency in children and pregnant women.

Decreased absorption is a much less common problem; however, it can be seen in patients who have had a complete gastrectomy or who have **celiac sprue,** a condition that results in severe chronic diarrhea because of sensitivity to the plant protein, gluten. Inflammatory bowel disease, particularly Crohn disease, may also result in decreased absorption of iron.

Clinical Features

Patients with iron-deficiency anemia that is severe enough to cause symptoms may complain of fatigue, easy tiring, palpitations, lightheadedness, and lack of energy. Some patients may develop cravings for nonfood substances, such as clay or ice, a condition known as *pica.* Oral manifestations include angular cheilitis and atrophic glossitis or generalized oral mucosal atrophy. The glossitis has been described as a diffuse or patchy atrophy of the dorsal tongue papillae, often accompanied by tenderness or a burning sensation. Such findings are also evident in oral candidiasis, and some investigators have suggested that iron deficiency predisposes the patient to candidal infection, which results in the changes seen at the corners of the mouth and on the tongue. Such lesions are rarely seen in the United States, perhaps because the anemia is usually detected relatively early before the oral mucosal changes have had a chance to develop.

Laboratory Findings

The diagnosis should be established by means of a complete blood count with RBC indices because many other conditions, such as hypothyroidism, other anemias, or chronic depression, may elicit similar systemic clinical complaints. The laboratory evaluation characteristically shows hypochromic microcytic RBCs, which may be reduced in numbers. Additional supporting evidence for iron deficiency includes the findings of low serum iron levels and ferritin concentration together with elevated total iron-binding capacity.

Treatment and Prognosis

Therapy for most cases of iron-deficiency anemia consists of dietary iron supplementation by means of oral ferrous sulfate. For patients with malabsorption problems or severe anemia, parenteral iron may be given periodically. The response to therapy is usually prompt, with red cell parameters returning to normal within 1–2 months. The underlying cause of the anemia should be identified so that it may be addressed, if feasible.

◆ PLUMMER-VINSON SYNDROME (PATERSON-KELLY SYNDROME; SIDEROPENIC DYSPHAGIA)

Plummer-Vinson syndrome is a rare condition characterized by iron-deficiency anemia, seen in conjunction with glossitis and dysphagia. Its prevalence in developed countries has been declining, probably as a result of the improved nutritional status of the populations. The condition is significant in that it has been associated with a high frequency of both oral and esophageal squamous cell carcinoma; therefore, it is considered a premalignant process.

Clinical and Radiographic Features

Most reported patients with Plummer-Vinson syndrome have been women of Scandinavian or Northern European background, between 30 and 50 years of age. Patients typically complain of a burning sensation associated with the tongue and oral mucosa. Sometimes this discomfort is so severe that dentures cannot be worn. Angular cheilitis is often present and may be severe (Fig. 17.15). Marked atrophy of the lingual papillae, which produces a smooth, red appearance of the dorsal tongue, is seen clinically (Fig. 17.16).

Patients also frequently complain of difficulty in swallowing **(dysphagia)** or pain on swallowing. An evaluation with endoscopy or esophageal barium contrast radiographic studies usually shows the presence of abnormal bands of tissue in the esophagus, called **esophageal webs.** Another sign is an alteration of the growth pattern of the nails, which results in a spoon-shaped configuration **(koilonychia)** (Fig. 17.17). The nails also may be brittle.

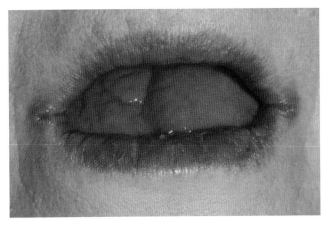

• **Fig. 17.15 Plummer-Vinson Syndrome.** Patients often show angular cheilitis.

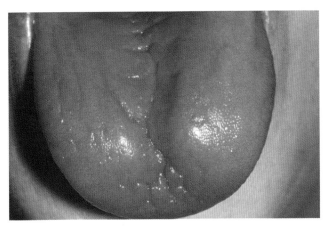

• **Fig. 17.16 Plummer-Vinson Syndrome.** The diffuse papillary atrophy of the dorsal tongue is characteristic of the oral changes. (From Neville BW, Damm DD, White DK: *Color atlas of clinical oral pathology,* ed. 2, Philadelphia, 1999, Lippincott Williams & Wilkins.)

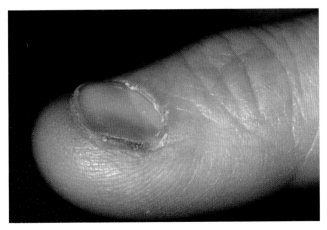

• **Fig. 17.17 Plummer-Vinson Syndrome.** The concave, "spoon-shaped" appearance of this patient's fingernails is a characteristic feature of chronic iron deficiency. (Courtesy of Dr. Ashleigh Briody.)

Symptoms of anemia may prompt patients with Plummer-Vinson syndrome to seek medical care. Fatigue, shortness of breath, and weakness are characteristic symptoms.

Laboratory Findings

Hematologic studies show a hypochromic microcytic anemia that is consistent with an iron-deficiency anemia.

Histopathologic Features

A biopsy specimen of involved mucosa from a patient with Plummer-Vinson syndrome typically shows epithelial atrophy with varying degrees of submucosal chronic inflammation. In advanced cases, evidence of epithelial atypia or dysplasia may be seen.

Treatment and Prognosis

Treatment of Plummer-Vinson syndrome is primarily directed at correcting the iron-deficiency anemia by means of dietary iron supplementation. This therapy usually resolves the anemia, relieves the glossodynia, and may reduce the severity of the esophageal symptoms. Occasionally, esophageal dilation is necessary to help improve the symptoms of dysphagia. Patients with Plummer-Vinson syndrome should be evaluated periodically for oral, hypopharyngeal, and esophageal cancer because a 5%–50% prevalence of upper aerodigestive tract malignancy has been reported in affected persons.

◆ PERNICIOUS ANEMIA

Pernicious anemia is an uncommon condition that occurs with greatest frequency among older patients of Northern European heritage, although recent studies have identified the disease in black and Hispanic populations as well. Asian populations seem to be affected much less frequently. The disease is a megaloblastic anemia caused by poor absorption of cobalamin (vitamin B_{12}, extrinsic factor). Intrinsic factor, which is produced by the parietal cells of the stomach lining, is needed for vitamin B_{12} absorption. Normally, when cobalamin is ingested, it binds to intrinsic factor in the duodenum. Because the lining cells of the intestine preferentially take up the cobalamin-intrinsic factor complex, significant amounts of the vitamin cannot be absorbed unless both components are present.

In the case of pernicious anemia, most patients lack intrinsic factor because of an autoimmune destruction of the parietal cells of the stomach; this results in decreased absorption of cobalamin. Antibodies directed against intrinsic factor are also found in the serum of these patients. Vitamin B_{12} deficiency may occur for other reasons, and although the resulting signs and symptoms may be identical to those of pernicious anemia, these should be considered as

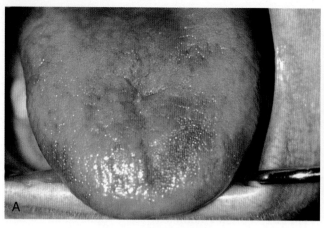
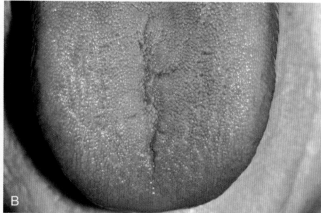

• **Fig. 17.18 Pernicious Anemia. A,** The dorsal tongue shows erythema and atrophy. **B,** After therapy with vitamin B$_{12}$, the mucosal alteration resolved.

distinctly different deficiency disorders. For example, a decreased ability to absorb cobalamin may also occur after gastrointestinal bypass operations. In addition, because cobalamin is primarily derived from animal sources, some strict vegetarians (vegans) may develop vitamin B$_{12}$ deficiency.

Because cobalamin is necessary for normal nucleic acid synthesis, anything that disrupts the absorption of the vitamin causes problems, especially for cells that are multiplying rapidly and, therefore, synthesizing large amounts of nucleic acids. The cells that are the most mitotically active are affected to the greatest degree, especially the hematopoietic cells and the gastrointestinal lining epithelial cells.

Clinical Features

With respect to systemic complaints, patients with pernicious anemia often report fatigue, weakness, shortness of breath, headache, and feeling faint. Such symptoms are associated with most anemias and probably reflect the reduced oxygen-carrying capacity of the blood. Vitamin B$_{12}$ also functions to maintain myelin throughout the nervous system; therefore, with reduced levels of the vitamin, many patients report paresthesia, tingling, or numbness of the extremities. Difficulty in walking and diminished vibratory and positional sense may be present. Psychiatric symptoms of memory loss, irritability, depression, and dementia have also been described.

Oral symptoms often consist of a burning sensation of the tongue, lips, buccal mucosa, or other mucosal sites. Clinical examination may show focal patchy areas of oral mucosal erythema and atrophy (Fig. 17.18), or the process may be more diffuse, depending on the severity and duration of the condition. The tongue may be affected in as many as 50%–60% of patients with pernicious anemia, but it may not show as much involvement as other areas of the oral mucosa in some instances. The atrophy and erythema may be easier to appreciate on the dorsal tongue than at other sites, however.

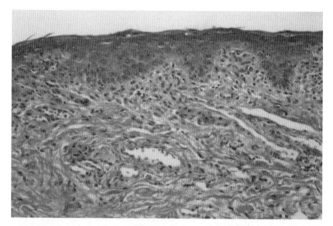

• **Fig. 17.19 Pernicious Anemia.** This medium-power photomicrograph shows epithelial atrophy and atypia with chronic inflammation of the underlying connective tissue. These features are characteristic of a megaloblastic anemia, such as pernicious anemia.

Histopathologic Features

Histopathologic examination of an erythematous portion of the oral mucosa shows marked epithelial atrophy with loss of rete ridges, an increased nuclear-to-cytoplasmic ratio of the surface epithelial cells, and prominent nucleoli (Fig. 17.19). This pattern can be misinterpreted as epithelial dysplasia at times, although the nuclei in pernicious anemia typically are pale staining and show peripheral chromatin clumping. A patchy diffuse chronic inflammatory cell infiltrate is usually noted in the underlying connective tissue.

Laboratory Findings

Hematologic evaluation of vitamin B$_{12}$ deficiency shows a macrocytic anemia and reduced serum cobalamin levels. The Schilling test for pernicious anemia has been used to determine the pathogenesis of the cobalamin deficiency by comparing absorption and excretion rates of radiolabeled cobalamin. However, this study is rather complicated to perform, and is now considered to be obsolete. The presence of serum antibodies directed against intrinsic factor is quite specific for pernicious anemia.

Treatment and Prognosis

Once the diagnosis of pernicious anemia is established, treatment traditionally has consisted of monthly intramuscular injections of cyanocobalamin. The condition responds rapidly once therapy is initiated, with reports of clearing of oral lesions within 5 days. High-dose oral cobalamin therapy has also been shown to be an equally effective treatment, however, with advantages being its cost-effectiveness and the elimination of painful injections. One systematic literature review has identified what appears to be an increased risk of gastric carcinoma, with pernicious anemia patients being seven times more likely to develop this tumor compared to the general population. Both vitamin B_{12} deficiency and folate deficiency will cause megaloblastic anemia. Folate deficiency is much less common today because many foods are enriched with folate. Nevertheless, it is important to distinguish between the two conditions. Treatment of vitamin B_{12} deficiency with folate will resolve the anemia and the oral mucosal atrophy, but reduced myelin production will continue, resulting in further CNS damage.

◆ PITUITARY DWARFISM

Pituitary dwarfism is a relatively rare condition that results from either the diminished production of growth hormone by the anterior pituitary gland, abnormalities of the growth hormone molecule, or a reduced capacity of the tissues to respond to growth hormone. Affected patients are typically much shorter than normal, although their body proportions are generally appropriate.

Several conditions may cause short stature, and a careful evaluation of the patient must be performed to rule out other possible causes, such as the following:
1. Intrinsic defects in the patient's tissues (e.g., certain skeletal dysplasias, chromosomal abnormalities, and idiopathic short stature)
2. Alterations in the environment of the growing tissues (e.g., malnutrition, hypothyroidism, and diabetes mellitus)

If a lack of growth hormone is detected, the cause should be determined. Sometimes the fault lies with the pituitary gland itself (e.g., aplasia or hypoplasia). In other instances, the problem may be related to destruction of the pituitary or hypothalamus by tumors, therapeutic radiation, or infection.

If the hypothalamus is affected, a deficiency in growth hormone–releasing hormone, which is produced by the hypothalamus, results in a deficiency of growth hormone. Often deficiencies in other hormones, such as thyroid hormone and cortisol, are also detected in patients with primary pituitary or hypothalamic disorders.

Some patients exhibit normal or even elevated levels of growth hormone, yet still show little evidence of growth. These individuals usually have inherited an autosomal recessive trait, resulting in abnormal and reduced growth hormone receptors on the patients' cells. Thus normal growth cannot proceed.

Clinical Features

Perhaps the most striking feature of pituitary dwarfism is the remarkably short stature of the affected patient. Sometimes this is not noticed until the early years of childhood, but a review of the patient's growth history should show a consistent pattern of failure to achieve the minimal height on the standard growth chart. Often the patient's height may be as much as three standard deviations below normal for a given age. Unlike the body proportions in many of the dysmorphic syndromes and skeletal dysplasias, the body proportions of patients affected by a lack of growth hormone are usually normal. One possible exception is the size of the skull, which is usually within normal limits. Because the facial skeleton does not keep pace with the skull, however, the face of an affected patient may appear smaller than it should be. Mental status is generally within normal limits.

The maxilla and mandible of affected patients are smaller than normal, and the teeth show a delayed pattern of eruption. The delay ranges from 1 to 3 years for teeth that normally erupt during the first decade of life and from 3 to 10 years for teeth that normally erupt in the second decade of life. Often the shedding of deciduous teeth is delayed by several years, and the development of the roots of the permanent teeth also appears to be delayed. A lack of development of the third molars seems to be a common finding. The size of the teeth is usually reduced in proportion to the other anatomic structures. One recent study suggested that growth hormone-deficient patients may exhibit more severe periodontal disease compared to a matched control population.

Laboratory Findings

Radioimmunoassay for human growth hormone shows levels that are markedly below normal.

Treatment and Prognosis

Replacement therapy with human growth hormone is the treatment of choice for patients with pituitary dwarfism if the disorder is detected before closure of the epiphyseal growth plates. In the past, growth hormone was extracted from cadaveric pituitary glands, which carried the very serious potential of prion-related Creutzfeldt-Jakob disease; since 1985, genetically engineered human growth hormone has been produced with recombinant DNA technology. For patients with a growth hormone deficiency caused by a hypothalamic defect, treatment with growth hormone–releasing hormone is appropriate. If patients are identified and treated at an early age, they can be expected to achieve a relatively normal height. The craniofacial bone structure also assumes a less childlike pattern. Evaluation of a series of patients who had been treated for long periods with growth hormone determined that up to half developed acromegalic features, including larger feet and a larger mandible. For patients who lack growth hormone receptors, no treatment is available.

◆ GIGANTISM

Gigantism is a rare condition caused by an increased production of growth hormone, usually related to a functional pituitary adenoma. Approximately 3 persons per million population are diagnosed each year. The increased production of growth hormone takes place before closure of the epiphyseal plates, and the affected person grows at a much more rapid pace, becoming abnormally tall. Although the average height of the population of the United States has been gradually increasing during the past several decades, individuals who exceed the mean height by more than three standard deviations may be considered candidates for endocrinologic evaluation. Familial examples of gigantism have also been described.

Clinical and Radiographic Features

Patients with gigantism usually show markedly accelerated growth during childhood, irrespective of normal growth spurts. Radiographic evaluation of the skull often shows an enlarged sella as a result of the presence of a pituitary adenoma. The adenoma may result in hormonal deficiencies, such as hypothyroidism and hypoadrenocorticism, if the remaining normal pituitary gland tissue is compressed and destroyed. **McCune-Albright syndrome** (polyostotic fibrous dysplasia and *café au lait* pigmentation with associated endocrinologic disturbances) (see page 663) may account for as many as 20% of the cases of gigantism.

If the condition remains uncorrected for a prolonged period, extreme height (more than 7 feet tall) will be achieved, and enlargement of the facial soft tissues, the mandible, and the hands and feet will become apparent. These changes often resemble those seen in **acromegaly** (discussed later). Another oral finding is true generalized macrodontia.

Treatment and Prognosis

Appropriate management of gigantism involves the surgical removal of the functioning pituitary adenoma, usually by a transsphenoidal approach. Radiation therapy may also be used, as well as one of the somatostatin analogues and a growth hormone receptor antagonist (discussed in the next topic, **acromegaly**).

The life span of patients with gigantism is usually markedly reduced. Complications associated with hypertension, peripheral neuropathy, osteoporosis, and pulmonary disease contribute to increased morbidity and mortality.

◆ ACROMEGALY

Acromegaly is an uncommon condition characterized by the excess production of growth hormone after closure of the epiphyseal plates in the affected patient. Usually, this increase in growth hormone is due to a functional pituitary adenoma. The incidence is estimated to be approximately two to eleven new cases diagnosed per million population per year, based on recent European data. The prevalence is now believed to be between 30 and 140 affected patients per million.

Clinical and Radiographic Features

Because most patients with acromegaly have a pituitary adenoma, symptoms related directly to the space-occupying mass of the tumor may be present. These symptoms include headaches, visual disturbances, and other signs of a brain tumor. Sometimes pressure atrophy of the residual normal pituitary by the adenoma results in diminished production of other pituitary hormones and causes other indirect endocrine problems. The direct effects of increased levels of growth hormone include a variety of problems, such as hypertension, heart disease, hyperhidrosis, arthritis, and peripheral neuropathy.

Renewed growth in the small bones of the hands and feet (Fig. 17.20) and in the membranous bones of the skull and jaws is typically observed. Patients may complain of gloves, rings, or hats becoming "too small." The soft tissue is also often affected, producing a coarse facial appearance (Fig. 17.21). Hypertrophy of the soft palatal tissues may cause or accentuate sleep apnea. Because these signs and symptoms are slow to develop and are vague at the onset, an average time of 6–10 years elapses from the onset of symptoms to the diagnosis of disease. The average age at diagnosis is 42 years, and no sex predilection is seen.

From a dental perspective, these patients have mandibular prognathism as a result of the increased growth of the mandible (Fig. 17.22), which may cause apertognathia (anterior open bite). Growth of the jaws also may cause spacing of the teeth, resulting in diastema formation. Soft tissue growth often produces uniform macroglossia in affected patients.

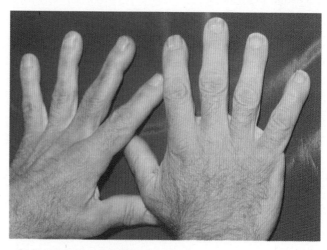

• **Fig. 17.20 Acromegaly.** Enlargement of the bones of the hands. (Courtesy of Dr. William Bruce.)

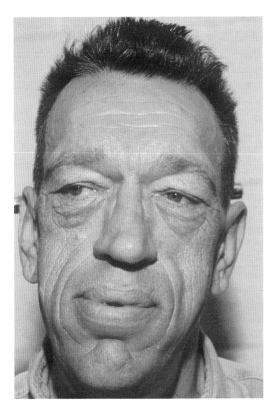

• **Fig. 17.21 Acromegaly.** This patient shows the typical coarse facial features. (Courtesy of Dr. William Bruce.)

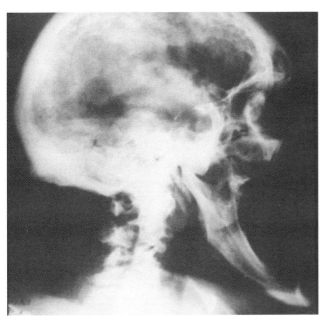

• **Fig. 17.22 Acromegaly.** This lateral skull film shows the dramatic degree of mandibular enlargement that may occur.

Laboratory Findings and Diagnosis

If acromegaly is suspected, measurement of serum growth hormone levels is done after giving the patient a measured quantity of glucose orally. Normally, this glucose challenge will reduce the production of growth hormone, but if the patient has acromegaly, growth hormone will not be suppressed. Usually magnetic resonance imaging (MRI) will identify the pituitary adenoma that is responsible for inappropriate growth hormone secretion.

Treatment and Prognosis

The treatment of a patient with acromegaly is typically directed at the removal of the pituitary tumor mass and the return of the growth hormone levels to normal. The most effective treatment with the least associated morbidity is surgical excision by a transsphenoidal approach. The prognosis for such a procedure is good, although a mortality rate of approximately 1% is still expected. The condition is usually controlled with this procedure, but patients with larger tumors and markedly elevated growth hormone levels are less likely to be controlled.

Radiation therapy may be used in some instances, but the return of the growth hormone levels to normal is not as rapid or as predictable as with surgery. Because some patients also experience hypopituitarism caused by radiation effects on the rest of the gland, some centers may offer radiation therapy as treatment only when surgery fails or is too risky. Pharmacotherapy with one of the somatostatin analogues (e.g., octreotide, lanreotide, and pasireotide) helps to control acromegaly if surgical treatment is unsuccessful or if surgery is contraindicated. A growth hormone receptor–blocking agent, pegvisomant, has also been developed and may be used in conjunction with one of the somatostatin analogues or by itself if the patient cannot tolerate the somatostatin analogue. Pegvisomant is injected daily and acts in the peripheral tissues to inhibit the action of growth hormone. These drugs are also used as an adjunct to radiation therapy during the prolonged period that is sometimes necessary for that treatment to take effect.

The prognosis for untreated patients is guarded, with an increased mortality rate compared with that of the general population. Hypertension, diabetes mellitus, coronary artery disease, congestive heart failure, respiratory disease, and colon cancer are seen with increased frequency in acromegalic patients, and each of these contributes to the increased mortality rate. Although treatment of the patient with acromegaly helps to control many of the other complicating problems and improves the prognosis, the life span of these patients still is shortened, particularly for those with persistent elevated growth hormone levels, cardiomyopathy, or hypertension.

◆ HYPOTHYROIDISM (CRETINISM; MYXEDEMA)

Hypothyroidism is a condition that is characterized by decreased levels of thyroid hormone. When this decrease occurs during infancy, the resulting clinical problem is known as **cretinism.** If an adult has markedly decreased thyroid hormone levels for a prolonged period, then deposition of a glycosaminoglycan ground substance is seen in the subcutaneous tissues, producing a nonpitting edema. Some call this severe form of hypothyroidism **myxedema;** others use the terms *myxedema* and *hypothyroidism* interchangeably.

Hypothyroidism may be classified as either **primary** or **secondary.** In primary hypothyroidism, the thyroid gland itself is in some way abnormal; in secondary hypothyroidism, the pituitary gland does not produce an adequate amount of thyroid-stimulating hormone (TSH), which is necessary for the appropriate release of thyroid hormone. Secondary hypothyroidism, for example, often develops after radiation therapy for brain tumors, resulting in unavoidable radiation damage to the pituitary gland. Most cases, however, represent the primary form of the disease.

Screening for this disorder is routinely carried out at birth, and the prevalence of congenital hypothyroidism in North America is approximately 1 in 4000 births. Usually, this is due to hypoplasia or agenesis of the thyroid gland. In other areas of the world, hypothyroidism in infancy is usually due to a lack of dietary iodine. In adults, hypothyroidism is often caused by autoimmune destruction of the thyroid gland (known as **Hashimoto thyroiditis**) or iatrogenic factors, such as radioactive iodine therapy or surgery for the treatment of hyperthyroidism. Because thyroid hormone is necessary for normal cellular metabolism, many of the clinical signs and symptoms of hypothyroidism can be related to the decreased metabolic rate in these patients.

Clinical Features

The most common features of hypothyroidism include such signs and symptoms as lethargy, dry and coarse skin, swelling of the face (Fig. 17.23) and extremities, huskiness of the voice, constipation, weakness, and fatigue. The heart rate is usually slowed **(bradycardia).** Reduced body temperature **(hypothermia)** may be present, and the skin often feels cool and dry to the touch. In the infant, these signs may not be readily apparent, and the failure to grow normally may be the first indication of the disease.

With respect to the oral findings, the lips may appear thickened because of the accumulation of glycosaminoglycans. Diffuse enlargement of the tongue occurs for the same reason (Fig. 17.24). If the condition develops during childhood, the teeth may fail to erupt, although tooth formation may not be impaired (Figs. 17.25 and 17.26).

Laboratory Findings

The diagnosis is made by assaying the free thyroxine (T_4) levels. If these levels are low, then TSH levels are measured to determine whether primary or secondary hypothyroidism is present. With primary thyroid disease, TSH levels are elevated. With secondary disease caused by pituitary dysfunction, TSH levels are normal or borderline.

Treatment and Prognosis

Thyroid replacement therapy, usually with levothyroxine, is indicated for confirmed cases of hypothyroidism. The prognosis is generally good for adult patients. If the condition is recognized within a reasonable time, the prognosis is also good for children. If the condition is not identified in a timely manner, however, permanent damage to the CNS may occur, resulting in intellectual disability. For affected children, thyroid hormone replacement therapy often results in a dramatic resolution of the condition (see Fig. 17.23).

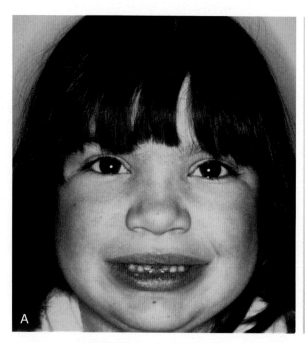
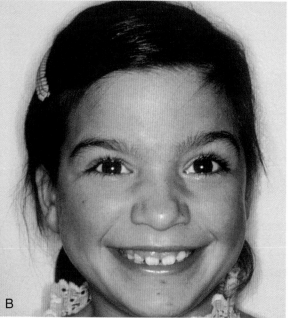

• **Fig. 17.23 Hypothyroidism. A,** The facial appearance of this 9-year-old child is due to the accumulation of tissue edema secondary to severe hypothyroidism. **B,** Same patient after 1 year of thyroid hormone replacement therapy. Note the eruption of the maxillary permanent teeth.

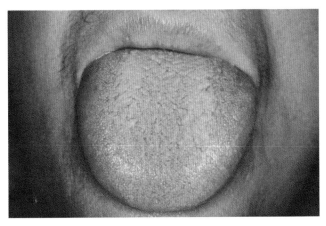

• **Fig. 17.24 Hypothyroidism.** The enlarged tongue (macroglossia) is secondary to edema associated with adult hypothyroidism (myxedema). (Courtesy of Dr. George Blozis.)

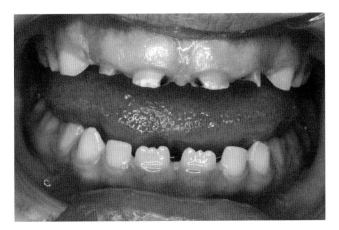

• **Fig. 17.25 Hypothyroidism.** Photograph of the same patient depicted in Fig. 17.23 before hormone replacement therapy. Note the retained deciduous teeth, for which the patient was initially referred.

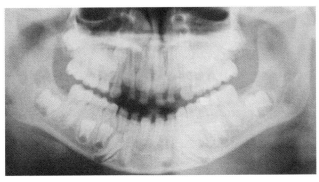

• **Fig. 17.26 Hypothyroidism.** Panoramic radiograph of the same patient in Figs. 17.23 and 17.25. Note the unerupted, yet fully developed permanent dentition.

◆ HYPERTHYROIDISM (THYROTOXICOSIS; GRAVES DISEASE)

Hyperthyroidism is a condition caused by excess production of thyroid hormone. This excess production results in a state of markedly increased metabolism in the affected patient. Most cases (60%–90%) are due to **Graves disease**, a condition that was initially described in the early nineteenth century. It is thought to be triggered by autoantibodies that are directed against receptors for thyroid-stimulating hormone (TSH) on the surface of the thyroid cells. When the autoantibodies bind to these receptors, they seem to stimulate the thyroid cells to release inappropriate thyroid hormone.

Other causes of hyperthyroidism include hyperplastic thyroid tissue and thyroid tumors, both benign and malignant, which secrete inappropriate thyroid hormone. Similarly, a pituitary adenoma may produce TSH, which can then stimulate the thyroid to secrete excess thyroid hormone.

Clinical Features

Graves disease is five to ten times more common in women than in men and is seen with some frequency. The overall prevalence of this condition is 1.2% in the population of the United States, with almost 2% of the adult female population affected. Graves disease is most commonly diagnosed in patients during the third and fourth decades of life.

Most patients with Graves disease exhibit diffuse thyroid enlargement. Many of the signs and symptoms of hyperthyroidism can be attributed to an increased metabolic rate caused by the excess thyroid hormone. Patients usually complain about nervousness, heart palpitations, heat intolerance, emotional lability, and muscle weakness. The following are often noted during the clinical evaluation:
• Weight loss despite increased appetite
• Tachycardia
• Excessive perspiration
• Widened pulse pressure (increased systolic and decreased diastolic pressures)
• Warm, smooth skin
• Tremor

Ocular involvement (also known as Graves' orbitopathy or thyroid eye disease), which develops in 20%–40% of affected patients, is perhaps the most striking feature of this disease. In the early stages of hyperthyroidism, patients have a characteristic stare with eyelid retraction and lid lag. With some forms of Graves disease, protrusion of the eyes (**exophthalmos** or **proptosis**) develops (Fig. 17.27). This bulging of the eyes is due to an accumulation of glycosaminoglycans in the retro-orbital connective tissues, and patients who smoke cigarettes are more frequently affected. Diplopia (double vision), dry eyes, and compression of the optic nerve may result in significant visual impairment.

Laboratory Findings

The diagnosis of hyperthyroidism is made by assaying free T_4 (thyroxine) and TSH levels in the serum. In affected patients, the T_4 levels should be elevated and the TSH concentration is typically depressed.

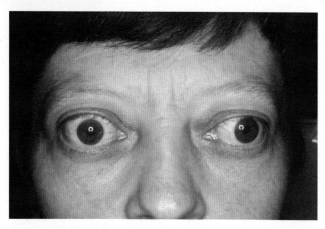

• **Fig. 17.27 Hyperthyroidism.** The prominent eyes are characteristic of the exophthalmos associated with Graves disease.

Histopathologic Features

Diffuse enlargement and hypercellularity of the thyroid gland are seen in patients with Graves disease, typically with hyperplastic thyroid epithelium and little apparent colloid production. Lymphocytic infiltration of the glandular parenchyma is also often noted.

Treatment and Prognosis

Initial treatment of hyperthyroidism often consists of one of the beta-blocking drugs, either atenolol or propranolol, which will reduce such uncomfortable symptoms as anxiety, nervousness, excessive sweating, heart palpitations, and tachycardia. The underlying cause of the excess circulating thyroid hormone then must be addressed.

In the United States, radioactive iodine (^{131}I) is the most commonly used form of therapy for adult patients with Graves disease, although it cannot be given if the patient is pregnant. The thyroid gland normally takes up iodine from the bloodstream because this element is a critical component of thyroid hormone. When radioactive iodine is given to a patient with Graves disease, the thyroid gland quickly removes it from the bloodstream and sequesters the radioactive material within the glandular tissue. The radioactivity then destroys the hyperactive thyroid tissue, bringing the thyroid hormone levels back to normal. Most of the radiation is received during the first few weeks because the half-life of ^{131}I is short.

Other techniques include drug therapy with agents that block the normal use of iodine by the thyroid gland, and this form of therapy is initially favored in most European centers. The two drugs that have been widely prescribed in the United States are propylthiouracil (PTU) and methimazole. PTU has been associated with liver toxicity in some patients, and the US Food and Drug Administration has recommended that its use should be limited to specific circumstances, such as methimazole allergy or during the first trimester of pregnancy. Methimazole should not be given to a patient who is in the first trimester of pregnancy because

it can cause fetal abnormalities. Sometimes methimazole may be administered chronically in the hope that a remission may be induced. In addition, the thyroid gland, or a significant portion of it, may be removed surgically, thereby reducing thyroid hormone production. Methimazole is often given prior to either surgical removal of the thyroid or treatment with radioactive iodine in order to bring thyroid hormone levels into the normal range.

Drug therapy alone is often unsuccessful in controlling hyperthyroidism, and approximately half of patients treated in this way will relapse. Unfortunately, with radioactive iodine and surgery, the risk of hypothyroidism is relatively great, and thyroid hormone replacement therapy is often needed.

Treatment of thyroid eye disease has been a challenge, with systemic corticosteroid therapy often used to reduce inflammation, and surgical intervention employed to decompress the orbit and restore eyelid function. Neither of these approaches was of significant benefit for patients with severe ocular disease. In 2020, a human monoclonal antibody, teprotumumab, was approved by the U.S. Food and Drug Administration to treat thyroid eye disease. This medication blocks the interaction of thyrotropin receptors and insulin-like growth factor I receptors, which are implicated in causing thyroid eye disease. The treatment results are impressive, although currently a 6-month course of treatment is estimated to cost $200,000.

In a patient with uncontrolled hyperthyroidism, a definite risk exists with respect to an inappropriate release of large amounts of thyroid hormone at one time, resulting in a relatively rare, but very serious, condition called a **thyroid storm.** A thyroid storm may be precipitated by infection, psychologic trauma, or stress. Clinically, patients may have delirium, convulsions, an elevated temperature (up to 106 °F), and tachycardia (sometimes more than 140 beats/minute). Such individuals should be hospitalized immediately because the mortality rate associated with thyroid storm is reported to range from 8% to 25%. The clinician should be aware of the potential for this problem, and patients with hyperthyroidism should ideally have the condition under control before dental treatment.

◆ HYPOPARATHYROIDISM

Calcium levels in extracellular tissues are normally regulated by parathyroid hormone (PTH) (parathormone) in conjunction with vitamin D. If calcium levels drop below a certain point, then the release of PTH is stimulated. The hormone then acts directly on the kidney and the osteoblasts of the bone to restore the calcium to normal levels. In the kidney, calcium reabsorption is promoted, phosphate excretion is enhanced, and the production of vitamin D is stimulated, which increases the absorption of calcium from the gut. Osteoblasts are stimulated to produce a variety of cytokines that subsequently increase osteoclastic differentiation and metabolically activate the osteoclasts to resorb bone, thus liberating calcium.

If a reduced amount of PTH is produced, the relatively rare condition known as **hypoparathyroidism** results. In the United States and Europe, approximately 75% of hypoparathyroidism cases are due to inadvertent surgical removal of the parathyroid glands when the thyroid gland is excised for other reasons, but sometimes it is the result of autoimmune destruction of the parathyroid tissue. Rare syndromes, such as **DiGeorge syndrome** and the **autoimmune polyendocrinopathy-candidiasis-ectodermal dystrophy syndrome (endocrine-candidiasis syndrome, autoimmune polyglandular syndrome, type 1)** (see page 207), also may be associated with hypoparathyroidism.

Clinical Features

With the loss of parathyroid function, the serum levels of calcium drop, resulting in hypocalcemia. Often the patient with chronic hypoparathyroidism adapts to the presence of hypocalcemia and is asymptomatic unless situations that further reduce the calcium levels are encountered. Such situations include metabolic alkalosis, as seen during hyperventilation, when a state of tetany may become evident.

Chvostek sign is an oral finding of significance, characterized by a twitching of the upper lip when the facial nerve is tapped just below the zygomatic process. A positive response suggests a latent degree of tetany. If the hypoparathyroidism develops early in life during odontogenesis, then a pitting enamel hypoplasia and failure of tooth eruption may occur (Fig. 17.28). The presence of persistent oral candidiasis in a young patient may signal the onset of autoimmune polyendocrinopathy-candidiasis-ectodermal dystrophy syndrome. Hypoparathyroidism may be only one of several endocrine deficiencies associated with this condition.

Laboratory Findings

PTH can be measured by means of a radioimmunoassay. If serum PTH levels are decreased in conjunction with a decreased serum calcium concentration, elevated serum phosphate level, and normal renal function, then a diagnosis of hypoparathyroidism can be made.

Treatment and Prognosis

Patients with hypoparathyroidism are usually treated with oral doses of an active form of vitamin D, calcitriol (1,25-dihydroxycholecalciferol, vitamin D_3). Additional supplements of dietary calcium are also typically necessary to maintain the proper serum calcium levels. With this regimen, patients can often live a fairly normal life, however problems with renal calculi and soft tissue calcifications frequently develop.

The search has continued for better treatment options for this disorder, focusing on molecular solutions. PTH is a linear protein that is composed of a chain of 84 amino acids, and recently a recombinant PTH composed of all 84 amino acids has been developed. This recombinant PTH has been approved by the FDA for daily subcutaneous injection to treat patients with hypoparathyroidism who have failed standard therapy.

◆ PSEUDOHYPOPARATHYROIDISM (ALBRIGHT HEREDITARY OSTEODYSTROPHY; ACRODYSOSTOSIS)

The rare condition known as **pseudohypoparathyroidism** represents at least two broad disorders in which normal parathyroid hormone (PTH) is present in adequate amounts but the biochemical pathways responsible for activating the target cells are not functioning properly. The clinical result is a patient who appears to have hypoparathyroidism.

In the case of pseudohypoparathyroidism type I, two subcategories have been defined. For type Ia, a molecular defect of a specific intracellular binding protein known as $G_s\alpha$ seems to prevent the formation of cyclic adenosine monophosphate (cAMP), a critical component in the activation of cell metabolism. Because other hormones also require binding with $G_s\alpha$ to carry out their functions, patients have multiple problems with other endocrine organs and functions. This condition is usually inherited as an autosomal dominant trait.

With respect to pseudohypoparathyroidism type Ib, the problem is thought to be caused by defective receptors for the PTH on the surface of the target cells (the proximal renal tubules). For this reason, no other endocrine tissues or functions are affected. An autosomal dominant mode of inheritance has been suggested for a few families affected by type Ib pseudohypoparathyroidism, but most cases are apparently sporadic.

Pseudohypoparathyroidism type II is characterized by the induction of cAMP by PTH in the target cells; however, a functional response by the cells is not invoked. All of the reported cases of this form of the disease appear to be sporadic.

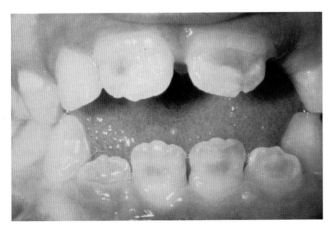

• **Fig. 17.28 Hypoparathyroidism.** Enamel hypoplasia has affected the dentition of this patient, who had hypoparathyroidism while the teeth were forming.

Clinical Features

Pseudohypoparathyroidism most commonly appears as type Ia disease. Patients affected by pseudohypoparathyroidism, type Ia, have a characteristic array of features that includes mild intellectual disability, early-onset obesity, round face, short neck, and markedly short stature. Midfacial hypoplasia is also commonly observed. The metacarpals and metatarsals are usually shortened, and the fingers appear short and thick. Subcutaneous calcifications (**osteoma cutis**) may be identified in some patients. Other endocrine abnormalities that are typically encountered include hypogonadism and hypothyroidism.

Patients with type Ib and II disease clinically appear normal, aside from their symptoms of hypocalcemia.

Dental manifestations of pseudohypoparathyroidism include generalized enamel hypoplasia, widened pulp chambers with intrapulpal calcifications, oligodontia, delayed eruption, shortened roots, and blunting of the apices of the teeth. The pulpal calcifications are often described as "dagger" shaped. A Class III occlusal relation is frequently identified in these patients, possibly related to maxillary hypoplasia.

The diagnosis of pseudohypoparathyroidism is made based on elevated serum levels of PTH seen concurrently with hypocalcemia, hyperphosphatemia, and otherwise normal renal function. More sophisticated studies are necessary to delineate the various subtypes.

Treatment and Prognosis

Pseudohypoparathyroidism is managed by the administration of vitamin D and calcium. The serum calcium levels and urinary calcium excretion are carefully monitored. Because of individual patient differences, the medication may need to be carefully adjusted; however, the prognosis is considered to be good. Annual or semiannual routine dental examinations, particularly during childhood, are usually advised for these patients.

◆ HYPERPARATHYROIDISM

Excess production of parathyroid hormone (PTH) results in the condition known as **hyperparathyroidism.** PTH normally is produced by the parathyroid glands in response to a decrease in serum calcium levels.

Primary hyperparathyroidism is the uncontrolled production of PTH, usually as a result of a parathyroid adenoma (80%–90% of cases) or parathyroid hyperplasia (10%–15% of cases). Rarely (approximately 1% of cases), a parathyroid carcinoma may be the cause of primary hyperparathyroidism. Infrequently this endocrine disturbance is caused by any one of several inherited syndromes, including **multiple endocrine neoplasia type 1** or **type 2a,** or **hyperparathyroidism–jaw tumor syndrome.** In the latter condition, affected patients develop multiple jaw lesions that histopathologically are consistent with central ossifying

fibroma (see page 652). In most cases, affected patients develop a single parathyroid adenoma that produces excess parathyroid hormone. There also appears to be an increased risk for these patients to develop parathyroid carcinoma.

Secondary hyperparathyroidism develops when PTH is continuously produced in response to chronic low levels of serum calcium, a situation usually associated with chronic renal disease. The kidney processes vitamin D, which is necessary for calcium absorption from the gut. Therefore, in a patient with chronic renal disease, active vitamin D is not produced and less calcium is absorbed from the gut, resulting in lowered serum calcium levels.

Clinical and Radiographic Features

Most patients with primary hyperparathyroidism are older than 60 years of age. Women have this condition two to four times more often than men do. In developed countries, the condition typically is identified on routine serologic testing, and the majority of patients are relatively asymptomatic.

Patients with the classic triad of signs and symptoms of hyperparathyroidism are described as having "stones, bones, and abdominal groans." Affected individuals are more likely to present with these signs and symptoms in economically less developed countries where serologic evaluation is not done on a routine basis.

"Stones" refers to the fact that these patients, particularly those with primary hyperparathyroidism, have a marked tendency to develop renal calculi (kidney stones, nephrolithiasis) because of the elevated serum calcium levels. Metastatic calcifications are also seen, frequently involving other soft tissues, such as blood vessel walls, subcutaneous soft tissues, the sclera, the dura, and the regions around the joints.

"Bones" refers to a variety of osseous changes that may occur in conjunction with hyperparathyroidism. One of the first clinical signs of this disease is seen radiographically as subperiosteal resorption of the phalanges of the index and middle fingers. Generalized loss of the lamina dura surrounding the roots of the teeth is also seen as an early manifestation of the condition (Fig. 17.29). Alterations in trabecular pattern characteristically develop next. A decrease in trabecular density and blurring of the normal trabecular pattern occur; often a "ground glass" appearance results.

With persistent disease, other osseous lesions develop, such as the so-called **brown tumor** of hyperparathyroidism. This lesion derives its name from the color of the tissue specimen, which is usually a dark red-brown because of the abundant hemorrhage and hemosiderin deposition within the tumor. These lesions appear radiographically as well-demarcated unilocular or multilocular radiolucencies (Fig. 17.30). They commonly affect the mandible, clavicles, ribs, and pelvis. They may be solitary but are often multiple, and long-standing lesions may produce significant cortical expansion. Typically, the other osseous changes are observable if brown tumors are present. The most severe skeletal manifestation of chronic hyperparathyroidism has been called **osteitis fibrosa cystica,** a condition that

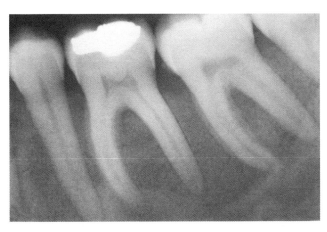

• **Fig. 17.29 Hyperparathyroidism.** This periapical radiograph reveals the "ground glass" appearance of the trabeculae and loss of lamina dura in a patient with secondary hyperparathyroidism. (Courtesy of Dr. Randy Anderson.)

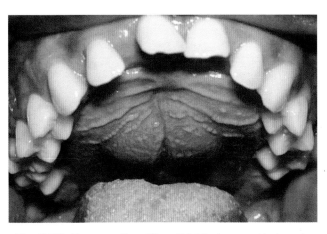

• **Fig. 17.31 Hyperparathyroidism.** Palatal enlargement is characteristic of the renal osteodystrophy associated with secondary hyperparathyroidism.

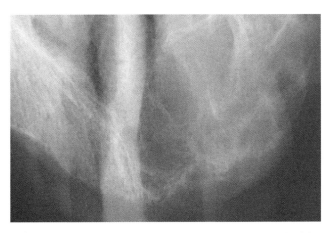

• **Fig. 17.30 Hyperparathyroidism.** This occlusal radiograph of the edentulous maxillary anterior region shows a multilocular radiolucency characteristic of a brown tumor of primary hyperparathyroidism. (Courtesy of Dr. Brian Blocher.)

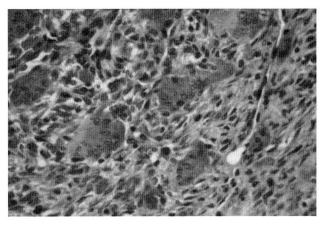

• **Fig. 17.32 Hyperparathyroidism.** This high-power photomicrograph of a brown tumor of hyperparathyroidism shows scattered multinucleated giant cells within a vascular and proliferative fibroblastic background.

develops from the central degeneration and fibrosis of long-standing brown tumors. In patients with secondary hyperparathyroidism caused by end-stage renal disease (**renal osteodystrophy; chronic kidney disease—mineral and bone disorder**), striking enlargement of the jaws has been known to occur (Fig. 17.31) and produce a "ground-glass" radiographic pattern (see Fig. 17.29).

"**Abdominal groans**" refers to the tendency for the development of duodenal ulcers. In addition, changes in mental status are often seen, ranging from lethargy and weakness to confusion or dementia.

Histopathologic Features

The brown tumor of hyperparathyroidism is histopathologically identical to the **central giant cell granuloma** of the jaws, a benign tumorlike lesion that usually affects teenagers and young adults (see page 631). Both lesions are characterized by a proliferation of exceedingly vascular granulation

tissue, which serves as a background for numerous multinucleated osteoclast-type giant cells (Fig. 17.32). Some lesions may also show a proliferative response characterized by a parallel arrangement of spicules of woven bone set in a cellular fibroblastic background with variable numbers of multinucleated giant cells (Fig. 17.33). This pattern is often associated with secondary hyperparathyroidism related to chronic renal disease (renal osteodystrophy).

Treatment and Prognosis

In **primary hyperparathyroidism,** the hyperplastic parathyroid tissue or the functional tumor must be removed surgically to reduce PTH levels to normal. Localization of the parathyroid adenoma is often facilitated by a sestamibi scan, which is a nuclear medicine technique using a technetium 99-labeled small protein that is preferentially taken up by the tumor. Ultrasonography is another technique that is often used to identify hyperplastic parathyroid glands or parathyroid adenomas. Such lesions are frequently removed

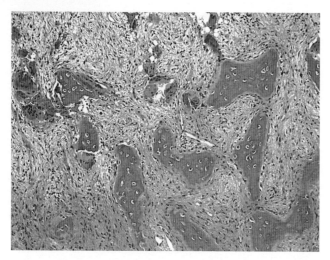

• **Fig. 17.33 Hyperparathyroidism.** This medium-power photomicrograph shows trabeculae of cellular woven bone and clusters of multinucleated giant cells within a background of cellular fibrous connective tissue. These features are characteristic of tissue changes seen in renal osteodystrophy.

by a minimally invasive surgical technique, and intraoperative assessment of the adequacy of excision can be determined by noting a drop in parathormone levels within 10 minutes of removing the adenoma.

Secondary hyperparathyroidism may evolve to produce signs and symptoms related to renal calculi or renal osteodystrophy. Restriction of dietary phosphate, use of phosphate-binding agents, and pharmacologic treatment with an active vitamin D metabolite (e.g., calcitriol) and a calcimimetic agent, such as cinacalcet, may avert problems. Cinacalcet sensitizes the calcium receptors of the parathyroid cells to extracellular calcium, causing the cells to reduce their output of parathormone. Exposure to aluminum salts, which inhibit bone mineralization, should be eliminated also. Patients who do not respond to medical therapy may require parathyroidectomy. Renal transplantation may restore the normal physiologic processing of vitamin D, as well as phosphorus and calcium reabsorption and excretion; however, this does not occur in every case.

♦ HYPERCORTISOLISM (CUSHING SYNDROME)

Hypercortisolism is a clinical condition that results from a sustained increase in glucocorticoid levels. In most cases this increase is due to corticosteroid therapy that is prescribed for other medical purposes. The increase is less commonly caused by an endogenous source, such as production of adrenocorticotropic hormone (ACTH) by an adrenal tumor or pituitary adenoma. If a pituitary adenoma is responsible, then the term **Cushing disease** is applied. This condition is rather rare and usually affects young adult women.

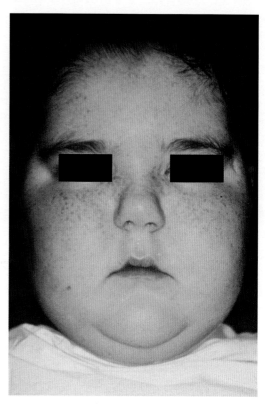

• **Fig. 17.34 Cushing Syndrome.** The rounded facial features ("moon facies") of this patient are due to the abnormal deposition of fat, which is induced by excess corticosteroid hormone. (Courtesy of Dr. George Blozis.)

Clinical Features

The signs of Cushing syndrome usually develop slowly. The most consistent clinical observation is weight gain, particularly in the central areas of the body. The accumulation of fat in the dorsocervical spine region results in a "buffalo hump" appearance; fatty tissue deposition in the facial area results in the characteristic rounded facial appearance known as *moon facies* (Fig. 17.34). Other common findings include the following:

* Red-purple abdominal striae
* Hirsutism
* Poor healing
* Osteoporosis
* Hypertension
* Mood changes (particularly depression)
* Hyperglycemia with thirst and polyuria
* Muscle wasting with weakness

Diagnosis

If the patient has been receiving large amounts of corticosteroids (greater than the equivalent of 20 mg of prednisone) on a daily basis for several months, then the diagnosis is rather obvious, given the classic signs and symptoms described earlier. The diagnosis may be more difficult to establish in patients with a functioning adrenal cortical tumor or an ACTH-secreting pituitary adenoma. Evaluation of these patients should include the measurement of free cortisol in the urine and an assay of the effect of dexamethasone (a potent artificial corticosteroid) on the serum ACTH and cortisol levels. In an unaffected patient, the levels of free cortisol should be within normal limits, and the administration of an exogenous corticosteroid, such as dexamethasone, should suppress the normal level of ACTH, with a concomitant decrease in the cortisol levels. Because functioning tumors do not respond to normal feedback mechanisms, the anticipated decreases in ACTH and cortisol would not be seen in a patient with such a tumor.

Treatment and Prognosis

The clinician should be aware of the signs and symptoms of hypercortisolism to refer affected patients for appropriate endocrinologic evaluation and diagnosis. Once the diagnosis is established and the cause is determined to be an adrenal or pituitary tumor, surgical removal of the lesion is the treatment of choice. Radiation therapy also may be effective, particularly in younger patients, however the reduction in ACTH production by the tumor may require several months to reach normal levels. For patients who are treated with radiation therapy or who have unresectable tumors, drugs that inhibit cortisol synthesis (such as, ketoconazole or metyrapone) may be used to help control the excess production of cortisol.

Most cases of hypercortisolism, however, are caused by systemic corticosteroid therapy that is given for a variety of immunologic reasons, including treatment of autoimmune diseases and allogeneic transplant recipients. Certain strategies, such as the use of corticosteroid-sparing agents or alternate-day therapy, may minimize the corticosteroid dose needed. The goal should be for patients to use the lowest dose possible to manage immunologic disease.

In normal situations, cortisol is critical to the function of the body, particularly in dealing with stress. As the hormone is metabolized and serum levels drop, feedback to the pituitary gland signals it to produce ACTH, which stimulates the adrenal gland to produce additional cortisol. Unfortunately, therapeutic corticosteroids suppress the production of ACTH by the pituitary gland to the extent that the pituitary gland may not be able to produce ACTH in response to stress, and an acute episode of hypoadrenocorticism (*addisonian crisis*) may be precipitated. Therefore, the clinician must be aware of the potential side effects of chronic high-dose corticosteroid use and must be able to adapt the treatment of the patient accordingly. For stressful dental and surgical procedures especially, it is often necessary to increase the corticosteroid dose because of the greater need of the body for cortisol. Consultation with the physician who is managing the corticosteroid therapy is advised to determine to what extent the dose should be adjusted.

◆ ADDISON DISEASE (HYPOADRENOCORTICISM)

Insufficient production of adrenal corticosteroid hormones caused by the destruction of the adrenal cortex results in the condition known as **Addison disease**, or **primary hypoadrenocorticism.** The incidence of new cases diagnosed in the Western hemisphere is approximately 6 per million population per year, while the prevalence is about 140 cases per million people. The causes are diverse and include the following:

- Autoimmune destruction (most common cause in Western societies)
- Infections (e.g., tuberculosis and deep fungal diseases, particularly in patients with acquired immunodeficiency syndrome [AIDS])
- Rarely, metastatic tumors, sarcoidosis, hemochromatosis, or amyloidosis

If the pituitary gland is not functioning properly, **secondary hypoadrenocorticism** may develop because of decreased production of ACTH, the hormone responsible for maintaining normal levels of serum cortisol.

Clinical Features

The clinical features of hypoadrenocorticism do not actually begin to appear until at least 90% of the glandular tissue has been destroyed. With gradual destruction of the adrenal cortex, an insidious onset of fatigue, irritability, depression, weakness, and hypotension is noted over a period of months. A generalized hyperpigmentation of the skin occurs, classically described as *bronzing.* The hyperpigmentation is generally more prominent on sun-exposed skin and over pressure points, such as the elbows and knees; it is caused by increased levels of beta-lipotropin or ACTH, each of which can stimulate melanocytes. The patient usually complains of gastrointestinal upset with anorexia, nausea, vomiting, diarrhea, weight loss, and a peculiar craving for salt, due to hyponatremia caused by lack of the mineralocorticoid, aldosterone. When hypoadrenocorticism is accompanied by hypoparathyroidism and mucocutaneous candidiasis, the possibility of autoimmune polyendocrinopathy-candidiasis-ectodermal dystrophy syndrome should be considered (see page 207).

The oral manifestations include diffuse or patchy, brown, macular pigmentation of the oral mucosa (particularly the lips, tongue, palate, and attached gingiva) caused by excess melanin production (Fig. 17.35). Often the oral mucosal changes are the first manifestation of the disease, with the skin hyperpigmentation occurring afterward. Sometimes the oral hypermelanosis may be difficult to distinguish from physiologic racial pigmentation, but a history of a recent onset of oral pigmentation should suggest the possibility of Addison disease.

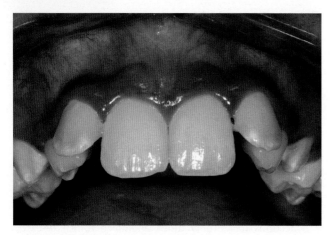

• **Fig. 17.35 Addison Disease.** Diffuse pigmentation of the maxillary facial gingiva in a patient with Addison disease. (Courtesy of Dr. John Kalmar.)

Laboratory Findings

The diagnosis of hypoadrenocorticism is confirmed by a rapid ACTH stimulation test and measurement of serum cortisol levels and plasma ACTH levels. If serum cortisol levels are below 16–18 µg/dL, then the patient has adrenal insufficiency. In primary hypoadrenocorticism, the plasma ACTH levels are high (>100 ng/L). In secondary hypoadrenocorticism, the levels are normal (9–52 ng/L) or low, as would be expected because the condition results from decreased ACTH production by the pituitary gland.

Treatment and Prognosis

Addison disease is managed with replacement therapy, including both a glucocorticoid (such as, hydrocortisone) and mineralocorticoid (such as, fludrocortisone). The physiologic dose of glucocorticoid is considered to be approximately 15–25 mg of hydrocortisone or its equivalent per day, usually given in divided doses. Because the body's need for corticosteroid hormones increases during stressful events, the patient must take this into account and increase the dose accordingly. This adjustment is generally not required for dental procedures performed using local anesthesia and lasting less than 1 hour, but an increased dose may be necessary for certain dental and oral surgical procedures that are more lengthy or are done under general anesthesia.

Before the availability of corticosteroids, the prognosis for patients with hypoadrenocorticism was poor, with most patients surviving less than 2 years. Even today, if the condition is not recognized promptly, death may result in a relatively short period of time. With proper diagnosis and management, most patients with hypoadrenocorticism can expect to have a normal life span, although a recent population-based study suggested an increased mortality rate related to malignancy and cardiovascular disease.

◆ DIABETES MELLITUS

Diabetes mellitus is a common disorder of carbohydrate metabolism that is thought to have several causes, although the basic problem is one of either decreased production of insulin or tissue resistance to the effects of insulin. The net result of this abnormal state is an increase in the blood glucose level (**hyperglycemia).**

Diabetes mellitus is usually divided into two presentations:
1. Type I—characterized by complete, or nearly complete, lack of insulin production
2. Type II—characterized by inadequate insulin production or resistance of target tissues to the effects of insulin

Type I diabetes mellitus was formerly known as insulin-dependent diabetes mellitus or juvenile-onset diabetes, but these terms are not considered to be accurate. Type II diabetics often require insulin injections in order to manage their disease, and from 5% to 10% of type 1 diabetics develop their disease after 30 years of age. Patients with type 1 diabetes mellitus usually exhibit severe hyperglycemia and ketoacidosis without treatment, and they require exogenous insulin injections to survive.

Type II diabetes mellitus is sometimes more difficult to diagnose. It usually occurs in older, obese adults, but it may be seen in obese adolescents as well. For this reason, the term "adult-onset diabetes" was abandoned. Although hyperglycemia is present, ketoacidosis rarely develops. Furthermore, patients can produce some endogenous insulin. Certain patients may require insulin to help control their disease; the insulin injections, however, are usually not necessary for the patient's survival.

With respect to epidemiology, in the United States diabetes mellitus affects approximately 7%–11% of the population, or slightly more than 30 million people, although approximately 8 million of these cases remain undiagnosed. More than 1.5 million new cases are identified each year in the United States. Of these affected patients, most have type II diabetes; only 5%–10% have type I.

Diabetes is an important disease when we consider the many complications associated with it and the economic effect it has on society. One of the main complications of diabetes is **peripheral vascular disease,** a problem that results in kidney failure, as well as ischemia and gangrenous involvement of the limbs. By some estimates, 25% of all new cases of kidney failure occur in diabetic patients. Thus diabetes is the leading cause of kidney failure in the United States. Each year more than 50,000 amputations are performed for the gangrenous complications of diabetes. This disease is the leading cause of lower limb amputations in the United States. Retinal involvement often results in blindness; thus the leading cause of new cases of blindness in working-age adults in the United States is diabetes, with more than 12,000 people affected annually. Complications because of diabetes are estimated to contribute to the deaths of more than 200,000 Americans each year.

The cause of diabetes mellitus is essentially unknown, although most cases of type I diabetes appear to be caused by autoimmune destruction of the pancreatic islet cells, and this immunologic attack may be precipitated by a viral infection in a genetically susceptible individual. Type II diabetes does not appear to have an autoimmune cause, however, because no destruction of the islet cells is seen microscopically. Instead, genetic abnormalities have been detected in patients with certain types of type II diabetes, which may explain why the condition occurs so often in families. If one parent is affected by type II diabetes, then the chances of a child having the disorder is about 40%. Similarly, if one identical twin has type II diabetes, then the chances are 90% that the disease will also develop in the other twin.

Clinical Features

Although a complete review of the pathophysiology of diabetes mellitus is beyond the scope of this text, the clinical signs and symptoms of a patient with this disease are easier to understand with some basic knowledge of the process. The hormone insulin, produced by the beta cells of the pancreatic islets of Langerhans, is necessary for the uptake of glucose by the cells of the body. When insulin binds to its specific cell surface receptor, a resulting cascade of intracellular molecular events causes the recruitment of intracellular glucose-binding proteins, which facilitate the uptake of glucose by each cell.

Type I Diabetes Mellitus

Because patients with type I diabetes have a deficiency in the amount of insulin, the body's cells cannot absorb glucose and it remains in the blood. Normal blood glucose levels are between 70 and 120 mg/dL; in diabetic patients, these levels are often between 200 and 400 mg/dL. Above 300 mg/dL, the kidneys can no longer reabsorb the glucose; therefore, it spills over into the urine. Because glucose is the main source of energy for the body, and because none of this energy can be used because glucose cannot be absorbed, the patient feels tired and lethargic. The body begins to use other energy sources, such as fat and protein, resulting in the production of ketones as a by-product of those energy consumption pathways. The patient often loses weight, despite increased food intake **(polyphagia).** With the hyperglycemia, the osmolarity of the blood and urine increases. The increased osmolarity results in frequent urination **(polyuria)** and thirst, which leads to increased water intake **(polydipsia).** Clinically, most patients with type I diabetes are younger (average age at diagnosis being 14 years), and they have a thin body habitus.

Type II Diabetes Mellitus

By contrast, patients with type II diabetes are usually older than 40 years of age at diagnosis, and 80%–90% of them are obese. In this situation, it is thought that a decrease in the number of insulin receptors or abnormal post-binding molecular events related to glucose uptake results in glucose not being absorbed by the body's cells. Thus patients are said to show "insulin resistance" because serum insulin levels are usually within normal limits or even elevated. If the hyperglycemia is taken into account, however, the amount of circulating insulin is typically not as much as would be present in a normal person with a similar level of blood glucose.

Therefore, many of these patients are described as having a relative lack of insulin.

The symptoms associated with type II diabetes are much more subtle in comparison to those seen with type I. The first sign of type II diabetes is often detected with routine hematologic examination rather than any specific patient complaint. Ketoacidosis is rarely seen in patients with type II diabetes. Nevertheless, many of the other complications of diabetes are still associated with this form of the disease.

Monitoring of either type of diabetes includes not only blood glucose measurement (showing the immediate levels of blood glucose), but also assessment of the percentage of glycated hemoglobin, which is a reflection of the overall control of blood glucose levels over the past 2–3 months. Glycated hemoglobin, commonly known as HbA_{1c}, develops with continuous exposure to blood glucose. Because erythrocytes (which contain hemoglobin) survive for about 120 days in the bloodstream, nonenzymatic glycation that occurs during the 2–3-month period immediately prior to the blood draw correlates with the average concentration of blood glucose during that time. For example, an HbA_{1c} reading of 6% would be consistent with an average blood glucose level of 126 mg/dL for the preceding 2–3 months.

Complications

Many complications of diabetes mellitus are directly related to the **microangiopathy** caused by the disease. The microangiopathy results in occlusion of the small blood vessels, producing peripheral vascular disease. The resultant decrease in tissue perfusion results in ischemia. The ischemia predisposes the patient to infection, particularly severe infections such as gangrene. Another contributing factor is the impairment of neutrophil function, particularly neutrophil chemotaxis.

Amputation of the lower extremity often is necessary because of the lack of tissue perfusion and the patient's inability to cope with infection. Similar vascular occlusion may affect the coronary arteries (which places the patient at risk for myocardial infarction) or the carotid arteries and their branches (predisposing the patient to cerebrovascular accident, or stroke). When microvascular occlusion affects the retinal vessels, blindness typically results. Kidney failure is the outcome of renal blood vessel involvement. If the ketoacidosis is not corrected in type I diabetes, the patient may lapse into a diabetic coma.

The oral manifestations of diabetes mellitus are generally limited to patients with type I diabetes. Problems include periodontal disease, which occurs more frequently and progresses more rapidly than in normal patients. Healing after surgery may be delayed, and the likelihood of infection is probably increased. Diffuse, nontender, bilateral enlargement of the parotid glands, called **diabetic sialadenosis** (see page 476), may be seen in patients with either form of diabetes. In uncontrolled or poorly controlled diabetic patients, a striking enlargement and erythema of the attached gingiva has been described (Fig. 17.36). In addition, these patients appear to be more susceptible to **oral candidiasis** in its various clinical forms (see page 201). Erythematous

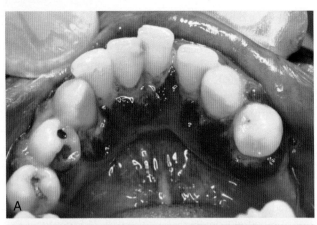

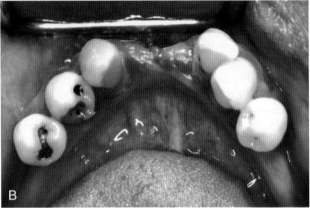

• **Fig. 17.36 Diabetes Mellitus. A,** This diffuse, erythematous enlargement of the gingival tissues developed in a diabetic patient who discontinued taking her insulin. **B,** The gingival tissues have greatly improved after reinstitution of regular insulin injections. Several incisors were extracted because of severe periodontal bone loss.

candidiasis, which appears as central papillary atrophy of the dorsal tongue papillae, is reported in up to 30% of these patients. **Mucormycosis** (see page 219) may occur in patients with poorly controlled type I diabetes. Some investigators have identified an increased prevalence of **benign migratory glossitis** (see page 784) in patients with type I diabetes; however, others have not been able to confirm this finding. **Xerostomia,** a subjective feeling of dryness of the oral mucosa, has been reported as a complaint in one-third of diabetic patients. Unfortunately, studies that attempt to confirm an actual decrease in salivary flow rate in diabetic patients have produced conflicting results. Some studies show a decrease in salivary flow; some, no difference from normal; and some, an increased salivary flow rate.

Treatment and Prognosis

For patients with type II diabetes, dietary modification coupled with exercise may be the only treatment necessary, with the goal being weight loss. The dietary and lifestyle changes may need to be coupled with one or more oral hypoglycemic agents. These drugs are designed to affect different pathophysiologic aspects of the disease. For example, secretagogues increase the insulin supply. These include the second-generation sulfonylurea medications, such as glipizide or glyburide, and nonsulfonylureas, such as mitiglinide and nateglinide. Metformin is a biguanide that increases glucose utilization and decreases insulin resistance and hepatic glucose production. Thiazolidinediones, such as rosiglitazone and pioglitazone, also reduce insulin resistance. Acarbose and miglitol are α-glucosidase inhibitors that reduce the absorption of glucose from the gastrointestinal tract by inhibiting enzymatic degradation of more complex sugars. Sodium-glucose cotransporter 2 inhibitors, including canagliflozin and dapagliflozin, increase glucose excretion from the kidneys. Newer agents also include the glucagon-like peptide 1 (GLP-1) receptor agonists, such as dulaglutide, semaglutide, and liraglutide, which are given parenterally and may contribute to weight loss. If these modalities do not control the blood glucose levels, then treatment with insulin is necessary.

For patients with type I diabetes, injections of insulin are required to control blood glucose levels. Different types of insulin are marketed, each type having different degrees of duration and times of peak activity. Insulin was previously extracted primarily from beef and pork pancreata. In some patients, however, antibodies developed to this foreign protein and rendered the insulin useless. To overcome this problem, pharmaceutical companies have developed brands of insulin that have the molecular structure of human insulin. Laboratories produce this human insulin with genetically engineered bacteria using recombinant DNA technology.

The patient's schedule of insulin injections must be carefully structured and monitored to provide optimal control of blood glucose levels. This schedule is carefully formulated by the patient's physician and takes into account such factors as the patient's activity level and the severity of the insulin deficiency. It is imperative that adequate dietary carbohydrates be ingested after the administration of the insulin; otherwise, a condition known as **insulin shock** may occur. If carbohydrates are not consumed after an insulin injection, then the blood glucose levels may fall to dangerously low levels. The brain is virtually dependent on blood glucose as its energy source. If the blood glucose level drops below 40 mg/dL, the patient may go into shock. This condition can be treated by administration of sublingual dextrose paste, IV infusion of a dextrose solution, or injection of glucagon.

In summary, diabetes mellitus is a common, complex medical problem with many complications. The prognosis is guarded. Studies suggest that strict control of blood glucose levels results in a slowing of the development of the late complications of type I diabetes (e.g., blindness, kidney damage, and neuropathy) and reduces the frequency of these complications. Health care practitioners should be aware of the problems these patients may have and should be prepared to deal with them. Consultation with the patient's physician may be necessary, particularly for patients with type I diabetes that show poor blood glucose control, have active infections, or require extensive oral surgical procedures.

◆ HYPOPHOSPHATASIA

Hypophosphatasia is a rare metabolic bone disease that is characterized by a deficiency of tissue-nonspecific alkaline phosphatase. Approximately 300 distinct mutations of the gene responsible for alkaline phosphatase production have been described. One of the first presenting signs of hypophosphatasia may be the premature loss of the primary teeth, presumably caused by a lack of cementum on the root surfaces. In the homozygous autosomal recessive form, there are rather severe manifestations, and many of these patients are identified in infancy. The milder forms of the disease are inherited in an autosomal dominant or recessive fashion, appearing in childhood or even adulthood, with variable degrees of expression. Generally, the younger the age of onset, the more severe the expression of the disease. The common factors in all types include the following:

- Reduced levels of the bone, liver, and kidney isozyme of alkaline phosphatase
- Increased levels of blood and urinary phosphoethanolamine
- Bone abnormalities that resemble rickets

Most authorities believe that the decreased alkaline phosphatase levels probably are responsible for the clinically observed abnormalities. Alkaline phosphatase is thought to play a role in the production of bone, but its precise mechanism of action is unknown.

Clinical and Radiographic Features

Six types of hypophosphatasia are now recognized, depending on the severity and the age of onset of the symptoms:
1. Perinatal lethal
2. Perinatal benign
3. Infantile
4. Childhood
5. Adult
6. Odontohypophosphatasia

Perinatal Lethal Hypophosphatasia

The **perinatal lethal** form has the most severe manifestations. It is usually diagnosed at birth, and the infant rarely survives for more than a few hours. Death is due to respiratory failure. Marked hypocalcification of the skeletal structures is observed.

Perinatal Benign Hypophosphatasia

The **perinatal benign** form of hypophosphatasia appears similar to the lethal form, but these infants have a clinical course similar to infantile hypophosphatasia. Some investigators have noted that skeletal calcification may be detected in some of these fetuses during the third trimester of pregnancy, in contrast to the lethal form.

Infantile Hypophosphatasia

Babies affected by **infantile** hypophosphatasia may appear normal up to 6 months of age; after this time, they begin to show a failure to grow. Vomiting and hypotonia may

develop as well. Skeletal malformations that suggest rickets are typically observed; these malformations include shortened, bowed limbs. Deformities of the ribs predispose these patients to pneumonia, and skull deformities cause increased intracranial pressure. Nephrocalcinosis and nephrolithiasis also produce problems for these infants. Radiographs show a markedly reduced degree of ossification with a preponderance of hypomineralized osteoid. If these infants survive, premature shedding of the deciduous teeth is often seen.

Childhood Hypophosphatasia

The **childhood** form is usually detected at a later age and has a wide range of clinical expression. One of the more consistent features is the premature loss of the primary teeth without evidence of a significant inflammatory response (Figs. 17.37 and 17.38). The deciduous incisor teeth are usually affected first and may be the only teeth involved. In some patients, this may be the only expression of the disease. The teeth may show enlarged pulp chambers in some instances, and a significant degree of alveolar bone loss may be seen. More severely affected patients may have open fontanelles with premature fusion of cranial sutures. This

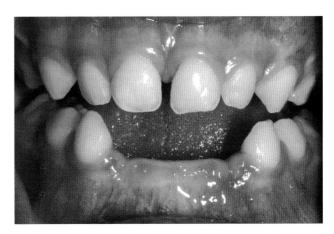

• **Fig. 17.37 Hypophosphatasia.** Premature loss of the mandibular anterior teeth. (Courtesy of Dr. Jackie Banahan.)

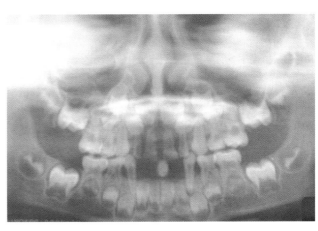

• **Fig. 17.38 Hypophosphatasia.** This panoramic radiograph shows the loss of the mandibular anterior teeth. (Courtesy of Dr. Jackie Banahan.)

early fusion occasionally leads to increased intracranial pressure and subsequent brain damage. Affected patients typically have a short stature, bowed legs, and a waddling gait. The development of motor skills is often delayed.

Radiographically, the skull of more severely affected individuals may show uniformly spaced, poorly defined, small radiolucencies, a pattern that has been described as resembling "beaten copper." This appearance may be the result of areas of thinning of the inner cortical plate produced by the cerebral gyri.

Adult Hypophosphatasia

The **adult** form is typically mild. Patients often have a history of premature loss of their primary or permanent dentition, and many of these patients are edentulous. Stress fractures that involve the metatarsal bones of the feet may be a presenting sign of the condition, or an increased number of fractures associated with relatively minor trauma may alert the clinician to this disorder.

Odontohypophosphatasia

This form of hypophosphatasia is perhaps the most controversial. Affected patients present with premature loss of the incisor teeth as the only clinical sign of disease, although serologic studies will be consistent with hypophosphatasia. Some investigators have suggested that this may simply represent a mild expression of the disorder.

Diagnosis

The diagnosis of hypophosphatasia is based on the clinical manifestations and the finding of decreased levels of serum alkaline phosphatase and increased amounts of phosphoethanolamine in both the urine and the blood. Interestingly, as some patients grow older, serum alkaline phosphatase levels may approach normal.

Histopathologic Features

The histopathologic evaluation of bone sampled from a patient affected with the **infantile** form of hypophosphatasia shows abundant production of poorly mineralized osteoid. In the **childhood** or **adult** form, the bone may appear relatively normal or it may show an increased amount of woven bone, which is a less mature form of osseous tissue.

The histopathologic examination of either a primary or permanent tooth that has been exfoliated from an affected patient often shows an absence or a marked reduction of cementum that covers the root's surface (Fig. 17.39). This reduced amount of cementum is thought to predispose to tooth loss because of the inability of periodontal ligament fibers to attach to the tooth and to maintain it in its normal position.

Treatment and Prognosis

In the past, the treatment of hypophosphatasia essentially consisted of symptomatic care because the lack of alkaline

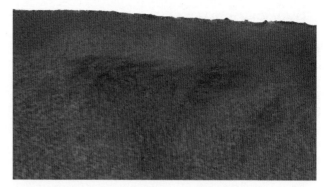

• **Fig. 17.39 Hypophosphatasia.** This medium-power photomicrograph of an exfoliated tooth shows no cementum associated with the root surface.

phosphatase could not be corrected. Attempts to treat this condition by infusing alkaline phosphatase were unsuccessful, presumably because the enzyme functions within the cell rather than in the extracellular environment. In 2015, however, the U.S. Food and Drug Administration approved a recombinant enzyme known as asfotase alfa for treatment of perinatal, infantile, and childhood hypophosphatasia. The medication is comprised of three components: the catalytic portion of tissue nonspecific alkaline phosphatase; the Fc portion of IgG; and a molecular configuration that increases binding to hydroxyapatite, an important calcium-containing component of bone. The results of this treatment are impressive, either halting or reversing most of the manifestations of hypophosphatasia; nevertheless, the treatment is quite expensive.

For those patients without access to asfotase alfa, the traditional treatment approaches remain an option. Basically, fractures are treated with orthopedic surgery, followed by rehabilitation. Prosthetic appliances are indicated to replace missing teeth, but satisfactory results are not always possible because the alveolar bone is hypoplastic. In patients who are skeletally mature, dental implants have also been used successfully in managing the edentulous spaces. Because mutational analysis of DNA can identify carriers of the defective gene, patients and their parents should be provided with genetic counseling. As stated earlier, the prognosis varies with the onset of symptoms; the perinatal and infantile types are associated with a rather poor outcome. The childhood and adult forms are usually compatible with a normal life span.

◆ VITAMIN D–RESISTANT RICKETS (HEREDITARY HYPOPHOSPHATEMIA; FAMILIAL HYPOPHOSPHATEMIC RICKETS)

After the use of vitamin D to treat rickets became widespread, it was recognized that some individuals with clinical features characteristic of rickets did not seem to respond to therapeutic doses of the vitamin. For this reason, this condition in these patients was called **vitamin D–resistant rickets**. Most cases of this rare condition appear to be inherited as an X-linked dominant trait; therefore, males are usually affected more severely than females, who presumably have attenuated features because of lyonization. In the United States, this condition occurs at a frequency of 1 in 20,000 births. In addition to the rachitic changes, these patients are also hypophosphatemic and show a decreased capacity for reabsorption of phosphate from the renal tubules. The disorder is caused by mutations in a zinc metalloproteinase gene known as *phosphate-regulating gene with endopeptidase activity on the X chromosome (PHEX)*. Although the precise mechanisms of action of this gene are unclear, it appears to play a role in vitamin D metabolism.

In contrast, patients affected by the rare autosomal recessive condition known as **vitamin D–dependent rickets** exhibit hypocalcification of the teeth, unlike those with vitamin D–resistant rickets. Otherwise, the two disorders have similar clinical features. Vitamin D–dependent rickets is caused by a lack of 1α-hydroxylase, the enzyme responsible for converting the relatively inactive vitamin D precursor, 25-hydroxycholecalciferol (calcifediol) to the active metabolite 1,25-dihydroxycholecalciferol (calcitriol) in the kidney. Therefore, these patients respond to replacement therapy with active vitamin D (calcitriol).

Clinical Features

Patients with vitamin D–resistant rickets have a short stature. The upper body segment appears more normal, but the lower body segment is shortened. The lower limbs are generally shortened and bowed.

Laboratory investigation reveals hypophosphatemia with diminished renal reabsorption of phosphate and decreased intestinal absorption of calcium. This typically results in rachitic changes that are unresponsive to vitamin D (calciferol). With aging, ankylosis of the spine frequently develops.

From a dental standpoint, the teeth have large pulp chambers, with pulp horns extending almost to the dentinoenamel junction (Figs. 17.40 and 17.41). In some cases

the cuspal enamel may be worn down by attrition to the level of the pulp horn, causing pulpal exposure and pulp death. The exposure may be so small that the resulting periapical abscesses and gingival sinus tracts seem to affect what appear to be otherwise normal teeth (Fig. 17.42). Studies have also shown that microclefts may develop in the enamel, giving the oral microflora access to the dentinal tubules and subsequently to the pulp. One study examined a series of affected children and found that 25% of these patients had multiple abscesses involving the primary dentition. Another report described 24 affected children with a mean age of 6 years, and 67% had a history of periapical abscess formation. Affected adults also have an increased frequency of endodontic problems, with an average of approximately seven endodontically treated teeth per person in people over 40 years of age, compared to two endodontically treated teeth per person in a matched control group. In addition, vitamin D-resistant rickets patients have been shown to have an increased risk of periodontal disease.

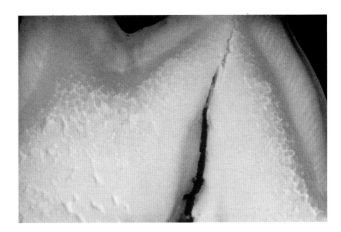

• **Fig. 17.41 Vitamin D–Resistant Rickets.** Ground section of the same tooth depicted in Fig. 17.39. A pulp horn extends to the dentinoenamel junction. (Courtesy of Dr. Carl Witkop.)

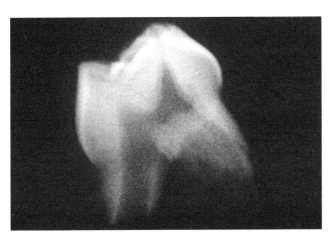

• **Fig. 17.40 Vitamin D–Resistant Rickets.** This radiograph of an extracted tooth shows a prominent pulp chamber with pulp horns extending out toward the dentinoenamel junction.

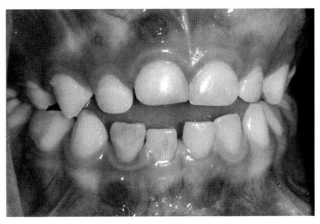

• **Fig. 17.42 Vitamin D–Resistant Rickets.** This patient exhibits multiple nonvital teeth with associated parulides. This arose in the absence of caries or trauma.

Histopathologic Features

Microscopic examination of an erupted tooth from a patient with vitamin D–resistant rickets usually shows markedly enlarged pulp horns. The dentin appears abnormal and is characterized by the deposition of globular dentin, which often exhibits clefting. The clefts may extend from the pulp chamber to the dentinoenamel junction. Microclefts are also seen within the enamel. The pulp frequently is nonvital, presumably because of the bacterial contamination associated with both the enamel and the dentinal clefts.

Treatment and Prognosis

For a normal stature to develop, patients with vitamin D-resistant rickets usually need early treatment with calcitriol and multiple daily doses of phosphate. In 2018, however, a monoclonal antibody, burosumab, was approved for treatment of this condition. This antibody targets a fibroblast growth factor 23 (FGF23), a cytokine that normally is regulated by PHEX. FGF23 helps regulate the degree to which phosphate is reabsorbed by the kidney, and excess levels of FGF23 decrease the reabsorption of phosphate, allowing it to be eliminated in the urine, therefore decreasing the amount in the blood. In addition, FGF23 appears to inactivate enzymes that normally convert vitamin D precursors to active vitamin D, thus reducing calcium absorption from the intestine.

With respect to the dental aspects of vitamin D-resistant rickets, endodontic therapy is necessary for the pulpally involved teeth. Initiating therapy in early childhood with a synthetic vitamin D compound (1α-hydroxycholecalciferol) appears to reduce dental problems in affected patients when compared with untreated historic controls. Interestingly, the radiographic dental abnormalities do not seem to be improved. Some investigators have suggested that application of the newer dental sealants may reduce the frequency of pulpal necrosis, but long-term follow-up studies will be necessary to confirm this. Standard systemic treatment with oral vitamin D and phosphate supplementation appears to reduce the severity of periodontitis.

Although serum and urine calcium levels must be monitored carefully to prevent nephrocalcinosis with its potential for kidney damage, patients generally have a normal life span.

◆ CROHN DISEASE (REGIONAL ILEITIS; REGIONAL ENTERITIS)

Crohn disease is an inflammatory and probably an immunologically mediated condition of unknown cause that primarily affects the distal portion of the small bowel and the proximal colon. It is now well established that the manifestations of Crohn disease may be seen anywhere in the gastrointestinal tract, from the mouth to the anus. In addition, other extraintestinal sites of disease involvement (such as, the skin, eyes, and joints) have also been identified. The oral

lesions are significant because they may precede the gastrointestinal lesions in as many as 30% of the cases that have both oral and gastrointestinal involvement. It is interesting that the prevalence of Crohn disease appears to be increasing, but the reasons for this increase have not been determined. The prevalence of Crohn disease in the United States is estimated to be 214 cases per 100,000 people. Familial clustering of cases has suggested that genetic factors play a role in the pathogenesis of this disease.

Clinical Features

Most patients with Crohn disease are teenagers when the disease first becomes evident, although another diagnostic peak of disease activity occurs in patients more than 60 years of age. Gastrointestinal signs and symptoms usually include abdominal cramping and pain, nausea, and diarrhea, occasionally accompanied by fever. Weight loss and malnutrition may develop, which can lead to anemia, decreased growth, and short stature.

A wide range of oral lesions has been clinically reported in Crohn disease; however, many of the abnormalities described are relatively nonspecific and may be associated with other conditions that cause **orofacial granulomatosis** (see page 330). The more prominent findings include diffuse or nodular swelling of the oral and perioral tissues, a cobblestone appearance of the mucosa, and deep, granulomatous-appearing ulcers. The ulcers are often linear and develop in the buccal vestibule (Fig. 17.43). Patchy erythematous macules and plaques involving the attached and unattached gingivae have been termed *mucogingivitis* and may represent one of the more common lesions related to Crohn disease. Soft tissue swellings that resemble denture-related fibrous hyperplasia may be seen, as well as smaller mucosal tags. Acquired lymphangiectasias of the buccal mucosa, buccal vestibule, and labial mucosa have been described, appearing similar to lymphangiomas, which typically are seen in early childhood. Another manifestation that

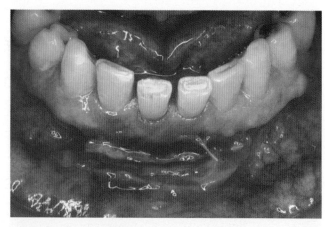

• **Fig. 17.43 Crohn Disease.** This patient has a linear ulceration of the mandibular vestibule. An adhesion between the alveolar and labial mucosae was caused by repeated ulceration and healing of the mucosa at this site.

has been reported is aphthous-like oral ulcerations, although the significance of this finding is uncertain because aphthous ulcerations are found rather frequently in the general population, including the same age group that is affected by Crohn disease. One large study showed no difference in the prevalence of aphthous ulcers in patients with Crohn disease compared with a control population. Less than 1% of patients with Crohn disease may develop diffuse stomatitis, with some cases apparently caused by *Staphylococcus aureus,* and others being nonspecific. In at least one instance, recurrent severe buccal space infections resulted in cutaneous salivary fistula formation. Infrequently, pyostomatitis vegetans (see next topic) has been associated with Crohn disease.

Histopathologic Features

Microscopic examination of lesional tissue obtained from the intestine or from the oral mucosa should show nonnecrotizing granulomatous inflammation within the submucosal connective tissue (Fig. 17.44). The severity of the granulomatous inflammation may vary tremendously from patient to patient and from various sites in the same patient. Therefore, a negative biopsy result at any one site and time may not necessarily rule out a diagnosis of Crohn disease. As with the clinical lesions, the histopathologic pattern is relatively nonspecific, resembling orofacial granulomatosis. Special stains should be performed to rule out the possibility of deep fungal infection, syphilis, or mycobacterial infection.

Treatment and Prognosis

Most patients with mild Crohn disease are initially treated medically with mesalamine (5-aminosalicylic acid) or sulfasalazine, a drug that is enzymatically broken down by bacteria in the colon to form sulfapyridine and 5-aminosalicylic acid. Some patients respond well to this medication, typically when it is combined with an antibiotic such as metronidazole. With moderate to severe involvement, systemic prednisone may be used and is often effective, particularly when

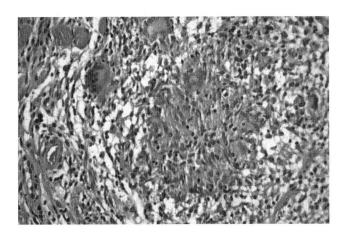

• **Fig. 17.44 Crohn Disease.** This medium-power photomicrograph of an oral lesion shows a nonnecrotizing granuloma in the submucosal connective tissue.

combined with an immunomodulating drug, such as azathioprine, methotrexate, or 6-mercaptopurine. For more severe or refractory cases of Crohn disease, one of the tumor necrosis factor-α inhibitors (such as, infliximab, adalimumab, golimumab, or certolizumab pegol) may be used. Ustekinumab, a monoclonal antibody that inibits IL12/IL23, has also been shown to be an effective medication for managing Crohn disease. If these medications fail to control the condition, an anti-adhesion monoclonal antibody known as vedolizumab can be used to help block the migration of inflammatory cells specifically into the lesional areas of the intestinal lining. Sometimes the disease cannot be maintained in remission by medical therapy, and complications develop that require surgical intervention. Complications may include bowel obstruction or fistula or abscess formation. If a significant segment of the terminal ileum has been removed surgically or is involved with the disease, then periodic injections of vitamin B_{12} may be necessary to prevent megaloblastic anemia secondary to the lack of ability to absorb the vitamin. Similar supplementation of magnesium, iron, the fat-soluble vitamins, and folate may also be required because of malabsorption. Cigarette smoking is known to exacerbate Crohn disease, and patients should be advised to stop this habit.

Oral lesions have been reported to clear with treatment of the gastrointestinal process in many cases. Occasionally persistent oral ulcerations will develop, and these may have to be treated with topical or intralesional corticosteroids. Systemic thalidomide and infliximab have been used successfully to manage refractory oral ulcers of Crohn disease.

◆ PYOSTOMATITIS VEGETANS

Pyostomatitis vegetans is a relatively rare condition that has a controversial history. It has been associated in the past with diseases such as pemphigus or pyodermatitis vegetans. Most investigators today, however, believe that pyostomatitis vegetans is an unusual oral expression of inflammatory bowel disease, particularly **ulcerative colitis** or **Crohn disease.** The pathogenesis of the condition, like that of inflammatory bowel disease, is poorly understood. A few patients with pyostomatitis vegetans have also been noted to have one of several concurrent liver abnormalities.

Clinical Features

Patients with pyostomatitis vegetans exhibit characteristic yellowish, slightly elevated, linear, serpentine pustules set on an erythematous oral mucosa. The lesions primarily affect the buccal and labial mucosa, soft palate, and ventral tongue (Figs. 17.45 and 17.46). These lesions have been called "snail track" ulcerations, although in most instances the lesions are probably not truly ulcerated. Oral discomfort is variable but can be surprisingly minimal in some patients. This variation in symptoms may be related to the number of pustules that have ruptured to form ulcerations. The oral lesions may

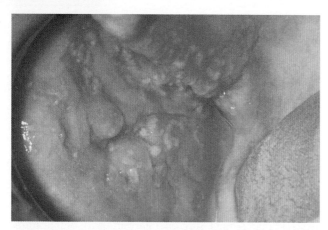

• **Fig. 17.45 Pyostomatitis Vegetans.** The characteristic lesions are seen on the buccal mucosa, appearing as yellow-white pustules.

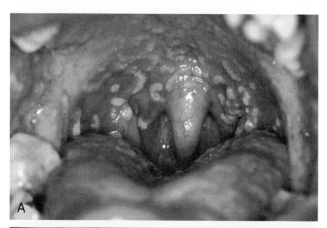

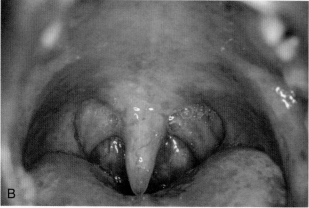

• **Fig. 17.46 Pyostomatitis Vegetans. A,** Characteristic "snail track" lesions involve the soft palate. **B,** Same patient after 5 days of prednisone therapy. (From Neville BW, Laden SA, Smith SE, et al: Pyostomatitis vegetans, *Am J Dermatopathol* 7:69–77, 1985.)

appear concurrently with the bowel symptoms, or they may precede the intestinal involvement.

Histopathologic Features

A biopsy specimen of an oral lesion of pyostomatitis vegetans usually shows marked edema, causing an acantholytic appearance of the involved epithelium. This may be the

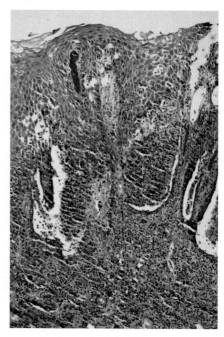

• **Fig. 17.47 Pyostomatitis Vegetans.** Medium-power photomicrograph showing intraepithelial abscesses composed of eosinophils.

result of the accumulation of numerous eosinophils within the spinous layer, often forming intraepithelial abscesses (Fig. 17.47). Subepithelial eosinophilic abscesses have been reported in some instances. The underlying connective tissue usually supports a dense mixed infiltrate of inflammatory cells that consists of eosinophils, neutrophils, and lymphocytes. Perivascular inflammation may also be present.

Treatment and Prognosis

Usually, the intestinal signs and symptoms of inflammatory bowel disease are of most concern for patients with pyostomatitis vegetans. Medical management of the bowel disease with sulfasalazine or systemic corticosteroids also produces clearing of the oral lesions (see Fig. 17.46). Often the oral lesions clear within days after systemic corticosteroid therapy has begun, and they may recur if the medication is withdrawn. If the bowel symptoms are relatively mild, then the oral lesions have been reported to respond to topical therapy with some of the more potent corticosteroid preparations.

♦ UREMIC STOMATITIS

Patients who have either acute or chronic renal failure typically show markedly elevated levels of urea and other nitrogenous wastes in the bloodstream. **Uremic stomatitis** represents a relatively uncommon complication of renal failure. In two series that included 562 patients with renal failure, only eight examples of this oral mucosal condition were documented. Nevertheless, for the patients in whom uremic stomatitis develops, this can be a painful disorder. The cause

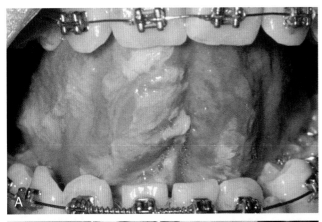

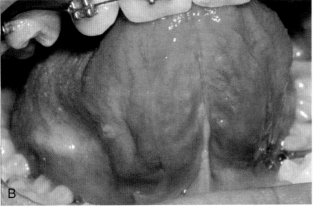

• **Fig. 17.48 Uremic Stomatitis. A,** Ragged white plaques affect the ventral tongue and floor of the mouth. **B,** Same patient after renal dialysis. (From Ross WF, Salisbury PL: Uremic stomatitis associated with undiagnosed renal failure, *Gen Dent* 42:410–412, 1994.)

of the oral lesions is unclear, but some investigators suggest that urease, an enzyme produced by the oral microflora, may degrade urea secreted in the saliva. This degradation results in the liberation of free ammonia, which presumably damages the oral mucosa.

Clinical Features

Most cases of uremic stomatitis have been reported in patients with acute renal failure. The onset may be abrupt, with white plaques distributed predominantly on the buccal mucosa, tongue, and floor of the mouth (Fig. 17.48). Patients may complain of unpleasant taste, oral pain, or a burning sensation with the lesions, and the clinician may detect an odor of ammonia or urine on the patient's breath. The clinical appearance occasionally has been known to mimic oral hairy leukoplakia.

Treatment and Prognosis

In some instances, uremic stomatitis may clear within a few days after renal dialysis, although such resolution may take place over 2–3 weeks. In other instances, treatment with a mildly acidic mouth rinse, such as diluted hydrogen peroxide, seems to clear the oral lesions. For control of pain while

the lesions heal, patients may be given palliative therapy with ice chips or a topical anesthetic, such as viscous lidocaine or dyclonine hydrochloride. Although renal failure itself is life threatening, at least one example of a uremic plaque that presumably caused a patient's death has been recorded. This event was thought to have been caused by the dislodging of the plaque with subsequent obstruction of the patient's airway.

Bibliography

Mucopolysaccharidosis

Alpöz AR, Çoker M, Çelen E, et al.: The oral manifestations of Maroteaux-Lamy syndrome (mucopolysaccharidosis VI): a case report, *Oral Surg Oral Med Oral Pathol Oral Radiol Endod* 101:632–637, 2006.

Benetó N, Vilageliu L, Grinberg D, et al.: Sanfilippo syndrome: molecular basis, disease models and therapeutic approaches, *Int J Mol Sci* 21:7819, 2020.

Bianchi PM, Gaini R, Vitale S: ENT and mucopolysaccharidoses, *Ital J Pediatr* 44(Suppl 2):127, 2018.

Downs AT, Crisp T, Ferretti G: Hunter's syndrome and oral manifestations: a review, *Pediatr Dent* 17:98–100, 1995.

Harmatz PR, Shediac R: Mucopolysaccharidosis VI: pathophysiology, diagnosis and treatment, *Front Biosci (Landmark Ed)* 22:385–406, 2017.

Kinirons MJ, Nelson J: Dental findings in mucopolysaccharidosis type IV A (Morquio's disease type A), *Oral Surg Oral Med Oral Pathol* 70:176–179, 1990.

Kubaski F, Vairo F, Baldo G, et al.: Therapeutic options for mucopolysaccharidosis II (Hunter disease), *Curr Pharm Des* 26:5100–5109, 2020.

McGovern E, Owens L, Nunn J, et al.: Oral features and dental health in Hurler Syndrome following hematopoietic stem cell transplantation, *Int J Paediatr Dent* 20:322–329, 2010.

Muenzer J: Overview of the mucopolysaccharidoses, *Rheumatology* 50: v4–v12, 2011.

Nakamura T, Miwa K, Kanda S, et al.: Rosette formation of impacted molar teeth in mucopolysaccharidoses and related disorders, *Dentomaxillofac Radiol* 21:45–49, 1992.

Oliveira-Torres R, Braga-Pintor AV, Ribeiro-Guedes F, et al.: Three-dimensional dental and craniofacial manifestations in patients with late diagnosis of mucopolysaccharidosis type II: report of 2 cases, *Oral Surg Oral Med Oral Pathol Oral Radiol* 126:e35–e39, 2018.

Oussoren E, Brands MMMG, Ruijter GJG, et al.: Bone, joint and tooth development in mucopolysaccharidoses: relevance to therapeutic options, *Biochim Biophys Acta* 1812:1542–1556, 2011.

Santana-Sarmento DJ, Gonçalves de Carvalho SH, Sousa-Melo SL, et al.: Mucopolysaccharidosis: radiographic findings in a series of 16 cases, *Oral Surg Oral Med Oral Pathol Oral Radiol* 120:e240–e246, 2015.

Sawamoto K, Álvarez-González JV, Piechnik M, et al.: Mucopolysaccharidosis IVA: diagnosis, treatment, and management, *Int J Mol Sci* 21:1517, 2020.

Sifuentes M, Doroshow R, Hoft R, et al.: A follow-up study of MPS I patients treated with laronidase enzyme replacement therapy for 6 years, *Mol Genet Metab* 90:171–180, 2007.

Smith KS, Hallett KB, Hall RK, et al.: Mucopolysaccharidosis: MPS VI and associated delayed tooth eruption, *Int J Oral Maxillofac Surg* 24:176–180, 1995.

Staba SL, Escolar ML, Poe M, et al.: Cord-blood transplants from unrelated donors in patients with Hurler's syndrome, *N Engl J Med* 350:1960–1969, 2004.

Stapleton M, Hoshina H, Sawamoto K, et al.: Critical review of current MPS guidelines and management, *Mol Genet Metab* 126:238–245, 2019.

Lipid Reticuloendothelioses

Anderson LJ, Henley W, Wyatt KM, et al.: Long-term effectiveness of enzyme replacement therapy in adults with Gaucher disease: results from the NCS-LSD cohort study, *J Inherit Metab Dis* 37:953–960, 2014.

Bender CV, da Silveira HLD, dos Santos NS, et al.: Oral, dental, and craniofacial features in chronic acid sphingomyelinase deficiency, *Am J Med Genet* 182A:2891–2901, 2020.

Beutler E: Lysosomal storage diseases: natural history and ethical and economic aspects, *Mol Genet Metab* 88:208–215, 2006.

Bley AE, Giannikopoulos OA, Hayden D, et al.: Natural history of infantile GM2 gangliosidosis, *Pediatrics* 128:e1233–e1241, 2011.

Cachón-González MB, Zaccariotto E, Cox TM: Genetics and therapies for GM2 gangliosidosis, *Curr Gene Ther* 18:68–89, 2018.

Dayan B, Elstein D, Zimran A, et al.: Decreased salivary output in patients with Gaucher disease, *Q J Med* 96:53–56, 2003.

Fernandes-Filho JA, Shapiro BE: Tay-Sachs disease, *Arch Neurol* 61:1466–1468, 2004.

Imrie J, Dasgupta S, Besley GTN, et al.: The natural history of Niemann-Pick disease type C in the UK, *J Inherit Metab Dis* 30:51–59, 2007.

Kolodny EH: Niemann-Pick disease, *Curr Opin Hematol* 7:48–52, 2000.

Levran O, Desnick RJ, Schuchman EH: Niemann-Pick disease: a frequent missense mutation in the acid sphingomyelinase gene of Ashkenazi Jewish type A and B patients, *Proc Natl Acad Sci U S A* 88:3748–3752, 1991.

McGovern MM, Aron A, Brodie SE, et al.: Natural history of type A Niemann-Pick disease: possible endpoints for therapeutic trials, *Neurology* 66:228–232, 2006.

Nobre RM, Ribeiro ALR, Alves-Junior SM, et al.: Dentomaxillofacial manifestations of Gaucher's disease: preliminary clinical and radiographic findings, *Dentomaxillofac Radiol* 41:541–547, 2012.

Revel-Vilk S, Szer J, Mehta A, et al.: How we manage Gaucher Disease in the era of choices, *Br J Haematol* 182:467–480, 2018.

Sam R, Ryan E, Daykin E, et al.: Current and emerging pharmacotherapy for Gaucher disease in pediatric populations, *Expert Opin Pharmacother* 22:1489–1503, 2021.

Saranjam HR, Sidransky E, Levine WZ, et al.: Mandibular and dental manifestations of Gaucher disease, *Oral Dis* 18:421–429, 2012.

Schultze H, Sandhoff K: Lysosomal lipid storage diseases, *Cold Spring Harb Perspect Biol* 3:a004804, 2011.

Sévin M, Lesca G, Baumann N, et al.: The adult form of Niemann-Pick disease type C, *Brain* 130:120–133, 2007.

Shiran A, Brenner B, Laor A, et al.: Increased risk of cancer in patients with Gaucher disease, *Cancer* 72:219–224, 1993.

Stirnemann J, Belmatoug N, Camou F, et al.: A review of Gaucher disease pathophysiology, clinical presentation and treatments, *Int J Mol Sci* 18:441, 2017.

Tamura H, Takahashi T, Ban N, et al.: Niemann-Pick type C disease: Novel *NPC1* mutations and characterization of the concomitant acid sphingomyelinase deficiency, *Mol Genet Metab* 87:113–121, 2006.

Vanier MT: Prenatal diagnosis of Niemann-Pick diseases types A, B and C, *Prenat Diagn* 22:630–632, 2002.

Zeevi I, Anavi Y, Kaplan I, et al.: Jaws features in type 1 Gaucher disease, *J Oral Maxillofac Surg* 71:694–701, 2013.

Lipoid Proteinosis

Akoglu G, Karaduman A, Ergin S, et al.: Clinical and histopathological response to acitretin therapy in lipoid proteinosis, *J Dermatolog Treat* 22:178–183, 2011.

Bahadir S, Çobanoğlu Ü, Kapicioğlu Z, et al.: Lipoid proteinosis: a case with ophthalmological and psychiatric findings, *J Dermatol* 3:215–218, 2006.

Bazopoulou-Kyrkanidou E, Tosios KI, Zabelis G, et al.: Hyalinosis cutis et mucosae: gingival involvement, *J Oral Pathol Med* 27:233–237, 1998.

Callizo M, Ibáñez-Flores N, Laue J, et al.: Eyelid lesions in lipoid proteinosis or Urbach-Wiethe disease: case report and review of the literature, *Orbit* 30:242–244, 2011.

Frenkel B, Vered M, Taicher S, et al.: Lipoid proteinosis unveiled by oral mucosal lesions: a comprehensive analysis of 137 cases, *Clin Oral Investig* 21:2245–2251, 2017.

Hamada T: Lipoid proteinosis, *Clin Exp Dermatol* 27:624–629, 2002.

Hamada T, Wessagowit V, South AP, et al.: Extracellular matrix protein 1 gene *(ECM1)* mutations in lipoid proteinosis and genotype-phenotype correlation, *J Invest Dermatol* 120:345–350, 2003.

Lee KC, Peters SM, Ko YCK, et al.: Oral manifestations of lipoid proteinosis in a 10-year-old female: A case report and literature update, *Oral Surg Oral Med Oral Pathol Oral Radiol* 126:e228–e232, 2018.

Loos E, Kerkhofs L, Laureyns G: Lipoid proteinosis: a rare cause of hoarseness, *J Voice* 33:155–158, 2019.

Nasir M, Latif A, Ajmal M, et al.: Molecular analysis of lipoid proteinosis: identification of a novel nonsense mutation in the *ECM1* gene in a Pakistani family, *Diagn Pathol* 6:69, 2011.

Xu W, Wang L, Zhang L, et al.: Otolaryngological manifestations and genetic characteristics of lipoid proteinosis, *Ann Otol Rhinol Laryngol* 119:767–771, 2010.

Jaundice

Cohen SM: Jaundice in the full-term newborn, *Pediatr Nurs* 32:202–208, 2006.

Fargo MV, Grogan SP, Saguil A: Evaluation of jaundice in adults, *Am Fam Physician* 95:164–168, 2017.

Hass PL: Differentiation and diagnosis of jaundice, *AACN Clin Issues* 10:433–441, 1999.

John S, Pratt DS: Jaundice, In Jameson JL, Fauci AS, Kasper DL, et al., editors: *Harrison's principles of internal medicine*, ed 20, New York, 2018, McGraw-Hill, pp 276–281.

Winger J, Michelfelder A: Diagnostic approach to the patient with jaundice, *Prim Care* 38:469–482, 2011.

Sullivan JI, Rockey DC: Diagnosis and evaluation of hyperbilirubinemia, *Curr Opin Gastroenterol* 33:164–170, 2017.

Amyloidosis

Adamo D, Gasparro R, Marenzi G, et al.: Amyloidoma of the tongue: case report, surgical management, and review of the literature, *J Oral Maxillofac Surg* 78:1572–1582, 2020.

Elad S, Czerninski R, Fischman S, et al.: Exceptional oral manifestations of amyloid light chain protein (AL) systemic amyloidosis, *Amyloid* 17:27–31, 2010.

Gertz MA: Immunoglobulin light chain amyloidosis: 2020 update on diagnosis, prognosis, and treatment, *Am J Hematol* 95:848–860, 2020.

Gertz MA, Mauermann ML, Grogan M, et al.: Advances in the treatment of hereditary transthyretin amyloidosis: a review, *Brain Behav* 9:e01371, 2019.

Gertz MA, Dispenzieri A: Systemic amyloidosis recognition, prognosis, and therapy - a systematic review, *JAMA* 324:79–89, 2020.

Hachulla E, Janin A, Flipo RM, et al.: Labial salivary gland biopsy as a reliable test for the diagnosis of primary and secondary amyloidosis: a prospective clinical and immunohistologic study in 59 patients, *Arthritis Rheum* 36:691–697, 1993.

Johansson I, Ryberg M, Steen L, et al.: Salivary hypofunction in patients with familial amyloidotic polyneuropathy, *Oral Surg Oral Med Oral Pathol* 74:742–748, 1992.

Leiba M, Jarjoura S, Abboud W, et al.: Role of oral examination in newly diagnosed multiple myeloma patients: A safe and simple way to detect light chain amyloidosis, *Oral Dis* 24:1343–1348, 2018.

Muchtar E, Gertz MA, Lacy MQ, et al.: Ten-year survivors in AL amyloidosis: characteristics and treatment pattern, *Br J Haematol* 187:588–594, 2019.

Papa R, Lachmann HJ, Secondary AA: Amyloidosis, *Rheum Dis Clin N Am* 44:585–603, 2018.

Pau M, Reinbacher KE, Feichtinger M, et al.: Surgical treatment of macroglossia caused by systemic primary amyloidosis, *Int J Oral Maxillofac Surg* 42:294–297, 2013.

Penner CR, Müller S: Head and neck amyloidosis: a clinicopathologic study of 15 cases, *Oral Oncol* 42:421–429, 2006.

Picken MM: The pathology of amyloidosis in classification: a review, *Acta Haematol* 143:322–334, 2020.

Rebelo Pontes HA, Lacerda de Souza L, Rodrigues-Fernandes CI, et al.: A nodule in the palatal mucosa, *Oral Surg Oral Med Oral Pathol Oral Radiol* 130:473–477, 2020.

Sharpley FA, Petrie A, Mahmood S, et al.: A 24-year experience of autologous stem cell transplantation for light chain amyloidosis patients in the United Kingdom, *Br J Haematol* 187:642–652, 2019.

Skinner M, Anderson JJ, Simms R, et al.: Treatment of 100 patients with primary amyloidosis: a randomized trial of melphalan, prednisone, and colchicine versus colchicine only, *Am J Med* 100:290–298, 1996.

Stoopler ET, Alawi F, Laudenbach JM, et al.: Bullous amyloidosis of the oral cavity: a rare clinical presentation and review, *Oral Surg Oral Med Oral Pathol Oral Radiol Endod* 101:734–740, 2006.

Xanthelasma

Baykal C, Ekinci AP, Yazganoglu KD, et al.: The clinical spectrum of xanthomatous lesions of the eyelids, *Int J Dermatol* 56:981–992, 2017.

Karsai S, Czarnecka A, Raulin C: Treatment of xanthelasma palpebrarum using a pulsed dye laser: a prospective clinical trial in 38 cases, *Dermatol Surg* 36:610–617, 2010.

Nguyen AH, Vaudreuil AM, Huerter CJ: Systematic review of laser therapy in xanthelasma palpebrarum, *Int J Dermatol* 56:e47–e55, 2017.

Nöel B: Premature atherosclerosis in patients with xanthelasma, *J Eur Acad Dermatol Venereol* 21:1244–1248, 2007.

Özdöl S, Şahin S, Tokgözoğlu L: Xanthelasma palpebrarum and its relation to atherosclerotic risk factors and lipoprotein (a), *Int J Dermatol* 47:785–789, 2008.

Pandhi D, Gupta P, Singal A, et al.: Xanthelasma palpebrarum: a marker of premature atherosclerosis (risk of atherosclerosis in xanthelasma), *Postgrad Med J* 88:198–204, 2012.

Vitamin Deficiency

Antonucci R, Locci C, Clemente MG, et al.: Vitamin D deficiency in childhood: old lessons and current challenges, *J Pediatr Endocrinol Metab* 31:247–260, 2018.

Ben-Zvi GT, Tidman MJ: Be vigilant for scurvy in high-risk groups, *Practitioner* 256:23–25, 2012.

Blanck HM, Bowman BA, Serdula MK, et al.: Angular stomatitis and riboflavin status among adolescent Bhutanese refugees living in southeastern Nepal, *Am J Clin Nutr* 76:430–435, 2002.

Campos-Outcalt D: Vitamin D: when it helps, when it hurts, *J Fam Pract* 62:368–370, 2013.

Carazo A, Macáková K, Matoušová K, et al.: Vitamin A update: forms, sources, kinetics, detection, function, deficiency, therapeutic use and toxicity, *Nutrients* 13:1703, 2021.

Golriz F, Donnelly LF, Devaraj S, et al.: Modern American scurvy — experience with vitamin C deficiency at a large children's hospital, *Pediatr Radiol* 47:214–220, 2017.

Gorey S, Canavan M, Robinson S, et al.: A review of vitamin D insufficiency and its management: a lack of evidence and consensus persists, *QJM* 112:165–167, 2019.

Heath ML, Sidbury R: Cutaneous manifestations of nutritional deficiency, *Curr Opin Pediatr* 18:417–422, 2006.

Kothari P, Tate A, Adewumi A, et al.: The risk for scurvy in children with neurodevelopmental disorders, *Spec Care Dentist* 40:251–259, 2020.

Polegato BF, Pereira AG, Azevedo PS, et al.: Role of thiamin in health and disease, *Nutr Clin Pract* 34:558–564, 2019.

Popovich D, McAlhany A, Adewumi AO, et al.: Scurvy: forgotten but definitely not gone, *J Pediatr Health Care* 23:405–415, 2009.

Powers HJ: Riboflavin (vitamin B_2) and health, *Am J Clin Nutr* 77:1352–1360, 2003.

Rivadeneira A, Moyer P, Salciccioli JD: Pellagra in the USA: unusual manifestations of a rare entity, *BMJ Case Rep* 12:e230972, 2019.

Suter PM, Russell RM: Vitamin and trace mineral deficiency and excess, In Jameson JL, Fauci AS, Kasper DL, et al., editors: *editors: Harrison's principles of internal medicine*, ed 20, New York, 2018, McGraw-Hill, pp 2309–2319.

Smith A, DiPrimio G, Humphrey-Murto S: Scurvy in the developed world, *Can Med Assoc J* 183:e752–e755, 2011.

Thacher TD, Fischer PR, Pettifor JM, et al.: A comparison of calcium, vitamin D, or both for nutritional rickets in Nigerian children, *N Engl J Med* 341:563–568, 1999.

Touyz LZG: Oral scurvy and periodontal disease, *J Can Dent Assoc* 63:837–845, 1997.

Van der Velden U: Vitamin C and its role in periodontal diseases – the past and the present: a narrative review, *Oral Health Prev Dent* 18:115–124, 2020.

Wilson RB: Pathophysiology, prevention, and treatment of beriberi after gastric surgery, *Nutr Rev* 78:1015–1029, 2020.

Iron-Deficiency Anemia

Camaschella C: Iron deficiency, *Blood* 133:30–39, 2019.

Cappellini MD, Musallam KM, Taher AT: Iron deficiency anaemia revisited, *J Intern Med* 287:153–170, 2020.

DeLoughery TG: Iron deficiency anemia, *Med Clin N Am* 101:319–332, 2017.

Goodnough LT: Iron deficiency syndromes and iron-restricted erythropoiesis, *Transfusion* 1584–1592, 2012.

Mirza FG, Abdul-Kadir R, Breymann C, et al.: Impact and management of iron deficiency and iron deficiency anemia in women's health, *Expert Rev Hematol* 11:727–736, 2018.

Osaki T, Ueta E, Arisawa K, et al.: The pathophysiology of glossal pain in patients with iron deficiency anemia, *Am J Med Sci* 318:324–329, 1999.

Pasricha S-R, Tye-Din J, Muckenthaler MU, et al.: Iron deficiency, *Lancet* 397:233–248, 2021.

Plummer-Vinson Syndrome

Bredenkamp JK, Castro DJ, Mickel RA: Importance of iron repletion in the management of Plummer-Vinson syndrome, *Ann Otol Rhinol Laryngol* 99:51–54, 1990.

Chen TSN, Chen PSY: Rise and fall of the Plummer-Vinson syndrome, *J Gastroenterol Hepatol* 9:654–658, 1994.

Dantas RO, Villanova MG: Esophageal motility impairment in Plummer-Vinson syndrome: correction by iron treatment, *Dig Dis Sci* 38:968–971, 1993.

Köklü S, Bulut M, Çakal B, et al.: Gastric cancer presenting with Plummer-Vinson syndrome, *J Am Geriatr Soc* 57:933–934, 2009.

Novacek G: Plummer-Vinson syndrome, *Orphanet J Rare Dis* 1:36, 2006.

Phatak S, Redkar N, Patil MA, et al.: Plummer-Vinson syndrome, *BMJ Case Rep*, 2012.

Seitz ML, Sabatino D: Plummer-Vinson syndrome in an adolescent, *J Adolesc Health* 12:279–281, 1991.

Wahlberg PCG, Andersson KEH, Biörklund AT, et al.: Carcinoma of the hypopharynx: analysis of incidence and survival in Sweden in over a 30-year period, *Head Neck* 20:714–719, 1998.

Walker J, Baran R, Velez N, et al.: Koilonychia: an update on pathophysiology, differential diagnosis and clinical relevance, *J Eur Acad Dermatol Venereol* 30:1985–1991, 2016.

Yukselen V, Karaoglu AO, Yasa MH: Plummer-Vinson syndrome: a report of three cases, *Int J Clin Pract* 57:646–648, 2003.

Pernicious Anemia

Drummond JF, White DK, Damm DD: Megaloblastic anemia with oral lesions: a consequence of gastric bypass surgery, *Oral Surg Oral Med Oral Pathol* 59:149–153, 1985.

Field EA, Speechley JA, Rugman FR, et al.: Oral signs and symptoms in patients with undiagnosed vitamin B_{12} deficiency, *J Oral Pathol Med* 24:468–470, 1995.

Green R: Vitamin B12 deficiency from the perspective of a practicing hematologist, *Blood* 129:2603–2611, 2017.

Green R, Mitra AD: Megaloblastic anemias - nutritional and other causes, *Med Clin N Am* 101:297–317, 2017.

Greenberg M: Clinical and histologic changes of the oral mucosa in pernicious anemia, *Oral Surg Oral Med Oral Pathol* 52:38–42, 1981.

Hall SN, Appelman HD: Autoimmune gastritis, *Arch Pathol Lab Med* 143:1327–1331, 2019.

Lehman JS, Bruce AJ, Rogers RS: Atrophic glossitis from vitamin B_{12} deficiency: a case misdiagnosed as burning mouth disorder, *J Periodontol* 77:2090–2092, 2006.

Rebelo Pontes HA, Conte Neto N, Bechara Ferreira K, et al.: Oral manifestations of vitamin B_{12} deficiency: a case report, *J Can Dent Assoc* 75:533–537, 2009.

Robinson AN, Loh JSP: Atrophic glossitis, *N Engl J Med* 381:1568, 2019.

Toh B-H: Pathophysiology and laboratory diagnosis of pernicious anemia, *Immunol Res* 65:326–330, 2017.

Vannella L, Lahner E, Osborn J, et al.: Systematic review: gastric cancer incidence in pernicious anaemia, *Aliment Pharmacol Ther* 37:375–382, 2013.

Pituitary Dwarfism

Britto IMPA, Aguiar-Oliveira MH, Oliveira-Neto LA, et al.: Periodontal disease in adults with untreated congenital growth hormone deficiency: a case-control study, *J Clin Periodontol* 38:525–531, 2011.

Buduneli N, Alpoz AR, Candan U, et al.: Dental management of isolated growth hormone deficiency: a case report, *J Clin Pediatr Dent* 29:263–266, 2005.

Carvalho LR, Justamante de Faria ME, Farah-Osorio MG, et al.: Acromegalic features in growth hormone (GH)-deficient patients after long-term GH therapy, *Clin Endocrinol (Oxf)* 59:788–792, 2003.

Funatsu M, Sato K, Mitani H: Effects of growth hormone on craniofacial growth, *Angle Orthod* 76:970–977, 2006.

Hodax JK, DiVall SA: Update on methods to enhance growth, *Curr Opin Endocrinol Diabetes Obes* 27:82–86, 2020.

Kosowicz J, Rzymski K: Abnormalities of tooth development in pituitary dwarfism, *Oral Surg Oral Med Oral Pathol* 44:853–863, 1977.

Mullis PE: Genetics of isolated growth hormone deficiency, *J Clin Res Pediatr Endocrinol* 2:52–62, 2010.

Richmond E, Rogol AD: Treatment of growth hormone deficiency in children, adolescents and at the transitional age, *Best Pract Res Clin Endocrinol Metab* 30:749–755, 2016.

Gigantism

Bendor-Samuel OM, Pal A, Cudlip S, et al.: Pituitary gigantism: a rare learning opportunity, *Arch Dis Child Educ Pract Ed* 105:111–116, 2020.

Creo AL, Lteif AN: Pituitary gigantism: a retrospective case series, *J Pediatr Endocrinol Metab* 29:597–602, 2016.

Daniel A, d'Emden M, Duncan E: Pituitary gigantism treated successfully with the growth hormone receptor antagonist, pegvisomant, *Intern Med J* 43:345–347, 2013.

Eugster EA, Pescovitz OH: Gigantism, *J Clin Endocrinol Metab* 84:4379–4384, 1999.

Marino AC, Taylor DG, Desai B, et al.: Surgery for pediatric pituitary adenomas, *Neurosurg Clin N Am* 30:465–471, 2019.

Shimatsu A, Teramoto A, Hizuka N, et al.: Efficacy, safety, and pharmacokinetics of sustained-release lanreotide (lanreotide Autogel) in Japanese patients with acromegaly or pituitary gigantism, *Endocr J* 60:651–663, 2013.

Tourtelot JB, Vesely DL: Pituitary tumor with gigantism, acromegaly and preclinical Cushing's disease diagnosed from the 10th row, *Am J Med Sci* 346:169–171, 2013.

Acromegaly

Anagnostis P, Efstathiadou ZA, Polyzos SA, et al.: Acromegaly: presentation, morbidity and treatment outcomes at a single centre, *Int J Clin Pract* 65:896–902, 2011.

Ben-Shlomo A, Melmed S: Skin manifestations in acromegaly, *Clin Dermatol* 24:256–259, 2006.

Cohen RB, Wilcox CW: A case of acromegaly identified after patient complaint of apertognathia, *Oral Surg Oral Med Oral Pathol* 75:583–586, 1993.

Dineen R, Stewart PM, Sherlock M: Acromegaly, *QJM* 110:411–420, 2017.

Farinazzo-Vital RW, Motohiro-Tanaka O, Reis-Fraga M, et al.: Acromegaly in an orthodontic patient, *Am J Orthod Dentofacial Orthop* 130:388–390, 2006.

Gadelha MR, Kasuki L, Lim DST, et al.: Systemic complications of acromegaly and the impact of the current treatment landscape: an update, *Endocr Rev* 40:268–332, 2019.

Kernen FR, Bidra AS: Dental implant therapy in a patient with acromegaly: a clinical report, *J Prosthodont* 28:355–360, 2019.

Kreitschmann-Andermahr I, Kohlmann J, Kleist B, et al.: Oro-dental pathologies in acromegaly, *Endocrine* 60:323–328, 2018.

Lavrentaki A, Paluzzi A, Wass JAH, et al.: Epidemiology of acromegaly: review of population studies, *Pituitary* 20:4–9, 2017.

Leonart LP, Ferreira VL, Tonin FS, et al.: Medical treatments for acromegaly: a systematic review and network meta-analysis, *Value Health* 21:874–880, 2018.

Pai F-Y, Chen C-J, Wang W-H, et al.: Low-dose gamma knife radiosurgery for acromegaly, *Neurosurgery* 85:e20–e30, 2019.

Hypothyroidism

Bauer AJ, Wassner AJ: Thyroid hormone therapy in congenital hypothyroidism and pediatric hypothyroidism, *Endocrine* 66:51–62, 2019.

Burman KD, McKinley-Grant L: Dermatologic aspects of thyroid disease, *Clin Dermatol* 24:247–255, 2006.

Chaker L, Bianco AC, Jonklaas J, et al.: Hypothyroidism, *Lancet* 390:1550–1562, 2017.

Duntas LH, Yen PM: Diagnosis and treatment of hypothyroidism in the elderly, *Endocrine* 66:63–69, 2019.

Mg'ang'a PM, Chindia ML: Dental and skeletal changes in juvenile hypothyroidism following treatment: case report, *Odontostomatol Trop* 13:25–27, 1990.

Rallia M, Angelettia D, Fiore M, et al.: Hashimoto's thyroiditis: An update on pathogenic mechanisms, diagnostic protocols, therapeutic strategies, and potential malignant transformation, *Autoimmun Rev* 19:102649, 2020.

Hyperthyroidism

De Leo S, Lee SY, Braverman LE: Hyperthyroidism, *Lancet* 388:906–918, 2016.

Douglas RS, Kahaly GJ, Patel A, et al.: Teprotumumab for the treatment of active thyroid eye disease, *N Engl J Med* 382:341–352, 2020.

Kravets I: Hyperthyroidism: diagnosis and treatment, *Am Fam Physician* 93:363–370, 2016.

McDermott MT: Hyperthyroidism, *Ann Intern Med* 157(1), 2012. ITC1–ITC16.

Pérusse R, Goulet J-P, Turcotte J-Y: Contraindications to vasoconstrictors in dentistry. Part II: hyperthyroidism, diabetes, sulfite sensitivity, cortico-dependent asthma, and pheochromocytoma, *Oral Surg Oral Med Oral Pathol* 74:687–691, 1992.

Sharma A, Stan MN: Thyrotoxicosis: diagnosis and management, *Mayo Clin Proc* 94:1048–1064, 2019.

Sundaresh V, Brito JP, Wang Z, et al.: Comparative effectiveness of therapies for Graves' hyperthyroidism: a systematic review and network meta-analysis, *J Clin Endocrinol Metab* 98:3671–3677, 2013.

Yeatts RP: Graves' ophthalmopathy, *Med Clin North Am* 79:195–209, 1995.

Hypoparathyroidism

Ahonen P, Myllärniemi S, Sipilä I, et al.: Clinical variation of autoimmune polyendocrinopathy-candidiasis-ectodermal dystrophy (APECED) in a series of 68 patients, *N Engl J Med* 322:1829–1836, 1990.

Bilezikian J: Hypoparathyroidism, *J Clin Endocrinol Metab* 105:1722–1736, 2020.

Cusano NE, Bilezikian JP: Signs and symptoms of hypoparathyroidism, *Endocrinol Metab Clin North Am* 47:759–770, 2018.

Gafni RI, Collins MT: Hypoparathyroidism, *N Engl J Med* 380:1738–1747, 2019.

Kelly A, Pomarico L: Pomarico Ribeiro de Souza I: Cessation of dental development in a child with idiopathic hypoparathyroidism: a 5-year follow-up, *Oral Surg Oral Med Oral Pathol Oral Radiol Endod* 107:673–677, 2009.

Lankisch TO, Jaeckel E, Strassburg CP: The autoimmune polyendocrinopathy-candidiasis-ectodermal dystrophy or autoimmune polyglandular syndrome, type 1, *Semin Liver Dis* 29:307–314, 2009.

Mitchell DM, Regan S, Cooley MR, et al.: Long-term follow-up of patients with hypoparathyroidism, *J Clin Endocrinol Metab* 97:4507–4514, 2012.

Siraj N, Hakami Y, Khan A: Medical hypoparathyroidism, *Endocrinol Metab Clin North Am* 47:797–808, 2018.

Walls AWG, Soames JV: Dental manifestations of autoimmune hypoparathyroidism, *Oral Surg Oral Med Oral Pathol* 75:452–454, 1993.

Pseudohypoparathyroidism

Gelfand IM, Eugster EA, DiMeglio LA: Presentation and clinical progression of pseudohypoparathyroidism with multi-hormone resistance and Albright hereditary osteodystrophy: a case series, *J Pediatr* 149:877–880, 2006.

Goeteyn V, De Potter CR, Naeyaert JM: Osteoma cutis in pseudohypoparathyroidism, *Dermatology* 198:209–211, 1999.

Hejlesen J, Underbjerg L, Gjørup H, et al.: Dental anomalies and orthodontic characteristics in patients with pseudohypoparathyroidism, *BMC Oral Health* 20:2, 2020.

Jüppner H, Linglart A, Fröhlich LF, et al.: Autosomal-dominant pseudohypoparathyroidism type Ib is caused by different microdeletions within or upstream of the GNAS locus, *Ann N Y Acad Sci* 1068:250–255, 2006.

Le Norcy E, Reggio-Paquet C, de Kerdanet M, et al.: Dental and craniofacial features associated with GNAS loss of function mutations, *Eur J Orthod* 42:525–533, 2020.

Mantovani G, Bastepe M, Monk D, et al.: Recommendations for diagnosis and treatment of pseudohypoparathyroidism and related disorders: an updated practical tool for physicians and patients, *Horm Res Paediatr* 93:182–196, 2020.

Potts JT, Jüppner H: Disorders of the parathyroid gland and calcium homeostasis, In Jameson JL, Fauci AS, Kasper DL, et al., editors: *Harrison's principles of internal medicine*, ed 20, New York, 2018, McGraw-Hill, pp 2921–2942.

Schlund M, Depeyre A, Kohler F, et al.: Cranio-maxillofacial and dental findings in Albright's hereditary osteodystrophy and pseudohypoparathyroidism, *Cleft Palate Craniofac J* 56:831–836, 2019.

Hyperparathyroidism

Aggunlu L, Akpek S, Coskun B: Leontiasis ossea in a patient with hyperparathyroidism secondary to chronic renal failure, *Pediatr Radiol* 34:630–632, 2004.

Gavaldá C, Bagán JV, Scully C, et al.: Renal hemodialysis patients: oral, salivary, dental and periodontal findings in 105 adult cases, *Oral Dis* 5:299–302, 1999.

Hata T, Irei I, Tanaka K, et al.: Macrognathia secondary to dialysis-related renal osteodystrophy treated successfully by parathyroidectomy, *Int J Oral Maxillofac Surg* 35:378–382, 2006.

Insogna KL: Primary hyperparathyroidism, *N Engl J Med* 379:1050–1059, 2018.

Lajolo C, Patini R, Limongelli L, et al.: Brown tumors of the oral cavity: presentation of 4 new cases and a systematic literature review, *Oral Surg Oral Med Oral Pathol Oral Radiol* 129:575–584, 2020.

Leal Rocha A, Mendes Nunes LF, Vieira Travassos D, et al.: A sessile nodule in the dorsum of the tongue, *Oral Surg Oral Med Oral Pathol Oral Radiol* 128:449–455, 2019.

Lerman MA, Do C, Gunaratnam L, et al.: Localized mandibular enlargement in end-stage renal disease: two case reports and a review of the literature, *Oral Surg Oral Med Oral Pathol Oral Radiol* 113:384–390, 2012.

Machado NN, Wilhelm SM: Diagnosis and evaluation of primary hyperparathyroidism, *Surg Clin N Am* 99:649–666, 2019.

Mainville G, Furchtgott N, Ing SW, et al.: A rapidly growing mandibular swelling, *J Am Dent Assoc* 144:45–48, 2013.

Palla B, Burian E, Fliefel R, et al.: Systematic review of oral manifestations related to hyperparathyroidism, *Clin Oral Investig* 22:1–27, 2018.

Silverman S Jr, Gordon G, Grant T, et al.: The dental structures in primary hyperparathyroidism. Studies in forty-two consecutive patients, *Oral Surg Oral Med Oral Pathol* 15:426–436, 1962.

Wasserman JD, Tomlinson GE, Druker H, et al.: Multiple endocrine neoplasia and hyperparathyroid-jaw tumor syndromes: clinical features, genetics and surveillance recommendations in childhood, *Clin Cancer Res* 23:e123–e132, 2017.

You M, Tang B, Wang Z-J, et al.: Radiological manifestations of renal osteodystrophy in the orofacial region: a case report and literature review, *Oral Radiol* 34:262–266, 2018.

Zhu CY, Sturgeon C, Yeh MW: Diagnosis and management of primary hyperparathyroidism, *JAMA* 323:1186–1187, 2020.

Hypercortisolism

Broersen LHA, Jha M, Biermasz NR, et al.: Effectiveness of medical treatment for Cushing's syndrome: a systematic review and meta-analysis, *Pituitary* 21:631–641, 2018.

Castinetti F, Morange I, Conte-Devolx B, et al.: Cushing's disease, *Orphanet J Rare Dis* 7:41, 2012.

Ferriere A, Tabarin A: Cushing's syndrome: treatment and new therapeutic approaches, *Best Pract Res Clin Endocrinol Metab* 34:101381, 2020.

Miller BS, Auchus RJ: Evaluation and treatment of patients with hypercortisolism—a review, *JAMA Surg* 155:1152–1159, 2020.

Molitch ME: Diagnosis and treatment of pituitary adenomas—a review, *JAMA* 317:516–524, 2017.

Nieman LK: Diagnosis of Cushing's syndrome in the modern era, *Endocrinol Metab Clin North Am* 47:259–273, 2018.

Tempark T, Phatarakijnirund V, Chatproedprai S, et al.: Exogenous Cushing's syndrome due to topical corticosteroid application: case report and review literature, *Endocrine* 38:328–334, 2010.

Addison Disease

Arlt W: Disorders of the adrenal cortex, In Jameson JL, Fauci AS, Kasper DL, et al., editors: *editors: Harrison's principles of internal medicine*, ed 20, New York, 2018, McGraw-Hill, pp 2719–2739.

Barthel A, Benker G, Berens K, et al.: An update on Addison's disease, *Exp Clin Endocrinol Diabetes* 127:165–170, 2019.

Bergthorsdottir R, Leonsson-Zachrisson M, Odén A, et al.: Premature mortality in patients with Addison's disease: a population-based study, *J Clin Endocrinol Metab* 91:4849–4853, 2006.

Betterle C, Presotto F, Furmaniak J: Epidemiology, pathogenesis, and diagnosis of Addison's disease in adults, *J Endocrinol Invest* 42:1407–1433, 2019.

Chakera AJ, Vaidya B: Addison disease in adults: diagnosis and management, *Am J Med* 123:409–413, 2010.

Milenkovic A, Markovic D, Zdravkovic D, et al.: Adrenal crisis provoked by dental infection: case report and review of the literature, *Oral Surg Oral Med Oral Pathol Oral Radiol Endod* 110:325–329, 2010.

Porter SR, Haria S, Scully C, et al.: Chronic candidiasis, enamel hypoplasia, and pigmentary anomalies, *Oral Surg Oral Med Oral Pathol* 74:312–314, 1992.

Saverino S, Falorn A: Autoimmune Addison's disease, *Best Pract Res Clin Endocrinol Metab* 34:101379, 2020.

Seeker P, Osswald S: Tongue discoloration, *N Engl J Med* 384:e102, 2021.

Shah SS, Oh CH, Coffin SE, et al.: Addisonian pigmentation of the oral mucosa, *Cutis* 76:97–99, 2005.

Diabetes Mellitus

D'Aiuto F, Gable D, Syed Z, et al.: Evidence summary: the relationship between oral diseases and diabetes, *Br Dent J* 222:944–948, 2017.

American Diabetes Association: 2. Classification and diagnosis of diabetes: Standards of Medical Care in Diabetes-2019, *Diabetes Care* 42(Suppl. 1):S13–S28, 2019.

Belazi M, Velegraki A, Fleva A, et al.: Candidal overgrowth in diabetic patients: potential predisposing factors, *Mycoses* 48:192–196, 2005.

Costa FO, Miranda Cota LO, Pereira Lages EJ, et al.: Progression of periodontitis and tooth loss associated with glycemic control in individuals undergoing periodontal maintenance therapy: a 5-year-follow-up study, *J Periodontol* 84:595–605, 2013.

Demmer RT, Holtfreter B, Desvarieux M, et al.: The influence of type 1 and type 2 diabetes on periodontal disease progression, *Diabetes Care* 35:2036–2042, 2012.

Franco OH, Steyerberg EW, Hu FB, et al.: Associations of diabetes mellitus with total life expectancy and life expectancy with and without cardiovascular disease, *Arch Intern Med* 167:1145–1151, 2007.

Genco RJ, Borgnakke WS: Diabetes as a potential risk for periodontitis: association studies, *Periodontology* 2000(83):40–45, 2020.

Guggenheimer J, Moore PA, Rossie K, et al.: Insulin-dependent diabetes mellitus and oral soft tissue pathologies: I. Prevalence and characteristics of non-candidal lesions, *Oral Surg Oral Med Oral Pathol Oral Radiol Endod* 89:563–569, 2000.

Guggenheimer J, Moore PA, Rossie K, et al.: Insulin-dependent diabetes mellitus and oral soft tissue pathologies: II. Prevalence and characteristics of *Candida* and candidal lesions, *Oral Surg Oral Med Oral Pathol Oral Radiol Endod* 89:570–576, 2000.

Mauri-Obradors E, Estrugo-Devesa A, Jané-Salas E, et al.: Oral manifestations of Diabetes Mellitus. A systematic review, *Med Oral Patol Oral Cir Bucal* 22:e586–e594, 2017.

Patel MH, Kumar JV, Moss ME: Diabetes and tooth loss: an analysis of data from the National Health and Nutrition Examination Survey, 2003–2004, *J Am Dent Assoc* 144:478–485, 2013.

Powers AC, Niswender KD, Evans-Molina C: Diabetes mellitus: diagnosis, classification, and pathophysiology, In Jameson JL, Fauci AS, Kasper DL, et al., editors: *Harrison's principles of internal medicine*, ed 20, New York, 2018, McGraw-Hill, pp 2850–2883.

Wysocki GP, Daley T: Benign migratory glossitis in patients with juvenile diabetes, *Oral Surg Oral Med Oral Pathol* 63:68–70, 1987.

Hypophosphatasia

Bangura A, Wright L, Shuler T: Hypophosphatasia: current literature for pathophysiology, clinical manifestations, diagnosis, and treatment, *Cureus* 12(6):e8594, 2020.

Bianchi ML, Bishop NJ, Guañabens N, et al.: Hypophosphatasia in adolescents and adults: overview of diagnosis and treatment, *Osteoporos Int* 31:1445–1460, 2020.

Biosse Duplan M, Coyac BR, Bardet C, et al.: Phosphate and vitamin D prevent periodontitis in X-linked hypophosphatemia, *J Dent Res* 96:388–395, 2017.

Bloch-Zupan A, Vaysse F: Hypophosphatasia: oral cavity and dental disorders, *Arch Pédiatr* 24:5S80–5S84, 2017.

Fenn JS, Lorde N, Ward JM, et al.: Hypophosphatasia, *J Clin Pathol* 74:635–640, 2021.

Khan AA, Josse R, Kannu P, et al.: Hypophosphatasia: Canadian update on diagnosis and management, *Osteoporos Int* 30:1713–1722, 2019.

Lynch CD, Ziada HM, Buckley LA, et al.: Prosthodontic rehabilitation of hypophosphatasia using dental implants: a review of the literature and two case reports, *J Oral Rehabil* 36:462–468, 2009.

Okawa R, Kadota T, Matayoshi S, et al.: Dental manifestations leading to the diagnosis of hypophosphatasia in two children, *J Dent Child* 87:179–183, 2020.

Okawa R, Kokomoto K, Nakano K: Dental effects of enzyme replacement therapy in case of childhood-type hypophosphatasia, *BMC Oral Health* 21:323, 2021.

Rush ET: Childhood hypophosphatasia: to treat or not to treat, *Orphanet J Rare Dis* 13:116, 2018.

Salles JP: Hypophosphatasia: biological and clinical aspects, avenues for therapy, *Clin Biochem Rev* 41:13–27, 2020.

Schroth RJ, Long C, Lee VHK, et al.: Dental outcomes for children receiving asfotase alfa for hypophosphatasia, *Bone* 152:116089, 2021.

Simon S, Resch H, Klaushofer K, et al.: Hypophosphatasia: from diagnosis to treatment, *Curr Rheumatol Rep* 20:69, 2018.

Van den Bos T, Handoko G, Niehof A, et al.: Cementum and dentin in hypophosphatasia, *J Dent Res* 84:1021–1025, 2005.

Villa-Suárez JM, García-Fontana C, Andújar-Vera F, et al.: Hypophosphatasia: a unique disorder of bone mineralization, *Int J Mol Sci* 22:4303, 2021.

Vitamin D–Resistant Rickets

Andersen MG, Beck-Nielsen SS, Haubek D, et al.: Periapical and endodontic status of permanent teeth in patients with hypophosphatemic rickets, *J Oral Rehabil* 39:144–150, 2012.

Archard HO, Witkop CJ: Hereditary hypophosphatemia (vitamin D-resistant rickets) presenting primary dental manifestations, *Oral Surg Oral Med Oral Pathol* 22:184–193, 1966.

Baroncelli GI, Zampollo E, Manca M, et al.: Pulp chamber features, prevalence of abscesses, disease severity, and PHEX mutation in X-linked hypophosphatemic rickets, *J Bone Miner Metab* 39:212–223, 2021.

Batra P, Tejani Z, Mars M: X-linked hypophosphatemia: dental and histologic findings, *J Can Dent Assoc* 72:69–72, 2006.

Beltes C, Zachou E: Endodontic management in a patient with vitamin D-resistant rickets, *J Endod* 38:255–258, 2012.

Bradley H, Dutta A, Philpott R: Presentation and non-surgical endodontic treatment of two patients with X-linked hypophosphatemia: a case report, *Int Endod J* 54:1403–1414, 2021.

Chaussin-Miller C, Sinding C, Wolikow M, et al.: Dental abnormalities in patients with familial hypophosphatemic vitamin D-resistant rickets: prevention by early treatment with 1-hydroxyvitamin D, *J Pediatr* 142:324–331, 2003.

Douyere D, Joseph C, Gaucher C, et al.: Familial hypophosphatemic vitamin D-resistant rickets—prevention of spontaneous dental abscesses on primary teeth: a case report, *Oral Surg Oral Med Oral Pathol Oral Radiol Endod* 107:525–530, 2009.

Haffner D, Emma F, Eastwood DM, et al.: Clinical practice recommendations for the diagnosis and management of X-linked hypophosphataemia, *Nat Rev Nephrol* 15:435–455, 2019.

McWhorter AG, Seale NS: Prevalence of dental abscess in a population of children with vitamin D-resistant rickets, *Pediatr Dent* 13:91–96, 1991.

Murayama T, Iwatsubo R, Akiyama S, et al.: Familial hypophosphatemic vitamin D-resistant rickets: dental findings and histologic study of teeth, *Oral Surg Oral Med Oral Pathol Oral Radiol Endod* 90:310–316, 2000.

Robinson M-E, AlQuorain H, Murshed M, et al.: Mineralized tissues in hypophosphatemic rickets, *Pediatr Nephrol* 35:1843–1854, 2020.

Saraff V, Nadar R, Högler W: New developments in the treatment of X-Linked hypophosphataemia: implications for clinical management, *Pediatr Drugs* 22:113–121, 2020.

Seow WK, Needleman HL, Holm IA: Effect of familial hypophosphatemic rickets on dental development: a controlled, longitudinal study, *Pediatr Dent* 17:346–350, 1995.

Yacarini Paredes SE, Bezerra Segato RA, Daher Moreira L, et al.: Dentoalveolar abscesses not associated with caries or trauma: a diagnostic hallmark of hypophosphatemic rickets initially misdiagnosed as hypochondroplasia, *Head Neck Pathol* 12:604–609, 2018.

Crohn Disease

Brunner B, Hirschi C, Weimann R, et al.: Treatment-resistant lingual Crohn's disease disappears after infliximab, *Scand J Gastroenterol* 40:1255–1259, 2005.

Cushing K, Higgins PDR: Management of Crohn disease - a review, *JAMA* 325:69–80, 2021.

Feuerstein JD, Cheifetz AS: Crohn disease: epidemiology, diagnosis, and management, *Mayo Clin Proc* 92:1088–1103, 2017.

Friedman S, Blumberg RS: Inflammatory bowel disease, In Jameson JL, Fauci AS, Kasper DL, et al., editors: *Harrison's principles of internal medicine*, ed 20, New York, 2018, McGraw-Hill, pp 2258–2276.

Gajendran M, Loganathan P, Catinella AP, et al.: A comprehensive review and update on Crohn's disease, *Dis Mon* 64:20–57, 2018.

Galvin S, Flint SR, Toner ME, et al.: Oral lymphangiectasias and Crohn's disease: two case reports, *Oral Surg Oral Med Oral Pathol Oral Radiol* 126:e31–e34, 2018.

Harty S, Fleming P, Rowland M, et al.: A prospective study of the oral manifestations of Crohn's disease, *Clin Gastroenterol Hepatol* 3:886–891, 2005.

Hegarty A, Hodgson T, Porter S: Thalidomide for the treatment of recalcitrant oral Crohn's disease and orofacial granulomatosis, *Oral Surg Oral Med Oral Pathol Oral Radiol Endod* 95:576–585, 2003.

Laube R, Liu K, Schifter M, et al.: Oral and upper gastrointestinal Crohn's disease, *J Gastroenterol Hepatol* 33:355–364, 2018.

Mills CC, Amin M, Manisali M: Salivary duct fistula and recurrent buccal space infection: a complication of Crohn's disease, *J Oral Maxillofac Surg* 61:1485–1487, 2003.

Müller S: Non-infectious granulomatous lesions of the orofacial region, *Head Neck Pathol* 13:449–456, 2019.

Plauth M, Jenss H, Meyle J: Oral manifestations of Crohn's disease: an analysis of 79 cases, *J Clin Gastroenterol* 13:29–37, 1991.

Sánchez AR, Rogers RS, Sheridan PJ: Oral ulcerations are associated with the loss of response to infliximab in Crohn's disease, *J Oral Pathol Med* 34:53–55, 2005.

Scully C, Cochran KM, Russell RI, et al.: Crohn's disease of the mouth: an indicator of intestinal involvement, *Gut* 23:198–201, 1982.

Tan CXW, Brand HS, de Boer NKH, et al.: Gastrointestinal diseases and their oro-dental manifestations: Part 1: Crohn's disease, *Br Dent J* 221:794–799, 2016.

Torres J, Mehandru S, Colombel J-F, et al.: Crohn's disease, *Lancet* 389:1741–1755, 2017.

Van de Scheur MR, van der Waal RIF, Völker-Dieben HJ, et al.: Orofacial granulomatosis in a patient with Crohn's disease, *J Am Acad Dermatol* 49:952–954, 2003.

Veauthier B, Hornecker JR: Crohn's disease: diagnosis and management, *Am Fam Physician* 98:661–669, 2018.

Pyostomatitis Vegetans

Ballo FS, Camisa C, Allen CM: Pyostomatitis vegetans: report of a case and review of the literature, *J Am Acad Dermatol* 21:381–387, 1989.

Chaudhry SI, Philpot NS, Odell EW, et al.: Pyostomatitis vegetans associated with asymptomatic ulcerative colitis: a case report, *Oral Surg Oral Med Oral Pathol Oral Radiol Endod* 87:327–330, 1999.

Clark LG, Tolkachjov SN, Bridges AG, et al.: Pyostomatitis vegetans (PSV)-pyodermatitis vegetans (PDV): A clinicopathologic study of 7 cases at a tertiary referral center, *J Am Acad Dermatol* 75:578–584, 2016.

Diaconescu S, Strat S, Balan GG, et al.: Dermatological manifestations in pediatric inflammatory bowel disease, *Medicina* 56:425, 2020.

Ficarra G, Baroni G, Massi D: Pyostomatitis vegetans: cellular profile and expression of IL-6, IL-8 and TNF-α, *Head Neck Pathol* 4:1–9, 2010.

Healy CM, Farthing PM, Williams DM, et al.: Pyostomatitis vegetans and associated systemic disease: a review and two case reports, *Oral Surg Oral Med Oral Pathol* 78:323–328, 1994.

Hegarty AM, Barrett AW, Scully C: Pyostomatitis vegetans, *Clin Exp Dermatol* 29:1–7, 2004.

Magliocca KR, Fitzpatrick SG: Autoimmune disease manifestations in the oral cavity, *Surg Pathol* 10:57–88, 2017.

Markiewicz M, Suresh L, Margarone J, et al.: Pyostomatitis vegetans: a clinical marker of silent ulcerative colitis, *J Oral Maxillofac Surg* 65:346–348, 2007.

Neville BW, Laden SA, Smith SE, et al.: Pyostomatitis vegetans, *Am J Dermatopathol* 7:69–77, 1985.

Tan CXW, Brand HS, de Boer NKH, et al.: Gastrointestinal diseases and their oro-dental manifestations: Part 2: Ulcerative colitis, *Br Dent J* 222:53–57, 2017.

Thornhill MH, Zakrzewska JM, Gilkes JJH: Pyostomatitis vegetans: report of three cases and review of the literature, *J Oral Pathol Med* 21:128–133, 1992.

Uremic Stomatitis

Halazonetis J, Harley A: Uremic stomatitis: report of a case, *Oral Surg Oral Med Oral Pathol* 23:573–577, 1967.

Hovinga J, Roodvoets AP, Gailliard J: Some findings in patients with uraemic stomatitis, *J Maxillofac Surg* 3:124–127, 1975.

Leão JC, Gueiros LAM, Segundo AVL, et al.: Uremic stomatitis in chronic renal failure, *Clinics* 60:259–262, 2005.

McCreary CE, Flint SR, McCartan BE, et al.: Uremic stomatitis mimicking oral hairy leukoplakia. Report of a case, *Oral Surg Oral Med Oral Pathol Oral Radiol Endod* 83:350–353, 1997.

Proctor R, Kumar N, Stein A, et al.: Oral and dental aspects of chronic renal failure, *J Dent Res* 84:199–208, 2005.

Ross WF, Salisbury PL: Uremic stomatitis associated with undiagnosed renal failure, *Gen Dent* 42:410–412, 1994.

Talish M, DiLorenzo AM: Uremic stomatitis, *N Engl J Med* 382:2556, 2020.

Yano H, Kinjo M: Uraemic stomatitis, *BMJ Case Rep* 12:e231948, 2019. https://doi.org/10.1136/bcr-2019-231948.

18

Facial Pain and Neuromuscular Diseases

REVISED BY N. LYN WILSON WESTMARK

◆ BELL PALSY (IDIOPATHIC SEVENTH NERVE PARALYSIS; IDIOPATHIC FACIAL PARALYSIS)

Bell palsy is an acute weakness or paralysis of the facial nerve without an identifiable cause. It is the most common cause of facial paralysis or paresis, but is a clinical diagnosis of exclusion limited to idiopathic cases with acute onset. Although the etiology is uncertain, evidence suggests that the condition may be related to either a viral infection (herpes simplex, varicella-zoster, or Epstein Barr virus) or cell-mediated autoimmune reaction resulting in demyelination of the nerve. Other proposed etiologies include anatomical factors, ischemia, and cold stimulation. Coronavirus infection (SARS-CoV-2) also has been suggested to increase prevalence of Bell palsy, but limited and conflicting epidemiological data are available. Ultimately, the mechanism is related to inflammation or compression of the facial nerve resulting in weakness or paralysis. According to Baugh et al., a variety of factors may increase the risk for developing Bell palsy, including:

- Pregnancy (especially third trimester)
- Preeclampsia
- Diabetes
- Hypertension
- Obesity
- Upper respiratory infections

Bell palsy can occur at any age, but it develops most frequently in individuals 15–45 years of age. Depending on the population studied, the annual incidence of Bell palsy ranges from 11.5 to 53.3 per 100,000 persons. The lifetime risk for developing this condition is 1 in 60. Other specific conditions may cause facial nerve paralysis which should be excluded by history or physical exam, including neoplasms, sarcoidosis, orofacial granulomatosis (Melkersson-Rosenthal syndrome), Lyme disease, congenital malformations, inappropriate administration of local anesthesia, trauma, and postsurgical damage.

Clinical Features

Bell palsy presents with an abrupt unilateral loss of facial muscle control resulting in inability to smile, close the eye, or raise the eyebrow (Fig. 18.1). Drooling, slurred speech, and abnormal taste also may occur. Full severity often is reached within 72 hours, and patients frequently may wake in the morning with a full-fledged case. In patients where the eye cannot close, conjunctival dryness or ulceration may cause permanent ocular damage. Some patients experience a prodromal sensation of pain or fullness on the affected side prior to onset of paralysis.

Infrequently, bilateral involvement is seen. However, rapid onset of bilateral facial weakness should alert the clinician to the possibility of other diseases, such as **Guillain-Barré syndrome** or a form of sarcoidosis known as *uveoparotid fever* (see Heerfordt syndrome, page 329). If multiple cranial nerve deficits accompany facial nerve paralysis, then central nervous system (CNS) infectious diseases and basilar skull tumors must be considered in the differential diagnosis. If the patient has symptoms of vertigo, tinnitus, or rash on the auricle, then a diagnosis of Ramsay Hunt syndrome must be suspected (see page 240).

Treatment and Prognosis

Bell palsy is a self-limiting condition, and most patients will recover over a 3–4 month period. Without treatment, complete facial nerve function will be restored in nearly three-quarters of patients with complete paralysis and in over 90% of patients with partial paralysis. However, as many as 20%–30% of patients will not recover completely. The most consistently effective treatment is systemic corticosteroid therapy, which has been shown to improve recovery rates and should be started within 72 hours of symptom onset. A 10-day tapering course of prednisone often is prescribed, beginning at a dosage of 60 mg per day. Antiviral therapy (acyclovir, famciclovir, or valacyclovir) may be associated with a modest improvement in recovery and potential

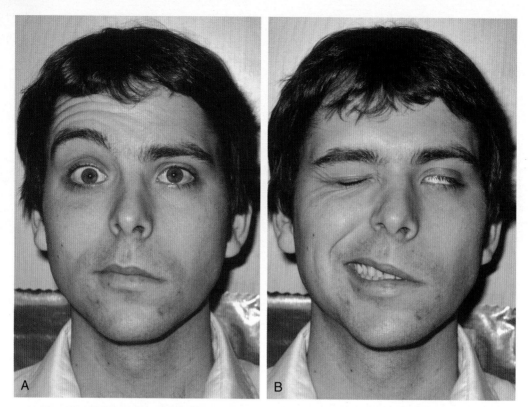

• **Fig. 18.1 Bell Palsy.** Paralysis of the facial muscles on the patient's left side. **A,** Patient is trying to raise the eyebrows. **B,** Patient is attempting to close the eyes and smile. (Courtesy of Dr. Bruce B. Brehm.)

avoidance of some long-term sequelae (abnormal lacrimation, muscle contracture), when given in combination with corticosteroids. However, antiviral therapy alone is not recommended. Surgical decompression of the facial nerve has been attempted, but evidence for the effectiveness of this approach is lacking. Electrodiagnostic testing may be helpful to assess the likelihood of recovery for patients with complete paralysis. Eye protection is critical for patients with impaired eye closure. Topical ocular antibiotics and artificial tears may be required to prevent corneal ulceration, and the eyelid may have to be taped shut. Patients without improvement or with worsening symptoms despite conventional therapy should undergo further workup for other causes of facial paralysis.

♦ FREY SYNDROME (AURICULOTEMPORAL SYNDROME; GUSTATORY SWEATING AND FLUSHING)

Named for Polish neurologist Łucja Frey, **Frey syndrome** typically is unilateral and characterized by facial flushing and sweating along the distribution of the auriculotemporal nerve in response to gustatory stimuli. This syndrome occurs after injury to the nerve, and signs begin to develop after nerve regeneration. The most widely accepted mechanism of Frey syndrome is aberrant neuronal regeneration.

The auriculotemporal nerve, in addition to supplying sensory fibers to the preauricular and temporal regions, carries parasympathetic fibers to the parotid gland and sympathetic vasomotor and sudomotor (sweat stimulating) fibers to the preauricular skin. After parotid abscess, trauma, facial surgery, neck dissection, or parotidectomy, the parasympathetic nerve fibers may be severed. In their attempt to reestablish innervation, these fibers occasionally become misdirected and regenerate along the sympathetic nerve pathways, establishing communication with the sympathetic nerve fibers of sweat glands and blood vessels of the facial skin. Subsequent to these aberrant neural connections, when salivation is stimulated, local sweat glands are activated inadvertently and the patient's cheek becomes flushed and moist.

Parotidectomies are the most common preceding cause, with 30%–60% of patients reporting subjective development of Frey syndrome 6–18 months after surgery, although a much higher frequency (70%–100%) can be documented if objective testing is performed (Minor starch-iodine test or infrared thermography). The condition is rare in infancy but has been seen after forceps delivery. Neonatal cases typically do not occur until the child begins to eat solid foods, at which time it may be interpreted as an allergy. Interestingly, bilateral gustatory sweating of the face and neck can be seen in diabetic patients, especially those with neuropathy or nephropathy.

Similar phenomena include sweating and flushing of the chin after submandibular gland surgery or injury (chorda tympani syndrome) or gustatory lacrimation (crocodile tears) after injury of the facial nerve proximal to the geniculate ganglion.

Clinical Features

The presenting signs and symptoms of Frey syndrome include sweating, flushing, warmth, and occasionally pain or itching in the preauricular and temporal regions during chewing or exposure to gustatory stimuli. Sweating and flushing become evident 2 months to 2 years (average 9 months) post nerve injury and may intensify over the course of several months before stabilizing. In children, Frey syndrome may be distinguished from allergy by repeated pattern of flushing, often unilateral, which resolves quickly after eating without intervention. When flushing occurs, the local skin temperature may be raised as much as 2°C. This may occur without sweating, especially in females. Pain, when present, is usually mild, and hypoesthesia or hyperesthesia are common features.

To detect sweating, a Minor starch-iodine test may be used. A 1% iodine solution is painted on the affected area of the skin. This solution is allowed to dry, and the area is then coated with a layer of starch. When the patient is given something to eat, the moisture of the sweat that is produced will mix with the iodine on the skin. This allows the iodine to react with the starch and produce a blue color (Fig. 18.2). Iodine-sublimated paper, which changes color when wet, also can be used, and thermography or surface thermometers will document the temperature changes of the skin.

Treatment and Prognosis

The initial risk for developing Frey syndrome is diminished greatly by positioning a musculofascial flap or allograft between the gland and the overlying skin of the cheek at the time of surgery, especially during parotidectomy. Use of temporoparietal fascia and acellular dermal matrix has been shown to reduce subjective and objective Frey syndrome, respectively. Most cases are mild enough that the patient may decide treatment is not required, although some patients may report a diminished quality of life. Additionally,

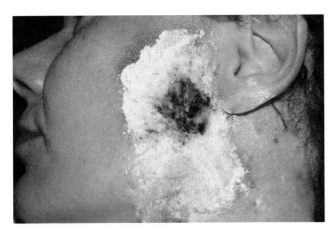

• **Fig. 18.2 Frey Syndrome.** This patient received an injury to her auriculotemporal nerve during orthognathic surgery 3 years earlier. Notice the region of sweating detected during mastication by a color change of the starch in the Minor starch-iodine test.

some adult patients may report spontaneous resolution, but this is much more common in infant Frey syndrome, which has an observed resolution rate of 69%.

If treatment is desired, intracutaneous injections of botulinum toxin A can provide long-term relief, although injections may need to be repeated. Topically applied medications, such as aluminum chloride or anticholinergics (e.g., scopolamine and glycopyrrolate), also have been used for short-term control. Surgical management may include insertion of various tissue barriers or tympanic neurectomy, but this rarely is indicated due to risk of injury to the facial nerve or a cosmetic defect. Therefore, surgery should be reserved for severe cases refractory to medical treatment.

HEAD AND NECK PAIN

Pain is a universal experience and is often a protective mechanism which alerts organisms to the possibility of harm. As pain is the primary motivation for the majority of health care encounters in our culture, it is prudent to consider pain in a wider context prior to discussing specific pain entities common to the head and neck region.

Pain can be characterized broadly as acute or chronic. Typically, acute pain is associated with a tissue injury of sudden onset and has a more predictable outcome. Chronic pain is ongoing and may become a disease entity by itself, requiring continued management, and it may affect an individual's physical, social, and psychological states. Estimates suggest that between 17% to 26% of the general population experience orofacial pain, and for 7%–12% that pain presentation will become chronic. The majority of acute pain presentations in dental practice are associated with the teeth and their supporting structures, and dentists usually diagnose and treat these conditions with relative ease. However, the diagnosis and management of non-odontogenic head and neck pain often presents a challenge to even the most skilled diagnosticians due to the complexity of the neural and vascular networks of the orofacial region.

Pain fibers from the orofacial region travel to the spinal nucleus caudalis of the trigeminal nerve in a process known as *trigeminal convergence.* Of note, nociceptive fibers from the cervical region also converge in this area, adding further complexity. This convergence often makes it virtually impossible for patients to distinguish the site of their pain from the source of their pain in a reliable fashion. For this reason, it is important that health care providers have a working knowledge of the myriad of diagnostic possibilities for those patients presenting with chronic orofacial pain. Although it is well beyond the scope of this chapter to discuss each of these entities, differential considerations related to chronic orofacial pain are summarized in Box 18.1. In general, if the pain is thought to be of nondental origin, then a comprehensive pain evaluation, complete with diagnostic anesthesia and appropriate laboratory testing, is warranted.

• BOX 18.1 Disorders Associated With Chronic Orofacial Pain

Temporomandibular Joint Disorders

Joint pain
  Arthralgia
  Arthritis
Joint disorders
  Disc-condyle complex disorders
    Disc displacement with reduction
    Disc displacement without reduction
  Hypomobility disorders
    Adhesions
    Ankylosis
  Hypermobility disorders
    Subluxation
    Luxation
Joint diseases
  Degenerative joint disease (osteoarthritis/osteoarthrosis)
  Condylysis (idiopathic condylar resorption)
  Osteochondritis dissecans
  Osteonecrosis
  Synovial chondromatosis
Congenital/developmental disorders of the condyle
  Aplasia
  Hypoplasia
  Hyperplasia

Masticatory Muscle Disorders

Muscle pain limited to the orofacial region
  Myalgia
  Myositis
  Spasm
Masticatory muscle pain attributed to systemic/central disorders
  Fibromyalgia
  Centrally mediated myalgia
Movement disorders affecting masticatory muscles
  Orofacial dyskinesia
  Oromandibular dystonia

Primary Headache Disorders

Migraine headache
Tension-type headache (TTH)
Trigeminal autonomic cephalalgias (TACS)
  Cluster headache
  Paroxysmal hemicrania
  Short-lasting unilateral neuralgia headache attacks with conjunctival injection and tearing (SUNCT)
  Short-lasting unilateral neuralgia headache attacks with cranial autonomic symptoms (SUNA)
  Hemicrania continua
Other primary headaches

Primary exertional headache
Primary thunderclap headache
Hypnic headache

Neuropathic Pain Disorders

Trigeminal neuralgia
Pretrigeminal neuralgia
Glossopharyngeal neuralgia
Nervus intermedius neuralgia
Superior laryngeal neuralgia
Occipital neuralgia
Painful ophthalmoplegia
Idiopathic (trigeminal) neuropathic pain
Post traumatic (trigeminal) neuropathy
Postherpetic (trigeminal) neuropathy
Anesthesia dolorosa
Persistent idiopathic facial pain
Complex regional pain syndrome
Burning mouth syndrome
Occlusal dysesthesia
Central neuropathic pain
  Central neuropathic pain due to multiple sclerosis
  Central poststroke pain

Cervical Pain Disorders

Cervicalgia
Sprain and strain of cervical spine
Cervical osteoarthritis
Radiculopathy
Cervical dystonia (Spasmodic torticollis)
Cervicogenic headache
Neck-tongue syndrome
Pain secondary to inflammation of the stylohyoid ligament (Eagle syndrome)

Systemic Causes of Orofacial Pain

Diabetes mellitus
Lyme disease
Multiple sclerosis
Neurodegenerative diseases
  Parkinson disease
Connective tissue diseases
  Systemic lupus erythematosus
  Rheumatoid arthritis (RA)
  Sjögren syndrome
  Systemic sclerosis
Giant cell arteritis
Primary malignancies

Modified from de Leeuw R, Klasser GD, editors: *Orofacial pain—guidelines for assessment, diagnosis and management*, ed 6, Chicago, 2018, Quintessence Publishing.

◆ TRIGEMINAL NEURALGIA (TIC DOULOUREUX; TIC)

The head and neck region is a common site for neuralgias (pain extending along the course of a nerve). Because facial neuralgias produce pain that often mimics pain of dental origin, the dental profession is frequently called on to rule out odontogenic or inflammatory causes. **Trigeminal neuralgia,** the most serious and the most common of the facial neuralgias, is characterized by a paroxysmal, extremely severe, electric shock-like or sharp, stabbing pain limited to one or more branches of the trigeminal nerve. The significance of this disorder is underscored by the fact that it has one of the highest suicide rates of any disease and is regarded as one of the most painful afflictions known. The pathogenesis of *classical* trigeminal neuralgia is not well understood but is thought to be secondary to vascular compression of the trigeminal nerve root, resulting in demyelination. *Secondary* trigeminal neuralgia occurs subsequent to a separate disease process such as multiple sclerosis or compression of the nerve by tumors or arteriovenous malformations. The condition may be termed *idiopathic* if no identifying disease process is found. Advanced imaging techniques such as magnetic resonance imaging have made subclassification of clinically diagnosed trigeminal neuralgia possible.

The incidence of trigeminal neuralgia in the general population is 4–29 per 100,000 person years annually. The condition is approximately 20 times more prevalent in patients with multiple sclerosis.

Clinical Features

Trigeminal neuralgia characteristically affects individuals older than 50 years of age (average onset 53–57 years), although it can develop at any age, including young children. Women are affected more often than men by a ratio of 3:1. One or more branches of the trigeminal nerve may be involved, with the majority of cases affecting the maxillary (V2) or mandibular (V3) distributions of the nerve. The ophthalmic division is reported to be affected in approximately 1%–4% of cases. The right side is affected more commonly, and bilateral involvement is unusual (3%–5% of cases). This may suggest the possibility of underlying multiple sclerosis. Trigeminal neuralgia associated with multiple sclerosis also tends to develop at a younger age and may be a presenting symptom. Multiple sclerosis should be ruled out when a diagnosis of trigeminal neuralgia is made in a person under the age of 40.

In the early stages, the pain of trigeminal neuralgia may be rather mild and is often described by the patient as a twinge, dull ache, or burning sensation. This clinical presentation may be attributed erroneously to disorders of the teeth, jaws, and paranasal sinuses, leading to inappropriate treatment. With time, the attacks occur at more frequent intervals and the pain becomes increasingly intense, sometimes being described as feeling like "an electric shock," "a bolt of lightning," or "being stabbed by an ice pick." Patients often clutch at the face and experience spasmodic contractions of the facial muscles during attacks, a feature that long ago led to the use of the term *tic douloureux* (i.e., painful jerking) for this disease.

For most patients, the pain will be provoked by stimulation of a specific trigger zone along the distribution of the trigeminal nerve, although spontaneous episodes of pain may occur. Continuous aching, burning, or throbbing pain in between episodes is reported by 24%–49% of patients. Extraoral and intraoral trigger zones are common, and the most frequently reported areas are the gingiva, chin, cheek, lips, and nasolabial fold. Stimulation of trigger areas, even by light sensation, may trigger an attack. Commonly reported trigger actions include toothbrushing, face washing, shaving, eating, or even exposure to a breeze.

• BOX 18.2 Clinical Features of Trigeminal Neuralgia

- Abrupt onset of pain often initiated by light touch to a consistent and specific trigger point.
- Pain is described as paroxysmal, severe, and shooting or shocking in nature
- Single episode duration is less than 2 minutes, but overall attack may consist of repeating episodes of short duration
- Pain is limited to the distribution of one or more branches of the trigeminal nerve and no motor deficits are present.
- A refractory period is present after an attack during which another episode generally cannot be triggered
- Severe episodes may be accompanied by ipsilateral muscle contraction
- Less common features
  - Continuous dull, aching pain between episodes may be present
  - Mild hypoesthesia may be present

Each painful episode typically lasts for no longer than 2 minutes, followed by a refractory period in which stimulation of the trigger zone will not elicit another attack. This refractory period can be clinically useful in distinguishing trigeminal neuralgia from stimulus-provoked odontogenic pain. Rarely autonomic signs may be present. If motor deficits, sensory loss, or ataxia are present, then a CNS tumor should be ruled out.

Variations in diagnostic criteria exist, with some experts including clinical criteria and others incorporating imaging findings, to distinguish between classical, secondary, and idiopathic trigeminal neuralgia. A summary of distinguishing clinical features of trigeminal neuralgia can be found in Box 18.2. If the pain pattern does not meet these criteria, then a different diagnosis should be considered, such as persistent idiopathic facial pain or one of the trigeminal autonomic cephalalgias.

Treatment and Prognosis

There have been rare reports of spontaneous permanent and intermittent remissions of trigeminal neuralgia. However, more often than not, this disease is characterized by a protracted clinical course with increasing frequency and severity of exacerbations. The initial treatment for trigeminal neuralgia is pharmacological, with carbamazepine (an anticonvulsant) being the first drug of choice, followed by oxcarbazepine. Over 80% of patients experience significant pain control on this regimen, but side effects are frequent and may be intolerable. Additionally, treatment response may wane over time, necessitating combination therapy. Other medications (phenytoin, gabapentin, lamotrigine, pregabalin, duloxetine, valproic acid, topiramate, and baclofen) also may be used in addition to first-line therapy, in combination, or as monotherapy. Side effects may still occur, and treatment may need to be modified. Botulinum toxin type A injections into trigger zones can be used as an adjunctive therapy and may lead to lasting (>1 year) symptom relief in some patients. Opioid medications are typically ineffective in managing the pain of trigeminal neuralgia.

If medical management fails, a variety of surgical treatments may be considered (Box 18.3). Microvascular decompression is an invasive, but nondestructive, surgical technique, which aims to address compression of the nerve by adjacent blood vessels. The mortality rate from this procedure is approximately 0.3%, but this approach is favored in cases with proven vascular compression as pain relief is achieved in 62%–89% of patients at long term follow up (3–11 years). Potential long-term complications include facial numbness and ipsilateral hearing loss.

A noninvasive but destructive technique is stereotactic radiosurgery (Gamma Knife) in which a portion of the trigeminal nerve is treated with a focused beam of radiation. Other ablative procedures that are less invasive but also involve destruction of affected portions of the trigeminal nerve by mechanical, thermal, and chemical means include balloon microcompression, radiofrequency thermocoagulation, and glycerol rhizotomy, respectively. Ablative therapies are recommended when vascular compression is not detected and, depending on the technique used, many patients may experience long-term (4–11 years) relief. As these procedures are ablative in nature, repeated procedures may be necessary, and there is a higher chance of sensory complications such as distorted sensations of the facial skin (**facial dysesthesia**) or a combination of anesthesia and spontaneous pain (**anesthesia dolorosa**). Anesthesia dolorosa is a dreaded form of central pain that can occur after any neurosurgical procedure that causes a variable amount of sensory loss, but this complication occurs more commonly with procedures that totally denervate a region.

◆ GLOSSOPHARYNGEAL NEURALGIA (VAGOGLOSSOPHARYNGEAL NEURALGIA)

Neuralgia of the ninth cranial nerve, **glossopharyngeal neuralgia,** is similar to trigeminal neuralgia (see previous topic) except in the anatomic location of the pain. In

glossopharyngeal neuralgia the pain is centered on the tonsil and the ear. The pain often radiates from the throat to the ear because of the involvement of the tympanic branch of the glossopharyngeal nerve. Some unfortunate individuals have a combination of glossopharyngeal neuralgia and trigeminal neuralgia (approximately 10%–12%).

Glossopharyngeal neuralgia is rare, representing only 0.2%–1.3% of facial pain syndromes, with an incidence of about 0.7 per 100,000 per year. The pain also may affect sensory areas supplied by the pharyngeal and auricular branches of the vagus nerve. As with trigeminal neuralgia, subtypes of glossopharyngeal neuralgia are recognized: *classical, secondary,* and *idiopathic.* Classical glossopharyngeal neuralgia is attributed to arterial compression of the nerve, usually the posterior inferior cerebellar artery. Secondary glossopharyngeal neuralgia occurs due to compression of the nerve by a specific lesion, such as intracranial or cranial base tumors, oropharyngeal tumors, pagetic bone, or calcified stylohyoid ligament (Eagle syndrome; see page 23). Idiopathic glossopharyngeal neuralgia is unassociated with any identifiable underlying disorder. Unlike trigeminal neuralgia, it is uncommon for glossopharyngeal neuralgia to be associated with multiple sclerosis.

Clinical Features

Glossopharyngeal neuralgia usually occurs in middle-aged and older adults. There is no sex predilection, and only rarely is there bilateral involvement. The paroxysmal pain may be felt in the ear (**tympanic plexus neuralgia),** infra-auricular area, tonsil, base of the tongue, posterior mandible, or lateral wall of the pharynx; however, the patient often has difficulty localizing the pain in the oropharynx.

The episodic pain in this unilateral neuralgia is sharp, lancinating (jabbing), and extremely intense. Attacks have an abrupt onset and a short duration (seconds to minutes). The pain typically radiates upward from the oropharynx to the ipsilateral ear, but pain referring to the nose, eye, chin, and shoulder also have been reported. Talking, chewing, swallowing, yawning, or touching a blunt instrument to the tonsil on the affected side may precipitate the pain, but a definite trigger zone is not easily identified. Because the pain is related to jaw movement, it may be confused with the pain of **temporomandibular joint dysfunction.**

Patients frequently point to the neck immediately below the angle of the mandible as the site of greatest pain, but trigger points are not found on the external skin, except within the ear canal. Excessive vagal effects will occur in approximately 10% of patients, resulting in cough, syncope, hypotension, seizures, bradycardia, or cardiac arrest (**vagoglossopharyngeal neuralgia).**

Treatment and Prognosis

As in trigeminal neuralgia, glossopharyngeal neuralgia is subject to unpredictable remissions and recurrences. It is not unusual during the early stages for remissions to last 6 months or more. Painful episodes are of varying severity but generally become more severe and more frequent with time. Some patients may report nearly continuous pain, but this is rare.

Many patients will experience pain relief when a topical anesthetic agent is applied to the tonsil and pharynx on the side of the pain. Because this relief lasts only 60–90 minutes, it is used more as a diagnostic tool and emergency measure than a long-term treatment. Repeated applications to a trigger point for 2 or 3 days may extend the pain-free episode enough to allow the patient to obtain much needed rest and nutrition.

For most patients with classical or idiopathic glossopharyngeal neuralgia, the first line of therapy is pharmacological, similar to trigeminal neuralgia (discussed above). For individuals with vagoglossopharyngeal neuralgia, atropine can be used to prevent the related cardiac phenomena. If a patient with glossopharyngeal neuralgia fails drug therapy, then surgical options should be considered. The preferred neurosurgical treatments are microvascular decompression or surgical sectioning of the glossopharyngeal nerve and the upper two rootlets of the vagus nerve, both of which have been shown to provide long term relief. Other possible procedures include radiofrequency nerve ablation, balloon compression, and stereotactic radiosurgery (Gamma Knife ablation). If the pain is secondary to another condition (e.g., tumor or Eagle syndrome), then management of the underlying lesion must be addressed.

◆ GIANT CELL ARTERITIS (TEMPORAL ARTERITIS; GRANULOMATOUS ARTERITIS)

Giant cell arteritis is an immune-mediated vasculitis that affects medium-sized and larger arteries, leading to vascular occlusion and ischemia. The condition also is termed **temporal arteritis** because the superficial temporal artery is the most commonly affected site. Although giant cell arteritis most often affects head and neck vessels, it is considered to be a systemic condition that can involve multiple vessels, including the aorta and its proximal branches. Although the exact cause is uncertain, there appears to be a strong genetic predisposition, with a higher frequency of disease in patients who express certain human leukocyte antigen (HLA) types, specifically the HLA-DRB1*0 allele. Because geographic and seasonal variations have been observed, an infectious etiology or trigger also has been suggested.

Giant cell arteritis occurs primarily in older individuals (average age = 70 years); the condition demonstrates an annual incidence rate of 20 per 100,000 population over the age of 50 years. There is an increased incidence associated with advancing age, with the highest rate observed in the eighth decade (average age, 70 years). The disease shows a predilection for individuals of Scandinavian and northern European descent. Women are affected more often than men (2:1 to 3:1 ratio).

Clinical Features

The disease most frequently involves the temporal artery, presenting with symptoms of new, severe headache and scalp tenderness. The superficial temporal artery often is exquisitely sensitive to palpation and eventually appears erythematous, swollen, tortuous, or sometimes ulcerated. A highly characteristic feature is jaw claudication, which is described as cramping pain due to ischemia of the masseter and temporalis muscles, which increases with usage (chewing or talking) but is relieved by rest. Jaw claudication and ocular involvement frequently coexist.

The most significant complication in the head and neck region is vision loss, which usually is due to vasculitis of the posterior ciliary artery and ischemic optic neuropathy. Permanent loss of vision occurs in 15% of patients. Visual disturbances (blurred vision with exercise, diplopia, transient vision loss) often are an early manifestation of giant cell arteritis, sometimes occurring before the onset of other symptoms.

Systemic signs and symptoms include fever, malaise, fatigue, anorexia, and weight loss. Many patients (40%) develop **polymyalgia rheumatica,** which is characterized by aching pain and morning stiffness in the neck, shoulders, and pelvic girdle. Giant cell arteritis may affect the aorta and other large vessels 30%–70% of cases, although such involvement often is asymptomatic. On occasion, however, undetected aortic inflammation may be associated with aortic aneurysm and rupture. Patients have an increased risk of cerebrovascular accidents, cardiac infarction, and limb claudication and vasculitis.

Histopathologic and Laboratory Features

Microscopic changes tend to be segmental and can be missed if the specimen is too small. At least 1 cm of the affected vessel must, therefore, be examined for proper evaluation.

The disease is characterized by chronic inflammation of the tunica intima and tunica media of the involved artery, with narrowing of the lumen from edema and proliferation of the tunica intima. Necrosis of the smooth muscle and elastic lamina is frequent. A variable number of multinucleated giant cells are mixed with macrophages and lymphocytes. Thrombosis or complete occlusion of the lumen is not unusual.

Clinical laboratory features often include an elevated erythrocyte sedimentation rate, increased C-reactive protein levels, and an elevated platelet count.

Diagnosis

Due the lower cost and less invasive procedure, ultrasound of the temporal artery is demonstrating a greater role in the early diagnosis of temporal arteritis, but this modality is highly operator sensitive. Imaging features include vessel wall thickening, occlusion, stenosis, and non-compressible arteries. Other imaging (MRI) may be recommended to evaluate for large vessel involvement. Despite imaging advances, temporal artery biopsy remains the preferred confirmatory test in the United States.

Treatment and Prognosis

Because of the risk for sudden and permanent loss of vision, prompt treatment of giant cell arteritis is critical. If diagnostic imaging or biopsy cannot be completed in a timely manner, treatment may need to be initiated. Initial treatment with high dose systemic corticosteroids and tocilizumab (monoclonal antibody against interleukin 6) is recommended. The disease typically responds well to high-dose systemic corticosteroid therapy, and symptoms often subside within a few days. However, many cases are chronic and require treatment for years. Additional steroid corticosteroid-sparing medications may include methotrexate or azathioprine.

◆ BURNING MOUTH DISORDER (BURNING MOUTH SYNDROME; ORAL DYSESTHESIA; ORAL SENSORY NEUROPATHY; STOMATOPYROSIS; STOMATODYNIA; GLOSSOPYROSIS; GLOSSODYNIA; BURNING TONGUE SYNDROME; BURNING MOUTH SYNDROME)

Burning mouth disorder (BMD) is one of the most common nondental orofacial pains encountered in the clinical practice, and it likely represents neuropathic pain, potentially with both peripheral and central nervous system components. Because taste disturbances (reduced ability to taste; altered taste; taste "phantoms") and altered perception of oral mucosal texture (xerostomia; swelling; gritty; slimy sensation) frequently accompany the onset of burning sensation, this condition has been referred to as *burning mouth syndrome.* Whether the presence of these additional clinical findings actually constitute a syndrome is a matter of much debate. Terms that are more inclusive of the various presenting symptoms are "*oral sensory neuropathy*" or "*oral dysesthesia.*"

Oral burning may be attributed to various local or systemic factors (Box 18.4), and if a local or systemic cause is found, the diagnosis of secondary BMD is applied. Primary BMD is limited to the presence of oral burning in the absence of both abnormal clinical and laboratory findings, meaning that the patient will have a clinically normal oral appearance.

The etiology and pathogenesis of primary BMD are not well established and are likely complex. Despite numerous investigations, no clear causative agent has been identified. Proposed theories include nerve damage, hormonal changes, psychological factors, and alteration of the peripheral and central nervous system. Specific proposed mechanisms include chorda tympani damage resulting in loss of central inhibition or dysregulation of the gustatory and sensory systems. Although patients with oral dysesthesias often present with psychological dysfunction such as depression,

Local Factors
- Clinically observable hyposalivation
- Chronic mechanical trauma
- Oral fungal, bacterial, or viral infection
- Contact stomatitis
- Geographic tongue
- Local manifestation of immune-mediated or autoimmune disease

Systemic Factors
- Vitamin B deficiency
  - Vitamin B_1 or B_2 deficiency
  - Pernicious anemia (B_{12})
  - Pellagra (niacin deficiency)
  - Folic acid deficiency
- Iron deficiency
- Diabetes mellitus
- Chronic gastritis or regurgitation

anxiety, or irritability, these findings are common in patients with chronic pain conditions, and there is no correlation between duration and intensity of the burning sensation and the amount of psychologic dysfunction. Potentially, the development of psychologic distress in some affected individuals may be caused by, or exacerbated by, the presence of chronic oral discomfort that is experienced by the patient.

Although BMD often is reported to affect women much more often than men, most of those reports are based on the gender of the patients who present to a particular center for treatment. However, this discrepancy in gender predilection may be explained by the increased tendency of women to seek medical care. The 1989 National Health Interview Survey, which interviewed thousands of adults over the age of 35, found no significant difference in the number men vs women with a complaint of burning mouth. This finding was replicated in a survey of elderly adults in Florida, with approximately 1.7% of both men and women affected. There seems to be increasing prevalence with advancing age, especially after age 55. The syndrome is rare before the age of 30 years.

Clinical Features

Burning mouth disorder (BMD) usually is described by the patient as a burning sensation of the oral mucosa. When asked, patients often will say that their mouth "feels like I scalded it with a hot cup of coffee." Although the anterior dorsal tongue is the most commonly affected site **(glossopyrosis),** other mucosal surfaces also may be symptomatic **(stomatopyrosis).** The anterior hard palate, as well as the maxillary and mandibular labial mucosa, frequently are involved, and the pain generally is bilateral and symmetric. Very infrequently unilateral involvement may occur.

Approximately 70% of patients also report taste disturbances, which can include an obtunded taste sensation, a distorted sense of taste, termed *dysgeusia*, or the development of taste "phantoms," in which a metallic, salty, sweet, "rotten," or bitter taste may be present. Patients have been known to seek dental care for removal of their amalgam restorations in an attempt (unsuccessfully) to relieve the metallic taste phantom.

At least 25% of these patients report having an altered texture of their oral mucosa, typically a dry mouth, although other textures (sandpaper, sliminess, swelling) also have been reported. The sensation of dry mouth mimics true *xerostomia* (see page 470); however, a normal degree of moisture will be present. None of the typical signs of decreased saliva will be evident. In other words, clear, copious saliva can be milked from the major salivary gland ducts. No significant plaque accumulation will be seen, and no Class V dental caries will be present. Actual reduction of salivary flow, as seen in patients with Sjögren syndrome (see page 472) or patients whose major salivary glands were located in the field of therapeutic radiation used to treat a head and neck/oral malignancy (see page 282) would result in extreme dental plaque accumulation and diffuse cervical dental caries.

Typically, this disorder has an abrupt onset, although much less frequently the onset is quite gradual. There are no proven etiologic triggers, but it is human nature to want to find a "cause and effect." For this reason, many patients may want to attribute their symptoms to anything new or different that occurred at the onset of the burning sensation, but no unifying precipitating event has been identified. The various "causative" factors actually are coincidental and unrelated to the BMD.

The report of irritation with foods is variable, with some patients reporting symptom relief when eating or drinking, whereas others report exacerbation, especially with hot or spicy foods. Mucosal changes are seldom visible, although some patients will show erythema of their anterior tongue because the abnormal sensation of BMD makes them want to rub the tongue against the teeth, resulting in removal of the keratin (which is white) associated with the filiform papillae. If the dorsum is diffusely erythematous and smooth, an underlying systemic or local infectious process, such as anemia or erythematous candidiasis, should be suspected.

The symptoms of BMD often fluctuate in intensity. One frequently described pattern is that of minimal discomfort on awakening, with increasing intensity throughout the day. Other affected patients describe a waxing and waning pattern that occurs over several days or weeks, and the symptoms of oral burning, taste or texture alterations, and xerostomia may change in prominence independently of one another over time. A minority describe a constant degree of discomfort. Some individuals with BMD report that their symptoms flare in the presence of increased personal stressors as is typical with many chronic pain conditions. Usually, the condition does not interfere with sleep.

Treatment and Prognosis

If an underlying systemic or local cause for the burning sensation can be identified and corrected, the burning symptoms should predictably disappear. Almost two-thirds of patients with idiopathic disease show at least some improvement of their symptoms with pharmacologic therapies including: anxiolytics, antioxidants, antidepressants, and/or anticonvulsants alone or in combination. Some of this apparent response may be attributed to the placebo effect. Because most patients see their health care provider when symptoms are at their peak, it is realistic to assume that any treatment provided at that point will appear to be effective because the symptoms will diminish following the peak. This scenario easily could explain the wide array of purported "treatments," which often have similar reported effectiveness, but totally unrelated mechanisms of action. In addition, a significant number of patients will undergo spontaneous resolution of their symptoms, and it may appear that a particular treatment was "effective," when in fact, the BMD would have resolved on its own. For these reasons, randomized double-blind, placebo-controlled trials are required in order to identify treatments that actually are effective in treating this condition. Many of the purported treatments have significant side effects or are expensive, which are not good features for a placebo.

Systematic reviews have shown the most evidence for use of systemic or topical benzodiazepines, specifically clonazepam, for both short- and long-term relief. Alpha-lipoic acid may convey some benefit when used in conjunction with other therapies, especially gabapentin, but the effectiveness of alpha-lipoic acid alone over placebo has not been confirmed. Capsaicin topical rinse may offer some benefit, but side effects (transient increased oral burning, gastric irritation) may be intolerable.

Non-pharmacologic approaches include cognitive behavioral therapy alone or in combination with the evidence-based pharmacologic management described above, and stress management, which may be useful in those patients with existing psychological factors affecting their pain experience.

The long-term prognosis for BMD is variable. It is reported that one-third to one-half of patients experience a spontaneous or gradual remission months or years after the onset of symptoms. However, other patients may be refractory to therapeutic interventions and continue to experience symptoms throughout the rest of their lives. Even though the condition is chronic and may not always respond to therapy, patients should be reassured that BMD is benign and not indicative of a more ominous disease.

◆ DYSGEUSIA AND HYPOGEUSIA (PHANTOM TASTE; DISTORTED TASTE)

Dysgeusia is defined as a persistent abnormal taste and this condition was mentioned briefly in the previous section on burning mouth disorder. However, dysgeusia occurs independently of this association and merits additional discussion

---

• BOX 18.5 **Local and Systemic Factors Associated With Altered Taste Sensations (Dysgeusia) or Diminished Taste Sensations (Hypogeusia)**

Local Factors

Oral candidiasis
Oral galvanism
Periodontitis or gingivitis
Chlorhexidine rinse
Xerostomia

Systemic Factors

Vitamin A deficiency
Vitamin B_{12} deficiency
Zinc deficiency
Iron deficiency
Nutritional overdose (zinc, vitamin A, or pyridoxine)
Food sensitivity or allergy
Sjögren syndrome
Chorda tympani nerve damage
Anorexia, cachexia, or bulimia
Severe vomiting during pregnancy
Liver dysfunction
Crohn disease

Cystic fibrosis
Familial dysautonomia
Addison disease
Turner syndrome
Alcoholism
Medications (200 types)
Psychosis or depression
Pesticide ingestion
Lead, copper, or mercury poisoning
Temporal arteritis
Brainstem ischemia or infarction
Migraine headaches
Temporal lobe central nervous system (CNS) tumor
Nerve trauma, gustatory nerves
Herpes zoster, geniculate ganglion
Upper respiratory tract infection
Chronic gastritis or regurgitation
Bell palsy
COVID-19 infection
Radiation therapy to head and neck

---

here. Interestingly, the majority of purported taste disorders are in fact disorders of smell, and deficiencies in one or both of these senses has a potentially significant impact on the patient's quality of life. Altered or phantom gustatory and olfactory function are less tolerated than hyposmia or hypogeusia, and these symptoms can be quite distressing. The COVID-19 pandemic brought new attention to the experience of alterations in taste and smell, as many infected individuals report chemosensory changes ranging from a decrease in sensation (hyposmia, anosmia, hypogeusia, ageusia) to altered perception (parosmia, phantosmia, dysgeusia.) Prior to this, estimated prevalence of taste disorders was 5%–20% and olfactory disorders was approximately 20%–30% in the general population. Higher rates of dysfunction are reported in individuals over the age of 70. In general, both taste and smell discriminatory capability decreases with advancing age.

Although dysgeusia can be associated with medications, local factors, an underlying systemic disorder, or after radiation therapy to the head and neck region (Box 18.5), many cases are idiopathic. Trauma, tumors, or inflammation of the peripheral nerves of the gustatory system usually produce transient hypogeusia rather than dysgeusia. In contrast, relatively common upper respiratory tract infections produce a temporary and mild dysgeusia in almost one-third of cases, although they seldom produce hypogeusia. Various mechanisms have been proposed in COVID-19 including both peripheral neurotropism and infection with inflammation of associated non-neuronal cells, but no clear etiology has been identified. CNS neoplasms predominantly produce dysgeusia, not hypogeusia or ageusia, and taste hallucinations are fairly common during migraine headaches, Bell palsy, or herpes zoster of the geniculate ganglion. Ischemia and infarction of the brainstem can lead to ageusia of only half of the

tongue (**hemiageusia**) on the same side as the brainstem lesion.

The perception of a particular taste depends on its concentration in a liquid environment; hence, persons with severe dry mouth may suffer from both hypogeusia and dysgeusia. In addition, more than 200 drugs are known to produce taste disturbances (Table 18.1), and more than 500 are associated with salivary hypofunction or xerostomia. Dysgeusia is also a common complaint in patients undergoing chemotherapy with standard chemotherapeutic regimens, which can affect not only quality of life but also treatment outcomes due to food aversion and weight loss. The clinician should be especially diligent in assessing local, intraoral causes of dysgeusia, such as periodontal or dental abscess, oral candidiasis, and routine gingivitis or periodontitis.

Clinical Features

In contrast to hypogeusia, dysgeusia is discerned promptly and distressingly by affected individuals. The clinician must be certain that the patient's alteration is, in fact, a taste disorder rather than an olfactory one, because 75% of "flavor" information (e.g., taste, aroma, texture, temperature, and irritating properties) is derived from smell. Abnormal taste function should be verified through formal taste testing by using standard tastants that are representative of each of the four primary taste qualities (i.e., sweet, sour, salty, and bitter) in a nonodorous solution. Taste testing is more technique sensitive than olfactory testing, and additional electrical and chemical analysis of taste bud function is frequently required. Because this is outside the scope of most general practices, patients are typically referred to a *taste and smell center*.

TABLE 18.1   Examples of Pharmaceutical Agents That May Be Associated With Altered Taste

Pharmaceutical Action	Examples
Anticoagulant	Phenindione
Antihistamine	Chlorpheniramine maleate
Antihypertensive or diuretic	Captopril, diazoxide, and ethacrynic acid
Antimicrobial	Amphotericin B, ampicillin, griseofulvin, idoxuridine, lincomycin, metronidazole, streptomycin, tetracycline, and tyrothricin
Antineoplastic or immunosuppressant	Doxorubicin, methotrexate, vincristine, azathioprine, and carmustine
Antiparkinsonian agent	Baclofen, chlormezanone, and levodopa
Antipsychotic or anticonvulsant	Carbamazepine, lithium, and phenytoin
Anti-rheumatic	Allopurinol, colchicine, gold, levamisole, penicillamine, and phenylbutazone
Antiseptic	Hexetidine and chlorhexidine
Antithyroid agent	Carbimazole, methimazole, and thiouracil
Hypoglycemic	Glipizide and phenformin
Opiate	Codeine and morphine
Sympathomimetic	Amphetamines and phenmetrazine
Vasodilator	Oxyfedrine and bamifylline

Affected patients may describe their altered taste as one of the primary tastes, but many describe the new taste as metallic, rotten, foul, or rancid. The latter two are more likely to be associated with aberrant odor perception (**parosmia**) than with dysgeusia, and this presentation is more common in COVID-19. The altered taste may require a stimulus, such as certain foods or liquids, in which case the taste is said to be distorted. If no stimulus is required, then the dysgeusia is classified as a *phantom taste*, as described in the discussion of burning mouth disorder above.

Treatment and Prognosis

If an underlying disease or process is identified and treated successfully, the taste function should return to normal. In cases related to COVID-19, two thirds of those affected will report complete recovery, approximately 20% report partial recovery, and most improvement occurs within 2 weeks after onset. For idiopathic cases there is no effective pharmacologic therapy. Dysgeusia in particular tends to affect lifestyles and interpersonal relationships significantly, perhaps leading to depression, anxiety, or nutritional deficiencies from altered eating habits. Fortunately, two-thirds of dysgeusia patients experience spontaneous resolution (average duration, 10 months). Idiopathic hypogeusia is less of a problem for the patient, but slowly tends to become worse over time. Fortunately, spontaneous resolution is still a possibility for idiopathic hypogeusia.

◆ OSTEOARTHRITIS (DEGENERATIVE ARTHRITIS; DEGENERATIVE JOINT DISEASE)

Osteoarthritis is a common degenerative and destructive alteration of the joints that traditionally was considered to be the inevitable result of simple wear and tear on aging anatomic structures, because almost every person older than 50 years is affected to some extent. This condition involves loss of articular cartilage, deterioration of subchondral bone, and also involves affiliated structures such as ligaments, muscles, synovium, and the joint capsule. Disease initiation and progression is influenced by mechanical, inflammatory, and metabolic processes. Articular cartilage becomes weakened with overload or overuse, metabolic alteration, or over time due to senescence of chondroblasts and chondrocytes. As the articular tissue is damaged, underlying bone can become exposed. Attempts at repair of both cartilage and bone also produce pro-inflammatory factors that contribute to abnormal remodeling, resulting in a dual process of degenerative destruction and proliferation.

The knee, hip, and hand are the most common sites of osteoarthritis, but this condition also affects the temporomandibular joint (TMJ). Patients with osteoarthritis of the TMJ tend to be younger than those with disease affecting the large weight-bearing joints. Prevalence of TMJ osteoarthritis is difficult to assess due to variability in diagnostic criteria and clinical assessment, but approximately 8%–16% of the population exhibit clinical signs.

Clinical and Radiographic Features

Osteoarthritis usually involves multiple joints, typically the large weight-bearing joints mentioned above. Clinical signs and symptoms include pain, restriction of joint movement, and joint sounds. The disease is characterized by a gradually intensifying deep ache and pain, usually worse in the evening than in the morning. Some degree of morning joint stiffness and stiffness after inactivity is present in 80% of cases. The affected joint may become swollen and warm to the touch, rarely with erythema of the overlying skin. Movement restriction can be due to inflammation or deformation of the joint due to degenerative changes. Joint sounds such as crepitation (i.e., crackling noise during motion) are a late sign of the disease and are associated with more pronounced damage.

These changes are seen also when the TMJ is affected, except that patients seldom experience stiffness of the TMJ. In addition, the muscles of mastication frequently exhibit tenderness because of the overactivation and fatigue associated with "muscle guarding" (i.e., attempting to keep the painful joint immobile).

Radiographically, joints affected by osteoarthritis demonstrate mild changes early in the course of the disease. However, as the disease progresses, the radiographic presentation becomes more characteristic of arthritic joints in general with some combination of the following: erosion of the cortical outline, narrowing or obliteration of the joint space, surface irregularities and protuberances (**exostoses, osteophytes**), flattening of the articular surface, osteosclerosis and osteolysis of bone beneath the cartilage, radiolucent **subchondral cysts,** and ossification within the synovial membrane (**ossicles**). More sensitive diagnostic techniques, such as computed tomography (CT), cone beam computed tomography (CBCT), magnetic resonance imaging (MRI), and arthroscopy, reveal the same features but in much more detail; hence, they are able to identify earlier changes. MRI is particularly useful in assessing joint effusion and the articular disc. Significant osseous imaging findings are often later complications of joint degeneration, and earlier evidence of the disease process often can be detected with arthroscopy before cartilage and bony surface changes are radiographically demonstrable. Of note, the degree of pain experience is not directly correlated with severity of radiographically evident osseous change.

Histopathologic Features

The articular disc of a joint affected by osteoarthritis can exhibit sclerotic change, calcifications, diminished number of chondrocytes, and alteration of the collagen matrix. The surface is proliferative in some areas and degenerative in others. The bone beneath the cartilage shows a loss of osteocytes, minimal osteoblastic or osteoclastic activity, fatty degeneration or necrosis of the marrow, marrow fibrosis, infiltration by chronic inflammatory cells, and perhaps the formation of a large degenerative space beneath the articular cartilage (**subchondral cyst**). Inflammation and thickening of the synovial membrane is seen, sometimes with the formation of metaplastic bone (**ossicles**) or hyaline cartilage granules (**chondral bodies**), which may number in the hundreds within a single joint. The synovial joint fluid typically contains inflammatory and degradation molecules, the levels of which have prognostic significance.

The TMJ is unique because of its fibrocartilage covering and its meniscus. The disk may be centrally destroyed, and there is little vertical clefting of the articular surface. All other features of TMJ osteoarthritis, however, are similar to those noted in other joints and are irreversible.

Treatment and Prognosis

The treatment of osteoarthritis is usually palliative and consists of analgesics and nonsteroidal anti-inflammatory drugs (NSAIDs) to reduce pain and inflammation. Occlusal splints may reduce TMJ symptoms by relieving the pressure on the joint surfaces, and orofacial physiotherapy and hot or cold packs may be helpful to relax involved muscles. Glucosamine and chondroitin sulfate oral supplements, common therapies for large joint arthritis, may offer some benefit.

Aggressive therapy might not be indicated for this disease except in its most severe form. A 30-year follow-up investigation found radiographic evidence of continued joint destruction, but the clinical signs and symptoms were no more severe than they had been initially. In general, surgical management of TMJ osteoarthritis is not recommended unless all conservative, nonsurgical means have failed and the patient's symptoms warrant an escalation of therapy. Surgical interventions are available such as arthrocentesis, arthroscopy, and open joint surgery or total joint replacement. Arthrocentesis is minimally invasive and involves lavage of the affected joint with physiological solution, with or without hyaluronic acid or corticosteroids. Arthroscopy is a more invasive technique which allows for visualization and manipulation of the joint tissues as well as lavage. Open joint surgery and total joint replacement are reserved for patients with significant destruction affecting function.

◆ RHEUMATOID ARTHRITIS

Rheumatoid arthritis (RA) is a chronic autoimmune disorder characterized by nonsuppurative inflammatory destruction of synovium and subsequent destruction of the affected joints due to autoantibody formation to immunoglobulin G (IgG). Specific antibodies include anti-citrullinated protein antibodies (APCAs) and rheumatoid factor, although individuals can have RA and be seronegative for these. The presentation and clinical course and presentation are variable, similar to many autoimmune diseases. Prevalence of RA in the United States is estimated to be about 0.6%–1%, or 1.3 million individuals. Higher prevalence (5%–6%) in individuals of Native American descent has been reported.

The etiology is multifactorial, and increased susceptibility is associated with female gender, genetics, and certain environmental factors. Genetic components are associated strongly with RA, specifically the human leukocyte antigen (HLA) locus DRβ1. However, other genetic associations also exist and vary, particularly amongst ACPA seropositive and seronegative individuals, although some variations are found in both groups. Environmental factors, such as smoking and silica exposure, as well as viral infection (Epstein-Barr virus) also have been shown to contribute to the development of RA in susceptible individuals. Of interest to oral health providers, periodontal disease also is associated with risk of developing RA; however current research does not prove causation. The proposed mechanisms are mediated by oral microbiota, specifically the induction of citrullination and formation of ACPAs by *P. gingivalis* and *A. actinomycetemcomitans*.

RA demonstrates both intra-articular and extra-articular features. Systemic manifestations are relatively common in RA and include: vasculitis, interstitial lung diseases, cardiovascular diseases, anemia, osteoporosis, and ocular involvement (scleritis, keratoconjunctivitis, and uveitis).

In contrast to osteoarthritis (see previous topic), RA begins as an attack against the periarticular structures, such as the synovial membrane **(synovitis).** A reactive macrophage-laden fibroblastic proliferation **(pannus)** from the synovium creeps onto the joint surface. This releases collagenases and other proteases, which destroy the cartilage and underlying bone. Attempted remodeling by the damaged bone results in a characteristic deformation of the joint.

Clinical and Radiographic Features

RA affects women two to three times more frequently than men. Women generally become symptomatic in middle age (40–60 years), whereas men often have later disease onset. The onset and course of the disease are extremely variable, and serology sometimes can be detectable up to 10 years before clinical manifestations of the disease. For many patients, only one or two joints become involved and significant pain or limitation of motion never develops. In others, the disease rapidly progresses to debilitating **polyarthralgia.**

Typically, the signs and symptoms become more severe over time and include swelling, stiffness, pain, joint deformity, and disability, with possible late term fibrous or bony fusion of opposing articular surfaces **(ankylosis).** Morning stiffness and joint swelling are particularly common, even in early disease. Periods of remission often are interspersed with periods of exacerbation. Symmetric polyarticular involvement of the small joints of the hands and feet almost always is present, but it is not unusual for the elbows, wrists, and knees to be affected. Involvement of the central (hips, shoulders) and axial joints, is less common, but still may occur. The hands often display a classic ulnar deviation with swan neck deformities of the fingers. **Rheumatoid nodules** are firm, partially moveable, nontender growths which occur beneath the skin near the affected joint. Although they are now less common due to earlier disease

intervention, they are considered pathognomonic for the disease.

Ideally, patients are identified and treated prior to developing radiographically evident joint disease, as manifestations can occur within the first 2 years after symptom presentation. Plain films are commonly utilized for routine monitoring and diagnosis, but ultrasound and MRI have utility as well. Initial radiographic findings include tissue edema and periarticular osteopenia, whereas later findings include bony erosion and decreased joint spaces. Up to 86% of RA patients are reported to have some level of TMJ involvement, although this is often subclinical. When present, TMJ involvement is usually bilateral and occurs late in the clinical course of the disease. The signs and symptoms include stiffness, crepitation, pain or ache, tenderness, or limitation of mouth opening. Severity is variable, but swelling is less obvious than with other joints. A joint click on opening frequently is reported.

Frequently, the pain of TMJ RA is not related to motion but rather to pressure on the joint. Clenching the teeth on one side produces pain of the contralateral joint. Subluxation or ankylosis is less frequent in the TMJs than in other joints, but gross destruction of the condylar heads may be so severe that a progressive class II malocclusion and anterior open bite develop. Permanent TMJ subluxation has been reported.

Radiographically, involved TMJs demonstrate a flattened condylar head with irregular surface features, an irregular temporal fossa surface, perhaps with remodeling of the fossa itself, and anterior displacement of the condyle. Several diagnostic techniques are available besides routine TMJ radiographs. CT scans, MRI, and arthroscopy are excellent tools for assessing TMJ damage. Ultrasonography is valuable for larger joints but has been used little in TMJ disease and has few studies to demonstrate its utility and reliability at this time. Nuclear medicine scans that use scintigraphy have been largely replaced by MRI scans due to the ability to image the soft and hard joint structures, as well as associated tissues, such as musculature.

Laboratory Values

Rheumatoid arthritis may be seropositive or seronegative, and laboratory studies may be normal in about 30% of patients. As a result, negative serology does not rule out RA. Studies of particular interest in RA include anti-citrullinated protein antibodies (ACPAs), rheumatoid factor (RF), and acute phase reactants such as C-reactive protein (CRP), and erythrocyte sedimentation rate (ESR). ACPAs have been identified as specific serological markers of RA. The presence of these antibodies leads to the formation of immune complexes and subsequent inflammation of the type seen in RA. Additionally 70%–80% of patients with RA exhibit significant elevations of rheumatoid factor (RF), an autoantibody thought to be directed toward an altered host IgG antibody that is no longer recognized by the body as "self." During active phases of the disease, elevations of ESR and CRP are common. These tests are not specific for

RA, but they are useful for distinguishing between inflammatory and non-inflammatory conditions, as well as monitoring the clinical course of RA. Additionally, antinuclear antibodies (ANAs) can be detected in many patients with RA, but this is not diagnostically specific because it also may be associated with other autoimmune diseases.

Histopathologic Features

Needle biopsy using guided techniques or arthroscopy is the most popular technique for obtaining diagnostic synovial material, and the arthroscopic technique gives the ability to directly visualize tissue being sampled. Aspiration and analysis of synovial fluid from the affected joint frequently are undertaken to rule out other forms of arthritis, but these techniques are used more commonly for large joints.

Microscopically, early cases of RA demonstrate hyperplasia of the synovial lining cells with deeper portions of the membrane showing hyperemia, edema, and infiltration by lymphocytes, macrophages, and occasional neutrophils. Older lesions show continued, often pronounced synovial proliferation and edema, with cholesterol crystals and fewer inflammatory cells. Typically, the membrane protrudes into the joint space as villi or fingerlike projections. These projections occasionally undergo necrosis, producing **rice bodies**—small whitish villi fragments composed of cellular debris admixed with fibrin and collagen. When the TMJ is severely involved, the meniscus is typically perforated or replaced completely by fibrous scar.

The rheumatoid nodule is represented by a moderately well-demarcated area of amorphous, eosinophilic necrosis surrounded by a thick layer of mononuclear cells. The mononuclear cells closest to the amorphous center are typically large and palisaded.

Treatment and Prognosis

No cure exists for RA and treatment is lifelong, focusing on strategies to suppress the disease process and prevent joint degeneration. Patient education, physical therapy, lifestyle modification, and exercise are important adjunct therapies, but the mainstay of treatment for many patients is the use of disease-modifying anti-rheumatic drugs (DMARDs). These medications are now recommended to be started as soon as the diagnosis is made. There are numerous agents available with varying side effect profiles that may necessitate treatment change. The classic and first-line DMARD is methotrexate, a folic acid antagonist. Other DMARDs include sulfasalazine, leflunomide, biologics (specifically tumor necrosis factor inhibitors), and targeted biologics such as janus kinase (JAK) inhibitors. Treatment with glucocorticoids sometimes is necessary to provide symptomatic relief or bridge therapy, but long-term use of corticosteroids is not ideal. Other adjunct therapies include NSAIDs, perhaps aided by occasional corticosteroid injections into the joint. The latter injections are used sparingly, however, because frequent use is associated with additional degenerative changes and fibrous ankylosis.

With the advent of biologic and targeted DMARDs, immunosuppressive drugs (such as azathioprine, cyclosporine, and cyclophosphamide) rarely are recommended today due to the risk of their side effect profile and increased risk for serious infections and potential induction of malignancy. However, immunosuppressive therapy may be indicated for patients who have failed all other efforts at disease modulation.

Severely damaged joints may require surgical replacement, with the goals of therapy being attenuation of pain and reduction of disability. Total joint replacement of the hips, knees, and shoulders are reported to have the highest satisfaction rates associated with surgical management of these patients. Due to the complex nature of temporomandibular joint disorders, as discussed in the next section, replacement of the TMJ may increase function but not necessarily result in resolution of pain.

◆ TEMPOROMANDIBULAR DISORDERS

Temporomandibular disorders (**TMDs**) are a group of musculoskeletal or neuromuscular conditions affecting the temporomandibular joint (TMJ), masticatory muscles, and associated structures. They are the most frequent cause of non-odontogenic orofacial pain. TMDs are generally myogenous (affecting muscle) or arthrogenous (affecting the joint) related, but at least half are considered myogenous in nature.

In the general population, prevalence of painful TMD is reported to be about 9%, and an estimated 3.6%–7% will need intervention for their condition. The OPPERA (Orofacial Pain: Prospective Evaluation and Risk Assessment) study, a large U.S. based multicenter prospective cohort study reported an annual 4% incidence of TMD, but the average descriptors of these cases were "slightly annoying" and "mild," so this number does not necessarily represent the incidence of clinically significant cases seeking treatment. Incidence is highest in the 20–40 year age range. TMDs are seen most commonly in young and middle-aged women, but this may be due to more frequent healthcare utilization among this group. Prevalence is highest in the 20–40 year age range. Of note, however, the OPPERA study has reported an equal distribution of TMD amongst male and female participants.

TMD is not an isolated facial pain, and multicenter studies have shown that there are underlying neurophysiologic mechanisms common to many chronic pain conditions. Additionally, individuals with sleep disordered breathing are reported to have a 40% increased risk of TMD development.

Although the etiology of TMD is not known, it is generally agreed that a variety of conditions may reduce the organic physiologic adaptive capacity of the masticatory system and result in TMDs. Implicated contributing conditions include trauma, systemic disease processes, skeletal morphology, joint laxity, and alterations in the peripheral and central nervous system (sensitization).

Classification of Temporomandibular Disorders

Muscular Disorders

- Hyperactivity, spasm, and trismus
- Inflammation (myositis)
- Trauma
- Myofascial pain and fibromyalgia
- Atrophy or hypertrophy

Joint Disorders

- Disc displacement (internal derangement)
- Hypomobility of the disc (adhesions or scars)
- Dislocation and subluxation
- Arthritis
- Infections
- Metabolic disease (gout, chondrocalcinosis)
- Capsulitis, synovitis
- Ankylosis (fibrous, bony)
- Fracture
- Condylar hyperplasia, hypoplasia, or aplasia
- Neoplasia

The classification of TMDs (Box 18.6) remains a challenge due to our limited understanding of their etiology and the lack of universally accepted diagnostic criteria for the myriad of conditions presenting as TMDs, although various classification systems such as the Research Diagnostic Criteria for Temporomandibular Disorders (DCRDC/TMD) and the International Classification of Orofacial Pain continue to be developed and validated to inform future scientific endeavors and improve patient outcomes. Our understanding of the TMDs has evolved as our understanding of the complex biopsychosocial nature of chronic pain has developed, and development of new diagnostic and treatment algorithms have improved management of chronic pain in general. Multi-center research efforts such as the long-running OPPERA clinical study attest to the idea that TMD is a complex multifactorial disease with genetic, physiological, and psychological implications.

Clinical and Radiographic Features

Pain is primary motivation for seeking treatment, but limitations in jaw movement during functional excursions, and restricted joint movement with or without associated joint noises, are frequent complaints. The pain usually is localized to the preauricular area but may radiate to the temporal, frontal, or occipital areas. The pain may present as a headache **(cephalalgia),** a ringing in the ears **(tinnitus),** an earache **(otalgia),** a toothache **(odontalgia),** or any combination of these symptoms. The pain usually is associated with the surrounding musculature and soft tissue more than the TMJ itself. Muscle splinting, a protective mechanism characterized by shortening and stiffening of muscle fibers meant to protect from further injury, can lead to involuntary CNS-induced muscular contractions **(myospasm),** or the muscle fibers themselves may become inflamed **(myositis).**

Myofascial trigger point pain is common in TMD, but it is seldom noted in other TMJ disorders. It is characterized by circumscribed regions, often referred to as taut bands within the muscle ("trigger points"), that elicit local or referred pain on palpation and may be a source of constant deep pain. In many instances, patients are aware only of the referred pain and not the trigger points themselves. The exact nature of the trigger points is not known, but they seem similar to small areas of myospasm and can, through their chronic nature, induce CNS excitatory effects. This hyperexcitability of the CNS produces the clinical findings of **hyperalgesia** (an exaggerated response to a painful stimulus) and **allodynia** (a painful response to a nonpainful stimulus), which are characteristic of chronic pain conditions.

Non-arthritic inflammatory disorders of the TMJ are characterized by continuous deep pain or ache. The pain is evoked by palpation of the affected joint or by mandibular movement, especially chewing and clenching. Both TMJs may be involved, at the same time or at differing times.

Derangements of the condyle and meniscus complex are more often associated with dysfunction **(arthropathy)** than with joint pain **(arthralgia).** Articular disc displacements can occur in an anterior, posterior, and mediolateral direction and are characterized by a variety of joint noises and limitations in jaw opening. Ligament laxity and elongation are thought to be major contributing factors to disc-condyle displacement disorders, and poor joint lubrication and osteoarthritis are implicated as well. Disc-condyle disorders include both disc displacement without reduction and disc displacement with reduction, of which the latter is more common. MRI of the TMJ complex reveals that up to 35% of asymptomatic individuals appear to have disc displacements.

Many systemic conditions are thought to contribute to the development of TMDs and must be included in the differential diagnosis of chronic orofacial pain. Inflammatory conditions of the musculoskeletal system and autoimmune-mediated connective tissue disorders (such as lupus erythematosus, rheumatoid arthritis, and progressive systemic sclerosis) are frequently co-morbid with TMDs. Similar to other chronic pain conditions, patients with TMD may report increased stress, anxiety, or depression. This is not causative but can be associated with symptom exacerbation.

The selection of imaging technique of the TMJ complex depends largely upon what type of information is needed from this adjunctive examination and how this information will affect patient management. Panoramic radiographs routinely are used as screening films for patients presenting with preauricular pain, and the interpretation of these films will influence the decision for the use of advanced imaging modalities such as CT and MRI. MRI imaging is preferred as it can assess not only bony components but also the disc and other associated structures.

• BOX 18.7 Examples of Medications Used to Treat the Symptoms of Temporomandibular Disorders

- Oral Medications
  - Acetaminophen (with or without codeine)
  - Nonsteroidal anti-inflammatory drugs (NSAIDs)
    - Ibuprofen, Naproxen, Diclofenac* (also available in topical formulation)
  - Muscle relaxants
    - Methocarbamol, cyclobenzaprine, metaxalone
  - Benzodiazepine derivatives
    - Diazepam
  - Glucocorticoids
    - Prednisone
- Injectable
  - Glucocorticoids
    - Triamcinolone
  - Botulinum toxin A
  - Local anesthetics

Treatment and Prognosis

The natural clinical course of the TMDs is poorly understood and we cannot reliably determine which conditions will progress to more significant long-term consequences such as chronic dysfunction and chronic pain. Many TMDs are transient and self-limiting, with resolution reported in a majority of cases in 6–15 months. Cohort studies vary, 51% of patients reporting resolution in 6 months and up to 90% having resolution or sustainable symptom reduction in 12–15 months post treatment. Therefore, reversible and conservative therapies are encouraged. Conservative interventions include patient education, simple rest or immobilization of the joint, soft diet, application of cold (usually reserved for acute injuries) or heat, occlusal splints, physical therapy, and elimination of parafunctional habits, if present. Appropriate management of concurrent psychological and social stressors may be of benefit, similar to other chronic pain conditions. Various medications also have been used for TMD with some success (Box 18.7), and other therapies include dry needling or injection of local anesthetic into muscular trigger points to relieve pain, as well as botulinum-A toxin injection into the temporalis and masseter muscles for pain relief and reduction of muscle activity. However, few TMD treatments have been examined in a blinded, controlled fashion.

Surgical intervention may be required for severely affected joints, especially those with internal meniscal derangements, condylar dislocation or fracture, ankylosis, and degenerative or developmental deformities. Usually, TMD is treated conservatively for several years without improvement before surgery is attempted, although there is emerging, but limited, evidence for minimally invasive arthroscopic procedures in early treatment. Due to the multifactorial influences on TMD and high prevalence of muscular dysfunction, joint surgery may not completely resolve symptomatic TMD.

Bibliography

Bell Palsy

Baugh RF, Basura GJ, Ishii LE, et al.: Clinical practice guideline: Bell's Palsy executive summary, *Otolaryngol Head Neck Surg* 149: 656–663, 2013.

de Almeida JR, Al Khabori M, Guyatt GH, et al.: Combined corticosteroid and antiviral treatment for Bell palsy: a systematic review and meta-analysis, *JAMA* 302:985–993, 2009.

de Almeida JR, Guyatt GH, Sud S, et al.: Management of Bell palsy: clinical practice guideline, *CMAJ* 186:917–922, 2014.

Gagyor I, Madhok VB, Daly F, et al.: Antiviral treatment for Bell's palsy (idiopathic facial paralysis), *Cochrane Database Syst Rev* 9: CD001869, 2019.

Kafle DR, Thakur SK: Evaluation of prognostic factors in patients with Bell's palsy, *Brain Behav* 11:e2385, 2021.

Kim TH, Yeo SG, Byun JY: Role of biomarkers as prognostic factors in acute peripheral facial palsy, *Int J Mol Sci* 23:307, 2021. https://doi.org/10.3390/ijms23010307.

Lee SY, Seong J, Kim YH: Clinical implication of facial nerve decompression in complete Bell's palsy: a systematic review and meta-analysis, *Clin Exp Otorhinolaryngol* 12:348–359, 2019.

Luu NN, Chorath KT, May BR, et al.: Clinical practice guidelines in idiopathic facial paralysis: systematic review using the appraisal of guidelines for research and evaluation (AGREE II) instrument, *J Neurol* 268:1847–1856, 2021.

Madhok VB, Gagyor I, Daly F, et al.: Corticosteroids for Bell's palsy (idiopathic facial paralysis), *Cochrane Database Syst Rev* 7: CD001942, 2016.

Menchetti I, McAllister K, Walker D, et al.: Surgical interventions for the early management of Bell's palsy, *Cochrane Database Syst Rev* 1: CD007468, 2021.

Mutlu A, Kalcioglu MT, Gunduz AY, et al.: Does the SARS-CoV-2 pandemic really increase the frequency of peripheral facial palsy? *Am J Otolaryngol* 42:103032, 2021.

TM O: Medical management of acute facial paralysis, *Otolaryngol Clin North Am* 51:1051–1075, 2018.

Peitersen E: Bell's palsy: the spontaneous course of 2,500 peripheral facial nerve palsies of different etiologies, *Acta Oto-Laryngologica Suppl* 549:4–30, 2002.

Schwartz SR, Jones SL, Getchius TS, et al.: Reconciling the clinical practice guidelines on Bell's palsy from the AAO-HNSF and the AAN, *Neurology* 82:1927–1929, 2014.

Tamaki A, Cabrera CI, Li S, et al.: Incidence of Bell palsy in patients with COVID-19, *JAMA Otolaryngol Head Neck Surg* 147:767–768, 2021.

Zhang W, Xu L, Luo T, et al.: The etiology of Bell's palsy: a review, *J Neurol* 267:1896–1905, 2020.

Zhao H, Zhang X, Tang YD, et al.: Bell's palsy: clinical analysis of 372 cases and review of related literature, *Eur Neurol* 77:168–172, 2017.

Frey Syndrome

Blanc S, Bourrier T, Boralevi F, et al.: Frey syndrome, *J Pediatr* 174:211–217, 2016.

Choi HG, Kwon SY, Won JY, et al.: Comparisons of three indicators for Frey's syndrome: subjective symptoms, minor's starch iodine test, and infrared thermography, *Clin Exp Otorhinolaryngol* 6:249–253, 2013.

Dizon MV, Fischer GJ, McKay A, et al.: Localized facial flushing in infancy. Auriculotemporal nerve (Frey) syndrome, *Arch Dermatol* 133:1143–1145, 1997.

Dulguerov P, Quinodoz D, Cosendai G, et al.: Prevention of Frey syndrome during parotidectomy, *Arch Otolaryngol Head Neck Surg* 125:833–839, 1999.

Guntinas-Lichius O, Gabriel B, Klussmann JP: Risk of facial palsy and severe Frey's syndrome after conservative parotidectomy for benign disease: analysis of 610 operations, *Acta Otolaryngol* 126:1104–1109, 2006.

Klarskov C, Kvon Rohden E, Thorsteinsson B, et al.: Gustatory sweating in people with type 1 and type 2 diabetes mellitus: prevalence and risk factors, *Endocrinol Diabetes Metab* 4:e00290, 2021.

Mantelakis A, Lafford G, Lee CW, et al.: Frey's syndrome: a review of aetiology and treatment, *Cureus* 13:e20107, 2021.

Mashrah MA, Aldhohrah T, Abdelrehem A, et al.: What is the best method for prevention of postparotidectomy Frey syndrome? Network meta-analysis, *Head Neck* 43:1345–1358, 2021.

Motz KM, Kim YJ: Auriculotemporal syndrome (Frey syndrome), *Otolaryngol Clin North Am* 49:501–509, 2016.

Shaw JE, Parker R, Hollis S, et al.: Gustatory sweating in diabetes mellitus, *Diabet Med* 13:1033–1037, 1996.

Tillman BN, Lesperance MM, Brinkmeier JV: Infantile Frey's syndrome, *Int J Pediatr Otorhinolaryngol* 79:929–931, 2015.

Xie S, Wang K, Xu T, et al.: Efficacy and safety of botulinum toxin type A for treatment of Frey's syndrome: evidence from 22 published articles, *Cancer Med* 4:1639–1650, 2015.

Trigeminal Neuralgia
Bendtsen L, Zakrzewska JM, Abbott J, et al.: European Academy of Neurology guideline on trigeminal neuralgia, *Eur J Neurol* 26:831–849, 2019.

Bendtsen L, Zakrzewska JM, Heinskou TB, et al.: Advances in diagnosis, classification, pathophysiology, and management of trigeminal neuralgia, *Lancet Neurol* 19:784–796, 2020.

Cruccu G, Di Stefano G, Truini A: Trigeminal neuralgia, *N Engl J Med* 383:754–762, 2020.

De Toledo IP, Conti Réus J, Fernandes M, et al.: Prevalence of trigeminal neuralgia: a systematic review, *J Am Dent Assoc* 147:570–576, 2016.

Di Stefano G, Maarbjerg S, Nurmikko T, et al.: Triggering trigeminal neuralgia, *Cephalalgia* 38:1049–1056, 2018.

Hall GC, Carroll D, Parry D, et al.: Epidemiology and treatment of neuropathic pain: the UK primary care perspective, *Pain* 122:156–162, 2006.

Headache Classification Committee of the International Headache Society (IHS): The International Classification of Headache Disorders, 3rd edition, *Cephalalgia* 38:1–211, 2018.

Heinskou TB, Rochat P, Maarbjerg S, et al.: Prognostic factors for outcome of microvascular decompression in trigeminal neuralgia: a prospective systematic study using independent assessors, *Cephalalgia* 39:197–208, 2019.

Holste K, Chan AY, Rolston JD, et al.: Pain outcomes following microvascular decompression for drug-resistant trigeminal neuralgia: a systematic review and meta-analysis, *Neurosurgery* 86:182–190, 2020.

International Classification of Orofacial Pain, 1st edition (ICOP), *Cephalalgia* 40:129–221, 2020.

Lambru G, Zakrzewska J, Matharu M: Trigeminal neuralgia: a practical guide, *Pract Neurol* 21:392–402, 2021.

Maarbjerg S, Gozalov A, Olesen J, et al.: Concomitant persistent pain in classical trigeminal neuralgia—evidence for different subtypes, *Headache* 54:1173–1183, 2014.

Maarbjerg S, Gozalov A, Olesen J, et al.: Trigeminal neuralgia—a prospective systematic study of clinical characteristics in 158 patients, *Headache* 54:1574–1582, 2014.

Maarbjerg S, Wolfram F, Gozalov A, et al.: Association between neurovascular contact and clinical characteristics in classical trigeminal neuralgia: a prospective clinical study using 3.0 Tesla MRI, *Cephalalgia* 35:1077–1084, 2015.

Mueller D, Obermann M, Yoon MS, et al.: Prevalence of trigeminal neuralgia and persistent idiopathic facial pain: a population-based study, *Cephalalgia* 31:1542–1548, 2011.

Noory N, Smilkov EA, Frederiksen JL, et al.: Neurovascular contact plays no role in trigeminal neuralgia secondary to multiple sclerosis, *Cephalalgia* 41:593–603, 2021.

O'Connor AB, Schwid SR, Herrmann DN, et al.: Pain associated with multiple sclerosis: systematic review and proposed classification, *Pain* 137:96–111, 2008.

Zakrzewska JM, Wu J, Mon-Williams M, et al.: Evaluating the impact of trigeminal neuralgia, *Pain* 158:1166–1174, 2017.

Glossopharyngeal Neuralgia
Blumenfeld A, Nikolskaya G: Glossopharyngeal neuralgia, *Curr Pain Headache Rep* 17:343, 2013.

Franzini A, Moosa S, D'Ammando A, et al.: The neurosurgical treatment of craniofacial pain syndromes: current surgical indications and techniques, *Neurol Sci* 40:159–168, 2019.

Headache Classification Committee of the International Headache Society (IHS): The International Classification of Headache Disorders, 3rd edition, *Cephalalgia* 38:1–211, 2018.

International Classification of Orofacial Pain, 1st edition (ICOP), *Cephalalgia* 40:129–221, 2020.

Katusic S, Williams DB, Beard CM, et al.: Incidence and clinical features of glossopharyngeal neuralgia, Rochester, Minnesota, 1945-1984, *Neuroepidemiology* 10:266–275, 1991.

Lu VM, Goyal A, Graffeo CS, et al.: Glossopharyngeal neuralgia treatment outcomes after nerve section, microvascular decompression, or stereotactic radiosurgery: a systematic review and meta-analysis, *World Neurosurg* 120:572–582, 2018.

Manzoni GC, Torelli P: Epidemiology of typical and atypical craniofacial neuralgias, *Neurol Sci* 26(Suppl. 2):s65–s67, 2005.

Teton ZE, Holste KG, Hardaway FA, et al.: Pain-free survival after vagoglossopharyngeal complex sectioning with or without microvascular decompression in glossopharyngeal neuralgia, *J Neurosurg* 132:232–238, 2019.

Giant Cell Arteritis
Cockey G, Shah SR, Hampton T: Giant cell arteritis presenting with a tongue lesion, *Am J Med* 132:576–578, 2019.

De Smit E, O'Sullivan E, Mackey DA, et al.: Giant cell arteritis: ophthalmic manifestations of a systemic disease, *Graefes Arch Clin Exp Ophthalmol* 254:2291–2306, 2016.

Dejaco C, Ramiro S, Duftner C, et al.: EULAR recommendations for the use of imaging in large vessel vasculitis in clinical practice, *Ann Rheum Dis* 77:636–643, 2018.

Fongaufier C, Guffroy A, Lutz JC: Tongue and scalp necrosis: simultaneous initial complications revealing giant cell arteritis, *J Rheumatol* 45:873–874, 2018.

Greigert H, Ramon A, Tarris G, et al.: Temporal artery vascular diseases, *J Clin Med* 11:275, 2022. https://doi.org/10.3390/jcm11010275.

Maz M, Chung SA, Abril A, et al.: 2021 American College of Rheumatology/Vasculitis Foundation Guideline for the Management of Giant Cell Arteritis and Takayasu Arteritis, *Arthritis Rheumatol* 73:1349–1365, 2021.

Prieto-Peña D, Castañeda S, Martínez-Rodríguez I, et al.: Imaging tests in the early diagnosis of giant cell arteritis, *J Clin Med* 10:3704, 2021. https://doi.org/10.3390/jcm10163704.

Soulages A, Sibon I, Vallat JM, et al.: Neurologic manifestations of giant cell arteritis, *J Neurol* 269:3430–3442, 2022.

Younger DS: Giant cell arteritis, *Neurol Clin* 37:335–344, 2019.

Burning Mouth Disorder

Bergdahl M, Bergdahl J: Burning mouth syndrome: prevalence and associated factors, *J Oral Pathol Med* 28:350–354, 1999.

de Souza FT, Teixeira AL, Amaral TM, et al.: Psychiatric disorders in burning mouth syndrome, *J Psychosom Res* 72:142–146, 2012.

Eliav E, Kamran B, Schaham R, et al.: Evidence of chorda tympani dysfunction in patients with burning mouth syndrome, *J Am Dent Assoc* 138:628–633, 2007.

Hartmann A, Seeberger R, Bittner M, et al.: Profiling intraoral neuropathic disturbances following lingual nerve injury and in burning mouth syndrome, *BMC Oral Health* 17:68, 2017.

Heckmann SM, Kirchner E, Grushka M, et al.: A double-blind study on clonazepam in patients with burning mouth syndrome, *Laryngoscope* 122:813–816, 2012.

Imura H, Shimada M, Yamazaki Y, et al.: Characteristic changes of saliva and taste in burning mouth syndrome patients, *J Oral Pathol Med* 45:231–236, 2016.

Klasser GD, Grushka M, Su N: Burning mouth syndrome, *Oral Maxillofac Surg Clin North Am* 28:381–396, 2016.

Kohorst JJ, Bruce AJ, Torgerson RR, et al.: A population-based study of the incidence of burning mouth syndrome, *Mayo Clin Proc* 89:1545–1552, 2014.

Kohorst JJ, Bruce AJ, Torgerson RR, et al.: The prevalence of burning mouth syndrome: a population-based study, *Br J Dermatol* 172:1654–1656, 2015.

Kolkka-Palomaa M, Jääskeläinen SK, Laine MA, et al.: Pathophysiology of primary burning mouth syndrome with special focus on taste dysfunction: a review, *Oral Dis* 21:937–948, 2015.

Liu YF, Kim Y, Yoo T, et al.: Burning mouth syndrome: a systematic review of treatments, *Oral Dis* 24:325–334, 2018.

López-Jornet P, Collado Y, Zambudio A, et al.: Chemosensory function in burning mouth syndrome a comparative cross-sectional study, *Nutrients* 13:722, 2021. https://doi.org/10.3390/nu13030722.

Lopez-Jornet P, Felipe CC, Pardo-Marin L, et al.: Salivary biomarkers and their correlation with pain and stress in patients with burning mouth syndrome, *J Clin Med* 9:929, 2020. https://doi.org/10.3390/jcm9040929.

McMillan R, Forssell H, Buchanan JA, et al.: Interventions for treating burning mouth syndrome, *Cochrane Database Syst Rev* 11: CD002779, 2016.

Orliaguet M, Misery L: Neuropathic and psychogenic components of burning mouth syndrome: a systematic review, *Biomolecules* 11:1237, 2021. https://doi.org/10.3390/biom11081237.

Poon R, Su N, Ching V, et al.: Reduction in unstimulated salivary flow rate in burning mouth syndrome, *Br Dent J* 217:E14, 2014.

Riley JL, Gilbert GH, Heft MW: Orofacial pain symptom prevalence: selective sex differences in the elderly? *Pain* 76:97–104, 1998.

Su N, Poon R, Liu C, et al.: Pain reduction in burning mouth syndrome (BMS) may be associated with selective improvement of taste: a retrospective study, *Oral Surg Oral Med Oral Pathol Oral Radiol* 129:461–467, 2020.

Dysgeusia and Hypogeusia

Brandão Neto D, Fornazieri MA, Dib C, et al.: Chemosensory dysfunction in COVID-19: prevalences, recovery rates, and clinical associations on a large Brazilian sample, *Otolaryngol Head Neck Surg* 164:512–518, 2021.

DeVere R: Disorders of taste and smell, *Continuum (Minneap Minn)* 23:421–446, 2017.

Doty RL: Epidemiology of smell and taste dysfunction, *Handb Clin Neurol* 164:3–13, 2019.

Doty RL: Treatments for smell and taste disorders: a critical review, *Handb Clin Neurol* 164:455–479, 2019.

Epstein JB, de Andrade E, Silva SM, et al.: Taste disorders following cancer treatment: report of a case series, *Support Care Cancer* 27:4587–4595, 2019.

Fornazieri MA, Garcia ECD, Lopes NMD, et al.: Adherence and efficacy of olfactory training as a treatment for persistent olfactory loss, *Am J Rhinol Allergy* 34:238–248, 2020.

Liu G, Zong G, Doty RL, et al.: Prevalence and risk factors of taste and smell impairment in a nationwide representative sample of the US population: a cross-sectional study, *BMJ Open* 6:e013246, 2016.

Lozada-Nur F, Chainani-Wu N, Fortuna G, et al.: Dysgeusia in COVID-19: possible mechanisms and implications, *Oral Surg Oral Med Oral Pathol Oral Radiol* 130:344–346, 2020.

Mahmoud MM, Abuohashish HM, Khairy DA, et al.: Pathogenesis of dysgeusia in COVID-19 patients: a scoping review, *Eur Rev Med Pharmacol Sci* 25:1114–1134, 2021.

Mastrangelo A, Bonato M, Cinque P: Smell and taste disorders in COVID-19: from pathogenesis to clinical features and outcomes, *Neurosci Lett* 748:135694, 2021.

Teaima AA, Salem OM, Teama MAEM, et al.: Patterns and clinical outcomes of olfactory and gustatory disorders in six months: prospective study of 1031 COVID-19 patients, *Am J Otolaryngol* 43:103259, 2022.

Osteoarthritis

Arayasantiparb R, Mitrirattanakul S, Kunasarapun P, et al.: Association of radiographic and clinical findings in patients with temporomandibular joints osseous alteration, *Clin Oral Investig* 24:221–227, 2020.

Bergstrand S, Ingstad HK, Møystad A, et al.: Long-term effectiveness of arthrocentesis with and without hyaluronic acid injection for treatment of temporomandibular joint osteoarthritis, *J Oral Sci* 61:82–88, 2019.

de Leeuw R, Boering G, van der Kuijl B, et al.: Hard and soft tissue imaging of the temporomandibular joint 30 years after diagnosis of osteoarthrosis and internal derangement, *J Oral Maxillofac Surg* 54:1270–1280, 1996. discussion 1280–1271.

Derwich M, Mitus-Kenig M, Pawlowska E: Interdisciplinary approach to the temporomandibular joint osteoarthritis-review of the literature, *Medicina (Kaunas)* 56:225, 2020. https://doi.org/10.3390/medicina56050225.

Derwich M, Mitus-Kenig M, Pawlowska E: Morphology of the temporomandibular joints regarding the presence of osteoarthritic changes, *Int J Environ Res Public Health* 17:2923, 2020. https://doi.org/10.3390/ijerph17082923.

Dijkgraaf LC, de Bont LG, Boering G, et al.: The structure, biochemistry, and metabolism of osteoarthritic cartilage: a review of the literature, *J Oral Maxillofac Surg* 53:1182–1192, 1995.

Dijkgraaf LC, Spijkervet FK, de Bont LG: Arthroscopic findings in osteoarthritic temporomandibular joints, *J Oral Maxillofac Surg* 57:255–268, 1999; discussion 269–270.

Guarda Nardini L, Meneghini M, Guido M, et al.: Histopathology of the temporomandibular joint disc: findings in 30 samples from joints with degenerative disease, *J Oral Rehabil* 48:1025–1034, 2021.

Hunter DJ, Bierma-Zeinstra S: Osteoarthritis, *Lancet* 393:1745–1759, 2019.

Jeon KJ, Lee C, Choi YJ, et al.: Analysis of three-dimensional imaging findings and clinical symptoms in patients with temporomandibular joint disorders, *Quant Imaging Med Surg* 11:1921–1931, 2021.

Kalladka M, Quek S, Heir G, et al.: Temporomandibular joint osteo-arthritis: diagnosis and long-term conservative management: a topic review, *J Indian Prosthodont Soc* 14:6–15, 2014.

Ong TK, Franklin CD: A clinical and histopathological study of osteoarthrosis of the temporomandibular joint, *Br J Oral Maxillofac Surg* 34:186–192, 1996.

Pantoja LLQ, de Toledo IP, Pupo YM, et al.: Prevalence of degener-ative joint disease of the temporomandibular joint: a systematic review, *Clin Oral Investig* 23:2475–2488, 2019.

Roberts WE, Stocum DL: Part II: temporomandibular joint (TMJ)-regeneration, degeneration, and adaptation, *Curr Osteoporos Rep* 16:369–379, 2018.

Rheumatoid Arthritis

Alamanos Y, Voulgari PV, Drosos AA: Incidence and prevalence of rheumatoid arthritis, based on the 1987 American College of Rheu-matology criteria: a systematic review, *Semin Arthritis Rheum* 36:182–188, 2006.

Burmester GR, Pope JE: Novel treatment strategies in rheumatoid arthritis, *Lancet* 389:2338–2348, 2017.

Covert L, Mater HV, Hechler BL: Comprehensive management of rheumatic diseases affecting the temporomandibular joint, *Diagnostics (Basel)* 11:409, 2021. https://doi.org/10.3390/diagnostics 11030409.

Hajishengallis G: Periodontitis: from microbial immune subversion to systemic inflammation, *Nat Rev Immunol* 15:30–44, 2015.

Hiz O, Ediz L, Ozkan Y, et al.: Clinical and magnetic resonance imag-ing findings of the temporomandibular joint in patients with rheu-matoid arthritis, *J Clin Med Res* 4:323–331, 2012.

Hunter TM, Boytsov NN, Zhang X, et al.: Prevalence of rheumatoid arthritis in the United States adult population in healthcare claims databases, 2004-2014, *Rheumatol Int* 37:1551–1557, 2017.

Ishikawa Y, Hashimoto M, Ito H, et al.: Anti-nuclear antibody devel-opment is associated with poor treatment response to biological disease-modifying anti-rheumatic drugs in patients with rheuma-toid arthritis, *Semin Arthritis Rheum* 49:204–210, 2019.

Ozcan I, Ozcan KM, Keskin D, et al.: Temporomandibular joint involvement in rheumatoid arthritis: correlation of clinical, labora-tory and magnetic resonance imaging findings, *B-ENT* 4:19–24, 2008.

Salaffi F, Carotti M, Beci G, et al.: Radiographic scoring methods in rheumatoid arthritis and psoriatic arthritis, *Radiol Med* 124:1071–1086, 2019.

Smolen JS, Aletaha D, Barton A, et al.: Rheumatoid arthritis, *Nat Rev Dis Primers* 4:18001, 2018.

Smolen JS, Landewé RBM, Bijlsma JWJ, et al.: EULAR recommenda-tions for the management of rheumatoid arthritis with synthetic and biological disease-modifying antirheumatic drugs: 2019 update, *Ann Rheum Dis* 79:685–699, 2020.

Sokka T, Pincus T: Erythrocyte sedimentation rate, C-reactive protein, or rheumatoid factor are normal at presentation in 35%-45% of patients with rheumatoid arthritis seen between 1980 and 2004: analyses from Finland and the United States, *J Rheumatol* 36:1387–1390, 2009.

Wechalekar MD, Najm A, Veale DJ, et al.: The 2018 OMERACT Synovial Tissue Biopsy Special Interest Group Report on Standard-ization of Synovial Biopsy Analysis, *J Rheumatol* 46:1365–1368, 2019.

Wechalekar MD, Smith MD: Arthroscopic guided synovial biopsy in rheumatology: current perspectives, *Int J Rheum Dis* 20:141–144, 2017.

Xu Y, Wu Q: Prevalence trend and disparities in rheumatoid arthritis among US adults, 2005–2018, *J Clin Med* 10(15):3289, 2021 July 26. https://doi.org/10.3390/jcm10153289.

Temporomandibular Disorders

Ahmad M, Schiffman EL: Temporomandibular joint disorders and orofacial pain, *Dent Clin N Am* 60:105–124, 2016.

Al-Moraissi EA, Alradom J, Aladashi O, et al.: Needling therapies in the management of myofascial pain of the masticatory muscles: a network meta-analysis of randomised clinical trials, *J Oral Rehabil* 47:910–922, 2020.

Al-Moraissi EA, Conti PCR, Alyahya A, et al.: The hierarchy of differ-ent treatments for myogenous temporomandibular disorders: a sys-tematic review and network meta-analysis of randomized clinical trials, *Oral Maxillofac Surg* 26:519–533, 2022. https://doi.org/10.3390/jcm10153289.

Al-Moraissi EA, Farea R, Qasem KA, et al.: Effectiveness of occlusal splint therapy in the management of temporomandibular disorders: network meta-analysis of randomized controlled trials, *Int J Oral Maxillofac Surg* 49:1042–1056, 2020.

Bueno CH, Pereira DD, Pattussi MP, et al.: Gender differences in tem-poromandibular disorders in adult populational studies: a system-atic review and meta-analysis, *J Oral Rehabil* 45:720–729, 2018.

De Kanter RJ, Truin GJ, Burgersdijk RC, et al.: Prevalence in the Dutch adult population and a meta-analysis of signs and symptoms of temporomandibular disorder, *J Dent Res* 72:1509–1518, 1993.

De Rossi SS, Greenberg MS, Liu F, et al.: Temporomandibular disor-ders: evaluation and management, *Med Clin North Am* 98:1353–1384, 2014.

Fillingim RB, Ohrbach R, Greenspan JD, et al.: Associations of psy-chologic factors with multiple chronic overlapping pain conditions, *J Oral Facial Pain Headache* 34:s85–s100, 2020.

Fillingim RB, Slade GD, Greenspan JD, et al.: Long-term changes in biopsychosocial characteristics related to temporomandibular dis-order: findings from the OPPERA study, *Pain* 159:2403–2413, 2018.

Guarda-Nardini L, De Almeida AM, Manfredini D: Arthrocentesis of the temporomandibular joint: systematic review and clinical impli-cations of research findings, *J Oral Facial Pain Headache* 35:17–29, 2021.

International Classification of Orofacial Pain, 1st edition (ICOP), *Cephalalgia* 40:129–221, 2020.

Jung W, Lee KE, Suh BJ: Influence of psychological factors on the prognosis of temporomandibular disorders pain, *J Dent Sci* 16:349–355, 2021.

Kapos FP, Exposto FG, Oyarzo JF, et al.: Temporomandibular disor-ders: a review of current concepts in aetiology, diagnosis and man-agement, *Oral Surg* 13:321–334, 2020.

Klasser GD, Manfredini D, Goulet JP, et al.: Oro-facial pain and tem-poromandibular disorders classification systems: a critical appraisal and future directions, *J Oral Rehabil* 45:258–268, 2018.

Larheim TA, Westesson P, Sano T: Temporomandibular joint disk displacement: comparison in asymptomatic volunteers and patients, *Radiology* 218:428–432, 2001.

Liu F, Steinkeler A: Epidemiology, diagnosis, and treatment of tempo-romandibular disorders, *Dent Clin N Am* 57:465–479, 2013.

Manfredini D: Occlusal equilibration for the management of tempo-romandibular disorders, *Oral Maxillofac Surg Clin North Am* 30:257–264, 2018.

Manfredini D, Favero L, Cocilovo F, et al.: A comparison trial between three treatment modalities for the management of myo-fascial pain of jaw muscles: a preliminary study, *Cranio* 36:327–331, 2018.

Manfredini D, Guarda-Nardini L, Winocur E, et al.: Research diag-nostic criteria for temporomandibular disorders: a systematic review of axis I epidemiologic findings, *Oral Surg Oral Med Oral Pathol Oral Radiol Endod* 112:453–462, 2011.

Manfredini D, Lombardo L, Siciliani G: Temporomandibular disorders and dental occlusion. A systematic review of association studies: end of an era? *J Oral Rehabil* 44:908–923, 2017.

Meloto CB, Slade GD, Lichtenwalter RN, et al.: Clinical predictors of persistent temporomandibular disorder in people with first-onset temporomandibular disorder: a prospective case-control study, *J Am Dent Assoc* 150:572–581, 2019.

Monaco A, Cattaneo R, Marci MC, et al.: Central sensitization-based classification for temporomandibular disorders: a pathogenetic hypothesis, *Pain Res Manag* 2017:5957076, 2017.

Patel J, Cardoso JA, Mehta S: A systematic review of botulinum toxin in the management of patients with temporomandibular disorders and bruxism, *Br Dent J* 226:667–672, 2019.

Schiffman E, Ohrbach R: Executive summary of the Diagnostic Criteria for Temporomandibular Disorders for clinical and research applications, *J Am Dent Assoc* 147:438–445, 2016.

Schiffman E, Ohrbach R, Truelove E, et al.: Diagnostic criteria for temporomandibular disorders (DC/TMD) for clinical and research applications: recommendations of the International RDC/TMD Consortium Network* and Orofacial Pain Special Interest Group†, *J Oral Facial Pain Headache* 28:6–27, 2014.

Shaffer SM, Brismée JM, Sizer PS, et al.: Temporomandibular disorders. Part 1: anatomy and examination/diagnosis, *J Man Manip Ther* 22:2–12, 2014.

Shaffer SM, Brismée JM, Sizer PS, et al.: Temporomandibular disorders. Part 2: conservative management, *J Man Manip Ther* 22:13–23, 2014.

Valesan LF, Da-Cas CD, Réus JC, et al.: Prevalence of temporomandibular joint disorders: a systematic review and meta-analysis, *Clin Oral Investig* 25:441–453, 2021.

19

Forensic Dentistry

EDWARD E. HERSCHAFT

Forensic dentistry, which is also referred to as *forensic odontology*, is the area of dentistry concerned with the correct management, examination, evaluation, and presentation of dental evidence in criminal or civil legal proceedings in the interest of justice. Thus, the forensic dentist must be knowledgeable in both dentistry and law.

Classically, forensic dentistry can be considered a subspecialty of oral and maxillofacial pathology. This is analogous to the relationship in medicine between forensic pathology and pathology. The requirements of forensic dental field work, however, often demand an interdisciplinary knowledge of dental science. This has resulted in other dental specialists and general dentists joining oral and maxillofacial pathologists in providing legal authorities with dental expertise.

Regardless of background, forensic dentists assist legal authorities by preparing dental evidence in the following situations:

- Management and maintenance of dental records that comply with the US Department of Health and Human Services (HHS) Health Insurance Portability and Accessibility (HIPAA) Act of 1996 and guidelines established by the HHS Occupational Safety and Health Administration (OSHA). The former regulations protect the privacy of an individual's health information obtained from electronic, written, or verbal exchange of records. The latter guidelines delineate legal requirements required to document all unique dental information and ensure that these data are the foundation on which dental identification of the patient is accomplished and potential malpractice litigation is reduced.
- Identification of human remains, through the comparison of antemortem and postmortem dental information, in cases that involve the death of an individual or numerous deaths in multiple fatality incident (MFI) situations. Collection and analysis of patterned marks (bite marks) in inanimate material or injured tissue that can be analyzed and potentially compared with a specific human or animal dentition.
- Recognition of the signs and symptoms of human abuse (including intimate partner violence [IPV], elder abuse, and child abuse) and the rights and responsibilities of the dental health care practitioner when reporting such abuse.

- Presentation of dental evidence as an expert witness in identification, bite mark, human abuse, malpractice, fraud, and personal injury cases.

◆ RECORD MANAGEMENT

The dental record is a legal document, owned by the dentist or an incorporated dental practice, which contains all subjective and objective information about the patient. In the United States, the Privacy Rule governing the use of protected health information (PHI) is regulated under the federal HIPAA act of 1996. Under this legislation the patient has the right to view original documents and obtain copies.

Despite the establishment of the Privacy Rule, the ability and necessity of forensic dentists, law enforcement personnel, medical examiners (MEs), and coroners to obtain released antemortem dental and medical records for forensic purposes without requiring consent of next-of-kin or a guardian was recognized and provided for in the HIPAA legislation—45 Code of Federal Regulations §164.512(g)(1).

Initially, demographic information is secured when the medical and dental history of the patient is obtained. Results of the physical examination of the dentition and supporting oral and para-oral structures are recorded.

In addition, the results of clinical laboratory tests, study casts, photographs, and radiographs become components of the record. With this database, the dentist can develop a thorough assessment of all of the patient's medical and dental problems. Subsequent documentation of this "problem list" facilitates the development of a plan of treatment and prognosis for the patient.

The treatment plan addresses the management of both systemic and oral problems. It can then be periodically revised and updated as problems resolve or as new ones develop. Supplemental material, such as dental laboratory authorizations, referral letters from other practitioners, statements of informed consent, written prescriptions, and insurance and financial statements, also is included and stored in the record.

The progress notes (i.e., daily log of actual treatment rendered) should contain information about restorative and therapeutic procedures provided. This information should include documentation of the specific brand of dental

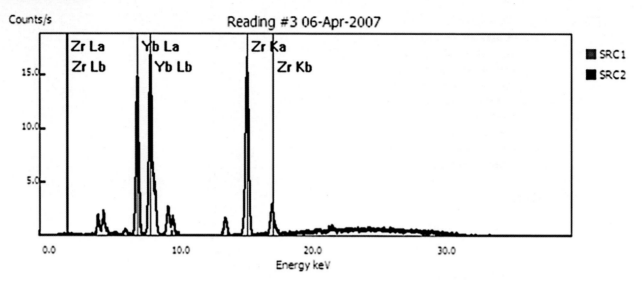

• **Fig. 19.1** The X-ray fluorescence (XRF) spectrum from a particle recovered from a cremation retort. The spectrum makes this a match for the restorative resin Four Seasons or Tetric Ceram (Ivoclar Vivadent, Amherst, NY). (Courtesy of Dr. Mary A. Bush and Peter J. Bush.)

material used in restorative procedures. This concept has forensic import because each dental restorative product contains inorganic materials, trace elements, and fillers that are unique to that product and can be detected by **X-ray fluorescence (XRF)** technology even after incineration. The XRF trace element and major element analysis of dental remains may be useful as an adjunct to traditional evaluation of dental information in some forensic settings, including cremation and dismemberment cases (Fig. 19.1). The technique was first used in an actual case to identify three victims of the Buffalo, New York Colgan Air flight 3402 accident in 2009.

Unusual physiologic and psychological reactions and the patient's comments concerning therapy are entered in the record. Summaries of telephone conversations with patients, consultants, insurance company representatives, or legal authorities should be noted. All entries should be signed or initialed by recording personnel. Changes in the record should not be erased but corrected by a single line drawn through the incorrect material. This method permits the original entry to remain readable and removes any questions concerning fraudulent intent to alter recorded information.

By 2015, medical and dental records in the United States were required to be maintained in an electronic format and numerous commercial and individually designed computer software programs have been marketed to assist physicians, dentists, health care facilities, hospitals, and insurance companies in collecting and preserving the medical and dental information of patients. The obvious advantage of electronic medical, health, or dental record (EMR, EHR, and EDR) systems is facilitation of networking and exchange of records among the different formats ("interoperability") for routine professional consultation or use in forensic identification cases requiring medical and dental records for comparison.

However, the increased use of EHRs and EDRs has also created legal, financial, and ethical issues concerning patient privacy as noted in the HIPAA regulations. Additionally, there may be a potential for insurance fraud associated with the computer enhancement of dental lesions or restorations on electronically generated dental radiographs.

The potential charge of insurance fraud associated with the enhancement of dental lesions or restorations on computer-generated or scanned **digital radiography (DR)** can be avoided if a clinician stores and maintains unaltered images. This is accomplished using programs with unchangeable, secure tagged block file extensions in their native file formats. When duplicates or copies are required, working images should be generated.

Computer-assisted management technology (e.g., WinID3 dental comparison software bridged with the Dexis DR program) has been an asset in expediting the comparison of antemortem and postmortem dental record information in MFI events, including the World Trade Center terrorist attack, the Indian Ocean tsunami disaster, the Hurricane Katrina recovery effort, and deaths caused by wildfires in the western United States. Additionally, Win ID3 is used to maintain missing person databases and is available as a free download in six different languages. Other software such as Adobe Photoshop and Mideo Systems CASEWORKSeis facilitates the superimposition of digitally scanned radiographs and photographs for comparison.

Whether preserved in written form or by using a computer database, the principles of record management describe a mechanism that ensures that dental information, which may be required to resolve a forensic problem, is properly maintained and retrievable. Additionally, records preserved in this manner are reliable evidentiary material if subpoenaed in peer review or malpractice litigation proceedings.

Time limits concerning how long records must be retained vary among the states. As a rule, states mandate that records be kept for 7–10 years. Federal legislation related to the problem of missing persons in the United States requires that records of pediatric dental patients be retained until the patient reaches the age of majority (adulthood). Depending on the jurisdiction, this can vary from 18 to 21 years of age.

The maintenance period for EHR and EDR patient data exceeds the duration of paper records and may vary from 20 to 100 years. Provisions for security and integrity of stored archival information in EHRs and EDRs must support ethical and legal principles regarding privacy because the technology used to input information will be unavailable to those who may need to examine this data in the future.

◆ IDENTIFICATION

Legal situations often revolve around the establishment of a person's proper identity. Any death not certified by an individual's own physician must be referred to the medical examiner (ME) or coroner for review. However, cases requiring an **autopsy** to determine the time, cause, and manner of death represent a small percentage of cases. When required, these tasks are the responsibility of a coroner or ME. These officials are charged with the role of establishing identification; determining the cause, mechanism, and mode or manner of death; and issuing a death certificate. Besides identification of the decedent, these key issues of death investigation for the coroner or ME are defined according to the following:

- **Cause of death.** The disease, injury, or chemical or physical agent responsible for initiating the lethal sequence of events (e.g., myocardial infarction, cancer, bullet, knife, poison, ligature, lightning, and infectious agents)
- **Mechanism of death.** The pathologic process that results in death (e.g., congestive heart failure, cardiac arrhythmias, asphyxia, sepsis, exsanguination, renal failure, and hepatic failure)
- **Mode or manner of death.** According to the **NASH** classification, the mode or manner of death is considered to be Natural, Accidental, Suicide, or Homicide. Natural deaths are caused exclusively by disease. Accidental deaths result from an environmental or human tragedy (e.g., lightning strike or vehicular incident).
- **Undetermined death.** Although the cause and mechanism of death may be resolved, the manner or mode may not be established because of decomposition, dismemberment, or postmortem destruction of the remains by insects or feral animals.

The coroner is an elected official and, depending on the laws of each state, does not necessarily have to be a physician or have advanced training in death investigation. An ME is an appointed official who is a pathologist specifically trained in forensic medicine. Many jurisdictions use forensic pathologists, and this trend has contributed to the professionalizing of a position increasingly involved with the interpretation of advanced scientific techniques requiring knowledge of toxicology, ballistics, anthropology, pharmacology, and criminalistics, as well as pathology.

A death certificate, identifying the decedent, is required before probation of a will, release of life insurance claims, or resolution of other affairs associated with the settlement of an estate. Criminal cases involving homicide, suicide, and fraudulent misidentification may also require the expertise of forensic dentists and other forensic scientists trained in identification techniques. These professionals act as consultants to the coroner or ME and assist in this aspect of a death investigation.

Besides analysis of the dentition, the most common methods of identification include personal recognition, fingerprinting (friction ridge analysis—dermatoglyphics), physical anthropologic examination of bones, and serologic and genetic (DNA) comparison techniques.

Additionally, the use of facial superimposition techniques (when the teeth are visible) and facial reconstruction techniques may also permit scientifically supported comparisons for identification. Each method has its advantages and disadvantages. However, all rely on the principle that identification is the positive correlation obtained by comparing known information about a suspect or victim with unique facts retrieved by physical examination of the suspect or victim.

Regardless of the method used to identify a decedent, the results of the antemortem and postmortem data comparison lead to one of the following four situations:

1. **Positive identification.** There is sufficient uniqueness among the comparable items in the antemortem and postmortem databases, and no major differences are observed.
2. **Presumptive (possible) identification.** There are commonalities among the comparable items in the antemortem and postmortem databases; however, enough information may be missing from either source to prevent the establishment of a positive identification.
3. **Insufficient identification evidence.** There is insufficient supportive evidence available to compare and arrive at a conclusion based on scientific principles.
4. **Exclusion of identification evidence.** Either explainable or unexplainable discrepancies exist among comparable items in the antemortem and postmortem databases. This results in inconsistencies that prevent the establishment of any identification. Exclusion may be just as important as a determination of positive identification.

Personal Recognition

Personal recognition is the least reliable method used to identify an individual. It is often based on the visual identification of a decedent by a family member, friend, or acquaintance. This process assesses artifactual material such as clothing, jewelry, keys, wallet contents, luggage, other personal effects, scars, and tattoos to determine identification. Evidence in this type of identification can be accidentally or purposely exchanged between bodies. This can occur in MFI situations or when there is criminal intent to create a misidentification in cases of identity theft or alias associated with criminal activity.

Even when a body is viewed shortly after death, distraught relatives can inadvertently misidentify the decedent. After the occurrence of postmortem changes associated with soft tissue decomposition, insect and burn artifact, skeletonization, or dismemberment, this method of identification may be precluded (Figs. 19.2–19.5).

Fingerprinting and Other Morphometric Means of Identification

• **Anthropometry** was the first "scientific" system police used to identify criminals. The French law enforcement officer, Alphonse Bertillon, developed this system in the latter part of the 19th century. The method was unreliable and flawed because it relied on biometric physical measurements of the head and body, individual markings including scars and tattoos, and other personal characteristics. Bertillon's anthropometry identification process was eventually replaced by analysis of the epidermal friction ridges of the fingers, palms, and feet unique to koala bears and all primates and commonly referred to as **fingerprinting.** Other evolving nondental morphometric identification techniques include:

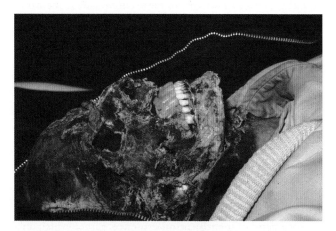

• **Fig. 19.2** Unrecognizable partially decomposed human remains with a maxillary removable partial denture in place. Notice that the skin tissue of the neck that has been protected by the windbreaker jacket has not reached the stage of decomposition of the tissues of the exposed face. (Courtesy of Dr. Raymond D. Rawson.)

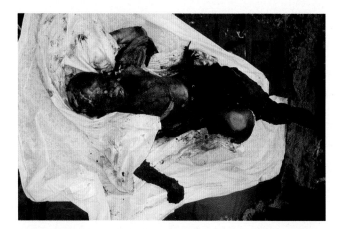

• **Fig. 19.3** A burn victim requiring identification by dental, DNA, or fingerprint methodology rather than personal recognition. (Courtesy of Dr. Raymond D. Rawson.)

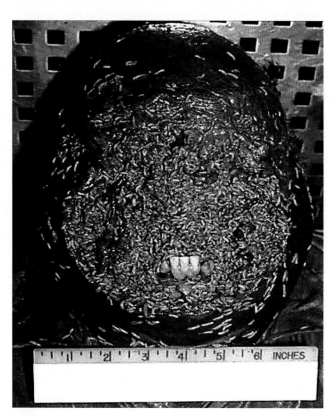

• **Fig. 19.4** Decomposing human remains with infestation of blue bottle fly (*Calliphora vomitoria*) larvae covering the face. These insect maggots are important forensically, and forensic entomology can be used to estimate time of death based on their egg and oviposition timing. Notice the mandibular removable partial denture replacing three incisors.

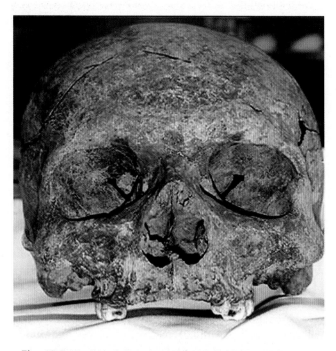

• **Fig. 19.5** The frontal view of a skeletonized human skull. The shape of the orbits and nasal borders may be helpful in determining into which ethnic group the remains should be assigned.

- Rugoscopy—analysis of the palatal rugae by computer-assisted photographic superimposition
- Cheiloscopy—comparison of lip prints
- Iris pattern evaluation for unique similarities.

These morphometric comparison methods, in addition to comparison of the radiographic outlines of the maxillary and frontal sinuses, are now considered unique and have become additional means of identification. By the beginning of the 20th century, forensic science had recognized that the ridge-like patterns on the fingertips and palms are unique for each person (dermatoglyphia). These friction ridges are genetically determined, and not even homozygous twins have the same patterns of loops, arches, and whorls. A principal variation in the fingerprints of twins is that they appear as mirror images of each other. The morphometric variation in combinations of the loops, arches, and whorls permits a scientific comparison of fingerprint records with the friction ridges of an unidentified decedent.

Because the fingerprint pattern is inherited, it is a static characteristic and remains unchanged throughout life. However, the friction ridges associated with a fingerprint may be missing through application of an acid or other caustic material for criminal intent. Several dermatological diseases may also result in alteration of these identifying morphometric markers. A very rare genetic mutation of the SMARCAD1 gene, which encodes only for a protein found in the skin, results in an absence of fingerprint patterns (adermatoglyphia) as well.

The inheritance of static dermatoglyphs is advantageous when one compares fingerprint identification with fluid characteristics associated with the teeth and their supporting structures. Dental patterns change as teeth erupt, exfoliate, decay, become restored, and, perhaps, are eventually extracted and replaced with implants or other prosthetic devices.

Unlike dental records, which are principally retained in private dental offices in the Americas and Western Europe, fingerprint information is maintained by governmental agencies. Several states retain records of non-criminals who work in sensitive occupations. In this regard, Nevada has a fingerprint database for employees in the gaming industry. The Criminal Justice Information Services (CJIS) Division of the Federal Bureau of Investigation (FBI) contains the largest biometric database in the world with over 130 million fingerprint records included in criminal, civil, and known and suspected terrorist formats.

Currently, these records are retained within the Integrated Automated Fingerprint Identification System (IAFIS). IAFIS permits input, matching, and retrieval of even a single fingerprint image for identification. Next-Generation Identification (NGI) technology is being developed for the FBI to expand the morphometric information contained in IAFIS to include palm print, iris, and facial identification data.

The establishment of the CJIS Division's IAFIS files permits automated computer data entry and search capabilities for matching and retrieval of fingerprint images. This information is available for electronic exchange among law enforcement agencies for identification purposes. Included in the IAFIS database are criminal and civil 10-print fingerprint records, latent fingerprint services, and subject and criminal history search capabilities. Information from this fingerprint repository is shared with international legal agencies, such as Interpol and the Royal Canadian Mounted Police.

Fingerprint nomenclature is standardized in IAFIS, and all fingerprint experts use the same terminology worldwide. This advantage is not observed in dental identification, in which numerous charting and tooth-numbering systems are used. Because soft tissues decompose shortly after death, the friction ridge patterns within the epidermis, and loss of other morphometric soft tissue structures in this tissue, may not be retrievable for comparison. This is the principal disadvantage of fingerprint, lip, rugae, and iris pattern analysis for identification.

Physical Anthropologic Examination of Bones and Teeth

Forensic anthropologists and forensic dentists often work together to resolve problems associated with identification. Both disciplines are concerned with analysis of calcified structures of the body—bones and teeth. Historically, this anatomic material has assisted forensic anthropologists and dentists in determining the ethnicity, age, and sex of a person (Table 19.1). These characteristics have become less distinct in some populations as individuals from different cultures and ethnic backgrounds have intermarried and blended these genetically determined features in their offspring.

In addition to the study of osseous material and despite variations in crown and root development within the dentition, the teeth can be studied clinically, radiographically, histologically, and biochemically to determine the age of a living individual or decedent.

Forensically, this information is essential in casework involving the need to establish legal age of majority (adulthood), medicolegal age at death, clarification of the age of undocumented immigrants, age estimation of unidentified remains, and separation of comingled remains in a multiple fatality incident among others.

From fetal development to adolescence, tooth maturation intervals are the principal method of dental age assessment. Lewis and Senn emphasize that dental age estimation of children becomes more accurate when teeth having less variance are used in these analyses and data derived from multiple teeth is considered. Studies also have been performed to assess differences in crown and root formation and eruption sequences among children of both genders and various ethnic populations. In 2010, AlQahtani et al. developed the London Atlas of Human Tooth Development and Eruption. This provides the forensic odontologist with "a comprehensive evidence-based atlas to estimate age using both tooth development and alveolar eruption for human individuals between 28 weeks in utero and 23 years" (Fig. 19.6). As one approaches adulthood, age estimation acquired by analysis of the dentition can be supplemented with radiographic data obtained from the calcification centers of the hand and

Skeletal Anthropologic Variations Associated With Ethnic and Sexual Characteristics of the Skull

	Ethnic Characteristics		
	European	African	Asian/Native American
Width	Narrow	Narrow	Broad
Height	High	Low	Intermediate
Profile	Straight	Prognathic	Intermediate
Orbit	Triangular/teardrop	Square	Circular
Nasal opening	Tapered	Wide	Rounded
Palate	Narrow	Wide	Intermediate

	Sexual Characteristics	
	Male	Female
Size	Large	Small
Glabellar (supraorbital) ridges	Pronounced	Not developed
Mastoid process	Large	Small
Occipital area	Pronounced muscle lines	Minimal muscle lines
Mandible	Larger, broader ramus	Smaller
Forehead	Steeper, slopes posteriorly	Rounded, more vertical

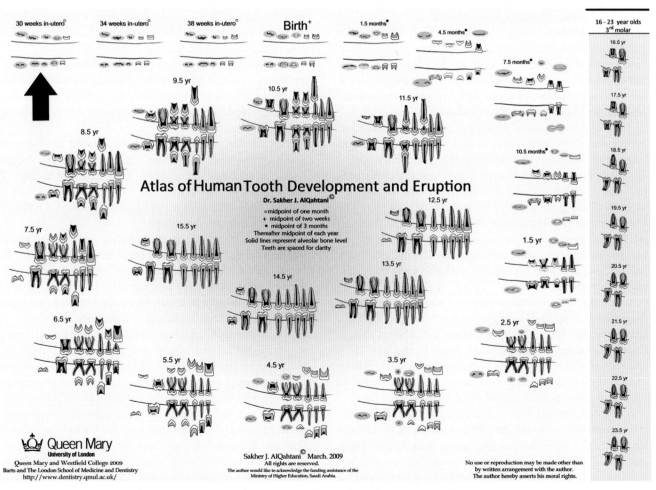

• **Fig. 19.6 Atlas of Human Tooth Development and Eruption**. The *arrow* indicates the starting point. The dentin is presented in *gray* for the deciduous teeth and in *green* for the permanent teeth. (Courtesy of Dr. Sakher J. AlQahtani.)

wrist, ribs, clavicles, and other bones to determine the precise age of a person younger than 20 years of age.

Biochemical laboratory procedures or assessment of dental post-formation changes are used to determine the age of adult individuals. Historically, dental post-formation changes of adult teeth included the study of their ground sections for variations in patterns of:

- Attrition
- Periodontal attachment
- Secondary dentin
- Cementum apposition
- Root resorption
- Transparency of root dentin

This approach, developed by Gustafson in 1947, has been modified to determine which of these factors are most significant—secondary dentin and transparency of root dentin.

Additionally, these contemporary methods of dental post-formation analysis have been supplemented by those relying on the following techniques:

- Evaluation of the rate of racemization of levels of metabolically stable aspartic acid enantiomers in enamel and dentin to determine an exact age.
- Occlusal tooth wear which can provide reliable estimates of age to within 3–5 years. Often, anthropologic analysis is helpful in arriving at a presumptive identification based on these criteria.

There are variations in the calcification and eruption patterns among various ethnic and cultural groups, and studies have been undertaken to delineate these differences further. After the third molars, long bones, and bones of the wrist and hand are completely developed, evaluation of biochemical components of the calcified structures and collagen is the most accurate method for determining chronologic age.

Methods that rely on an analysis of the rate of racemization of the stereoisomers of aspartic acid in enamel and dentin can be used to determine an accurate chronologic age. This is related to the fact that the change from the L-form of this amino acid to its mirror image D-form occurs over time. Thus, the ratio of the L- to D-forms of aspartic acid in the dentition is directly related to the age of the individual. Often, anthropologic and dental age analysis is helpful in arriving at a presumptive identification based on the criteria noted previously.

In 2022, after rigorous review, the Organization of Scientific Area Committees for Forensic Science (OSAC) Registry, administered by the National Institute of Standards and Technology (NIST), accepted the ADA Technical Report No. 1077 for Human Age Assessment by Dental Analysis.

Positive identification may be achievable when the skull and facial bones are used as a foundation to reconstruct the facial soft tissues (Figs. 19.7–19.9). Three-dimensional (3D) computer images, computed tomography (CT) images, and radiographs have even been used in the replication of the face of Europe's oldest mummified human, a male dubbed Ötzi, whose 5300-year-old remains were removed from glacial ice in the Ötztal Alps on the Austrian-Italian border.

With knowledge of the anatomic relationships between the skull and face, antemortem facial photographs or

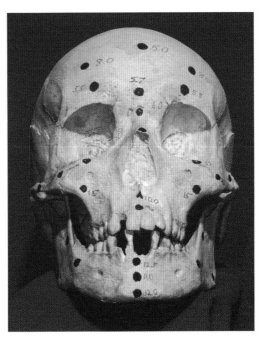

• **Fig. 19.7** Reconstruction of the facial soft tissue uses predetermined, standard anthropologic thickness measurements for specific points around the face. These measurements are based on variables that are related to ethnic and sexual characteristics. (Courtesy of Dr. Cleve Smith.)

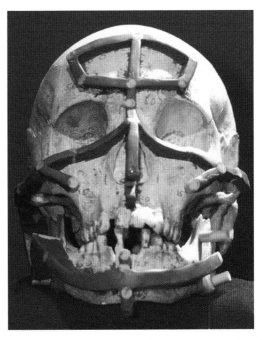

• **Fig. 19.8** The soft tissue thickness points can be connected with sculpting clay or digitized on a computer screen. The ultimate result of these techniques is a re-creation of the contour of the soft tissue features that permits a visual identification. (Courtesy of Dr. Cleve Smith.)

radiographs can be superimposed for comparison with the skull of an unknown. Video superimposition with two television cameras and an electronic mixing device has been used successfully to overlay a photograph of a human face on an image of a skull for identification. The development of

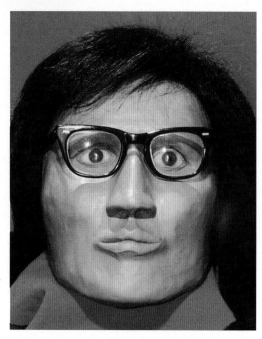

• **Fig. 19.9** The width of the mouth is related to the interpupillary distance. The length and shape of the nose are determined by the relationship between the inferior and superior nasal spines. If known, then the addition of a specific hairstyle, eyeglasses, and eye color can further individualize a facial reconstruction. (Courtesy of Dr. Cleve Smith.)

computer software programs capable of superimposition has further facilitated the process.

The anterior dentition of the skull can be overlaid and compared with a smiling antemortem photograph. The shapes and positions of the individual teeth and their relationships to each other have been considered distinctive enough features on which to base identification, as have certain significant cranial and facial landmarks, including the orbits, nasal openings, malar eminence, and chin. Prosthetic joint replacements, intraosseous and dental implants, and radiographic signs of prior bone fracture are other anthropologic findings that can be used to facilitate identification.

Additionally, prosthetic devices, implanted defibrillators and pacemakers, and osseous implants, with the exception of dental implants, are designated with individual identification code numbers provided by their manufacturers. These codes can be visualized in the various devices and are useful in identifying individuals in cremation and dismemberment scenarios when the teeth and fingerprints are not available for evaluation.

Serologic and Genetic (DNA) Comparison

Every individual is unique by virtue of his or her chromosomal DNA—a polymer structured as a double helix and composed of four different nucleotides. The polymorphic sequencing of these nucleotides along the two strands of the DNA molecule accounts for the genetic diversity of all living things. This "ultimate identification material" was first used forensically to obtain a conviction in a criminal case in 1986, and DNA comparison has since become an accepted forensic method to resolve problems of identification.

Before 1986, comparison of antigenic markers found on red blood cells (RBCs) and in body fluids of secretors of these markers among the human population was traditionally used as a means of *exclusionary* (*exculpatory*) evidence. Because the ABH antigenic surface markers of RBCs are not discriminatory, this type of evidence was primarily used to exclude a suspect or victim when negative comparative results were achieved. Positive comparisons were justified only to place the suspect or victim in a population of individuals having similar serologic antigens.

Although DNA has become the principal biologic substance used to effect a positive identification, antigenic surface markers A, B, and H of the ABO blood group system, as well as various components of the rhesus (Rh) and Lewis systems, continue to be accepted for medicolegal comparison. The ability to secrete the ABH antigens in saliva and other body fluids is genetically determined, and more than 80% of individuals are secretors. With appropriate laboratory tests, even dried samples of fluid and blood can be analyzed for these markers.

DNA found in human cells is composed of chromosomal and mitochondrial DNA (mtDNA). Two copies of chromosomal DNA are incorporated into the nuclei of a person's cells by DNA provided from both parents. However, hundreds of copies of mtDNA are contained in the cytoplasm of these cells. This DNA is only maternally transferred and can be isolated from cells without nuclei, such as RBCs. Unlike nuclear DNA, mtDNA is single stranded and circular. Because there is no mixing of sequence types from generation to generation in maternally transferred mtDNA, it can be compared with that of distant maternal relatives to effect identification when other reference sources are unavailable.

Restriction fragment length polymorphism (RFLP) and polymerase chain reaction (PCR) analyses are the principal laboratory techniques used to compare and evaluate fragments of DNA material from a suspect or victim's biologic forensic specimens (e.g., semen, vaginal fluid, teeth, soft tissues, and saliva). Both are extremely accurate, precise, and reproducible; these methods are used when the conditions of the sample DNA presented dictate the need for their respective advantages.

RFLP methods result in splitting source DNA into thousands of fragments using "biologic scissors" known as *restriction enzymes*. Fragment size varies among individuals related to the variable number of tandem repeats (VNTR) of base pairs. These short segments of DNA contain a number of repeat units that differ among individuals. After gel separation of the fragments and transfer to a nylon mesh, specific DNA fragments are identified using oligonucleotides labeled with radioisotopes. Analysis of a series of different VNTR loci permits generation of an individual DNA profile.

A match of four or more VNTR loci is consistent with a positive match between DNA evidence gathered from suspect, victim, or crime scene evidence. The RFLP method requires large amounts of high molecular weight DNA, a major disadvantage. Small DNA samples (<100 ng) or degraded evidence in which the DNA has become denatured because of extreme heat or pH variation requires an analytic method other than RFLP.

The evaluation of minute quantities of DNA or DNA that has undergone degradation can be accomplished with the highly sensitive PCR test. Using this laboratory technique, smaller VNTR loci of a specific DNA sequence can be amplified into enough copies for sufficient analysis. Because of its high degree of sensitivity, PCR analysis has been used to evaluate small amounts of DNA from a suspect's clothing left at the scene of a crime, as well as from bone fragments from the Vietnam War. DNA amplification of microsatellite loci (referred to as *STRs*) and minisatellite loci (or *LTRs*) using PCR, is referred to as *AmpFLP analysis.*

The hard and soft tissues of the oral cavity and saliva are often good sources for DNA material. However, if the teeth or other hard structures of the mouth are to be used for the collection of DNA evidence, then the identification value of these structures should be considered (beyond their ability to yield a harvest DNA). A tooth or jaw fragment capriciously destroyed can result in the loss of valuable radiographic and anatomic sources for eventual dental identification. Besides the obvious source of DNA from human tissues, the forensic dentist often considers the evaluation of chewed gum, cigarette remains, licked envelopes, stamps, or similar inanimate objects as potential sources for DNA evidence using PCR analysis described previously.

Regardless of the surface from which DNA evidence may be harvested, the two-swab protocol developed by Dr. David Sweet and others at the Bureau of Legal Dentistry, University of British Columbia is the recovery method of choice:

- A sterile cotton swab is moistened with distilled water and rolled over the surface of the skin or object using moderate pressure and circular motion.
- This swab is air dried.
- A second *dry* cotton swab is rolled over the *same* surface of the skin or object using moderate pressure and circular motion *to absorb all moisture left by the first swab.*
- This swab is also air dried.
- Both swabs are placed in properly labeled storage containers and submitted to the laboratory for frozen storage at −20°C (−4°F).

Control samples may be collected from whole blood, autopsy tissue samples or oral buccal swabs from a living individual.

Passage of the DNA Identification Act of 1994 and the establishment of the FBI's National DNA Index System (NDIS) in 1998 have facilitated the exchange and comparison of DNA profiles among federal, state, and local crime laboratories in the United States. This is accomplished electronically through the FBI Laboratory's Combined DNA Index System (CODIS). Through the CODIS computer program's forensic and offender indexes, biologic evidence from crime scenes can be linked to DNA profiles of individuals convicted of sex offenses and other felonies.

As of April 2021, the total number of DNA profiles contained in the FBI CODIS databases reached 20 million. Since its inception, approximately 550,000 successful comparisons ("hits") have been made among cases in which the CODIS system was activated. This represents a 98% success rate linking DNA from a crime scene with similar material from the convicted offender profiles. CODIS software has also been helpful in the identification of missing and unidentified individuals.

The US Department of Defense has initiated a policy of obtaining DNA samples on all military personnel. This DNA "fingerprint" has significantly reduced the possibility of another unknown soldier among future military casualties. Despite the positive effects of DNA evidence in resolving questions of identity, the technique is not without controversy. Challenges have been made by population geneticists, concerned about random matching and variations among ethnic subgroups.

Dental Evaluation

Basic Principles

In an identification case, the principal advantage of dental evidence is that, like other hard tissue, it is often preserved indefinitely after death. Although the status of a person's teeth changes throughout life, the combination of decayed, missing, and filled teeth is measurable, reproducible, and comparable at any fixed point in time. Therefore, like the comparison of unique patterns in a fingerprint and other soft tissue morphometric structures, a scientific, objective analysis of antemortem and postmortem dental variables is achievable through an assessment of the presence and position of individual teeth. Thus, these respective anatomic, restorative, and pathologic dental components provide the database for the antemortem and postmortem comparison of dental structures (Fig. 19.10). For example, a unique dental restoration, such as seen in Fig. 19.11, might provide an important clue in making an identification. In addition, the legal community accepts the fact that dentists can recognize procedures that they have performed. Morphometric soft tissue patterns and the outline of the maxillary and frontal sinuses are also considered unique and can support the

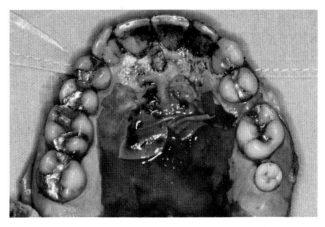

• **Fig. 19.10** The combination of decayed, missing, and filled teeth, along with unique anatomic and pathologic findings, provides the database for comparison in a dental identification. Note the microdont in the maxillary left quadrant.

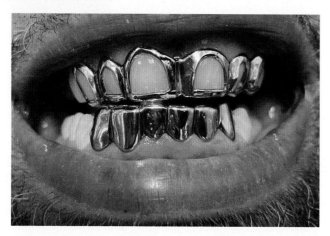

• **Fig. 19.11** Unique dental restorations or prostheses may contribute important information allowing the identification of an individual.

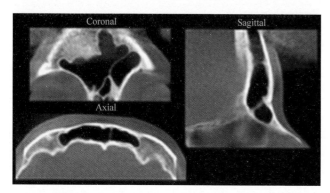

• **Fig. 19.12** The outline shape of the frontal sinus is a unique morphometric factor that may be used in human identification when comparing cone-beam computed tomography (CBCT) and anterior-posterior radiographs of a known individual with those of an unknown person or decedent. (Courtesy of Dr. Robert Danforth.)

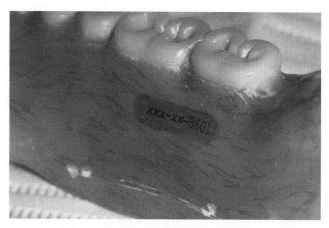

• **Fig. 19.13** Denture identification is accomplished by inserting a typed name or code number (i.e., Social Security number or hospital patient number) in an area of the denture that will not interfere with the aesthetics of the prosthesis. This procedure is performed in the laboratory during the final acrylic pack. Information also can be engraved in the framework of an all-metal appliance.

rationale for comparison of ante- and postmortem radiographs of the head (Fig. 19.12).

Problems associated with dental identification information are often related to acquiring and interpreting antemortem records. Most antemortem dental records are retrieved from private sector dental providers. However, dental records may be recovered from insurance carriers, dental schools, hospitals, clinics, state and federal prisons, military files, and the FBI National Crime Information Center (NCIC) databases.

To initiate a request for antemortem records, a putative (suspected) identification is required. Reports of missing and unidentified persons, obtained from law enforcement agencies, are the principal source for this material. Thousands of victims who cannot be identified by fingerprint methods remain unidentified because a putative identification has not been established.

The FBI-NCIC computer registry of missing and unidentified persons was established to help rectify this problem. This computer system maintains demographic, dental, and medical information on missing persons. It attempts to match these data with similar facts obtained from unidentified bodies. The latter information is submitted by various investigative and legal agencies. Potentially, the otherwise unidentifiable victims of random violence, serial homicides, terrorist acts, and child abduction can now be identified without the need to determine a putative identification. A disadvantage of the NCIC computer identification system is that it does not have the capability to identify possible decedents based solely on dental information.

The National Dental Image Repository (NDIR) has been established to address this issue. Law enforcement agencies can voluntarily post supplemental dental images related to NCIC Missing, Unidentified, and Wanted Person records on the NDIR secure website. Thus, access, retrieval, and review of dental information by qualified forensic odontologists who are members of the NDIR Review Panel can facilitate dental comparisons. The NDIR website is located at Law Enforcement Online (LEO) at http://cgate.leo.gov. This repository permits law enforcement, criminal justice, and public safety authorities to maintain a national and international method of electronic communication, education, and sharing of dental information.

The Armed Forces, Department of Veterans Affairs, and many states require that identifying markings be placed on removable dental prostheses (Fig. 19.13). The American Dental Association and the National Association of Dental Laboratories (NADL) also support dental prosthetics identification (DPid). DPid also links with the US Food and Drug Administration's (FDA) Unique Device Identification (UDI) requirements. It is an attempt to provide a basis for identification among the substantial population of completely or partially edentulous individuals in the United States and internationally.

Identifying markings in dental prostheses are important because even if dental records of an edentulous person can be obtained, they may not reflect the current status of the ridges and alveolar bone. Commonly used information for identifying removable dental prostheses should include the following UDI documentation requirements:

- A unique identification number
- Country of origin
- Dentist/Dental Laboratory contact information
- Patient identification
- Manufacturing date and subsequent changes
- Brand names of components.

This information is linked to a secure database via a 2D Code (Data Matrix) for comparison.

Even when a suspected identification is achieved, it may still be difficult to secure antemortem dental records. The family or acquaintances of the victim may not know where dental treatment was sought. Reviewing the putative victim's canceled bank checks or medical deductions on tax records may be helpful in locating antemortem dental records in such cases.

Although records obtained from institutional or governmental dental facilities routinely indicate all restored teeth, this is not true of charts forwarded from private dentists. In these instances, previously restored teeth often are not charted unless the current dentist intends to re-treat them. Therefore, in these records, the antemortem radiographs and progress notes become the principal sources for dental information.

Unfortunately, the nomenclature associated with dental charting systems is not standardized (Table 19.2). In 1984, the American Dental Association adopted the Universal Tooth Numbering System. All insurance companies, the Armed Forces, dental schools, and most dentists in the United States now use this system. It should be used in all forensic dental cases.

In the Universal Numbering System, a consecutive number from 1 to 32 is assigned to the adult dentition. It begins with the maxillary right third molar and ends with the mandibular right third molar. The deciduous dentition is identified by letters from A to T, beginning with the maxillary right deciduous second molar and ending with the mandibular right deciduous second molar. Thus, the quadrants are identified in a clockwise direction, beginning with the maxillary right.

Other tooth-numbering methods include the Zsigmondy/Palmer System and the Federation Dentaire Internationale (FDI) Two-Digit System. Each uses a different coding technique to identify dental quadrants and specific teeth.

The Zsigmondy/Palmer System stresses the anatomic likeness of the eight tooth types in each symbolically identified dental quadrant. Homologous permanent teeth are assigned the same number from 1 to 8. Deciduous teeth are assigned letters *A* through *E*.

The FDI Two-Digit System is endorsed by the World Health Organization (WHO) and is used in most developed countries, except the United States. The first digit represents the quadrant. Quadrants 1 to 4 are assigned for permanent teeth; 5 to 8 represent quadrants for the primary dentition. As in the Universal Numbering System, the quadrants are identified in a clockwise direction, beginning with the maxillary right. The second digit designates the permanent tooth type from 1 to 8, or deciduous tooth type from 1 to 5.

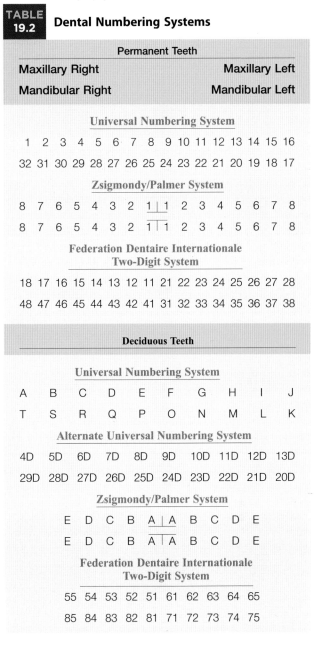

TABLE 19.2 Dental Numbering Systems

Permanent Teeth	
Maxillary Right	Maxillary Left
Mandibular Right	Mandibular Left

Universal Numbering System

1 2 3 4 5 6 7 8 9 10 11 12 13 14 15 16
32 31 30 29 28 27 26 25 24 23 22 21 20 19 18 17

Zsigmondy/Palmer System

8 7 6 5 4 3 2 1 | 1 2 3 4 5 6 7 8
8 7 6 5 4 3 2 1 | 1 2 3 4 5 6 7 8

Federation Dentaire Internationale Two-Digit System

18 17 16 15 14 13 12 11 21 22 23 24 25 26 27 28
48 47 46 45 44 43 42 41 31 32 33 34 35 36 37 38

Deciduous Teeth

Universal Numbering System

A B C D E F G H I J
T S R Q P O N M L K

Alternate Universal Numbering System

4D 5D 6D 7D 8D 9D 10D 11D 12D 13D
29D 28D 27D 26D 25D 24D 23D 22D 21D 20D

Zsigmondy/Palmer System

E D C B A | A B C D E
E D C B A | A B C D E

Federation Dentaire Internationale Two-Digit System

55 54 53 52 51 61 62 63 64 65
85 84 83 82 81 71 72 73 74 75

Thus, in the Universal Numbering System, tooth 12 is the maxillary left first bicuspid. In the FDI Two-Digit System, tooth 12 (one-two) is the maxillary right lateral incisor. In the Zsigmondy/Palmer System, all lateral incisors are designated with a No. 2 code. The position of a specific No. 2 tooth is diagrammatically indicated by a symbolic quadrant.

Unless the forensic dentist knows which system has been used to encode the teeth in the antemortem record, all teeth should be referred to by their actual names. This method will prevent errors because all dentists use the same anatomic nomenclature when referring to individual teeth.

Dental identification problems may be further compounded because dental radiographs can be mounted and viewed from right to left or vice versa. Intraoral radiographic duplicating film does not contain a raised dot to assist the dentist in orienting the film for mounting. The lack of this orienting device can lead to transposition of dental evidence and potential misidentification based on an incorrect comparison. Besides the lack of a raised dot, panoramic radiographic duplicating film can be detected because of its single-sided emulsion and series of notches on one edge to indicate that the image is not an original (Fig. 19.14, *A*).

Additionally, when using intraoral digital sensors, the operator must be careful not to inadvertently expose the device from the wrong side. This orientation error can remain undetected because the "**a**" placed on the sensor (which serves the same function as the raised dot on radiographic film) always appears in the same position after processing regardless of which side of the sensor has been exposed (see Fig. 19.14, *B*).

With the advent of aesthetic materials for posterior restorations and the reduction in the prevalence of caries, it may be difficult for the forensic dentist to determine whether restorations are present by simple visual assessment of the teeth. In addition, the postmortem dental evaluation is often performed in an autopsy room, temporary morgue, or funeral home. In these locations, proper lighting and access to dental instruments, supplies, and equipment that can facilitate analysis of the oral structures, are not readily available for detailed examination.

Often, there are additional demands for immediacy in providing a coroner, ME, or other legal agent with the results of a dental identification. These demands further compound the forensic dentist's technical and stress-related problems while performing the tasks related to this discipline. Because

of the previous caveats, the forensic dentist should prepare an equipment kit (Box 19.1). The kit should be portable, containing instruments, supplies, and equipment specifically required for the performance of dental procedures in an autopsy room environment.

Guidelines for Dental Identification

Although dental information can support the identification of a visually recognizable body, identification of dental remains is especially helpful when a decedent is skeletonized, decomposed, burned, or dismembered. Because each of these forensic situations presents different technical problems to the dentist, Body Identification Guidelines have been established by the American Board of Forensic Odontology (ABFO). The purpose of delineating these criteria is to assist dentists in comparing antemortem and postmortem dental information. Furthermore, the possibility of misidentification is reduced in both routine and mass-disaster cases.

Under the Body Identification Guidelines, provisions are made for the following:

- Examination of the postmortem dental remains in compliance with infection control and Occupational Safety and Health Administration (OSHA) requirements

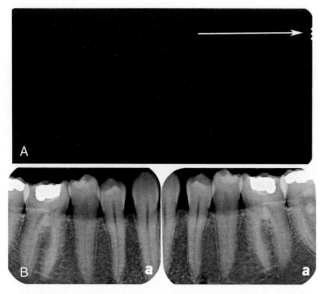

• **Fig. 19.14 A,** Panoramic duplicating film has a series of notches (*arrow*) on one edge to indicate that the image is not an original. **B,** When phosphor digital plates are inadvertently exposed from the wrong side, the error may not be detected because the "**a**" position marker always appears in the same location after processing regardless of which side of the sensor has been exposed. This problem can be prevented by placing a metal indicator on the side of the device that should not be exposed. (Courtesy of Dr. Richard A. Weems.)

• BOX 19.1 Suggested Instrument Kit for Forensic Identification

Dental explorers
Dental mirrors
Periodontal probes
Bite blocks
Tissue scissors
Osteotome
Rubber air/water syringe
Cotton swabs
Gauze
Flashlight or headlamp
Specimen containers
Scalpels and blades
Cheek retractors
ABFO No. 2 ruler
Bone mallet
Photographic mirrors
SLR film-based camera
Digital camera
Photographic film, digital memory card
Radiographic film and digital sensors
Rubber, latex, and nitrile gloves
Tissue forceps
Tissue clamp
Tongue clamp
Disclosing solution
Stryker saw
Writing instruments
Case labels
Appropriate charts
Masks and HEPA filter
Handheld portable radiation emitting device

ABFO, American Board of Forensic Odontology; *HEPA,* high-efficiency particulate air; *SLR,* single-lens reflex.

- Examination of antemortem dental records
- Comparison of all dental and paradental information from the two databases
- Development of a written report listing conclusions and an opinion regarding the strength of the identification, for example positive, presumptive, insufficient, or exculpatory (Exculpatory evidence is favorable to the defendant in a criminal trial, clearing the defendant of guilt.)

Postmortem Examination

The postmortem dental evidence is gathered by photographic, radiographic, and charting techniques. All records should include the case number, date, demographic and anthropologic information, the name of the authority that is requesting the dental examination, the location of the examination, and the name of the examining dentist.

Photographs should be taken of full head and face views. Images of the occlusal planes of both dental arches and individual views of unusual pathologic or restorative findings are also obtained. A digital 35-mm single-lens reflex (DSLR) camera and appropriate electronic flash and lens systems for close-up photography should be used. Basic digital images should include color exposures which can also be converted to black and white images for analysis.

Jaw resection is no longer a commonly accepted method employed to facilitate access to the postmortem dentition. This change in practice has resulted from ethical and medicolegal challenges and concerns regarding its use. However, postmortem examination, dental impressions, and radiographs can be obtained by relieving the mandibular muscle attachments and those of the temporomandibular joint (TMJ). This procedure permits access to the oral structures by 180-degree reflection of the lower jaw. If requested by the coroner or ME, then the dental specimens from the autopsy may have to be retained and preserved in a 10% formalin solution.

The guidelines for body identification recognize that the dentist and dental auxiliary personnel involved in performing forensic dental procedures do so at the request and direction of a legal authority, such as a coroner or ME. Therefore, it is only with the permission of these individuals that techniques involving postmortem facial dissection or jaw resection are performed by the forensic dentist to achieve complete access to dental tissues.

These measures are used most often in decomposed, dismembered, or incinerated bodies to make postmortem dental charting and radiographic examination easier. Mandibular reflection or soft tissue dissection may be necessary in visually recognizable (viewable) bodies when the oral cavity is inaccessible because of rigor mortis. In this situation the procedure is performed from an inframandibular approach.

In those rare instances when the forensic dentist is authorized to remove the jaws this task is accomplished with a reciprocating (Stryker) saw or osteotome and mallet, causing a Le Fort I fracture of the maxilla. The dissection instruments are placed above the inferior nasal spine and malar processes to ensure that the apices of the maxillary teeth are not transected. Similarly, if the mandible is not removed by disarticulation, then cuts into the mandibular rami should be high enough to prevent damage to impacted third molars.

While obtaining postmortem radiographic evidence, the forensic dentist may encounter technical obstacles that need to be addressed. It often is difficult to place intraoral radiographic film or digital radiographic sensors securely against the mandible or maxilla of a deceased individual. A modified Rinn XCP self-supporting film holder, which does not require active participation from the examinee, has been developed for postmortem identification. Because all dental evidence may eventually be required to be relinquished in court, the use of double-pack intraoral radiographs permits the forensic dentist to retain a set of films. Digital radiographic exposure and storage of images precludes this problem.

When the jaws cannot be resected postmortem changes in rigor mortis cases and in bodies that are partially decomposed may prevent the positioning of intraoral periapical radiographic films or digital sensors. Occlusal films, 5X7 lateral plates, and panoramic radiographs are often used in these situations. Additionally, charting of dental evidence in fourth-degree burn cases, in which charring of soft tissues results in contraction of the muscles of mastication, may preclude the placement of these devices. With the coroner or ME's permission, the entire skull can be removed from the rest of the remains and placed in a panoramic radiographic machine.

Fifth-degree burn cases result in cremation (sometimes referred to as **cremains**). Dental evidence may be lost or compromised in these cases as temperatures range between 870 and 980°C (1600 and 1800°F). Most cremated skeletal and dental remains are structurally recognizable, and it is only the processing of these structures in commercial crematoria that creates the ash most associated with this process. The composition of bone and teeth is principally inorganic calcium hydroxyapatite. Thus, these structures can become very fragile, can crumble easily, and require extreme care when handled in severely burned remains.

Fragmentation of dental structures in dismemberment cases and total loss of soft tissues in skeletonized remains necessitate alterations in routine radiation exposure settings. Generally, when radiographs of this type of material are taken, 10-mA and 65-kVp exposure settings are used. Because there is little or no soft tissue, standard exposure times or impulse settings are halved to prevent overexposure of the radiograph.

The maxilla can be split along the midsagittal suture, and each half can be placed horizontally on an occlusal film. This projection can be used to simulate antemortem panoramic radiographs or bite-wing views. Similar exposures can be obtained from the mandible by mounting the jaw on the edge of a table or bracket tray and placing an occlusal film under the supporting half. Exposures of the opposite side of the arch are made by simply flipping the mandible and repeating the procedure.

Databases have been created from elemental analysis or chemical characterization of various dental restorative and endodontic materials using scanning electron microscopic/energy-dispersive X-ray spectroscopy (SEM/EDS) and X-ray fluorescence (XRF) techniques. Referral to these resources may assist the forensic odontologist in the postmortem analysis of dental restorations when severe destruction of the dentition or cremation precludes the efficacy of using more traditional analytical methods.

The charting (odontogram) of the postmortem dentition should provide for situations in which teeth are missing after death. If such a discrepancy remains unexplained, then it may preclude the positive identification of the body. Scavenging animals or poor investigation of a crime or disaster scene can cause postmortem loss of teeth. Environmental conditions at or around the time of death, such as tidal action in a saltwater drowning, can also contribute to perimortem loss of teeth. When teeth are lost in this manner, the crest of the alveolar bone remains intact. In addition, there is no reossification of the socket (Fig. 19.15). This pattern is inconsistent with what is observed after extraction of a tooth.

Postmortem tooth loss is associated with decomposition of the periodontal ligament. Thus, the tooth simply falls out when the body is moved by feral or wild animals or during crime scene recovery efforts.

Antemortem Record Examination

Antemortem records are usually obtained directly from the police, coroner, or ME. Before accepting this evidence, the forensic dentist should determine that the records indicate the name of the person to be identified and the name and address of the submitting dentist. In addition, most jurisdictions require an evidence transfer document to be signed. This form indicates that the continuity of evidence has been maintained by specifying where and when the evidence was obtained, who secured the evidence, and who was in control or currently in possession of this material.

Several antemortem records of the same person may be submitted from different dental practices for comparison with postmortem dental evidence. It is not uncommon for the general dental records of a decedent and those obtained from the oral and maxillofacial surgeon, endodontist,

orthodontist, and other dental specialty practices to be forwarded for forensic analysis. Even if only one antemortem record is sent, the forensic dentist should rechart all information obtained from the radiographs, progress notes, and odontograms on a standardized form or computer-generated dental chart. This record should be identical to the one on which the postmortem information was documented. All of this material should be appropriately labeled as the antemortem record.

The use of computer software, such as the WinID3 program, in MFI situations accomplishes this same principle by entering all antemortem and postmortem dental information into the respective identification program. Besides making the comparison of records easier to manage, the creation of similar antemortem and postmortem analytic material is easier to present in court.

Comparison of Antemortem and Postmortem Records and Written Conclusions

After all dental information has been collected from the antemortem and postmortem databases it is compared for similarities and discrepancies. Comparison of dental evidence is unique among the techniques used to identify a decedent. A positive identification may still be established, even when some reconcilable discrepancies are observed.

Various codes and symbols have been used to chart the antemortem and postmortem status of the jaws. Currently in the United States, the WinID3 and Unified Victim Identification System/UVIS Dental Identification Module (UVIS/UDIM) dental identification software programs are most commonly used to compare dental records of missing individuals to those of unknown human remains and have been used similarly in MFI situations. The odontogram charting codes employed in WinID3 are presented in Table 19.3.

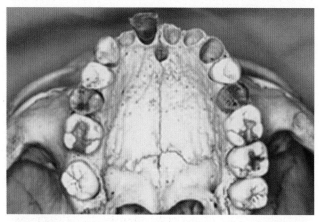

• **Fig. 19.15** Postmortem tooth loss results in an alveolar socket with unfractured margins and no reossification. In this example, teeth Nos. 7, 9, 10, and 11 represent postmortem tooth loss. Tooth No. 2 is a result of antemortem loss. Teeth Nos. 4, 8, and 13 were found near the body and reinserted into their respective sockets.

TABLE 19.3 WinID3 Charting Codes

Primary Codes	Secondary Codes
M—Mesial	A—Annotation
O—Occlusal	B—Deciduous
D—Distal	C—Crown
F—Facial	E—Resin
L—Lingual	G—Gold
I—Incisal	H—Porcelain
U—Unerupted	N—Nonprecious
V—Virgin	P—Pontic
X—Missing	R—Root canal
J—Missing crown	S—Silver amalgam
I—No data	T—Denture tooth
	Z—Temporary

The UVIS/UDIM software and Plass Data DVI System International software have been employed by forensic odontologists in the office of the New York medical examiner and the International Organization (INTERPOL) National Central Bureau, respectively. Although these computer programs can facilitate the process of comparison among the numerous antemortem and postmortem dental records presented in MFI or individual unknown/missing identification cases, the ultimate decision regarding the concordance of information between the antemortem and postmortem records rests with the forensic odontologist not the computer program.

Furthermore, the forensic dentist must routinely rely on the belief that antemortem records are truly those of the person they are purported to represent. The latter problem is best exemplified by the controversy associated with the antemortem dental records used to identify the bodies of Adolph Hitler and Eva Braun. Until recently, there was uncertainty concerning the reliability of those records. This uncertainty was based on the possibility that the records had been falsified to encourage the misidentification of Hitler and his wife. However, among other comparable dental evidence, the presence of an unusual and easily recognizable solid metal fixed prosthesis replacing the mandibular right cuspid and second bicuspid teeth was observed in the antemortem dental records obtained from Hitler's dentist, Dr. Hugo Blaschke. This bridge, resembling a telephone receiver, was also found in the postmortem jaws recovered from the partially burned human remains (Hitler) in the garden of the Reich Chancellery ruins (Fig. 19.16).

The case demonstrated in Fig. 19.17 shows that all teeth, restorations, and anatomic structures are identical, except that deciduous tooth K is still present in the antemortem radiograph. Tooth No. 20 is erupted in the postmortem film. This difference could not support a positive identification if it were a component of fingerprint or DNA evidence. The facts that the deciduous tooth has exfoliated and the permanent tooth erupted before death are acceptable discrepancies in comparable dental evidence.

Comparison of dental evidence is often complicated by the quality of the evidence submitted. The physical status of the postmortem dental material can be compromised when teeth have fractured or are avulsed secondary to trauma. Often, only fragments of the jaws may be presented for comparison, and there may have been postmortem loss of teeth.

Dental restorations can be separated from the teeth or melted in a fire. Acrylic restorative material melts in temperatures less than 540°C (1000°F), gold and amalgam melt at 870°C (1600°F), and porcelain can withstand temperatures greater than 1100°C (2010°F). In addition, extreme temperature in a fire can cause the teeth to explode or appear shrunken. Although the principal role of the dentition of a fire victim is to provide data for identification, studies indicate that morphologic and microscopic tissue alterations of the teeth may assist forensic scientists, such as arson investigators, in determining temperature and duration of exposure to fire.

The problems associated with incomplete antemortem records are compounded when radiographs are of poor quality as a result of exposure and developing errors. Mischarted information in the antemortem record can also be considered a reconcilable discrepancy. This error often occurs when teeth have been extracted and adjoining teeth have moved into the position of the extraction site. Restorations may be inadvertently indicated on the wrong tooth when the clinician is charting or entering information into the progress record.

Regardless of the difficulties encountered when dental evidence is compared, the final conclusions must be based on an objective analysis of the data presented. The conclusions must be supportable and defensible when they are presented under oath in a court of law.

HITLER'S DENTAL STATUS - 1945

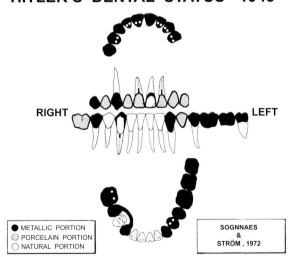

RIGHT   LEFT

● METALLIC PORTION
◐ PORCELAIN PORTION
○ NATURAL PORTION

SOGNNAES
&
STRÖM, 1972

• **Fig. 19.16** Antemortem dental record of Adolph Hitler obtained from his dentist, Dr. Hugo Blaschke, by the Allies at the end of WWII. Note the "telephone bridge." (From Sognnaes RF, Ström F: The odontological identification of Adolf Hitler. Definitive documentation by X-rays, interrogations and autopsy findings, *Acta Odont Scand* 31:43–69, 1973.)

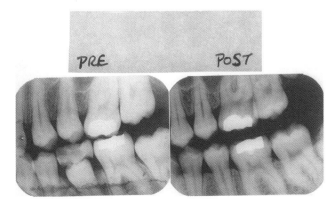

PRE   POST

• **Fig. 19.17** Antemortem and postmortem radiographs demonstrating the fluid, changing nature of dental information.

Dentistry's Role in Multiple (Mass) Fatality Incident Identification

The term *multiple (mass) fatality incident (MFI)* evokes images of a chaotic event, initiated by a destructive force, which results in numerous deaths necessitating identification. These mass disaster events resulting in MFIs can be classified in one of three ways:

1. Natural
2. Accidental
3. Criminal (e.g., serial homicide, mass suicide, and acts of terrorism)

Each type of MFI event results in the death of numerous victims. However, the problems faced by the forensic dental team responsible for identifying the decedents may vary, depending on the type of MFI encountered.

Natural Disasters

Natural MFIs include earthquakes, tornadoes, hurricanes, volcanic eruptions, fire storms, tsunamis, and floods. These may occur over relatively short periods or may be protracted over days or weeks. Victims may be scattered throughout broad areas, extending for miles. In addition, many victims in natural MFI situations may be unknowns who cannot be presumptively identified. Transients, homeless individuals, and tourists who are visiting an area involved in a natural MFI are often difficult to identify. Several countries or states can be affected, as in the 2004 Indian Ocean tsunami event and the 2021 western states forest fires in the United States.

In a natural disaster involving multiple fatalities, the principal problem for the dental identification team is that the environmental infrastructure is often compromised. For example, after the Category 5 Hurricane Katrina in 2005, medical and dental offices and hospital facilities containing antemortem records had been destroyed by tornadic activity and flooding. In addition, communication lines and roads were damaged, preventing the retrieval of most available antemortem records. Concurrently, many bodies from cemeteries in the affected areas were disinterred by the storm. All of these factors compounded, delayed, or precluded the prompt identification of many victims.

Accidents

Accidental MFI events are most often associated with transportation accidents, building fires, industrial and mining accidents, and military accidents. These situations usually occur over short time periods and are associated with defined populations (e.g., airplane, bus, or train passengers; mine, mill, or factory workers; residents in an affected structure).

Airlines maintain passenger logs of individuals who are registered on specific flights. However, it has been estimated that at any given time as many as 10% of air travelers may purchase their tickets using an alias for identification. This occurred among the passengers of Malaysia Airlines Flight MH370 when it was determined that two of the victims of this accident were traveling with stolen passports.

The mining company, mill, or industrial plant can document those who have reported for work. In these examples, the victims of accidents should logically come from the defined population of employees on that shift. Therefore, antemortem records are first solicited from the families and health care providers of these individuals. Another source of medical and dental records in these cases is the occupational health files of workers, which are maintained by the employer.

Problems can be associated with the identification of victims of industrial and military accidents because these populations may be of similar age, sex, and ethnicity. Commonly, individuals working in industrial or military settings wear similar clothing. Thus, military uniforms and protective industrial clothing decrease the potential use of personal recognition as an identification aid in these cases.

Criminal Disasters

Unlike natural and accidental MFIs, criminal situations resulting in multiple deaths may occur over extremely long time periods (years) and wide ranges of territory (e.g., different cities, states, or countries). This was the pattern of the rapes and murders committed by Ted Bundy, whose victims included young women residing in states from Washington to Florida from 1974 to 1978. The remains of the victims of serial killers can be hidden, as in the Green River homicides in the Pacific Northwest and the murders of young men committed by John Wayne Gacy in Chicago. Dismemberment and mutilation of victims is exemplified by the Jeffrey Dahmer case. Dental structures in these situations may not always be available for postmortem review.

Law enforcement agencies are often unaware of the victims of serial killers from other jurisdictions. Each agency may be investigating an individual homicide without recognizing a pattern of broader criminal involvement. Until the development of the FBI-NCIC computer registry, coordinated efforts at identification were hampered.

The rise in national and international terrorism in the 21st century has changed the paradigm associated with the traditional participation of the dental profession in an MFI setting. Until recently, forensic odontologists and other dental professionals were simply tasked as experts in the identification of the decedents. Currently, there are ongoing efforts within organized dentistry to develop effective responses to acts of bioterrorism. These efforts are exemplified by the profession's encouragement of legislation authorizing dental professionals, in federally declared emergencies, to perform various procedures that are routinely not within the practice of the profession. Under these provisions, dentists registered and trained in emerging medical diseases, bioterrorism, and emergency medical care would be indemnified for actions taken in the performance of these humanitarian services.

Acts of terrorism may include exposure to biologic agents, chemical toxins, and the discharge of nuclear devices. Thus, the dentist involved in MFI recovery and identification after an act of terrorism may additionally be required to assist medical workers in providing care for the injured. In these scenarios, dentists must consider their personal safety and that of their families. Civil defense and emergency preparedness organizational plans are beginning to include dentists among those charged with triaging the injured. Additional roles for the dental professional in future acts of bioterrorism and nuclear or chemical attack include providing first aid care and immunizations to injured and exposed survivors.

Responsibilities

In the United States, the National Response Framework (NRF) provides a comprehensive, risk-based, emergency management plan to respond to any hazardous event. The NRF establishes guidelines to manage domestic response to radiological, technical, natural, or terrorist incidents by developing 15 emergency support functions and delineating the agencies charged with performing specific tasks in a response (Table 19.4).

As part of the presidential directive that created the US Department of Homeland Security after the September 11, 2001 terrorist attacks, the National Incident Management System (NIMS) was also developed. The overall objective of this system is coordination of governmental agencies, nongovernmental organizations, and the private sector in the resolution of nationally significant incidents.

Regardless of the type of MFI, the local coroner or ME is ultimately responsible for performing the autopsies and identifying the victims. In accidents that involve modes of public transportation, the National Transportation Safety Board (NTSB) is empowered to investigate and determine the cause of the crash. Other agencies with jurisdiction at a disaster scene may represent local police, public safety, and funeral home personnel. In addition, there may be representatives of the Federal Emergency Management Agency (FEMA), members of the FBI fingerprint team, representatives of the United States Department of Health and Human Services (DHHS) National Disaster Medical System (NDMS) division personnel mobilized with a federal Disaster Mortuary Operational Response Team (DMORT) or Disaster Medical Assistance Team (DMAT), the clergy, and community volunteer organizations.

Although DMORT and DMAT units include dental personnel, these teams may not be mobilized in all MFIs. In these situations, forensic dentists and support staff responsible for identification or care of the injured should also be organized into teams. Several state dental associations (including California, Washington, Michigan, New York, South Carolina, Nevada, and Iowa) have developed,

supplied, and trained such groups in preparation for emergencies requiring their expertise. Training sessions include mock MFI exercises. These drills can prepare the dental team members for dealing with the technical problems of cases involving multiple fatalities.

In addition, training sessions can be used to counsel the dental team and to inform members of the posttraumatic stress often associated with this type of forensic work. This delayed stress is a result of the sensory and psychological insults encountered by the dentist, hygienist, or dental assistant who is dealing with human death on a large scale.

During an MFI the NDMS, under its emergency support functions, is authorized and has responsibility to assist local authorities by establishing temporary morgue facilities; identifying victims using scientific techniques; and processing, preparing, and disposing of victims' remains to families, funeral homes, or proper legal representatives. This mission has been accomplished through the development of ten regional DMORTs administered by the DHHS. Each DMORT is composed of funeral directors, MEs, coroners, pathologists, forensic anthropologists, medical records technicians and transcribers, fingerprint specialists, forensic dentists, dental hygienists, dental assistants, radiology technicians, mental health specialists, computer professionals, administrative support staff, and security and investigative personnel.

These individuals are private citizens, each with a specific field of expertise, who are mobilized during a disaster. The licensure and certification of the DMORT members is recognized by all states because they are considered temporary federal employees during the emergency response.

Working with the authorization of the local coroner or ME, a local dental disaster team or dental component of a federally deployed DMORT is responsible for antemortem record assembly and interpretation, postmortem physical and dental radiographic examination, and final comparison of dental information. These are the same principles used to establish an individual identification. Yet, when numerous victims need to be identified in a short time, problems of identification are compounded exponentially.

No remains have been found for one-third of the 3000 victims who died in the World Trade Center terrorist attack in 2001. Fewer than 300 victims were found intact, although

TABLE 19.4	**Organization of the US National Response Framework**	
US National Response Framework (NRF)		
Emergency Support Functions		
Transportation	Mass Care, Emergency Assistance, Housing, and Human Services	Agriculture and Natural Resources
Communications	Logistics	Energy
Public Works and Engineering	Public Health and Medical Services*	Public Safety and Security
Firefighting	Search and Rescue	Cross-Sector Business and Infrastructure
Information and Planning	Oil and Hazardous Materials Response	External Affairs

*Dental services (including forensics) is included in this section of the NRF.

tens of thousands of fragmentary human remains and personal effects have been recovered and processed through the Staten Island landfill that has been used as a temporary sorting facility. Many of these remains have yet to be linked to a victim.

Dividing the forensic dental team into subsections responsible for each of the three identification domains (antemortem, postmortem, and record comparison) permits a division of labor among the team members. This division reduces errors in identification, in that specific tasks in the identification process are assigned to separate subsections. A chain of command should be established, and the team leader of each shift should be directly responsible to the local coroner or ME. This person is the only member of the team authorized to release the results of the dental identification process to appropriate investigative agencies.

Technologic Aids in Multiple Fatality Incident Analysis

Advances in photographic, radiographic, and computer technology have provided the forensic dental team with additional resources to enable recovery, documentation, storage, and comparison of forensic dental evidence in MFIs, as well as in other situations requiring forensic dental expertise (e.g., bite mark analysis and documentation of human abuse). Among these advances are developments in the following:

- **Digital photography.** The basic digital camera used for forensic evidence documentation should include a through-the-lens (TTL), light-metering, SLR, 35-mm digital camera body with interchangeable lenses or an adjustable lens capable of normal range (30–50 mm) to macro range (90–100 mm) focal length. A removable flash memory card with adequate storage capacity is also required. The Scientific Working Group on Imaging Technology (SWGIT) imaging guidelines provide the forensic odontologist with information regarding the limitations and parameters imposed by the judicial system regarding the manipulation and presentation of digital photographic evidence.
- **Digital radiography (DR) equipment.** Electronically generated and stored radiographic imaging can be accomplished by the following:
  - Scanning normally processed radiographic film into a computer
  - Using a phosphor substrate shaped and used like radiographic film to expose and scan radiographic information into the computer by a special proprietary device
  - Using a sensor sized and shaped like a radiographic film that is made of a scintillation screen and a charge-coupled device (CCD) or complementary metal oxide semiconductor (CMOS)
- **Direct digital radiography (DDR).** When energized by radiation, this device creates a direct image on the pixels of its CCD or CMOS. This radiographic image is then sent to a computer through wire or wireless technology. Thus, because of its ability to save time, DDR technology is recommended for clinical and forensic casework. Additionally, DDR procedures reduce exposure times by

requiring 90% less radiation than that required to expose a standard type D film radiograph and 50% less radiation than that required in exposure of type E film radiographs. The parameters by which the quality of a radiograph is evaluated include resolution and contrast sensitivity. Image resolution describes the detail an image holds. In film-based radiographs, this is expressed as a function of how close lines can be to each other and still be visibly distinguished. Digital imaging measures resolution as pixel counts. The contrast sensitivity is a measure of the smallest percentage change in an object's base thickness (density) that can be detected in a radiograph. The high resolution of the image produced by the DDR sensor is one of its most advantageous properties.

- **Cone-beam computed tomography (CBCT).** CBCT provides a 3D imaging modality to collect a complete maxillo-mandibular-facial anatomic volume of data. Computer software can be used to analyze the obtained image, and the diagnostic interpretation provided can be used for treatment planning, assessment of pathologic conditions, and evaluation of dental implants. Application of CBCT in forensic dental situations can overcome intraoral access problems with some specimens (e.g., fourth-degree burn cases).
- **Portable hand-held X-ray generation devices** (e.g., Kavo Nomad™ Pro 2 Intraoral X-Ray System, Genoray Handheld Portable Dental X-Ray Unit, Rextar X Portable X-Ray Generator, and the MinXray HF 120/60HPPWV PowerPlus™ Portable X-Ray Unit, among others). With these devices, the forensic dentist is able to expose film or digital radiographs quickly and effortlessly with a battery-powered unit that can be carried to the body on the gurney in the morgue. Additional applications for the use of these devices in special care dental settings include exposure of radiographs on pediatric or sedated patients, those having endodontic therapy, or individuals receiving dental treatment in a hospital operating room. These devices have been used in the identification of MFI victims in numerous disasters worldwide. However, they are still not licensed for use by Radiation Safety Boards in every state in the United States.
- **X-ray fluorescence (XRF) methodology.** As discussed previously, analysis of dental materials in cremation and other difficult forensic identification cases may be facilitated by analysis of specimens with this technology.
- **Computer software technology.** The advent of computer software has assisted MFI dental identification teams in filing, storing, sorting, and matching bits of antemortem and postmortem information. Computer assistance has proved beneficial in disasters involving hundreds of victims. Commonly used programs include the following:
  - The FBI-NCIC program, based on the California Dental Identification System, developed by Dr. Norman Sperber and Dr. Robert Siegel (San Diego, CA)
  - CAPMI-4 (Computer-Assisted Postmortem identification—version 4.0), developed by Dr. Lewis

Lorton of the US Army Institute of Dental Research (It was first used in 1985 in support of the Arrow Air-US military charter aviation runway accident in Gander, Newfoundland.)

- WinID3 dental comparison software, developed by Dr. James McGivney (St Louis, MO) (Bridged with the Dexis DR program, WinID3 facilitated comparison of antemortem and postmortem dental records in Hurricane Katrina recovery efforts and various transportation and industrial MFI events.)
- UDIM (UVIS Dental Identification Module), the dental recording/search component of the UVIS system, developed by Dr. Kenneth Aschheim (New York, NY)

Each of these computer software systems is user friendly, can be run on readily available and accessible hardware, is automated and capable of networking, and relies on objective data entry and storage of antemortem and postmortem dental records, digital radiographs, and digital images. The use of these computer software programs in MFI situations reduces the time and effort that had to be expended in past events. Before their use, an examiner in the dental identification team walked along tables with a postmortem record comparing the dental data and radiographs at each station containing an antemortem record.

Despite the fact that these technologic advances have facilitated forensic casework, the caveat for the forensic dentist remains that identification is the result of human thought processes and not the highly technical supportive procedures that provide the material being evaluated. To arrive at correct comparative conclusions based on the evidence, individual dental team members must evaluate the computer-generated matches for definitive identification.

◆ BITE PATTERN EVIDENCE

Basic Principles

A bite mark is a patterned injury or surface disturbance produced by teeth on the skin of an individual or inanimate object. Historically, analysis of this type of evidence presumes that the dentition of the biter (animal or human) is unique (being the only one of its kind) and can be compared scientifically and related to the resultant patterned mark on the surface of a victim or inanimate object. Initial studies indicated the uniqueness of the human dentition. However, because of the similar size and shape of the dental structures among humans, there evolved a debate among forensic odontologists and those in the legal profession related to the ability of these "unique" features to be transferred into skin, which is acknowledged as a poor impression material.

Because it is reasonable to consider the teeth as cutting or mashing tools, the basis for accepting bite pattern evidence can be supported on the same scientific principles used to evaluate tool marks. However, it is now believed that although individual human dentitions may have distinctive features, the patterned marks left by the teeth may not be unique for each person as once thought. Variations in tooth size, wear, fractures, and position in the dental arch, diastemata, and restored surfaces contribute to the principle of distinctiveness within an individual dentition, but not uniqueness among human dentitions.

Thus, issues related to the validity, reliability, and admissibility of bite mark evidence continue to rest with the judicial system and its various rules pertaining to the introduction of scientific evidence in court. The Innocence Project, founded in 1992, has brought significant legal appeals regarding bite mark evidence, which has resulted in this evidence being overturned in several jurisdictions. Because bite mark pattern evidence is often questionable, as of 2020, 26 incarcerated individuals have been released when DNA revealed that bite mark analysis resulted in a wrongful conviction.

Based on these legal decisions and a 2009 report from the National Academy of Sciences critical of this use of bite mark evidence, it has become the most controversial component of the forensic dental discipline. This has resulted in the current philosophy regarding the significance of bite mark evidence resting in its *exculpatory* rather than *inculpatory* power when comparing the dentition of a putative suspect to a bite mark on an inanimate object or bite mark patterned injury (BMPI) in most cases.

Victims of mammalian animal bites account for most bite injuries reported annually. Bite-related injuries represent approximately 1% of all hospital emergency visits that require medical attention. Of these, >1.6 million dog bites were recorded by the National Emergency Department Sample (NEDS) between 2010 and 2014. This represented 26% of all bite-related admissions to emergency rooms in the United States. The second and third most likely mammalian biters are cats and humans, respectively. Each represents from 5% to 20% of cases reporting to urban emergency rooms.

As the habitats of wild animals in North America continue to recede, humans are more likely to come in contact with these dangerous carnivores. This is reflected in the increase in attacks on humans by mountain lions and brown, black, and grizzly bears, resulting in biting injuries or death from biting and clawing. In 2020, the International Shark Attack File (ISAF) of the Florida Museum of Natural History reported 57 unprovoked shark bites on humans and 39 provoked bites worldwide.

Animal bites may be observed postmortem when a body has not been buried or discovered quickly. Commonly, insect bites are made by ants and roaches, which leave patterned injuries that can be mistakenly interpreted as antemortem human BMPIs or trauma (Fig. 19.18). Postmortem bites from rats and scavenging feral and wild dogs and cats are often avulsive and of narrower or smaller diameter than human bites.

Injuries caused by human bites are routinely related to either aggressive or sexual behavior. Ironically, it is not uncommon for the perpetrator of an aggressive act to be bitten by the victim (as a means of self-defense). In children, biting is a form of expression that occurs when verbal communication fails. Biting injuries in children can result from

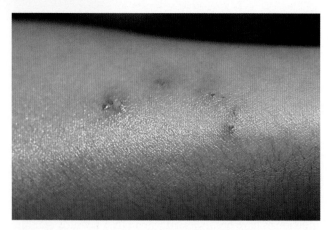

• **Fig. 19.18** Insect bites on the skin that mimic the pattern injury associated with bite mark trauma. In a decedent, this pattern may additionally be mistakenly interpreted as antemortem trauma. (Courtesy of Dr. David K. Ord.)

playground altercations or sports competition and are especially common among 13- to 30-month-old children who attend day care centers. The resultant injuries in this population are usually mild, requiring only washing, cold compresses, and comforting the victim.

Self-inflicted bites are observed in **Lesch-Nyhan syndrome.** This syndrome is an X-linked, recessively transmitted disease manifesting insensitivity to pain and self-mutilation (among other signs) by chewing away the lips. This disease is rare, and self-inflicted bites are more commonly seen in adults and children who are victims of physical abuse or sexual assault. These individuals may bite their own forearms or hands in anguish or to prevent themselves from crying out while they are being traumatized.

Injuries resulting from animal or human bites may become septic or may progress to systemic infections. Secondary bacterial infections are more commonly associated with human bites than with animal bites, although 80% of domestic cat bites become infected because bacteria are injected into the deep puncture wounds inflicted by their needlelike, carnassial teeth. Infectious complications include tetanus, tuberculosis, syphilis, actinomycosis, cat-scratch disease (caused by *Bartonella henselae*), and those infectious complications related to streptococcal and staphylococcal organisms. Anaerobic organisms associated with bite injuries may eventually result in complications, such as osteomyelitis, septic arthritis, tenosynovitis, meningitis, and infections of the lymphatic system.

Viral complications, including hepatitis B virus, herpes simplex, and cytomegalovirus, have resulted from transmission through human bites. The human immunodeficiency virus (HIV) can also potentially be transmitted through the exchange of blood and saliva in a bite injury. The risk of seroconversion from this mode of HIV transmission, however, is believed to be extremely low. An immunocompromised individual who is already infected with the HIV virus is at increased risk of secondary infection when bitten by a cat.

Rabies is the most serious infectious complication that results from mammalian animal bites. Rabid dogs account for approximately 90% of cases worldwide, whereas in the United States bats have become the major cause of rabies related human fatalities. It is often necessary to identify the specific offending animal for rabies control or potential litigation. This identification is not routinely done by matching the animal's teeth to the pattern injury. When humans bite, however, the marks left in injured tissue or inanimate objects are often analyzed and compared with the alleged perpetrator's dentition.

Historical and Legal Issues

References to biting during acts of passion or aggression can be found in the *Bible, Kama Sutra,* and Old English law. In colonial America, the Reverend George Burroughs was charged with the crime of biting one of the women accused of witchcraft during the Salem, Massachusetts witch hunt incidents in 1692. He was hanged for this offense. Bite mark evidence was provided in expert dental testimony in the 1870 Ohio trial of Ansil L. Robinson, who was accused of murdering his mistress. Although the defendant was eventually acquitted, the expert dental presentation by Dr. Jonathan Taft regarding the pattern injury on the victim's arm became a benchmark for future experts in the discipline.

The concept of accepting evidence related to the analysis of patterns created by the dentition was first accepted by the appellate level courts of the United States justice system in 1954. At that time, *Doyle vs State of Texas* became the first modern case in which a criminal conviction was based on evidence relating a suspect's dentition to pattern marks in an inanimate object (a piece of cheese). Because of the *Doyle* case, more than 260 decisions involving bite mark evidence have been entered into the case law records of the appellate courts of the United States.

The legal community has recognized tool mark and fingerprint pattern analysis as scientifically acceptable forensic disciplines for some time. The evidence presented by experts in these areas has been accepted in 20% of state courts under the *Frye* standard *(Frye vs United States),* and the remaining 80% of state courts and all federal courts under the Federal Rules of Evidence 702–705. These are special rules dealing with the admissibility of scientific evidence in the American judicial system. Thus, they are also applicable to bite mark information.

The *Frye* test had been the standard for scientific admissibility or acceptance in most state and federal courts since 1923. The three components of scientific evidence admissibility that are considered under the *Frye* test include the following:
1. The scientific principle must be recognizable.
2. The scientific principle must be sufficiently established.
3. The scientific principle must have gained general acceptance within the scientific discipline to which it belongs.

Among the three requirements, only the concept of "general acceptance" must be met to satisfy the *Frye* test of admissibility.

Evidentiary use of genomic DNA profiling has undermined the general acceptance of bite mark evidence although according to Forensic Science Reform, there is "inordinate resistance (by the legal community) to create fair pathways towards exoneration because of its systemic structure of 'Stare Decisis' and its resistance to correct mistakes in both its own system and the forensic science communities." *Stare Decisis* is the legal doctrine which bases current court decisions regarding an issue on prior rulings concerning the same issue. Therefore, courts in the United States have been hesitant to rule against the "general acceptance" of bite mark evidence as scientific in recent legal decisions.

In 2013, Texas legislators passed the Texas Junk Science Law (SB 344). This legislation provides prisoners the right to challenge their conviction due to any uncertainty related to forensic science evidence used to obtain the conviction (e.g., fingerprint, bite mark, blood splatter, shoe print, tire track patterns, etc.).

In 1993, the US Supreme Court ruled on the admissibility of scientific evidence in *Daubert vs Merrell Dow Pharmaceuticals*. It was the Court's decision in this case that the general acceptance aspect of the *Frye* test should no longer be the sole, determining factor used in considering admissibility of scientific evidence. Essentially, the Court replaced this principle with one that stresses scientific validity. This decision removes the responsibility of determining sound scientific evidence from the scientific community in which it has gained general acceptance.

Instead, the *Daubert* ruling gives great latitude to the trial judge in considering the admissibility of scientific evidence. Trial judges often have limited knowledge of scientific methodology; however, under *Daubert* they are required to determine if the weight and admissibility of expert testimony is not only scientifically valid but also relevant and germane to the issues in individual cases. Thus, the results of the Supreme Court's decision in *Daubert* are to make the judge a "gatekeeper" to ensure that the expert witness is providing scientifically valid evidence.

The "general acceptance" concept is no longer the sole determinant of admissibility in *Daubert*. It becomes one of several factors that must be met for scientific evidence to be admissible. These factors include the following:
- Techniques used must be testable and tested.
  - Peer review and publication of results are not required but may persuade the judge in admitting evidence.
  - Standards should be established for evaluation of the scientific methods and error rates associated with the techniques used.
  - Consideration is given to acceptance of scientific principles that have gained general acceptance within the scientific discipline to which they belong.

Bite mark evidence is currently admissible under the *Frye* standard and Federal Rules of Evidence as determined by the *Daubert* decision. Although some legal experts believe the Federal Rules of Evidence provide better guidelines for admissibility decisions, challenges to the scientific basis of bite mark evidence may be averted under either set of standards. Currently, this evidence is used more routinely in an *exculpatory* manner to exclude rather than include a suspect as the perpetrator.

Characteristics of Bite Marks

To evaluate a patterned mark, its characteristics must be recognizable and distinguishable. Reasonably, the mark should be consistent with the face of the instrument from which it was generated. Specific teeth can create representative patterns that are recognizable. These are described as individual characteristics of the entire bite mark. Human incisors make rectangular marks. Depending on the amount of attrition observed on the incisal edges of cuspids, these surfaces may be associated with point or triangular patterns. Unlike mandibular bicuspid teeth, which have a diminutive lingual cusp, maxillary bicuspids often mark in a pattern that resembles a "figure eight."

Class characteristics of a human bite mark are related to the shapes that are created when groups of teeth from both dental arches are impressed into a bitten surface. Semicircular, ovoid, or elliptical patterns are usually observed, but variations may be associated with tapered, square, and U-shaped arches. Typically, bite marks are composed of two arc-shaped areas corresponding to the maxillary and mandibular arches and their respective teeth. When only one arch contacts a surface, a crescent pattern may be formed. The greatest dimensions of an adult human bite mark do not usually exceed 4 cm (Fig. 19.19).

Individual and class characteristics of bite patterns are generated by groups of specific teeth. The dynamics of occlusion and muscle function must also be accounted for when variations in individual and class characteristics of a bite mark are considered. Such variations can be caused by malocclusion, individual tooth mobility associated with periodontal disease, and movement of facial muscles during biting. Class II malocclusion can cause the palatal surfaces of the maxillary anterior teeth, rather than their incisal edges, to contact the material being bitten. Shield-like imprints of the palatal surfaces are generated in the bite mark rather than the rectangular patterns routinely associated with these teeth.

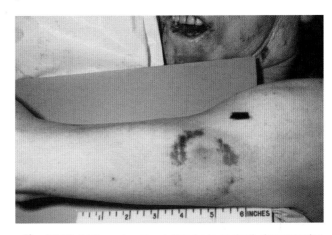

• **Fig. 19.19** A bite mark pattern inflicted prior to death demonstrating the individual and class characteristics associated with impressions made by the human dentition. An ecchymotic area in the center of the ovoid pattern is observed, which is not always related to the sucking action of a sexual bite. Therefore, this finding should not be over-interpreted to imply sexual intent on the part of the biter. The impressions made by the teeth of the mandibular arch are more delicate.

Aberrant muscle forces associated with tongue thrusting can alter the way the teeth contact a bitten surface. Temporomandibular joint dysfunction can also contribute to variations in bite patterns. It can be associated with midline shifts or inability to achieve maximum opening while biting. Periodontal disease may result in individual tooth mobility, which could affect the bite mark pattern.

When bitten, many inanimate objects tend to act like dental-impression material, retaining the marks of the teeth. Such cases have involved bite marks in foods, chewing gum, paper toweling, and a roll of masking tape. Unlike inanimate material, the skin is a dynamic tissue that can change after it is injured. Swelling, caused by the acute inflammatory response of the tissue, can distort and affect the interpretation of the pattern. Bleeding into the area of a bite mark can mask the pattern.

The age of an injury is the time elapsed from its infliction to the analysis of the damaged tissue. Reliable determination of the age of antemortem skin injuries requires histopathologic and histochemical analysis to relate the injury to the time of the alleged incident (Table 19.5). Color changes in the bitten tissue, associated with the degradation of hemoglobin from lysed RBCs, can be used only to broadly estimate the time of occurrence and qualify the age of a bruise as recent or old. Environmental factors, including seasonal temperature, location of the body, and presence or absence of clothing, may additionally act as important variables requiring consideration when attempting to determine the age of injury patterns.

Contusions and areas of ecchymosis are not unusual in bite marks made in living tissue. The absence of bleeding into the injury may imply that it was inflicted after death. Additional postmortem soft tissue changes that can affect the quality of a bite pattern injury and its eventual weight as evidence include artifacts created by lividity (caused by the settling of blood pigments in dependent body areas), decomposition, and embalming.

Bite marks from sexual attacks are commonly found on the neck, breasts, arms, buttocks, genitalia, and thighs. Axillary bites and bite patterns on the back, shoulder, penis, and scrotum are often associated with homosexual activity. Abused children may be bitten in areas of the face, particularly the cheek, ear, and nose. Assailants also can be bitten. The analysis of these bite pattern injuries may be just as incriminating as those found on the victim of a violent act.

A review of 778 bite mark injuries concerning the anatomic locations most often bitten, victim and biter demographics, the type of crimes in which biting occurred, and legal disposition of cases revealed the following information:
- Females were bitten more often than males.
- Perpetrators were male more often than female.
- The most common sites bitten were the arms. Bites in these locations occurred more commonly among males.
- Females were bitten on the breast more often than males. This location accounted for the second most commonly bitten area of the body.
- The type of crime and the age of the victim were related to patterns in location, distribution, and number of bites.

Guidelines for Bite Mark Analysis

In 1984, the American Board of Forensic Odontology (ABFO) established Guidelines for Bite Mark Analysis. Additional workshops of the Board have provided further insight into the techniques available to recover, store, analyze and evaluate bite mark evidence based on the Guidelines. The development of the Guidelines also created a scientific approach to the description of the bite mark, collection of evidence from suspect and victim, and subsequent analysis of the evidence.

The Guidelines do not mandate specific analytic methods for comparison. Through their careful use, however, the

TABLE 19.5	Histopathologic and Clinical Changes Used to Monitor the Time Elapsed (Aging) in Skin Injuries Associated With Bite Marks			
Time	**Predominant Cellular Infiltrate and Deposits**	**Healing**	**Variable Clinical Color**
Hours			
4–8	Polymorphonuclear leukocytes with a peripheral front		Red-blue-purple
12	Polymorphonuclear leukocytes		
16–24	Macrophages peak		Blue-black
24–36	Polymorphonuclear leukocytes peak	Peripheral fibroblasts	
Days			
1–3	Central necrosis		
3+	Hemosiderin		Green-blue
4		Collagen fibers	
4–5		Capillary growth	Brown-yellow-green
6		Lymphocytes peak at periphery	
10–14		Granulation tissue	Tan-yellow

quality of the investigation and conclusions based on bite mark evidence follow customary procedures. Thus, with these guidelines, it should be possible to determine the weight of bite mark evidence required to establish the validity of bite mark comparison. According to the current Guidelines, *bite mark, suggestive of a bite mark,* and *not a bite mark* are the terms used to indicate the confidence level of the odontologist that a patterned mark represents a bite mark.

Description of the Bite Mark

Demographic information (i.e., age, ethnicity, sex, and name of the victim; examination date; referring agency; case number) is obtained in cases involving both living and deceased victims. The names of the forensic dental examiner and referring agency contact person should also be included.

The location of the bite is then described. Attention is directed to the anatomic location, surface contour, and tissue characteristics of the bitten area. Underlying structures, such as bone or fat, may influence the analytic quality of the pattern injury. Relative skin mobility is also evaluated.

The shape, color, size, and type of injury are recorded. Metric measurements of the horizontal and vertical dimensions of the bite mark are determined. Irregularities and variations from the standard semicircular, ovoid, and crescent shapes associated with human bite marks are noted. Injury types include abrasion, laceration, ecchymotic and petechial hemorrhage, incision, and avulsion. Artifactual injuries, such as proximate stab and bullet wounds, should be recorded because these may distort the pattern by separating anatomic cleavage lines of the skin **(Langer lines)**.

Evidence Collection

Examination of the Victim and the Suspect

Both the victim and the suspect are examined, and evidence from each is gathered for comparative study and evaluation. Collection of evidence must be performed in a manner that protects the rights of the person who is providing the evidence and that permits the eventual acceptance of the evidence in court. Therefore, to ensure objective analysis, it is recommended that dental impressions, photographs, and demographic information obtained from the putative suspected biter be collected by a dentist other than the odontologist making the comparison.

A standard health history and informed consent are obtained before any evidence recovery procedure regarding the suspect is performed. An intraoral and extraoral examination of the suspect is completed, which includes dental charting, soft tissue and tongue evaluation, and probing of the periodontium. Therefore, knowledge of the medical history of the suspect relative to systemic problems associated with cardiovascular disease, allergy, seizure disorder, diabetes, and respiratory disease or requirements for antibiotic prophylaxis has medicolegal importance in forensic casework, as well as in traditional patient evaluation.

A search warrant, court order, or legal consent may be required before evidence is collected from a suspect. A specific list of the dental-related evidence desired should be recorded in the legal document. This list usually includes facial and oral photographs, impressions of the teeth, occlusal registrations and bite exemplars, and saliva samples. These documents protect the rights of the suspect against unreasonable search and seizure and provide for due process, as guaranteed by the Fourth and Fourteenth Amendments, respectively, to the US Constitution.

Bite marks are considered similar to such physical evidence as fingerprints, hair, blood, and semen samples, as well as to sobriety tests. Therefore, this material is not protected under provisions of the Fifth Amendment, which deals with self-incrimination.

Evidence collection from the victim entails non-invasive and invasive techniques. The former includes photography, saliva trace evidence collection, fabrication of study casts of the bite mark, and stereolithography (SLA) to create 3D models of the BMPI. The latter may involve tissue incision, excision, and preservation of a BMPI in a decedent. Preservation of this tissue permits analysis of the injury by transillumination and observation of the area from the side opposite the light source.

Photography

Because evidence associated with bite marks, human abuse, and sexual and physical assault is transitory, there is an immediacy associated with the collection of physical evidence in these cases. Initial photographs of the pattern mark should be taken before any investigative procedures that may alter the pristine bite mark evidence (e.g., touching, removing, impressing, swabbing, and cleansing).

Ideally, standard visible light photographic techniques include the use of a 35-mm DSLR camera with a flat-field macro lens and dedicated electronic flash. Numerous images using different camera and lighting positions, exposure settings, and color and black-and-white exposures should be obtained. Additional legal considerations and protocols related to the documentation of image enhancement, restoration, compression, and analysis have been established for digital bite mark images.

Orientation positions and close-up views with a reference scale are required. A reference scale permits the bite mark images to be measured and prepared as life-size (i.e., 1:1) representations of the pattern injury. Ultimately, these images can then be compared with casts and other exemplars obtained from the suspect. The scale should be stabilized and positioned next to, and in the same plane as, the bite mark to eliminate potential distortion artifacts in the resultant images. It should never be hand-held. The scale should be omitted from at least one image to document that no marks or other injuries have been intentionally hidden by it.

The ABFO No. 2 photomacrographic reference scale (Lightning Powder Company, Inc.; Salem, OR) was developed by the ABFO for use in bite mark photography (Fig. 19.20). This standardized, L-shaped, rigid, accurate scale has become the gold standard in bite mark photographic analysis. Variations of it have eventually come to be used in all varieties of forensic casework requiring accurate measurement of evidence at crime scenes or in the laboratory (e.g., analysis of shoe print, tire track, and blood splatter patterns).

This nonflexible instrument contains two metric scales, an 18% color gray scale, three circular symbols, and rectifying grids. Each of these components is used to account for photographic distortions, which can negate the value of the photographic evidence. Techniques using Adobe Photoshop and Mideo Systems CASEWORKSeis computer software have been used to rectify distortions observed in the ABFO No. 2 reference scale and ultimately to eliminate these from a bite mark image being analyzed.

With living victims, serial pictures of the BMPI are taken over several days. This series provides documentation of the color changes associated with healing and age of the wound. In addition, special advanced photographic techniques, using nonvisible energy sources at the extremes of the electromagnetic spectrum and fluorescent alternative light sources, can be used to identify latent images of the teeth that may remain after the bite mark has clinically disappeared. These techniques require special films and illumination sources, bracketing of aperture (f-stop) openings, variations in shutter speeds, and/or lens filters to work within the desired wavelengths and include the following (Table 19.6):

- **Reflective ultraviolet (UV) photography.** This technique enhances the bite mark image by selectively identifying photoactive **chromophores,** such as melanin and hemoglobin pigment in the superficial layers of the injured tissue. Variations in the amount of these natural light–absorbing organic pigments in the traumatized tissue are observable in images exposed with this energy source. This is based on the fluorescence created when the skin is exposed to UV light in the 200–400-nm wavelength range. Although there may be focusing problems associated with UV photography and exposures *must* be made with a tripod-mounted camera, the fact that this technique may permit recovery of latent evidence, even months after all clinical signs of a bite mark injury have disappeared, makes the effort worthwhile.
- **Infrared (IR) photography.** Tungsten lamps and quartz-halogen lamps are good sources of IR radiation when attempting to expose IR images from unfiltered light sources. To expose images specifically within the IR wavelengths of 750–1000 nm, a filter must be placed in front of the lens to absorb visible light. The Kodak 87 gel filter accomplishes this task by limiting all transmittance of

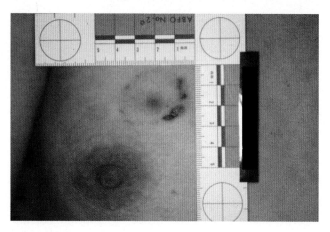

• **Fig. 19.20** The American Board of Forensic Odontology (ABFO) No. 2 Reference Scale.

TABLE 19.6	Comparison of Photographic Electromagnetic Energy Spectrum Sources and Their Forensic Imaging Capabilities			
	Visible Light	Ultraviolet Light	Infrared Light	Alternate Light Imaging Fluorescence
Light wavelength	400–700 nm	200–400 nm	700–1000 nm	450 nm
Filter	None	Kodak Wratten Filter No. 18A gel (visibly opaque glass filter)	Kodak Gel 87	Kodak Gel 15
Target Pigment or Material				
Hemoglobin in pattern injuries and vessels	+	+	+	+
Melanin	+	+		+
Tattoos	+	+	+	+
Ink variations in document forgeries			+	+
Gunshot residues			+	+
Latent fingerprints				+
Serologic fluids (saliva, semen, and blood)				+
Residual fibers				+

light except at the designated wavelengths. Additionally, IR photography requires that the camera lens be refocused (focus shift) after initial focusing under visible light and before exposure of the image. Like alternate light source photography, the focal plane for IR photography lies below the skin surface. The deeper focal depth permits visualization of faded tattoos and wound damage within a blood stain. This technique is not the best for identifying individual characteristics in bite mark injuries.

- **Alternate light source (alternate light imaging [ALI]) photography.** This technique is also referred to as *fluorescent photography.* It is advantageous in assisting investigators to locate and document evidence involving the presence of ink residues, fingerprint patterns, and the chromophores previously indicated. ALI enhances visualization of pigments derived from chromophores that may be found within evidence involving latent serologic fluids and subdermal bruises or pattern injuries of victims of violent or sexual crimes. ALI techniques illuminate deeper tissue targets by using a predominantly monochromatic band of light between the wavelengths of 430 and 460 nm. To accomplish the visualization of the weak fluorescent glow from the desired pigments, ALI photography must be performed by eliminating all other sources of light from striking the imaging surface (film or digital sensor). This requires that ALI techniques be performed in total darkness with yellow filters, such as the Kodak gelatin No. 15. Because longer exposure times are also required, images exposed using ALI *must* be made with a tripod-mounted camera.

As previously stated, photographs of the suspect should involve the same attention to technical quality control. Extraoral, intraoral, and occlusal photographs are taken. Additional images of wax or acrylic test bites and measurements of maximum interincisal opening are also recorded.

Saliva Evidence

Although the forensic dentist is concerned principally with the analysis of the physical evidence associated with a bite mark, biologic evidence in the form of serologic and DNA material is also of probative importance. To ensure that the DNA sample has not been contaminated, collection of saliva trace evidence from the surface of the bite injury of the victim is performed before other evidence-gathering manipulation of the injury. There is an increase in the yield of recovered DNA for analysis when this procedure is carried out according to the two-swab protocol described previously.

Using this technique, a saliva sample is collected by first rubbing the bitten area with a cotton swab that has been moistened in sterile, distilled water. The swab should contain no preservatives. The bite mark is subsequently rolled with a second, dry, cotton swab. Both samples can be considered a single exhibit because they have been collected from the center of the pattern injury. They are placed in an evidence box and permitted to air-dry before submission to the laboratory. No control swabs are required from adjacent areas of the victim's skin.

DNA from the victim of a BMPI should be obtained from whole blood samples or buccal swabs. Additionally, autopsy tissue samples can be obtained from decedent victims. All samples can be used for DNA comparison with bodily fluid or tissue samples obtained from the suspect.

Because a victim may be bitten through the clothing, areas of garments that approximate a BMPI should also be retained and evaluated for saliva. Many victims of sexual abuse wash the area of a bite mark before reporting for treatment. This is unfortunate because biologic evidence associated with DNA recovery can be lost. In this regard, emergency room personnel should be trained to recognize potential BMPIs and be instructed not to wash or disinfect these areas until saliva evidence can be obtained.

Impressions and Study Casts

When a bite injury exhibits indentations that can be related to the dentition of an alleged biter, accurate, 3D, life-size exemplars (casts) can be obtained from molds of the area. Dental impression materials are used to create the molds that are then reinforced to prevent dimensional changes and distortions.

The Guidelines for Bite Mark Analysis deliberately do not dictate which impression materials should be used to create exemplars of a bite mark. Low- and medium-viscosity vinyl polysiloxane (VPS) impression materials are dimensionally stable, meet American Dental Association specifications, and are all acceptable. Hydrocolloid, polysulfide, polyether, and alginate materials are not recommended because of problems associated with long-term stability.

Orthopedic cast materials, heavy-body VPS materials, and non-exothermic resins have been used to create the rigid, stable trays for bite mark impressions. All impression trays and study casts should be appropriately labeled with demographic information for the specific case. Additionally, anatomic direction markers should be added to the impression tray before its removal from the skin surface. This will ensure that the impression is correctly oriented relative to the actual pattern injury.

Original impression trays and study casts are retained for eventual presentation in court. Working casts and models should be duplicated from the original impression or master casts. It is recommended that master casts be poured in type IV stone, according to the manufacturer's specifications, and that these casts remain pristine.

Tissue Samples

Tissue samples of a bite mark can be retained from decedents. With the permission of the ME or coroner, the epidermis, dermis, and underlying muscle and adipose tissue can be removed for transillumination analysis. Before excision, an acrylic ring or stent must be secured within 1 inch of the borders of the injured tissue sample. The ring or stent prevents shrinkage and distortion of the specimen when it is placed into a 4% formalin solution for fixation. The acrylic material is bound to the skin surface with cyanoacrylate and sutures (Fig. 19.21). These tissue samples can be transilluminated by backlighting. This process permits observation of the pattern

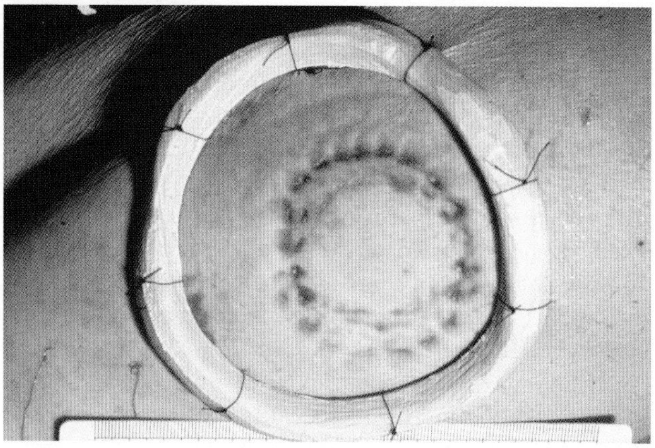

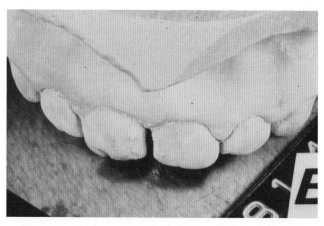

• **Fig. 19.21** An experimental bite pattern injury on a cadaver. This bite mark has had an acrylic stent glued and sutured around its circumference before dissection and fixation in 4% formalin. (Courtesy of Dr. E. Steven Smith.)

• **Fig. 19.22** An overlay of the maxillary cast of a suspect's dentition on a photograph of a bite pattern injury. Note the diastema between the central incisor teeth. The distal incisal surfaces of the lateral incisor teeth are not in the plane of occlusion.

injury in the bruised skin by a manner that is not possible when the tissue is *in situ*.

Evidence Analysis and Comparison

The responsibility of comparing the photographs of the bite pattern injury with the dentition of the suspect rests with the forensic dentist. As an expert in the analysis of these patterns, this person objectively evaluates the evidence. The forensic dentist first determines whether the pattern is truly a result of biting or whether it is an artifact. Patterns of blood splatter around a wound, other tool marks, or insect artifacts unrelated to the teeth may be mistaken for bite marks in photographs provided for evaluation by crime scene investigators, police, and emergency room or autopsy personnel.

Once it is established that the pattern is related to the teeth, it can be compared to the dentition of the suspect for *inclusionary* or *exclusionary* purposes. An expert opinion is then made according to the results of the relationship of the bite pattern and suspect's teeth. According to the ABFO Guidelines for Investigative and Final Bite Mark Reports, *the biter, the probable biter, not excluded as the biter, excluded as the biter,* and *inconclusive* are the terms used to indicate the confidence level of the odontologist that the dentition of the putative suspect is concordant with a bite patterned mark observed on an inanimate object or victim.

To accomplish these goals, the dentist uses numerous methods that have been accepted in the courts. Images of the bite mark and the teeth can be digitized in a computer. This information can then be enhanced and subsequently overlaid for matching purposes.

Historically, a clear overlay of the chewing surfaces of the teeth was made by simply tracing these surfaces on a sheet of transparent acetate. Placing the incisal edges of the study casts on the glass of an office photocopier and duplicating on special paper achieved the same end. A similar effect was obtained by placing an opaque powder, such as barium sulfate, into wax or acrylic test bites and by obtaining radiographs of these exemplars. All of these overlays were then superimposed over the bite mark for comparison.

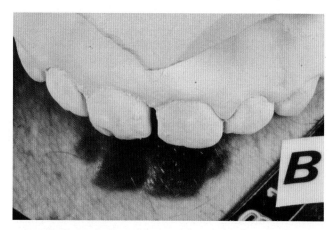

• **Fig. 19.23** A repositioned overlay of the maxillary cast of a suspect's dentition on a photograph of a bite pattern injury (same case as depicted in Fig. 19.22). The drag marks, diastema space, and mesial contact points of the lateral incisor teeth become apparent in the pattern. (From Nuckles DB, Herschaft EE, Whatmough LN: Forensic odontology in solving crimes: dental techniques and bite-mark evidence, *Gen Dent* 42:210–214, 1994. Published with permission by the Academy of General Dentistry. © 1994 by the Academy of General Dentistry. All rights reserved.)

Studies indicate that there are limitations to the accuracy of these potentially subjective, biased overlay techniques and it has been suggested that hand-traced overlay methods be discontinued. Additionally, a stone cast exemplar of the dentition of a suspect has been placed over a 1:1 image of a BMPI for comparison (Figs. 19.22 and 19.23). This method of comparison may have limitations as well considering that current computer based technology, intended to assist the odontologist more objectively in bite mark casework, also may possess foundational constraints.

Presently, images of the bite mark and the incisal edges of the teeth of the suspect are routinely digitized and computer-generated hollow volume overlays are fabricated, enhanced, and subsequently compared using Adobe Photoshop or other graphics editing programs (Fig. 19.24).

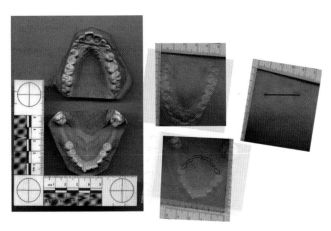

• **Fig. 19.24** On the left side, dental casts of an alleged suspect are being scanned and scaled to 1:1 before digitizing their image. The right half of the illustration shows three photographs of bite marks on the victim. Transparent overlays of the teeth of the alleged suspect have been digitally superimposed over 1:1 digital images of the victim's bite mark using a software program developed by Mideo Systems, Inc. (Huntington Beach, CA). (Courtesy of Dr. David K. Ord.)

In court, bite mark evidence must be able to withstand legal challenges based on its scientific validity and the credibility of the expert witness who presents the evidence. This is true regardless of the techniques used to retrieve, compare, and determine a conclusion based on the evidence. When the Guidelines for Bite Mark Analysis are used, such challenges can be minimized.

◆ HUMAN ABUSE

Epidemiology and Classification

Dental professionals are likely to encounter more victims of physical, neglective, sexual, and psychological abuse as the scope of the problems associated with violent human behavior become more recognized and openly discussed. Currently in the United States, statistics reveal more than 3.5 million cases of child abuse were investigated in 2018. Of these, almost 700,000 were confirmed to be victims of abuse or neglect. This figure represents approximately 1% of all children in the United States. In addition, 1809 cases of child abuse in 2019 resulted in death.

A 2017 report indicated that, worldwide, approximately 1 in 6 people (16%) 60 years of age and older had their human rights violated through the following forms of abuse:

- Physical
- Sexual
- Psychological and emotional
- Financial and material
- Abandonment
- Neglect
- Serious loss of dignity and respect.

In the United States, more than 10 million adult victims experience intimate partner violence (IPV) annually. This represents one incident of IPV occurring every three seconds.

Child abuse is the non-accidental, physical, mental, emotional, or sexual trauma; exploitation; or neglect endured by a child younger than 18 years of age while under the care of a responsible person, such as a parent, sibling, babysitter, teacher, or other person acting *in loco parentis.* The latter term refers to "the legal responsibility of a person or organization to take on some of the functions and responsibilities of a parent."

Elder abuse and abuse of the disabled are similar in all regards to child abuse, except that they deal with geriatric victims or individuals who are physically and/or mentally impaired or disabled. These populations often require special care or have been institutionalized. Staff members in facilities where these patients reside may perpetrate this form of human abuse on occupants.

Victims of IPV are unique and differ from those of child, elder, or disabled abuse because they often have autonomy to choose their circumstances. It is estimated that 1 in 4 women and 1 in 10 men have experienced sexual, physical violence, and/or stalking by an intimate partner. However, unlike the abused child, or geriatric or disabled resident in a nursing home, an abused intimate partner can make choices to leave the traumatic, violent environment. However, many do not and remain committed to the relationship!

The National Child Abuse and Neglect Data System (NCANDS) is a federally sponsored program directed by the Department of Health and Human Services to collect and analyze annual data on child abuse and neglect. Recognizing the global problem, in 2020 the World Health Organization (WHO) released a *Global Status Report on Preventing Violence Against Children.* This document addresses violence against children in the home, school, workplace, community, and other settings. The project is a comprehensive, global study conducted by the WHO on all forms of violence against children (Box 19.2).

More than 200 million girls between infancy and age 15, and women have undergone some form of female genital mutilation (FGM), which has no health benefits. Cutting and partial or total removal of external female genitalia or other injury to the female genital organs occurs principally in African, Middle Eastern, and Asian countries.

It is estimated that 218 million children between the ages of 5 and 17 years old are employed. Among these, 160 million are child labor or child slavery victims required to perform hazardous work. This represents an increase of 8.4 million child labor victims since 2016. Boys are more likely to be involved and, worldwide, agricultural production accounts for the largest number of children employed. Over 40 million individuals have been forced into prostitution and pornography, and 10 million children were victims of human trafficking.

Victims and their abusers come from all ethnic, religious, socioeconomic, and educational backgrounds. Reports concerning the distribution of cases among the different types of abuse vary widely. Up to 70% of child abuse cases may be the result of physical trauma. Some studies relate 15%–25% of the cases to sexual abuse and 50% to neglect. Neglective abuse is subclassified by the caretaker's neglect of the child's

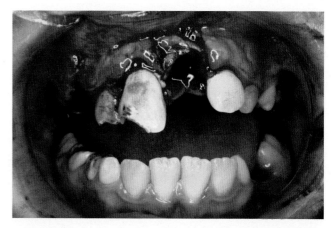

• **Fig. 19.25** An avulsed tooth, a fractured tooth, and a torn labial frenum associated with oral facial injuries in physical child abuse.

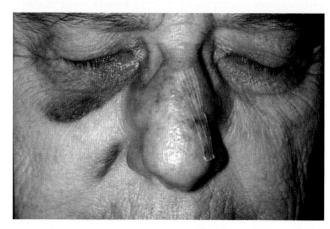

• **Fig. 19.26** Bilateral periorbital ecchymoses (raccoon mask) and fractured nasal bone in a 77-year-old white female victim of physical elder abuse. (Courtesy of Dr. John D. McDowell.)

medical, dental, and safety needs; physical well-being; or education.

Intentional drugging or poisoning and failure to thrive are additional types of maltreatment classified as abusive. Munchausen syndrome by proxy is a form of child abuse in which the caregiver intentionally overstates, contrives, and/or creates a physical, emotional, or behavioral problem in the child. The victim is made to appear sick or is harmed in some other way to deceive health care professionals and others in order to gain attention and sympathy for the caregiver.

It should be recalled that there are numerous metabolic, cutaneous, and congenital diseases that may mimic the signs and symptoms associated with child abuse. These include hemophilia, various vitamin deficiencies, Ehlers-Danlos syndrome, incontinentia pigmenti, Fanconi syndrome, and osteogenesis imperfecta among others.

Many abusive individuals were themselves abused as children. Criminal charges are often lodged against an abusing caretaker. It is recognized, however, that counseling and psychological and emotional support can also help to stabilize a violent, dysfunctional family unit.

Signs and Symptoms

Regardless of the overall statistical variations in subclassification of the problem of abuse, the dentist is most likely to encounter physical and sexual abuse, as well as health care and safety neglect among pediatric, older adult, and disabled dental patients. Of the children and older adults who are physically abused, 50% manifest orofacial and scalp injuries

(Figs. 19.25 and 19.26). These unexplained injuries are inappropriately reported by the caretaker or are inconsistent with the history provided. Abusive trauma to the face, mouth and skull includes the following:

- Laceration of the labial or lingual frenum, which results from a blow to the lip or forceful feeding
- Repeated fracture or the avulsion of teeth
- Zygomatic arch and nasal fractures
- Bilateral contusions of the lip commissures from the placement of a gag
- Bilateral periorbital ecchymoses (raccoon mask)
- Mastoid ecchymosis (Battle sign) indicating fracture of the middle cranial fossa and related traumatic brain injury (Fig. 19.27)
- Traumatic alopecia secondary to grabbing the head hair of the victim while throwing them.

Pattern injuries can be associated with the semicircular or crescent shape of bite marks. Other instruments that contact the skin may leave parallel linear patterns; these include injuries made by a hanger, strap, belt, or ruler. Multiple parallel lines are associated with finger marks after an open-handed slap. Multiple circular, punched out, or ulcerated areas are caused by intentional burning with a cigarette or cigar. Loop patterns are created by electrical cord, rope, and wire (Figs. 19.28 and 19.29).

Other characteristics of child and elder abuse injuries are related to their multiplicity and repetitive nature. They often

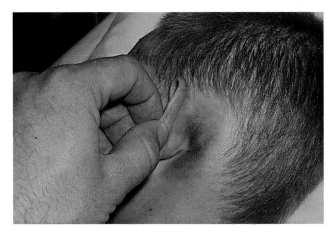

• **Fig. 19.27** Battle sign—mastoid ecchymosis.

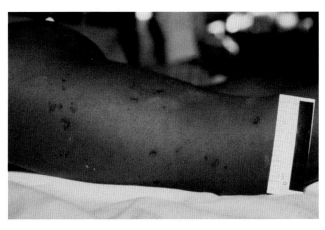

• **Fig. 19.28** Multiple circular ulcerated injuries are associated with intentional burns from a cigarette. When a child is accidentally burned by a cigarette, only one elliptic ulcer is observed.

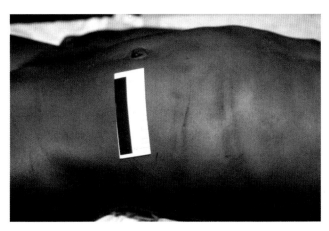

• **Fig. 19.29** Parallel linear ("railroad track") patterns are associated with blows to the skin with such straight-edged objects as a belt, a hanger, an electrical cord, and a ruler.

appear in various stages of resolution. Some injuries are acute; others are healing or even scarred. Therefore, the dentist should examine the skin of the pediatric, geriatric, or disabled dental patient. Suspicion of abuse is increased when the child or older patient appears overdressed for seasonal conditions; overdressing may be an attempt to mask or hide the physical signs of abuse.

By adulthood, 10% of men and 25% of women are the victims of sexual abuse. Oral infections associated with sexually transmitted diseases (STDs) are obviously signs of sexual abuse when they are observed in a minor. Erythematous or petechial lesions of the palate or ulceration of the sublingual area should be noted because these findings can result from the physical trauma associated with performing fellatio or cunnilingus (see page 297).

Among siblings, nursing or "baby bottle caries" is a sign of neglective abuse and indicates the caretaker's inattention to the dental needs of the children. When infants and toddlers are placed to bed with a nursing bottle filled with cariogenic solutions (e.g., milk, soft drinks, and sweet juices), the maxillary incisors are bathed in the sugary solution and can manifest severe caries. The mandibular teeth, protected from the cariogenic material by the position of the tongue and nipple during sucking, are spared the destructive effects, and the child takes on the appearance of a pseudoprognathism or pseudo-Class III malocclusion (Fig. 19.30).

The dentist may become aware of other abusive behavior directed to a child or older patient by a responsible caretaker. Abusive behavior can involve refusal or delay in seeking treatment for serious medical or dental problems, abandonment, refusal to cooperate with planned treatment, and failure to return to the same physician or dentist for treatment.

Role of Dentistry in Recognizing and Reporting Human Abuse

Awareness of the signs and symptoms of abuse among individuals of all ages should be a goal for every dentist. As a component of the dental relicensure process, the state of New

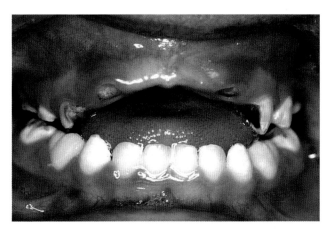

• **Fig. 19.30** Pseudoprognathism or pseudo-Class III malocclusion observed in a neglected child with nursing bottle (baby bottle) decay. (Courtesy of Dr. Cynthia Hipp.)

York requires documentation of continuing education credits in the area of child abuse recognition and the dental professional's responsibility to report such cases.

By statute, all states require that dental personnel, other health care professionals, teachers, and day care and nursing home employees report suspected cases of child and elder abuse. Unfortunately, the reporting of IPV is limited in most jurisdictions to cases involving the use of a weapon while committing a violent act. Unlike the requirement for dental professionals to report child and elder abuse, the dentist has no legal requirement to report IPV because these victims are autonomous. However, the American Dental Association's Principles of Ethics and Code of Professional Conduct indicate a responsibility on behalf of dental professionals to intercede in cases involving family violence.

The agency to which the report is made varies among the different jurisdictions. Commonly, the police, social service, child welfare, senior services agencies, or family services departments are the governmental offices designated to accept reports. When a report is made in good faith, the dentist is immune from any counter prosecution or civil liability that might stem from a false report. Failure to report is considered a misdemeanor in most states. In addition, the dentist may be subject to license revocation or malpractice litigation by failing to make a report.

When a dentist determines that a report of child or elder abuse should be made, documentation of the physical evidence to support the charge is mandatory. All evidence is collected according to the principles described for identification and bite mark cases. Descriptions of the injuries and their locations, supporting photographs and radiographs, and information stating the basis for suspicion of abuse are included in the report. When abuse is considered, the dentist should examine the patient and assess the problem separately from the abusive caregiver. Parental consent is not required to obtain appropriate physical evidence from victims younger than the age of majority.

Therefore, all parents and accompanying siblings should be directed to remain in the office waiting area while a minor patient is being treated. This policy should be maintained whether abuse is suspected or not so that the dentist, acting *in loco parentis*, can examine each patient for signs and symptoms of abuse and obtain the child's report concerning the findings without influence or pressure from the caregiver.

◆ DENTISTS AS EXPERT WITNESSES

Observational, or lay, witnesses testify only to the facts known to them. They are referred to as *witnesses of fact*. Such witnesses are permitted to make inferences about physical facts based on ordinary experience. The witness of fact is not entitled to present hearsay evidence related by another person.

The judicial system recognizes that people with a scientific background or specialized field of study that is admissible under the *Frye* rule or Federal Rules of Evidence can provide the courts with analyses or explanations relative to that discipline. The facts and opinions offered by such a

witness are beyond the scope of information that could be expected to be provided by a lay person or witness of fact. A witness who is qualified to testify under this standard is acknowledged as an "expert."

Members of the dental profession are experts. They are qualified to testify by the judge, who bases his or her opinion on educational background, dental and forensic expertise, publications, and other professional qualifications. Dentists who have additional training in one of the dental specialties may be called on to present specific information from that discipline.

Dental experts assist attorneys and, ultimately, the triers of fact (judges and juries) in understanding the scope and complexities of dental science and practice in relation to questions of law. The dentist should not become an advocate for either side in a case but should strive to be an educator and friend of the court.

In addition to their expertise in criminal trials involving bite marks, human abuse, and/or identification of homicide victims, dentists may be required to testify as experts in civil litigation cases that involve the following situations:

- **Malpractice based on negligence.** This category includes battery (e.g., extraction of the wrong tooth); misdiagnosis; and failure to diagnose, refer, or inform. All of these actions fall outside the standard of care for the profession.
- **Personal injury.** TMJ damage or dental trauma suffered in vehicular, home, sports, recreational, and work-related accidents fall under this category.
- **Dental fraud.** Charging for materials or procedures that were not used or performed are examples of fraud.
- **Identification of multiple fatality incident victims.** These may include casualties of natural disasters and accidents that are adjudicated civilly or criminal acts in which an offender is brought before the criminal judicial system.

Dentists are often unfamiliar with, and may be intimidated by, the adversarial nature of courtroom procedure and protocol. When presenting evidence, the dental expert should remember that his or her role in the legal process is to help the trier of fact understand the dental issues in the case. To this end, and as a scientist, the dental expert witness should present the evidence confidently, accurately, and objectively, relating information in nontechnical terms.

When cross-examined by the opposing attorney, the dental expert witness should remain composed and confident. As an expert, the dentist has the right to refer to records and exemplars prepared for the case. The dentist is entitled to read and review any books or articles proffered by the opposing attorney with the intent of discrediting the testimony.

Pretrial preparation is required if the dental expert and the attorney who has retained his or her services are to develop the evidence to be presented in court. Both must be aware of the strengths and weaknesses of the material and decide how best to provide the jury with this information. Adequate time must be allotted to prepare exhibits for court. It is also advantageous to attempt to determine the position that will be taken by dental experts called by the opposing side.

◆ SUMMARY

Each practitioner has a responsibility to understand the forensic implications associated with the practice of his or her profession. This understanding should include more than ethics and jurisprudence, which were traditionally the only aspects of knowledge of the law acquired by dental professionals. Appreciation of forensic dental problems involving body identification, dental age estimation methods, recognition and reporting of human abuse, and bite mark analysis permits clinicians to maintain legally acceptable records and assist legal authorities in the identification of victims of individual or multiple fatality incidents and criminal acts.

The pursuit of justice in cases of rape, homicide, and human abuse often relies on dental testimony to interpret bite marks or BMPIs. The development of UV and IR wavelength photographic techniques and equipment has given forensic dentists the opportunity to provide objective scientific evidence in these types of cases. Evidence gathered using these resources can be analyzed and assessed with computer software, laboratory, and clinical procedures that also enhance the ability of the forensic odontologist to interpret results.

The reliance of the legal community on the dental profession to continue to provide expertise in civil and criminal proceedings ensures that forensic dentistry will remain a viable component of the forensic sciences and the practice of dentistry.

Bibliography

Al-Amad SH, Clement JG, McCullough MJ, et al.: Evaluation of two dental identification computer systems: DAVID and WinID3, *J Forensic Odontostomatol* 25(1):23–29, 2007.

AlQahtani SJ, Hector MP, Liversidge HM: Brief communication: the London atlas of human tooth development and eruption, *Am J Phys Anthropol* 142(3):481–490, 2010.

American Board of Forensic Odontology: Bite mark methodology guidelines, In *ABFO diplomates reference manual (revised 01/22/13), section III: policies, procedures, guidelines & standards*, 2013, pp 109–121. PDF available online: http://www.abfo.org/resources/abfo-manual/. (Accessed 8 August 2013.)

American Board of Forensic Odontology: Body identification guidelines, In *ABFO diplomates reference manual (revised 01/22/13), section III: policies, procedures, guidelines & standards*, 2013, pp 122–174. PDF available online: http://www.abfo.org/rsources/abfo-manual/. (Accessed 8 August 2013.)

American Dental Association: *American Dental Association technical report no. 1077 for human age assessment by dental analysis*, 2020, Organization of Scientific Area Committees for Forensic Science (OSAC) Registry. https://www.ada.org/publications/ada-news. (Accessed 7 March 2022.)

American Dental Association, Department of Informatics: *Electronic health records (EHRs)*, 2014 http://www.ada.org/en/member-center/member-benefits/practice-resources/dental-informatics/electronic-health-records. (Accessed 21 October 2014.)

Anon: Guidelines for bite mark analysis. American Board of Forensic Odontology, Inc., *J Am Dent Assoc* 112(3):383–386, 1986.

Arany S, Ohtani S, Yoshioka N, et al.: Age estimation from aspartic racemization of root dentin by internal standard method, *Forensic Sci Int* 141:127–130, 2004.

Aschheim KW, Adams B: Computerized dental coding and sorting algorithms: is there a best? *J Forensic Odontostomatol* 31(Suppl 1):113–114, 2013.

Austin-Smith D, Maples WR: The reliability of skull/photograph superimposition individual identification, *J Forensic Sci* 39:446–455, 1994.

Bang G, Ramm E: Determination of age in humans from root dentin transparency, *Acta Odontol Scand* 56:238–244, 1970.

Barsley RE: Forensic and legal issues in oral diagnosis, *Dent Clin North Am* 37:143–144, 1993.

Berger MA: Evidentiary framework, In Cecil JS, et al., editors: *Shepard's reference manual on scientific evidence*, New York, 1994, McGraw-Hill, pp 39–117.

Blankenship JA, Mincer HH, Anderson KM, et al.: Third molar development in the estimation of chronologic age in American blacks as compared with whites, *J Forensic Sci* 52:428–433, 2007.

Bowers CM, Johansen RJ: Photographic evidence protocol: the use of digital imaging methods to rectify angular distortion and create life size reproductions of bite mark evidence, *J Forensic Sci* 47:179–186, 2002.

Bush MA, Miller RG: The crash of Colgan Air flight 3407: advanced techniques in victim identification, *J Am Dent Assoc* 142:1325–1356, 2011.

Bush MA, Bush PJ, Miller RG: Detection and classification of composite resins in incinerated teeth for forensic purposes, *J Forensic Sci* 51:636–642, 2006.

Bush MA, Miller RG, Prutsman-Pfeiffer J, et al.: Identification through XRF analysis of dental restorative resin materials: a comprehensive study of non-cremated, and processed cremated individuals, *J Forensic Sci* 52:157–165, 2007.

Bush MA, Miller RG, Norrlander AL, et al.: Analytical survey of restorative resins by SEM/EDS and XRF: databases for forensic purposes, *J Forensic Sci* 53:419–425, 2008.

Calliphora vomitoria. https://en.wikipedia.org/wiki/Calliphora_vomitoria. (Accessed 12 August 2021.)

Child Abuse Prevention and Treatment Act of 1974 (PL93-247), DHEW Pub No 78-30137, 42 USCS Section 5106 g (4), Washington, DC, 1988.

Child Liberation Foundation n.d.: Child trafficking statistics. https://liberatechildren.org/child-trafficking-statistics.

Chiodo GT, Tolle SW, Tilden VP: The dentist and family violence, *Gen Dent* 46:20–25, 1998.

Christian CW: *Metabolic and genetic mimics of child abuse*, 2014 https://champprogram.com/pdf/Metabolic-Mimickers-feb-12-2014-handout.pdf. (Accessed 12 December 2020.)

Cottone JA, Standish SM: *Outline of forensic dentistry*, Chicago, 1982, Year Book Medical Publishers.

Covell K. The rights of the child part three: child sexual exploitation and the age of consent, *aboutkidshealth: trusted answers from The Hospital for Sick Children* http://www.aboutkidshealth.ca/en/news/series/rightsofchildren/pages/the-rights-of-children-part-three-child-sexual-exploitation-and-the-age-of-consent.aspx. (Accessed 21 October 2014.)

da Fonseca MA, Feigal RJ, ten Bensel RW: Dental aspects of 1248 cases of child maltreatment on file at a major county hospital, *Pediatr Dent* 14:152–157, 1992.

Danforth RA, Herschaft EE, Weems RA: Dental, oral, and maxillofacial radiographic features of forensic interest, In Senn DR, Weems RA, editors: *American Society of Forensic Odontology manual of forensic odontology*, ed 5, Boca Raton, FL, 2013, CRC Press, pp 131–160.

Daubert v. Merrell Dow Pharmaceuticals, Inc., 113 S. Ct. 2786 (1993). http://law.harvard.edu/publications/evidenceiii/cases/daubert.htm. (Accessed 21 October 2014.)

Dental prosthetics identification: http://www.denture-id.com/ Regulations.

De Valck E: Major incident response: collecting antemortem data, *Forensic Sci Int* 159:15–19, 2006.

DiMaio DJ, DiMaio VJM: *Forensic pathology*, Boca Raton, FL, 1993, CRC Press.

Dorion RBJ, editor: *Bitemark evidence: a color atlas and text*, Boca Raton, FL, 2011, CRC Press.

Doyle v. State, 159 Texas, C.R. 310, 263 S.W. 2d 779 (January 20, 1954). https://forensicdentis.wpengine.com/doyle-v-state/. (Accessed 21 October 2014.)

Epstein JB, Scully C: Mammalian bites: risk and management, *Am J Dent* 5:167–172, 1992.

Federal Bureau of Investigation: *FBI announces contract award for Next Generation Identification system*, Washington, DC, 2008, FBI National Press Office. http://www.fbi.gov/news/pressrel/ press-releases/fbi-announces-contract-award-for-next-generation-identification-system. (Accessed 21 October 2014.)

Federal Bureau of Investigation Integrated automated fingerprint identification system. www.fbi.gov/hq/cjisd/iafis.htm#main. (Accessed 21 October 2014.)

Federal Bureau of Investigation: Laboratory services, Combined DNA Index System (CODIS). http://www.fbi.gov/about-us/lab/ biometric-analysis/codis. (Accessed October 21, 2014.)

Federal Bureau of Investigation National Press Office: *The FBI's Combined DNA Index System (CODIS) hits major milestone*, 2021 https://www.fbi.gov/news/pressrel/press-releases/the-fbis-combined-dna-index-system-codis-hits-major-milestone.

Florida Museum. Yearly worldwide shark attack summary: the ISAF 2020 shark attack report. https://www.floridamuseum.ufl.edu/ shark-attacks/yearly-worldwide-summary/.

Forrester JD, et al.: Mortality, hospital admission, and healthcare cost due to injury from venomous and non-venomous animal encounters in the USA: 5-year analysis of the National Emergency Department sample, *Trauma Surg Acute Care Open* 3(1):e0000250, 2018. https://doi.org/10.1136/tsaco-2018-000250.eCollection 2018.

Frair J, West MH: Ultraviolet forensic photography, *Kodak Tech Bits* 2:311, 1989.

Freeman AJ, Senn DR, Arendt DM: Seven hundred seventy eight bite marks: analysis by anatomical location, victim and biter demographics, type of crime, and legal disposition, *J Forensic Sci* 50:1436–1443, 2005.

Frye v. United States, 293 F. 1013 (D.C. Cir 1923). http://www.law. ufl.edu/_pdf/faculty/little/topic8.pdf. (Accessed 21 October 2014).

Golden GS: Use of alternative light source illumination in bite mark photography, *J Forensic Sci* 39:815–823, 1994.

Golden GS: Lessons learned from the WTC disaster: a first-person account, *J Can Dent Assoc* 32:675–680, 2004.

Gorlin RJ, Cohen MM, Levin LS: *Syndromes of the head and neck*, ed 3, New York, 1990, Oxford University Press.

Gustafson G: Age determination on teeth, *J Am Dent Assoc* 41:445–454, 1950.

Health Information Privacy, U.S. Department of Health and Human Services. https://www.hhs.gov/hipaa/for-professionals/privacy/ laws-regulations/index.html.

Herschaft EE, Alder ME, Ord DK, et al., editors: *American Society of Forensic Odontology—manual of forensic odontology*, ed 4, Albany, NY, 2007, ImPress Printing.

Hopper J: *Child abuse: statistics, research, and resources*, 1998. www. jimhopper.com. www.jimhopper.com/abstats/. (Accessed 21 October 2014.)

Hyzer WG, Krauss TC: The bite mark standard reference scale ABFO no. 2, *J Forensic Sci* 33:498–506, 1988.

Institute of Medicine: *The computer-based patient record: an essential technology for health care*, Revised Edition, Washington, DC, 1997, The National Academies Press. https://doi.org/ 10.17226/5306.

International Labour Organization: *Child labour*, 2020. https://www. ilo.org/global/topics/child-labour/lang- -en/index.htm.

Jakush J: Forensic dentistry, *J Am Dent Assoc* 119:355–368, 1989.

Johansen R, Bowers CM: *Digital analysis of bite mark evidence using Adobe Photoshop*, 2000, Forensic Imaging Institute.

Kim YK, Kho HS, Lee KH: Age estimation by occlusal wear, *J Forensic Sci* 45:303–309, 2000.

Koen WJ, Bowers CMC: *Forensic science reform: protecting the innocent*, ed 1, St. Louis, MO, 2012, Elsevier. https://www.sciencedirect. com/science/article/pii/B9780128027196000054.

Koen WJ, Bowers CM, editors: Bite mark evidence, In *Forensic science reform*, 2017, Academic Press, pp 137–165. https://www. sciencedirect.com/science/article/pii/B9780128027196000054.

Laser-Maira J.A., Hounmenou C.E., Peach D.: Global commercial and sexual exploitation of children. Oxford encyclopedia of criminology and criminal justice. https://oxfordre.com/criminology/ view/10.1093/acrefore/9780190264079.001.0001/acrefore-9780 190264079-e-592.

Lewis JM, Senn DR: Dental age estimation, In Senn DR, Weems RA, editors: *American Society of Forensic Odontology manual of forensic odontology*, ed 5, Boca Raton, FL, 2013, CRC Press, pp 211–255.

Lewis LM, Levine MD, Dribben WH: Bites and stings, In Dale DC, Federman DD, editors: *Interdisciplinary medicine*, New York, 2000, WebMD Inc.

Lorton L, Rethman M, Friedman R: The computer-assisted postmortem identification (CAPMI) system: a computer-based identification program, *J Forensic Sci* 33(4):977–984, 1988.

Maples WR: An improved technique using dental histology for estimation of adult age, *J Forensic Sci* 23:764–770, 1978.

Miller RG, Bush PJ, Dorion RB, et al.: Uniqueness of the dentition as impressed in human skin: a cadaver model, *J Forensic Sci* 54:909–914, 2009.

Mincer HH, Harris EF, Berryman HE: The ABFO study of third molar development and its use as an estimator of chronological age, *J Forensic Sci* 38:379–390, 1993.

Moenssens AA, Inbau FE, Slam JE: *Scientific evidence in criminal cases*, ed 3, Mineola, NY, 1986, Foundation Press.

Mohammed RB, et al.: Rugoscopy: human identification by computer-assisted photographic superimposition technique, *J Forensic Dent Sci* 5(2):90–95, 2013. https://doi.org/ 10.4103/0975-1475.119771.

Moorrees CF, Fanning EA, Hunt EE: Age variations of formation stages for ten permanent teeth, *J Dent Res* 42:1490, 1963.

Myers SL, Williams JM, Hodges JS: Effects of extreme heat on teeth with implications for histologic processing, *J Forensic Sci* 44:805–809, 1999.

National Academy of Sciences: *Strengthening forensic sciences in the United States: a path forward*, Washington, DC, 2009, The National Academies Press.

National Statistics: Domestic violence fact sheet, National Coalition Against Domestic Violence. https://assets.speakcdn.com/assets/2497/ domestic_violence-2020080709350855.pdf?1596828650457.

National Statistics on Child Abuse, National Children's Alliance. https://www.nationalchildrensalliance.org/media-room/national-statistics-on-child-abuse/.

Oeschger MP, Hubar JS: Modified intraoral film holders for postmortem identification, *J Forensic Sci* 44:846–848, 1999.

Ohtani S, Yamamoto T: Strategy for the estimation of chronological age using the aspartic acid racemization method with special reference to coefficient of correlation between D/L ratios and ages, *J Forensic Sci* 50:1020–1027, 2005.

Pear R: Standards issued for electronic health records, *The New York Times*, 2010. http://www.nytimes.com/2010/07/14/health/policy/14health.html?_r=0. (Accessed 21 October 2014.)

Pierce L: Early history of bitemarks, In Averill D, editor: *Manual of forensic odontology*, ed 2, Colorado Springs, 1991, American Society of Forensic Odontology, pp 127–128.

Pinheiro PS: *World report on violence against children*, Geneva, Switzerland, 2006, United Nations Publishing Services.

Pitluck HM, Barsley RE: 364 Bitemark case citations, In Herschaft EE, Alder ME, Ord DK, et al., editors: *American Society of Forensic Odontology manual of forensic odontology*, ed 4, Albany, NY, 2007, ImPress Printing.

Pretty IA: A web-based survey of odontologists' opinions concerning bitemark analysis, *J Forensic Sci* 48:1117–1120, 2003.

Pretty IA: The use of dental aging techniques in forensic odontological practice, *J Forensic Sci* 48:1127–1132, 2003.

Pretty IA, Sweet DJ: A look at forensic dentistry—part 1: the role of teeth in the determination of human identity, *Br Dent J* 190:359–366, 2001.

Pretty IA, Sweet DJ: The scientific basis for human bitemark analysis—a critical review, *Sci Justice* 41:85–92, 2001.

Quarterehomme G, Işcan MY: Gunshot wounds to the skull: comparison of entries and exits, *Forensic Sci Int* 94(1–2):141–146, 1998.

Ramsland K: *The C.S.I. effect*, New York, 2006, Berkley Publishing Group.

Regan JD, Parrish JA: *The science of photomedicine*, New York, 1982, Plenum Press.

Rextar Portable X-Ray Generator: GoodDrs. https://www.gooddrs.us/radiography/rextar-x-portable-x-ray-generator/.

Roberts D: The iceman: lone voyager from the copper age, *Natl Geogr Mag* 183:36–67, 1993.

Sanger RG, Bross DC: *Clinical management of child abuse and neglect: a guide for the professional*, Chicago, 1984, Quintessence Publishing.

Schrader BA, Senn DR: Dental identification of human remains from orthopedic metallic fixation devices, In *Proceedings of the American Academy of Forensic Sciences*, vol 7, 2006, p 198.

Siderits R, Birkenstamm J, Khani F, et al.: Three-dimensional laser scanning of "Crime Scene Gum" as a forensic method demonstrating the creation of virtual tooth surface contour and web-based rapid model fabrication, *Forensic Sci Commun* 12:1–6, 2010.

Sinclair K, McKechnie VM: DNA extraction from stamps and envelope flaps using QIA amp and QIA shredder, *J Forensic Sci* 45:229–230, 2000.

Sittig DF, Singh H: Legal, ethical, and financial dilemmas in electronic health record adoption and use, *Pediatrics* 127(4):e1042–e1047, 2011.

Smith ES, Rawson RD: *Proceedings of the first national symposium on dentistry's role and responsibility in mass disaster identification*, Chicago, 1988, American Dental Association.

Sognnaes RF, Ström F: The odontological identification of Adolph Hitler. Definitive documentation by x-rays, interrogation and autopsy findings, *Acta Odont Scand* 31:43–69, 1973.

Solomons HC, Elardo R: Biting in day care centers: incidence, prevention, and intervention, *J Pediatr Health Care* 5(4):191–196, 1991. https://doi.org/10.1016/0891-5245(91)90060-4.

Soomer H, Ranta H, Lincoln MJ, et al.: Reliability and validity of eight dental age estimation methods for adults, *J Forensic Sci* 48:149–152, 2003.

Spitz WU, Spitz DJ: *Spitz and Fischer's medicolegal investigation of death: guidelines for the application of pathology to criminal investigation*, ed 4, Springfield, IL, 2006, Charles C Thomas.

Standish SM, Stimson PG, editors: Forensic dentistry: legal obligations and methods of identification for the practitioner, *Dent Clin North Am* 21:1–196, 1977.

Stirling J Jr, American Academy of Pediatrics Committee on Child Abuse Neglect: Beyond Munchausen syndrome by proxy: identification and treatment of child abuse in a medical setting, *Pediatrics* 119:1026–1030, 2007.

Sweet DJ, Bowers CM: Accuracy of bite mark overlays: a comparison of five common methods to produce exemplars from a suspect's dentition, *J Forensic Sci* 43:362–367, 1998.

Sweet DJ, Hildebrand D: Recovery of DNA from human teeth by cryogenic grinding, *J Forensic Sci* 43(6):1199–1202, 1998.

Sweet DJ, Lorente M, Lorente JA, et al.: An improved method to recover saliva from human skin: the double swab technique, *J Forensic Sci* 42:320–322, 1997.

Talon DA, Citron DM, Abrahamian FM, et al.: Bacteriologic analysis of infected dog and cat bites: Emergency Medicine Animal Bite Infection Study Group, *N Engl J Med* 340:85–92, 1999.

Texas Junk Science Law (SB 346): https://www.shanephelpslaw.com/the-atticus-files/2019/february/texas-junk-science-law/.

The Innocence Project. Description of bite mark exonerations. https://www.innocenceproject.org/wp-content/uploads/2020/04/Description-of-bite-mark-exonerations-and-statistical-analysis_UPDATED-04.09.2020.pdf.

US Department of Health and Human Services Centers for Medicare & Medicaid Services: 42 CFR Parts 412, 413, and 495, Medicare and Medicaid Programs; Electronic Health Record Incentive Program—stage 2: final rule. http://www.gpo.gov/fdsys/pkg/FR-2012-09-04/pdf/2012-21050.pdf. (Accessed 21 October 2014.)

US Federal Emergency Management Agency (FEMA): National Response Framework. 2021. https://www.fema.gov/emergencymanagers/national-preparedness/frameworks/response. (Accessed 5 February 2023.)

Vale GL: Identification by dental evidence: basic and beyond, *J Can Dent Assoc* 32:665–672, 2004.

Vale GL: History of bitemark evidence, In Dorion RBJ, editor: *Bitemark evidence*, New York, 2005, Marcel Dekker.

Villacorta N: The mystery of the missing fingerprints, *Science*, 2011. https://www.sciencemag.org/news/2011/08/mystery-missing-fingerprints.

Warnick AJ: *Forensic dental identification team manual*, Detroit, 1989, Detroit Dental Association.

Willems G: A review of the most commonly used dental age estimation techniques, *J Forensic Odontostomatol* 19:9–17, 2001.

Word CJ, Sawosik TM, Bing DH: Summary of validation studies from twenty-six forensic laboratories in the United States and Canada on the use of the AmpliType PM PCR amplification and typing kit, *J Forensic Sci* 42:39–48, 1997.

World Health Organization: *Global status report on preventing violence against children 2020*, 2020. https://www.who.int/publications/i/item/9789240004191.

World Health Organization: Female genital mutilation. https://www.who.int/news-room/fact-sheets/detail/female-genital-mutilation.

World Health Organization Rabies. https://www.who.int/news-room/fact-sheets/detail/rabies.

Wright FD, Golden G: Forensic photography, In Stimson P, Mertz C, editors: *Forensic dentistry*, Boca Raton, FL, 1997, CRC Press.

Yon Y, Mikton CR, Gassoumis ZD, Wilber KH: Elder abuse prevalence in community settings: a systematic review and meta-analysis, *Lancet Glob Health* 5(2):e147–e156, 2017. https://www.ncbi.nlm.nih.gov/pubmed/28104184.

Zarkowski P: Bite mark evidence: its worth in the eyes of the expert, *J Law Ethics Dent* 1:47–57, 1988.

Zelditch ML, Swiderski DL, Sheets HD: *Geometric morphometrics for biologists: a primer*, ed 2, St. Louis, MO, 2012, Elsevier.

Appendix

Differential Diagnosis of Oral and Maxillofacial Diseases

The most important aspect of patient care is the accurate diagnosis of the patient's disease. Unfortunately, the clinical presentation of many disease processes can be strikingly similar, despite their vast differences in etiology and pathogenesis. Because treatment and, ultimately, prognosis are based on the diagnosis, the diagnostic process is critical in optimal patient management. This appendix provides some guidelines for expediting and facilitating the diagnostic process from a clinical perspective.

The first step in gathering information is the acquisition of a thorough history of the disease process. This step typically includes items such as the onset, severity, location, duration, character, and course of the signs and symptoms being experienced by the patient. Additional information regarding medical, social, and family history may be necessary. With this information, the clinician can often start the process of formulating a list of possible diagnoses, even before performing an examination.

The information obtained during the clinical examination is also important because many lesions have characteristic appearances. By evaluating these characteristics in conjunction with the patient's history, often the clinician can narrow the list of diagnostic possibilities. This list, known as a *differential diagnosis*, essentially includes possible pathologic entities, usually ranked in order from most likely to least likely.

DEFINITIONS

To better describe the appearances of lesions and communicate these features to colleagues, the clinician should be familiar with the following terms:

Macule. Focal area of color change that is not elevated or depressed in relation to its surroundings.

Papule. Solid, raised lesion that is less than 5 mm in diameter.

Nodule. Solid, raised lesion that is greater than 5 mm in diameter.

Sessile. Describing a tumor or growth whose base is the widest part of the lesion.

Pedunculated. Describing a tumor or growth whose base is narrower than the widest part of the lesion.

Papillary. Describing a tumor or growth exhibiting numerous surface projections.

Verrucous. Describing a tumor or growth exhibiting a rough, warty surface.

Vesicle. Superficial blister, 5 mm or less in diameter, usually filled with clear fluid.

Bulla. Large blister, greater than 5 mm in diameter.

Pustule. Blister filled with purulent exudate.

Ulcer. Lesion characterized by loss of the surface epithelium and frequently some of the underlying connective tissue. It often appears depressed or excavated.

Erosion. Superficial lesion, often arising secondary to rupture of a vesicle or bulla, that is characterized by partial or total loss of the surface epithelium.

Fissure. Narrow, slitlike ulceration or groove.

Plaque. Lesion that is slightly elevated and is flat on its surface.

Petechia. Round, pinpoint area of hemorrhage.

Ecchymosis. Nonelevated area of hemorrhage, larger than a petechia.

Telangiectasia. Vascular lesion caused by dilatation of a small, superficial blood vessel.

Cyst. Pathologic epithelium-lined cavity, often filled with liquid or semi-solid contents.

Unilocular. Describing a radiolucent lesion having a single compartment.

Multilocular. Describing a radiolucent lesion having several or many compartments.

By using these terms, the clinician can describe the characteristics of lesions efficiently and uniformly. Applying these clinical descriptors to the lesions also can help categorize them with respect to the differential diagnosis. By adding additional characteristics such as prevalence, patient race or nationality, patient age at diagnosis, patient sex, and sites of predilection, the clinician can hone the differential diagnosis list considerably.

HOW TO USE THIS APPENDIX

This appendix is designed to help the clinician formulate a differential diagnosis by organizing and categorizing disease entities according to their most prominent or identifiable clinical features. Under each "clinical feature" heading is a list of lesions with that clinical feature as a prominent component. Diseases are listed according to estimated frequency relative to similar diseases or lesions.

The most common lesions are marked with triple asterisks (***), less common lesions are marked with double asterisks (**), and rare lesions are marked with a single asterisk (*). Such estimated frequency indicators should not be compared between lists; they are intended only for the single differential diagnosis list in which they occur.

Clinical features that most readily distinguish the lesions are listed with each disease process to help focus the clinician's search for the most accurate diagnosis. Finally, the corresponding page number in the book is provided for each disease entity so that the reader can refer to the text for a more detailed discussion.

INDEX TO THE APPENDIX: DIFFERENTIAL DIAGNOSIS LISTS

Part 1: Mucosal and Soft Tissue Pathology: Color Changes

A. White Lesions: Can Be Scraped Off — 916
B. White Lesions: Cannot Be Scraped Off — 916
C. White and Red Lesions — 917
D. Red Lesions — 917
E. Petechial, Ecchymotic, and Telangiectatic Lesions — 918
F. Blue and/or Purple Lesions — 918
G. Brown, Gray, and/or Black Lesions — 918
H. Yellow Lesions — 919

Part 2: Mucosal and Soft Tissue Pathology: Surface Alterations

A. Vesiculoerosive and Ulcerative Lesions: Acute (Short Duration and Sudden Onset) — 920
B. Vesiculoerosive and Ulcerative Lesions: Chronic (Long Duration) — 920
C. Papillary Growths: Focal or Diffuse — 921

Part 3: Mucosal and Soft Tissue Pathology: Masses or Enlargements

A. Soft Tissue Masses (Lumps and Bumps): Lower Lip — 922
B. Soft Tissue Masses (Lumps and Bumps): Upper Lip — 922
C. Soft Tissue Masses (Lumps and Bumps): Buccal Mucosa — 922
D. Soft Tissue Masses (Lumps and Bumps): Gingiva/Alveolar Mucosa — 922
E. Soft Tissue Masses (Lumps and Bumps): Floor of Mouth — 923
F. Soft Tissue Masses (Lumps and Bumps): Tongue — 923
G. Soft Tissue Masses (Lumps and Bumps): Hard or Soft Palate — 923
H. Soft Tissue Masses (Lumps and Bumps): Multiple Lesions — 924
I. Soft Tissue Masses (Lumps and Bumps): Midline Neck Lesions — 924
J. Soft Tissue Masses (Lumps and Bumps): Lateral Neck Lesions — 924
K. Generalized Gingival Enlargement — 925

Part 4: Radiographic Pathology

A. Unilocular Radiolucencies: Pericoronal Location — 926
B. Unilocular Radiolucencies: Periapical Location — 926
C. Unilocular Radiolucencies: Other Locations — 926
D. Multilocular Radiolucencies — 927
E. Radiolucencies: Poorly Defined or Ragged Borders — 927
F. Radiolucencies: Multifocal or Generalized — 928
G. Radiopacities: Well-Demarcated Borders — 928
H. Radiopacities: Poorly Demarcated Borders — 929
I. Radiopacities: Multifocal or Generalized — 929
J. Mixed Radiolucent/Radiopaque Lesions: Well-Demarcated Borders — 929
K. Mixed Radiolucent/Radiopaque Lesions: Poorly Demarcated Borders — 930
L. Mixed Radiolucent/Radiopaque Lesions: Multifocal or Generalized — 930
M. Unique Radiographic Appearances: "Ground Glass" (Frosted Glass) Radiopacities — 930
N. Unique Radiographic Appearances: "Cotton Wool" Radiopacities — 930
O. Unique Radiographic Appearances: "Sunburst" Radiopacities — 930
P. Unique Radiographic Appearances: "Onion-Skin" Radiopacities — 930
Q. Soft Tissue Radiopacities — 931

Part 5: Pathology of Teeth

A. Hyperdontia (Extra Teeth) — 932
B. Hypodontia (Missing Teeth) — 932
C. Macrodontia (Larger Than Normal Teeth) — 932
D. Microdontia (Smaller Than Normal Teeth) — 932
E. Malformed Crown — 932
F. Enamel Loss After Tooth Formation — 933
G. Extrinsic Staining of Teeth — 933
H. Intrinsic Discoloration ("Staining") of Teeth — 933
I. Abnormally Shaped Roots — 933
J. Enlarged Pulp Chamber or Canal — 934
K. Pulpal Calcification — 934
L. Thickened Periodontal Ligament — 934
M. Generalized Loss of Lamina Dura — 934
N. Premature Exfoliation of Teeth — 935

Part 1: Mucosal and Soft Tissue Pathology: Color Changes

Frequency of Occurrence	Lesion or Condition	Comments or Special Characteristics	Page
A. White Lesions: Can Be Scraped Off			
***	White-coated tongue	May be scraped off slightly, with difficulty	12
***	Pseudomembranous candidiasis	"Milk curd" or "cottage cheese" appearance; may leave red base when rubbed off	201
***	Morsicatio	Surface may appear to be peeling off	272
***	Toothpaste or mouthwash reaction	Filmy whiteness; leaves normal appearing mucosa when rubbed off	342
**	Thermal burn	Example: pizza burn	276
**	Sloughing traumatic lesion	Example: cotton roll "burn"	280
**	Chemical burn	Example: aspirin burn secondary to direct application for toothache	278
*	Secondary syphilis	Mucous patch; may be only partially scraped off	179
*	Diphtheria	Gray-white pseudomembrane of oropharynx	177
B. White Lesions: Cannot Be Scraped Off			
***	Linea alba	Buccal mucosa along occlusal plane	272
***	Leukoedema	Primarily in blacks; milky white alteration of buccal mucosa bilaterally; disappears when stretched	7
***	Leukoplakia	May show benign hyperkeratosis, epithelial dysplasia, or invasive carcinoma	381
***	Tobacco pouch keratosis	Usually in mandibular vestibule; associated with use of snuff or chewing tobacco	391
***	White-coated tongue	Diffuse involvement of dorsal tongue	12
**	Lichen planus	Wickham's striae; typically bilateral on buccal mucosa	787
**	Morsicatio	Most common on anterior buccal mucosa, labial mucosa, and lateral border of tongue; exhibits ragged surface	272
**	Actinic cheilosis	Pale, gray-white, scaly alteration of lower lip; usually in older men with history of chronic sun exposure; precancerous	395
*	Nicotine stomatitis	Usually associated with pipe smoking; occurs on hard palate	397
*	Hairy leukoplakia	Usually lateral border of tongue; rough surface with vertical fissures; usually associated with HIV infection	253
*	Hyperplastic candidiasis	Most commonly affects anterior buccal mucosa	206
*	Lupus erythematosus	Most common on buccal mucosa; may mimic lichen planus or leukoplakia; associated skin lesions usually present	798
*	Skin graft	History of previous surgery	—
*	Submucous fibrosis	More common in South Asia; associated with betel quid chewing	393
*	White sponge nevus	Hereditary; onset in childhood; generalized lesions, especially buccal mucosa	748
*	Hereditary benign intraepithelial dyskeratosis	Hereditary; onset in childhood; generalized lesions, especially buccal mucosa; ocular involvement possible	749
*	Pachyonychia congenita	Hereditary; onset in childhood; most common on dorsal tongue and areas of trauma; nail, palmar, and plantar changes also present	750

Part 1: Mucosal and Soft Tissue Pathology: Color Changes—cont'd

Frequency of Occurrence	Lesion or Condition	Comments or Special Characteristics	Page
*	Dyskeratosis congenita	Hereditary; onset in childhood; dystrophic nail changes	752
*	Uremic stomatitis	Renal failure	852
C. White and Red Lesions			
***	Erythema migrans	Geographic tongue; continually changing pattern; rarely involves other oral mucosal sites	784
***	Candidiasis	White component may be rubbed off	201
**	Lichen planus	Atrophic or erosive forms; Wickham's striae; typically bilateral on buccal mucosa	787
**	Burns	Examples: pizza burn, aspirin burn, other chemical burns; white component may be rubbed off	276
**	Actinic cheilosis	Pale, gray-white and red alteration to lower lip; usually in older men with history of chronic sun exposure	395
**	Erythroleukoplakia	Usually shows epithelial dysplasia or carcinoma	390
**	Cinnamon reaction	Related to cinnamon-flavored gum; typically on buccal mucosa and lateral tongue	344
*	Nicotine stomatitis	Usually associated with pipe smoking; occurs on hard palate	397
*	Lupus erythematosus	Most common on buccal mucosa; may mimic lichen planus or leukoplakia; associated skin lesions usually present	798
*	Scarlet fever	Secondary to β-hemolytic streptococcal infection; strawberry/raspberry tongue	175
*	Verruciform xanthoma	Most common on gingiva and hard palate; surface may be papillary	365
D. Red Lesions			
***	Pharyngitis	Examples: strep throat, viral pharyngitis	174
***	Traumatic erythema	Caused by local irritation	—
***	Denture stomatitis	Denture-bearing palatal mucosa	205
***	Erythematous candidiasis	Example: central papillary atrophy (median rhomboid glossitis)	202
***	Erythema migrans	Geographic tongue (cases with absence of white borders); continually changing pattern; rarely involves other mucosal sites	784
***	Angular cheilitis	Erythema and cracking at labial commissures	204
**	Thermal burns	Example: caused by hot liquids	276
**	Erythroplakia	Usually shows epithelial dysplasia or carcinoma	390
**	Lichenoid and granulomatous stomatitis	Most common on the upper labial mucosa	336
*	Anemia	Atrophic, red tongue; can be due to pernicious anemia, iron-deficiency anemia, hypovitaminosis B	582
*	Hemangioma	Develops in younger patients; may blanch; may show bluish hue	547
*	Lupus erythematosus	Usually with associated skin lesions	798
*	Scarlet fever	Secondary to β-hemolytic streptococcal infection; strawberry/raspberry tongue	175
*	Plasma cell gingivitis	Allergic reaction usually related to flavoring agents	152
*	Radiation mucositis	Patient currently undergoing radiotherapy	281

(Continued)

Part 1: Mucosal and Soft Tissue Pathology: Color Changes—cont'd

Frequency of Occurrence	Lesion or Condition	Comments or Special Characteristics	Page
E. Petechial, Ecchymotic, and Telangiectatic Lesions			
***	Nonspecific trauma	History of injury to lesional site	296
**	Upper respiratory infections	Soft palate petechiae	296
*	Infectious mononucleosis	Soft palate petechiae; tonsillitis and/or pharyngitis may be present	241
*	Idiopathic thrombocytopenic purpura	Areas of trauma; gingival bleeding possibly present	590
*	Trauma from fellatio	Posterior palatal petechiae or ecchymosis	297
*	Hemophilia	Hereditary; childhood onset; gingival bleeding may be present	579
*	Leukemia	Caused by secondary thrombocytopenia; gingival bleeding may be present	593
*	Hereditary hemorrhagic telangiectasia	Multiple, pinhead-sized telangiectasias; possible history of nosebleeds or gastrointestinal bleeding	759
*	CREST syndrome	Multiple, pinhead-sized telangiectasias; **C**alcinosis cutis, **R**aynaud's phenomenon, **E**sophageal motility defect, **S**clerodactyly, **T**elangiectasias	805
F. Blue and/or Purple Lesions			
***	Varicosities	Especially after 45 years of age; most common on ventral tongue and lips	13
***	Submucosal hemorrhage	Also see Appendix List, Part 1, E. (previous topic) Petechial, Ecchymotic, and Telangiectatic Lesions	296
***	Amalgam tattoo	Most common on gingiva; blue-gray; radiopaque amalgam particles sometimes discovered on radiographs	298
***	Mucocele	Especially on lower labial mucosa; typically pale blue; cyclic swelling and rupturing often exhibited	460
**	Eruption cyst	Overlying an erupting tooth	688
**	Salivary duct cyst	Usually pale blue	463
**	Hemangioma	Usually red-purple; may blanch under pressure; onset in younger patients	547
**	Ranula	Pale blue, fluctuant swelling of lateral floor of mouth	462
*	Kaposi sarcoma	Especially in AIDS patients; usually purple; most common on palate and maxillary gingiva	564
*	Nasopalatine duct cyst	Midline of anterior palate	27
*	Salivary gland tumors	Especially mucoepidermoid carcinoma and pleomorphic adenoma; usually pale blue; most common on posterior lateral palate	Chapter 11
*	Gingival cyst of the adult	Most common in mandibular bicuspid-cuspid region	698
*	Blue nevus	Most common on hard palate	377
*	Melanoma	Most common on hard palate and maxillary gingiva; may show mixture of deep blue, brown, black, and other colors	434
G. Brown, Gray, and/or Black Lesions			
***	Racial pigmentation	Most common on attached gingiva in darker complexioned patients	—
***	Amalgam tattoo	Most common on gingiva; usually slate-gray to black; opaque amalgam particles may be found on radiographs	298

Part 1: Mucosal and Soft Tissue Pathology: Color Changes—cont'd

Frequency of Occurrence	Lesion or Condition	Comments or Special Characteristics	Page
***	Black/brown hairy tongue	Discoloration and elongation of filiform papillae	12
***	Melanotic macule	Brown; most common on lower lip	372
**	Smoker's melanosis	Most common on anterior facial gingiva	306
**	Non-amalgam tattoos	Example: graphite from pencil	298
*	Melanocytic nevus	Most common on hard palate; can be flat or raised	374
*	Melanoma	Most common on hard palate and maxillary gingiva; may show mixture of deep blue, brown, black, and other colors	434
*	Oral melanoacanthoma	Rapidly enlarging pigmented lesion; usually occurs in blacks	373
*	Drug ingestion	Examples: chloroquine, chlorpromazine, minocycline; especially on hard palate	307
*	Peutz-Jeghers syndrome	Freckle-like lesions of vermilion and perioral skin; intestinal polyps; hereditary	758
*	Addison disease	Chronic adrenal insufficiency; associated with bronzing of skin	843
*	Neurofibromatosis type I	*Café au lait* pigmentation; cutaneous neurofibromas	537
*	McCune-Albright syndrome	*Café au lait* pigmentation; polyostotic fibrous dysplasia; endocrine disorders	643
*	Heavy metal poisoning	Typically along marginal gingiva (e.g., lead, bismuth, silver)	304
*	Melanotic neuroectodermal tumor of infancy	Anterior maxilla; destroys underlying bone	541

H. Yellow Lesions

Frequency of Occurrence	Lesion or Condition	Comments or Special Characteristics	Page
***	Fordyce granules	Sebaceous glands; usually multiple submucosal papules on buccal mucosa or upper lip vermilion	6
**	Superficial abscess	Example: parulis from nonvital tooth	129
**	Accessory lymphoid aggregate	Most common in oropharynx and floor of mouth; may exhibit orange hue	578
**	Lymphoepithelial cyst	Most common on lingual and palatine tonsils, and floor of mouth; may be yellow-white	36
**	Lipoma	Most common on buccal mucosa; soft to palpation	530
*	Jaundice	Generalized discoloration, especially involving soft palate and floor of mouth; sclera usually affected also	823
*	Verruciform xanthoma	Most common on gingiva and hard palate; surface may be rough or papillary	365
*	Pyostomatitis vegetans	"Snail-track" pustules; associated with inflammatory bowel disease	851

Part 2: Mucosal and Soft Tissue Pathology: Surface Alterations

Frequency of Occurrence	Lesion or Condition	Comments or Special Characteristics	Page
A. Vesiculoerosive and Ulcerative Lesions: Acute (Short Duration and Sudden Onset)			
***	Traumatic ulcer	Mild-to-moderate pain; history of local trauma	273
***	Aphthous stomatitis	Extremely painful; may be single or multiple; nonkeratinized movable mucosa; often recurs	321
***	Recurrent herpes labialis	Vermilion and labial skin; begins as multiple vesicles; often recurs	231
**	Primary herpetic gingivostomatitis	Fever and malaise; children and young adults; multiple vesicles; gingiva consistently affected	230
**	Necrotizing (ulcerative) gingivitis (NUG)	Painful destruction of gingival papillae; fetid odor; mostly in teenagers and young adults	151
**	Mucosal burns	Chemical or thermal	276
**	Recurrent intraoral herpes simplex	Gingiva or hard palate (except in immunocompromised); focal cluster of vesicles and shallow ulcers	232
**	Allergic reactions	Example: Caused by topical medications or dental materials; erythema and vesicles	342
**	Erythema multiforme / Stevens-Johnson syndrome	Predominantly in children and young adults; multiple blisters and ulcers; often crusting, hemorrhagic lip lesions; may have associated "target" skin lesions or involvement of ocular and genital mucosa	781
**	Herpangina	Especially in children; multiple small ulcers on soft palate and tonsillar pillars	244
*	Varicella (chickenpox)	Associated with skin eruption; few oral vesicles and ulcers; usually in children	235
*	Herpes zoster	Unilateral involvement along nerve distribution; usually middle-aged and older adults; painful vesicles and ulcers	238
*	Hand-foot-and-mouth disease	Especially in children; multiple vesicles and ulcers; associated vesicles on hands and feet	244
*	Necrotizing sialometaplasia	Usually posterior lateral hard palate; prior swelling may be present; deep crater-like ulcer; may be only minimal pain	477
*	Anesthetic necrosis	Usually at site of palatal injection	294
*	Primary syphilis	Chancre at site of inoculation; usually painless with clean ulcer bed	179
*	Behçet syndrome	Aphthous-like ulcers; genital ulcers and ocular inflammation	326
B. Vesiculoerosive and Ulcerative Lesions: Chronic (Long Duration)			
***	Erosive lichen planus	Associated with white striae; usually in middle-aged and older adults; most common on buccal mucosa and gingiva ("desquamative gingivitis")	787
**	Traumatic granuloma	Solitary, non-healing ulcer	273
**	Squamous cell carcinoma	Usually in middle-aged and older adults; usually indurated and may have rolled border; may be painless	401
**	Mucous membrane pemphigoid	Most common in middle-aged and older women; most commonly presents as a "desquamative gingivitis"; may involve ocular and genital mucosa	775
*	Lupus erythematosus	May have associated red and white change; usually with skin involvement	798
*	Pemphigus vulgaris	Usually in middle-aged and older patients; multiple oral blisters and ulcers usually precede skin lesions	769
*	Deep fungal infections	Examples: histoplasmosis, blastomycosis; may be painless	Chapter 6
*	Tuberculosis	Associated mass may be present; may be painless	185

Part 2: Mucosal and Soft Tissue Pathology: Surface Alterations—cont'd

Frequency of Occurrence	Lesion or Condition	Comments or Special Characteristics	Page
*	Sarcoidosis	May be associated with erythematous macules or plaques; may be painless	328
*	Epidermolysis bullosa	Hereditary (except epidermolysis bullosa acquisita); onset in infancy and childhood; multiple skin and oral blisters or ulcers in areas of trauma; may result in extensive scarring	766
*	Pyostomatitis vegetans	Yellowish "snail-track" pustules; associated with inflammatory bowel disease	851
*	Granulomatosis with polyangiitis (Wegener granulomatosis)	Usually palatal ulceration and destruction; associated lung and kidney involvement may be present; may show "strawberry gingivitis"	333
*	Extranodal NK/T-cell lymphoma, nasal-type (midline lethal granuloma)	Palatal lymphoma with ulceration and destruction of underlying bone; may be painless	607
*	Noma	Gangrenous necrosis secondary to necrotizing ulcerative gingivitis; usually in malnourished children or immunocompromised individuals	191
*	Tertiary syphilis	Gumma; associated mass may be present; may be painless; may perforate palate	180
C. Papillary Growths: Focal or Diffuse			
***	Hairy tongue	Usually brown or black discoloration; hyperkeratotic elongation of filiform papillae on posterior dorsal tongue	12
***	Papilloma	Can be white or pink; most common on soft palate and tongue; usually pedunculated	355
***	Inflammatory papillary hyperplasia	Usually involves midportion of hard palate beneath denture	519
**	Leukoplakia (some variants)	Examples: proliferative verrucous leukoplakia, granular or nodular leukoplakia	381
**	Squamous cell carcinoma	Examples with papillary surface changes	401
**	Giant cell fibroma	Usually in children and young adults; most common on gingiva	514
*	Spongiotic gingival hyperplasia	Usually in children; some examples appear papillary	150
*	Verruca vulgaris	Common wart; especially in younger patients; most common on labial mucosa	357
*	Hairy leukoplakia	Usually lateral border of tongue; rough surface with vertical fissures; usually associated with HIV infection	253
*	Verruciform xanthoma	Most common on gingiva and hard palate	365
*	Verrucous carcinoma	Especially in older patients with long history of snuff or chewing tobacco use; especially in mandibular vestibule and buccal mucosa; may be white or red	421
*	Condyloma acuminatum	Venereal wart; broad-based lesions with blunted projections; frequently multiple	358
*	Multifocal epithelial hyperplasia	Usually multiple, flat-topped papular lesions; usually in children; most common in Native Americans and Inuit; color may vary from normal to white	360
*	Darier's disease	Most commonly appears as pebbly appearance of hard palate; associated crusty, greasy skin lesions; hereditary	756
*	Acanthosis nigricans (malignant type)	Most commonly appears as generalized pebbly alteration of upper lip; pigmented, pebbly skin changes in flexural areas; associated gastrointestinal malignancy	806

Part 3: Mucosal and Soft Tissue Pathology: Masses Or Enlargements

Frequency of Occurrence	Lesion or Condition	Comments or Special Characteristics	Page
A. Soft Tissue Masses (Lumps and Bumps): Lower Lip			
***	Mucocele	Typically pale blue; often exhibits cyclic swelling and rupturing; labial mucosa only	460
***	Fibroma	Usually normal in color	514
**	Pyogenic granuloma	Red, ulcerated, bleeds easily; usually on vermilion border	525
**	Squamous cell carcinoma	Tumor with rough, granular, irregular surface; usually on vermilion border	401
*	Other mesenchymal tumors	Examples: hemangioma, neurofibroma, lipoma	Chapter 12
*	Salivary duct cyst	May be bluish; labial mucosa only	463
*	Salivary gland tumor	Usually mucoepidermoid carcinoma	Chapter 11
*	Keratoacanthoma	Volcano-shaped mass with central keratin plug; rapid development; vermilion border only	398
B. Soft Tissue Masses (Lumps and Bumps): Upper Lip			
**	Fibroma	Usually normal in color	514
**	Minor gland sialolith	Small, hard submucosal mass: may be tender	465
**	Salivary gland tumor	Usually canalicular adenoma (older than age 40) or pleomorphic adenoma (younger than age 40)	Chapter 11
*	Salivary duct cyst	May be bluish	463
*	Other mesenchymal tumors	Examples: hemangioma, neurofibroma, schwannoma	Chapter 12
*	Nasolabial cyst	Fluctuant swelling of lateral labial vestibule	26
C. Soft Tissue Masses (Lumps and Bumps): Buccal Mucosa			
***	Fibroma	Usually normal in color; along occlusal plane	514
**	Lipoma	May be yellow; soft to palpation	530
**	Mucocele	Typically pale blue; often exhibits cyclic swelling and rupturing	460
*	Hyperplastic lymph node	Usually buccinator node; movable submucosal mass	578
*	Other mesenchymal tumors	Examples: hemangioma, neurofibroma	Chapter 12
*	Squamous cell carcinoma	Tumor with rough, granular, irregular surface	401
*	Salivary gland tumor	Pleomorphic adenoma and mucoepidermoid carcinoma most common	Chapter 11
D. Soft Tissue Masses (Lumps and Bumps): Gingiva/Alveolar Mucosa			
***	Parulis	Fistula from nonvital tooth	130
***	Epulis fissuratum	Ill-fitting denture	517
***	Pyogenic granuloma	Usually red, ulcerated, easily bleeding; increased frequency in pregnant women	525
***	Peripheral ossifying fibroma	May be red or normal in color; may be ulcerated	529
***	Fibroma	Usually normal in color	514
***	Peripheral giant cell granuloma	Reddish purple; frequently ulcerated	527
**	Spongiotic gingival hyperplasia	Usually in children; most common on maxillary anterior facial gingiva	150
**	Squamous cell carcinoma	Tumor with rough, granular, irregular surface	401
*	Metastatic tumors	May be painful and destroy bone	569

Part 3: Mucosal and Soft Tissue Pathology: Masses Or Enlargements—cont'd

Frequency of Occurrence	Lesion or Condition	Comments or Special Characteristics	Page
*	Gingival cyst of the adult	Most common in mandibular bicuspid-cuspid region; may be blue	698
*	Traumatic neuroma	Edentulous mandible in mental foramen area; often painful to palpation	532
*	Kaposi sarcoma	Especially in AIDS patients; usually purple	254
*	Peripheral odontogenic tumors	Example: peripheral ameloblastoma	715
*	Congenital epulis	Usually in females; especially anterior maxilla	546
*	Melanotic neuroectodermal tumor of infancy	Anterior maxilla; destroys underlying bone; may be pigmented	541
*	Other mesenchymal tumors	Examples: hemangioma, neurofibroma	Chapter 12

E. Soft Tissue Masses (Lumps and Bumps): Floor of Mouth

***	Ranula/mucocele	Typically a pale blue, fluctuant swelling	462
**	Sialolith	Usually hard mass in submandibular duct; may be associated with tender swelling of affected gland; radiopaque mass	465
**	Lymphoepithelial cyst	Small, yellow-white submucosal lesion	36
**	Squamous cell carcinoma	Tumor with rough, granular, irregular surface	401
*	Epidermoid or dermoid cyst	Midline yellow-white submucosal lesion	32
*	Salivary gland tumors	Especially mucoepidermoid carcinoma	Chapter 11
*	Mesenchymal tumors	Examples: lipoma, neurofibroma, hemangioma	Chapter 12

F. Soft Tissue Masses (Lumps and Bumps): Tongue

***	Fibroma	Usually normal in color; most common on margins of tongue	514
**	Squamous cell carcinoma	Tumor with rough, granular, irregular surface; usually lateral or ventral border	401
**	Mucocele	Usually anterior ventral surface; usually bluish or clear color	460
**	Pyogenic granuloma	Usually red, ulcerated, easily bleeding	525
*	Granular cell tumor	Dome-shaped; usually on dorsum of tongue	544
*	Other mesenchymal tumors	Examples: lymphangioma, hemangioma, neurofibroma, osseous choristoma	Chapter 12
*	Salivary gland tumors	Especially mucoepidermoid carcinoma and adenoid cystic carcinoma	Chapter 11
*	Lingual thyroid	Usually posterior midline of dorsal surface; usually in women	10

G. Soft Tissue Masses (Lumps and Bumps): Hard or Soft Palate

***	Palatal abscess	Associated with nonvital tooth	129
***	Leaf-like denture fibroma	Pedunculated hyperplastic growth beneath ill-fitting denture	517
**	Salivary gland tumors	Especially pleomorphic adenoma, mucoepidermoid carcinoma, adenoid cystic carcinoma, polymorphous low-grade adenocarcinoma; may have bluish hue	Chapter 11
**	Nasopalatine duct cyst	Fluctuant swelling of anterior midline palate	27
*	Lymphoma	Often boggy and edematous; may have bluish hue; may be bilateral	600
*	Kaposi sarcoma	Usually purple; may be multiple; usually associated with AIDS	254
*	Other mesenchymal tumors	Examples: fibroma, hemangioma, neurofibroma	Chapter 12
*	Squamous cell carcinoma	Tumor with rough, granular, irregular surface; occasionally arises from maxillary sinus	401

(Continued)

Part 3: Mucosal and Soft Tissue Pathology: Masses Or Enlargements—cont'd

Frequency of Occurrence	Lesion or Condition	Comments or Special Characteristics	Page
*	Mucocele/salivary duct cyst	Usually has bluish hue	460
*	Melanocytic nevus/melanoma	Usually pigmented	374, 434
*	Necrotizing sialometaplasia	Early stage lesion; often associated with pain or paresthesia	477
*	Adenomatoid hyperplasia of minor salivary glands	Asymptomatic, painless mass	477
H. Soft Tissue Masses (Lumps and Bumps): Multiple Lesions			
**	Multiple fibromas	Some patients may develop more than one fibroma on the oral mucosa	514
*	Kaposi sarcoma	Usually purple lesions of palate and maxillary gingiva; usually associated with AIDS	254
*	Neurofibromatosis type I	Oral and skin neurofibromas; *café au lait* skin pigmentation	537
*	Multifocal epithelial hyperplasia	Usually flat-topped papular lesions; usually in children; most common in Native Americans and Inuit; color may vary from normal to white	360
*	Amyloidosis	Pale, firm deposits, especially in tongue; periocular cutaneous lesions frequently present; most often associated with multiple myeloma	824
*	Granulomatous diseases	Examples: sarcoidosis, Crohn disease, leprosy	328
*	Multiple endocrine neoplasia type 2B	Mucosal neuromas of lips and tongue; adrenal pheochromocytomas; medullary thyroid carcinoma; marfanoid body build	540
*	Tuberous sclerosis	Small fibroma-like growths on gingiva; angiofibromas of face; epilepsy; intellectual disability	762
*	Multiple hamartoma syndrome	Cowden syndrome; small fibroma-like growths on gingiva; multiple hamartomas of various tissues; breast cancer in affected women	765
I. Soft Tissue Masses (Lumps and Bumps): Midline Neck Lesions			
**	Thyroid gland enlargement	Examples: goiter, thyroid tumor	—
*	Thyroglossal duct cyst	May move up and down with tongue motion	33
*	Dermoid cyst	Soft and fluctuant	32
*	Plunging ranula	Soft and compressible	462
J. Soft Tissue Masses (Lumps and Bumps): Lateral Neck Lesions			
***	Reactive lymphadenopathy	Secondary to oral and maxillofacial infection; often tender to palpation	578
**	Epidermoid cyst	Soft and movable	31
**	Lipoma	Soft mass	530
**	Metastatic carcinoma	Deposits from oral and pharyngeal carcinomas; usually indurated and painless; may be fixed	410
**	Lymphoma	May be unilateral or bilateral; usually painless; Hodgkin and non-Hodgkin types	598
*	Infectious mononucleosis	Fatigue; sore throat; tender lymph nodes	241
*	Salivary gland tumors	Arising from submandibular gland or tail of parotid gland	Chapter 11
*	Submandibular sialadenitis	Example: secondary to sialolithiasis	467
*	Branchial cleft cyst	Soft and fluctuant; most common in young adults	35
*	Granulomatous diseases	Examples: tuberculosis, sarcoidosis	185, 328

Part 3: Mucosal and Soft Tissue Pathology: Masses Or Enlargements—cont'd

Frequency of Occurrence	Lesion or Condition	Comments or Special Characteristics	Page
*	Cat-scratch disease	History of exposure to cat	194
*	Cystic hygroma	Infants; soft and fluctuant	553
*	Plunging ranula	Soft and compressible	462
*	Other mesenchymal tumors	Examples: neurofibroma, carotid body tumor	Chapter 12
K. Generalized Gingival Enlargement			
***	Hyperplastic gingivitis	Examples: associated with puberty, pregnancy, diabetes	147
**	Drug-related gingival hyperplasia	Examples: phenytoin, calcium-channel blockers, cyclosporine; may be fibrotic	156
*	Gingival fibromatosis	May be hereditary; onset in childhood	158
*	Leukemic infiltrate	Usually boggy and hemorrhagic	593
*	Granulomatosis with polyangiitis (Wegener granulomatosis)	"Strawberry" gingivitis; may have palatal ulceration and destruction; lung and kidney involvement	333
*	Scurvy	Vitamin C deficiency	828

Part 4: Radiographic Pathology

Frequency of Occurrence	Lesion or Condition	Comments or Special Characteristics	Page
A. Unilocular Radiolucencies: Pericoronal Location			
***	Hyperplastic dental follicle	<5 mm in thickness	687
***	Dentigerous cyst	>5 mm in thickness	685
**	Eruption cyst	Bluish swelling overlying erupting tooth	688
**	Odontogenic keratocyst	—	689
*	Orthokeratinized odontogenic cyst	—	693
*	Ameloblastoma	Especially unicystic type	707
*	Ameloblastic fibroma	Usually in younger patients	724
*	Adenomatoid odontogenic tumor	Usually in anterior region of jaws; most often with maxillary canine; usually in teenagers	718
*	Calcifying odontogenic cyst	Gorlin cyst	701
*	Carcinoma arising in dentigerous cyst	Mostly in older adults	705
*	Intraosseous mucoepidermoid carcinoma	Mostly in posterior mandible	496
*	Other odontogenic lesions	Examples: calcifying epithelial odontogenic tumor, odontogenic myxoma, central odontogenic fibroma	Chapter 15
B. Unilocular Radiolucencies: Periapical Location			
***	Periapical granuloma	Nonvital tooth	123
***	Periapical cyst	Nonvital tooth	126
**	Periapical cemento-osseous dysplasia (early)	Especially in black females; usually apical to mandibular anteriors; teeth are vital	646
*	Periapical scar	Usually endodontically treated tooth with destruction of cortical plate	125
*	Radicular dentin dysplasia (Dentin dysplasia type I)	Multiple periapical granulomas or cysts; shortened, malformed roots	108
C. Unilocular Radiolucencies: Other Locations			
***	Developing tooth bud	Within alveolar bone	—
**	Lateral radicular cyst	Nonvital tooth; lateral canal	126
**	Nasopalatine duct cyst	Between and apical to maxillary central incisors; palatal swelling may occur	27
**	Lateral periodontal cyst	Especially in mandibular bicuspid-cuspid region	699
**	Residual (periapical) cyst	Edentulous area	126
**	Odontogenic keratocyst	—	689
**	Central giant cell granuloma	Especially in anterior mandible	631
**	Stafne bone defect	Angle of mandible below mandibular canal	23
*	Cemento-osseous dysplasia	Early stage; usually in young adult and middle-aged black women; usually in mandible	645
*	Central ossifying fibroma	Early-stage lesion	652
*	Ameloblastoma	Especially unicystic type	707

Part 4: Radiographic Pathology—cont'd

Frequency of Occurrence	Lesion or Condition	Comments or Special Characteristics	Page
*	Buccal bifurcation cyst	Buccal aspect of erupting mandibular first or second molar	704
*	Other odontogenic cysts and tumors	Examples: ameloblastic fibroma, central odontogenic fibroma, calcifying odontogenic cyst	Chapter 15
*	Langerhans cell histiocytosis	"Histiocytosis X"; usually in children or young adults	596
*	Melanotic neuroectodermal tumor of infancy	Anterior maxilla; may be pigmented	541
*	Median palatal cyst	Clinical midline swelling of hard palate	30
*	Schwannoma/ neurofibroma	Usually associated with mandibular nerve	534
D. Multilocular Radiolucencies			
***	Odontogenic keratocyst	—	689
***	Ameloblastoma	Especially in posterior mandible; often associated with impacted tooth	707
**	Central giant cell granuloma	Especially in anterior mandible	631
*	Ameloblastic fibroma	Especially in young patients	724
*	Odontogenic myxoma	"Cobweb" trabeculation	735
*	Central odontogenic fibroma	—	731
*	Calcifying epithelial odontogenic tumor	Often associated with impacted tooth	720
*	Orthokeratinized odontogenic cyst	Often associated with impacted tooth	693
*	Lateral periodontal cyst (botryoid type)	Especially in mandibular bicuspid-cuspid region	699
*	Calcifying odontogenic cyst	Especially in cases with minimal or no calcifications; often associated with impacted tooth	701
*	Central hemangioma/ arteriovenous malformation	Especially in younger patients; may have honeycombed radiographic appearance; may pulsate	549
*	Aneurysmal bone cyst	Especially in younger patients	638
*	Cherubism	Hereditary; onset in childhood; multiple quadrants involved	634
*	Hyperparathyroidism (brown tumor)	Usually elevated serum calcium levels	840
*	Intraosseous mucoepidermoid carcinoma	Usually in posterior mandible	496
*	Fibrous dysplasia	Very rarely on panoramic films of mandibular lesions	641
E. Radiolucencies: Poorly Defined or Ragged Borders			
***	Periapical granuloma or cyst	Nonvital tooth	123
***	Focal osteoporotic marrow defect	Especially edentulous areas in posterior mandible; more common in females	625
**	Osteomyelitis	Usually painful or tender	134

(Continued)

Part 4: Radiographic Pathology—cont'd

Frequency of Occurrence	Lesion or Condition	Comments or Special Characteristics	Page
**	Medication-related osteonecrosis of the jaw (MRONJ)	Exposed necrotic bone; most often associated with bisphosphonate drugs	286
*	Simple bone cyst	Mandibular lesion that scallops up between roots of teeth; usually in younger patients	636
*	Metastatic tumors	Painful; paresthesia; usually in older adults	673
*	Osteoradionecrosis	History of radiation therapy; painful	283
*	Multiple myeloma	May be painful; in older adults	609
*	Primary intraosseous carcinomas	Odontogenic or salivary origin	716
*	Osteosarcoma	Often painful; usually in young adults	665
*	Chondrosarcoma	—	669
*	Ewing sarcoma	Usually in children	671
*	Other primary bone malignancies	Examples: fibrosarcoma, lymphoma	—
*	Desmoplastic fibroma of bone	Especially in younger patients	663
*	Massive osteolysis	Phantom (vanishing) bone disease	627

F. Radiolucencies: Multifocal or Generalized

***	Cemento-osseous dysplasia	Early stage lesions; usually in black females; usually in mandible	645
**	Nevoid basal cell carcinoma syndrome	Odontogenic keratocysts	694
**	Multiple myeloma	Painful; in older adults; "punched-out" lesions	609
*	Cherubism	Usually multilocular; onset in childhood; hereditary	634
*	Hyperparathyroidism	Multiple brown tumors	840
*	Langerhans cell histiocytosis	"Histiocytosis X"; in children and young adults; teeth "floating in air"	596

G. Radiopacities: Well-Demarcated Borders

***	Torus or exostosis	Associated with bony surface mass	19
***	Retained root tip	Remnants of periodontal ligament usually seen	—
***	Idiopathic osteosclerosis	Most commonly associated with roots of posterior teeth; no apparent inflammatory etiology	626
***	Pseudocyst of the maxillary sinus	Homogeneous, dome-shaped relative opacity rising above bony floor of maxillary sinus	310
**	Condensing osteitis	Usually at apex of nonvital tooth	141
**	Odontoma, compound	Toothlike structures with thin, radiolucent rim at junction with surrounding bone; may prevent eruption of teeth; more common in anterior segments of jaws	729
**	Odontoma, complex	Amorphous mass with thin, radiolucent rim at junction with surrounding bone; may prevent eruption of teeth; more common in posterior segments of jaws	729
**	Cemento-osseous dysplasia	Late-stage lesions; especially in middle-aged and older black women; usually in mandible	645

Part 4: Radiographic Pathology—cont'd

Frequency of Occurrence	Lesion or Condition	Comments or Special Characteristics	Page
**	Soft tissue radiopacity superimposed on bone	Examples: sialoliths, calcified nodes, phleboliths, bullet fragments, shotgun pellets, amalgam tattoos (See also Appendix List, Part 4, Q, page XXX)	—
*	Intraosseous foreign body	—	—
*	Osteoma	Associated with bony surface mass	655
*	Enamel pearl	Furcation area of molar tooth	90
*	Osteoblastoma/osteoid osteoma/ cementoblastoma	Late-stage lesions	658
H. Radiopacities: Poorly Demarcated Borders			
**	Cemento-osseous dysplasia	Late stage lesions; especially in middle-aged and older black women; usually in mandible	645
**	Medication-related osteonecrosis of the jaw (MRONJ)	Sclerosis of alveolar crestal bone; exposed necrotic bone; most often associated with bisphosphonate drugs	286
**	Condensing osteitis	Usually at apex of nonvital tooth	141
**	Sclerosing osteomyelitis	May be painful	137
*	Fibrous dysplasia	"Ground glass" appearance; onset usually in younger patients	641
*	Paget disease of bone	"Cotton wool" appearance; late-stage lesions; in older patients	628
*	Proliferative periostitis	"Onion-skin" cortical change; in younger patients; often associated with nonvital tooth	141
*	Osteosarcoma	May have "sunburst" cortical change; frequently painful; usually in young adults	665
*	Chondrosarcoma	—	669
I. Radiopacities: Multifocal or Generalized			
**	Florid cemento-osseous dysplasia	Late-stage lesions; especially in middle-aged and older black women; usually in mandible	647
**	Medication-related osteonecrosis of the jaw (MRONJ)	Multifocal sites of involvement; sclerosis of alveolar crestal bone; exposed necrotic bone; most often associated with bisphosphonate drugs	286
*	Idiopathic osteosclerosis	Occasionally may be multifocal	626
*	Paget disease of bone	"Cotton wool" appearance; late-stage lesions; in older patients; more common in maxilla	628
*	Gardner syndrome	Multiple osteomas; epidermoid cysts; gastrointestinal polyps with high tendency toward malignant transformation; hereditary	656
*	Polyostotic fibrous dysplasia	"Ground glass" appearance; onset usually in younger patients; may be associated with café au lait skin pigmentation and endocrine abnormalities (McCune-Albright syndrome)	641
*	Osteopetrosis	Hereditary; recessive form may be associated with secondary osteomyelitis, visual and hearing impairment	620
J. Mixed Radiolucent/Radiopaque Lesions: Well-Demarcated Borders			
***	Developing tooth	—	—
***	Cemento-osseous dysplasia	Intermediate-stage lesions; especially in middle-aged black women; usually in mandible	645
**	Odontoma	Compound or complex type; in younger patients; may prevent eruption of teeth	729

(Continued)

Part 4: Radiographic Pathology—cont'd

Frequency of Occurrence	Lesion or Condition	Comments or Special Characteristics	Page
*	Central ossifying fibroma	—	652
*	Ameloblastic fibro-odontoma	Usually in children	725
*	Adenomatoid odontogenic tumor	Usually in anterior region of jaws; most often with maxillary canine; usually in teenagers	718
*	Calcifying epithelial odontogenic tumor	Pindborg tumor; often associated with impacted tooth; may show "driven snow" opacities	720
*	Calcifying odontogenic cyst	Gorlin cyst; may be associated with odontoma	701
*	Osteoblastoma/osteoid osteoma	Intermediate-stage lesion; usually in younger patients; often painful	658
*	Cementoblastoma	Intermediate-stage lesion; attached to tooth root	659
K. Mixed Radiolucent/Radiopaque Lesions: Poorly Demarcated borders			
**	Medication-related osteonecrosis of the jaw (MRONJ)	Exposed necrotic bone; most often associated with bisphosphonate drugs	286
**	Osteomyelitis	With sequestrum formation or with sclerosing type; often painful	134
*	Metastatic carcinoma	Especially prostate and breast carcinomas; may be painful	673
*	Osteosarcoma/chondrosarcoma	May be painful	665
L. Mixed Radiolucent/Radiopaque Lesions: Multifocal or Generalized			
**	Florid cemento-osseous dysplasia	Intermediate-stage lesions; especially in middle-aged black women; usually in mandible	647
**	Medication-related osteonecrosis of the jaw (MRONJ)	Exposed necrotic bone; most often associated with bisphosphonate drugs	286
*	Paget disease of bone	In older patients; more common in maxilla	628
M. Unique Radiographic Appearances: "Ground Glass" (Frosted Glass) Radiopacities			
*	Fibrous dysplasia	Onset usually in younger patients	641
*	Hyperparathyroidism	May cause loss of lamina dura	840
N. Unique Radiographic Appearances: "Cotton Wool" Radiopacities			
**	Cemento-osseous dysplasia	Especially in middle-aged black women; usually in mandible	645
*	Paget disease of bone	In older patients; more common in maxilla	628
*	Gardner syndrome	Multiple osteomas; epidermoid cysts; gastrointestinal polyps with high tendency toward malignant transformation; hereditary	656
*	Gigantiform cementoma	Hereditary; facial enlargement may be present	650
O. Unique Radiographic Appearances: "Sunburst" Radiopacities			
*	Osteosarcoma	Often painful; usually in young adults	665
*	Intraosseous hemangioma	Especially in younger patients	549
P. Unique Radiographic Appearances: "Onion-Skin" Radiopacities			
*	Proliferative periostitis	In younger patients; often associated with nonvital tooth; best seen with occlusal radiograph	141
*	Ewing sarcoma	In young children	671
*	Langerhans cell histiocytosis	"Histiocytosis X"; usually in children or young adults	596

Part 4: Radiographic Pathology—cont'd

Frequency of Occurrence	Lesion or Condition	Comments or Special Characteristics	Page
Q. Soft Tissue Radiopacities			
***	Amalgam tattoo	Markedly radiopaque; associated with surface discoloration	298
**	Other foreign bodies	Examples: bullet fragments, shotgun pellets	—
**	Sialolith	Glandular pain may be present while patient is eating	465
**	Tonsilloliths	Superimposed on mandibular ramus	176
*	Phlebolith	May occur in varicosities or hemangiomas	14
*	Calcified lymph nodes	Example: tuberculosis	185
*	Osseous and cartilaginous choristomas	Most common on tongue	559
*	Calcinosis cutis	May be seen with systemic sclerosis (especially CREST syndrome)	805
*	Myositis ossificans	Reactive calcification in muscle	—

Part 5: Pathology of Teeth

Frequency of Occurrence	Lesion or Condition	Comments or Special Characteristics	Page
A. Hyperdontia (Extra Teeth)			
***	Idiopathic supernumerary teeth	Mesiodens, paramolar, distomolar	75
**	Cleft lip and palate	Extra lateral incisor or canine	1
*	Gardner syndrome	Osteomas and gastrointestinal polyps	656
*	Cleidocranial dysplasia	Hypoplastic or missing clavicles; failure of tooth eruption	623
B. Hypodontia (Missing Teeth)			
***	Idiopathic hypodontia	Missing third molars, lateral incisors	75
**	Cleft lip and palate	Missing lateral incisor or canine	1
*	Hereditary hypohidrotic ectodermal dysplasia	Cone-shaped teeth	747
*	Incontinentia pigmenti	Cone-shaped teeth	755
*	Radiotherapy during childhood	Stunted tooth development	56
C. Macrodontia (Larger Than Normal Teeth)			
**	Fusion	Joining of two tooth germs	82
**	Gemination	Incomplete splitting of a tooth germ	82
*	Idiopathic macrodontia	—	81
*	Facial hemihyperplasia	Affected side only; nondental tissues also enlarged	37
*	Gigantism	Abnormally tall stature	834
D. Microdontia (Smaller Than Normal Teeth)			
***	Supernumerary teeth	Mesiodens; fourth molars	75
***	Peg-shaped lateral incisors	Cone-shaped teeth	81
**	Dens invaginatus	Cone-shaped teeth; tendency for pulpal death and periapical pathosis	88
*	Idiopathic microdontia	Usually generalized	81
*	Hereditary hypohidrotic ectodermal dysplasia	Cone-shaped teeth; sparse, blond hair; diminished sweating	747
*	Radiotherapy during childhood	Stunted tooth development	56
*	Congenital syphilis	Hutchinson's incisors	181
*	Hypopituitarism	Associated dwarfism	833
E. Malformed Crown			
***	Mesiodens and other supernumeraries	Cone-shaped teeth or microdont	75
**	Environmental enamel hypoplasia	Example: high fever during tooth development	51
**	Peg-shaped lateral incisors	Cone-shaped teeth	81
**	Dens invaginatus	Cone-shaped teeth; tendency toward pulpal death and periapical pathosis	88
**	Turner tooth	Infection or trauma to associated primary tooth	53
**	Fusion or gemination	"Double" tooth	82
*	Talon cusp	Extra cusp on lingual of anterior tooth	85
*	Dens evaginatus	Extra cusp on occlusal of premolar tooth	86
*	Amelogenesis imperfecta	Hereditary defect in enamel formation	98

Part 5: Pathology of Teeth—cont'd

Frequency of Occurrence	Lesion or Condition	Comments or Special Characteristics	Page
*	Dentinogenesis imperfecta	Fracturing away of enamel due to hereditary defect in dentin formation; gray-yellow opalescent teeth; calcified pulp chambers	104
*	Regional odontodysplasia	Poor tooth formation in a focal area; "ghost teeth"	110
*	Congenital syphilis	Hutchinson's incisors; mulberry molars	181
*	Vitamin D–resistant rickets	Hereditary condition; high pulp horns	848
*	Renal osteodystrophy	Abnormal calcium and phosphate metabolism	841
*	Hypoparathyroidism	Possible associated endocrine-candidiasis syndrome	838
*	Pseudohypoparathyroidism	—	839
*	Epidermolysis bullosa	Hereditary blistering skin disease	766
*	Radiotherapy during childhood	Stunted tooth development	56
*	Globodontia	Associated with otodental syndrome	96
*	Lobodontia	Cusp anatomy resembles teeth of carnivores	97

F. Enamel Loss After Tooth Formation

***	Caries	—	—
***	Trauma	Fractured tooth	—
***	Attrition	Physiologic loss of tooth structure	58
***	Abrasion	Pathologic loss of tooth structure	58
**	Erosion	Chemical loss of tooth structure	58
*	Dentinogenesis imperfecta	Hereditary defect in dentin formation; poor junction between enamel and dentin	104
*	Amelogenesis imperfecta	Hereditary defect in enamel formation; especially hypocalcified types	98

G. Extrinsic Staining of Teeth

***	Tobacco	Black or brown	67
***	Coffee, tea, and cola drinks	Brown or black	67
**	Chromogenic bacteria	Brown, black, green, or orange	67
**	Chlorhexidine	Yellow-brown	67

H. Intrinsic Discoloration ("Staining") of Teeth

***	Aging	Yellow-brown; less translucency	—
***	Death of pulp	Gray-black; less translucency	118
**	Fluorosis	White; yellow-brown; brown; mottled	57
**	Tetracycline	Yellow-brown; yellow fluorescence	70
**	Internal resorption	"Pink tooth of Mummery"	62
*	Calcific metamorphosis	Yellow	120
*	Dentinogenesis imperfecta	Blue-gray; translucent	104
*	Amelogenesis imperfecta	Yellow-brown	98
*	Congenital erythropoietic porphyria	Yellow; brown-red; red fluorescence	68
*	Erythroblastosis fetalis	Yellow; green	69

I. Abnormally Shaped Roots

***	External root resorption	Secondary to infection, cyst, tumor	62
***	Dilaceration	Abnormal curvature	94

(Continued)

Part 5: Pathology of Teeth—cont'd

Frequency of Occurrence	Lesion or Condition	Comments or Special Characteristics	Page
**	Hypercementosis	Excessive cementum production	93
**	Supernumerary roots	—	96
**	Concrescence	Joining of teeth by cementum	82
**	Taurodontism	Enlarged pulp chambers; shortened roots	92
**	Enamel pearl	Ectopic enamel in furcation	90
*	Benign cementoblastoma	Tumor attached to root	659
*	Radiotherapy during childhood	Stunted root development	56
*	Dentinogenesis imperfecta	Shortened roots; obliterated pulps	104
*	Radicular dentin dysplasia (Dentin dysplasia type I)	Shortened, pointed roots ("rootless teeth"); obliterated pulps; periapical pathosis	108
J. Enlarged Pulp Chamber or Canal			
**	Internal resorption	Secondary to caries or trauma	62
**	Taurodontism	Enlarged pulp chambers; shortened roots	92
*	Severe form of dentinogenesis imperfecta	"Shell teeth"	104
*	Regional odontodysplasia	"Ghost teeth"	110
*	Vitamin D–resistant rickets	High pulp horns	848
*	Hypophosphatasia	—	847
*	Mild form of dentinogenesis imperfecta ("Dentin dysplasia type II")	"Thistle-tube" pulps with pulp stone formation in permanent dentition	104
K. Pulpal Calcification			
***	Pulp stones	Asymptomatic radiographic finding	121
***	Secondary dentin	Response to caries	119
**	Calcific metamorphosis	Pulpal obliteration secondary to aging or trauma	120
*	Dentinogenesis imperfecta (moderate form)	Pulpal obliteration by excess dentin	104
*	Radicular dentin dysplasia (Dentin dysplasia type I)	Pulpal obliteration by excess dentin; "chevron"-shaped pulp chambers	108
*	Mild form of dentinogenesis imperfecta ("Dentin dysplasia type II")	Pulpal obliteration of primary teeth; pulp stones in permanent teeth	104
L. Thickened Periodontal Ligament			
***	Periapical abscess	Focal thickening at apex of nonvital tooth; painful, especially on percussion of involved tooth	129
***	Current orthodontic therapy	—	—
**	Increased occlusal function	—	—
*	Systemic sclerosis (scleroderma)	Generalized widening	801
*	Sarcoma or carcinoma infiltration	Especially osteosarcoma; localized to teeth in area of tumor	667, 673
M. Generalized Loss of Lamina Dura			
*	Hyperparathyroidism	Calcium removed from bones; bone may have "ground glass" appearance	840
*	Osteomalacia	Vitamin D deficiency in adults	829
*	Paget disease of bone	"Cotton wool" change hides lamina dura	628

Part 5: Pathology of Teeth—cont'd

Frequency of Occurrence	Lesion or Condition	Comments or Special Characteristics	Page
*	Fibrous dysplasia	"Ground glass" change hides lamina dura	641
N. Premature Exfoliation of Teeth			
***	Trauma	Avulsed tooth	—
**	Aggressive periodontitis	Premature alveolar bone loss	160
**	Immunocompromised states	AIDS, leukemia, chemotherapy	257
**	Diabetes mellitus	Increased susceptibility to infection and severity of periodontitis	844
*	Osteomyelitis	Bone destruction loosening teeth	134
*	Cyclic or chronic neutropenia	Increased susceptibility to infection; premature alveolar bone loss	589
*	Langerhans cell histiocytosis	"Histiocytosis X"; eosinophilic granuloma; premature alveolar bone loss	596
*	Radicular dentin dysplasia (Dentin dysplasia type I)	"Rootless teeth"	108
*	Regional odontodysplasia	"Ghost teeth"	110
*	Papillon-Lefèvre syndrome	Palmar and plantar hyperkeratosis; premature periodontitis	167
*	Down syndrome	Premature periodontitis	—
*	Hypophosphatasia	Lack of cementum production in primary teeth	847
*	Scurvy	Vitamin C deficiency	828

Index

Note: Page numbers followed by *f* indicate figures, *t* indicate tables, and *b* indicate boxes.

A

"Abdominal groans", in
    hyperparathyroidism, 841
ABFO No. 2 photomacrographic reference
    scale, 903, 904*t*
Abfraction, tooth wear due to, 61, 61*f*
Abscess(es)
  gingival, 164
  Munro
    in erythema migrans, 785–786, 786*f*
    in psoriasis, 797
  periapical, 129–132
    classification of, 129–130
    clinical and radiographic features of,
      129–131, 130*f*
    with cutaneous sinus, 130–131, 131*f*
    defined, 129
    parulis (gum boil) as, 130–131,
      130–132*f*
    pathogenesis of, 130
    periapical granuloma after, 123
    phoenix, 129
    treatment and prognosis for, 132
  periodontal, 164–165, 164–165*f*
  phoenix, 123
ABVD regimen for Hodgkin lymphoma,
    600
Acantholysis
  in Darier disease, 757
  in pemphigus vulgaris, 770–772, 773*f*
Acantholytic dyskeratosis, focal, 757–758,
    757*f*
Acanthomatous ameloblastoma, 710, 712*f*
Acanthosis
  in granular cell tumor, 545
  nigricans, 806–807
    benign, 806
    clinical features of, 806–807, 806*f*
    histopathologic features of, 807, 807*f*
    malignant, 806
    pseudo-, 806
    treatment and prognosis for, 807
Acanthotic form of seborrheic keratosis, 366,
    367*f*
Accessory cusps, 85–88
  clinical and radiographic features of,
    85–87

Accessory cusps *(Continued)*
  cusp of Carabelli as, 85
  dens evaginatus as, 86–87, 87*f*
  with shovel-shaped incisors, 87, 87*f*
  talon cusp as, 85–86
Accidents, 896
ACE (angiotensin-converting enzyme)
    inhibitors, angioedema due to,
    348, 350
Acinic cell carcinoma, 497–498, 497–498*f*
Acinic cell tumor, 497
Ackerman's tumor, 421–423, 422–423*f*
Acquired immunodeficiency syndrome
    (AIDS). *See* Human
    immunodeficiency virus (HIV)
Acquired melanocytic nevus(i)
  clinical features of, 375–376, 375–376*f*
  histopathologic features of, 376,
    376–377*f*
  treatment and prognosis for, 376–377
Acral keratosis in multiple hamartoma
    syndrome, 765
Acral lentiginous melanoma, 436
Acral melanoma, 436
Acrobrachycephaly, 41, 42*f*
Acrocephalosyndactyly, 41–43, 42*f*
Acrodynia, 305
Acrodysostosis, 839–840
Acromegaly, 834–835
  clinical and radiographic features of, 834,
    834–835*f*
  laboratory findings and diagnosis of, 835
  treatment and prognosis for, 835
  vs. gigantism, 834
Acro-osteolysis in systemic sclerosis, 802,
    802*f*
Acrosclerosis, 805–806, 805–806*f*
Actinic cheilitis. *See* Actinic cheilosis
  clinical features of, 395, 395*f*
  histopathologic features of, 395, 396*f*
  treatment and prognosis of, 396,
    396*f*
Actinic cheilosis, 395–396
  and actinic keratosis, 396
  clinical features of, 395, 395*f*
  histopathologic features of, 395, 396*f*
  treatment and prognosis of, 396, 396*f*

Actinic keratosis, 396–397, 396–397*f*
  in xeroderma pigmentosum, 753
Actinic lentigo(igines), 369–370, 370*f*
  vs. seborrheic keratosis, 366
Actinomycosis, 192–194
  clinical features of, 193, 193*f*
  diagnosis of, 194
  histopathologic features of, 193–194,
    194*f*
  pathogenesis of, 192
  treatment and prognosis for, 194
Acute chest syndrome, 583
Acute lymphonodular pharyngitis, 244
Acute necrotizing ulcerative gingivitis
    (ANUG), 151
Acute retroviral syndrome, 252
Adamantiades, Benedict, 326–328
Adamantiades syndrome. *See* Behçet
    syndrome
Addison disease, 843–844, 844*f*
  due to histoplasmosis, 212
  due to paracoccidioidomycosis, 216
Adenoid cystic carcinoma, 501–503
  clinical and radiographic features of,
    501–502, 501–502*f*
  histopathologic features of, 502–503
    cribriform pattern as, 502, 503*f*
    perineural invasion as, 503, 503*f*
    solid variant as, 502–503
    tubular pattern as, 502
  treatment and prognosis for, 503
Adenoid form of seborrheic keratosis,
    367–368
Adenolymphoma, 488–489
Adenoma(s)
  basal cell, 491–492, 492*f*
  canalicular, 490–491, 490*f*
  monomorphic, 490
  oxyphilic, 487–488, 487*f*
  pleomorphic (*see* Pleomorphic adenoma)
  sebaceum, in tuberous sclerosis, 763, 763*f*
Adenomatoid hyperplasia of minor salivary
    glands, 477
Adenomatoid odontogenic tumor, 718–720
  calcifying odontogenic cyst with, 701
  clinical and radiographic features of,
    718–719, 718–719*f*

Adenomatoid odontogenic tumor
    (*Continued*)
  epidemiology of, 718
  histopathologic features of, 720, 720*f*
  relative distribution of, 721, 721*f*
  treatment and prognosis for, 720
Adenosquamous carcinoma, 424–425
Age spot, 369–370, 370*f*
Ageusia, 870
Aggressive ossifying fibroma, 653–655
Aglossia, 8
Agranulocytosis, 589
  congenital, 589
AIDS. *See* Human immunodeficiency virus
AIDS-dementia complex, 252
AIDS-related complex (ARC), 252
Albers-Schönberg disease. *See* Osteopetrosis
Albright hereditary osteodystrophy,
    839–840
Alcohol, and squamous cell carcinoma, 403
ALI (alternate light imaging) photography,
    905
Allergic contact stomatitis, 342–343, 343*f*
Allergic disease(s)
  allergic contact stomatitis as, 342–343,
      343*f*
  angioedema as, 348–350, 348–349*f*
  contact stomatitis from artificial
      cinnamon flavoring as, 344–346
  lichenoid and granulomatous stomatitis
      as, 336–337
  lichenoid contact reaction from dental
      restorative materials as, 346–347,
      347*f*
  mucosal reactions to systemic drug
      administration as, 337–342
  perioral dermatitis as, 343–344, 344*f*
Allergic gingivostomatitis, 152–154, 153*f*
Alternate light imaging (ALI) photography,
    905
Alternative light source photography, 905
Aluminum chloride, allergic contact
    stomatitis to, 343*f*
Alveolar cyst of newborn, 697–698, 698*f*
Alveolar masses, differential diagnosis of,
    922–925*t*
Alveolar osteitis, 143–144
Alveolar ridge keratosis, 383, 383*f*
Alveolar soft-part sarcoma, 568–569, 569*f*
Alveolitis, fibrinolytic, 143–144
Amalgam discoloration, 69, 70*f*
Amalgam, lichenoid reaction to, 346–347,
    347*f*, 791
Amalgam tattoo, 298–300
  clinical and radiographic features of, 299,
      299–300*f*
  from endodontic-related implantation,
      298, 298*f*
  from floss-related implantation, 298, 298*f*
  histopathologic features of, 300, 300*f*
  treatment and prognosis for, 300
Amelanotic melanoma, 436

Ameloblastic carcinoma, 716–717,
    716–717*f*
Ameloblastic carcinosarcoma, 728
Ameloblastic dentinosarcomas, 728
Ameloblastic fibroma, 724–725, 724–725*f*
Ameloblastic fibro-odontoma, 725–727,
    726–727*f*
Ameloblastic fibro-odontosarcomas, 728
Ameloblastic fibrosarcoma, 727–728, 728*f*
Ameloblastic odontoma, 728–729
Ameloblastic sarcoma, 727–728, 728*f*
Ameloblastoma, 707–716
  acanthomatous, 710, 712*f*
  calcifying odontogenic cyst with, 701
  conventional solid or multicystic
      acanthomatous pattern in, 710, 712*f*
      basal cell pattern in, 712, 712*f*
      desmoplastic, 711–712, 712*f*
      granular cell pattern in, 711, 712*f*
      treatment and prognosis for, 712–713,
          713*f*
  conventional solid or multicystic
      intraosseous, 708–713
      clinical features of, 708–709, 708–710*f*
      desmoplastic, 709, 711*f*
      epidemiology of, 708
      follicular pattern in, 709–712, 711*f*
      histopathologic features of, 709
      plexiform pattern in, 709–710, 711*f*
      radiographic features of, 708–709,
          708–710*f*
      relative distribution of, 708, 708*f*
      vs. lateral periodontal cyst, 708, 711*f*
  desmoplastic, 709, 711–712, 711–712*f*
  granular cell, 711, 712*f*
  malignant, 716–717, 716–717*f*
  mural, 714, 715*f*
  pathogenesis of, 707
  peripheral (extraosseous), 715–716, 715*f*
  pigmented, 541–543, 542*f*
  transformation of dentigerous cyst to, 688
  treatment and prognosis for, 715
  unicystic, 713–715
      clinical and radiographic features of,
          713–714, 713–714*f*
      histopathologic features of, 714,
          714*f*
      intraluminal (plexiform), 714, 714*f*
      luminal, 714, 714*f*
Amelogenesis imperfecta, 98–104
  classification of, 98*t*
  clinical and radiographic features of,
      100–103
  defined, 51, 98
  genetic basis for, 99*t*, 100–103
  histopathologic features of, 103
  hypocalcification, 101–102, 103*f*
  hypocalcified, 98
  hypomaturation, 98, 101–102
      pigmented, 102
      snow-capped, 102, 102*f*
      X-linked, 102, 102*f*

Amelogenesis imperfecta (*Continued*)
  hypomineralization, 101–102
  hypomineralized, 98
  hypoplastic, 98, 100–101
      generalized pattern of, 100, 100*f*
      generalized thin variants of, 100,
          101*f*
      localized pattern of, 100
  with taurodontism (hypomaturation/
      hypoplastic), 102–103, 103*f*
  tooth discoloration due to, 67
AMELX gene, 99*t*, 100
AmpFLP analysis, 889
Amphotericin B for candidiasis, 209, 211*t*
Amputation neuroma, 532, 532–533*f*
Amyloid, 824
Amyloidosis, 824–827
  clinical features of, 824–826, 825*f*
  defined, 824
  diagnosis of, 826
  hemodialysis-associated, 825
  heredofamilial, 825–826
  histopathologic features of, 826, 826*f*
  macroglossia in, 9
  myeloma-associated, 825, 825*f*
  organ-limited, 824
  pathogenesis of, 824
  primary, 825
  secondary, 825
  systemic, 825
  treatment and prognosis for, 826–827
ANCA (antineutrophil cytoplasm
    antibodies) in Wegener
    granulomatosis, 336
Anemia, 582–583
  aplastic, 586–587, 587*f*
  associated with chronic disorders, 583*b*
  clinical features of, 582–583
  defined, 582
  with disturbed iron metabolism, 583*b*
  etiology of, 582, 583*b*
  Fanconi, 587
  hemolytic, 583*b*
      jaundice in autoimmune, 823
  iron-deficiency, 830
  megaloblastic, 583*b*
  myelophthisic, 593
  pernicious, 831–833, 832*f*
  sickle cell, 583–585, 584*f*
      jaundice in, 823
  treatment and prognosis for, 583
Anesthesia dolorosa, 866
Anesthetic necrosis, 294, 294*f*
Aneurysmal bone cyst, 638–640, 639*f*
Angiitis, granulomatous, 240
Angina
  bullosa hemorrhagica, vs. mucous
      membrane pemphigoid, 778, 779*f*
  Ludwig
      clinical features of, 133, 133*f*
      pathogenesis of, 132
      treatment and prognosis for, 134

Angiocentric immunoproliferative lesion, 607–609, 608f
Angiocentric T-cell lymphoma, 607–609, 608f
Angioedema, 348–350, 348–349f
Angiofibroma(s)
  facial, in tuberous sclerosis, 763, 763f
  nasopharyngeal, 552–553, 553f
Angiogenesis, 416
Angiolipoma, 531
Angiomas, leptomeningeal, 551
Angiomatosis
  bacillary, 195
  encephalotrigeminal (Sturge-Weber), 551–552, 551–552f
  meningeal, 551
Angiomyolipoma in tuberous sclerosis, 764
Angiomyoma, 556, 556f
Angioneurotic edema, 348–350, 348–349f
Angiosarcoma, 563–564, 563f
Angiotensin-converting enzyme (ACE) inhibitors, angioedema due to, 348, 350
Angular cheilitis, 202t, 204–205, 204f
  exfoliative vs., 294
  in Plummer-Vinson syndrome, 830, 831f
Animal bites, 899
Ankyloglossia, 10, 10f
Ankylosis, 873
  of tooth, 73–74, 74f
Anodontia, 75, 77
  in ectodermal dysplasia, 747
Anosmia, 870
Antemortem records
  comparison of postmortem and, 894–895, 894t, 895f
  examination of, 894
  request for, 890
Anthropologic examination of bones and teeth, 885–888, 886t, 886f
Anthropometry, 884
Antiangiogenic agents, osteonecrosis of jaw due to, 286, 286b
Antibiotic sore mouth, 202–203, 203f
Antigenic markers, 888
Antimalarial medications, oral mucosal discoloration due to, 308–309, 308f
Antineoplastic therapy
  enamel hypoplasia due to, 56, 56f
  noninfectious oral complications of, 280–286
    clinical features of, 281–284
    dermatitis as, 282, 282f
    developmental abnormalities as, 284
    hemorrhage as, 281
    mucositis as, 281, 281–282f, 284–285
    osteoradionecrosis as, 283–284, 283–284f
    taste disorders as, 283, 285
    treatment and prognosis for, 284–286
    trismus as, 284
    xerostomia as, 282–283, 283f, 285

Antineutrophil cytoplasm antibodies (ANCA) in Wegener granulomatosis, 336
Antiresorptive osteonecrosis of the jaw (ARONJ), 286, 286b, 288f
Antiretroviral therapy, 264
Antoni A pattern, 534, 536f
Antoni B pattern, 534, 536f
Antral pseudocysts, 310–312, 311–312f
Antrolith, 197
ANUG (acute necrotizing ulcerative gingivitis), 151
APECED (autoimmune polyendocrinopathy-candidiasis ectodermal dystrophy) syndrome, 206–207, 208f
  and hypoparathyroidism, 839
Apert syndrome, 41–43, 42f
Aphthosis
  complex, 324–325
  simple, 324–325
Aphthous stomatitis, recurrent. See Recurrent aphthous stomatitis
Aphthous ulcerations, recurrent. See Recurrent aphthous stomatitis
Apical periodontal cyst. See Periapical cyst
Apical periodontitis, chronic. See Periapical granuloma
Aplastic anemia, 586–587, 587f
Aquamid (polyacrylamide), oral lesions associated with, 302
ARC (AIDS-related complex), 252
Arc burn, 276
Argyria, 305, 306f
Argyrosis, localized, 298
ARONJ (antiresorptive osteonecrosis of the jaw), 286, 286b, 303f
Arsenic intoxication, 305
Artecoll (polymethylmethacrylate), oral lesions associated with, 302, 303f
ArteFill (polymethylmethacrylate), oral lesions associated with, 302, 303f
Arteriovenous malformations, 549
Arteritis, giant cell (temporal, granulomatous), 867–868
Arthralgia due to temporomandibular disorders, 875
Arthritis
  degenerative, 871–872
  psoriatic, 797
  reactive, 786–787
  rheumatoid, 872–874
Arthropathy due to temporomandibular disorders, 875
Artificial cinnamon flavoring, contact stomatitis from, 344–346
  clinical features of, 344, 345f
  diagnosis of, 345–346
  histopathologic features of, 345, 345f
  treatment and prognosis for, 346
Ascher syndrome, 5, 6f
Ascorbic acid deficiency, 827

Ash-leaf spots in tuberous sclerosis, 763
Aspergilloma, 221, 221f
Aspergillosis, 221–222
  clinical features of, 219–220, 221f
  diagnosis of, 222
  disseminated, 221–222
  histopathologic features of, 222, 222f
  pathogenesis of, 221
  treatment and prognosis for, 222
Aspirin, chemical injury due to, 278, 278f
Asteroid bodies, 329, 330f
Astrocytoma, subependymal giant cell, in tuberous sclerosis, 763
Attrition, tooth wear due to, 58–59, 59f, 61
Atypical eosinophilic ulcerations, 275, 275f
Atypical Spitz tumor, 378
Auriculotemporal syndrome, 862–863, 863f
Autoantibodies, molecular sites of attack of, 768–769, 769f
Autoimmune hemolytic anemia, jaundice in, 823
Autoimmune polyendocrinopathy candidiasis-ectodermal dystrophy (APECED) syndrome
  and hypoparathyroidism, 839
Autoimmune polyendocrinopathy syndrome, type 1, 206–207, 208f
Autoimmune polyglandular syndrome, type 1 and hypoparathyroidism, 839
Autopsy, 883

B
"Baby bottle caries", 909, 909f
Bacillary angiomatosis, 195
Bacillary peliosis hepatis, 195
Bacille Calmette-Guérin (BCG) vaccine, 185
Bacteria and squamous cell carcinoma, 404
Bacterial infection(s), 172–200
  actinomycosis as, 192–194, 193–194f
  cat-scratch disease as, 194–196, 195f
  diphtheria as, 177–179
  erysipelas as, 173–174, 174f
  gonorrhea as, 184–185
  impetigo as, 172–173
  leprosy as, 188–191
  noma as, 191
  scarlet fever as, 175–176, 175f
  sinusitis as, 196–198, 196f, 198f
  streptococcal tonsillitis and pharyngitis as, 174–175, 174f
  syphilis as, 179–184
  tonsillar plugs and tonsillolithiasis as, 176–177, 177f
  tuberculosis as, 185–188
Bacterial stains, tooth discoloration due to, 67–68
Balanitis circinata in reactive arthritis, 786
Ballooning degeneration in herpes simplex virus, 233–234, 233f
Banal nevus, 375

Bannayan-Riley-Ruvalcaba syndrome, multiple hamartoma syndrome and, 765

Barbell, 301, 301*f*

Bartonella henselae, 194

Basal cell adenocarcinoma, 492

Basal cell adenoma, 491–492, 492*f*

Basal cell carcinoma, 430–432, 431–432*f*
  in nevoid basal cell carcinoma syndrome, 694, 695*f*
  vs. peripheral ameloblastoma, 715–716
  in xeroderma pigmentosum, 753

Basal cell cytoplasmic antibody, 341

Basaloid squamous carcinoma, 425, 425*f*

Basaloid squamous cell carcinoma, 425, 425*f*

Basic multicellular unit (BMU), 287–288, 288*f*

Basosquamous carcinoma, 432

Bathing trunk nevus, 379

Batson plexus in metastasis, 569

BCG (bacille Calmette-Guérin) vaccine, 185

BCR-ABL fusion gene, 593

Beckwith-Wiedemann syndrome, 9

Behçet disease. *See* Behçet syndrome

Behçet, Hulusi, 326

Behçet syndrome, 326–328
  clinical features of, 326–327, 327*f*
  diagnosis of, 327, 328*t*
  histopathologic features of, 328
  pathogenesis of, 326
  treatment and prognosis for, 328

Bell palsy, 861–862, 862*f*

Bence Jones protein, 609

Benign juvenile melanoma, 378–379

Benign lymphoepithelial lesion, 475, 475*f*

Benign migratory glossitis in diabetes mellitus, 846

Benign mixed tumor. *See* Pleomorphic adenoma

Beriberi, 828

Bertillon, Alphonse, 884

β-hemolytic streptococci
  erysipelas due to, 173
  scarlet fever due to, 175

Betel chewer's mucosa, 394
  vs. morsicatio mucosae oris, 272–273

Betel quid
  oral submucous fibrosis due to, 393–395, 394*f*
  and squamous cell carcinoma, 403

Betel quid lichenoid lesions, 394

Bifid condyle, 19, 19*f*

Bifid tongue, 300–301, 301*f*

Bifid uvula, 2, 3*f*

Bilateral ossifying fibromas, 650

Biofilm, 161

Birbeck granules, 597, 598*f*

Bismuth intoxication, 305

Bisphosphonate-related osteonecrosis of the jaw (BRONJ), 286, 286*b*, 288*f*
  clinical and radiographic features of, 288–289, 288–289*f*
  histopathologic features of, 289, 290*f*
  treatment and prognosis for, 289–292

Bite(s)
  infectious complications of, 900
  self-inflicted, 900

Bite mark(s)
  characteristics of, 901–902, 901*f*, 902*t*
  defined, 899
  description of, 903

Bite mark evidence
  for animal bites, 899
  for insect bites, 899

Bite mark patterned injury (BMPI), 899
  saliva evidence from, 905
  serial pictures of, 904–905

Bite pattern evidence, 899–907
  basic principles of, 899–900, 900*f*
  characteristics of bite marks in, 901–902, 901*f*, 902*t*
  description of bite mark in, 903
  evidence analysis and comparison in, 906–907, 906–907*f*
  evidence collection in, 903–906
  examination of victim and suspect in, 903
  guidelines for bite mark analysis in, 902–907
  historical and legal issues with, 900–901
  impressions and study casts in, 905
  photography in, 903–905, 904*t*, 904*f*
  saliva evidence in, 905
  tissue samples in, 905–906, 906*f*

Black hairy tongue, 12–13
  clinical features of, 12–13, 12*f*
  histopathologic features of, 13, 13*f*
  treatment and prognosis for, 13

Black lesions, differential diagnosis of, 916–919*t*

Blastomycosis, 214–216
  acute, 214
  chronic, 214
  clinical and radiographic features of, 214–215, 214–215*f*
  cutaneous lesions of, 214, 214*f*
  diagnosis of, 215
  epidemiology of, 214
  histopathologic features of, 215, 215*f*
  oral lesions of, 215, 215*f*
  pathogenesis of, 214
  South American, 216–217, 216*f*
  treatment and prognosis for, 217

Blast transformation, 595

Bloch-Sulzberger syndrome, 755–756, 755–756*f*

Blue lesions, differential diagnosis of, 916–919*t*

Blue nevus, 377–378, 377–378*f*

Blue sclerae in osteogenesis imperfecta, 618, 619*f*

BMD (burning mouth disorder), 868–869, 868*b*

BMPI (bite mark patterned injury), 899
  saliva evidence from, 905
  serial pictures of, 904–905

BMU (basic multicellular unit), 287–288, 288*f*

Bohn's nodules, 25–27, 26*f*, 698

Bone(s)
  in hyperparathyroidism, 840, 841*f*
  physical anthropologic examination of, 885–888, 886*t*, 886*f*

Bone cavity, idiopathic, 636–638, 637*f*

Bone cyst
  aneurysmal, 638–640, 639*f*
  simple (traumatic, hemorrhagic, solitary, unicameral), 636–638, 637*f*
  Stafne (latent, static), 23–25, 24–25*f*

Bone eburnation, 626–627, 626*f*

Bone pathology, 618–684
  bone cyst as
    aneurysmal, 638–640, 639*f*
    simple, 636–638, 637*f*
  cementoblastoma (true cementoma) as, 659–661, 660–661*f*
  central giant cell granuloma as, 631–633, 632–633*f*
  central xanthoma of jaws, 640–641
  cherubism as, 634–635, 634–636*f*
  chondroma as, 661
  chondrosarcoma as, 669–671, 669*f*
    mesenchymal, 670–671, 671*f*
  cleidocranial dysplasia (cleidocranial dysostosis) as, 623–625, 623*t*, 624*f*
  fibroma as
    chondromyxoid, 661–662, 662*f*
    desmoplastic, 663–665, 664*f*
    ossifying, 652–653, 652–653*f*
    juvenile, 653–655, 654–655*f*
  fibro-osseous lesions of jaws as, 641–674
    cemento-osseous (osseous) dysplasia, 645–650
    familial gigantiform cementoma as, 650–651, 651*f*
    fibrous dysplasia as, 641–645
    juvenile ossifying fibroma as, 653–655, 654–655*f*
    ossifying fibroma as, 652–653, 652–653*f*
  fibrous xanthoma of bone, 640–641
  fibroxanthoma of bone, 640–641
  focal osteoporotic marrow defect as, 625, 625*f*
  giant cell tumor ("true giant cell tumor") as, 633, 633*f*
  idiopathic osteosclerosis as, 626–627, 626*f*
  massive osteolysis as, 627–628, 627–628*f*

Bone pathology *(Continued)*
    metastatic tumors to jaws as, 673–674, 673–674*f*
    osteoblastoma as, 658–659, 658–659*f*
    osteogenesis imperfecta ("brittle bone disease") as, 618–620, 619*f*, 619*t*
    osteoma as, 655–656, 656*f*
        giant osteoid (osteoid), 658–659, 658–659*f*
    osteopetrosis as, 620–623, 621–622*f*, 621*t*
    osteosarcoma (osteogenic sarcoma) as, 665–669
        postirradiation, 669
        surface (juxtacortical), 668, 668*f*
    Paget disease of bone (osteitis deformans) as, 628–630, 629–630*f*
    primary intraosseous xanthoma, 640–641
    primary xanthoma of bone, 640–641
    sarcoma as
        Ewing, 671–673, 672*f*
        postirradiation bone, 669
    synovial chondromatosis (chondrometaplasia) as, 662–663, 663*f*
Bone scar, 141, 141*f*, 626–627, 626*f*
Bone sequestration, oral ulceration with, 310, 310*f*
Bone whorl, 626–627, 626*f*
Botryoid odontogenic cysts, 699–700, 700*f*
Botryomycosis, 193
Bourneville-Pringle syndrome. *See* Tuberous sclerosis
Bowenoid actinic keratosis, 397
BP180 (bullous pemphigoid antigen), 780
BP230 (bullous pemphigoid antigen), 780
Brachycephaly, 41
Bradycardia in hypothyroidism, 836
Branchial cleft cyst, 35–36, 35–36*f*
Brandywine isolate, 105
Braun, Eva, 895
"Brittle bone disease", 618–620, 619*f*, 619*t*
Bronchiolitis obliterans in paraneoplastic pemphigus, 775
BRONJ. *See* Bisphosphonate-related osteonecrosis of the jaw (BRONJ)
Brown lesions, differential diagnosis of, 916–919*t*
Brown tumor in hyperparathyroidism, 840–841, 841*f*
Buccal bifurcation cyst(s), 704–705, 705*f*
    cervical enamel extensions and, 91
Buccal exostoses, 19, 19*f*
Buccal mucosa, differential diagnosis of soft tissue masses of, 922–925*t*
Bulky hyperkeratotic epithelial proliferation, 388
Bulla, defined, 914
Bull neck, 178
Bullous impetigo, 172
Bullous lichen planus, 788

Bullous pemphigoid, 771*t*, 779–781, 780*f*
Bullous pemphigoid antigens (BP180 and BP230), 780
Bundy, Ted, 896
Burkitt lymphoma, 606–607
    African (endemic), 606
    American (sporadic), 606
    clinical and radiographic features of, 606, 606*f*
    defined, 606
    histopathologic features of, 607, 607*f*
    immunodeficiency-associated, 606
    treatment and prognosis for, 607
Burn(s)
    cotton roll, 280, 280*f*
    electrical and thermal, 276–278
Burning mouth disorder (BMD), 868–869, 868*b*
Burning tongue syndrome, 868–869, 868*b*
Burroughs, George, 900
Burton line, 305

C
Café au lait pigmentation
    in fibrous dysplasia, 643, 644*f*
    in neurofibromatosis type I, 538, 538*f*
Calcific metamorphosis, 69, 120
    clinical and radiographic features of, 120, 120–121*f*
    treatment and prognosis for, 121
Calcifying cystic odontogenic tumor. *See* Calcifying odontogenic cyst
Calcifying epithelial odontogenic tumor, 720–722
    clinical and radiographic features of, 721, 721*f*
    epidemiology of, 720–721
    histopathologic features of, 721–722, 722*f*
    pathogenesis of, 720–721
    relative distribution of, 721, 721*f*
    treatment and prognosis for, 722
Calcifying odontogenic cyst, 701–703
    association of other odontogenic tumors with, 701
    categories of, 701
    central, 701, 701*f*
    clinical and radiographic features of, 701–702
    extraosseous (peripheral), 701, 702*f*
    histopathologic features of, 702–703, 702–703*f*
    intraosseous, 701, 701*f*, 703
    pathogenesis of, 701
    treatment and prognosis for, 703
Calcinosis cutis, 805, 805*f*
Calculi
    renal, in hyperparathyroidism, 840
    salivary (*see* Sialolithiasis)
Caliber-persistent artery, 14–15, 14–15*f*

Canalicular adenoma, 490–491, 490*f*
Canals of Scarpa, 27
Cancrum oris, 151–152, 191–192, 192*f*
Candida and squamous cell carcinoma, 404
Candidal hyperplasia, 382
Candidal leukoplakia, 202*t*
    clinical features of, 206, 206–207*f*, 382, 382*f*
Candidiasis, 201–212
    acute atrophic, 202–203, 203*f*
    chronic
        atrophic, 205
        in endocrine-candidiasis syndrome, 202–206, 203*f*
        hyperplastic, 202*t*, 206, 206–207*f*
        multifocal, 202*t*, 203–204, 204*f*
    clinical features of, 201–207, 202*t*
    diabetic, 845–846
    diagnosis of, 209
    erythematous, 202–206, 202*t*, 203*f*
    histopathologic features of, 207–208, 208*f*
    HIV-associated, 252–253, 252*f*
    mucocutaneous, 202*t*, 206–207, 208*f*
    pathogenesis of, 201
    pseudomembranous, 201–202, 202*t*, 202–203*f*
    treatment and prognosis for, 209–212, 211*t*, 212*f*
Candidosis. *See* Candidiasis
Canker sores. *See* Recurrent aphthous stomatitis
Cannon disease. *See* White sponge nevus
Capdepont's, 105
Capillary hemangioma, 549, 550*f*
CAPMI-4 (Computer-Assisted Postmortem indentification–version 4.0), 898
Carcinoma ex mixed tumor. *See* Carcinoma ex pleomorphic adenoma
Carcinoma ex papillary cystadenoma lymphomatosum, 490
Carcinoma ex pleomorphic adenoma, 499–501
    clinical features of, 499–500, 500*f*
    histopathologic features of, 500–501, 500*f*
    intracapsular, 501
    treatment and prognosis for, 501
Carcinoma *in situ*
    ex mixed tumor, 501
    in leukoplakia, 387–388, 388*f*
Carcinosarcoma, 423–424, 423–424*f*
    ameloblastic, 728
    of salivary gland, 499–501
Cardiac rhabdomyoma in tuberous sclerosis, 763
Caries
    "baby bottle", 909, 909*f*
    due to drug abuse, 293, 293*f*
    xerostomia-related (radiation-induced), 282, 283*f*, 471

Carotid body paraganglioma, 543–544, 543–544*f*
Cartilage-hair syndrome, 588
Cartilaginous choristoma, 559
Castleman disease, 229
Cat-scratch disease, 194–196, 195*f*
Cause of death, 883
Cavernous sinus thrombosis
　clinical features of, 133, 134*f*
　pathogenesis of, 132
　treatment and prognosis for, 134
CBCT (cone-beam computed tomography) in multiple fatality incident analysis, 898
CCLE (chronic cutaneous lupus erythematosus), 798–799, 799–800*f*
CD30+ lymphoproliferative disorder, primary cutaneous, 274
Celiac sprue, iron-deficiency anemia due to, 830
Cellular blue nevus, 377
Cellular hemangioma, 549, 550*f*
Cellulitis, 132–134
　clinical features of, 133, 133–134*f*
　defined, 132
　pathogenesis of, 132
　from periapical abscess, 130
　treatment and prognosis for, 134
Cell-within-a-cell phenomenon, 750
Cemental dysplasia, periapical, 646–647, 647*f*
Cemental hyperplasia, 93–94, 93*b*, 94*f*
Cemental tear, 164–165
Cementifying fibromas. *See* Ossifying fibroma(s)
Cementoblastoma, 659–661, 660–661*f*, 737
　"true", 737
Cementoma
　gigantiform
　　familial, 650–651, 651*f*
　　nonfamilial, 650
　periapical, 646–647, 647*f*
　"true", 659–661, 660–661*f*
Cemento-osseous dysplasia, 645–650
　clinical and radiographic features of, 646–648
　defined, 645
　diagnosis of, 648–649
　florid, 647–648, 648–649*f*
　focal, 646, 646*f*
　histopathologic features of, 648, 649*f*
　pathogenesis of, 645
　periapical, 646–647, 647*f*
　treatment and prognosis for, 649–650, 650*f*
Cemento-ossifying fibromas. *See* Ossifying fibroma(s)
Central giant cell granuloma, 631–633
　clinical features of, 631–632, 632*f*
　defined, 631

Central giant cell granuloma *(Continued)*
　etiology and pathogenesis of, 631
　histopathologic features of, 632–633, 633*f*
　radiographic features of, 631–632, 632*f*
　treatment and prognosis for, 633
　vs. brown tumor, 841
Central mucoepidermoid carcinoma, 496–497, 497*f*
Central papillary atrophy of tongue, 202*t*, 203, 203*f*
Central xanthoma of jaws, 640–641
　clinical and radiographic features of, 640, 640*f*
　histopathologic features of, 640–641, 640*f*
　treatment and prognosis for, 641
Cephalalgia due to temporomandibular disorders, 875
Cerebriform nucleus, 605, 605*f*
Cervical enamel extensions
　clinical and radiographic features of, 91, 91*f*
　defined, 90–91
　treatment and prognosis for, 91–92
Cervical enamel projections, 90
Cervical lymphoepithelial cyst, 35–36, 35–36*f*
Cervical pain disorders, 864*b*
Cervical ranula, 463, 463*f*
Cervicofacial emphysema, 314–315, 314*f*
C1 esterase inhibitors (C1-INH) deficiency, angioedema due to, 348–349, 348*f*
Chancre, 179, 179*f*
Charm needle implantation, 301, 302*f*
Cheilitis
　actinic
　　clinical features of, 395, 395*f*
　　histopathologic features of, 395, 396*f*
　　treatment and prognosis of, 396, 396*f*
　angular, 202*t*, 204–205, 204*f*
　　exfoliative vs., 294
　　in Plummer-Vinson syndrome, 830, 831*f*
　exfoliative, 294–296, 295*f*
　factitious, 294
　glandularis, 468–469, 469*f*
　granulomatosa of Miescher, 330–331, 331*f*
Cheilocandidiasis, 204–205, 205*f*
　exfoliative cheilitis vs, 294
Cheiloscopy, 885
Cheilosis
　actinic, 395–396
　　clinical features of, 395, 395*f*
　　histopathologic features of, 395, 396*f*
　　treatment and prognosis of, 396, 396*f*
　solar, 395–396
　　clinical features of, 395, 395*f*
　　histopathologic features of, 395, 396*f*
　　treatment and prognosis of, 396, 396*f*

Chemical injury(ies), 278–280
　clinical features of, 280, 280*f*
　due to aspirin, 278, 278*f*
　due to hydrogen peroxide, 278–279, 279*f*
　due to phenol, 279, 279*f*
　due to silver nitrate, 279
　due to tooth whitening strips, 278, 278*f*
　histopathologic features of, 280
Chemodectoma, 543–544, 543–544*f*
Chemotherapy
　diagnosis of, 594–595
　histopathologic features of, 594
　induction for leukemia, 595
　maintenance, for leukemia, 595
　treatment and prognosis for, 595
Chemotherapy-related epithelial necrosis, 281, 281*f*
Chemotherapy-related ulceration, 281*f*
Cherubism, 634–635, 634–636*f*
Chevrons in tobacco pouch keratosis, 392–393, 392*f*
Chewing tobacco. *See* Smokeless tobacco
Chickenpox, 235–238
　breakthrough infection with, 236
　clinical features of, 236–237, 236–237*f*
　complications of, 237
　diagnosis of, 237
　epidemiology of, 235–236
　histopathologic features of, 237
　in immunocompromised patients, 237
　during pregnancy, 237
　treatment and prognosis for, 237–238
Child abuse, 907, 908*f*
Chloasma, 371–372, 371*f*
Chlorodontia, 69, 69*f*
Chondral bodies in osteoarthritis, 872
Chondroid appearance in pleomorphic adenoma, 486, 486*f*
Chondroma(s), 661
　periosteal, 661
　soft tissue, 559
Chondromatosis, synovial, 662–663, 663*f*
Chondromatous metaplasia, reactive, 309–310, 309*f*
Chondrometaplasia, 662–663, 663*f*
Chondromyxoid fibroma, 661–662, 662*f*
Chondrosarcoma, 669–671
　clear cell, 670
　clinical and radiographic findings in, 669–670, 669*f*
　dedifferentiated, 670
　defined, 669
　epidemiology of, 669
　etiology and pathogenesis of, 669
　histopathologic features of, 670, 670*f*
　mesenchymal, 670–671, 671*f*
　myxoid, 670
　primary, 669
　secondary, 669
　treatment and prognosis for, 670
　variants of, 670

Chorda tympani syndrome, 862
Choristomas, osseous and cartilaginous, 559, 559f
Christmas disease, 579, 579t
Chromophores, 904
Chromosomal DNA, 888
Chronic apical periodontitis. See Periapical granuloma
Chronic cutaneous lupus erythematosus (CCLE), 798–799, 799–800f
Chronic fatigue syndrome, 242
Chronic kidney disease–mineral and bone disorder, hyperparathyroidism due to, 841
Chronic recurrent multifocal osteomyelitis (CRMO), 138
   clinical and radiographic features of, 139–140
   histopathologic features of, 140
   treatment and prognosis for, 140–141
Chronic sclerosing sialadenitis, 468, 468f
Chronic ulcerative stomatitis, 792–794, 793–794f
Chrysiasis, 306
Chvostek sign, 839
Cicatricial pemphigoid. See Mucous membrane pemphigoid
Cigarette smoking and squamous cell carcinoma, 402
CIMDL (cocaine-induced midline destructive lesion), 292
Cinnamon flavoring, artificial, contact stomatitis from, 344–346
   clinical features of, 344, 345f
   diagnosis of, 345–346
   histopathologic features of, 345, 345f
   treatment and prognosis for, 346
Ciprofloxacin, tooth discoloration due to, 70
Circumoral dermatitis, 295, 295f
Civatte bodies in lichen planus, 790
CJIS (Criminal Justice Information Services), 885
CL (cleft lip), 1, 2f
Clear cell chondrosarcoma, 670
Clear cell odontogenic carcinoma, 717–718, 717–718f
Clear cell odontogenic tumor, 717–718, 717–718f
Cleft(s). See Orofacial clefts
Cleft lip (CL), 1, 2f
Cleft palate (CP), 1, 2f
Cleft uvula, 2, 3f
Cleidocranial dysostosis, 623–625, 623t, 624f
Cleidocranial dysplasia, 623–625, 623t, 624f
Clotrimazole for candidiasis, 209, 211t
"Cloverleaf" skull, 41
CMV (cytomegalovirus), 229, 242–244, 243f

Coated tongue, 12–13
   clinical features of, 12–13, 12f
   histopathologic features of, 13, 13f
   treatment and prognosis for, 13
Cobalamin malabsorption, pernicious anemia due to, 831–832, 832f
Cocaine-induced midline destructive lesion (CIMDL), 292
Cocaine, orofacial complications of, 292, 293f
Cocci, 217–218, 217f
Coccidioidomycosis, 217–218, 217f
   chronic progressive pulmonary, 217
   disseminated, 217
CODIS (Combined DNA Index System), 889
Codman triangle, 665–666
Coffee, tooth discoloration due to, 68
"Cold sore", 231–232, 232f
Cole-Engman syndrome, 752–753, 752f
Colitis, ulcerative, and pyostomatitis vegetans, 851
Collagen, oral lesions associated with, 302
Colloid bodies in lichen planus, 790
Coloboma, 43
Colon adenocarcinoma, metastatic, 570f
Color changes, differential diagnosis of, 916–919t
Combined DNA Index System (CODIS), 889
Commissural lip pits, 4, 4f
Common acquired nevus, 375
Common blue nevus, 377
Common mole
   clinical features of, 375–376, 375–376f
   histopathologic features of, 376, 376–377f
   treatment and prognosis for, 376–377
Compound nevus, 375
Computer-assisted management technology, 882
Computer-Assisted Postmortem Identification–version 4.0 (CAPMI- 4), 898
Computer software technology in multiple fatality incident analysis, 898
Concrescence, double teeth due to, 82–85
   clinical features of, 84, 84–85f
   defined, 82
   treatment and prognosis for, 84–85
Condensing osteitis, 141, 141f, 626
Condylar hyperplasia, 16–17, 17t, 17f
Condylar hypoplasia, 17–19, 18f
Condyle, bifid, 19, 19f
Condyloma
   acuminatum, 358–360
      clinical features of, 358–359, 359f
      epidemiology of, 358
      histopathologic features of, 359, 359f
      treatment and prognosis for, 359–360

Condyloma (Continued)
   with HIV infection, 260
   latum, 180, 181f
Cone-beam computed tomography (CBCT) in multiple fatality incident analysis, 898
"Confetti" spots, 763
Congenital epulis, 546–547, 546f
Congenital erythropoietic porphyria, tooth discoloration due to, 68–69, 68f
Congenital fistulas of lower lip, 4–5, 4–5f
Congenital granular cell lesion, 546
Congenital hemangioma, 547
Congenital lip pits, 4–5, 4–5f
Congenital melanocytic nevus, 379–380, 380f
Congenital rubella syndrome (CRS), 248
Conjunctivitis, ligneous, 581–582, 582f
Contact burn, 276
Contact stomatitis
   allergic, 342–343, 343f
   from artificial cinnamon flavoring, 344–346
      clinical features of, 344, 345f
      diagnosis of, 345–346
      histopathologic features of, 345, 345f
      treatment and prognosis for, 346
Conventional acquired melanocytic nevus, 375, 375f
C4orf26 gene, 99t, 100
Coronal dentin dysplasia
   classification of, 104–105, 104t
   clinical and radiographic features of, 106–107, 107f
   histopathologic features of, 107, 107f
   treatment and prognosis for, 107–108
Coronavirus disease 2019 (COVID-19), 265–266, 266f
Coroner, 883
Coronoid hyperplasia, 15–16, 16f
Corps ronds in Darier disease, 757
Corynebacterium diphtheriae, 174
Cosmetic fillers, oral lesions associated with, 302–304, 303f
Cosmetic tattooing, 299
Cotton roll burn, 280, 280f
Cotton roll stomatitis, 280, 280f
"Cotton wool" radiopacities, differential diagnosis of, 926–931t
COVID-19 pandemic, 870–871
Cowden syndrome, 765–766, 765–766f
Coxa vara, 643
CP (cleft palate), 1, 2f
Crack cocaine, orofacial complications of, 292, 293f
Craniofacial dysostosis, 40–41, 41f
Craniofacial fibrous dysplasia, 642
Cremains, 893
Cremation, 893
CREST syndrome, 805–806, 805–806f
Cretinism, 835–836, 836–837f

Cribriform pattern of adenoid cystic carcinoma, 502, 503*f*
Criminal disasters, 896–897
Criminal Justice Information Services (CJIS), 885
CRMO. *See* Chronic recurrent multifocal osteomyelitis (CRMO)
"Crocodile tears", 862
Crohn disease, 850–851, 850–851*f*
and pyostomatitis vegetans, 851
Crouzon syndrome, 40–41, 41*f*
Crowe sign, 538
Crown, differential diagnosis of malformed, 932–935*t*
CRS (congenital rubella syndrome), 248
Cryptococcosis, 218–219, 219*f*
Cunnilingus, fibrous hyperplasia from, 297, 298*f*
Cushing disease, 842
Cushing syndrome, 842–843, 842*f*
Cusp(s)
accessory, 85–88
of Carabelli, 87
clinical and radiographic features of, 85–87
cusp of Carabelli as, 85, 85*f*, 87
dens evaginatus as, 86–87, 87*f*
with shovel-shaped incisors, 87, 87*f*
talon cusp as, 85–86, 86*f*
treatment and prognosis for, 87–88
of Carabelli, 85, 85*f*
talon, 85–86, 86*f*
Cutaneous horns, 357–358, 396–397, 397*f*
Cutaneous lupus erythematosus
chronic, 798–799, 799–800*f*
subacute, 800
Cutaneous sinus, periapical abscess with, 130–131, 131*f*
Cutaneous T-cell lymphoma. *See* Mycosis fungoides
Cutright lesion, 309–310, 309*f*
Cyclic hematopoiesis, 589–590, 590*f*
Cyclosporine-related gingival hyperplasia, 156, 156*f*
Cylindrical cell papilloma, 363–364
Cylindromas
dermal, 491
salivary gland, 501
Cyst(s)
alveolar, of newborn, 697–698, 698*f*
bone
aneurysmal, 638–640, 639*f*
simple, 636–638, 637*f*
Stafne (latent, static), 23–25, 24–25*f*
buccal bifurcation, 704–705, 705*f*
cervical enamel extensions and, 91
defined, 25, 914
dentigerous (*see* Dentigerous cyst)
dermoid (dysontogenic), 32–33
developmental (*see* Developmental cyst(s))
epidermal inclusion (implantation), 31

Cyst(s) *(Continued)*
epidermoid, 33
of skin (infundibular), 31
clinical features of, 31, 31*f*
histopathologic features of, 32, 32*f*
epithelial inclusion, 698
eruption, 688–689, 689*f*
fissural, 25
follicular
dentigerous (*see* Dentigerous cyst)
of skin, 31–32
clinical features of, 31–32, 31–32*f*
histopathologic features of, 32, 32*f*
treatment and prognosis for, 32
gingival
of adult, 698, 699*f*
of newborn, 697–698, 698*f*
"globulomaxillary", 27
heterotopic oral gastrointestinal (enteric duplication), 33
horn (pseudo-horn), 367, 367*f*
of incisive papilla, 28, 29*f*
lateral periodontal, 27, 31, 126
lateral radicular, 127, 127–128*f*
lymphoepithelial
cervical, 35–36, 35–36*f*
oral, 36–37, 36–37*f*
"median mandibular", 31
nasolabial (nasoalveolar, Klestadt), 26–27, 26–27*f*
nasopalatine duct (incisive canal), 27–30
clinical and radiographic features of, 28, 28–29*f*
histopathologic features of, 28–29, 29*f*
treatment and prognosis for, 30
odontogenic (*see* Odontogenic cyst(s))
palatal
median (palatine), 30–31
of newborn, 25–26, 26*f*
paradental, 685, 704
periapical (radicular, apical periodontal), 126–129
clinical and radiographic features of, 126–127, 126–128*f*
defined, 126
etiology and pathogenesis of, 126
"globulomaxillary cyst" as, 27
histopathologic features of, 127–129, 128–129*f*
"median mandibular" as, 31
periapical granuloma after, 123
pocket, 126
residual, 127, 128*f*, 129
treatment and prognosis for, 129
true, 126
pilar (trichilemmal, isthmus-catagen), 31
clinical features of, 31, 31*f*
histopathologic features of, 32, 32*f*
primordial, 689, 689*f*
residual carcinomatous transformation of, 706

Cyst(s) *(Continued)*
salivary duct (mucus retention, mucus duct), 460, 463–465, 464*f*
sebaceous, 31
sinus retention, 312–313
subchondral, in osteoarthritis, 872
teratoid, 33
thyroglossal duct (thyroglossal tract), 33–34, 34*f*
Cystadenoma, papillary, 465
Cystic hygroma, 553–555, 554*f*
Cytoid bodies in lichen planus, 790
Cytomegalovirus (CMV), 229, 242–244, 243*f*

D
Dahmer, Jeffrey, 896
Darier disease, 756–757, 756–757*f*
isolated, 757–758, 757*f*
Darier-White disease, 756–757, 756–757*f*
Daubert vs. Merrell Dow Pharmaceuticals (1993), 901
DDR (direct digital radiography) in multiple fatality incident analysis, 898
Death
cause of, 883
mechanism of, 883
mode or manner of, 883
undetermined, 883
Death certificate, 883
Dedifferentiated chondrosarcoma, 670
Dedifferentiation, 423
Degenerative arthritis, 871–872
Degenerative joint disease, 871–872
Demarcated opacities, 51–58
Denosumab, osteonecrosis of jaw due to, 287, 287*b*
Dense bone island, 626–627, 626*f*
Dens evaginatus, 86–87, 87*f*
Dens in dente. *See* Dens invaginatus
Dens invaginatus, 88–90
clinical and radiographic features of, 88–90
coronal, 88–89, 88*f*
type II, 88–89, 88–89*f*
type III, 88–89, 89*f*
defined, 88
radicular, 89–90
treatment and prognosis for, 90
Dental. *See also under* Teeth and Tooth
Dental corrosion
clinical features of, 59–60, 60–61*f*
treatment and prognosis for, 61–62
Dental erosion
clinical features of, 59–60, 60–61*f*
treatment and prognosis for, 61–62
Dental evaluation for identification, 889–899
antemortem record examination in, 894
basic principles of, 889–892

Dental evaluation for identification (Continued)
comparison of antemortem and postmortem records and written conclusions in, 894–895, 894t, 895f
dental numbering systems in, 891, 891t
dental prostheses in, 890–891, 890f
guidelines for, 892–895
instrument kit for, 892, 892b
in multiple (mass) fatality incident, 896–899
panoramic radiographs in, 892, 892f
postmortem examination in, 893–894, 894f
presence and position of individual teeth in, 889–890, 889f
requesting antemortem records for, 893
Dental fluorosis, 57–58, 57f
tooth discoloration due to, 67
Dental fraud, 910
Dental numbering systems, 891, 891t
Dental prostheses, identifying marks on, 890–891, 890f
Dental prosthetics identification (DPid), 890
Dental record in forensic dentistry, 881–883, 882f
Dental restorative materials
lichenoid contact reaction from, 346–347, 347f
tooth discoloration due to, 69, 70f
Denticles, 122
Dentigerous cyst, 685–688
central type, 686–687, 687f
circumferential type, 686–687, 687f
clinical and radiographic features of, 685–687
defined, 685
gross appearance of, 685, 686f
histopathologic features of, 687–688, 688f
inflamed, 687–688, 688f
lateral type, 686–687, 687f
neoplastic transformation of, 688, 706f
noninflamed, 687–688, 688f
pathogenesis of, 685
treatment and prognosis for, 688
vs. enlarged follicle, 687, 687f
Dentin
dentin dysplasia type II as
clinical and radiographic features of, 106–107, 107f
histopathologic features of, 107, 107f
treatment and prognosis for, 107–108
dentinogenesis imperfecta as
classification of, 104–105, 104t
clinical features of, 105, 105f
histopathologic features of, 107, 107f
prevalence of, 105
radiographic features of, 105–107, 105–107f
treatment and prognosis for, 107–108

Dentin (Continued)
dentin sialophosphoprotein-associated dentin defects as, 105–108
clinical and radiographic features of, 105–107
histopathologic features of, 107
treatment and prognosis for, 107–108
fibrous dysplasia of, 109
hereditary disorders of, 104–105, 104t
classification of, 104–105, 104t
dentin dysplasia type I as, 108–110
clinical features of, 108–109, 108–109f
histopathologic features of, 109, 110f
radiographic features of, 109, 109f
subclassification of, 109, 109b
treatment and prognosis for, 109–110
hereditary opalescent, 105
interface, 120
primary, 119–120
secondary, 119–121
clinical and radiographic features of, 120, 120–121f
pathogenesis of, 119–120
physiologic, 119–120, 120–121f
shell teeth as, 106, 106f
tertiary (reactionary, reparative, irregular, irritation), 120
histopathologic features of, 120, 120–121f
pathogenesis of, 120
Dentin dysplasia
type I, 108–110
classification of, 104–105, 104t
clinical features of, 108–109, 108–109f
histopathologic features of, 109, 110f
radiographic features of, 109, 109f
subclassification of, 109, 109b
treatment and prognosis for, 109–110
type II
classification of, 105, 105t
clinical and radiographic features of, 106–107, 107f
histopathologic features of, 107, 107f
treatment and prognosis for, 107–108
Dentin dysplasia–like alterations, systemic diseases correlated with, 108, 108b
Dentinogenesis imperfecta (DGI)
classification of, 105, 105t
defined, 618
histopathologic features of, 107, 107f
prevalence of, 105
radiographic features of, 105–107, 105–107f
tooth discoloration due to, 67
treatment and prognosis for, 107–108
Dentinogenic ghost cell tumor, 701
Dentinoma, peripheral fibroameloblastic, 733
Dentinosarcomas, ameloblastic, 728

Dentin sensitivity, 117
Dentin sialophosphoprotein (DSPP)-associated dentin defects, 105–108
clinical and radiographic features of, 105–107
histopathologic features of, 107
treatment and prognosis for, 107–108
Denture epulis, 517–519
clinical features of, 517–518, 518f
histopathologic features of, 518–519, 519f
treatment and prognosis for, 519
Denture fibroma, leaflike, 517–518, 518f
Denture injury tumor, 517–519
clinical features of, 517–518, 518f
histopathologic features of, 518–519, 519f
treatment and prognosis for, 519
Denture papillomatosis, 519–520, 519–520f
Denture stomatitis, 202t, 205, 205–206f
Dermal analogue tumors, 491
Dermal cylindromas, 491
Dermal melanocytoma, 377–378, 377–378f
Dermatitis
circumoral, 295, 295f
due to antineoplastic therapy, 282, 282f
impetiginized, 172
lichenoid, 787
perioral (periorificial), 343–344, 344f
Dermatofibroma, 520, 521f
Dermatologic disease(s), 747–818
acanthosis nigricans as, 806–807
Darier disease as, 756–757, 756–757f
dyskeratosis congenita as, 752–753, 752f
ectodermal dysplasia as, 747–748, 748f
Ehlers-Danlos syndromes as, 760–762, 761t, 762f
epidermolysis bullosa as, 766–769
hereditary benign intraepithelial dyskeratosis (Witkop–von Sallmann syndrome) as, 749–750, 750f
hereditary hemorrhagic telangiectasia (Osler-Weber-Rendu syndrome) as, 759–760, 759–760f
hereditary mucoepithelial dysplasia as, 754–755, 754–755f
immune-mediated, 768–769
chronic ulcerative stomatitis, 792–794, 793–794f
CREST syndrome, 805–806, 805–806f
erythema migrans as, 784–786
erythema multiforme as, 781–783
evaluation of, 768–769, 769f
graft-versus-host disease as, 794–796, 795f
immunopathologic features of, 748f, 761t, 768–769
lichen planus as, 787–792
lupus erythematosus as, 798–801

Dermatologic disease(s) *(Continued)*
  pemphigoid as
    bullous, 779–781
    mucous membrane, 775–779
  pemphigus as paraneoplastic, 774–775
  psoriasis as, 796–798, 796–797*f*
  reactive arthritis (Reiter syndrome) as, 786–787
  Stevens-Johnson syndrome and toxic epidermal necrolysis as, 783–784
  systemic sclerosis as, 801–805
  incontinentia pigmenti (Bloch-Sulzberger syndrome) as, 755–756, 755–756*f*
  multiple hamartoma syndrome as, 765–766, 765–766*f*
  pachyonychia congenita as, 750–752, 751–752*f*
  pemphigus as vulgaris, 769–773
  Peutz-Jeghers syndrome as, 758–759, 758*f*
  tuberous sclerosis as, 762–765
  warty dyskeratoma as, 757–758, 757*f*
  white sponge nevus as, 748–749
  xeroderma pigmentosum as, 753–754, 753*f*
Dermatosis papulosa nigra, 366–367, 367*f*
Dermoid cyst, 32–33, 33–34*f*
Desmoids, extraabdominal, 523
Desmoid-type fibromatosis, 523
Desmoplasia, 416
Desmoplastic ameloblastoma, 709, 711–712, 711–712*f*
Desmoplastic fibroma, 663–665, 664*f*
  of soft tissue, 523
Desmosomes, 769–770
Desquamative gingivitis
  in erosive lichen planus, 788
  in mucous membrane pemphigoid, 776, 777*f*
Developmental alterations
  due to antineoplastic therapy, 284
  of teeth, 74–111
    in number, 75–81
    in shape, 82–98
    in size, 81–82
    in structure, 98–111
Developmental cyst(s), 25–37
  branchial cleft (cervical lymphoepithelial), 35–36, 35–36*f*
  dermoid (dysontogenic), 32–33, 33–34*f*
  follicular, of skin, 31–32
    clinical features of, 31–32, 31–32*f*
    histopathologic features of, 32, 32*f*
    treatment and prognosis for, 32
  "globulomaxillary", 27
  hemihyperplasia (hemihypertrophy) as, 38–39, 39*f*
  medial palatal (palatine), 30–31, 30*f*
  "median mandibular", 31
  nasolabial (nasoalveolar, Klestadt), 26–27, 26–27*f*
  nasopalatine duct (incisive canal), 27–30

Developmental cyst(s) *(Continued)*
  clinical and radiographic features of, 28, 28–29*f*
  histopathologic features of, 28–29, 29*f*
  treatment and prognosis for, 30
  palatal, of newborn, 25–26, 26*f*
  progressive hemifacial atrophy as, 38–39, 39*f*
  segmental odontomaxillary dysplasia (hemimaxillofacial dysplasia) as, 39–40, 40*f*
  thyroglossal duct (thyroglossal tract), 33–34, 34*f*
Developmental defect(s), 1–50
  ankyloglossia (tongue-tie) as, 10, 10*f*
  Apert syndrome (acrocephalosyndactyly) as, 41–43, 42*f*
  bifid condyle as, 19, 19*f*
  caliber-persistent artery as, 14–15, 14–15*f*
  condylar hypoplasia as, 17–19, 18*f*
  coronoid hyperplasia as, 15–16, 16*f*
  Crouzon syndrome (craniofacial dysostosis) as, 40–41, 41*f*
  cysts as (*see* Developmental cyst(s))
  double lip as, 5–6, 5–6*f*
  Eagle syndrome as, 23
  fissured (scrotal) tongue as, 11–12, 11*f*
  Fordyce granules as, 6–7, 6*f*
  hairy tongue as, 12–13
    clinical features of, 12–13, 12*f*
    histopathologic features of, 13, 13*f*
    treatment and prognosis for, 13
  lateral soft palate fistulas as, 15, 15*f*
  leukoedema as, 7–8, 7–8*f*
  lingual thyroid as, 10–11, 11*f*
  lip pits as
    commissural, 4, 4*f*
    paramedian, 4, 4–5*f*
  macroglossia as, 8–9, 8*b*, 9*f*
  mandibulofacial dysostosis as, 43–44, 43*f*
  microglossia (hypoglossia) as, 8, 8*f*
  orofacial clefts as, 1–4, 2–3*f*
  Stafne defect as, 23–25, 24–25*f*
  torus mandibularis as, 21–23
    clinical and radiographic features of, 21–22, 22*f*
    histopathologic features of, 22, 22*f*
    treatment and prognosis for, 23
  torus palatinus as, 20–21, 21*f*
  varicosities (varices) as, 13–14, 14*f*
DGI. *See* Dentinogenesis imperfecta (DGI)
Diabetes mellitus, 844–846, 846*f*
  type I, 844–845
  type II, 844–845
Diabetic sialadenosis, 845–846
Dietary factors, and squamous cell carcinoma, 404
Differential diagnosis
  defined, 914
  of mucosal and soft tissue pathology with color changes, 916–919*t*

Differential diagnosis *(Continued)*
  with masses or enlargements, 922–925*t*
  with surface alterations, 920–921*t*
  of radiographic pathology, 926–931*t*
  of tooth pathology, 932–935*t*
Diffuse cutaneous systemic sclerosis, 801–805
Diffuse infiltrative lymphocytosis syndrome (DILS), 259
Diffuse linear calcifications, 123, 123*f*
DiGeorge syndrome and hypoparathyroidism, 839
Digital photography in multiple fatality incident analysis, 898
Digital radiography (DR), 882
  in multiple fatality incident analysis, 898
Dilaceration, 54, 94–96, 95*f*
Dilated odontome, 89, 90*f*
DILS (diffuse infiltrative lymphocytosis syndrome), 259
Dimorphism, 201
Diphtheria, 177–179
Direct digital radiography (DDR) in multiple fatality incident analysis, 898
Direct immunofluorescence, 769, 769*f*
Disaster Medical Assistance Team (DMAT), 897
Disaster Mortuary Operational Response Team (DMORT), 897
Discoid lupus erythematosus, 799, 799*f*
Discolorations, drug-related, 307–309, 308–309*f*
Disease-modifying antirheumatic drugs (DMARDs), 874
Dismemberment, 893
Distodens, 79, 79*f*
Distomolar, 79, 79*f*
Distorted taste, 869–871, 870*b*, 871*t*
DLX3 gene, 99*t*, 100
DMAT (Disaster Medical Assistance Team), 897
DMORT (Disaster Mortuary Operational Response Team), 897
DNA comparison, 888–889
DNA "fingerprint", 889
DNA Identification Act (1994), 889
Double lip, 5–6, 5–6*f*
Down syndrome, 9, 9*f*
Doyle vs. State of Texas (1954), 900
DR (digital radiography), 882
  in multiple fatality incident analysis, 898
Drooling, 469
Drug abuse, orofacial complications of, 292–294, 293*f*
Drug-induced xerostomia, 470–471, 470*t*
Drug reactions, 337–342
  anaphylactic stomatitis as, 338
  augmented, 338
  bizarre, 338
  clinical features of, 339–341
  diagnosis of, 341–342

Drug reactions *(Continued)*
  fixed, 338–339, 338*b*
  lichenoid, 338, 338–339*b*
  lupus erythematosus–like, 338–339, 339*b*
  mucosal pemphigoid-like, 338, 340*b*
  nonspecific, 338
  pemphigus-like, 338, 340*b*
  treatment and prognosis for, 342
Drug-related discolorations of oral mucosa,
    307–309, 308–309*f*
Drug-related gingival hyperplasia,
    156–158
  clinical features of, 157–158
  cyclosporine-related, 156, 156*f*
  defined, 156
  in edentulous areas, 157, 158*f*
  extensive, 157, 157*f*
  histopathologic features of, 158
  medications associated with, 156, 156*b*
  mild, 157, 157*f*
  nifedipine-related, 156, 156*f*
  oral hygiene and, 157
  phenytoin-related, 157, 157*f*
  prevalence of, 157
  treatment and prognosis for, 158
Drug-related gingival overgrowth.
          See Drug-related gingival
          hyperplasia
Dry mouth, 470–471, 470*t*
Dry socket, 143
DSPP-associated dentin defects. *See* Dentin
          sialophosphoprotein (DSPP)-
          associated dentin defects
DSPP gene, 105
Ductal dysplasia in leukoplakia, 387,
    387*f*
Ductal papillomas, 492–493
  clinical features of, 492, 492–493*f*
  histopathologic features of, 492–493,
    493*f*
  treatment and prognosis for, 493
Duodenal ulcers in hyperparathyroidism,
    841
Dwarfism, pituitary, 833–834
Dysgeusia, 869–871, 870*b*, 871*t*
  due to antineoplastic therapy, 283, 285
Dyskeratoma, warty (follicular), 757–758,
    757*f*
Dyskeratosis
  congenita, 752–753, 752*f*
    and aplastic anemia, 587
  focal acantholytic, 757–758, 757*f*
  follicularis, 756–757, 756–757*f*
    isolated, 757–758, 757*f*
  hereditary benign intraepithelial,
    749–750, 750*f*
Dysontogenic cyst, 32–33, 33–34*f*
Dyspareunia in mucous membrane
          pemphigoid, 777
Dysphagia, 410
  in Plummer-Vinson syndrome, 830
  sideropenic, 830–831, 831*f*

E
Eagle syndrome, 23, 23*f*
EBV. *See* Epstein-Barr virus (EBV)
Ecchymosis
  defined, 296, 914
  differential diagnosis of, 916–919*t*
  due to sequestration in spleen, 591, 591*f*
Echinocandins for candidiasis, 210–211,
    211*t*
Ecthyma, 172
Ectodermal dysplasia, 747–748, 748*f*
  hypohidrotic, 747
Ectomesenchymal chondromyxoid tumor,
    558
  clinical features of, 558, 558*f*
  histopathologic features of, 558, 559*f*
  treatment and prognosis for, 558
Ectopic enamel, 90–92, 91*f*
Eczema herpeticum, 232–233
Edema, angioneurotic, 348–350,
    348–349*f*
EDR (electronic dental record), 882
Ehlers-Danlos syndromes, 760–762
  classic, 760–761, 761*t*, 762*f*
  clinical features of, 760–762, 762*f*
  forms of, 760, 761*t*
  hypermobility type, 761, 761*t*
  treatment and prognosis for, 762
  vascular type, 761, 761*t*
EHR (electronic health record), 882
Elder abuse, 907, 908*f*
Electrical burns, 276–278, 277*f*
Electronic dental record (EDR), 882
Electronic health record (EHR), 882
Electronic medical record (EMR), 882
Elephantiasis
  gingivae (*see* Gingival fibromatosis)
  neuromatosa, 538, 538*f*
Elephantiasis neuromatosa, 538
Elephant Man, 539
Emphysema, cervicofacial, 314–315, 314*f*
EMR (electronic medical record), 882
Enamel
  development of, 51
  ectopic, 90–92, 91*f*
  mottled, 57, 57*f*
Enamel defects, environmental, 51–74
  clinical and radiographic features of,
    51–58, 52–53*f*
  dental fluorosis as, 57–58, 57*f*
  due to antineoplastic therapy, 56, 56*f*
  factors associated with, 51, 52*b*
  molar-incisor hypomineralization as, 55
  molar root-incisor malformation as,
    55–56, 55–56*f*
  pathogenesis of, 72
  syphilitic hypoplasia as, 58
  timing of insult in, 51
  Turner hypoplasia as, 53–54, 53*f*
Enamel hypoplasia
  clinical and radiographic features of,
    51–58, 52–53*f*

Enamel hypoplasia *(Continued)*
  defined, 51–52
  syphilitic, 58
  Turner, 53–54, 53*f*
Enamel loss, differential diagnosis of,
    932–935*t*
Enameloid conglomerates, 111, 111*f*
Enamel opacities, 51–52
Enamel pearls
  clinical and radiographic features of,
    90–91, 91*f*
  defined, 90
  treatment and prognosis for, 91–92
ENAM gene, 99*t*, 100
Encephalotrigeminal angiomatosis,
    551–552, 551–552*f*
Enchondromas, 661
Endocarditis, Libman-Sacks, 798
Endocrine-candidiasis syndrome, 202*t*,
    206–207, 208*f*
  and hypoparathyroidism, 839
Endodontic-related amalgam implantation,
    298, 298*f*
Endophytic papilloma, 362–363
Endophytic sinonasal papilloma, 362–363,
    362–363*f*
Enlargements, differential diagnosis of,
    922–925*t*
Enostosis, 626–627, 626*f*
Enteric duplication cysts, 33
Enteritis, regional, 850–851, 850–851*f*
Enterocystomas, 33
Enterovirus(es), 244–246
  acute lymphonodular pharyngitis due to,
    245, 246*f*
  classification of, 244
  clinical features of, 244–245
  diagnosis of, 246
  hand-foot-and-mouth disease due to,
    244–245, 245*f*
  herpangina due to, 244, 245*f*
  histopathologic features of, 245–246
  treatment and prognosis for, 246
Entropion in mucous membrane
          pemphigoid, 776–777, 777*f*
Environmental alterations of teeth, 51–74,
    52*b*
  environmental effects on tooth structure
          development as, 51–58, 52*b*
  localized disturbances in eruption as,
    71–74
  postdevelopmental loss of tooth structure
          as, 58–67
Environmental discoloration of teeth,
    67–71, 67*b*
  clinical features of, 67–70, 68*f*
  extrinsic, 67
    clinical features of, 67–70, 68*f*
    due to bacterial stains, 67–68
    due to tobacco products, tea, or coffee,
      68, 68*f*
    treatment and prognosis for, 70–71

Environmental discoloration of teeth
(Continued)
    intrinsic, 67
        due to congenital erythropoietic
            porphyria, 68–69, 68f
        due to hyperbilirubinemia, 69
        due to lepromatous leprosy, 69
        due to medications, 69–70
        due to restorative materials, 69, 70f
        due to trauma, 69
        treatment and prognosis for, 71
Eosinophilic granuloma. See Langerhans cell
    histiocytosis
Eosinophilic, hyalinized change in
    pleomorphic adenoma, 486, 486f
Eosinophilic ulcerations, 273–274
    atypical, 275, 275f
Ephelis, 368–369, 371f
Epidemic parotitis, 249–250, 250f
Epidermal inclusion cyst, 31
Epidermoid cyst(s), 33
    in Gardner syndrome, 31, 657, 657f
    of skin, 31
        clinical features of, 31, 31f
        histopathologic features of, 32, 32f
Epidermolysis bullosa, 766–769
    acquisita, 766
        vs. mucous membrane pemphigoid,
            778–779
    categories of, 766, 767t
    clinical features of, 766–768, 767f
    defined, 766
    dystrophic, 766, 767t
        dominant, 766–767, 767f, 767t
        recessive, 767–768, 767f, 767t
    histopathologic features of, 768, 768f
    junctional, 767t, 768, 768f
    pathogenesis of, 766
    simplex, 767t, 768
    treatment and prognosis for, 768
Epidermotropism, 604
Epiloia. See Tuberous sclerosis
Epithelial attachment apparatus, 769,
    770f
Epithelial dysplasia, in lichen planus, 790
Epithelial inclusion cysts, 698
Epithelial necrosis, chemotherapy-related,
    281f
Epithelial pathology, 354–459
    acquired melanocytic nevus as, 375–380
    actinic cheilosis as, 395–396
    actinic keratosis as, 396–397, 396–397f
    actinic lentigo as, 369–370, 370f
    basal cell carcinoma as, 430–432,
        431–432f
    basaloid squamous carcinoma as, 425,
        425f
    benign HPV-associated lesions as,
        354–364, 355t
        condyloma acuminatum (venereal
            wart) as, 358–360
        cylindrical cell papilloma as, 363–364

Epithelial pathology (Continued)
        exophytic sinonasal papilloma as,
            361–362
        fungiform papilloma as, 361–362, 362f
        inverted papilloma as, 362–363
        multifocal epithelial hyperplasia as,
            360–361
        sinonasal papillomas as, 361
        squamous papilloma as, 361
    blue nevus as, 377–378, 377–378f
    carcinoma of maxillary sinus as, 426, 426f
    congenital melanocytic nevus as,
        377–378, 377–378f
    ephelis (freckle) as, 368–369, 371f
    erythroplakia as, 390–391, 390f
    keratoacanthoma as, 398–401
    lentigo simplex as, 370–371, 371f
    leukoplakia as, 381–390
    melanoma as, 434–442
    melasma as, 371–372, 371f
    Merkel cell carcinoma as, 432–434, 433f
    molluscum contagiosum as, 364–365,
        364–365f
    nasopharyngeal carcinoma as, 428–430,
        429f
    nicotine stomatitis as, 397–398, 398f
    oral melanoacanthoma
        (melanoacanthosis) as, 373–374,
        374f
    oral melanotic macule (focal melanosis)
        as, 372–373, 372–373f, 373b
    oral potentially malignant disorders,
        380–381, 380–381b
    oral submucous fibrosis as, 393–395,
        394f
    sebaceous hyperplasia as, 368, 368–369f
    seborrheic keratosis as, 366–368
    sinonasal undifferentiated carcinoma as,
        426–428, 427f
    spindle cell carcinoma as, 423–424,
        423–424f
    verruca vulgaris (common wart) as,
        357–358
    verruciform xanthoma as, 365–366,
        365–366f
    verrucous carcinoma as, 421–423,
        422–423f
Epithelial rests of Malassez in periapical
    granuloma, 124–125
Epithelioid multinodular osteoblastoma,
    659
Epstein-Barr virus (EBV), 229
    infectious mononucleosis due to,
        241–242, 241f
Epstein-Barr virus (EBV)-associated
    lymphoproliferative disorders,
    601, 602f
Epstein's pearls, 25–26, 26f, 698
Epulis
    congenital, 546–547, 546f
    fissuratum (denture), 517–519
        clinical features of, 517–518, 518f

Epulis (Continued)
        histopathologic features of, 518–519,
            519f
        treatment and prognosis for, 519
    giant cell, 527–529, 528f
    granulomatosa, 526, 527f
    ossifying fibroid, 529–530, 529–530f
Erethism, 305
Erlenmeyer flask deformities, 821
Erosion
    defined, 914
    tooth wear due to
        clinical features of, 59–60, 60–61f
        treatment and prognosis for, 61–62
Erosive lichen planus
    clinical features of, 788, 789–790f
    diagnosis of, 791
    treatment and prognosis for, 791–792,
        792f
Eruption cyst, 688–689, 689f
Eruption hematoma, 688–689, 689f
Eruption sequestrum, 72, 73f
Erysipelas, 173–174, 174f
Erythema
    migrans, 784–786
        clinical features of, 784–785
            on sites other than tongue, 785, 785f
            on tongue, 785, 785f
        in diabetes mellitus, 845–846
        epidemiology of, 784
        etiopathogenesis of, 784
        fissured tongue in, 11–12, 11f, 785
        histopathologic features of, 785–786,
            785–786f
        and reactive arthritis, 786
        treatment and prognosis for, 786
    multiforme, 230, 771t, 781–783
        clinical features of, 781
        etiopathogenesis of, 781
        histopathologic features of, 782,
            782f
        major, 781, 782f
        minor, 781, 781f
        treatment and prognosis for,
            782–783
    nodosum, 328–329
Erythematous candidiasis, 202–206, 202t,
    203f
Erythroblastosis fetalis, tooth discoloration
    due to, 69
Erythrocytosis, primary acquired, 592
Erythroleukoplakia, 384, 384f, 390
Erythromelalgia, 592
Erythroplakia, 384, 390–391
Erythroplasia of Queyrat, 390–391
Erythropoietic porphyria, tooth
    discoloration due to congenital,
    68–69, 68f
Esophageal dysfunction in CREST
    syndrome, 805
Esophageal webs, 404
    in Plummer-Vinson syndrome, 830

Esthesioneuroblastoma, 562–563, 562–563f
Ewing sarcoma, 671–673, 672f
Exanthema subitum, 229
Exclusion of identification evidence, 883
Exfoliative cheilitis, 294–296, 295f
Exophthalmos, 837, 838f
Exophytic papilloma, 361–362, 362f
Exostosis(es), 19–20
    buccal, 19, 19f
    clinical and radiographic features of, 19–20, 19–20f
    histopathologic features of, 20
    in osteoarthritis, 872
    palatal, 19–20, 20f
    reactive subpontine, 20, 20f
    solitary, 20
    torus mandibularis as, 21–23
        clinical and radiographic features of, 21–22, 22f
        histopathologic features of, 22, 22f
        treatment and prognosis for, 23
    torus palatinus as, 20–21, 21f
    treatment and prognosis for, 20
Expansive osseous dysplasia, 650
Expert witnesses, dentists as, 910
Extraabdominal desmoids, 523
Extramedullary myeloid tumor, 594
Extranodal extension, 411
Extranodal marginal zone B-cell lymphoma, Sjögren syndrome and, 476
Extranodal NK/T-cell lymphoma, nasal-type, 607–609, 608f
Extrinsic factor malabsorption, pernicious anemia due to, 831

F
Facial angiofibromas in tuberous sclerosis, 763, 763f
Facial bones, physical anthropologic examination of, 885–888, 886t, 886f
Facial cleft
    lateral, 2
    oblique, 2
Facial dysesthesia, 866
Facial pain. See also Head and neck pain
    persistent idiopathic, 865
Facial paralysis, idiopathic, 861–862, 862f
Facial reconstruction techniques, 883
Facial superimposition techniques, 883
Facies leprosa, 190
Factitious cheilitis, 294
FAM83H gene, 99t, 100
Familial adenomatous polyposis, 656
Familial expansive osseous dysplasia, 650–651, 650f
Familial fibrous dysplasia, 634
Familial gigantiform cementoma, 650–651, 651f
Familial hypophosphatemic rickets, 848–850, 849f

Familial Mediterranean fever, 825–826
Familial white folded dysplasia. See White sponge nevus
Fanconi anemia, 587
FBI–National Crime Information Center (NCIC) data base, 890, 898
Federal Emergency Management Agency (FEMA), 897
Federation Dentaire Internationale (FDI) Two-Digit System, 891, 891t
Fellatio, palatal petechiae from, 297, 297f
Ferguson-Smith syndrome, 399
"Fever blister", 231–232, 232f
Fibrinolytic alveolitis, 143–144
Fibroameloblastic dentinoma, peripheral, 733
Fibrodentin, 120
Fibroepithelial papules in multiple hamartoma syndrome, 765f, 766
Fibroepithelial polyp, 517–518, 518f
Fibrolipoma, 531
Fibroma(s), 514
    aggressive ossifying, 653–655
    ameloblastic, 724–725, 724–725f
    chondromyxoid, 661–662, 662f
    clinical features of, 514, 515f
    desmoplastic, 663–665, 664f
        of soft tissue, 523
    giant cell, 514–517
        clinical features of, 515–516, 516f
        histopathologic features of, 516–517, 517f
        treatment and prognosis for, 517
    histopathologic features of, 514, 516f
    irritation (traumatic), 514
    leaflike denture, 517–518, 518f
    in nevoid basal cell carcinoma syndrome, 695
    odontogenic (see Odontogenic fibroma)
    ossifying (cementifying, cementoossifying), 652–653, 652–653f
        clinical and radiographic features of, 652–653, 652f
        defined, 652
        etiology and pathogenesis of, 652
        histopathologic features of, 653, 653f
        juvenile, 653–655, 654–655f
            clinical and radiographic features of, 654, 654f
            etiopathogenesis of, 654
            histopathologic features of, 654–655, 654–655f
            psammomatoid, 653, 655f
            trabecular, 654, 654f
            treatment and prognosis for, 655
        multiple (bilateral), 650
        peripheral, 529–530, 529–530f
        treatment and prognosis for, 653
    periungual, in tuberous sclerosis, 763, 763f
    treatment and prognosis for, 514
    ungual, in tuberous sclerosis, 763, 763f

Fibromatosis, 523, 523f
    gingivae (see Gingival fibromatosis)
    juvenile aggressive, 523
Fibromyxomas, 736
Fibro-odontoma, ameloblastic, 725–727, 726–727f
Fibro-odontosarcomas, ameloblastic, 728
Fibro-osseous lesions of jaws, 641–674
    cemento-osseous dysplasia as, 645–650
    familial gigantiform cementoma as, 650–651, 651f
    fibrous dysplasia as, 641–645
    juvenile ossifying fibroma as, 653–655, 654–655f
    ossifying fibroma as, 652–653, 652–653f
Fibrosarcoma, 559–560, 560f
    ameloblastic, 727–728, 728f
Fibrosis, oral submucous, 393–395, 394f
Fibrous dysplasia, 641–645
    clinical and radiographic features of, 641–643
    craniofacial, 642
    defined, 641
    of dentin, 109
    etiology and pathogenesis of, 641
    familial, 634
    histopathologic features of, 644, 645f
    monostotic, 641–642
    polyostotic, 643, 644f
    treatment and prognosis for, 645
Fibrous histiocytoma, 520–521, 521f
    malignant, 560–561, 561f
Fibrous hyperplasia, inflammatory, 517–519
    clinical features of, 517–518, 518f
    histopathologic features of, 518–519, 519f
    treatment and prognosis for, 519
Fibrous nodule. See Fibroma
Fibrous papules in tuberous sclerosis, 764, 764f
Fibrous tumor, solitary, 521–522, 522f
Fibroxanthoma, 520–521, 521f
Fingerprinting, 884
Fingertip ulceration in systemic sclerosis, 802, 802f
Fissural cysts, 25
Fissure, defined, 914
Fissured tongue, 11–12, 11f
Fistulas
    congenital, of lower lip, 4–5, 4–5f
    lateral soft palate, 15, 15f
Fixed drug eruptions, 338–339, 338b
Flame-shaped pulp chambers, 106–107, 107f
Flat torus, 21
Floor of mouth, differential diagnosis of soft tissue masses of, 922–925t
Florid cemento-osseous dysplasia, 647–648, 648–649f
Florid papillomatosis, oral, 422

Floss-related amalgam implantation, 298, 298*f*

Fluconazole for candidiasis, 209, 211*t*

Fluorescence in situ hybridization (FISH), 659

Fluorescent photography, 905

Fluorosis, dental, 57–58, 57*f*

Foam cells, 640

Focal acantholytic dyskeratosis, 757–758, 757*f*

Focal cemento-osseous dysplasia, 646, 646*f*
vs. condensing osteitis, 141

Focal epithelial hyperplasia360–361.
See Multifocal epithelial hyperplasia

Focal fibrous hyperplasia. *See* Fibroma

Focal melanosis, 372–373, 372–373*f*, 373*b*

Focal mucinosis, oral, 524–525, 525*f*

Focal osteoporotic marrow defect, 625, 625*f*

Focal periapical osteopetrosis, 626–627, 626*f*

Focal sclerosing osteomyelitis, 141, 141*f*, 626–627, 626*f*

Follicular cysts
dentigerous (*see* Dentigerous cyst)
of skin, 31–32
clinical features of, 31–32, 31–32*f*
histopathologic features of, 32, 32*f*
treatment and prognosis for, 32

Follicular dyskeratoma, 757–758, 757*f*

Forchheimer sign, 249

Fordyce granules, 6–7, 6*f*

Foreign body gingivitis, 154–155
clinical features of, 154, 154–155*f*
histopathologic features of, 155, 155*f*
lichenoid, 787
treatment and prognosis for, 155

Forensic dentistry, 881–913
autopsy in, 883
bite pattern evidence in, 899–907
basic principles of, 899–900, 900*f*
characteristics of bite marks in, 901–902, 901*f*, 902*t*
description of bite mark in, 903
evidence analysis and comparison in, 906–907, 906–907*f*
evidence collection in, 903–906
examination of victim and suspect in, 903
guidelines for bite mark analysis in, 902–907
historical and legal issues with, 900–901
impressions and study casts in, 905
photography in, 903–905, 904*t*, 904*f*
saliva evidence in, 905
tissue samples in, 905–906, 906*f*
cause of death in, 883
defined, 881
dentists as expert witnesses in, 910
fingerprinting for, 884–885

Forensic dentistry (*Continued*)
for human abuse, 907–910
epidemiology and classification of, 907–908, 908*b*
role of dentistry in recognizing and reporting, 909–910
signs and symptoms of, 908–909, 908–909*f*
identification in, 883–899
dental evaluation for, 889–899
antemortem record examination in, 894
basic principles of, 889–892
comparison of antemortem and postmortem records and written conclusions in, 894–895, 894*t*, 895*f*
dental numbering systems, 891, 891*t*
dental prostheses in, 890–891, 890*f*
guidelines for, 892–895
instrument kit for, 892, 892*b*
in multiple (mass) fatality incident, 896–899
panoramic radiographs in, 892, 892*f*
postmortem examination in, 893–894, 894*f*
presence and position of individual teeth in, 889–890, 889*f*
requesting antemortem records for, 893
exclusion evidence for, 883
insufficient evidence for, 883
personal recognition for, 883–884, 884*f*
physical anthropologic examination of bones and teeth for, 885–888, 886*t*, 886*f*
positive, 883
presumptive (possible), 883
serologic and genetic (DNA) comparison for, 888–889
indications for, 881
mechanism of death in, 883
mode or manner of death in, 883
morphometric means of identification, 884–885
record management in, 881–883, 882*f*
undetermined death in, 883

Forensic odontology. *See* Forensic dentistry

Forensic pathologists, 883

Forked tongue, 300–301, 301*f*

Formication due to drug abuse, 293

Formocresol, mucosal burn due to, 279, 279*f*

Fournier molars, 182

Franceschetti-Zwahlen-Klein syndrome, 43–44, 43*f*

Fraud, 910

Freckle, 369
Hutchinson, 436

Frenal tag, 514, 516*f*

Frey, Lucja, 862

Frey syndrome, 862–863, 863*f*

Frosted glass radiopacities, differential diagnosis of, 926–931*t*

Fruiting bodies in aspergillosis, 222, 222*f*

Frye vs. United States (1923), 900

Fungal disease(s)
aspergillosis as, 221–222
blastomycosis as, 214–216
candidiasis as, 201–212
coccidioidomycosis as, 217–218, 217*f*
cryptococcosis as, 218–219, 219*f*
histoplasmosis as, 212–214
mucormycosis as, 219–221
paracoccidioidomycosis as, 216–217, 216*f*

Fungiform papilloma, 361–362, 362*f*

Fungus ball, 221, 221*f*

Fusion, double teeth due to, 83–84
clinical features of, 83–85, 83–84*f*
defined, 82–83
treatment and prognosis for, 84–85

G

Gacy, John Wayne, 896

Gangrene, orofacial, 191–192, 192*f*

Gangrenous stomatitis, 191–192, 192*f*

Gardasil (human papillomavirus vaccine), 355

Gardner syndrome, 656–658
clinical and radiographic features of, 656–657, 656–657*f*
epidermoid cysts in, 31, 657, 657*f*
histopathologic features of, 658
treatment and prognosis for, 658

Gardner syndrome as, 656–658, 656–657*f*

Garment nevus, 379

Garrè, Carl, 142

Gaucher disease, 821

Gemination, double teeth due to, 82–85
clinical features of, 83–84, 83*f*
defined, 82–83
treatment and prognosis for, 84–85

Generalized eruptive keratoacanthomas, 399

Genetic comparison, 888–889

German measles, 248–249

Germinal centers, 578

Ggranulomatous stomatitis, as allergic disease, 336–337, 337*f*

Ghost cell(s), 702, 702*f*

Ghost cell odontogenic carcinoma, 702

Ghost cell tumor, dentinogenic, 701

Ghost teeth, 110–111, 110*b*, 111*f*

Giant cell arteritis, 867–868

Giant cell epulis, 527–529, 528*f*

Giant cell fibroma, 514–517
clinical features of, 515–516, 516*f*
histopathologic features of, 516–517, 517*f*
treatment and prognosis for, 517

Giant cell granuloma
central, 631–633, 632–633*f*
vs. brown tumor, 841

Giant cell granuloma (Continued)
    odontogenic fibroma with, 733, 733f
    peripheral, 527–529, 528f
Giant-cell hyaline angiopathy in periapical
        cyst, 129, 129f
Giant cell lesion, 527–529, 528f
Giant cell tumor, 633, 633f
Giant hairy nevus, 379
Giant osteoid osteoma, 658–659, 658–659f
Gigantiform cementoma
    familial, 650–651, 651f
    nonfamilial, 650
Gigantism, 834
Gilbert syndrome, jaundice in, 823
Gingival abscess, 164
Gingival cyst
    of adult, 698, 699f
    of newborn, 697–698, 698f
Gingival enlargement, differential diagnosis
        of, 922–925t
Gingival erythema, linear, 257, 257f
Gingival fibromatosis, 158–160
    clinical features of, 159–160, 159–160f
    defined, 158
    histopathologic features of, 160, 160f
    hypertrichosis associated with, 158, 159f
    isolated, 158
    localized, 160, 160f
    syndromes associated with, 158, 159b
    treatment and prognosis for, 160
Gingival granular cell tumor of the newborn,
        546
Gingival hemorrhage, tooth discoloration
        due to, 68
Gingival hyperplasia
    drug-related (see Drug-related gingival
        hyperplasia)
    localized juvenile spongiotic, 150–151,
        150f
    in tuberous sclerosis, 764–765, 764f
Gingival masses, differential diagnosis of,
        922–925t
Gingival overgrowth. See Gingival
        hyperplasia
Gingival recession, smokeless tobacco–
        related, 391, 391f
Gingivitis, 147–150
    chronic, 148–149, 149f
        hyperplastic, 148–149, 149f
    clinical features of, 147–149
    defined, 147
    desquamative, 155
        in erosive lichen planus, 788
        in mucous membrane pemphigoid,
            776, 777f
    epidemiology of, 147
    foreign body, 154–155
        clinical features of, 154, 154–155f
        histopathologic features of, 155, 155f
        treatment and prognosis for, 155
    histopathologic features of, 149, 149f
    HIV-related, 257, 257f

Gingivitis (Continued)
    hyperplastic
        chronic, 148–149, 149f
        with pyogenic granuloma, 148–149,
            149f
    lichenoid foreign body, 787
    local factors associated with, 147, 148b
    localized juvenile spongiotic, 150–151,
        150f
    marginal, 148–149, 148f
    mouth breathing–related, 147, 148f
    necrotizing vs. gonorrhea, 184
    necrotizing ulcerative, 151–152, 152f
        HIV-associated, 257, 258f
        in infectious mononucleosis, 241–242
    papillary, 148–149
    plasma cell, 152–154, 153f
        vs. contact stomatitis from artificial
            cinnamon flavoring, 344
    puberty, 147
    scorbutic, 829, 829f
    spongiotic, 150–151, 150f
    strawberry, 334, 334–335f
    systemic factors associated with, 147,
        148b
    treatment and prognosis for, 149–150
    types of, 147, 148b
Gingivostomatitis
    acute herpetic, 230, 231f
    allergic, 152–154, 153f
    atypical, 152–154, 153f
    necrotizing, 152
Glandular fever, 241–242, 241f
Glandular odontogenic cyst, 31, 703–704,
        704f
Globodontia, 96–97, 96–97f
"Globulomaxillary cyst", 27
Globus sensation, 410
Glomangiopericytoma, 521
Glomus jugulare tumor, 543–544
Glomus tympanicum tumor, 543–544
Glossitis
    interstitial, 180–181
    luetic, 180–181
    median rhomboid, 202t, 203, 203f
Glossodynia, 868–869, 868b
Glossopharyngeal neuralgia, 866–867
Glossopyrosis, 868–869, 868b
Glycosaminoglycans, 819
Gnathodiaphyseal dysplasia, 619, 651
Goldenhar syndrome, condylar hypoplasia
        with, 17
Gold intoxication, 305
Gonococcal ophthalmia neonatorum, 185
Gonorrhea, 184–185, 184f
Gorham disease, 627–628, 627–628f
Gorham-Stout syndrome, 627–628,
        627–628f
Gorlin cyst. See Calcifying odontogenic cyst
Gorlin sign, 761–762, 762f
Gorlin syndrome. See Nevoid basal cell
        carcinoma syndrome

Graft-versus-host disease (GVHD),
        794–796, 795f
    acute, 794
    chronic, 794
    clinical features of, 794–795, 795f
    cyclosporine-related nongingival
        hyperplasia in, 157, 158f
    diagnosis of, 795–796
    etiopathogenesis of, 794
    histopathologic features of, 795
    squamous cell carcinoma arising in, 795
    treatment and prognosis for, 796
Graft-versus-leukemia effect, 794
Grains in Darier disease, 757
Granular cell ameloblastoma, 711, 712f
Granular cell lesion, congenital, 546
Granular cell odontogenic fibroma, 734–735
Granular cell odontogenic tumor, 734–735
Granular cell tumor, 544–546, 545f
    gingival, of newborn, 546
Granulocytic sarcoma, 594
Granuloma
    calcifying fibroblastic, 529–530,
        529–530f
    eosinophilic (see Langerhans cell
        histiocytosis)
    giant cell
        central, 631–633, 632–633f
            vs. brown tumor, 841
        odontogenic fibroma with, 733,
            733f
        peripheral, 527–529, 528f
    gravidarum, 526
    midline lethal, 607–609, 608f
    periapical, 123–125
        clinical and radiographic features of,
            123–124, 124f
        defined, 123
        etiology and pathogenesis of, 123
        histopathologic features of, 124–125,
            124f
        treatment and prognosis for, 125, 125f
    pulse, in periapical cyst, 129, 129f
    pyogenic, 525–527
        clinical features of, 525–526, 526f
        gingival, 148–149, 149f
        histopathologic features of, 526, 527f
        during pregnancy, 526, 527f
        treatment and prognosis for, 527
    traumatic, 273–274, 274f
Granulomatosis
    interventions to rule out local causes of,
        330, 331t
    Langerhans cell (see Langerhans cell
        histiocytosis)
    lymphomatoid, 608
    orofacial, 155, 330, 331f
        clinical features of, 330–332, 331–332f
        in Crohn disease, 850–851
        diagnosis of, 332–333
        histopathologic features of, 332, 332f
        systemic evaluation of, 330, 331t

Granulomatosis (Continued)
    treatment and prognosis for, 333,
        333–334f
    with polyangitis, 333–336
    Wegener, 333–336
        clinical features of, 333–335, 334–335f
        diagnosis of, 335–336, 336b
        generalized, 333
        histopathologic features of, 335, 335f
        limited, 333–334
        superficial, 333–334
        treatment and prognosis for, 336
Granulomatous angiitis, 240
Granulomatous arteritis, 867–868
Grave's disease, 837–838, 838f
Gray lesions, differential diagnosis of,
    916–919t
"Ground glass" radiopacities, differential
    diagnosis of, 926–931t
Grzybowski syndrome, 399
Guillain-Barré syndrome, 861
Gum boil, 130–131, 130–132f
Gumma, 180–181
Günther disease, tooth discoloration due to,
    68–69, 68f
Gustatory lacrimation syndrome, 862
Gustatory sweating and flushing, 862–863,
    863f
GVHD. See Graft-versus-host disease
    (GVHD)

H
Hailey-Hailey disease, 770
Hairy tongue, 12–13
    clinical features of, 12–13, 12f
    histopathologic features of, 13, 13f
    treatment and prognosis for, 13
Halo nevus, 379, 379f
Hamartoma(s)
    intracranial, in tuberous sclerosis, 763f,
        764–765
    in multiple hamartoma syndrome,
        765–766, 765–766f
    odontogenic epithelial, 733
    odontomas as, 729
Hamman's crunch, 314
Hand-foot and-mouth disease, 244–245,
    245f
Hand-Schüller-Christian disease, 596
Hansen disease. See Leprosy
Hard palate, differential diagnosis of soft
    tissue masses of, 922–925t
Hashimoto thyroiditis, 836
HBID (hereditary benign intraepithelial
    dyskeratosis), 749–750, 750f
Headache disorders, primary, 864b
Head and neck pain, 863, 864b
    due to burning mouth disorder, 868–869,
        868b
    due to giant cell arteritis, 867–868
    due to glossopharyngeal neuralgia,
        866–867

Head and neck pain (Continued)
    due to trigeminal neuralgia, 864–866,
        865b
Health Insurance Portability and
    Accountability Act (HIPAA,
    1996), 881
Heck disease360–361. See Multifocal
    epithelial hyperplasia
Heerfordt syndrome, 329, 861
Hemangioendothelioma, 563
    juvenile, 549
    kaposiform, 548
Hemangioma(s), 547–551
    capillary, 549, 550f
    clinical and radiographic features of,
        547–548, 548f
    congenital, 547
    defined, 547
    histopathologic features of, 549–551,
        550f
    of infancy, 547, 548f
    juvenile (cellular), 549, 550f
    lobular capillary (see Pyogenic granuloma)
    in multiple hamartoma syndrome, 765
    in PHACE(S) syndrome, 548
    sclerosing, 520–521, 521f
    "strawberry", 547–548, 548f
    treatment and prognosis for, 550–551
    tufted, 548
Hemangiopericytoma, 521
    sinonasal-type, 521
Hemarthrosis, 580, 580f
Hematologic disorder(s), 578–617
    agranulocytosis as, 589
    anemia as, 582–583, 583b
        aplastic, 586–587, 587f
        sickle cell, 583–585, 584f
    cyclic neutropenia (cyclic hematopoiesis)
        as, 589–590, 590f
    hemophilia as, 579–581, 579t, 580f
    Langerhans cell histiocytosis as, 596–598
    leukemia as, 593–595, 594f
    lymphoid hyperplasia as, 578, 579f
    lymphoma as
        Burkitt, 606–607
        cutaneous T-cell, 604–606
        extranodal NK/T-cell, nasal-type,
            607–609, 608f
        Hodgkin, 579t, 598–600, 599f
        non-Hodgkin, 600–604
    multiple myeloma as, 609–611,
        609–610f
    mycosis fungoides as, 604–606
    neutropenia as, 587–589
    plasmacytoma as, 611, 611f
    plasminogen deficiency as, 581–582,
        582f
    polycythemia vera as, 592
    thalassemia as, 585–586, 585–586f
    thrombocytopenia as, 590–592, 591f
Hematoma, 296, 297f, 591, 591f
    eruption, 688–689, 689f

Hematopoiesis, cyclic, 589–590, 590f
Hematopoietic cell transplantation,
    nonmyeloablative allogenic, 794
Hemiageusia, 870
Hemiatrophy, progressive facial, 38–39, 39f
Hemidesmosomes in bullous pemphigoid,
    780
Hemifacial hyperplasia, 37
    complex vs. simple, 37
    condylar hyperplasia vs., 16
    macroglossia in, 9
Hemifacial microsomia, condylar hypoplasia
    with, 17
Hemihyperplasia, 37–38, 37b, 38f
    complex vs. simple, 37
Hemihypertrophy, 37–38, 37b, 38f
Hemimaxillofacial dysplasia, 39–40, 40f
Hemochromatosis, 586
Hemodialysis-associated amyloidosis, 825
Hemoglobinopathies, 583
Hemolytic anemia, 583b
    jaundice in autoimmune, 823
Hemophilia, 579–581
    clinical features of, 580, 580f
    defined, 579
    dental care with, 581
    and HIV, 581
    most common forms of, 579, 579t
    pseudotumor of, 580
    treatment and prognosis for, 580–581
Hemophilia A, 579, 579t
Hemophilia B, 579, 579t
Hemorrhage
    due to antineoplastic therapy, 281
    submucosal, 296–297, 296–297f
    tooth discoloration due to gingival, 68
Hemorrhagic bone cyst, 636–638, 637f
Henderson-Paterson bodies, 364, 365f
Hereditary angioedema with normal C1-
    INH (HAE-nC1-INH),
    348–349
Hereditary benign intraepithelial
    dyskeratosis (HBID), 749–750,
    750f
Hereditary hemorrhagic telangiectasia
    (HHT), 759–760, 759–760f
Hereditary hypophosphatemia, 848–850,
    849f
Hereditary mucoepithelial dysplasia,
    754–755, 754–755f
Hereditary opalescent dentin, 105
Hereditary transthyretin amyloidosis,
    825–826
Heredofamilial amyloidosis, 825–826
Herpangina, 244, 245f
Herpes, 229
Herpes barbae, 232–233
Herpes gladiatorum, 232–233
Herpes labialis, 231–232, 232f
Herpes simplex virus (HSV), 229–235
    acute herpetic gingivostomatitis due to,
        230, 231f

Herpes simplex virus (HSV) *(Continued)*
    chronic infection with, 232–233, 233*f*
    clinical features of, 230–233
    diagnosis of, 234
    eczema herpeticum (Kaposi varicelliform eruption) due to, 232–233
    herpes barbae due to, 232–233
    herpes gladiatorum (scrumpox) due to, 232–233
    herpes labialis ("cold sore", "fever blister") due to, 231–232, 232*f*
    herpetic whitlow (herpetic paronychia) due to, 232, 233*f*
    histopathologic features of, 233–234, 233–234*f*
    HIV-associated, 260, 260*f*
    in immunocompromised host, 233, 233*f*, 235
    pathogenesis of, 229
    pharyngotonsillitis due to, 231
    primary infection with, 229–230, 231*f*
    recurrent (secondary, recrudescent) infection with, 230, 232*f*
    treatment and prognosis for, 234–235
Herpes simplex virus type 1 (HSV-1), 229
Herpes simplex virus type 2 (HSV-2), 229
Herpes zoster, 238–241, 238–239*f*
    with HIV infection, 260
Herpes zoster vaccine (Zostavax), 240–241
Herpetic paronychia, 232, 233*f*
Herpetic whitlow, 232, 233*f*
Herpetiform aphthous stomatitis, 324–325, 324*f*
Herpetoviridae, 229
Heterotopic oral gastrointestinal cysts, 33
HHT (hereditary hemorrhagic telangiectasia), 759–760, 759–760*f*
HHVs. *See* Human herpesvirus(es) (HHVs)
Hide-bound disease. *See* Systemic sclerosis
HIPAA (Health Insurance Portability and Accountability Act, 1996), 881
Histiocytoma, fibrous, 520–521, 521*f*
    malignant, 560–561, 561*f*
Histiocytosis, Langerhans cell (idiopathic), 596–598
    classification of, 596
    clinical and radiographic features of, 596, 597*f*
    histopathologic features of, 597, 597–598*f*
    of tongue, 273–274
    treatment and prognosis for, 597–598
Histiocytosis X. *See* Histiocytosis, Langerhans cell
Histocompatibility antigen B-51 (HLAB51) in Behçet syndrome, 326
Histoplasmosis, 212–214
    acute, 212
    chronic, 212

Histoplasmosis *(Continued)*
    clinical and radiographic features of, 212, 213*f*
    diagnosis of, 213
    disseminated, 212
    histopathologic features of, 212–213, 213*f*
    HIV-associated, 212
    pathogenesis of, 212
    treatment and prognosis for, 213–214
Hitler, Adolph, 895
HIV. *See* Human immunodeficiency virus (HIV)
HIV-associated periodontitis, 257, 258*f*
HIV-related gingivitis, 257, 257*f*
HLA-B51 (histocompatibility antigen B-51) in Behçet syndrome, 326
Hockey stick deformity, 643
Hodgkin disease. *See* Hodgkin lymphoma
Hodgkin lymphoma, 598–600
    classical, 599–600
    clinical features of, 598–599, 599*f*
    histopathologic features of, 599–600, 599*f*
    lymphocyte depletion subtype of, 600
    lymphocyte-rich, 600
    mixed cellularity form of, 600
    nodular lymphocyte–predominant, 600
    nodular sclerosis subtype of, 600
    staging of, 599–600, 599*t*
    treatment and prognosis for, 600
    unclassifiable, 600
Homogeneous leukoplakia, 383–384
Homogeneous thick leukoplakia, 383–384, 384*f*
Homogeneous thin leukoplakia, 383–384
Horn cysts, 367, 367*f*
Hperchromatic nuclei, 416
HPV. *See* Human papillomavirus (HPV)
HSV. *See* Herpes simplex virus (HSV)
HTLV-1 (T-cell leukemia/lymphoma virus type 1), 593
Human abuse, 907–910
    epidemiology and classification of, 907–908, 908*b*
    role of dentistry in recognizing and reporting, 909–910
    signs and symptoms of, 908–909, 908–909*f*
Human herpesvirus(es) (HHVs), 229
    cytomegalovirus as, 242–244
    herpes simplex virus as, 229–235
    herpes zoster (shingles) due to, 238–241
    infectious mononucleosis due to, 241–242
    varicella (chickenpox) due to, 235–238
Human herpesvirus type 1 (HHV-1), 229
Human herpesvirus type 2 (HHV-2), 229
Human herpesvirus type 3 (HHV-3), 229
Human herpesvirus type 4 (HHV-4), 229
    infectious mononucleosis due to, 241
Human herpesvirus type 5 (HHV-5), 229

Human herpesvirus type 6 (HHV-6), 229
Human herpesvirus type 7 (HHV-7), 229
Human herpesvirus type 8 (HHV-8), 229, 254
Human immunodeficiency virus (HIV), 250–265
    blood screening for, 251
    clinical features of, 252–263
    diagnosis of, 263–264, 264*b*
    hemophilia and, 581
    histoplasmosis as, 212
    hyperpigmentation as, 259
    Kaposi sarcoma as, 254–256, 255*f*
    mycobacterial infection as, 258–259
    non-Hodgkin lymphoma as, 256–257, 257*f*
    oral hairy leukoplakia as, 253–254, 254*f*
    oral manifestations of, 252
        aphthous stomatitis as, 262, 262–263*f*
        candidiasis as, 252–253, 252–253*f*
        cytomegalovirus as, 243
        herpes simplex virus as, 260, 260*f*
        histoplasmosis as, 262, 262*f*
        human papillomavirus as, 260–262, 261*f*
        molluscum contagiosum as, 262–263, 263*f*
        varicella-zoster virus as, 260
    pathogenesis of, 251
    periodontal disease as, 257, 258*f*
    persistent generalized lymphadenopathy as, 256, 256*f*
    prevalence of, 252
    salivary gland disease, 259
    squamous cell carcinoma as, 263, 263*f*
    thrombocytopenia as, 259–260
    treatment and prognosis for, 264–265
Human papillomavirus (HPV)
    alveolar ridge, 383, 383*f*
    benign lesions associated with, 354–364, 355*t*
        condyloma acuminatum (venereal wart) as, 358–360
        cylindrical cell papilloma as, 363–364
        exophytic sinonasal papilloma as, 361–362
        fungiform papilloma as, 361–362, 362*f*
        inverted papilloma as, 362–363
        modes of transmission of, 354
        multifocal epithelial hyperplasia as, 360–361
        natural history of, 354
        prevalence of, 354
        sinonasal papillomas as, 361
        squamous papilloma as, 355–357, 361
        verruca vulgaris (common wart) as, 357–358
    HIV-associated, 260–262, 261*f*
    leukoplakia due to, 382
Human papillomavirus (HPV) vaccines (Gardasil), 355

Hunter disease, 820t
Hurler disease, 820t
Hutchinson freckle, 436
Hutchinson incisors, 58, 182, 182f
Hutchinson, Jonathan, 181, 328
Hutchinson triad, 181
Hyaline bodies
  in lichen planus, 790
  in periapical cyst, 129, 129f
Hyalinized, eosinophilic change in
    pleomorphic adenoma, 486, 486f
Hyalinosis cutis et mucosae, 822–823,
    822–823f
Hyaluronic acid (Restylane, Juvederm), oral
    lesions associated with, 302
Hydrogen peroxide, chemical injury due to,
    278–279, 279f
Hydropic degeneration in lichen planus, 790
Hydrops fetalis, 586
Hydroxyapatite (Radiesse), oral lesions
    associated with, 302, 303f
Hygroma, cystic, 553–555, 554f
Hyperbilirubinemia, tooth discoloration due
    to, 69
Hypercarotenemia, 824
Hypercementosis, 93–94, 93b, 94f
Hypercortisolism, 842–843, 842f
Hyperdontia
  clinical features of, 78–80, 78–79f
  defined, 75
  differential diagnosis of, 932–935t
  with mesiodens, 78f
  with multiple supernumerary teeth, 78,
    78f
  syndromes associated with, 75, 76b
Hyperglycemia, 844
Hyperkeratosis in leukoplakia, 385
Hyperkeratotic form of seborrheic keratosis,
    367–368
Hyperorthokeratosis in leukoplakia,
    385–386, 386f
Hyperostoses, 655
Hyperparakeratosis in leukoplakia,
    385–386, 386f
Hyperparathyroidism, 840–842
  clinical and radiographic features of,
    840–841, 841f
  histopathologic features of, 841,
    841–842f
  primary, 840–842
  secondary, 840, 842
  treatment and prognosis for, 841–842
Hyperparathyroidism-jaw tumor syndrome,
    652, 840
Hyperpigmentation with HIV infection,
    256
Hyperplasia
  condylar, 16–17, 17t, 17f
  coronoid, 15–16, 16f
  hemifacial, 37
    condylar hyperplasia vs., 16
    macroglossia in, 9

Hyperplasia (Continued)
  subpontic osseous, 20, 20f
Hyperplastic candidiasis, 202t, 206,
    206–207f
Hyperplastic gingivitis
  chronic, 148–149, 149f
  with pyogenic granuloma, 148–149, 149f
Hypertaurodontism, 92, 93f
Hyperthyroidism, 837–838, 838f
Hypertrichosis, 379
Hypoadrenocorticism, 843–844, 844f
  due to paracoccidioidomycosis, 216
  histoplasmosis as, 212
  primary, 843
  secondary, 843
Hypocalcified amelogenesis imperfecta, 98
Hypodactylia, 8
Hypodontia
  defined, 75
  differential diagnosis of, 932–935t
  in ectodermal dysplasia, 747, 748f
  in incontinentia pigmenti, 755, 756f
  treatment and prognosis for, 80
Hypogeusia, 869–871, 870b, 871t
  due to antineoplastic therapy, 283, 285
Hypoglossia, 8, 8f
Hypohyperdontia, 79
Hypomaturation amelogenesis imperfecta,
    98
Hypomelia, 8
Hypoparathyroidism, 838–839, 839f
  pseudo-, 839–840
Hypophosphatasia, 847–848
  adult, 848
  childhood, 847–848, 847f
  clinical and radiographic features of,
    847–848, 847f
  diagnosis of, 848
  histopathologic features of, 848, 848f
  infantile, 847
  perinatal
    benign, 847
    lethal, 847
  treatment and prognosis for, 848
Hypophosphatemia, hereditary, 848–850,
    849f
Hypoplasia, 460
Hypoplasminogenemia, 581–582, 582f
Hypoplastic amelogenesis imperfecta, 98
Hyposmia, 870
Hypotaurodontism, 92, 93f
Hypothermia in hypothyroidism, 836
Hypothyroidism, 9, 835–836, 836–837f

I
IAFIS (Integrated Automated Fingerprint
    Identification System), 885
Icterus, 823–824, 824f
Identification, 883–899
  dental evaluation for, 889–899
    antemortem record examination in,
    894

Identification (Continued)
  basic principles of, 889–892
  comparison of antemortem and
    postmortem records and written
    conclusions in, 894–895, 894t,
    895f
  dental numbering systems in, 891,
    891t
  dental prostheses in, 890–891, 890f
  guidelines for, 892–895
  instrument kit for, 892, 892b
  in multiple (mass) fatality incident,
    896–899
  panoramic radiographs in, 892, 892f
  postmortem examination in, 893–894,
    894f
  presence and position of individual
    teeth in, 889–890, 889f
  requesting antemortem records for,
    893
  exclusion evidence for, 883
  fingerprinting for, 884–885
  insufficient evidence for, 883
  morphometric means of, 884–885
  personal recognition for, 883–884, 884f
  physical anthropologic examination of
    bones and teeth for, 885–888,
    886t, 886f
  positive, 883
  presumptive (possible), 883
  serologic and genetic (DNA) comparison
    for, 888–889
Idiopathic bone cavity, 636–638, 637f
Idiopathic facial paralysis, 861–862, 862f
Idiopathic midline destructive disease,
    607–609, 608f
Idiopathic osteolysis, 627–628, 627–628f
Idiopathic osteosclerosis, 626–627, 626f
  vs. condensing osteitis, 141
Idiopathic seventh nerve paralysis, 861–862,
    862f
IgG4-related disease, 471–472
Ileitis, regional, 850–851, 850–851f
Imidazole agents for candidiasis, 209,
    211t
Immune-mediated dermatologic disease(s),
    768–769
  chronic ulcerative stomatitis, 792–794,
    793–794f
  CREST syndrome, 805–806, 805–806f
  erythema as
    migrans, 784–786
    multiforme, 781–783
  evaluation of, 768–769, 769f
  graft-versus-host disease, 794–796, 795f
  immunopathologic features of, 748f,
    761t, 768–769
  lichen planus as, 787–792
  lupus erythematosus as, 798–801
  pemphigoid as
    bullous, 779–781
    mucous membrane, 775–779

Immune-mediated dermatologic disease(s) (*Continued*)
  pemphigus as
    paraneoplastic, 774–775
    vulgaris, 769–773
  psoriasis as, 796–798, 796–797*f*
  reactive arthritis (Reiter syndrome) as, 786–787
  Stevens-Johnson syndrome and toxic epidermal necrolysis as, 783–784
  systemic sclerosis as, 801–805
Immune reconstitution syndrome, 264
Immune thrombocytopenic purpura (ITP), 591
Immunobullous disease, 769
Immunocompromised patients
  herpes zoster in, 240
  HSV recurrence in, 233, 233*f*
  varicella in, 237
Immunofluorescence techniques, 769, 769*f*
Immunologic disease(s)
  Behçet syndrome as, 326–328
  orofacial granulomatosis as, 330–333
  recurrent aphthous stomatitis as, 321–326
  sarcoidosis as, 328–330
  transient lingual papillitis as, 321, 322*f*
  Wegener granulomatosis as, 333–336
Immunosuppression, and squamous cell carcinoma, 406
Impaction, tooth, 72–73, 73*f*
Impetiginized dermatitis, 172
Impetigo, 172–173
  bullous (staphylococcal), 172
  clinical features of, 172, 173*f*
  defined, 172
  diagnosis of, 172
  nonbullous (contagiosa), 172, 173*f*
  treatment and prognosis for, 172–173
Implantation cyst, 31
Impressions of bite mark injury, 905
IMRT (Intensity-modulated radiation therapy), 419
Incisive canal, 27
Incisive canal cyst, 27–30
  clinical and radiographic features of, 28, 28–29*f*
  histopathologic features of, 28–29, 29*f*
  treatment and prognosis for, 30
Incisive papilla, cysts of, 28, 29*f*
Incisors
  Hutchinson, 58, 182, 182*f*
  shovel-shaped, 87, 87*f*
Incontinentia pigmenti, 755–756, 755–756*f*
Indirect immunofluorescence, 769, 769*f*
Induction chemotherapy, for leukemia, 595
Infantile hemangioma, 547, 548*f*
Infectious mononucleosis (mono), 241–242, 241*f*

Infiltrating lipoma, 531
Inflammatory collateral cyst, 704–705
Inflammatory fibrous hyperplasia, 517–519
  clinical features of, 517–518, 518*f*
  histopathologic features of, 518–519, 519*f*
  treatment and prognosis for, 519
Inflammatory papillary hyperplasia, 519–520, 519–520*f*
Infraocclusion of tooth, 73, 74*f*
Infrared (IR) photography, 904
Infundibular cyst, 31
  clinical features of, 31, 31–32*f*
  histopathologic features of, 32, 32*f*
Insect bites, 899, 900*f*
Insufficient identification evidence, 883
"Insulin resistance", 845
Insulin shock, 846
Integrase inhibitors, 264
Integrated Automated Fingerprint Identification System (IAFIS), 885
Intensity-modulated radiation therapy (IMRT), 419
Interstitial glossitis, 180–181
Intimate partner violence (IPV), 907
Intrabony vascular malformations, 549, 549*f*
Intracapsular carcinoma ex pleomorphic adenoma, 501
Intracranial hamartoma in tuberous sclerosis, 763*f*, 764–765
Intradermal nevus, 375–376*f*, 376
Intraductal papillomas, 492–493
  clinical features of, 492
  histopathologic features of, 492–493
  treatment and prognosis for, 493
Intraepithelial vesicle in herpes simplex virus, 233–234, 233*f*
Intramucosal melanocytic nevus, 376, 377*f*
Intramuscular lipoma, 531
Intraoral cacinoma and squamous cell carcinoma, 407*f*, 408–410, 409–410*f*
Intraoral psoriasis, 797
Intraosseous mucoepidermoid carcinoma, 496, 497*f*
  malignant transformation of dentigerous cyst to, 688
Inverted follicular keratosis of Helwig, 368
Inverted papilloma, 362–363, 362–363*f*
  ductal, 492–493
    clinical features of, 492, 492–493*f*
    histopathologic features of, 492–493, 493*f*
    treatment and prognosis for, 493
  Schneiderian, 361, 362–363*f*
Involucrum, acute osteomyelitis with, 135
Iodoquinol for candidiasis, 211–212
IPV (intimate partner violence), 907
Iron deficiency and squamous cell carcinoma, 404
Iron-deficiency anemia, 830

IR (infrared) photography, 904
Irritation and squamous cell carcinoma, 406
Irritation fibroma. *See* Fibroma
Isthmus-catagen cyst, 31
  clinical features of, 31–32, 31–32*f*
  histopathologic features of, 32, 32*f*
ITP (immune thrombocytopenic purpura), 591
Itraconazole for candidiasis, 209, 211*t*

J
Jackson-Lawler type pachyonychia congenita, 750–752
Jacobson's organ, 27
Jadassohn-Lewandowsky type pachyonychia congenita, 750–752
Jadassohn-Tièche nevus, 377–378, 377–378*f*
Jaffe-Lichtenstein syndrome, 643
Jaundice, 69, 823–824, 824*f*
Jaw(s)
  fibro-osseous lesions of, 641–674
    cemento-osseous (osseous) dysplasia as, 645–650
    familial gigantiform cementoma as, 650–651, 651*f*
    fibrous dysplasia as, 641–645
    juvenile ossifying fibroma as, 653–655, 654–655*f*
    ossifying fibroma as, 652–653, 652–653*f*
  metastatic tumors to, 673–674, 673–674*f*
Jaw cysts in nevoid basal cell carcinoma syndrome, 695–696, 696*f*
"Joint mice", 662
Jugular paragangliomas, 543–544
Junctional nevus, 376, 376*f*
Juvederm (hyaluronic acid), oral lesions associated with, 302
Juvenile aggressive fibromatosis, 523
Juvenile hemangioendothelioma, 549
Juvenile hemangioma, 549, 550*f*
Juvenile nasopharyngeal angiofibroma, 552
Juvenile ossifying fibroma, 653–655
  clinical and radiographic features of, 654, 654*f*
  etiopathogenesis of, 654
  histopathologic features of, 654–655, 654–655*f*
  psammomatoid, 653, 655*f*
  trabecular, 654, 654*f*
  treatment and prognosis for, 655
Juvenile recurrent parotitis, 468

K
Kabuki syndrome, 5
Kala-azar, 224
Kaposiform hemangioendothelioma, 548
Kaposi sarcoma (KS), 564–565
  classic (chronic) type, 564, 564*f*
  clinical features of, 564, 564*f*

Kaposi sarcoma (KS) *(Continued)*
  defined, 564
  endemic type, 564
  epidemiology of, 564
  etiology of, 229, 564
  histopathologic features of, 564
    in nodular stage, 564, 565*f*
    in patch stage, 564
    in plaque stage, 564
  HIV-associated, 254–256, 255*f*
  iatrogenic type (transplant-associated),
      564
  treatment and prognosis for, 565
Kaposi sarcoma–associated herpesvirus
    (KSHV), 229, 254
Kaposi varicelliform eruption, 232–233
Kasabach-Merritt phenomenon, 548
KCOT (keratocystic odontogenic tumor),
    690
Keratin horn, 357–358, 396–397, 397*f*
Keratinizing squamous cell carcinoma, 429
Keratin pearls, 416
Keratoacanthoma, 398–401
  clinical features of, 399, 399–400*f*
  histopathologic features of, 400, 400*f*
  treatment and prognosis for, 400–401
Keratocarcinoma. *See* Keratoacanthoma
Keratoconjunctivitis sicca, 472
Keratocystic odontogenic tumor (KCOT),
    690
Keratocyst(s), odontogenic.
    See Odontogenic keratocyst(s)
    (OKC)
Keratosis
  actinic (solar), 396–397, 396–397*f*
    in xeroderma pigmentosum, 753
  alveolar ridge, 383, 383*f*
  follicularis, 756–757, 756–757*f*
  frictional, 383, 383*f*
  sanguinaria-associated, 381–382, 382*f*
  seborrheic, 366–368
    clinical features of, 366–367, 367*f*
    histopathologic features of, 367–368,
        367*f*
    irritated, 368
    treatment and prognosis for, 368
  smokeless tobacco (tobacco pouch, spit
      tobacco), 381, 391–393
    clinical features of, 391–392, 391*f*
    histopathologic features of, 392–393,
        392*f*
    treatment and prognosis for, 393, 393*f*
  solar, 396–397, 396–397*f*
Ketoconazole for candidiasis, 209, 211*t*
Kindler syndrome, 766
"Kissing disease", 241–242, 241*f*
Kissing tonsils, 578
Kleeblattschädel deformity, 41
Klestadt cyst, 26–27, 26*f*
Koilocytes, 356–357
Koilonychia in Plummer-Vinson syndrome,
    830

Koplik spots, 247, 247*f*
Kostmann syndrome, 589
KS. *See* Kaposi sarcoma (KS)
KSHV (Kaposi sarcoma–associated
    herpesvirus), 229, 254
Küttner tumor, 472
Kveim test, 330

L
Labial melanotic macule, 372
Labial piercing, 301, 301*f*
Labial salivary gland tumors, 483*t*
Labret, 301, 301*f*
Lacunar cells, 600
LADD syndrome, 460
Lamina dura, differential diagnosis of
    generalized loss of, 932–935*t*
Langerhans cell disease. *See* Langerhans cell
    histiocytosis
Langerhans cell granulomatosis.
    See Langerhans cell histiocytosis
Langerhans cell histiocytosis, 596–598
  classification of, 596
  clinical and radiographic features of, 596,
      597*f*
  histopathologic features of, 597,
      597–598*f*
  treatment and prognosis for, 597–598
Langer lines, 903
Laryngeal paragangliomas, 543
Latent bone cyst, 23–25, 24–25*f*
Lateral facial cleft, 2
Lateral neck lesions, differential diagnosis of,
    922–925*t*
Lateral periodontal cyst(s), 699–701
  carcinoma arising from, 706*f*
  clinical and radiographic features of,
      699–700, 699–700*f*
  defined, 699
  "globulomaxillary cyst" as, 27
  histopathologic features of, 700, 700*f*
  "median mandibular cyst" as, 31
  pathogenesis of, 699
  treatment and prognosis for, 700–701
  vs. conventional solid or multicystic
      intraosseous ameloblastoma, 708,
      711*f*
  vs. lateral radicular cyst, 127
Lateral radicular cyst, 127, 127–128*f*
Lateral soft palate fistulas, 15, 15*f*
Lay witnesses, 910
LE. *See* Lupus erythematosus (LE)
Lead poisoning, 304
Leiomyoma, 555–557
  clinical and radiographic features of,
      555–556, 556*f*
  defined, 555
  histopathologic features of, 556–557,
      556–557*f*
  treatment and prognosis for, 557
  types of, 555
Leiomyosarcoma, 565–566, 565–566*f*

Leishmaniasis, 224–225, 224*f*
  cutaneous, 224
  mucocutaneous, 224, 224*f*
  visceral, 224
Lentigo(igines)
  actinic (solar, senile), 369–370, 370*f*
  maligna, 436
  simplex, 370–371, 371*f*
Lentigo maligna melanoma, 436, 436*f*
Leonine facies, 189
Leontiasis ossea, 629
Lepra cells, 190, 190*f*
Leprosy, 188–191
  diagnosis of, 191
  histopathologic features of, 190, 190*f*
  lepromatous (multibacillary)
    clinical features of, 189, 189*f*
    histopathologic features of, 189, 190*f*
    pathogenesis of, 189
    tooth discoloration due to, 69
    treatment and prognosis for, 191
  treatment and prognosis for, 191
  tuberculoid (paucibacillary)
    clinical features of, 189
    histopathologic features of, 189, 190*f*
    pathogenesis of, 189
    treatment and prognosis for, 191
Leptomeningeal angiomas, 551
Lesch-Nyhan syndrome, self-inflicted bites
    in, 900
Leser-Trélat sign, 367
Letterer-Siwe disease, 596
Leukemia, 593–595
  acute, 593
    lymphoblastic, 593, 595
    myeloid, 593, 595
  chronic, 593
    lymphocytic, 593
      paraneoplastic pemphigus due to,
          774
    myeloid, 593, 595
  classification of, 593
  clinical features of, 593–594
  defined, 593
  environmental agents associated with, 593
  genetic disorders associated with, 593
  lymphocytic/lymphoblastic, 593
    acute, 593, 595
    chronic, 593, 774
  myeloid, 593
    acute, 593, 595
    chronic, 593, 595
Leukocytoclastic vasculitis, 328
Leukoderma acquisitum centrifugum, 379,
    379*f*
Leukoedema, 7–8, 7–8*f*
Leukokeratosis. *See* Leukoplakia
Leukoplakia, 381–390, 422
  candidal, 202*t*
    clinical features of, 206, 206–207*f*,
        382, 382*f*
  cause of

Leukoplakia (Continued)
    due to alcohol, 381
    due to microorganisms, 382, 382f
    due to sanguinaria, 381–382, 382f
    due to tobacco, 381
    due to trauma, 383, 383f
    due to ultraviolet radiation, 382
  chemoprevention for, 389
  clinical features of, 383–385
  defined, 381
  etiology of, 381
  histopathologic features of, 385–388
    acanthosis as, 385
    carcinoma in situ as, 387–388, 388f
    epithelial dysplasia as, 387
      ductal, 387, 387f
      mild, 387, 387f
      moderate, 387, 387f
      severe, 387, 387f
    hyperkeratosis as, 385
    hyperorthokeratosis as, 385–386, 386f
    hyperparakeratosis as, 385–386, 386f
  mixture of phases or subtypes of, 386f
  oral hairy, 241
    HIV-associated, 253–254, 254f
    vs. hairy tongue, 13
    vs. morsicatio mucosae oris, 272–273
  in oral submucous fibrosis, 394
  prevalence of, 381
  smokeless tobacco use and smokeless
        tobacco keratosis as, 391–393
  speckled, 384, 384f
  thin or smooth, 386f
  treatment and prognosis for, 388–390
  vs. erythroplakia, 384
Lhermitte-Duclos disease, multiple
        hamartoma syndrome and, 765
Libman-Sacks endocarditis, 798
Lichenoid, 336–337, 337f
Lichenoid amalgam reaction, 788
Lichenoid contact reaction from dental
        restorative materials, 346–347,
        347f
Lichenoid dermatitis, 787
Lichenoid drug eruptions, 338, 338–339b
Lichenoid foreign body gingivitis, 787
Lichenoid mucositis, 787
Lichenoid reaction to amalgam, 346–347,
        347f, 791
Lichen planus, 149–150, 771t, 787–792
  bullous, 788
  clinical features of, 787–788, 787f
  diagnosis of, 791, 792f
  erosive
    clinical features of, 788, 789–790f
    diagnosis of, 791
    treatment and prognosis for, 791–792,
        792f
  etiopathogenesis of, 787
  histopathologic features of, 788–790,
        790f
  malignant potential of, 791–792

Lichen planus (Continued)
  reticular
    diagnosis of, 791, 792f
    clinical features of, 788, 788–789f
    treatment and prognosis for, 791–792
  treatment and prognosis for, 791–792
Lie bumps, 321
Liesegang ring calcifications, 722, 722f
Ligneous conjunctivitis, 581–582, 582f
Limited scleroderma, 805–806, 805–806f
Linea alba, 272, 273f
Linear gingival erythema, 257, 257f
Linear IgA bullous dermatosis vs. mucous
        membrane pemphigoid, 778
Linear scleroderma "en coup de sabre", 39
Lingual cortical mandibular defect, 23–25,
        24–25f
Lingual mandibular salivary gland
        depression, 23–25, 24–25f
Lingual papillitis, transient, 321, 322f
Lingual piercing, 301, 301f
Lingual thyroid, 10–11, 11f
Lip(s)
  cleft, 1, 2f
  congenital fistulas of lower, 4–5, 4–5f
  differential diagnosis of soft tissue masses
        of, 922–925t
  double, 5–6, 5–6f
  median cleft of upper, 2
Lip fissures, 295–296
Lipid reticuloendothelioses, 821–822
Lipoid proteinosis, 822–823, 822–823f
Lipoma(s), 530–532
  clinical features of, 530–531, 531f
  histopathologic features of, 531, 531f
  intramuscular (infiltrating), 531
  in multiple hamartoma syndrome, 765
  pleomorphic, 531
  spindle cell, 531
  treatment and prognosis for, 531–532
Liposarcoma, 561, 561f
  dedifferentiated, 561
  myxoid, 561
  pleomorphic, 561
  round cell, 561
  well-differentiated, 561
Lip pits
  commissural, 4, 4f
  paramedian (congenital), 4, 4–5f
Lip vermilion carcinoma, and squamous cell
        carcinoma, 408, 408f
Lisch nodules, 538
Liver spot, 369–370, 370f
Lobodontia, 97–98, 97f
Lobular capillary hemangiomas, 525.
        See also Pyogenic granuloma
Lobular torus, 21
Localized argyrosis, 298
Localized juvenile spongiotic gingivitis,
        150–151, 150f
Localized scleroderma, 803, 804f
Löfgren syndrome, 329

Loose bodies, 662
LTRs (minisatellite loci), 889
Ludwig angina
  clinical features of, 133, 133f
  pathogenesis of, 132
  treatment and prognosis for, 134
Lues. See Syphilis
Luetic glossitis, 180–181
Lung carcinoma, metastatic, 570f
Lupus band test, positive, 800–801
Lupus cheilitis, 798
Lupus erythematosus (LE), 798–801
  cutaneous
    chronic, 798–799, 799–800f
    subacute, 800
  diagnosis of, 800–801, 801t
  discoid, 799, 799f
  histopathologic features of, 800, 800f
  systemic, clinical features of, 798, 798f,
        799t
  treatment and prognosis for, 801
Lupus erythematosus (LE)–like drug
        eruptions, 338–339, 339b
Lupus pernio, 328–329, 329f
Lupus vu, 186
Lyell disease, 781
Lymphadenopathy, HIV-associated
        persistent generalized, 256, 256f
Lymphangiomas, 9
Lymphatic malformations, 553–555
  classification of, 553
  clinical features of, 553–554, 554f
  defined, 553
  histopathologic features of, 554–555,
        554–555f
  macrocystic, 553, 555f
  microcystic, 553, 555f
  mixed, 553
  treatment and prognosis for, 555
Lymphoepithelial carcinoma, 429
Lymphoepithelial cyst
  cervical, 35–36, 35–36f
  oral, 36–37, 36–37f
Lymphoepithelial lesion, benign, 475, 475f
Lymphoepithelioma carcinoma, 429
Lymphoid hyperplasia, 578, 579f
Lymphoma
  angiocentric T-cell, 607–609, 608f
  Burkitt, 606–607
  cutaneous T-cell, 604–606
  extranodal NK/T-cell, nasal-type,
        607–609, 608f
  Hodgkin (see Hodgkin lymphoma)
  mucosa-associated lymphoid tissue
        (MALT), 601
  non-Hodgkin, 600–604
    HIV-associated, 256–257, 257f
  paraneoplastic pemphigus due to, 774
  Sjögren syndrome and, 476
Lymphomatoid granulomatosis, 608
Lymphoproliferative disorder(s)
  EBV-associated, 601, 602f

Lymphoproliferative disorder(s) *(Continued)*
  primary cutaneous CD30+, 274
Lyon hypothesis, 747

M
Macrodontia, 82, 82*f*
  differential diagnosis of, 932–935*t*
Macroglossia, 8–9, 8*b*, 9*f*
  in hemihyperplasia, 38
Macrognathia, 81
Macule
  defined, 914
  melanotic
    labial, 372
    oral, 372–373, 372–373*f*, 373*b*
Maffucci syndrome, 661, 669
Maintenance chemotherapy for leukemia, 595
Malignant disorders, oral potentially, 380–381, 380–381*b*
Malignant fibrous histiocytoma, 560–561, 561*f*
Malignant melanoma. *See* Melanoma
Malignant mixed tumors, 499–501, 500*f*
Malignant odontogenic myxoma, 737
Malignant peripheral nerve sheath tumor, 562
  in neurofibromatosis type I, 539, 539*f*
Malignant schwannoma, in neurofibromatosis type I, 539, 539*f*
Malignant Triton tumor, 562
Malpractice, 910
MALT (mucosa-associated lymphoid tissue) lymphoma, 601
MALT lymphoma, Sjögren syndrome and, 476
Mammary analogue secretory carcinoma, 498–499, 498*f*
Mandibular cyst, median, 31
Mandibulofacial dysostosis, 43–44, 43*f*
  condylar hypoplasia with, 17
Manner of death, 883
Marble bone disease. *See* Osteopetrosis
Marginal gingivitis, 148–149, 148*f*
Marie-Sainton syndrome, 623–625
Maroteaux-Lamy disease, 820*t*
Mask of pregnancy, 371–372, 371*f*
Mass(es), differential diagnosis of, 922–925*t*
Mass fatality incident (MFI) identification. *See* Multiple fatality incident (MFI) identification
Massive osteolysis, 627–628, 627–628*f*
Masticatory muscle disorders, 864*b*
Matrix formation in enamel development, 51
Maturation in enamel development, 51
Maxillary sinus carcinoma, 426, 426*f*
Mazabraud syndrome, 643
McCune-Albright syndrome, 643
  gigantism due to, 834
McGivney, James, 899

MCV (molluscum contagiosum virus), 364–365, 364–365*f*
ME (medical examiner), 883
Measles, 246–248, 247*f*
  mumps, rubella, and varicella virus (MMRV) vaccine (ProQuad), 238
Mechanism of death, 883
Medial palatal cyst, 30–31, 30*f*
Median cleft of upper lip, 2
"Median mandibular cyst", 31
Median rhomboid glossitis, 202*t*, 203, 203*f*
Medical examiner (ME), 883
Medication(s). *See also under* Drug
  tooth discoloration due to
    extrinsic, 68
    intrinsic, 69–70, 70*f*
Medication-related osteonecrosis of the jaw (MRONJ), 286–292
  case definition of, 286, 286*b*
  clinical and radiographic features of, 288–289, 288–289*f*
  due to antiangiogenic agents, 286, 286–287*b*
  due to antiresorptive agents, 286–287, 286*b*, 288*f*
  histopathologic features of, 289, 290*f*
  treatment and prognosis for, 289–292
Mediterranean fever, familial, 825–826
Medullary thyroid carcinoma (MTC) syndrome, 535*t*
  in multiple endocrine neoplasia type 2B, 540
Megadontia, 82
Megalodontia, 82
Melanin incontinen, 372
Melanin pigmentation of oral mucosa, associations with, 372–373, 373*b*
Melanoacanthoma, 373–374, 374*f*
Melanoacanthosis, 373–374, 374*f*
Melanocarcinoma. *See* Melanoma
Melanocytic nevi, 374–375
Melanocytic nevus(i), 374–375
  acquired, 375–380
    clinical features of, 375–376, 375–376*f*
    histopathologic features of, 376, 376–377*f*
    pathogenesis of, 375
    treatment and prognosis for, 376–377
Melanocytoma, dermal, 377–378, 377–378*f*
Melanoma, 434–442
  acral, 436
  amelanotic, 436
  benign juven, 378–379
  clinical features of, 435–437, 435*b*, 436–437*f*
  histopathologic features of, 437–438, 438*f*
  lentigo maligna, 436, 436*f*
  metastatic, 569*f*
  mucosal, 436–437, 436–437*f*

Melanoma *(Continued)*
  nodular, 436, 438*f*
  pagetoid spread of, 437, 438*f*
  radial growth phase, 436
  in situ, 436
  superficial spreading, 436, 436*f*
  treatment and prognosis for, 438–442, 438–442*t*
  vertical growth phase, 436
Melanosis
  focal, 372–373, 372–373*f*, 373*b*
  smoker's, 306–307, 307*f*
Melanotic macule
  labial, 372
  oral, 372–373, 372–373*f*, 373*b*
Melanotic neuroectodermal tumor of infancy, 541–543, 542*f*
Melanotic progonoma, 541–543, 542*f*
Melasma, 371–372, 371*f*
Melkersson-Rosenthal syndrome, 12, 330–331, 331–332*f*
Membranous basal cell adenoma, 491
MEN. *See* Multiple endocrine neoplasia (MEN) syndromes
Mendelian Inheritance of Man (MIM) database, 104–105
Meningeal angiomatosis, 551
Menorrhagia due to iron-deficiency anemia, 830
Mercury poisoning, 304
Merkel cell carcinoma, 432–434, 433*f*
Merrick, Joseph, 539
Mesenchymal chondrosarcoma, 670–671, 671*f*
Mesiodens, 78*f*
Mesotaurodontism, 92, 93*f*
Metallic intoxication, 304–306
  with arsenic, 306
  with bismuth, 306
  clinical features of, 305–306, 306*f*
  with gold, 306
  with lead, 304
  with mercury, 304
  with silver, 304–305
  treatment and prognosis for, 306
Metastasis(es)
  to jaws, 673–674, 673–674*f*
  to oral soft tissues, 569–570
    clinical features of, 569–570, 569–570*f*
    histopathologic features of, 570, 570*f*
    treatment and prognosis for, 570
Metastasis and squamous cell carcinoma, 408–410, 411*f*
Metastasizing mixed tumor, 499–501
Methamphetamine, orofacial complications of, 292, 293*f*
Methicillin-resistant *Staphylococcus aureus* (MRSA), 172–173
MFI identification. *See* Multiple fatality incident (MFI) identification
Microangiopathy due to diabetes mellitus, 845

Microdontia, 81, 81f
  differential diagnosis of, 932–935t
Microglossia, 8, 8f
Microorganisms, leukoplakia due to, 382, 382f
Microsatellite loci (STRs), 889
Microstomia in systemic sclerosis, 803f, 804–805
Middle ear paragangliomas, 543
Midline destructive disease, idiopathic, 607–609, 608f
Midline lethal granuloma, 607–609, 608f
Midline malignant reticulosis, 607–609, 608f
Midline neck lesions, differential diagnosis of, 922–925t
MIH (molar-incisor hypomineralizaion), 55
Mikulicz aphthae, minor, 323
Mikulicz disease, 471
Mikulicz syndrome, 471
Mild epithelial dysplasia, 387, 387f
Milium(ia), 32, 32f
MIM (Mendelian Inheritance of Man) database, 104–105
Mineral deficiencies and squamous cell carcinoma, 404
Mineralization in enamel development, 51
Minisatellite loci (LTRs), 889
Minocycline hydrochloride
  oral mucosal discoloration due to, 308, 308f
  tooth discoloration due to, 70
Minor salivary gland(s)
  adenomatoid hyperplasia of, 477
  sialolithiasis of, 465, 466f
  tumors of, 481, 482t
    location of, 481, 482t
    percentage malignant by site of, 484t
Mitochondrial DNA (mtDNA), 888
Mitosoid cell, 360–361
Mittenlike deformity in epidermolysis bullosa, 767, 767f
Mixed radiolucent/radiopaque lesions, differential diagnosis of, 926–931t
Mixed tumor
  malignant, 499–501, 500f
  metastasizing, 499–501
MMP20 gene, 99t, 100
MMRV (measles, mumps, rubella, and varicella virus) vaccine (ProQuad), 238
Mode of death, 883
Moderate epithelial dysplasia, 387, 387f
Mohs micrographic surgery, 432
Molar(s)
  Fournier, 182
  Moon, 182
  mulberry, 58, 182, 182f
Molar-incisor hypomineralization (MIH), 55
Mole, 374–375
  pathogenesis of, 374–375

Molluscum bodies, 364, 365f
Molluscum contagiosum, 364–365, 364–365f
  HIV-associated, 262–263, 263f
Molluscum contagiosum virus (MCV), 364–365, 364–365f
Moniliasis, 201
Monoclonal gammopathy, 610
Monomorphic adenoma, 490
Mononucleosis, infectious, 241–242, 241f
Moon facies in hypercortisolism, 842, 842f
Moon molars, 182
MOPP regimen for Hodgkin lymphoma, 600
Morphea, 803, 804f
Morphometric means of identification, 884–885
Morquio-A disease, 820t
Morquio-B disease, 820t
Morsicatio
  buccarum, 272, 273f
  labiorum, 272
  linguarum, 272, 273f
  mucosae oris, 272–273, 273f
Mottled enamel, 57, 57f
Mouse facies in systemic sclerosis, 802, 802f
Mouth breathing–related gingivitis, 147, 148f
MRIM (molar root-incisor malformation), 55–56, 55–56f
MRONJ. See Medication-related osteonecrosis of the jaw (MRONJ)
MRSA (methicillin-resistant Staphylococcus aureus), 172–173
MSBP (Munchausen syndrome by proxy), 908
MTC (medullary thyroid carcinoma) syndrome, 535t
  in multiple endocrine neoplasia type 2B, 540
mtDNA (mitochondrial DNA), 888
Mucinosis, oral focal, 524–525, 525f
Mucocele, 460–462
  clinical features of, 460–462, 461f
  histopathologic features of, 462, 462f
  location of, 461–462, 461t
  pathogenesis of, 460
  ranula as, 462–463, 463f
  retention, 460
  sinus, 312–313
  superficial, 461–462, 462f
  treatment and prognosis for, 462
Mucocutaneous candidiasis, 202t, 206–207, 208f
Mucoepidermoid carcinoma, 424, 493–496
  clear cell, 495, 495f
  clinical features of, 494, 494f
  grading of, 495, 496t
    high-grade, 495, 495f
    intermediate-grade, 495
    low-grade, 495, 495f

Mucoepidermoid carcinoma (Continued)
  histopathologic features of, 494–495, 494–495f
  intraosseous (central), 496, 497f
  pathogenesis of, 494
  treatment and prognosis for, 495–496
Mucoepidermoid tumor, 493
Mucoepithelial dysplasia, hereditary, 754–755, 754–755f
Mucogingivitis in Crohn disease, 850–851
Mucopolysaccharides, 819
Mucopolysaccharidosis, 819–820, 820t, 820f
Mucormycosis, 219–221
  clinical features of, 219–220, 220f
  diagnosis of, 220
  histopathologic features of, 220, 220f
  pathogenesis of, 219
  radiographic features of, 219–220, 220f
  treatment and prognosis for, 220–221
Mucosa-associated lymphoid tissue (MALT) lymphoma, 601
Mucosal burns
  due to chemicals, 278–280, 278f
    from aspirin, 278, 278f
    from hydrogen peroxide, 278–279, 279f
    from phenol, 279, 279f
    from silver nitrate, 279
  electrical and thermal, 276–278, 278f
Mucosal burns due to chemicals from tooth whitening strips, 278–280, 278f
Mucosal chewing, chronic, 272–273, 273f
Mucosal lentiginous melanoma, 437, 438f
Mucosal melanoma, 436–437, 436–437f
Mucosal pathology, differential diagnosis of
  with color changes, 916–919t
  with masses or enlargements, 922–925t
  with surface alterations, 920–921t
Mucosal pemphigoid-like eruptions, 338, 340b
Mucositis
  due to antineoplastic therapy, 281, 281–282f, 284–285
  lichenoid, 787
  necrotizing, 151–152, 152f
  necrotizing ulcerative, 191–192, 192f
  peri-implant, 147
  psoriasiform, 785–786
Mucous membrane pemphigoid, 771t, 775–779
  clinical features of, 776–777
    desquamative gingivitis as, 776, 777f
    dyspareunia as, 777
    entropion as, 776–777, 777f
    laryngeal lesions as, 777
    ocular adhesions as, 776–777, 777f
    symblepharons as, 776–777, 777f
    trichiasis as, 776–777, 777f
    ulcerations as, 776, 776f
    vesicles as, 776, 776f

Mucous membrane pemphigoid (Continued)
  epidemiology of, 776
  histopathologic features of, 777–779
  pathogenesis of, 776
  treatment and prognosis for, 779
  vs. angina bullosa hemorrhagica, 778, 779f
  vs. epidermolysis bullosa acquisita, 778–779
  vs. linear IgA bullous dermatosis, 778
Mucous patches, 180, 180f
Mucus duct cyst, 463–465, 464f
Mucus escape reaction. See Mucocele
Mucus extravasation phenomenon. See Mucocele
Mucus retention cyst, 460, 463–465, 464f
Muir-Torre syndrome, 399
  sebaceous hyperplasia in, 368
Mulberry molars, 58, 182, 182f
Multifocal epithelial hyperplasia, 360–361
  clinical features of, 360, 360f
  epidemiology of, 360
  histopathologic features of, 360–361, 361f
  with HIV infection, 260
  treatment and prognosis for, 361
Multifocal papilloma virus epithelial hyperplasia. See Multifocal epithelial hyperplasia
Multifocal radiopacities, differential diagnosis of, 926–931t
Multilocular, defined, 914
Multilocular radiolucencies, differential diagnosis of, 926–931t
Multinodular oncocytic hyperplasia, 488, 488f
Multiple cemento-ossifying fibromas, 650
Multiple endocrine neoplasia (MEN) syndromes, 9, 540
Multiple endocrine neoplasia type 1 (MEN 1), 535t
  hyperparathyroidism in, 840
Multiple endocrine neoplasia type 2A (MEN 2A), 535t
  hyperparathyroidism in, 840
Multiple endocrine neoplasia type 2B (MEN 2B), 540–541
  clinical features of, 540–541, 540–541f
  genetic basis for, 535t, 540
  histopathologic features of, 541, 541f
  laboratory values in, 541
  treatment and prognosis for, 541
Multiple fatality incident (MFI) identification, 896–899
  for accidents, 896
  for criminal disasters, 896–897
  dentist as expert witness for, 910
  for natural disasters, 896
  responsibilities in, 897–898
  technologic aids for, 898–899

Multiple hamartoma syndrome, 765–766, 765–766f
Multiple myeloma, 609–611, 609–610f
Multiple ossifying fibromas, 650
Multiple sclerosis, trigeminal neuralgia due to, 865
Multiple self-healing squamous epitheliomas, 399
Mumps, 249–250, 250f
  surgical, 467
Munchausen syndrome by proxy (MSBP), 908
Munro abscesses
  in erythema migrans, 785–786, 786f
  in psoriasis, 797
Mutifocal papilloma virus epithelial hyperplasia, 360–361
Mycetoma, 221, 221f
Mycobacterial disease
  with HIV infection, 258–259
  nontuberculous, 185, 187
Mycobacterium leprae, 188–189
Mycobacterium tuberculosis, 185
Mycosis cells, 605
Mycosis fungoides, 604–606
  clinical features of, 604–605, 604f
  eczematous (erythematous) stage of, 605
  histopathologic features of, 605–606, 605f
  plaque stage of, 605, 605f
  treatment and prognosis for, 605–606
  tumor stage of, 605
Myelodysplasia syndromes, 593
Myeloid sarcoma, 594
Myeloid tumor, extramedullary, 594
Myeloma-associated amyloidosis, 825, 825f
Myeloma, multiple, 609–611, 609–610f
Myelophthisic anemia, 593
Myoblastoma, granular cell, 544
Myoepithelial cells in pleomorphic adenoma, 486, 486f
Myoepithelial sialadenitis, 475, 475f
Myoepitheliomas, 486–487
Myofascial trigger point pain due to temporomandibular disorders, 875
Myofibroma, 523–524, 524f
Myofibromatosis, 523–524, 524f
Myopericytoma, 521
Myositis due to temporomandibular disorders, 875
Myospasm due to temporomandibular disorders, 875
Myospherulosis, 315, 315f
Myxedema, 835–836, 836–837f
Myxofibromas, 736
Myxoid chondrosarcoma, 670
Myxoid liposarcoma, 561
Myxoma
  odontogenic, 735–737
    clinical and radiographic features of, 735–736, 735–736f

Myxoma (Continued)
    histopathologic features of, 736, 736–737f
    malignant, 737
    pathogenesis of, 735
    relative distribution of, 735, 735f
    treatment and prognosis for, 736–737
  osteogenic, 735
Myxomatous background in pleomorphic adenoma, 486, 486f
Myxosarcomas, 737

N
NASH classification, 883
Nasoalveolar cyst, 26–27, 26–27f
Nasolabial cyst, 26–27, 26–27f
Nasopalatine duct cyst, 27–30
  clinical and radiographic features of, 28, 28–29f
  histopathologic features of, 28–29, 29f
  treatment and prognosis for, 30
Nasopalatine ducts, 27
Nasopharyngeal angiofibroma, 552–553, 553f
Nasopharyngeal carcinoma, 428–430, 429f
Natal teeth, 79–81, 80f
National Association of Dental Laboratories (NADL), 890
National Child Abuse and Neglect Data System (NCANDS), 907
National Crime Information Center (NCIC) data base, 890, 898
National Dental Image Repository (NDIR), 890
National Disaster Medical System (NDMS), 897
National DNA Index System (NDIS), 889
National Incident Management System (NIMS), 897
National Institute of Standards and Technology (NIST), 887
National Response Plan (NRP), 897, 897t
National Transportation Safety Board (NTSB), 897
Natural disasters, 896
Natural killer (NK)/T-cell lymphoma, extranodal, nasal-type, 607–609, 608f
NCANDS (National Child Abuse and Neglect Data System), 907
NCIC (National Crime Information Center) data base, 890, 898
NDIR (National Dental Image Repository), 890
NDIS (National DNA Index System), 889
NDMS (National Disaster Medical System), 897
Necrotizing gingivitis (NG), 151–152, 152f
  vs. gonorrhea, 184
Necrotizing gingivostomatitis, 152
Necrotizing mucositis, 151–152, 152f

Necrotizing periodontitis (NP), 161, 163–164
Necrotizing sialometaplasia, 477–479, 478f
Necrotizing stomatitis, 151–152, 191–192, 192f
Necrotizing ulcerative gingivitis (NUG), 151–152, 152f
  in infectious mononucleosis, 241–242
Necrotizing ulcerative mucositis, 191–192, 192f
Necrotizing ulcerative periodontitis (NUP), 151–152, 257, 258f
Negligence, malpractice based on, 910
Neisseria gonorrhoeae, 174
NEMO (nuclear factor-κB essential modulator) in incontinentia pigmenti, 755
Neonatal teeth, 79–80
Neuralgia
  glossopharyngeal (vagoglossopharyngeal), 866–867
  postherpetic, 240
  trigeminal, 864–866, 865b
  tympanic plexus, 866
Neural syndromes, hereditary, 535t
Neurilemoma, 534, 536f
Neuroblastoma, olfactory, 562–563, 562–563f
Neurocutaneous melanosis, 379
Neuroendocrine carcinoma of skin, 432–434, 433f
Neuroendocrine syndromes, hereditary, 535t
Neurofibroma, 534–537, 536–537f
  granular cell, 544
Neurofibromatosis (NF), 9, 534–537
Neurofibromatosis type I (NF1), 537–539
  clinical and radiographic features of, 537–539, 538f
  diagnostic criteria for, 537–538, 537b
  genetic basis for, 535t, 537–538
  malignant peripheral nerve sheath tumor in, 539, 539f
  treatment and prognosis for, 539
Neurofibromatosis type II (NF2), 534, 535t
Neurofibrosarcoma in neurofibromatosis type I, 539
Neuroma(s)
  in multiple endocrine neoplasia type 2B, 541, 541f
  in multiple hamartoma syndrome, 765
  palisaded encapsulated (solitary circumscribed), 533–534, 533–534f
  traumatic (amputation), 531f, 532, 533f
Neuromuscular disease(s)
  Bell palsy as, 861–862, 862f
  dysgeusia and hypogeusia as, 869–871, 870b, 871t
  Frey syndrome as, 862–863, 863f
  osteoarthritis as, 871–872
  rheumatoid arthritis as, 872–874

Neuromuscular disease(s) (Continued)
  temporomandibular disorders as, 864b, 874–876, 875–876b
Neuronopathic features of Niemann-Pick disease, 821
Neuropathic pain disorders, 864b
Neutropenia, 587–589
  benign ethnic, 588
  cyclic, 589–590, 590f
  severe congenital, 588
Nevocellular nevus, 374–375
  pathogenesis of, 375
Nevoid basal cell carcinoma syndrome, 431, 694–697
  clinical and radiographic features of, 694–696, 694b
    basal cell carcinomas as, 694, 696f
    hypertelorism and mandibular swelling as, 694, 695f
    odontogenic keratocysts as, 690, 697, 697f
    ovarian cysts and fibromas as, 695
    palmar and plantar pits as, 694–695, 695f
    skeletal anomalies as, 695, 695f
  defined, 694
  diagnostic criteria for, 696, 697b
  etiology and pathogenesis of, 694
  histopathologic features of, 696, 697f
  treatment and prognosis for, 696–697, 697f
Nevus(i)
  blue (Jadassohn-Tièche), 377–378, 377–378f
  compound, 375
  defined, 374–375
  flammeus, 551, 551f
  halo (Sutton), 379, 379f
  intradermal, 375–376f, 376
  junctional, 376, 376f
  melanocytic (nevocellular)
    acquired, 375–380
      clinical features of, 375–376, 375–376f
      histopathologic features of, 376, 376–377f
      treatment and prognosis for, 376–377
    pathogenesis of, 374–375
  types of, 375b
  white sponge, 748–749
    clinical features of, 748, 748f
    histopathologic features of, 749, 749f
    pathogenesis of, 748
    treatment and prognosis for, 749
Nevus cells, 374–375
Newborn
  congenital epulis of, 546–547, 546f
  gingival (alveolar) cyst of, 697–698, 698f
  gingival granular cell tumor of, 546
  palatal cysts of, 25–26, 26f
NF. See Neurofibromatosis (NF)

NHL. See Non-Hodgkin lymphoma (NHL)
Niacin deficiency, 828
NICH (noninvoluting congenital hemangioma), 547
Nicotine palatinus, 397–398, 398f
Nicotine stomatitis, 397–398, 398f
Niemann-Pick disease, 821
Nifedipine-related gingival hyperplasia, 156, 156f
NIMS (National Incident Management System), 897
NK (natural killer)/T-cell lymphoma, extranodal, nasal-type, 607–609, 608f
Nodular (noduloulcerative) basal cell carcinoma, 430
Nodular melanoma, 436, 438f
Nodular subepidermal fibrosis, 520–521, 521f
Nodular torus, 21
Nodule, defined, 914
Noma, 151–152, 191–192, 192f
Nonfamilial gigantiform cementoma, 650
Non-Hodgkin lymphoma (NHL), 600–604
  classification of, 600–601, 601b
  clinical and radiographic features of, 601–603, 602–603f
  defined, 600
  epidemiology of, 600
  high-grade (aggressive), 604
  histopathologic features of, 603, 603f
  HIV-associated, 256–257, 257f
  low-grade (indolent), 603–604
  pathogenesis of, 601
  treatment and prognosis for, 603–604
Nonhomogeneousleukoplakia, 384, 384f
Noninvoluting congenital hemangioma (NICH), 547
Nonkeratinizing squamous cell carcinoma, 429
Nonmyeloablative allogenic hematopoietic cell transplantation, 794
Nonnucleoside reverse transcriptase inhibitors, 264
Nontuberculous mycobacterial disease, 185, 187
Nosocomial infection, 221
NP (necrotizing periodontitis), 161, 163–164
NRP (National Response Plan), 897, 897t
NTSB (National Transportation Safety Board), 897
Nuclear factor-κB essential modulator (NEMO) in incontinentia pigmenti, 755
Nucleoside reverse transcriptase inhibitors, 264
NUG. See Necrotizing ulcerative gingivitis (NUG)
Numb-chin syndrome, 673

NUP (necrotizing ulcerative periodontitis), 151–152
HIV-associated, 257, 258f
Nystatin for candidiasis, 209, 211t

O
Oblique facial cleft, 2
Observational witnesses, 910
Occupational exposures and environmental pollutants, and squamous cell carcinoma, 403
Occupational Safety and Health Administration (OSHA), 881
Ochronosis, 69
Oculoauriculovertebral syndrome, condylar hypoplasia with, 17
Oculo-facio-cardio-dental (OFCD) syndrome, 82
Odontalgia due to temporomandibular disorders, 875
Odontoameloblastoma, 728–729
Odontodysplasia, regional, 110–111, 110b, 111f
Odontogenic carcinoma, 705–707
clear cell, 717–718, 717–718f
clinical and radiographic features of, 705–706, 706f
ghost cell, 702
histopathologic features of, 706, 706–707f
pathogenesis of, 705
treatment and prognosis for, 707
Odontogenic cyst(s), 685–707
botryoid, 699–700, 700f
buccal bifurcation, 704–705, 705f
calcifying, 701–703
carcinoma arising in, 705–707, 706–707f
classification of, 685, 686b
defined, 685
dentigerous (follicular), 685–688
developmental, 685
eruption, 688–689, 689f
gingival (alveolar)
of adult, 698, 699f
of newborn, 697–698, 698f
glandular (sialo-), 31, 703–704, 704f
inflammatory, 685
keratocyst as, 689–693
lateral periodontal, 699–701
in nevoid basal cell carcinoma syndrome (Gorlin syndrome), 694–697
orthokeratinized, 693–694, 693f
carcinoma arising from, 706
primordial, 689, 689f
squamous odontogenic tumorlike proliferations in, 723–724
Odontogenic epithelial hamartoma, 733
Odontogenic fibroma
central (intraosseous), 731–733
clinical and radiographic features of, 731–732, 732f

Odontogenic fibroma (Continued)
histopathologic features of, 732–733, 733f
relative distribution of, 731–732, 732f
treatment and prognosis for, 733
with giant cell granuloma, 733, 733f
granular cell, 734–735
peripheral, 733–734, 734f
vs. peripheral ameloblastoma, 715–716
simple, 732, 732f
WHO (epithelium-rich), 732, 733f
Odontogenic keratocyst(s) (OKC), 689–693
carcinoma arising from, 706
clinical and radiographic features of, 690–691, 690–691f
differential diagnosis of, 690–691, 691f
"globulomaxillary cyst" as, 27, 31
histopathologic features of, 691–692, 692f
in nevoid basal cell carcinoma syndrome, 690, 697, 697f
pathogenesis of, 689
relative distribution of, 690, 690f
treatment and prognosis for, 692–693, 693f
vs. primordial cyst, 689
Odontogenic myxoma
clinical and radiographic features of, 735–736, 735–736f
histopathologic features of, 736, 736–737f
malignant, 737
pathogenesis of, 735
relative distribution of, 735, 735f
treatment and prognosis for, 736–737
Odontogenic tumor(s), 707
adenomatoid, 718–720
calcifying odontogenic cyst with, 701
clinical and radiographic features of, 718–719, 718–719f
epidemiology of, 718
histopathologic features of, 720, 720f
relative distribution of, 721, 721f
treatment and prognosis for, 720
ameloblastic carcinoma as, 716–717, 716–717f
ameloblastic fibroma as, 724–725, 724–725f
ameloblastic fibro-odontoma as, 725–727, 726–727f
ameloblastic fibrosarcoma (ameloblastic sarcoma) as, 727–728, 728f
ameloblastoma as, 707–716
conventional solid or multicystic intraosseous, 708–713
malignant, 716–717
peripheral (extraosseous), 715–716, 715f
unicystic, 713–715
calcifying cystic (see Calcifying odontogenic cyst)

Odontogenic tumor(s) (Continued)
calcifying epithelial, 720–722
clinical and radiographic features of, 721, 721f
epidemiology of, 720–721
histopathologic features of, 721–722, 722f
pathogenesis of, 720–721
relative distribution of, 721, 721f
treatment and prognosis for, 722
cementoblastoma ("true cementoma") as, 737
clear cell, 717–718, 717–718f
granular cell, 734–735, 734f
keratocystic, 690
mixed, 707, 707b, 724–731
odontoameloblastoma as, 728–729
of odontogenic ectomesenchyme, 707, 707b, 731–737
of odontogenic epithelium, 707, 707b
odontogenic fibroma as
central, 731–733
granular cell, 734–735, 734f
peripheral, 733–734, 734f
odontogenic myxoma as, 735–737
odontoma as, 729–730
primordial, 731
squamous, 723–724, 723f
Odontohypophosphatasia, 848
Odontoma(s), 729–730
ameloblastic, 728–729
calcifying odontogenic cyst with, 701–702
clinical and radiographic features of, 729–730, 729–730f
complex, 729–730
clinical and radiographic features of, 729–730, 729–730f
compound, 730f
compound, 729–730
clinical and radiographic features of, 729–730, 729–730f
histopathologic features of, 730, 730f
histopathologic features of, 730, 730f
pathogenesis of, 729
treatment and prognosis for, 730
Odontomaxillary dysplasia, segmental, 39–40, 40f
Odontome, dilated, 89, 90f
Odynophagia, 410
OHL. See Oral hairy leukoplakia (OHL)
OKC. See Odontogenic keratocyst(s) (OKC)
Olfactory neuroblastoma, 562–563, 562–563f
Oligodontia, 75
in ectodermal dysplasia, 747, 748f
in incontinentia pigmenti, 755, 756f
Ollier disease, 661, 669
Oncocytes, 487
Oncocytic carcinoma, 488

Oncocytic hyperplasia, multinodular, 488, 488f
Oncocytic metaplasia, 488
Oncocytic salivary duct ectasia, 464–465, 464f
Oncocytic Schneiderian papilloma, 363–364
Oncocytoma, 487–488, 487f
Oncocytosis, 488, 488f
  diffuse hyperplastic, 488
Oncogenes and tumor suppressor genes, and squamous cell carcinoma, 406
Oncogenic viruses and squamous cell carcinoma, 404–406
"Onion-skin" radiopacities, differential diagnosis of, 926–931t
Online Mendelian Inheritance in Man (OMIM) database, 618
Opalescent teeth in osteogenesis imperfecta, 618, 619f
Ophthalmia neonatorum, gonococcal, 185
Oral burning, 868
Oral cavity and pharyngeal cancers by SEER stage, survival rates, 416t
Oral dysesthesia, 868
Oral epithelial dysplasia, 386
Oral florid papillomatosis, 422
Oral focal mucinosis, 524–525, 525f
Oral hairy leukoplakia (OHL), 241
  HIV-associated, 253–254, 254f
  vs. hairy tongue, 13
  vs. morsicatio mucosae oris, 272–273
Oral lymphoepithelial cyst, 36–37, 36–37f
Oral melanoacanthoma, 373–374, 374f
Oral melanotic macule, 372–373, 372–373f, 373b
Oral potentially malignant disorders, 380–381, 380–381b
Oral sensory neuropathy, 868
Oral squamous papilloma with HIV infection, 260
Oral submucous fibrosis, 393–395, 394f
Organization of Scientific Area Committees for Forensic Science (OSAC) Registry, 887
Organ of Jacobson, 27
ORN (osteoradionecrosis), 134–135, 283–284, 283–284f
  clinical features of, 281–284, 283–284f
  treatment and prognosis for, 285–286
Orofacial clefts, 1–4
  bifid uvula as, 2, 3f
  cleft lip as, 1, 2f
  cleft palate as, 1, 2f
  clinical and radiographic features of, 2–3
  etiology and pathogenesis of, 1–4
  lateral facial cleft as, 2
  median cleft of upper lip as, 2
  oblique facial cleft as, 2
  in Pierre Robin sequence, 3, 3f
  submucous palatal cleft as, 3, 3f
  treatment and prognosis for, 3–4

Orofacial gangrene, 191–192, 192f
Orofacial granulomatosis, 330–333
  clinical features of, 330–332, 331–332f
  in Crohn disease, 850–851
  histopathologic features of, 332, 332f
  interventions to rule out local causes of, 330, 331t
  systemic evaluation of, 330, 331t
Orofacial pain. See Head and neck pain
Orogenital sexual practices, oral trauma from, 297–298, 297–298f
Oromandibular-limb hypogenesis syndromes, 8
Oropharyngeal carcinoma and squamous cell carcinoma, 408–410, 410–411f
Orthokeratinized odontogenic cyst, 693–694, 693f
  carcinoma arising from, 706
Osseous and chondromatous metaplasia, 519
Osseous choristoma, 559, 559f
Osseous dysplasia, 645–650, 647f
  expansive, 650
Osseous metaplasia, reactive, 309–310, 309f
Ossicles in osteoarthritis, 872
Ossifying fibroid epulis, 529–530, 529–530f
Ossifying fibroma(s), 652–653, 652–653f
  clinical and radiographic features of, 652–653, 652f
  defined, 652
  etiology and pathogenesis of, 652
  histopathologic features of, 653, 653f
  juvenile, 653–655
    clinical and radiographic features of, 654, 654f
    etiopathogenesis of, 654
    histopathologic features of, 654–655, 654–655f
    psammomatoid, 653, 655f
    trabecular, 654, 654f
    treatment and prognosis for, 655
  multiple (bilateral), 650
  peripheral, 529–530, 529–530f
  treatment and prognosis for, 653
Osteitis
  alveolar, 143–144
  condensing, 141, 141f, 626
  deformans (see Paget disease, of bone)
  fibrosa cystica in hyperparathyroidism, 840–841
Osteoarthritis, 871–872
Osteoblastoma(s), 658–659, 658–659f
  aggressive, 658
Osteodystrophy
  Albright hereditary, 839–840
  hyperparathyroidism due to renal, 841, 841f
Osteogenesis imperfecta, 618–620, 619f, 619t
  and dentinogenesis imperfecta, 104–105
Osteogenic myxoma, 735

Osteogenic sarcoma. See Osteosarcoma
Osteoid osteoma, 658–659, 658–659f
Osteolysis, massive (idiopathic), 627–628, 627–628f
Osteoma(s), 655–656
  cancellous, 656
  clinical and radiographic features of, 655–656, 656f
  compact, 656, 656f
  cutis, 655, 840
  endosteal or central, 655
  extraskeletal, 655
  histopathologic features of, 656, 656f
  osteoid, 658–659, 658–659f
  periosteal, peripheral, or exophytic, 655
  soft tissue, 559
  treatment and prognosis for, 656
Osteomalacia, 829
Osteomyelitis, 134–137
  chronic
    primary, 134–135, 138
      clinical and radiographic features of, 138
      histopathologic features of, 140, 140f
      treatment and prognosis for, 140–141
    recurrent multifocal, 138
      clinical and radiographic features of, 139–140
      histopathologic features of, 140
      treatment and prognosis for, 140–141
    suppurative
      clinical and radiographic features of, 135, 135–136f
      histopathologic features of, 136, 137f
      pathogenesis of, 134–135
      treatment and prognosis for, 136–137
  clinical and radiographic features of, 135
  defined, 134
  etiology and pathogenesis of, 134–135
  from periapical abscess, 130
  predisposing factors for, 135
  with proliferative periostitis, 141–143, 142–143f
  sclerosing
    diffuse, 134–135, 137–138
      clinical and radiographic features of, 137
      histopathologic features of, 137
      treatment and prognosis for, 138
    focal, 141, 141f, 626–627, 626f
  suppurative (bacterial, secondary), 134–135
    acute
      clinical and radiographic features, 135–136
      histopathologic features of, 136, 137f

Osteomyelitis *(Continued)*
        with involucrum, 135
        pathogenesis of, 135
        with sequestrum, 135, 136*f*
        treatment and prognosis for, 136
    chronic
        clinical and radiographic features of,
            135–136, 136*f*
        histopathologic features of, 136,
            137*f*
        pathogenesis of, 135–136
        treatment and prognosis for, 137
Osteonecrosis of jaw, medication-related,
        286–292
    case definition of, 286, 286*b*
    clinical and radiographic features of,
        288–289, 288–289*f*
    due to antiangiogenic agents, 286, 286*b*
    due to antiresorptive agents, 286–287,
        286–287*b*, 288*f*
    histopathologic features of, 289, 290*f*
    treatment and prognosis for, 289–292
Osteopetrosis, 620–623
    autosomal dominant adult ("benign")
        type, 620, 621*t*
    autosomal recessive
        infantile ("malignant") type, 620,
            621–622*f*, 621*t*
        intermediate type, 620, 621*t*
    classification of, 620–621, 621*t*
    defined, 620
    focal periapical, 626–627, 626*f*
    genetic basis for, 620
    histopathologic features of, 622, 622*f*
    treatment and prognosis for, 623
    types of, 620
Osteophytes in osteoarthritis, 872
Osteoporosis circumscripta, 629
Osteoporotic marrow defect, focal, 625,
        625*f*
Osteoradionecrosis (ORN), 134–135,
        281–284, 283–284*f*
    clinical features of, 281–284, 283–284*f*
    treatment and prognosis for, 285–286
Osteosarcoma, 665–669
    central (intramedullary)
        classification of, 665
        clinical features of, 665–666,
            666–667*f*
        histopathologic features of, 666–667,
            667*f*
        radiographic features of, 665–666, 666*f*
        treatment and prognosis for, 668
    chondroblastic, 667
    classification of, 665, 665*t*
    defined, 665
    etiology of, 665
    extraskeletal, 665
    gnathic, 665
    low-grade, 667
    parosteal, 668, 668*f*
    periosteal, 668, 668*f*

Osteosarcoma *(Continued)*
    postirradiation, 669
    surface (juxtacortical, peripheral), 665,
        665*t*, 668, 668*f*
        high-grade, 668
Osteosclerosis, idiopathic, 626–627,
        626*f*
    vs. condensing osteitis, 141
Ostia, 196
Otalgia due to temporomandibular
        disorders, 875
Otodental syndrome, 96
Ovarian cysts in nevoid basal cell carcinoma
        syndrome, 695
"Owl eye" cells, 243, 243*f*
Oxaprozin, allergic mucosal reaction to,
        341*f*
Oxycodone, orofacial complications of, 292,
        293*f*
Oxyphilic adenoma, 487–488, 487*f*

P
Paan, oral submucous fibrosis due to,
        393–395, 394*f*
Pachyonychia congenita, 750–752,
        751–752*f*
Paget disease
    of bone, 628–630
        clinical and radiographic features of,
            629–630, 629*f*
        defined, 628
        diagnosis of, 630
        epidemiology of, 628
        etiology and pathogenesis of, 628
        histopathologic features of, 630,
            630*f*
        hypercementosis in, 93
        malignant transformation of, 630
        treatment and prognosis for, 630
    of skin, 437
Pagetoid spread of melanoma, 437, 438*f*
Pain. *See* Head and neck pain
Palatal cyst(s)
    median, 30–31, 30*f*
    of newborn, 25–26, 26*f*
Palatal exostoses, 19–20, 20*f*
Palatal perforation, oxycodone-related, 292,
        293*f*
Palatal salivary gland tumors, 483*t*
Palatal shelves, 1
Palatal tori, 21, 21*f*
Palatal tubercles, 19–20, 20*f*
Palate
    cleft, 1, 2*f*
    pleomorphic adenoma of, 485, 485*f*
    primary and secondary, 1, 27
    smoker's, 397–398, 398*f*
Palatine cyst, 30–31, 30*f*
Palisaded encapsulated neuroma, 533–534,
        533–534*f*
Palmar pits in nevoid basal cell carcinoma
        syndrome, 694–695, 695*f*

Palmoplantar keratosis in multiple
        hamartoma syndrome, 765
Panencephalitis, subacute sclerosing, 247
Pannus, 873
Panoramic radiographs in identification,
        892, 892*f*
Papilla, retrocuspid, 516
Papillary atrophy in Plummer-Vinson
        syndrome, 830, 831*f*
Papillary cystadenoma, 465
    lymphomatosum, 488–490, 489*f*
        carcinoma ex, 490
Papillary, defined, 914
Papillary gingivitis, 148–149
Papillary growths, differential diagnosis of,
        920–921*t*
Papillary hyperplasia, inflammatory,
        519–520, 519–520*f*
Papillitis, transient lingual, 321, 322*f*
Papilloma(s)
    cylindrical cell, 363–364
    ductal (intraductal, inverted ductal),
        492–493
        clinical features of, 492, 492–493*f*
        histopathologic features of, 492–493,
            493*f*
        treatment and prognosis for, 493
    fungiform (septal, squamous, exophytic),
        361–362, 362*f*
    inverted (endophytic), 362–363,
        362–363*f*
    Schneiderian
        inverted, 361, 362–363*f*
        sinonasal, 361
    squamous, 355–357
        clinical features of, 356, 356*f*
        defined, 355
        epidemiology of, 355
        histopathologic features of, 356–357,
            356*f*
        sinonasal, 361–362
        treatment and prognosis for, 357
Papillomatosis, 356
    denture, 519–520, 519–520*f*
    oral florid, 422
    recurrent respiratory, 356
Papillon-Lefèvre syndrome, 167–169,
        168*f*
Papule, defined, 914
Papulokeratotic variant of transient lingual
        papillitis, 321, 322*f*
Papyraceous scarring, 761
Paracoccidioidomycosis, 216–217, 216*f*
Paradental cyst, 685, 704
Paraganglioma, 543–544, 543–544*f*
Parakeratin clefts, 422
Paramedian lip pits, 4, 4–5*f*
Paramolar, 79, 79*f*
Paranasal sinuses, 196, 196*f*
Paraneoplastic pemphigus, 771*t*, 774–775
    clinical features of, 774–775, 774*f*
    epidemiology of, 774

Paraneoplastic pemphigus *(Continued)*
  histopathologic features of, 775, 775*f*
  pathogenesis of, 770, 774
  treatment and prognosis for, 775
Parasitosis due to drug abuse, 293
Parent body, 315
Paronychia, herpetic, 232, 233*f*
Parosmia, 871
Parosteal osteosarcoma, 668, 668*f*
Parotid gland, pleomorphic adenoma of
        deep lobe of, 484*f*, 485
Parotid tumors, 479, 480*t*
Parotitis
  epidemic, 249–250, 250*f*
  juvenile recurrent, 468
Parry-Romberg syndrome, 38–39, 39*f*
Parulis, 130–131, 130–132*f*
Pastia lines, 175–176
Patched *(PTCH)* gene, 694
Paterson-Kelly syndrome, 404, 830–831,
        831*f*
Pattern injuries, 908–909, 909*f*
Pautrier microabscesses, 605, 605*f*
PCR (polymerase chain reaction), 888
Pedunculated, defined, 914
Peliosis hepatis, bacillary, 195
Pellagra, 828, 828*f*
Pelvic inflammatory disease (PID), 184
Pemphigoid
  bullous, 771*t*, 779–781, 780*f*
  mucous membrane (cicatricial), Mucous
        membrane pemphigoid
Pemphigus
  chronic benign familial, 770
  paraneoplastic, 771*t*, 774–775
    clinical features of, 774–775, 774*f*
    epidemiology of, 774
    histopathologic features of, 775, 775*f*
    pathogenesis of, 770, 774
    treatment and prognosis for, 775
  vegetans, 769
  vulgaris, 769–773, 771*t*
    clinical features of, 770, 772*f*
    epidemiology of, 769
    histopathologic features of, 770–773,
        772–773*f*
    pathogenesis of, 769–770
    treatment and prognosis for, 773
Pemphigus-like drug reactions, 338, 340*b*
Periadenitis mucosa necrotica recurrens
        (PMNR), 323, 323–325*f*, 327*f*
Periapical abscess, 129–132
  classification of, 129–130
  clinical and radiographic features of,
        129–131, 130*f*
  with cutaneous sinus, 130–131, 131*f*
  defined, 129
  parulis (gum boil) as, 130–131, 130–132*f*
  pathogenesis of, 130
  periapical granuloma after, 123
  phoenix, 129
  treatment and prognosis for, 132

Periapical cemental dysplasia, 646–647,
        647*f*
Periapical cementoma, 646–647, 647*f*
Periapical cemento-osseous dysplasia,
        646–647, 647*f*
Periapical cyst, 126–129
  clinical and radiographic features of,
        126–127, 126–128*f*
  defined, 126
  etiology and pathogenesis of, 126
  "globulomaxillary cyst" as, 27, 31
  histopathologic features of, 127–129,
        128–129*f*
  periapical granuloma after, 123
  pocket, 126
  residual, 127, 128*f*, 129
    carcinomatous transformation of, 706
  treatment and prognosis for, 129
  true, 126
Periapical fibrous scars, 125, 125*f*
Periapical granuloma, 123–125
  clinical and radiographic features of,
        123–124, 124*f*
  defined, 123
  etiology and pathogenesis of, 123
  histopathologic features of, 124–125,
        124*f*
  treatment and prognosis for, 125, 125*f*
Periapical osteopetrosis, focal, 626–627,
        626*f*
Periapical radiolucency, differential
        diagnosis of, 926–931*t*
Pericoronal radiolucency, differential
        diagnosis of, 926–931*t*
Pericoronitis, 165, 165*f*
  treatment and prognosis for, 166–167
Peri-implant diseases, 167
Peri-implantitis, 167, 167*f*
Peri-implant mucositis, 147, 167
Perineural invasion, 416
  by adenoid cystic carcinoma, 503, 503*f*
  by polymorphous low-grade
        adenocarcinoma, 503–505, 504*f*
Periodontal abscess, 164–165, 164–165*f*
  treatment and prognosis for, 166
Periodontal cysts
  apical *(see* Periapical cyst)
  lateral *(see* Lateral periodontal cyst(s))
Periodontal disease(s), 147–171
  COVID-19 as, 265–266, 266*f*
  gingival fibromatosis as, 158–160
  gingival hyperplasia as
    drug-related, 156–158
    localized juvenile spongiotic, 150–151
    spongiotic, 150–151, 150*f*
  gingivitis as, 147–150
    desquamative, 155
    foreign body, 154–155
    localized juvenile spongiotic, 150–151
    necrotizing ulcerative, 151–152, 152*f*
    plasma cell, 152–154, 153*f*
    spongiotic, 150–151, 150*f*

Periodontal disease(s) *(Continued)*
  HIV-associated, 257–258, 258*f*
  Papillon-Lefèvre syndrome as, 167–169,
        168*f*
  periodontitis as, 160–167
Periodontal ligament, differential diagnosis
        of thickened, 932–935*t*
Periodontal ligament space in systemic
        sclerosis, 803, 803*f*
Periodontitis, 160–167
  acute apical, 123, 129
  aggressive, 161
  associated with systemic disease, 161,
        161*b*
  chronic, 161, 162*f*
    apical *(see* Periapical granuloma)
  classification of, 161
  clinical and radiographic features of,
        161–165
  defined, 160
  histopathologic features of, 165
  HIV-associated, 257, 258*f*
  necrotizing, 161, 163–164
    treatment and prognosis for, 166
  necrotizing ulcerative, 151–152
    HIV-associated, 257, 258*f*
  pathogenesis of, 161
  refractory, 166
  treatment and prognosis for, 166–167
Perioral dermatitis, 343–344, 344*f*
Periorificial dermatitis, 343–344, 344*f*
Periosteal chondromas, 661
Periosteal osteosarcoma, 668, 668*f*
Periostitis
  ossificans, 141–143, 142–143*f*
  osteomyelitis with proliferative, 141–143,
        142–143*f*
Peripheral fibroameloblastic dentinoma, 733
Peripheral fibroma with calcification,
        529–530, 529–530*f*
Peripheral giant cell granuloma, 527–529,
        528*f*
  histopathologic features of, 526, 527*f*
  treatment and prognosis for, 527
Peripheral nerve sheath tumor, malignant,
        562
  in neurofibromatosis type I, 539, 539*f*
Peripheral ossifying fibroma, 529–530,
        529–530*f*
Peripheral vascular disease due to diabetes
        mellitus, 844
Periungual fibromas in tuberous sclerosis,
        763, 763*f*
Perlèche, 202*t*, 204–205, 204*f*
Pernicious anemia, 831–833, 832*f*
Persistent generalized lymphadenopathy
        (PGL), HIV-associated, 256, 256*f*
Personal injury, 910
Personal recognition, 883–884, 884*f*
Petechiae, 296, 296*f*, 591
  defined, 914
  differential diagnosis of, 916–919*t*

Peutz-Jeghers syndrome, 758–759, 758*f*

PGL (persistent generalized lymphadenopathy), HIV-associated, 256, 256*f*

PHACE(S) syndrome, 548

Phantom bone disease, 627–628, 627–628*f*

Phantom taste, 869–871, 870*b*, 871*t*

Pharyngitis
  acute lymphonodular, 245, 246*f*
  streptococcal, 174–175, 174*f*

Pharyngotonsillitis, 231

Phenol, chemical injury due to, 279, 279*f*

Phenolphthalein, oral mucosal discoloration due to, 308

Phenytoin-related gingival hyperplasia, 157, 157*f*

Pheochromocytomas in multiple endocrine neoplasia type 2B, 541

PHI (protected health information), 881

Philadelphia chromosome, 593

Phlebolith, 14

Phoenix abscess, 123, 129

Phosphate-regulating gene with endopeptidase activity on the X chromosome *(PHEX)*, 849

Photography
  alternative light source (alternate light imaging, fluorescent), 905
  of bite marks, 903–905, 904*t*, 904*f*
  infrared, 904
  reflective ultraviolet, 904

Phycomycosis, 219–221
  clinical features of, 219–220, 220*f*
  diagnosis of, 220
  histopathologic features of, 220, 220*f*
  pathogenesis of, 219
  radiographic features of, 219–220, 220*f*
  treatment and prognosis for, 220–221

Physical anthropologic examination of bones and teeth, 885–888, 886*t*, 886*f*

Physical injury(ies), 272–320
  anesthetic necrosis as, 294, 294*f*
  antral pseudocysts due to, 310–312, 311–312*f*
  cervicofacial emphysema due to, 314–315, 314*f*
  drug-related discolorations of oral mucosa as, 307–309, 308–309*f*
  due to amalgam tattoo and other localized exogenous pigmentations, 298–300
  due to antineoplastic therapy, 280–286
  due to chemicals, 278–280, 278*f*
  due to cosmetic fillers, 302–304, 303*f*
  due to drug abuse, 292–294, 293*f*
  due to endodontic materials, 279–280, 279*f*
  due to oral piercings and other body modifications, 300–302, 301–302*f*
  due to sexual practices, 297–298, 297–298*f*
  due to systemic metallic intoxication, 304–306

Physical injury(ies) *(Continued)*
  electrical and thermal burns as, 276–278, 277–278*f*
  exfoliative cheilitis as, 294–296, 295*f*
  linea alba as, 272, 273*f*
  medication-related osteonecrosis of jaw as, 286–292
  morsicatio mucosae oris as, 272–273, 273*f*
  myospherulosis as, 315, 315*f*
  oral ulceration with bone sequestration as, 310, 310*f*
  reactive osseous and chondromatous metaplasia (Cutright lesion) as, 309–310, 309*f*
  smoker's melanosis as, 306–307, 307*f*
  submucosal hemorrhage due to, 296–297, 296–297*f*
  traumatic ulcerations as, 273–275
  true cysts of sinuses due to, 312–313, 313*f*

PID (pelvic inflammatory disease), 184

Piercings, 300–302, 301–302*f*

Pierre Robin sequence, orofacial clefts in, 3, 3*f*

Pigmented ameloblastoma, 541–543, 542*f*

Pigmented basal cell carcinoma, 431

Pilar cyst, 31
  clinical features of, 31, 31*f*

Pindborg tumor, 720–722
  clinical and radiographic features of, 721, 721*f*
  epidemiology of, 720–721
  histopathologic features of, 721–722, 722*f*
  pathogenesis of, 720–721
  relative distribution of, 721, 721*f*
  treatment and prognosis for, 722

Pink disease, 305

Pink tooth of Mummery, 62–63, 63*f*

Pituitary dwarfism, 833–834

Plantar pits in nevoid basal cell carcinoma syndrome, 694–695, 695*f*

Plaque, defined, 914

Plasma cell gingivitis, 152–154, 153*f*
  vs. contact stomatitis from artificial cinnamon flavoring, 344

Plasmacytoma, 611, 611*f*
  extramedullary, 611

Plasminogen deficiency, 581–582, 582*f*

Plass Data DVI System International software, 895

Platelet destruction, increased, 590–591

Platelet production, reduced, 590

Pleomorphic adenoma, 483–487
  carcinoma ex, 499–501
    clinical features of, 499–500, 500*f*
    histopathologic features of, 500–501, 500*f*
    intracapsular, 501
    treatment and prognosis for, 501

Pleomorphic adenoma *(Continued)*
  clinical and radiographic features of, 483–485, 484*f*
  of deep lobe of parotid gland, 485, 485*f*
  epidemiology of, 483
  histopathologic features of, 485–487, 486*f*
    chondroid appearance as, 486, 486*f*
    eosinophilic, hyalinized change as, 486, 486*f*
    myoepithelial cells as, 486, 486*f*
    myxomatous background as, 486, 486*f*
  of palate, 485, 485*f*
  pathogenesis of, 483
  treatment and prognosis for, 487

Pleomorphic lipoma, 531

Pleomorphic liposarcoma, 561

Plumbism, 304–306

Plummer-Vinson syndrome, 404, 830–831, 831*f*

Plunging ranula, 463*f*

PMNR (periadenitis mucosa necrotica recurrens), 323, 323–325*f*, 327*f*

Pneumoparotid, 314

Polyarthralgia, 873

Polycythemia vera (primary, rubra vera), 592

Polydipsia in diabetes mellitus, 845

Polyethylene agents for candidiasis, 209, 211*t*

Poly-L-lactic acid (Sculptra), oral lesions associated with, 302

Polymerase chain reaction (PCR), 888

Polymethylmethacrylate (Artecoll, ArteFill), oral lesions associated with, 302, 303*f*

Polymorphic reticulosis, 607–609, 608*f*

Polymorphous low-grade adenocarcinoma, 503–505
  clinical features of, 504, 504*f*
  histopathologic features of, 504–505, 504–505*f*
  treatment and prognosis for, 505

Polymyalgia rheumatica, 867

Polyp
  fibroepithelial, 517–518, 518*f*
  pulp
    clinical features of, 118
    histopathologic features of, 118–119
    treatment and prognosis for, 119

Polyphagia in diabetes mellitus, 845

Polypoid squamous cell carcinoma, 423–424, 423–424*f*

Polyuria in diabetes mellitus, 845

Poorly defined borders, differential diagnosis of radiolucencies with, 926–931*t*

Poorly demarcated borders
  differential diagnosis of mixed radiolucent/radiopaque lesions with, 926–931*t*
  differential diagnosis of radiopacities with, 926–931*t*

Popliteal pterygium syndrome, 5
Porphyria, tooth discoloration due to congenital erythropoietic, 68–69, 68f
Port wine stain, 551–552, 551f
Posaconazole for candidiasis, 210
Positive identification, 883
Possible identification, 883
Postherpetic neuralgia, 240
Postirradiation bone sarcoma, 669
Postmortem examination, 893–894, 894f
Postmortem records, comparison of antemortem and, 894–895, 894t, 895f
Postoperative maxillary cyst, 312–313, 313f
Potentially malignant disorder, 381
Pregnancy
    mask of, 371–372, 371f
    pyogenic granuloma during, 526, 527f
Pregnancy tumor, 526, 527f
Presumptive identification, 883
Prevotella intermedia, 191
Primary cutaneous CD30+ lymphoproliferative disorder, 274
Primary palate, 1, 27
Primordial cyst, 689, 689f
Primordial odontogenic tumor, 731
    clinical and radiographic features of, 731, 731f
    histopathologic features of, 731, 731f
    treatment and prognosis for, 731
Privacy Rule, 881
Progeria, 120
Prognastic staging classification
    for oral cavity carcinoma and cutaneous carcinoma, of head and neck, 415t
    for oropharyngeal carcinoma, 415–416t
Progonoma, melanotic, 541–543, 542f
Progressive facial hemiatrophy, 38–39, 39f
Progressive hemifacial atrophy, 38–39, 39f
Progressive systemic sclerosis. See Systemic sclerosis
Proliferative periostitis, osteomyelitis with, 141–143, 142–143f
Proliferative verrucous leukoplakia (PVL), 149–150, 384, 385f, 788
Proptosis, 837, 838f
ProQuad (measles, mumps, rubella, and varicella virus vaccine), 238
Prosoplasia, 127–129
Protease inhibitors, 264
Protected health information (PHI), 881
Proteinosis, lipoid, 822–823, 822–823f
Proteus-like syndrome, multiple hamartoma syndrome and, 765
Proteus syndrome, 539
Protostylid, 85
Protozoal disease(s)
    leishmaniasis as, 224–225, 224f
    toxoplasmosis as, 222–224, 223f
Pseudoacanthosis nigricans, 806

Pseudocarcinoma. See Keratoacanthoma
Pseudocarcinomatous hyperplasia, 215
    in granular cell tumor, 545, 545f
Pseudocysts, antral, 310–312, 311–312f
Pseudoepitheliomatous hyperplasia, 215
    in granular cell tumor, 545, 545f
Pseudo-horn cysts, 367, 367f
Pseudohypoparathyroidism, 839–840
Pseudomembranous candidiasis, 201–202, 202t, 202–203f
Pseudosarcoma, 423–424, 423–424f
Pseudotumor of hemophilia, 580
Psoriasiform mucositis, 785–786
Psoriasis, 796–798, 796–797f
    intraoral, 797
    and reactive arthritis, 786
Psoriatic arthritis, 797
PTCH (patched) gene, 694
PTEN hamartoma-tumor syndrome, 765–766, 765–766f
Ptyalism, 469–470
Puberty gingivitis, 147
Pulpal calcifications, 121–123
    clinical and radiographic features of, 122, 122f
    differential diagnosis of, 932–935t
    epidemiology of, 121–122
    factors associated with, 121–122
    histopathologic features of, 122–123, 122–123f
    treatment and prognosis for, 123
    types of, 122
Pulpalgia, 117
Pulpal necrosis, 118
Pulpal pain, 117
Pulp chambers
    differential diagnosis of enlarged, 932–935t
    thistle tube-shaped or flame-shaped, 106–107, 107f
Pulp, clinically normal, 117
Pulpitis, 117–119
    chronic hyperplastic
        clinical features of, 118, 118f
        histopathologic features of, 119
        treatment and prognosis for, 119
    clinical features of, 117–118
    defined, 117
    etiology and pathogenesis of, 117
    histopathologic features of, 118–119, 119f
    irreversible, 118
        clinical features of, 118
        histopathologic features of, 119, 119f
        treatment and prognosis for, 119
    reversible
        clinical features of, 117
        defined, 117
        histopathologic features of, 119, 119f
        treatment and prognosis for, 119

Pulp polyp
    histopathologic features of, 118–119
    treatment and prognosis for, 119
Pulp stones, 122
Pulse granuloma in periapical cyst, 129, 129f
Purple lesions, differential diagnosis of, 916–919t
Purpura, 296, 296f
    thrombocytopenic
        immune, 591
        thrombotic, 591
Pustule, defined, 914
PUVA therapy
    for mycosis fungoides, 605
    for psoriasis, 796
PVL (proliferative verrucous leukoplakia), 384, 385f
Pyogenic granuloma, 525–527
    clinical features of, 525–526, 526f
    gingival, 148–149, 149f
    during pregnancy, 526, 527f
Pyostomatitis vegetans, 851–852, 852f
Pyridoxine deficiency, 828
Pyronine bodies in periapical granuloma, 124–125

Q
Quincke disease, 348–350, 348–349f

R
RA (rheumatoid arthritis), 872–874
Rabies, 900
Rachitic rosary, 829
Radiation, and squamous cell carcinoma, 403–404
Radiation dermatitis, 282, 282f
Radiation-induced caries, 282, 283f, 471
Radiation mucositis, 281, 282f
Radiation-related xerostomia, 282, 283f
Radical neck dissection, 419
    modified, 419
    selective, 419
    for squamous cell carcinoma
Radicular cyst (see Periapical cyst)
Radicular cyst, lateral, 127, 127–128f
Radicular dentin dysplasia, 108–110
    classification of, 105, 105t
    clinical features of, 108–109, 108–109f
    radiographic features of, 109, 109f
    subclassification of, 109, 109b
Radiculomegaly, 82
Radiographic pathology, differential diagnosis of, 926–931t
Radiolucencies, differential diagnosis of, 926–931t
Radiopacities, differential diagnosis of, 926–931t
Ragged borders, differential diagnosis of radiolucencies with, 926–931t
Ramsay Hunt syndrome, 240

Ranula, 462–463, 463*f*
Rapidly involuting congenital hemangioma (RICH), 547
Raynaud phenomenon
 in CREST syndrome, 805
 in systemic sclerosis, 802
Reactive arthritis, 786–787
Reactive osseous and chondromatous metaplasia, 309–310, 309*f*
Reactive subpontine exostoses, 20, 20*f*
Record management in forensic dentistry, 881–883, 882*f*
Recurrent aphthous stomatitis, 321–326
 diagnosis of, 323*b*, 325
 epidemiology of, 321–322
 histopathologic features of, 325
 treatment and prognosis for, 325–326, 325*f*
Recurrent aphthous ulcerations.
   See Recurrent aphthous stomatitis
Recurrent respiratory papillomatosis (RRP), 356
Red lesions, differential diagnosis of, 916–919*t*
Red strawberry tongue, 175
Reed-Sternberg cells, 599–600, 599*f*
Reflective ultraviolet photography, 904
Regional enteritis, 850–851, 850–851*f*
Regional ileitis, 850–851, 850–851*f*
Regional odontodysplasia, 110–111, 110*b*, 111*f*
Reimpaction of tooth, 73, 74*f*
Reinclusion of tooth, 73, 74*f*
Reiter syndrome, 786–787
Relative risk, 381
Renal calculi in hyperparathyroidism, 840
Renal carcinoma, metastatic, 569*f*
Renal osteodystrophy, hyperparathyroidism due to, 841, 841*f*
Residual periapical cyst, 127, 128*f*, 129
 carcinomatous transformation of, 706
Resorption, tooth. *See* Tooth resorption
Restriction enzymes, 888
Restriction fragment length polymorphism (RFLP), 888
Restylane (hyaluronic acid), oral lesions associated with, 302
Retention cyst, sinus, 312–313, 313*f*
Retention mucocele, 460
Reticular lichen planus
 clinical features of, 788, 788–789*f*
 diagnosis of, 791, 792*f*
 treatment and prognosis for, 791–792
Reticuloendothelioses, lipid, 821–822
Reticulosis, polymorphic (midline malignant), 607–609, 608*f*
Retinal anlage tumor, 541–543, 542*f*
Retinal pigment epithelium, congenital hypertrophy of, 657
Retinol deficiency, 827
Retrocuspid papilla, 516, 517*f*
Reverse polarity, 714

Reverse smoker's palate, 397–398
RFLP (restriction fragment length polymorphism), 888
Rhabdomyoma, 557–558
 adult
  clinical features of, 557, 557*f*
  histopathologic features of, 557, 558*f*
 cardiac, in tuberous sclerosis, 763
 clinical features of, 557, 557*f*
 defined, 557
 fetal, 557
 histopathologic features of, 557–558, 558*f*
 treatment and prognosis for, 558
Rhabdomyosarcoma, 566–567
 alveolar, 566–567
 botryoid, 567
 classification of, 566
 clinical features of, 566–567, 566–567*f*
 defined, 566
 embryonal
  clinical features of, 566, 566*f*
  histopathologic features of, 567, 567*f*
 epidemiology of, 566
 histopathologic features of, 567, 567*f*
 pleomorphic, 566
 treatment and prognosis for, 567
Rheumatoid arthritis (RA), 872–874
Rheumatoid nodules, 873
Riboflavin deficiency, 828
Rice bodies, 874
RICH (rapidly involuting congenital hemangioma), 547
Rickets, 829
 familial hypophosphatemic, 848–850, 849*f*
 vitamin D–dependent, 849
 vitamin D–resistant, 848–850, 849*f*
Riga-Fede disease, 81, 273–274, 275*f*
Robinson, Ansil L., 900
Romberg syndrome, 38–39, 39*f*
Root(s)
 differential diagnosis of abnormally shaped, 932–935*t*
 supernumerary, 96, 96*f*
Root canal, differential diagnosis of enlarged, 932–935*t*
Rootless teeth, 108–109
 classification of, 105*t*, 108–109
 clinical features of, 108–109, 108–109*f*
 radiographic features of, 109, 109*f*
 subclassification of, 109, 109*b*
Root resorption due to periapical granuloma, 123–124, 124*f*
Roseola, 229
Round cell liposarcoma, 561
RRP (recurrent respiratory papillomatosis), 356
Rubella, 248–249
Rubeola, 246–248, 247*f*
Rugoscopy, 885

Rushton bodies in periapical cyst, 127–129, 128*f*
Russell bodies in periapical granuloma, 124–125

S
Saddle nose deformity, drug-related, 292, 293*f*
Saint Anthony's fire, 173
Saliva evidence, 905
Salivary adenocarcinoma, not otherwise specified (NOS), 505–506, 505–506*f*
Salivary calculi. *See* Sialolithiasis
Salivary duct cyst, 460, 463–465, 464*f*
Salivary duct ectasia, oncocytic, 464–465, 464*f*
Salivary gland aplasia, 460
Salivary gland pathology, 460–513
 adenomatoid hyperplasia of minor salivary glands as, 477
 cheilitis glandularis as, 468–469, 469*f*
 HIV-associated, 259
 IgG4-related disease as, 471–472
 mucocele as, 460–462
 necrotizing sialometaplasia as, 477–479, 478*f*
 ranula as, 462–463, 463*f*
 salivary duct cyst as, 463–465, 464*f*
 salivary gland aplasia as, 460, 461*f*
 sialadenitis as, 467–468
 sialadenosis (sialosis) as, 476–477, 477*f*
 sialolithiasis as, 465–467
 sialorrhea as, 469–470
 Sjögren syndrome as, 472–476
 tumors as (*see* Salivary gland tumor(s))
 xerostomia as, 470–471, 470*t*
Salivary gland tumor(s), 479–506
 acinic cell carcinoma as, 497–498, 497–498*f*
 adenoid cystic carcinoma as, 501–503
 basal cell adenoma as, 491–492, 492*f*
 canalicular adenoma as, 490–491, 490*f*
 carcinoma ex pleomorphic adenoma as, 499–501
 carcinosarcoma as, 499–501
 classification of, 479
 ductal papillomas as, 492–493
 frequency of malignancy by site for, 479, 480*t*
 general considerations with, 479–482
 incidence of, 479
 intraosseous mucoepidermoid carcinoma (central mucoepidermoid carcinoma) as, 496, 497*f*
 labial, 481, 483*t*
 malignant mixed tumors as, 499–501, 500*f*
 mammary analogue secretory carcinoma as, 498–499, 498*f*
 metastasizing mixed tumor as, 499–501
 of minor salivary glands, 481, 484*t*

Salivary gland tumor(s) *(Continued)*
  location of, 481, 483*t*
    percentage malignant by site of, 484*t*
  monomorphic adenoma as, 490
  mucoepidermoid carcinoma as, 493–496
  oncocytoma (oxyphilic adenoma) as,
    487–488, 487*f*
  palatal, 483*t*
  parotid, 479, 480*t*
  pleomorphic adenoma (benign mixed
    tumor) as, 483–487
  polymorphous low-grade adenocarcinoma
    as, 503–505
  salivary adenocarcinoma, not otherwise
    specified as, 505–506, 505–506*f*
  sites of, 479, 480*t*
  sublingual, 481
  submandibular, 479–481, 481*t*
  Warthin tumor (papillary cystadenoma
    lymphomatosum) as, 488–490,
    489*f*
Salivary stones. *See* Sialolithiasis
Salivation, excessive, 469–470
Sanfilippo-A disease, 820*t*
Sanfilippo-B disease, 820*t*
Sanguinaria-associated keratosis, 381–382,
  382*f*
San Joaquin Valley fever, 217, 217*f*
SAPHO syndrome, 138
  clinical and radiographic features of,
    139–140
  histopathologic features of, 140
  treatment and prognosis for, 140–141
Sarcoidosis, 328–330
  clinical features of, 328–329, 329*f*
  histopathologic features of, 329, 330*f*
  treatment and prognosis for, 330
Sarcoma(s)
  alveolar soft-part, 568–569, 569*f*
  ameloblastic, 727–728, 728*f*
  etiology of, 229
  Ewing, 671–673, 672*f*
  histopathologic features of
    HIV-associated, 254–256, 255*f*
  Kaposi, 564–565
    classic (chronic) type, 564, 564*f*
    clinical features of, 564, 564*f*
    defined, 564
    endemic type, 564
    epidemiology of, 564
    etiology of, 564
    histopathologic features of, 564
      in nodular stage, 564, 565*f*
      in patch stage, 564
      in plaque stage, 564
    iatrogenic type (transplant-associated),
      564
    treatment and prognosis for, 565
  myeloid (granulocytic), 594
  osteogenic (*see* Osteosarcoma)
  postirradiation bone, 669
  soft tissue, 559

Sarcoma(s) *(Continued)*
  synovial, 567–568, 568*f*
  undifferentiated pleomorphic, 560–561,
    561*f*
Sarcomatoid squamous cell carcinoma,
  423–424, 423–424*f*
Scaphocephaly, 41
Scarlatina, 175–176, 175*f*
Scarlet fever, 175
Scarring, papyraceous, 761
Schaumann bodies, 329, 330*f*
Scheie disease, 820*t*
Scheuthauer-Marie-Sainton syndrome,
  623–625
Schneiderian, oncocytic, 363–364
Schneiderian papilloma
  inverted, 361, 362–363*f*
  oncocytic, 363–364
Schwachman-Diamond syndrome, 588
Schwannoma(s), 534, 536*f*
  ancient, 534
  granular cell, 544
  malignant, in neurofibromatosis type I,
    539, 539*f*
  plexiform, 534
Schwannomatosis, 534, 535*t*
Scirrhous change, 416
SCLE (subacute cutaneous lupus
    erythematosus), 800
Sclerae, blue, in osteogenesis imperfecta,
  618, 619*f*
Sclerodactyly in CREST syndrome, 805,
  805*f*
Scleroderma. *See also* Systemic sclerosis
  limited, 805–806, 805–806*f*
  linear "en coup de sabre", 39
  localized, 803, 804*f*
Sclerosing (morpheaform) basal cell
    carcinoma, 431
Sclerosing hemangioma, 520–521, 521*f*
Sclerosing osteomyelitis, focal, 141, 141*f*,
  626–627, 626*f*
Scorbutic gingivitis, 829, 829*f*
Scrofula, 187, 187*f*
Scrotal tongue, 11–12, 11*f*
  in erythema migrans, 12
Scrumpox, 232–233
Sculptra (poly-L-lactic acid), oral lesions
    associated with, 302
Scurvy, 828, 829*f*
Sebaceous cyst, 31
Sebaceous hyperplasia, 368, 368–369*f*
Seborrheic keratosis, 366–368
  clinical features of, 366–367, 367*f*
  histopathologic features of, 367–368,
    367*f*
  irritated, 368
  treatment and prognosis for, 368
Secondary palate, 1, 27
Secondary retention of tooth, 73, 74*f*
Segmental odontomaxillary dysplasia,
  39–40, 40*f*

Selective neck dissection, 419
"Self-healing" carcinoma.
    See Keratoacanthoma
Senile lentigo, 369–370, 370*f*
Sentinel-node biopsy, 419
Septal papilloma, 361–362, 362*f*
Sequestration
  in spleen, 591–592
  spontaneous or traumatic, 310, 310*f*
Sequestrum, acute osteomyelitis with, 135,
  136*f*
Serial killers, 896
Serologic comparison, 888–889
Sessile, defined, 914
Seventh nerve paralysis, idiopathic,
  861–862, 862*f*
Severe epithelial dysplasia, 387, 387*f*
Sexual practices, oral trauma from, 297–298,
  297–298*f*
Sézary cells, 605
Sézary syndrome, 605
Shagreen patches in tuberous sclerosis, 763
Shell teeth, 106, 106*f*
Shepherd's crook deformity, 643
Shield system for classification of hereditary
    dentin disorders, 104–105, 105*t*
Shingles, 238–241, 238–239*f*
  with HIV infection, 260
Shovel-shaped incisors, 87, 87*f*
Sialadenitis, 467–468
  acute bacterial, 467, 467*f*
  chronic, 467–468, 467*f*
    sclerosing, 468, 468*f*
  clinical and radiographic features of,
    467–468, 467*f*
  defined, 467
  etiology and pathogenesis of, 467
  histopathologic features of, 468, 468*f*
  juvenile recurrent parotitis as, 468
  myoepithelial, 475, 475*f*
  subacute necrotizing, 468
  treatment and prognosis for, 468
Sialadenoma papilliferum, 492–493
  clinical features of, 492, 492–493*f*
  histopathologic features of, 492–493,
    493*f*
  treatment and prognosis for, 493
Sialadenosis, 476–477, 477*f*
  diabetic, 845–846
Sialocyst, 463–465, 464*f*
Sialolipoma, 531
Sialolithiasis, 465–467
  clinical features of, 465, 465–466*f*
  defined, 465
  histopathologic features of, 465–466,
    466*f*
  of minor salivary gland, 465, 466*f*
  pathogenesis of, 465
  radiographic features of, 465, 465–466*f*
  treatment and prognosis for, 466–467
Sialometaplasia, necrotizing, 477–479,
  478*f*

Sialo-odontogenic cyst, 703–704, 704f
Sialorrhea, 469–470
Sialosis, 476–477, 477f
Sicca syndrome, 472
Sickle cell anemia, 583–585, 584f
    jaundice in, 823
Sickle cell crisis, 583
Sickle cell disease, 583
Sickle cell trait, 583
Sideropenic dysphagia, 830–831, 831f
Silver intoxication, 304–305, 306f
Silver nitrate, chemical injury due to,
    279
Simple bone cyst, 636–638, 637f
Simvastatin, allergic mucosal reaction to,
    340f
Sinonasal papillomas, 361
Sinonasal-type hemangiopericytoma, 521
Sinonasal undifferentiated carcinoma
    (SNUC), 426–428, 427f
Sinusitis, 196–198, 196f, 198f
    allergic fungal, 221
Sinus mucocele, 312–313, 313f
Sinus retention cyst, 312–313
Sixth disease, 229
Sjögren syndrome, 472–476, 869
    classification of, 472
    clinical and radiographic features of,
        473–474, 474f
    defined, 472
    etiology and pathogenesis of, 472
    histopathologic features of, 475–476,
        475–476f
    keratoconjunctivitis sicca in, 472
    laboratory values in, 474–475
    and lymphoma, 476
    primary, 472
    secondary, 472
    treatment and prognosis for, 476
Skeletal anomalies in nevoid basal cell
        carcinoma syndrome, 695, 695f
Skeletal anthropologic variations, 885–888,
        886t, 886f
Skin
    clinical features of, 31–32, 31–32f
    epidermoid cyst of, 31
        clinical features of, 31, 31–32f
        histopathologic features of, 32, 32f
    follicular cysts of, 31–32
        histopathologic features of, 32, 32f
        treatment and prognosis for, 32
Skull, physical anthropologic examination
        of, 885–888, 886t, 886f
SLE (systemic lupus erythematosus), clinical
        features of, 798, 798f, 799t
Small cell carcinoma of skin, 432–434,
        433f
Smokeless tobacco and squamous cell
        carcinoma, 402–403
Smokeless tobacco keratosis, 391–393
    clinical features of, 391–392, 391f
    defined, 381

Smokeless tobacco keratosis (Continued)
    histopathologic features of, 392–393,
        392f
    treatment and prognosis for, 393, 393f
Smokeless tobacco–related gingival
        recession, 391, 391f
Smokeless tobacco use
    epidemiology, 391
    types of, 391
Smoker's melanosis, 306–307, 307f
Smoker's palate, 397–398, 398f
SNUC (sinonasal undifferentiated
        carcinoma), 426–428, 427f
Snuff dipper's cancer, 393, 421–423,
        422–423f
Snuff dipper's lesion. See Smokeless tobacco
        keratosis
Snuff pouch, 391
Soft palate, differential diagnosis of soft
        tissue masses of, 922–925t
Soft palate fistulas, lateral, 15, 15f
Soft tissue chondromas, 559
Soft tissue masses, differential diagnosis of,
        922–925t
Soft tissue osteomas, 559
Soft tissue pathology, differential diagnosis
        of
    with color changes, 916–919t
    with masses or enlargements, 922–925t
    with surface alterations, 920–921t
Soft tissue radiopacities, differential
        diagnosis of, 926–931t
Soft tissue sarcoma(s), 559
    alveolar soft-part sarcoma as, 568–569,
        569f
    angiosarcoma as, 563–564, 563f
    ectomesenchymal chondromyxoid tumor
        as, 558
    fibrosarcoma, 559–560, 560f
    Kaposi sarcoma as, 564–565
    leiomyosarcoma as, 565–566, 565–566f
    liposarcoma as, 561, 561f
    malignant peripheral nerve sheath tumor
        as, 562
    olfactory neuroblastoma
        (esthesioneuroblastoma) as,
        562–563, 562–563f
    rhabdomyosarcoma as, 566–567
    synovial sarcoma as, 567–568, 568f
    undifferentiated pleomorphic sarcoma
        (malignant fibrous histiocytoma)
        as, 560–561, 561f
Soft tissue tumor(s), 514–577
    congenital epulis as, 546–547, 546f
    epulis fissuratum as, 517–519
    fibroma as, 514
        giant cell, 514–517
        irritation (traumatic), 514
        peripheral ossifying, 529–530,
            529–530f
    fibromatosis as, 523, 523f
    fibrous histiocytoma as, 520–521, 521f

Soft tissue tumor(s) (Continued)
    genetic abnormalities of various, 515t
    granular cell tumor as, 544–546
    hemangioma and vascular malformations
        as, 547–551
    inflammatory papillary hyperplasia
        (denture papillomatosis) as,
        519–520, 519–520f
    leiomyoma as, 555–557
    lipoma as, 530–531
    lymphatic malformations as, 553–555
    melanotic neuroectodermal tumor of
        infancy as, 541–543
    metastases as, 569–570
    multiple endocrine neoplasia type 2B as,
        540–541
    myofibromatosis as, 523–524, 524f
    nasopharyngeal angiofibroma as,
        552–553, 553f
    neurofibroma as, 534–537, 536–537f
    neurofibromatosis type I (von
        Recklinghausen disease of the
        skin) as, 537–539
    neuroma as
        palisaded encapsulated (solitary
            circumscribed), 533–534,
            533–534f
        traumatic (amputation), 531f, 532,
            533f
    oral focal mucinosis as, 524–525, 525f
    osseous and cartilaginous choristomas as,
        559, 559f
    paraganglioma as, 543–544, 543–544f
    peripheral giant cell granuloma (giant cell
        epulis) as, 527–529, 528f
    pyogenic granuloma (lobular capillary
        hemangioma) as, 525–527
    rhabdomyoma as, 557–558
    sarcomas as (see Soft tissue sarcoma(s))
    schwannoma (neurilemoma), 534, 535t,
        536f
    solitary fibrous tumor
        (hemangiopericytoma) as,
        521–522, 522f
    Sturge-Weber syndrome as, 551–552,
        551–552f
Solar cheilosis, 395–396
Solar elastosis, 395, 397, 431–432
Solar keratosis, 396–397, 396–397f
    in xeroderma pigmentosum, 753
Solar lentigo, 369–370, 370f
Solid variant of adenoid cystic carcinoma,
    502–503
Solitary bone cyst, 636–638, 637f
Solitary circumscribed neuroma, 533–534,
    533–534f
Solitary exostoses, 20
Solitary fibrous tumor, 521–522, 522f
South American blastomycosis, 216–217,
    216f
Speckled leukoplakia, 384, 384f
Spindle and epithelioid cell nevus, 378–379

Spindle cell carcinoma, 423–424, 423–424f
Spindle cell lipoma, 531
Spindle torus, 21
Spit tobacco keratosis. *See* Smokeless tobacco keratosis
Spitz (spindle and epithelioid), 378–379
Spitz nevus, 378–379
Spleen, sequestration in, 591–592
Split papules, 179–180, 180f
Split tongue, 300–301
Spongiotic gingival hyperplasia, 150–151, 150f
Squamous cell carcinoma, 398–421
  adenosquamous, 424–425
  arising in graft-versus-host disease, 795, 795f
  basal cell, 430–432, 431–432f
  basaloid, 425, 425f
  clinical and radiographic features of, 406–410
    intraoral cacinoma, 407f, 408–410, 409–410f
    lip vermilion carcinoma, 408, 408f
    metastasis, 408–410, 411f
    oral cavity carcinoma, 406–408, 406–408f
    oropharyngeal carcinoma, 408–410, 410–411f
  epidermolysis bullosa and, 768
  etiology of, 402–406
    due to alcohol, 403
    due to bacteria, 404
    due to betel quid, 403
    due to *Candida*, 404
    due to chronic trauma or irritation, 406
    due to dietary factors, 404
    due to immunosuppression, 406
    due to occupational exposures and environmental pollutants, 403
    due to oncogenes and tumor suppressor genes, 406
    due to oncogenic viruses, 404–406
    due to radiation, 403–404
    due to smokeless tobacco, 402–403
    due to tobacco smoking, 402
    due to vitamin/mineral deficiencies, 404
  histopathologic features of, 416–418, 417–418f
  histopathologic grading of, 417
  HIV-associated, 263, 263f
  keratinizing, 429
  malignant transformation of dentigerous cyst to, 688
  of maxillary sinus, 426, 426f
  multiple, 420–421
  nasopharyngeal, 428–430, 429f
  nonkeratinizing, 429
    differentiated, 429
    undifferentiated, 429

Squamous cell carcinoma *(Continued)*
  proliferative verrucous leukoplakia and, 384
  sinonasal undifferentiated, 426–428, 427f
  spindle cell (sarcomatoid, polypoid), 423–424, 423–424f
  treatment and prognosis for, 418–420
  verrucous, 421–423, 422–423f
  in xeroderma pigmentosum, 753
Squamous ed, 368
Squamous odontogenic tumor, 723–724, 723f
Squamous odontogenic tumorlike proliferations, 723–724
Squamous papilloma, 355–357
  clinical features of, 356, 356f
  defined, 355
  epidemiology of, 355
  histopathologic features of, 356–357, 356f
  sinonasal, 361–362
  treatment and prognosis for, 357
SSPE (subacute sclerosing panencephalitis), 247
Stafne bone cyst, 23–25, 24–25f
Stafne defect, 23–25, 24–25f
Staging, of melanoma, 438–442t
Stannous fluoride, tooth discoloration due to, 68
Staphylococcal impetigo, 172
Staphylococcus aureus
  impetigo due, 172
  methicillin-resistant, 172–173
Stare Decisis, 901
Static bone cyst, 23–25, 24–25f
Static bone defect, 23–25, 24–25f
Stevens-Johnson syndrome, 781, 783–784, 783f
Stomatitis
  anaphylactic, 338
  aphthous
    herpetiform, 324–325, 324f
    HIV-associated, 262, 262–263f
    major, 324, 324f
    minor, 323–324, 323–324f
  chronic ulcerative, 792–794, 793–794f
  contact
    allergic, 342–343, 343f
    from artificial cinnamon flavoring, 344–346
      clinical features of, 344, 345f
      diagnosis of, 345–346
      histopathologic features of, 345, 345f
      treatment and prognosis for, 346
  cotton roll, 280, 280f
  denture, 202t, 205, 205–206f
  gangrenous (necrotizing), 151–152, 191–192, 192f
    HIV-associated, 257–258, 258f
  granulomatous, as allergic disease, 336–337, 337f

Stomatitis *(Continued)*
  medicamentosa, 338
  nicotine, 397–398, 398f
  recurrent aphthous (*see* Recurrent aphthous stomatitis)
  uremic, 852–853, 853f
    vs. morsicatio mucosae oris, 272–273
  venenata, 342–343, 343f
Stomatodynia, 868–869, 868b
Stomatopyrosis, 868–869, 868b
  due to oral submucous fibrosis, 394
"Stones" in hyperparathyroidism, 840
STR(s) (microsatellite loci), 889
Strawberry gingivitis, 334, 334–335f
Streptococcal pharyngitis, 174–175, 174f
Streptococcal tonsillitis, 174–175, 174f
Streptococcus pyogenes, impetigo due to, 172
String of pearls, 341
Study casts of bite mark injury, 905
Sturge-Weber syndrome, 551–552, 551–552f
Stylalgia, 23, 23f
Stylocarotid syndrome., 23, 23f
Stylohyoid syndrome, 23, 23f
Subacute cutaneous lupus erythematosus (SCLE), 800
Subacute necrosing sialadenitis, 468
Subacute sclerosing panencephalitis (SSPE), 247
Subchondral cysts in osteoarthritis, 872
Subependymal giant cell astrocytoma in tuberous sclerosis, 763
Sublingual gland tumors, 481
Sublingual varix, 14
Submandibular tumors, 479–481, 481t
Submergence of tooth, 73, 74f
Submucosal hemorrhage, 296–297, 296–297f
Submucous fibrosis, 393–395, 394f
Submucous palatal cleft, 3, 3f
Subpontic osseous hyperplasia, 20, 20f
Subpontic osseous proliferation, 20, 20f
Sulfur granules, 193
"Sunburst" radiopacities, differential diagnosis of, 926–931t
Superficial basal cell carcinoma, 431
Superficial mucocele, 461–462, 462f
Superficial spreading melanoma, 436, 436f
Supernumerary roots, 96, 96f
Supernumerary teeth
  clinical features of, 79
  conical, 79
  defined, 75, 82–83
  distomolar or distodens as, 79, 79f
  mesiodens as, 78f
  molariform, 79
  multiple, 78, 78–79f
  paramolar as, 79, 79f
  rudimentary, 79
  supplemental, 79
  syndromes associated with, 75, 76b

Supernumerary teeth *(Continued)*
  treatment and prognosis for, 80
  tuberculate, 79
Surface alterations, differential diagnosis of, 920–921*t*
Surgical ciliated cyst, 312–313, 313*f*
Surgical mumps, 467
Susuk, implantation of, 301, 302*f*
Sutton nevus, 379, 379*f*
Sweet, David, 889
Swift-Feer disease, 305
Symblepharons in mucous membrane pemphigoid, 776–777, 777*f*
Syndactyly, 42, 42*f*
Syngnathia, 5
Synovial chondromatosis, 662–663, 663*f*
Synovial sarcoma, 567–568, 568*f*
Synovitis, 873
Syphilis, 179–184
  clinical features of, 179–182
  congenital, 179, 181–182, 181*t*, 182*f*
  diagnosis of, 181–182
  epidemiology of, 179
  etiology and pathogenesis of, 179
  histopathologic features of, 182–183, 182–183*f*
  latent, 180–181
  primary, 179, 179*f*
  secondary (disseminated), 179–180, 180–181*f*
  tertiary, 180–181, 181*f*
  treatment and prognosis for, 183–184
Syphilitic hypoplasia, 58
Systemic disease(s) with oral manifestations, 819–860
  acromegaly as, 834–835, 834–835*f*
  Addison disease (hypoadrenocorticism) as, 843–844, 844*f*
  amyloidosis as, 824–827, 825–826*f*
  anemia as
    iron-deficiency, 830
    pernicious, 831–833, 832*f*
  Crohn disease as, 850–851, 850–851*f*
  diabetes mellitus as, 844–846, 846*f*
  gigantism as, 834
  hypercortisolism (Cushing syndrome) as, 842–843, 842*f*
  hyperparathyroidism as, 840–842
  hyperthyroidism as, 837–838, 838*f*
  hypoparathyroidism as, 838–839, 839*f*
  hypophosphatasia as, 847–848, 847–848*f*
  hypothyroidism as, 835–836, 836–837*f*
  jaundice (icterus) as, 823–824, 824*f*
  lipid reticuloendothelioses as, 821–822
  lipoid proteinosis as, 822–823, 822–823*f*
  mucopolysaccharidosis as, 819–820, 820*t*, 820*f*
  orofacial pain due to, 864*b*
  pituitary dwarfism as, 833–834
  Plummer-Vinson syndrome as, 830–831, 831*f*
  pseudohypoparathyroidism as, 839–840

Systemic disease(s) with oral manifestations *(Continued)*
  pyostomatitis vegetans as, 851–852, 852*f*
  uremic stomatitis as, 852–853, 853*f*
  vitamin deficiency as, 827–829, 828–829*f*
  vitamin D–resistant rickets as, 848–850, 849*f*
  xanthelasma as, 827, 827*f*
Systemic lupus erythematosus (SLE), 798
Systemic sclerosis, 801–805
  clinical features of, 802–803, 802*f*
  diagnosis of, 803
  diffuse cutaneous, 802
  histopathologic features of, 803, 804*f*
  limited cutaneous, 802
  pathogenesis of, 802
  radiographic features of, 802–803, 802*f*
  treatment and prognosis for, 803–805

T
Taft, Jonathan, 900
Talisman, implantation of, 301
Talon cusp, 85–86, 86*f*
Target lesions in erythema multiforme, 781, 781*f*
Taste
  disorders, due to antineoplastic therapy, 283, 285
  phantom (distorted), 869–871, 870*b*, 871*t*
Tattoos and tattooing
  amalgam, 298–300
    clinical and radiographic features of, 299, 299–300*f*
    from endodontic-related implantation, 298, 298*f*
    from floss-related implantation, 298, 298*f*
    histopathologic features of, 300, 300*f*
    treatment and prognosis for, 300, 302
  cosmetic, 299
Taurodontism, 92, 92–93*f*, 93*b*
  amelogenesis imperfecta with, 102–103, 103*f*
Taurodonts, 819
Tay-Sachs disease, 821
TB. *See* Tuberculosis (TB)
T-cell leukemia/lymphoma virus type 1 (HTLV-1), 593
T-cell lymphoma
  angiocentric, 607–609, 608*f*
  cutaneous (*see* Mycosis fungoides)
Tea, tooth discoloration due to, 68
Teeth, 51–116. *See also under* Dental and Tooth
  abnormal number of, 75
    anodontia as, 75, 77
    clinical features of, 77–80
    genetic basis for, 75, 76*b*
    hyperdontia as
      clinical features of, 78–80
      defined, 75

Teeth *(Continued)*
    with distomolar or distodens, 79, 79*f*
    with mesiodens, 78*f*
    with multiple supernumerary teeth, 78, 78–79*f*
    with paramolar, 79, 79*f*
    syndromes associated with, 75, 76*b*
  hypodontia as
    defined, 75
    genetic basis for, 75, 76*b*
  oligodontia as, 75
  supernumerary, syndromes associated with, 75, 76*b*
  treatment and prognosis for, 80–81
  abnormal shape of, 82–98
    accessory cusps as, 85–88
      clinical and radiographic features of, 85–87
      cusp of Carabelli as, 85, 85*f*
      talon cusp as, 85–86, 86*f*
    concrescence as, 82–85
      defined, 82–83
      treatment and prognosis for, 84–85
    cusp of Carabelli as, 87
    dens evaginatus as, 86–87, 87*f*
    dens invaginatus (dens in dente) as, 88–90
      defined, 88
    dilaceration as, 94–96, 95*f*
    due to hypercementosis, 93–94, 93*b*, 94*f*
    due to supernumerary roots, 96, 96*f*
    fusion as, 82–85
      clinical features of, 83–84, 83–84*f*
      defined, 82–83
      treatment and prognosis for, 84–85
    gemination as, 82–85
      clinical features of, 83–84, 83*f*
      defined, 82–83
      treatment and prognosis for, 84–85
    globodontia as, 96–97, 96–97*f*
    lobodontia as, 97–98, 97*f*
    with shovel-shaped incisors, 87, 87*f*
  abnormal size of, 81–82, 81–82*f*
  with accessory cusps, 85–88
    clinical and radiographic features of, 85–87
    cusp of Carabelli as, 85, 85*f*, 87
    dens evaginatus as, 86–87, 87*f*
    with shovel-shaped incisors, 87, 87*f*
    talon cusp as, 85–86, 86*f*
    treatment and prognosis for, 87–88
  agencies, treatment and prognosis for, 80
  dens invaginatus (dens in dente) as
    clinical and radiographic features of, 88–90
    coronal, 88–89, 88–90*f*
    radicular, 89–90
    treatment and prognosis for, 90
  developmental alterations of, 74–111
    in number, 75–81
    in shape, 82–98
    in size, 81–82

Teeth *(Continued)*
  in structure, 98–111
  double (connate, conjoined), 82
    defined, 82
    due to concrescence, 82–85
      clinical features of, 84, 84–85*f*
      treatment and prognosis for, 85
    due to fusion, 82–85
      clinical features of, 83–84, 83–84*f*
      defined, 82–83
      treatment and prognosis for, 84–85
    due to gemination, 82–85
      clinical features of, 83–84, 83*f*
      defined, 82–83
      treatment and prognosis for, 84–85
  due to ectopic enamel, 90–92, 91*f*
  environmental alterations of, 51–74,
      52*b*
    environmental effects on tooth
        structure development as, 51–58,
        52*b*
    localized disturbances in eruption as,
        71–74
  environmental discoloration of, 67–71,
      67*b*
  ghost, 110–111, 110*b*, 111*f*
  hypodontia as, treatment and prognosis
      for, 80
  hypohyperdontia as, 79
  natal, 79–81, 80*f*
  neonatal, 79–80
  opalescent, 618, 619*f*
  physical anthropologic examination of,
      885–888, 886*t*, 886*f*
  postdevelopmental loss of tooth structure
      as, 58–67
  rootless, 108–109
    classification of, 105*t*, 108–109
    clinical features of, 108–109, 108–109*f*
    radiographic features of, 109, 109*f*
    subclassification of, 109, 109*b*
  shell, 106, 106*f*
  supernumerary
    clinical features of, 78
    conical, 79
    defined, 75, 82–83
    distomolar or distodens as, 79, 79*f*
    mesiodens as, 78*f*
    molariform, 79
    multiple, 78–79*f*, 79
    paramolar as, 79, 79*f*
    rudimentary, 79
    supplemental, 79
    treatment and prognosis for, 80
    tuberculate, 79
  taurodontism as, 92, 92–93*f*, 93*b*
  transposition of, 79, 80*f*
  treatment and prognosis for, 80–81
Teeth structure, environmental effects on
    development of, 51–58, 52*b*
Telangiectasia
  in CREST syndrome, 805, 806*f*

Telangiectasia *(Continued)*
  defined, 914
  differential diagnosis of, 916–919*t*
  hereditary hemorrhagic, 759–760,
      759–760*f*
  in Merkel cell carcinoma, 433
Temporal arteritis, 867–868
Temporomandibular disorders (TMDs),
    864*b*
  classification of, 875, 875*b*
  clinical and radiographic features of, 875
  defined, 874
  epidemiology of, 874
  etiopathogenesis of, 874, 875*b*
  treatment and prognosis for, 876, 876*b*
  vs. glossopharyngeal neuralgia, 866
Temporomandibular joint (TMJ)
  osteoarthritis of, 871–872
  rheumatoid arthritis of, 873
Tendoperiostitis, chronic, 138
  clinical and radiographic features of, 139
  histopathologic features of, 140
  treatment and prognosis for, 140–141
Teratoid cyst, 33
Teratoma, 32
Terrorism, 896
Tetracycline, tooth discoloration due to, 70,
    70*f*
Texas Junk Science Law (SB 344), 901
Thalassemia, 585–586, 585–586*f*
  α-, 586
  β-, 585–586, 585*f*
  clinical and radiographic features of,
      585–586, 585*f*
  defined, 585
  major, 585
  minor, 585
  pathogenesis of, 585
  treatment and prognosis for, 586
α-Thalassemia trait, 586
Thèques, 376
Thermal burns, 276–278, 277–278*f*
Thiamin deficiency, 828
Thistle tube–shaped pulp chambers,
    106–107, 107*f*
Thrombocytopenia, 590–592, 591*f*
  in anemia, 594
  with HIV infection, 259–260
Thrombocytopenic purpura
  immune, 591
  thrombotic, 591
Thrombotic thrombocytopenic purpura
    (TTP), 591
Thrush, 201, 202*t*, 202–203*f*
Thyroglossal duct cyst, 33–34, 34*f*
Thyroglossal tract cyst, 33–34, 34*f*
Thyroglossal tract remnants, 34
Thyroiditis, Hashimoto, 836
Thyroid, lingual, 10–11, 11*f*
Thyroid storm, 838
Thyrotoxicosis, 837–838, 838*f*
Tic douloureux, 864–866, 865*b*

Tingible bodies, 578
Tinnitus due to temporomandibular
    disorders, 875
Tissue samples of bite mark, 905–906, 906*f*
TMDs. *See* Temporomandibular disorders
    (TMDs)
TMJ (temporomandibular joint)
  osteoarthritis of, 871–872
  rheumatoid arthritis of, 873
TNM (tumor-node-metastasis) staging
  of melanoma, 438–442*t*
  of squamous cell carcinoma
    for cutaneous carcinoma of the head
        and neck (including lip vermilion
        carcinoma), 413*t*
    for HPV-mediated (p16-positive)
        oropharyngeal carcinoma, 414*t*
    for oral cavity carcinoma (including lip
        mucosa), 412*t*
    for p16-negative oropharyngeal
        carcinoma, 414*t*
Tobacco, 381
  vs. leukoplakia, 381
Tobacco pouch, 391
Tobacco pouch keratosis, 391–393, 422
  clinical features of, 391–392, 391*f*
  histopathologic features of, 392–393, 392*f*
  treatment and prognosis for, 393, 393*f*
  and verrucous carcinoma, 393
Tobacco products
  leukoplakia due to, 381
  tooth discoloration due to, 68, 68*f*
α–Tocopherol deficiency, 827
Tongue
  ankyloglossia of, 10, 10*f*
  central papillary atrophy of, 202*t*, 203,
      203*f*
  differential diagnosis of soft tissue masses
      of, 922–925*t*
  eosinophilic granuloma of, 273–274
  fissured (scrotal), 11–12, 11*f*
    in erythema migrans, 12
  forked (split, bifid), 300–301
  hairy (black hairy, coated), 12–13
    clinical features of, 12–13, 12*f*
    histopathologic features of, 13, 13*f*
    treatment and prognosis for, 13
  macroglossia of, 8–9, 8*b*, 9*f*
  microglossia of, 8, 8*f*
  red strawberry, 175
  white strawberry, 175, 175*f*
Tongue-tie, 10, 10*f*
Tongue torches, 321
Tonsil(s)
  kissing, 578
  in lymphoid hyperplasia, 578, 579*f*
Tonsillar plugs, 176–177, 177*f*
Tonsillitis, streptococcal, 174–175, 174*f*
Tonsillolithiasis, 176–177, 177*f*
Tooth. *See also under* Dental and Teeth
  dilaceration of, 54
  Turner, 53–54, 53*f*

Tooth agenesis
  clinical features of, 77–78, 77f
  treatment and prognosis for, 80
Tooth discoloration, environmental, 67–71,
    67b
  clinical features of, 67–70, 68f
  extrinsic, 67
    clinical features of, 67–70, 68f
    differential diagnosis of, 932–935t
    due to bacterial stains, 67–68
    due to gingival hemorrhage, 68
    due to medications, 68
    due to stannous fluoride and
        chlorhexidine, 68
    due to tobacco products, tea, or coffee,
        68, 68f
    treatment and prognosis for, 70–71
  intrinsic, 67
    clinical features of, 68–70
    differential diagnosis of, 932–935t
    due to alkaptonuria, 69
    due to congenital erythropoietic
        porphyria, 68–69, 68f
    due to hyperbilirubinemia, 69, 69f
    due to lepromatous leprosy, 69
    due to medications, 69–70, 70f
    due to restorative materials, 69, 70f
    due to trauma, 69
    treatment and prognosis for, 71
  treatment and prognosis for, 70–71
Tooth emergence, 71
Tooth enamel. See Enamel
Tooth eruption
  defined, 71
  delayed, 71–72, 71b, 72f
  localized disturbances in, 71–74
    ankylosis as, 73–74, 74f
    impaction as, 72–73, 73f
Tooth exfoliation, differential diagnosis of
    premature, 932–935t
Tooth impaction, 72–73, 73f
Toothpaste, allergic contact stomatitis to,
    342, 343f
Tooth pathology, differential diagnosis of,
    932–935t
Tooth resorption, 62–67
  clinical and radiographic features of,
    62–66
  external, 62–67
    clinical and radiographic features of,
      63, 64–65f
    before eruption, 65, 66f
    factors associated with, 62, 62b
    idiopathic, 62
    idiopathic apical, 65, 66f
    internal, 66, 67f
    invasive cervical, 64–65, 65f
    multiple idiopathic root, 64–65, 66f
    during orthodontics, 64
    treatment and prognosis for, 67
  histopathologic features of, 66, 67f
  inflammatory, 63, 64f

Tooth resorption (Continued)
  internal, 62–67
    clinical and radiographic features of,
        62–63, 63–64f
    histopathologic features of, 66, 67f
    treatment and prognosis for, 67
  in reimplanted avulsed teeth, 64,
      65f, 67
  replacement or metaplastic, 63, 63f
  treatment and prognosis for, 67
Tooth structure
  developmental alterations of, 98–111
    amelogenesis imperfecta as, 98–104
    due to hereditary disorders of dentin,
        104–105, 105t
    regional odontodysplasia as, 110–111,
        110b, 111f
  postdevelopmental loss of, 58–67
    due to internal and external resorption,
        62–67
    due to tooth wear, 58–62
Tooth surface loss. See Tooth wear
Tooth wear, 58–62
  due to abfraction, 61, 61f
  due to abrasion, 59, 59–60f
  due to attrition, 59, 59f, 61
  due to erosion, 59–60
    clinical features of, 59–62, 60–61f
    treatment and prognosis for, 61–62
  etiology of, 58
  treatment and prognosis for, 61–62
Tooth whitening strips, mucosal burn from,
    278–280, 278f
Torus
  flat, 21
  lobular, 21
  mandibularis, 21–23
    clinical and radiographic features of,
      21–22, 22f
    histopathologic features of, 22, 22f
    treatment and prognosis for, 23
  nodular, 21
  palatinus, 21, 21f
  spindle, 21
Tower skull, 41, 42f
Toxic epidermal necrolysis, 781, 783–784,
    783f
Toxoplasmosis, 222–224, 223f
  congenital, 223
Trabecular carcinoma of skin, 432–434,
    433f
"Tramline" calcifications, 551, 552f
Transient lingual papillitis, 321, 322f
Transplant-associated Kaposi sarcoma, 564
Trauma
  leukoplakia due to, 383, 383f
  and squamous cell carcinoma, 406
  tooth discoloration due to, 69
Traumatic bone cyst, 636–638, 637f
Traumatic ciliated cyst, 312–313, 313f
Traumatic fibroma. See Fibroma(s)
Traumatic granuloma, 273–274, 274f

Traumatic neuroma, 531f, 532, 533f
Traumatic ulcerations, 273–275
  clinical features of, 274–275, 274–275f
  histopathologic features of, 275
  treatment and prognosis for, 275, 276f
Traumatic ulcerative granuloma with
    stromal eosinophilia (TUGSE),
    273–274
Traumatized oral lipomas, 531
Treacher Collins syndrome, 43–44, 43f
Trench mouth, 151–152, 152f
Treponema pallidum, 179
Triazoles for candidiasis, 209–211, 211t
Trichiasis in mucous membrane
    pemphigoid, 776–777, 777f
Trichilemmal cyst, 31
  clinical features of, 31, 31f
  histopathologic features of, 32, 32f
Trichilemmomas in multiple hamartoma
    syndrome, 765, 765f
Tricho-dento-osseous syndrome, 103,
    103f
Trichoepitheliomas, 491
Trigeminal convergence, 863
Trigeminal neuralgia, 864–866, 865b
Trigonocephaly, 41
Trismus
  due to antineoplastic therapy, 284
  due to oral submucous fibrosis, 394
Triton tumor, malignant, 562
TTP (thrombotic thrombocytopenic
    purpura), 591
Tubercle in tuberculosis, 187
Tuberculosis (TB), 185–188
  clinical and radiographic features of,
      186–187, 186–187f
  diagnosis of, 187–188
  epidemiology of, 185
  extrapulmonary, 186
  histopathologic features of, 187, 188f
  with HIV infection, 258–259
  pathogenesis of, 185
  primary, 185
  scrofula due to, 187, 187f
  secondary, 186
  treatment and prognosis for, 188
  tubercle in, 187
Tuberous sclerosis, 762–765
  clinical features of, 763–764
    angiomyolipoma as, 764
    cardiac rhabdomyoma as, 763–764
    CNS manifestations as, 763, 763f
    facial angiofibromas as, 763, 763f
    oral manifestations as, 764, 764f
    shagreen patches and ash-leaf spots as,
        763
    ungual or periungual fibromas as, 763,
        763f
  histopathologic features of, 764
  treatment and prognosis for, 764–765
Tubular pattern of adenoid cystic carcinoma,
    502

Tufted hemangioma, 548
TUGSE (traumatic ulcerative granuloma with stromal eosinophilia), 273–274
Tumor-node-metastasis (TNM) staging of melanoma, 438–442t
    of squamous cell carcinoma, 412
Tumor suppressor genes and squamous cell carcinoma, 406
Turner hypoplasia, 53–54, 53f
Turner tooth, 53–54, 53f
Tympanic paragangliomas, 543
Tympanic plexus neuralgia, 866
Tyndall effect, 377
Type II hereditary angioedema (HAE II), 348–349
Tzanck cells
    in herpes simplex virus, 233–234
    in pemphigus vulgaris, 770–772

U
UDIM (UVIS Dental Identification Module), 895, 899
Ulcer(s) and ulcerations
    aphthous, recurrent (see Recurrent aphthous stomatitis)
    with bone sequestration, 310, 310f
    chemotherapy-related, 281f
    defined, 914
    eosinophilic, 273–274
        atypical, 275, 275f
    of fingertips in systemic sclerosis, 802, 802f
    traumatic, 273–275
        clinical features of, 274–275, 274–275f
        histopathologic features of, 275
        treatment and prognosis for, 275, 276f
Ulcerative colitis and pyostomatitis vegetans, 851
Ulcerative lesions, differential diagnosis of, 920–921t
Ulcerative stomatitis, chronic, 792–794, 793–794f
Ultraviolet (UV) photography, reflective, 904
Ultraviolet (UV) radiation, leukoplakia due to, 382
Undetermined death, 883
Undifferentiated pleomorphic sarcoma, 560–561, 561f
Ungual fibromas in tuberous sclerosis, 763, 763f
Unicameral bone cyst, 636–638, 637f
Unified Victim Identification System (UVIS), 894
Unified Victim Identification System (UVIS) Dental Identification Module (UDIM), 894, 899
Unilocular, defined, 914
Unilocular radiolucencies, differential diagnosis of, 926–931t
Unique Device Identification (UDI), 890

Universal Numbering System, 891, 891t
Urbach-Wiethe syndrome, 822–823, 822–823f
Uremic stomatitis, 852–853, 853f
    vs. morsicatio mucosae oris, 272–273
US Department of Health and Human Services (HHS), 881
US Food and Drug Administration's (FDA), 890
Uveoparotid fever, 329, 861
UVIS (Unified Victim Identification System), 894
UVIS (Unified Victim Identification System) Dental Identification Module (UDIM), 894, 899
UV (ultraviolet) photography, reflective, 904
UV (ultraviolet) radiation, leukoplakia due to, 382
Uvula, bifid (cleft), 2, 3f

V
Vagal paragangliomas, 543
Vagoglossopharyngeal neuralgia, 866–867
Valley fever, 217, 217f
van der Woude syndrome, 5, 5f
Vanishing bone disease, 627–628, 627–628f
Variable number of tandem repeats (VNTR), 888
Varicella, 235–238
    breakthrough infection with, 236
    clinical features of, 236–237, 236–237f
    complications of, 237
    diagnosis of, 237
    epidemiology of, 235–236
    histopathologic features of, 237
    in immunocompromised patients, 237
    during pregnancy, 237
    treatment and prognosis for, 237–238
Varicella virus vaccine (Varivax), 238
Varicella-zoster immune globulin (VariZIG), 238
Varicella-zoster virus (VZV), 229
    herpes zoster due to, 238–241, 238–239f
    with HIV infection, 260
    varicella due to, 235–238, 236–237f
Varices, 13–14
Varicosities, 13–14, 14f
Varivax (varicella virus vaccine), 238
VariZIG (varicella-zoster immune globulin), 238
Vascular anomalies, classification of, 547, 547b
Vascular invasion, 416
Vascular malformations, 547–551
    arteriovenous, 549
    clinical and radiographic features of, 548–549, 548f
    defined, 547
    histopathologic features of, 549, 550f
    intrabony, 549, 549f
    treatment and prognosis for, 550–551
    venous, 548–549f, 549

Vasculitis, leukocytoclastic, 328
Venereal wart, 357–358
    clinical features of, 358–359, 359f
    epidemiology of, 358
    histopathologic features of, 359, 359f
    with HIV infection, 260
    treatment and prognosis for, 359–360
Venous malformations, 548–549f, 549
Vermilionectomy, 396
Verocay bodies, 534, 536f
Verruca vulgaris, 357–358
    clinical features of, 357–358, 357f
    histopathologic features of, 358, 358f
    with HIV infection, 260
    treatment and prognosis for, 358
Verruciform leukoplakia. See Verrucous leukoplakia
Verruciform xanthoma, 365–366, 365–366f
Verrucous carcinoma, 384, 393, 421–423, 422–423f
    vs. proliferative verrucous leukoplakia, 384, 385f
Verrucous, defined, 914
Verrucous leukoplakia, 384
    proliferative, 384, 385f
Vesicle, 914
Vesiculoerosive lesions, differential diagnosis of, 920–921t
Vincent infection, 151–152, 152f
Vincent, Jean Hyacinthe, 151
Viral infection(s), 229–271
    cytomegalovirus as, 229
    enteroviruses as, 244–246
    herpes simplex virus as, 229–235
    herpes zoster (shingles) as, 238–241, 238–239f
    HIV and AIDS as, 250–265
    human herpesviruses as, 229
    infectious mononucleosis as, 241–242
    measles (rubeola) as, 246–248, 247f
    mumps (epidemic parotitis) as, 249–250, 250f
    rubella (German measles) as, 248–249
    varicella (chickenpox) as, 235–238
Visceral signs of Niemann-Pick disease, 821
Vitamin A deficiency, 828
Vitamin-A deficiency, 404
Vitamin B_1 deficiency, 827
Vitamin B_2 deficiency, 827
Vitamin B_3 deficiency, 827
Vitamin B_6 deficiency, 827
Vitamin B_{12} malabsorption, pernicious anemia due to, 831
Vitamin C deficiency, 828–829
Vitamin D deficiency, 827, 829, 829f
Vitamin D–dependent rickets, 849
Vitamin deficiency(ies), 827–829
    clinical features of, 828–829, 828–829f
    and squamous cell carcinoma, 404
    treatment and prognosis for, 829
Vitamin D–resistant rickets, 848–850, 849f
Vitamin E deficiency, 827, 829

Vitamin K deficiency, 827, 829
VNTR (variable number of tandem repeats), 888
von Behring, Emil, 177
von Mikulicz-Radecki, Johann, 471
von Recklinghausen disease of the skin. *See* Neurofibromatosis type I (NF1)
von Willebrand disease, 579*t*
von Willebrand factor, 591
VZV. *See* Varicella-zoster virus (VZV)

W
Waldeyer ring, 36, 428
Waldeyer tonsillar tissue, 428
Wart
  common, 357–358
    clinical features of, 357–358, 357*f*
    histopathologic features of, 358, 358*f*
    with HIV infection, 260
    treatment and prognosis for, 358
  venereal, 357–358
    clinical features of, 358–359, 359*f*
    epidemiology of, 358
    histopathologic features of, 359, 359*f*
    treatment and prognosis for, 359–360
Warthin-Finkeldey giant cells, 247–248, 247*f*
Warthin tumor, 488–490, 489*f*
Warty dyskeratoma, 757–758, 757*f*
"Water brash", 469
WDR72 gene, 99*t*, 100
Wegener, generalized, 333–336
Wegener granulomatosis, 333–336
  clinical features of, 333–335, 334–335*f*
  generalized, 333
  histopathologic features of, 335, 335*f*
  limited, 333–334

Wegener granulomatosis *(Continued)*
  superficial, 333–334
  treatment and prognosis for, 336
Wegner
  limited, 333–334
  superficial, 333–334
Well-demarcated borders
  differential diagnosis of mixed radiolucent/radiopaque lesions with, 926–931*t*
  differential diagnosis of radiopacities with, 926–931*t*
Well-differentiated liposarcoma, 561
White lesions, differential diagnosis of, 916–919*t*
White sponge nevus, 748–749
  clinical features of, 748, 748*f*
  histopathologic features of, 749, 749*f*
  pathogenesis of, 748
  treatment and prognosis for, 749
White strawberry tongue, 175, 175*f*
Whitlow, herpetic, 232, 233*f*
Whole-exome sequencing, 99
Whole-genome sequencing, 99
Wickham striae, 787, 787*f*
Wilson, Erasmus, 787
WinID3 program, 894, 894*t*, 899
Witkop–von Sallmann syndrome, 749–750, 750*f*
Witnesses of fact, 910
Witten-Zak syndrome, 399

X
Xanthelasma, 827, 827*f*
Xanthoma(s)
  in multiple hamartoma syndrome, 765
  verruciform, 365–366, 365–366*f*

Xanthoma cells, 365–366, 366*f*, 640
Xeroderma pigmentosum, 399, 753–754, 753*f*
Xerostomia, 470–471, 470*t*, 869
  in diabetes mellitus, 846
  due to antineoplastic therapy, 282–283, 283*f*
  in graft-versus-host disease, 795
Xerostomia-related caries, 282, 283*f*, 471
X-irradiation, and squamous cell carcinoma, 403–404
X-ray fluorescence (XRF), 882, 882*f*
  in multiple fatality incident analysis, 898
X-ray generation devices, multiple fatality incident analysis portable hand-held in, 898

Y
Yellow lesions, differential diagnosis of, 916–919*t*

Z
Zellballen, 544, 544*f*
Zinsser-Cole-Engman syndrome, 752–753, 752*f*
Zostavax (herpes zoster vaccine), 240–241
Zoster sine herpete, 238–239
Zsigmondy/Palmer System, 891, 891*t*
Zygomycosis, 219–221
  clinical features of, 219–220, 220*f*
  diagnosis of, 220
  histopathologic features of, 220, 220*f*
  pathogenesis of, 219
  radiographic features of, 219–220, 220*f*
  treatment and prognosis for, 220–221